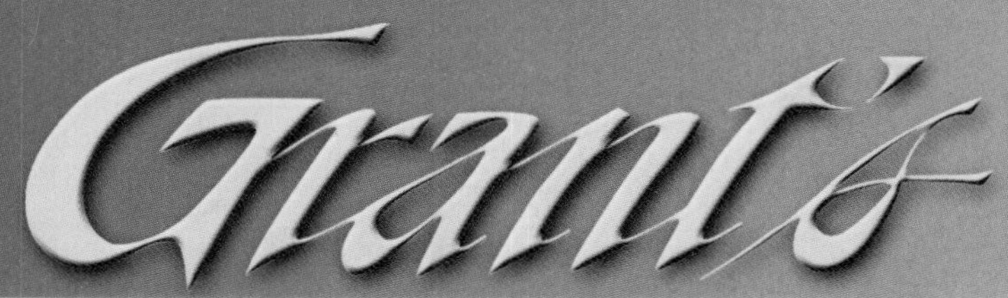
Grant's



# Atlas of Anatomy

Twelfth Edition


1 THORAX 1

2 ABDOMEN 95

3 PELVIS AND PERINEUM 193

4 BACK 285

5 LOWER LIMB 353

6 UPPER LIMB 475

7 HEAD 607

8 NECK 745

9 CRANIAL NERVES 811

INDEX 845

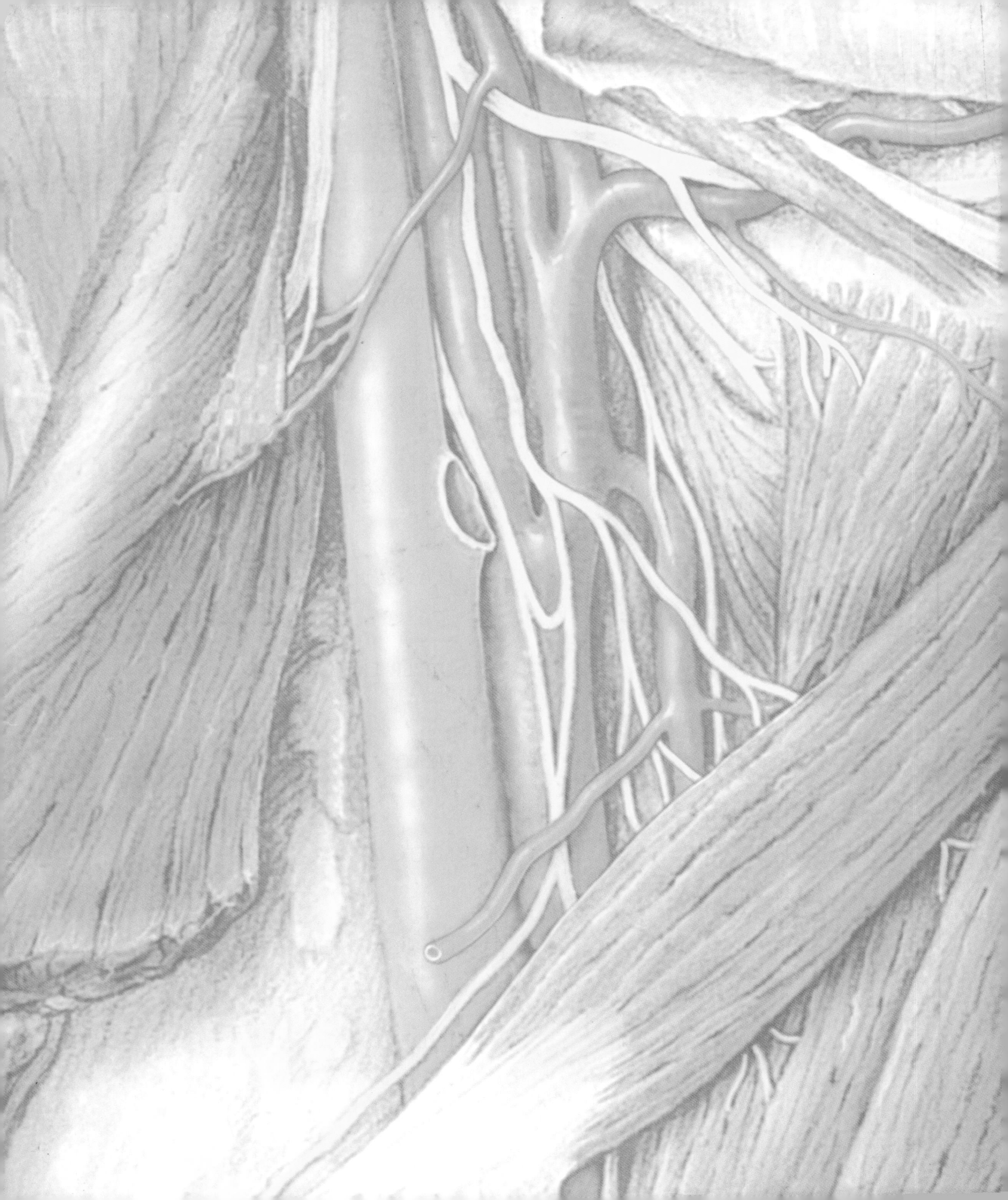

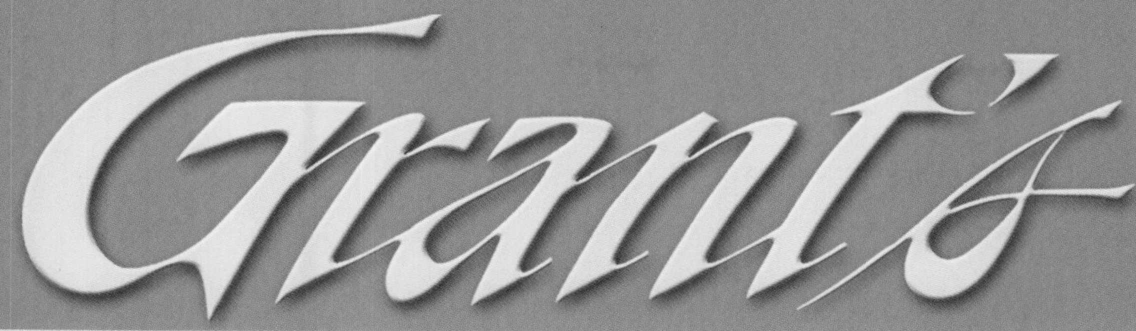

# Atlas of Anatomy
Twelfth Edition

**Anne M.R. Agur, B.Sc. (OT), M.Sc., Ph.D**

Professor, Division of Anatomy, Department of Surgery, Faculty of Medicine
Department of Physical Therapy, Department of Occupational Therapy,
Division of Biomedical Communications, Institute of Medical Science
Graduate Department of Rehabilitation Science, Graduate Department of Dentistry
University of Toronto
Toronto, Ontario, Canada

**Arthur F. Dalley II, Ph.D.**

Professor, Department of Cell & Developmental Biology
Adjunct Professor, Department of Orthopaedics and Rehabilitation
Vanderbilt University School of Medicine
Adjunct Professor of Anatomy
Belmont University School of Physical Therapy
Nashville, Tennessee, U.S.A.

Wolters Kluwer | Lippincott Williams & Wilkins
Health

Philadelphia • Baltimore • New York • London
Buenos Aires • Hong Kong • Sydney • Tokyo

Acquisitions Editor: Crystal Taylor
Senior Developmental Editor: Kathleen H. Scogna
Marketing Manager: Valerie Sanders
Creative Director: Doug Smock
Managing Editor, Production: Eve Malakoff-Klein
Compositor: Maryland Composition, Inc.
Printer: C&C Offset Printing

Twelfth Edition



*By J.C.B. Grant:*
First Edition, 1943 Second Edition, 1947
Third Edition, 1951 Fourth Edition, 1956
Fifth Edition, 1962 Sixth Edition, 1972
*By J.E. Anderson:*
Seventh Edition, 1978 Eighth Edition, 1983
*By A.M.R. Agur:*
Ninth Edition, 1991 Tenth Edition, 1999
Eleventh Edition, 2005

351 West Camden Street
Baltimore, Maryland 21201-2436 USA

530 Walnut Street
Philadelphia, Pennsylvania 19106-3621 USA

Printed in China

9 8 7 6 5 4 3 2



Library of Congress Cataloging-in-Publication Data

Agur, A. M. R.
Grant's atlas of anatomy/Anne M.R. Agur, Arthur F. Dalley II.—12th ed.
p. ; cm.
Includes bibliographical references and index.
ISBN 978-0-7817-9604-0 (hardcover ed.)—ISBN 978-0-7817-7055-2 (softcover ed.) 1. Human anatomy—Atlases. I. Dalley, Arthur F. II. Title. III. Title: Atlas of anatomy.
[DNLM: 1. Anatomy, Regional—Atlases. QS 17 A284g 2009]
QM25.A38 2009
611.0022'2—dc22

2007043565

## DISCLAIMER

Care has been taken to confirm the accuracy of the information presented and to describe generally accepted practices. However, the authors, editors, and publisher are not responsible for errors or omissions or for any consequences from application of the information in this book and make no warranty, expressed or implied, with respect to the currency, completeness, or accuracy of the contents of the publication. Application of this information in a particular situation remains the professional responsibility of the practitioner; the clinical treatments described and recommended may not be considered absolute and universal recommendations.

The authors, editors, and publisher have exerted every effort to ensure that drug selection and dosage set forth in this text are in accordance with the current recommendations and practice at the time of publication. However, in view of ongoing research, changes in government regulations, and the constant flow of information relating to drug therapy and drug reactions, the reader is urged to check the package insert for each drug for any change in indications and dosage and for added warnings and precautions. This is particularly important when the recommended agent is a new or infrequently employed drug.

Some drugs and medical devices presented in this publication have Food and Drug Administration (FDA) clearance for limited use in restricted research settings. It is the responsibility of the health care provider to ascertain the FDA status of each drug or device planned for use in their clinical practice.

To purchase additional copies of this book, call our customer service department at **(800) 638-3030** or fax orders to **(301) 223-2320**. International customers should call (301) 223-2300.

Visit Lippincott Williams & Wilkins on the Internet: http://www.lww.com. Lippincott Williams & Wilkins customer service representatives are available from 8:30 am to 6:00 pm, EST.

CCS0409

*To my husband Enno and my children Erik and Kristina*
*for their support and encouragement*
*(A.M.R.A.)*

*To Muriel*
*My bride, best friend, counselor, and mother of our sons;*
*To my family*
*Tristan, Lana, Elijah Grey, and Finley*
*Denver and Skyler*
*With great appreciation for their support, humor and patience*
*(A.F.D.)*

# DR. JOHN CHARLES BOILEAU GRANT
# 1886—1973

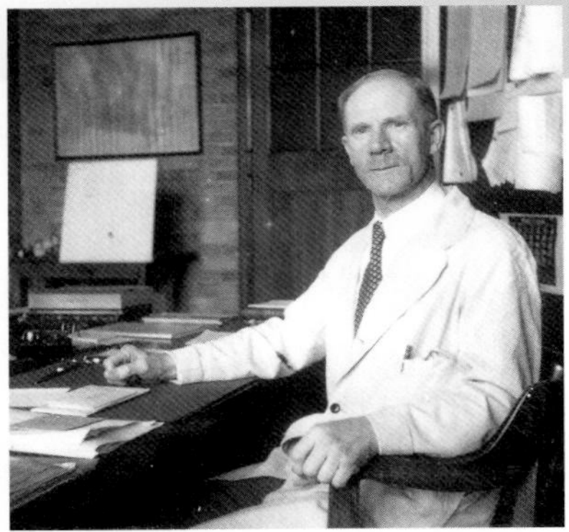

*Dr. J.C.B. Grant in his office, McMurrich Building, University of Toronto, 1946. Through his textbooks, Dr. Grant made an indelible impression on the teaching of anatomy throughout the world.*

by **Dr. Carlton G. Smith, M.D., Ph.D. (1905–2003)**
Professor Emeritus, Division of Anatomy, Department of Surgery
Faculty of Medicine
University of Toronto, Canada

The life of J.C. Boileau Grant has been likened to the course of the seventh cranial nerve as it passes out of the skull: complicated, but purposeful.[1] He was born in the parish of Lasswade in Edinburgh, Scotland, on February 6, 1886. Dr. Grant studied medicine at the University of Edinburgh from 1903 to 1908. Here, his skill as a dissector in the laboratory of the renowned anatomist, Dr. Daniel John Cunningham (1850–1909), earned him a number of awards.

Following graduation, Dr. Grant was appointed the resident house officer at the Infirmary in Whitehaven, Cumberland. From 1909 to 1911, Dr. Grant demonstrated anatomy in the University of Edinburgh, followed by two years at the University of Durham, at Newcastle-on-Tyne in England, in the laboratory of Professor Robert Howden, editor of *Gray's Anatomy*.

With the outbreak of World War I in 1914, Dr. Grant joined the Royal Army Medical Corps and served with distinction. He was mentioned in dispatches in September 1916, received the Military Cross in September 1917 for "conspicuous gallantry and devotion to duty during attack," and received a bar to the Military Cross in August 1918.[1]

In October 1919, released from the Royal Army, he accepted the position of Professor of Anatomy at the University of Manitoba in Winnipeg, Canada. With the frontline medical practitioner in mind, he endeavored to "bring up a generation of surgeons who knew exactly what they were doing once an operation had begun."[1] Devoted to research and learning, Dr. Grant took interest in other projects, such as performing anthropometric studies of Indian tribes in northern Manitoba during the 1920s. In Winnipeg, Dr. Grant met Catriona Christie, whom he married in 1922.

Dr. Grant was known for his reliance on logic, analysis, and deduction as opposed to rote memory. While at the University of Manitoba, Dr. Grant began writing *A Method of Anatomy, Descriptive and Deductive*, which was published in 1937.[2]

In 1930, Dr. Grant accepted the position of Chair of Anatomy at the University of Toronto. He stressed the value of a "clean" dissection, with the structures well defined. This required the delicate touch of a sharp scalpel, and students soon learned that a dull tool was anathema. Instructive dissections were made available in the Anatomy Museum, a means of student review on which Dr. Grant placed a high priority. Many of these illustrations have been included in *Grant's Atlas of Anatomy*.

The first edition of the *Atlas*, published in 1943, was the first anatomical atlas to be published in North America.[3] *Grant's Dissector* preceded the *Atlas* in 1940.[4]

Dr. Grant remained at the University of Toronto until his retirement in 1956. At that time, he became Curator of the Anatomy Museum in the University. He also served as Visiting Professor of Anatomy at the University of California at Los Angeles, where he taught for 10 years.

Dr. Grant died in 1973 of cancer. Through his teaching method, still presented in the Grant's textbooks, Dr. Grant's life interest—human anatomy—lives on. In their eulogy, colleagues and friends Ross MacKenzie and J. S. Thompson said: "Dr. Grant's knowledge of anatomical fact was encyclopedic, and he enjoyed nothing better than sharing his knowledge with others, whether they were junior students or senior staff. While somewhat strict as a teacher, his quiet wit and boundless humanity never failed to impress. He was, in the very finest sense, a scholar and a gentleman."[1]

# PREFACE

This edition of *Grant's Atlas* has, like its predecessors, required intense research, market input, and creativity. It is not enough to rely on a solid reputation; with each new edition, we have adapted and changed many aspects of the *Atlas* while maintaining the commitment to pedagogical excellence and anatomical realism that has enriched its long history. Medical and health sciences education, and the role of anatomy instruction and application within it, continually evolve to reflect new teaching approaches and educational models. The health care system itself is changing, and the skills and knowledge that future health care practitioners must master are changing along with it. Finally, technologic advances in publishing, particularly in online resources and electronic media, have transformed the way students access content and the methods by which educators teach content. All of these developments have shaped the vision and directed the execution of this twelfth edition of *Grant's Atlas*, as evidenced by the following key features:

**Classic "Grant's" images updated for today's students.** A unique feature of *Grant's Atlas* is that, rather than providing an idealized view of human anatomy, the classic illustrations represent actual dissections that the student can directly compare with specimens in the lab. Because the original models used for these illustrations were real cadavers, the accuracy of these illustrations is unparalleled, offering students the best introduction to anatomy possible. Over the years we have made many changes to the illustrations to match the shifting expectations of students, adding more vibrant colors and updating the style from the original carbon-dust renderings. In this edition, at the suggestion of reviewers, we have continued this trend by introducing more lifelike skin tones to provide a more realistic—but no less accurate--depiction of anatomy. In addition, almost all of these dissection figures were carefully analyzed to ensure that label placement remained effective and that the illustration's relevance was still clear. Almost every figure in this edition of *Grant's Atlas* was altered, from simple label changes to full-scale revision.

**Schematic illustrations to facilitate learning.** Full-color schematic illustrations supplement the dissection figures to clarify anatomical concepts, show the relationships of structures, and give an overview of the body region being studied. Many new schematic illustrations have been added to this edition; others have been revised to refine their pedagogical aspects. All conform to Dr. Grant's admonition to "keep it simple": extraneous labels were deleted, and some labels were added to identify key structures and make the illustrations as useful as possible to students. In addition, many new, simple orientation drawings were added for ease of identifying dissected regions.

**Legends with easy-to find clinical applications.** Admittedly, artwork is the focus of any atlas; however, the *Grant's* legends have long been considered a unique and valuable feature of the *Atlas*. The observations and comments that accompany the illustrations draw attention to salient points and significant structures that might otherwise escape notice. Their purpose is to interpret the illustrations without providing exhaustive description. Readability, clarity, and practicality were emphasized in the editing of this edition. For the first time, clinical comments, which deliver practical "pearls" that link anatomic features with their significance in health care practice, are highlighted in blue within the figure legends. The clinical comments have also been expanded in this edition, providing even more relevance for students searching for medical application of anatomical concepts.

**Enhanced diagnostic and surface anatomy and images.** Because medical imaging have taken on increased importance in the diagnosis and treatment of injuries and illnesses, diagnostic images are used liberally throughout the chapters, and a special imaging section appears at the end of each chapter. Over 100 clinically relevant magnetic resonance images (MRIs), computed tomography (CT) scans, ultrasound scans, and corresponding orientation drawings are included in this edition. We have also increased the number of labeled surface anatomy photographs and introduced greater ethnic diversity in the surface anatomy representations.

**Tables—updated, expanded, and improved.** Another feature unique to *Grant's Atlas* is the use of tables to help students organize complex information in an easy-to-use format ideal for review and study. The eleventh edition saw the introduction of muscle tables. In this edition, we have expanded the tables to include those for nerves, arteries, veins, and other relevant structures. The table format in this edition also received a substantial update; a consistent color code is used to clearly demarcate columns. Many tables are also strategically placed on the same page as the illustrations that demonstrate the structures listed in the tables.

**Logical organization and layout.** The organization and layout of the *Atlas* has always been determined with ease-of-use as the goal. Although the basic organization by body region was maintained in this edition, the order of plates within every chapter was scrutinized to ensure that it is logical and pedagogically effective. Sections within each chapter further organize the region into discrete subregions; these subregions appear as "titles" on the pages. Readers need only glance at these titles to orient themselves to the region and subregion that the figures on the page belong to. All sections also appear as a "table of contents" on the first page of each chapter.

**Helpful learning and teaching tools.** For the first time in its history, the twelfth edition of *Grant's Atlas* offers a wide range of electronic ancillaries for both student and teacher on Lippincott Williams & Wilkins' online ancillary site "thePoint" (http://thepoint.lww.com/grantsatlas). Students are given access to an interactive electronic atlas containing all of the atlas images with full search capabilities as well as zoom and compare features, as well as selected video clips from the best-selling *Acland's DVD Atlas of Human Anatomy* collection. Students can test themselves with 300 multiple choice questions, 95 "drag-and-drop" labeling exercises, and a sampling of *Clinical Anatomy Flash Cards*. For instructors, electronic ancillaries include an interactive atlas with slideshow and image-export functions, an image bank, and selected "dissection sequences" of plates.

We hope that you enjoy using this twelfth edition of *Grant's Atlas* and that it becomes a trusted partner in your educational experience. We believe that this new edition safeguards the *Atlas's* historical strengths while enhancing its usefulness to today's students.

*Anne M.R. Agur*
*Arthur F. Dalley II*

# ACKNOWLEDGMENTS

Starting with the first edition of this *Atlas* published in 1943, many people have given generously of their talents and expertise and we acknowledge their participation with heartfelt gratitude. Most of the original carbon-dust halftones on which this book is based were created by **Dorothy Foster Chubb,** a pupil of Max Brödel and one of Canada's first professionally trained medical illustrators. She was later joined by **Nancy Joy**, who is Professor Emeritus in the Division of Biomedical Communications, University of Toronto. Mrs. Chubb was mainly responsible for the artwork of the first two editions and the sixth edition; Miss Joy for those in between. In subsequent editions, additional line and half-tone illustrations by **Elizabeth Blackstock, Elia Hopper Ross,** and **Marguerite Drummond** were added. In recent editions, the artwork of Valerie Oxorn, Caitlin Duckwall, and Rob Duckwall, and the surface anatomy photography of Anne Rayner of Vanderbilt University Medical Center's Medical Art Group, have augmented the modern look and feel of the atlas.

Much credit is also due to Charles E. Storton for his role in the preparation of the majority of the original dissections and preliminary photographic work. We also wish to acknowledge the work of Dr. James Anderson, a pupil of Dr. Grant, under whose stewardship the seventh and eighth editions were published.

The following individuals also provided invaluable contributions to previous editions of the atlas, and are gratefully acknowledged: C.A. Armstrong, P.G. Ashmore, D. Baker, D.A. Barr, J.V. Basmajian, S. Bensley, D. Bilbey, J. Bottos, W. Boyd, J. Callagan, H.A. Cates, S.A. Crooks, M. Dickie, J.W.A. Duckworth, F.B. Fallis, J.B. Francis, J.S. Fraser, P. George, R.K. George, M.G. Gray, B.L. Guyatt, C.W. Hill, W.J. Horsey, B.S. Jaden, M.J. Lee, G.F. Lewis, I.B. MacDonald, D.L. MacIntosh, R.G. MacKenzie, S. Mader, K.O. McCuaig, D. Mazierski, W.R. Mitchell, K. Nancekivell, A.J.A. Noronha, S. O'Sullivan, W. Pallie, W.M. Paul, D. Rini, C. Sandone, C.H. Sawyer, A.I. Scott, J.S. Simpkins, J.S. Simpson, C.G. Smith, I.M. Thompson, J.S. Thompson, N.A. Watters, R.W. Wilson, B. Vallecoccia, and K. Yu.

## Twelfth Edition

We are indebted to our colleagues and former professors for their encouragement—especially Dr. Keith L. Moore for his expert advice and Drs. Daniel O. Graney, Lawrence Ross, Warwick Gorman, and Douglas J. Gould for their invaluable input.

We extend our gratitude to the medical artists who worked on this edition: Valerie Oxorn, and Caitlin and Rob Duckwall of Dragonfly Media Group, who contributed new and modified illustrations. We would also like to acknowledge Wayne Hubbel, former Art Coordinator at Lippincott Williams & Wilkins and now a freelancer, who helped size and label art for this edition.

Special thanks go to everyone at **Lippincott Williams & Wilkins**—especially Crystal Taylor, Acquisitions Editor; Kathleen Scogna, Senior Developmental Editor; and Eve Malakoff-Klein, Managing Editor, Production. All of your efforts and expertise are much appreciated.

We would like to thank the hundreds of instructors and students who have over the years communicated via the publisher and directly with the editor their suggestions for how this *Atlas* might be improved. Finally, we would like to acknowledge the reviewers who reviewed previous editions of the *Atlas* as well as the following reviewers who reviewed the eleventh edition and provided expert advice on the development of this edition in particular:

### Faculty Reviewers

Diana Alagna, BS, Branford Hall Career Institute, Southington, Connecticut

Gary Allen, PhD, Dalhousie University, Halifax, Nova Scotia, Canada

Gail Amort-Larson, MS, University of Alberta, Edmonton, Alberta, Canada

Alan W. Budenz, DDS, MS, MBA, Arthur A. Dugoni School of Dentistry, University of the Pacific, San Francisco, California

Anne Burrows, PhD, Duquesne University, Pittsburgh, Pennsylvania

Donald Fletcher, PhD, The Brody School of Medicine, East Carolina University, Greenville, South Carolina

Patricia Jordan, PhD, St. George's University, Grenada, West Indies

Elizabeth Julian, Augusta Technical Institute, Augusta, Georgia

H. Wayne Lambert, PhD, University Of Louisville, Louisville, Kentucky

Hector Lopez, DO, University of North Texas Health Science Center, Texas College of Osteopathic Medicine, Fort Worth, Texas

Brian MacPherson, PhD, University of Kentucky College of Medicine, Lexington, Kentucky

Helen Pearson, PhD, Temple University School of Medicine, Philadelphia, Pennsylvania

Chellapilla Rao, PhD, St. George's University School of Medicine, Grenada, West Indies

Darlene Redenbach, PhD, University of British Columbia, Vancouver, Canada

Heather Roberts, PhD, Sierra College, Rocklin, California

R. Shane Tubbs, PhD, University of Alabama, Birmingham, Alabama

Brad Wright, PhD, University of Vermont College of Medicine, Burlington, Vermont

### Student Reviewers

Geoffrey Berbary, Texas A and M University, College Station, Texas

Himanshu Bhatia, University Of Texas Health Sciences, Houston, Texas

Joseph Feuerstein, Boston University School of Medicine, Boston, Massachusetts

David Ficco, Life University, Marietta, Georgia

Eric Gross, Medical College of Wisconsin, Milwaukee, Wisconsin

Kathleen Hong, Boston University School of Medicine, Boston, Massachusetts

Patricia Johnson, Southwest College, Tempe, Arizona

Richy Lee, Medical University of the Americas, Charlestown, Nevis, West Indies

Sharon Phillips, University of Massachusetts Medical School, Worcester, Massachusetts

Karen Weinshelbaum, Mount Sinai School of Medicine, New York, New York

Joshua Weissman, Boston University School of Medicine, Boston, Massachusetts

Heather Willis, The Brody School of Medicine, East Carolina University, Greenville, South Carolina

We hope that readers and reviewers will find many of their suggestions incorporated into the twelfth edition and will continue to provide their valuable input.

*Anne M.R. Agur*
*Arthur F. Dalley II*

# CONTENTS

Dr. John Charles Boileau Grant **vi**
Preface **vii**
Acknowledgments **ix**
List of Tables **xiii**
Table and Figure Credits **xiv**
References **xvi**

1 THORAX **1**
Pectoral Region 2
Breast 4
Bony Thorax and Joints 10
Thoracic Wall 17
Thoracic Contents 25
Pleural Cavities 28
Mediastinum 29
Lungs and Pleura 30
Bronchi and Bronchopulmonary Segments 36
Innervation and Lymphatic Drainage of Lungs 42
External Heart 44
Coronary Vessels 52
Internal Heart and Valves 56
Conducting System of Heart 64
Pericardial Sac 65
Superior Mediastinum and Great Vessels 66
Diaphragm 73
Posterior Thorax 74
Overview of Autonomic Innervation 84
Overview of Lymphatic Drainage of Thorax 86
Sectional Anatomy and Imaging 88

2 ABDOMEN **95**
Overview 96
Anterolateral Abdominal Wall 98
Inguinal Region 106
Testis 116
Peritoneum and Peritoneal Cavity 118
Digestive System 128
Stomach 129
Pancreas, Duodenum, and Spleen 131
Intestines 136
Liver and Gallbladder 146
Biliary Ducts 156
Portal Venous System 160
Posterior Abdominal Wall 162
Kidneys 164
Lumbar Plexus 172
Diaphragm 174
Abdominal Aorta and Inferior Vena Cava 175
Autonomic Innervation 176
Lymphatic Drainage 182
Sectional Anatomy and Imaging 186

3 PELVIS AND PERINEUM **193**
Pelvic Girdle 194
Ligaments of Pelvic Girdle 200
Floor and Walls of Pelvis 202
Sacral and Coccygeal Plexuses 206
Peritoneal Reflections in Pelvis 208
Rectum and Anal Canal 210
Organs of Male Pelvis 216
Vessels of Male Pelvis 224
Lymphatic Drainage of Male Pelvis and Perineum 228
Innervation of Male Pelvic Organs 230
Organs of Female Pelvis 232
Vessels of Female Pelvis 240
Lymphatic Drainage of Female Pelvis and Perineum 244
Innervation of Female Pelvic Organs 246
Subperitoneal Region of Pelvis 250
Surface Anatomy of Perineum 252
Overview of Male and Female Perineum 254
Male Perineum 261
Female Perineum 269
Imaging of Pelvis and Perineum 276

4 BACK **285**
Overview of Vertebral Column 286
Cervical Spine 294
Craniovertebral Joints 298
Thoracic Spine 300
Lumbar Spine 302
Ligaments and Intervertebral Discs 304
Vertebral Venous Plexuses 309
Bones, Joints, and Ligaments of Pelvic Girdle 310
Anomalies of Vertebrae 318
Muscles of Back 320
Suboccipital Region 330
Spinal Cord and Meninges 334
Components of Spinal Nerves 343
Dermatomes and Myotomes 348
Imaging of Vertebral Column 350

## 5 LOWER LIMB 353
Systemic Overview of Lower Limb 354
Bones 355
Nerves 356
Blood Vessels 362
Lymphatics 366
Musculofascial Compartments 368
Retroinguinal Passage and Femoral Triangle 370
Anterior and Medial Compartments of Thigh 374
Lateral Thigh 383
Gluteal Region and Posterior Compartment of Thigh 384
Hip Joint 394
Knee Region 402
Knee Joint 408
Anterior and Lateral Compartments of Leg, Dorsum of Foot 422
Posterior Compartment of Leg 432
Tibiofibular Joints 442
Sole of Foot 443
Ankle, Subtalar, and Foot Joints 448
Arches of Foot 466
Bony Anomalies 467
Imaging and Sectional Anatomy 468

## 6 UPPER LIMB 475
Systemic Overview of Upper Limb 476
Bones 476
Nerves 480
Blood Vessels 486
Musculofascial Compartments 492
Pectoral Region 494
Axilla, Axillary Vessels, and Brachial Plexus 501
Scapular Region and Superficial Back 512
Arm and Rotator Cuff 516
Joints of Shoulder Region 530
Elbow Region 538
Elbow Joint 544
Anterior Aspect of Forearm 550
Anterior Aspect of Wrist and Palm of Hand 558
Posterior Aspect of Forearm 574
Posterior Aspect of Wrist and Dorsum of Hand 578
Lateral Aspect of Wrist and Hand 584
Medial Aspect of Wrist and Hand 587
Bones and Joints of Wrist and Hand 588
Function of Hand: Grips, Pinches, and Thumb Movements 596
Imaging and Sectional Anatomy 598

## 7 HEAD 607
Cranium 608
Face and Scalp 626
Circulation and Innervation of Cranial Cavity 632
Meninges and Meningeal Spaces 636
Cranial Base and Cranial Nerves 640
Blood Supply of Brain 646
Orbit and Eyeball 650
Parotid Region 662
Temporal Region and Infratemporal Fossa 664
Temporomandibular Joint 672
Tongue 676
Palate 682
Teeth 685
Nose, Paranasal Sinuses, and Pterygopalatine Fossa 690
Ear 703
Lymphatic Drainage of Head 716
Autonomic Innervation of Head 717
Imaging of Head 718
Neuroanatomy: Overview and Ventricular System 722
Telencephalon (Cerebrum) and Diencephalon 725
Brainstem and Cerebellum 734
Imaging of Brain 740

## 8 NECK 745
Subcutaneous Structures and Cervical Fascia 746
Skeleton of Neck 750
Regions of Neck 752
Lateral Region (Posterior Triangle) of Neck 754
Anterior Region (Anterior Triangle) of Neck 758
Neurovascular Structures of Neck 762
Visceral Compartment of Neck 768
Root and Prevertebral Region of Neck 772
Submandibular Region and Floor of Mouth 778
Posterior Cervical Region 783
Pharynx 786
Isthmus of Fauces 792
Larynx 798
Sectional Anatomy and Imaging of Neck 806

## 9 CRANIAL NERVES 811
Overview of Cranial Nerves 812
Cranial Nerve Nuclei 816
Cranial Nerve I: Olfactory 818
Cranial Nerve II: Optic 819
Cranial Nerves III, IV, and VI: Oculomotor, Trochlear, and Abducent 821
Cranial Nerve V: Trigeminal 824
Cranial Nerve VII: Facial 830
Cranial Nerve VIII: Vestibulocochlear 832
Cranial Nerve IX: Glossopharyngeal 834
Cranial Nerve X: Vagus 836
Cranial Nerve XI: Spinal Accessory 838
Cranial Nerve XII: Hypoglossal 839
Summary of Autonomic Ganglia of Head 840
Summary of Cranial Nerve Lesions 841
Sectional Imaging of Cranial Nerves 842

## INDEX 845

# LIST OF TABLES


## 1 THORAX
1.1 Muscles of Thoracic Wall **21**
1.2 Muscles of Respiration **24**
1.3 Surface Markings of Parietal Pleura and Surface Markings of Lungs Covered with Visceral Pleura **31**

## 2 ABDOMEN
2.1 Principal Muscles of Anterolateral Abdominal Wall **104**
2.2 Structures Forming the Inguinal Canal **108**
2.3 Parts and Relationships of Duodenum **133**
2.4 Schema of Terminology for Subdivisions of the Liver **151**
2.5 Principal Muscles of Posterior Abdominal Wall **172**
2.6 Autonomic Innervation of the Abdominal Viscera (Splanchnic Nerves) **179**

## 3 PELVIS AND PERINEUM
3.1 Differences Between Male and Female Pelves **198**
3.2 Muscles of Pelvic Walls and Floor **203**
3.3 Nerves of Sacral and Coccygeal Plexuses **207**
3.4 Arteries of Male Pelvis **225**
3.5 Lymphatic Drainage of the Male Pelvis and Perineum **229**
3.6 Effect of Sympathetic and Parasympathetic Stimulation on the Urinary Tract, Genital System, and Rectum **230**
3.7 Arteries of Female Pelvis **243**
3.8 Lymphatic Drainage of the Structures of the Female Pelvis and Perineum **245**
3.9 Muscles of Perineum **256**

## 4 BACK
4.1 Typical Cervical Vertebrae (C3-C7) **294**
4.2 Thoracic Vertebrae **300**
4.3 Lumbar Vertebrae **302**
4.4 Intrinsic Back Muscles **329**
4.5 Muscles of the Atlanto-Occipital and Atlantoaxial Joints **332**

## 5 LOWER LIMB
5.1 Motor Nerves of Lower Limb **358**
5.2 Muscles of Anterior Thigh **377**
5.3 Muscles of Medial Thigh **378**
5.4 Muscles of Gluteal Region **386**
5.5 Muscles of Posterior Thigh (Hamstring) **387**
5.6 Nerves of Gluteal Region **392**
5.7 Arteries of Gluteal Region and Posterior Thigh **393**
5.8 Bursae Around Knee **415**
5.9 Muscles of the Anterior Compartment of Leg **423**
5.10 Common, Superficial, and Deep Fibular Nerves **424**
5.11 Arterial Supply to Dorsum of Foot **427**
5.12 Muscles of the Lateral Compartment of Leg **429**
5.13 Muscles of the Posterior Compartment of Leg **432**
5.14 Arterial Supply of Leg and Foot **441**
5.15 Muscles in Sole of Foot—First Layer **444**
5.16 Muscles in Sole of Foot—Second Layer **445**
5.17 Muscles in Sole of Foot—Third Layer **446**
5.18 Muscles in Sole of Foot—Fourth Layer **447**
5.19 Joints of Foot **460**

## 6 UPPER LIMB
6.1 Cutaneous Nerves of Upper Limb **485**
6.2 Anterior Axioappendicular Muscles **499**
6.3 Arteries of Proximal Upper Limb (Shoulder Region and Arm) **505**
6.4 Axilla, Axillary Vessels, and Brachial Plexus **507**
6.5 Superficial Back (Posterior Axioappendicular) and Deltoid Muscles **513**
6.6 Movements of Scapula **515**
6.7 Deep Scapulohumeral/Shoulder Muscles **517**
6.8 Arm Muscles **520**
6.9 Arteries of Forearm **550**
6.10 Muscles of Anterior Surface of the Forearm **553**
6.11 Muscles of Hand **565**
6.12 Arteries of Hand **573**
6.13 Muscles of Posterior Surface of the Forearm **575**

## 7 HEAD
7.1 Main Muscles of Facial Expression **629**
7.2 Nerves of Face and Scalp **631**
7.3 Arteries of Face and Scalp **632**
7.4 Veins of Face **633**
7.5 Arterial Supply to the Brain **647**
7.6 Arteries of Orbit **657**
7.7 Muscles of Orbit **658**
7.8 Actions of Muscles of the Orbit Starting From Primary Position **659**
7.9 Muscles of Mastication (Acting on Temporomandibular Joint) **672**
7.10 Movements of the Temporomandibular Joint **673**
7.11 Muscles of Tongue **677**
7.12 Muscles of Soft Palate **684**
7.13 Primary and Secondary Dentition **689**

## 8 NECK
8.1 Platysma **746**
8.2 Cervical Regions and Contents **752**
8.3 Sternocleidomastoid and Trapezius **753**
8.4 Suprahyoid and Infrahyoid Muscles **761**
8.5 Arteries of the Neck **764**
8.6 Anterior Vertebral Muscles **774**
8.7 Lateral Vertebral Muscles **777**
8.8 Muscles of Posterior Cervical Region **783**
8.9 Muscles of Pharynx **788**
8.10 Muscles of Larynx **802**

## 9 CRANIAL NERVES
9.1 Summary of Cranial Nerves **815**
9.2 Olfactory Nerve (CN I) **818**
9.3 Optic Nerve (CN II) **819**
9.4 Oculomotor (CN III), Trochlear (CN IV), and Abducent (CN VI) Nerves **822**
9.5 Trigeminal Nerve (CN V) **824**
9.6 Branches of Ophthalmic Nerve (CN $V^1$) **825**
9.7 Branches of Maxillary Nerve (CN $V^2$) **826**
9.8 Branches of Mandibular Nerve (CN $V^3$) **828**
9.9 Facial Nerve (CN VII), Including Motor Root and Intermediate Nerve **830**
9.10 Vestibulocochlear Nerve (CN VIII) **832**
9.11 Glossopharyngeal Nerve (CN IX) **834**
9.12 Vagus Nerve (CN X) **837**
9.13 Spinal Accessory Nerve (CN XI) **838**
9.14 Hypoglossal Nerve (CN XII) **839**
9.15 Autonomic Ganglia of the Head **840**
9.16 Summary of Cranial Nerve Lesions **841**

# TABLE AND FIGURE CREDITS

**Note:** A list of the table and figure sources for this book from previous editions of *Clinically Oriented Anatomy*, *Grant's Atlas*, and *Essential Clinical Anatomy* can be found online at http://thepoint.lww.com/grantsatlas.

**Chapter 1**

**1.5AB** Courtesy of Dr. K. Bukhanov, University of Toronto, Canada
**1.5C** Dean D, Herbener TE. Cross-Sectional Human Anatomy, 2000:25 (Plate 2.9).
**1.23** Courtesy of Dr. E.L. Lansdown, University of Toronto, Canada
**1.33A** Courtesy of Dr. D.E. Sanders, University of Toronto, Canada
**1.33B** Courtesy of Dr. S. Herman, University of Toronto, Canada
**1.33C** Courtesy of Dr. E.L. Lansdown, University of Toronto, Canada
**1.36** Courtesy of I. Verschuur, Joint Department of Medical Imaging, UHN/Mount Sinai Hospital, Toronto, Canada
**1.41B&D** Courtesy of I. Verschuur, Joint Department of Medical Imaging, UHN/Mount Sinai Hospital, Toronto, Canada
**1.46C** Courtesy of I. Verschuur, Joint Department of Medical Imaging, UHN/Mount Sinai Hospital, Toronto, Canada
**1.47B&D** Courtesy of I. Morrow, University of Manitoba, Canada
**1.48B** Courtesy of Dr. J. Heslin, Toronto, Canada
**1.52B** Courtesy of I. Verschuur, Joint Department of Medical Imaging, UHN/Mount Sinai Hospital, Toronto, Canada
**1.55AB** Moore KL, Dalley AF. Clinically Oriented Anatomy. 5th ed, 2006:170 (Fig. 1.55). A is based on Torrent-Guasp F, Buckberg GD, Clemente C et al. The Structure and Function of the Helical Heart and Its Buttress Wrapping. I. The normal macroscopic structure of the heart. Sem. Thor. Cardiovasc Surgery. 13 (4): 301-319, 2001.
**1.58B** Feigenbaum H, Armstrong WF, Ryan T. Feigenbaum's Echocardiography. 5th ed, 2005:116.
**1.66B** Courtesy of Dr. E.L. Lansdown, University of Toronto, Canada
**1.81A-F** MRIs courtesy of Dr. M.A. Haider, University of Toronto, Canada
**1.82A-C** MRIs courtesy of Dr. M.A. Haider, University of Toronto, Canada
**1.83AB** MRIs courtesy of Dr. M.A. Haider, University of Toronto, Canada
**1.85A-F** Courtesy of I. Verschuur, Joint Department of Medical Imaging, UHN/Mount Sinai Hospital, Toronto, Canada

**Chapter 2**
**2.22B** MRI courtesy of Dr. M.A. Haider, University of Toronto, Canada
**2.31** Courtesy of Dr. J. Heslin, Toronto, Canada
**2.32A, C, D** Courtesy of Dr. E.L. Lansdown, University of Toronto, Canada
**2.32B** Courtesy of Dr. J. Heslin, Toronto, Canada
**2.37A** Courtesy of Dr. C.S. Ho, University of Toronto, Canada
**2.37B** Courtesy of Dr. E.L. Lansdown, University of Toronto, Canada
**2.40A** Courtesy of Dr. E.L. Lansdown, University of Toronto, Canada
**2.40B** Courtesy of Dr. J. Heslin, Toronto, Canada
**2.42** Courtesy of Dr. K. Sniderman, University of Toronto, Canada
**2.48B** Courtesy of A. M. Arenson, University of Toronto, Canada
**2.54D** Courtesy of Dr. G.B. Haber, University of Toronto, Canada
**2.56AB** Courtesy of Dr. J. Heslin, Toronto, Canada
**2.58AB** Courtesy of Dr. G.B. Haber, University of Toronto, Canada
**2.61B** Radiograph courtesy of G.B.Haber, University of Toronto, Canada; photo courtesy of Mission Hospital Regional Center, Mission Viejo, California
**2.65B** Courtesy of M. Asch, University of Toronto, Canada
**2.67B** Courtesy of E.L. Lansdown, University of Toronto, Canada
**2.68B (right)** Courtesy of M. Asch, University of Toronto, Canada
**2.85A, C, D** Courtesy of Dr. M.A. Haider, University of Toronto, Canada
**2.85B** The Visible Human Project; National Library of Medicine; Visible Man Image number 1499.
**2.86A, B, C** Courtesy of Dr. M.A. Haider, University of Toronto, Canada
**2.86D** The Visible Human Project; National Library of Medicine; Visible Man Image number 1625.
**2.87A-D** Courtesy of Dr. M.A. Haider, University of Toronto, Canada
**2.88A-D** Courtesy of Dr. M.A. Haider, University of Toronto, Canada
**2.89A-C** Ultrasounds courtesy of A.M. Arenson, University of Toronto, Canada.
**2.89D, F** Courtesy of J. Lai, University of Toronto, Canada
**2.86E, G** Dean D, Herbener TE. Cross Sectional Human Anatomy, 2000:45,53 (Plates 3.9, 3.13)

**Chapter 3**
**3.26A-C** Ultrasounds courtesy of Dr. A. Toi, University of Toronto, Canada
**3.36D** Courtesy of E.L. Lansdown, University of Toronto, Canada
**3.36E** From Sadler TW. Langman's Medical Embryology. 10th ed, 2006:92 (Fig. 7.5)
**3.66A-D** Courtesy of Dr. M.A. Haider, University of Toronto, Canada
**3.66E** Courtesy of The Visible Human Project; National Library of Medicine; Visible Man Image number 1940
**3.67** Uflacker R. Atlas of Vascular Anatomy: An Angiographic Approach, 1997:611.
**3.68A-C** Courtesy of Dr. M.A. Haider, University of Toronto, Canada
**3.69** MRIs courtesy of Dr. M.A. Haider, University of Toronto, Canada
**3.70A-G** MRIs courtesy of Dr. M.A. Haider, University of Toronto, Canada; sectioned specimens from The Visible Human Project; National Library of Medicine; Visible Woman Image numbers 1870 and 1895
**3.71AB** Courtesy of Dr. M.A. Haider, University of Toronto, Canada.
**3.72A-D** Ultrasounds courtesy of A.M. Arenson, University of Toronto, Canada
**3.73D** Reprinted with permission from Stuart GCE, Reid DF. Diagnostic studies. In Copeland LJ (ed.): Textbook of Gynecology. Philadelphia, WB Saunders, 1993.

**Chapter 4**
**4.1B** Courtesy of D. Salonen, University of Toronto, Canada
**4.7B, D, F, 4.8E** Courtesy of Drs. E. Becker and P. Bobechko, University of Toronto, Canada
**4.8C&D** Courtesy of E. Becker, University of Toronto, Canada
**4.11A, B** Courtesy of J. Heslin, Unitersity of Toronto, Canada
**4.11C, D** Courtesy of D. Armstrong, University of Toronto, Canada
**4.12C** Courtesy of D. Salonen, University of Toronto, Canada
**4.40C** Clay JH, Pounds DM. Basic Clinical Massage Therapy: Integrating Anatomy and Treatment. 2003:92 (Fig. 3.40)
**4.49B** Courtesy of D. Salonen, University of Toronto, Canada
**4.54AB** Courtesy of The Visible Human Project; National Library of Medicine; Visible Man 1168.
**4.54C** Courtesy of D. Armstrong, University of Toronto, Canada
**4.55A, B** Courtesy of The Visible Human Project; National Library of Medicine; Visible Man 1715.
**4.56A, B** Courtesy of The Visible Human Project; National Library of Medicine; Visible Man 1805.
**4.57A-D** Courtesy of D. Salonen, University of Toronto, Canada

**Chapter 5**
**5.7A-D** A and B are based on Fender FA. Foerster's scheme of the dermatomes. Arch Neurol Psychiatry 1939; 41:699. C and D are based on Keefan JJ, Garrett FD. The segmental distribution of the cutaneous nerves in the limbs of man. Anat Rec 1948;102:409
**5.11B** Rassner: Dermatologie. Lehrbuch und Atlas © Urban & Schwarzenberg Verlag München. (Appeared in Moore KL, Dalley AF. Clincally Oriented Anatomy. 4th Ed., 1999:527.)
**5.13B** Courtesy of Dr. E.L. Lansdown, University of Toronto, Canada
**5.32A** Courtesy of E. Becker, University of Toronto, Canada
**5.32 C** Daffner RH. Clinical Radiology: The Essentials. Baltimore: Williams & Wilkins, 1993:491 (Fig. 11.99)
**5.33B** Courtesy of Dr. D. Salonen, University of Toronto, Canada
**5.46** (inset at page bottom) Roche Lexicon Medizin. 4th Ed. Munich: Urban & Schwarzenberg, 1998.

(Appeared in Moore KL, Dalley AF. and Clincally Oriented Anatomy. 5 Ed., 2006:699.)
**5.49A, B** Courtesy of Dr. P. Bobechko, University of Toronto, Canada
**5.49C** Courtesy of Dr. D. Salonen, University of Toronto, Canada
**5.50B&C** Courtesy of Dr. D. Salonen, University of Toronto, Canada
**5.51** Courtesy of Dr. P. Bobechko, University of Toronto, Canada
**5.52B, C** Courtesy of Dr. D. Salonen, University of Toronto, Canada
**5.57C, D** Clay JH, Pounds DM. Basic Clinical Massage Therapy: Integrating Anatomy and Treatment. 2002:352,354 (Figs. 10.16 & 10.18)
**5.64A** Courtesy of Dr. D. K. Sniderman, University of Toronto, Canada
**5.71B, 5.76A** Courtesy of Dr. E. Becker, University of Toronto, Canada
**5.76B** Courtesy of Dr. P. Bobechko, University of Toronto, Canada
**5.77B** Courtesy of E. Becker, University of Toronto, Canada
**5.79B** Courtesy of Dr. W. Kucharczyk, University of Toronto, Canada
**5.80B** Courtesy of Dr. W. Kucharczyk, University of Toronto, Canada
**5.88C** Courtesy of Dr. P. Bobechko, University of Toronto, Canada
**5.89B, D** Courtesy of P. Babyn, University of Toronto, Canada
**5.90C** Courtesy of The Visible Human Project; National Library of Medicine; Visible Man 2105.
**5.90D, E, F** MRIs courtesy of Dr. D. Salonen, University of Toronto, Canada
**5.91C** Courtesy of The Visible Human Project; National Library of Medicine; Visible Man 2551.
**5.91D, E, F** MRIs courtesy of Dr. D. Salonen, University of Toronto, Canada
**Table 5.2 A-D** Modified from Clay JH, Pounds DM. Basic Clinical Massage Therapy: Integrating Anatomy and Treatment. 2002:301 (Plate 9.2).
**Table 5.2 E, H** Modified from Clay JH, Pounds DM. Basic Clinical Massage Therapy: Integrating Anatomy and Treatment. 2002:280,312 (Figs. 8.10, 9.10)
**Table 5.13** Clay JH and Pounds DM. Basic Clinical Massage Therapy: Integrating Anatomy and Treatment. 2002:362,364 (Figs. 10.28, 10.30)

### Chapter 6

**6.5A, B** Based on Fender FA. Foerster's scheme of the dermatomes. Arch Neurol Psychiatry 1939;41:688. (Appeared in Moore KL, Dalley AF. Clinically Oriented Anatomy. 4th ed, 1999:682,683.)
**6.5C, D** Based on Keegan JJ, Garrett FD. The segmental distribution of the cutaneous nerves in the limbs of man. Anat Rec 1948;102:409
**6.17A-E** Modified from Clay JH, Pounds DM. Basic Clinical Massage Therapy: Integrating Anatomy and Treatment. 2002:120,124,119,149 (Figs. 4.4, 4.9, 4.1, 4.49)
**6.22C** Courtesy of D. Armstrong, University of Toronto, Canada
**6.30B&D** Clay JH, Pounds DM. Basic Clinical Massage Therapy: Integrating Anatomy and Treatment. 2002:144,138 (Figs. 4.44, 4.33)
**6.44A** Courtesy of E. Becker, University of Toronto, Canada
**6.44 C, E** Courtesy of D. Salonen, University of Toronto, Canada
**6.44 D** Courtesy of R. Leekam, University of Toronto and West End Diagnostic Imaging, Canada
**6.49C** Courtesy of E. Becker, University of Toronto, Canada
**6.50** Radiographs courtesy of J. Heslin, Toronto, Canada;
**6.51B** Courtesy of D. Salonen, University of Toronto, Canada
**6.52B** Courtesy of E. Becker, University of Toronto, Canada
**6.55A** Courtesy of K. Sniderman, University of Toronto, Canada
**6.57A, 6.58A, 6.59A, 6.60A** Clay JH, Pounds DM. Basic Clinical Massage Therapy: Integrating Anatomy and Treatment. 2002:170 (Plate 5.3)
**6.66ABCD** Clay JH, Pounds DM. Basic Clinical Massage Therapy: Integrating Anatomy and Treatment. 2002:174 (Plate 5.55)
**6.72A** Courtesy of D. Armstrong, University of Toronto, Canada
**6.78F** Courtesy of E. Becker, University of Toronto, Canada
**6.81A, B** Courtesy of E. Becker, University of Toronto, Canada
**6.82B** Courtesy of D. Armstrong, University of Toronto, Canada
**6.89L** Courtesy of D. Armstrong, University of Toronto, Canada
**6.90B-D** Courtesy of D. Salonen, University of Toronto, Canada
**6.91C-E** Courtesy of D. Salonen, University of Toronto, Canada
**6.92A-C** Courtesy of D. Salonen, University of Toronto, Canada
**6.93 B** Courtesy of R. Leekam, University of Toronto and West End Diagnostic Imaging, Canada
**Table 6.5** Clay JH, Pounds DM. Basic Clinical Massage Therapy: Integrating Anatomy and Treatment. 2002:113,136,132 (Plates 4.4, 4.31, 4.24)
**Table 6.8** Clay JH, Pounds DM. Basic Clinical Massage Therapy: Integrating Anatomy and Treatment. 2002:170,171,173,179 (Plates 5.3, 5.4, 5.6, and Fig. 5.1)
**Table 6.13 3&4** Clay JH, Pounds DM. Basic Clinical Massage Therapy: Integrating Anatomy and Treatment. 2002:127 (Plate 5.5)

### Chapter 7

**7.1B, E&F** Courtesy of Dr. D. Armstrong, University of Toronto, Canada
**7.7A, B** Courtesy of Dr. E. Becker, University of Toronto, Canada
**7.29A-C** Courtesy of Dr. D. Armstrong, University of Toronto, Canada
**7.30A&B** Courtesy of I. Verschuur, Joint Department of Medical Imaging, UHN/Mount Sinai Hospital, Toronto, Canada
**7.33C** Courtesy of Dr. W. Kucharczyk, University of Toronto, Canada
**7.35C** Courtesy of Dr. W. Kucharczyk, University of Toronto, Canada
**7.38A** Courtesy of J.R. Buncic, University of Toronto, Canada
**7.46** CTs and MRIs from Langland OE, Langlais RP, Preece JW. Principles of Dental Imaging, 2002:278 (Figs. 11.32A, B; 11.33A, B).
**7.53A** Langland OE, Langlais RP, Preece JW. Principles of Dental Imaging, 2002:334 (Fig. 14.1).
**7.53B** Courtesy of M.J. Phatoah, University of Toronto, Canada.
**7.54E** Courtesy of Dr. B. Libgott, Division of Anatomy/Department of Surgery, University of Toronto, Ontario, Canada
**7.55B, C** Woelfel JB, Scheid RC. Dental Anatomy: Its Relevance to Dentistry. 6th ed, 2002:86,46 (Figs. 3.5, 1.29).
**7.64B** Courtesy of D. Armstrong, University of Toronto, Canada
**7.64C** Courtesy of E. Becker, University of Toronto, Canada
**7.65C** Courtesy of E. Becker, University of Toronto, Canada
**7.67D** Courtesy of Dr. E. Becker, University of Toronto, Canada
**7.71D** Courtesy of Welch Allen, Inc. Skaneateles Falls, NY. (Appeared in Moore KL, Dalley AF. Clinically Oriented Anatomy. 4th ed, 1999:966 (Fig. 8.2)
**7.81B** Courtesy of W. Kucharczyk, University of Toronto, Canada
**7.81C, D** Courtesy of W. Kucharczyk, University of Toronto, Canada
**7.82B** Courtesy of Dr. W. Kucharczyk, University of Toronto, Canada
**7.83A-E** All photos courtesy of The Visible Human Project; National Library of Medicine; Visible Man 1107 and 1168.
**7.86–7.89, 7.91, 7.92B, C, 7.93** Colorized from photographs provided courtesy of Dr. C.G. Smith, which appears in Smith CG. Serial Dissections of the Human Brain. Baltimore: Urban & Schwarzenber, Inc. and Toronto: Gage Publishing Ltd., 1981 (© Carlton G. Smith)
**7.90A-F** MRIs courtesy of Dr. D. Armstrong, University of Toronto, Canada
**7.94A-E** MRIs courtesy of Dr. D. Armstrong, University of Toronto, Canada
**7.95A-F** MRIs courtesy of Dr. D. Armstrong, University of Toronto, Canada
**7.96A-C** MRIs courtesy of Dr. D. Armstrong, University of Toronto, Canada
**Table 7.9** Illustrations from Clay JH, Pounds DM. Basic Clinical Massage Therapy: Integrating Anatomy and Treatment. 2002:76,74,79 (Figs.3.17, 3.15, 3.19).
**Table 7.12** (bottom left illustration) Clay JH, Pounds DM. Basic Clinical Massage Therapy: Integrating Anatomy and Treatment, 2002:80 (Fig. 3.22).

### Chapter 8

**8.4B** Courtesy of J. Heslin, University of Toronto, Canada
**8.18B** Modified from Clay JH, Pounds DM. Basic Clinical Massage Therapy: Integrating Anatomy and Treatment. 2003:92 (Fig. 3.40)
**8.25B** From Liebgott B. The Anatomical Basis of Dentistry. Philadelphia, PA: Mosby, 1982.
**8.31A** Rohen JW, Yokochi C, Lutjen-DrecollE, Romrell LJ. Color Atlas of Anatomy: A Photographic Study of the Human Body. 5th ed, 2002.
**8.31C** Courtesy of Dr. D. Salonen, University of Toronto, Canada.
**8.34A-C** Courtesy of Dr. D. Salonen, University of Toronto, Canada;
**8.36B** Courtesy of Dr. E. Becker, University of Toronto, Canada
**8.37** Photo courtesy of Acuson Corporation, Mt. View, California
**Table 8.3** Modified from Clay JH, Pounds DM. Basic Clinical Massage Therapy: Integrating Anatomy and Treatment. 2003:90,91 (Figs. 3.36, 3.48)
**Table 8.4** Modified from Clay JH, Pounds DM. Basic Clinical Massage Therapy: Integrating Anatomy and Treatment. 2003:88 (Fig. 3.34)
**Table 8.5B** Courtesy of Dr. D. Armstrong, University of Toronto, Canada
**Table 8.7** Clay JH, Pounds DM. Basic Clinical Massage Therapy: Integrating Anatomy and Treatment. 2003:101,128 (Figs. 3.53, 4.17)
**Table 8.8A-D** Clay JH, Pounds DM. Basic Clinical Massage Therapy: Integrating Anatomy and Treatment. 2003:96,100,104 (Figs. 3.48, 3.52, 3.56)

### Chapter 9

**9.6A-F** Courtesy of Dr. W. Kucharczyk, University of Toronto, Canada
**9.7A-C** Photos courtesy of Dr. W. Kucharczyk, University of Toronto, Canada

# REFERENCES

Photograph of Dr. J. C. B. Grant courtesy of Dr. C. G. Smith.

## REFERENCES


### Tribute to Dr. Grant

1. Robinson C. Canadian Medical Lives: J.C. Boileau Grant: Anatomist Extraordinary. Markham, Ontario, Canada: Associated Medical Services Inc./Fithzenry & Whiteside, 1993.
2. Grant JCB. A Method of Anatomy, Descriptive and Deductive. Baltimore: Williams & Wilkins Co., 1937. (11th edition, J. Basmajian and C. Slonecker, 1989)
3. Grant JCB. Grant's Atlas of Anatomy. Baltimore: Williams & Wilkins Co., 1943 (10th Edition, A. Agur and L. Ming, 1999)
4. Grant JCB, Cates HA. Grant's Dissector (A Handbook for Dissectors). Baltimore: Williams & Wilkins Co., 1940 (12th edition, E.K. Sauerland, 1999)

### Chapter 1

(Fig. 1.51) Anson BH. The aortic arch and its branches. *Cardiology*. New York: McGraw-Hill, vol 1: 1963.

### Chapter 2

(Fig. 2.49) Couinaud C. Lobes et segments hepatiques: Note sur l'architecture anatomique et chirurgicale du foie. *Presse Med* 1954;62:709.

(Fig. 2.49) Healy JE, Schroy PC. Anatomy of the biliary ducts within the human liver: Analysis of the prevailing pattern of branchings and the major variations of the biliary ducts. *Arch Surg* 1953;66:599.

(Fig. 2.89B) Campbell M. Ureteral reduplication (double ureter). *Urology*. Vol.1. Philadelphia: WB Saunders, 1954:309.

### Chapter 3

(Fig. 3.43A) Oelrich TM. The urethral sphincter muscle in the male. *Am J Anat* 1980;158:229.

(Fig. 3.43B) Oelrich TM. The striated urogenital sphincter muscle in the female. *Anat Rec* 1983;205:223.

### Chapter 4

(Fig. 4.48A) Jit I, Charnakia VM. The vertebral level of the termination of the spinal cord. *J Anat Soc India* 1959;8:93.

CHAPTER 1

# THORAX

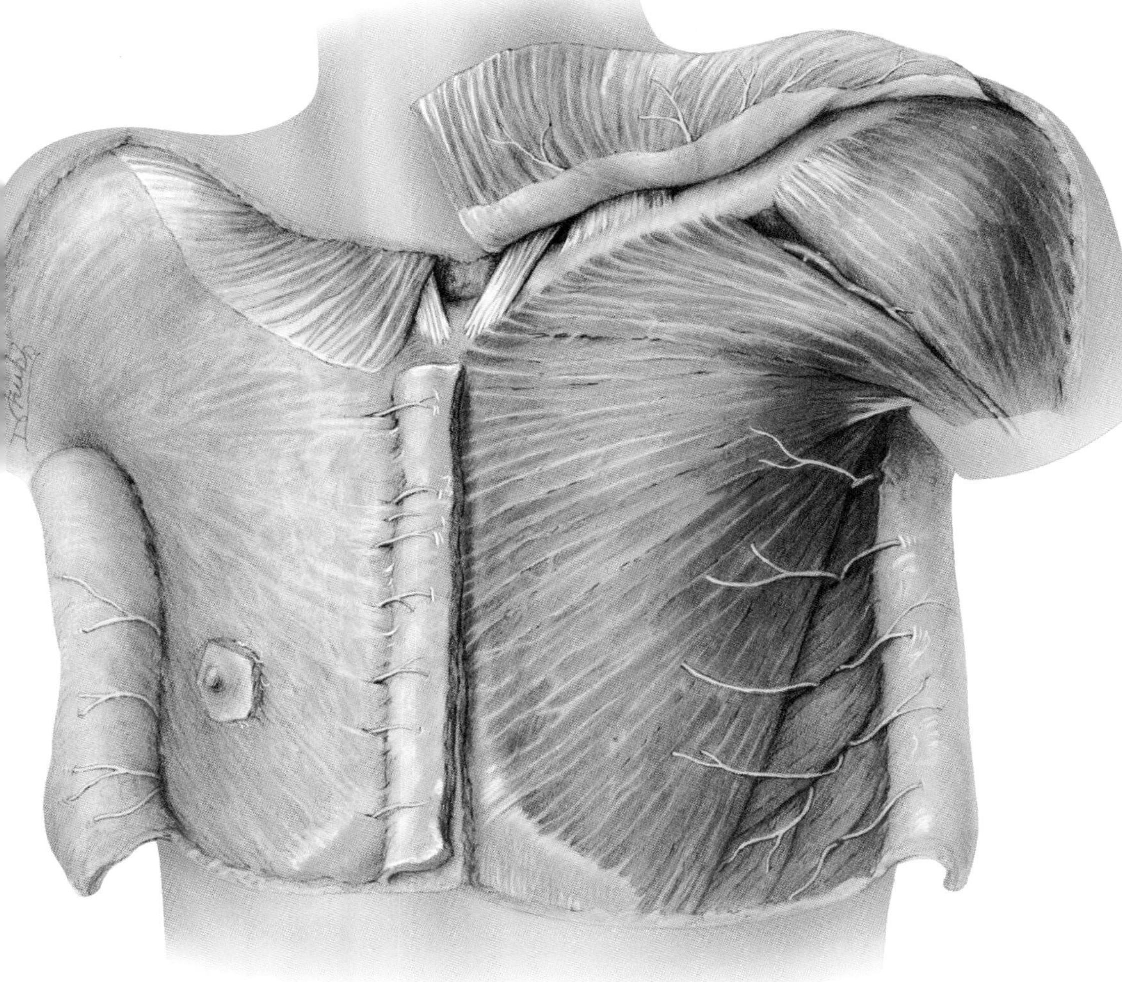


- Pectoral Region **2**
- Breast **4**
- Bony Thorax and Joints **10**
- Thoracic Wall **17**
- Thoracic Contents **25**
- Pleural Cavities **28**
- Mediastinum **29**
- Lungs and Pleura **30**
- Bronchi and Bronchopulmonary Segments **36**
- Innervation and Lymphatic Drainage of Lungs **42**
- External Heart **44**
- Coronary Vessels **52**
- Internal Heart and Valves **56**
- Conduction System of Heart **64**
- Pericardial Sac **65**
- Superior Mediastinum and Great Vessels **66**
- Diaphragm **73**
- Posterior Thorax **74**
- Overview of Autonomic Innervation **84**
- Overview of Lymphatic Drainage of Thorax **86**
- Sectional Anatomy and Imaging **88**

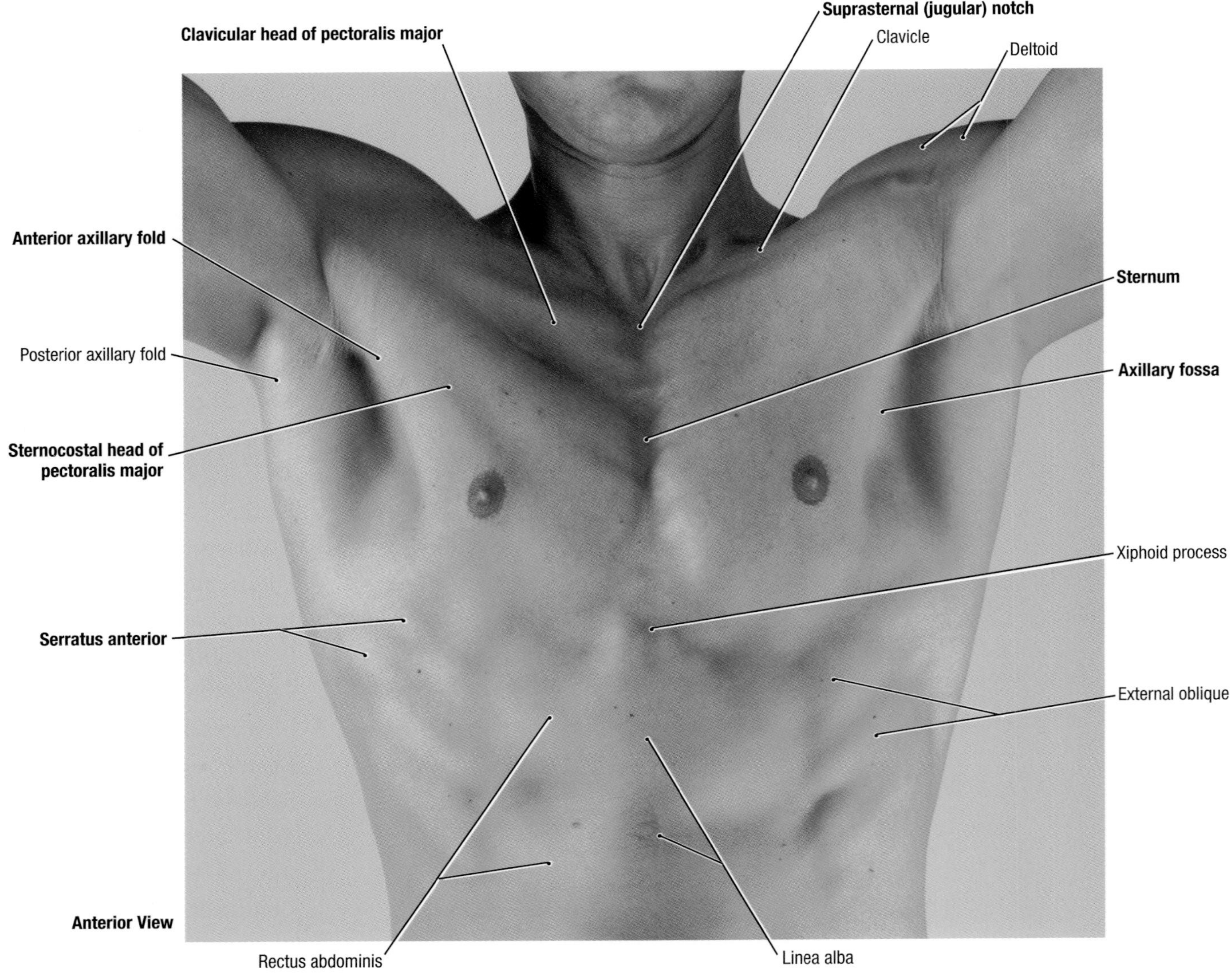
Clavicular head of pectoralis major
Suprasternal (jugular) notch
Clavicle
Deltoid
Anterior axillary fold
Sternum
Posterior axillary fold
Axillary fossa
Sternocostal head of pectoralis major
Xiphoid process
Serratus anterior
External oblique
Anterior View
Rectus abdominis
Linea alba

## 1.1 Surface anatomy of male pectoral region

- The subject is adducting the shoulders against resistance to demonstrate the pectoralis major muscle.
- The pectoralis major muscle has two parts, the sternocostal and clavicular heads.
- The anterior axillary fold is formed by the inferior border of the sternocostal head of the pectoralis major muscle.
- The axillary fossa ("armpit") is a surface feature overlying a fat-filled space, the axilla.

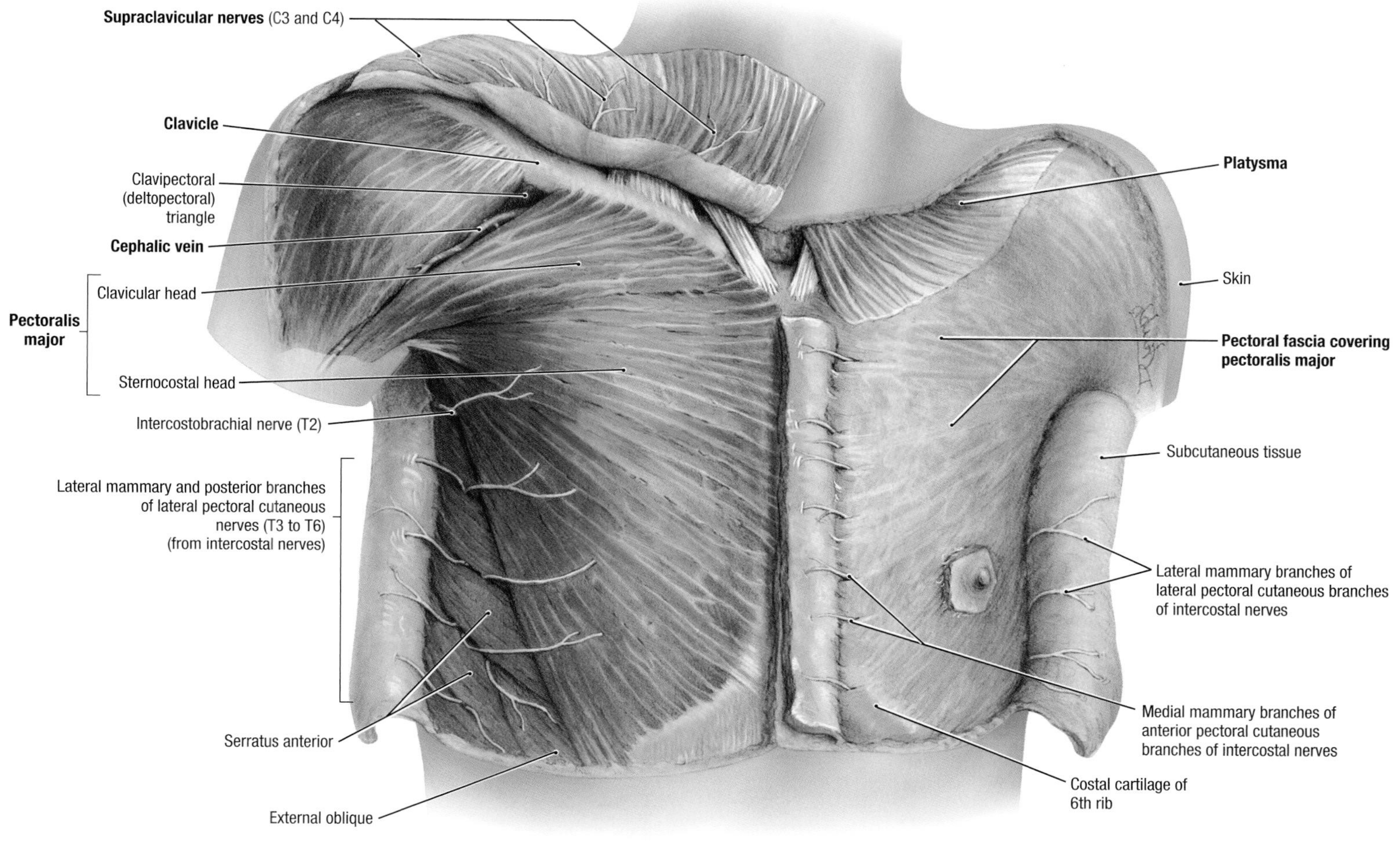
Supraclavicular nerves (C3 and C4)
Clavicle
Clavipectoral (deltopectoral) triangle
Cephalic vein
Pectoralis major
Clavicular head
Sternocostal head
Intercostobrachial nerve (T2)
Lateral mammary and posterior branches of lateral pectoral cutaneous nerves (T3 to T6) (from intercostal nerves)
Serratus anterior
External oblique
Platysma
Skin
Pectoral fascia covering pectoralis major
Subcutaneous tissue
Lateral mammary branches of lateral pectoral cutaneous branches of intercostal nerves
Medial mammary branches of anterior pectoral cutaneous branches of intercostal nerves
Costal cartilage of 6th rib
Anterior View

## 1.2 Superficial dissection, male pectoral region

- The platysma muscle, which descends to the 2nd or 3rd rib, is cut short on the right side of the specimen; together with the supraclavicular nerves, it is reflected on the left side.
- The thin pectoral fascia covers the pectoralis major.
- The clavicle lies deep to the subcutaneous tissue and the platysma muscle.
- The cephalic vein passes deeply in the clavipectoral (deltopectoral) triangle to join the axillary vein.
- Supraclavicular (C3 and C4) and upper thoracic nerves (T2 to T6) supply cutaneous innervation to the pectoral region.
- The clavipectoral (deltopectoral) triangle, bounded by the clavicle superiorly, the deltoid muscle laterally, and the clavicular head of the pectoralis major muscle medially, underlies a surface depression called the infraclavicular fossa.

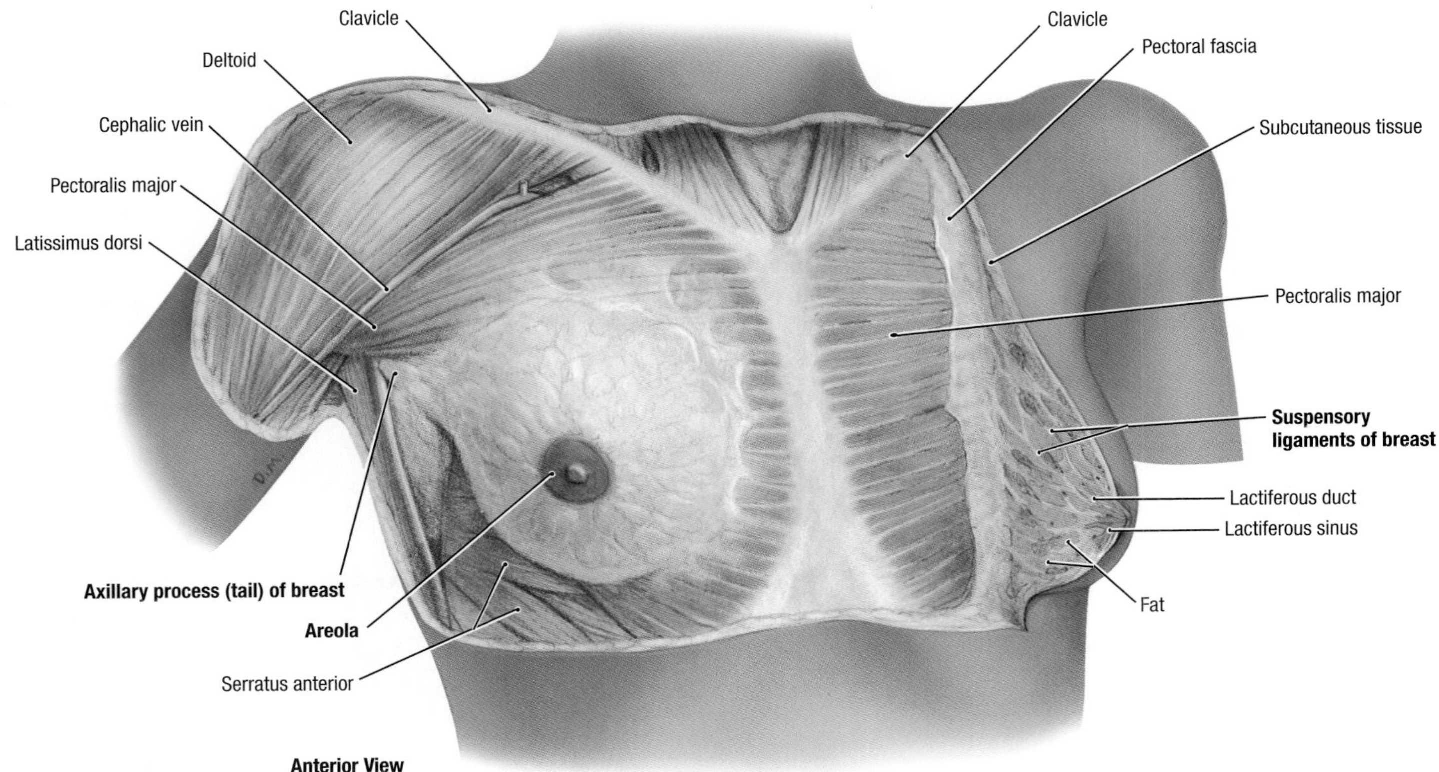
Clavicle
Deltoid
Cephalic vein
Pectoralis major
Latissimus dorsi
Axillary process (tail) of breast
Areola
Serratus anterior
Anterior View
Clavicle
Pectoral fascia
Subcutaneous tissue
Pectoralis major
Suspensory ligaments of breast
Lactiferous duct
Lactiferous sinus
Fat

## 1.3 Superficial dissection, female pectoral region

- On the specimen's right side, the skin is removed; on the left side, the breast is sagittally sectioned.
- The breast extends from the 2nd to the 6th ribs. The axillary process (tail) of the breast consists of glandular tissue projecting toward the axilla.
- The region of loose connective tissue between the pectoral fascia and the deep surface of the breast, the retromammary bursa, permits the breast to move on the deep fascia.

- Interference with the lymphatic drainage by cancer may cause lymphedema (edema, excess fluid in the subcutaneous tissue), which in turn may result in deviation of the nipple and a leathery, thickened appearance of the breast skin. Prominent (puffy) skin between dimpled pores may develop, which gives the skin an orange-peel appearance ***(peau d'orange sign)***. Larger dimples may form if pulled by cancerous invasion of the suspensory ligaments of the breast.

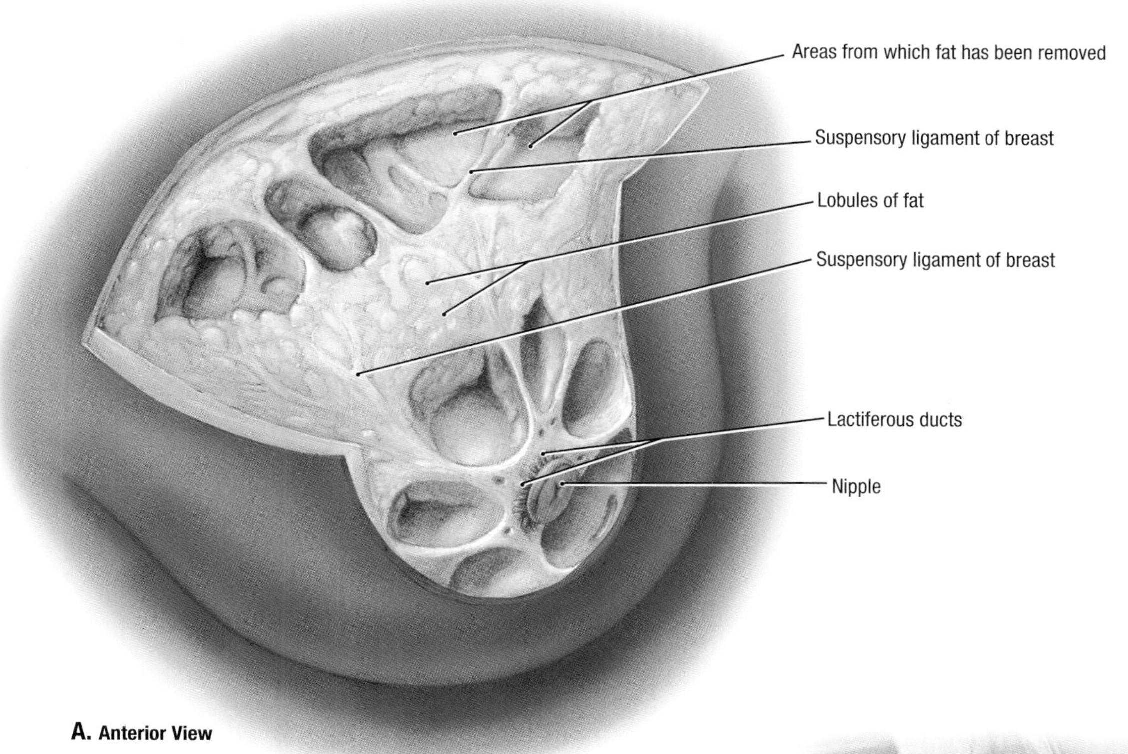
Areas from which fat has been removed
Suspensory ligament of breast
Lobules of fat
Suspensory ligament of breast
Lactiferous ducts
Nipple

**A.** **Anterior View**

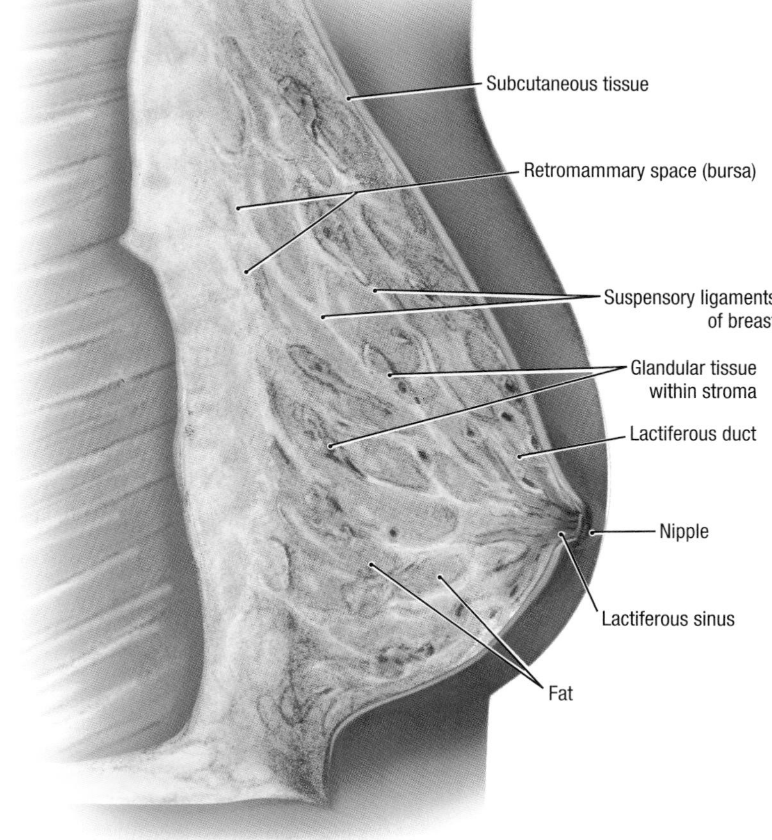
Subcutaneous tissue
Retromammary space (bursa)
Suspensory ligaments of breast
Glandular tissue within stroma
Lactiferous duct
Nipple
Lactiferous sinus
Fat

**B.** **Sagittal Section of Breast**

## 1.4 Female mammary gland

**A.** The breast consists primarily of fat compartmentalized between connective and glandular tissue septa. The lactiferous ducts (usually 15 to 20 in number) expand to form subareolar lactiferous sinuses and then open on the nipple; the glandular tissue lies within a dense (fibro-) areolar stroma, from which suspensory ligaments extend to the deeper layers of the skin. Areas of superficial fat were scooped out from some compartments between the septa. **B.** Structure of the breast revealed by sagittal section. Cancer can spread by contiguity (invasion of adjacent tissue). When breast cancer cells invade the retromammary space, attach to or invade the pectoral fascia overlaying the pectoralis major muscle, or metastasize to the interpectoral nodes (Fig. 1.8), the breast elevates when the muscle contracts. This movement is a clinical sign of advanced breast cancer.

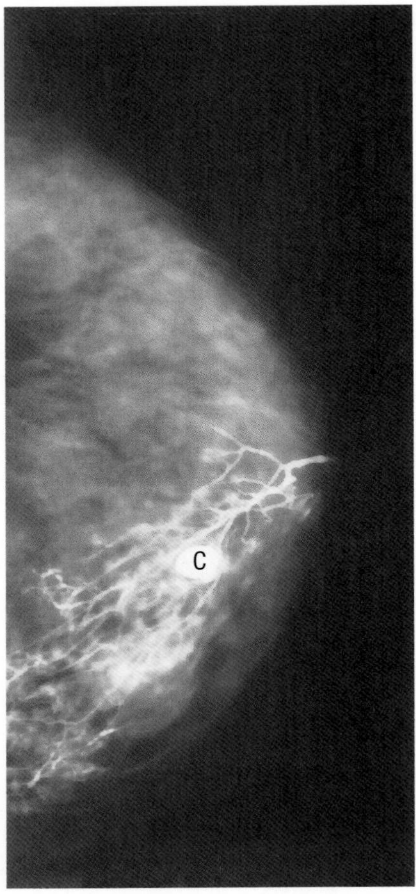
C

**A.** **Superior View**

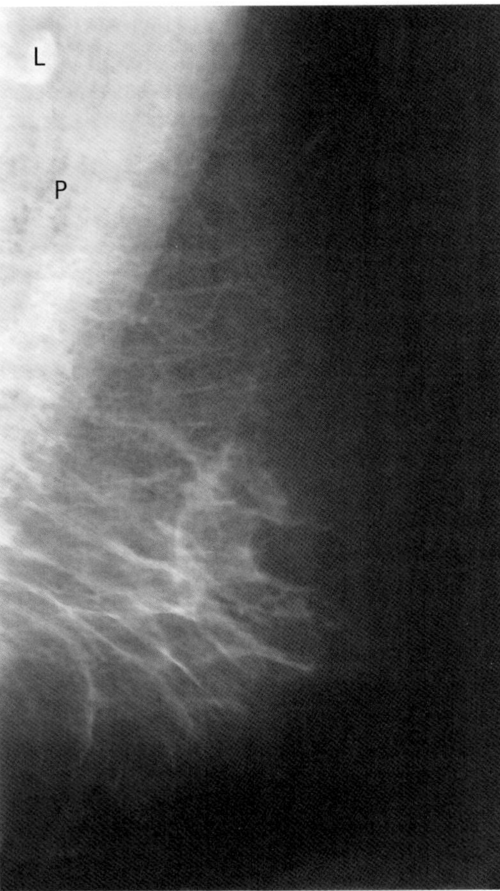
L
P

**B.** **Lateral View**

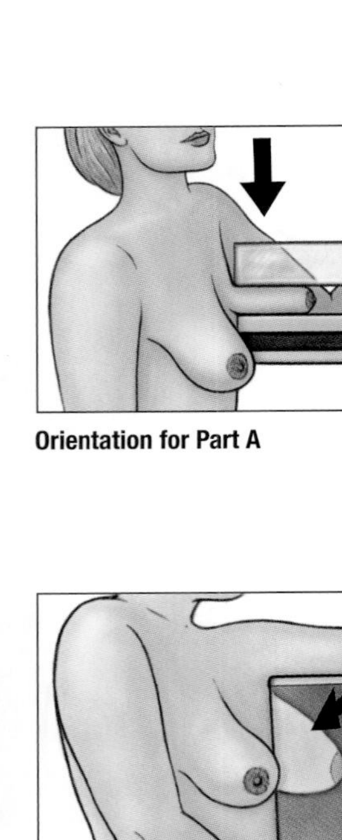

**Orientation for Part A**

**Orientation for Part B**

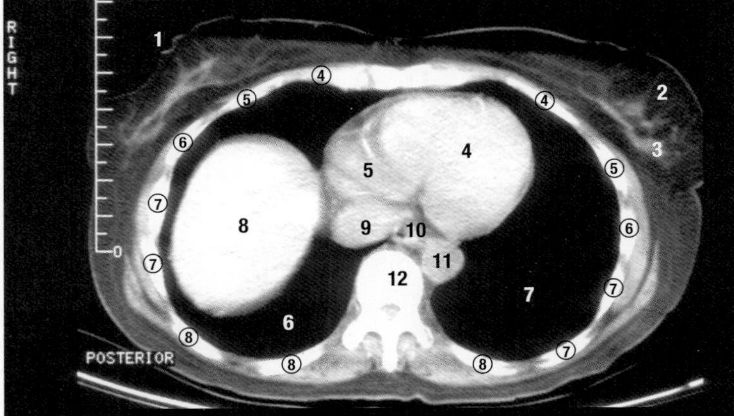
RIGHT
POSTERIOR
1
2
3
4
5
6
7
8
9
10
11
12

**C.** **Inferior View**

**Structures in Part C:**

1 Nipple
2 Lactiferous ducts
3 Suspensory ligaments
4 Left ventricle
5 Right atrium
6 Right lung
7 Left lung
8 Liver
9 Inferior vena cava
10 Esophagus
11 Descending aorta
12 T9 vertebra
⑦ Corresponding rib numbers

## 1.5 Imaging of breast

**A.** Galactogram. Contrast has been injected into a lactiferous duct, outlining the branching pattern of its tributaries. Note the presence of a ductal cyst *(C)*. **B.** Normal mammogram. Observe the connective tissue network of the breast. The stroma is radiopaque and changes with age and during lactation. Pectoralis major muscle *(P)* and an axillary lymph node *(L)* can also be seen. **C.** Axial computed tomographic (CT) scan at the level of the female breasts (T9 level).

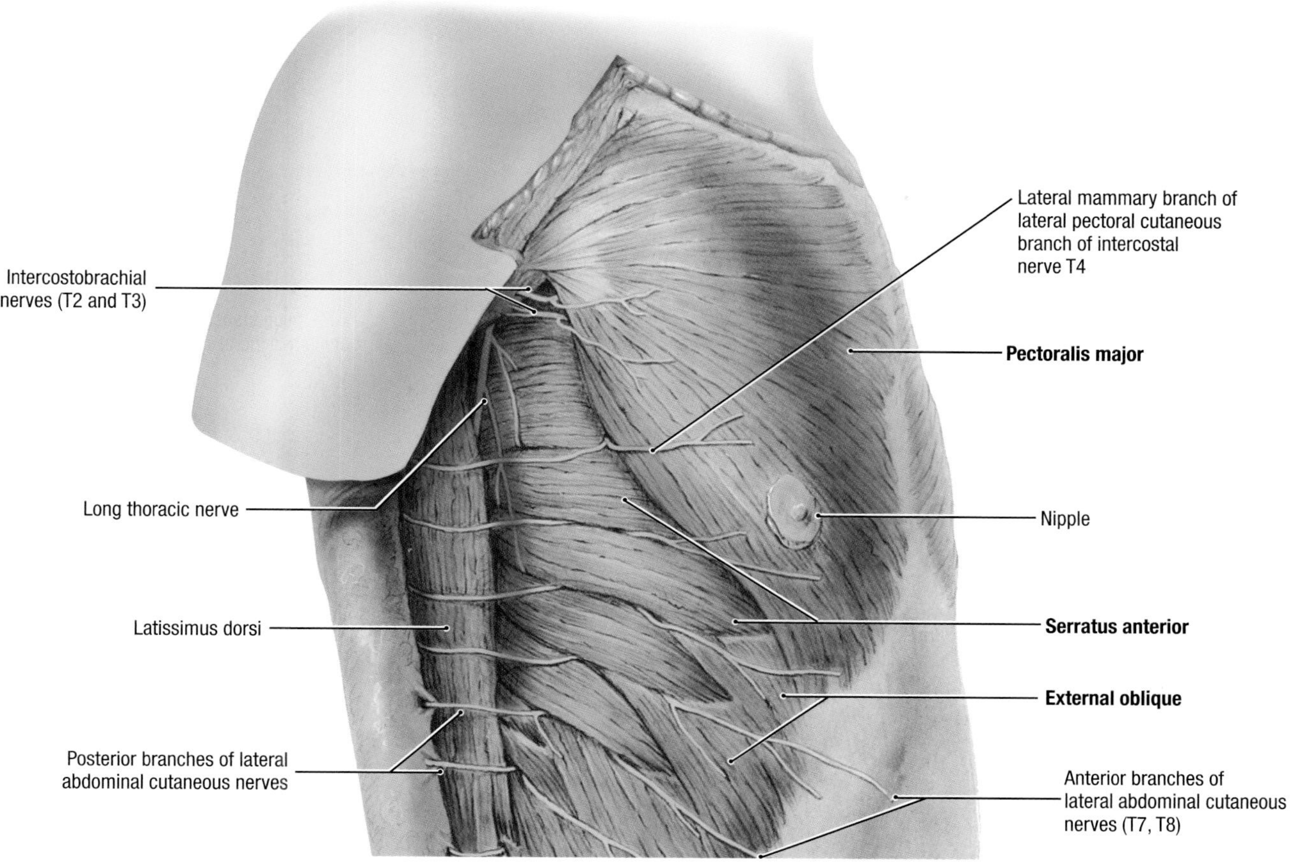
Intercostobrachial nerves (T2 and T3)
Lateral mammary branch of lateral pectoral cutaneous branch of intercostal nerve T4
Pectoralis major
Long thoracic nerve
Nipple
Latissimus dorsi
Serratus anterior
External oblique
Posterior branches of lateral abdominal cutaneous nerves
Anterior branches of lateral abdominal cutaneous nerves (T7, T8)

**A.** **Anterolateral View**

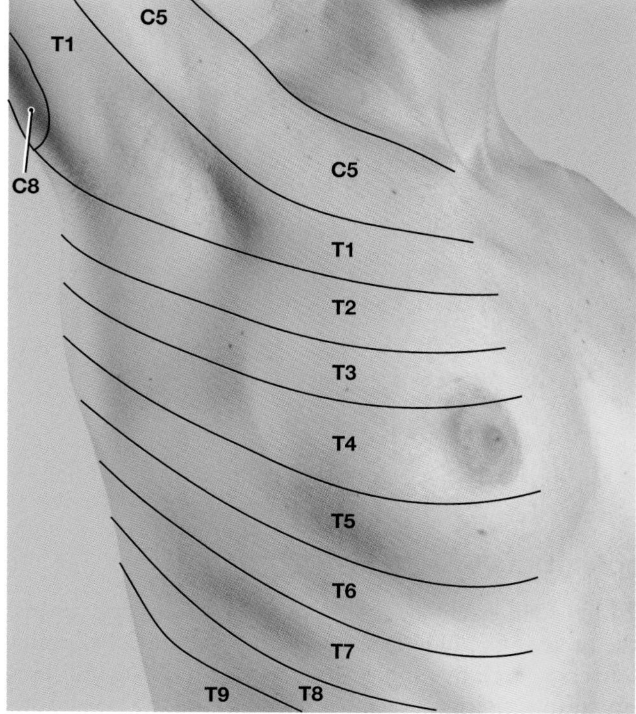
C5
T1
C8
C5
T1
T2
T3
T4
T5
T6
T7
T9
T8

**B.** **Anterolateral View**

## 1.6 Bed of breast

**A.** Muscles comprising bed of breast and cutaneous nerves. **B.** Dermatomes extending across bed of breast. Local anesthesia of an intercostal space (intercostal nerve block) is produced by injecting a local anesthetic agent around the intercostal nerves between the paravertebral line and the area of required anesthesia. Because any particular area of skin usually receives innervation from two adjacent nerves, considerable overlapping of contiguous dermatomes occurs. Therefore, complete loss of sensation usually does not occur unless two or more intercostal nerves are anesthetized.

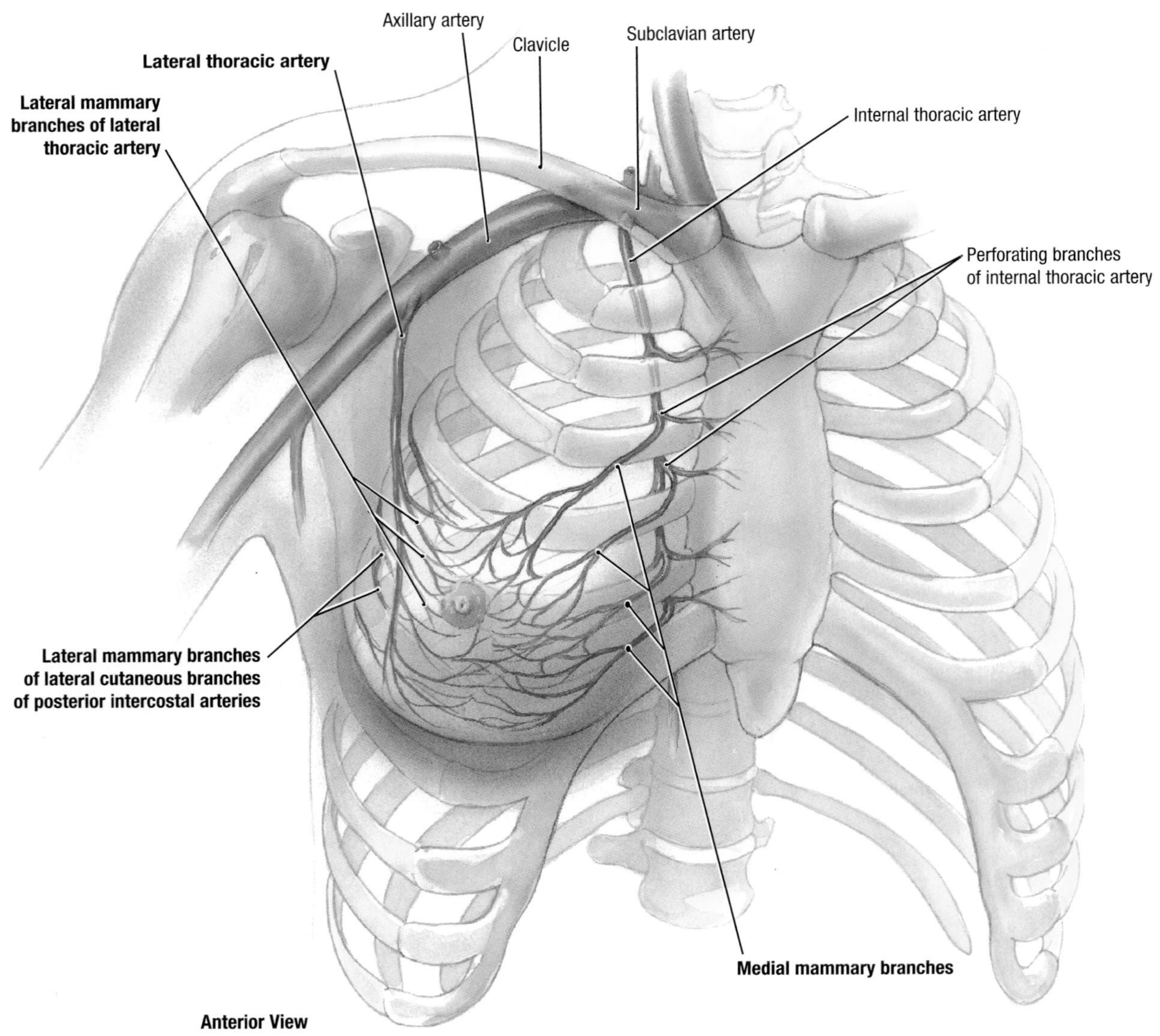
Axillary artery
Clavicle
Subclavian artery
Lateral thoracic artery
Lateral mammary branches of lateral thoracic artery
Internal thoracic artery
Perforating branches of internal thoracic artery
Lateral mammary branches of lateral cutaneous branches of posterior intercostal arteries
Medial mammary branches
Anterior View

## 1.7 Arterial supply of the breast

Arteries enter the breast from its superomedial and superolateral aspects; vessels also penetrate the deep surface of the breast. The blood supply is from the medial mammary branches of the internal thoracic artery, lateral mammary branches from the lateral thoracic artery, and lateral mammary branches of lateral cutaneous branches of the posterior intercostal arteries. The arteries branch profusely and anastomose with each other.

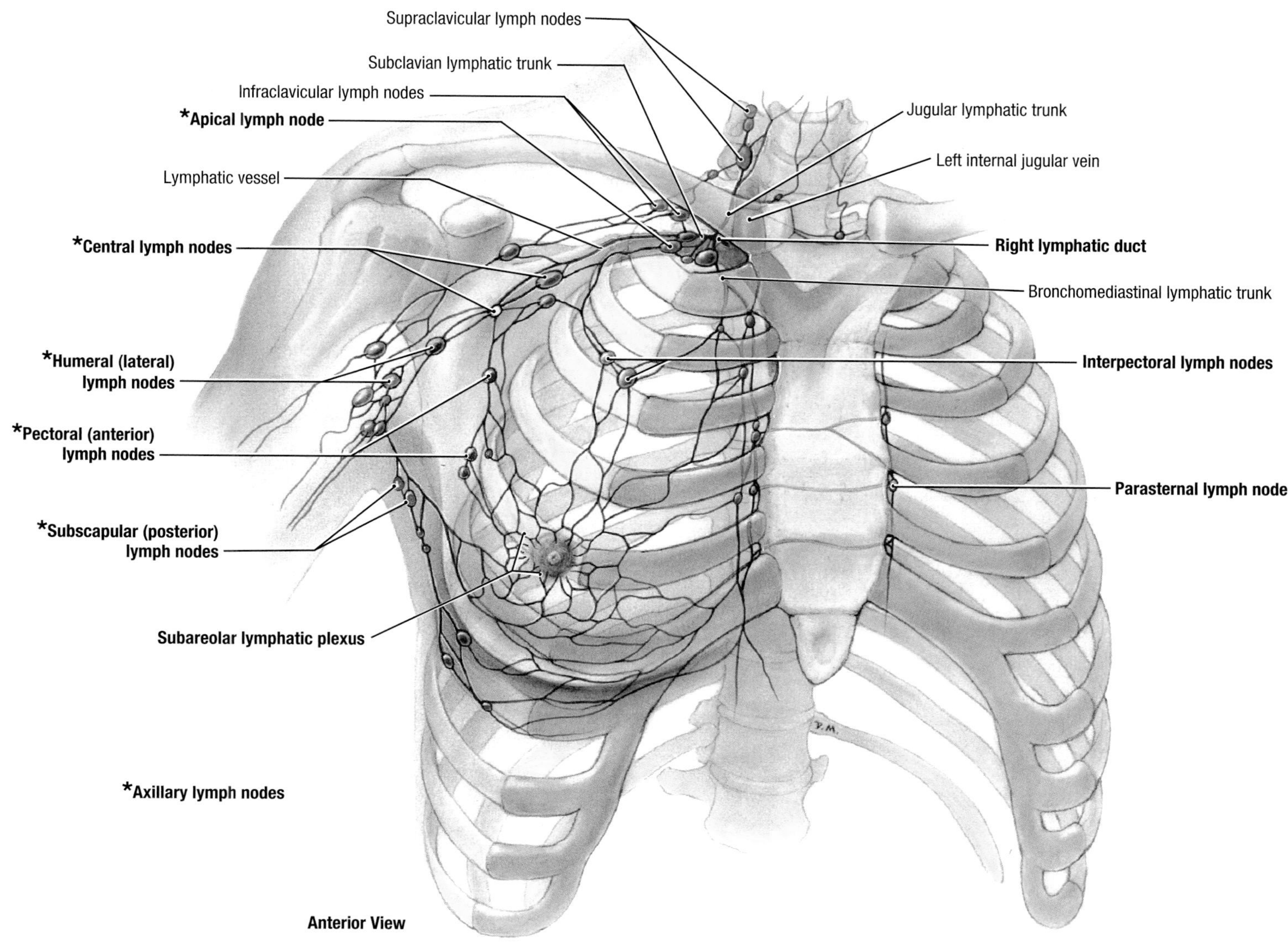
Supraclavicular lymph nodes
Subclavian lymphatic trunk
Infraclavicular lymph nodes
*Apical lymph node
Lymphatic vessel
*Central lymph nodes
*Humeral (lateral) lymph nodes
*Pectoral (anterior) lymph nodes
*Subscapular (posterior) lymph nodes
Subareolar lymphatic plexus
*Axillary lymph nodes
Anterior View
Jugular lymphatic trunk
Left internal jugular vein
Right lymphatic duct
Bronchomediastinal lymphatic trunk
Interpectoral lymph nodes
Parasternal lymph node

## 1.8 Lymphatic drainage of breast

Lymph drained from the upper limb and breast passes through nodes arranged irregularly in groups of axillary lymph nodes: (a) pectoral, along the inferior border of the pectoralis minor muscle; (b) subscapular, along the subscapular artery and veins; (c) humeral, along the distal part of the axillary vein; (d) central, at the base of the axilla, embedded in axillary fat; and (e) apical, along the axillary vein between the clavicle and the pectoralis minor muscle. Most of the breast drains via the pectoral, central, and apical axillary nodes to the subclavian lymph trunk, which joins the venous system at the junction of the subclavian and internal jugular veins. The medial part of the breast drains to the parasternal nodes, which are located along the internal thoracic vessels.

Breast cancer typically spreads by means of lymphatic vessels (lymphogenic metastasis), which carry cancer cells from the breast to the lymph nodes, chiefly those in the axilla. The cells lodge in the nodes, producing nests of tumor cells (metastases). Abundant communications among lymphatic pathways and among axillary, cervical, and parasternal nodes may also cause metastases from the breast to develop in the supraclavicular lymph nodes, the opposite breast, or the abdomen.

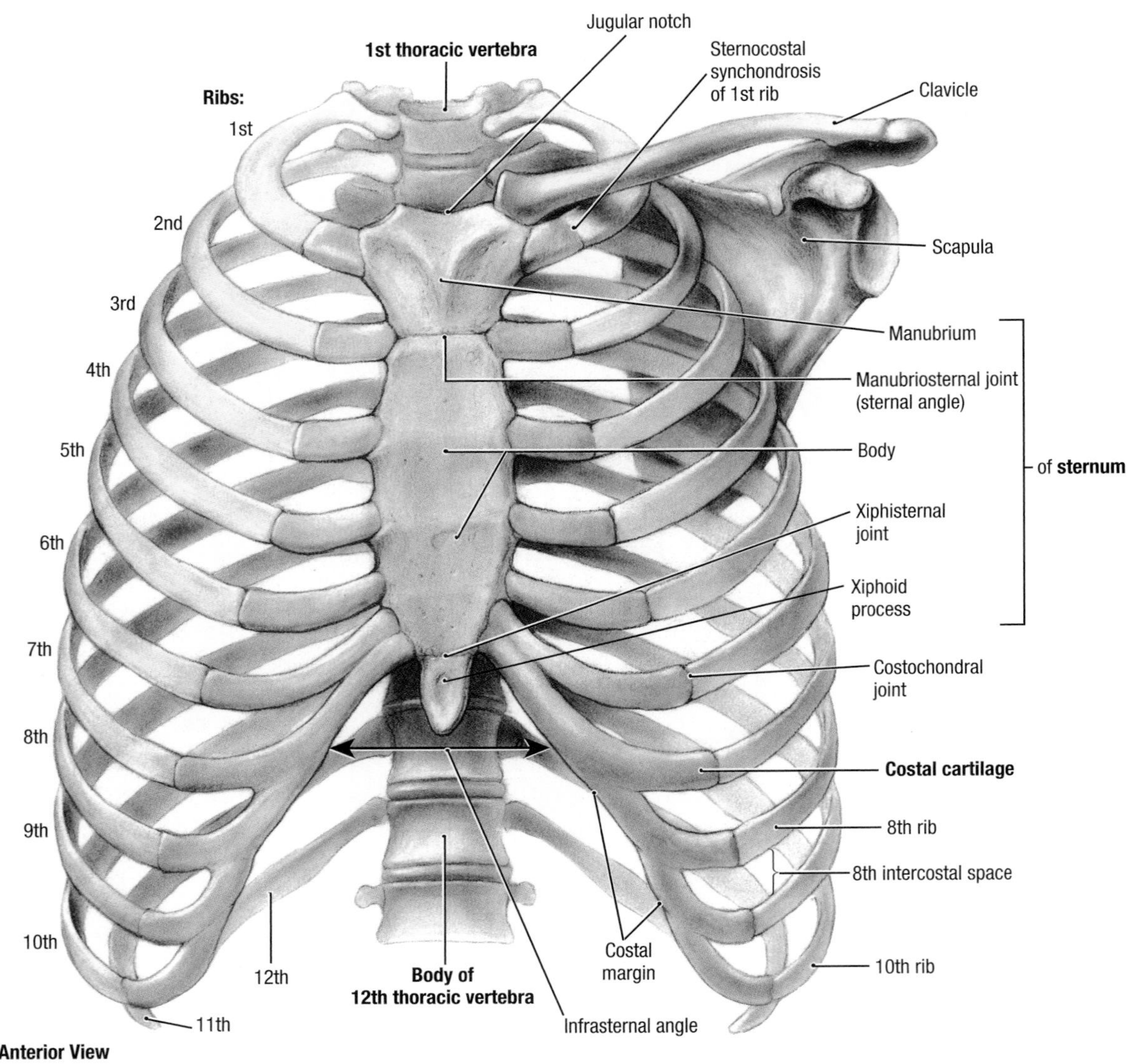
1st thoracic vertebra
Jugular notch
Sternocostal synchondrosis of 1st rib
Clavicle
Ribs:
1st
2nd
3rd
4th
5th
6th
7th
8th
9th
10th
11th
12th
Scapula
Manubrium
Manubriosternal joint (sternal angle)
Body
Xiphisternal joint
Xiphoid process
of sternum
Costochondral joint
Costal cartilage
8th rib
8th intercostal space
10th rib
Costal margin
Body of 12th thoracic vertebra
Infrasternal angle

A. Anterior View

## 1.9 Bony thorax

- The skeleton of the thorax consists of 12 thoracic vertebrae, 12 pairs of ribs and costal cartilages, and the sternum.
- Anteriorly, forming the costal margin, the superior seven costal cartilages articulate with the sternum; the 8th, 9th, and 10th cartilages articulate with the cartilage above; the 11th and 12th are "floating" ribs, i.e., their cartilages do not articulate anteriorly.
- The clavicle lies over the anterosuperior aspect of the 1st rib, making it difficult to palpate.
- The 2nd rib is easy to locate because its costal cartilage articulates with the sternum at the sternal angle, located at the junction of the manubrium and body of the sternum.
- The 3rd to 10th ribs can be palpated in sequence inferolaterally from the 2nd rib; the fused costal cartilages of the 7th to 10th ribs form the costal arch (margin), and the tips of the 11th and 12th ribs can be palpated posterolaterally.

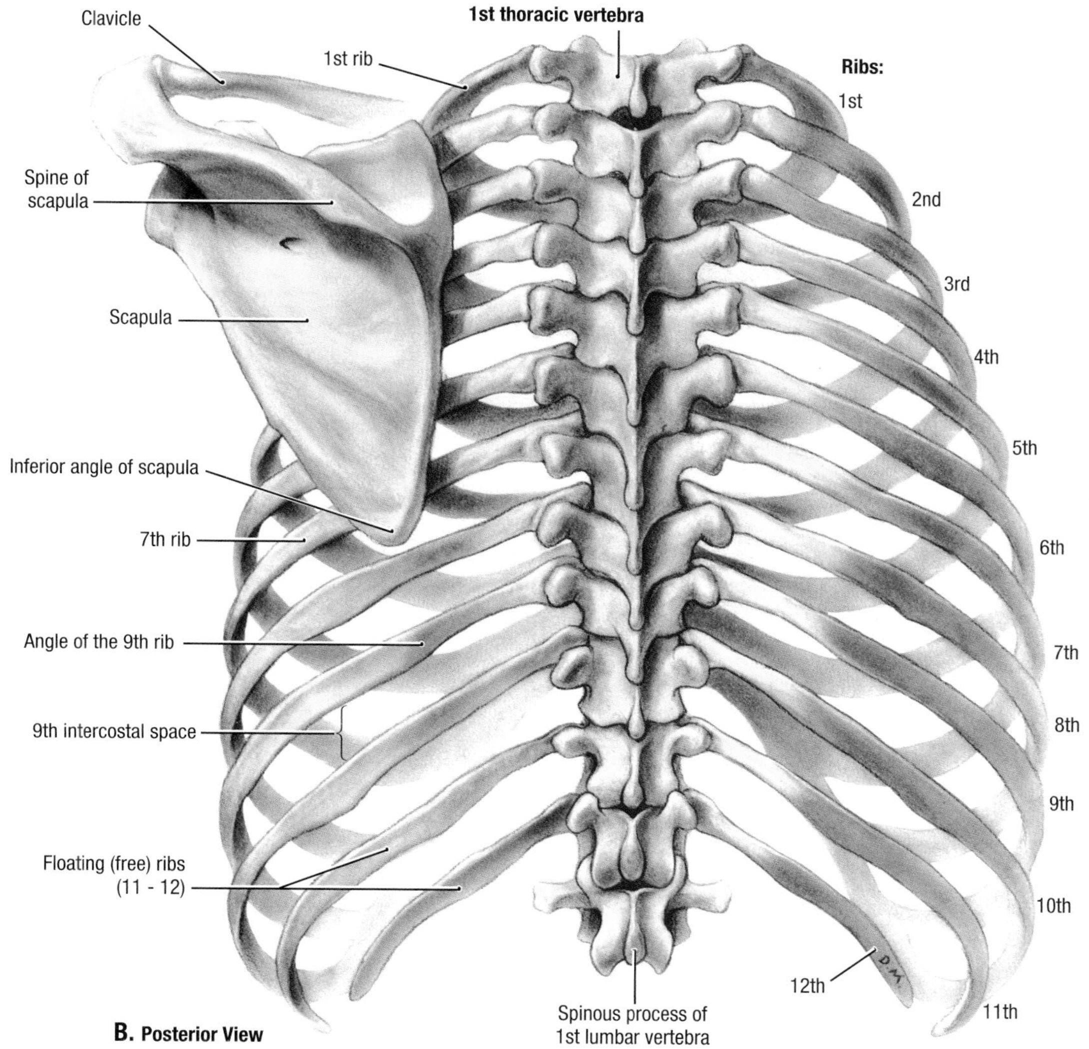
Clavicle
1st rib
1st thoracic vertebra
Ribs:
1st
2nd
3rd
4th
5th
6th
7th
8th
9th
10th
11th
12th
Spine of scapula
Scapula
Inferior angle of scapula
7th rib
Angle of the 9th rib
9th intercostal space
Floating (free) ribs (11 - 12)
Spinous process of 1st lumbar vertebra

**B. Posterior View**

## 1.9 Bony thorax *(continued)*

- The superior thoracic aperture (thoracic inlet) is the doorway between the thoracic cavity and the neck region; it is bounded by the 1st thoracic vertebra, the 1st ribs and their cartilages, and the manubrium of the sternum.
- Each rib articulates posteriorly with the vertebral column.
- Posteriorly, all ribs angle inferiorly; anteriorly, the 3rd to 10th costal cartilages angle superiorly.
- The scapula is suspended from the clavicle and crosses the 2nd to 7th ribs.

- When clinicians refer to the superior thoracic aperture as the thoracic "outlet," they are emphasizing the important nerves and arteries that pass through this aperture into the lower neck and upper limb. Hence, various types of thoracic outlet syndromes exist, such as the costoclavicular syndrome—pallor and coldness of the skin of the upper limb and diminished radial pulse—resulting from compression of the subclavian artery between the clavicle and the 1st rib.

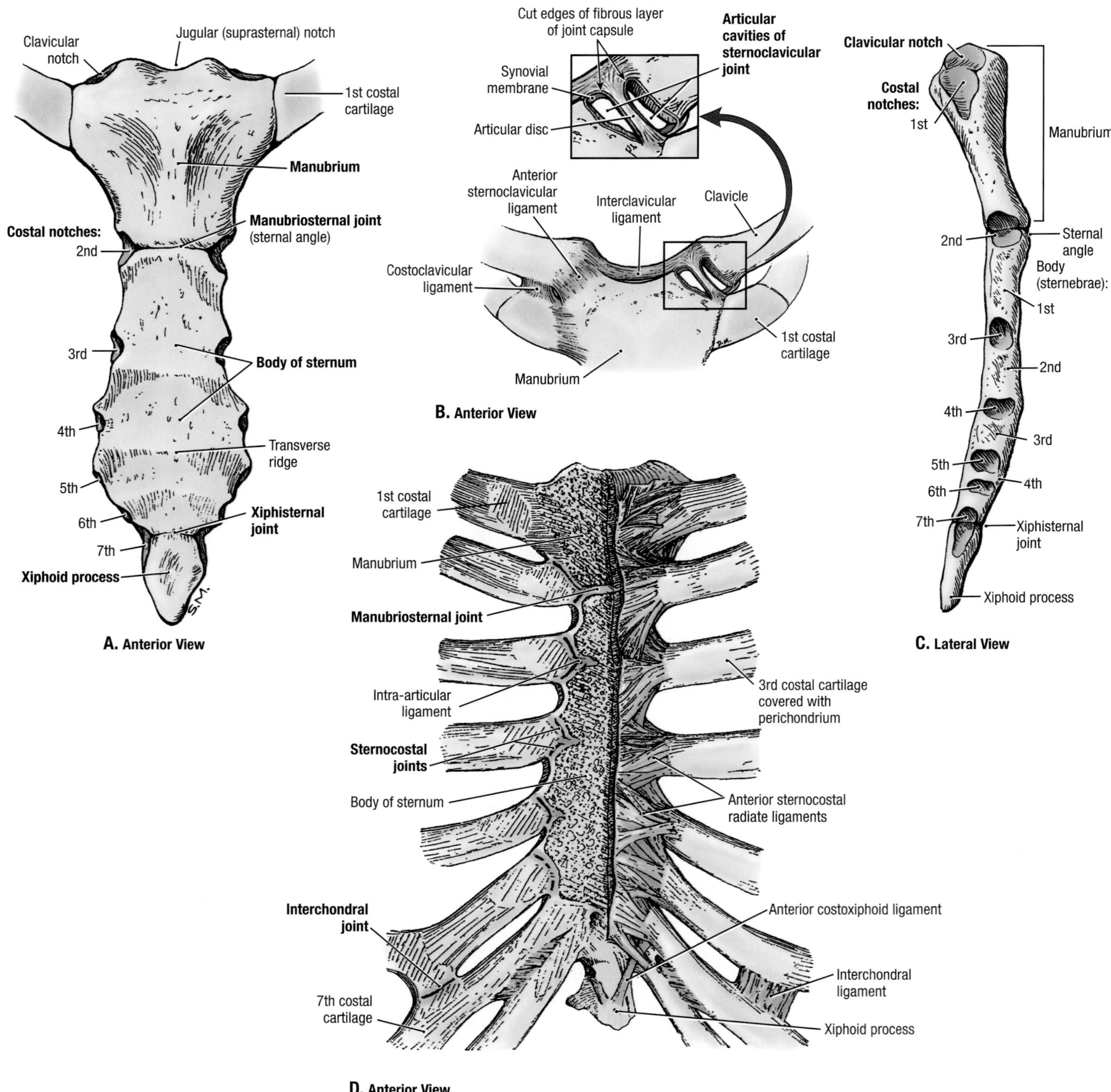
Clavicular notch
Jugular (suprasternal) notch
1st costal cartilage
Manubrium
Costal notches:
2nd
Manubriosternal joint (sternal angle)
3rd
Body of sternum
4th
Transverse ridge
5th
6th
Xiphisternal joint
7th
Xiphoid process
A. Anterior View
Cut edges of fibrous layer of joint capsule
Articular cavities of sternoclavicular joint
Synovial membrane
Articular disc
Anterior sternoclavicular ligament
Interclavicular ligament
Clavicle
Costoclavicular ligament
1st costal cartilage
Manubrium
B. Anterior View
Clavicular notch
Costal notches:
1st
Manubrium
2nd
Sternal angle
Body (sternebrae):
1st
3rd
2nd
4th
3rd
5th
6th
4th
7th
Xiphisternal joint
Xiphoid process
C. Lateral View
1st costal cartilage
Manubrium
Manubriosternal joint
Intra-articular ligament
3rd costal cartilage covered with perichondrium
Sternocostal joints
Body of sternum
Anterior sternocostal radiate ligaments
Interchondral joint
Anterior costoxiphoid ligament
Interchondral ligament
7th costal cartilage
Xiphoid process
D. Anterior View

## 1.10 Sternum and associated joints

**A.** Parts of the anterior aspect of the sternum. **B.** Sternoclavicular joint. **C.** Features of the lateral aspect of the sternum. **D.** Sternocostal, manubriosternal, and interchondral joints. On the right side of the specimen, the cortex of the sternum and the external surface of the costal cartilages have been shaved away.

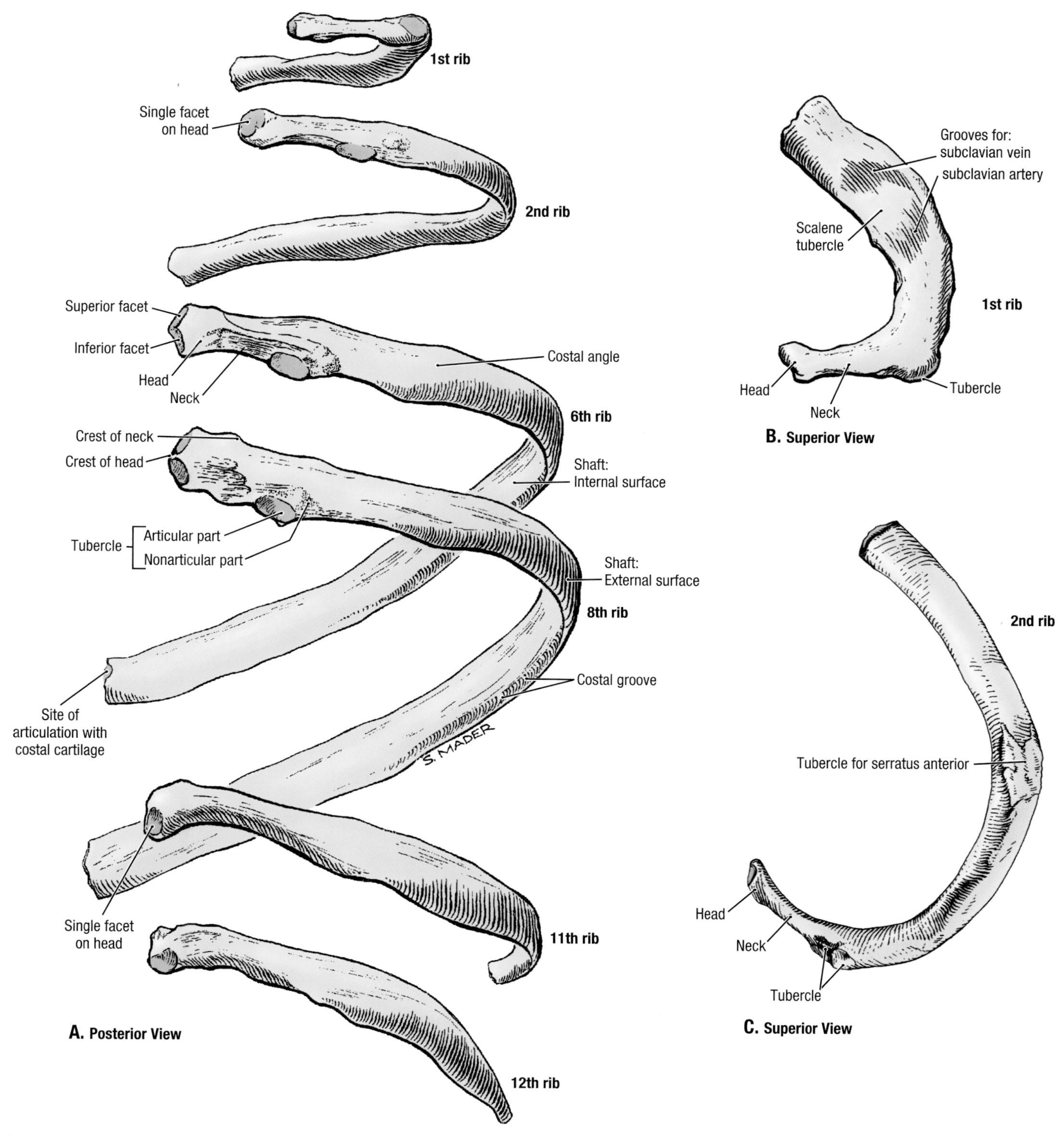
1st rib
Single facet on head
2nd rib
Superior facet
Inferior facet
Head
Neck
Costal angle
6th rib
Crest of neck
Crest of head
Shaft: Internal surface
Tubercle
Articular part
Nonarticular part
Shaft: External surface
8th rib
Costal groove
Site of articulation with costal cartilage
S. MADER
Single facet on head
11th rib
12th rib
A. Posterior View
Grooves for:
subclavian vein
subclavian artery
Scalene tubercle
1st rib
Head
Neck
Tubercle
B. Superior View
2nd rib
Tubercle for serratus anterior
Head
Neck
Tubercle
C. Superior View

## 1.11 Ribs

**A.** "Typical" (6th and 8th) and "atypical" (1st and 2nd, 11th and 12th) ribs. **B.** First rib. **C.** Second rib.

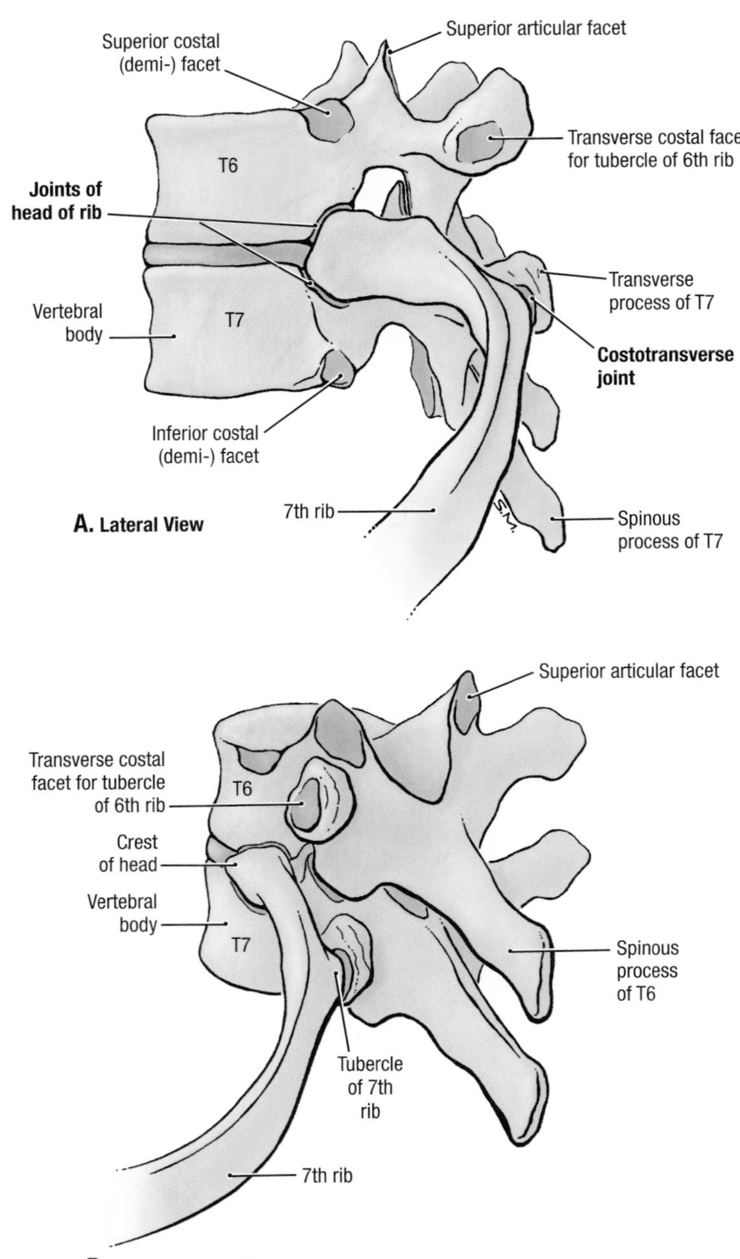
Superior costal
(demi-) facet
Superior articular facet
Transverse costal facet
for tubercle of 6th rib
T6
Joints of
head of rib
Vertebral
body
T7
Transverse
process of T7
Costotransverse
joint
Inferior costal
(demi-) facet
7th rib
Spinous
process of T7
A. Lateral View
Superior articular facet
Transverse costal
facet for tubercle
of 6th rib
T6
Crest
of head
Vertebral
body
T7
Spinous
process
of T6
Tubercle
of 7th
rib
7th rib
B. Posterolateral View

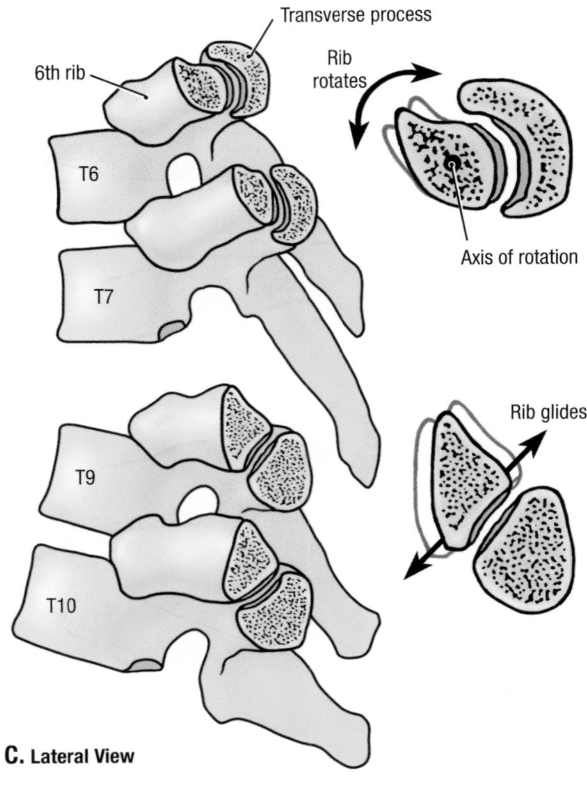
Transverse process
6th rib
Rib
rotates
T6
Axis of rotation
T7
Rib glides
T9
T10
C. Lateral View

## 1.12 Costovertebral articulations

**A** and **B.** Articulating structures

- The costovertebral articulations include the joints of the head of the rib with two adjacent vertebral bodies and the tubercle of the rib with the transverse process of a vertebra.
- There are two articular facets on the head of the rib: a larger, inferior costal facet for articulation with the vertebral body of its own number, and a smaller, superior costal facet for articulation with the vertebral body of the vertebra superior to the rib.
- The crest of the head of the rib separates the superior and inferior costal facets.
- The smooth articular part of the tubercle of the rib, the transverse costal facet, articulates with the transverse process of the same numbered vertebra at the costotransverse joint.

**C.** Movements at the costotransverse joints: At the 1st to 7th costotransverse joints, the ribs rotate, increasing the anteroposterior diameter of the thorax; at the 8th, 9th, and 10th, they glide, increasing the transverse diameter of the upper abdomen.

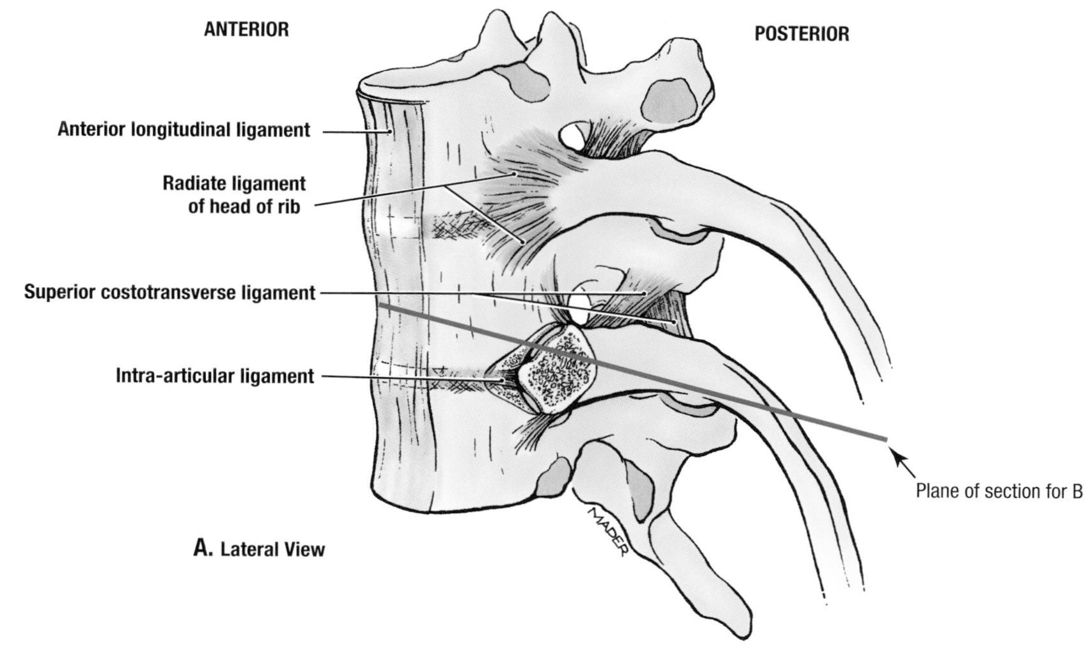
ANTERIOR
POSTERIOR
Anterior longitudinal ligament
Radiate ligament of head of rib
Superior costotransverse ligament
Intra-articular ligament
Plane of section for B
MADER
A. Lateral View

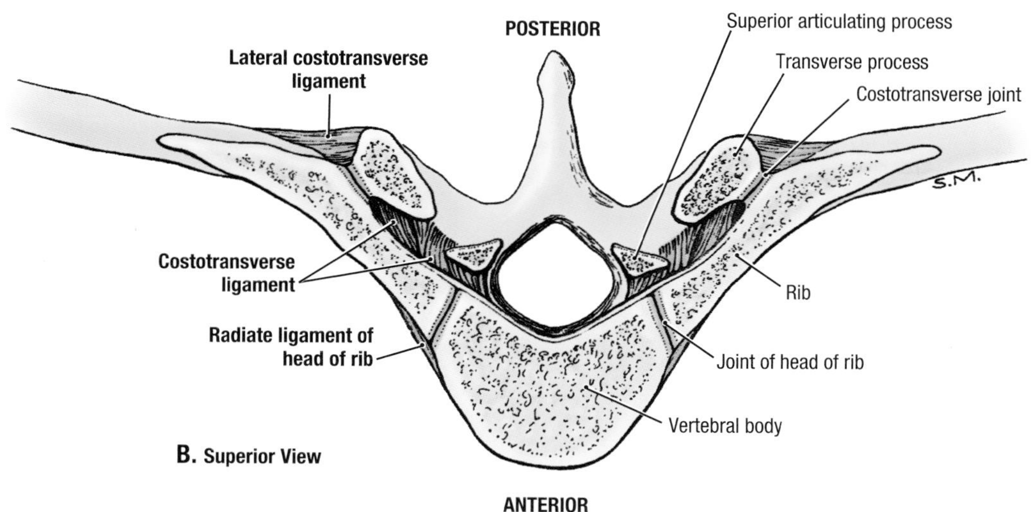
POSTERIOR
Superior articulating process
Transverse process
Costotransverse joint
Lateral costotransverse ligament
S.M.
Costotransverse ligament
Rib
Radiate ligament of head of rib
Joint of head of rib
Vertebral body
B. Superior View
ANTERIOR

## 1.13 Ligaments of costovertebral articulations

**A.**

- The radiate ligament joins the head of the rib to two vertebral bodies and the interposed intervertebral disc.
- The superior costotransverse ligament joins the crest of the neck of the rib to the transverse process above.
- The intra-articular ligament joins the crest of the head of the rib to the intervertebral disc.

**B.**

- The vertebral body, transverse processes, superior articulating processes, and posterior elements of the articulating ribs have been transversely sectioned to visualize the joint surfaces and ligaments.
- The costotransverse ligament joins the posterior aspect of the neck of the rib to the adjacent transverse process.
- The lateral costotransverse ligament joins the nonarticulating part of the tubercle of the rib to the tip (apex) of the transverse process.
- The articular surfaces of the synovial plane costovertebral joints are colored blue.

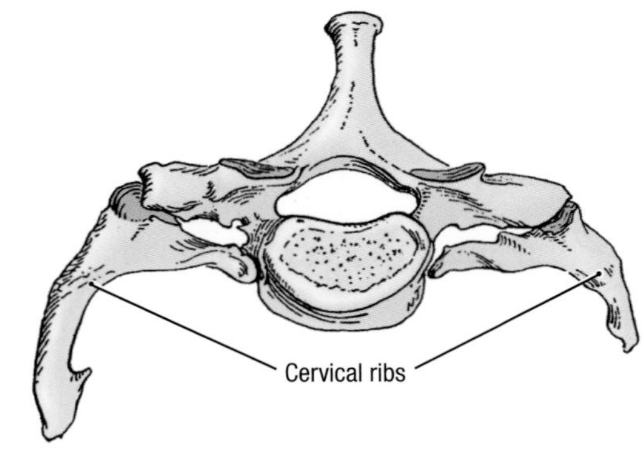
Cervical ribs

**A.** Superior View

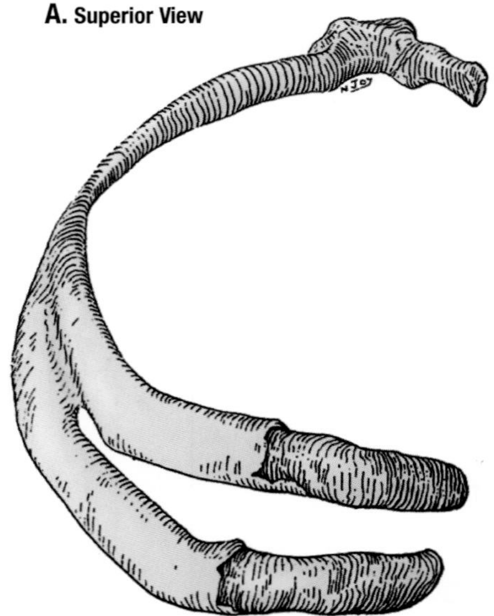

**B.** Anterior View

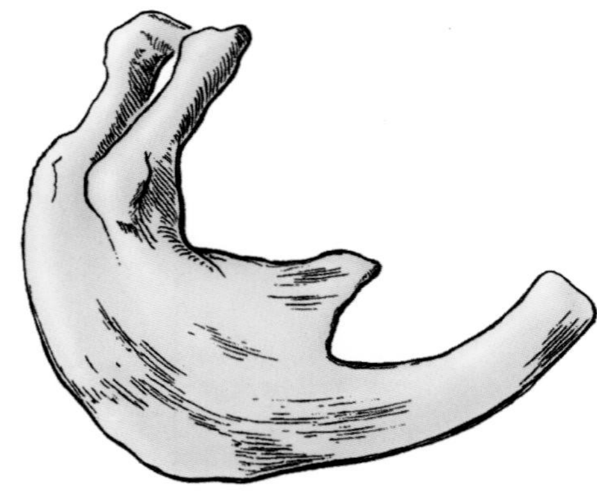

**C.** Superior View

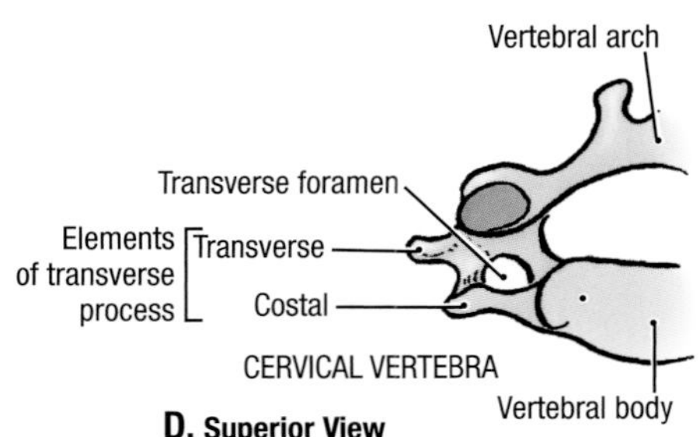
Vertebral arch
Transverse foramen
Elements of transverse process
Transverse
Costal
CERVICAL VERTEBRA
Vertebral body

**D.** Superior View

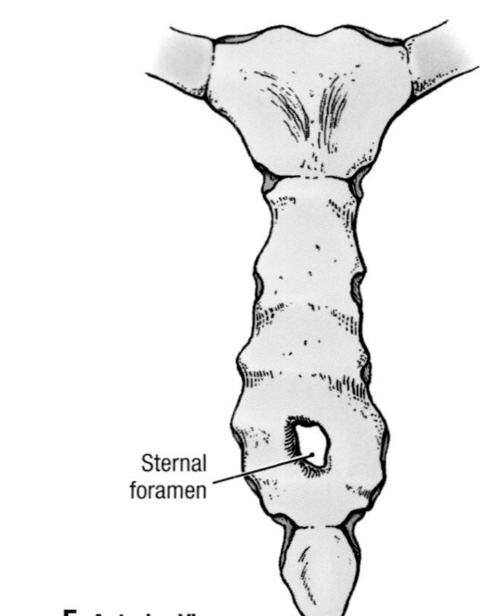
Sternal foramen

**E.** Anterior View

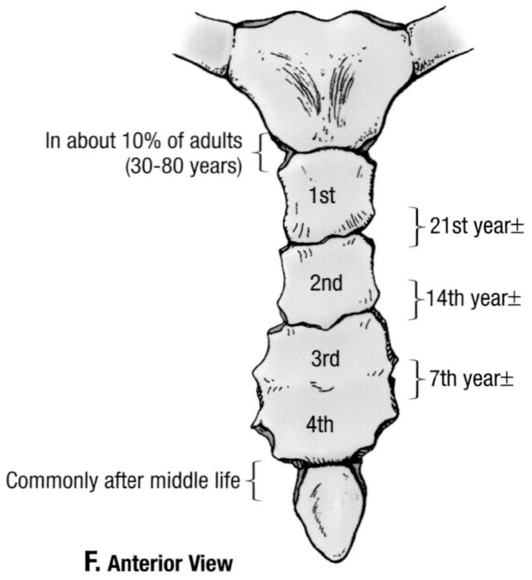
In about 10% of adults (30-80 years)
1st
2nd
3rd
4th
21st year±
14th year±
7th year±
Commonly after middle life

**F.** Anterior View

## 1.14 Rib and sternum anomalies

**A.** Cervical ribs. This is an enlarged costal element of the 7th cervical vertebra. (Compare with diagrammatic cervical vertebra in **D.**) Cervical ribs can be unilateral or bilateral, and large and palpable or detectable only radiologically. It can be asymptomatic or, through pressure on the most inferior root of the brachial plexus, can produce sensory and motor changes over the distribution of the ulnar nerve. **B.** Bifid rib. The superior component of this 3rd rib is supernumerary and articulated with the lateral aspect of the 1st sternebra. The inferior component articulated at the junction of the 1st and 2nd sternebrae. **C.** Bicipital rib. In this specimen, there has been partial fusion of the first two thoracic ribs. **E.** Sternal foramen. **F.** Ossification of sternum.

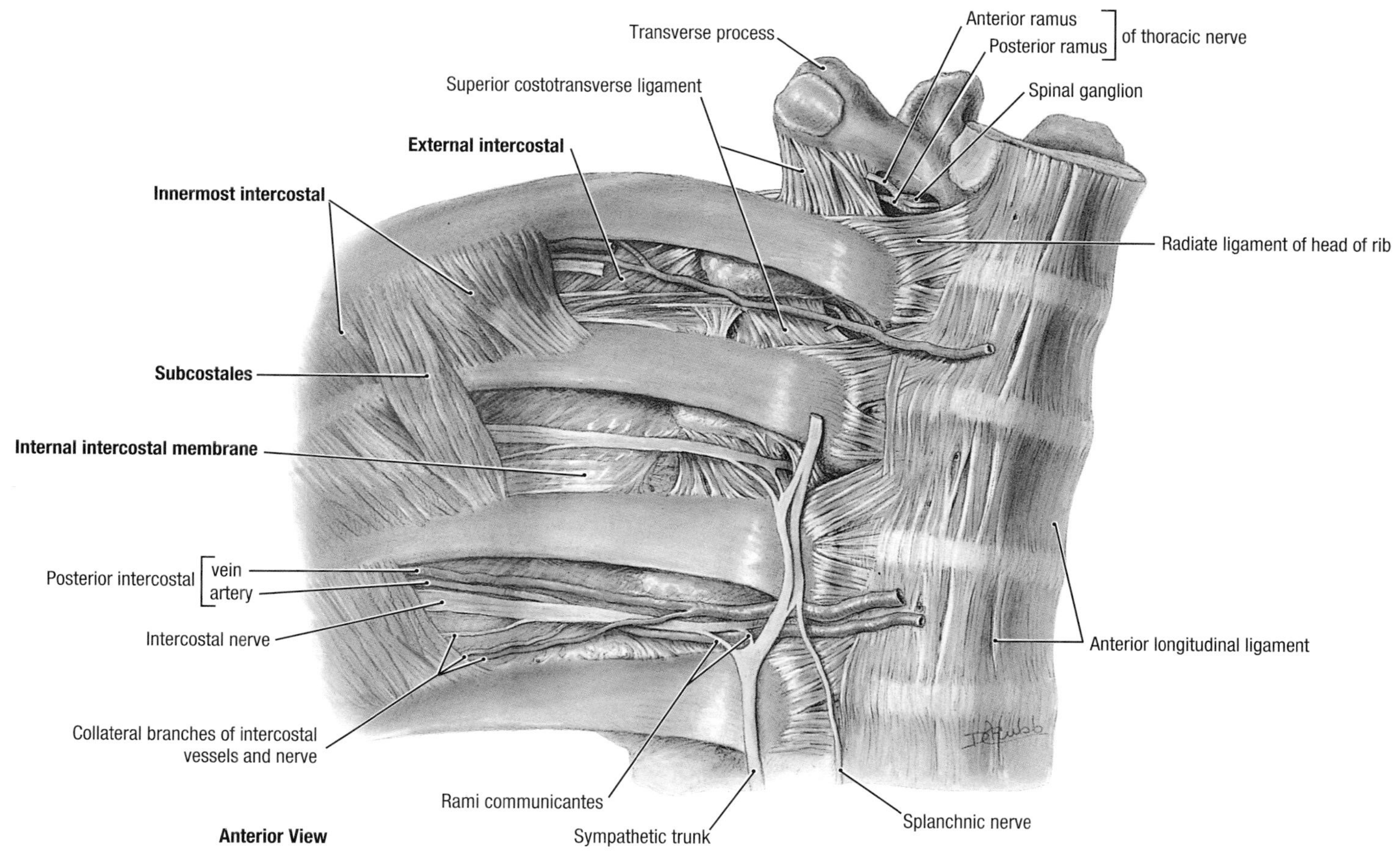
Transverse process
Anterior ramus
Posterior ramus
of thoracic nerve
Superior costotransverse ligament
Spinal ganglion
External intercostal
Innermost intercostal
Radiate ligament of head of rib
Subcostales
Internal intercostal membrane
Posterior intercostal
vein
artery
Intercostal nerve
Anterior longitudinal ligament
Collateral branches of intercostal vessels and nerve
Rami communicantes
Splanchnic nerve
Anterior View
Sympathetic trunk

## 1.15 Vertebral ends of internal aspect of intercostal spaces

- Portions of the innermost intercostal muscle that bridge two intercostal spaces are called subcostales muscles.
- The internal intercostal membrane, in the middle space, is continuous medially with the superior costotransverse ligament.
- Note the order of the structures in the most inferior space: posterior intercostal vein and artery, and intercostal nerve; note also their collateral branches.
- The anterior ramus crosses anterior to the superior costotransverse ligament; the posterior ramus is posterior to it.
- The intercostal nerves attach to the sympathetic trunk by rami communicantes; the splanchnic nerve is a visceral branch of the trunk.

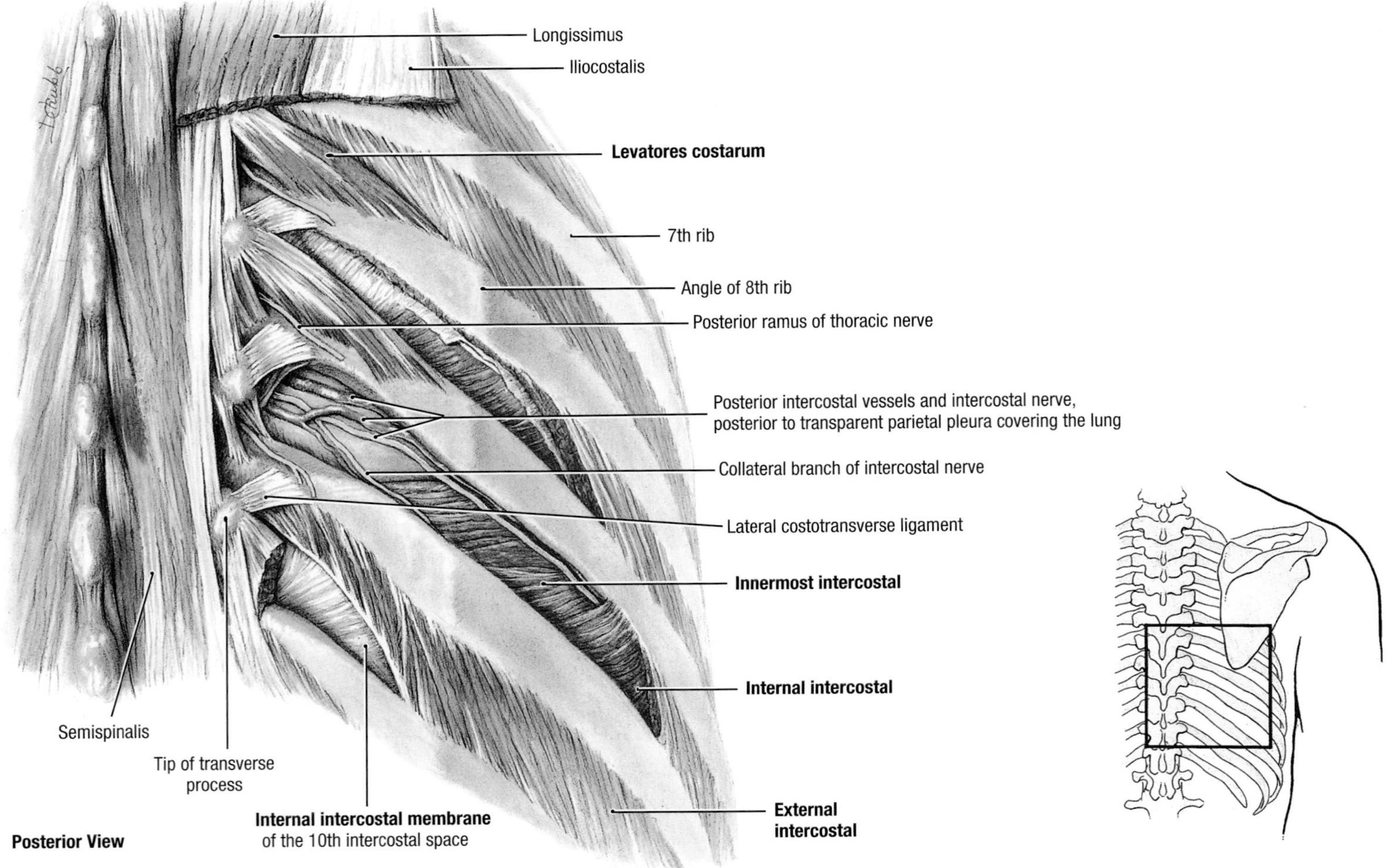
Longissimus
Iliocostalis
Levatores costarum
7th rib
Angle of 8th rib
Posterior ramus of thoracic nerve
Posterior intercostal vessels and intercostal nerve, posterior to transparent parietal pleura covering the lung
Collateral branch of intercostal nerve
Lateral costotransverse ligament
Innermost intercostal
Internal intercostal
External intercostal
Semispinalis
Tip of transverse process
Internal intercostal membrane of the 10th intercostal space
Posterior View

## 1.16 Vertebral ends of external aspect of inferior intercostal spaces

- The iliocostalis and longissimus muscles have been removed, exposing the levatores costarum muscle. Of the five intercostal spaces shown, the superior two (6th and 7th) are intact. In the 8th and 10th spaces, varying portions of the external intercostal muscle have been removed to reveal the underlying internal intercostal membrane, which is continuous with the internal intercostal muscle. In the 9th space, the levatores costarum muscle has been removed to show the posterior intercostal vessels and intercostal nerve.
- The intercostal vessels and nerve disappear laterally between the internal and innermost intercostal muscles.
- The intercostal nerve is the most inferior of the neurovascular trio (posterior intercostal vein and artery and intercostal nerve) and the least sheltered in the intercostal groove; a collateral branch arises near the angle of the rib.

- Sometimes it is necessary to insert a hypodermic needle through an intercostal space into the pleural cavity (See Fig. 1.24) to obtain a sample of pleural fluid or to remove blood or pus (thoracocentesis). To avoid damage to the intercostal nerve and vessels, the needle is inserted superior to the rib, high enough to avoid the collateral branches.

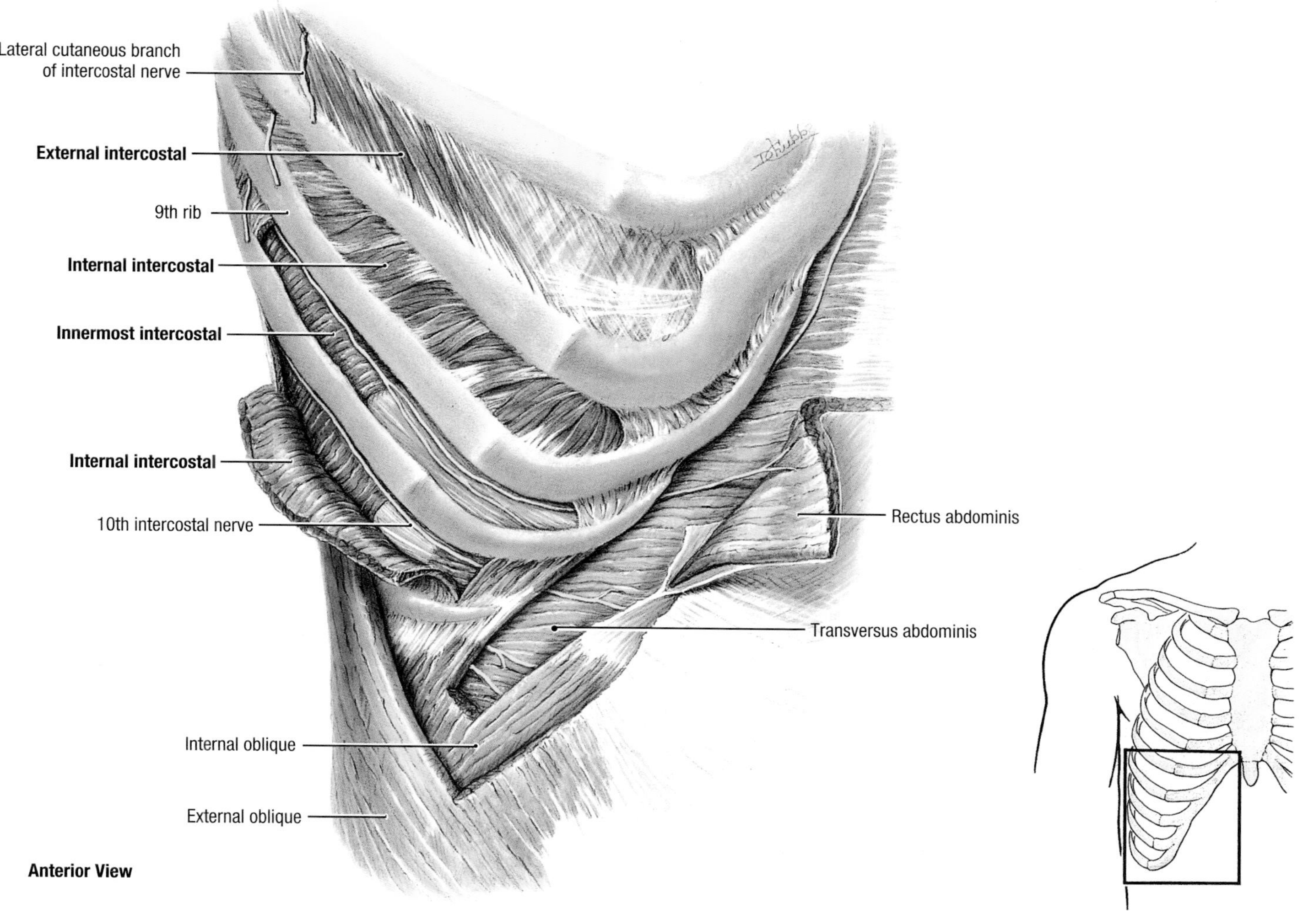
Lateral cutaneous branch of intercostal nerve
External intercostal
9th rib
Internal intercostal
Innermost intercostal
Internal intercostal
10th intercostal nerve
Rectus abdominis
Transversus abdominis
Internal oblique
External oblique
Anterior View

## 1.17 Anterior ends of inferior intercostal spaces

- The fibers of the external intercostal and external oblique muscles run inferomedially.
- The internal intercostal and internal oblique muscles are in continuity at the ends of the 9th, 10th, and 11th intercostal spaces.
- The intercostal nerves lie deep to the internal intercostal muscle but superficial to the innermost intercostal muscle; anteriorly, these nerves lie superficial to the transversus thoracis or transversus abdominis muscles.
- Intercostal nerves run parallel to the ribs and costal cartilages; on reaching the abdominal wall, nerves T7 and T8 continue superiorly, T9 continues nearly horizontally, and T10 continues inferomedially toward the umbilicus. These nerves provide cutaneous innervation in overlapping segmental bands.

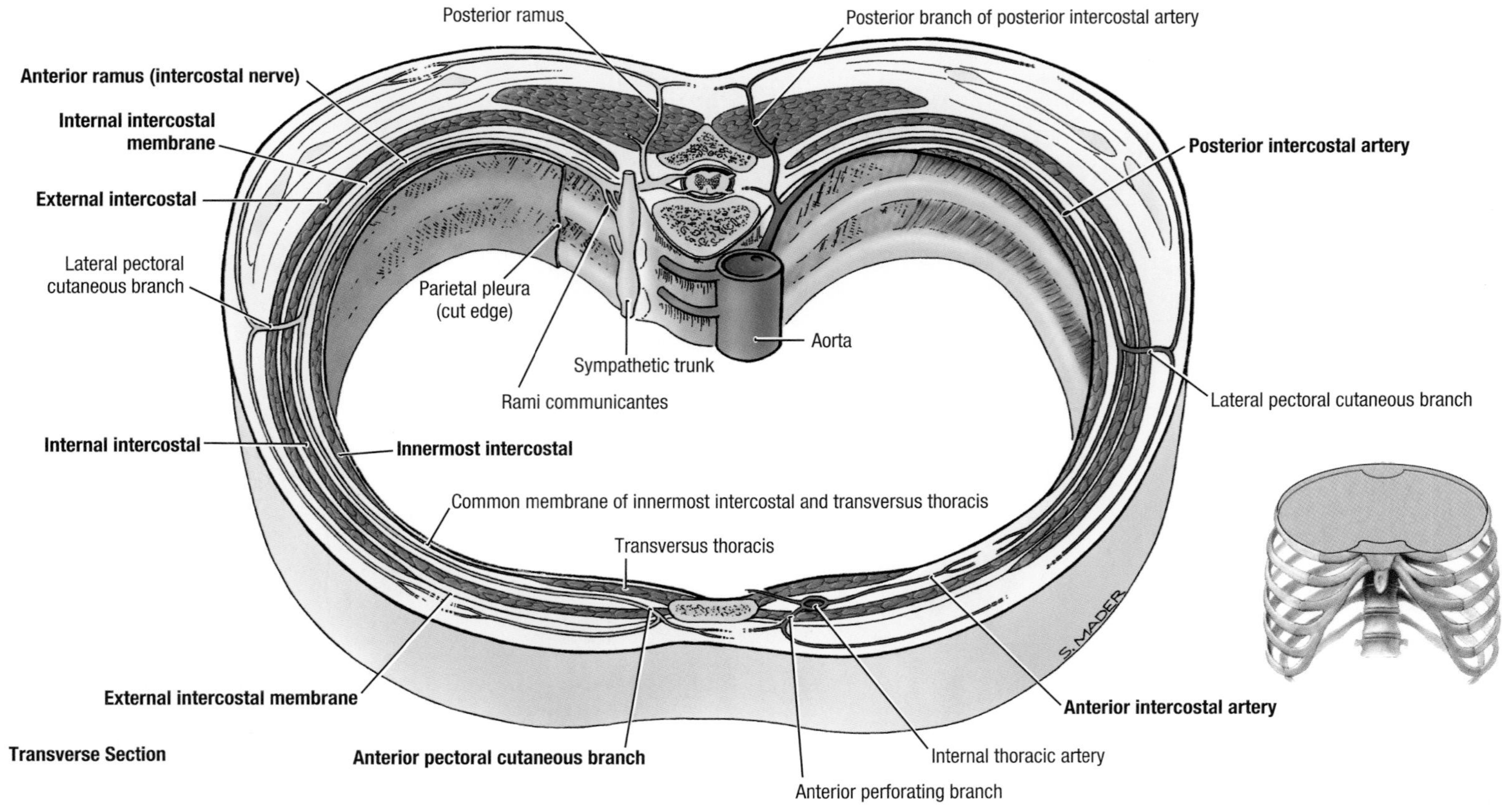
Posterior ramus
Posterior branch of posterior intercostal artery
Anterior ramus (intercostal nerve)
Internal intercostal membrane
Posterior intercostal artery
External intercostal
Lateral pectoral cutaneous branch
Parietal pleura (cut edge)
Aorta
Sympathetic trunk
Rami communicantes
Lateral pectoral cutaneous branch
Internal intercostal
Innermost intercostal
Common membrane of innermost intercostal and transversus thoracis
Transversus thoracis
S. MADER
External intercostal membrane
Anterior intercostal artery
Transverse Section
Anterior pectoral cutaneous branch
Internal thoracic artery
Anterior perforating branch

## 1.18 Contents of intercostal space, transverse section

- The diagram is simplified by showing nerves on the right and arteries on the left.
- The three musculomembranous layers are the external intercostal muscle and membrane, internal intercostal muscle and membrane, and the innermost intercostal muscle, transversus thoracis muscle, and the membrane connecting them.
- The intercostal nerves are the anterior rami of spinal nerves T1 to T11; the anterior ramus of T12 is the subcostal nerve.
- Posterior intercostal arteries are branches of the aorta (the superior two spaces are supplied from the superior intercostal branch of the costocervical trunk); the anterior intercostal arteries are branches of the internal thoracic artery or its branch, the musculophrenic artery.
- The posterior rami innervate the deep back muscles and skin adjacent to the vertebral column.

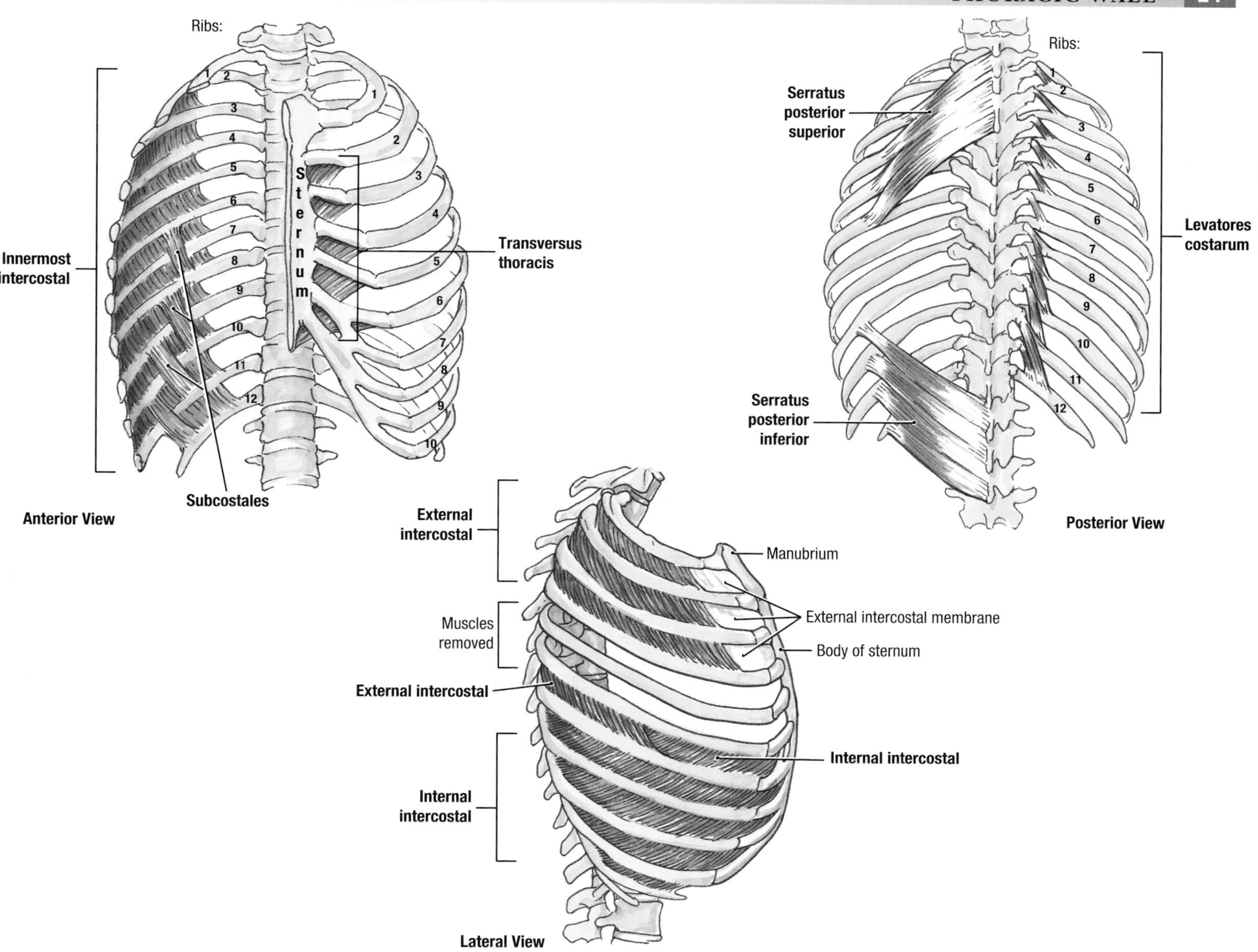
Ribs:
Innermost intercostal
Sternum
Transversus thoracis
Subcostales
Anterior View
Serratus posterior superior
Ribs:
Levatores costarum
Serratus posterior inferior
Posterior View
External intercostal
Muscles removed
External intercostal
Internal intercostal
Manubrium
External intercostal membrane
Body of sternum
Internal intercostal
Lateral View

## TABLE 1.1 MUSCLES OF THORACIC WALL

| Muscle | Superior attachment | Inferior attachment | Innervation | Action[a] |
|---|---|---|---|---|
| External intercostal | Inferior border of ribs | Superior border of ribs below | Intercostal nerve | Elevate ribs |
| Internal intercostal | | | | Depress ribs |
| Innermost intercostal | | | | Probably elevate ribs |
| Transversus thoracis | Posterior surface of lower sternum | Internal surface of costal cartilages 2–6 | | Depress ribs |
| Subcostales | Internal surface of lower ribs near their angles | Superior borders of 2nd or 3rd ribs below | | Elevate ribs |
| Levatores costarum | Transverse processes of T7–T11 | Subjacent ribs between tubercle and angle | Posterior rami of C8–T11 nerves | |
| Serratus posterior superior | Nuchal ligament, spinous processes of C7–T3 | Superior borders of 2nd–4th ribs | Second to fifth intercostal nerves | |
| Serratus posterior inferior | Spinous processes of T11–L2 | Inferior borders of 8th–12th ribs near their angles | Anterior rami of T9-T12 nerves | Depress ribs |

[a] All intercostal muscles keep intercostal spaces rigid, thereby preventing them from bulging out during expiration and from being drawn in during inspiration. Role of individual intercostal muscles and accessory muscles of respiration in moving the ribs is difficult to interpret despite many electromyographic studies.

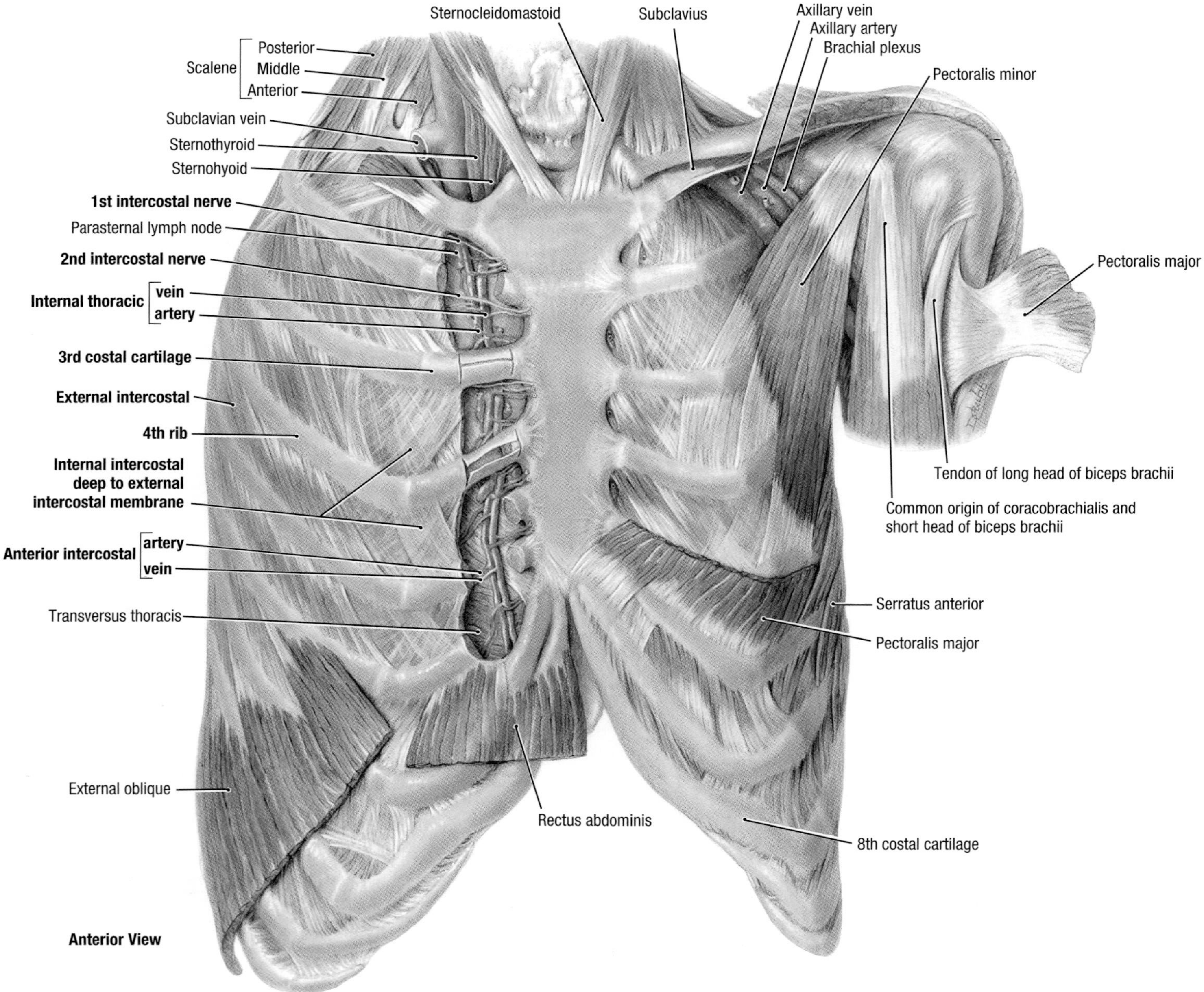
Sternocleidomastoid
Subclavius
Axillary vein
Axillary artery
Brachial plexus
Pectoralis minor
Scalene
Posterior
Middle
Anterior
Subclavian vein
Sternothyroid
Sternohyoid
1st intercostal nerve
Parasternal lymph node
2nd intercostal nerve
Internal thoracic
vein
artery
Pectoralis major
3rd costal cartilage
External intercostal
4th rib
Internal intercostal deep to external intercostal membrane
Tendon of long head of biceps brachii
Common origin of coracobrachialis and short head of biceps brachii
Anterior intercostal
artery
vein
Serratus anterior
Transversus thoracis
Pectoralis major
External oblique
Rectus abdominis
8th costal cartilage
Anterior View

## 1.19 External aspect of thoracic wall

- H-shaped cuts were made through the perichondrium of the 3rd and 4th costal cartilages to shell out segments of cartilage.
- The internal thoracic (internal mammary) vessels run inferiorly deep to the costal cartilages and just lateral to the edge of the sternum, providing anterior intercostal branches.
- The parasternal lymph nodes *(green)* receive lymphatic vessels from the anterior parts of intercostal spaces, the costal pleura and diaphragm, and the medial part of the breast.
- The subclavian vessels are "sandwiched" between the 1st rib and clavicle and are "padded" by the subclavius.

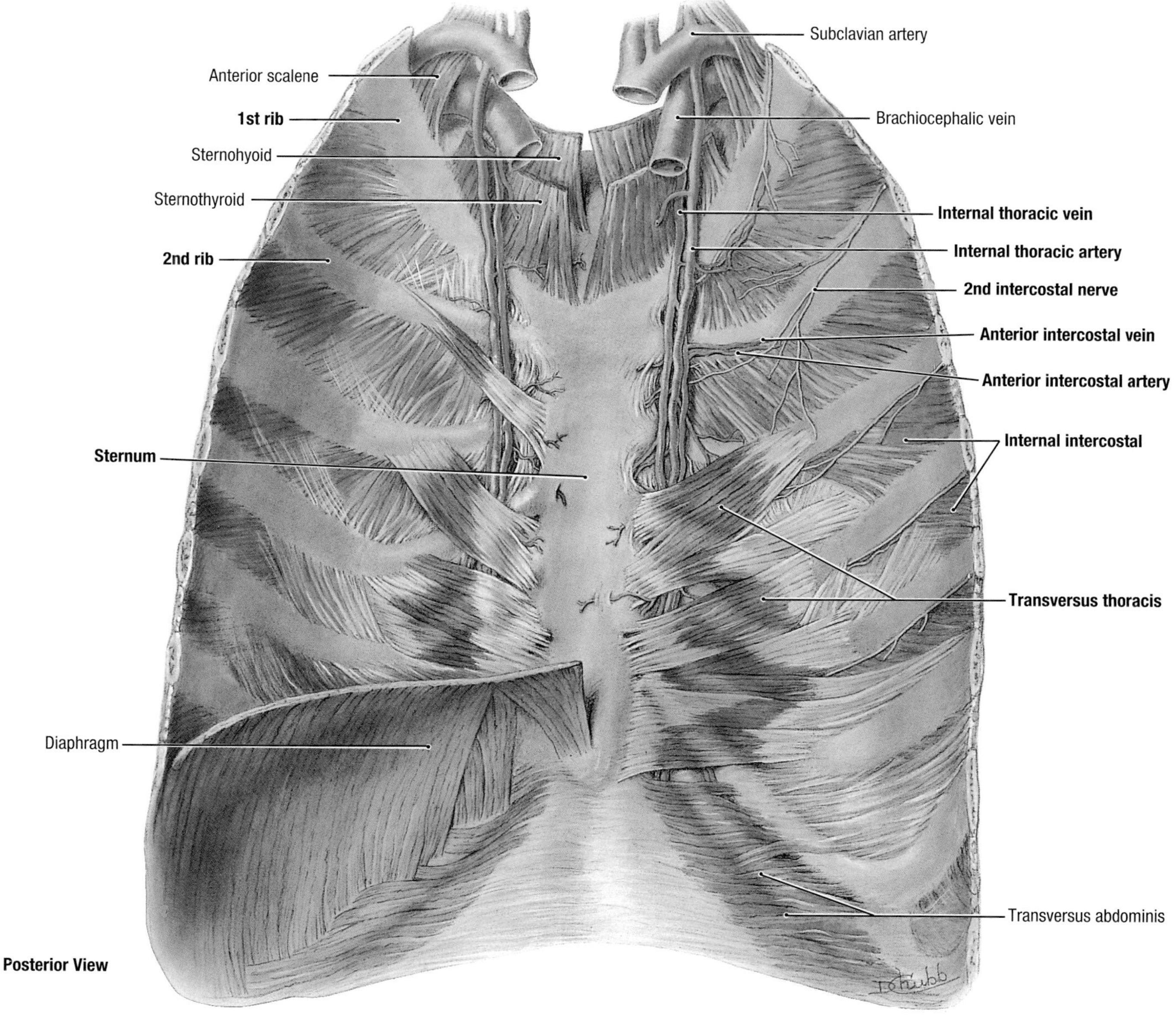
Subclavian artery
Anterior scalene
1st rib
Brachiocephalic vein
Sternohyoid
Sternothyroid
Internal thoracic vein
2nd rib
Internal thoracic artery
2nd intercostal nerve
Anterior intercostal vein
Anterior intercostal artery
Internal intercostal
Sternum
Transversus thoracis
Diaphragm
Transversus abdominis
Posterior View

## 1.20 Internal aspect of the anterior thoracic wall

- The inferior portions of the internal thoracic vessels are covered posteriorly by the transversus thoracis muscle; the superior portions are in contact with the parietal pleura (removed).
- The transversus thoracis muscle is continuous with the transversus abdominis muscle; these form the innermost layer of the three flat muscles of the thoracoabdominal wall.
- The internal thoracic (internal mammary) artery arises from the subclavian artery and is accompanied by two venae comitantes up to the 2nd costal cartilage in this specimen and, superior to this, by the single internal thoracic vein, which drains into the brachiocephalic vein.

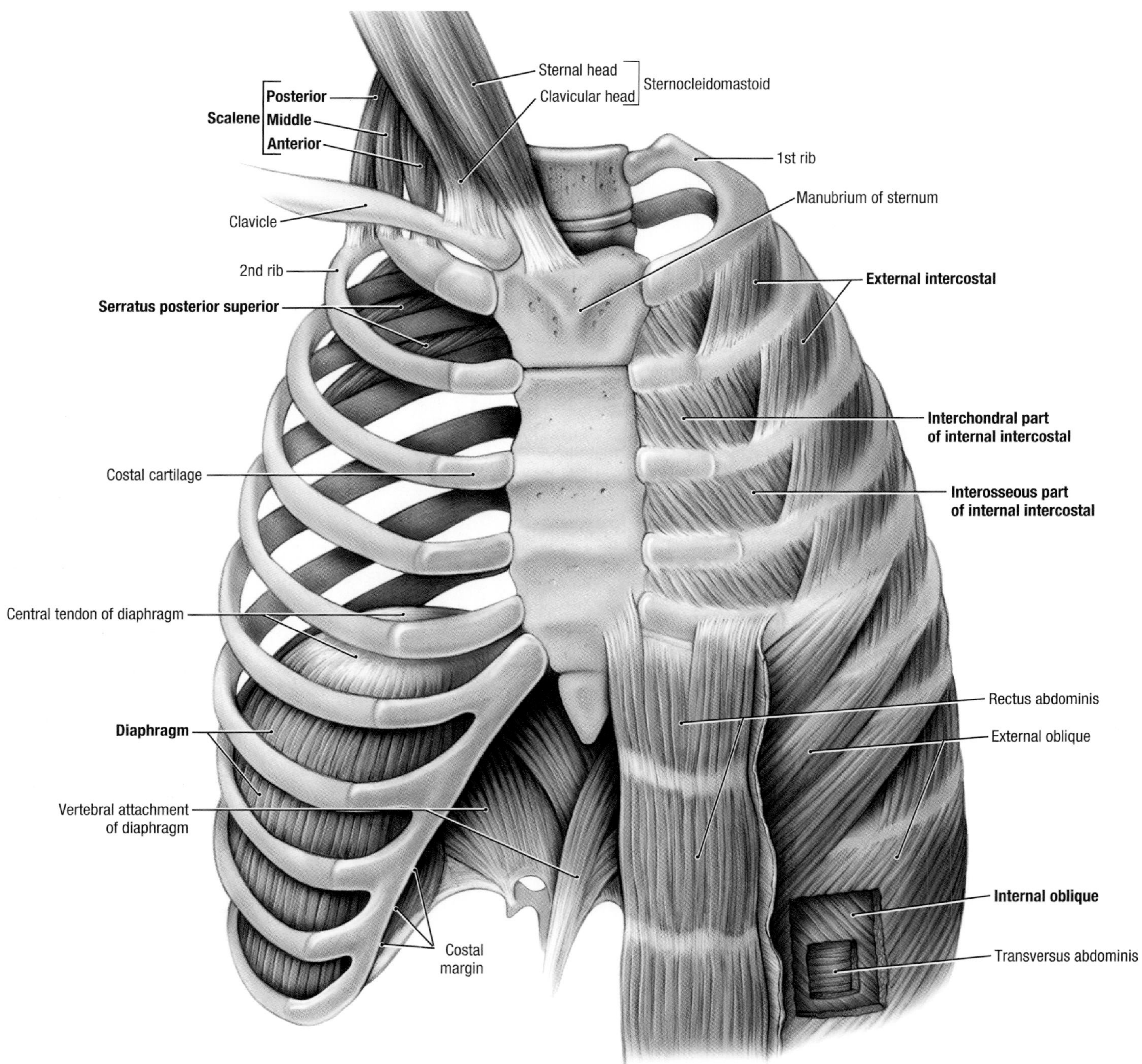

Sternal head
Clavicular head
Sternocleidomastoid
Posterior
Scalene
Middle
Anterior
1st rib
Manubrium of sternum
Clavicle
2nd rib
External intercostal
Serratus posterior superior
Interchondral part of internal intercostal
Costal cartilage
Interosseous part of internal intercostal
Central tendon of diaphragm
Rectus abdominis
Diaphragm
External oblique
Vertebral attachment of diaphragm
Internal oblique
Costal margin
Transversus abdominis


## TABLE 1.2 MUSCLES OF RESPIRATION

| Inspiration | | | Expiration |
|---|---|---|---|
| Normal (Quiet) | Major | Diaphragm (active contraction) | Passive (elastic) recoil of lungs and thoracic cage |
| | Minor | *Tonic contraction* of external intercostals and interchondral portion of internal intercostals to resist negative pressure | *Tonic contraction* of muscles of anterolateral abdominal walls (rectus abdominis, external and internal obliques, transversus abdominis) to antagonize diaphragm by maintaining intra-abdominal pressure |
| Active (Forced) | | In addition to the above, *active contraction* of | In addition to the above, *active contraction* of |
| | | Sternocleidomastoid, descending (superior) trapezius, pectoralis minor, and scalenes, to elevate and fix upper rib cage | Muscles of anterolateral abdominal wall (antagonizing diaphragm by increasing intra-abdominal pressure and by pulling inferiorly and fixing inferior costal margin): rectus abdominis, external and internal obliques, and transversus abdominis |
| | | External intercostals, interchondral portion of internal intercostals, subcostales, levatores costarum, and serratus posterior superior[a] to elevate ribs | Internal intercostal (interosseous part) and serratus posterior inferior[a] to depress ribs |

[a] Recent studies indicate that the serratus posterior superior and inferior muscles may serve primarily as organs of proprioception rather than motion.

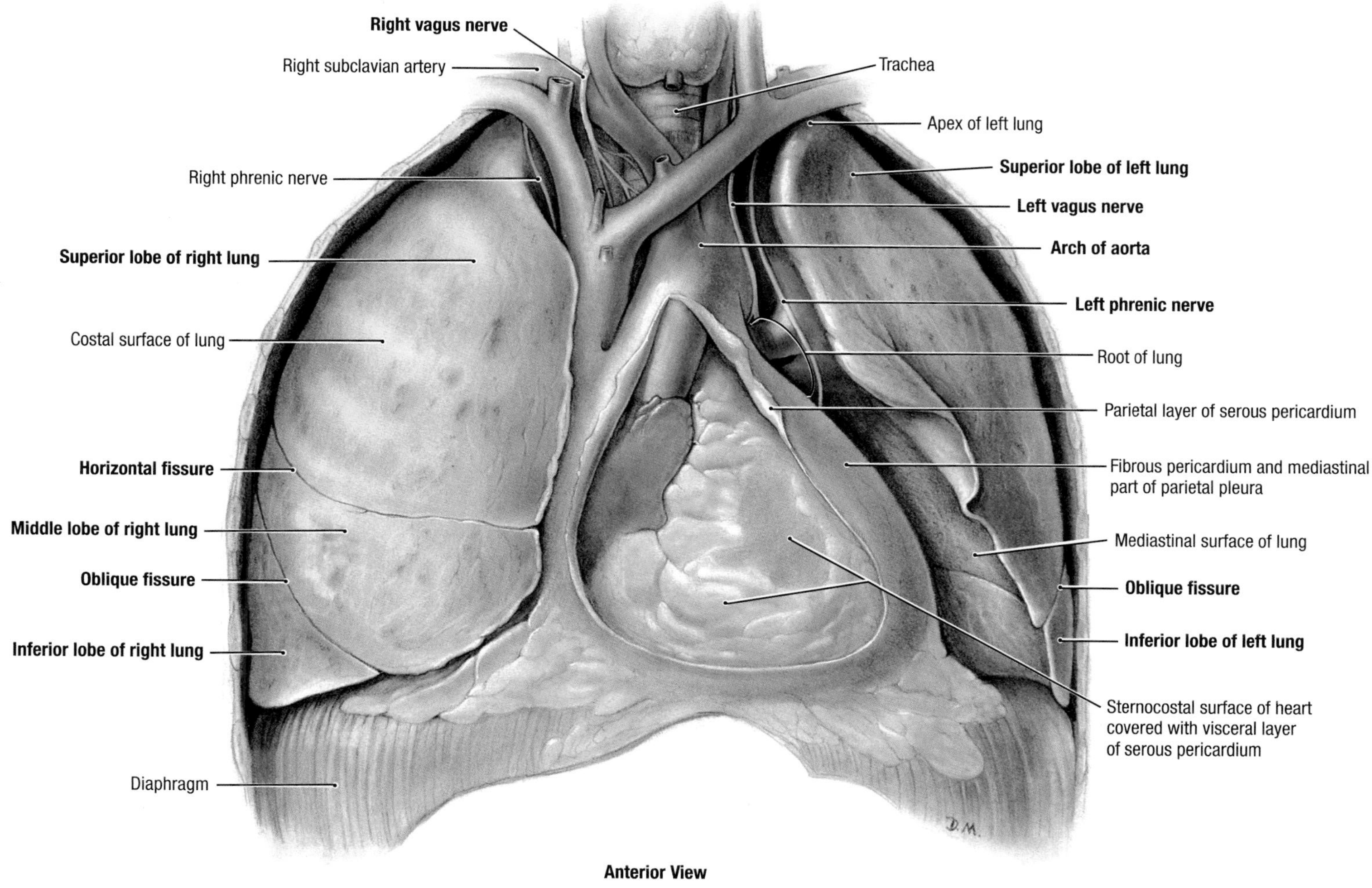
Right vagus nerve
Right subclavian artery
Trachea
Apex of left lung
Superior lobe of left lung
Right phrenic nerve
Left vagus nerve
Superior lobe of right lung
Arch of aorta
Left phrenic nerve
Costal surface of lung
Root of lung
Parietal layer of serous pericardium
Horizontal fissure
Fibrous pericardium and mediastinal part of parietal pleura
Middle lobe of right lung
Mediastinal surface of lung
Oblique fissure
Oblique fissure
Inferior lobe of right lung
Inferior lobe of left lung
Sternocostal surface of heart covered with visceral layer of serous pericardium
Diaphragm
D.M.
Anterior View

## 1.21 Thoracic contents in situ

- The fibrous pericardium, lined by the parietal layer of serous pericardium, is removed anteriorly to expose the heart and great vessels.
- The right lung has three lobes; the superior lobe is separated from the middle lobe by the horizontal fissure, and the middle lobe is separated from the inferior lobe by the oblique fissure. The left lung has two lobes, superior and inferior, separated by the oblique fissure.
- The anterior border of the left lung is reflected laterally to visualize the phrenic nerve passing anterior to the root of the lung and the vagus nerve lying anterior to the arch of the aorta and then passing posterior to the root of the lung.
- As the right vagus nerve passes anterior to the right subclavian artery, it gives rise to the recurrent branch and then divides to contribute fibers to the esophageal, cardiac, and pulmonary plexuses.

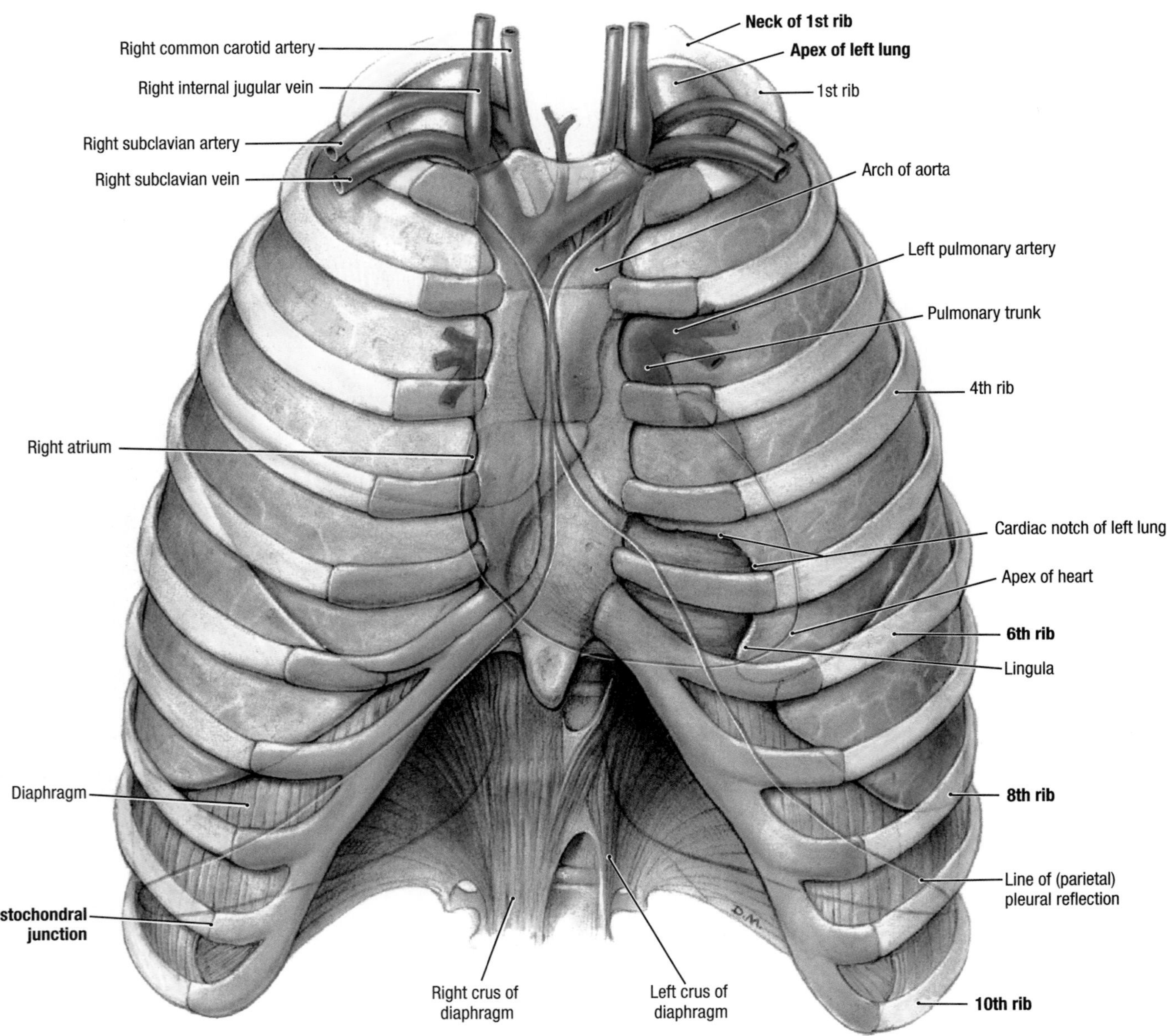
Right common carotid artery
Right internal jugular vein
Right subclavian artery
Right subclavian vein
Right atrium
Diaphragm
Costochondral junction
Right crus of diaphragm
Left crus of diaphragm
Neck of 1st rib
Apex of left lung
1st rib
Arch of aorta
Left pulmonary artery
Pulmonary trunk
4th rib
Cardiac notch of left lung
Apex of heart
6th rib
Lingula
8th rib
Line of (parietal) pleural reflection
10th rib

## 1.22 Topography of the lungs and mediastinum

- The mediastinum is located between the pleural cavities and is occupied by the heart and the tissues anterior, posterior, and superior to the heart.
- The apex of the lungs is at the level of the neck of the 1st rib, and the inferior border of the lungs is at the 6th rib in the left midclavicular line and the 8th rib at the lateral aspect of the bony thorax at the midaxillary line.
- The cardiac notch of the left lung and the deviation of the parietal pleura is away from the median plane toward the left side in the region of the cardiac notch.
- The inferior reflection of parietal pleura is at the 8th costochondral junction in the midclavicular line, at the 10th rib in the midaxillary line.
- The apex of the heart is in the 5th intercostal space at the left midclavicular line.
- The right atrium forms the right border of the heart and extends just beyond the lateral margin of the sternum.
- The branches of the great vessels pass through the superior thoracic aperture.

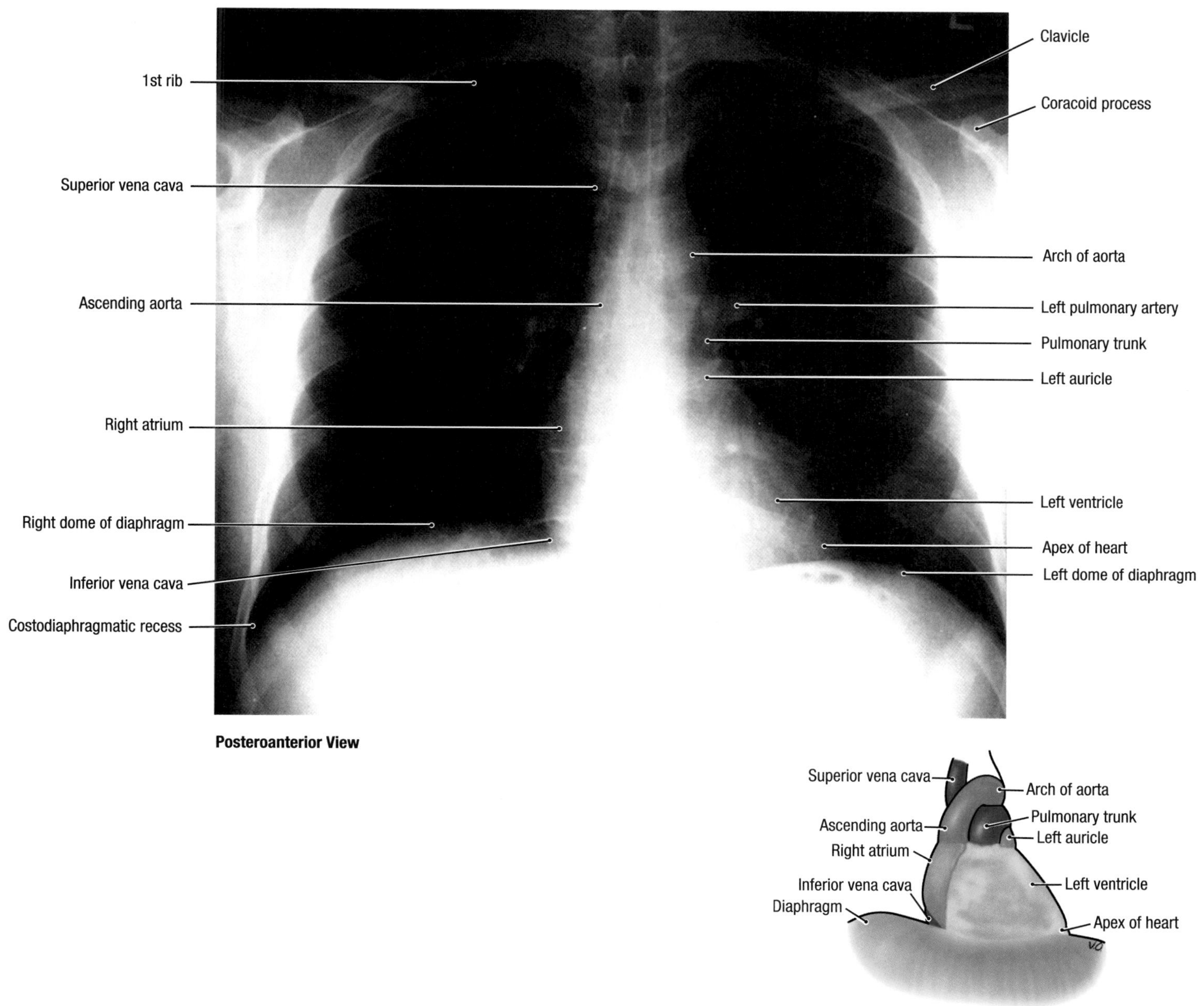
1st rib
Superior vena cava
Ascending aorta
Right atrium
Right dome of diaphragm
Inferior vena cava
Costodiaphragmatic recess
Clavicle
Coracoid process
Arch of aorta
Left pulmonary artery
Pulmonary trunk
Left auricle
Left ventricle
Apex of heart
Left dome of diaphragm
Posteroanterior View
Superior vena cava
Ascending aorta
Right atrium
Inferior vena cava
Diaphragm
Arch of aorta
Pulmonary trunk
Left auricle
Left ventricle
Apex of heart

## 1.23 Radiograph of chest

- The right dome of the diaphragm is higher than the left dome due primarily to the large underlying liver.
- The convex right mediastinal border of the heart is formed by the right atrium; above this, the superior vena cava and ascending aorta produce less convex borders.
- The left border of the mediastinal silhouette is formed by the arch of the aorta, pulmonary trunk, left auricle (normally not prominent), and left ventricle.
- Follow the 1st rib to where it curves laterally and then medially to cross the clavicle.

- Any structure in the mediastinum may contribute to pathological widening of the mediastinal silhouette. It is often observed after trauma resulting from a head-on collision, for example, which produces hemorrhage into the mediastinum from lacerated great vessels such as the aorta or SVC. Frequently, malignant lymphoma (cancer of lymphatic tissue) produces massive enlargement of mediastinal lymph nodes and widening of the mediastinum. Enlargement (hypertrophy) of the heart (occurring with congestive heart failure) is a common cause of widening of the inferior mediastinum.

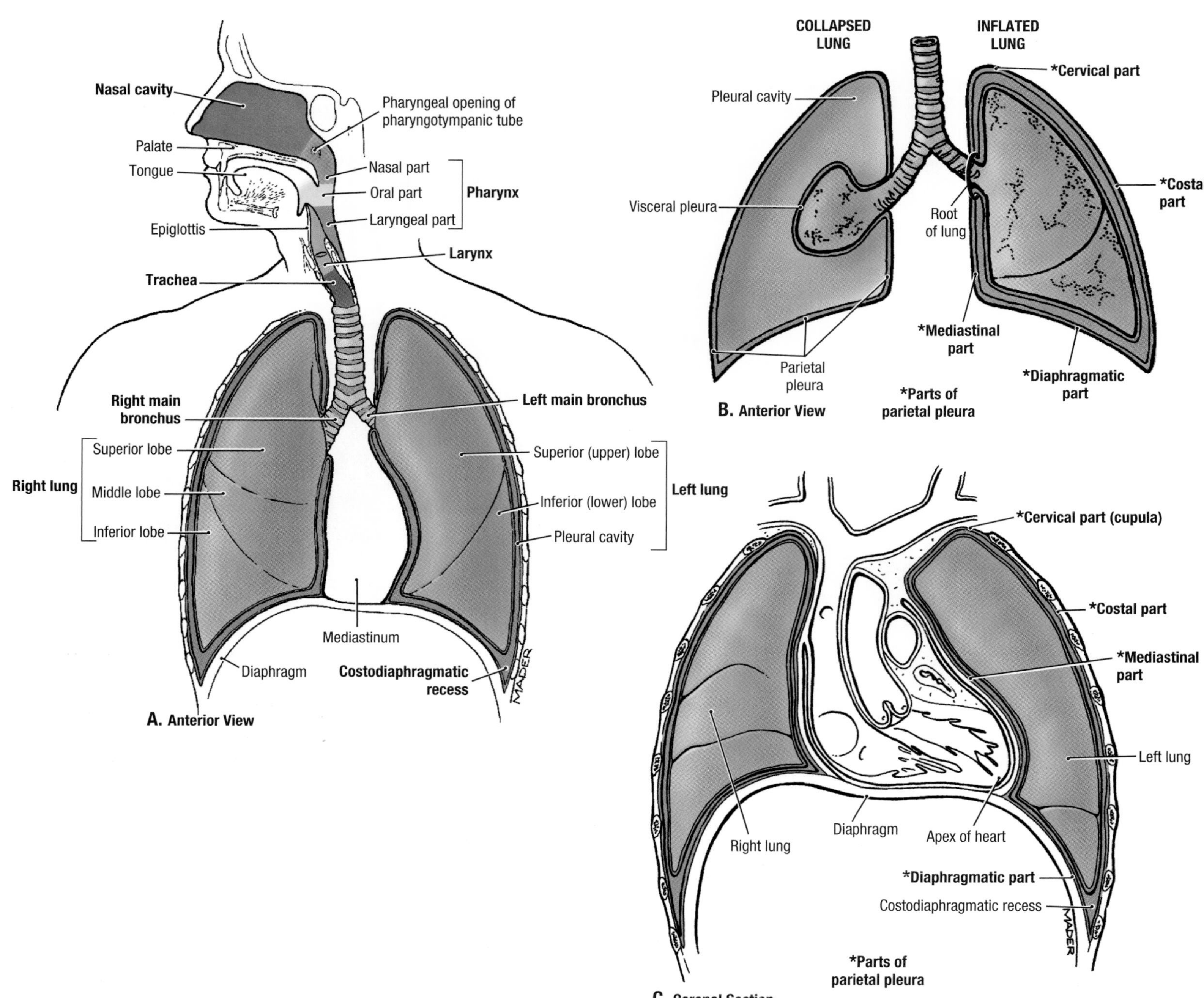
Nasal cavity
Palate
Tongue
Epiglottis
Trachea
Pharyngeal opening of pharyngotympanic tube
Nasal part
Oral part
Laryngeal part
Pharynx
Larynx
Right main bronchus
Left main bronchus
Right lung
Superior lobe
Middle lobe
Inferior lobe
Superior (upper) lobe
Inferior (lower) lobe
Pleural cavity
Left lung
Mediastinum
Diaphragm
Costodiaphragmatic recess
MADER
A. Anterior View
COLLAPSED LUNG
INFLATED LUNG
Pleural cavity
*Cervical part
Visceral pleura
Root of lung
*Costal part
*Mediastinal part
Parietal pleura
*Diaphragmatic part
*Parts of parietal pleura
B. Anterior View
*Cervical part (cupula)
*Costal part
*Mediastinal part
Left lung
Right lung
Diaphragm
Apex of heart
*Diaphragmatic part
Costodiaphragmatic recess
MADER
*Parts of parietal pleura
C. Coronal Section

## 1.24 Respiratory system

**A.** Overview. **B.** Pleural cavity and pleura. **C.** Coronal section through heart and lungs.

- The lungs invaginate a continuous membranous pleural sac; the visceral (pulmonary) pleura covers the lungs, and the parietal pleura lines the thoracic cavity; the visceral and parietal pleurae are continuous around the root of the lung.
- The parietal pleura can be divided regionally into the costal, diaphragmatic, mediastinal, and cervical parts; note the costodiaphragmatic recess.

- The pleural cavity is a potential space between the visceral and parietal pleurae that contains a thin layer of fluid. If a sufficient amount of air enters the pleural cavity, the surface tension adhering visceral to parietal pleura (lung to thoracic wall) is broken, and the lung collapses because of its inherent elasticity (elastic recoil). When a lung collapses, the pleural cavity—normally a potential space—becomes a real space (**B**) and may contain air (pneumothorax), blood (hemothorax), etc.

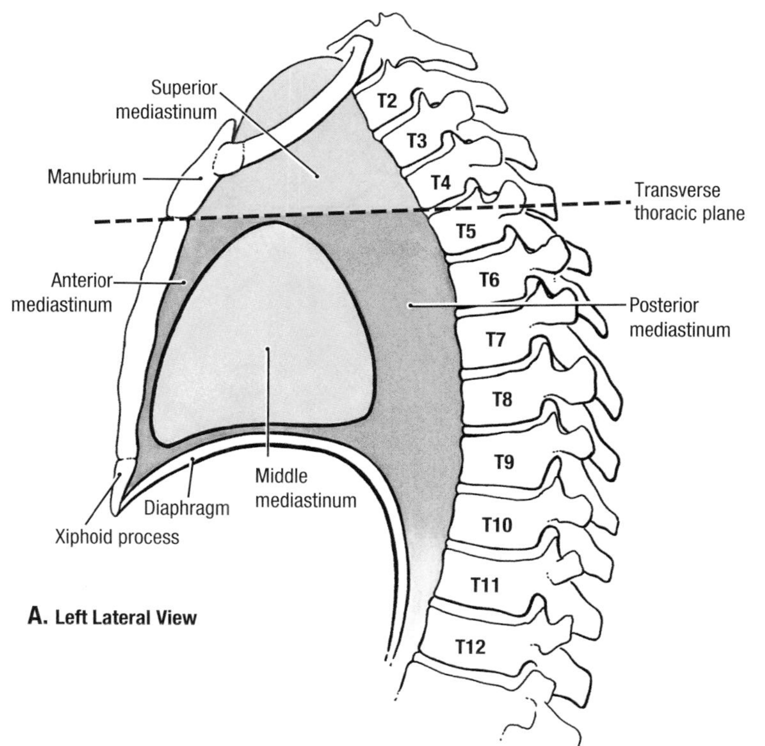
Superior mediastinum
Manubrium
T2
T3
T4
Transverse thoracic plane
T5
Anterior mediastinum
T6
Posterior mediastinum
T7
T8
T9
Middle mediastinum
Diaphragm
Xiphoid process
T10
T11
T12

**A. Left Lateral View**

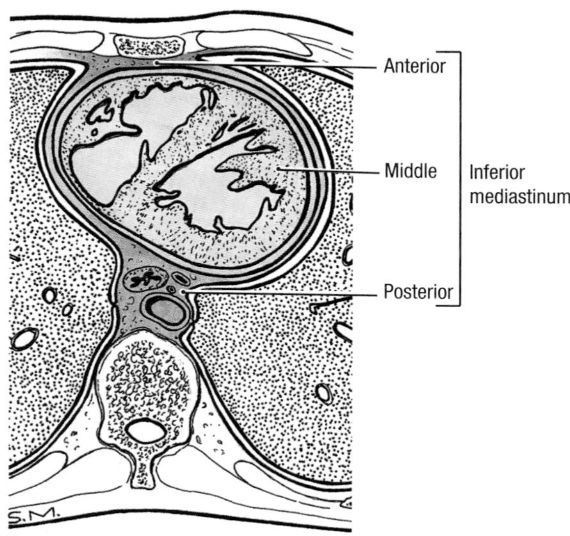
Anterior
Middle
Inferior mediastinum
Posterior
S.M.

**B. Transverse Section, Inferior View**

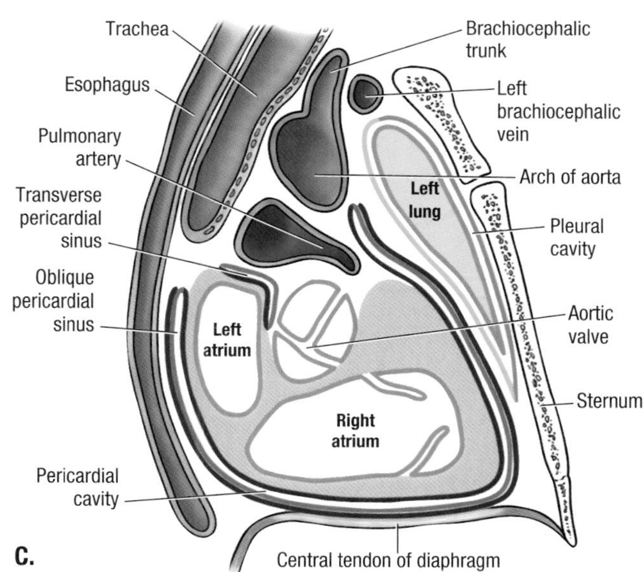
Trachea
Esophagus
Pulmonary artery
Transverse pericardial sinus
Oblique pericardial sinus
Brachiocephalic trunk
Left brachiocephalic vein
Arch of aorta
Left lung
Pleural cavity
Aortic valve
Left atrium
Right atrium
Sternum
Pericardial cavity
Central tendon of diaphragm

**C. Median Section, Right Lateral View**

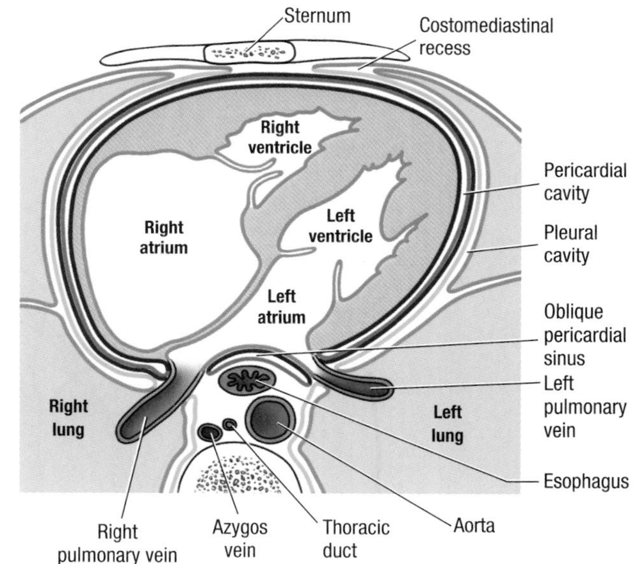
Sternum
Costomediastinal recess
Right ventricle
Pericardial cavity
Right atrium
Left ventricle
Pleural cavity
Left atrium
Oblique pericardial sinus
Left pulmonary vein
Right lung
Left lung
Esophagus
Right pulmonary vein
Azygos vein
Thoracic duct
Aorta

**Transverse Section, Inferior View**

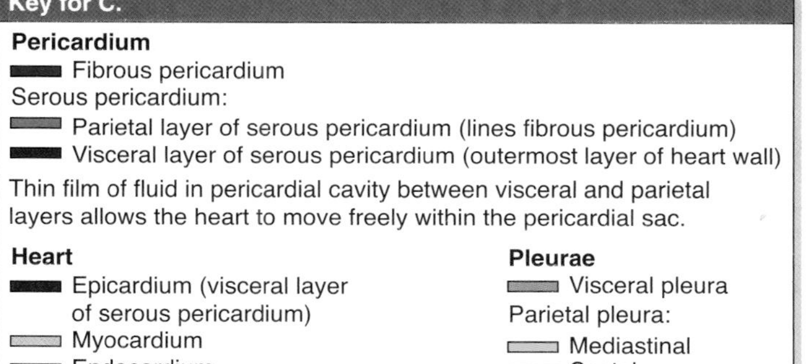
Key for C.
Pericardium
Fibrous pericardium
Serous pericardium:
Parietal layer of serous pericardium (lines fibrous pericardium)
Visceral layer of serous pericardium (outermost layer of heart wall)
Thin film of fluid in pericardial cavity between visceral and parietal layers allows the heart to move freely within the pericardial sac.
Heart
Epicardium (visceral layer of serous pericardium)
Myocardium
Endocardium
Pleurae
Visceral pleura
Parietal pleura:
Mediastinal
Costal

## 1.25 Mediastinum and pericardium

**A** and **B.** Subdivisions of mediastinum. **C.** Layers of pericardium and heart.

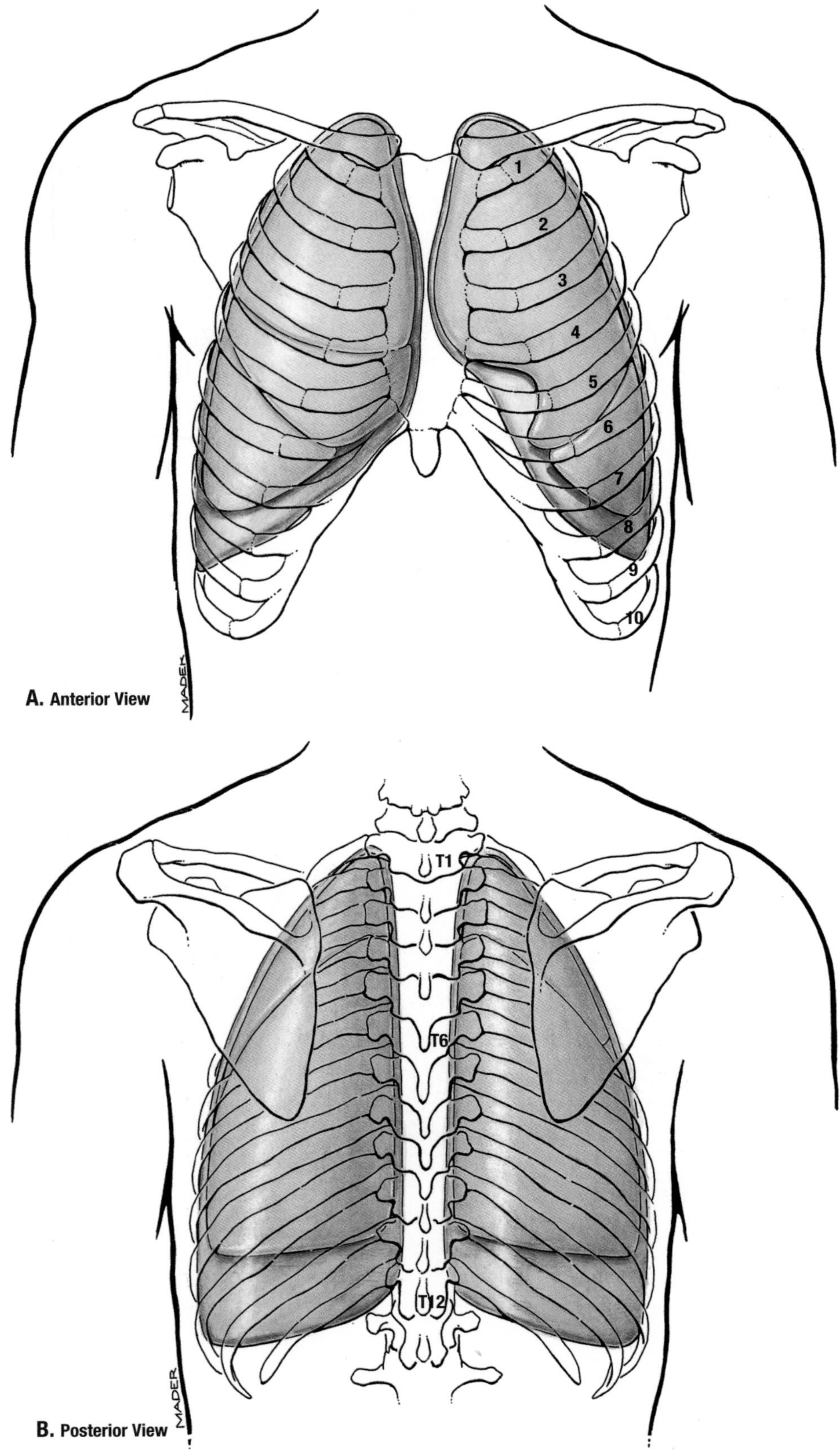
1
2
3
4
5
6
7
8
9
10
MADER
A. Anterior View
T1
T6
T12
MADER
B. Posterior View

**1.26 Extent of parietal pleura and lungs**

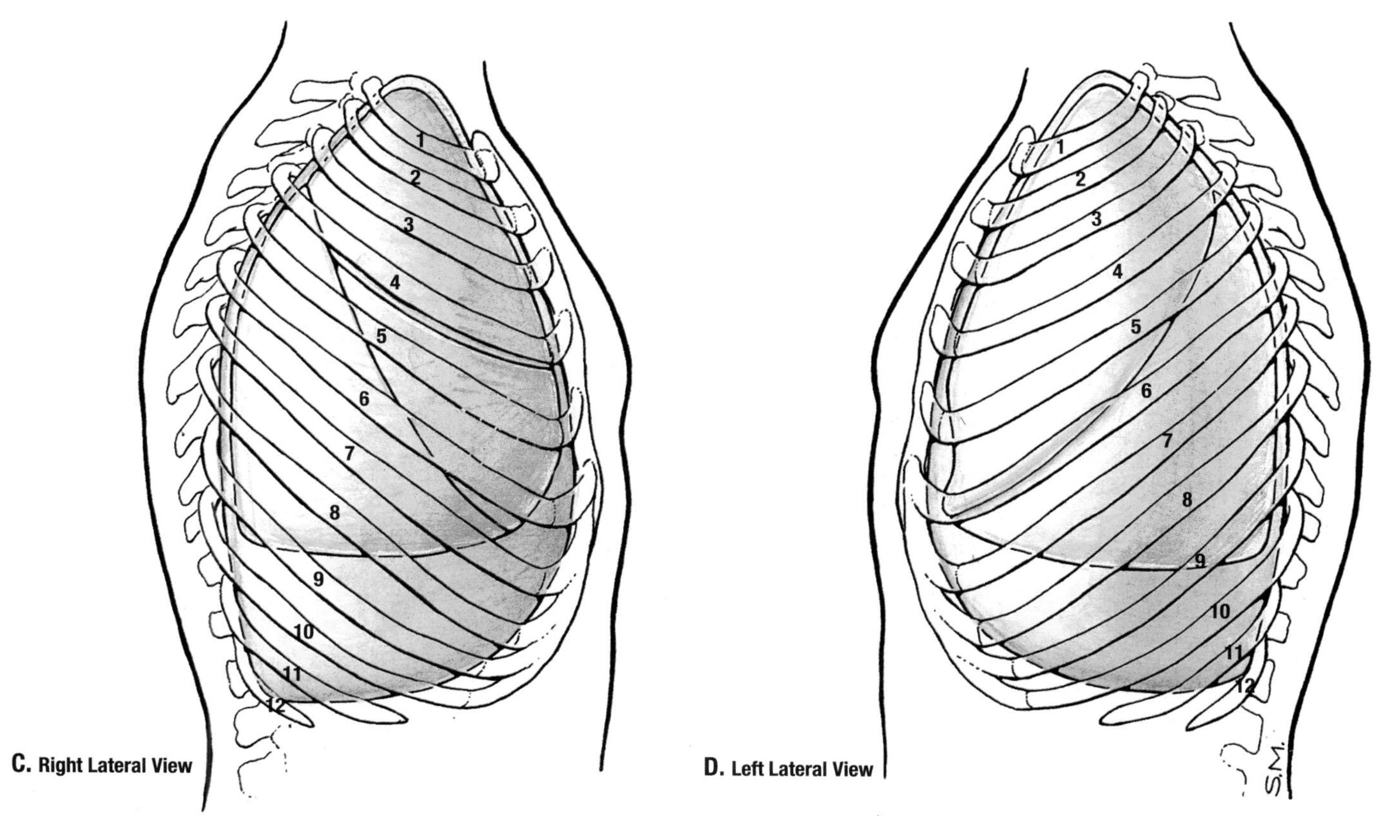
1
2
3
4
5
6
7
8
9
10
11
12
C. Right Lateral View
D. Left Lateral View
S.M.

**1.26** **Extent of parietal pleura and lungs *(continued)***

**TABLE 1.3 SURFACE MARKINGS OF PARIETAL PLEURA (BLUE)**

| Level | Left Pleura | Right Pleura |
|---|---|---|
| Apex | About 4 cm superior to middle of clavicle | About 4 cm superior to middle of clavicle |
| 4th costal cartilage | Midline (anteriorly) | Midline (anteriorly) |
| 6th costal cartilage | Lateral margin of sternum | Midline (anteriorly) |
| 8th costal cartilage | Midclavicular line | Midclavicular line |
| 10th rib | Midaxillary line | Midaxillary line |
| 11th rib | Line of inferior angle of scapula | Line of inferior angle of scapula |
| 12th rib | Lateral border of erector spinae to T12 spinous process (slightly lower level than right pleura) | Lateral border of erector spinae to T12 spinous process |

**SURFACE MARKINGS OF LUNGS COVERED WITH VISCERAL PLEURA (PINK)**

| Level | Left Lung | Right Lung |
|---|---|---|
| Apex | About 4 cm superior to middle of clavicle | About 4 cm superior to middle of clavicle |
| 2nd costal cartilage | Midline (anteriorly) | Midline (anteriorly) |
| 4th costal cartilage | Lateral margin of sternum | Lateral margin of sternum |
| 6th costal cartilage | Follows 4th costal cartilage, turns inferiorly to 6th costal cartilage in the midclavicular line (cardiac notch) | Midclavicular line |
| 8th rib | Midaxillary line | Midaxillary line |
| 10th rib | Line of inferior angle of scapula to T10 spinous process | Line of inferior angle of scapula to T10 spinous process |

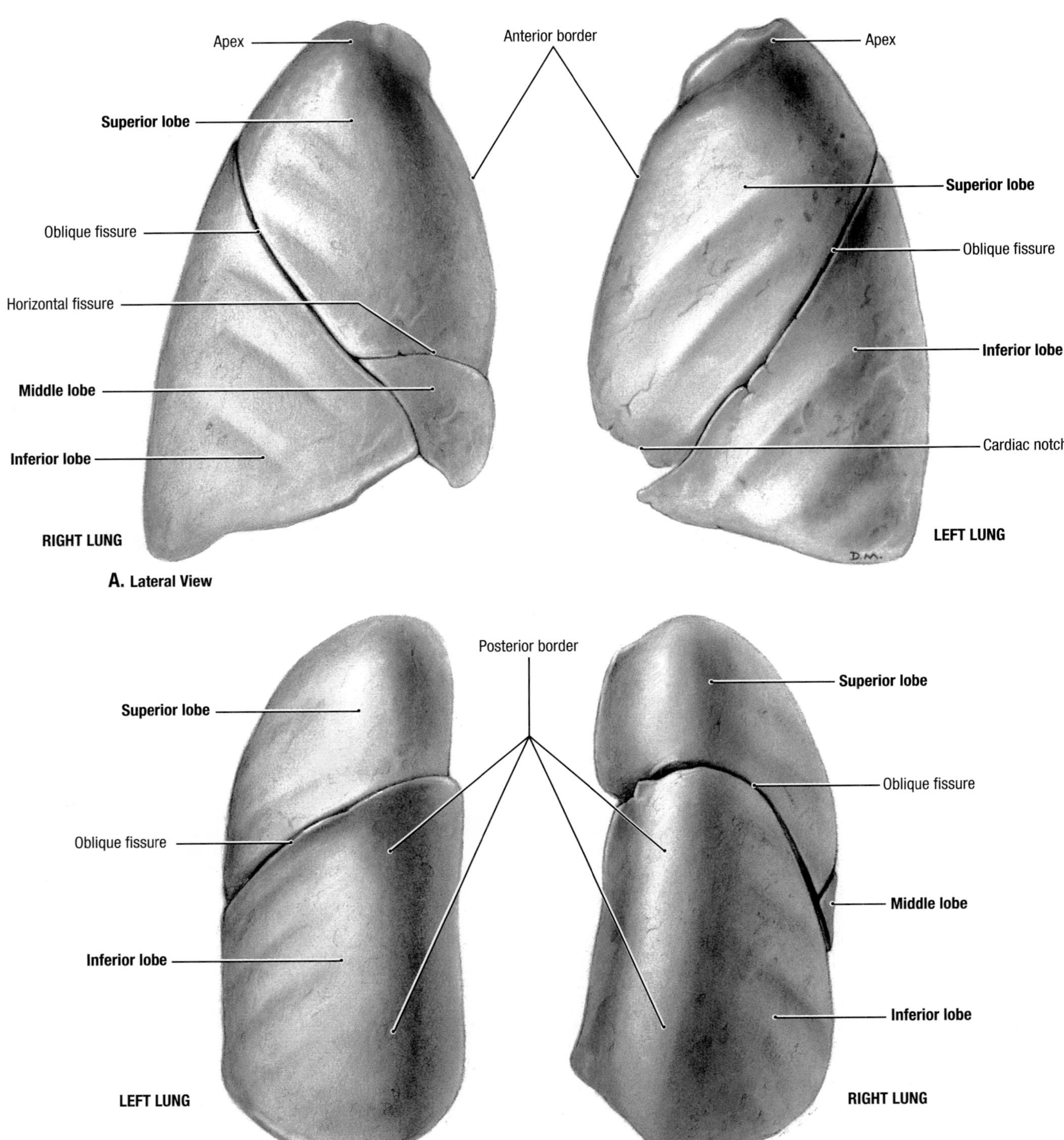
Apex
Anterior border
Apex
Superior lobe
Superior lobe
Oblique fissure
Oblique fissure
Horizontal fissure
Inferior lobe
Middle lobe
Cardiac notch
Inferior lobe
RIGHT LUNG
LEFT LUNG
A. Lateral View
Posterior border
Superior lobe
Superior lobe
Oblique fissure
Oblique fissure
Middle lobe
Inferior lobe
Inferior lobe
LEFT LUNG
RIGHT LUNG
B. Posterior View

## 1.27 Lungs

The right lung usually has three lobes, and the left lung, two lobes. The oblique and horizontal fissures of the right lung and the oblique fissure of the left lung may be incomplete or absent in some specimens.

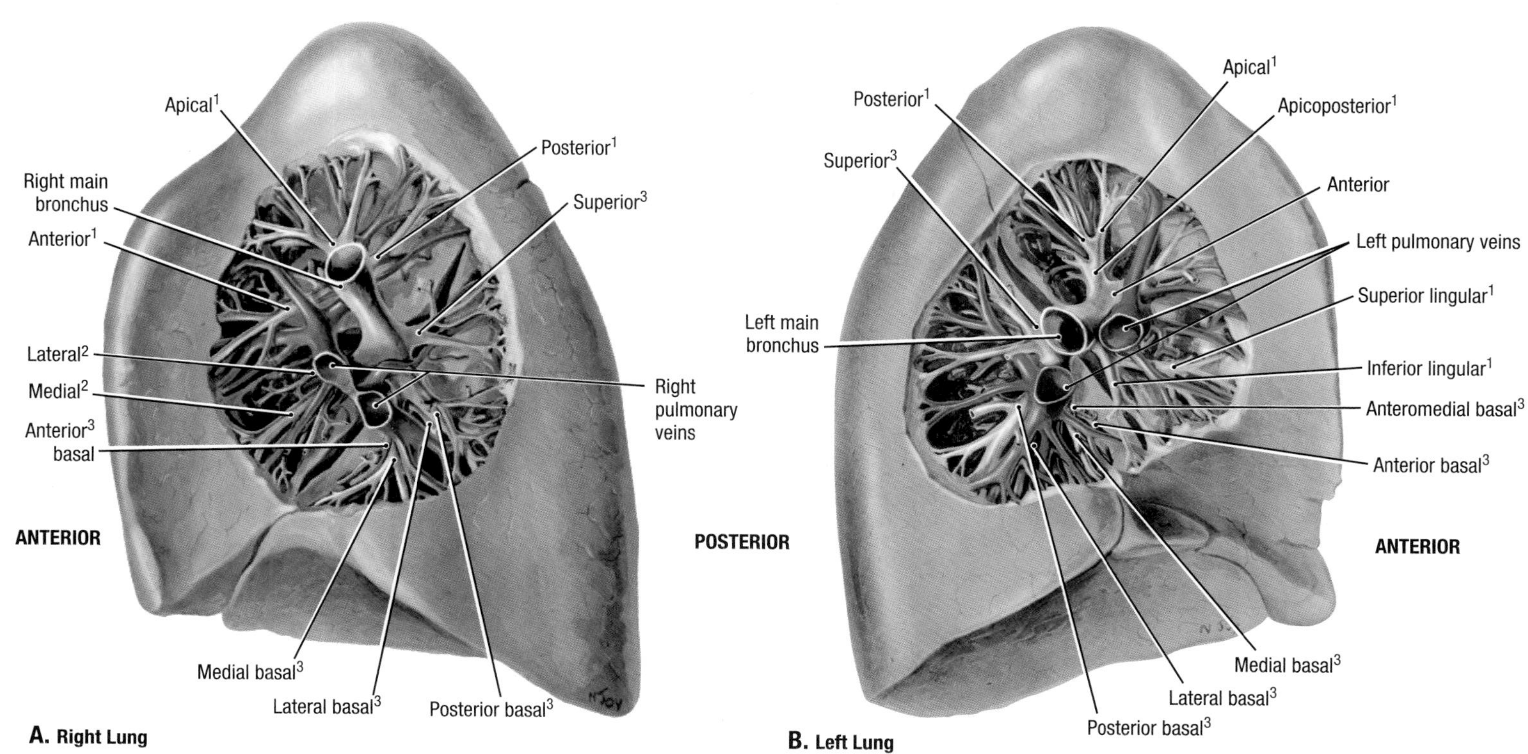
Apical1
Right main bronchus
Anterior1
Posterior1
Superior3
Lateral2
Medial2
Anterior3 basal
Right pulmonary veins
ANTERIOR
Medial basal3
Lateral basal3
Posterior basal3
A. Right Lung
Posterior1
Apical1
Apicoposterior1
Superior3
Anterior
Left pulmonary veins
Superior lingular1
Left main bronchus
Inferior lingular1
Anteromedial basal3
Anterior basal3
POSTERIOR
ANTERIOR
Medial basal3
Lateral basal3
Posterior basal3
B. Left Lung

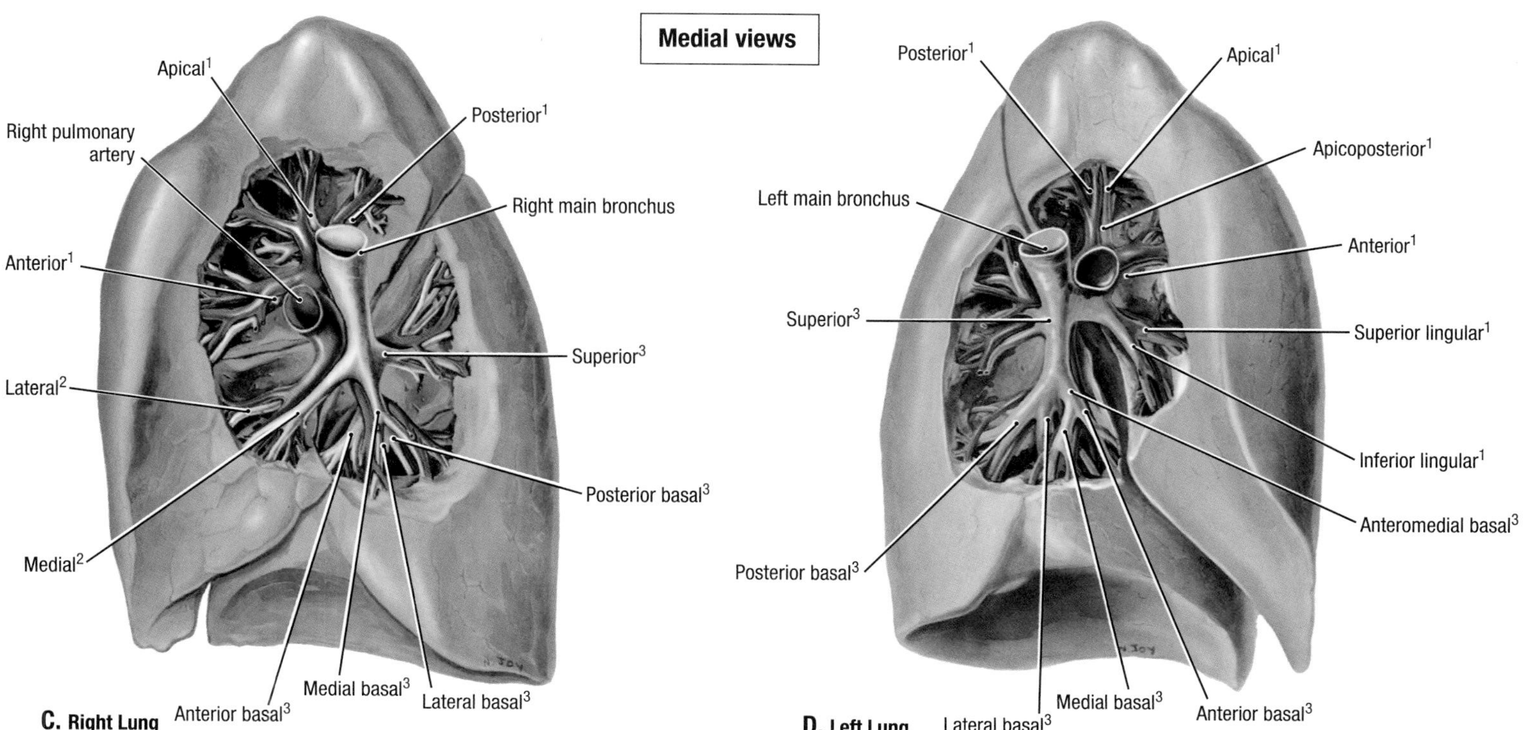
Medial views
Apical1
Right pulmonary artery
Posterior1
Right main bronchus
Anterior1
Superior3
Lateral2
Posterior basal3
Medial2
Medial basal3
Lateral basal3
Anterior basal3
C. Right Lung
Posterior1
Apical1
Apicoposterior1
Left main bronchus
Anterior1
Superior3
Superior lingular1
Inferior lingular1
Anteromedial basal3
Posterior basal3
Medial basal3
Anterior basal3
Lateral basal3
D. Left Lung

## 1.28 Bronchi, pulmonary veins, and pulmonary arteries

**A** and **C.** Right lungs. **B** and **D.** Left lungs. Superscripts indicate segmental bronchi to the [1]superior lobe, [2]middle lobe, and [3]inferior lobe. The pulmonary veins and arteries of fresh lungs were filled with latex, the bronchi were inflated with air. The tissues surrounding the bronchi and vessels were removed.

Obstruction of a pulmonary artery by a blood clot (embolism) results in partial or complete obstruction of blood flow to the lung.

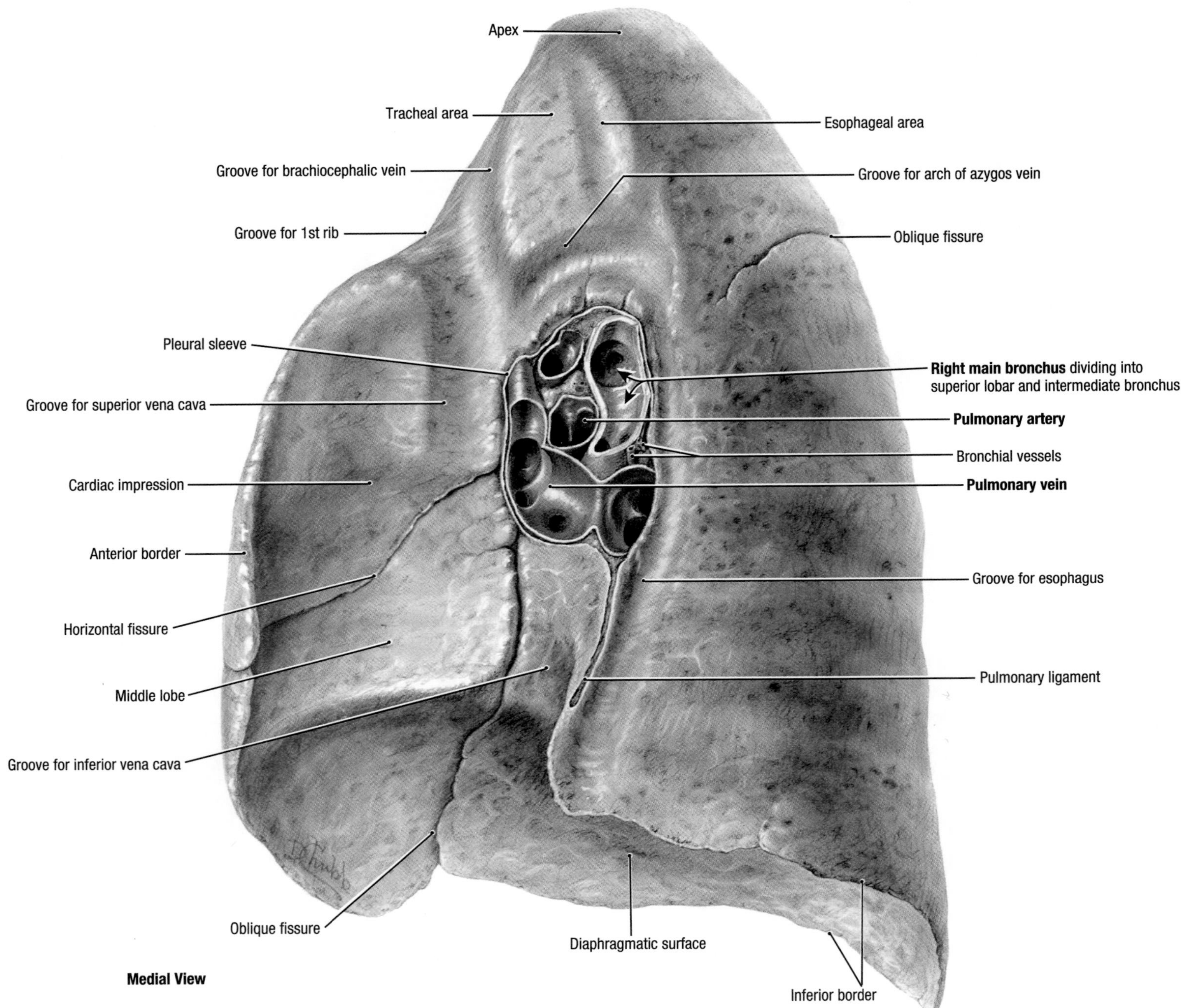
Apex
Tracheal area
Esophageal area
Groove for brachiocephalic vein
Groove for arch of azygos vein
Groove for 1st rib
Oblique fissure
Pleural sleeve
**Right main bronchus** dividing into superior lobar and intermediate bronchus
Groove for superior vena cava
**Pulmonary artery**
Bronchial vessels
Cardiac impression
**Pulmonary vein**
Anterior border
Groove for esophagus
Horizontal fissure
Middle lobe
Pulmonary ligament
Groove for inferior vena cava
Oblique fissure
Diaphragmatic surface
Inferior border
Medial View

## 1.29 Mediastinal (medial) surface and hilum of right lung

The embalmed lung shows impressions of the structures with which it comes into contact, clearly demarcated as surface features; the base is contoured by the domes of the diaphragm; the costal surface bears the impressions of the ribs; distended vessels leave their mark, but nerves do not. The oblique fissure is incomplete here.

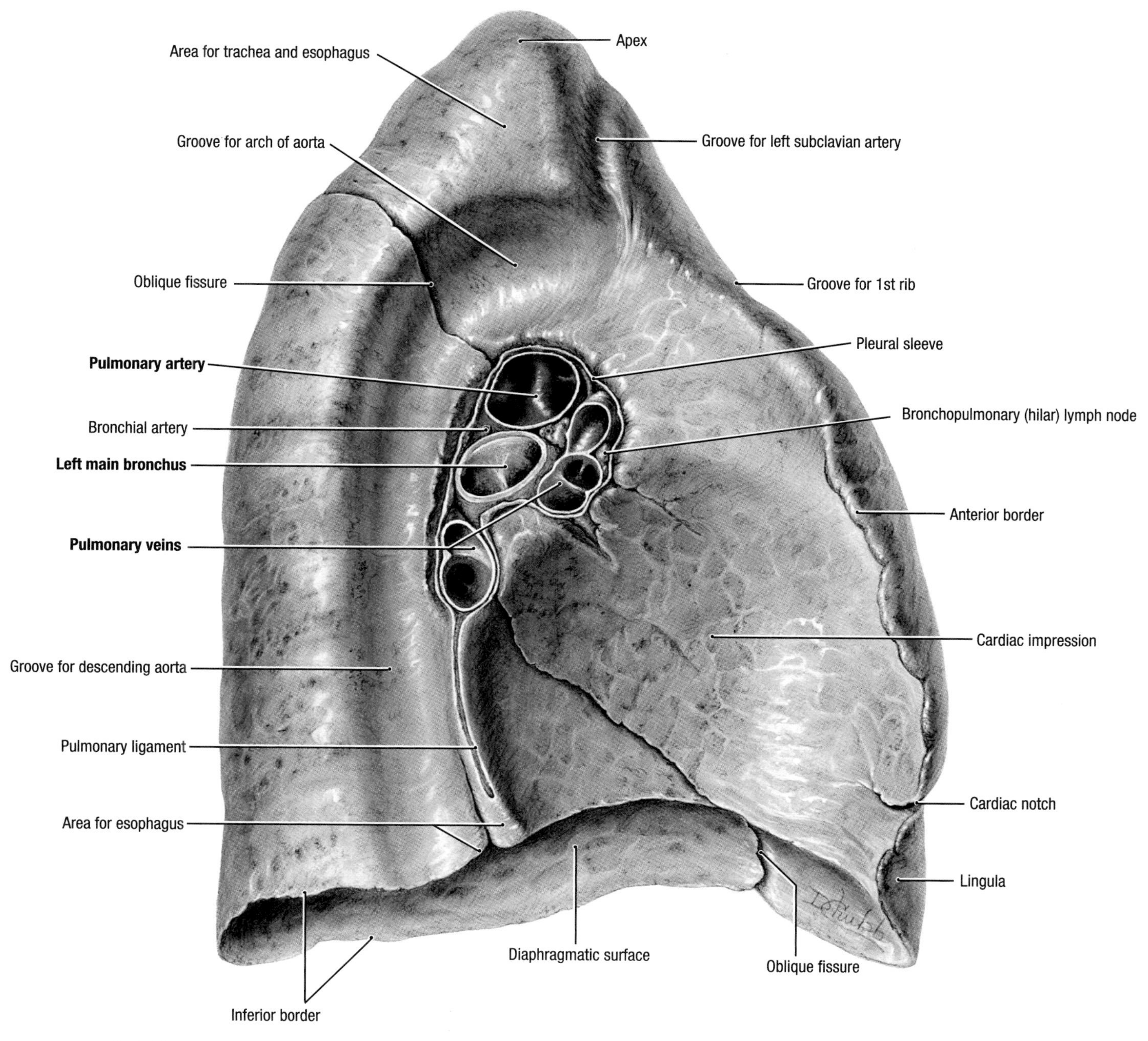
Apex
Area for trachea and esophagus
Groove for left subclavian artery
Groove for arch of aorta
Oblique fissure
Groove for 1st rib
Pleural sleeve
Pulmonary artery
Bronchial artery
Bronchopulmonary (hilar) lymph node
Left main bronchus
Anterior border
Pulmonary veins
Cardiac impression
Groove for descending aorta
Pulmonary ligament
Cardiac notch
Area for esophagus
Lingula
Diaphragmatic surface
Oblique fissure
Inferior border
Medial View

## 1.30 Mediastinal (medial) surface and hilum of left lung

Note the site of contact with esophagus, between the descending aorta and the inferior end of the pulmonary ligament. In the right and left roots, the artery is superior, the bronchus is posterior, one vein is anterior, and the other is inferior; in the right root, the bronchus to the superior lobe (also called the *eparterial bronchus*) is the most superior structure.

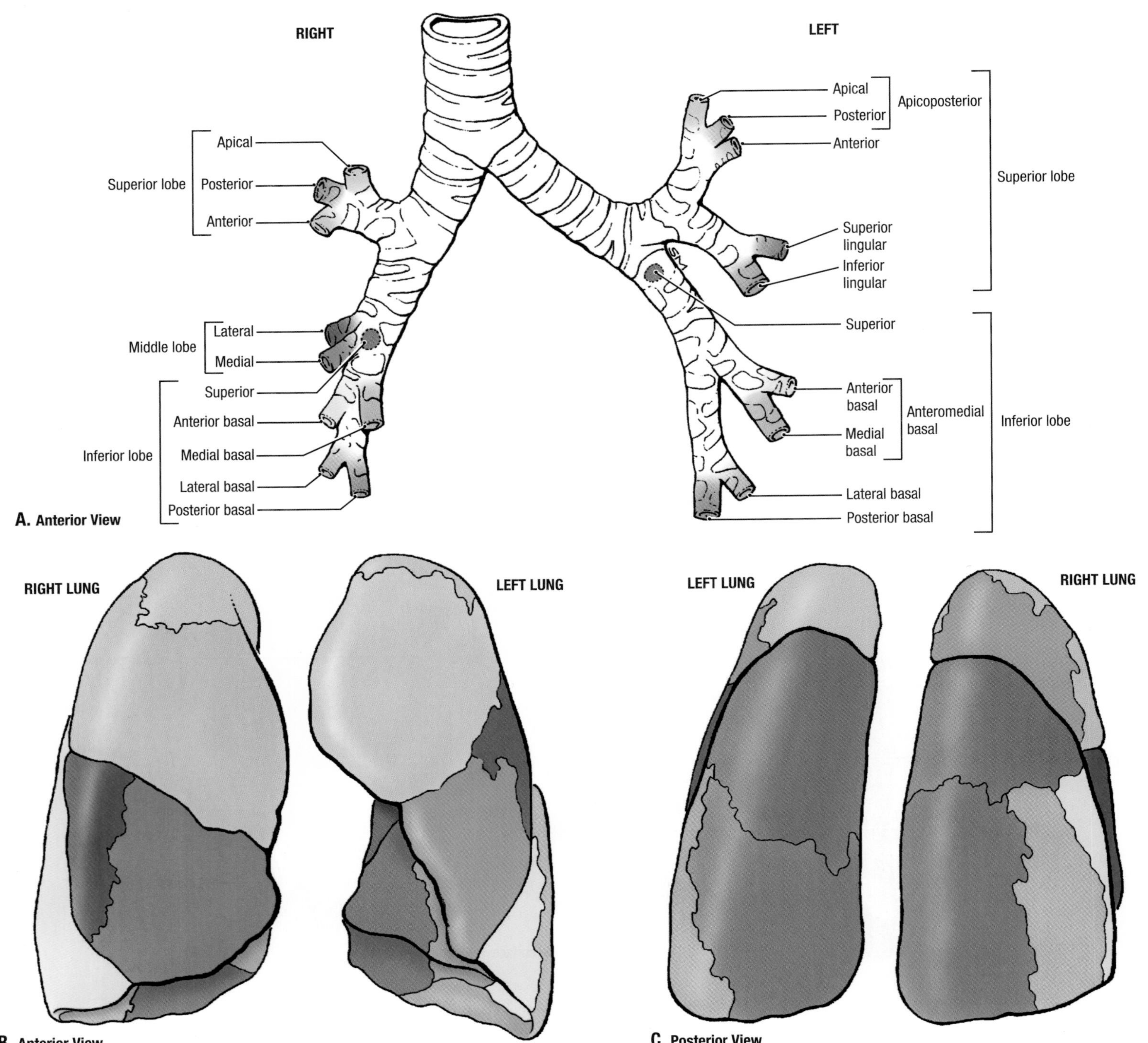
RIGHT
LEFT
Apical
Posterior
Apicoposterior
Anterior
Superior lobe
Apical
Superior lobe
Posterior
Anterior
Superior lingular
Inferior lingular
Superior
Lateral
Middle lobe
Medial
Superior
Anterior basal
Anterior basal
Anteromedial basal
Inferior lobe
Inferior lobe
Medial basal
Medial basal
Lateral basal
Lateral basal
Posterior basal
Posterior basal
A. Anterior View
RIGHT LUNG
LEFT LUNG
LEFT LUNG
RIGHT LUNG
B. Anterior View
C. Posterior View

## 1.31 Segmental bronchi and bronchopulmonary segments

**A.** There are 10 tertiary or segmental bronchi on the right, and 8 on the left. Note that on the left, the apical and posterior bronchi arise from a single stem, as do the anterior basal and medial basal. **B** to **F.** A bronchopulmonary segment consists of a tertiary bronchus, pulmonary vein and artery, and the portion of lung they serve. These structures are surgically separable to allow segmental resection of the lung. To prepare these specimens, the tertiary bronchi of fresh lungs were isolated within the hilum and injected with latex of various colors. Minor variations in the branching of the bronchi result in variations in the surface patterns.

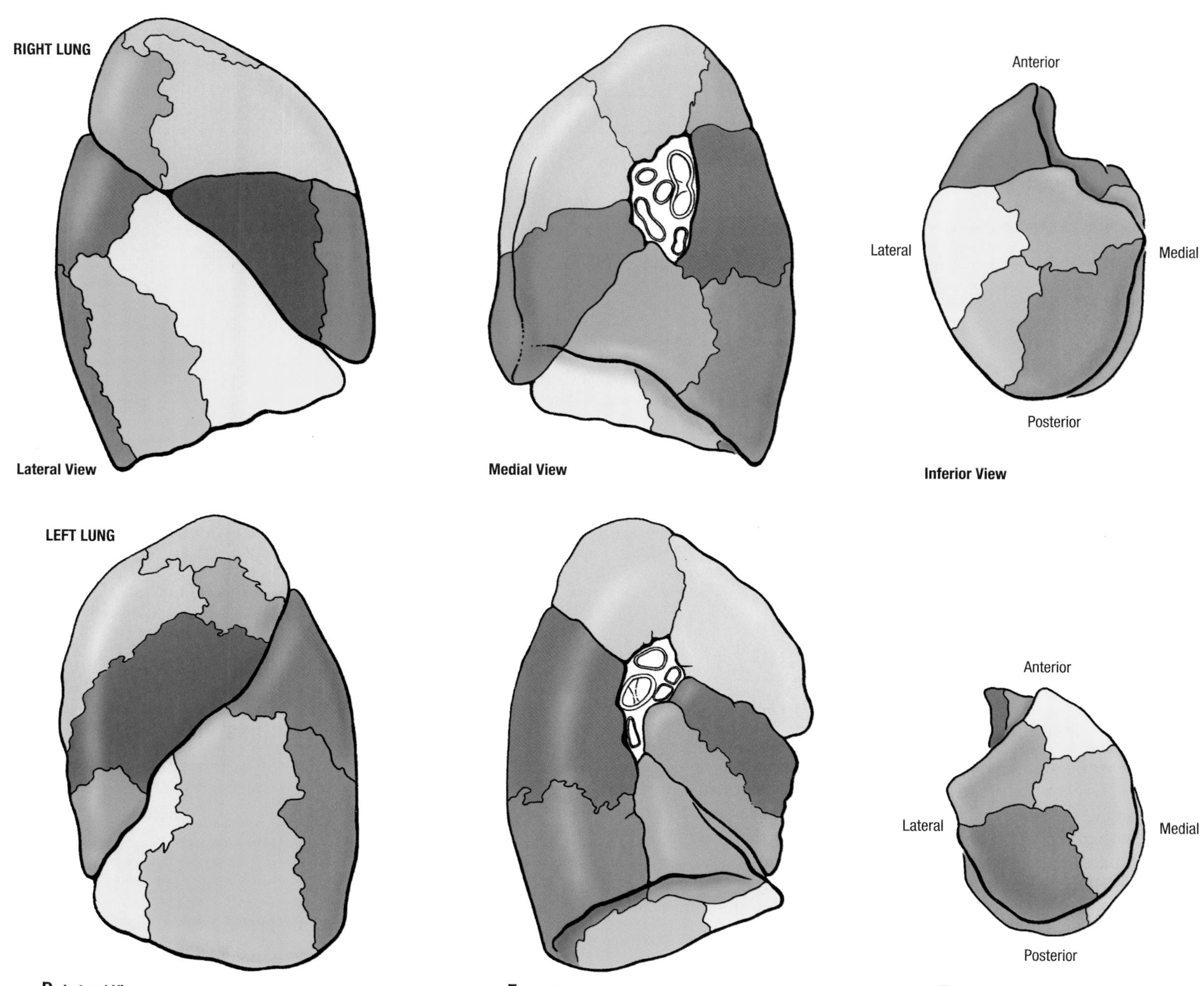
RIGHT LUNG
Lateral View
Medial View
Anterior
Lateral
Medial
Posterior
Inferior View
LEFT LUNG
D. Lateral View
E. Medial View
Anterior
Lateral
Medial
Posterior
F. Inferior View

## 1.31 Segmental bronchi and bronchopulmonary segments *(continued)*

Knowledge of the anatomy of the bronchopulmonary segments is essential for precise interpretations of diagnostic images of the lungs and for surgical resection (removal) of diseased segments. During the treatment of lung cancer, the surgeon may remove a whole lung *(pneumonectomy)*, a lobe *(lobectomy)*, or one or more bronchopulmonary segments *(segmentectomy)*. Knowledge and understanding of the bronchopulmonary segments and their relationship to the bronchial tree are also essential for planning drainage and clearance techniques used in physical therapy for enhancing drainage from specific areas (e.g., in patients with pneumonia or cystic fibrosis).

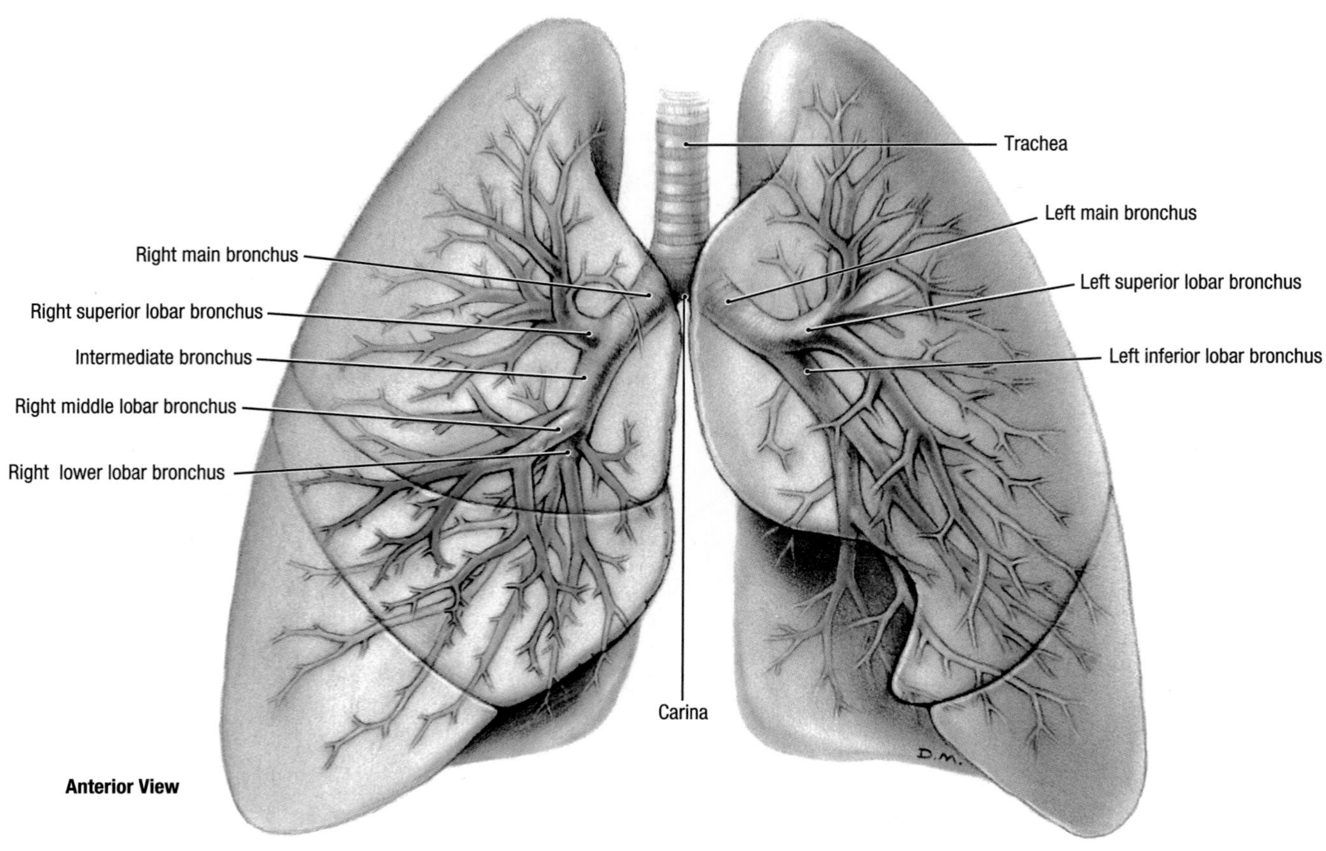
Trachea
Left main bronchus
Left superior lobar bronchus
Left inferior lobar bronchus
Right main bronchus
Right superior lobar bronchus
Intermediate bronchus
Right middle lobar bronchus
Right lower lobar bronchus
Carina
D.M.
Anterior View

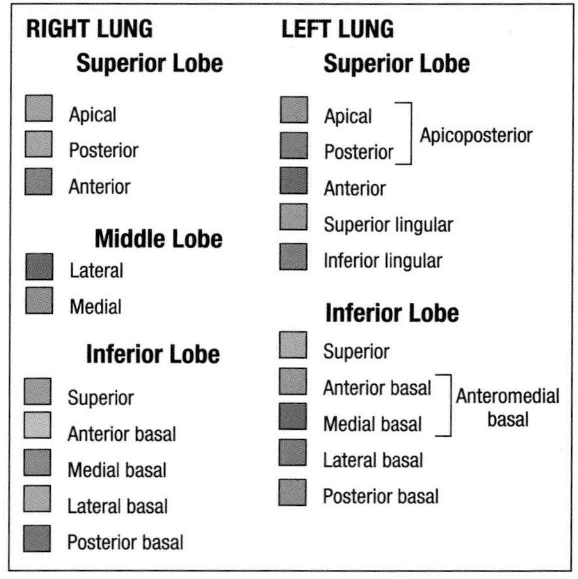
Segmental bronchi:
RIGHT LUNG
Superior Lobe
Apical
Posterior
Anterior
Middle Lobe
Lateral
Medial
Inferior Lobe
Superior
Anterior basal
Medial basal
Lateral basal
Posterior basal
LEFT LUNG
Superior Lobe
Apical
Posterior
Apicoposterior
Anterior
Superior lingular
Inferior lingular
Inferior Lobe
Superior
Anterior basal
Medial basal
Anteromedial basal
Lateral basal
Posterior basal

## 1.32 Trachea and bronchi in situ

- The segmental (tertiary) bronchi are color coded.
- The trachea bifurcates into right and left main (primary) bronchi; the right main bronchus is shorter, wider, and more vertical than the left. Therefore, it is more likely that foreign objects will become lodged in the right main bronchus.
- The right main bronchus gives off the right superior lobe bronchus (eparterial bronchus) before entering the hilum (hilus) of the lung; after entering the hilum, the right middle and inferior lobar bronchi branch off.
- The left main bronchus divides into the left superior and left inferior lobar bronchi; the lobar bronchi further divide into segmental (tertiary) bronchi.

- When examining the bronchi with a *bronchoscope*—an endoscope for inspecting the interior of the tracheobronchial tree for diagnostic purposes—one can observe a ridge, the *carina*, between the orifices of the main bronchi. If the tracheobronchial lymph nodes in the angle between the main bronchi are enlarged because cancer cells have metastasized from a bronchogenic carcinoma, for example, the carina is distorted, widened posteriorly, and immobile.

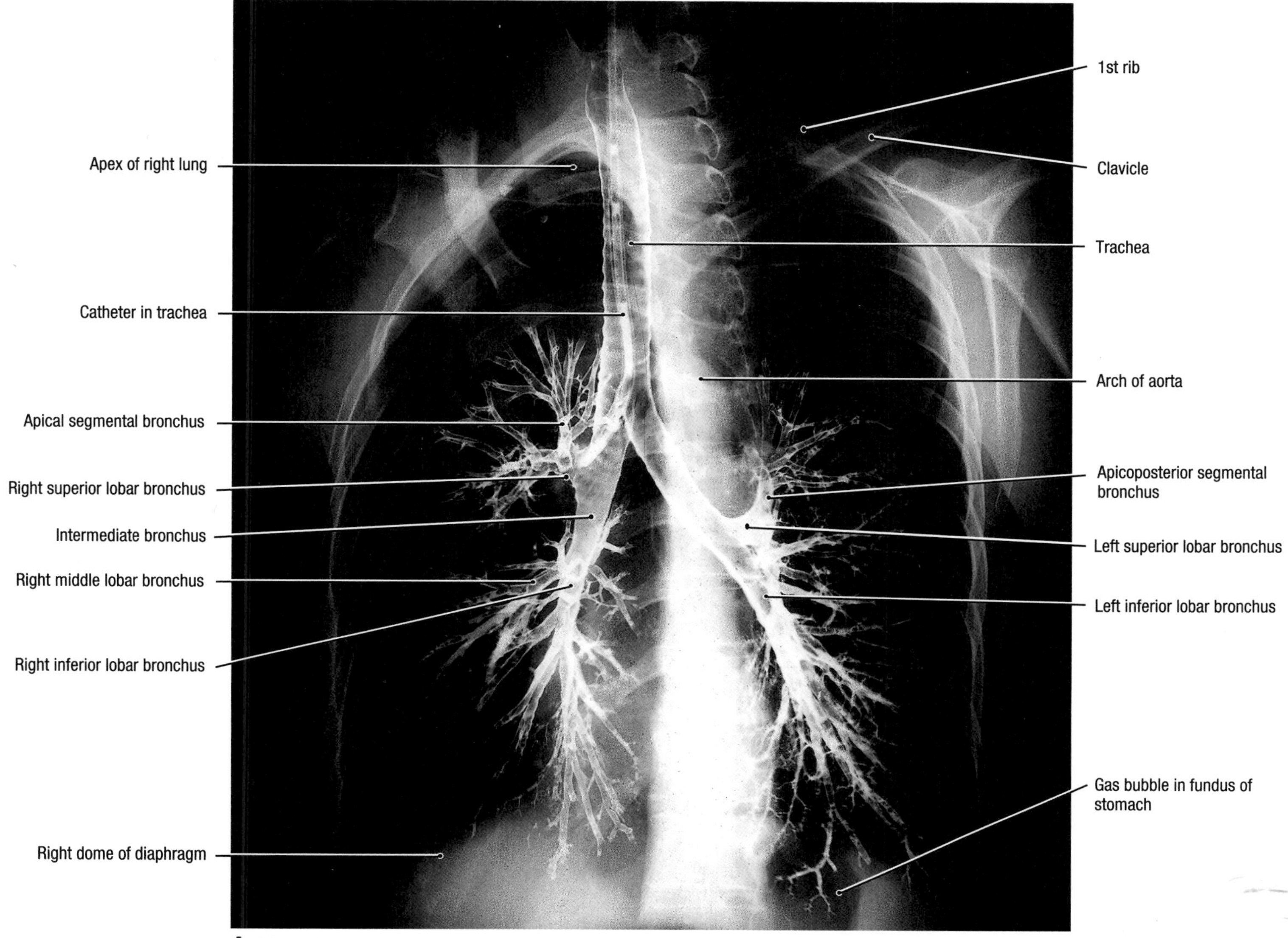
1st rib
Apex of right lung
Clavicle
Trachea
Catheter in trachea
Arch of aorta
Apical segmental bronchus
Apicoposterior segmental bronchus
Right superior lobar bronchus
Intermediate bronchus
Left superior lobar bronchus
Right middle lobar bronchus
Left inferior lobar bronchus
Right inferior lobar bronchus
Gas bubble in fundus of stomach
Right dome of diaphragm

**A.** Slightly Oblique Anteroposterior View

## 1.33 Bronchograms

**A.** Bronchogram of tracheobronchial tree.

Because the right bronchus is wider and shorter and runs more vertically than the left bronchus, aspirated foreign bodies are more likely to enter and lodge in it or one of its branches. A potential hazard encountered by dentists is an aspirated foreign body, such as a piece of tooth, filling material, or a small instrument. Such objects are also most likely to enter the right main bronchus.

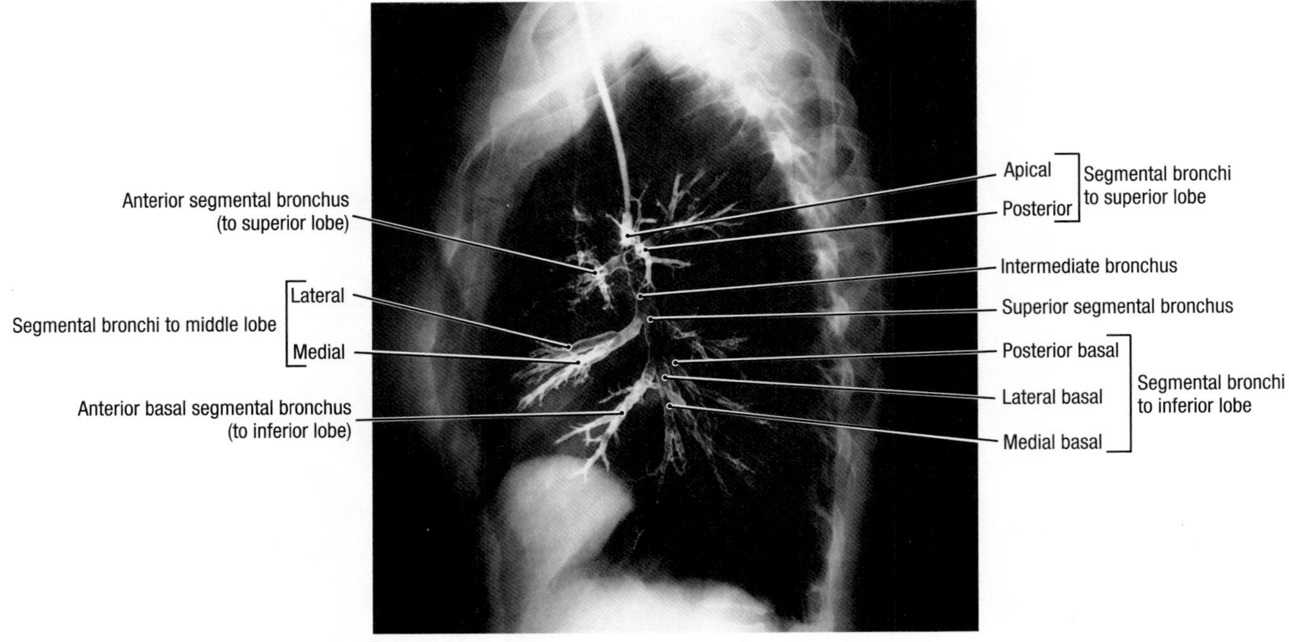
Anterior segmental bronchus
(to superior lobe)
Lateral
Segmental bronchi to middle lobe
Medial
Anterior basal segmental bronchus
(to inferior lobe)
Apical
Posterior
Segmental bronchi
to superior lobe
Intermediate bronchus
Superior segmental bronchus
Posterior basal
Lateral basal
Medial basal
Segmental bronchi
to inferior lobe

**B. Right Segmental Bronchi, Right Lateral View**

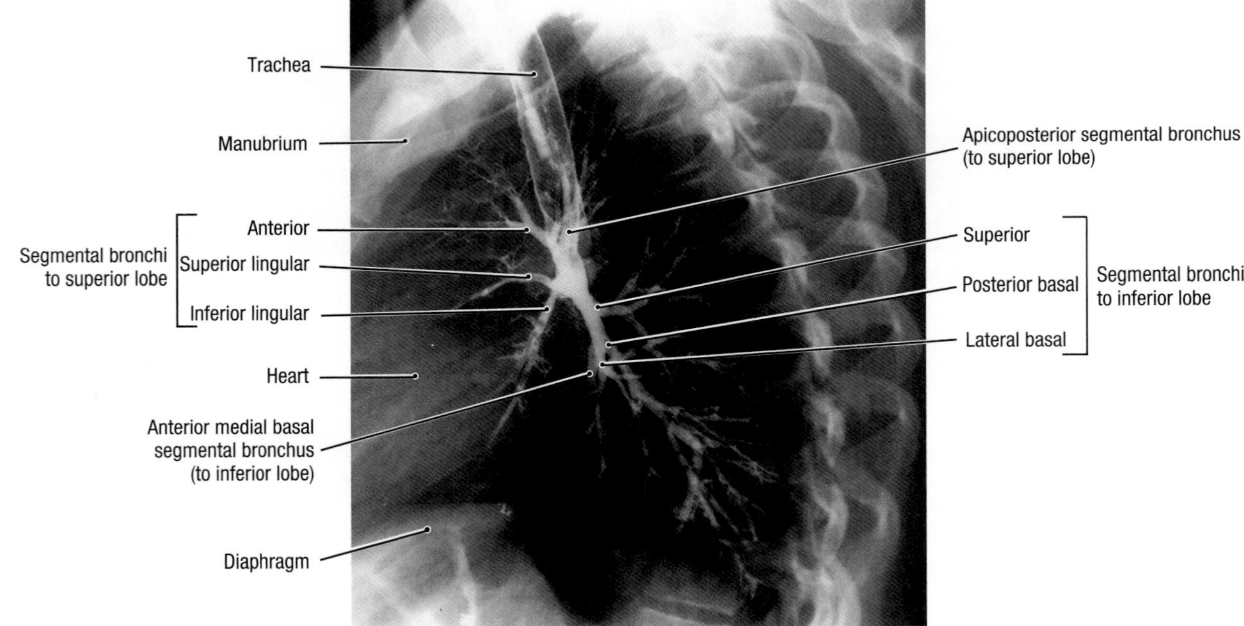
Trachea
Manubrium
Anterior
Segmental bronchi
to superior lobe
Superior lingular
Inferior lingular
Heart
Anterior medial basal
segmental bronchus
(to inferior lobe)
Diaphragm
Apicoposterior segmental bronchus
(to superior lobe)
Superior
Posterior basal
Lateral basal
Segmental bronchi
to inferior lobe

**C. Left Segmental Bronchi, Left Lateral View**

## 1.33 Bronchograms *(continued)*

**B.** Right lateral bronchogram, showing segmental bronchi. **C.** Left lateral bronchogram, showing segmental bronchi.

Superior lobe of right lung
Trachea
Superior lobe of left lung
Apical segmental bronchus
Segmental bronchi: Apical, Posterior, Anterior
Ligamentum arteriosum
Left pulmonary artery
Anterior segmental bronchus
Left superior pulmonary vein
Right pulmonary artery
Superior lingular segmental bronchus
Middle lobar bronchus
Segmental bronchi: Lateral, Medial
Inferior lingular segmental bronchus
Right superior pulmonary vein
Lingula
Superior vena cava
Middle lobe of right lung
Ascending aorta
Pulmonary trunk
Anterior View

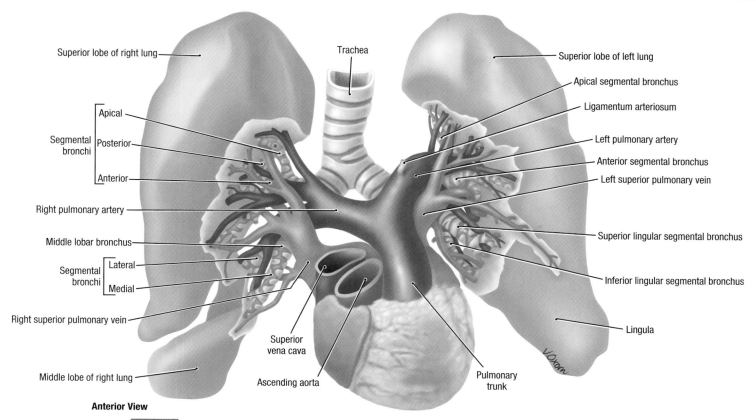

**1.34 Pulmonary artery, lungs retracted (inferior lobes not included)**

The middle lobe of the right lung is drained by the right superior pulmonary vein.

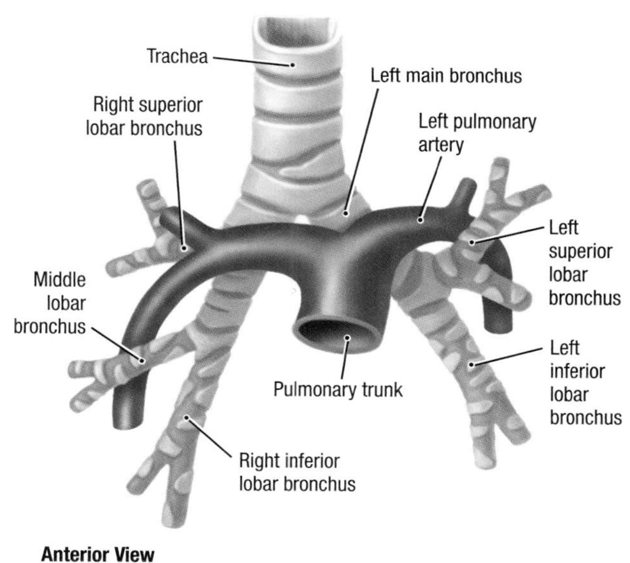
Trachea
Left main bronchus
Right superior lobar bronchus
Left pulmonary artery
Left superior lobar bronchus
Middle lobar bronchus
Left inferior lobar bronchus
Pulmonary trunk
Right inferior lobar bronchus
Anterior View

**1.35 Relationship of bronchi and pulmonary arteries**

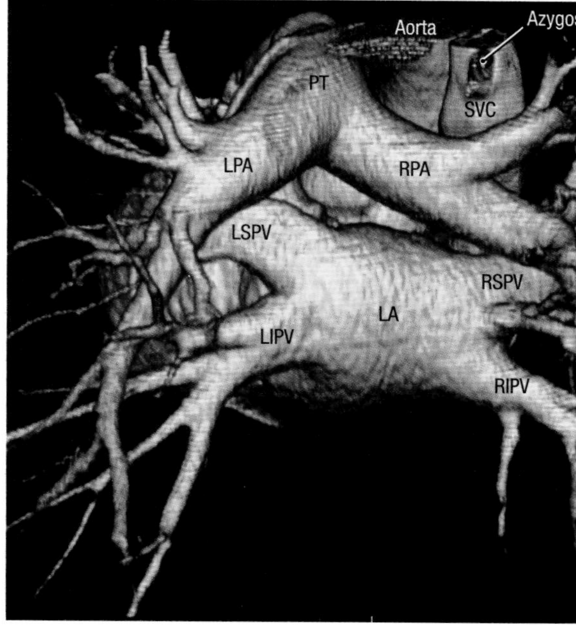
Aorta
Azygos
PT
SVC
LPA
RPA
LSPV
RSPV
LA
LIPV
RIPV
Posterior View

**1.36 3-D volume reconstruction (3DVR) of pulmonary arteries and veins and left atrium**

The pulmonary trunk *(PT)* divides into a longer right pulmonary artery *(RPA)* and shorter left pulmonary artery *(LPA);* the left superior *(LSPV)* and inferior *(LIPV)* and the right superior *(RSPV)* and inferior *(RIPV)* pulmonary veins drain into the left atrium *(LA)*. Superior vena cava *(SVC)*.

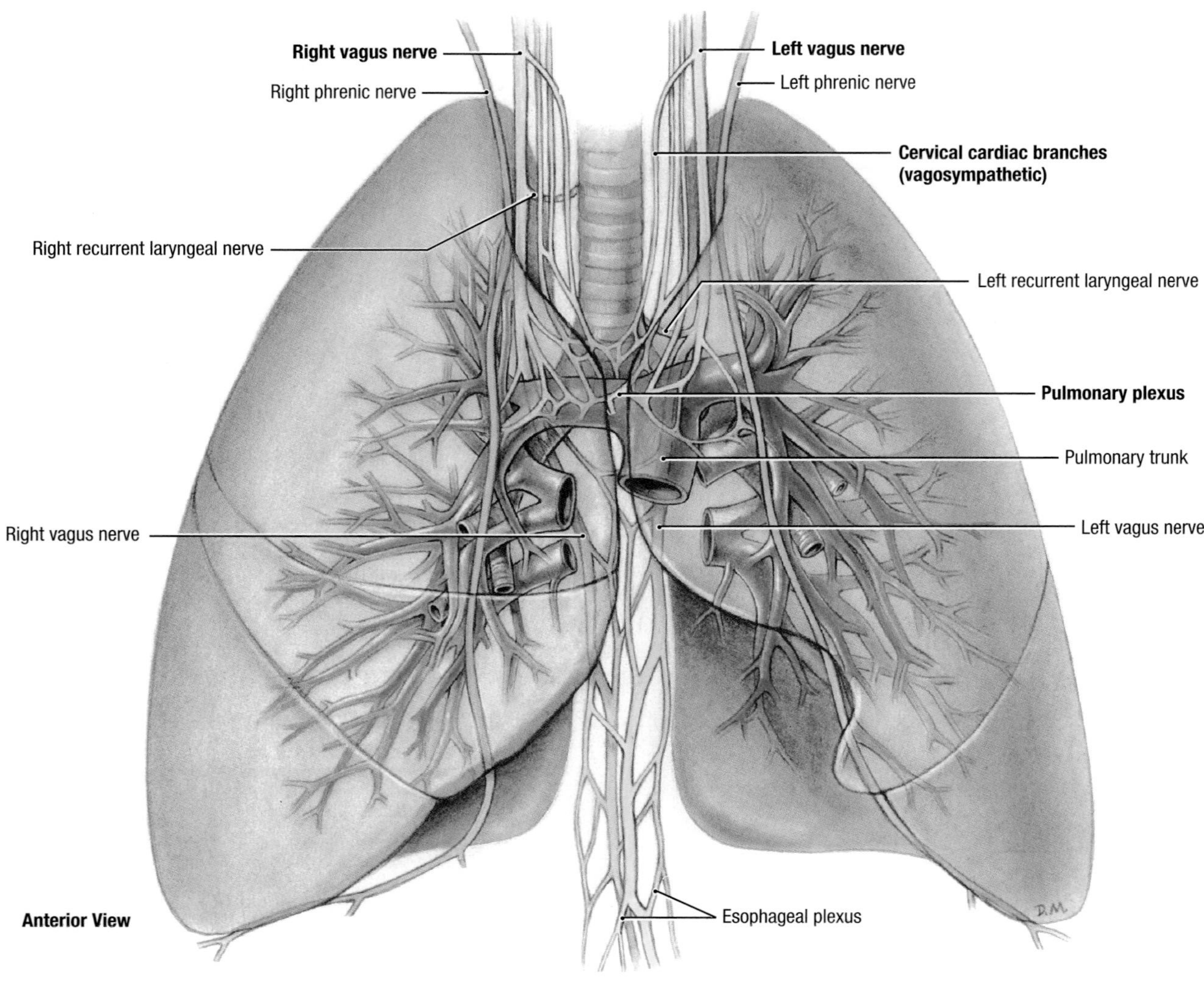
Right vagus nerve
Right phrenic nerve
Left vagus nerve
Left phrenic nerve
Cervical cardiac branches (vagosympathetic)
Right recurrent laryngeal nerve
Left recurrent laryngeal nerve
Pulmonary plexus
Pulmonary trunk
Right vagus nerve
Left vagus nerve
Anterior View
Esophageal plexus
D.M.

## 1.37 Innervation of lungs

- The pulmonary plexuses, located anterior and posterior to the roots of the lungs, receive sympathetic contributions from the right and left sympathetic trunks (2nd to 5th thoracic ganglia, not shown) and parasympathetic contributions from the right and left vagus nerves; cell bodies of postsynaptic parasympathetic neurons are in the pulmonary plexuses and along the branches of the pulmonary tree.
- The right and left vagus nerves continue inferiorly from the posterior pulmonary plexus to contribute fibers to the esophageal plexus.
- The phrenic nerves pass anterior to the root of the lung on their way to the diaphragm.

- The visceral pleura is insensitive to pain because its innervation is autonomic. The autonomic nerves reach the visceral pleura in company with the bronchial vessels. The visceral pleura receives no nerves of general sensation.
- The parietal pleura is sensitive to pain because it is richly supplied by branches of the somatic intercostal and phrenic nerves. Irritation of the parietal pleura produces local pain and referred pain to the areas sharing innervation by the same segments of the spinal cord.

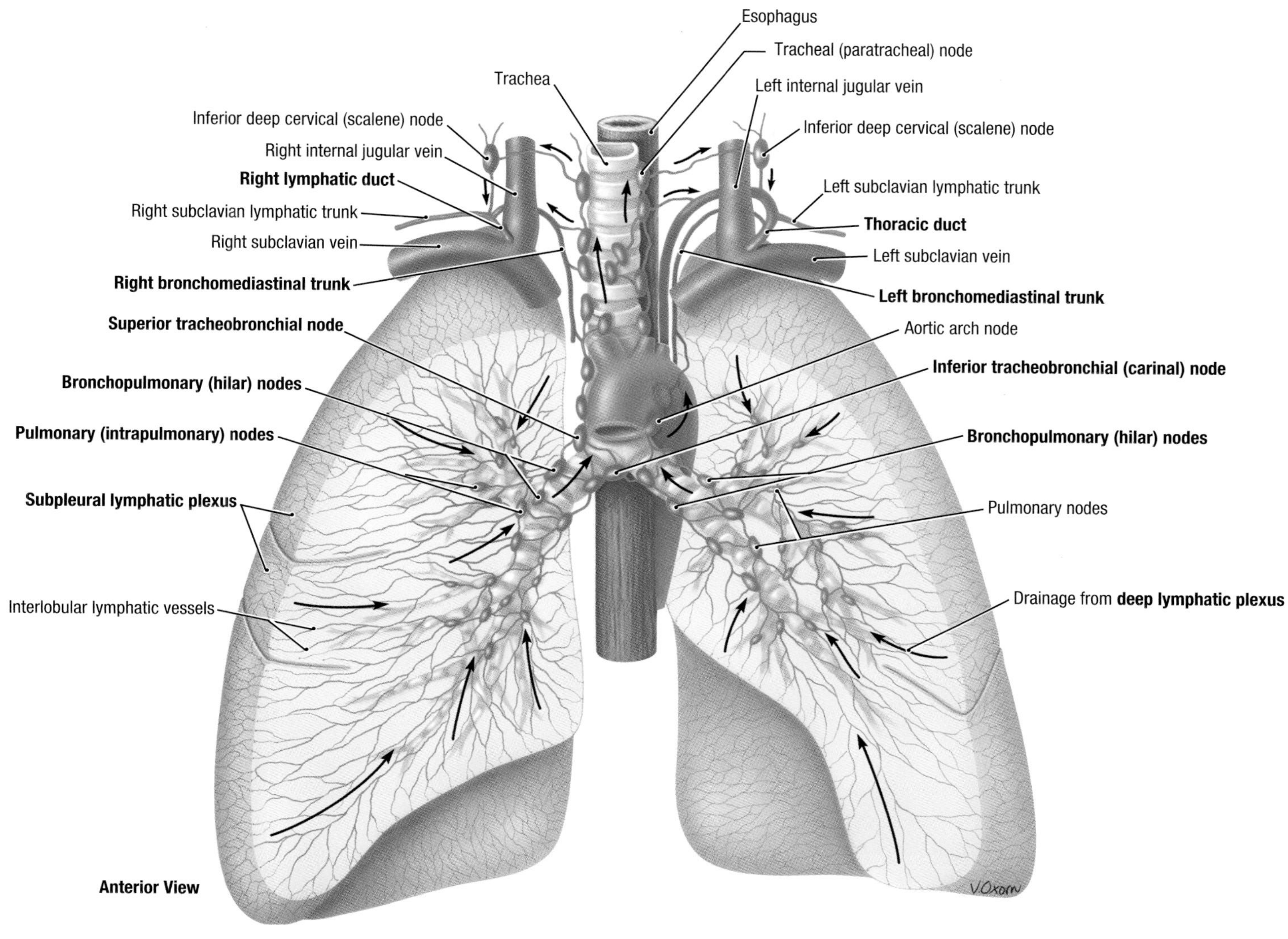
Esophagus
Tracheal (paratracheal) node
Trachea
Left internal jugular vein
Inferior deep cervical (scalene) node
Right internal jugular vein
Inferior deep cervical (scalene) node
Right lymphatic duct
Left subclavian lymphatic trunk
Right subclavian lymphatic trunk
Thoracic duct
Right subclavian vein
Left subclavian vein
Right bronchomediastinal trunk
Left bronchomediastinal trunk
Superior tracheobronchial node
Aortic arch node
Inferior tracheobronchial (carinal) node
Bronchopulmonary (hilar) nodes
Pulmonary (intrapulmonary) nodes
Bronchopulmonary (hilar) nodes
Subpleural lymphatic plexus
Pulmonary nodes
Interlobular lymphatic vessels
Drainage from deep lymphatic plexus
Anterior View

## 1.38 Lymphatic drainage of lungs

- Lymphatic vessels originate in the subpleural (superficial) and deep lymphatic plexuses.
- The subpleural lymphatic plexus is superficial, lying deep to the visceral pleura, and drains lymph from the surface of the lung to the bronchopulmonary (hilar) nodes.
- The deep lymphatic plexus is in the lung and follows the bronchi and pulmonary vessels to the pulmonary, and then bronchopulmonary, nodes located at the root of the lung.
- All lymph from the lungs enters the inferior (carinal) and superior tracheobronchial nodes and then continues to the right and left bronchomediastinal trunks to drain into the venous system via the right lymphatic and thoracic ducts; lymph from the left inferior lobe passes largely to the right side.
- Lymph from the parietal pleura drains into lymph nodes of the thoracic wall (Fig. 1.74).

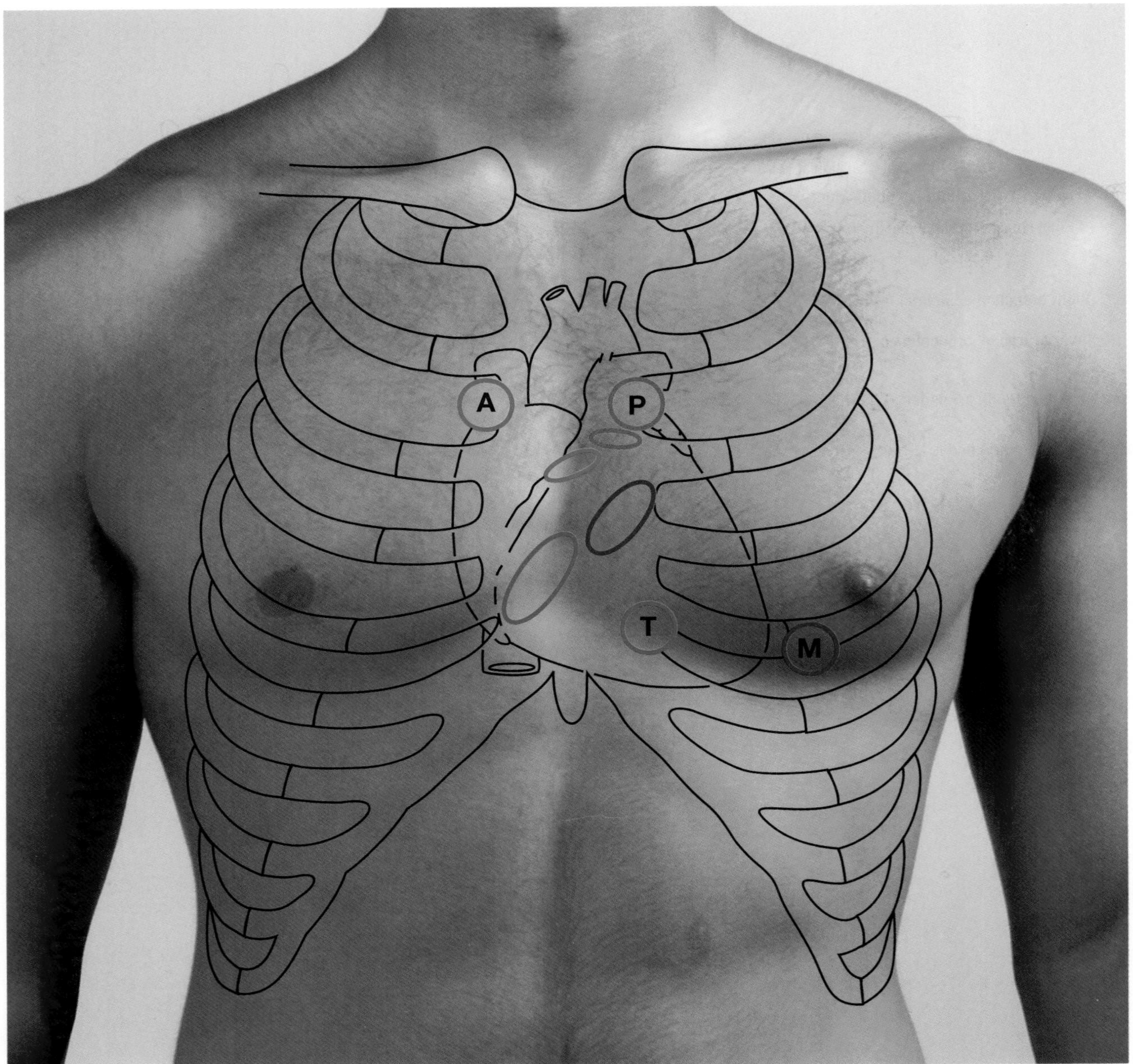
A
P
T
M

Anterior View

## 1.39 Surface markings of the heart, heart valves, and their auscultation areas

- The location of each heart valve in situ is indicated by a colored oval and the area of auscultation of the valve is indicated as a circle of the same color containing the first letter of the valve name: the tricuspid valve *(T)* is green, the mitral valve *(M)* is purple, the pulmonary valve *(P)* is pink and the aortic valve *(A)* is blue.
- The auscultation areas are sites where the sounds of each of the heart's valves can be heard most distinctly through a stethoscope.
- The aortic *(A)* and pulmonary *(P)* auscultation areas are in the 2nd intercostal space to the right and left of the sternal border; the tricuspid area *(T)* is near the left sternal border in the 5th or 6th intercostal space; the mitral valve *(M)* is heard best near the apex of the heart in the 5th intercostal space in the midclavicular line.

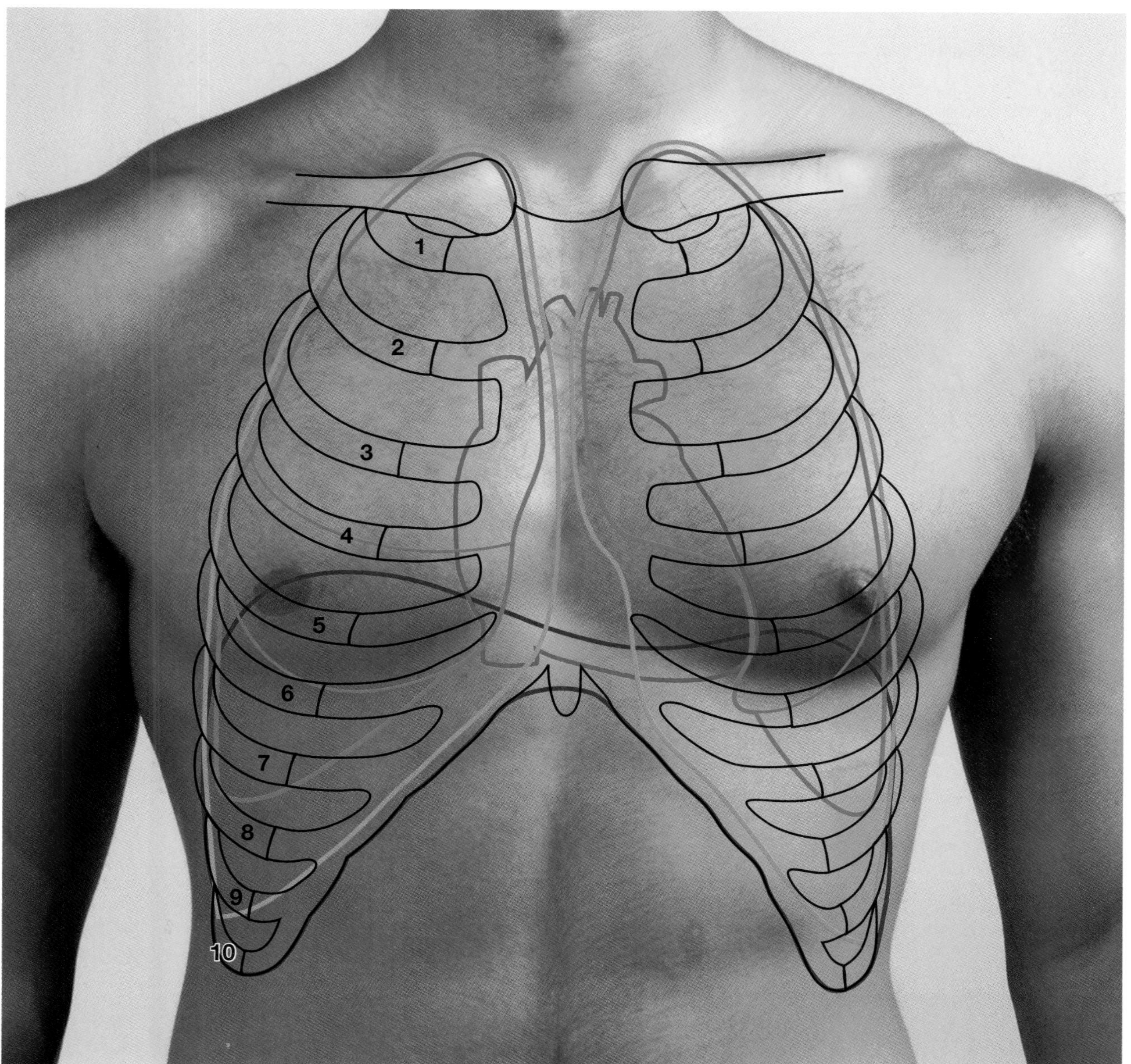
1
2
3
4
5
6
7
8
9
10

Anterior View

## 1.40 Surface markings of the heart, lungs, and diaphragm

- Outlined are the heart *(red)*, lungs *(green)*, parietal pleura *(blue)*, and diaphragm *(purple)*.
- The superior border of the heart is represented by a slightly oblique line joining the 3rd costal cartilages; the convex right side of the heart projects lateral to the sternum and inferiorly, lying at the 6th or 7th costochondral junction; the inferior border of the heart lying superior to the central tendon of the diaphragm and sloping slightly inferiorly to the apex at the 5th interspace at the midclavicular line.
- The right dome of the diaphragm is higher than the left because of the large size of the liver inferior to the dome; during expiration the right dome reaches as high as the 5th rib and the left dome ascends to the 5th intercostal space.
- The left pleural cavity is smaller than the right because of the projection of the heart to the left side.

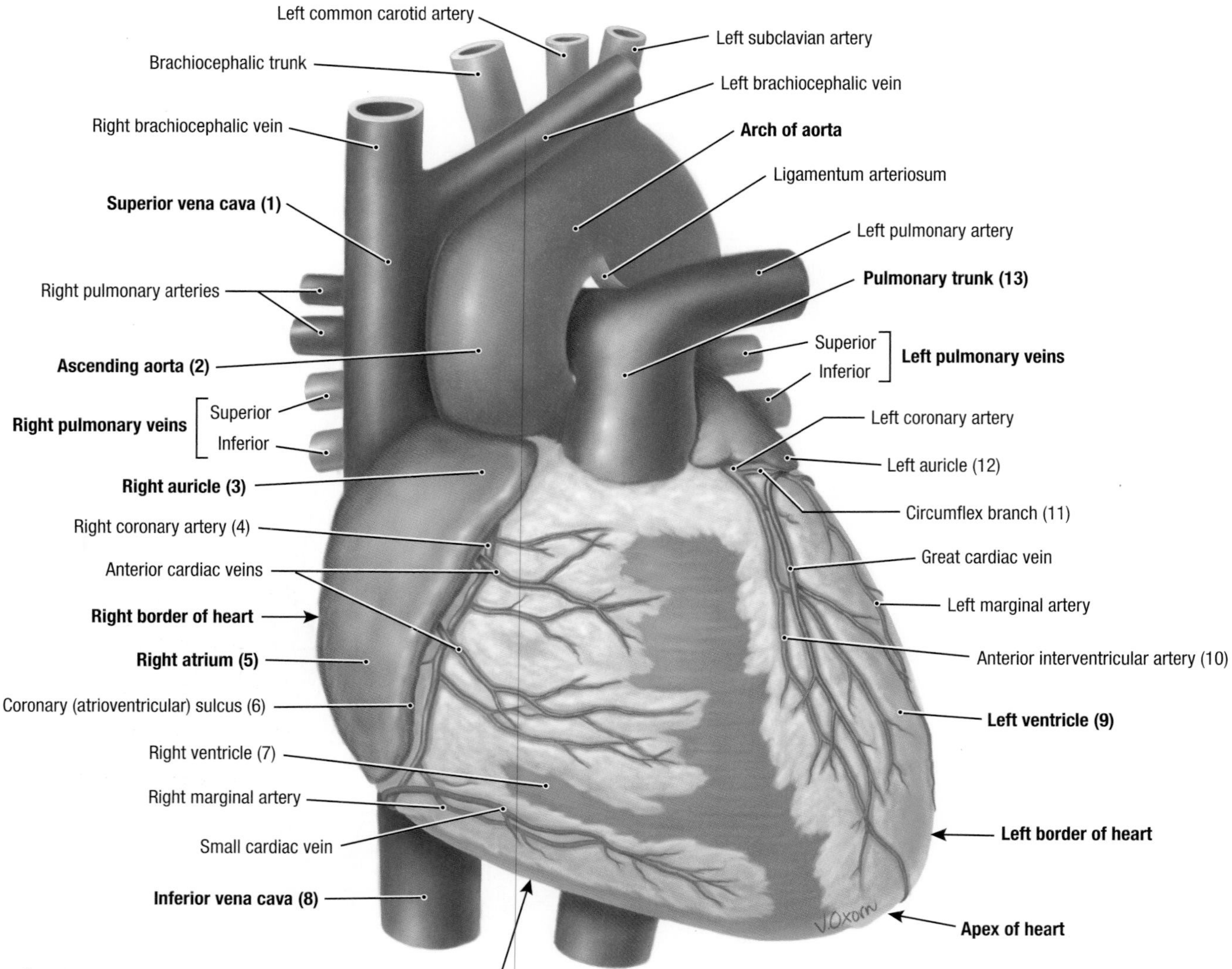

Left common carotid artery
Brachiocephalic trunk
Right brachiocephalic vein
**Superior vena cava (1)**
Right pulmonary arteries
**Ascending aorta (2)**
**Right pulmonary veins** Superior / Inferior
**Right auricle (3)**
Right coronary artery (4)
Anterior cardiac veins
**Right border of heart**
**Right atrium (5)**
Coronary (atrioventricular) sulcus (6)
Right ventricle (7)
Right marginal artery
Small cardiac vein
**Inferior vena cava (8)**
Left subclavian artery
Left brachiocephalic vein
**Arch of aorta**
Ligamentum arteriosum
Left pulmonary artery
**Pulmonary trunk (13)**
**Left pulmonary veins** Superior / Inferior
Left coronary artery
Left auricle (12)
Circumflex branch (11)
Great cardiac vein
Left marginal artery
Anterior interventricular artery (10)
**Left ventricle (9)**
**Left border of heart**
**Apex of heart**
**Inferior border of heart**
V.Oxorn

**A. Anterior View**

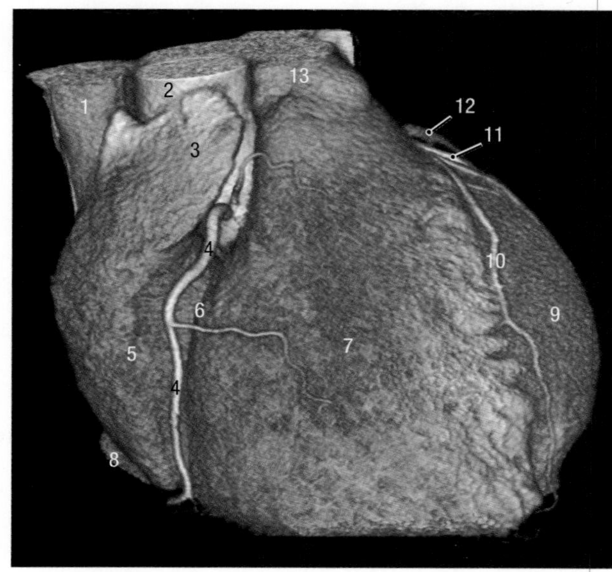
1
2
13
12
11
3
4
10
9
6
5
7
4
8

**B. Anterior View**

## 1.41 Heart and great vessels

**A.**

- The right border of the heart, formed by the right atrium, is slightly convex and almost in line with the superior vena cava.
- The inferior border is formed primarily by the right ventricle and part of the left ventricle.
- The left border is formed primarily by the left ventricle and part of the left auricle.

**B.**

- 3-D volume reconstruction of heart and coronary vessels. Numbers refer to structures in **A.**

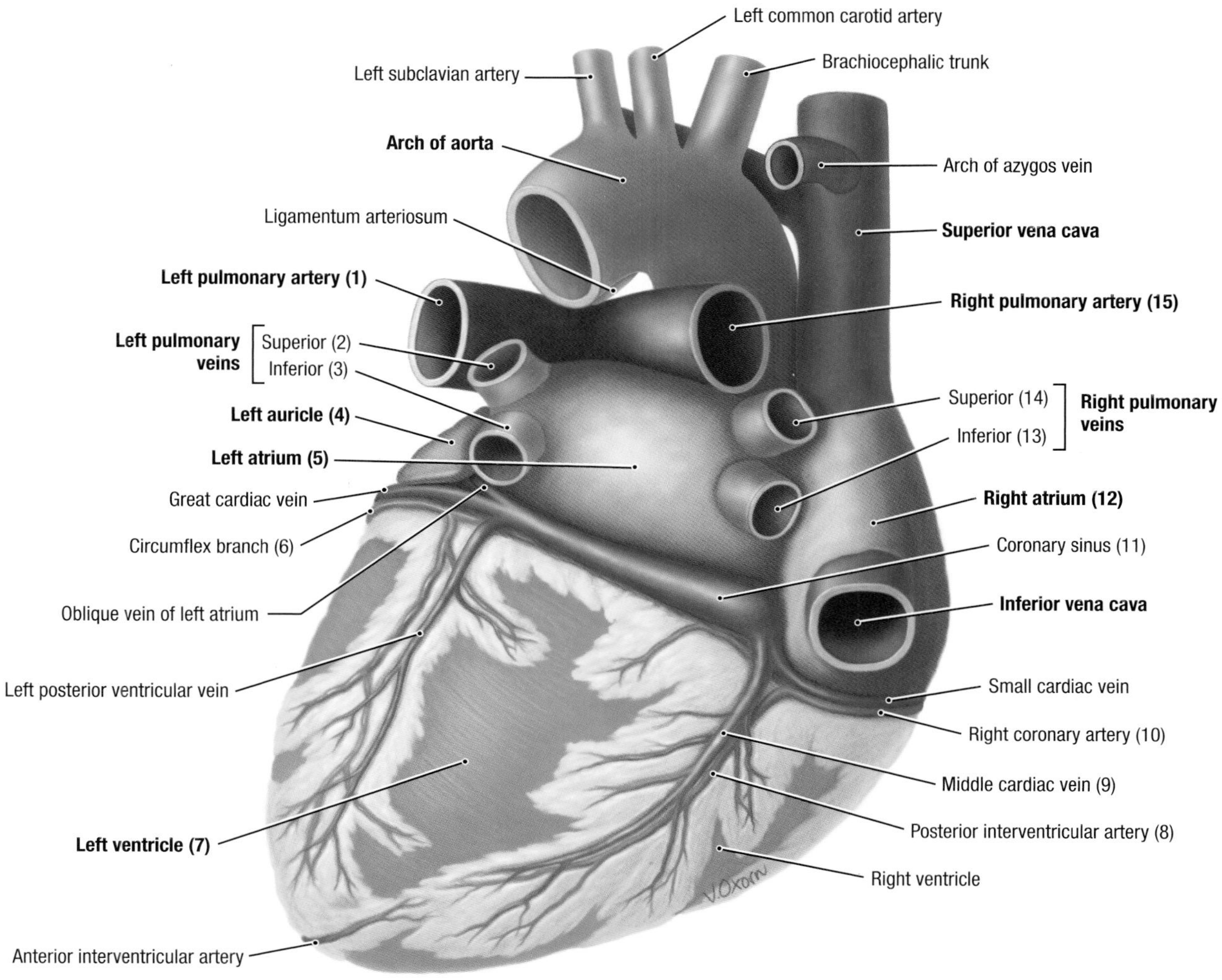

Left common carotid artery
Brachiocephalic trunk
Left subclavian artery
**Arch of aorta**
Arch of azygos vein
**Superior vena cava**
Ligamentum arteriosum
**Left pulmonary artery (1)**
**Right pulmonary artery (15)**
**Left pulmonary veins** Superior (2) Inferior (3)
Superior (14) Inferior (13) **Right pulmonary veins**
**Left auricle (4)**
**Left atrium (5)**
**Right atrium (12)**
Great cardiac vein
Circumflex branch (6)
Coronary sinus (11)
Oblique vein of left atrium
**Inferior vena cava**
Left posterior ventricular vein
Small cardiac vein
Right coronary artery (10)
Middle cardiac vein (9)
Posterior interventricular artery (8)
**Left ventricle (7)**
Right ventricle
Anterior interventricular artery

**C. Posteroinferior View**

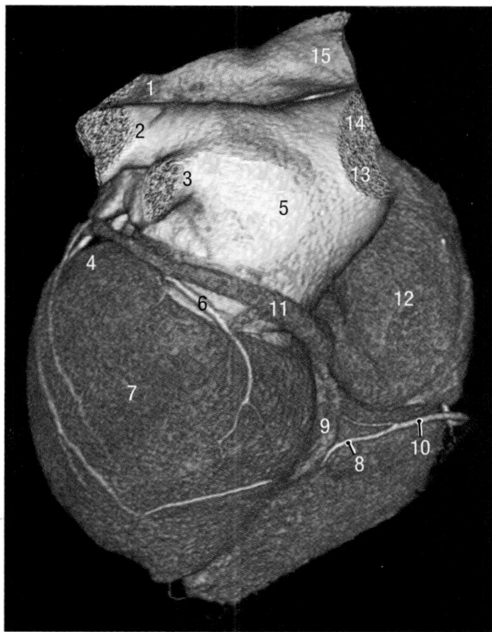
15
1
2
14
13
3
5
4
6
11
12
7
9
8
10

**D. Posteroinferior View**

## 1.41 Heart and great vessels *(continued)*

**C.**

- Most of the left atrium and left ventricle are visible in this posteroinferior view.
- The right and left pulmonary veins open into the left atrium.
- The right and left pulmonary arteries are just superior and parallel to the pulmonary veins.
- The arch of the aorta is arched in two planes: superiorly and to the left.
- The azygos vein arches over the right pulmonary vessels (and bronchus).

**D.**

- 3-D volume reconstruction of heart and coronary vessels. Numbers refer to structures in C.

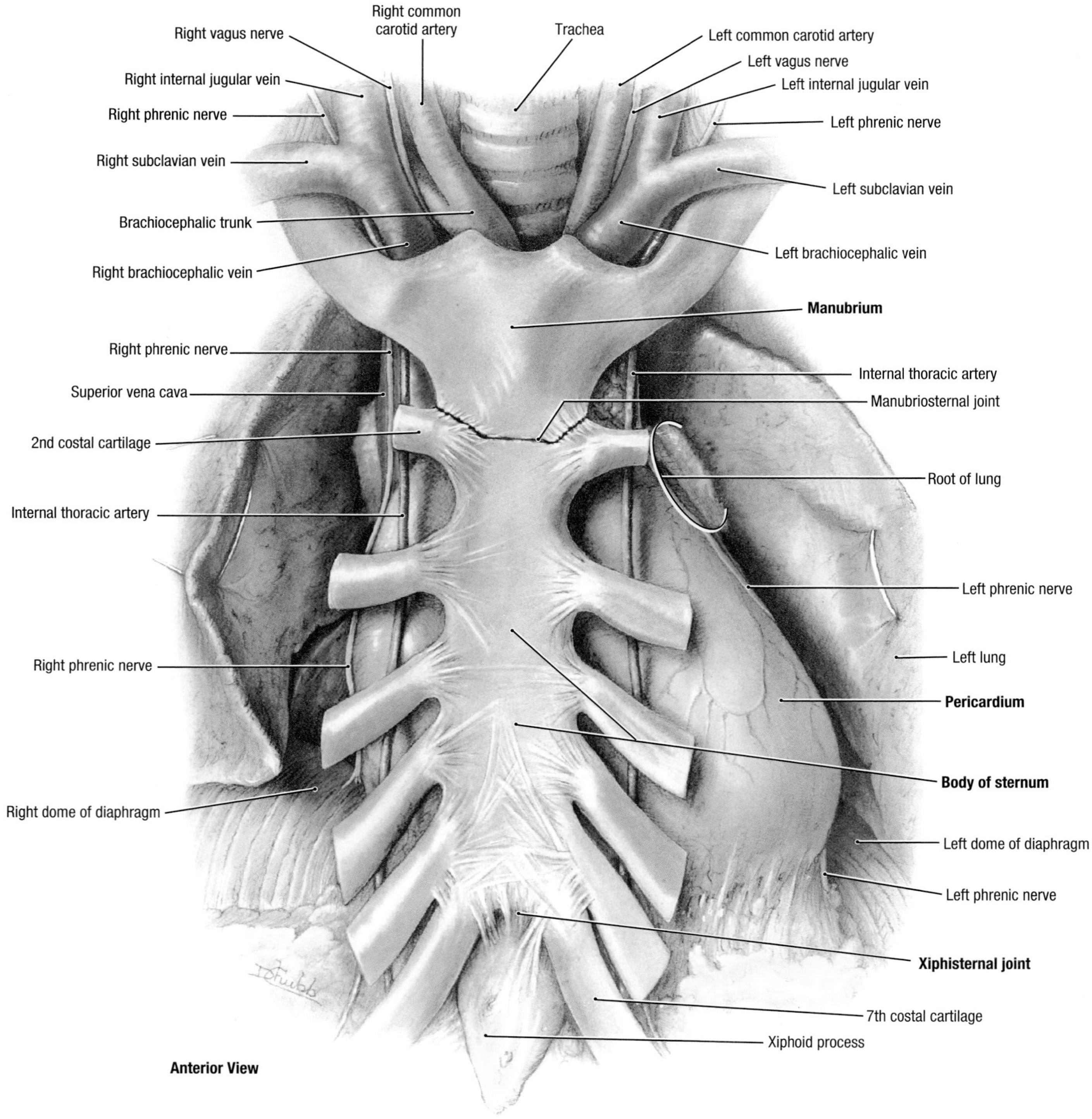
Right vagus nerve
Right common carotid artery
Trachea
Left common carotid artery
Left vagus nerve
Left internal jugular vein
Right internal jugular vein
Right phrenic nerve
Left phrenic nerve
Right subclavian vein
Left subclavian vein
Brachiocephalic trunk
Left brachiocephalic vein
Right brachiocephalic vein
Manubrium
Right phrenic nerve
Internal thoracic artery
Superior vena cava
Manubriosternal joint
2nd costal cartilage
Root of lung
Internal thoracic artery
Left phrenic nerve
Left lung
Right phrenic nerve
Pericardium
Body of sternum
Right dome of diaphragm
Left dome of diaphragm
Left phrenic nerve
Xiphisternal joint
7th costal cartilage
Xiphoid process
Anterior View

## 1.42 Pericardium in relation to sternum

- The pericardium lies posterior to the body of the sternum, extending from just superior to the sternal angle to the level of the xiphisternal joint; approximately two thirds lies to the left of the median plane.
- The heart lies between the sternum and the anterior mediastinum anteriorly and the vertebral column and the posterior mediastinum posteriorly; in cardiac compression, the sternum is depressed 4 to 5 cm, forcing blood out of the heart and into the great vessels.
- Internal thoracic arteries arise from the subclavian arteries and descend posterior to the costal cartilages, running lateral to the sternum and anterior to the pleura.

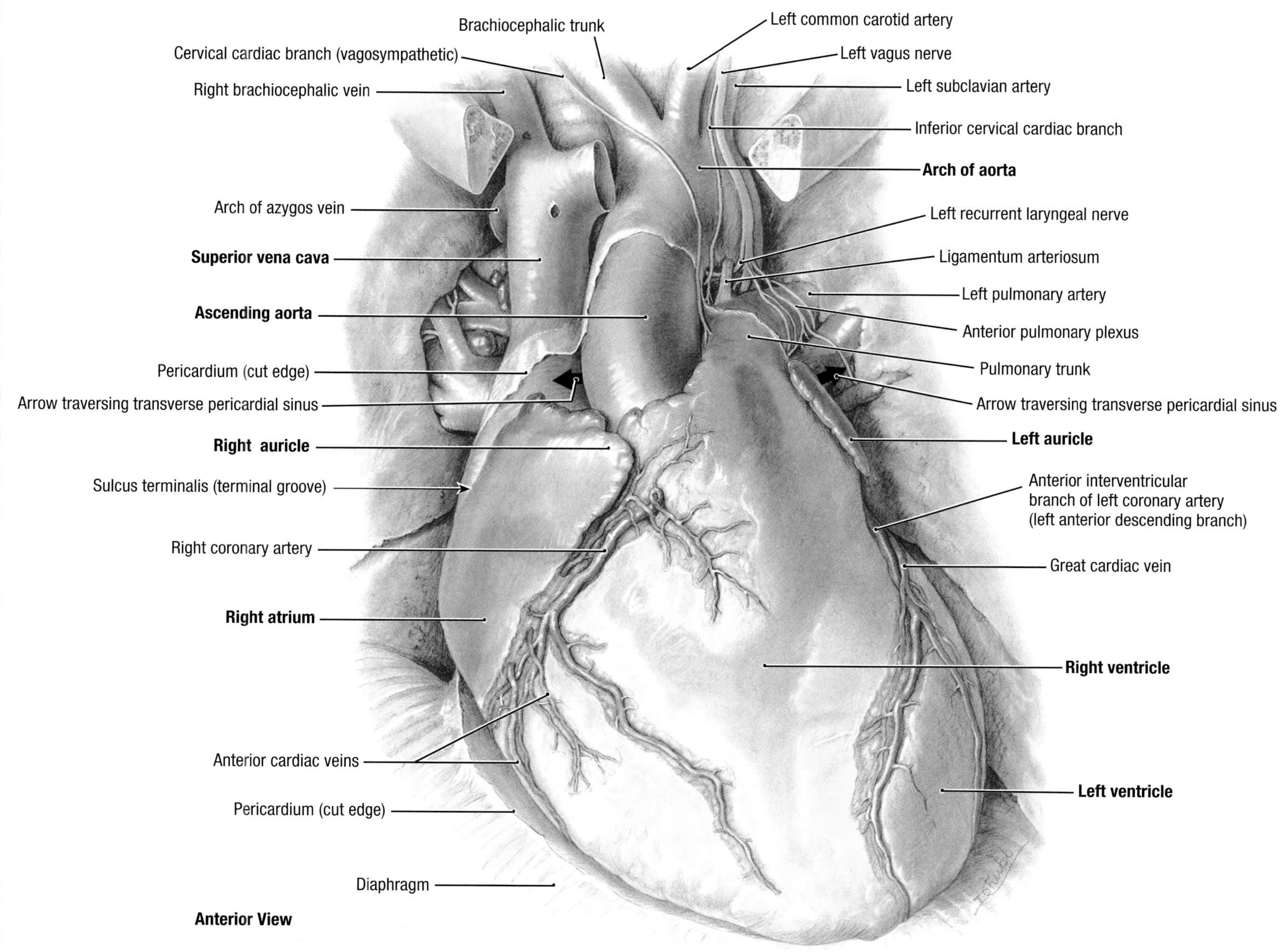
Brachiocephalic trunk
Cervical cardiac branch (vagosympathetic)
Right brachiocephalic vein
Arch of azygos vein
Superior vena cava
Ascending aorta
Pericardium (cut edge)
Arrow traversing transverse pericardial sinus
Right auricle
Sulcus terminalis (terminal groove)
Right coronary artery
Right atrium
Anterior cardiac veins
Pericardium (cut edge)
Diaphragm
Anterior View
Left common carotid artery
Left vagus nerve
Left subclavian artery
Inferior cervical cardiac branch
Arch of aorta
Left recurrent laryngeal nerve
Ligamentum arteriosum
Left pulmonary artery
Anterior pulmonary plexus
Pulmonary trunk
Arrow traversing transverse pericardial sinus
Left auricle
Anterior interventricular
branch of left coronary artery
(left anterior descending branch)
Great cardiac vein
Right ventricle
Left ventricle

## 1.43 Sternocostal (anterior) surface of heart and great vessels in situ

- The right ventricle forms most of the sternocostal surface.
- The entire right auricle and much of the right atrium are visible anteriorly, but only a small portion of the left auricle is visible; the auricles, like a closing claw, grasp the origins of the pulmonary trunk and ascending aorta from a posterior approach.
- The ligamentum arteriosum passes from the origin of the left pulmonary artery to the arch of the aorta.
- The right coronary artery courses in the anterior atrioventricular groove, and the anterior interventricular branch of the left coronary artery (anterior descending branch) courses in the anterior interventricular groove.
- The left vagus nerve passes lateral to the arch of the aorta and then posterior to the root of the lung; the left recurrent laryngeal nerve passes inferior to the arch of the aorta posterior to the ligamentum arteriosum.
- The great cardiac vein ascends beside the anterior interventricular branch of the left coronary artery to drain into the coronary sinus posteriorly.

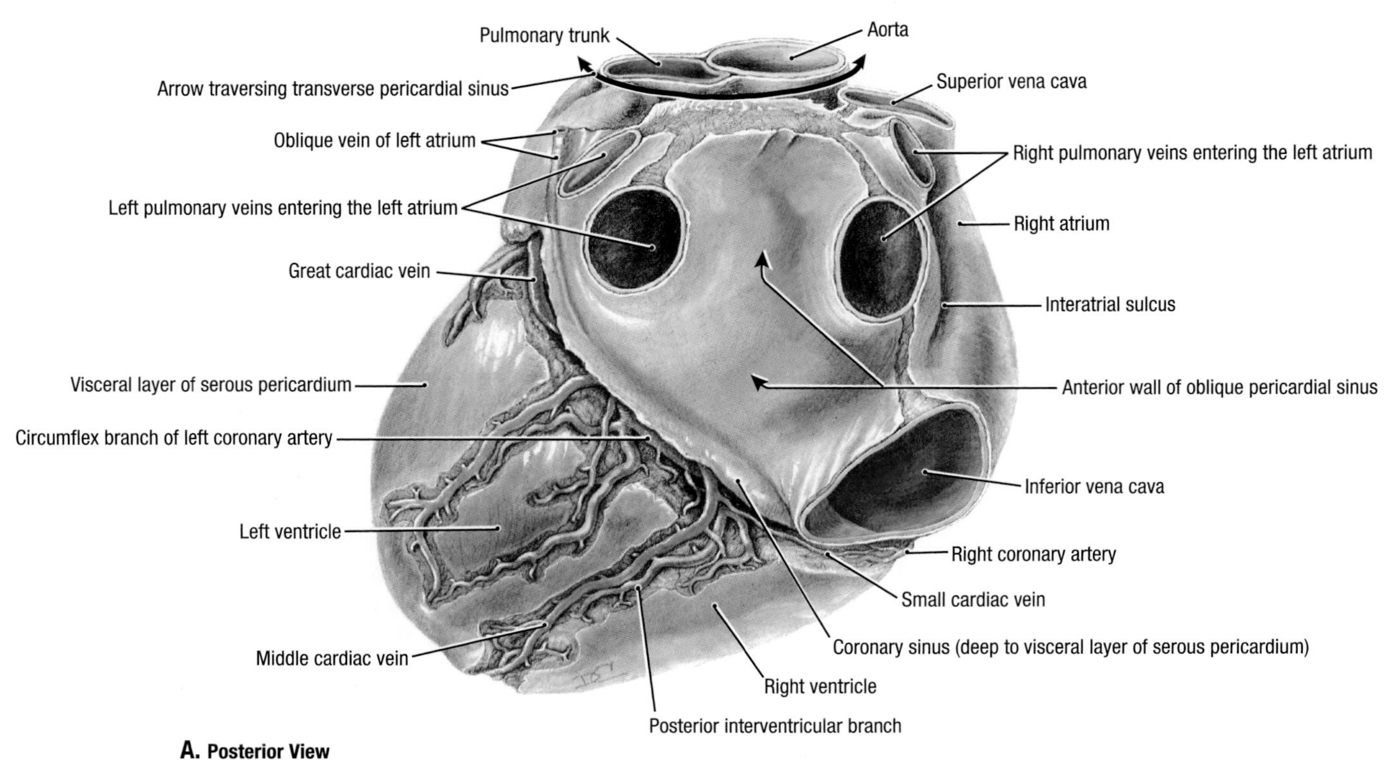
Pulmonary trunk
Aorta
Arrow traversing transverse pericardial sinus
Superior vena cava
Oblique vein of left atrium
Right pulmonary veins entering the left atrium
Left pulmonary veins entering the left atrium
Right atrium
Great cardiac vein
Interatrial sulcus
Visceral layer of serous pericardium
Anterior wall of oblique pericardial sinus
Circumflex branch of left coronary artery
Inferior vena cava
Left ventricle
Right coronary artery
Small cardiac vein
Middle cardiac vein
Coronary sinus (deep to visceral layer of serous pericardium)
Right ventricle
Posterior interventricular branch

**A. Posterior View**

## 1.44 Heart and pericardium

- This heart **(A)** was removed from the interior of the pericardial sac **(B).**
- The entire base, or posterior surface, and part of the diaphragmatic or inferior surface of the heart are in view.
- The superior vena cava and larger inferior vena cava join the superior and inferior aspects of the right atrium.
- The left atrium forms the greater part of the base (posterior surface) of the heart.
- The left coronary artery in this specimen is dominant, since it supplies the posterior interventricular branch.
- Most branches of cardiac veins cross branches of the coronary arteries superficially.
- The visceral layer of serous pericardium (epicardium) covers the surface of the heart and reflects onto the great vessels; from around the great vessels, the serous pericardium reflects to line the internal aspect of the fibrous pericardium as the parietal layer of serous pericardium. The fibrous pericardium and the parietal layer of serous pericardium form the pericardial sac that encases the heart.
- Note the cut edges of the reflections of serous pericardia around the arterial vessels (the pulmonary trunk and aorta) and venous vessels (the superior and inferior venae cavae and the pulmonary veins).

- The transverse pericardial sinus is especially important to cardiac surgeons. After the pericardial sac has been opened anteriorly, a finger can be passed through the transverse pericardial sinus posterior to the aorta and pulmonary trunk. By passing a surgical clamp or placing a ligature around these vessels, inserting the tubes of a coronary bypass machine, and then tightening the ligature, surgeons can stop or divert the circulation of blood in these large arteries while performing cardiac surgery.

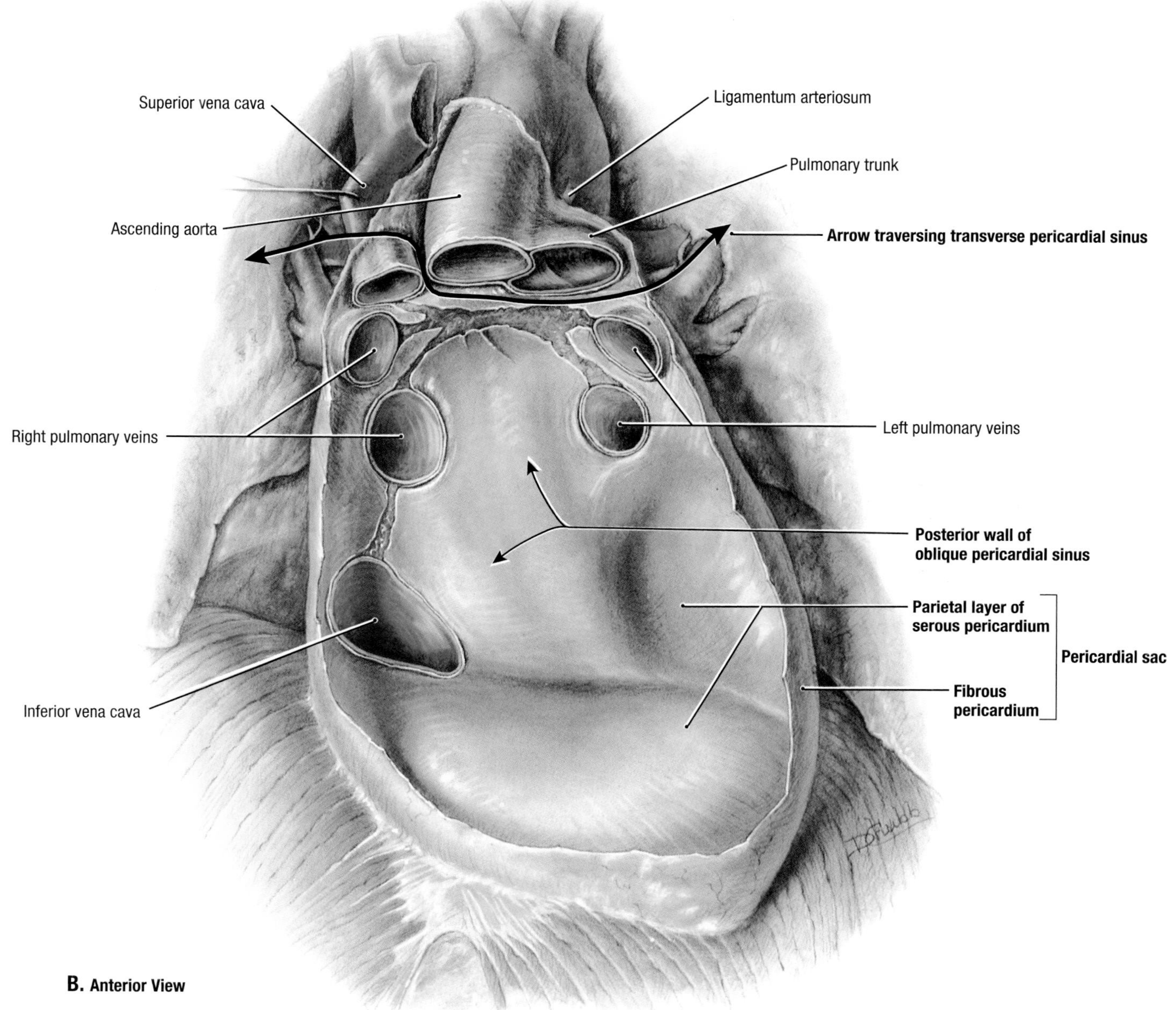
Superior vena cava
Ligamentum arteriosum
Pulmonary trunk
Ascending aorta
Arrow traversing transverse pericardial sinus
Right pulmonary veins
Left pulmonary veins
Posterior wall of oblique pericardial sinus
Parietal layer of serous pericardium
Pericardial sac
Fibrous pericardium
Inferior vena cava

**B. Anterior View**

## 1.44 Heart and pericardium *(continued)*

- Interior of pericardial sac. Eight vessels were severed to excise the heart: superior and inferior venae cavae, four pulmonary veins, and two pulmonary arteries.
- The oblique sinus is bounded anteriorly by the visceral layer of serous pericardium covering the left atrium (Fig. 1.44**A**), posteriorly by the parietal layer of serous pericardium lining the fibrous pericardium, and superiorly and laterally by the reflection of serous pericardium around the four pulmonary veins and the superior and inferior venae cavae (Fig. 1.44**B**).
- The transverse sinus is bounded anteriorly by the serous pericardium covering the posterior aspect of the pulmonary trunk and aorta, and posteriorly by the visceral pericardium covering the atria **(A)**.
- Cardiac tamponade (heart compression) is due to critically increased volume of fluid outside the heart but inside the pericardial cavity; e.g., due to stab wounds or from perforation of a weakened area of the heart muscle after heart attack (hemopericardium).

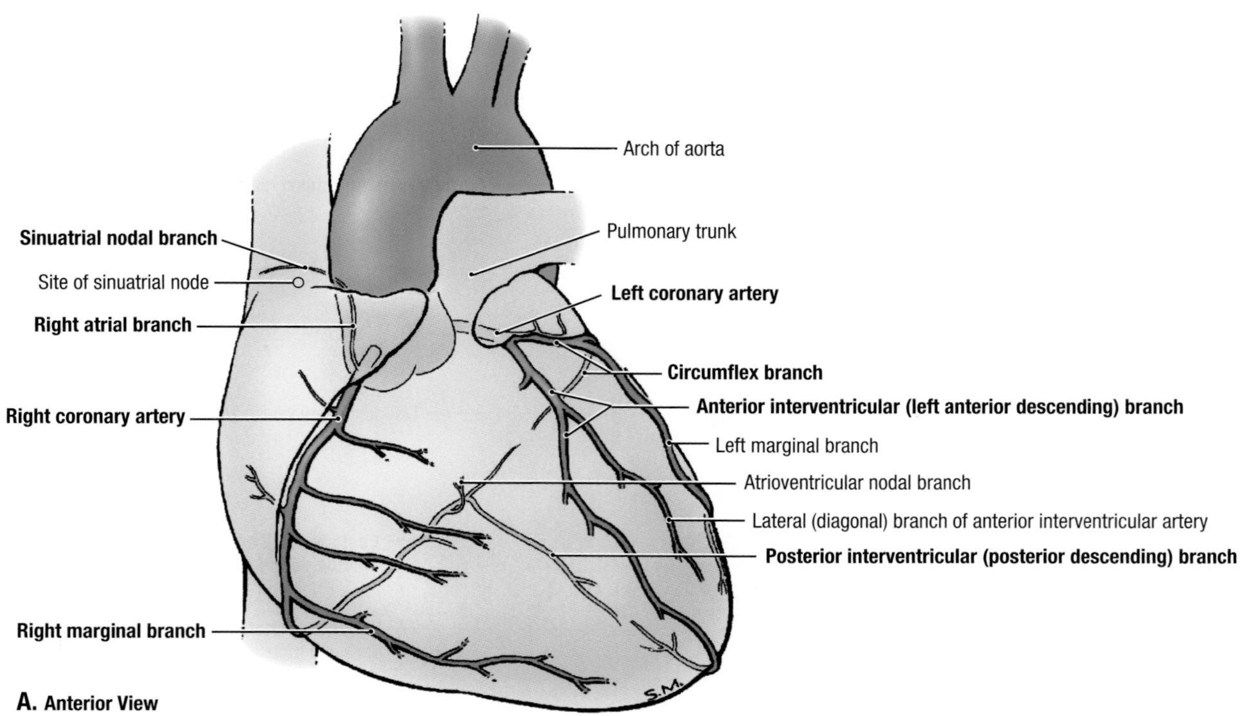
Arch of aorta
Pulmonary trunk
Sinuatrial nodal branch
Site of sinuatrial node
Right atrial branch
Left coronary artery
Circumflex branch
Anterior interventricular (left anterior descending) branch
Right coronary artery
Left marginal branch
Atrioventricular nodal branch
Lateral (diagonal) branch of anterior interventricular artery
Posterior interventricular (posterior descending) branch
Right marginal branch
S.M.

**A.** Anterior View

## 1.45 Coronary arteries

- The right coronary artery travels in the coronary sulcus to reach the posterior surface of the heart, where it anastomoses with the circumflex branch of the left coronary artery. Early in its course, it gives off the right atrial branch, which supplies the sinuatrial (SA) node via the sinuatrial nodal artery; major branches are a marginal branch supplying much of the anterior wall of the right ventricle, an atrioventricular (AV) nodal artery given off near the posterior border of the interventricular septum, and a posterior interventricular artery in the interventricular groove that anastomoses with the anterior interventricular artery, a branch of the left coronary artery.
- The left coronary artery divides into a circumflex branch that passes posteriorly to anastomose with the right coronary on the posterior aspect of the heart and an anterior descending branch in the interventricular groove; the origin of the SA nodal artery is variable and may be a branch of the left coronary artery.
- The interventricular septum receives its blood supply from septal branches of the two interventricular (descending) branches: typically the anterior two thirds from the left coronary, and the posterior one third from the right (see Fig. 1.48**A**).

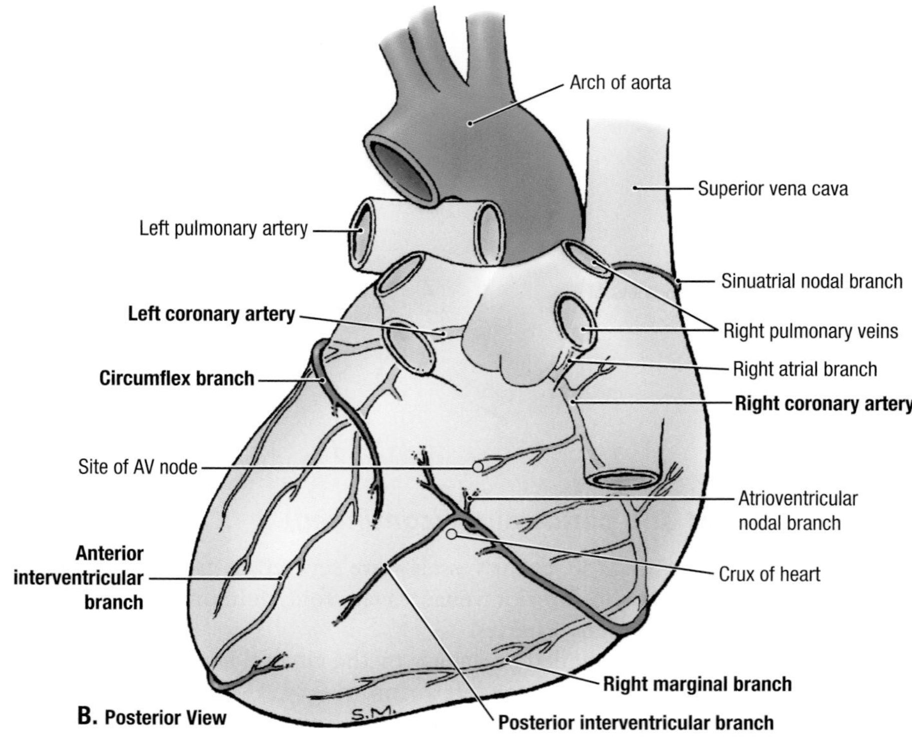
Arch of aorta
Superior vena cava
Left pulmonary artery
Sinuatrial nodal branch
Left coronary artery
Right pulmonary veins
Circumflex branch
Right atrial branch
Right coronary artery
Site of AV node
Atrioventricular nodal branch
Anterior interventricular branch
Crux of heart
Right marginal branch
Posterior interventricular branch
S.M.

**B.** Posterior View

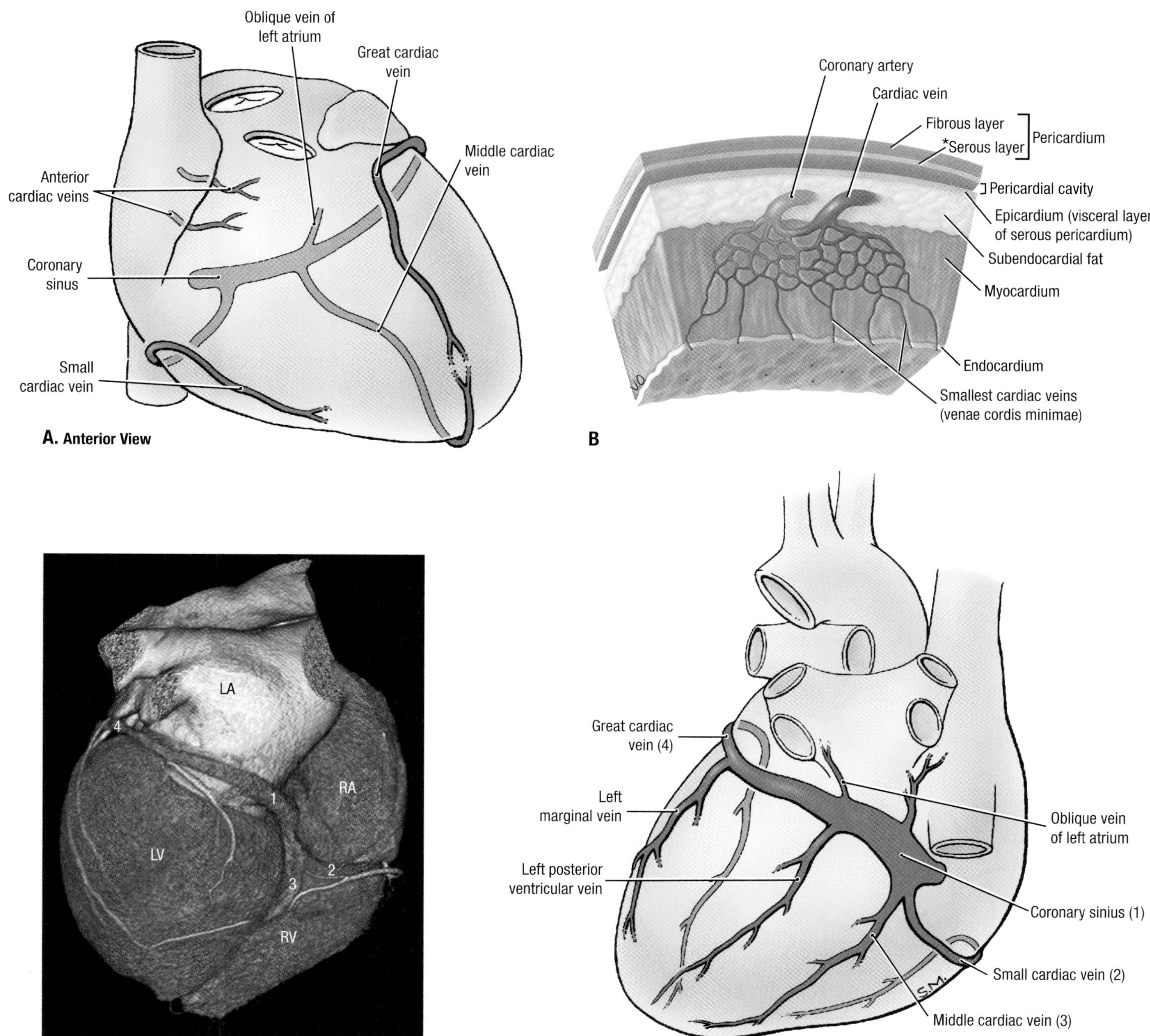
Oblique vein of left atrium
Great cardiac vein
Middle cardiac vein
Anterior cardiac veins
Coronary sinus
Small cardiac vein
A. Anterior View
Coronary artery
Cardiac vein
Fibrous layer
*Serous layer
Pericardium
Pericardial cavity
Epicardium (visceral layer of serous pericardium)
Subendocardial fat
Myocardium
Endocardium
Smallest cardiac veins (venae cordis minimae)
B
LA
RA
LV
RV
1
2
3
4
C. Posteroinferior View
Great cardiac vein (4)
Left marginal vein
Left posterior ventricular vein
Oblique vein of left atrium
Coronary sinius (1)
Small cardiac vein (2)
Middle cardiac vein (3)
D. Posteroinferior View

## 1.46 Cardiac veins

**A.** Anterior aspect. **B.** Smallest cardiac veins. **C.** 3-D volume reconstruction. Numbers refer to veins in **D.** Left atrium *(LA)*. Right atrium *(RA)*. Left ventricle *(LV)*; right ventricle *(RV)*. **D.** Posteroinferior aspect.

The coronary sinus is the major venous drainage vessel of the heart; it is located posteriorly in the atrioventricular (coronary) groove and drains into the right atrium. The great, middle, and small cardiac veins; the oblique vein of the left atrium; and the posterior vein of the left ventricle are the principal vessels draining into the coronary sinus. The anterior cardiac veins drain directly into the right atrium. The smallest cardiac veins (venae cordis minimae) drain the myocardium directly into the atria and ventricles **(B).** In **B,** the *asterisk* (*) indicates the parietal layer of serous pericardium (epicardium). The cardiac veins accompany the coronary arteries and their branches.

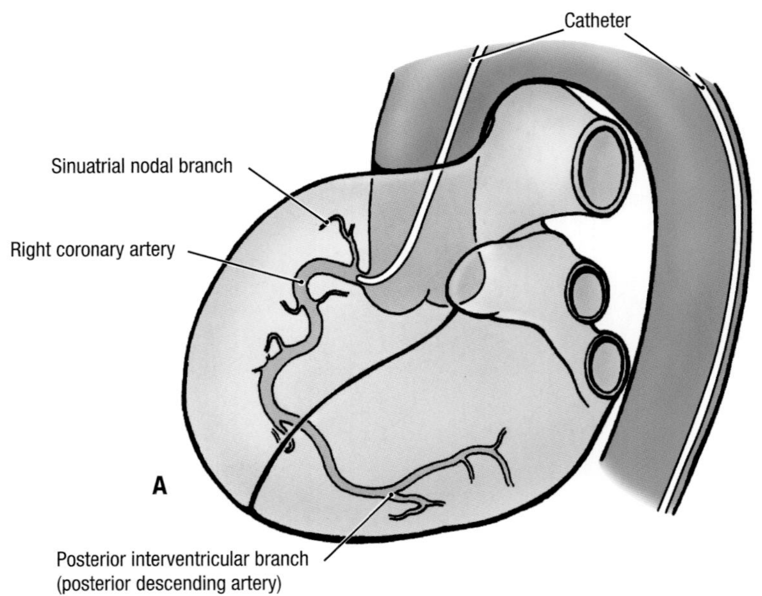
Catheter
Sinuatrial nodal branch
Right coronary artery
A
Posterior interventricular branch
(posterior descending artery)

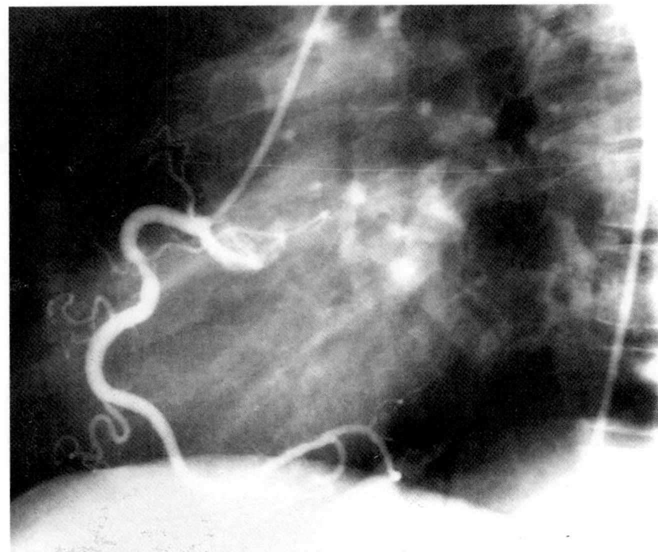

**B.** **Left Anterior Oblique View**

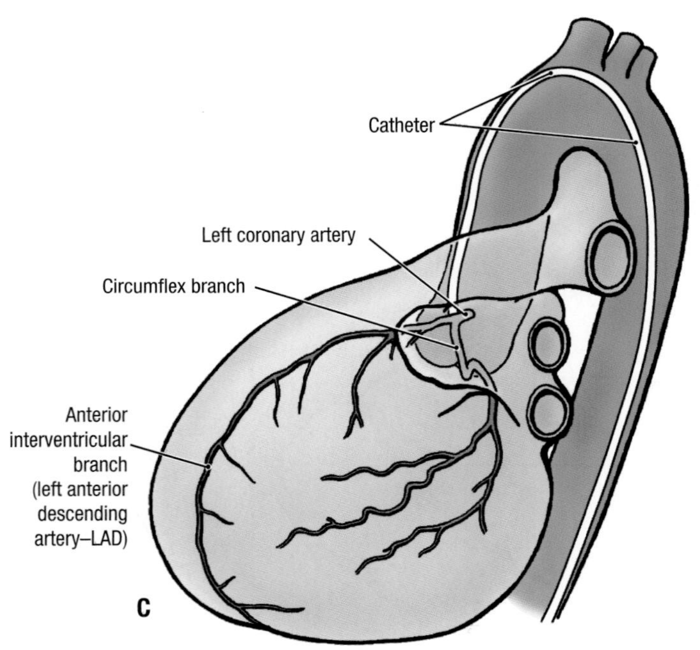
Catheter
Left coronary artery
Circumflex branch
Anterior
interventricular
branch
(left anterior
descending
artery–LAD)
C

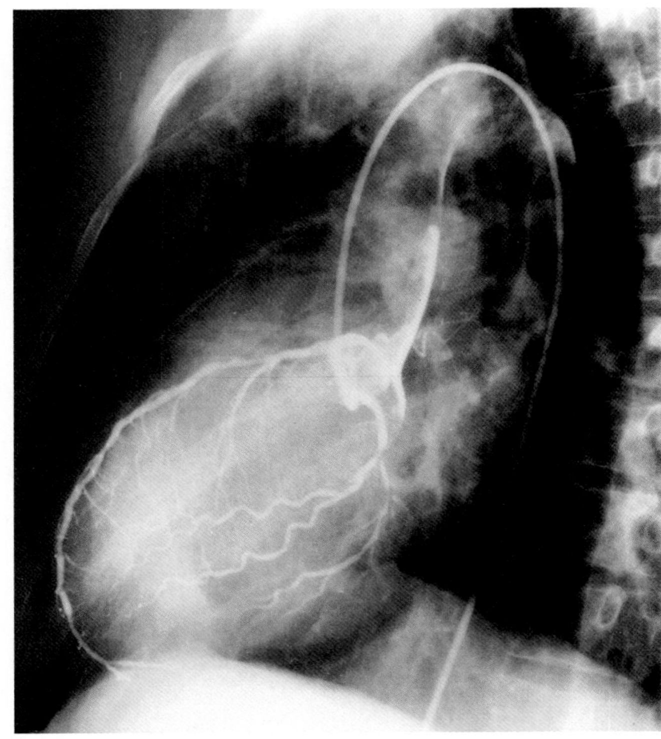

**D.** **Left Anterior Oblique View**

## 1.47 Coronary arteriograms with orientation drawings

Right (**A** and **B**) and left (**C** and **D**) coronary arteriograms.

Coronary artery disease (CAD) is one of the leading causes of death. CAD has many causes, all of which result in a reduced blood supply to the vital myocardial tissue. The three most common sites of coronary artery occlusion and the percentage of occlusions involving each artery are the (1) Anterior interventricular (clinically referred to as LAD) branch of the left coronary artery (LCA) (40–50%); (2) Right coronary artery (RCA), (30–40%); (3) Circumflex branch of the LCA (15–20%).

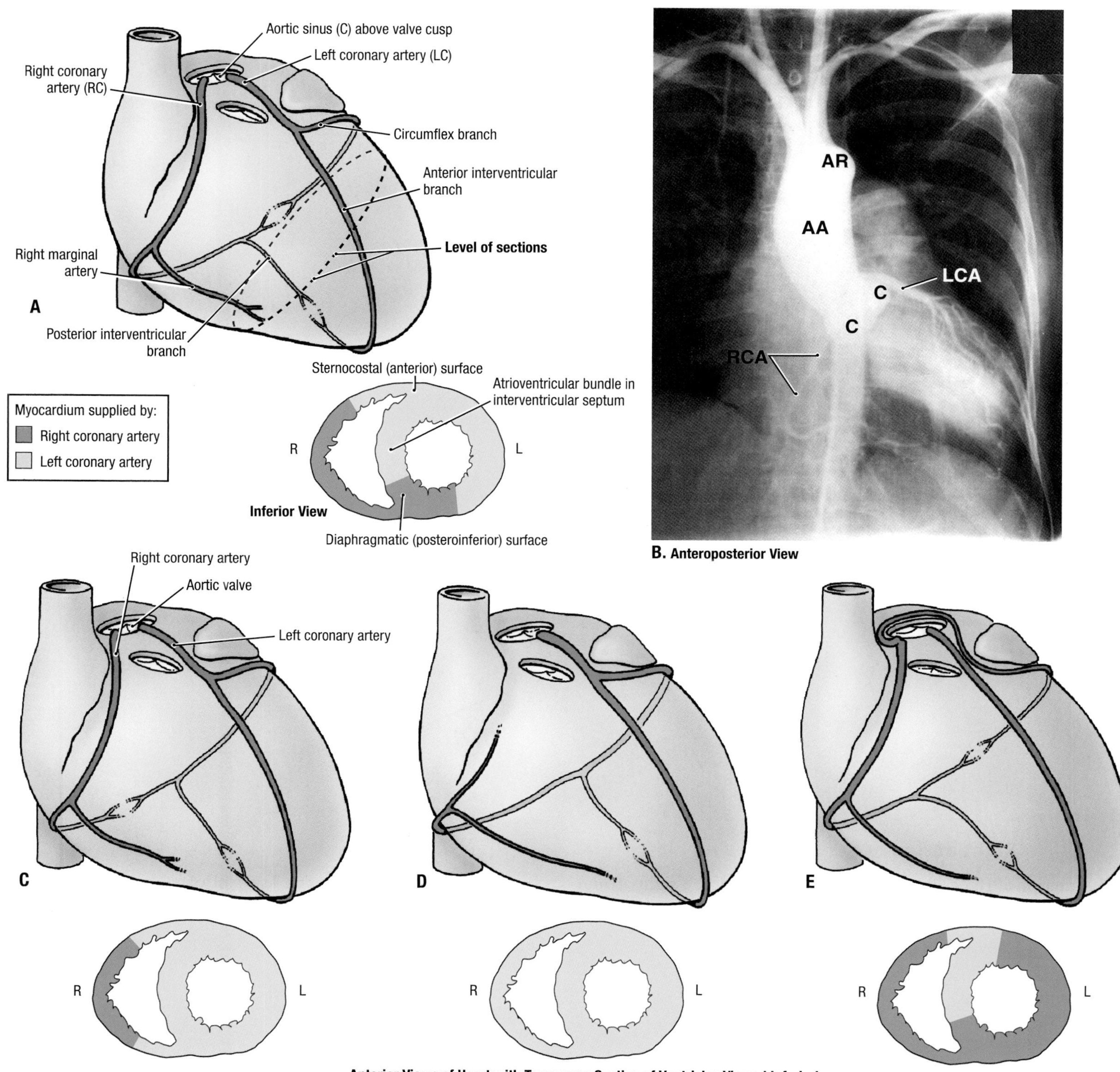
Aortic sinus (C) above valve cusp
Left coronary artery (LC)
Right coronary artery (RC)
Circumflex branch
Anterior interventricular branch
Level of sections
Right marginal artery
A
Posterior interventricular branch
Sternocostal (anterior) surface
Atrioventricular bundle in interventricular septum
Myocardium supplied by:
Right coronary artery
Left coronary artery
R
L
Inferior View
Diaphragmatic (posteroinferior) surface
AR
AA
LCA
C
C
RCA
B. Anteroposterior View
Right coronary artery
Aortic valve
Left coronary artery
C
D
E
R
L
R
L
R
L
Anterior Views of Heart with Transverse Section of Ventricles Viewed Inferiorly

## 1.48 Coronary circulation

**A.** In most cases, the right and left coronary arteries share equally in the blood supply to the heart. The *dotted line* indicates the plane of the cross-section demonstrating the parts of the myocardium supplied by the right and left coronary arteries. **B.** Aortic angiogram. Observe arch of aorta *(AR)*, ascending aorta *(AA)*, cusp of aortic valve *(C)*, left coronary artery *(LCA)*, and right coronary artery *(RCA)*. **C.** Dominant left coronary artery (about 15% of hearts). The posterior interventicular branch comes off the circumflex branch. **D.** Single coronary artery. **E.** Circumflex branch emerging from the right coronary sinus.

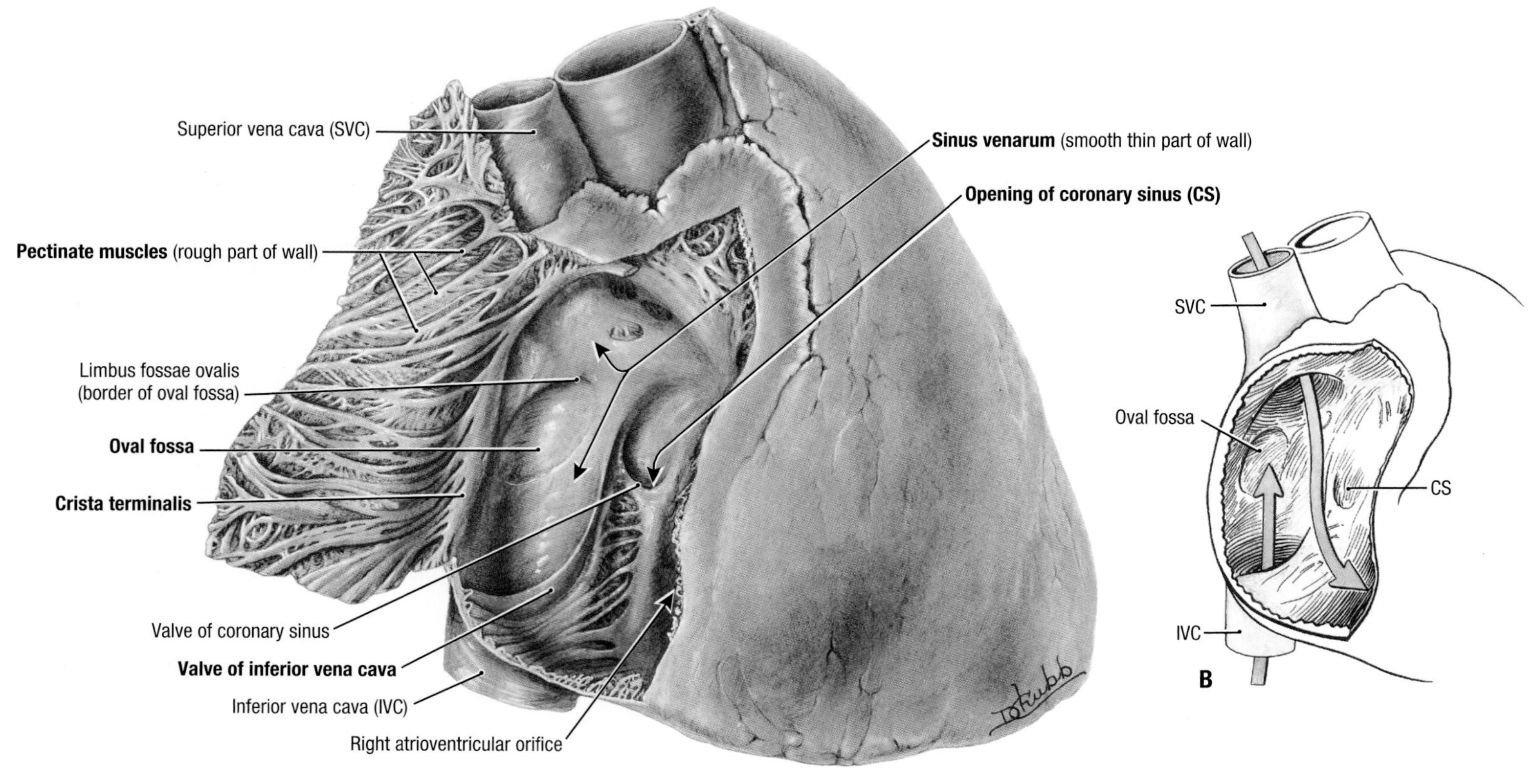
Superior vena cava (SVC)
Pectinate muscles (rough part of wall)
Limbus fossae ovalis
(border of oval fossa)
Oval fossa
Crista terminalis
Valve of coronary sinus
Valve of inferior vena cava
Inferior vena cava (IVC)
Right atrioventricular orifice
Sinus venarum (smooth thin part of wall)
Opening of coronary sinus (CS)
A. Anterior View
SVC
Oval fossa
CS
IVC
B

## 1.49 Right atrium

**A.** Interior of right atrium. The anterior wall of the right atrium is reflected. **B.** Blood flow into atrium from the superior and inferior vena cavae.

- The smooth part of the atrial wall is formed by the absorption of the right horn of the sinus venosus, and the rough part is formed from the primitive atrium.
- Crista terminalis, the valve of the inferior vena cava, and the valve of the coronary sinus separate the smooth part from the rough part.
- The pectinate muscle passes anteriorly from the crista terminalis; the crista underlies the sulcus terminalis (not shown), a groove visible externally on the posterolateral surface of the right atrium between the superior and inferior venae cavae.
- The superior and inferior venae cavae and the coronary sinus open onto the smooth part of the right atrium; the anterior cardiac veins and venae cordis minimae (not visible) also open into the atrium.
- The floor of the fossa is the remnant of the fetal septum primum; the crescent-shaped ridge (limbus fossae ovalis) partially surrounding the fossa is the remnant of the septum secundum.
- In **B,** the inflow from the superior vena cava is directed toward the tricuspid orifice, whereas blood from the inferior vena cava is directed toward the fossa ovalis.

- A congenital anomaly of the interatrial septum, usually incomplete closure of the oval foramen, is an atrial septal defect (ASD). A probe-size patency is present in the superior part of the oval fossa in 15–25% of adults (Moore and Persaud, 2003). These small openings, by themselves, cause no hemodynamic abnormalities. Large ASDs allow oxygenated blood from the lungs to be shunted from the left atrium through the ASD into the right atrium, causing enlargement of the right atrium and ventricle and dilation of the pulmonary trunk.

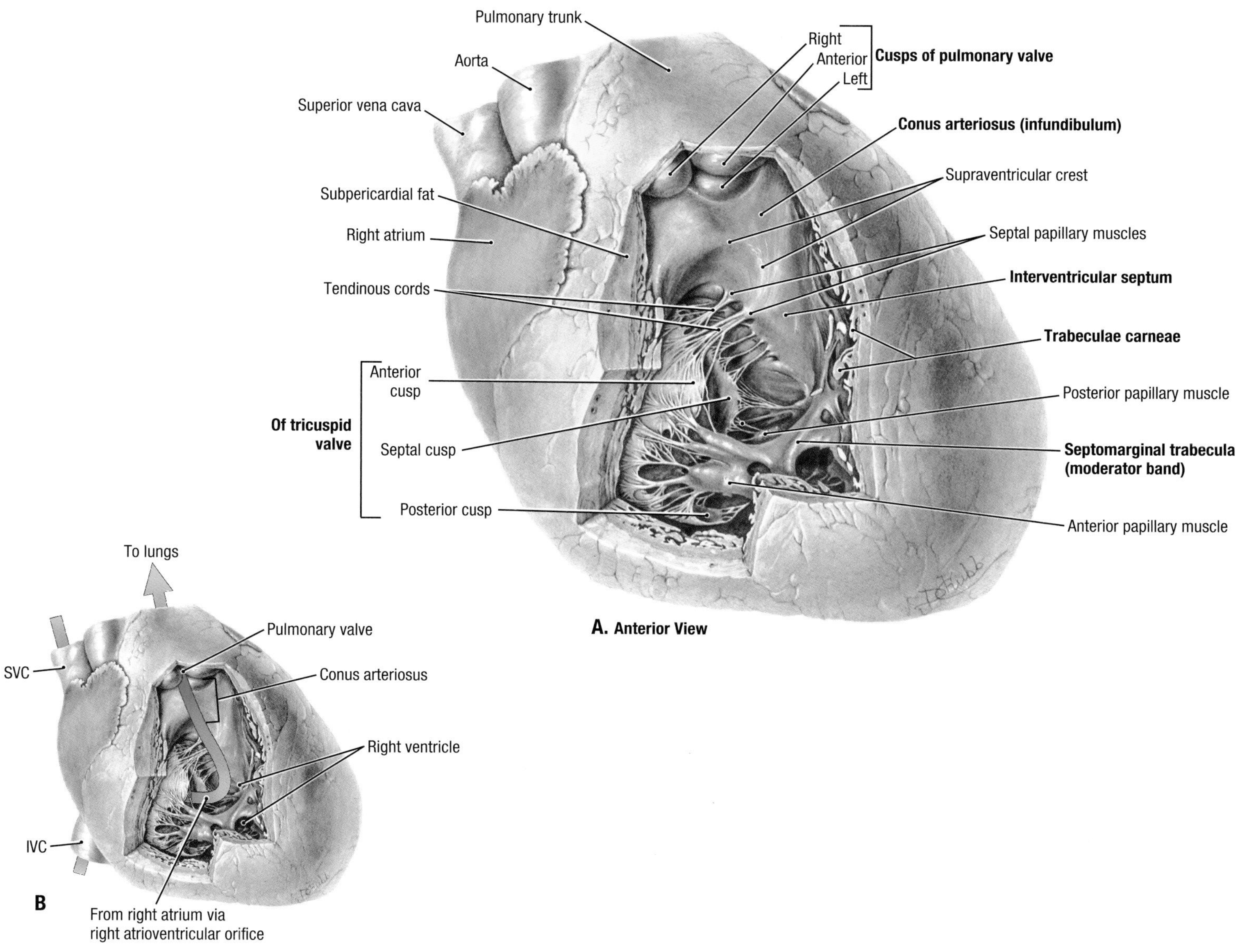
Pulmonary trunk
Aorta
Superior vena cava
Right
Anterior
Left
Cusps of pulmonary valve
Conus arteriosus (infundibulum)
Supraventricular crest
Subpericardial fat
Right atrium
Septal papillary muscles
Interventricular septum
Tendinous cords
Trabeculae carneae
Anterior cusp
Of tricuspid valve
Septal cusp
Posterior cusp
Posterior papillary muscle
Septomarginal trabecula (moderator band)
Anterior papillary muscle
A. Anterior View
To lungs
Pulmonary valve
SVC
Conus arteriosus
Right ventricle
IVC
B
From right atrium via right atrioventricular orifice

## 1.50 Right ventricle

**A.** Interior of right ventricle. **B.** Blood flow through right heart.

- The entrance to this chamber, the right atrioventricular or tricuspid orifice, is situated posteriorly; the exit, the orifice of the pulmonary trunk, is superior.
- The outflow portion of the chamber inferior to the pulmonary orifice (conus arteriosus or infundibulum) has a smooth, funnel-shaped wall; the remainder of the ventricle is rough with fleshy trabeculae.
- There are three types of trabeculae: mere ridges, bridges attached only at each end, and fingerlike projections called papillary muscles. The anterior papillary muscle rises from the anterior wall, the posterior (papillary muscle) from the posterior wall, and a series of small septal papillae from the septal wall.
- The septomarginal trabecula, here thick, extends from the septum to the base of the anterior papillary muscle.

- The membranous part of the interventricular septum develops separately from the muscular part and has a complex embryological origin (Moore and Persaud, 2003). Consequently, this part is the common site of ventricular septal defects (VSDs), although defects also occur in the muscular part, VSDs rank first on all lists of cardiac defects. The size of the defect varies from 1 to 25 mm. A VSD causes a left-to-right shunt of blood through the defect. A large shunt increases pulmonary blood flow, which causes severe pulmonary disease (*hypertension*, or increased blood pressure) and may cause *cardiac failure*.

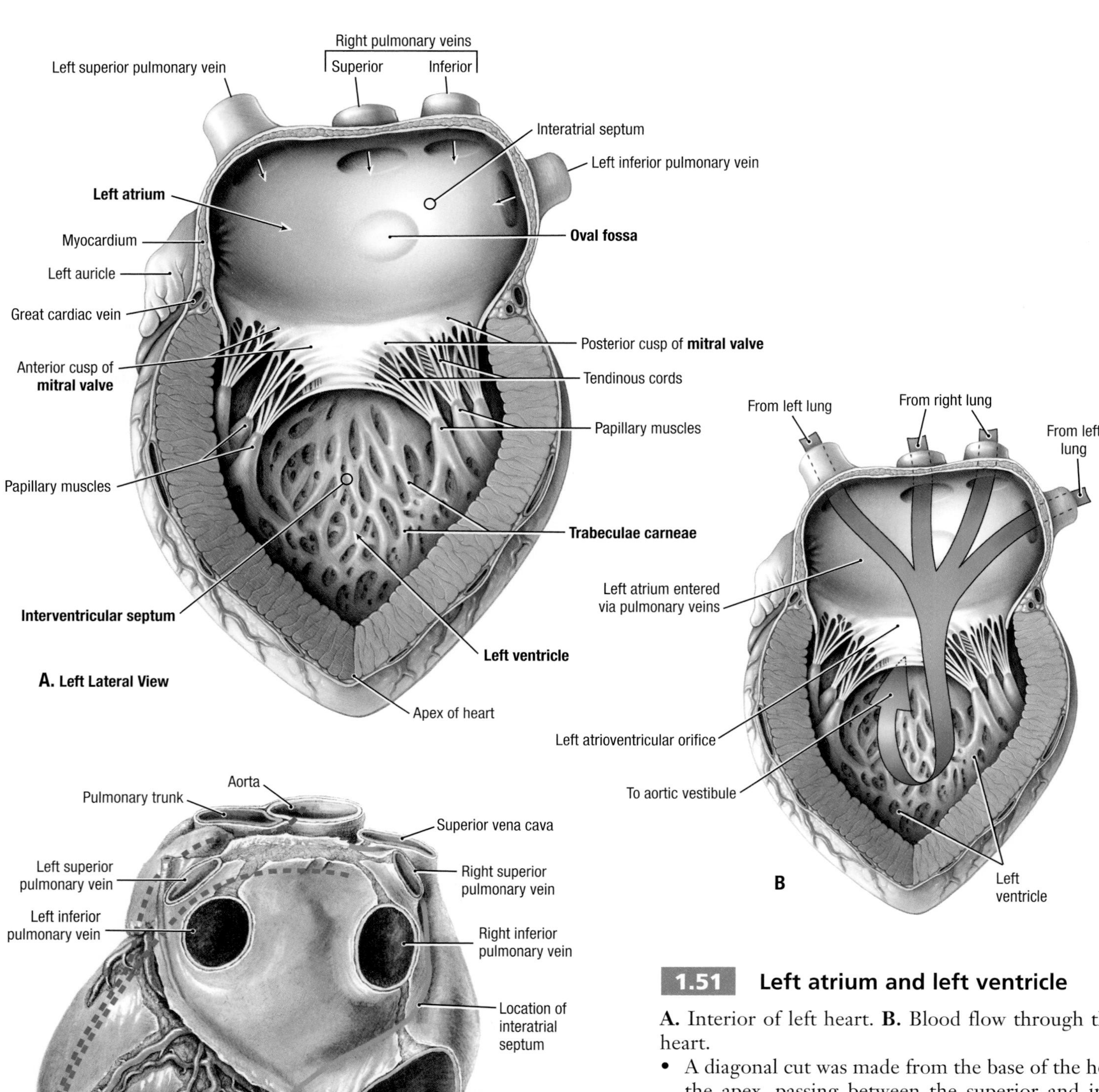
Right pulmonary veins
Superior
Inferior
Left superior pulmonary vein
Interatrial septum
Left inferior pulmonary vein
Left atrium
Oval fossa
Myocardium
Left auricle
Great cardiac vein
Posterior cusp of mitral valve
Anterior cusp of mitral valve
Tendinous cords
Papillary muscles
Papillary muscles
Trabeculae carneae
Interventricular septum
Left ventricle
A. Left Lateral View
Apex of heart
From left lung
From right lung
From left lung
Left atrium entered via pulmonary veins
Left atrioventricular orifice
To aortic vestibule
B
Left ventricle
Aorta
Pulmonary trunk
Superior vena cava
Left superior pulmonary vein
Right superior pulmonary vein
Left inferior pulmonary vein
Right inferior pulmonary vein
Location of interatrial septum
Inferior vena cava
Location of interventricular septum
Lines of incision:
Figure 1.51 A & B
Figure 1.52 A & B

## 1.51 Left atrium and left ventricle

**A.** Interior of left heart. **B.** Blood flow through the left heart.

- A diagonal cut was made from the base of the heart to the apex, passing between the superior and inferior pulmonary veins and through the posterior cusp of the mitral valve, followed by retraction (spreading) of the left heart wall on each side of the incision.
- The entrances (pulmonary veins) to the left atrium are posterior, and the exit (left atrioventricular or mitral orifice) is anterior.
- The left side of the oval fossa is also seen on the left side of the interatrial septum, although the left side is not usually as distinct as the right side is within the right atrium.
- Except for that of the auricle, the atrial wall is smooth.

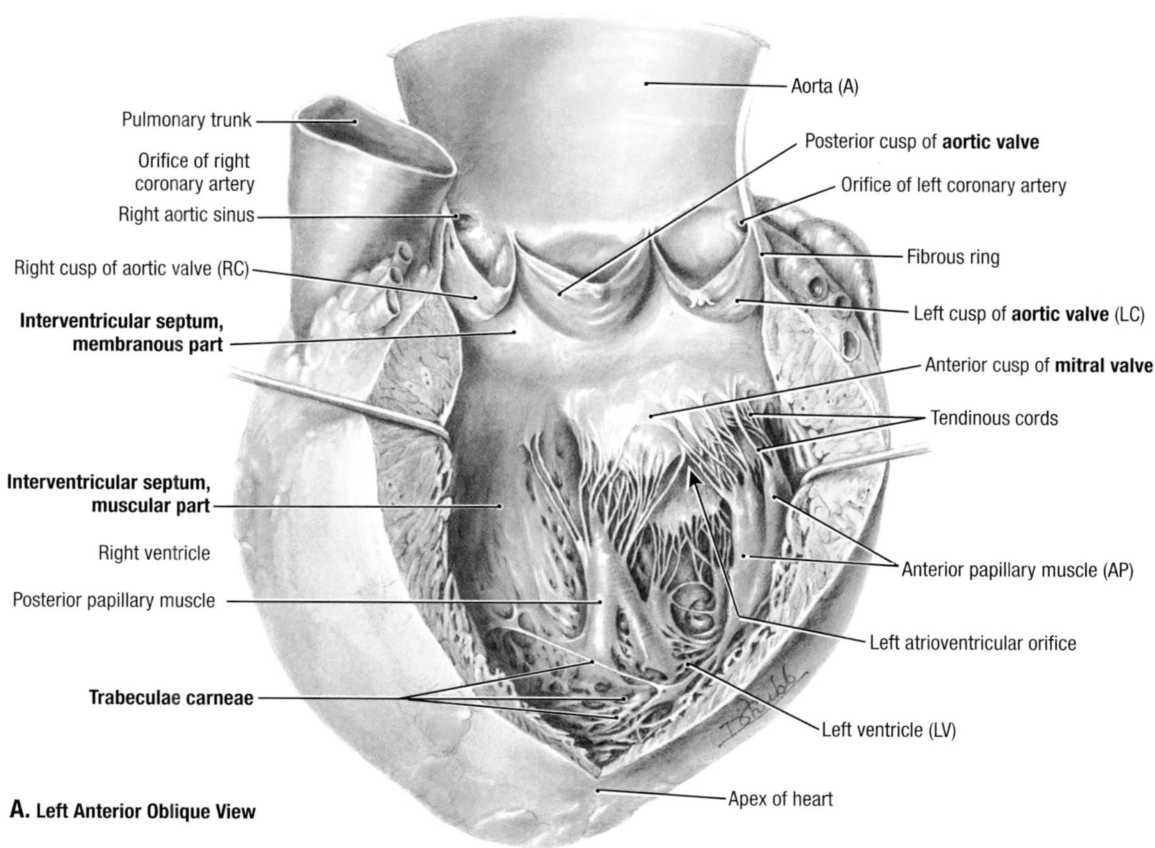
Aorta (A)
Pulmonary trunk
Posterior cusp of aortic valve
Orifice of right coronary artery
Orifice of left coronary artery
Right aortic sinus
Fibrous ring
Right cusp of aortic valve (RC)
Left cusp of aortic valve (LC)
Interventricular septum, membranous part
Anterior cusp of mitral valve
Tendinous cords
Interventricular septum, muscular part
Right ventricle
Anterior papillary muscle (AP)
Posterior papillary muscle
Left atrioventricular orifice
Trabeculae carneae
Left ventricle (LV)
Apex of heart

**A.** Left Anterior Oblique View

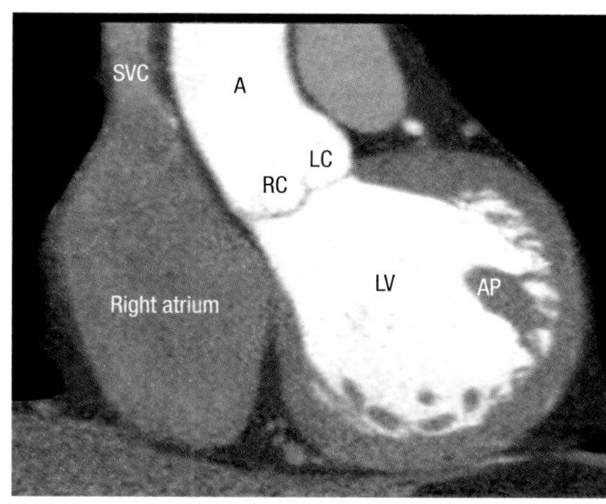
SVC
A
LC
RC
LV
AP
Right atrium

**B.** Anterior View

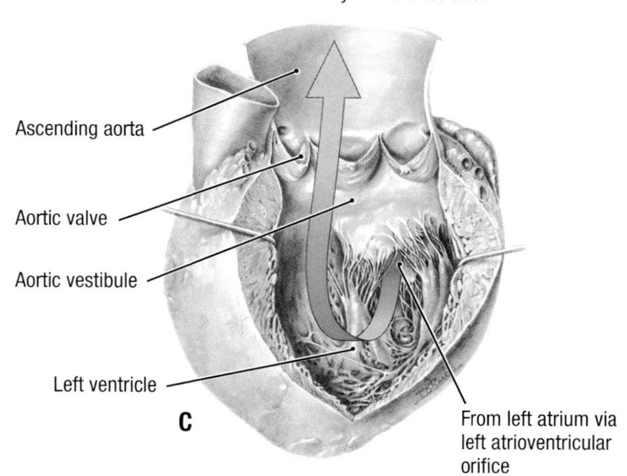
To systemic circulation
Ascending aorta
Aortic valve
Aortic vestibule
Left ventricle
C
From left atrium via left atrioventricular orifice

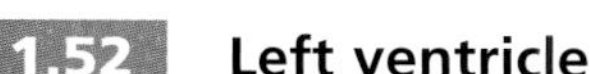

## 1.52 Left ventricle

A cut was made from the apex along the left margin of the heart, passing posterior to the pulmonary trunk, to open the aortic vestibule and ascending aorta.

**A.** Interior of left ventricle. **B.** Coronal CT angiogram. Letters refer to structures in **A. C.** Blood flow through the left ventricle.

- The chamber has a conical shape.
- The entrance (left atrioventricular, bicuspid, or mitral orifice) is situated posteriorly, and the exit (aortic orifice) is superior.
- The left ventricular wall is thin and muscular near the apex, thick and muscular superiorly, and thin and fibrous (nonelastic) at the aortic orifice.
- Two large papillary muscles, the anterior from the anterior wall and the posterior from the posterior wall, control the adjacent halves of two cusps of the mitral valve with tendinous cords (chordae tendineae).
- The anterior cusp of the mitral valve lies between the inlet (mitral orifice) and the outlet (aortic orifice).

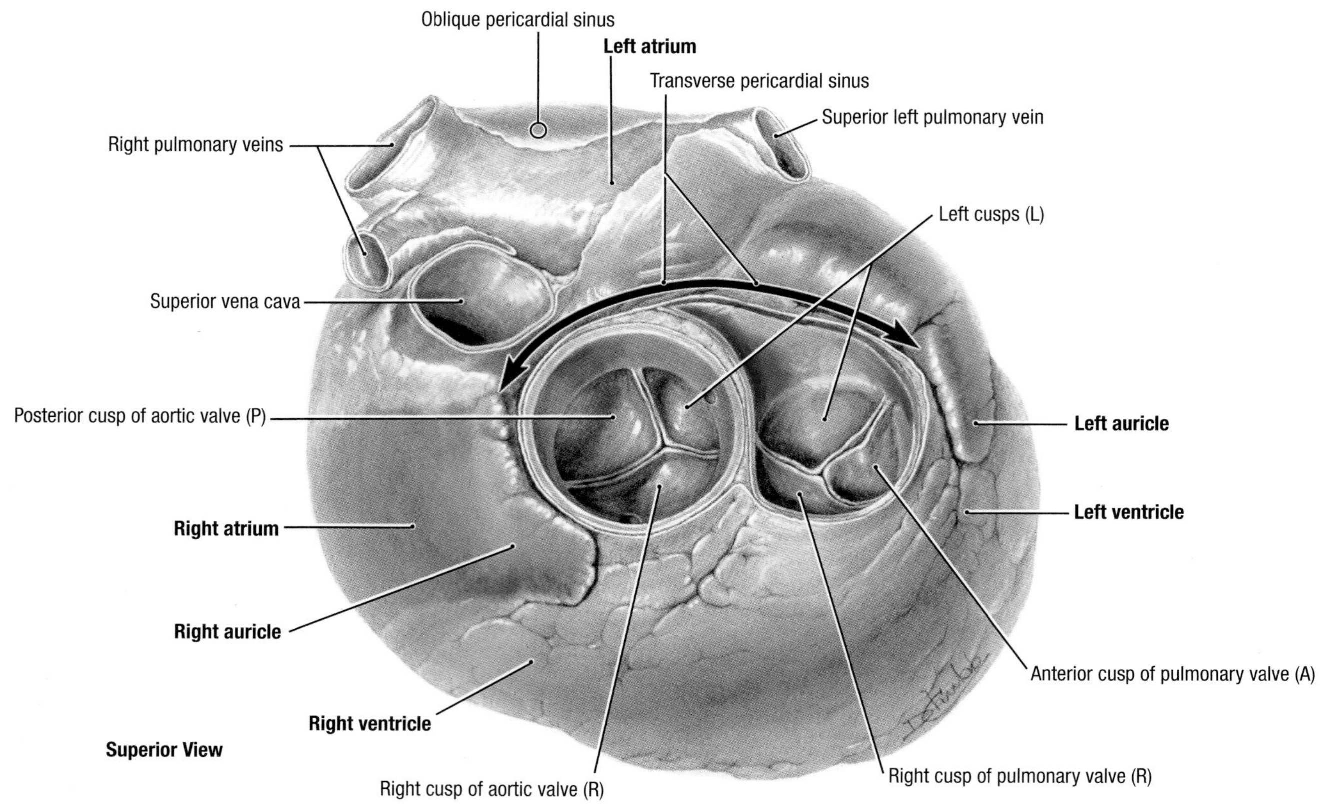
Oblique pericardial sinus
Left atrium
Transverse pericardial sinus
Superior left pulmonary vein
Right pulmonary veins
Left cusps (L)
Superior vena cava
Posterior cusp of aortic valve (P)
Left auricle
Left ventricle
Right atrium
Right auricle
Anterior cusp of pulmonary valve (A)
Right ventricle
Superior View
Right cusp of aortic valve (R)
Right cusp of pulmonary valve (R)

## 1.53 Excised heart

- The ventricles are positioned anteriorly and to the left, the atria posteriorly and to the right.
- The roots of the aorta and pulmonary artery, which conduct blood from the ventricles, are placed anterior to the atria and their incoming blood vessels (the superior vena cava and pulmonary veins).
- The aorta and pulmonary artery are enclosed within a common tube of serous pericardium and partly embraced by the auricles of the atria.
- The transverse pericardial sinus curves posterior to the enclosed stems of the aorta and pulmonary trunk and anterior to the superior vena cava and upper limits of the atria.
- The three cusps of the aortic and pulmonary valves—and the names of the cusps—have a developmental origin, as explained in Figure 1.54.

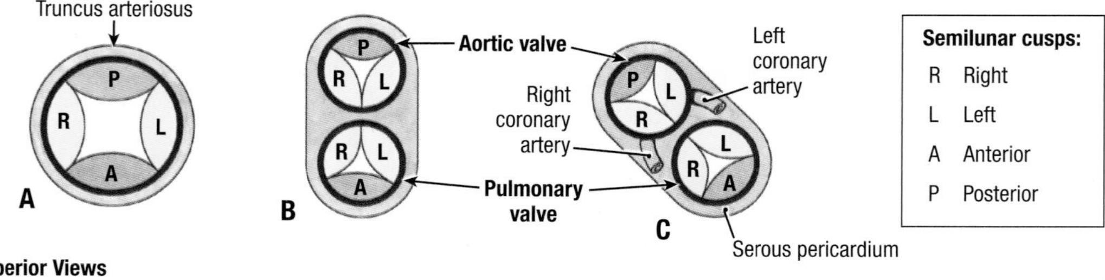
Truncus arteriosus
P
R
L
A
A
Aortic valve
P
R
L
R
L
A
B
Right
coronary
artery
Pulmonary
valve
Left
coronary
artery
P
L
R
L
R
A
C
Serous pericardium
Semilunar cusps:
R Right
L Left
A Anterior
P Posterior
Superior Views

## 1.54 Pulmonary and aortic valve names

The names of these cusps have a developmental origin: the truncus arteriosus with four cusps **(A)** splits to form two valves, each with three cusps **(B).** The heart undergoes partial rotation to the left on its axis, resulting in the arrangement of cusps shown in **C** and in Figure 1.53.

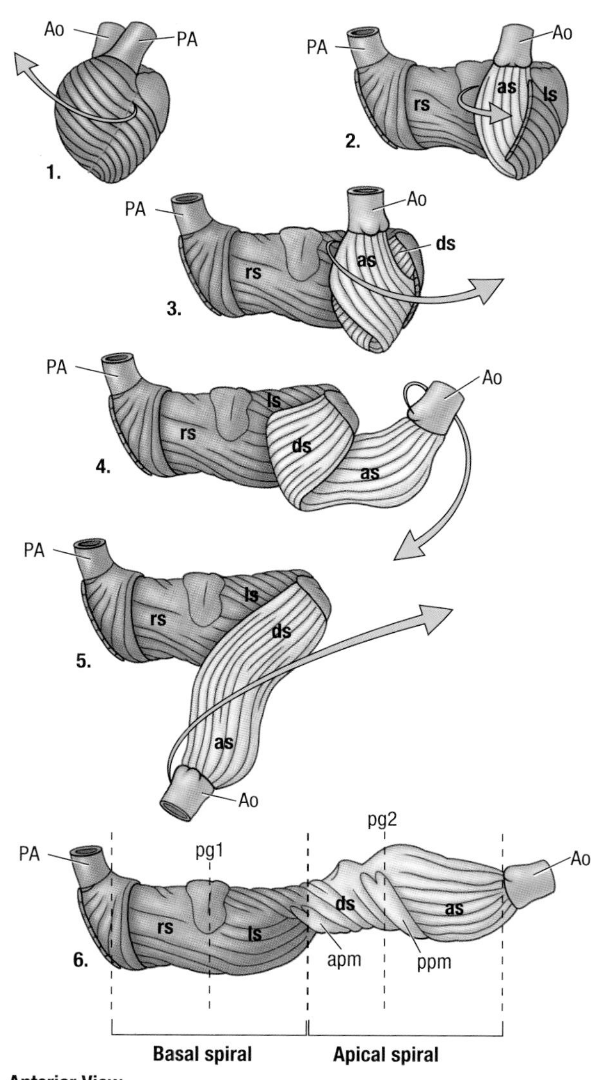
Ao
PA
1.
PA
as
rs
ls
Ao
2.
PA
Ao
ds
as
rs
3.
PA
Ao
ls
rs
ds
as
4.
PA
ls
rs
ds
5.
as
Ao
PA
pg1
pg2
Ao
ds
as
rs
ls
6.
apm
ppm
Basal spiral
Apical spiral
A. Anterior View

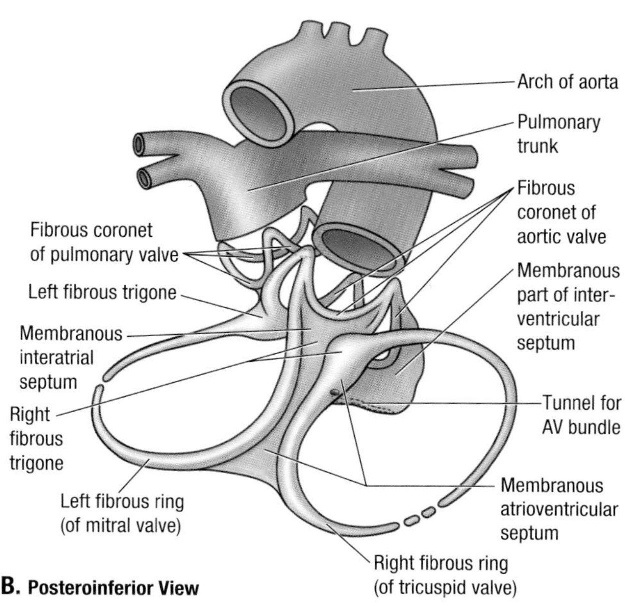
Arch of aorta
Pulmonary trunk
Fibrous coronet of aortic valve
Membranous part of interventricular septum
Tunnel for AV bundle
Membranous atrioventricular septum
Right fibrous ring (of tricuspid valve)
Fibrous coronet of pulmonary valve
Left fibrous trigone
Membranous interatrial septum
Right fibrous trigone
Left fibrous ring (of mitral valve)
B. Posteroinferior View

## 1.55 Arrangement of the myocardium and the fibrous skeleton of the heart.

**A.** The helical (double spiral) arrangement of the myocardium. (Modified from Torrent-Guasp et al., 2001). *1.* When the superficial myocardium is incised along the anterior interventricular groove *(dashed red line)* and peeled back starting at its origin from the fibrous ring of the pulmonary artery *(PA)*, the thick double spirals of the ventricular myocardial band are revealed *2.* A band of nearly horizontal fibers forms an outer basal spiral *(dark brown)* that comprises the outer wall of the right ventricle (right segment; *rs*) and an external layer of the outer wall of the left ventricle (left segment; *Ls*). *3.* When the left ventricle is rotated to bring the interventricular septum anteriorly, it can be seen that the myocardium then abruptly turns more vertically, descending to the apex (descending segment; *ds*) and then ascends (ascending segment; *as*) to insert onto the fibrous ring of the aorta *(Ao)*. The *ds* and *as* form the deeper apical spiral *(light brown)*, which comprises the internal layer of the outer wall of the left ventricle, while the crisscrossing *as* and *ds* fibers make up the interventricular septum. Thus the septum, like the outer wall of the left ventricle, is also double layered. *4* and *5.* The ventricular myocardial band is progressively unwrapped. *6.* The myocardium is completely uncoiled, and its segments are identified. The sequential contraction of the myocardial band enables the ventricles to function as parallel sucking and propelling pumps; on contraction, the ventricles do not merely collapse inward but rather wring themselves out. *apm*, anterior papillary muscles; *pg1* and *pg2*, posterior interventricular groove; *ppm*, posterior papillary muscles. **B.** The isolated fibrous skeleton is composed of four fibrous rings (or two rings and two "coronets"), each encircling a valve; two trigones; and the membranous portions of the interatrial, interventricular, and atrioventricular septa.

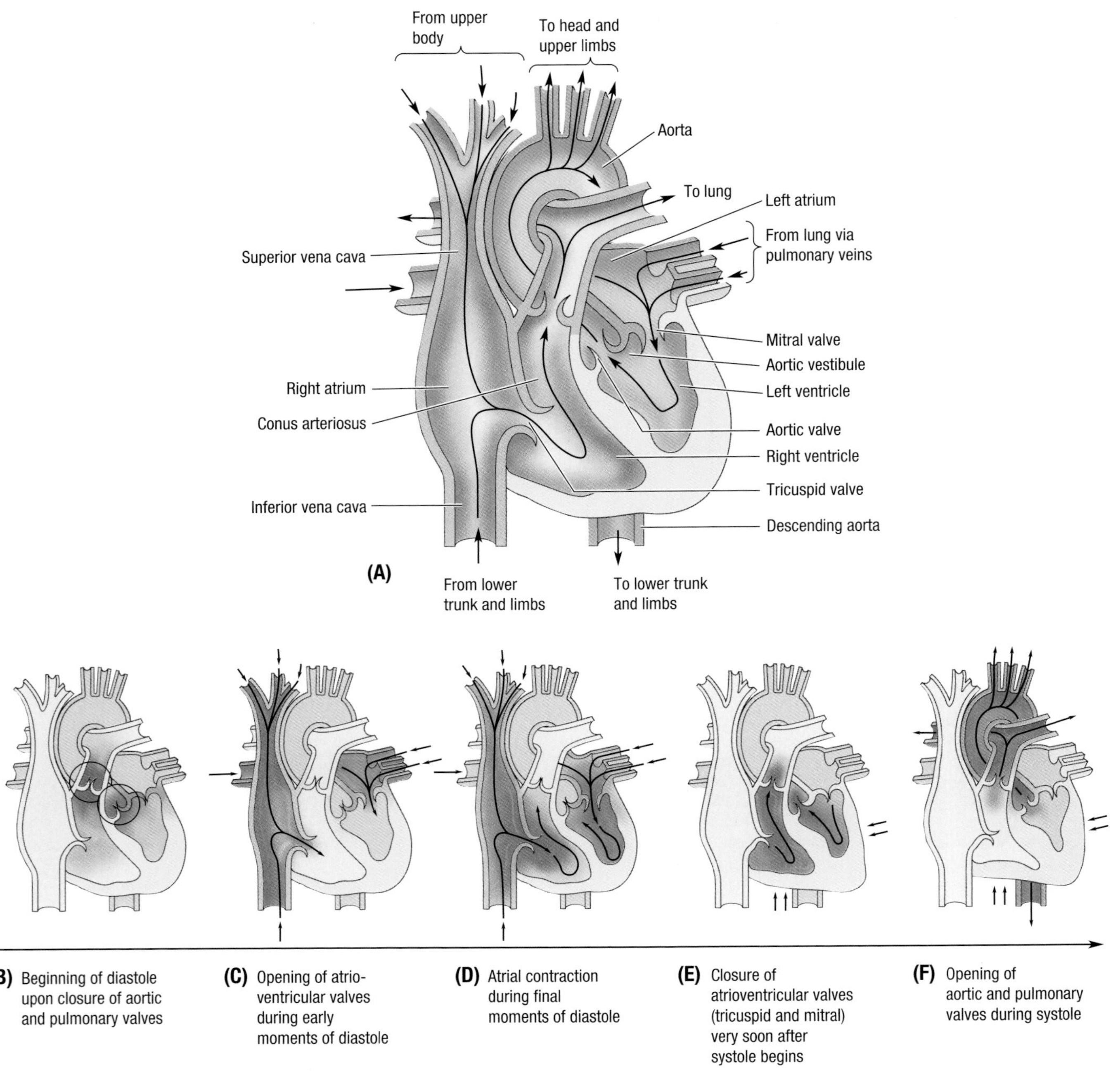

From upper body
To head and upper limbs
Aorta
To lung
Left atrium
From lung via pulmonary veins
Superior vena cava
Mitral valve
Aortic vestibule
Left ventricle
Right atrium
Conus arteriosus
Aortic valve
Right ventricle
Tricuspid valve
Inferior vena cava
Descending aorta
(A)
From lower trunk and limbs
To lower trunk and limbs
(B) Beginning of diastole upon closure of aortic and pulmonary valves
(C) Opening of atrio-ventricular valves during early moments of diastole
(D) Atrial contraction during final moments of diastole
(E) Closure of atrioventricular valves (tricuspid and mitral) very soon after systole begins
(F) Opening of aortic and pulmonary valves during systole
Anterior views


## 1.56 Cardiac cycle

The cardiac cycle describes the complete movement of the heart or heartbeat and includes the period from the beginning of one heartbeat to the beginning of the next one. The cycle consists of diastole (ventricular relaxation and filling) and systole (ventricular contraction and emptying). The right heart *(blue side)* is the pump for the pulmonary circuit; the left heart *(red side)* is the pump for the systemic circuit.

Disorders involving the valves of the heart disturb the pumping efficiency of the heart. Valvular heart disease produces either stenosis (narrowing) or insufficiency. Valvular stenosis is the failure of a valve to open fully, slowing blood flow from a chamber. Valvular insufficiency, or regurgitation, on the other hand, is failure of the valve to close completely, usually owing to nodule formation on (or scarring and contraction of) the cusps so that the edges do not meet or align. This allows a variable amount of blood (depending on the severity) to flow back into the chamber it was just ejected from. Both stenosis and insufficiency result in an increased workload for the heart. Because valvular diseases are mechanical problems, damaged or defective cardiac valves are often replaced surgically in a procedure called valvuloplasty. Most commonly, artificial valve prostheses made of synthetic materials are used in these valve replacement procedures, but xenografted valves (valves transplanted from other species, such as pigs) are also used.

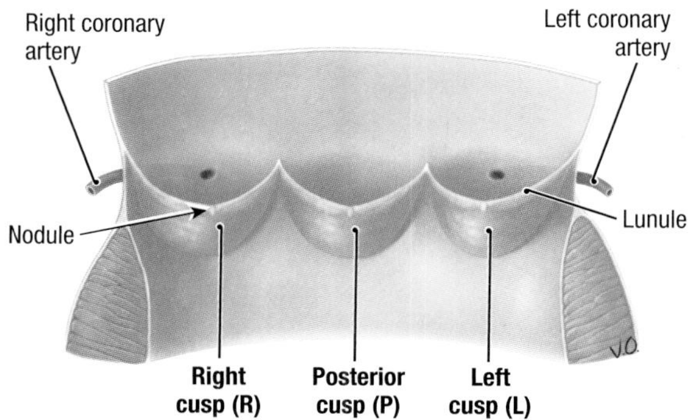
Right coronary artery
Left coronary artery
Nodule
Lunule
Right cusp (R)
Posterior cusp (P)
Left cusp (L)

**A.** **Left Posterior Oblique View of Aortic Valve**

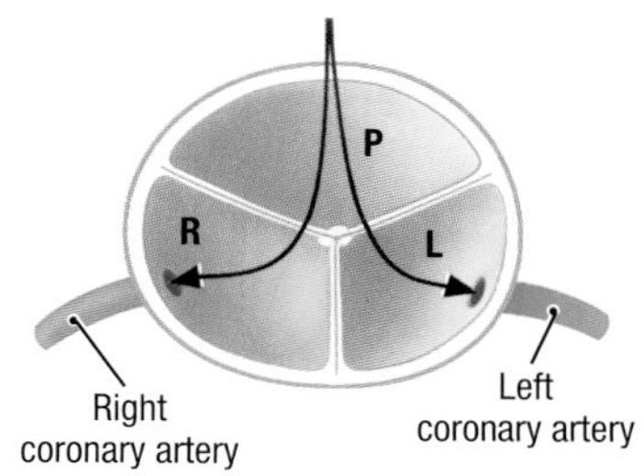
P
R
L
Right coronary artery
Left coronary artery

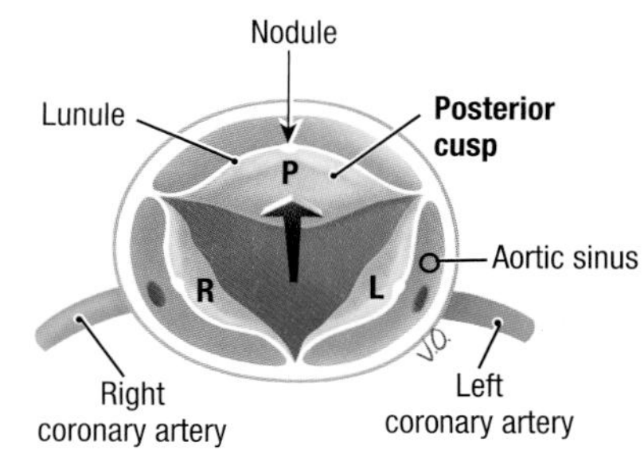
Nodule
Lunule
Posterior cusp
P
Aortic sinus
R
L
Right coronary artery
Left coronary artery

**B.** **Superior Views of Aortic Valve** (Arrows indicate direction of blood flow)

Septal cusp
Posterior cusp
Tendinous cords
Anterior papillary muscle (sectioned)
Membranous septum, atrioventricular part
Membranous septum, interventricular part (behind valve)
Anterior cusp
Anterior papillary muscle (sectioned)
Septal band of septomarginal trabecula
Posterior papillary muscle
Septal papillary muscle

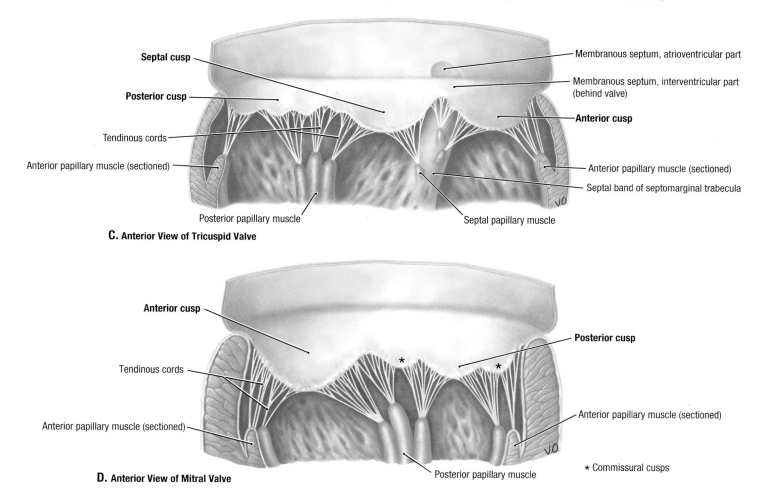

**C.** **Anterior View of Tricuspid Valve**

Anterior cusp
Tendinous cords
Anterior papillary muscle (sectioned)
Posterior cusp
*
*
Anterior papillary muscle (sectioned)
Posterior papillary muscle
* Commissural cusps

**D.** **Anterior View of Mitral Valve**

## 1.57 Valves of the heart

**A** and **B.** Semilunar valves. **C** and **D.** Atrioventricular valves.

In **(A),** as in Figure 1.52**A,** the anulus of the aortic valve has been incised between the right and left cusps and spread open. Each cusp of the semilunar valves bears a nodule in the midpoint of its free edge, flanked by thin connective tissue areas (lunules). When the ventricles relax to fill (diastole), backflow of blood from aortic recoil or pulmonary resistance fills the sinus (space between cusp and dilated part of the aortic or pulmonary wall), causing the nodules and lunules to meet centrally, closing the valve **(B).** Filling of the coronary arteries occurs during diastole (when ventricular walls are relaxed) as backflow "inflates" the cusps to close the valve. Tendinous cords pass from the tips of the papillary muscles to the free margins and ventricular surfaces of the cusps of the tricuspid **(C)** and mitral **(D)** valves. Each papillary muscle or muscle group controls the adjacent sides of two cusps, resisting valve prolapse during systole.

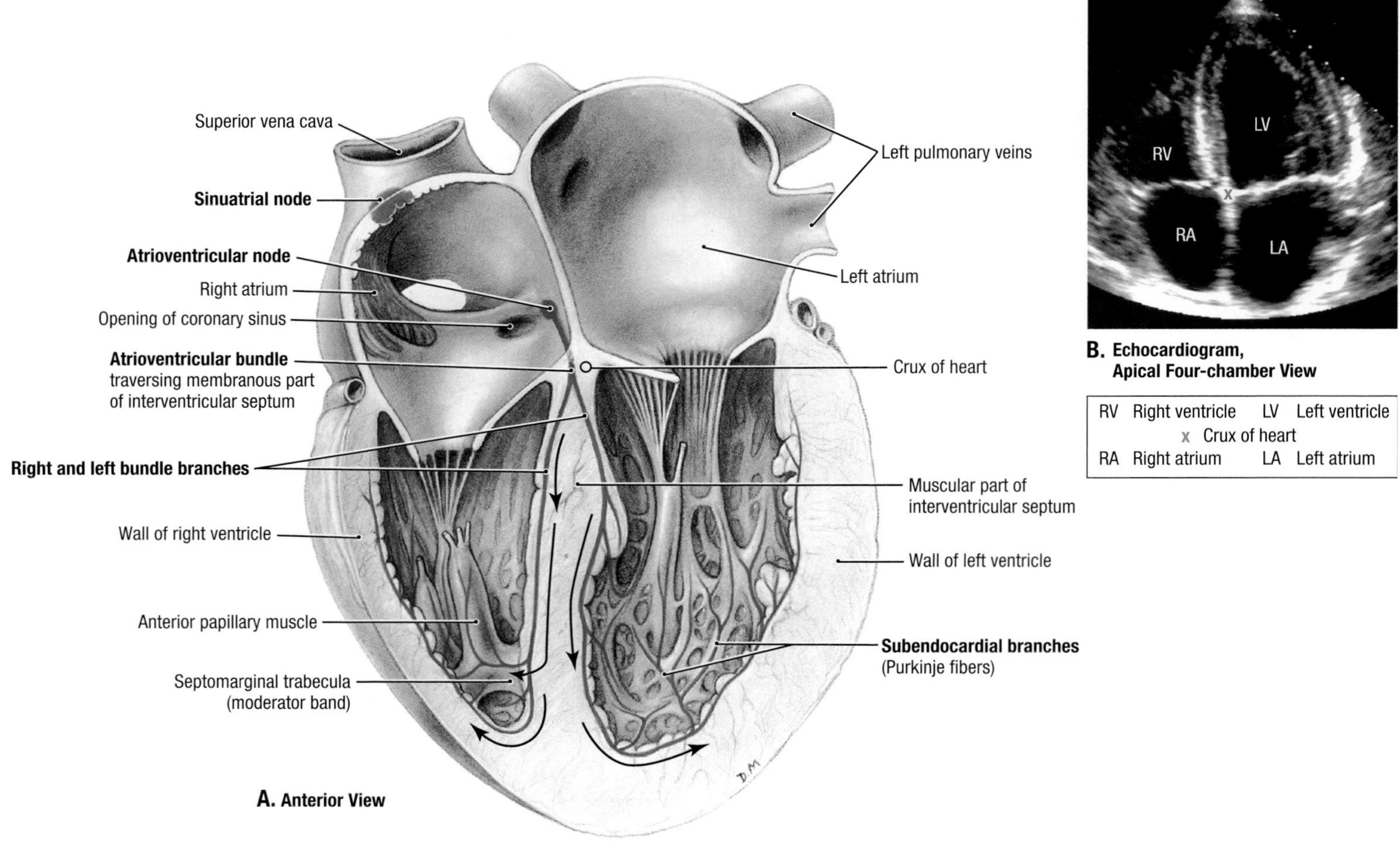
Superior vena cava
Sinuatrial node
Atrioventricular node
Right atrium
Opening of coronary sinus
Atrioventricular bundle traversing membranous part of interventricular septum
Right and left bundle branches
Wall of right ventricle
Anterior papillary muscle
Septomarginal trabecula (moderator band)
Left pulmonary veins
Left atrium
Crux of heart
Muscular part of interventricular septum
Wall of left ventricle
Subendocardial branches (Purkinje fibers)
RV
LV
RA
LA
x

**A.** Anterior View

**B.** Echocardiogram, Apical Four-chamber View

| RV Right ventricle | LV Left ventricle |
|---|---|
| x Crux of heart | |
| RA Right atrium | LA Left atrium |

## 1.58 Conduction system of heart, coronal section

- The sinuatrial (SA) node in the wall of the right atrium near the superior end of the sulcus terminalis extends over the opening of the superior vena cava. The SA node is the "pacemaker" of the heart because it initiates muscle contraction and determines the heart rate. It is supplied by the sinuatrial nodal artery, usually a branch of the right atrial branch of the right coronary artery (see Fig. 1.45**A–B**), but it may arise from the left coronary artery.
- Contraction spreads through the atrial wall (myogenic induction) until it reaches the atrioventricular (AV) node in the interatrial septum superomedial to the opening of the coronary sinus. The AV node is supplied by the atrioventricular nodal artery, usually arising from the right coronary artery posteriorly at the inferior margin of the interatrial septum.
- The AV bundle, usually supplied by the right coronary artery, passes from the AV node in the membranous part of the interventricular septum, dividing into right and left bundle branches on either side of the muscular part of the interventricular septum.
- The right bundle branch travels inferiorly in the interventricular septum to the anterior wall of the ventricle, with part passing via the septomarginal trabecula to the anterior papillary muscle; excitation spreads throughout the right ventricular wall through a network of subendocardial branches from the right bundle (Purkinje fibers).
- The left bundle branch lies beneath the endocardium on the left side of the interventricular septum and branches to enter the anterior and posterior papillary muscles and the wall of the left ventricle; further branching into a plexus of subendocardial branches (Purkinje fibers) allows the impulses to be conveyed throughout the left ventricular wall. The bundle branches are mostly supplied by the left coronary, except the posterior limb of the left bundle branch, which is supplied by both coronary arteries.

- Damage to the cardiac conduction system (often by compromised blood supply as in coronary artery disease) leads to disturbances of muscle contraction. Damage to the AV node results in "heart block" because the atrial excitation wave does not reach the ventricles, which begin to contract independently at their own slower rate. Damage to one of the branches results in "bundle branch block," in which excitation goes down the unaffected branch to cause systole of that ventricle; the impulse then spreads to the other ventricle, producing later, asynchronous contraction.

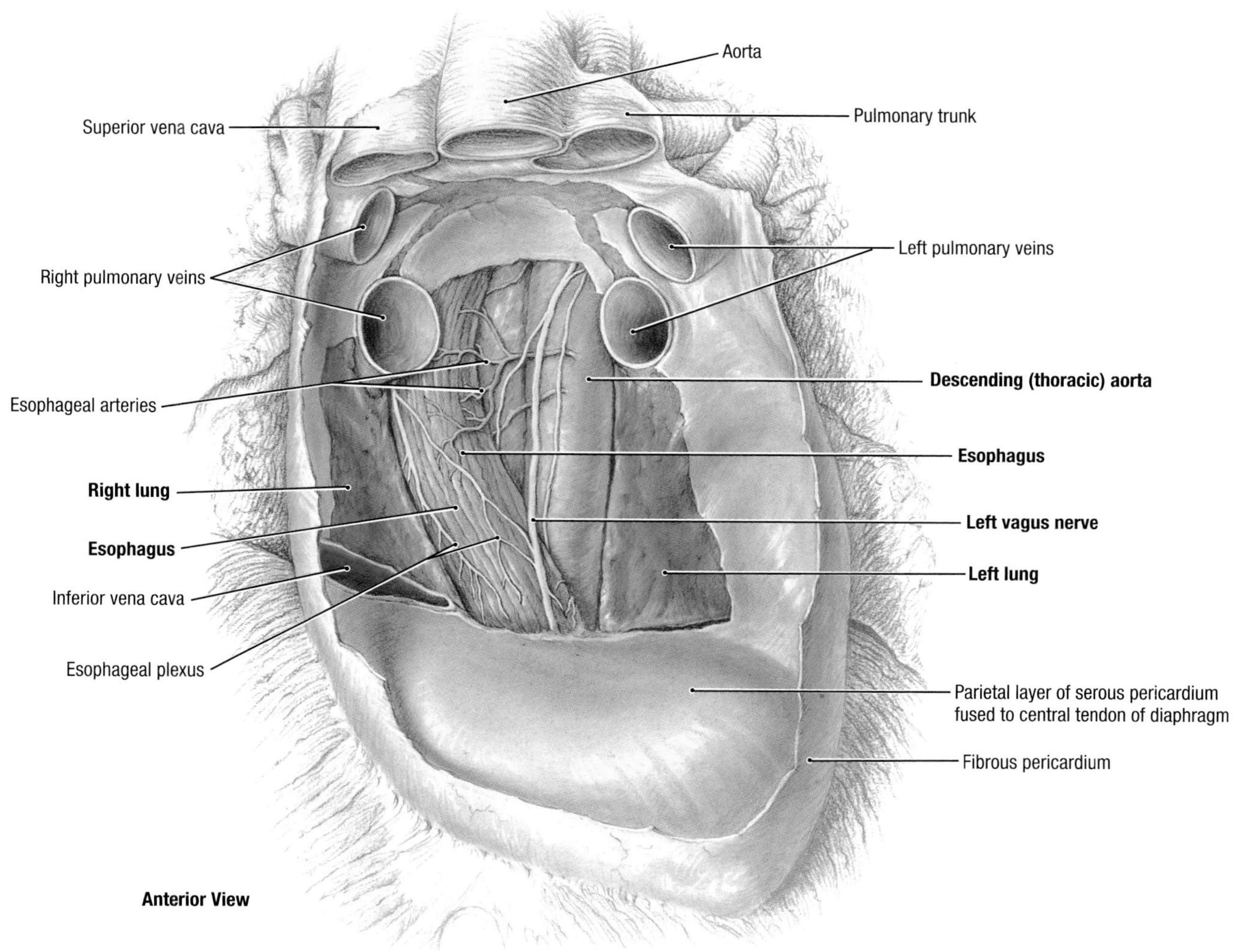
Aorta
Superior vena cava
Pulmonary trunk
Right pulmonary veins
Left pulmonary veins
Descending (thoracic) aorta
Esophageal arteries
Esophagus
Right lung
Left vagus nerve
Esophagus
Left lung
Inferior vena cava
Esophageal plexus
Parietal layer of serous pericardium
fused to central tendon of diaphragm
Fibrous pericardium
Anterior View

**1.59 Posterior relationships of heart and pericardium**

Posterior relationships. The fibrous and parietal layers of serous pericardium have been removed from posterior and lateral to the oblique sinus. The esophagus in this specimen is deflected to the right; it usually lies in contact with the aorta. Compare with Figure 1.44.

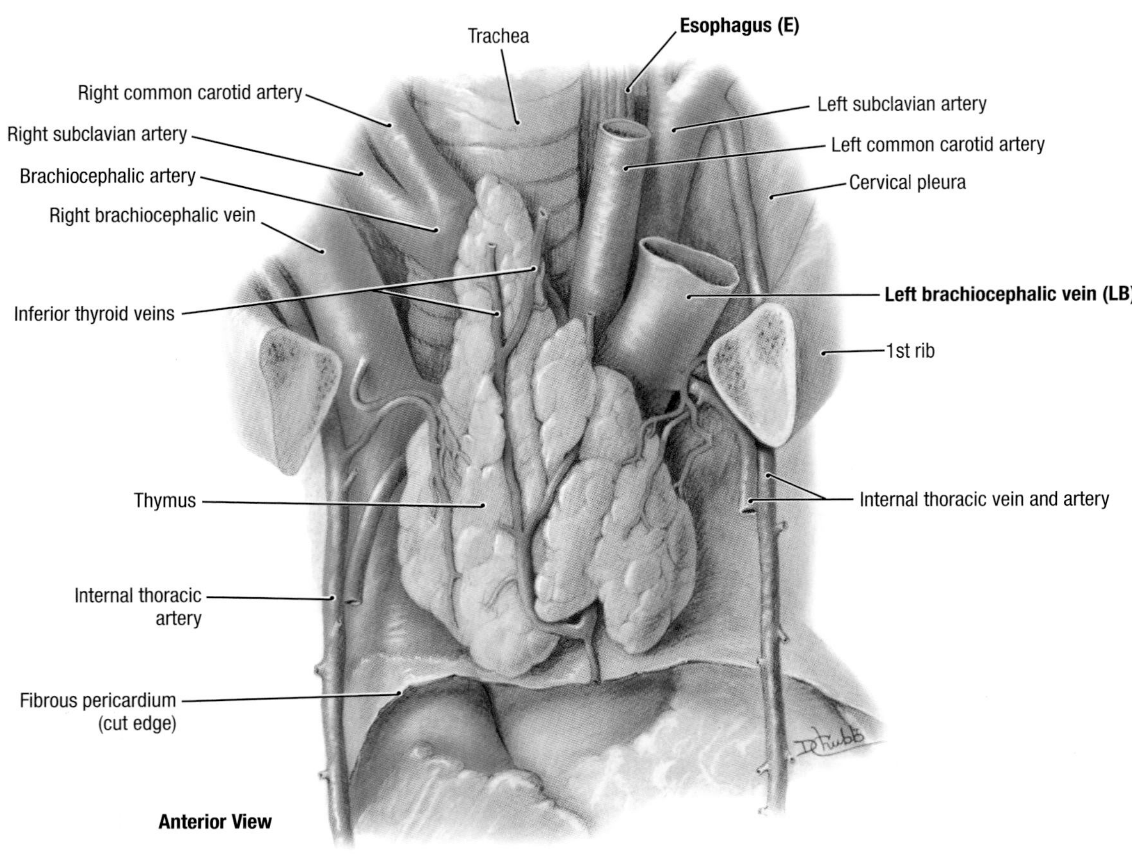
Trachea
Esophagus (E)
Right common carotid artery
Right subclavian artery
Brachiocephalic artery
Right brachiocephalic vein
Left subclavian artery
Left common carotid artery
Cervical pleura
Left brachiocephalic vein (LB)
Inferior thyroid veins
1st rib
Thymus
Internal thoracic vein and artery
Internal thoracic artery
Fibrous pericardium (cut edge)
Anterior View

## 1.60 Superior mediastinum I: superficial dissection

The sternum and ribs have been excised and the pleurae removed. It is unusual in an adult to see such a discrete thymus, which is impressive during puberty but subsequently regresses and is largely replaced by fat and fibrous tissue.

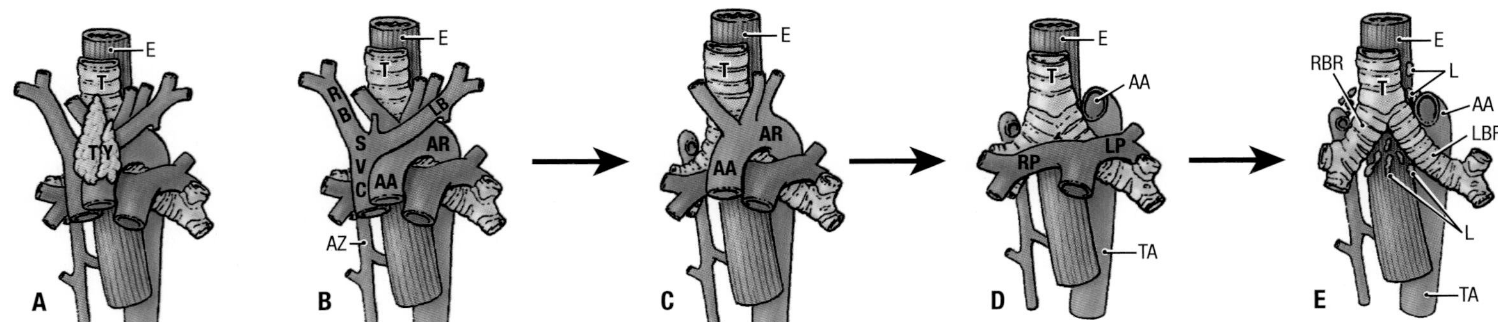
E
T
TY
A
RB
LB
S
V
C
AR
AA
AZ
B
C
AA
TA
RP
LP
D
RBR
L
LBR
E

## 1.61 Relations of great vessels and trachea

Observe, from superficial to deep: **(A)** Thymus *(TY)*; **(B)** the right *(RB)* and left *(LB)* brachiocephalic veins form the superior vena cava *(SVC)* and receive the arch of the azygos vein *(AZ)* posteriorly; **(C)** the ascending aorta *(AA)* and arch of the aorta *(AR)* arch over the right pulmonary artery and left main bronchus; **(D)** the pulmonary arteries (*RP* and *LP*); and **(E)** the tracheobronchial lymph nodes *(L)* at the tracheal bifurcation *(T)*.

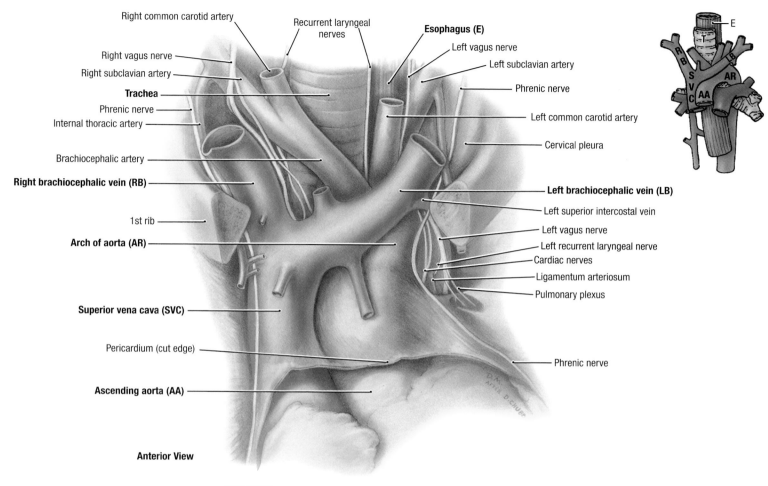

Right common carotid artery
Recurrent laryngeal nerves
Esophagus (E)
Left vagus nerve
Right vagus nerve
Left subclavian artery
Right subclavian artery
Trachea
Phrenic nerve
Phrenic nerve
Internal thoracic artery
Left common carotid artery
Cervical pleura
Brachiocephalic artery
Right brachiocephalic vein (RB)
Left brachiocephalic vein (LB)
Left superior intercostal vein
1st rib
Left vagus nerve
Arch of aorta (AR)
Left recurrent laryngeal nerve
Cardiac nerves
Ligamentum arteriosum
Pulmonary plexus
Superior vena cava (SVC)
Pericardium (cut edge)
Phrenic nerve
Ascending aorta (AA)
E
T
RB
LB
SVC
AA
AR
Anterior View

**1.62 Superior mediastinum II: root of neck**

The thymus gland has been removed.

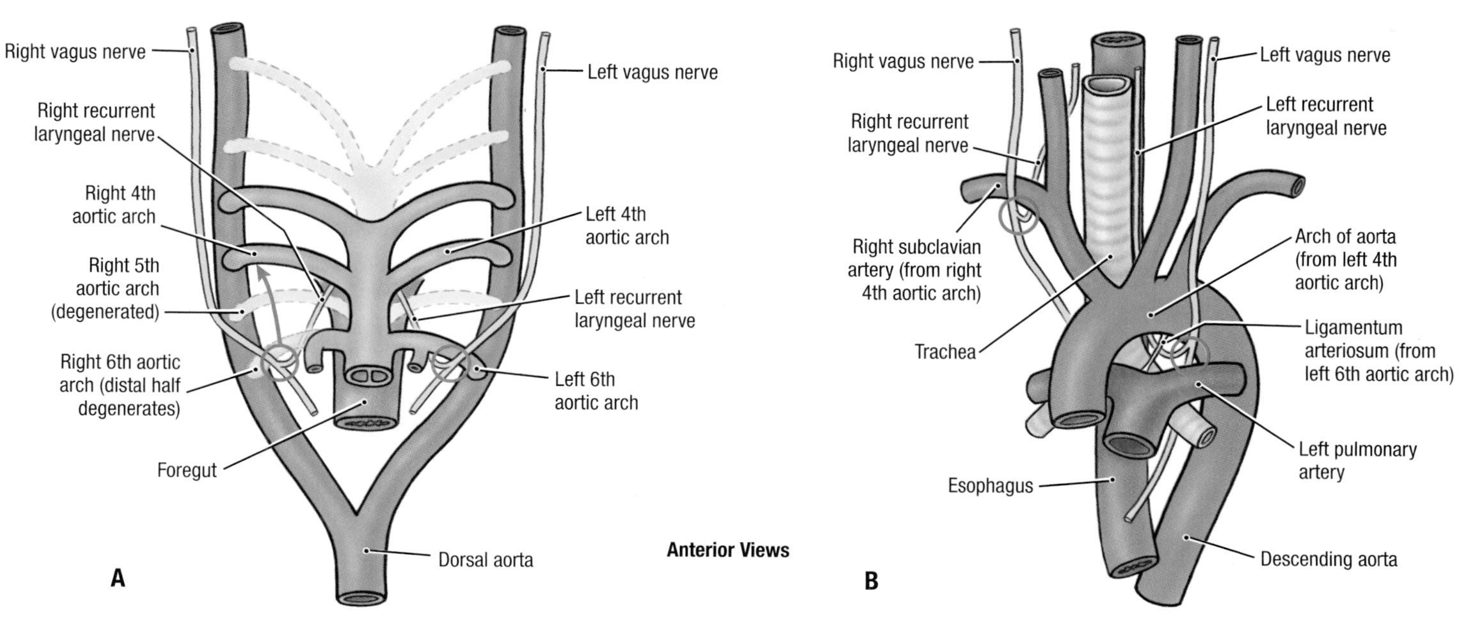
Right vagus nerve
Left vagus nerve
Right recurrent laryngeal nerve
Right 4th aortic arch
Left 4th aortic arch
Right 5th aortic arch (degenerated)
Left recurrent laryngeal nerve
Right 6th aortic arch (distal half degenerates)
Left 6th aortic arch
Foregut
Dorsal aorta
A
Anterior Views
Right vagus nerve
Left vagus nerve
Right recurrent laryngeal nerve
Left recurrent laryngeal nerve
Right subclavian artery (from right 4th aortic arch)
Arch of aorta (from left 4th aortic arch)
Trachea
Ligamentum arteriosum (from left 6th aortic arch)
Left pulmonary artery
Esophagus
Descending aorta
B

**1.63 Relationship of recurrent laryngeal nerve to the aortic arches**

**A.** Six weeks. **B.** Child.

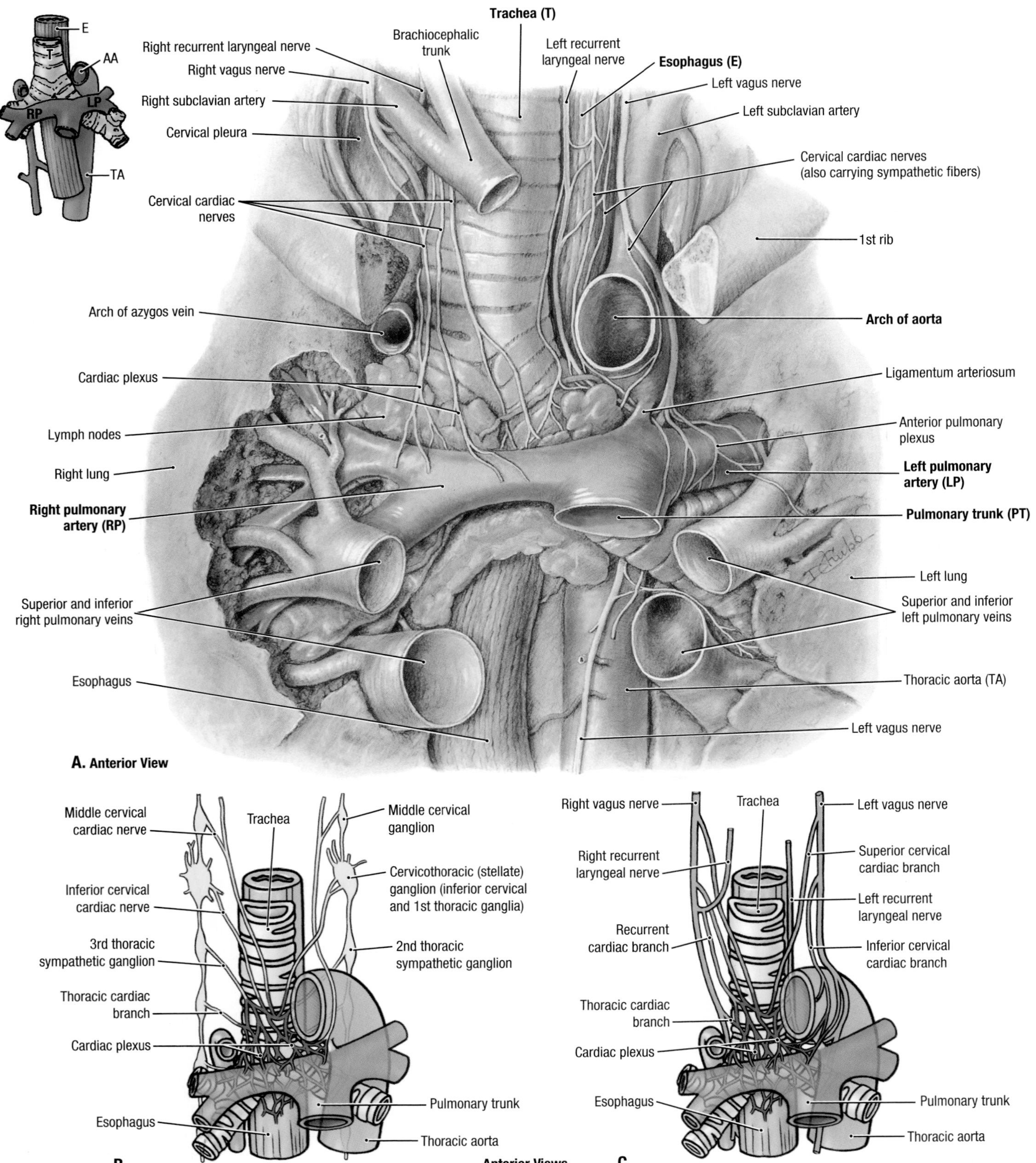

E
AA
T
RP
LP
TA
Trachea (T)
Brachiocephalic trunk
Right recurrent laryngeal nerve
Right vagus nerve
Right subclavian artery
Cervical pleura
Left recurrent laryngeal nerve
Esophagus (E)
Left vagus nerve
Left subclavian artery
Cervical cardiac nerves (also carrying sympathetic fibers)
Cervical cardiac nerves
1st rib
Arch of azygos vein
Arch of aorta
Cardiac plexus
Ligamentum arteriosum
Lymph nodes
Anterior pulmonary plexus
Right lung
Left pulmonary artery (LP)
Right pulmonary artery (RP)
Pulmonary trunk (PT)
Left lung
Superior and inferior right pulmonary veins
Superior and inferior left pulmonary veins
Thoracic aorta (TA)
Esophagus
Left vagus nerve
A. Anterior View
Middle cervical cardiac nerve
Trachea
Middle cervical ganglion
Inferior cervical cardiac nerve
Cervicothoracic (stellate) ganglion (inferior cervical and 1st thoracic ganglia)
3rd thoracic sympathetic ganglion
2nd thoracic sympathetic ganglion
Thoracic cardiac branch
Cardiac plexus
Pulmonary trunk
Esophagus
Thoracic aorta
B
Anterior Views
Right vagus nerve
Trachea
Left vagus nerve
Right recurrent laryngeal nerve
Superior cervical cardiac branch
Left recurrent laryngeal nerve
Recurrent cardiac branch
Inferior cervical cardiac branch
Thoracic cardiac branch
Cardiac plexus
Esophagus
Pulmonary trunk
Thoracic aorta
C


**1.64 Superior mediastinum III: cardiac plexus and pulmonary arteries**

**A.** Dissection. **B.** Sympathetic and **(C)** parasympathetic contribution to the cardiac plexus. *Yellow*, sympathetic; *blue*, parasympathetic; *green*, mixed sympathetic and parasympathetic nerves.

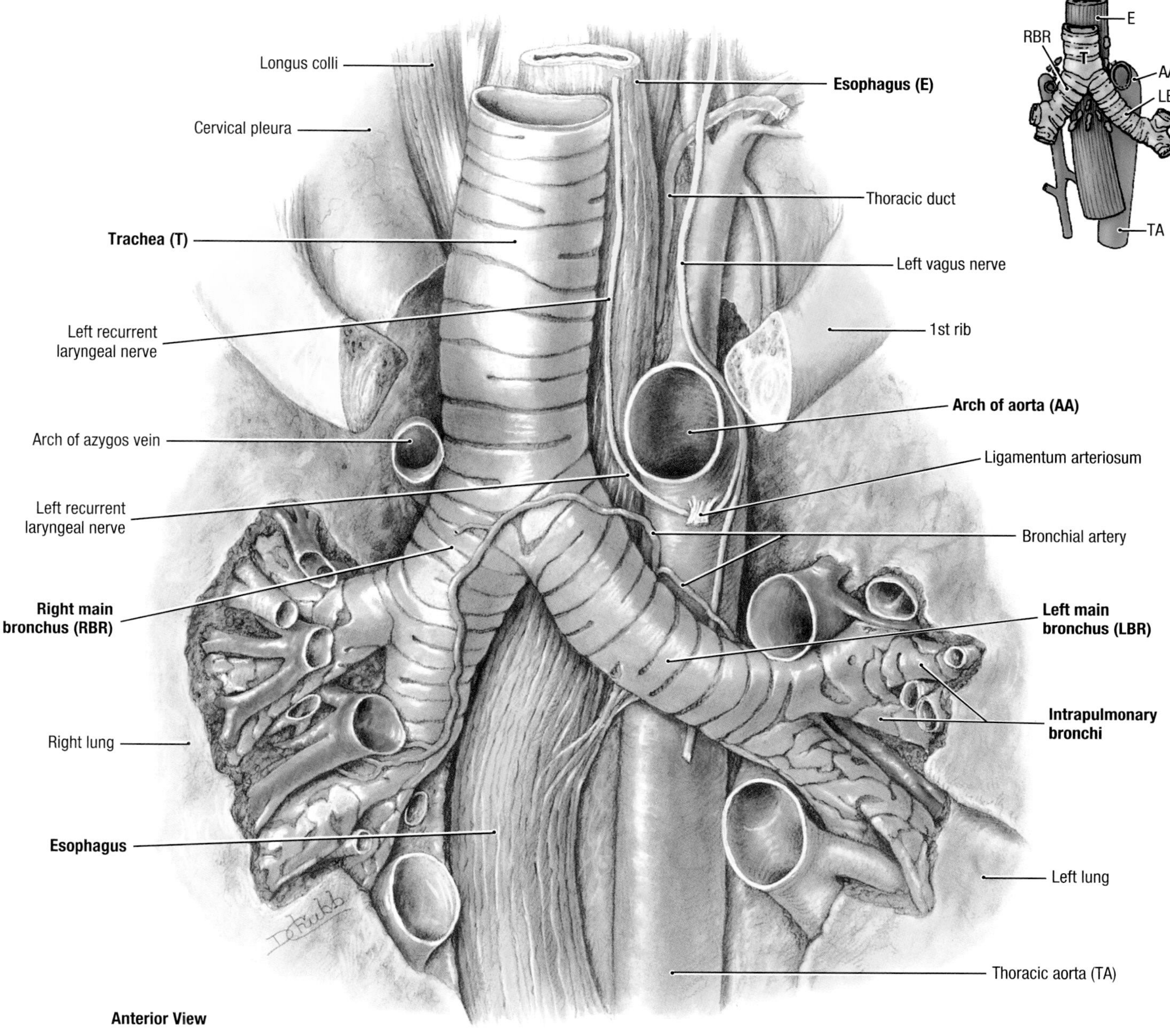

Longus colli
Cervical pleura
Trachea (T)
Left recurrent laryngeal nerve
Arch of azygos vein
Left recurrent laryngeal nerve
Right main bronchus (RBR)
Right lung
Esophagus
Esophagus (E)
Thoracic duct
Left vagus nerve
1st rib
Arch of aorta (AA)
Ligamentum arteriosum
Bronchial artery
Left main bronchus (LBR)
Intrapulmonary bronchi
Left lung
Thoracic aorta (TA)
Anterior View
E
RBR
T
AA
LBR
TA


## 1.65 Superior mediastinum IV: tracheal bifurcation and bronchi

- Note the four parallel structures: the trachea, esophagus, left recurrent laryngeal nerve, and thoracic duct. The esophagus bulges to the left of the trachea, the recurrent nerve lies in the angle between the trachea and esophagus, and the duct is at the left side of the esophagus. The trachea bifurcates at the level of the sternal angle.
- The arch of the aorta passes posterior to the left of these four structures as it arches over the left main bronchus; the arch of the azygos vein passes anterior to their right as it arches over the right main bronchus.
- The right main bronchus is (1) more vertical, (2) of greater caliber, and (3) shorter than the left main bronchus.

- The recurrent laryngeal nerves supply all the intrinsic muscles of the larynx, except one. Consequently, any investigative procedure or disease process in the superior mediastinum may involve these nerves and affect the voice. Because the left recurrent laryngeal nerve hooks around the arch of the aorta and ascends between the trachea and the esophagus, it may be involved when there is a bronchial or esophageal carcinoma, enlargement of mediastinal lymph nodes, or an aneurysm of the arch of the aorta.

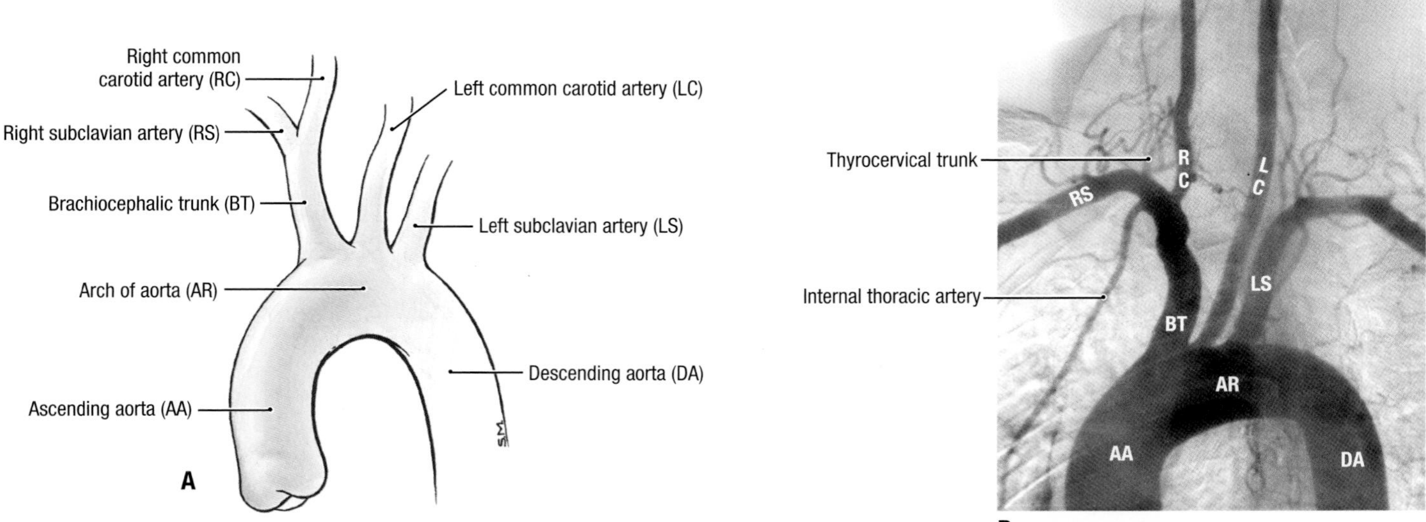
Right common carotid artery (RC)
Right subclavian artery (RS)
Brachiocephalic trunk (BT)
Arch of aorta (AR)
Ascending aorta (AA)
Left common carotid artery (LC)
Left subclavian artery (LS)
Descending aorta (DA)
A
Thyrocervical trunk
Internal thoracic artery
RS
RC
LC
LS
BT
AR
AA
DA
B. Left Anterior Oblique View

## 1.66 Branches of aortic arch

**A.** Aortic arch. **B.** Aortic angiogram. Observe the ascending aorta *(AA)*, the arch of the aorta *(AR)*, the descending aorta *(DA)*, the brachiocephalic *(BT)* trunk (artery) branching into the right subclavian *(RS)* and right common carotid *(RC)* arteries, and the left subclavian *(LS)* and left common carotid *(LC)* arteries arising directly from the aorta.

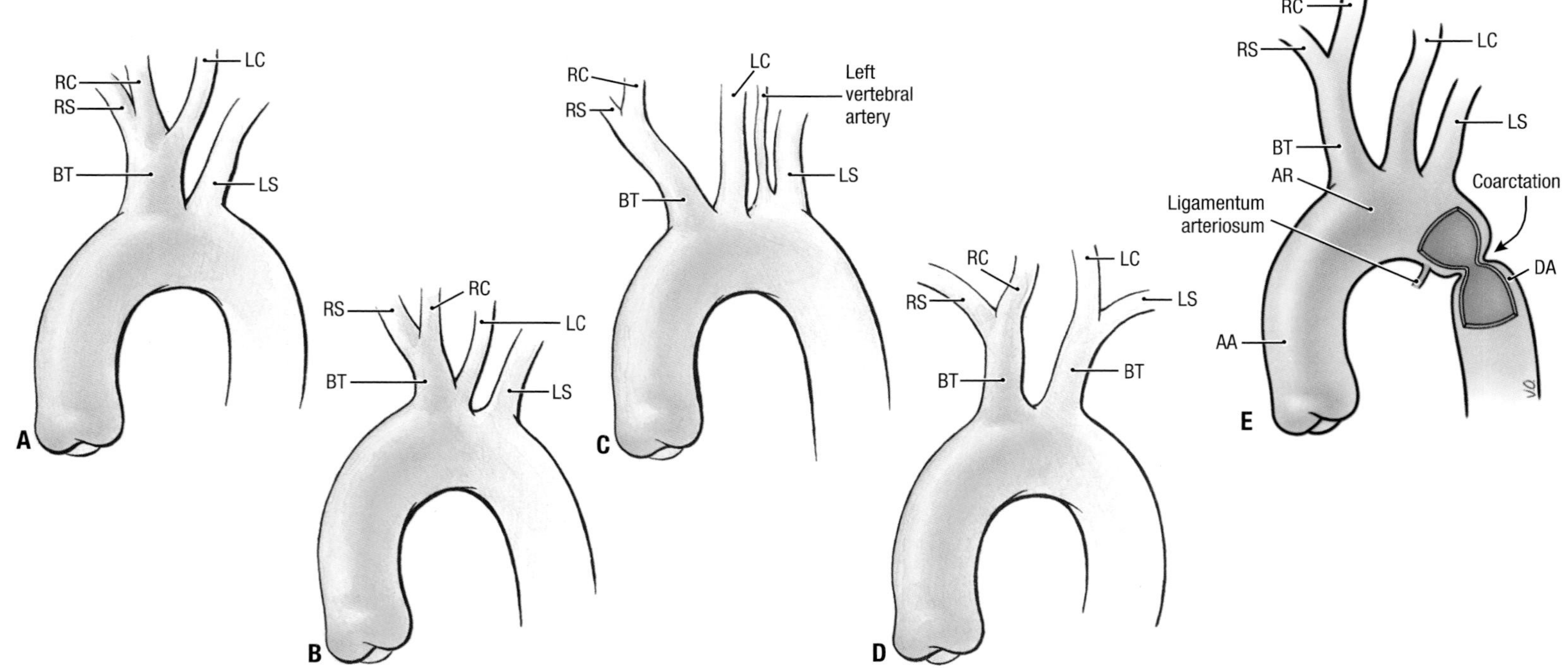
A
RC
RS
BT
LC
LS
B
RS
RC
BT
LC
LS
C
RC
RS
BT
LC
Left vertebral artery
LS
D
RC
RS
BT
LC
LS
BT
E
RC
RS
BT
AR
LC
LS
Coarctation
Ligamentum arteriosum
DA
AA

## 1.67 Variations in origins of branches of aortic arch

The most common pattern (65%) is shown in Figure 1.66. Less common variations include (**A** and **B**) left common carotid artery originating from the brachiocephalic trunk (27%); **(C)** each of the four arteries originating independently from the arch of the aorta (2.5%); **(D)** right and left brachiocephalic trunks originating from the arch of the aorta (1.2%); **(E)** Coarctation of aorta. In coarctation of the aorta, the arch or descending aorta has an abnormal narrowing (stenosis) that diminishes the caliber of the aortic lumen, producing an obstruction to blood flow. The most common site is near the ligamentum arteriosum. When the coarctation is inferior to this site (postuctal coarctation), a good collateral circulation usually develops between the proximal and distal parts of the aorta through the intercostal and internal thoracic arteries.

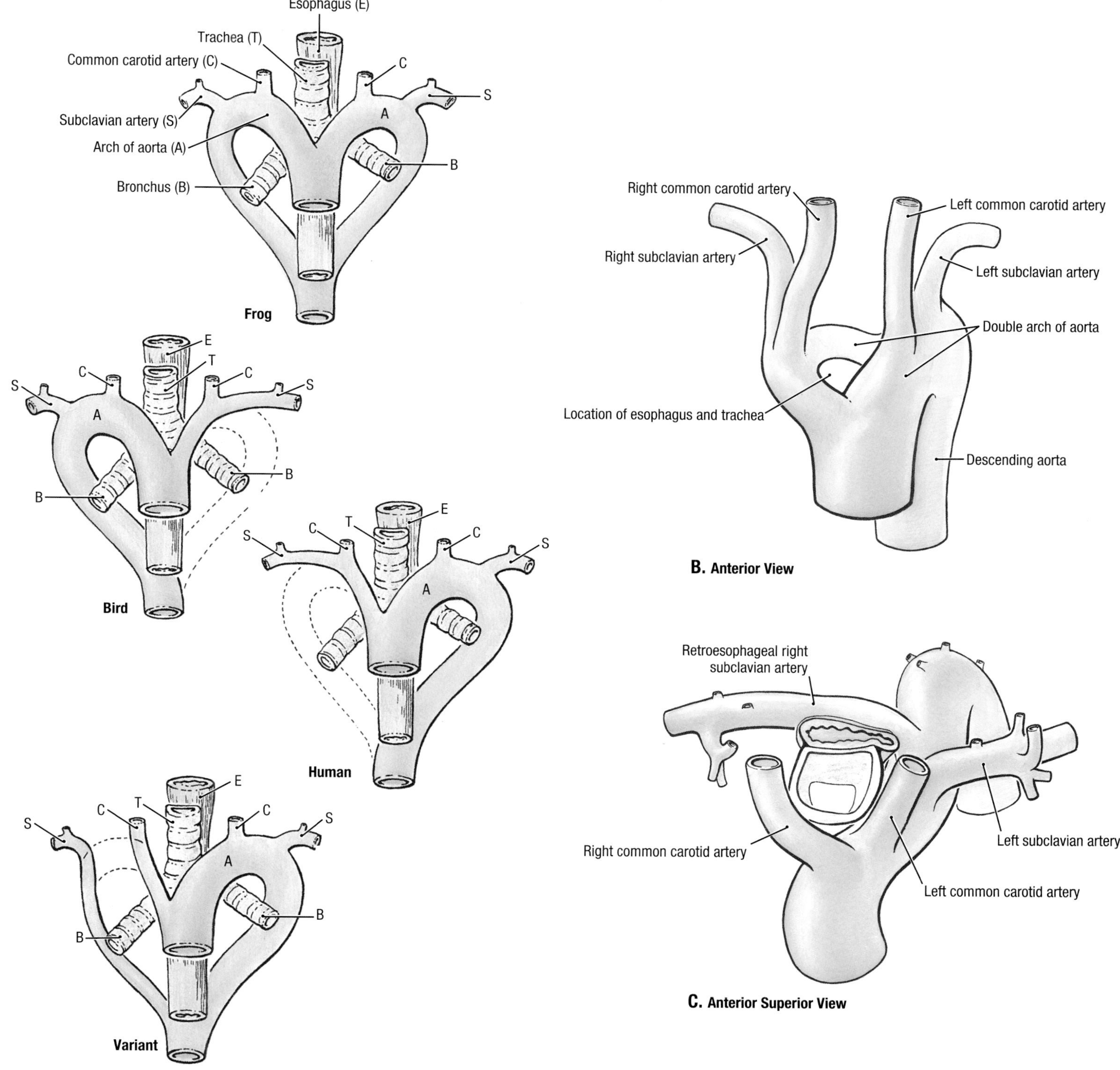
Esophagus (E)
Trachea (T)
Common carotid artery (C)
C
S
Subclavian artery (S)
A
Arch of aorta (A)
B
Bronchus (B)
Frog
E
T
C
C
S
S
A
B
B
Bird
E
T
C
C
S
S
A
Human
E
T
C
C
S
S
A
B
B
Variant
A. Anterior Views
Right common carotid artery
Left common carotid artery
Right subclavian artery
Left subclavian artery
Double arch of aorta
Location of esophagus and trachea
Descending aorta
B. Anterior View
Retroesophageal right subclavian artery
Right common carotid artery
Left subclavian artery
Left common carotid artery
C. Anterior Superior View

## 1.68 Scheme of varieties of aortic arches

**A.** Comparative anatomy. The double aortic arch of the frog; the right aortic arch of the bird; the left aortic arch of the mammal, including man, and a variant. **B.** Double aortic arch. The right and left aortic arches persist completely, as in the frog. In this rare condition, the esophagus and trachea pass through the so-formed "aortic ring." **C.** Retroesophageal right subclavian artery. The artery arises as the last branch of the arch of the aorta, passing posterior to the esophagus and trachea.

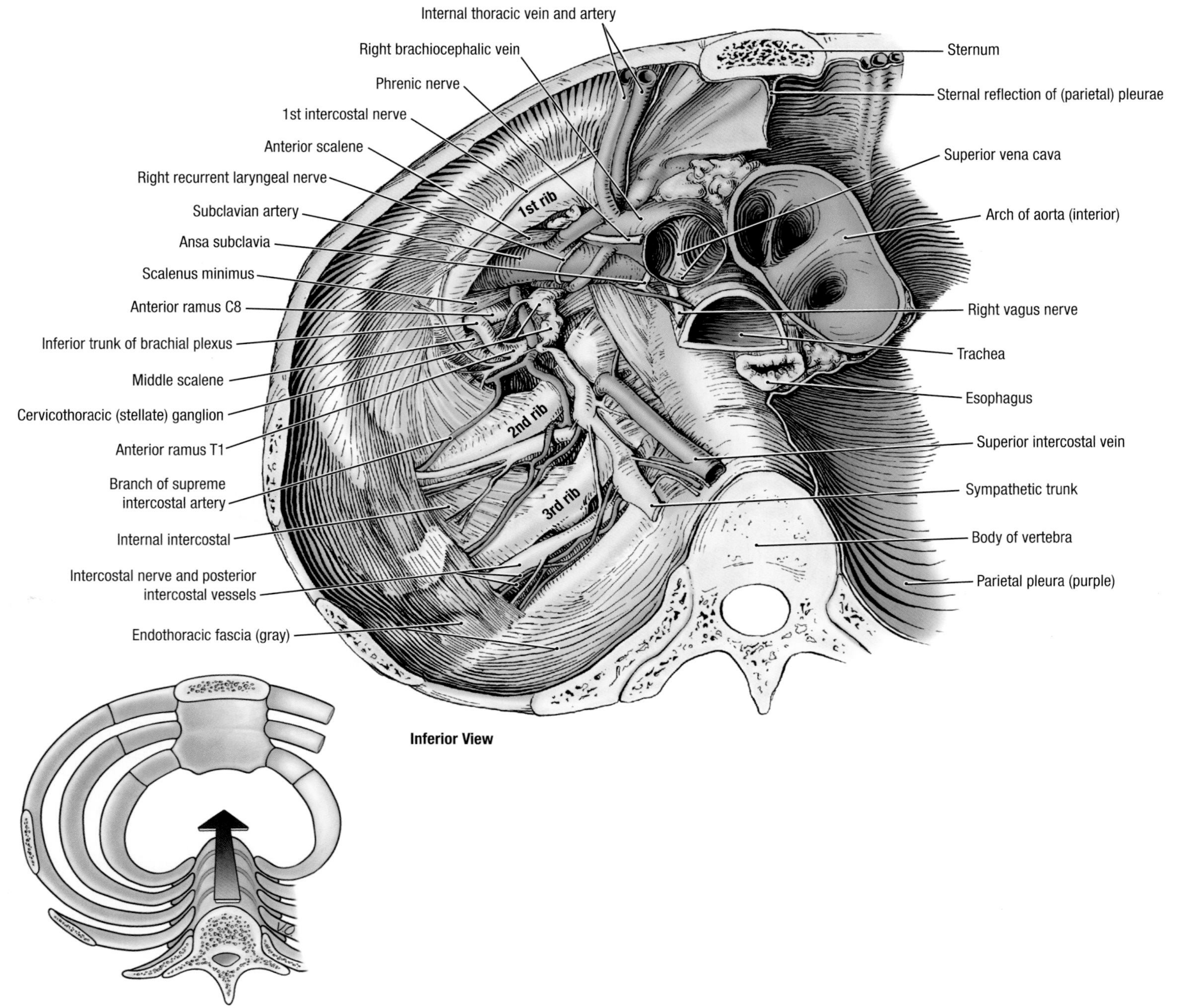
Internal thoracic vein and artery
Right brachiocephalic vein
Phrenic nerve
1st intercostal nerve
Anterior scalene
Right recurrent laryngeal nerve
Subclavian artery
Ansa subclavia
Scalenus minimus
Anterior ramus C8
Inferior trunk of brachial plexus
Middle scalene
Cervicothoracic (stellate) ganglion
Anterior ramus T1
Branch of supreme intercostal artery
Internal intercostal
Intercostal nerve and posterior intercostal vessels
Endothoracic fascia (gray)
1st rib
2nd rib
3rd rib
Sternum
Sternal reflection of (parietal) pleurae
Superior vena cava
Arch of aorta (interior)
Right vagus nerve
Trachea
Esophagus
Superior intercostal vein
Sympathetic trunk
Body of vertebra
Parietal pleura (purple)
Inferior View

## 1.69 Superior mediastinum and roof of pleural cavity

- The cervical, costal, and mediastinal parietal pleura *(purple)* and portions of the endothoracic fascia *(gray)* have been removed from the right side of the specimen to demonstrate structures traversing the superior thoracic aperture.
- The first part of the subclavian artery disappears as it crosses the first rib anterior to the anterior scalene muscle.
- The ansa subclavian from the sympathetic trunk and right recurrent laryngeal nerve from the vagus are seen looping inferior to the subclavian artery.
- The anterior rami of C8 and T1 merge to form the inferior trunk of the brachial plexus, which crosses the first rib posterior to the anterior scalene muscle.

Sternal reflection of left pleura
**Pericardial sac**
Sternal reflection of right pleura
Costomediastinal recess
Internal thoracic artery
Fatpad
Transversus thoracis
Left phrenic nerve
External oblique
**Muscular part of diaphagm**
Right phrenic nerve
Inferior vena cava
Esophagus
**Central tendon of diaphragm**
**Central tendon of diaphragm**
Mesoesophagus
Diaphragmatic pleura
Latissimus dorsi
Costodiaphragmatic recess
Serratus posterior inferior
Costal pleura
Aorta
Thoracic duct
Azygos vein
Greater (thoracic) splanchnic nerve
Sympathetic trunk

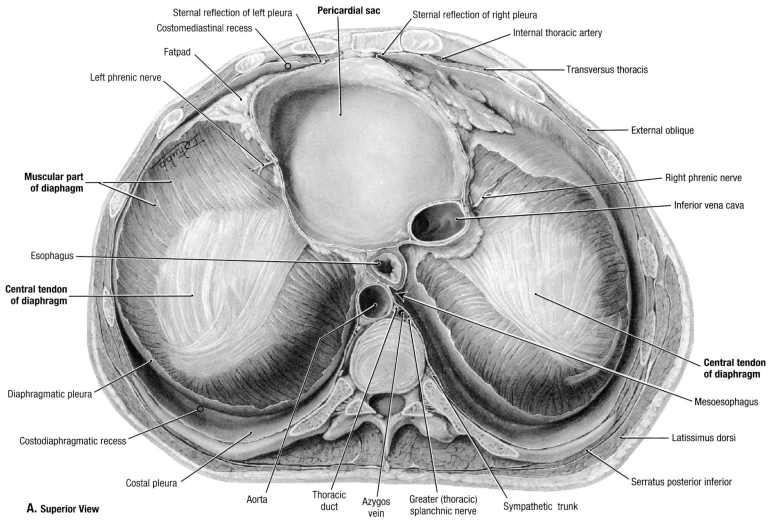

**A.** **Superior View**

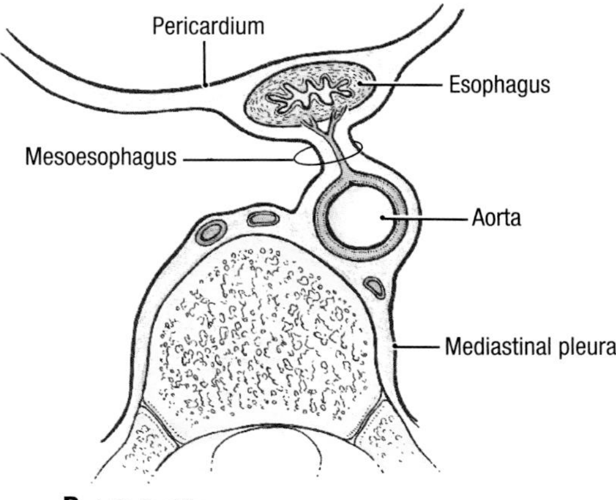
Pericardium
Esophagus
Mesoesophagus
Aorta
Mediastinal pleura

**B.** **Inferior View**

## 1.70 Diaphragm and pericardial sac

**A.** The diaphragmatic pleura is mostly removed. The pericardial sac is situated on the anterior half of the diaphragm; one third is to the right of the median plane, and two thirds to the left. Note also that anterior to the pericardium, the sternal reflection of the left pleural sac approaches but fails to meet that of the right sac in the median plane; and on reaching the vertebral column, the costal pleura becomes the mediastinal pleura. Irritation of the parietal pleura produces local pain and referred pain to the areas sharing innervation by the same segments of the spinal cord. Irritation of the costal and peripheral parts of the diaphragmatic pleura results in local pain and referred pain along the intercostal nerves to the thoracic and abdominal walls. Irritation of the mediastinal and central diaphragmatic areas of the parietal pleura results in pain that is referred to the root of the neck and over the shoulder (C3–C5 dermatomes). **B.** Between the inferior part of the esophagus and the aorta, the right and left layers of mediastinal pleura form a dorsal mesoesophagus.

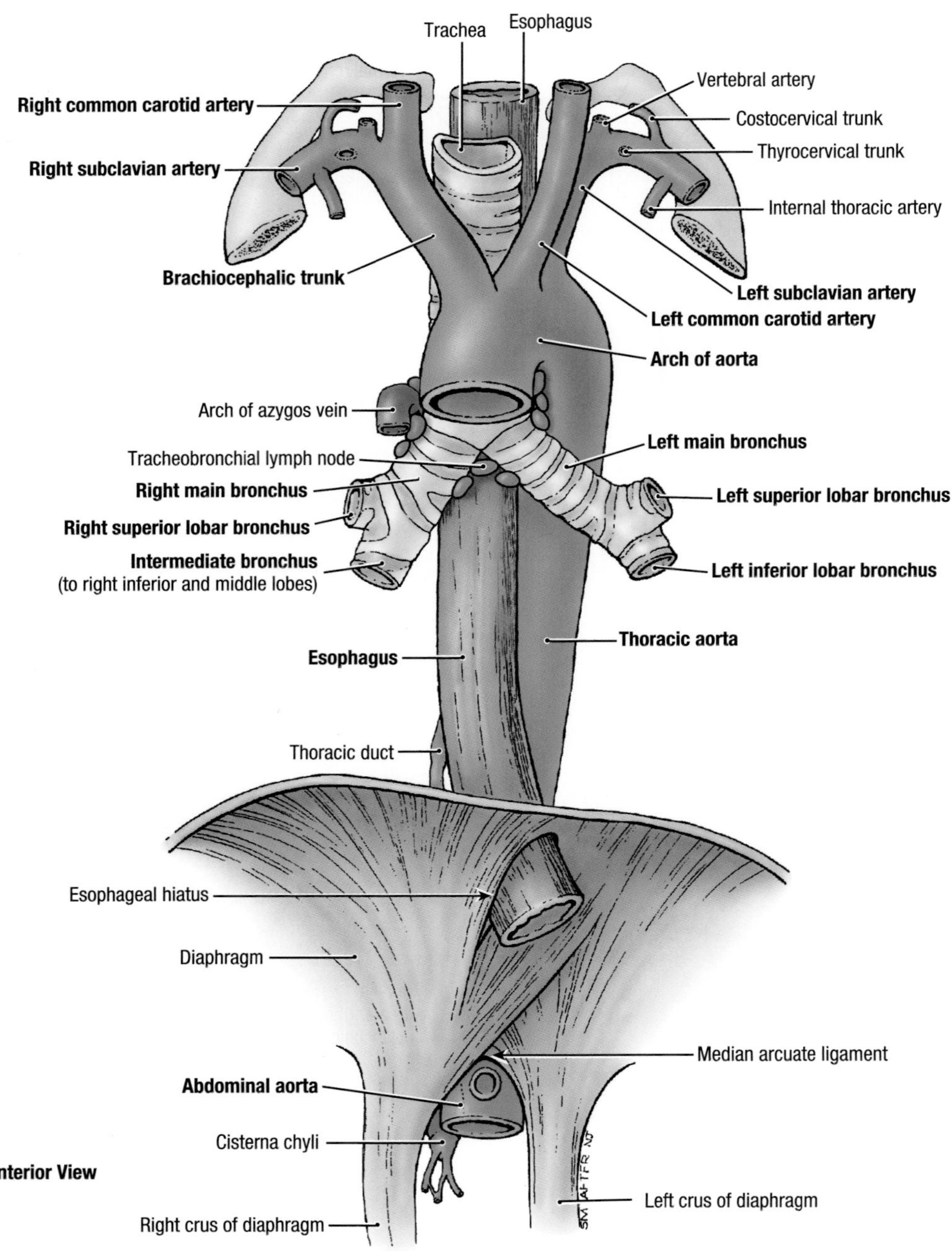
Trachea
Esophagus
Vertebral artery
Right common carotid artery
Costocervical trunk
Thyrocervical trunk
Right subclavian artery
Internal thoracic artery
Brachiocephalic trunk
Left subclavian artery
Left common carotid artery
Arch of aorta
Arch of azygos vein
Left main bronchus
Tracheobronchial lymph node
Right main bronchus
Left superior lobar bronchus
Right superior lobar bronchus
Intermediate bronchus
(to right inferior and middle lobes)
Left inferior lobar bronchus
Thoracic aorta
Esophagus
Thoracic duct
Esophageal hiatus
Diaphragm
Median arcuate ligament
Abdominal aorta
Cisterna chyli
Anterior View
Left crus of diaphragm
Right crus of diaphragm

## 1.71 Esophagus, trachea, and aorta

- The anterior relations of the thoracic part of the esophagus from superior to inferior are the trachea (from origin at cricoid cartilage to bifurcation), right and left bronchi, inferior tracheobronchial lymph nodes, pericardium (not shown) and, finally, the diaphragm.
- The arch of the aorta passes posterior to the left of these four structures as it arches over the left main bronchus; the arch of the azygos vein passes anterior to their right as it arches over the right main bronchus.
- The impressions produced in the esophagus by adjacent structures (aorta, left main bronchus) are of clinical interest because of the slower passage of substances at these sites. The impressions indicate where swallowed foreign objects are most likely to lodge and where a stricture may develop after the accidental drinking of a caustic liquid such as lye.

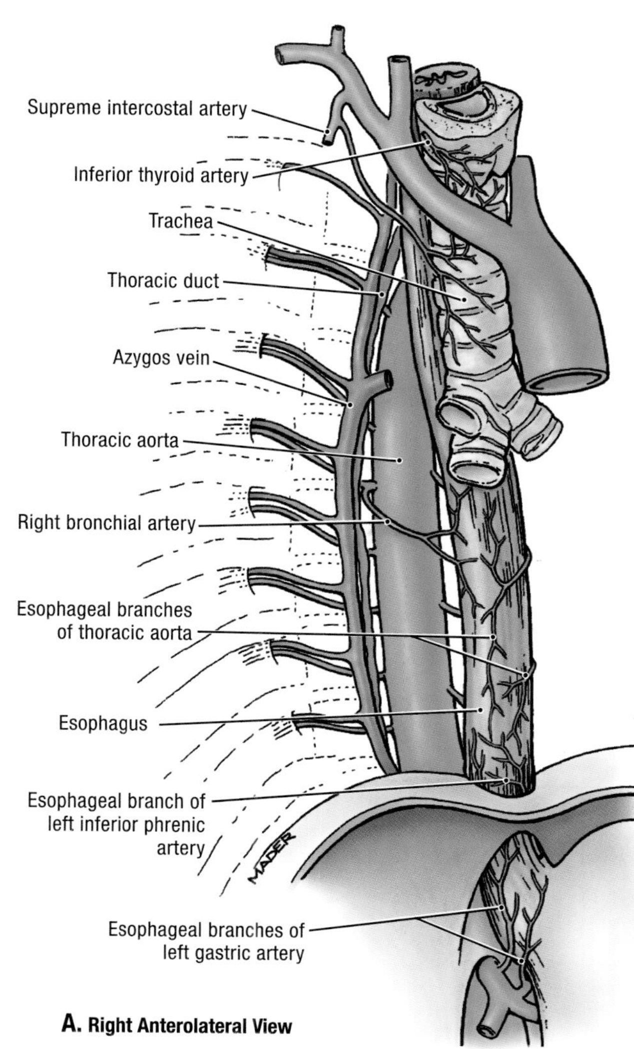
Supreme intercostal artery
Inferior thyroid artery
Trachea
Thoracic duct
Azygos vein
Thoracic aorta
Right bronchial artery
Esophageal branches of thoracic aorta
Esophagus
Esophageal branch of left inferior phrenic artery
Esophageal branches of left gastric artery
MADER

**A. Right Anterolateral View**

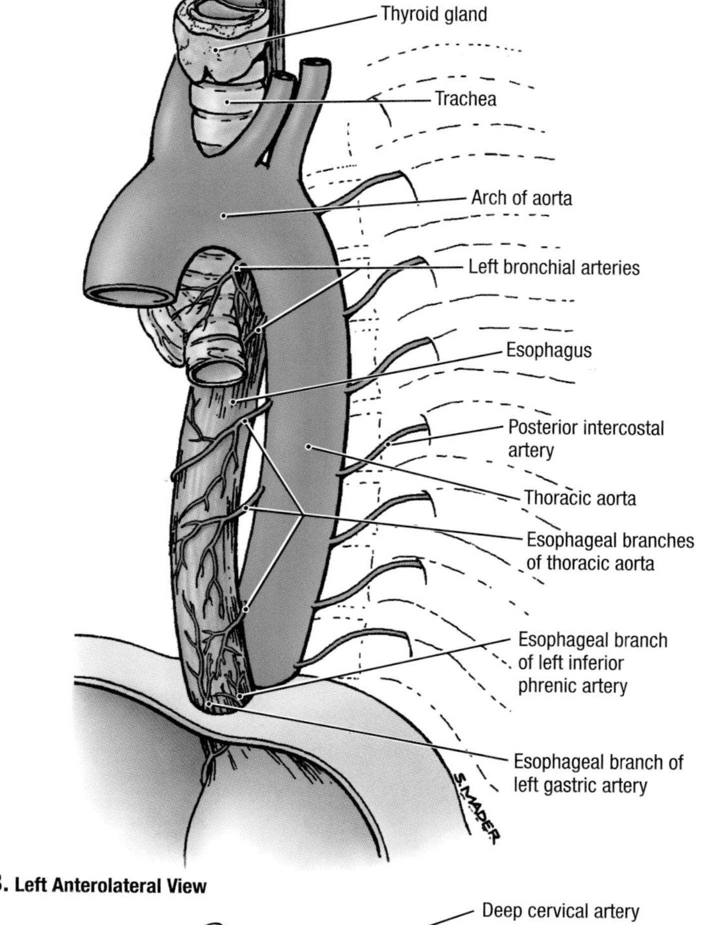
Thyroid gland
Trachea
Arch of aorta
Left bronchial arteries
Esophagus
Posterior intercostal artery
Thoracic aorta
Esophageal branches of thoracic aorta
Esophageal branch of left inferior phrenic artery
Esophageal branch of left gastric artery
S.MADER

**B. Left Anterolateral View**

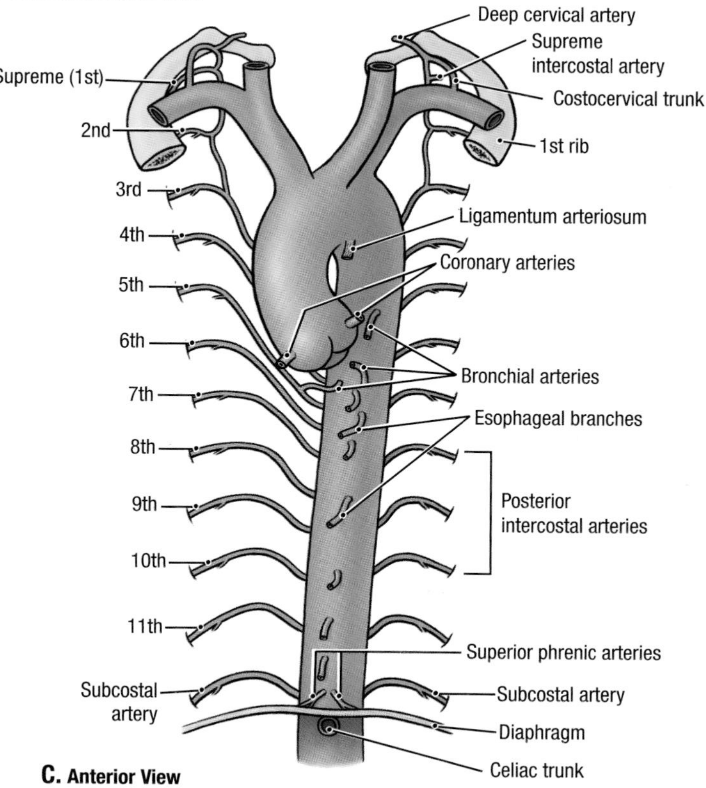
Deep cervical artery
Supreme intercostal artery
Costocervical trunk
1st rib
Supreme (1st)
2nd
3rd
4th
5th
6th
7th
8th
9th
10th
11th
Subcostal artery
Ligamentum arteriosum
Coronary arteries
Bronchial arteries
Esophageal branches
Posterior intercostal arteries
Superior phrenic arteries
Subcostal artery
Diaphragm
Celiac trunk

**C. Anterior View**

## 1.72 Arterial supply to trachea and esophagus

**A** and **B.** The continuous anastomotic chain of arteries on the esophagus is formed (a) by branches of the right and left inferior thyroid and right supreme intercostal arteries superiorly, (b) by the unpaired median aortic (bronchial and esophageal) branches, and (c) by branches of the left gastric and left inferior phrenic arteries inferiorly. The right bronchial artery usually arises from the superior left bronchial or 3rd right posterior intercostal artery (here the 5th) or from the aorta directly. The unpaired median aortic branches also supply the trachea and bronchi. **C.** Branches of the thoracic aorta.

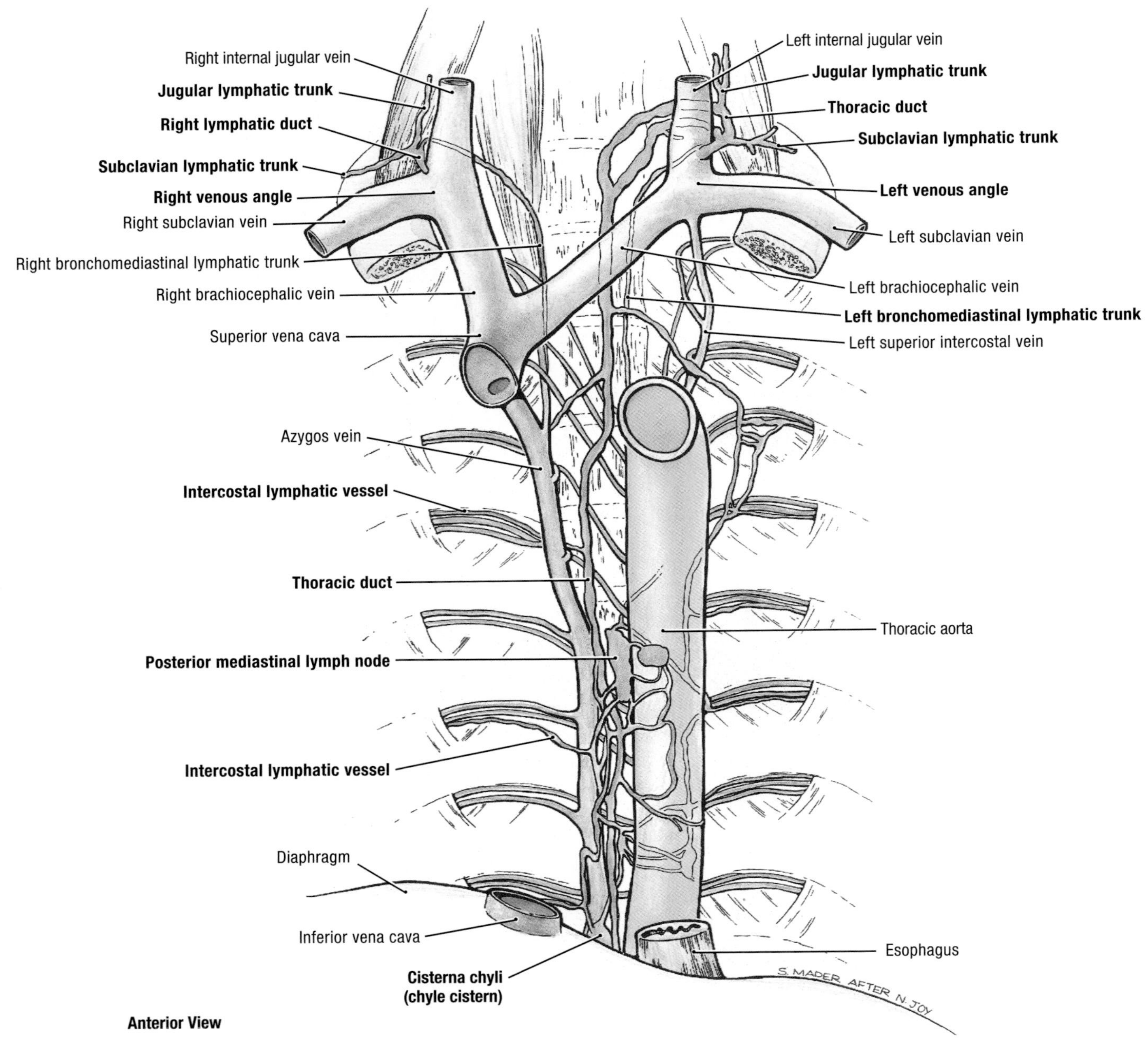
Right internal jugular vein
Jugular lymphatic trunk
Right lymphatic duct
Subclavian lymphatic trunk
Right venous angle
Right subclavian vein
Right bronchomediastinal lymphatic trunk
Right brachiocephalic vein
Superior vena cava
Azygos vein
Intercostal lymphatic vessel
Thoracic duct
Posterior mediastinal lymph node
Intercostal lymphatic vessel
Diaphragm
Inferior vena cava
Cisterna chyli (chyle cistern)
Anterior View
Left internal jugular vein
Jugular lymphatic trunk
Thoracic duct
Subclavian lymphatic trunk
Left venous angle
Left subclavian vein
Left brachiocephalic vein
Left bronchomediastinal lymphatic trunk
Left superior intercostal vein
Thoracic aorta
Esophagus
S. MADER AFTER N. JOY

## 1.73 Thoracic duct

- The descending aorta is located to the left, and the azygos vein slightly to the right of the midline.
- The thoracic duct (a) originates from the cisterna chyli at the T12 vertebral level, (b) ascends on the vertebral column between the azygos vein and the descending aorta, (c) passes to the left at the junction of the posterior and superior mediastina, and continues its ascent to the neck, where (d) it arches laterally to enter the venous system near or at the angle of union of the left internal jugular and subclavian veins (left venous angle).
- The thoracic duct is commonly plexiform (resembling a network) in the posterior mediastinum.
- The termination of the thoracic duct typically receives the jugular, subclavian, and bronchomediastinal trunks.
- The right lymph duct is short and formed by the union of the right jugular, subclavian, and bronchomediastinal trunks.

- Because the thoracic duct is thin walled and may be colorless, it may not be easily identified. Consequently, it is vulnerable to inadvertent injury during investigative and/or surgical procedures in the posterior mediastinum. Laceration of the thoracic duct results in chyle escaping into the thoracic cavity. Chyle may also enter the pleural cavity, producing chylothorax.

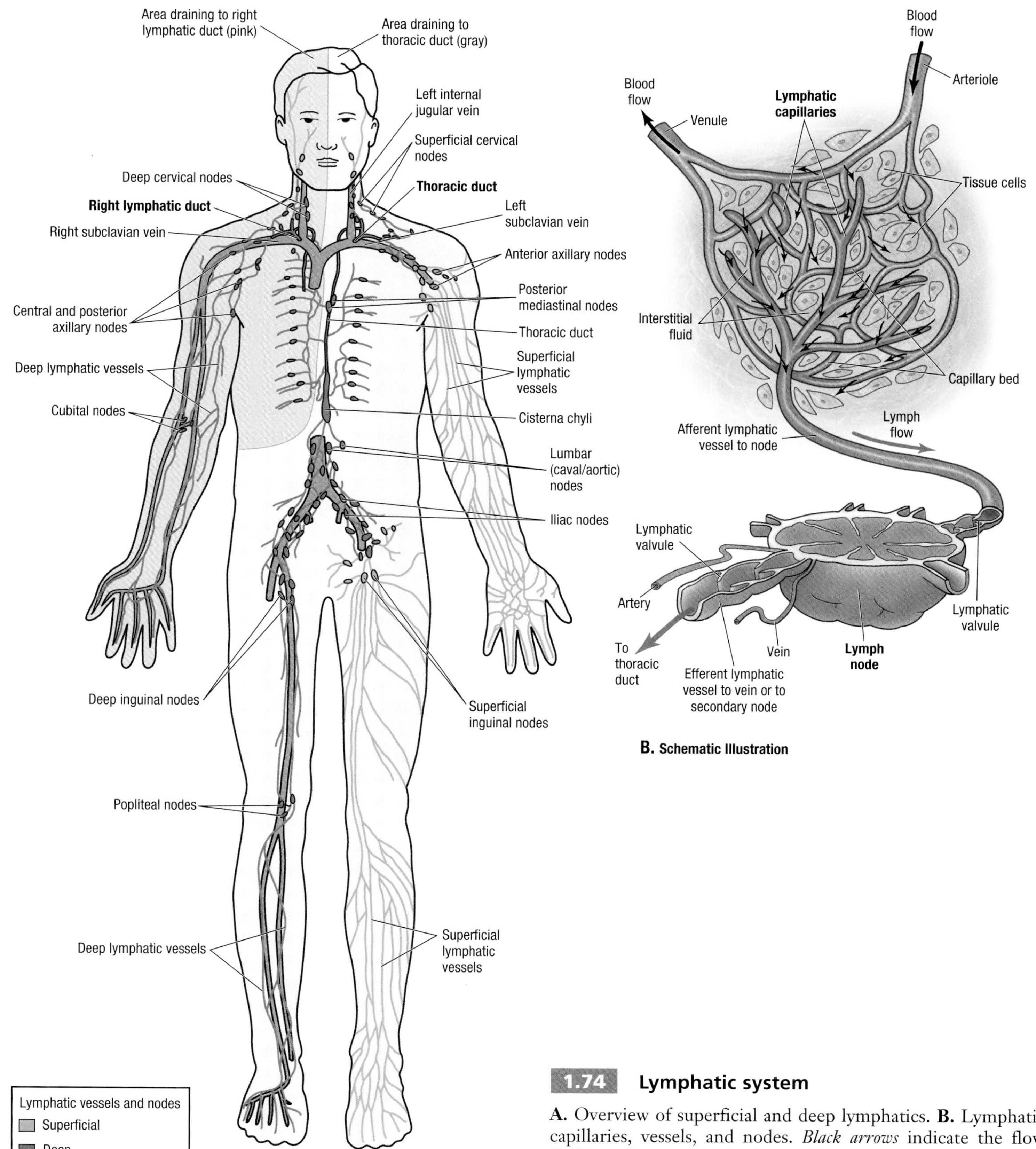
Area draining to right lymphatic duct (pink)
Area draining to thoracic duct (gray)
Left internal jugular vein
Superficial cervical nodes
Deep cervical nodes
Thoracic duct
Right lymphatic duct
Left subclavian vein
Right subclavian vein
Anterior axillary nodes
Posterior mediastinal nodes
Central and posterior axillary nodes
Thoracic duct
Deep lymphatic vessels
Superficial lymphatic vessels
Cubital nodes
Cisterna chyli
Lumbar (caval/aortic) nodes
Iliac nodes
Deep inguinal nodes
Superficial inguinal nodes
Popliteal nodes
Deep lymphatic vessels
Superficial lymphatic vessels
Lymphatic vessels and nodes
Superficial
Deep
A. Anterior View
Blood flow
Blood flow
Arteriole
Venule
Lymphatic capillaries
Tissue cells
Interstitial fluid
Capillary bed
Lymph flow
Afferent lymphatic vessel to node
Lymphatic valvule
Artery
Lymphatic valvule
To thoracic duct
Vein
Lymph node
Efferent lymphatic vessel to vein or to secondary node
B. Schematic Illustration

## 1.74 Lymphatic system

**A.** Overview of superficial and deep lymphatics. **B.** Lymphatic capillaries, vessels, and nodes. *Black arrows* indicate the flow (leaking of interstitial fluid out of blood vessels and absorption) into the lymphatic capillaries.

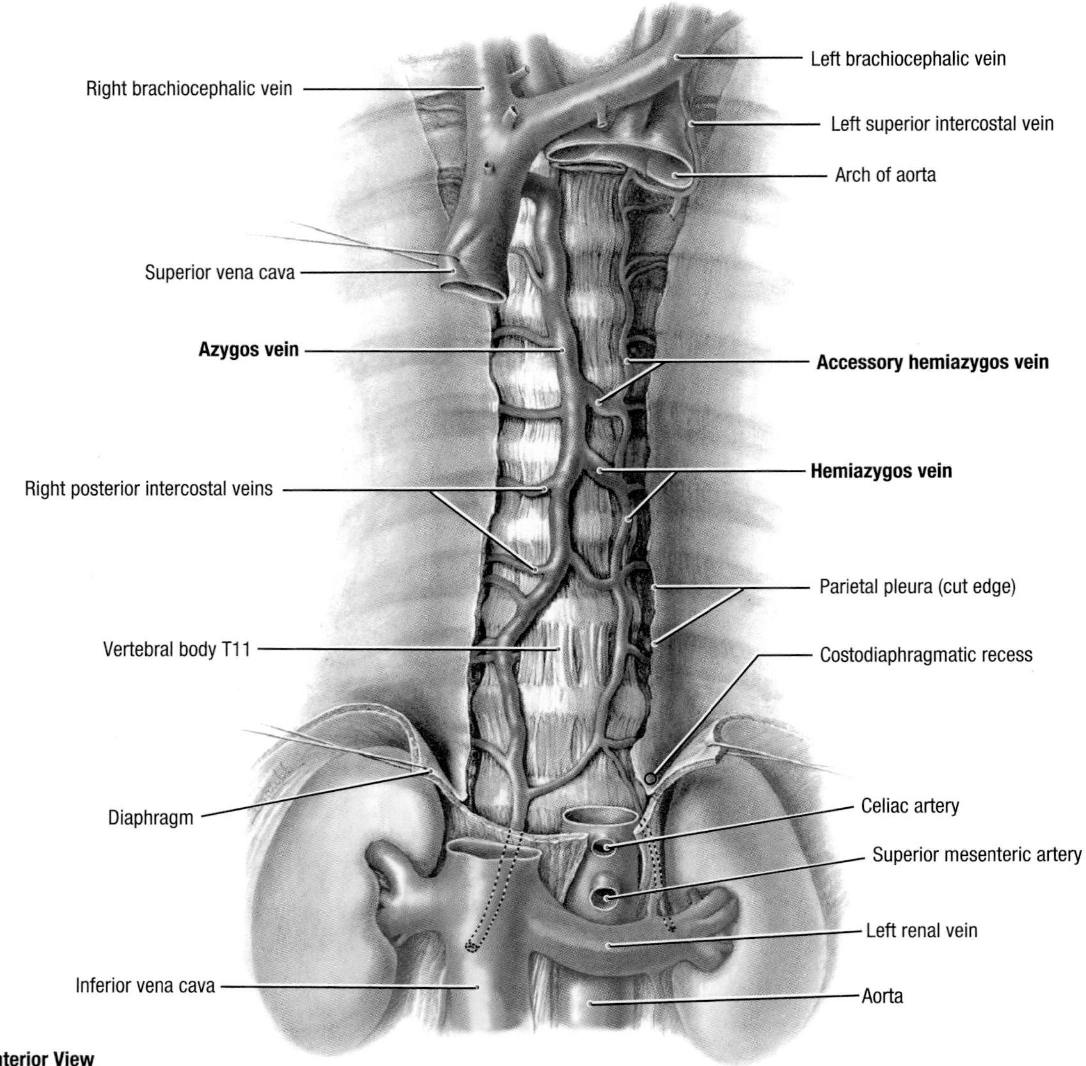
Right brachiocephalic vein
Left brachiocephalic vein
Left superior intercostal vein
Arch of aorta
Superior vena cava
Azygos vein
Accessory hemiazygos vein
Hemiazygos vein
Right posterior intercostal veins
Parietal pleura (cut edge)
Vertebral body T11
Costodiaphragmatic recess
Diaphragm
Celiac artery
Superior mesenteric artery
Left renal vein
Inferior vena cava
Aorta

**A. Anterior View**

## 1.75 Azygos system of veins

The ascending lumbar veins connect the common iliac veins to the lumbar veins and join the subcostal veins to become the lateral roots of the azygos and hemiazygos veins; the medial roots of the azygos and hemiazygos veins are usually from the inferior vena cava and left renal vein, if present. Typically the upper four left posterior intercostal veins drain into the left brachiocephalic vein, directly and via the left superior intercostal veins.

In **A,** the hemiazygos, accessory hemiazygos, and left superior intercostals veins are continuous, but commonly they are discontinuous. The hemiazygos vein crosses the vertebral column at approximately T9, and the accessory hemiazygos vein crosses at T8, to enter the azygos vein. In **A,** there are four cross-connecting channels between the azygos and hemiazygos systems. The azygos vein arches superior to the root of the right lung at T4 to drain into the superior vena cava.

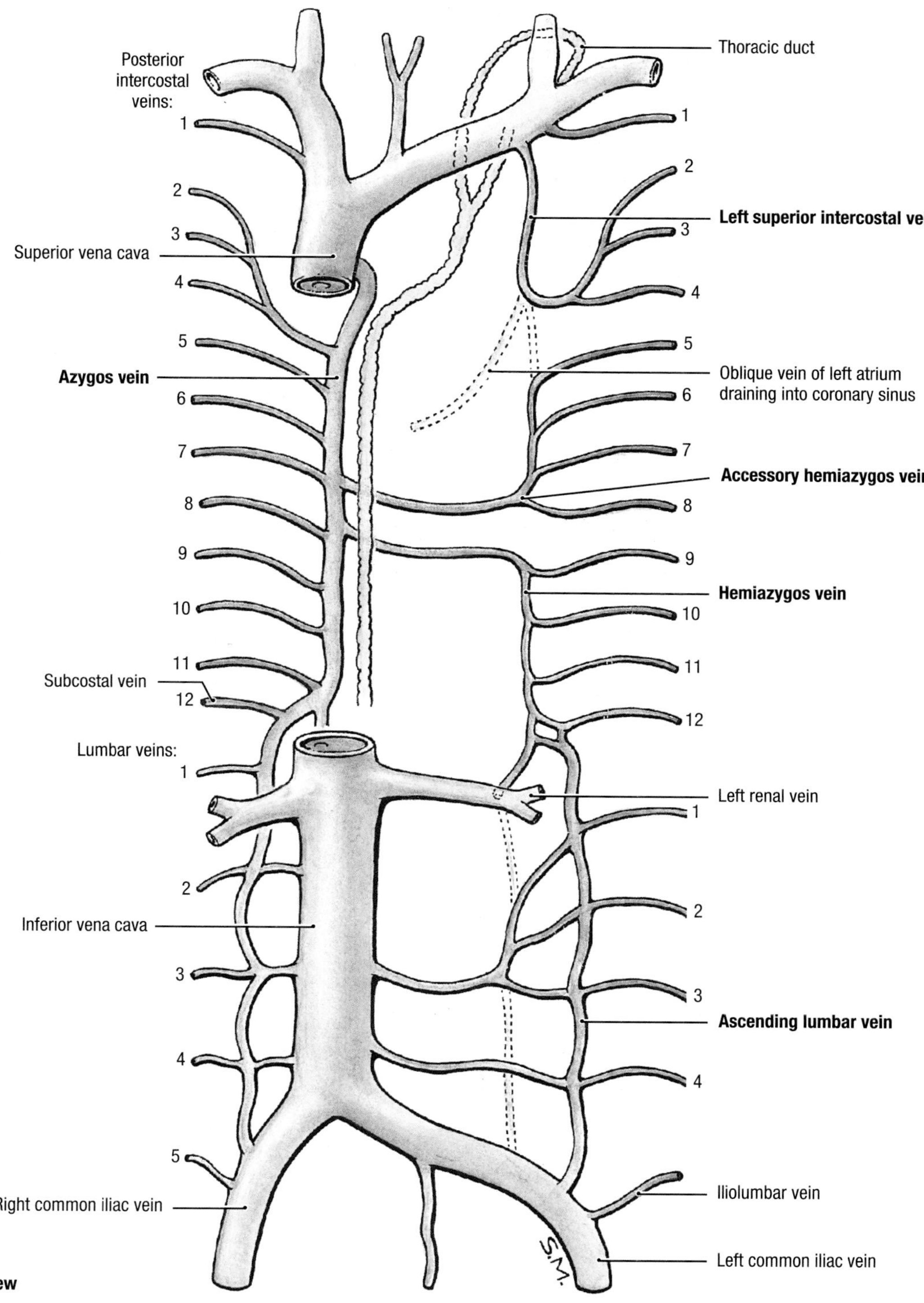
Posterior intercostal veins:
1
2
3
4
5
6
7
8
9
10
11
12
Superior vena cava
Azygos vein
Subcostal vein
Lumbar veins:
1
2
3
4
5
Inferior vena cava
Right common iliac vein
Thoracic duct
1
2
Left superior intercostal vein
3
4
5
Oblique vein of left atrium draining into coronary sinus
6
7
Accessory hemiazygos vein
8
9
Hemiazygos vein
10
11
12
Left renal vein
1
2
3
Ascending lumbar vein
4
Iliolumbar vein
Left common iliac vein
S.M.

**B.** Anterior View

## 1.75 Azygos system of veins *(continued)*

The azygos, hemiazygos, and accessory hemiazygos veins offer alternate means of venous drainage from the thoracic, abdominal, and back regions when ***obstruction of the IVC*** occurs. In some people, an accessory azygos vein parallels the main azygos vein on the right side. Other people have no hemiazygos system of veins. A clinically important variation, although uncommon, is when the azygos system receives all the blood from the IVC, except that from the liver. In these people, the azygos system drains nearly all the blood inferior to the diaphragm, except that from the digestive tract. When ***obstruction of the SVC*** occurs superior to the entrance of the azygos vein, blood can drain inferiorly into the veins of the abdominal wall and return to the right atrium through the IVC and azygos system of veins.

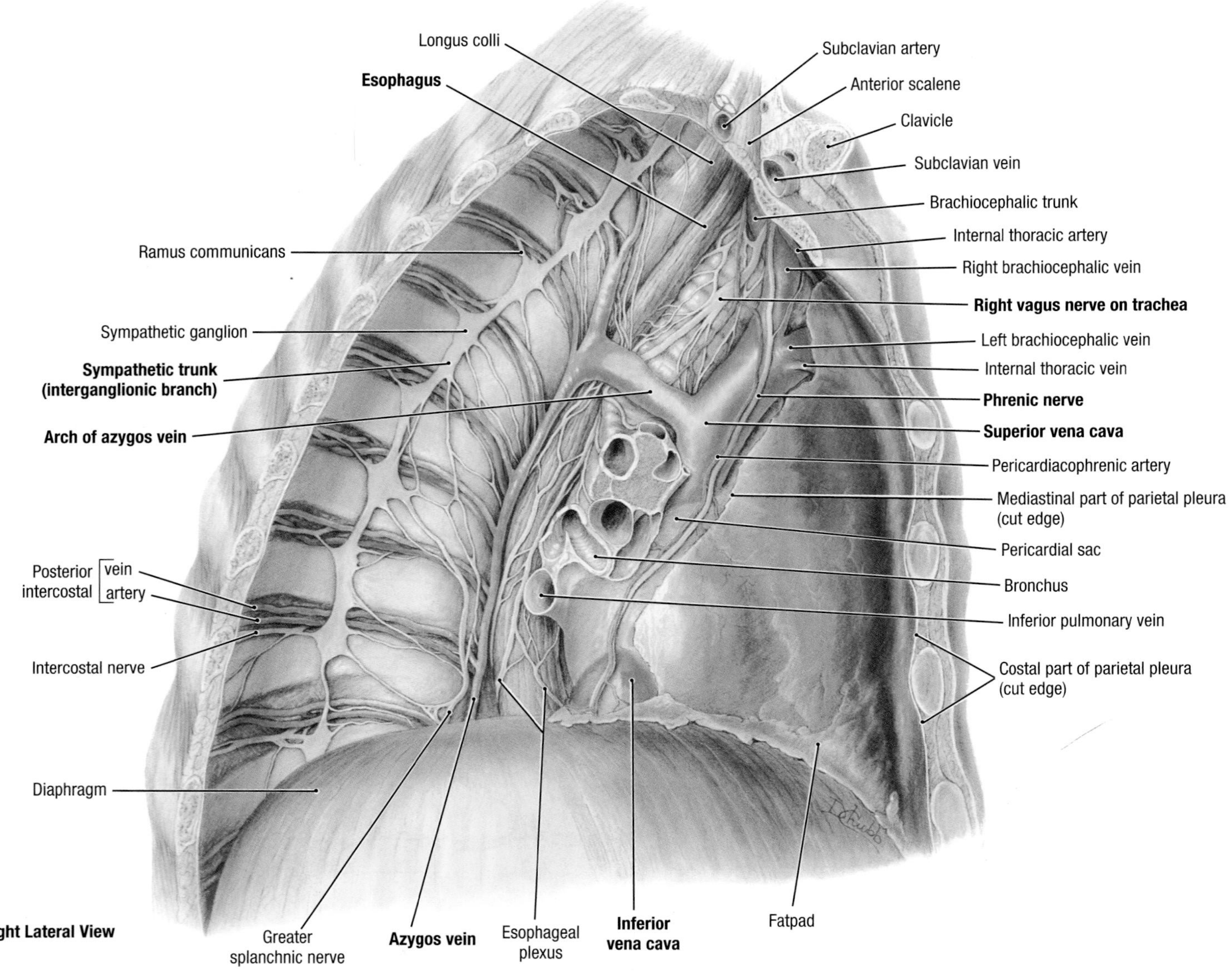
Longus colli
Esophagus
Subclavian artery
Anterior scalene
Clavicle
Subclavian vein
Brachiocephalic trunk
Internal thoracic artery
Right brachiocephalic vein
Right vagus nerve on trachea
Left brachiocephalic vein
Internal thoracic vein
Phrenic nerve
Superior vena cava
Pericardiacophrenic artery
Mediastinal part of parietal pleura (cut edge)
Pericardial sac
Bronchus
Inferior pulmonary vein
Costal part of parietal pleura (cut edge)
Ramus communicans
Sympathetic ganglion
Sympathetic trunk (interganglionic branch)
Arch of azygos vein
Posterior intercostal vein
artery
Intercostal nerve
Diaphragm
Right Lateral View
Greater splanchnic nerve
Azygos vein
Esophageal plexus
Inferior vena cava
Fatpad

## 1.76 Mediastinum, right side

- The costal and mediastinal pleurae have mostly been removed, exposing the underlying structures. Compare with the mediastinal surface of the right lung in Figure 1.29.
- The right side of the mediastinum is the "blue side," dominated by the arch of the azygos vein and the superior vena cava.
- Both the trachea and the esophagus are visible from the right side.
- The right vagus nerve descends on the medial surface of the trachea, passes medial to the arch of the azygos vein, posterior to the root of the lung, and then enters the esophageal plexus.
- The right phrenic nerve passes anterior to the root of the lung lateral to both venae cavae.

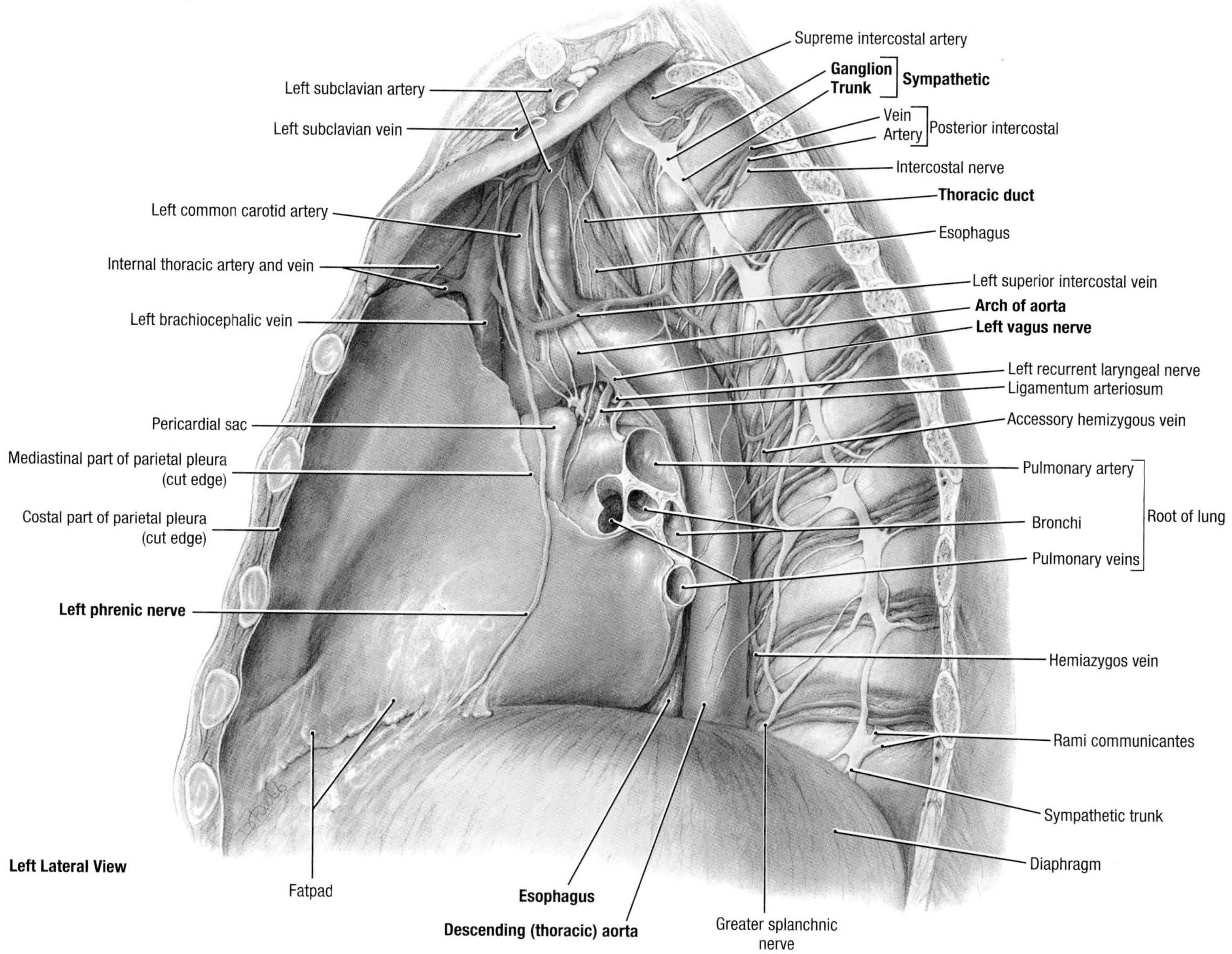
Supreme intercostal artery
Ganglion
Trunk
Sympathetic
Left subclavian artery
Left subclavian vein
Vein
Artery
Posterior intercostal
Intercostal nerve
Thoracic duct
Left common carotid artery
Esophagus
Internal thoracic artery and vein
Left superior intercostal vein
Arch of aorta
Left brachiocephalic vein
Left vagus nerve
Left recurrent laryngeal nerve
Ligamentum arteriosum
Pericardial sac
Accessory hemizygous vein
Mediastinal part of parietal pleura (cut edge)
Pulmonary artery
Costal part of parietal pleura (cut edge)
Bronchi
Root of lung
Pulmonary veins
Left phrenic nerve
Hemiazygos vein
Rami communicantes
Sympathetic trunk
Diaphragm
Left Lateral View
Fatpad
Esophagus
Descending (thoracic) aorta
Greater splanchnic nerve

## 1.77 Mediastinum, left side

- Compare with the mediastinal surface of the left lung in Figure 1.30.
- The left side of the mediastinum is the "red side," dominated by the arch and descending portion of the aorta, the left common carotid and subclavian arteries; the latter obscure the trachea from view.
- The thoracic duct can be seen on the left side of the esophagus.
- The left vagus nerve passes posterior to the root of the lung, sending its recurrent laryngeal branch around the ligamentum arteriosum inferior, then medial to the aortic arch.
- The phrenic nerve passes anterior to the root of the lung and penetrates the diaphragm more anteriorly than on the right side.

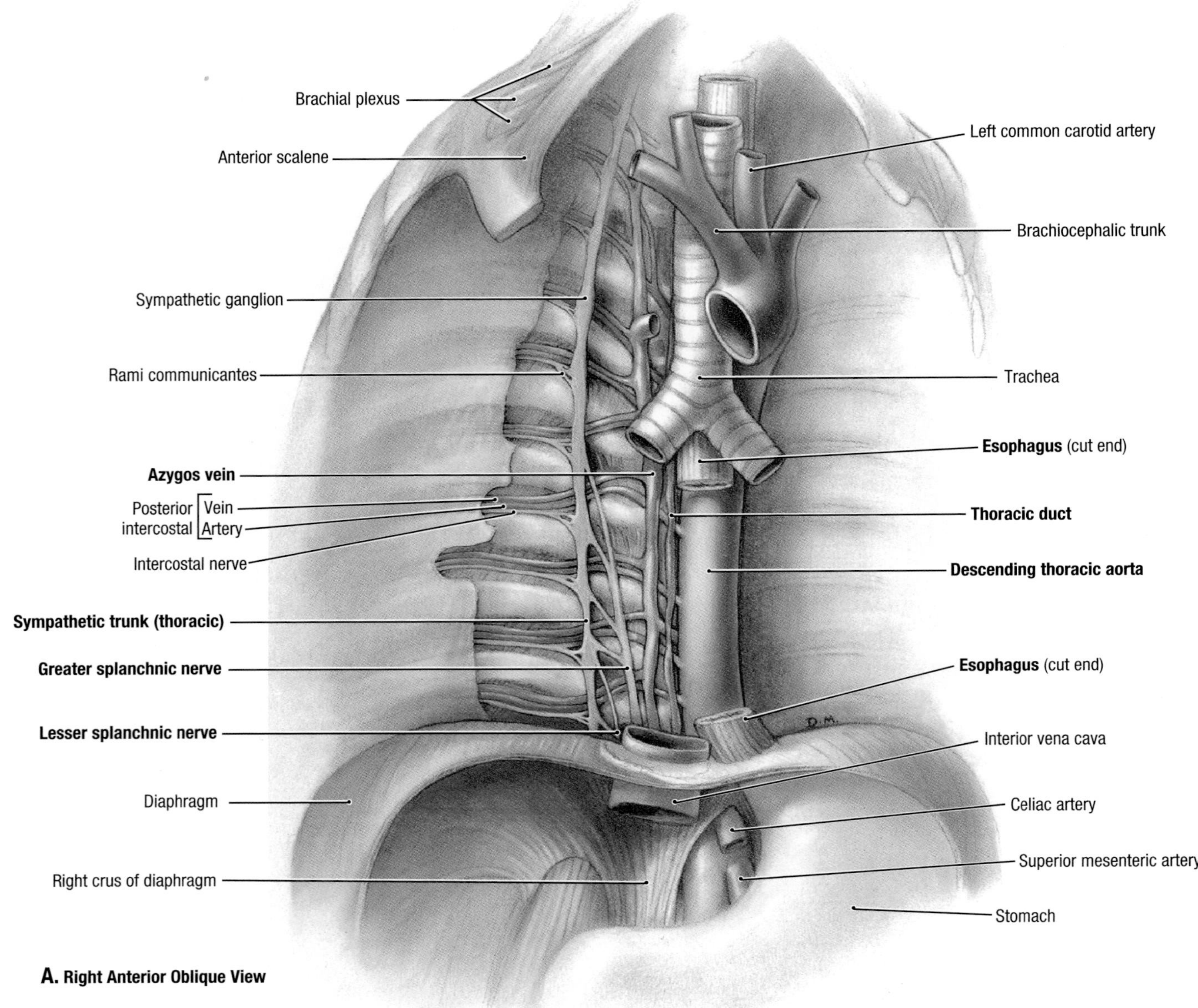
Brachial plexus
Anterior scalene
Sympathetic ganglion
Rami communicantes
Azygos vein
Posterior intercostal Vein
Posterior intercostal Artery
Intercostal nerve
Sympathetic trunk (thoracic)
Greater splanchnic nerve
Lesser splanchnic nerve
Diaphragm
Right crus of diaphragm
Left common carotid artery
Brachiocephalic trunk
Trachea
Esophagus (cut end)
Thoracic duct
Descending thoracic aorta
Esophagus (cut end)
Interior vena cava
Celiac artery
Superior mesenteric artery
Stomach
A. Right Anterior Oblique View

## 1.78 Structures of posterior mediastinum

- In this specimen, the parietal pleura is intact on the left side and partially removed on the right side. A portion of the esophagus, between the bifurcation of the trachea and the diaphragm, is also removed.
- The thoracic sympathetic trunk is connected to each intercostal nerve by rami communicantes.
- The greater splanchnic nerve is formed by fibers from the 5th to 10th thoracic ganglia, and the lesser splanchnic nerve receives fibers from the 10th and 11th thoracic ganglia. Both nerves contain presynaptic and visceral afferent fibers.
- The azygos vein ascends anterior to the intercostal vessels and to the right of the thoracic duct and aorta.

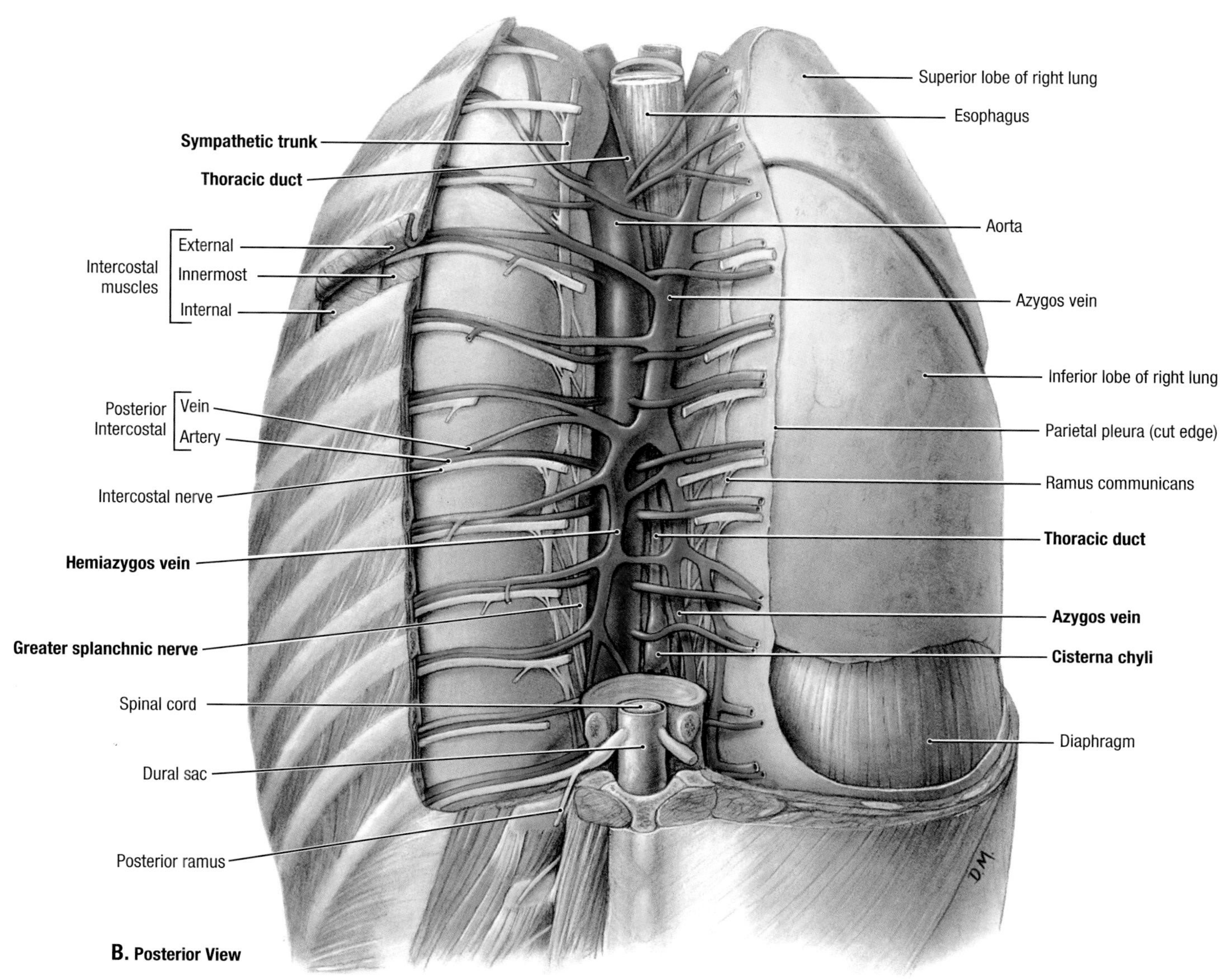
Superior lobe of right lung
Esophagus
Sympathetic trunk
Thoracic duct
Intercostal muscles
External
Innermost
Internal
Aorta
Azygos vein
Inferior lobe of right lung
Posterior Intercostal
Vein
Artery
Parietal pleura (cut edge)
Ramus communicans
Intercostal nerve
Thoracic duct
Hemiazygos vein
Azygos vein
Greater splanchnic nerve
Cisterna chyli
Spinal cord
Diaphragm
Dural sac
Posterior ramus
D.M.

**B.** Posterior View

## 1.78 Structures of posterior mediastinum *(continued)*

- The thoracic vertebral column and thoracic cage are removed on the right. On the left, the ribs and intercostal musculature are removed posteriorly as far laterally as the angles of the ribs. The parietal pleura is intact on the left side but partially removed on the right to reveal the visceral pleura covering the right lung.
- The azygos vein is on the right side, and the hemiazygos vein is on the left, crossing the midline (usually at T9, but higher in this specimen) to join the azygos vein. The accessory hemiazygos vein is absent in this specimen; instead, three most superior posterior intercostal veins drain directly into the azygos vein.

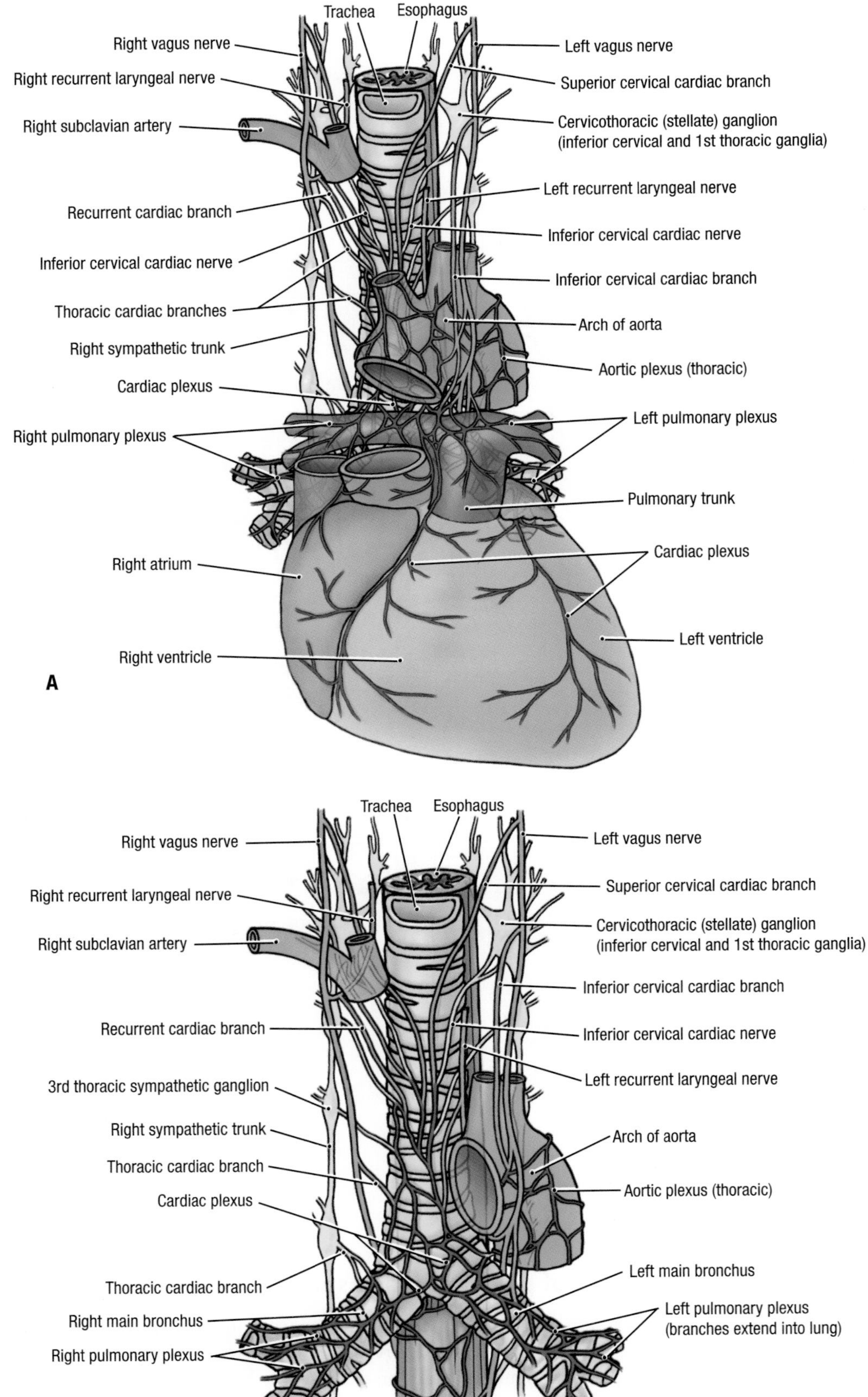
Trachea
Esophagus
Right vagus nerve
Right recurrent laryngeal nerve
Right subclavian artery
Recurrent cardiac branch
Inferior cervical cardiac nerve
Thoracic cardiac branches
Right sympathetic trunk
Cardiac plexus
Right pulmonary plexus
Right atrium
Right ventricle
A
Left vagus nerve
Superior cervical cardiac branch
Cervicothoracic (stellate) ganglion
(inferior cervical and 1st thoracic ganglia)
Left recurrent laryngeal nerve
Inferior cervical cardiac nerve
Inferior cervical cardiac branch
Arch of aorta
Aortic plexus (thoracic)
Left pulmonary plexus
Pulmonary trunk
Cardiac plexus
Left ventricle
Trachea
Esophagus
Right vagus nerve
Right recurrent laryngeal nerve
Right subclavian artery
Recurrent cardiac branch
3rd thoracic sympathetic ganglion
Right sympathetic trunk
Thoracic cardiac branch
Cardiac plexus
Thoracic cardiac branch
Right main bronchus
Right pulmonary plexus
B
Left vagus nerve
Superior cervical cardiac branch
Cervicothoracic (stellate) ganglion
(inferior cervical and 1st thoracic ganglia)
Inferior cervical cardiac branch
Inferior cervical cardiac nerve
Left recurrent laryngeal nerve
Arch of aorta
Aortic plexus (thoracic)
Left main bronchus
Left pulmonary plexus
(branches extend into lung)
Anterior Views

**1.79 Overview of autonomic innervation of thorax**

**A.** Innervation of heart. **B.** Innervation of trachea and bronchial tree.

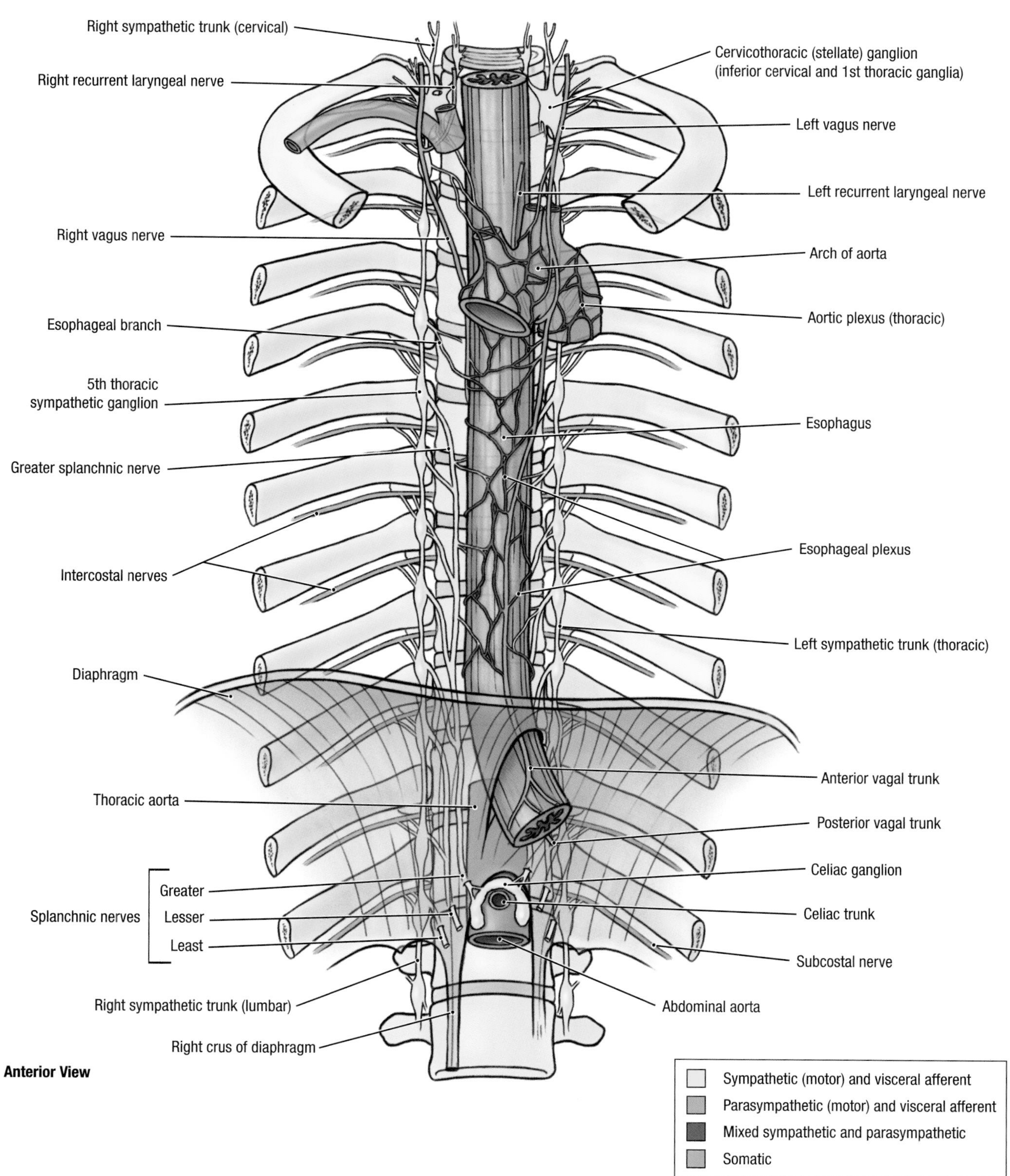
Right sympathetic trunk (cervical)
Right recurrent laryngeal nerve
Cervicothoracic (stellate) ganglion (inferior cervical and 1st thoracic ganglia)
Left vagus nerve
Left recurrent laryngeal nerve
Right vagus nerve
Arch of aorta
Aortic plexus (thoracic)
Esophageal branch
5th thoracic sympathetic ganglion
Esophagus
Greater splanchnic nerve
Esophageal plexus
Intercostal nerves
Left sympathetic trunk (thoracic)
Diaphragm
Anterior vagal trunk
Thoracic aorta
Posterior vagal trunk
Celiac ganglion
Splanchnic nerves
Greater
Lesser
Least
Celiac trunk
Subcostal nerve
Right sympathetic trunk (lumbar)
Abdominal aorta
Right crus of diaphragm
C. Anterior View
Sympathetic (motor) and visceral afferent
Parasympathetic (motor) and visceral afferent
Mixed sympathetic and parasympathetic
Somatic

**1.79 Overview of autonomic innervation of thorax *(continued)***

**C.** Innervation of posterior and superior mediastina.

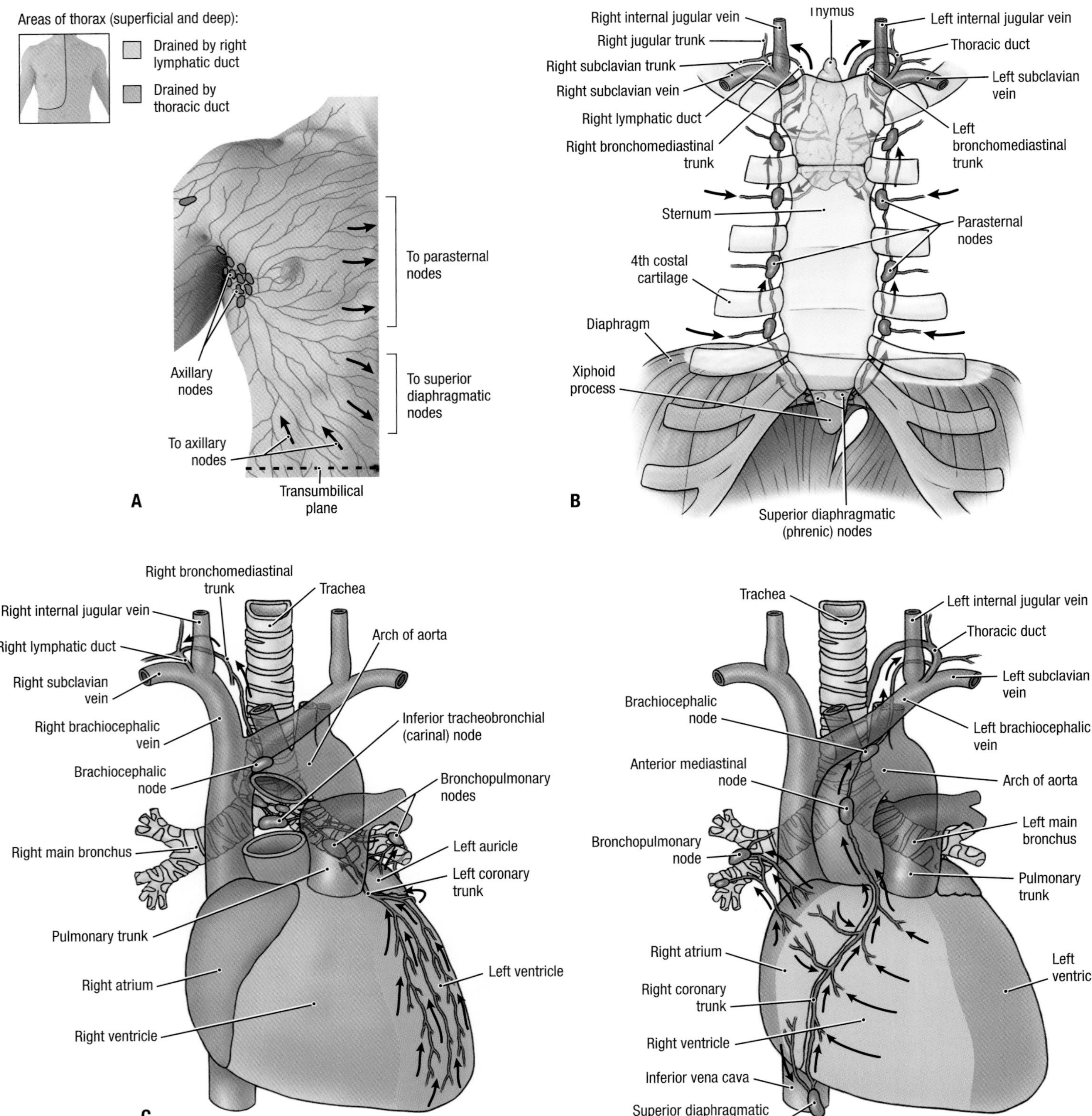
Areas of thorax (superficial and deep):
Drained by right lymphatic duct
Drained by thoracic duct
To parasternal nodes
To superior diaphragmatic nodes
Axillary nodes
To axillary nodes
Transumbilical plane
A
Right internal jugular vein
Right jugular trunk
Right subclavian trunk
Right subclavian vein
Right lymphatic duct
Right bronchomediastinal trunk
Thymus
Left internal jugular vein
Thoracic duct
Left subclavian vein
Left bronchomediastinal trunk
Sternum
Parasternal nodes
4th costal cartilage
Diaphragm
Xiphoid process
Superior diaphragmatic (phrenic) nodes
B
Right bronchomediastinal trunk
Trachea
Right internal jugular vein
Right lymphatic duct
Arch of aorta
Right subclavian vein
Right brachiocephalic vein
Inferior tracheobronchial (carinal) node
Brachiocephalic node
Bronchopulmonary nodes
Right main bronchus
Left auricle
Left coronary trunk
Pulmonary trunk
Left ventricle
Right atrium
Right ventricle
C
Area drained by left coronary trunk
Anterior Views
Trachea
Left internal jugular vein
Thoracic duct
Left subclavian vein
Brachiocephalic node
Left brachiocephalic vein
Anterior mediastinal node
Arch of aorta
Left main bronchus
Bronchopulmonary node
Pulmonary trunk
Right atrium
Left ventricle
Right coronary trunk
Right ventricle
Inferior vena cava
Superior diaphragmatic (phrenic) node
D
Area drained by right coronary trunk

## 1.80 Overview of lymphatic drainage of thorax

**A.** Superficial lymphatic drainage. **B.** Lymphatic drainage of parasternal nodes. **C.** Lymphatic drainage of left side of heart. **D.** Lymphatic drainage of right side of heart.

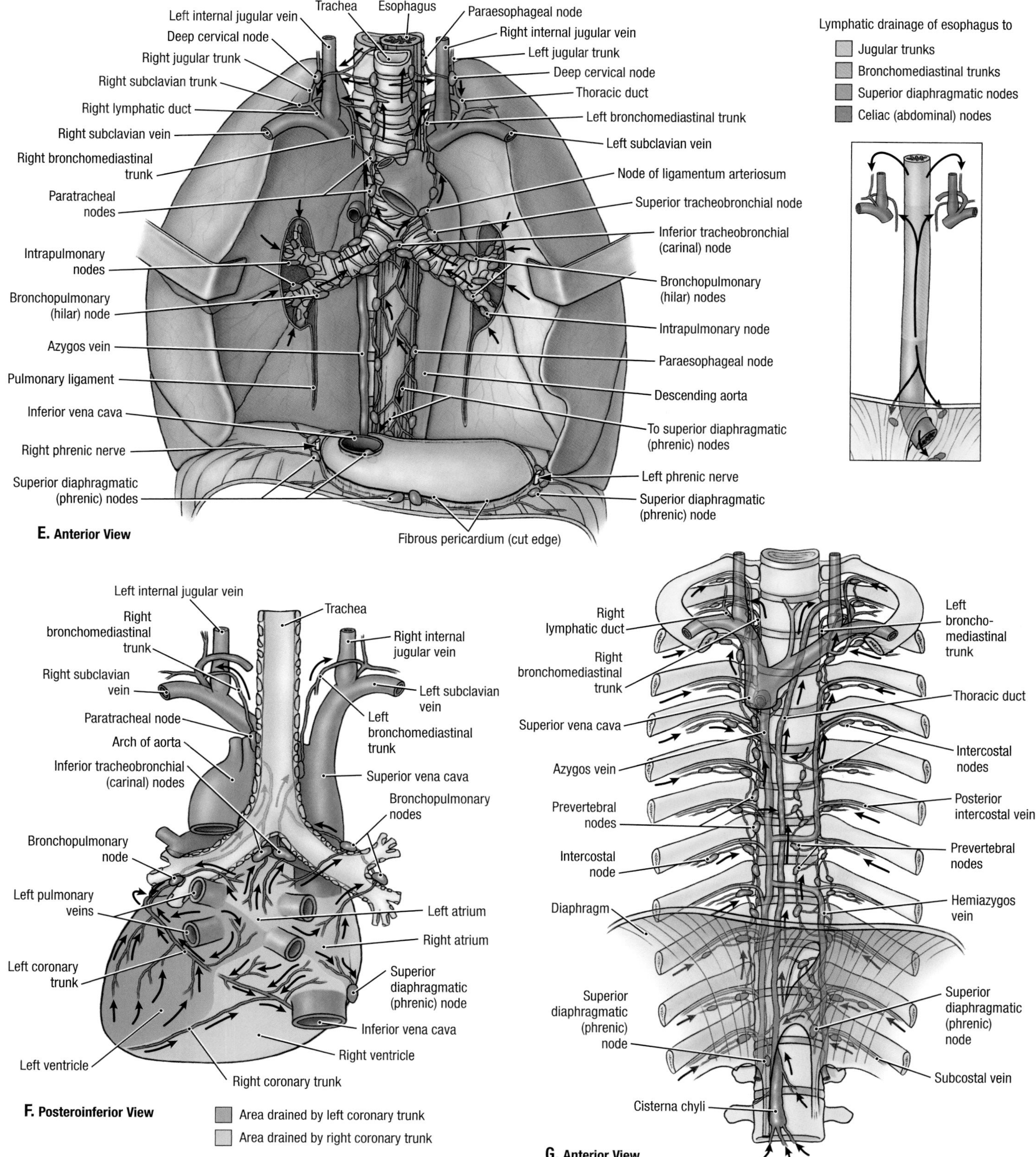
Left internal jugular vein
Trachea
Esophagus
Paraesophageal node
Deep cervical node
Right internal jugular vein
Right jugular trunk
Left jugular trunk
Right subclavian trunk
Deep cervical node
Thoracic duct
Right lymphatic duct
Left bronchomediastinal trunk
Right subclavian vein
Left subclavian vein
Right bronchomediastinal trunk
Node of ligamentum arteriosum
Paratracheal nodes
Superior tracheobronchial node
Inferior tracheobronchial (carinal) node
Intrapulmonary nodes
Bronchopulmonary (hilar) nodes
Bronchopulmonary (hilar) node
Intrapulmonary node
Azygos vein
Paraesophageal node
Pulmonary ligament
Descending aorta
Inferior vena cava
To superior diaphragmatic (phrenic) nodes
Right phrenic nerve
Left phrenic nerve
Superior diaphragmatic (phrenic) nodes
Superior diaphragmatic (phrenic) node
Fibrous pericardium (cut edge)
E. Anterior View
Lymphatic drainage of esophagus to
Jugular trunks
Bronchomediastinal trunks
Superior diaphragmatic nodes
Celiac (abdominal) nodes
Left internal jugular vein
Trachea
Right bronchomediastinal trunk
Right internal jugular vein
Right subclavian vein
Left subclavian vein
Paratracheal node
Left bronchomediastinal trunk
Arch of aorta
Inferior tracheobronchial (carinal) nodes
Superior vena cava
Bronchopulmonary nodes
Bronchopulmonary node
Left pulmonary veins
Left atrium
Right atrium
Left coronary trunk
Superior diaphragmatic (phrenic) node
Inferior vena cava
Right ventricle
Left ventricle
Right coronary trunk
F. Posteroinferior View
Area drained by left coronary trunk
Area drained by right coronary trunk
Right lymphatic duct
Left broncho-mediastinal trunk
Right bronchomediastinal trunk
Thoracic duct
Superior vena cava
Intercostal nodes
Azygos vein
Prevertebral nodes
Posterior intercostal vein
Prevertebral nodes
Intercostal node
Diaphragm
Hemiazygos vein
Superior diaphragmatic (phrenic) node
Superior diaphragmatic (phrenic) node
Subcostal vein
Cisterna chyli
G. Anterior View
Lymphatic drainage from abdomen and lower limbs

## 1.80 Overview of lymphatic drainage of thorax *(continued)*

**E.** Lymphatic drainage of lungs, esophagus, and superior surface of diaphragm. **F.** Lymphatic drainage of posterior and inferior surfaces of heart. **G.** Lymphatic drainage of posterior mediastinum.

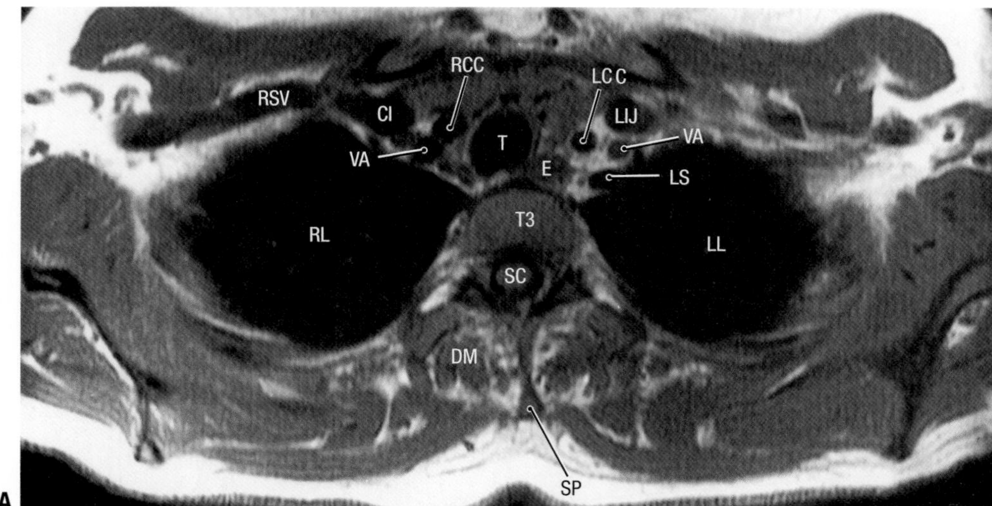
A
RCC
LCC
RSV
CI
LIJ
VA
T
VA
E
LS
T3
RL
LL
SC
DM
SP

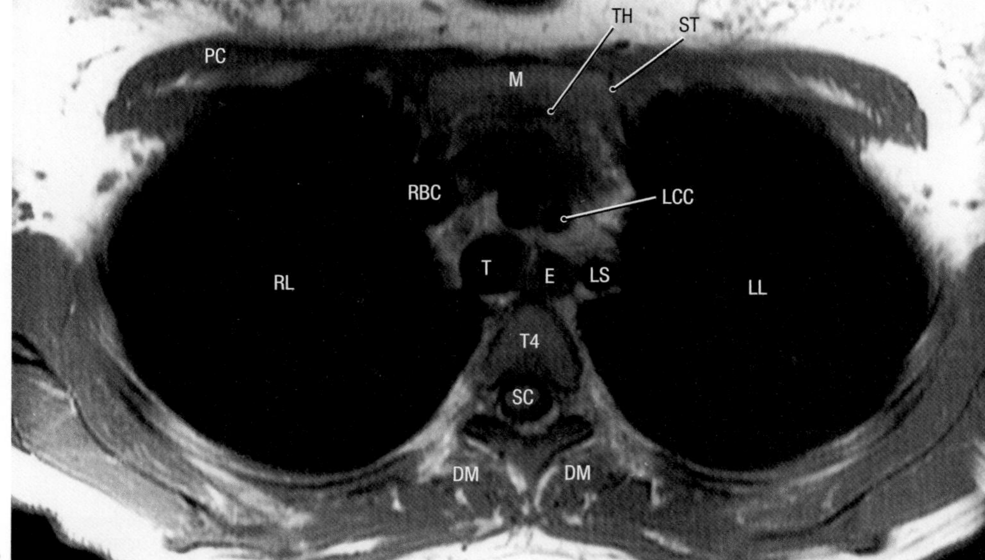
B
TH
ST
PC
M
RBC
LCC
T
E
LS
RL
LL
T4
SC
DM
DM

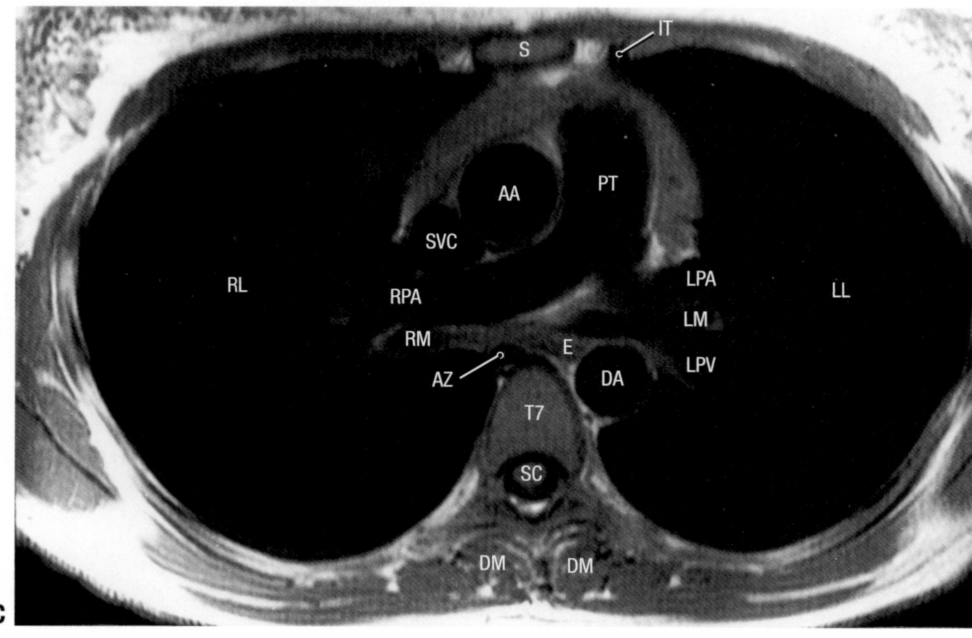
C
IT
S
AA
PT
SVC
RL
RPA
LPA
LL
LM
RM
E
LPV
AZ
DA
T7
SC
DM
DM

| | |
|---|---|
| AA | Ascending aorta |
| AI | Anterior interventricular artery |
| AZ | Azygos vein |
| CA | Cusp of aortic valve |
| CI | Confluence of internal jugular vein |
| DA | Descending aorta |
| DM | Deep back muscles |
| E | Esophagus |
| HR | Head of rib |
| HZ | Hemiazygos vein |
| IT | Internal thoracic vessels |
| IVS | Interventricular septum |
| LA | Left atrium |
| LC | Left coronary artery |
| LCC | Left common carotid artery |
| LIJ | Left internal jugular vein |
| LL | Left lung |
| LM | Left main bronchus |
| LPA | Left pulmonary artery |
| LPV | Left pulmonary vein |
| LS | Left subclavian artery |
| LV | Left vertebral artery |
| M | Manubrium |
| P | Pericardium |
| PC | Pectoralis major |
| PI | Pulmonary infundibulum |
| PM | Papillary muscle |
| PT | Pulmonary trunk |
| RA | Right atrium |
| RBC | Right brachiocephalic vein |
| RCC | Right common carotid artery |
| RL | Right lung |
| RM | Right middle lobar bronchus |
| RPA | Right pulmonary artery |
| RPV | Right pulmonary vein |
| RSV | Right subclavian vein |
| RV | Right vertebral artery |
| S | Sternum |
| SC | Spinal cord |
| SP | Spinous process |
| ST | Sternoclavicular joint |
| SVC | Superior vena cava |
| T3-T10 | Vertebral body |
| T | Trachea |
| TH | Thymus |
| VA | Vertebral artery |

**1.81 Transverse (axial) MRIs of the thorax (A–F)**

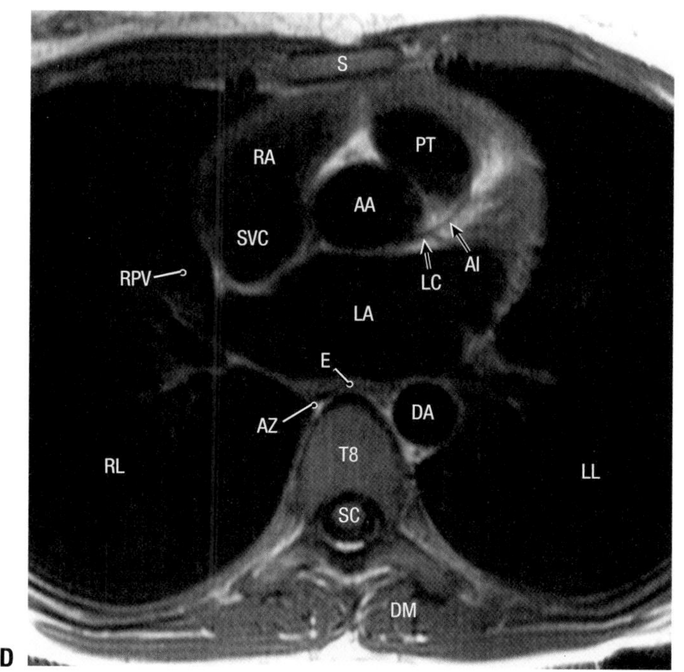
S
RA
PT
AA
SVC
RPV
LC
AI
LA
E
AZ
DA
T8
RL
LL
SC
DM
D

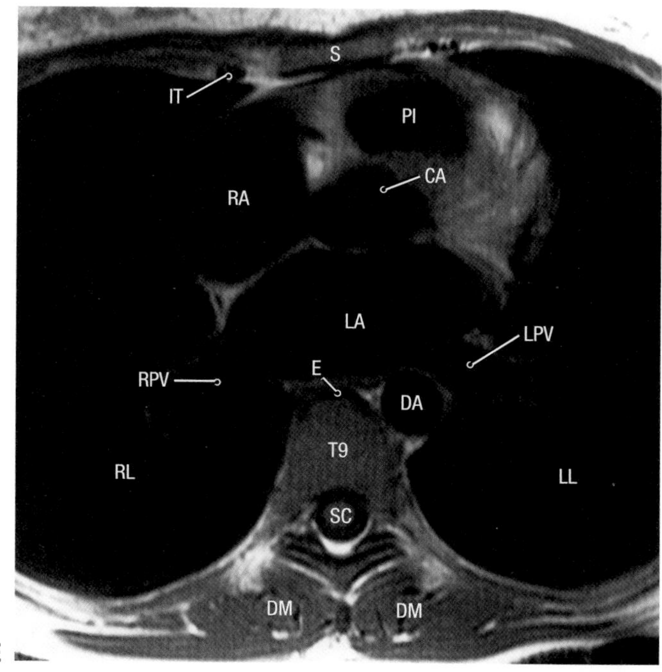
S
IT
PI
CA
RA
LA
LPV
RPV
E
DA
T9
RL
LL
SC
DM
DM
E

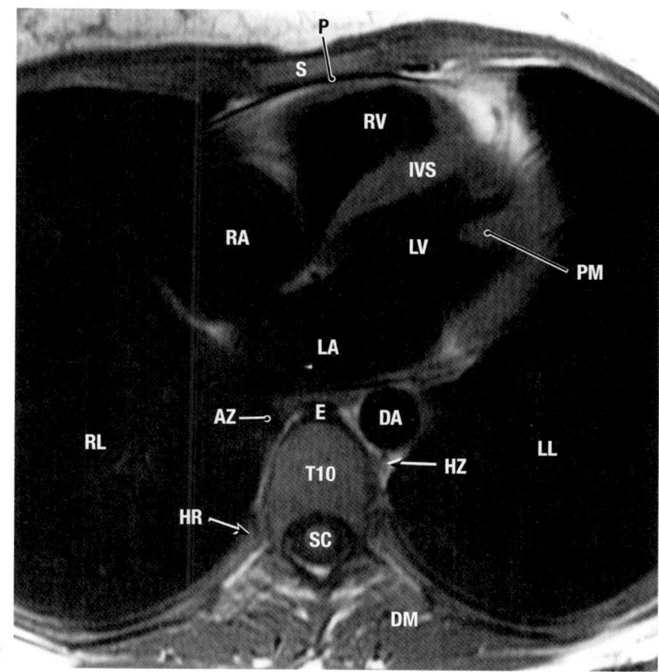
P
S
RV
IVS
RA
LV
PM
LA
AZ
E
DA
RL
LL
HZ
T10
HR
SC
DM
F

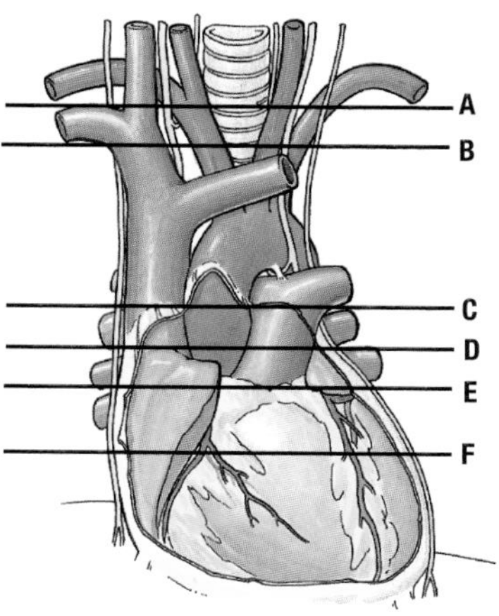
A
B
C
D
E
F

**1.81** Transverse (axial) MRIs of the thorax *(continued)*

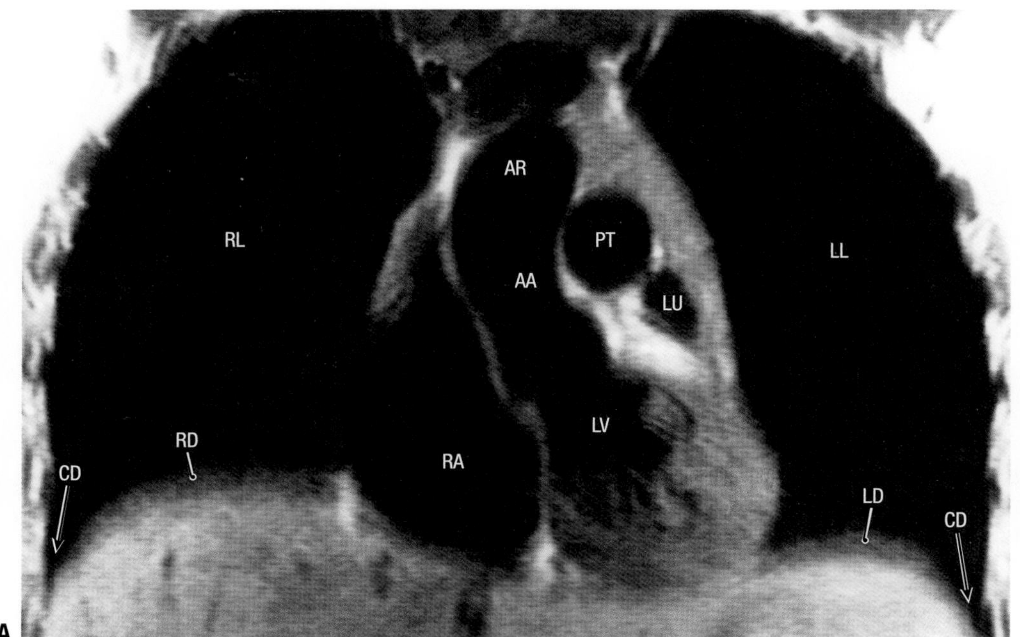
AR
PT
RL
LL
AA
LU
LV
RD
RA
CD
LD
CD
A

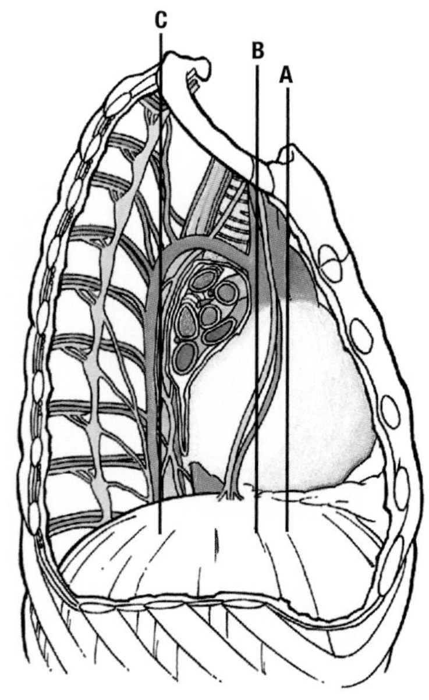
C
B
A

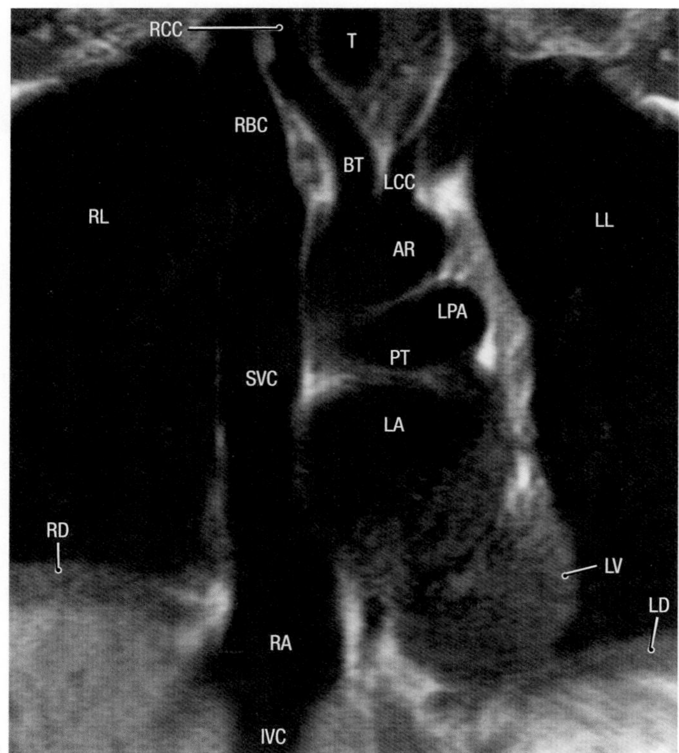
RCC
T
RBC
BT
LCC
RL
LL
AR
LPA
PT
SVC
LA
RD
LV
LD
RA
IVC
B

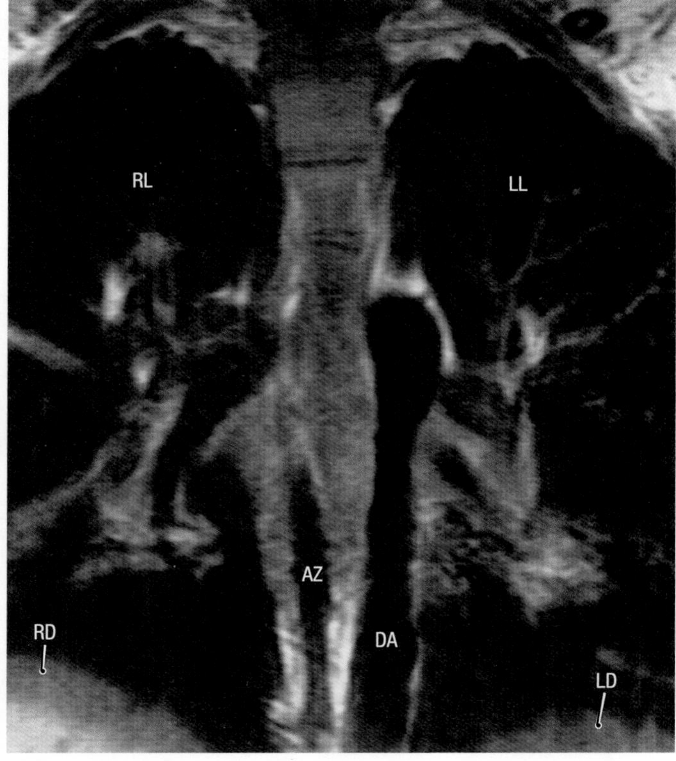
RL
LL
AZ
RD
DA
LD
C

| | | | | | | | |
|---|---|---|---|---|---|---|---|
| AA | Ascending aorta | IVC | Inferior vena cava | LU | Left auricle | RD | Right dome of diaphragm |
| AR | Arch of aorta | LA | Left atrium | LV | Left ventricle | RL | Right lung |
| AZ | Azygos vein | LCC | Left common carotid artery | PT | Pulmonary trunk | RV | Right ventricle |
| BT | Brachiocephalic trunk | LD | Left dome of diaphragm | RA | Right atrium | SVC | Superior vena cava |
| CD | Costodiaphragmatic recess | LL | Left lung | RBC | Right brachiocephalic vein | T | Trachea |
| DA | Descending aorta | LPA | Left pulmonary artery | RCC | Right common carotid artery | V | Vertebral body |

**1.82 Coronal MRIs of the thorax**

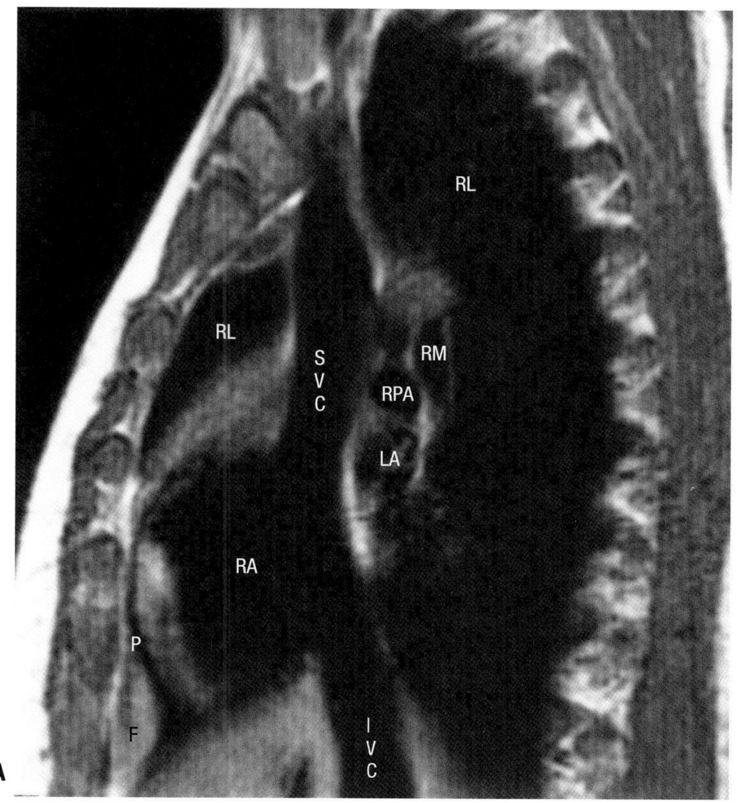
A
RL
RL
S
V
C
RM
RPA
LA
RA
P
F
I
V
C

| | |
|---|---|
| AR | Arch of aorta |
| AA | Ascending aorta |
| DA | Descending aorta |
| F | Fat |
| IVC | Inferior vena cava |
| LA | Left atrium |
| LBC | Left brachiocephalic vein |
| LCC | Left common carotid artery |
| LL | Left lung |
| LS | Left subclavian artery |
| LV | Left ventricle |
| P | Pericardium |
| RA | Right atrium |
| RL | Right lung |
| RM | Right main bronchus |
| RPA | Right pulmonary artery |
| RV | Right ventricle |
| SVC | Superior vena cava |

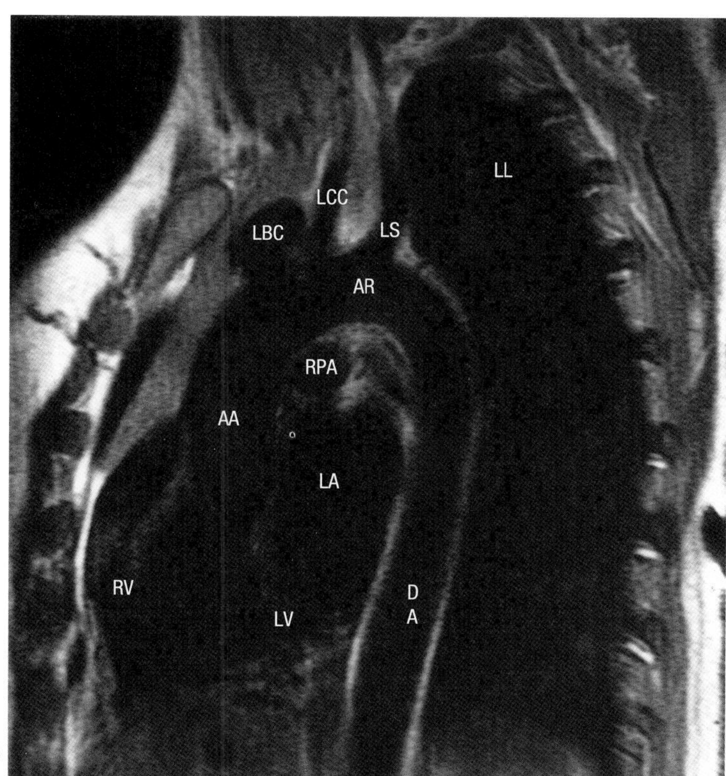
B
LL
LCC
LBC
LS
AR
RPA
AA
LA
RV
LV
D
A

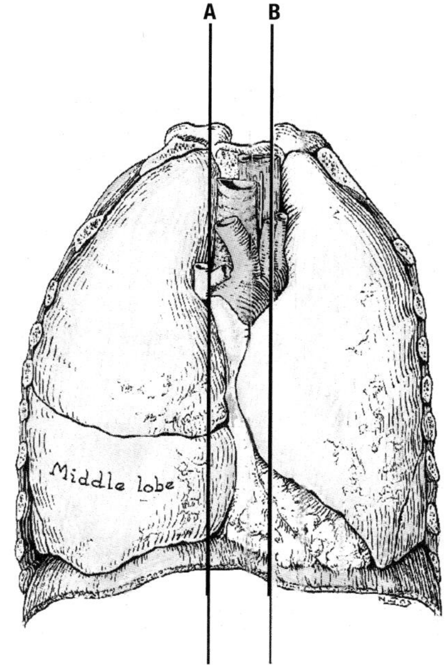
A
B
Middle lobe

**1.83 Sagittal MRIs of the thorax**

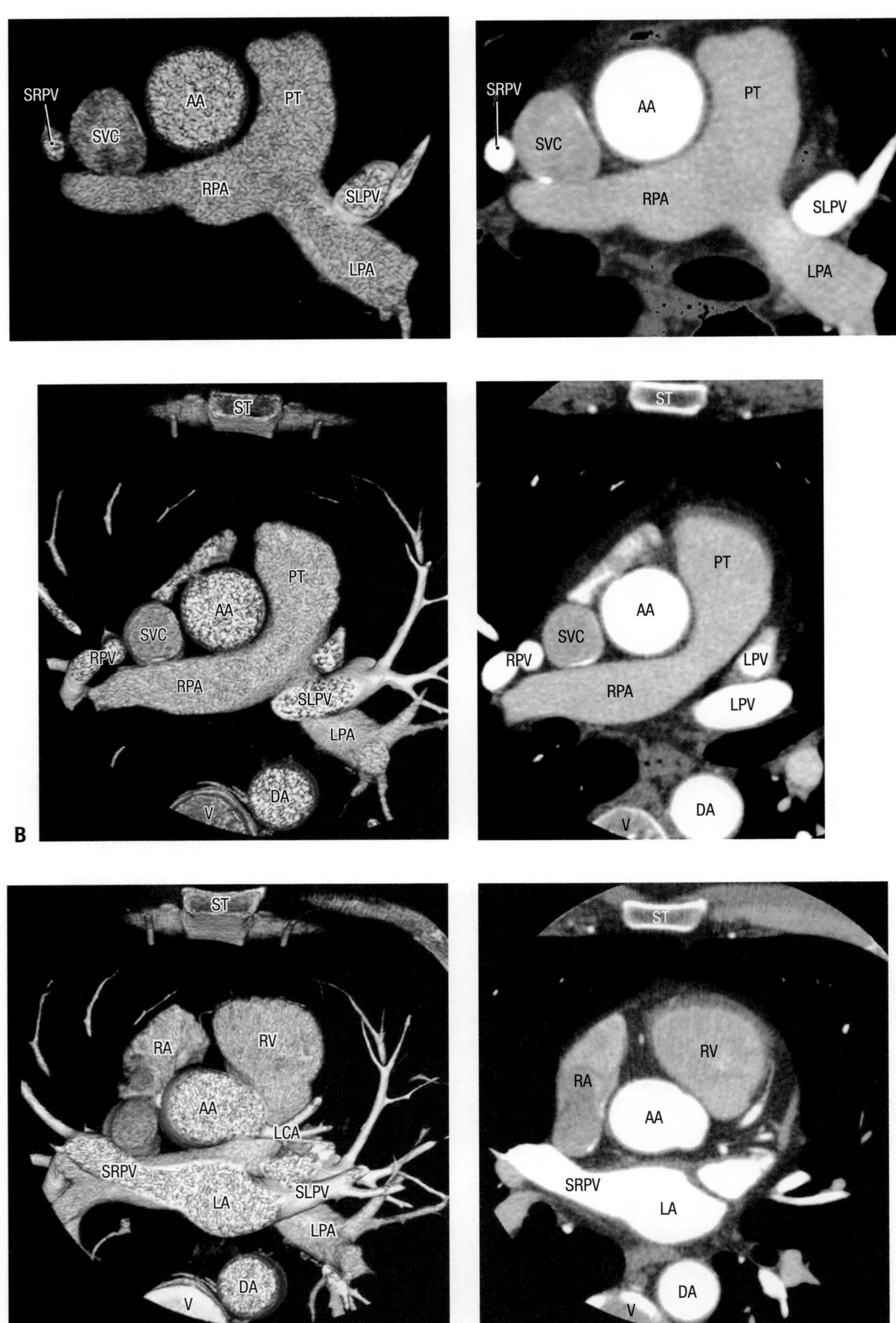
A
SRPV
AA
PT
SVC
RPA
SLPV
LPA
SRPV
AA
PT
SVC
RPA
SLPV
LPA
B
ST
PT
AA
SVC
RPV
RPA
SLPV
LPA
DA
V
ST
PT
AA
SVC
RPV
LPV
RPA
LPV
DA
V
C
ST
RA
RV
AA
LCA
SRPV
SLPV
LA
LPA
DA
V
ST
RV
RA
AA
SRPV
LA
DA
V

| | |
|---|---|
| AA | Ascending aorta |
| AZ | Azygos vein |
| DA | Descending aorta |
| E | Esophagus |
| ILPV | Inferior left pulmonary vein |
| IRPV | Inferior right pulmonary vein |
| IS | Interventricular septum |
| LA | Left atrium |
| LCA | Left coronary artery |
| LPA | Left pulmonary artery |
| LPV | Left pulmonary vein |
| LV | Left ventricle |
| MV | Mitral valve |
| PT | Pulmonary trunk |
| RA | Right atrium |
| RCA | Right coronary artery |
| RPA | Right pulmonary artery |
| RPV | Right pulmonary vein |
| RV | Right ventricle |
| SLPV | Superior left pulmonary vein |
| SRPV | Superior right pulmonary vein |
| SVC | Superior vena cava |
| V | Vertebra |
| ST | Sternum |

**1.84 Transverse or horizontal (axial) 3-D volume reconstructions (on left side of page) and CT angiograms of the thorax (A–F)** ***(continued)***

D

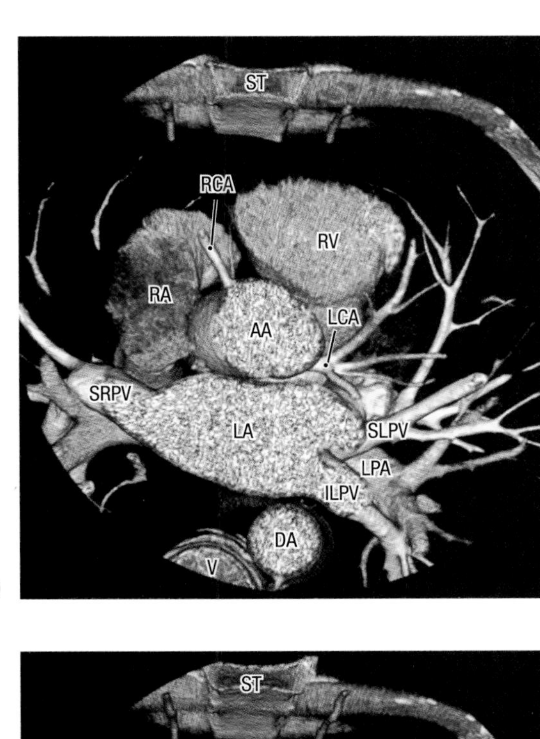
ST
RCA
RV
RA
AA
LCA
SRPV
LA
SLPV
LPA
ILPV
DA
V

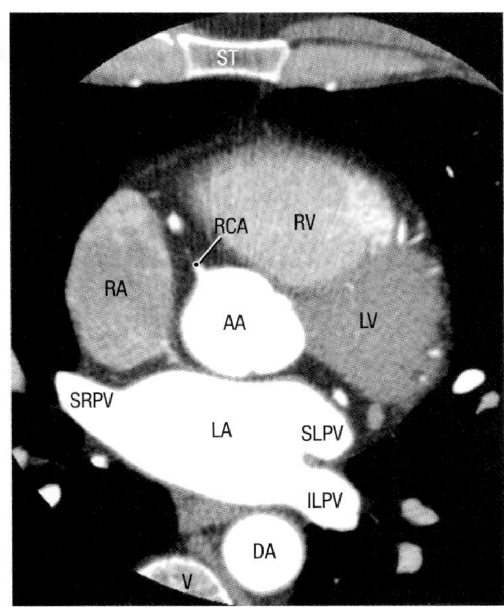
ST
RCA
RV
RA
AA
LV
SRPV
LA
SLPV
ILPV
DA
V

E

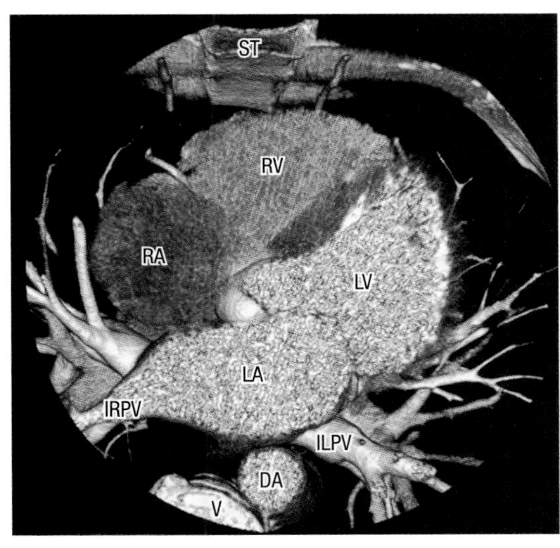
ST
RV
RA
LV
LA
IRPV
ILPV
DA
V

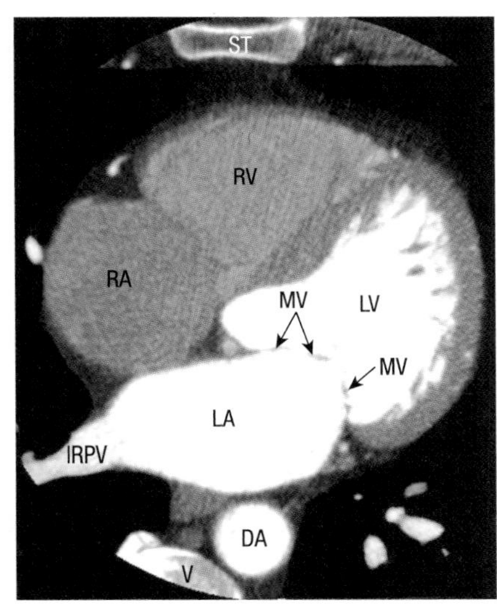
ST
RV
RA
MV
LV
MV
LA
IRPV
DA
V

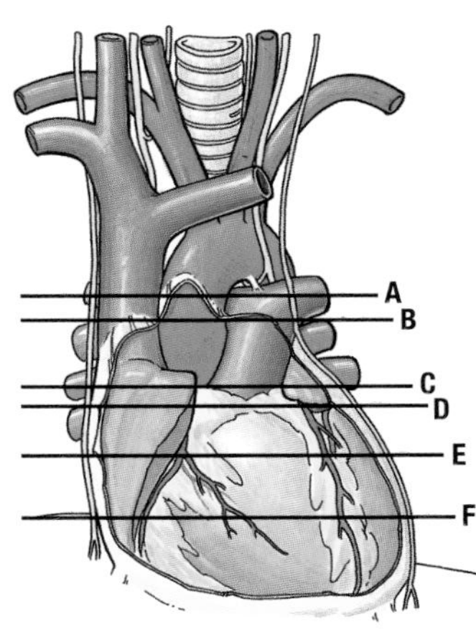
A
B
C
D
E
F

F

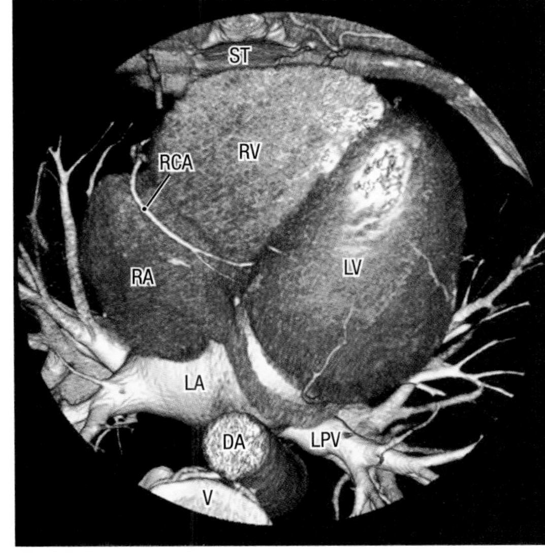
ST
RCA
RV
RA
LV
LA
DA
LPV
V

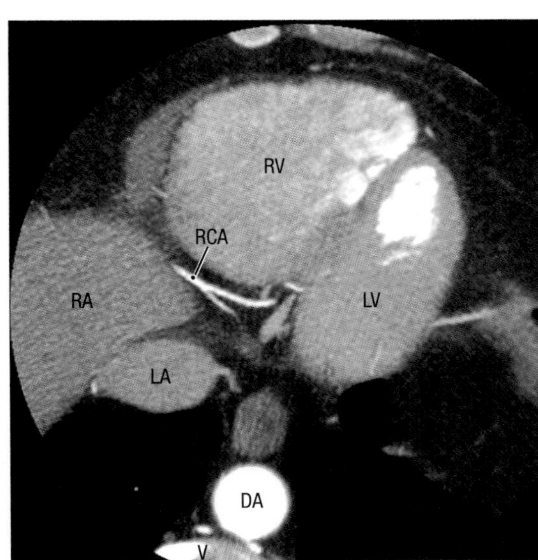
RV
RCA
RA
LV
LA
DA
V

**1.84** ***(continued)***

CHAPTER 2

# ABDOMEN

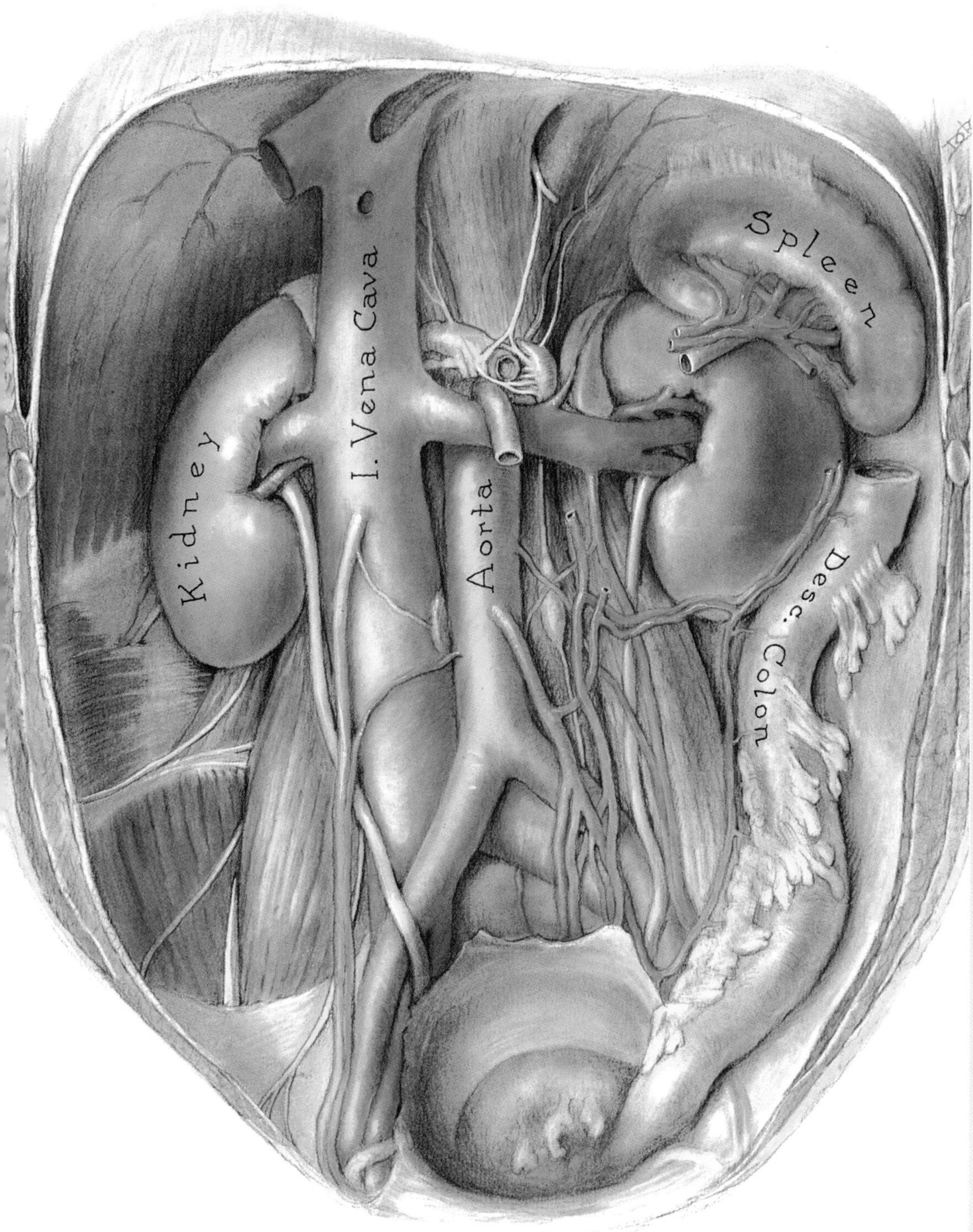
Spleen
Kidney
I. Vena Cava
Aorta
Desc. Colon


- Overview **96**
- Anterolateral Abdominal Wall **98**
- Inguinal Region **106**
- Testis **116**
- Peritoneum and Peritoneal Cavity **118**
- Digestive System **128**
- Stomach **129**
- Pancreas, Duodenum, and Spleen **131**
- Intestines **136**
- Liver and Gallbladder **146**
- Biliary Ducts **156**
- Portal Venous System **160**
- Posterior Abdominal Wall **162**
- Kidneys **164**
- Lumbar Plexus **172**
- Diaphragm **174**
- Abdominal Aorta and Inferior Vena Cava **175**
- Autonomic Innervation **176**
- Lymphatic Drainage **182**
- Sectional Anatomy and Imaging **186**

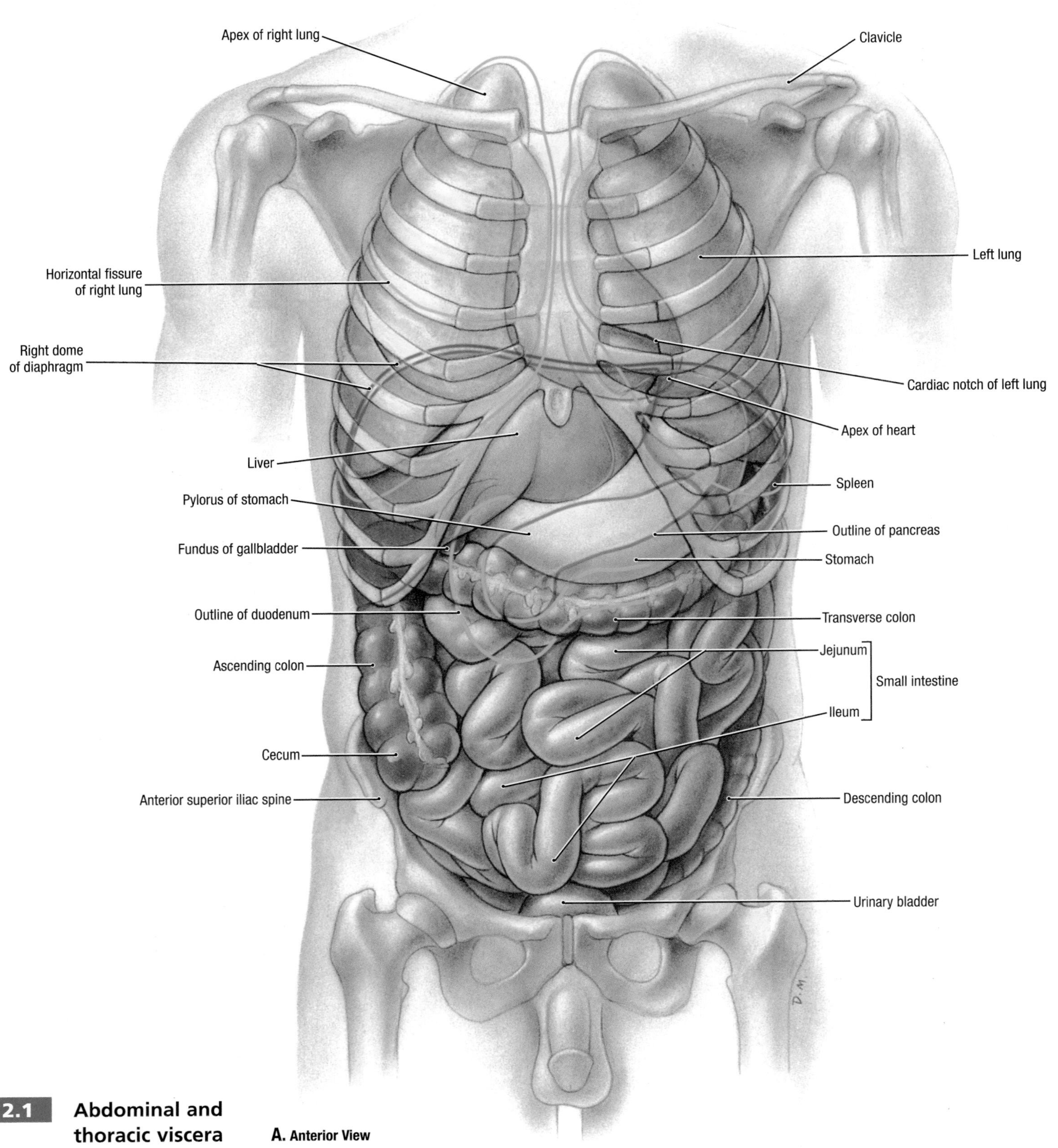
Apex of right lung
Clavicle
Left lung
Horizontal fissure of right lung
Right dome of diaphragm
Cardiac notch of left lung
Apex of heart
Liver
Spleen
Pylorus of stomach
Outline of pancreas
Fundus of gallbladder
Stomach
Outline of duodenum
Transverse colon
Jejunum
Ascending colon
Small intestine
Ileum
Cecum
Anterior superior iliac spine
Descending colon
Urinary bladder
D.M.

## 2.1 Abdominal and thoracic viscera in situ

**A. Anterior View**

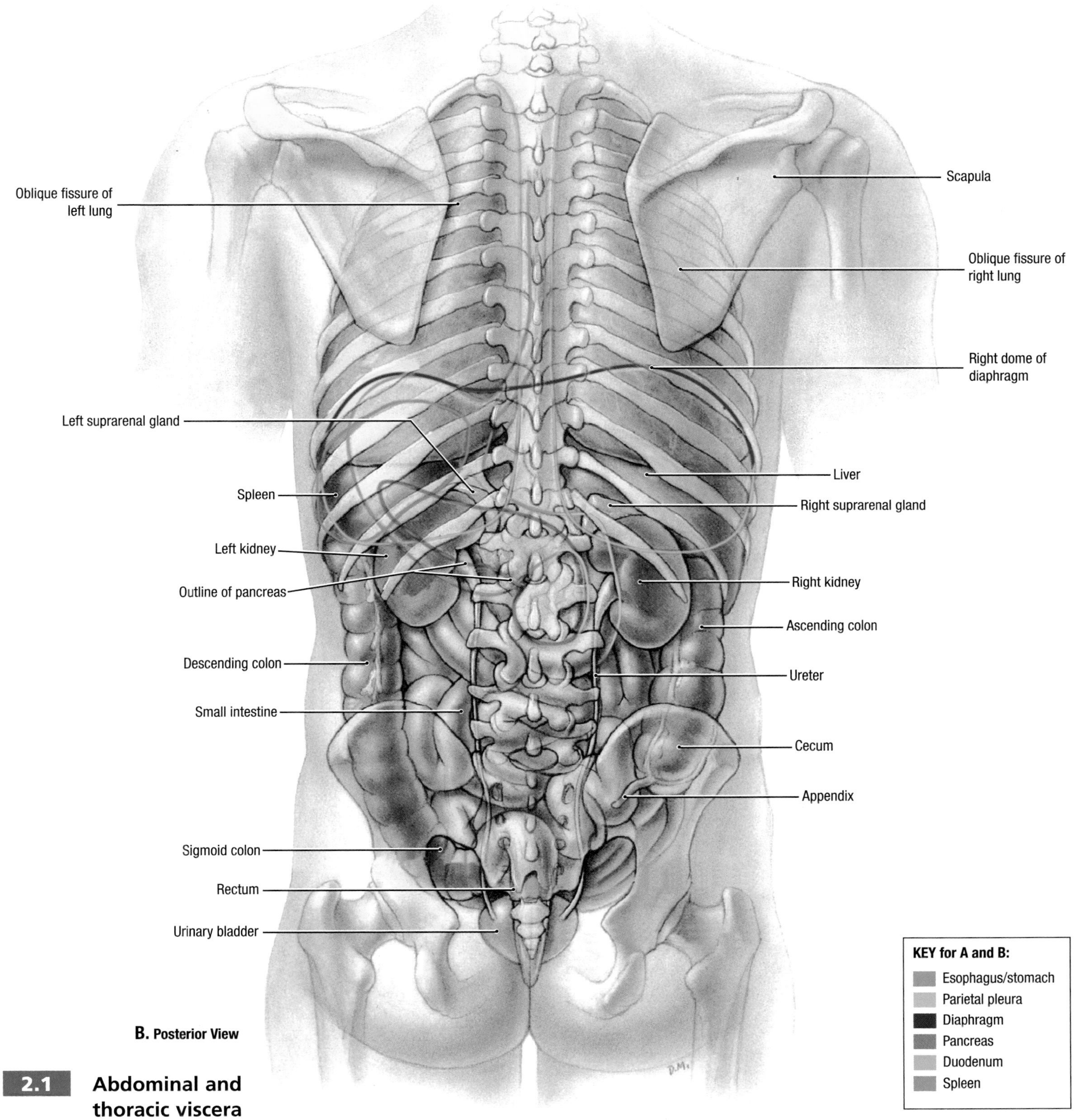

Oblique fissure of left lung
Scapula
Oblique fissure of right lung
Right dome of diaphragm
Left suprarenal gland
Liver
Spleen
Right suprarenal gland
Left kidney
Outline of pancreas
Right kidney
Ascending colon
Descending colon
Ureter
Small intestine
Cecum
Appendix
Sigmoid colon
Rectum
Urinary bladder
KEY for A and B:
Esophagus/stomach
Parietal pleura
Diaphragm
Pancreas
Duodenum
Spleen

**B.** **Posterior View**

## 2.1 Abdominal and thoracic viscera in situ *(continued)*

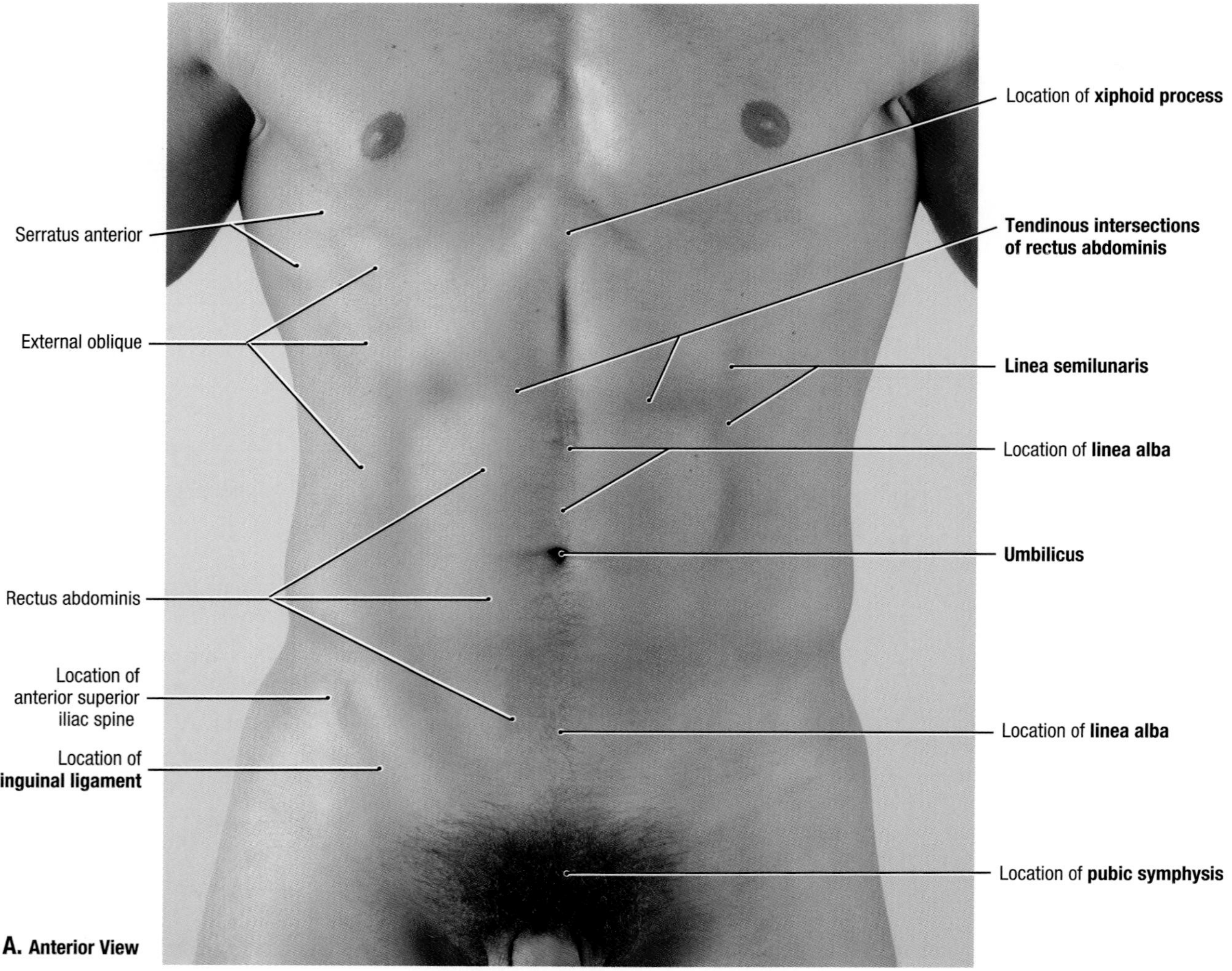
Location of **xiphoid process**
Serratus anterior
**Tendinous intersections of rectus abdominis**
External oblique
**Linea semilunaris**
Location of **linea alba**
**Umbilicus**
Rectus abdominis
Location of anterior superior iliac spine
Location of **linea alba**
Location of **inguinal ligament**
Location of **pubic symphysis**
**A.** Anterior View

## 2.2 Surface anatomy

**A.** Surface features.

- The umbilicus is where the umbilical cord entered into the fetus and indicates the level of the T10 dermatome, typically at the level of the IV disc between the L3 and L4 vertebrae.
- The linea alba is a subcutaneous fibrous band extending from the xiphoid process to the pubic symphysis that is demarcated by a midline vertical skin groove as far inferiorly as the umbilicus.
- Curved skin grooves, the linea semilunaris, demarcate the lateral borders of the rectus abdominis muscle and rectus sheath.
- Three transverse skin grooves overlie the tendinous intersections of the rectus abdominis muscle.
- The site of the inguinal ligament is indicated by a skin crease, the inguinal groove, just inferior and parallel to the ligament, marking the division between the anterolateral abdominal wall and the thigh.

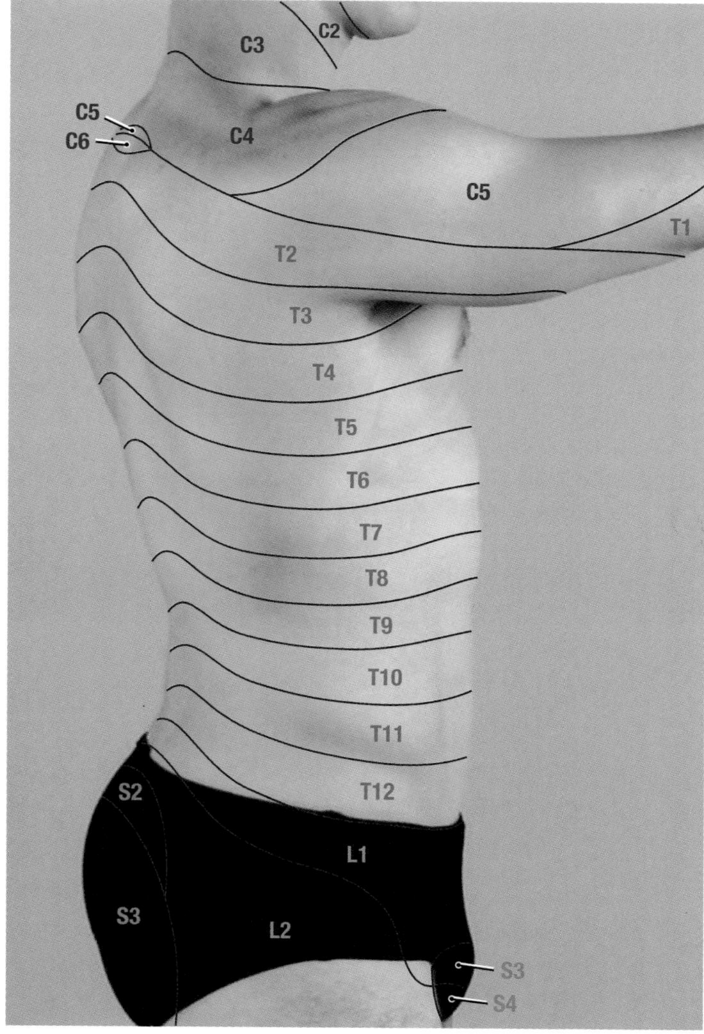
C2
C3
C5
C6
C4
C5
T1
T2
T3
T4
T5
T6
T7
T8
T9
T10
T11
T12
S2
L1
S3
L2
S3
S4

B. Lateral View

## 2.2 Surface anatomy *(continued)*

**B.** Dermatomes. The thoracoabdominal (T7–T11) nerves run between the external and internal oblique muscles to supply sensory innervation to the overlying skin. The T10 nerve supplies the region of the umbilicus. The subcostal nerve (T12) runs along the inferior border of the 12th rib to supply the skin over the anterior superior iliac spine and hip. The iliohypogastric nerve (L1) innervates the skin over the iliac crest and hypogastric region and the ilioinguinal nerve (L1), the skin of the medial aspect of the thigh, the scrotum or labium majus and mons pubis.

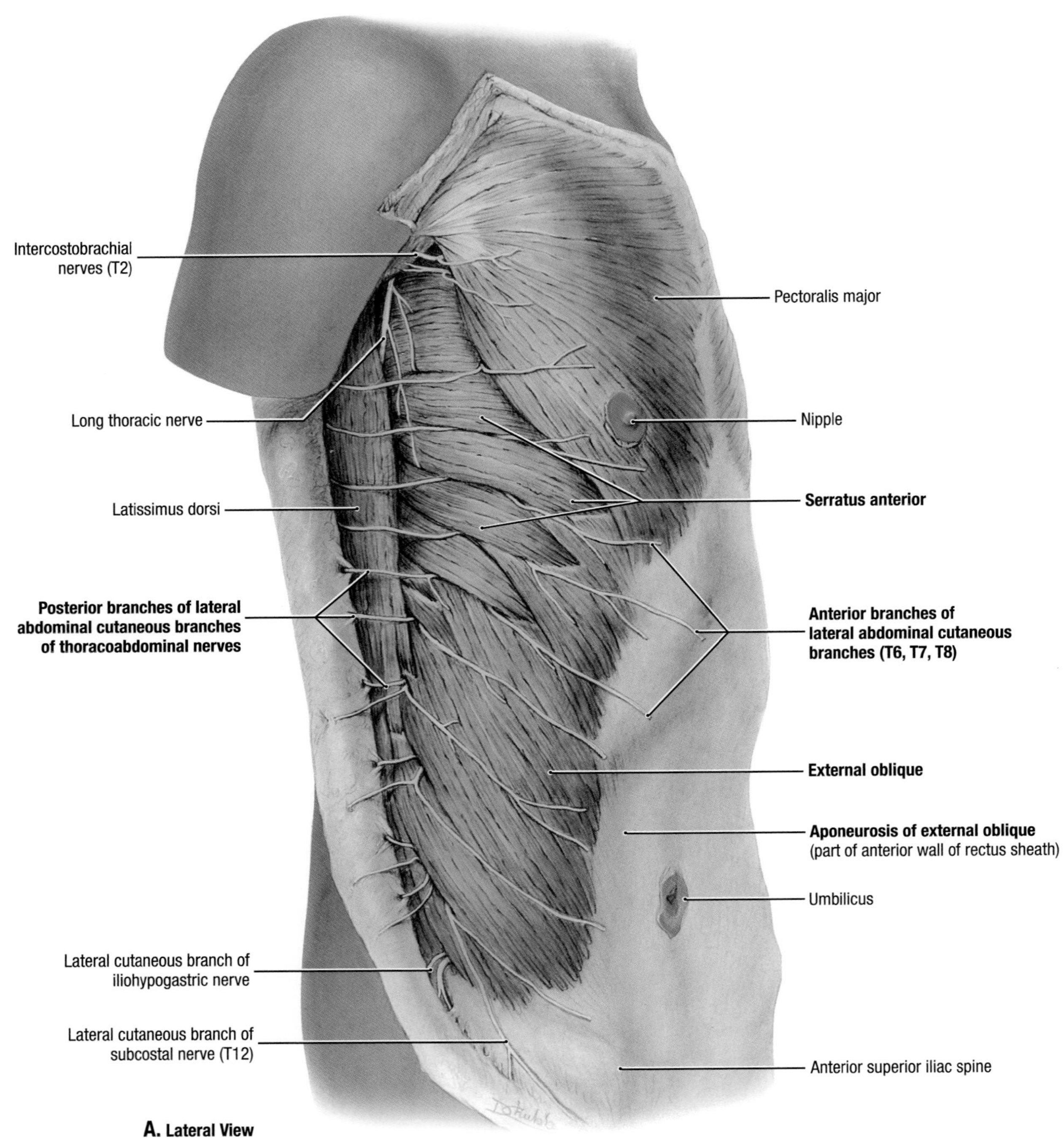
Intercostobrachial nerves (T2)
Pectoralis major
Long thoracic nerve
Nipple
Latissimus dorsi
Serratus anterior
Posterior branches of lateral abdominal cutaneous branches of thoracoabdominal nerves
Anterior branches of lateral abdominal cutaneous branches (T6, T7, T8)
External oblique
Aponeurosis of external oblique (part of anterior wall of rectus sheath)
Umbilicus
Lateral cutaneous branch of iliohypogastric nerve
Lateral cutaneous branch of subcostal nerve (T12)
Anterior superior iliac spine

**A. Lateral View**

## 2.3 Anterolateral abdominal wall, superficial dissection

The muscular portion of the external oblique muscle interdigitates with slips of the serratus anterior muscle, and the aponeurotic portion contributes to the anterior wall of the rectus sheath. The anterior and posterior branches of the lateral abdominal cutaneous branches of the thoracoabdominal nerves course superficially in the subcutaneous tissue.

- Umbilical hernias are usually small protrusions of extraperitoneal fat and/or peritoneum and omentum and sometimes bowel. They result from increased intraabdominal pressure in the presence of weakness or incomplete closure of the anterior abdominal wall after ligation of the umbilical cord at birth, or may be acquired later, most commonly in women and obese people.
- The lines along which the fibers of the abdominal aponeurosis interlace (see Fig. 2.6**A, B** & **D**) are also potential sites of herniation. These gaps may be congenital, the result of the stresses of obesity and aging, or the consequence of surgical or traumatic wounds.

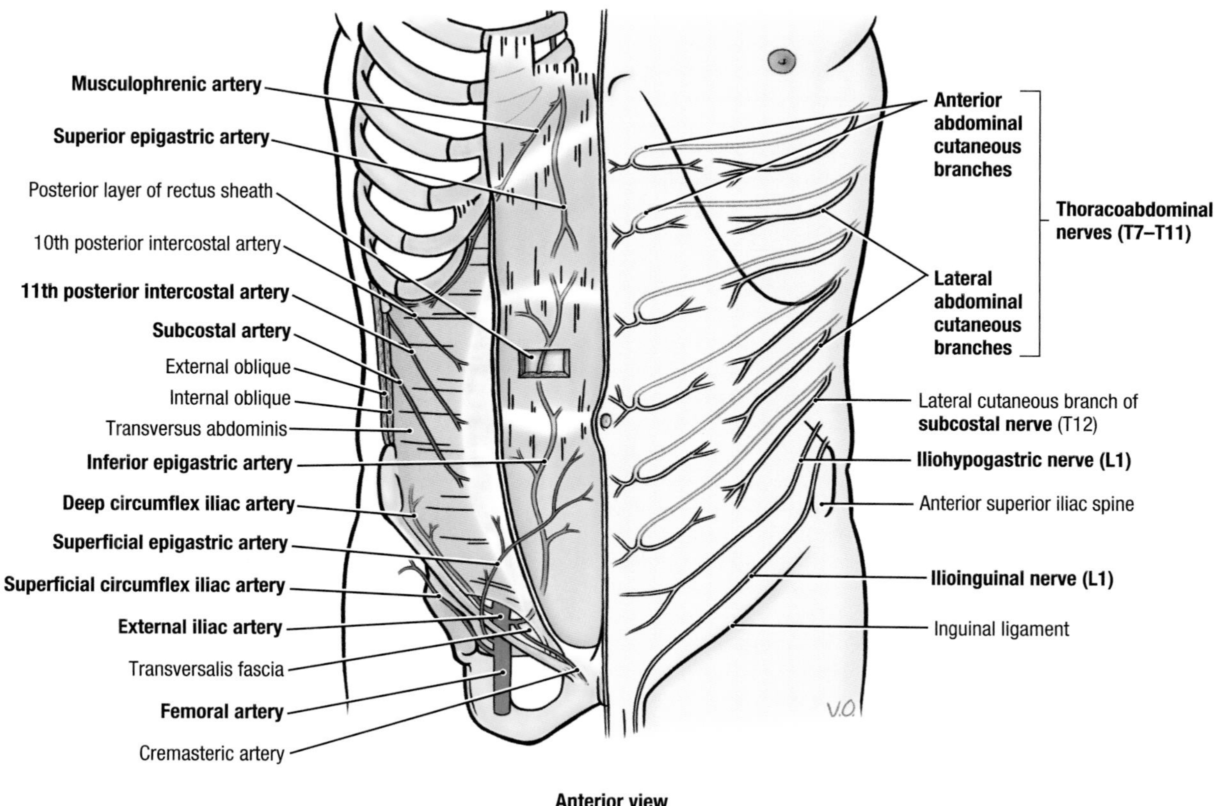
Musculophrenic artery
Superior epigastric artery
Posterior layer of rectus sheath
10th posterior intercostal artery
11th posterior intercostal artery
Subcostal artery
External oblique
Internal oblique
Transversus abdominis
Inferior epigastric artery
Deep circumflex iliac artery
Superficial epigastric artery
Superficial circumflex iliac artery
External iliac artery
Transversalis fascia
Femoral artery
Cremasteric artery
Anterior abdominal cutaneous branches
Thoracoabdominal nerves (T7–T11)
Lateral abdominal cutaneous branches
Lateral cutaneous branch of subcostal nerve (T12)
Iliohypogastric nerve (L1)
Anterior superior iliac spine
Ilioinguinal nerve (L1)
Inguinal ligament
V.O.
Anterior view

## 2.4 Arteries and nerves of anterolateral abdominal wall

The skin and muscles of the anterolateral abdominal wall are supplied mainly by the:

- Thoracoabdominal nerves: distal, abdominal parts of the anterior rami of the inferior six thoracic spinal nerves (T7–T11), which have muscular branches and anterior and lateral abdominal cutaneous branches. The anterior abdominal cutaneous branches pierce the rectus sheath a short distance from the median plane, after the rectus abdominis muscle has been supplied. Spinal nerves T7–T9 supply the skin superior to the umbilicus; T10 innervates the skin around the umbilicus.
- Subcostal nerve: large anterior ramus of spinal nerve T12.
- Iliohypogastric and ilioinguinal nerves: terminal branches of the anterior ramus of spinal nerve L1.
- Spinal nerve T11, plus the cutaneous branches of the subcostal (T12), iliohypogastric, and ilioinguinal (L1) nerves: supply the skin inferior to the umbilicus.

The blood vessels of the anterolateral abdominal wall are the:

- Superior epigastric vessels and branches of the musculophrenic vessels from the internal thoracic vessels.
- Inferior epigastric and deep circumflex iliac vessels from the external iliac vessels.
- Superficial circumflex iliac and superficial epigastric vessels from the femoral artery and great saphenous vein.
- Posterior intercostal vessels in the 11th intercostal space and anterior branches of subcostal vessels.

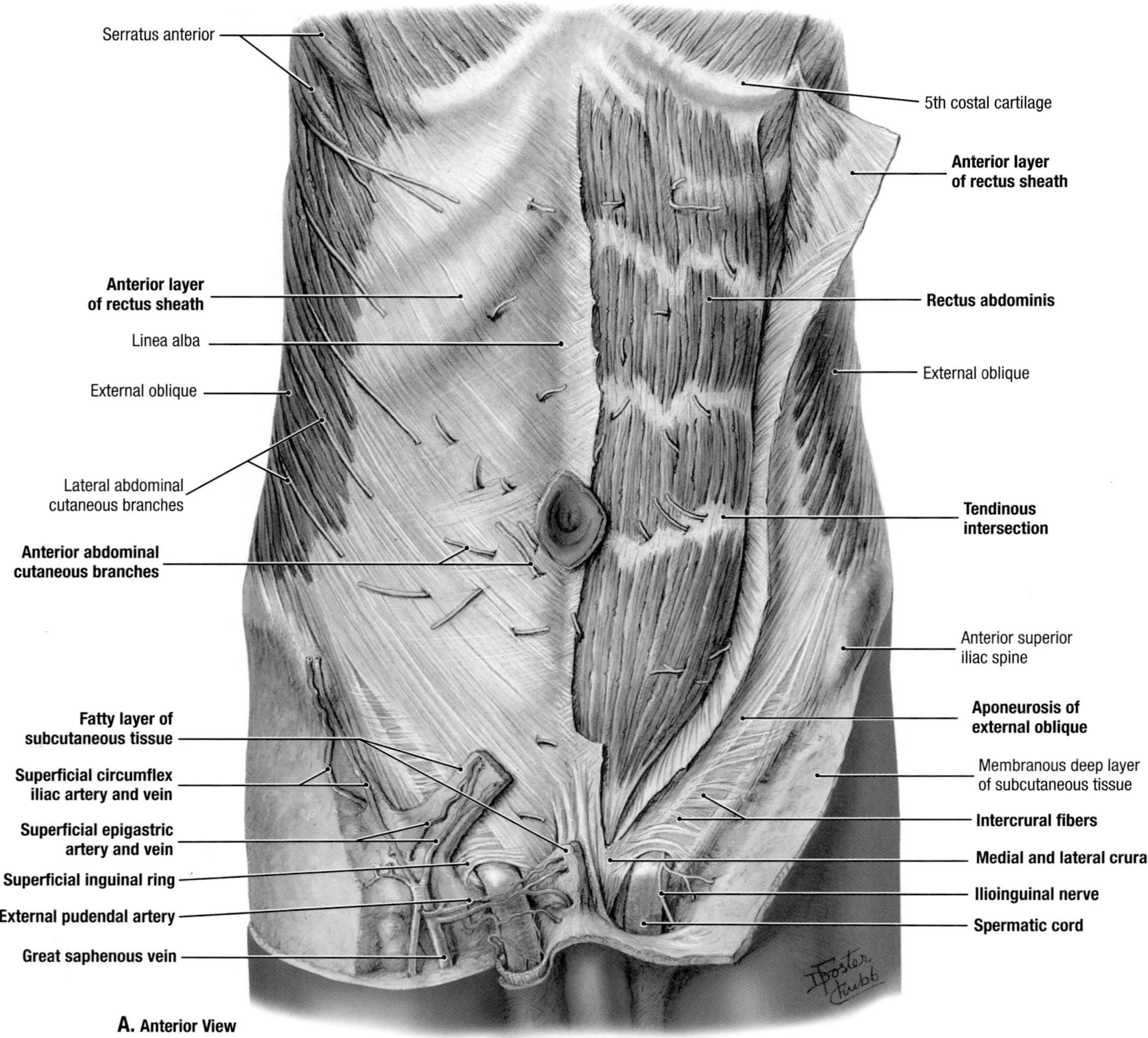
Serratus anterior
5th costal cartilage
Anterior layer of rectus sheath
Anterior layer of rectus sheath
Rectus abdominis
Linea alba
External oblique
External oblique
Lateral abdominal cutaneous branches
Tendinous intersection
Anterior abdominal cutaneous branches
Anterior superior iliac spine
Aponeurosis of external oblique
Fatty layer of subcutaneous tissue
Membranous deep layer of subcutaneous tissue
Superficial circumflex iliac artery and vein
Intercrural fibers
Superficial epigastric artery and vein
Medial and lateral crura
Superficial inguinal ring
Ilioinguinal nerve
External pudendal artery
Spermatic cord
Great saphenous vein

**A.** Anterior View

## 2.5 Anterior abdominal wall

**A.** Superficial dissection demonstrating the relationship of the cutaneous nerves and superficial vessels to the musculoaponeurotic structures. The anterior wall of the left rectus sheath is reflected, revealing the rectus abdominis muscle, segmented by tendinous intersections.

- After the T7 to T12 spinal nerves supply the muscles, their anterior abdominal cutaneous branches emerge from the rectus abdominis muscle and pierce the anterior wall of its sheath.
- The three superficial inguinal branches of the femoral artery (superficial circumflex iliac artery, superficial epigastric artery, and external pudendal artery) and the great saphenous vein lie in the fatty layer of subcutaneous tissue.
- The fibers of the external oblique aponeurosis separate into medial and lateral crura which, with the intercrural fibers that unite them, form the superficial inguinal ring. The spermatic cord of the male (shown here), or round ligament of the female, exit the inguinal canal through the superficial inguinal ring along with the ilioinguinal nerve.

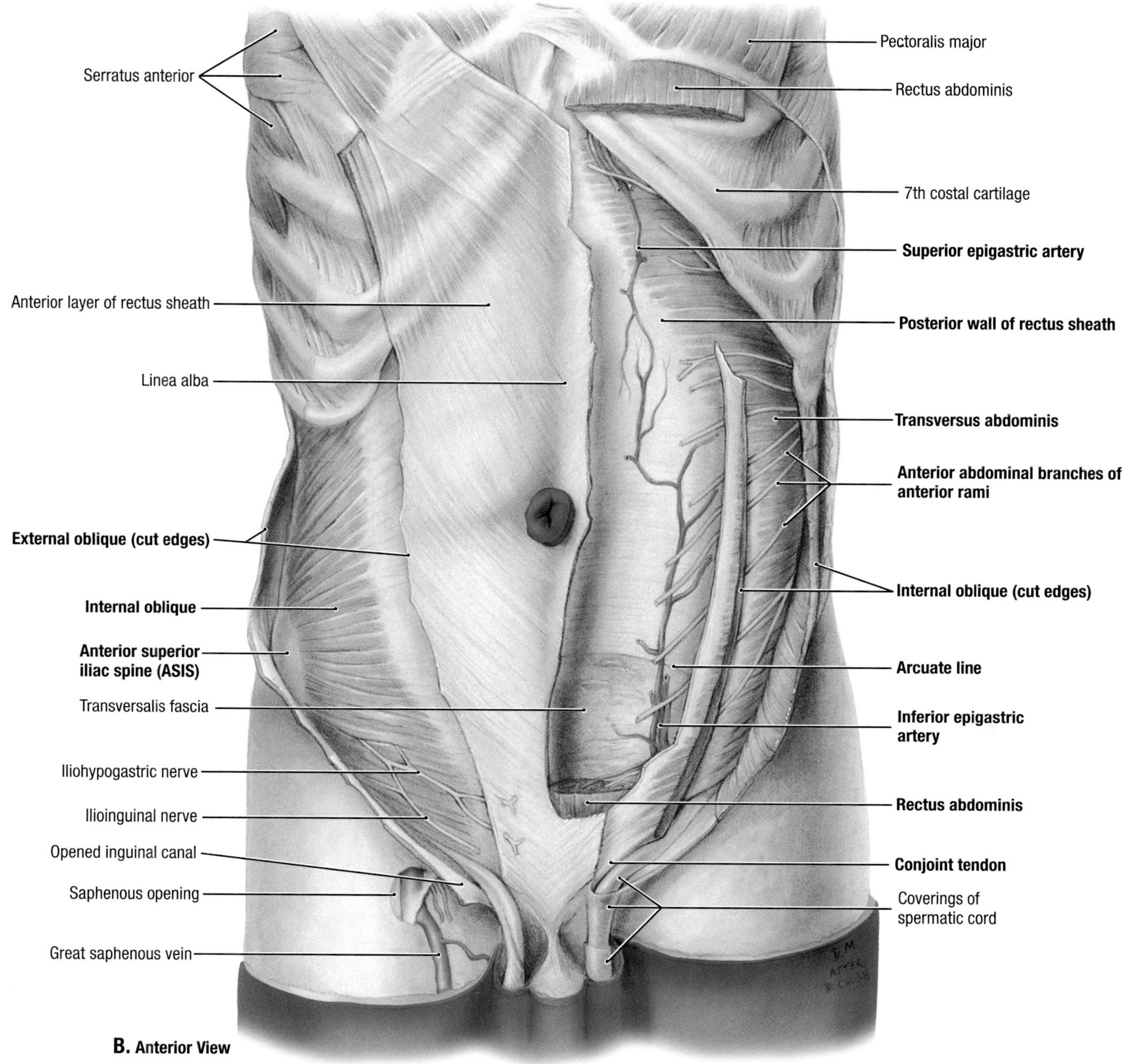
Serratus anterior
Anterior layer of rectus sheath
Linea alba
External oblique (cut edges)
Internal oblique
Anterior superior iliac spine (ASIS)
Transversalis fascia
Iliohypogastric nerve
Ilioinguinal nerve
Opened inguinal canal
Saphenous opening
Great saphenous vein
Pectoralis major
Rectus abdominis
7th costal cartilage
Superior epigastric artery
Posterior wall of rectus sheath
Transversus abdominis
Anterior abdominal branches of anterior rami
Internal oblique (cut edges)
Arcuate line
Inferior epigastric artery
Rectus abdominis
Conjoint tendon
Coverings of spermatic cord

**B.** Anterior View

## 2.5 Anterior abdominal wall *(continued)*

**B.** Deep dissection. On the right side of the specimen, most of the external oblique muscle is excised. On the left, the internal oblique muscle is divided and the rectus abdominis muscle is excised, revealing the posterior wall of the rectus sheath.

- The fibers of the internal oblique muscle run horizontally at the level of the anterior superior iliac spine (ASIS), obliquely upward superior to the ASIS, and obliquely downward inferior to the ASIS.
- The arcuate line is at the level of the ASIS; inferior to the line, only transversalis fascia lies posterior to the rectus abdominis muscle.
- Initially, the anterior abdominal branches of the anterior rami course between the internal oblique and transversus abdominis muscles.
- The anastomosis between the superior and inferior epigastric arteries indirectly unites the subclavian artery of the upper limb to the external iliac arteries of the lower limb. The anastomosis can become functionally patent in response to slowly developing occlusion of the aorta.

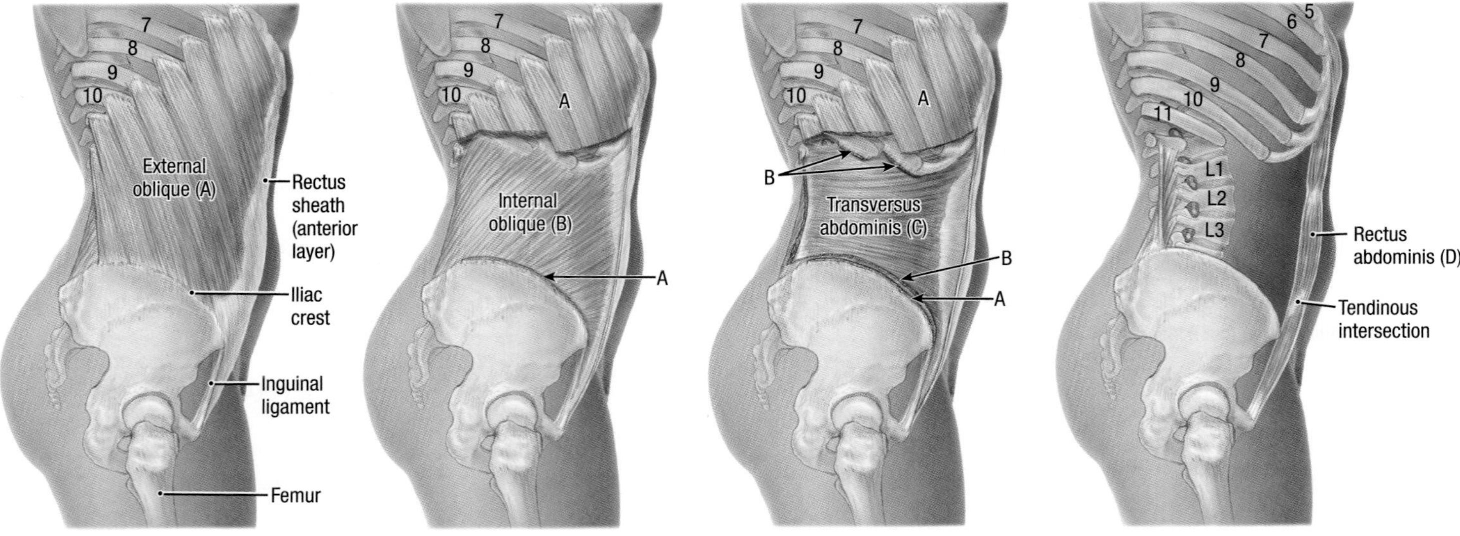
7
8
9
10
External oblique (A)
Rectus sheath (anterior layer)
Iliac crest
Inguinal ligament
Femur
7
8
9
10
A
Internal oblique (B)
A
7
8
9
10
A
B
Transversus abdominis (C)
B
A
5
6
7
8
9
10
11
L1
L2
L3
Rectus abdominis (D)
Tendinous intersection

**TABLE 2.1 PRINCIPAL MUSCLES OF ANTEROLATERAL ABDOMINAL WALL**

| Muscles[a] | Origin | Insertion | Innervation | Action(s) |
|---|---|---|---|---|
| External oblique (A) | External surfaces of 5th–12th ribs | Linea alba, pubic tubercle, and anterior half of iliac crest | Thoracoabdominal nerves (T7–T11) and subcostal nerve | Compresses and supports abdominal viscera[b]; flexes and rotates trunk |
| Internal oblique (B) | Thoracolumbar fascia, anterior two thirds of iliac crest | Inferior borders of 10th–12th ribs, linea alba, and pubis via conjoint tendon | | |
| Transversus abdominis (C) | Internal surfaces of 7th–12th costal cartilages, thoracolumbar fascia, iliac crest, and lateral third of inguinal ligament | Linea alba with aponeurosis of internal oblique, pubic crest, and pecten pubis via conjoint tendon | Thoracoabdominal (T7–T11), subcostal and first lumbar nerves | Compresses and supports abdominal viscera[b] |
| Rectus abdominis (D) | Pubic symphysis and pubic crest | Xiphoid process and 5th–7th costal cartilages | Thoracoabdominal nerves and anterior rami of inferior thoracic nerves | Flexes trunk (lumbar vertebrae) and compresses abdominal viscera[b]; stabilizes and controls tilt of pelvis (antilordosis) |

[a]Approximately 80% of people have a pyramidal muscle, which is located in the rectus sheath anterior to the most inferior part of the rectus abdominis. It extends from the pubic crest of the hip bone to the linea alba. This small muscle draws down on the linea alba.

[b]In so doing, these muscles act as antagonists of the diaphragm to produce expiration.

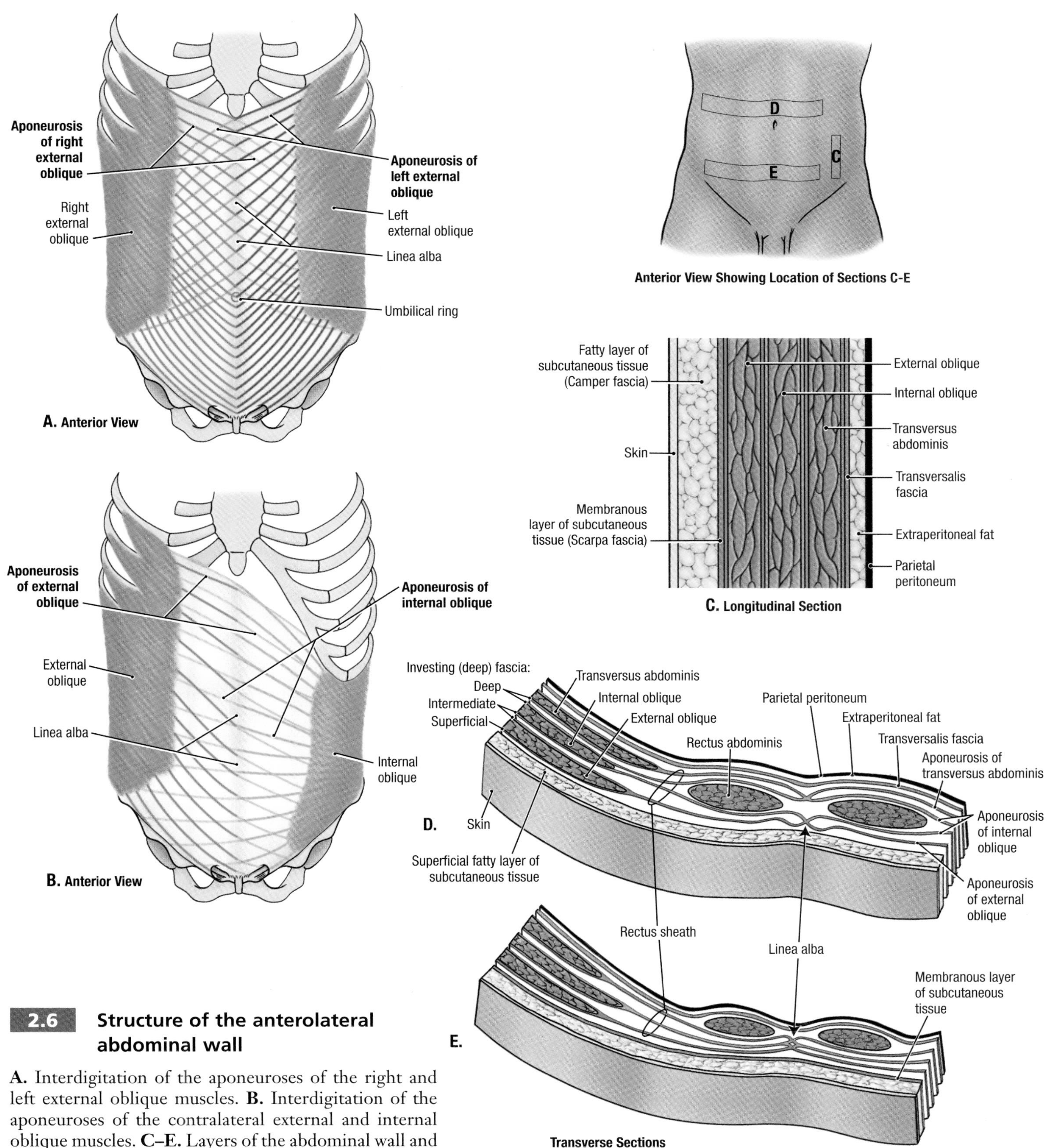
Aponeurosis of right external oblique
Aponeurosis of left external oblique
Right external oblique
Left external oblique
Linea alba
Umbilical ring
A. Anterior View
D
C
E
Anterior View Showing Location of Sections C-E
Fatty layer of subcutaneous tissue (Camper fascia)
Skin
Membranous layer of subcutaneous tissue (Scarpa fascia)
External oblique
Internal oblique
Transversus abdominis
Transversalis fascia
Extraperitoneal fat
Parietal peritoneum
C. Longitudinal Section
Aponeurosis of external oblique
Aponeurosis of internal oblique
External oblique
Linea alba
Internal oblique
B. Anterior View
Investing (deep) fascia:
Deep
Intermediate
Superficial
Transversus abdominis
Internal oblique
External oblique
Parietal peritoneum
Extraperitoneal fat
Rectus abdominis
Transversalis fascia
Aponeurosis of transversus abdominis
Aponeurosis of internal oblique
Aponeurosis of external oblique
D.
Skin
Superficial fatty layer of subcutaneous tissue
Rectus sheath
Linea alba
Membranous layer of subcutaneous tissue
E.
Transverse Sections

## 2.6 Structure of the anterolateral abdominal wall

**A.** Interdigitation of the aponeuroses of the right and left external oblique muscles. **B.** Interdigitation of the aponeuroses of the contralateral external and internal oblique muscles. **C–E.** Layers of the abdominal wall and the rectus sheath.

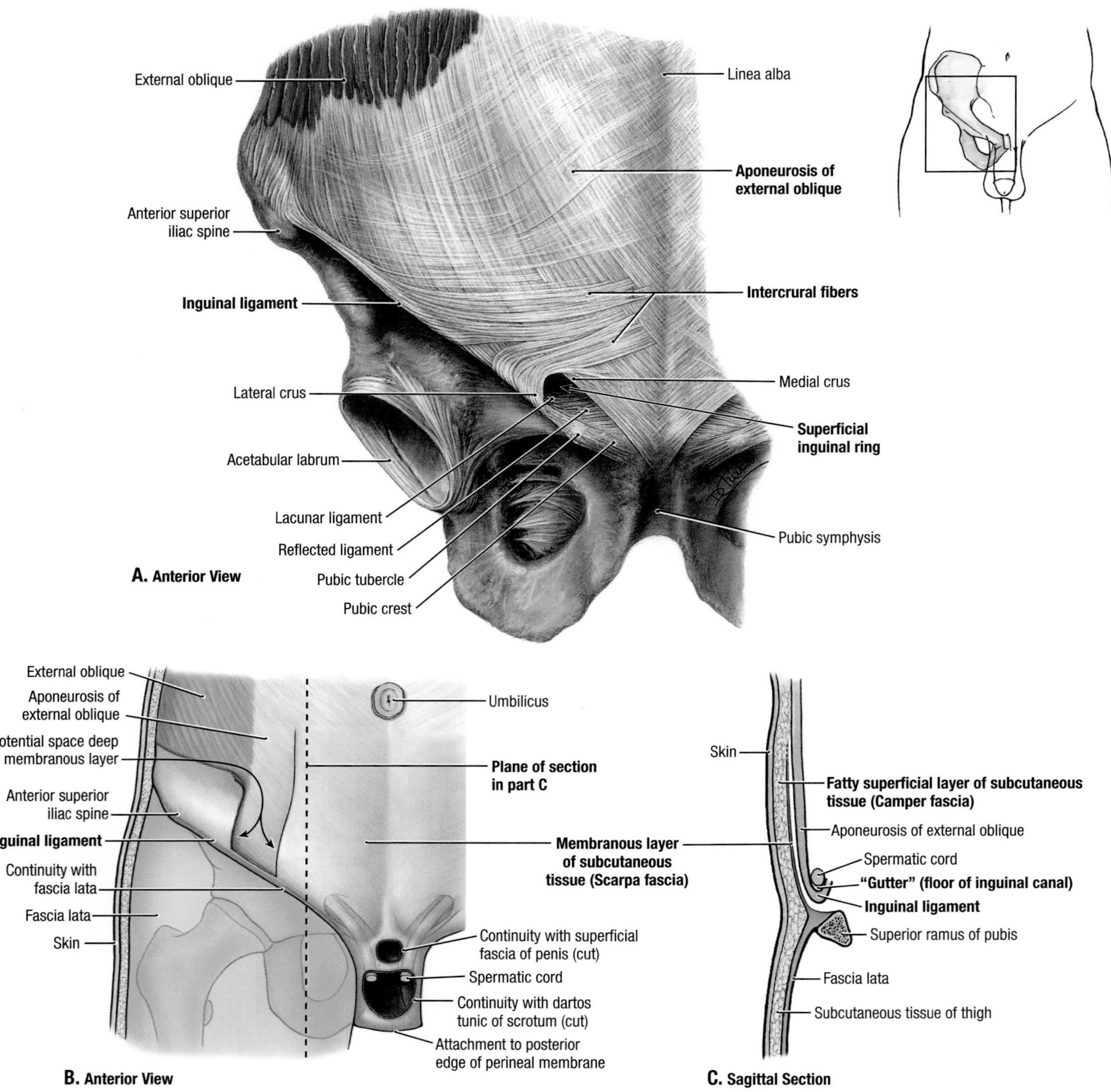
External oblique
Linea alba
Aponeurosis of external oblique
Anterior superior iliac spine
Inguinal ligament
Intercrural fibers
Medial crus
Lateral crus
Superficial inguinal ring
Acetabular labrum
Lacunar ligament
Reflected ligament
Pubic tubercle
Pubic crest
Pubic symphysis
A. Anterior View
External oblique
Aponeurosis of external oblique
Potential space deep to membranous layer
Anterior superior iliac spine
Inguinal ligament
Continuity with fascia lata
Fascia lata
Skin
Umbilicus
Plane of section in part C
Membranous layer of subcutaneous tissue (Scarpa fascia)
Continuity with superficial fascia of penis (cut)
Spermatic cord
Continuity with dartos tunic of scrotum (cut)
Attachment to posterior edge of perineal membrane
B. Anterior View
Skin
Fatty superficial layer of subcutaneous tissue (Camper fascia)
Aponeurosis of external oblique
Spermatic cord
"Gutter" (floor of inguinal canal)
Inguinal ligament
Superior ramus of pubis
Fascia lata
Subcutaneous tissue of thigh
C. Sagittal Section

## 2.7 Inguinal region of male-I

**A.** Formations of the aponeurosis of the external oblique muscle. **B** and **C.** Membranous (deep) layer of subcutaneous tissue. Inferior to the umbilicus, the subcutaneous tissue is composed of two layers: a superficial fatty layer and a deep membranous layer. Laterally, the membranous layer fuses with the fascia lata of the thigh about a finger's breadth inferior to the inguinal ligament. Medially, it fuses with the linea alba and pubic symphysis in the midline, and inferiorly, it continues as the membranous layer of the subcutaneous tissue of the perineum and penis and the dartos fascia of the scrotum. The inferior margin of the external oblique aponeurosis is thickened and turned internally forming the inguinal ligament. The superior surface of the in-turning inguinal ligament forms a shallow trough or "gutter" that is the floor of the inguinal canal.

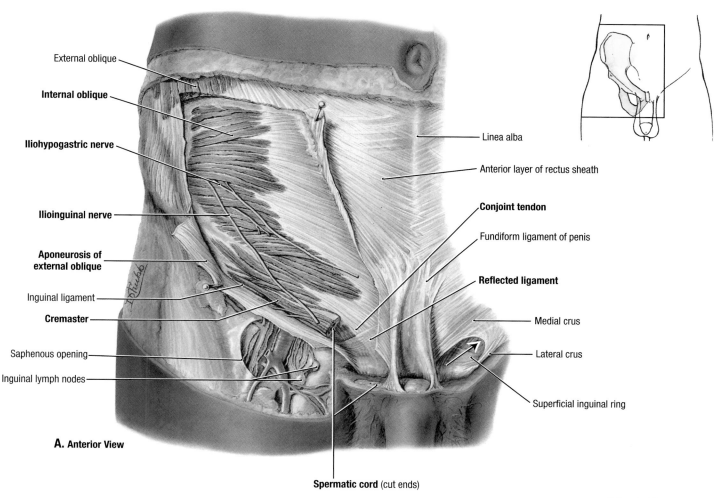

External oblique
Internal oblique
Iliohypogastric nerve
Ilioinguinal nerve
Aponeurosis of external oblique
Inguinal ligament
Cremaster
Saphenous opening
Inguinal lymph nodes
Linea alba
Anterior layer of rectus sheath
Conjoint tendon
Fundiform ligament of penis
Reflected ligament
Medial crus
Lateral crus
Superficial inguinal ring
Spermatic cord (cut ends)

**A.** Anterior View

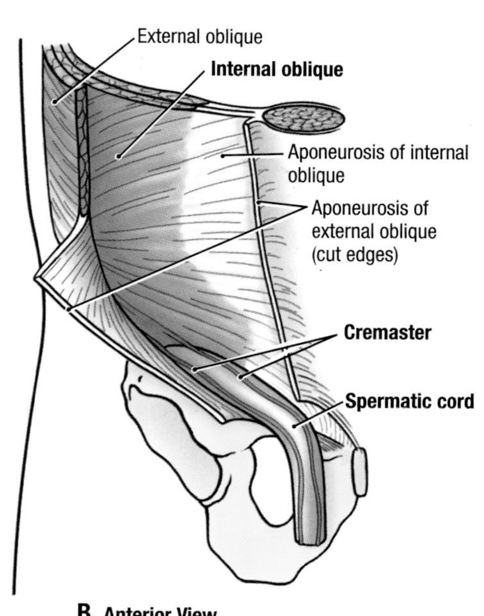
External oblique
Internal oblique
Aponeurosis of internal oblique
Aponeurosis of external oblique (cut edges)
Cremaster
Spermatic cord

**B.** Anterior View

## 2.8 Inguinal region of male—II

**A.** Internal oblique and cremaster muscle. Part of the aponeurosis of the external oblique muscle is cut away, and the spermatic cord is cut short. **B.** Schematic illustration.

- The cremaster muscle covers the spermatic cord.
- The reflected ligament is formed by aponeurotic fibers of the external oblique muscle and lies anterior to the conjoint tendon. The conjoint tendon is formed by the fusion of the aponeurosis of the internal oblique and transversus abdominis muscles.

- The cutaneous branches of the iliohypogastric and ilioinguinal nerves (L1) course between the internal and external oblique muscles and must be avoided when an appendectomy incision is made in this region.

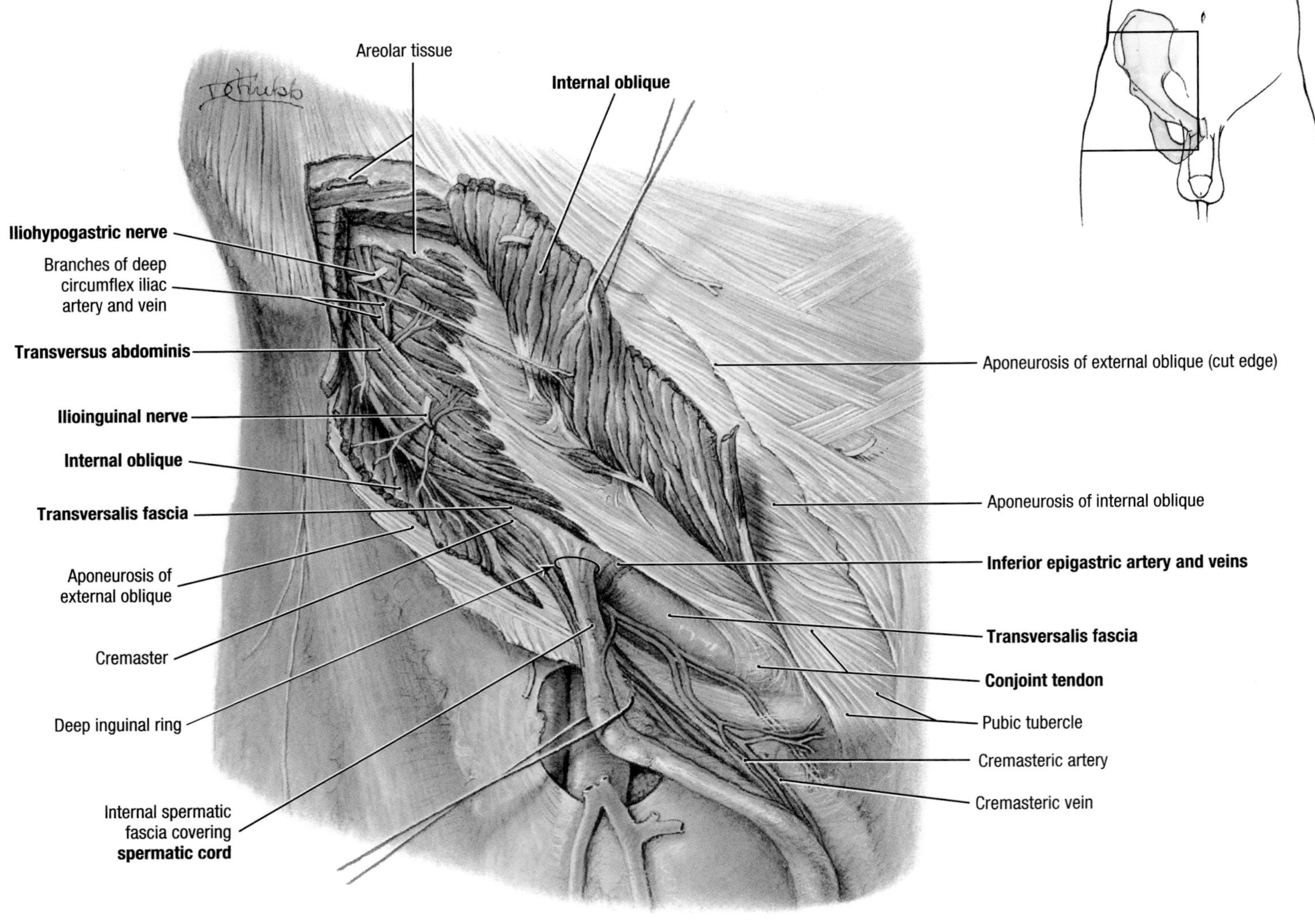
Areolar tissue
Internal oblique
Iliohypogastric nerve
Branches of deep circumflex iliac artery and vein
Transversus abdominis
Ilioinguinal nerve
Internal oblique
Transversalis fascia
Aponeurosis of external oblique
Cremaster
Deep inguinal ring
Internal spermatic fascia covering spermatic cord
Aponeurosis of external oblique (cut edge)
Aponeurosis of internal oblique
Inferior epigastric artery and veins
Transversalis fascia
Conjoint tendon
Pubic tubercle
Cremasteric artery
Cremasteric vein

**Anterior View**

## 2.9 Inguinal region of male—III

The internal oblique muscle is reflected, and the spermatic cord is retracted.

- The internal oblique muscle portion of the conjoint tendon is attached to the pubic crest, and the transversus abdominis portion to the pectineal line.
- The iliohypogastric and ilioinguinal nerves (L1) supply the internal oblique and transversus abdominis muscles.
- The transversalis fascia is evaginated to form the tubular internal spermatic fascia. The mouth of the tube, called the deep inguinal ring, is situated lateral to the inferior epigastric vessels.

**TABLE 2.2 STRUCTURES FORMING THE INGUINAL CANAL**

| Boundaries | Lateral Third | Middle Third | Medial Third |
|---|---|---|---|
| Posterior wall | Transversalis fascia including deep inguinal ring | Transversalis fascia | Transversalis fascia<br>Conjoint tendon |
| Anterior wall | Aponeurosis of external oblique<br>Internal oblique | Aponeurosis of external oblique | Aponeurosis of external oblique<br>Superficial inguinal ring |
| Roof | Arching fibers of internal oblique and transversus abdominis | | |
| Floor | Inguinal ligament | Inguinal ligament | Inguinal ligament<br>Lacunar ligament |

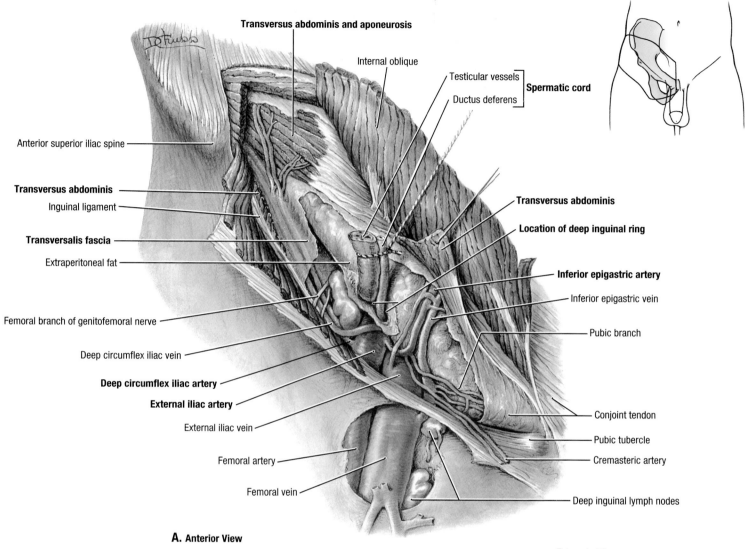

Transversus abdominis and aponeurosis
Internal oblique
Testicular vessels
Ductus deferens
Spermatic cord
Anterior superior iliac spine
Transversus abdominis
Inguinal ligament
Transversalis fascia
Extraperitoneal fat
Transversus abdominis
Location of deep inguinal ring
Inferior epigastric artery
Inferior epigastric vein
Femoral branch of genitofemoral nerve
Pubic branch
Deep circumflex iliac vein
Deep circumflex iliac artery
External iliac artery
External iliac vein
Conjoint tendon
Pubic tubercle
Cremasteric artery
Femoral artery
Femoral vein
Deep inguinal lymph nodes

**A.** Anterior View

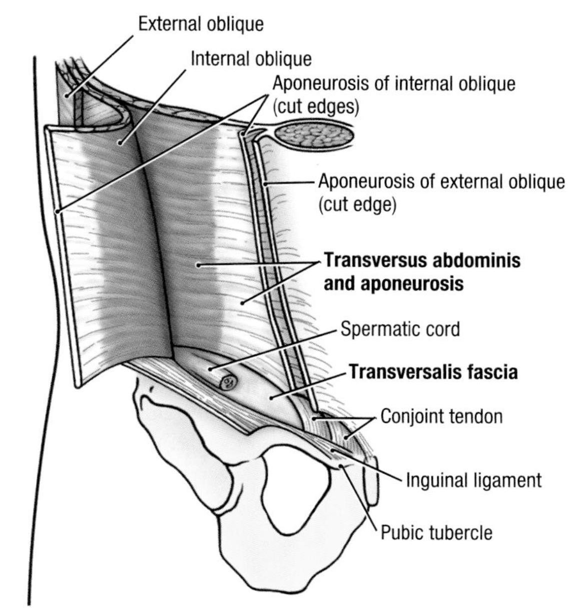
External oblique
Internal oblique
Aponeurosis of internal oblique (cut edges)
Aponeurosis of external oblique (cut edge)
Transversus abdominis and aponeurosis
Spermatic cord
Transversalis fascia
Conjoint tendon
Inguinal ligament
Pubic tubercle

**B.** Anterior View

## 2.10 Inguinal region of male—IV

**A.** The inguinal part of the transversus abdominis muscle and transversalis fascia is partially cut away, the spermatic cord is excised, and the ductus deferens is retracted. **B.** Schematic illustration.

- The deep inguinal ring is located superior to the inguinal ligament at the midpoint between the anterior superior iliac spine and pubic tubercle.
- The external iliac artery has two branches, the deep circumflex iliac and inferior epigastric arteries. Note also the cremasteric artery and pubic branch arising from the latter.

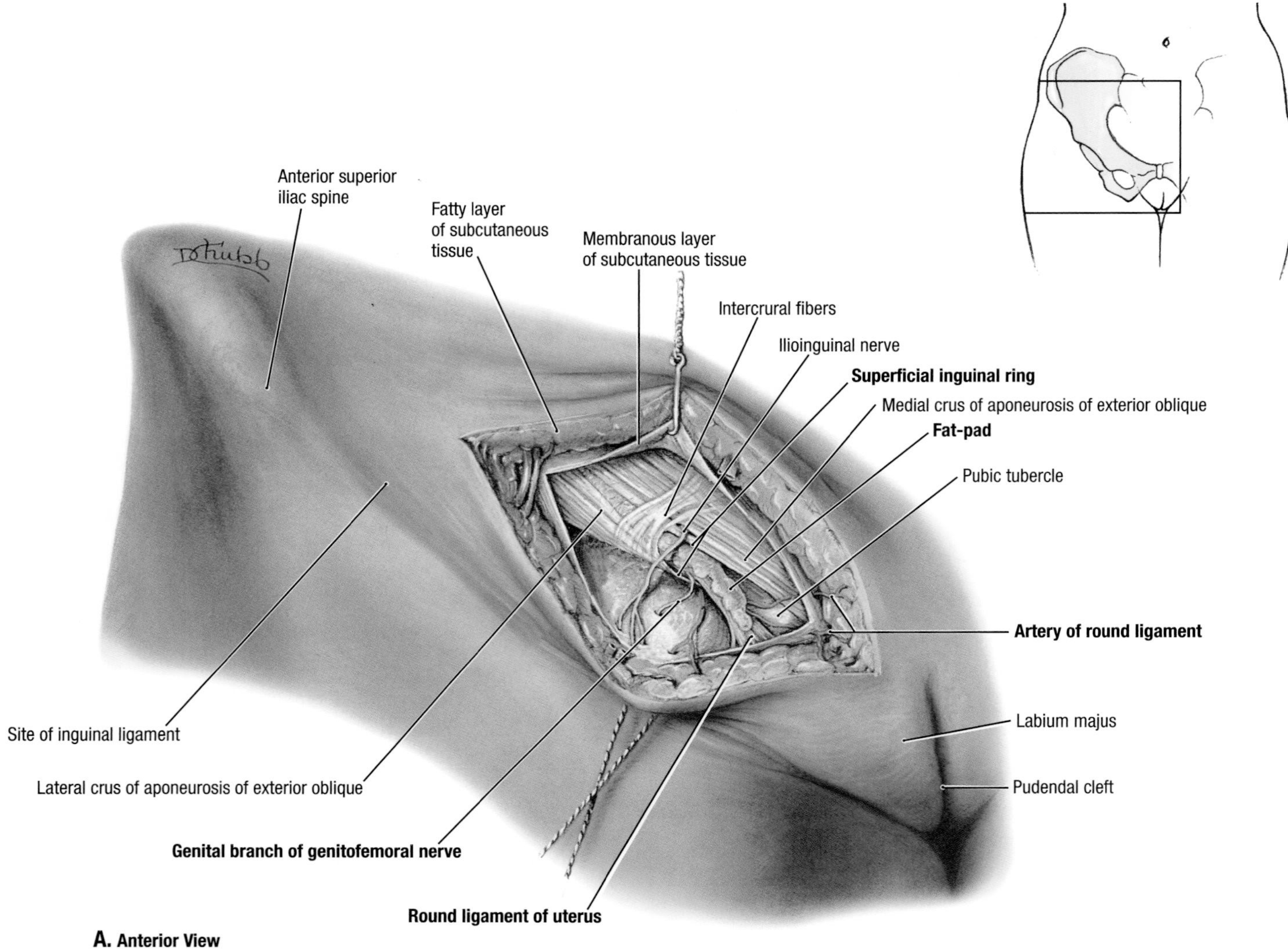

Anterior superior iliac spine
Fatty layer of subcutaneous tissue
Membranous layer of subcutaneous tissue
Intercrural fibers
Ilioinguinal nerve
Superficial inguinal ring
Medial crus of aponeurosis of exterior oblique
Fat-pad
Pubic tubercle
Artery of round ligament
Labium majus
Pudendal cleft
Site of inguinal ligament
Lateral crus of aponeurosis of exterior oblique
Genital branch of genitofemoral nerve
Round ligament of uterus


**A. Anterior View**

## 2.11 Inguinal canal of female

Progressive dissections of the female inguinal canal **(A–D).**

- In **A,** the superficial inguinal ring is small. Passing through the superficial inguinal ring are the round ligament of the uterus, a closely applied fat-pad, the genital branch of the genitofemoral nerve, and the artery of the round ligament of the uterus. The ilioinguinal nerve may also pass through the ring.
- The cremaster muscle does not extend beyond the superficial inguinal ring **(B).**
- The round ligament breaks up into strands as it leaves the inguinal canal and approaches the labium majus **(C).**
- The external iliac artery and vein are exposed deep to the inguinal canal by excising the transversalis fascia **(D).**

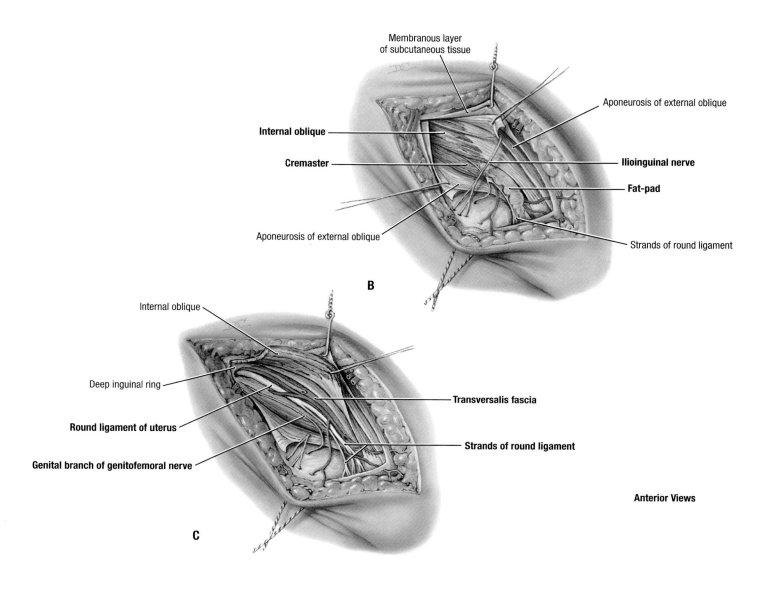

Membranous layer of subcutaneous tissue
Aponeurosis of external oblique
**Internal oblique**
**Cremaster**
**Ilioinguinal nerve**
**Fat-pad**
Aponeurosis of external oblique
Strands of round ligament

**B**

Internal oblique
Deep inguinal ring
**Transversalis fascia**
**Round ligament of uterus**
**Strands of round ligament**
**Genital branch of genitofemoral nerve**

**C**

**Anterior Views**

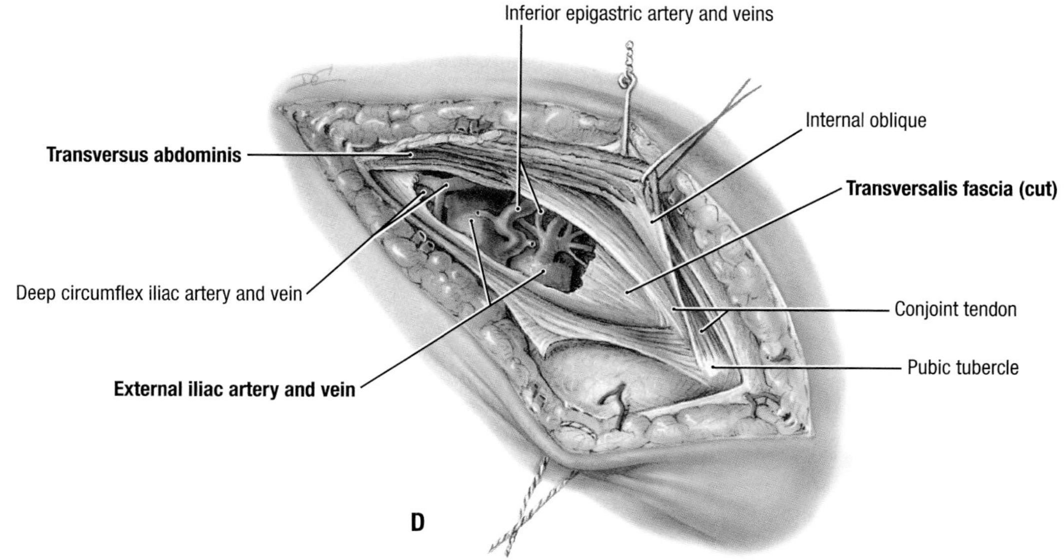
Inferior epigastric artery and veins
Internal oblique
Transversus abdominis
Transversalis fascia (cut)
Deep circumflex iliac artery and vein
Conjoint tendon
Pubic tubercle
External iliac artery and vein
D

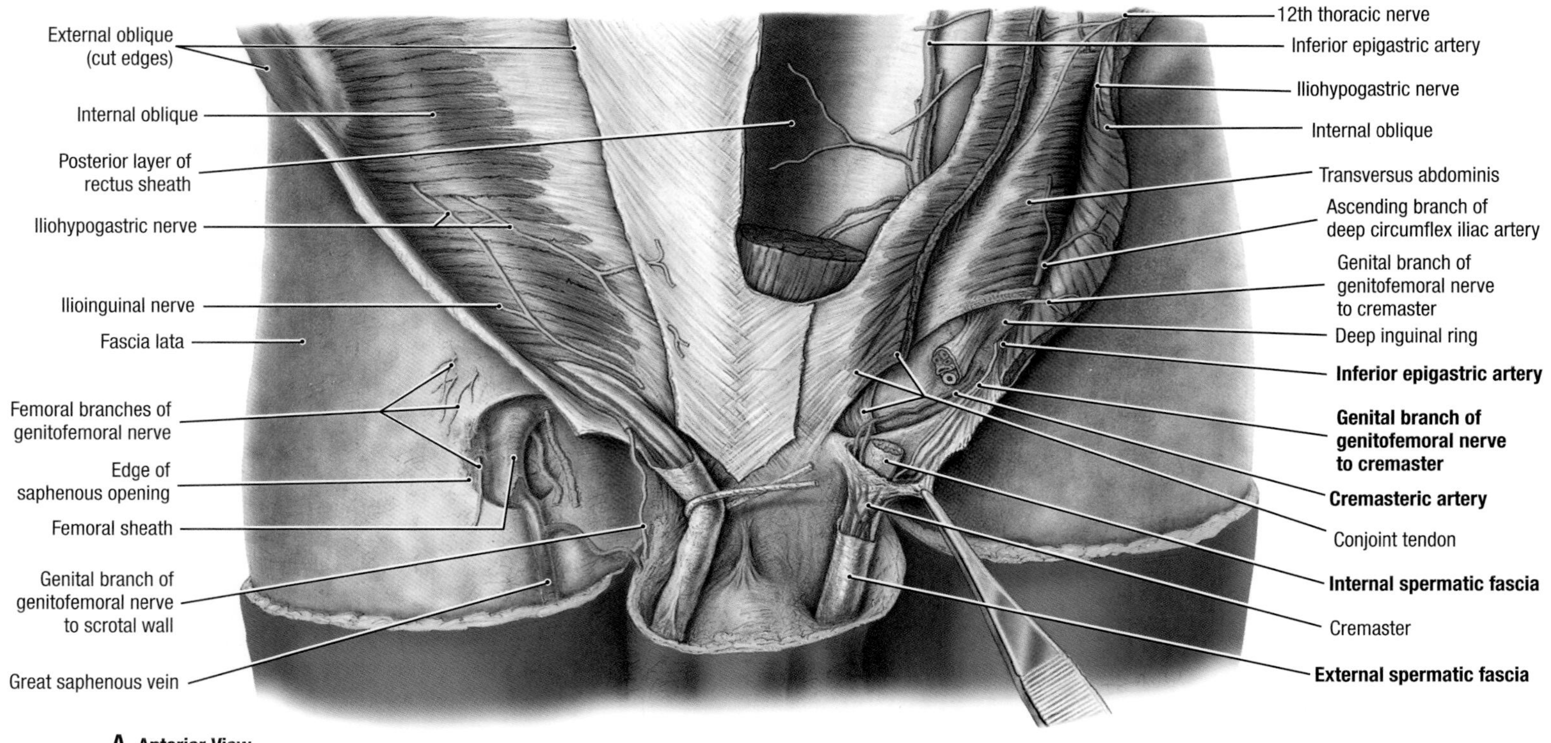

External oblique (cut edges)
Internal oblique
Posterior layer of rectus sheath
Iliohypogastric nerve
Ilioinguinal nerve
Fascia lata
Femoral branches of genitofemoral nerve
Edge of saphenous opening
Femoral sheath
Genital branch of genitofemoral nerve to scrotal wall
Great saphenous vein
12th thoracic nerve
Inferior epigastric artery
Iliohypogastric nerve
Internal oblique
Transversus abdominis
Ascending branch of deep circumflex iliac artery
Genital branch of genitofemoral nerve to cremaster
Deep inguinal ring
**Inferior epigastric artery**
**Genital branch of genitofemoral nerve to cremaster**
**Cremasteric artery**
Conjoint tendon
**Internal spermatic fascia**
Cremaster
**External spermatic fascia**


**A. Anterior View**

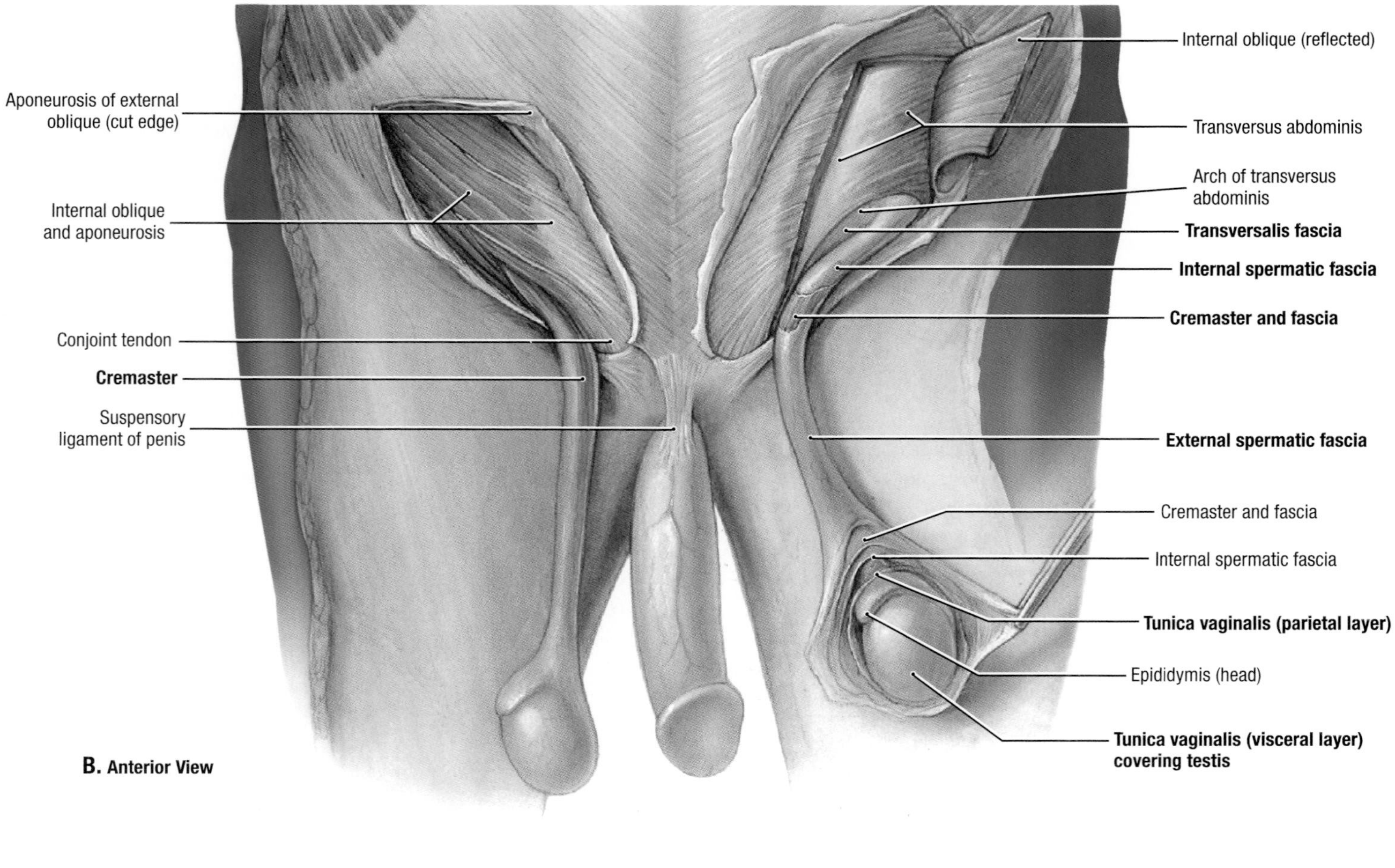

Aponeurosis of external oblique (cut edge)
Internal oblique and aponeurosis
Conjoint tendon
**Cremaster**
Suspensory ligament of penis
Internal oblique (reflected)
Transversus abdominis
Arch of transversus abdominis
**Transversalis fascia**
**Internal spermatic fascia**
**Cremaster and fascia**
**External spermatic fascia**
Cremaster and fascia
Internal spermatic fascia
**Tunica vaginalis (parietal layer)**
Epididymis (head)
**Tunica vaginalis (visceral layer) covering testis**

**B. Anterior View**

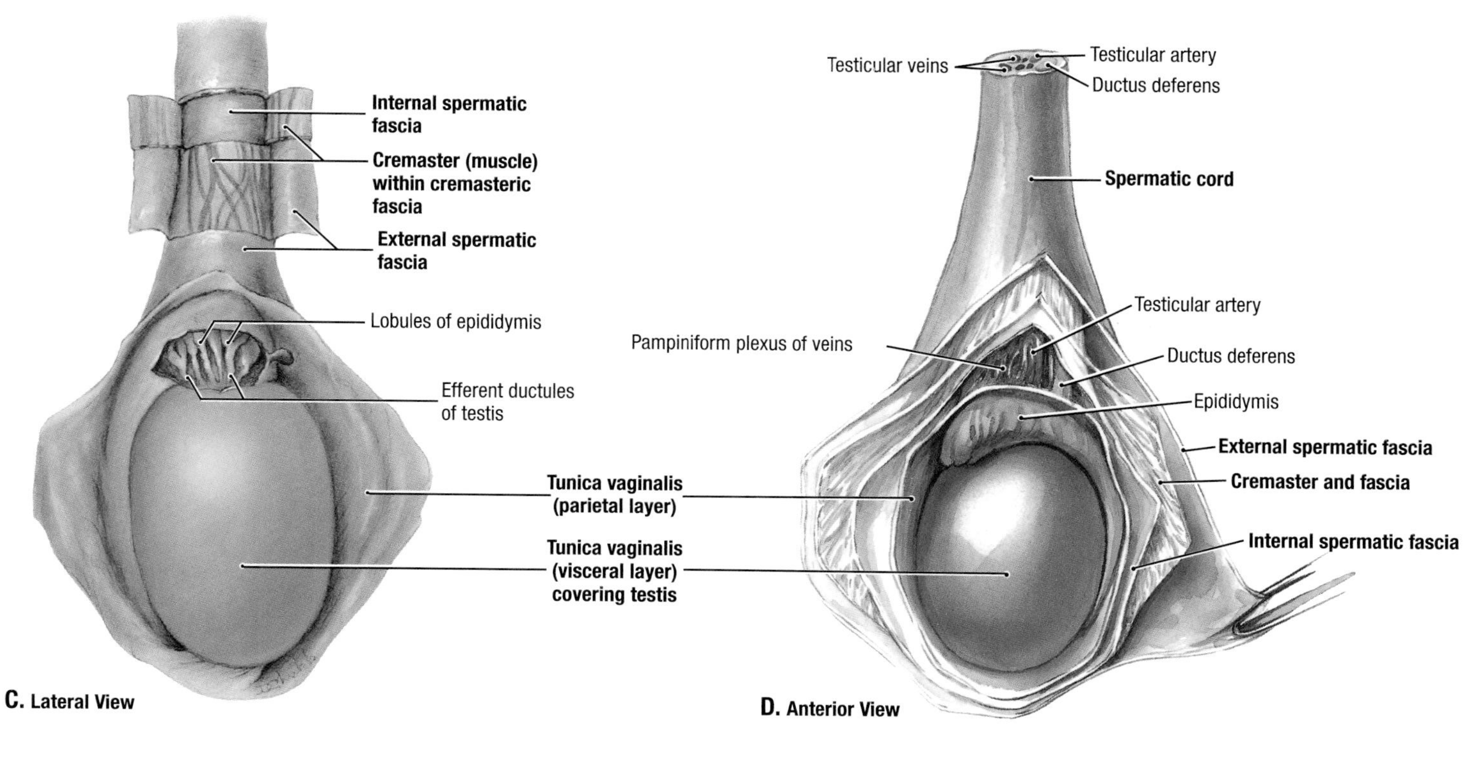
Internal spermatic fascia
Cremaster (muscle) within cremasteric fascia
External spermatic fascia
Lobules of epididymis
Efferent ductules of testis
Tunica vaginalis (parietal layer)
Tunica vaginalis (visceral layer) covering testis
C. Lateral View
Testicular veins
Testicular artery
Ductus deferens
Spermatic cord
Testicular artery
Pampiniform plexus of veins
Ductus deferens
Epididymis
External spermatic fascia
Cremaster and fascia
Internal spermatic fascia
D. Anterior View

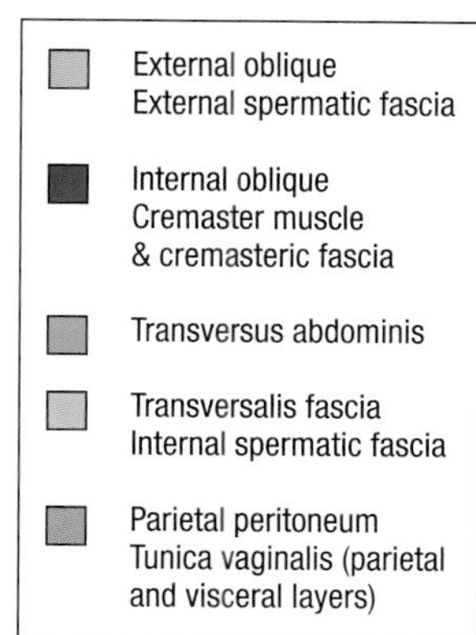
External oblique
External spermatic fascia
Internal oblique
Cremaster muscle
& cremasteric fascia
Transversus abdominis
Transversalis fascia
Internal spermatic fascia
Parietal peritoneum
Tunica vaginalis (parietal and visceral layers)

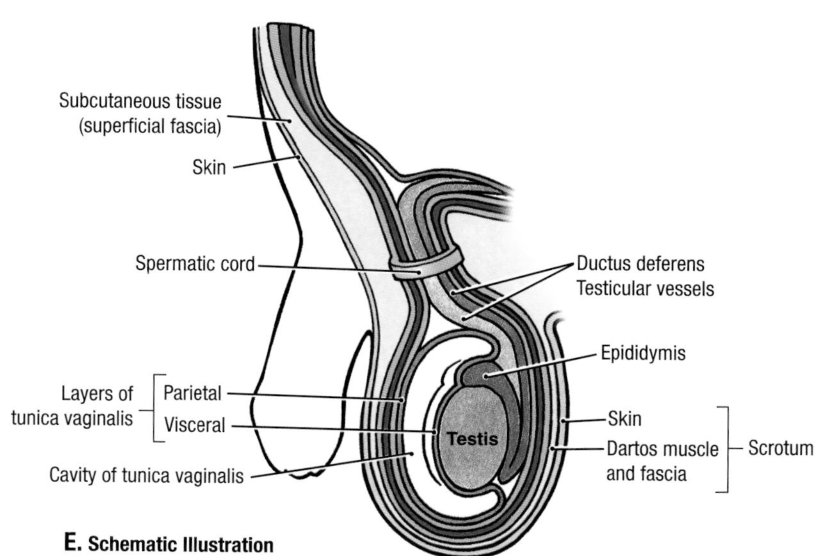
Subcutaneous tissue (superficial fascia)
Skin
Spermatic cord
Ductus deferens
Testicular vessels
Epididymis
Layers of tunica vaginalis
Parietal
Visceral
Testis
Cavity of tunica vaginalis
Skin
Dartos muscle and fascia
Scrotum
E. Schematic Illustration

## 2.12 Inguinal canal, spermatic cord, and testis

**A.** Dissection of inguinal canal. **B.** Dissection of inguinal region and coverings of the spermatic cord and testis. **C–E.** Coverings of spermatic cord and testis.

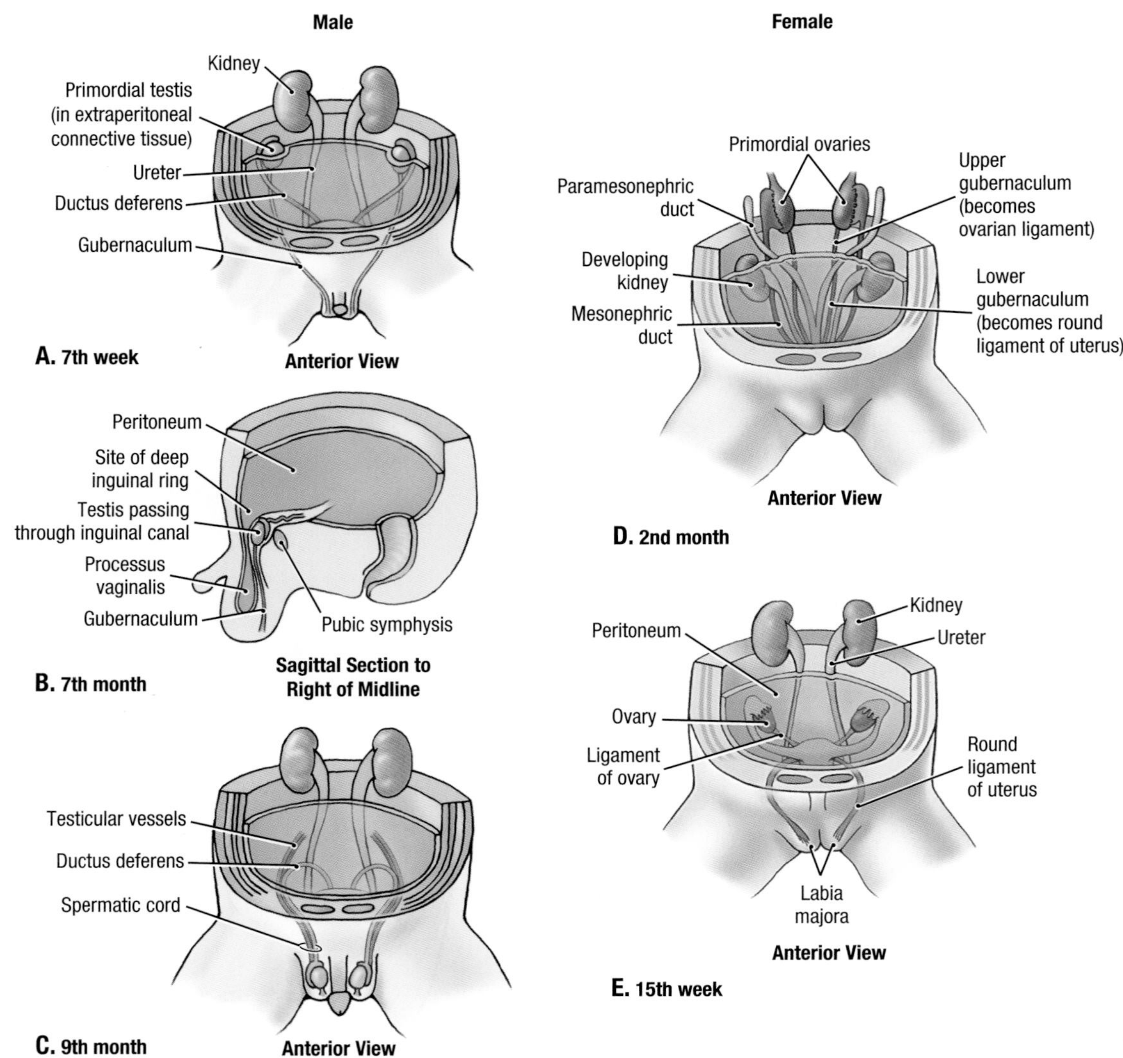
Male
Kidney
Primordial testis (in extraperitoneal connective tissue)
Ureter
Ductus deferens
Gubernaculum
A. 7th week
Anterior View
Peritoneum
Site of deep inguinal ring
Testis passing through inguinal canal
Processus vaginalis
Gubernaculum
Pubic symphysis
B. 7th month
Sagittal Section to Right of Midline
Testicular vessels
Ductus deferens
Spermatic cord
C. 9th month
Anterior View
Female
Primordial ovaries
Paramesonephric duct
Upper gubernaculum (becomes ovarian ligament)
Developing kidney
Mesonephric duct
Lower gubernaculum (becomes round ligament of uterus)
Anterior View
D. 2nd month
Peritoneum
Kidney
Ureter
Ovary
Ligament of ovary
Round ligament of uterus
Labia majora
Anterior View
E. 15th week

## 2.13 Descent of gonads

The inguinal canals in females are narrower than those in males, and the canals in infants of both sexes are shorter and much less oblique than in adults. For a complete description of the embryology of the inguinal region, see Moore and Persaud (2003).

The fetal testes descend from the dorsal abdominal wall in the superior lumbar region to the deep inguinal rings during the 9th–12th fetal weeks. This movement probably results from growth of the vertebral column and pelvis. The male gubernaculum, attached to the caudal pole of the testis and accompanied by an outpouching of peritoneum, the processus vaginalis, projects into the scrotum. The testis descends posterior to the processus vaginalis. The inferior remnant of the processus vaginalis forms the tunica vaginalis covering the testis. The ductus deferens, testicular vessels, nerves, and lymphatics accompany the testis. The final descent of the testis usually occurs before or shortly after birth.

The fetal ovaries also descend from the dorsal abdominal wall in the superior lumbar region during the 12th week but pass into the lesser pelvis. The female gubernaculum attaches to the caudal pole of the ovary and projects into the labia majora, attaching en route to the uterus; the part passing from the uterus to the ovary forms the ovarian ligament, and the remainder of it becomes the round ligament of the uterus. Because of the attachment of the ovarian ligaments to the uterus, the ovaries do not descend to the inguinal region; however, the round ligament passes through the inguinal canal and attaches to the subcutaneous tissue of the labium majus.

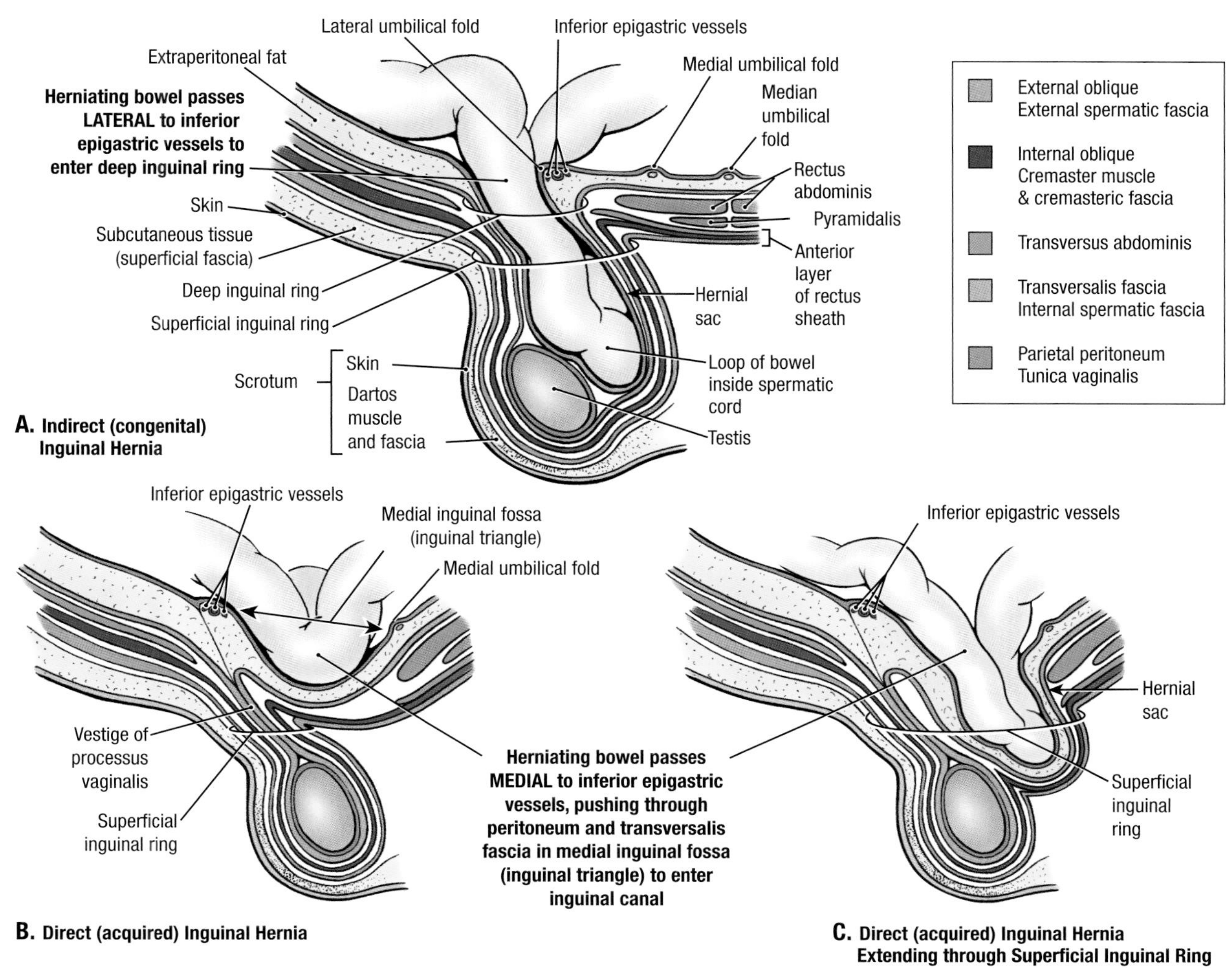
Lateral umbilical fold
Inferior epigastric vessels
Extraperitoneal fat
Medial umbilical fold
Median umbilical fold
Herniating bowel passes LATERAL to inferior epigastric vessels to enter deep inguinal ring
Rectus abdominis
Skin
Pyramidalis
Subcutaneous tissue (superficial fascia)
Anterior layer of rectus sheath
Deep inguinal ring
Hernial sac
Superficial inguinal ring
Scrotum
Skin
Dartos muscle and fascia
Loop of bowel inside spermatic cord
Testis
A. Indirect (congenital) Inguinal Hernia
External oblique
External spermatic fascia
Internal oblique
Cremaster muscle
& cremasteric fascia
Transversus abdominis
Transversalis fascia
Internal spermatic fascia
Parietal peritoneum
Tunica vaginalis
Inferior epigastric vessels
Medial inguinal fossa (inguinal triangle)
Medial umbilical fold
Vestige of processus vaginalis
Superficial inguinal ring
Herniating bowel passes MEDIAL to inferior epigastric vessels, pushing through peritoneum and transversalis fascia in medial inguinal fossa (inguinal triangle) to enter inguinal canal
Inferior epigastric vessels
Hernial sac
Superficial inguinal ring

**B.** Direct (acquired) Inguinal Hernia

**C.** Direct (acquired) Inguinal Hernia Extending through Superficial Inguinal Ring

## 2.14 Inguinal hernias

An inguinal hernia is a protrusion of parietal peritoneum and viscera, such as the small intestine, through the abdominal wall in the inguinal region. There are two major categories of inguinal hernia: indirect and direct. More than two-thirds are indirect hernias, most commonly occurring in males.

| Characteristics[a] | Direct (Acquired) | Indirect (Congenital) |
|---|---|---|
| Predisposing factors | Weakness of anterior abdominal wall in inguinal triangle (e.g., owing to distended superficial ring, narrow conjoint tendon, or attenuation of aponeurosis in males > 40 years of age) | Patency of processus vaginalis (complete or at least of superior part) in younger persons, the great majority of whom are males |
| Frequency | Less common (1/3 to 1/4 of inguinal hernias) | More common (2/3 to 3/4 of inguinal hernias) |
| Coverings at exit from abdominal cavity (**A** and **B**) | Peritoneum plus transversalis fascia (lies outside inner one or two fascial coverings of cord) | Peritoneum of persistent processus vaginalis plus all three fascial coverings of cord/round ligament |
| Course (**C**) | Usually traverses only medial third of inguinal canal, external and parallel to vestige of processus vaginalis | Traverses inguinal canal (entire canal if it is sufficient size) within processus vaginalis |
| Exit from anterior abdominal wall | Via superficial ring, lateral to cord; rarely enters scrotum | Via superficial ring inside cord, commonly passing into scrotum/labium majus |

[a]Letters in parentheses refer to the figure parts.

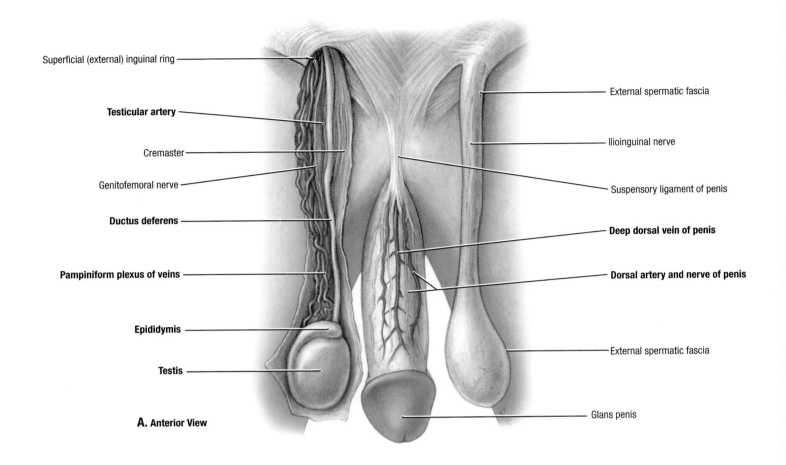

Superficial (external) inguinal ring
Testicular artery
Cremaster
Genitofemoral nerve
Ductus deferens
Pampiniform plexus of veins
Epididymis
Testis
External spermatic fascia
Ilioinguinal nerve
Suspensory ligament of penis
Deep dorsal vein of penis
Dorsal artery and nerve of penis
External spermatic fascia
Glans penis

**A. Anterior View**

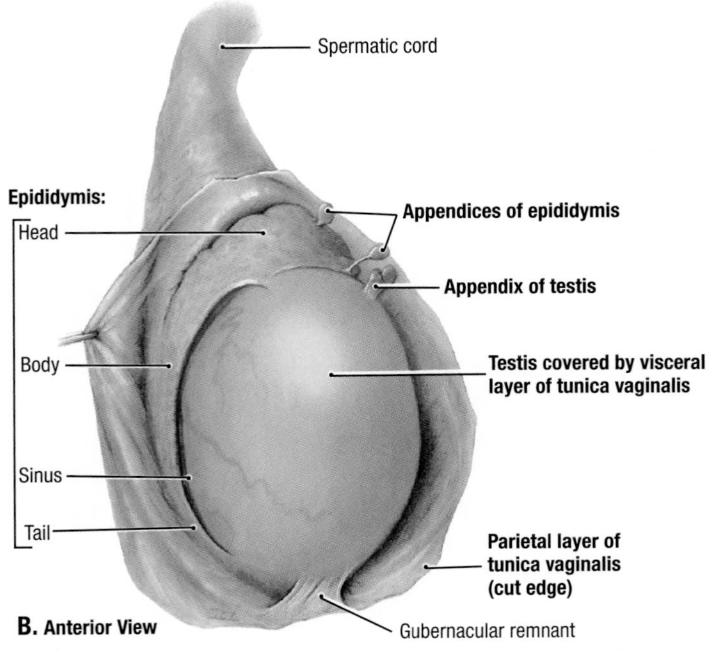
Spermatic cord
Epididymis:
Head
Body
Sinus
Tail
Appendices of epididymis
Appendix of testis
Testis covered by visceral layer of tunica vaginalis
Parietal layer of tunica vaginalis (cut edge)
Gubernacular remnant

**B. Anterior View**

## 2.15 Spermatic cord, testis, and epididymis

**A.** Dissection of spermatic cord. The subcutaneous tissue (dartos fascia) covering the penis has been removed and the deep fascia rendered transparent to demonstrate the median deep dorsal vein and the bilateral dorsal arteries and nerves of the penis. On the specimen's right, the coverings of the spermatic cord and testis are reflected, and the contents of the cord are separated. The testicular artery has been separated from the pampiniform plexus of veins that surrounds it as it courses parallel to the ductus deferens. Lymphatic vessels and autonomic nerve fibers (not shown) are also present. **B.** The tunica vaginalis has been incised longitudinally to expose its cavity, surrounding the testis anteriorly and laterally, and extending between the testis and epididymis at the sinus of the epididymis. The epididymis is located posterolateral to the left testis, i.e., on the right side of the right testis and on the left side of the left testis. The appendices of the testis and epididymis may be observed in some specimens. These structures are small remnants of the embryonic genital (paramesonephric) duct.

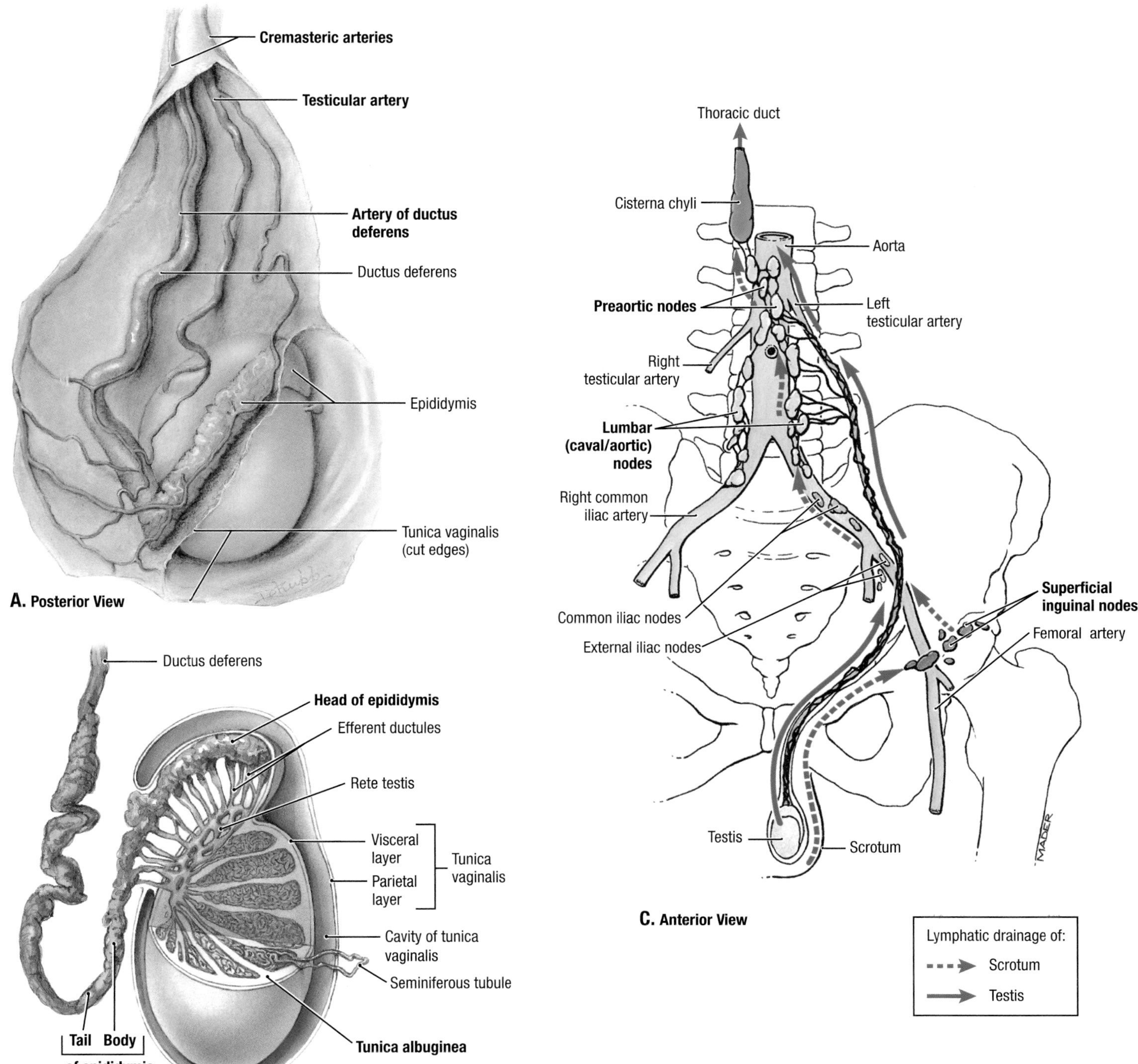
Cremasteric arteries
Testicular artery
Artery of ductus deferens
Ductus deferens
Epididymis
Tunica vaginalis (cut edges)
A. Posterior View
Ductus deferens
Head of epididymis
Efferent ductules
Rete testis
Visceral layer
Parietal layer
Tunica vaginalis
Cavity of tunica vaginalis
Seminiferous tubule
Tunica albuginea
Tail Body of epididymis
B. Longitinal Section of Tunica Vaginalis; Testis Sectioned in Sagittal and Transverse Planes
Thoracic duct
Cisterna chyli
Aorta
Preaortic nodes
Left testicular artery
Right testicular artery
Lumbar (caval/aortic) nodes
Right common iliac artery
Common iliac nodes
External iliac nodes
Superficial inguinal nodes
Femoral artery
Testis
Scrotum
C. Anterior View
Lymphatic drainage of:
Scrotum
Testis

## 2.16 Blood supply and lymphatic drainage of testis

**A.** Blood supply. **B.** Internal structure. **C.** Lymphatic drainage. Because the testes descend from the posterior abdominal wall into the scrotum during fetal development, their lymphatic drainage differs from that of the scrotum, which is an outpouching of the abdominal skin. Consequently, cancer of the testis metastasizes initially to the lumbar lymph nodes and cancer of the scrotum metastasizes initially to the superficial inguinal lymph nodes.

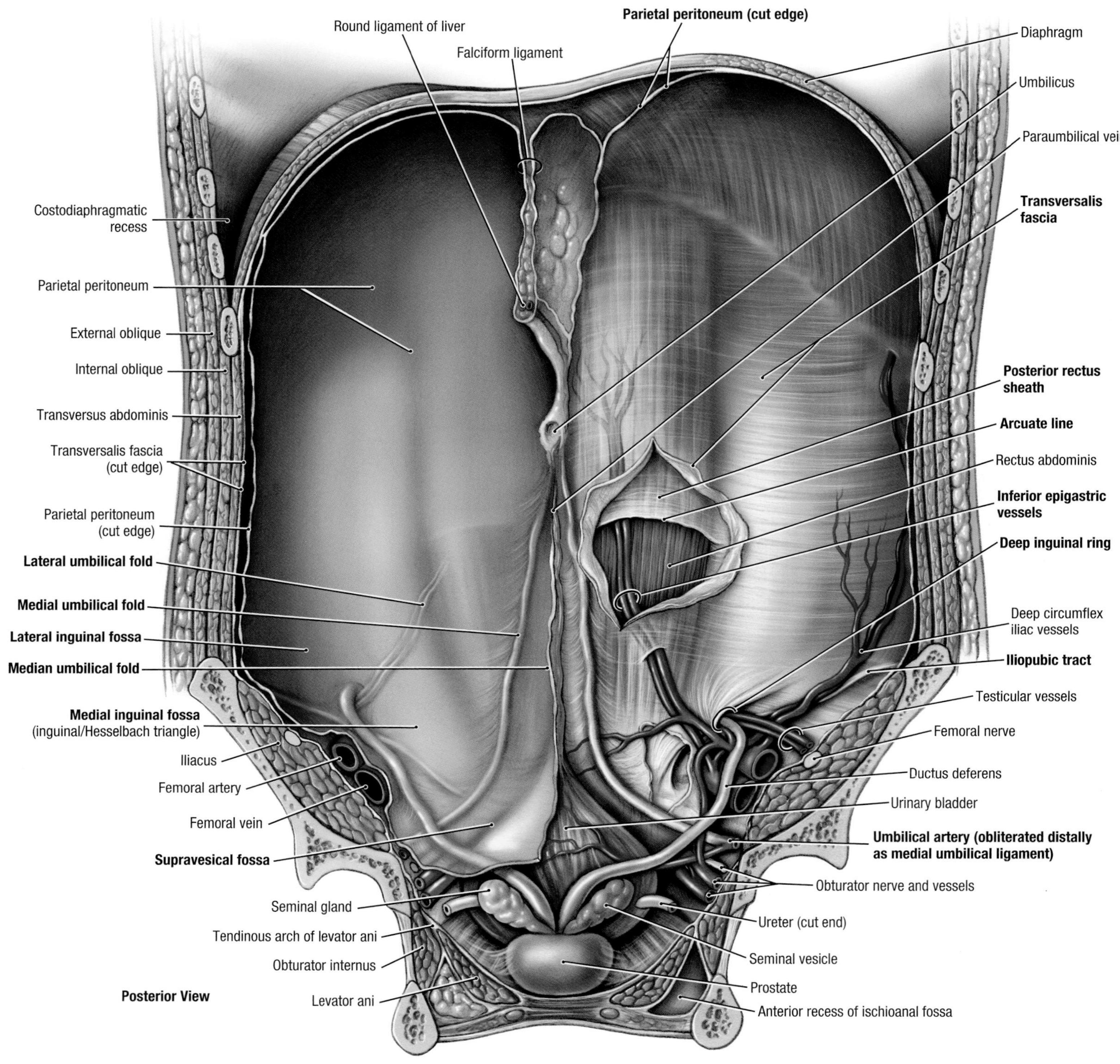
Round ligament of liver
Falciform ligament
Parietal peritoneum (cut edge)
Diaphragm
Umbilicus
Paraumbilical vein
Transversalis fascia
Costodiaphragmatic recess
Parietal peritoneum
External oblique
Internal oblique
Transversus abdominis
Transversalis fascia (cut edge)
Parietal peritoneum (cut edge)
Lateral umbilical fold
Medial umbilical fold
Lateral inguinal fossa
Median umbilical fold
Medial inguinal fossa (inguinal/Hesselbach triangle)
Iliacus
Femoral artery
Femoral vein
Supravesical fossa
Seminal gland
Tendinous arch of levator ani
Obturator internus
Levator ani
Posterior View
Posterior rectus sheath
Arcuate line
Rectus abdominis
Inferior epigastric vessels
Deep inguinal ring
Deep circumflex iliac vessels
Iliopubic tract
Testicular vessels
Femoral nerve
Ductus deferens
Urinary bladder
Umbilical artery (obliterated distally as medial umbilical ligament)
Obturator nerve and vessels
Ureter (cut end)
Seminal vesicle
Prostate
Anterior recess of ischioanal fossa

## 2.17 Posterior aspect of the anterolateral abdominal wall

Umbilical folds (median, medial, and lateral) are reflections of the parietal peritoneum that are raised from the body wall by underlying structures. The median umbilical fold extends from the urinary bladder to the umbilicus and covers the median umbilical ligament (the remnant of the urachus). The two medial umbilical folds cover the medial umbilical ligaments (occluded remnants of the fetal umbilical arteries). Two lateral umbilical folds cover the inferior epigastric vessels. The supravesical fossae are between the median and medial umbilical folds, the medial inguinal fossae (inguinal triangles) are between the medial and lateral umbilical folds, and the lateral inguinal fossae and deep inguinal rings are lateral to the lateral umbilical folds.

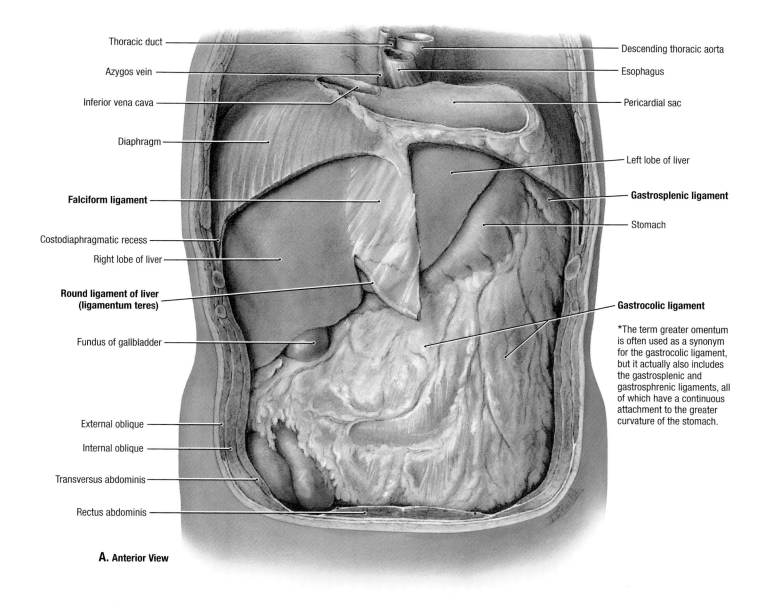

Thoracic duct
Azygos vein
Inferior vena cava
Diaphragm
**Falciform ligament**
Costodiaphragmatic recess
Right lobe of liver
**Round ligament of liver (ligamentum teres)**
Fundus of gallbladder
External oblique
Internal oblique
Transversus abdominis
Rectus abdominis
Descending thoracic aorta
Esophagus
Pericardial sac
Left lobe of liver
**Gastrosplenic ligament**
Stomach
**Gastrocolic ligament**

*The term greater omentum is often used as a synonym for the gastrocolic ligament, but it actually also includes the gastrosplenic and gastrosphrenic ligaments, all of which have a continuous attachment to the greater curvature of the stomach.

**A. Anterior View**

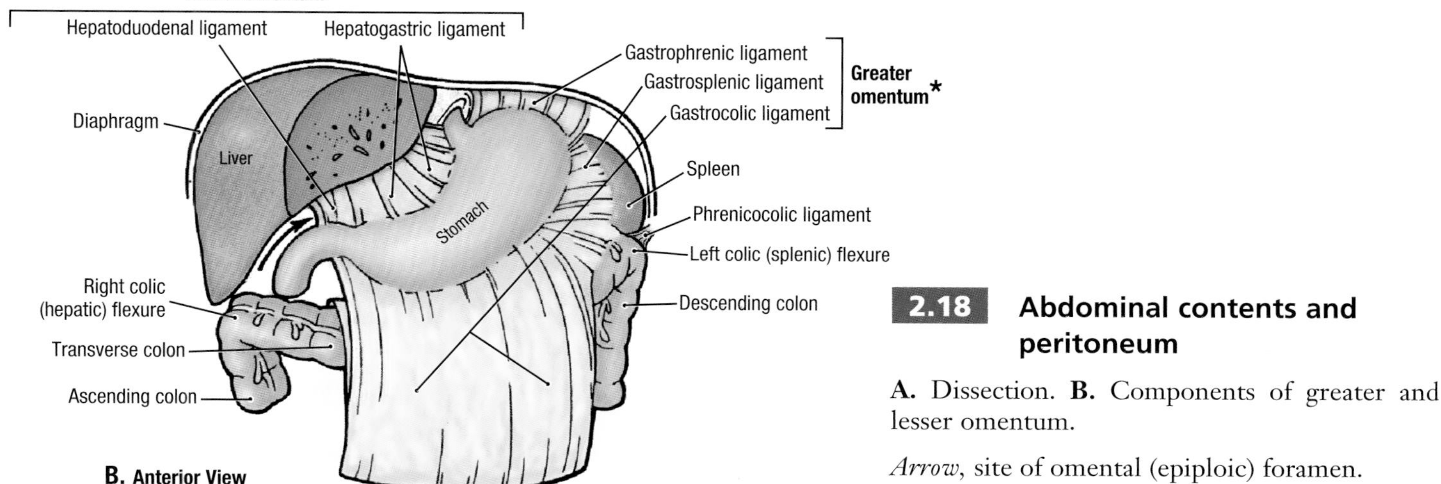
Lesser omentum
Hepatoduodenal ligament
Hepatogastric ligament
Gastrophrenic ligament
Gastrosplenic ligament
Gastrocolic ligament
Greater omentum*
Diaphragm
Liver
Stomach
Spleen
Phrenicocolic ligament
Left colic (splenic) flexure
Descending colon
Right colic (hepatic) flexure
Transverse colon
Ascending colon

**B. Anterior View**

## 2.18 Abdominal contents and peritoneum

**A.** Dissection. **B.** Components of greater and lesser omentum.

*Arrow*, site of omental (epiploic) foramen.

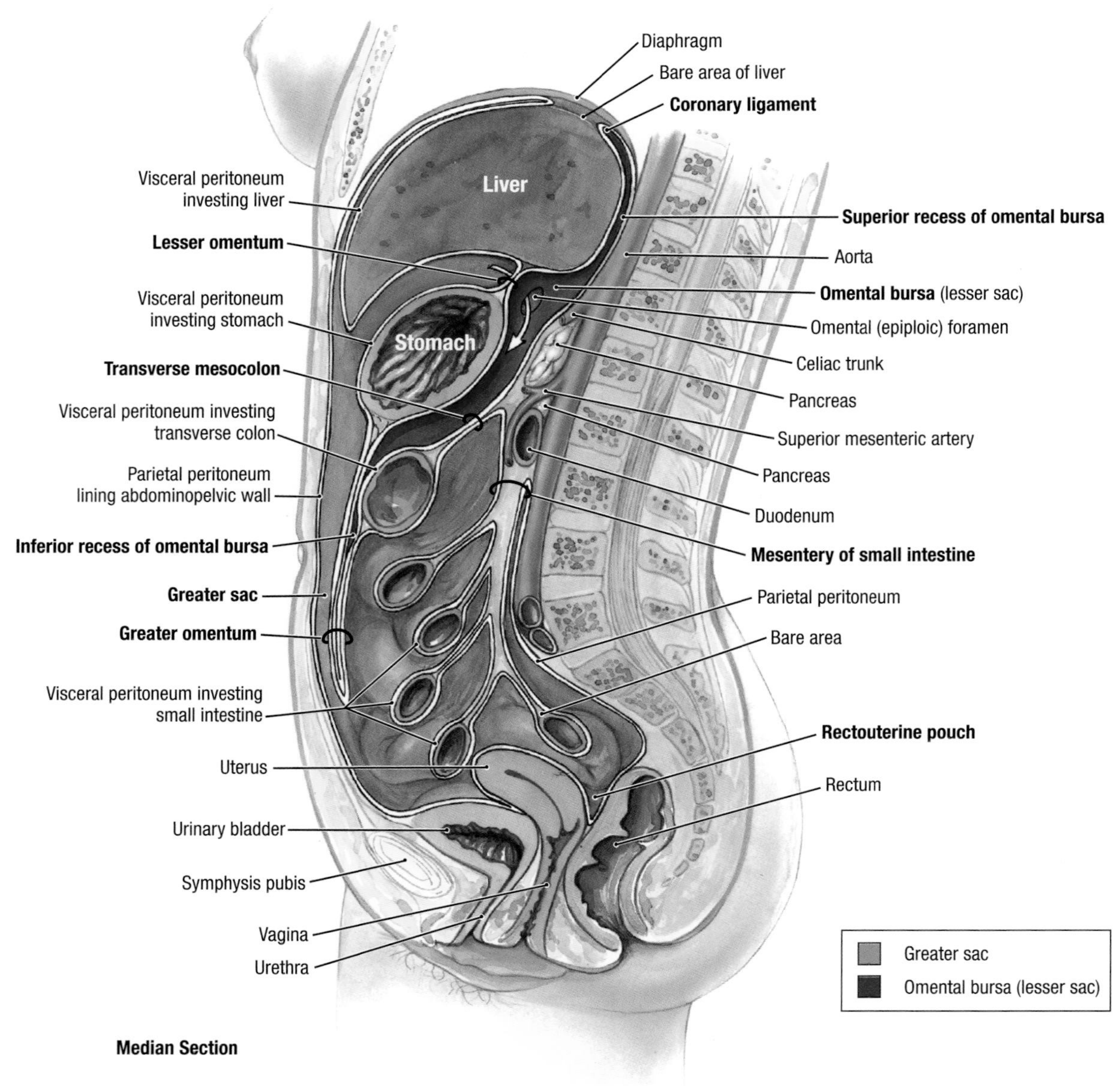
Diaphragm
Bare area of liver
Coronary ligament
Liver
Visceral peritoneum investing liver
Superior recess of omental bursa
Lesser omentum
Aorta
Omental bursa (lesser sac)
Visceral peritoneum investing stomach
Omental (epiploic) foramen
Stomach
Celiac trunk
Transverse mesocolon
Pancreas
Visceral peritoneum investing transverse colon
Superior mesenteric artery
Pancreas
Parietal peritoneum lining abdominopelvic wall
Duodenum
Inferior recess of omental bursa
Mesentery of small intestine
Greater sac
Parietal peritoneum
Greater omentum
Bare area
Visceral peritoneum investing small intestine
Rectouterine pouch
Uterus
Rectum
Urinary bladder
Symphysis pubis
Vagina
Urethra
Greater sac
Omental bursa (lesser sac)
Median Section

## 2.19 Peritoneal formations and bare areas

Various terms are used to describe the parts of the peritoneum that connect organs with other organs or to the abdominal wall, and to describe the compartments and recesses that are formed as a consequence. The *arrow* passes through the omental (epiploic) foramen.

| Term | Definition |
|---|---|
| **Peritoneal ligament** | Double layer of peritoneum that connects an organ with another organ or to the abdominal wall. |
| **Mesentery** | Double layer of peritoneum that occurs as a result of the invagination of the peritoneum by an organ and constitutes a continuity of the visceral and parietal peritoneum. |
| **Omentum** | Double-layered extension of peritoneum passing from the stomach and proximal part of the duodenum to adjacent organs. The greater omentum extends from the greater curvature of the stomach and the proximal duodenum; the lesser omentum from the lesser curvature. |
| **Bare area** | Every organ must have an area, the bare area, that is not covered with visceral peritoneum, to allow the entrance and exit of neurovascular structures. Bare areas are formed in relation to the attachments of mesenteries, omenta, and ligaments. |

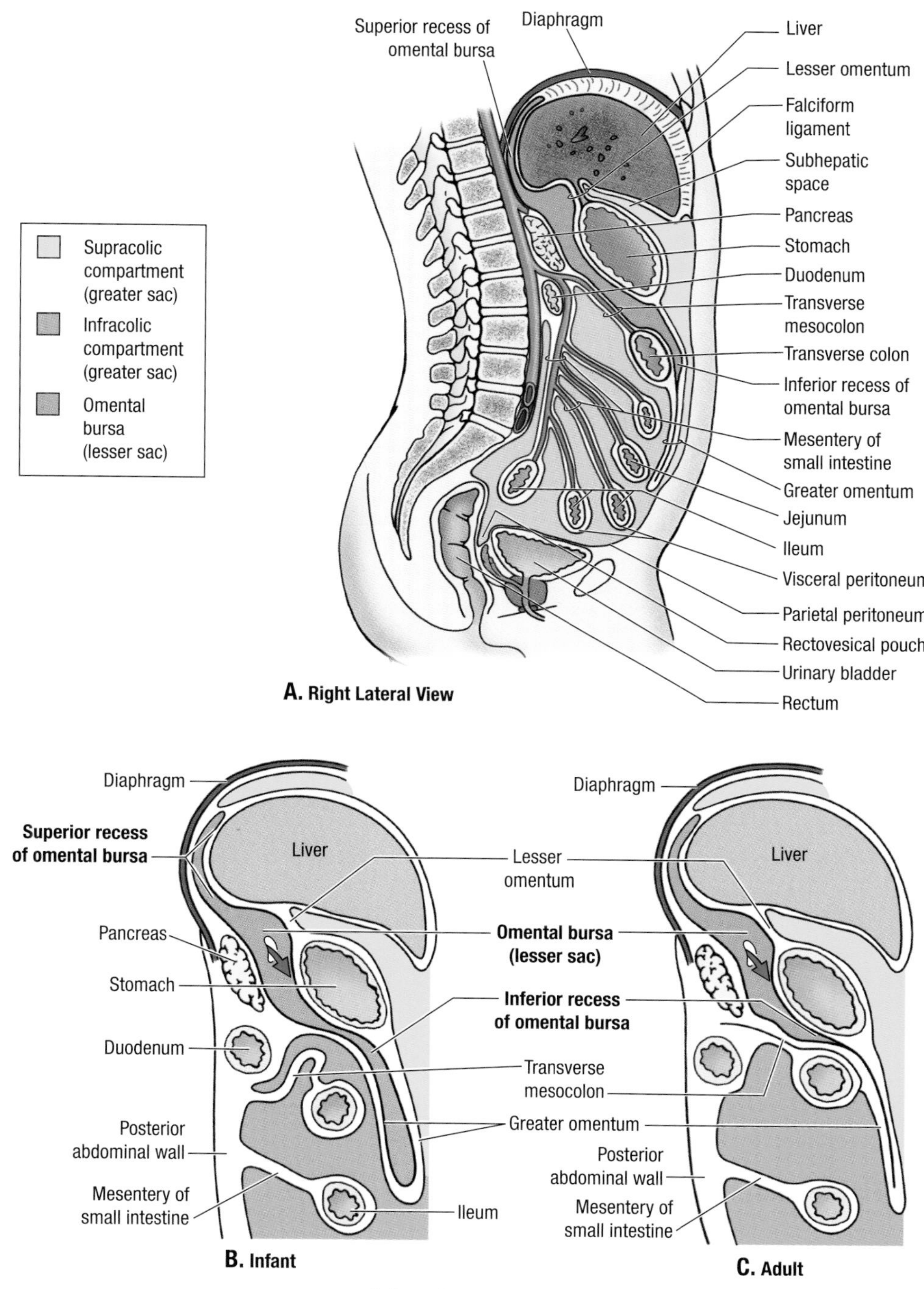
Supracolic compartment (greater sac)
Infracolic compartment (greater sac)
Omental bursa (lesser sac)
Superior recess of omental bursa
Diaphragm
Liver
Lesser omentum
Falciform ligament
Subhepatic space
Pancreas
Stomach
Duodenum
Transverse mesocolon
Transverse colon
Inferior recess of omental bursa
Mesentery of small intestine
Greater omentum
Jejunum
Ileum
Visceral peritoneum
Parietal peritoneum
Rectovesical pouch
Urinary bladder
Rectum
A. Right Lateral View
Diaphragm
Superior recess of omental bursa
Liver
Lesser omentum
Pancreas
Stomach
Omental bursa (lesser sac)
Inferior recess of omental bursa
Duodenum
Transverse mesocolon
Greater omentum
Posterior abdominal wall
Mesentery of small intestine
Ileum
B. Infant
C. Adult
Schematic Sagittal Sections, Lateral View

## 2.20 Subdivisions of peritoneal cavity

**A.** Sagittal section. **B.** In an infant, the omental bursa (lesser sac) is an isolated part of the peritoneal cavity, lying dorsal to the stomach and extending superiorly to the liver and diaphragm (superior recess of the omental bursa) and inferiorly between the layers of the greater omentum (inferior recess of the omental bursa). **C.** In an adult, after fusion of the layers of the greater omentum, the inferior recess of the omental bursa now extends inferiorly only as far as the transverse colon. The *red arrows* pass from the greater sac through the omental (epiploic) foramen into the omental bursa.

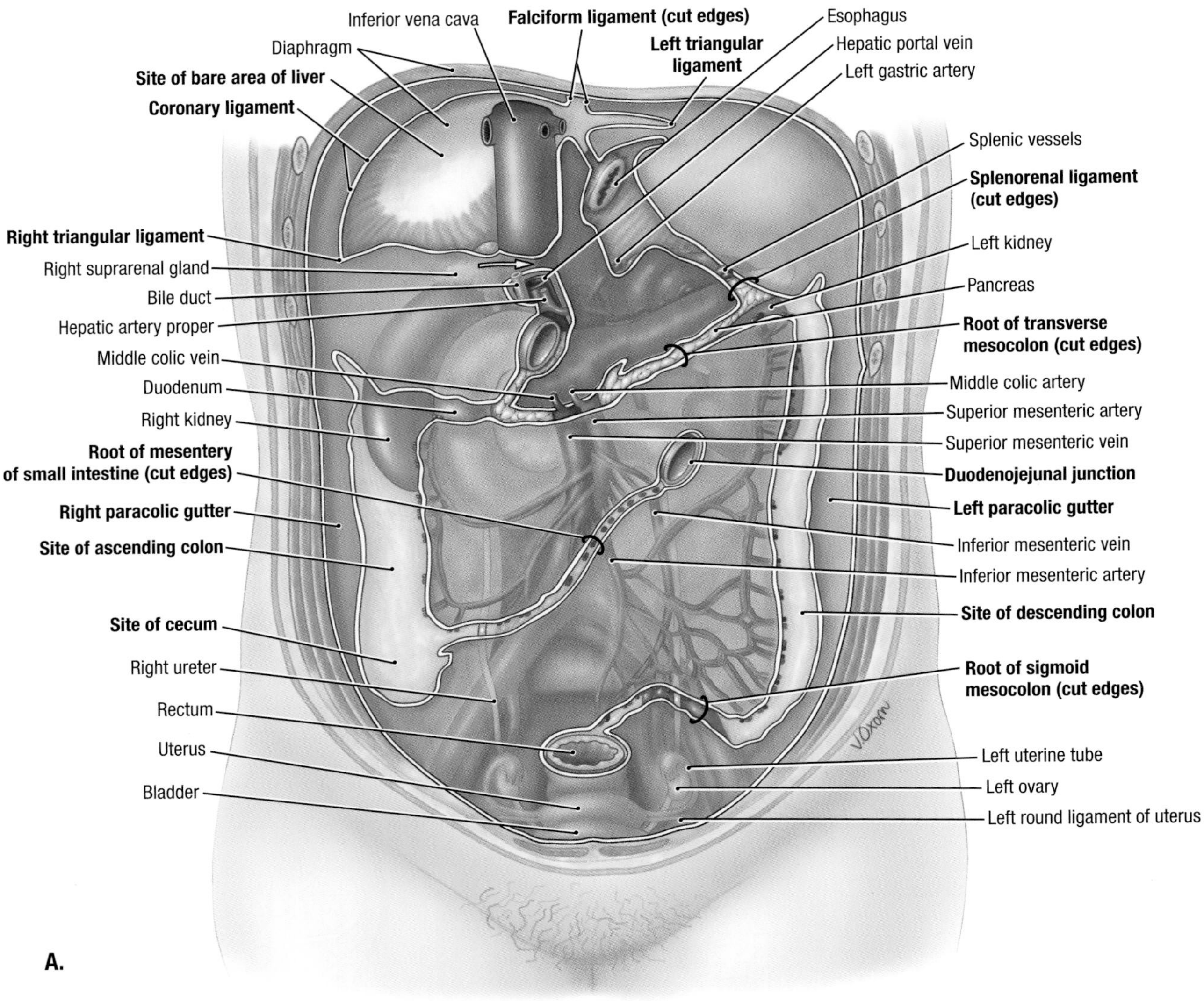

Inferior vena cava
Falciform ligament (cut edges)
Esophagus
Diaphragm
Left triangular ligament
Hepatic portal vein
Site of bare area of liver
Left gastric artery
Coronary ligament
Splenic vessels
Splenorenal ligament (cut edges)
Right triangular ligament
Left kidney
Right suprarenal gland
Bile duct
Pancreas
Hepatic artery proper
Root of transverse mesocolon (cut edges)
Middle colic vein
Middle colic artery
Duodenum
Superior mesenteric artery
Right kidney
Superior mesenteric vein
Root of mesentery of small intestine (cut edges)
Duodenojejunal junction
Right paracolic gutter
Left paracolic gutter
Site of ascending colon
Inferior mesenteric vein
Inferior mesenteric artery
Site of descending colon
Site of cecum
Right ureter
Root of sigmoid mesocolon (cut edges)
Rectum
Uterus
Left uterine tube
Left ovary
Bladder
Left round ligament of uterus

A.

Anterior Views

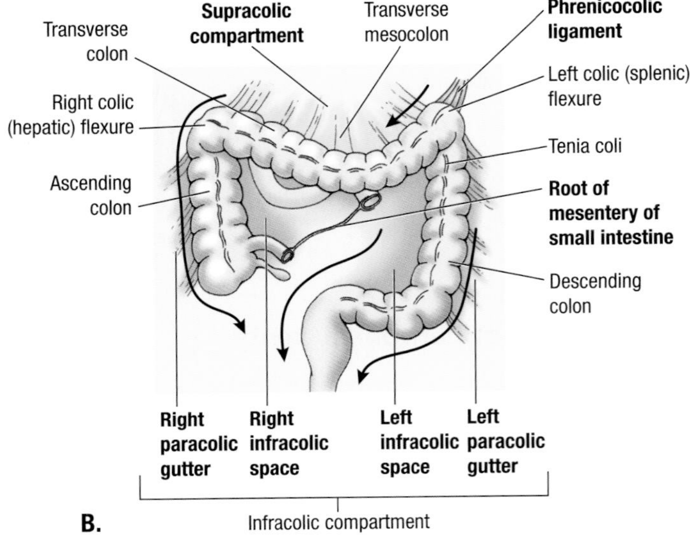
Transverse colon
Supracolic compartment
Transverse mesocolon
Phrenicocolic ligament
Left colic (splenic) flexure
Right colic (hepatic) flexure
Tenia coli
Ascending colon
Root of mesentery of small intestine
Descending colon
Right paracolic gutter
Right infracolic space
Left infracolic space
Left paracolic gutter
Infracolic compartment

B.

## 2.21 Posterior wall of peritoneal cavity

**A.** Roots of the peritoneal reflections. The peritoneal reflections from the posterior abdominal wall (mesenteries and reflections surrounding bare areas of liver and secondarily retroperitoneal organs) have been cut at their roots, and the intraperitoneal and secondarily retroperitoneal viscera have been removed. The *white arrow* passes through the omental (epiploic) foramen. **B.** Supracolic and infracolic compartments of the greater sac. The infracolic spaces and paracolic gutters are of clinical importance because they determine the paths (*black arrows*) for the flow of ascetic fluid with changes in position, and the spread of intraperitoneal reflections.

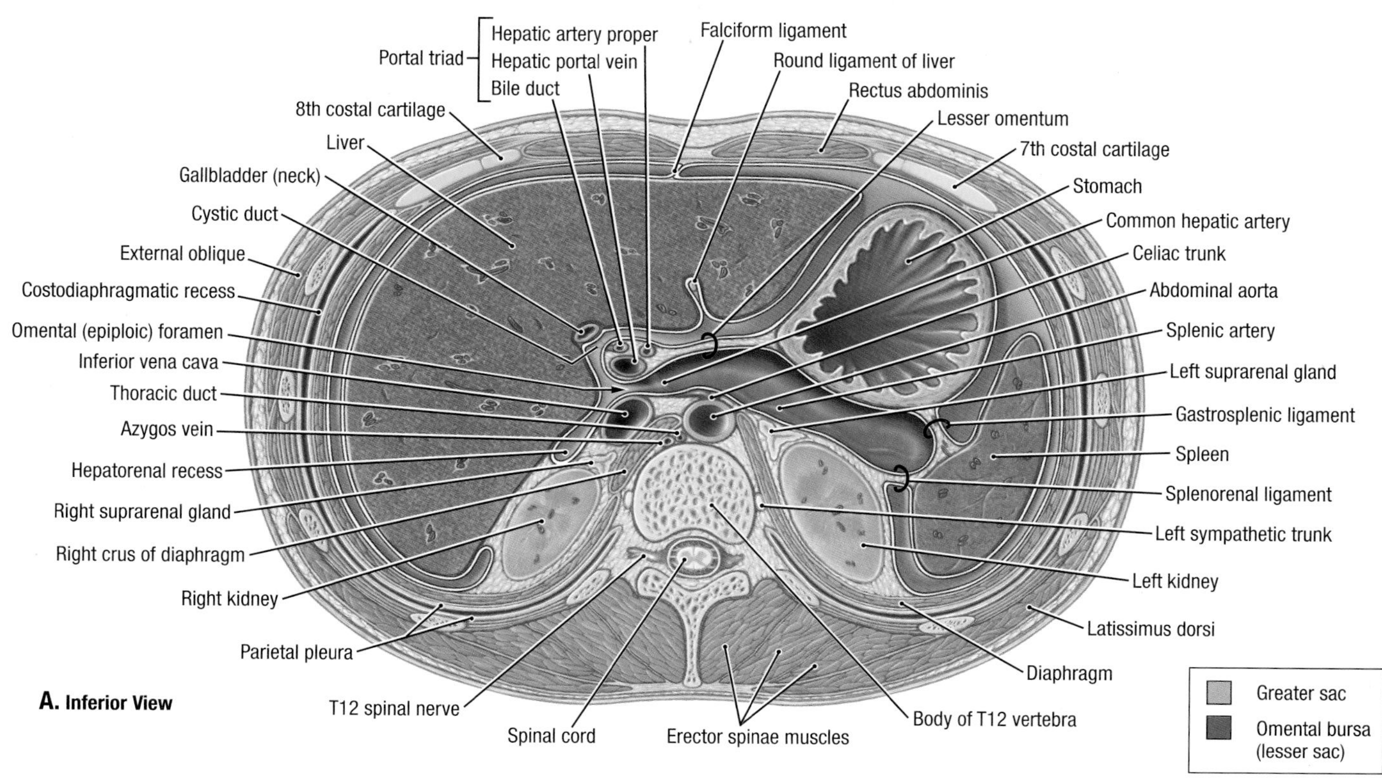
Portal triad
Hepatic artery proper
Hepatic portal vein
Bile duct
Falciform ligament
Round ligament of liver
Rectus abdominis
Lesser omentum
8th costal cartilage
Liver
7th costal cartilage
Gallbladder (neck)
Stomach
Cystic duct
Common hepatic artery
External oblique
Celiac trunk
Costodiaphragmatic recess
Abdominal aorta
Omental (epiploic) foramen
Splenic artery
Inferior vena cava
Left suprarenal gland
Thoracic duct
Gastrosplenic ligament
Azygos vein
Spleen
Hepatorenal recess
Splenorenal ligament
Right suprarenal gland
Left sympathetic trunk
Right crus of diaphragm
Left kidney
Right kidney
Latissimus dorsi
Parietal pleura
Diaphragm
T12 spinal nerve
Spinal cord
Erector spinae muscles
Body of T12 vertebra
Greater sac
Omental bursa (lesser sac)

**A.** Inferior View

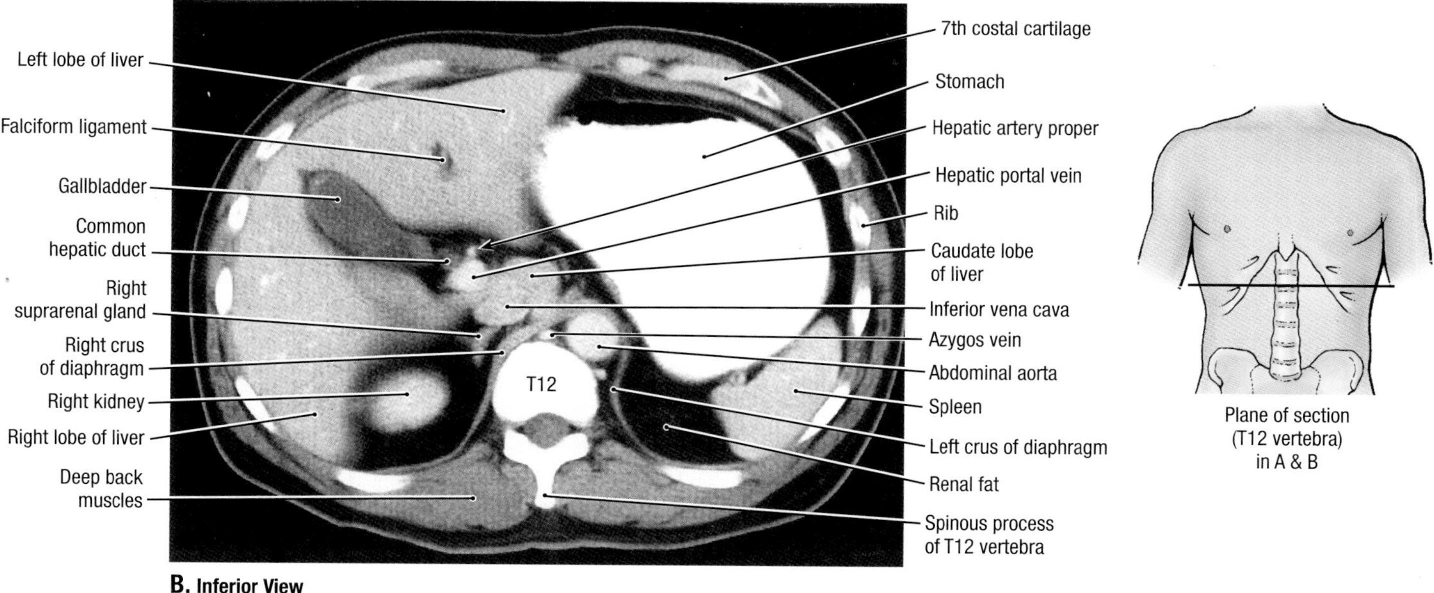
Left lobe of liver
Falciform ligament
Gallbladder
Common hepatic duct
Right suprarenal gland
Right crus of diaphragm
Right kidney
Right lobe of liver
Deep back muscles
T12
7th costal cartilage
Stomach
Hepatic artery proper
Hepatic portal vein
Rib
Caudate lobe of liver
Inferior vena cava
Azygos vein
Abdominal aorta
Spleen
Left crus of diaphragm
Renal fat
Spinous process of T12 vertebra
Plane of section (T12 vertebra) in A & B

**B.** Inferior View

## 2.22 Transverse sections through greater sac and omental bursa.

- When bacterial contamination occurs or when the gut is traumatically penetrated or ruptured as the result of infection and inflammation, gas, fecal matter, and bacteria enter the peritoneal cavity. The result is infection and inflammation of the peritoneum, called peritonitis.
- Under certain pathological conditions such as peritonitis, the peritoneal cavity may be distended with abnormal fluid (ascites). Widespread metastases (spread) of cancer cells to the abdominal viscera cause exudation (escape) of fluid that is often blood stained. Thus the peritoneal cavity may be distended with several liters of abnormal fluid. Surgical puncture of the peritoneal cavity for the aspiration of drainage of fluid is called paracentesis.

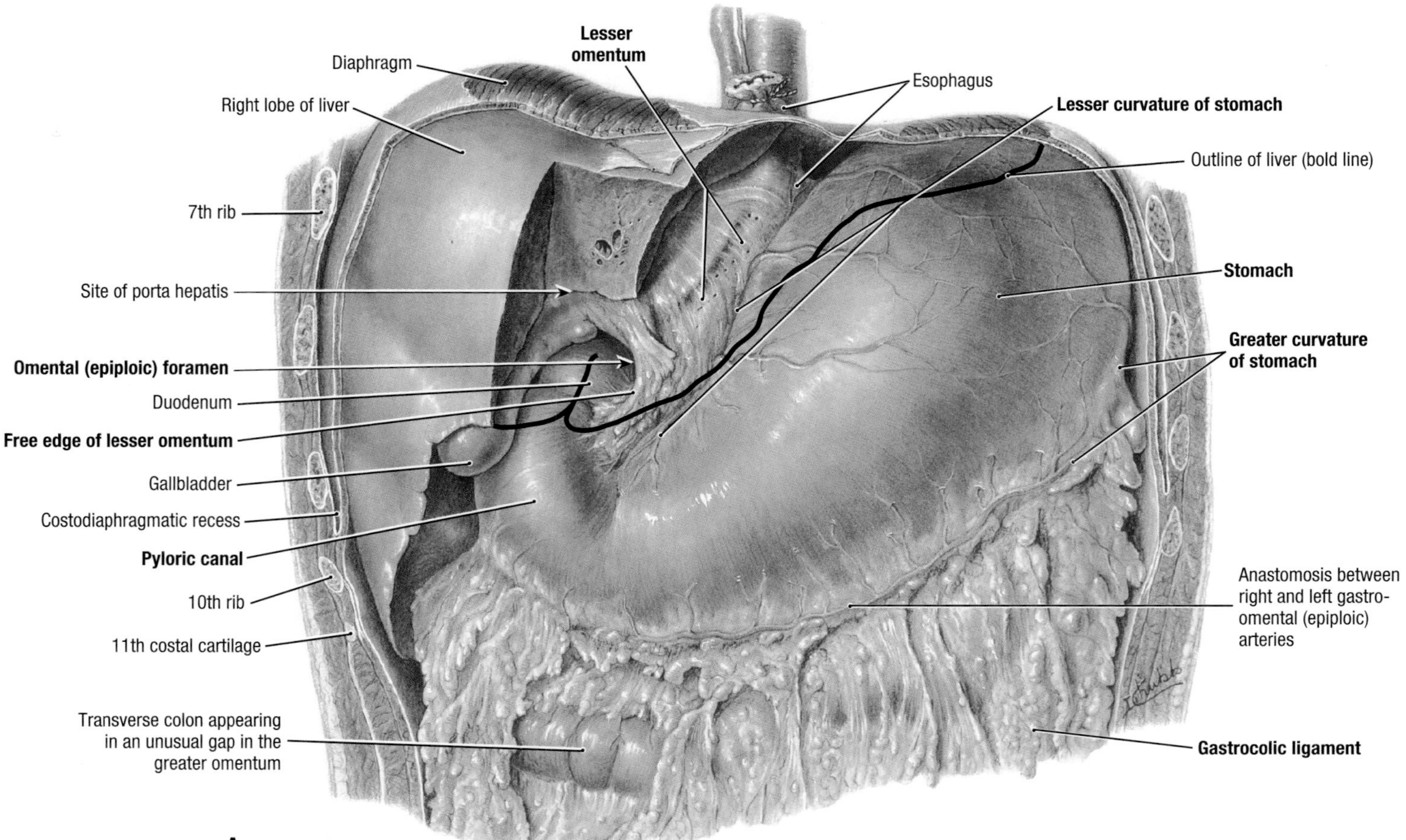

Diaphragm
Right lobe of liver
Lesser omentum
Esophagus
Lesser curvature of stomach
Outline of liver (bold line)
7th rib
Stomach
Site of porta hepatis
Greater curvature of stomach
Omental (epiploic) foramen
Duodenum
Free edge of lesser omentum
Gallbladder
Costodiaphragmatic recess
Pyloric canal
10th rib
Anastomosis between right and left gastro-omental (epiploic) arteries
11th costal cartilage
Transverse colon appearing in an unusual gap in the greater omentum
Gastrocolic ligament

**A. Anterior View**

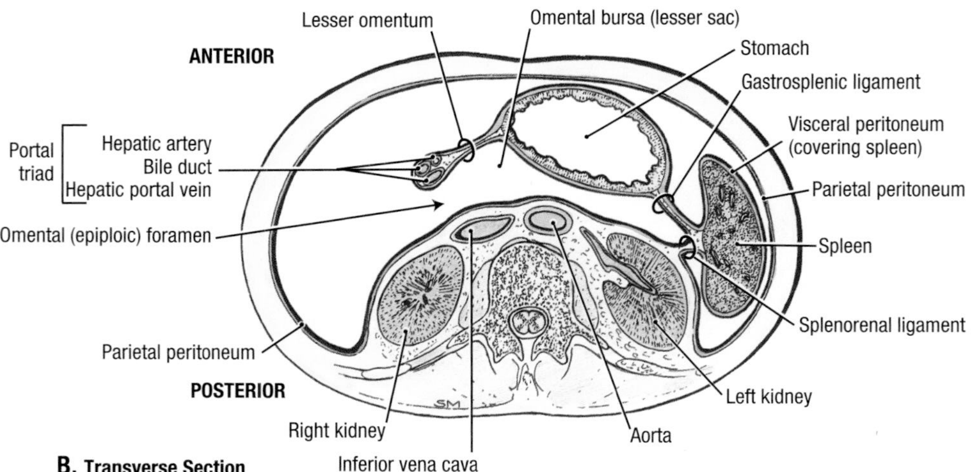
Lesser omentum
Omental bursa (lesser sac)
ANTERIOR
Stomach
Gastrosplenic ligament
Visceral peritoneum (covering spleen)
Portal triad
Hepatic artery
Bile duct
Hepatic portal vein
Parietal peritoneum
Omental (epiploic) foramen
Spleen
Splenorenal ligament
Parietal peritoneum
POSTERIOR
Left kidney
Right kidney
Aorta
Inferior vena cava

**B. Transverse Section**

## 2.23 Stomach and omenta

**A.** Lesser and greater omenta. The stomach is inflated with air, and the left part of the liver is cut away. The gallbladder, followed superiorly, leads to the free margin of the lesser omentum and serves as a guide to the omental epiploic foramen, which lies posterior to that free margin. **B.** Omental bursa (lesser sac), schematic transverse section.

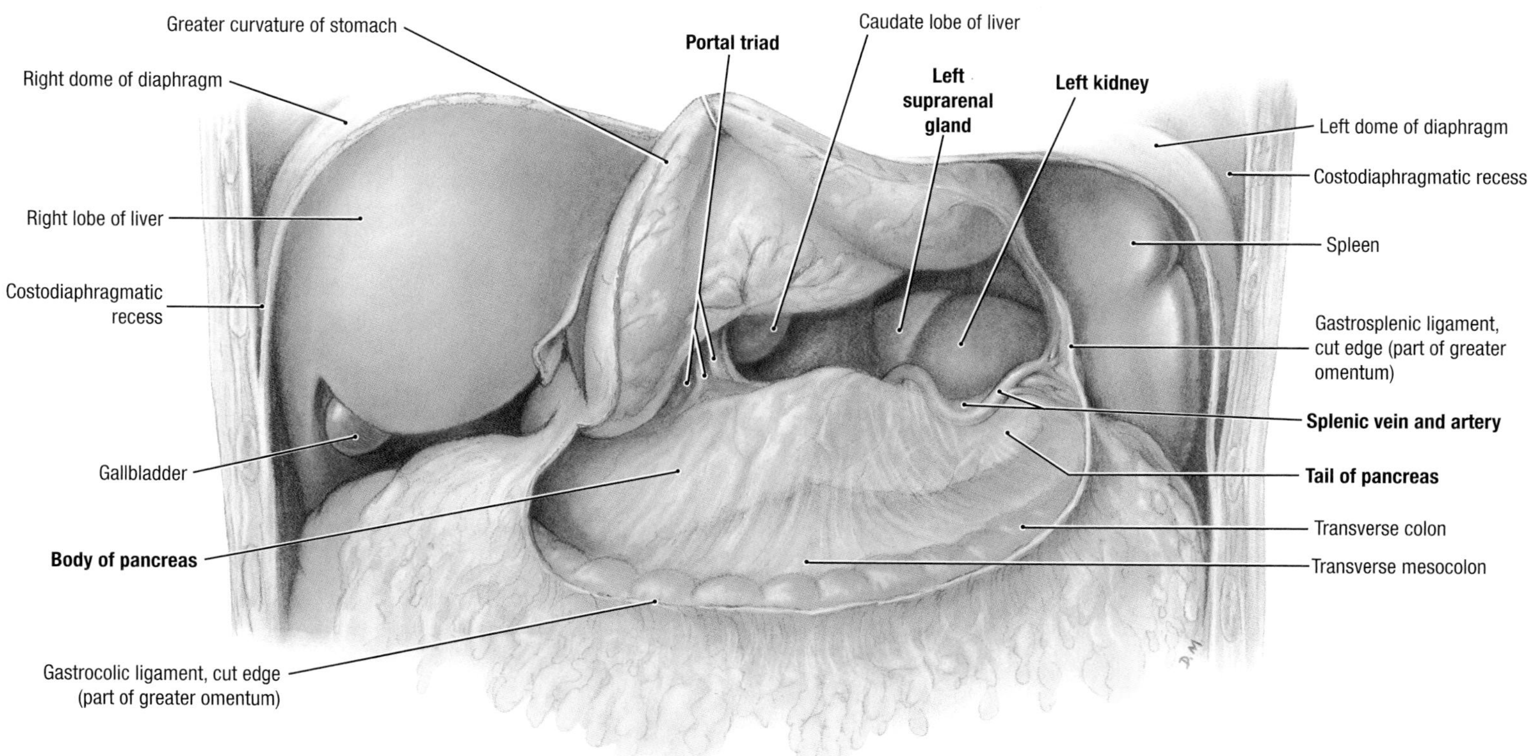
Greater curvature of stomach
Portal triad
Caudate lobe of liver
Right dome of diaphragm
Left suprarenal gland
Left kidney
Left dome of diaphragm
Costodiaphragmatic recess
Right lobe of liver
Spleen
Costodiaphragmatic recess
Gastrosplenic ligament, cut edge (part of greater omentum)
Splenic vein and artery
Gallbladder
Tail of pancreas
Transverse colon
Body of pancreas
Transverse mesocolon
Gastrocolic ligament, cut edge (part of greater omentum)

**A.** Anterior View

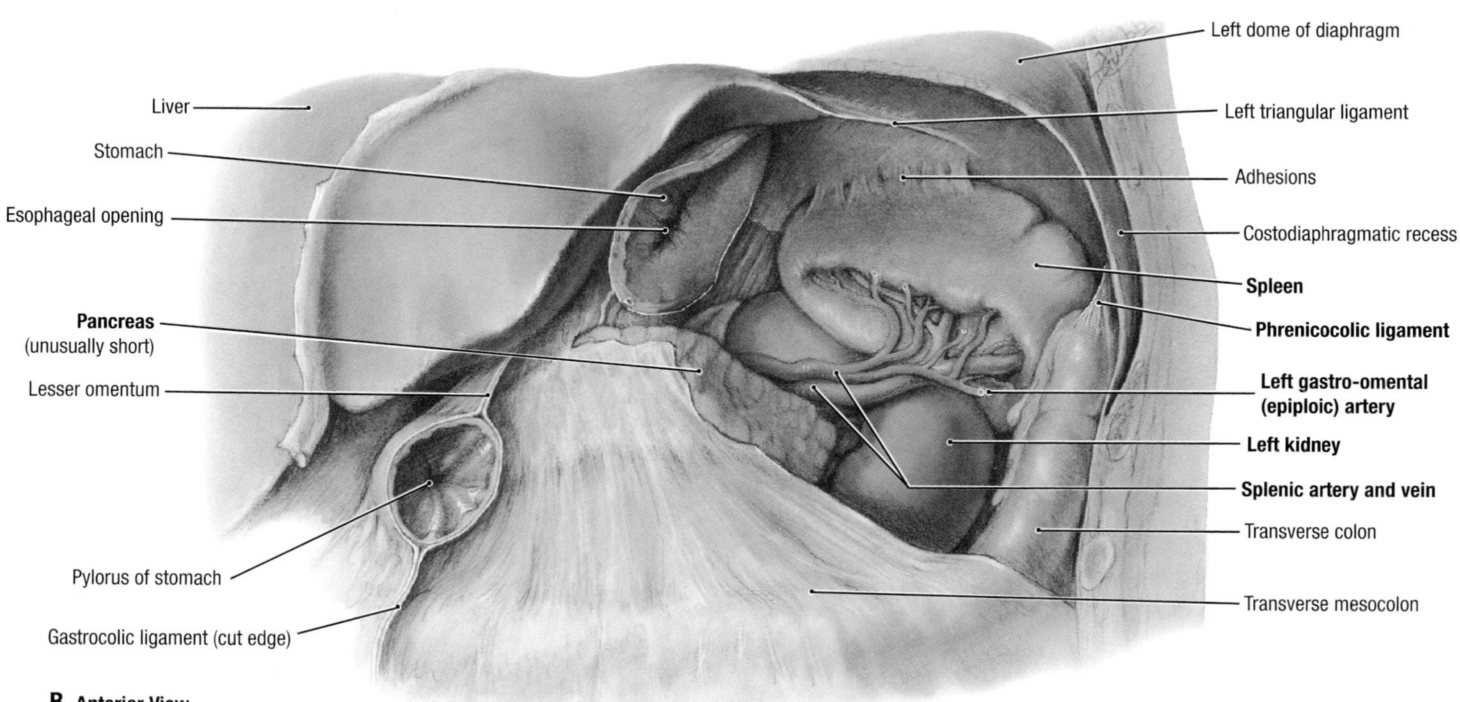
Left dome of diaphragm
Liver
Left triangular ligament
Stomach
Adhesions
Esophageal opening
Costodiaphragmatic recess
Spleen
Pancreas (unusually short)
Phrenicocolic ligament
Lesser omentum
Left gastro-omental (epiploic) artery
Left kidney
Splenic artery and vein
Transverse colon
Pylorus of stomach
Transverse mesocolon
Gastrocolic ligament (cut edge)

**B.** Anterior View

## 2.24 Posterior relationships of omental bursa (lesser sac)

**A.** Opened omental bursa. The greater omentum has been cut along the greater curvature of the stomach; the stomach is reflected superiorly. Peritoneum of the stomach bed is partially removed. **B.** Stomach bed. The stomach is excised. Peritoneum covering the stomach bed and inferior part of the kidney and pancreas is largely removed. Adhesions binding the spleen to the diaphragm are pathological, but not unusual.

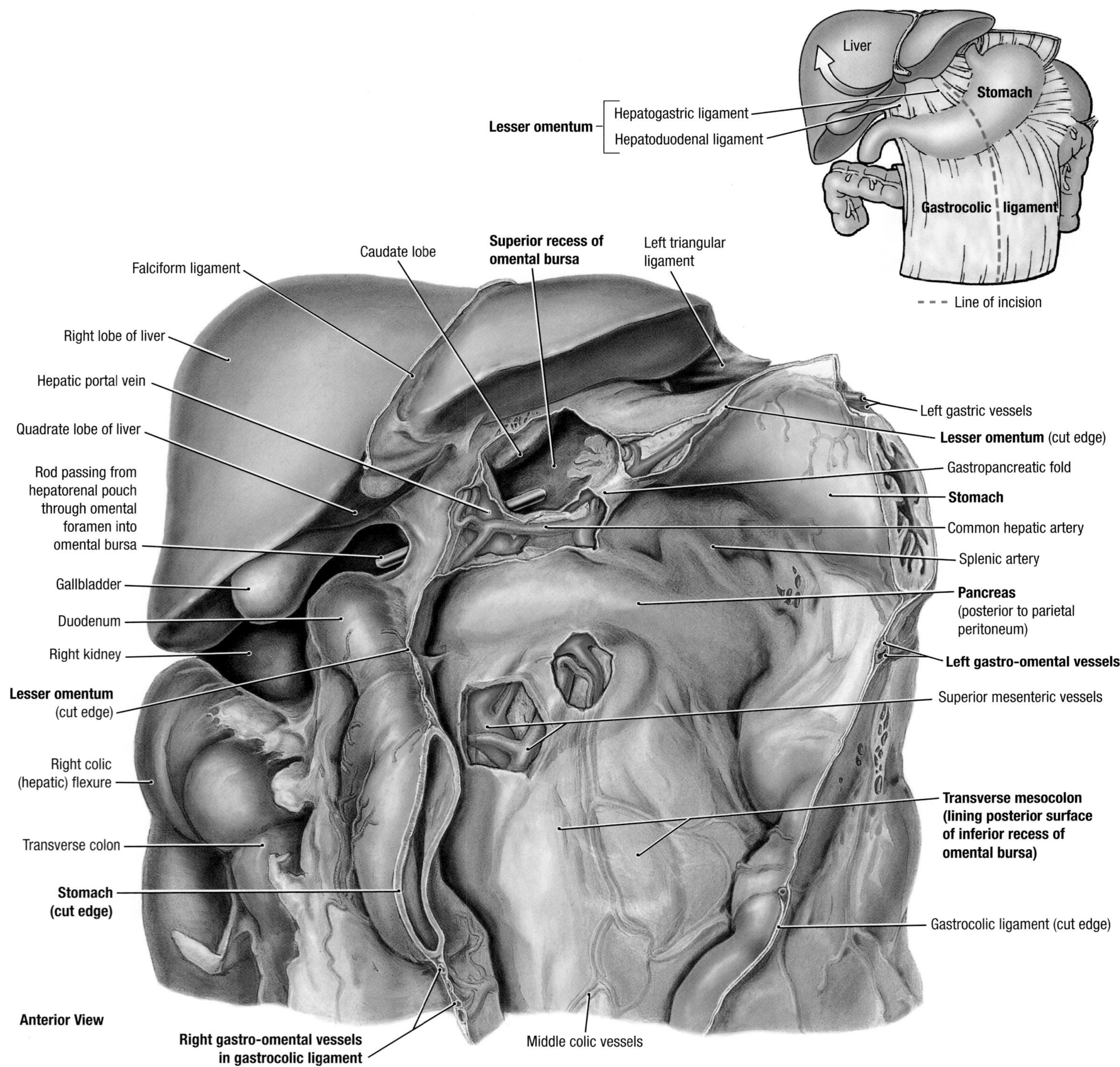
Liver
Stomach
Lesser omentum
Hepatogastric ligament
Hepatoduodenal ligament
Gastrocolic ligament
Line of incision
Falciform ligament
Caudate lobe
Superior recess of omental bursa
Left triangular ligament
Right lobe of liver
Hepatic portal vein
Quadrate lobe of liver
Rod passing from hepatorenal pouch through omental foramen into omental bursa
Gallbladder
Duodenum
Right kidney
Lesser omentum (cut edge)
Right colic (hepatic) flexure
Transverse colon
Stomach (cut edge)
Anterior View
Right gastro-omental vessels in gastrocolic ligament
Middle colic vessels
Left gastric vessels
Lesser omentum (cut edge)
Gastropancreatic fold
Stomach
Common hepatic artery
Splenic artery
Pancreas (posterior to parietal peritoneum)
Left gastro-omental vessels
Superior mesenteric vessels
Transverse mesocolon (lining posterior surface of inferior recess of omental bursa)
Gastrocolic ligament (cut edge)

## 2.25 Omental bursa (lesser sac), opened

The anterior wall of the omental bursa, consisting of the stomach, lesser omentum, anterior layer of the greater omentum, and vessels along the curvatures of the stomach, has been sectioned sagittally. The two halves have been retracted to the left and right: the body of the stomach on the left side, and the pyloric part of the stomach and first part of the duodenum on the right. The right kidney forms the posterior wall of the hepatorenal pouch (part of greater sac), and the pancreas lies horizontally on the posterior wall of the main compartment of the omental bursa (lesser sac). The gastrocolic ligament forms the anterior wall and the lower part of the posterior wall of the inferior recess of the omental bursa. The transverse mesocolon forms the upper part of the posterior wall of the inferior recess of the omental bursa.

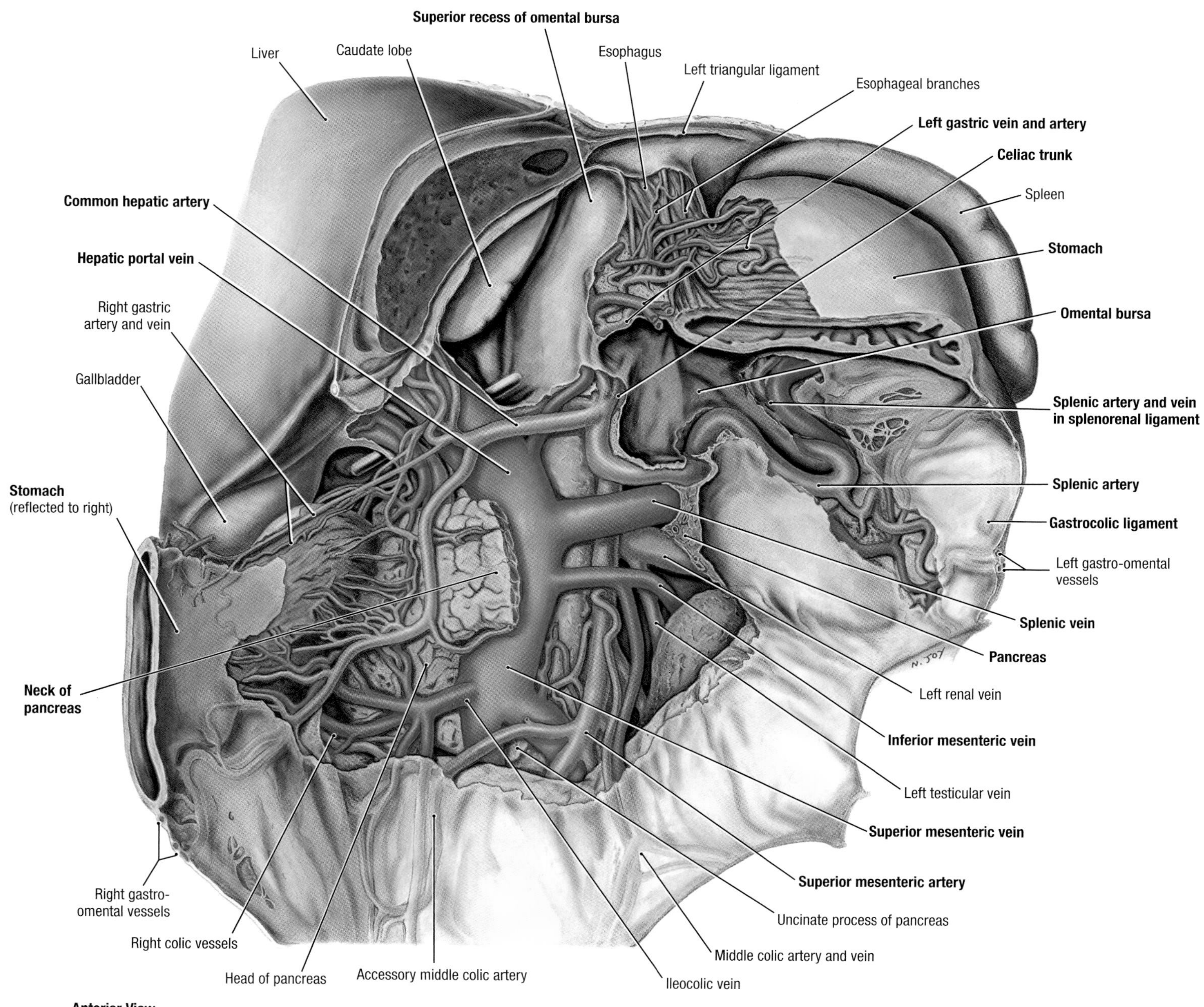
Superior recess of omental bursa
Liver
Caudate lobe
Esophagus
Left triangular ligament
Esophageal branches
Left gastric vein and artery
Celiac trunk
Spleen
Stomach
Omental bursa
Common hepatic artery
Hepatic portal vein
Right gastric artery and vein
Gallbladder
Stomach (reflected to right)
Neck of pancreas
Splenic artery and vein in splenorenal ligament
Splenic artery
Gastrocolic ligament
Left gastro-omental vessels
Splenic vein
Pancreas
Left renal vein
Inferior mesenteric vein
Left testicular vein
Superior mesenteric vein
Superior mesenteric artery
Uncinate process of pancreas
Middle colic artery and vein
Ileocolic vein
Accessory middle colic artery
Head of pancreas
Right colic vessels
Right gastro-omental vessels
Anterior View

## 2.26 Posterior wall of omental bursa

The parietal peritoneum of the posterior wall of the omental bursa has been mostly removed, and a section of the pancreas has been excised. The rod passes through the omental foramen.

- The celiac trunk gives rise to the left gastric artery, the splenic artery that runs tortuously to the left, and the common hepatic artery that runs to the right, passing anterior to the hepatic portal vein.
- The hepatic portal vein is formed posterior to the neck of the pancreas by the union of the superior mesenteric and splenic veins, with the inferior mesenteric vein joining at or near the angle of union.
- The left testicular vein usually drains into the left renal vein. Both are systemic veins.

Oral cavity
Lips
Tongue
Larynx
Trachea
Nasopharynx
Oropharynx
Laryngopharynx
Pharynx
Thoracic part
Abdominal part
Esophagus
Liver
Gallbladder
Pylorus
Duodenum
Stomach
Pancreas
Transverse colon
Ascending colon
Descending colon
Jejunum
Ileum
Cecum
Appendix
Sigmoid colon
Rectum
Anus

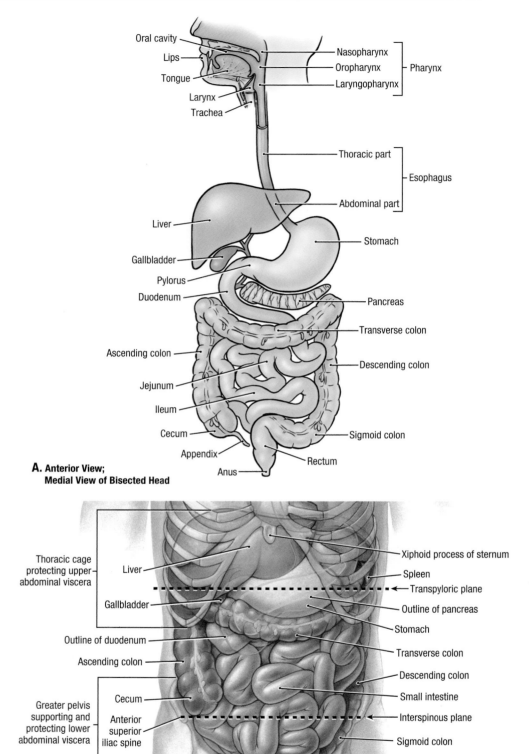

**A. Anterior View; Medial View of Bisected Head**

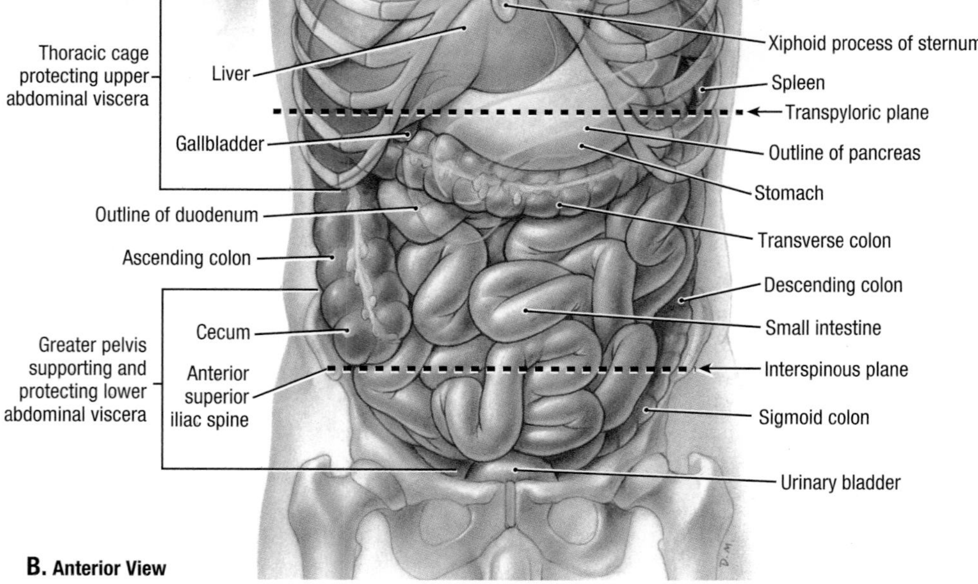
Thoracic cage protecting upper abdominal viscera
Liver
Gallbladder
Xiphoid process of sternum
Spleen
Transpyloric plane
Outline of pancreas
Stomach
Outline of duodenum
Ascending colon
Transverse colon
Descending colon
Greater pelvis supporting and protecting lower abdominal viscera
Cecum
Anterior superior iliac spine
Small intestine
Interspinous plane
Sigmoid colon
Urinary bladder

**B. Anterior View**

## 2.27 Digestive system

**A.** Schematic illustration. **B.** Abdominal portion. The digestive system extends from the lips to the anus. Associated organs include the liver, gallbladder, and pancreas.

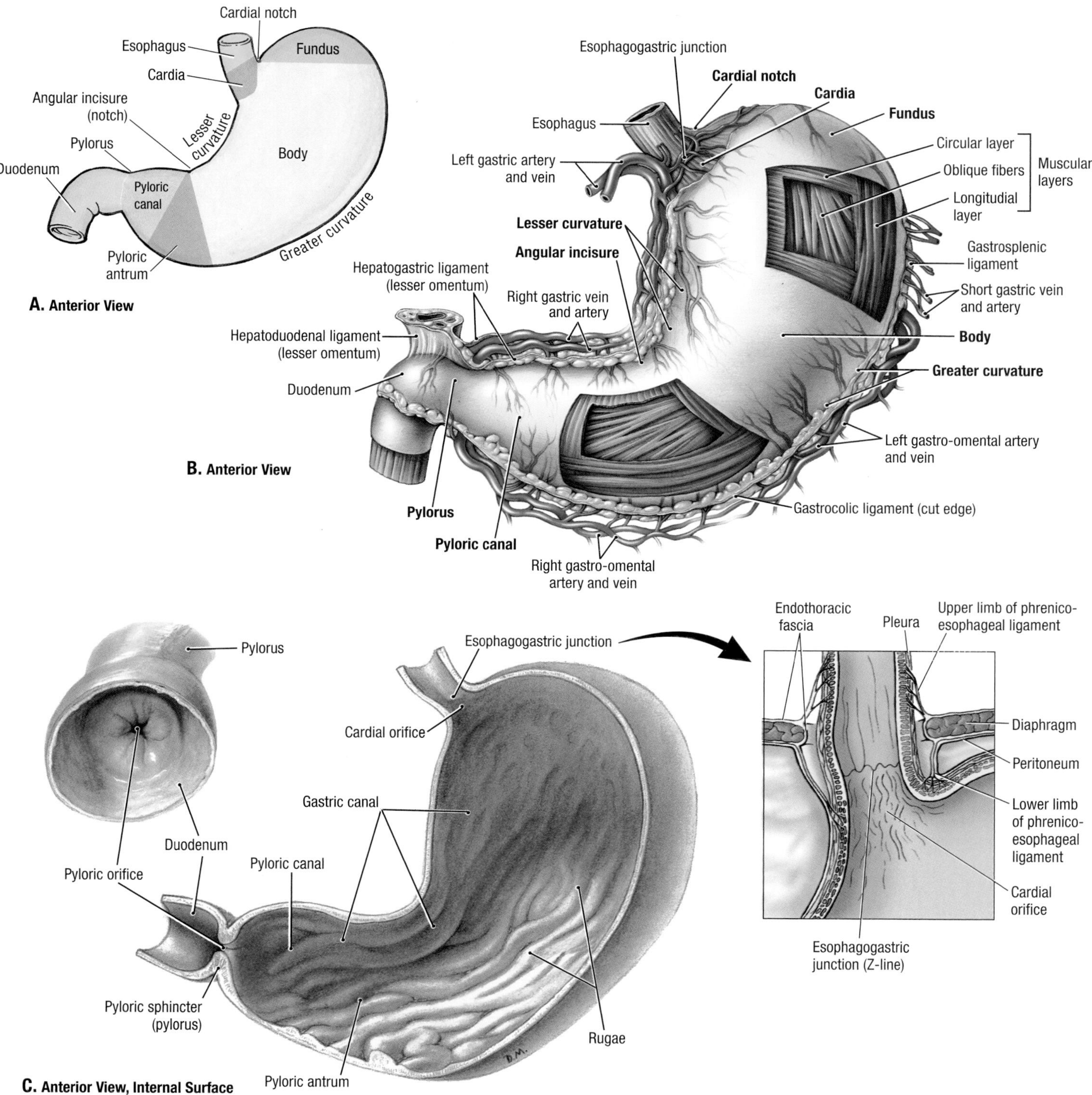
Cardial notch
Esophagus
Fundus
Cardia
Angular incisure (notch)
Lesser curvature
Pylorus
Body
Duodenum
Pyloric canal
Greater curvature
Pyloric antrum
A. Anterior View
Esophagogastric junction
Cardial notch
Cardia
Fundus
Esophagus
Circular layer
Oblique fibers
Longitudial layer
Muscular layers
Left gastric artery and vein
Lesser curvature
Angular incisure
Gastrosplenic ligament
Hepatogastric ligament (lesser omentum)
Short gastric vein and artery
Right gastric vein and artery
Hepatoduodenal ligament (lesser omentum)
Body
Greater curvature
Duodenum
Left gastro-omental artery and vein
B. Anterior View
Gastrocolic ligament (cut edge)
Pylorus
Pyloric canal
Right gastro-omental artery and vein
Endothoracic fascia
Pleura
Upper limb of phrenico-esophageal ligament
Pylorus
Esophagogastric junction
Cardial orifice
Diaphragm
Peritoneum
Gastric canal
Lower limb of phrenico-esophageal ligament
Duodenum
Pyloric canal
Pyloric orifice
Cardial orifice
Esophagogastric junction (Z-line)
Pyloric sphincter (pylorus)
Rugae
Pyloric antrum
C. Anterior View, Internal Surface

## 2.28 Stomach

**A.** Parts. **B.** External surface. **C.** Internal surface (mucous membrane), anterior wall removed. Insets: Left side of page—pylorus, viewed from the duodenum. Right side of page—details of the esophagogastric junction.

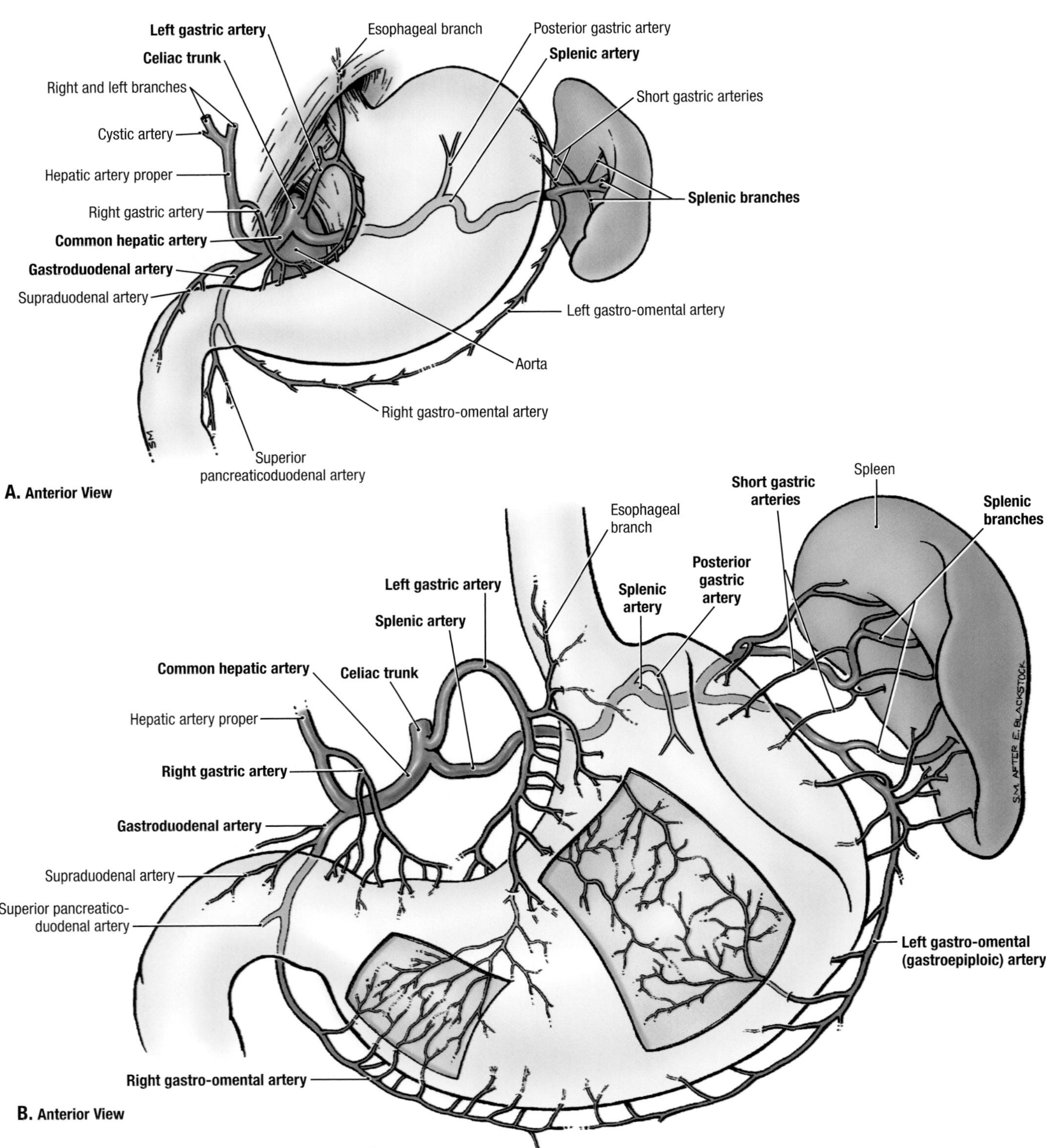
Left gastric artery
Celiac trunk
Right and left branches
Cystic artery
Hepatic artery proper
Right gastric artery
Common hepatic artery
Gastroduodenal artery
Supraduodenal artery
Esophageal branch
Posterior gastric artery
Splenic artery
Short gastric arteries
Splenic branches
Left gastro-omental artery
Aorta
Right gastro-omental artery
Superior pancreaticoduodenal artery
A. Anterior View
Spleen
Short gastric arteries
Splenic branches
Esophageal branch
Posterior gastric artery
Splenic artery
Left gastric artery
Splenic artery
Common hepatic artery
Celiac trunk
Hepatic artery proper
Right gastric artery
Gastroduodenal artery
Supraduodenal artery
Superior pancreatico-duodenal artery
Left gastro-omental (gastroepiploic) artery
Right gastro-omental artery
B. Anterior View

## 2.29 Celiac artery

**A.** Branches of celiac trunk. The celiac trunk is a branch of the abdominal aorta, arising immediately inferior to the aortic hiatus of the diaphragm (T12 vertebral level). The vessel is usually 1 to 2 cm long and divides into the left gastric, common hepatic, and splenic arteries. The celiac trunk supplies the liver, gall bladder, inferior esophagus, stomach, pancreas, spleen, and duodenum. **B.** Arteries of stomach and spleen. The serous and muscular coats are removed from two areas of the stomach, revealing anastomotic networks in the submucous coat.

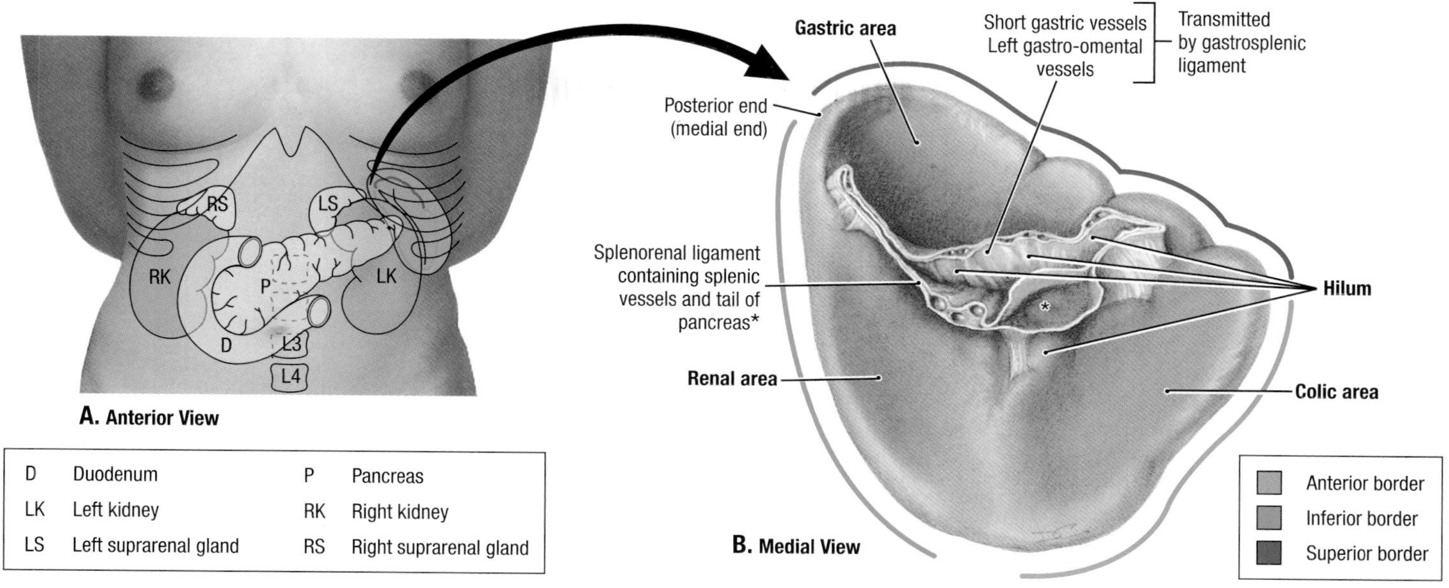
RS
LS
RK
P
LK
D
L3
L4
A. Anterior View
D Duodenum
LK Left kidney
LS Left suprarenal gland
P Pancreas
RK Right kidney
RS Right suprarenal gland
Gastric area
Short gastric vessels
Left gastro-omental vessels
Transmitted by gastrosplenic ligament
Posterior end (medial end)
Splenorenal ligament containing splenic vessels and tail of pancreas*
Hilum
Renal area
Colic area
Anterior border
Inferior border
Superior border
B. Medial View

## 2.30 Spleen

**A.** The surface anatomy of the spleen. The spleen lies superficially in the left upper abdominal quadrant between the 9th and 11th ribs. **B.** Note the impressions (colic, renal and gastric areas) made by structures in contact with its visceral surface. The superior border is notched.

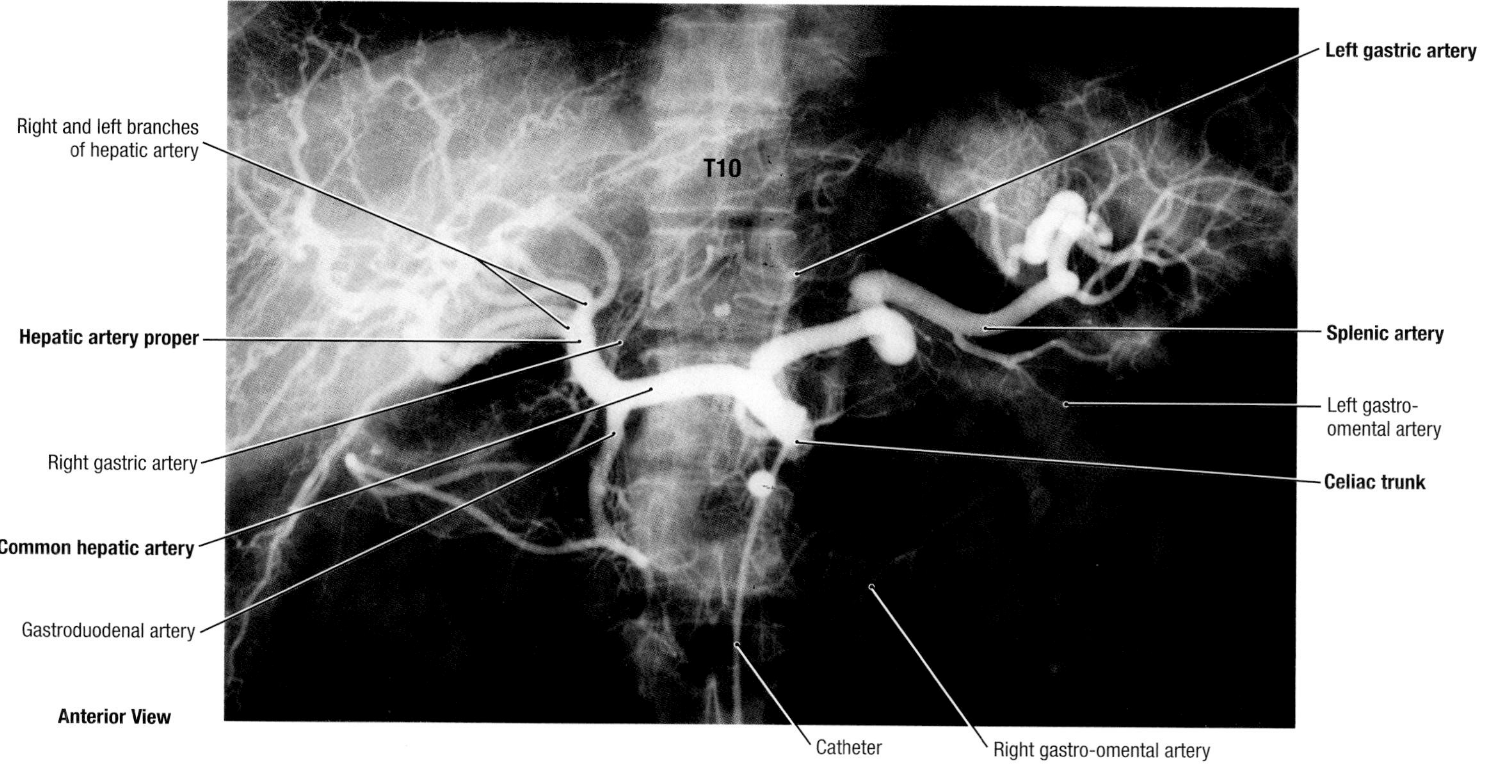
Left gastric artery
Right and left branches of hepatic artery
T10
Hepatic artery proper
Splenic artery
Left gastro-omental artery
Right gastric artery
Celiac trunk
Common hepatic artery
Gastroduodenal artery
Anterior View
Catheter
Right gastro-omental artery

## 2.31 Celiac arteriogram

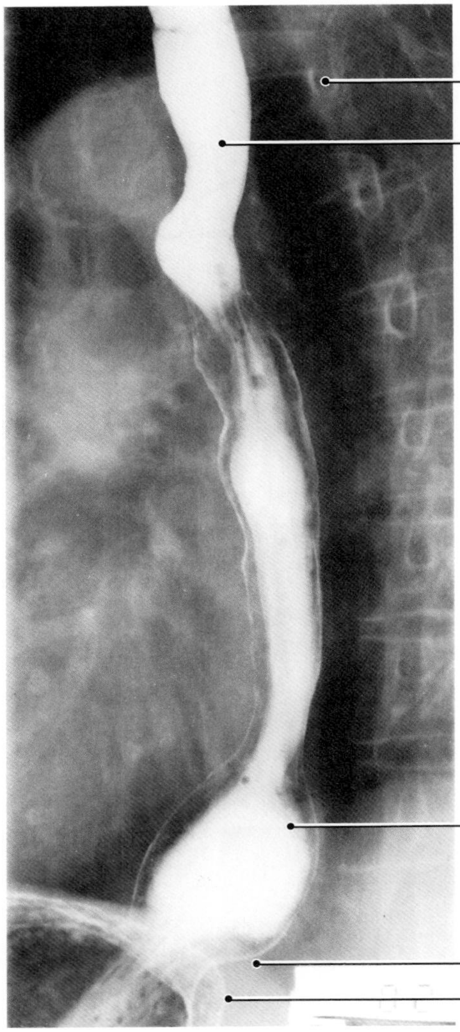

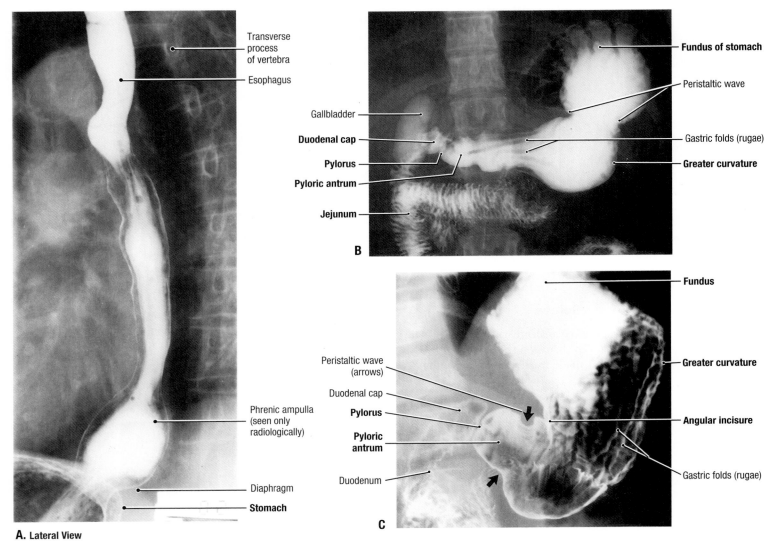

Transverse process of vertebra
Esophagus
Phrenic ampulla (seen only radiologically)
Diaphragm
Stomach
A. Lateral View

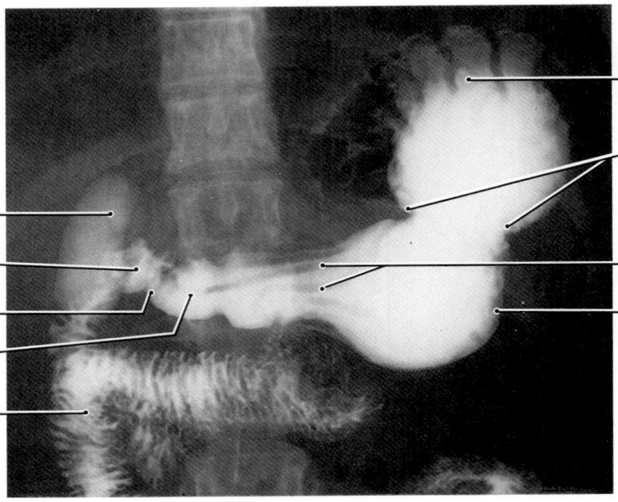

Fundus of stomach
Peristaltic wave
Gallbladder
Duodenal cap
Gastric folds (rugae)
Pylorus
Greater curvature
Pyloric antrum
Jejunum
B

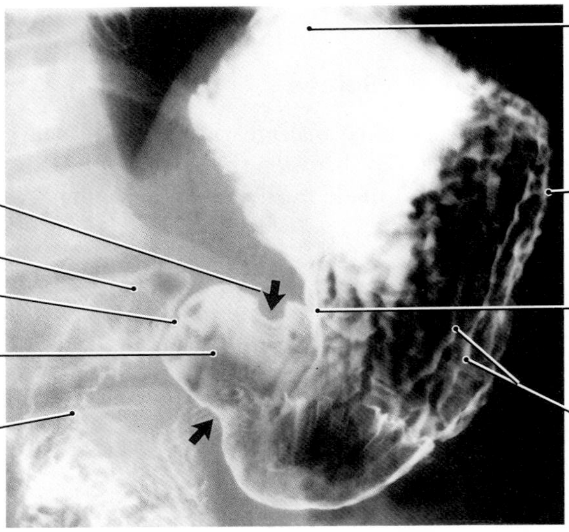

Fundus
Greater curvature
Peristaltic wave (arrows)
Duodenal cap
Pylorus
Angular incisure
Pyloric antrum
Gastric folds (rugae)
Duodenum
C

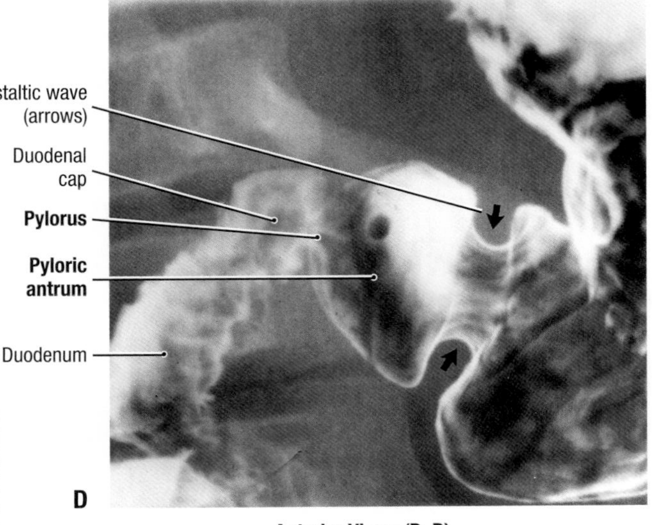
Peristaltic wave (arrows)
Duodenal cap
Pylorus
Pyloric antrum
Duodenum
D
Anterior Views (B–D)

## 2.32 Radiographs of esophagus, stomach, duodenum (barium swallow)

**A.** Esophagus. The esophageal (phrenic) ampulla is the distensible portion of the esophagus seen only radiologically. **B.** Stomach, small intestine, and gallbladder. Note additional contrast medium in gallbladder. **C.** Stomach and duodenum. **D.** Pyloric antrum and duodenal cap.

A hiatal—or hiatus—hernia is a protrusion of a part of the stomach into the mediastinum through the esophageal hiatus of the diaphragm. The hernias occur most often in people after middle age, possibly because of weakening of the muscular part of the diaphragm and widening of the esophageal hiatus.

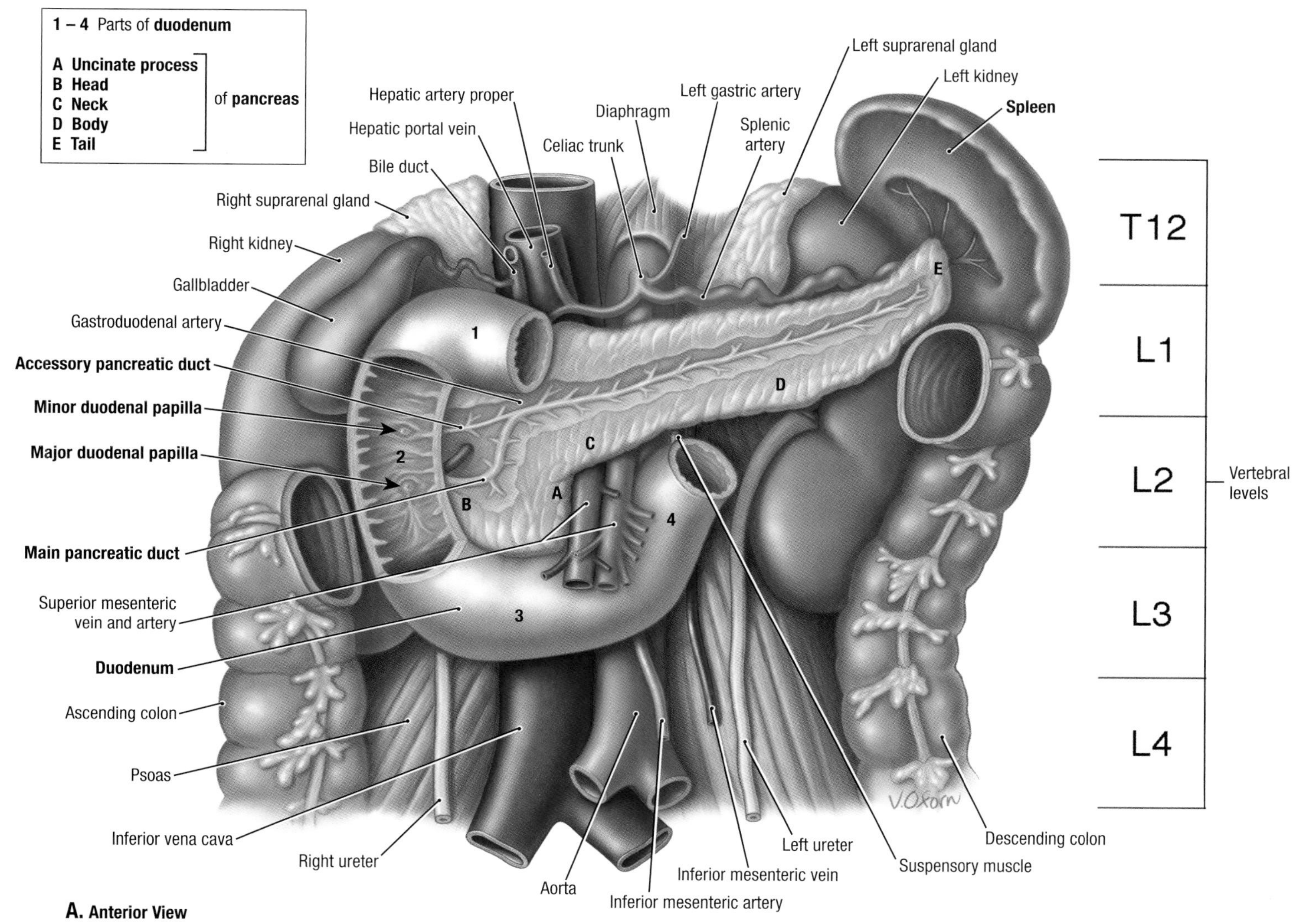
1 – 4 Parts of duodenum
A Uncinate process
B Head
C Neck
D Body
E Tail
of pancreas
Hepatic artery proper
Hepatic portal vein
Bile duct
Right suprarenal gland
Right kidney
Gallbladder
Gastroduodenal artery
Accessory pancreatic duct
Minor duodenal papilla
Major duodenal papilla
Main pancreatic duct
Superior mesenteric vein and artery
Duodenum
Ascending colon
Psoas
Inferior vena cava
Right ureter
Aorta
Inferior mesenteric artery
Inferior mesenteric vein
Left ureter
Suspensory muscle
Descending colon
Celiac trunk
Diaphragm
Left gastric artery
Splenic artery
Left suprarenal gland
Left kidney
Spleen
T12
L1
L2
L3
L4
Vertebral levels
A. Anterior View

**2.33 Parts and relationships of pancreas and duodenum**

**A.** Pancreas and duodenum in situ.

### TABLE 2.3 PARTS AND RELATIONSHIPS OF DUODENUM

| Part of Duodenum | Anterior | Posterior | Medial | Superior | Inferior | Vertebral Level |
|---|---|---|---|---|---|---|
| Superior (**1**st part) | Peritoneum<br>Gallbladder<br>Quadrate lobe of liver | Bile duct<br>Gastroduodenal artery<br>Hepatic portal vein<br>Inferior vena cava | | Neck of gallbladder | Neck of pancreas | Anterolateral to L1 vertebra |
| Descending (**2**nd part) | Transverse colon<br>Transverse mesocolon<br>Coils of small intestine | Hilum of right kidney<br>Renal vessels<br>Ureter<br>Psoas major | Head of pancreas<br>Pancreatic duct<br>Bile duct | | | Right of L2–L3 vertebrae |
| Inferior (horizontal or **3**rd part) | Superior mesenteric artery<br>Superior mesenteric vein<br>Coils of small intestine | Right psoas major<br>Inferior vena cava<br>Aorta<br>Right ureter | | Head and uncinate process of pancreas<br>Superior mesenteric artery and vein | | Anterior to L3 vertebra |
| Ascending (**4**th part) | Beginning of root of mesentery<br>Coils of jejunum | Left psoas major<br>Left margin of aorta | Superior mesenteric artery and vein | Body of pancreas | | Left of L3 vertebra |

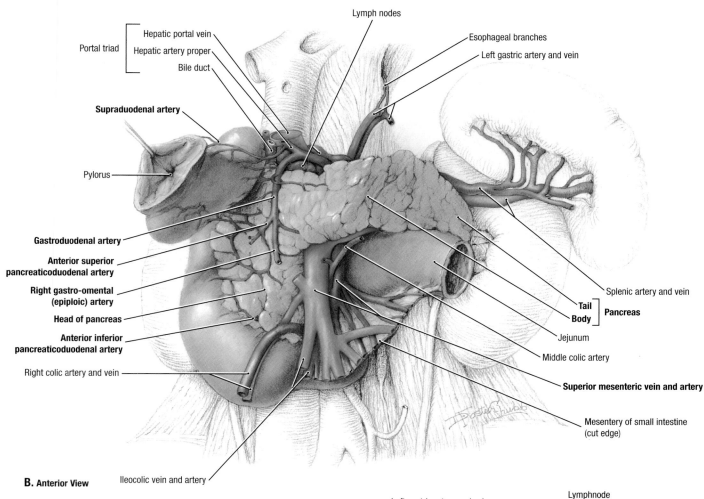

Lymph nodes
Portal triad
Hepatic portal vein
Hepatic artery proper
Bile duct
Esophageal branches
Left gastric artery and vein
Supraduodenal artery
Pylorus
Gastroduodenal artery
Anterior superior pancreaticoduodenal artery
Right gastro-omental (epiploic) artery
Head of pancreas
Anterior inferior pancreaticoduodenal artery
Right colic artery and vein
Splenic artery and vein
Tail
Body
Pancreas
Jejunum
Middle colic artery
Superior mesenteric vein and artery
Mesentery of small intestine (cut edge)
Ileocolic vein and artery

**B. Anterior View**

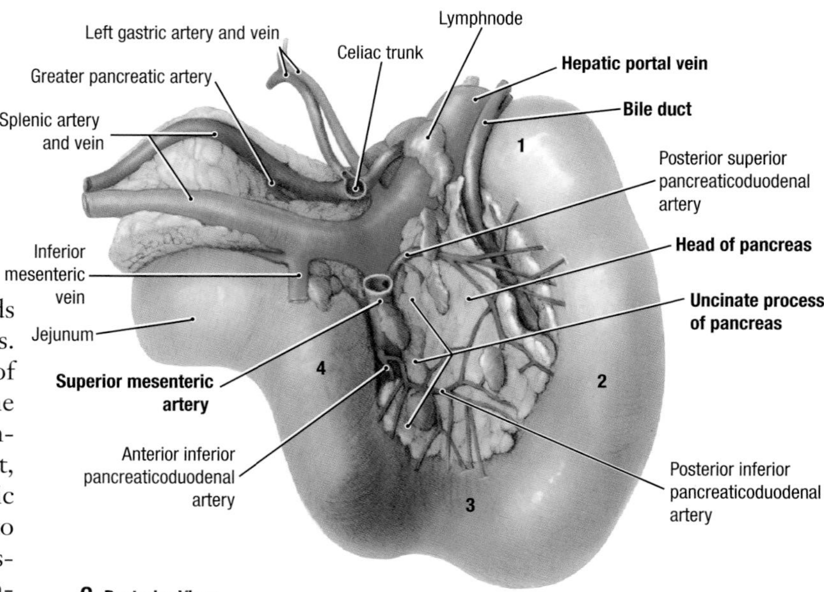
Left gastric artery and vein
Lymphnode
Celiac trunk
Hepatic portal vein
Greater pancreatic artery
Bile duct
Splenic artery and vein
1
Posterior superior pancreaticoduodenal artery
Head of pancreas
Inferior mesenteric vein
Uncinate process of pancreas
Jejunum
4
2
Superior mesenteric artery
Anterior inferior pancreaticoduodenal artery
Posterior inferior pancreaticoduodenal artery
3

**C. Posterior View**

## 2.33 Parts and relationships of the duodenum and pancreas *(continued)*

**B.** Anterior relationships. The gastroduodenal artery descends anterior to the neck of the pancreas. **C.** Posterior relationships. The splenic artery and vein course on the posterior aspect of the pancreatic tail, which usually extends to the spleen. The pancreas "loops" around the right side of the superior mesenteric vessels so that its neck is anterior, its head is to the right, and its uncinate process is posterior to the vessels. The splenic and superior mesenteric veins unite posterior to the neck to form the hepatic portal vein. The bile duct descends in a fissure (opened up) in the posterior part of the head of the pancreas. Most inflammatory erosions of the duodenal wall, duodenal (peptic) ulcers, are in the posterior wall of the superior (1st) part of the duodenum within 3 cm of the pylorus.

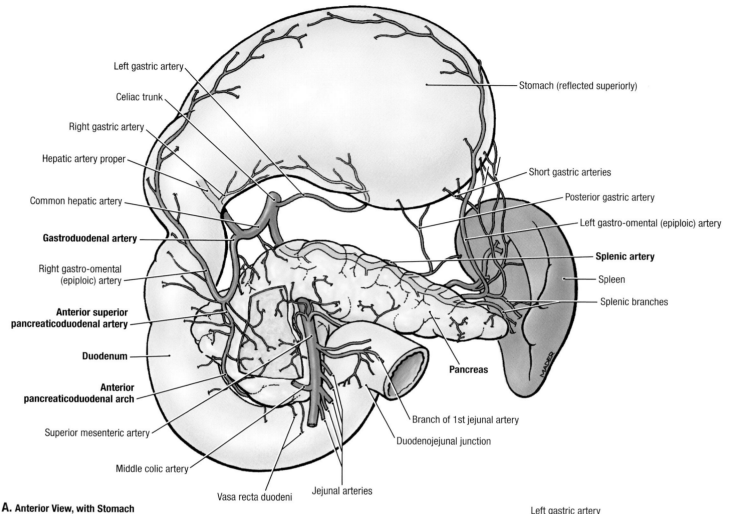

Left gastric artery
Celiac trunk
Right gastric artery
Hepatic artery proper
Common hepatic artery
**Gastroduodenal artery**
Right gastro-omental (epiploic) artery
**Anterior superior pancreaticoduodenal artery**
**Duodenum**
**Anterior pancreaticoduodenal arch**
Superior mesenteric artery
Middle colic artery
Vasa recta duodeni
Jejunal arteries
Stomach (reflected superiorly)
Short gastric arteries
Posterior gastric artery
Left gastro-omental (epiploic) artery
**Splenic artery**
Spleen
Splenic branches
**Pancreas**
Branch of 1st jejunal artery
Duodenojejunal junction
MADER

**A.** **Anterior View, with Stomach Reflected Superiorly**

## 2.34 Blood supply to the pancreas, duodenum, and spleen

**A.** Celiac trunk and superior mesenteric artery. **B.** Pancreatic and pancreaticoduodenal arteries.

- The anterior superior pancreaticoduodenal artery from the gastroduodenal artery and the anterior inferior pancreaticoduodenal artery of the superior mesenteric artery form the anterior pancreaticoduodenal arch anterior to the head of the pancreas. The posterior superior and posterior inferior branches of the same two arteries form the posterior pancreaticoduodenal arch posterior to the pancreas. The anterior and posterior inferior arteries often arise from a common stem.
- Arteries supplying the pancreas are derived from the common hepatic artery, gastroduodenal artery, pancreaticoduodenal arches, splenic artery, and superior mesenteric artery.

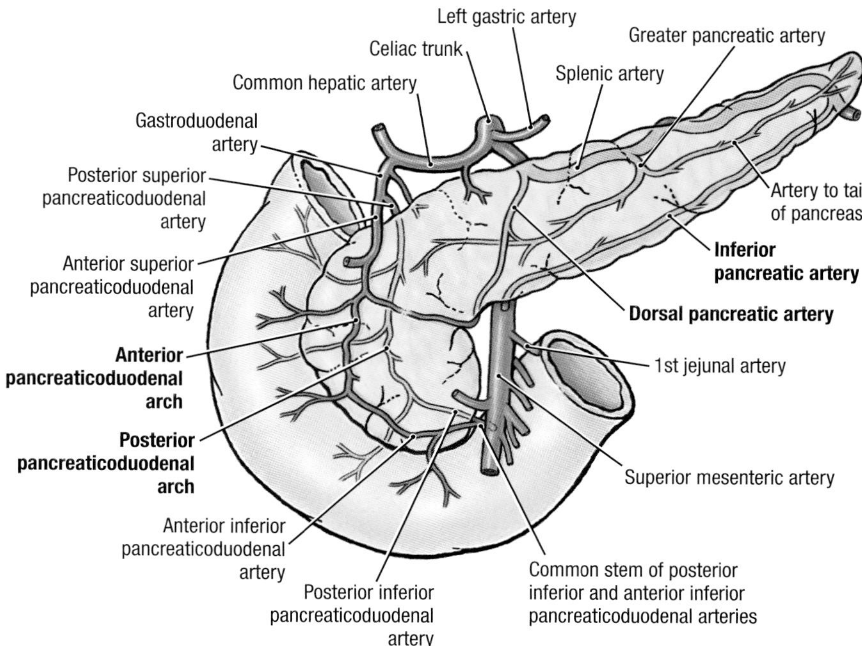
Left gastric artery
Celiac trunk
Greater pancreatic artery
Common hepatic artery
Splenic artery
Gastroduodenal artery
Posterior superior pancreaticoduodenal artery
Artery to tail of pancreas
Anterior superior pancreaticoduodenal artery
Inferior pancreatic artery
Dorsal pancreatic artery
Anterior pancreaticoduodenal arch
1st jejunal artery
Posterior pancreaticoduodenal arch
Superior mesenteric artery
Anterior inferior pancreaticoduodenal artery
Posterior inferior pancreaticoduodenal artery
Common stem of posterior inferior and anterior inferior pancreaticoduodenal arteries

**B.** **Anterior View**

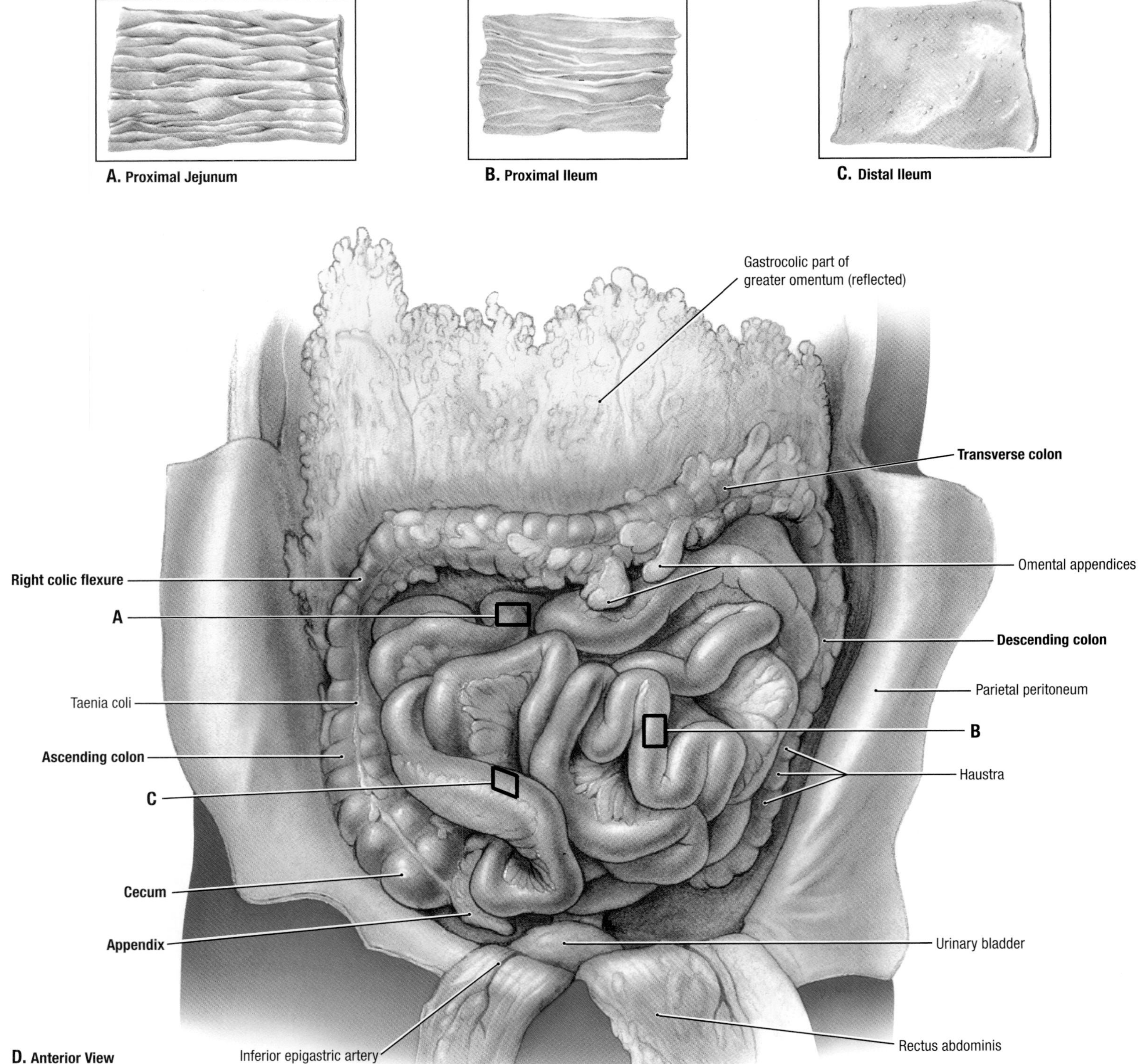
A. Proximal Jejunum
B. Proximal Ileum
C. Distal Ileum
Gastrocolic part of greater omentum (reflected)
Transverse colon
Right colic flexure
Omental appendices
A
Descending colon
Taenia coli
Parietal peritoneum
B
Ascending colon
Haustra
C
Cecum
Appendix
Urinary bladder
D. Anterior View
Inferior epigastric artery
Rectus abdominis

## 2.35 Intestines in situ, interior of small intestine

**A.** Proximal jejunum. The circular folds are tall, closely packed, and commonly branched. **B.** Proximal ileum. The circular folds are low and becoming sparse. The caliber of the gut is reduced, and the wall is thinner. **C.** Distal ileum. Circular folds are absent, and solitary lymph nodules stud the wall. **D.** Intestines in situ, greater omentum reflected. The ileum is reflected to expose the appendix. The appendix usually lies posterior to the cecum (retrocecal) or, as in this case, projects over the pelvic brim. The features of the large intestines are the taeniae coli; haustra; and omental appendices.

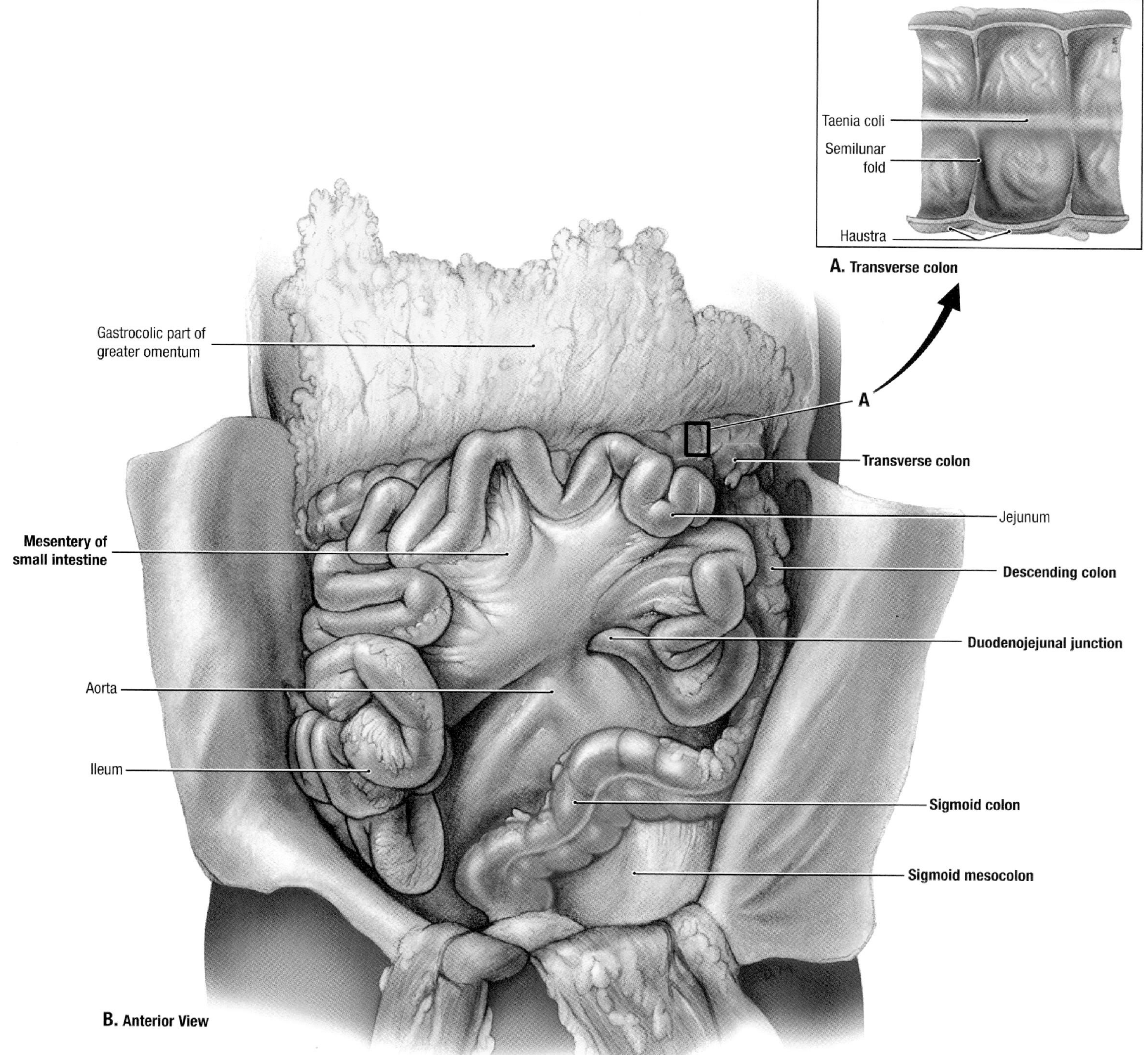
Taenia coli
Semilunar fold
Haustra
A. Transverse colon
A
Gastrocolic part of greater omentum
Transverse colon
Jejunum
Mesentery of small intestine
Descending colon
Duodenojejunal junction
Aorta
Ileum
Sigmoid colon
Sigmoid mesocolon
B. Anterior View

## 2.36 Sigmoid mesocolon and mesentry of small intestine, interior of transverse colon

**A.** Transverse colon. The semilunar folds and taeniae coli form prominent features on the smooth-surfaced wall. **B.** Sigmoid mesocolon and mesentry of the small intestine.

- The duodenojejunal junction is situated to the left of the median plane.
- The mesentery of the small intestine fans out extensively from its short root to accommodate the length of jejunum and ileum (approximately 6m).
- The descending colon is the narrowest part of the large intestine and is retroperitoneal. The sigmoid colon has a mesentery, the sigmoid mesocolon; the sigmoid colon is continuous with the rectum at the point at which the sigmoid mesocolon ends.

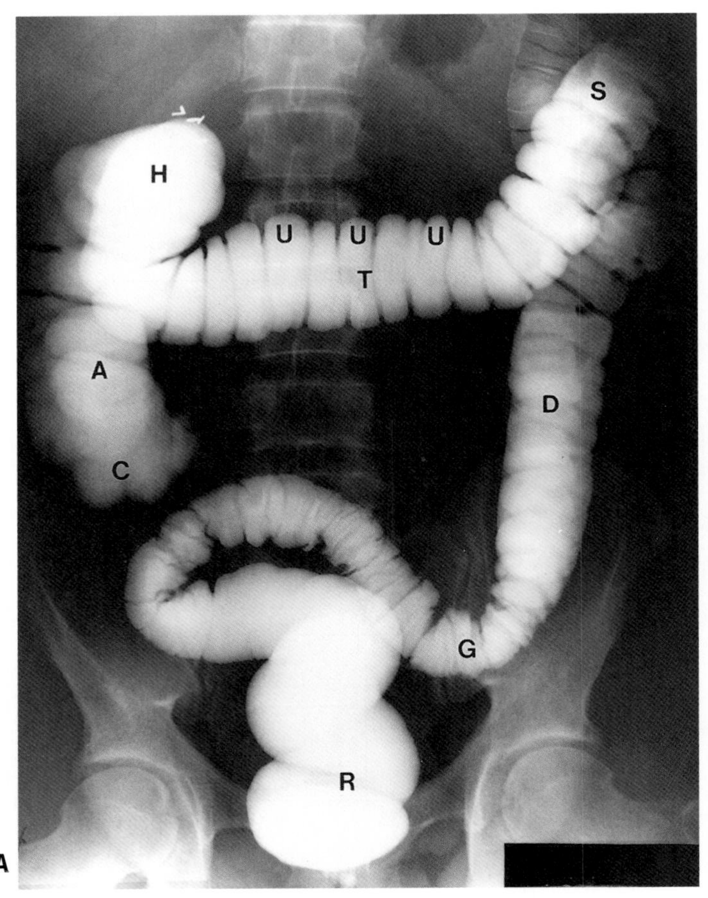
S
H
U
U
U
T
A
D
C
G
R
A

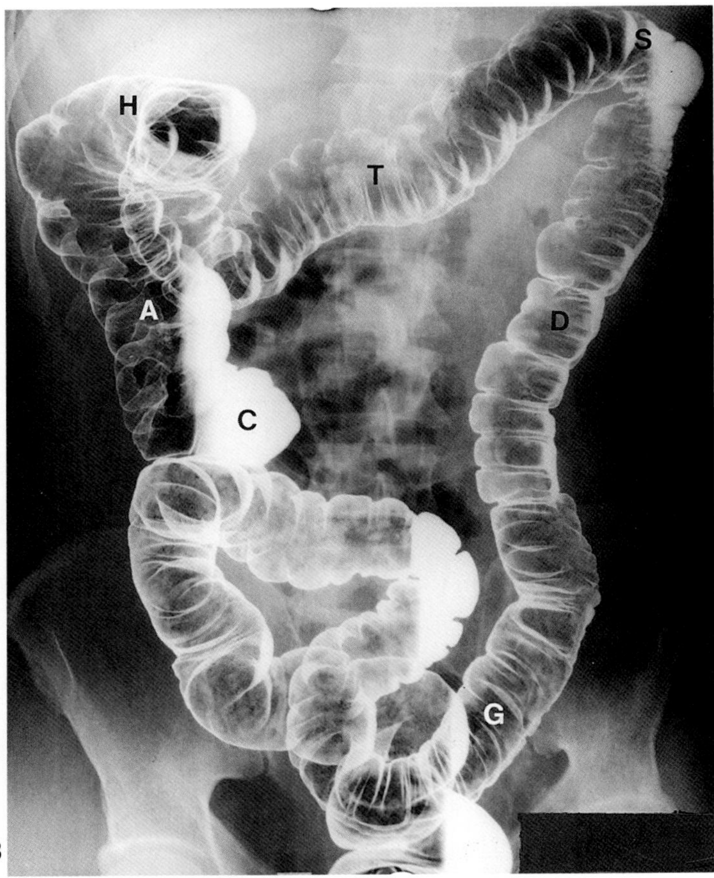
S
H
T
A
D
C
G
B

Posteroanterior Radiographs

| | | | | | |
|---|---|---|---|---|---|
| A | Ascending colon | G | Sigmoid colon | S | Splenic flexure |
| C | Cecum | H | Hepatic flexure | T | Transverse colon |
| D | Descending colon | R | Rectum | U | Haustra |

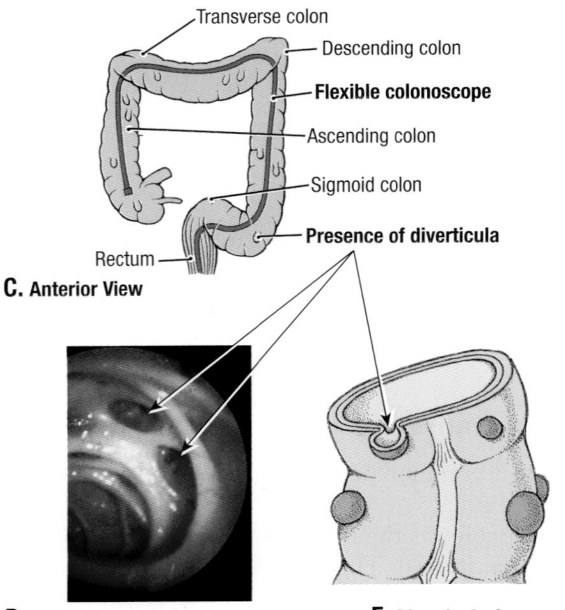
Transverse colon
Descending colon
Flexible colonoscope
Ascending colon
Sigmoid colon
Presence of diverticula
Rectum

C. Anterior View

D. Colonoscopic View

E. Diverticulosis

## 2.37 Barium enema and colonoscopy of colon

**A.** Single-contrast study. A barium enema has filled the colon. **B.** Double-contrast study. Barium can be seen coating the walls of the colon, which is distended with air, providing a vivid view of the mucosal relief and haustra. **C.** The interior of the colon can be observed with an elongated endoscope, usually a fiberoptic flexible colonoscope. The endoscope is a tube that inserts into the colon through the anus and rectum. **D.** Diverticulosis of the colon can be photographed through a colonoscope.

**E.** Diverticulosis is a disorder in which multiple false diverticula (external evaginations or out-pocketings of the mucosa of the colon) develop along the intestine. It primarily affects middle-aged and elderly people. Diverticulosis is commonly (60%) found in the sigmoid colon. Diverticula are subject to infection and rupture, leading to diverticulitis, and they can distort and erode the nutrient arteries, leading to hemorrhage.

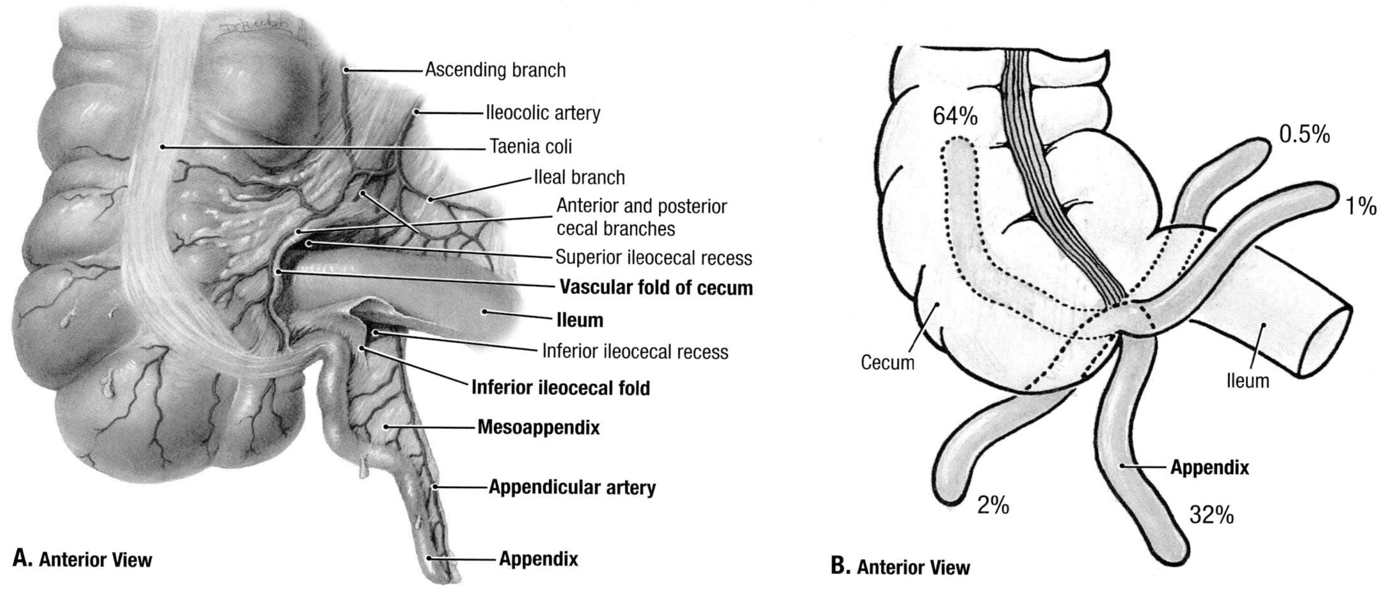
Ascending branch
Ileocolic artery
Taenia coli
Ileal branch
Anterior and posterior cecal branches
Superior ileocecal recess
Vascular fold of cecum
Ileum
Inferior ileocecal recess
Inferior ileocecal fold
Mesoappendix
Appendicular artery
Appendix
A. Anterior View
64%
0.5%
1%
Cecum
Ileum
Appendix
2%
32%
B. Anterior View

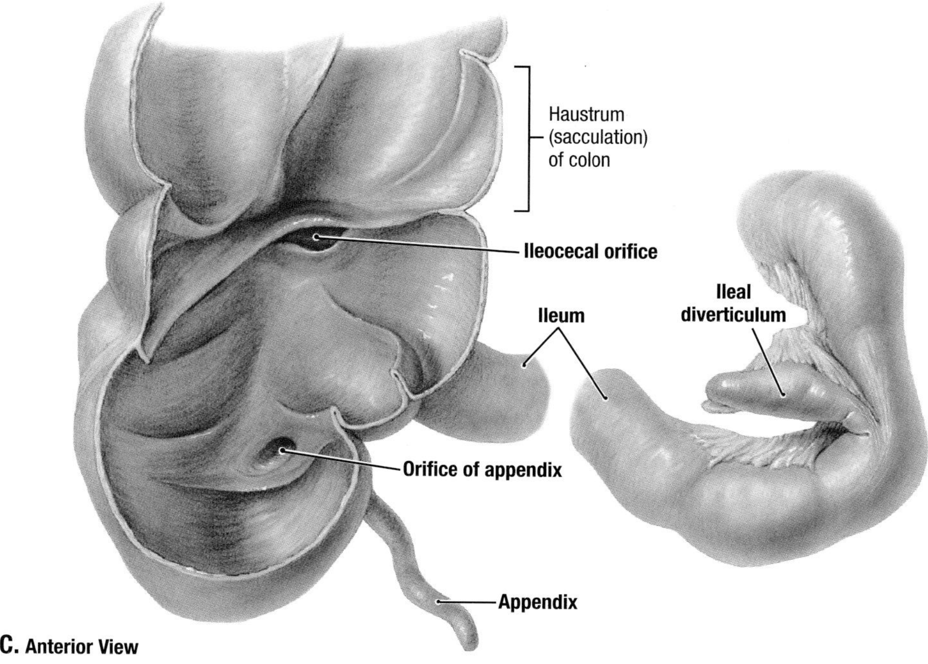
Haustrum (sacculation) of colon
Ileocecal orifice
Ileum
Ileal diverticulum
Orifice of appendix
Appendix
C. Anterior View

## 2.38 Ileocecal region and appendix

**A.** Blood supply. The appendicular artery is located in the free edge of the mesoappendix. The inferior ileocecal fold is bloodless, whereas the superior ileocecal fold is called the vascular fold of the cecum. **B.** The approximate incidence of various locations of the appendix. **C.** Interior of a dried cecum and ileal diverticulum (of Meckel). This cecum was filled with air until dry, opened, and varnished. Ileal diverticulum is a congenital anomaly that occurs in 1 to 2% of persons. It is a pouchlike remnant (3–6 cm long) of the proximal part of the yolk stalk, typically within 50 cm of the ileocecal junction. It sometimes becomes inflamed and produces pain that may mimic that produced by appendicitis.

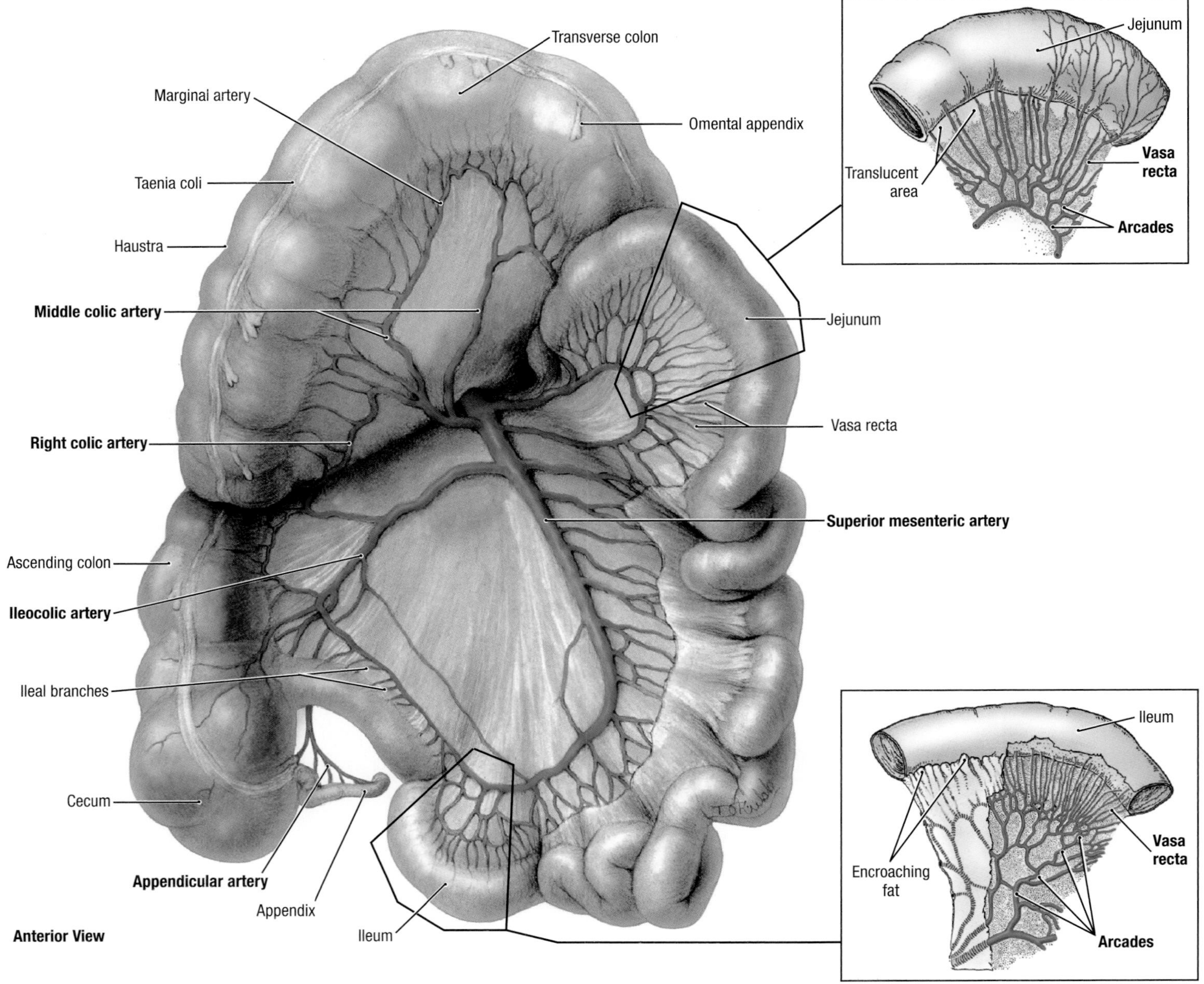
Transverse colon
Marginal artery
Omental appendix
Taenia coli
Haustra
Middle colic artery
Right colic artery
Ascending colon
Ileocolic artery
Ileal branches
Cecum
Appendicular artery
Appendix
Ileum
Anterior View
Jejunum
Vasa recta
Superior mesenteric artery
Jejunum
Translucent area
Vasa recta
Arcades
Ileum
Encroaching fat
Vasa recta
Arcades

## 2.39 Superior mesenteric artery and arterial arcades

The peritoneum is partially stripped off.

- The superior mesenteric artery ends by anastomosing with one of its own branches, the ileal branch of the ileocolic artery.
- On the inset drawings of jejunum and ileum compare the diameter, thickness of wall, number of arterial arcades, long or short vasa recta, presence of translucent (fat free) areas at the mesenteric border, and fat encroaching on the wall of the gut between the jejunum and ileum.

- Acute inflammation of the appendix is a common cause of an acute abdomen (severe abdominal pain arising suddenly). The pain of appendicitis usually commences as a vague pain in the periumbilical region because afferent pain fibers enter the spinal cord at the T10 level. Later, severe pain in the right lower quadrant results from irritation of the parietal peritoneum lining the posterior abdominal wall.

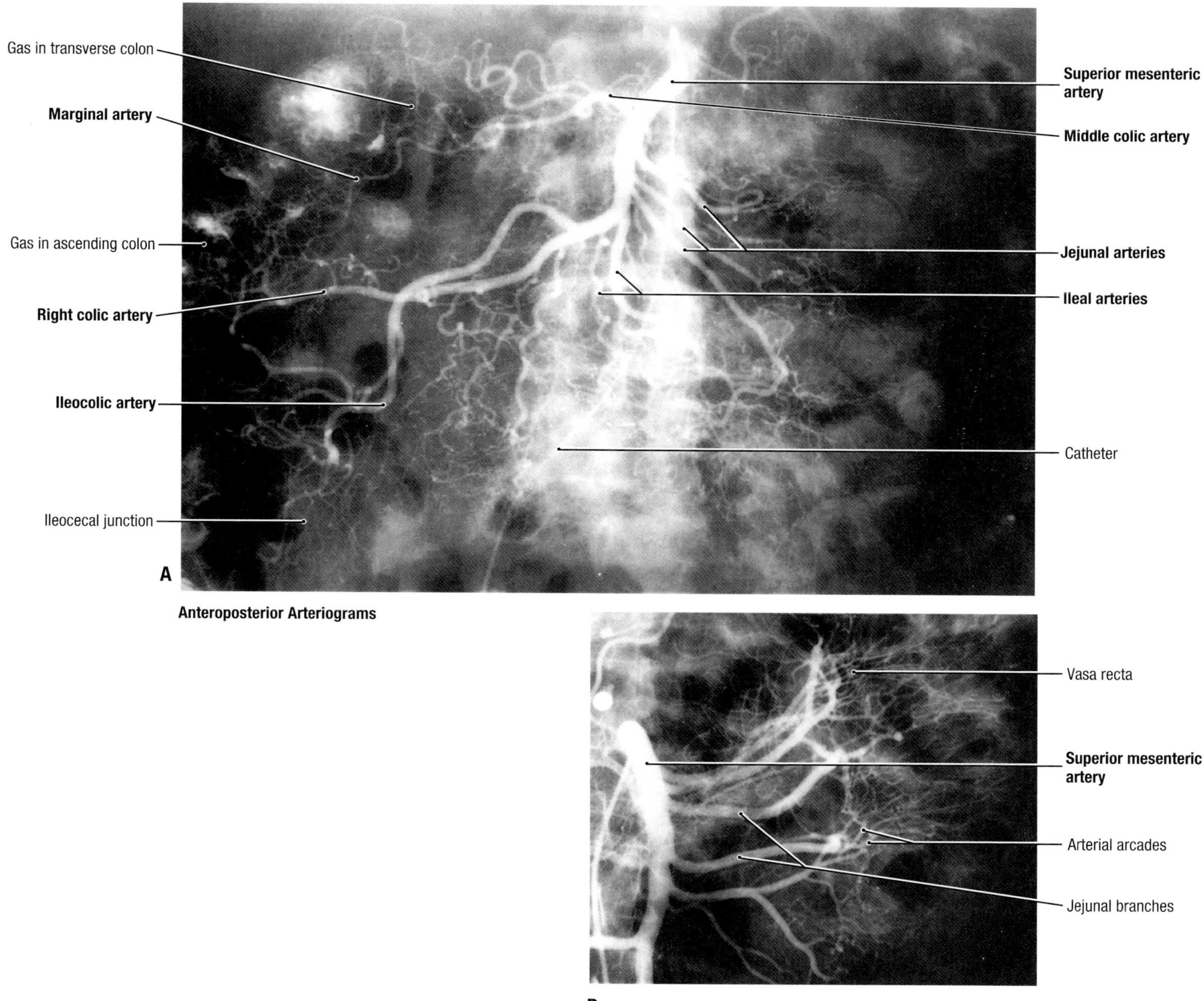
Gas in transverse colon
Marginal artery
Gas in ascending colon
Right colic artery
Ileocolic artery
Ileocecal junction
A
Superior mesenteric artery
Middle colic artery
Jejunal arteries
Ileal arteries
Catheter
Anteroposterior Arteriograms
Vasa recta
Superior mesenteric artery
Arterial arcades
Jejunal branches
B

## 2.40 Superior mesenteric arteriograms

**A.** Branches of superior mesenteric artery. Consult Figure 2.39 to identify the branches. **B.** Enlargement to show the jejunal branches, arterial arcades, and vasa recta.

- The branches of the superior mesenteric artery include, from its left side, 12 or more jejunal and ileal branches that anastomose to form arcades from which vasa recta pass to the small intestine and, from its right side, the middle colic, ileocolic, and commonly (but not here) an independent right colic artery that anastomose to form a marginal artery that parallels the mesenteric border at the colon and from which vasa recta pass to the large intestine.

Occlusion of the vasa recta by emboli results in ischemia of the part of the intestine concerned. If the ischemia is severe, necrosis of the involved segment results and ileus (obstruction of the intestine) of the paralytic type occurs. Ileus is accompanied by a severe colicky pain, along with abdominal distension, vomiting, and often fever and dehydration. If the condition is diagnosed early (e.g., using a superior mesenteric arteriogram), the obstructed part of the vessel may be cleared surgically

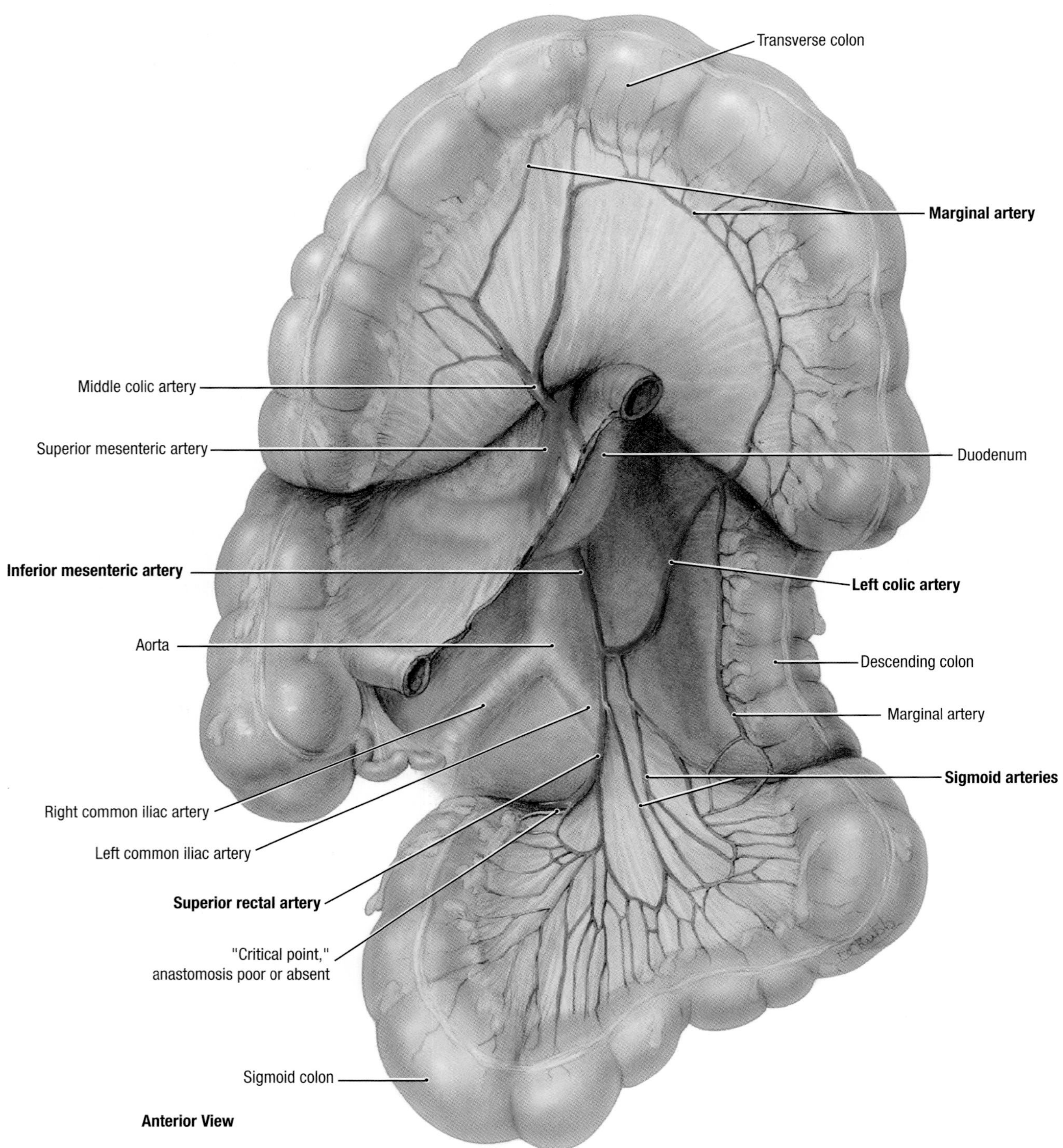
Transverse colon
Marginal artery
Middle colic artery
Superior mesenteric artery
Duodenum
Inferior mesenteric artery
Left colic artery
Aorta
Descending colon
Marginal artery
Sigmoid arteries
Right common iliac artery
Left common iliac artery
Superior rectal artery
"Critical point," anastomosis poor or absent
Sigmoid colon
Anterior View

## 2.41 Inferior mesenteric artery

The mesentery of the small intestine has been cut at its root.

- The inferior mesenteric artery arises posterior to the ascending part of the duodenum, about 4 cm superior to the bifurcation of the aorta; on crossing the left common iliac artery, it becomes the superior rectal artery.
- The branches of the inferior mesenteric artery include the left colic artery and several sigmoid arteries; the inferior two sigmoid arteries branch from the superior rectal artery.
- The point at which the last artery to the colon branches from the superior rectal artery is known as the "critical point"; this branch has poor or no anastomotic connections with the superior rectal artery.

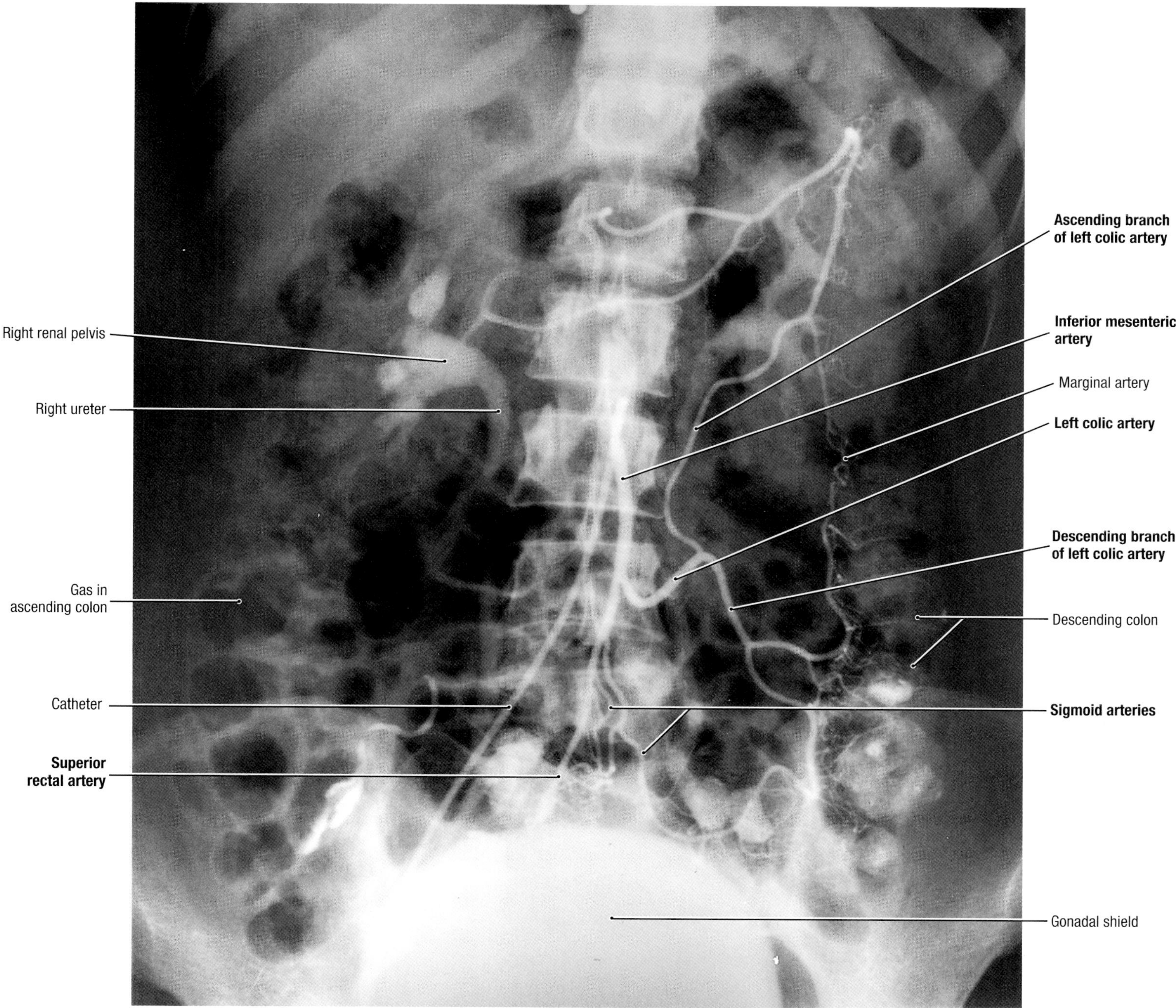
Ascending branch of left colic artery
Inferior mesenteric artery
Marginal artery
Left colic artery
Descending branch of left colic artery
Descending colon
Sigmoid arteries
Gonadal shield
Right renal pelvis
Right ureter
Gas in ascending colon
Catheter
Superior rectal artery

**Posteroanterior Arteriogram**

## 2.42 Inferior mesenteric arteriogram

- The left colic artery courses to the left toward the descending colon and splits into ascending and descending branches.
- The sigmoid arteries, two to four in number, supply the sigmoid colon.
- The superior rectal artery, which is the continuation of the inferior mesenteric artery, supplies the rectum; the superior rectal anastomoses is formed by branches of the middle and inferior rectal arteries (from the internal iliac artery).

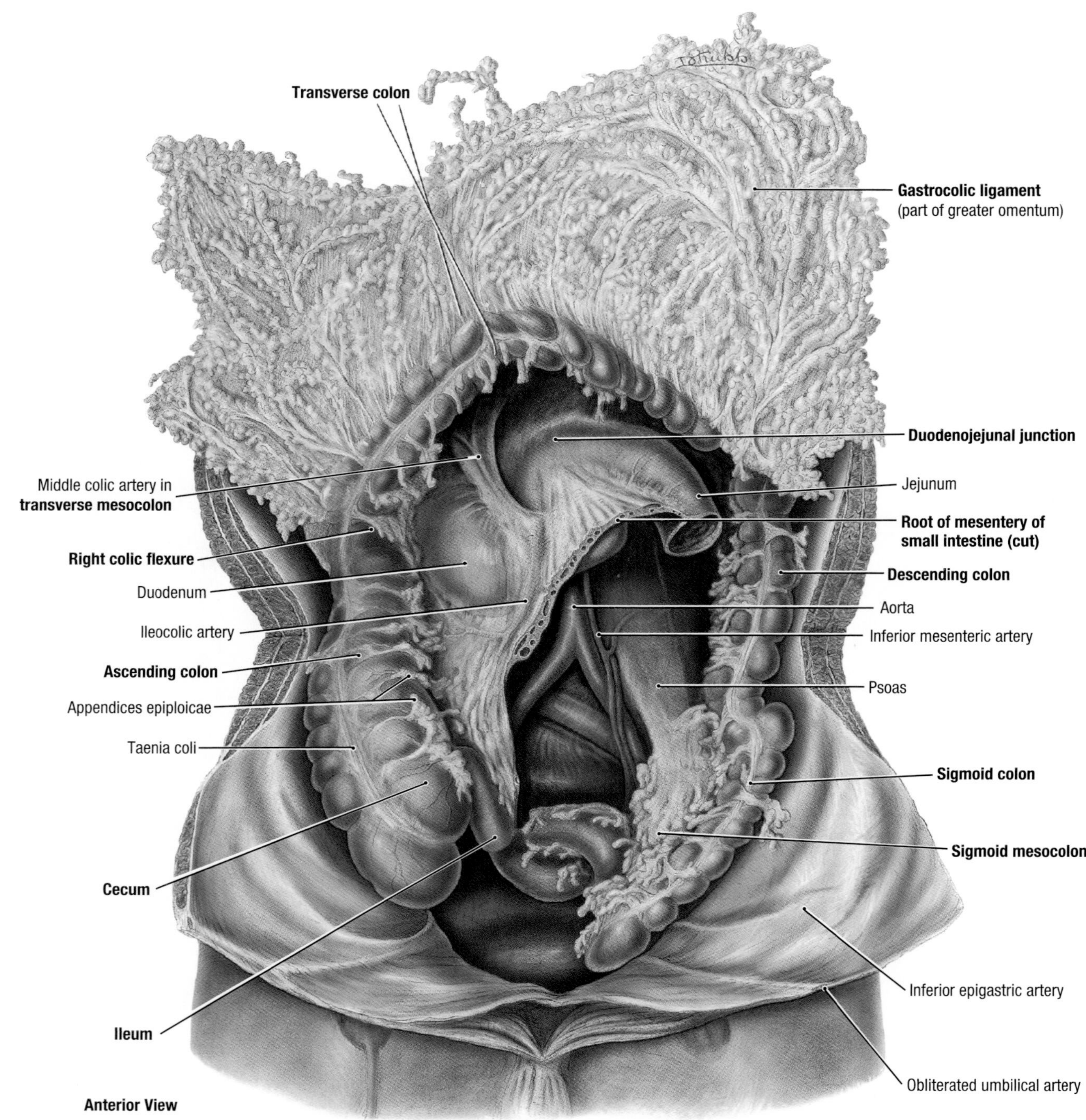

Transverse colon
Gastrocolic ligament
(part of greater omentum)
Duodenojejunal junction
Middle colic artery in
transverse mesocolon
Jejunum
Root of mesentery of
small intestine (cut)
Right colic flexure
Descending colon
Duodenum
Aorta
Ileocolic artery
Inferior mesenteric artery
Ascending colon
Appendices epiploicae
Psoas
Taenia coli
Sigmoid colon
Sigmoid mesocolon
Cecum
Inferior epigastric artery
Ileum
Obliterated umbilical artery
Anterior View


## 2.43 Peritoneum of posterior abdominal cavity

The gastrocolic ligament is retracted superiorly, along with the transverse colon and transverse mesocolon. The appendix had been surgically removed. This dissection is continued in Figure 2.44.

- The root of the mesentery of the small intestine, approximately 15 to 20 cm in length, extends between the duodenojejunal junction and ileocecal junction.
- The large intestine forms 3½ sides of a square around the jejunum and ileum. On the right are the cecum and ascending colon, superior is the transverse colon, on the left is the descending and sigmoid colon, inferiorly is the sigmoid colon.

- Chronic inflammation of the colon (ulcerative colitis, Crohn disease) is characterized by severe inflammation and ulceration of the colon and rectum. In some patients, a colectomy is performed, during which the terminal ileum and colon as well as the rectum and anal canal are removed. An ileostomy is then constructed to establish an artificial cutaneous opening between the ileum and the skin of the anterolateral abdominal wall.

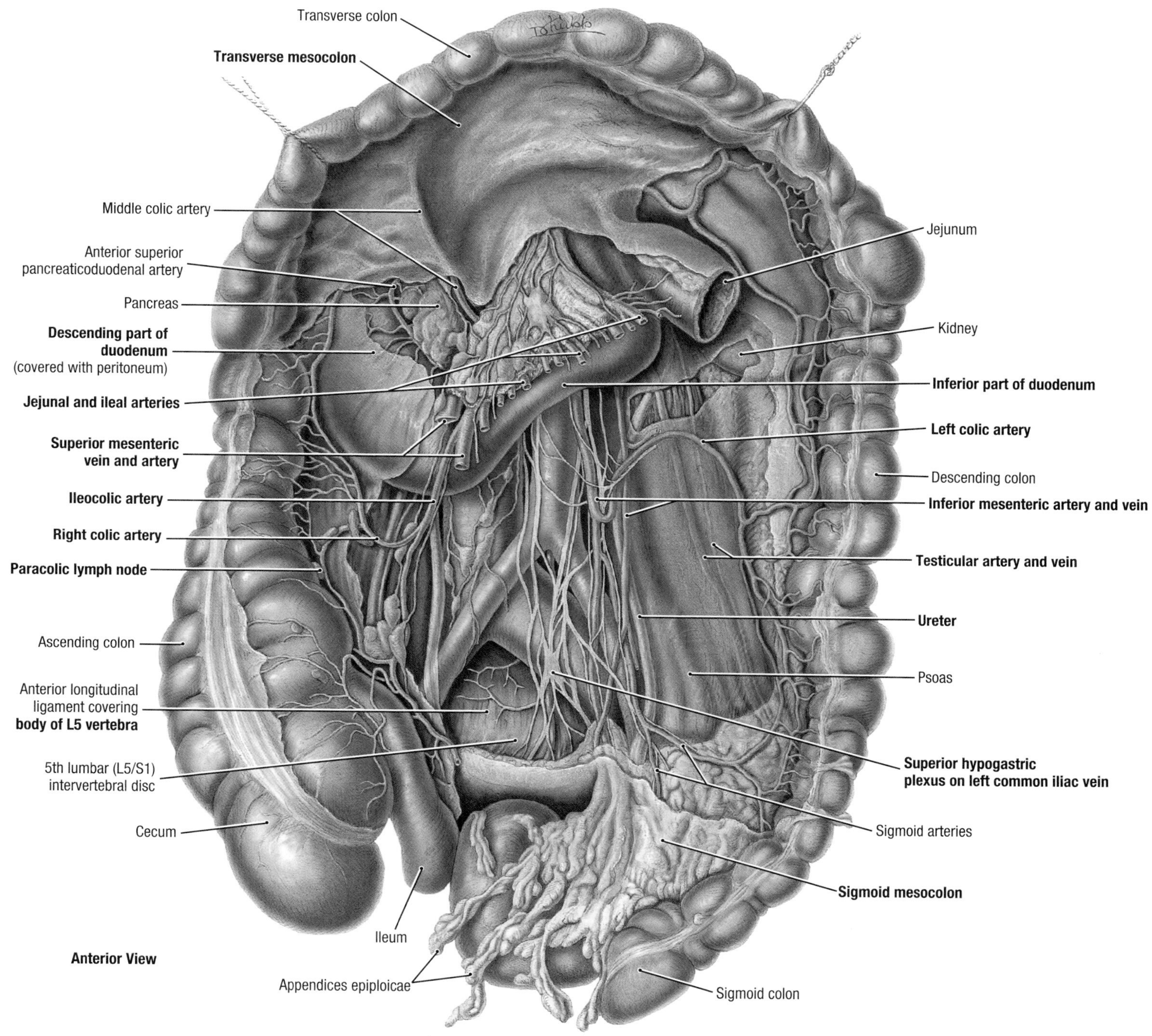
Transverse colon
Transverse mesocolon
Middle colic artery
Anterior superior pancreaticoduodenal artery
Pancreas
Descending part of duodenum (covered with peritoneum)
Jejunal and ileal arteries
Superior mesenteric vein and artery
Ileocolic artery
Right colic artery
Paracolic lymph node
Ascending colon
Anterior longitudinal ligament covering body of L5 vertebra
5th lumbar (L5/S1) intervertebral disc
Cecum
Ileum
Anterior View
Appendices epiploicae
Sigmoid colon
Jejunum
Kidney
Inferior part of duodenum
Left colic artery
Descending colon
Inferior mesenteric artery and vein
Testicular artery and vein
Ureter
Psoas
Superior hypogastric plexus on left common iliac vein
Sigmoid arteries
Sigmoid mesocolon

## 2.44 Posterior abdominal cavity with peritoneum removed

The jejunal and ileal branches (cut) pass from the left side of the superior mesenteric artery. The right colic artery here is a branch of the ileocolic artery. This is the same specimen as in Figure 2.43.

- The duodenum is large in diameter before crossing the superior mesenteric vessels and narrow afterward.
- On the right side, there are lymph nodes on the colon, paracolic nodes beside the colon, and nodes along the ileocolic artery, which drain into nodes anterior to the pancreas.
- The intestines and intestinal vessels lie on a resectable plane anterior to that of the testicular vessels; these in turn lie anterior to the plane of the kidney, its vessels, and the ureter.
- The superior hypogastric plexus lies within the bifurcation of the aorta and anterior to the left common iliac vein, the body of the 5th lumbar vertebra, and the 5th intervertebral disc.

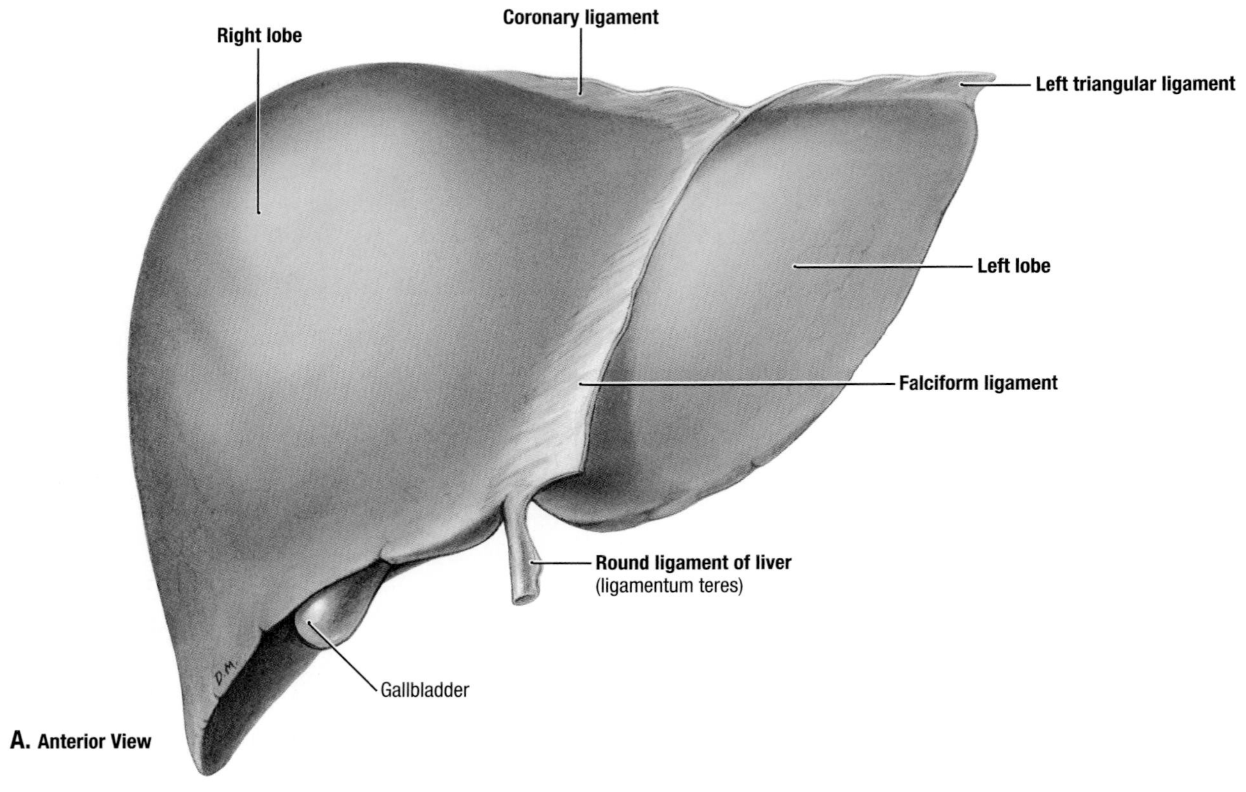
Right lobe
Coronary ligament
Left triangular ligament
Left lobe
Falciform ligament
Round ligament of liver
(ligamentum teres)
Gallbladder
A. Anterior View

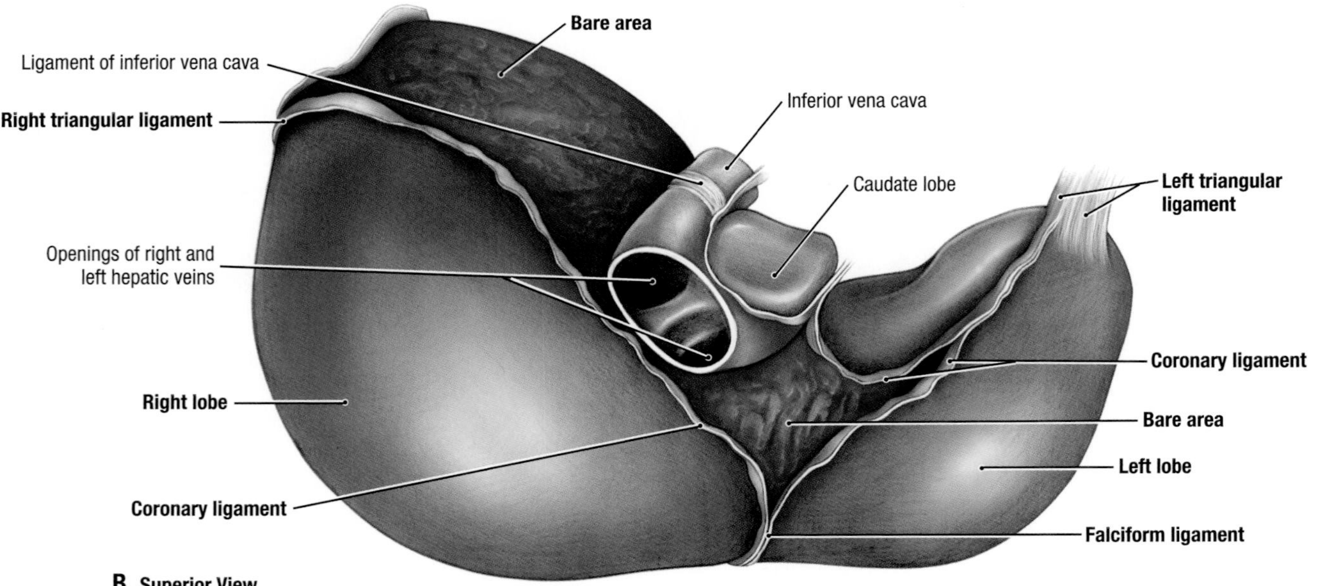
Bare area
Ligament of inferior vena cava
Right triangular ligament
Inferior vena cava
Caudate lobe
Left triangular
ligament
Openings of right and
left hepatic veins
Coronary ligament
Right lobe
Bare area
Left lobe
Coronary ligament
Falciform ligament
B. Superior View

## 2.45 Diaphragmatic (anterior and superior) surface of liver

**A.** The falciform ligament has been severed close to its attachment to the diaphragm and anterior abdominal wall and demarcates the right and left lobes of the liver. The round ligament of the liver (ligamentum teres) lies within the free edge of the falciform ligament. **B.** The two layers of peritoneum that form the falciform ligament separate over the superior aspect (surrounding the bare area) of the liver to form the superior layer of the coronary ligament and the right and left triangular ligaments.

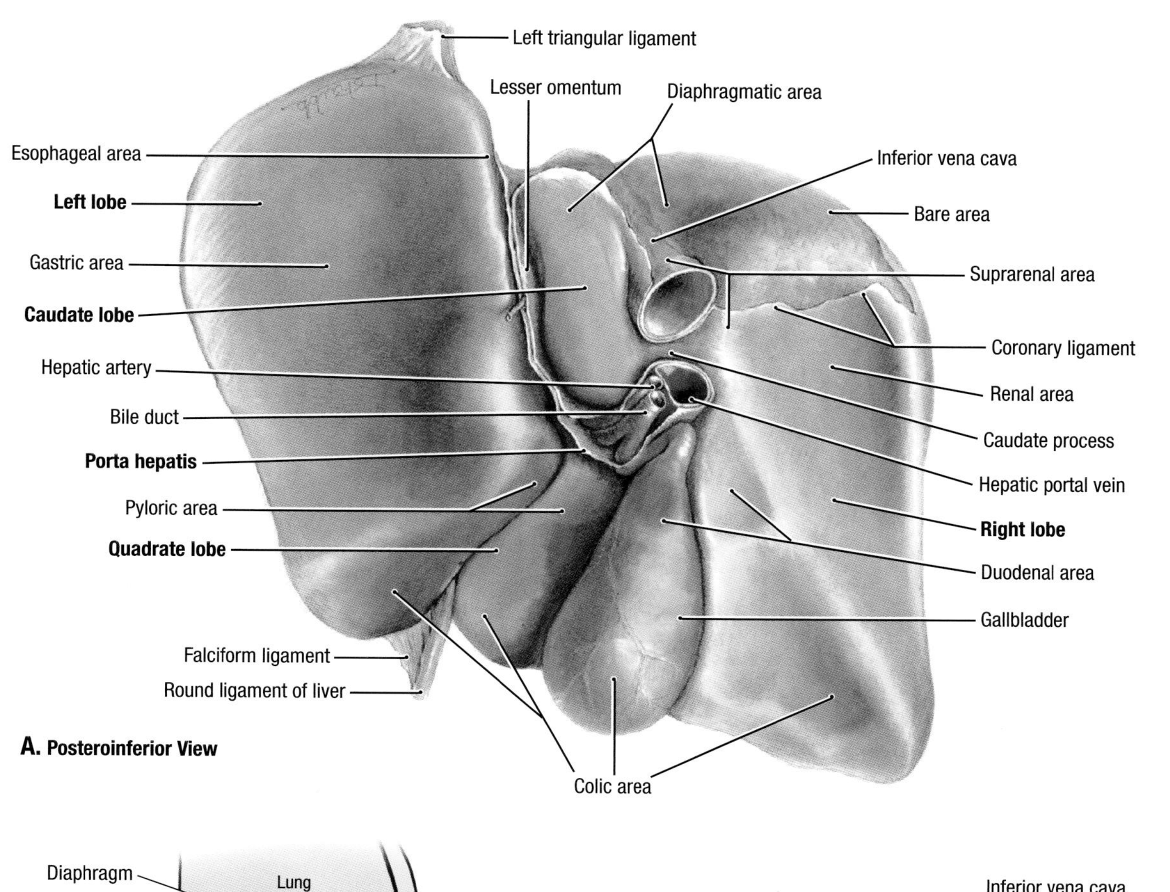
Left triangular ligament
Lesser omentum
Diaphragmatic area
Esophageal area
Inferior vena cava
Left lobe
Bare area
Gastric area
Suprarenal area
Caudate lobe
Coronary ligament
Hepatic artery
Renal area
Bile duct
Caudate process
Porta hepatis
Hepatic portal vein
Pyloric area
Right lobe
Quadrate lobe
Duodenal area
Gallbladder
Falciform ligament
Round ligament of liver
A. Posteroinferior View
Colic area

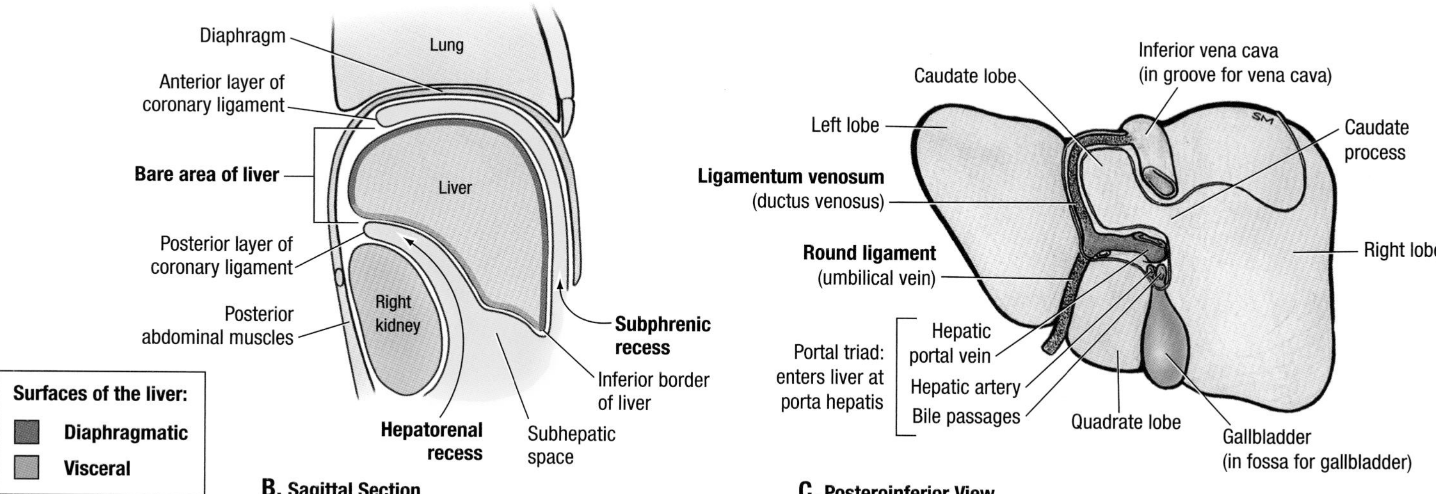
Diaphragm
Lung
Anterior layer of coronary ligament
Bare area of liver
Liver
Posterior layer of coronary ligament
Posterior abdominal muscles
Right kidney
Subphrenic recess
Inferior border of liver
Surfaces of the liver:
Diaphragmatic
Visceral
Hepatorenal recess
Subhepatic space
B. Sagittal Section
Inferior vena cava (in groove for vena cava)
Caudate lobe
Left lobe
Caudate process
Ligamentum venosum (ductus venosus)
Right lobe
Round ligament (umbilical vein)
Portal triad: enters liver at porta hepatis
Hepatic portal vein
Hepatic artery
Bile passages
Quadrate lobe
Gallbladder (in fossa for gallbladder)
C. Posteroinferior View

## 2.46 Visceral (posteroinferior) surface of liver

**A.** Isolated specimen demonstrating lobes, and impressions of adjacent viscera. **B.** Hepatic surfaces and peritoneal recesses. **C.** Round ligament of liver and ligamentum venosum. The round ligament of liver includes the obliterated remains of the umbilical vein that carried well-oxygenated blood from the placenta to the fetus. The ligamentum venosum is the fibrous remnant of the fetal ductus venosus that shunted blood from the umbilical vein to the inferior vena cava, short circuiting the liver. Hepatic tissue may be obtained for diagnostic purposes by liver biopsy. The needle puncture is commonly made through the right 10th intercostal space in the midaxillary line. Before the physician takes the biopsy, the person is asked to hold his or her breath in full expiration to reduce the costodiaphragmatic recess and to lessen the possibility of damaging the lung and contaminating the pleural cavity.

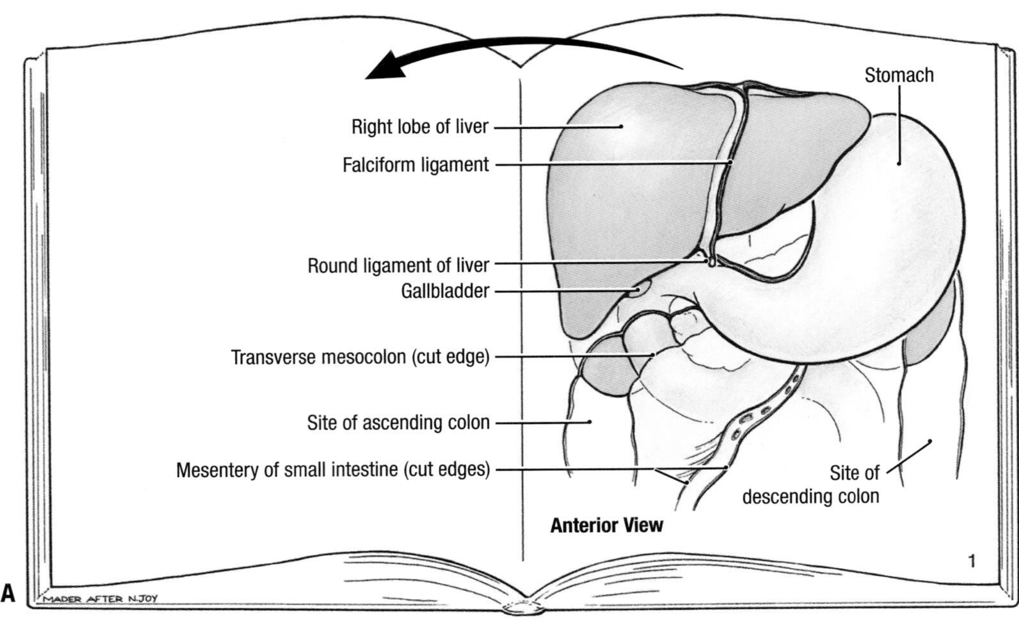
Stomach
Right lobe of liver
Falciform ligament
Round ligament of liver
Gallbladder
Transverse mesocolon (cut edge)
Site of ascending colon
Mesentery of small intestine (cut edges)
Site of descending colon
Anterior View
1
A
MADER AFTER N.JOY

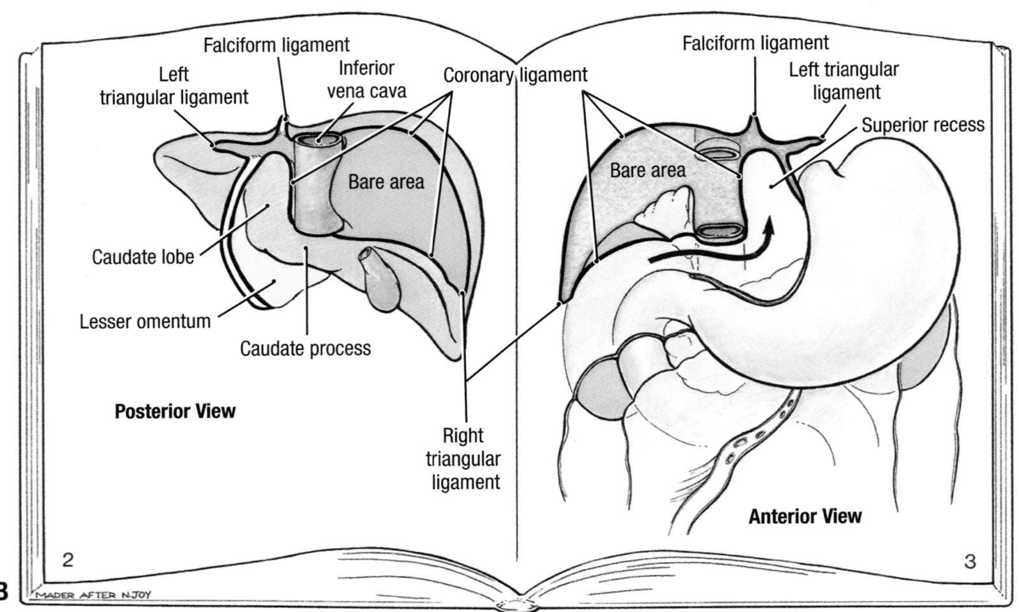
Falciform ligament
Left triangular ligament
Inferior vena cava
Coronary ligament
Bare area
Caudate lobe
Lesser omentum
Caudate process
Posterior View
Right triangular ligament
Falciform ligament
Left triangular ligament
Superior recess
Bare area
Anterior View
2
3
B
MADER AFTER N.JOY

## 2.47 Liver and its posterior relations, schematic illustration

**A.** Liver in situ. The jejunum, ileum, and the ascending, transverse, and descending colon have been removed. **B.** The liver is drawn schematically on a page in a book, so that as the page is turned (*arrow in A*), the liver is reflected to the right to reveal its posterior surface, and on the facing page, the posterior relations that compose the bed of the liver are viewed. The *arrow in B* traverses the site of the omental (epiploic) foramen. The bare area is triangular, hence the coronary ligament that surrounds it is three-sided; its left side, or base, is between the inferior vena cava and caudate lobe, and its apex is at the right triangular ligament, where the superior and inferior layers of the coronary ligament meet.

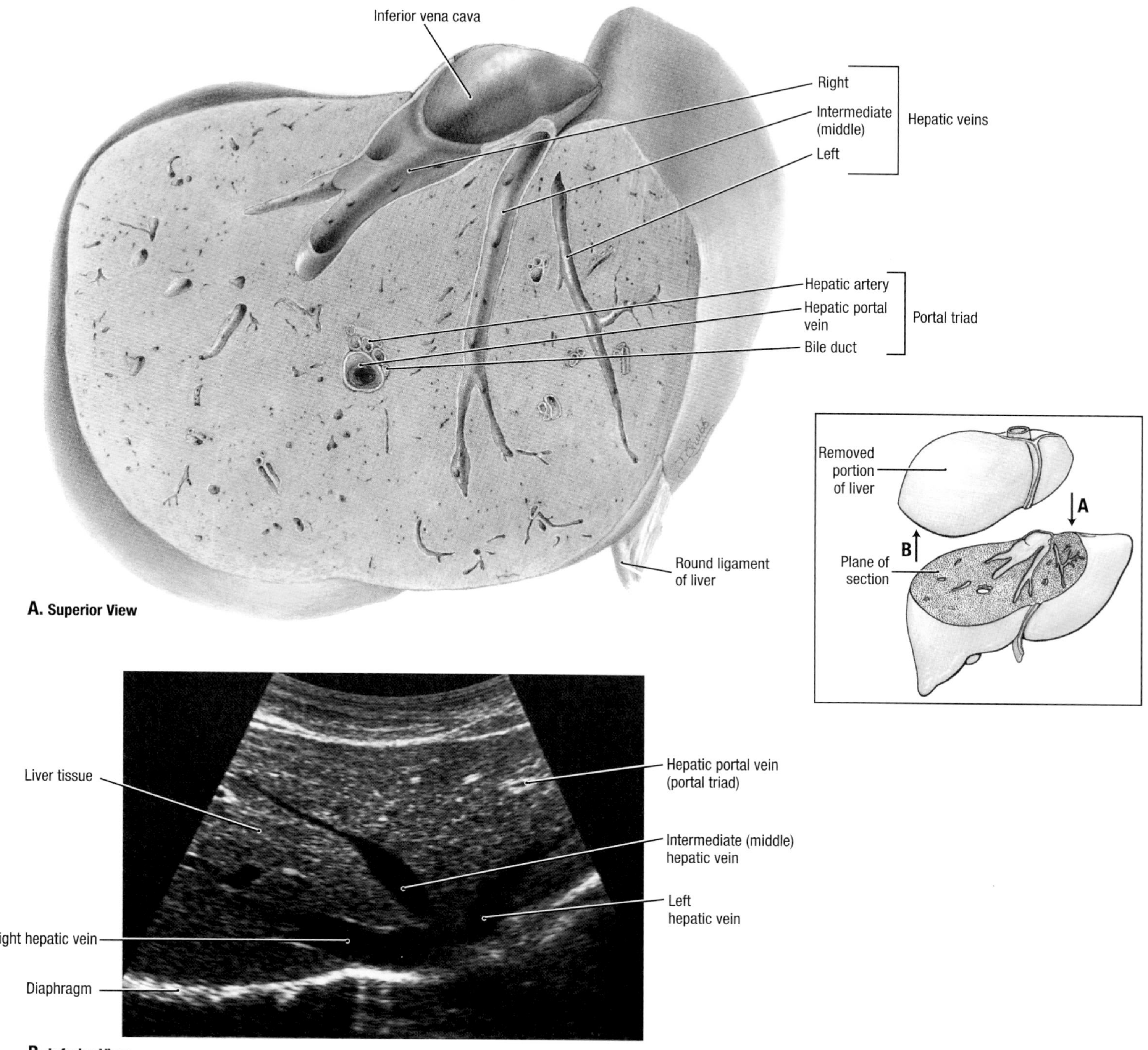
Inferior vena cava
Right
Intermediate (middle)
Left
Hepatic veins
Hepatic artery
Hepatic portal vein
Bile duct
Portal triad
Round ligament of liver
A. Superior View
Removed portion of liver
Plane of section
A
B
Liver tissue
Hepatic portal vein (portal triad)
Intermediate (middle) hepatic vein
Left hepatic vein
Right hepatic vein
Diaphragm
B. Inferior View

## 2.48 Hepatic veins

**A.** Approximately horizontal section of liver with the posterior aspect at top of page. Note the multiple perivascular fibrous capsules sectioned throughout the cut surface, each containing a portal triad (the hepatic portal vein, hepatic artery, bile ductules) plus lymph vessels. Interdigitating with these are branches of the three main hepatic veins (right, intermediate, and left), which, unaccompanied and lacking capsules, converge on the inferior vena cava. **B.** Ultrasound scan. The transducer was placed under the costal margin, and directed posteriorly producing an inverted image corresponding to **A.**

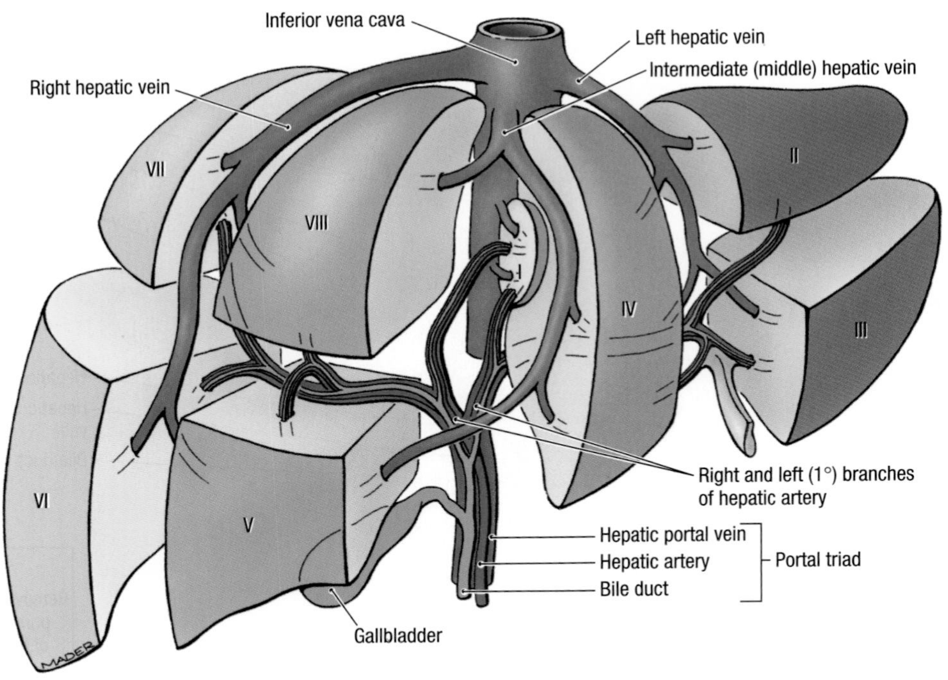
Inferior vena cava
Left hepatic vein
Intermediate (middle) hepatic vein
Right hepatic vein
VII
VIII
II
IV
III
VI
V
Right and left (1°) branches of hepatic artery
Hepatic portal vein
Hepatic artery
Bile duct
Portal triad
Gallbladder
A. Anterior View

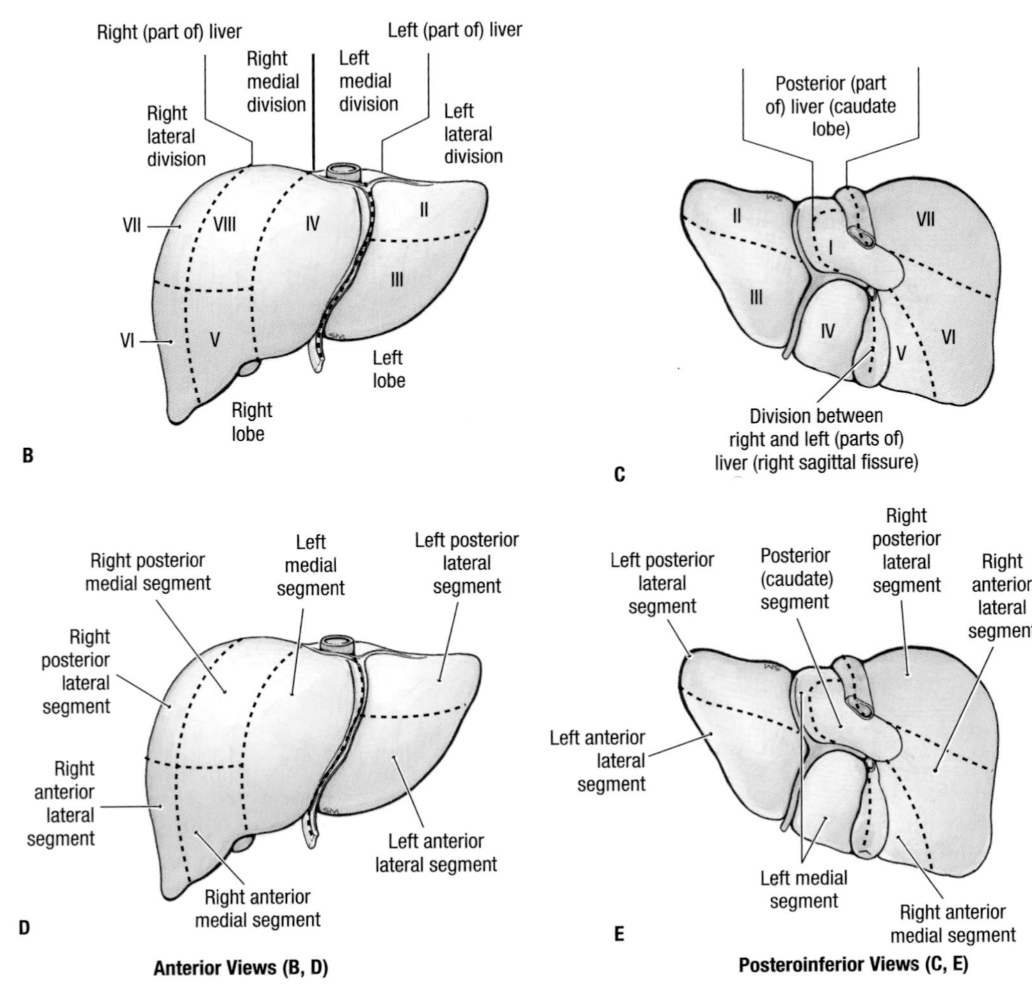
Right (part of) liver
Left (part of) liver
Right medial division
Left medial division
Right lateral division
Left lateral division
VII
VIII
IV
II
III
VI
V
Left lobe
Right lobe
B
Posterior (part of) liver (caudate lobe)
II
VII
I
III
IV
V
VI
Division between right and left (parts of) liver (right sagittal fissure)
C
Right posterior medial segment
Left medial segment
Left posterior lateral segment
Right posterior lateral segment
Right anterior lateral segment
Left anterior lateral segment
Right anterior medial segment
D
Left posterior lateral segment
Posterior (caudate) segment
Right posterior lateral segment
Right anterior lateral segment
Left anterior lateral segment
Left medial segment
Right anterior medial segment
E

Anterior Views (B, D)

Posteroinferior Views (C, E)

## 2.49 Hepatic segmentation

Each segment is supplied by a secondary or tertiary branch of the hepatic artery, bile duct, and portal vein. The hepatic veins interdigitate between the structures of the portal triad and are intersegmental in that they drain adjacent segments. Since the right and left hepatic arteries and ducts and branches of the right and left portal veins do not communicate, it is possible to perform hepatic lobectomies (removal of the right or left part of the liver) and segmentectomies. Each segment can be identified numerically or by name (Table 2.4).

**TABLE 2.4 SCHEMA OF TERMINOLOGY FOR SUBDIVISIONS OF THE LIVER**

| Anatomical Term | Right Lobe | | Left Lobe | | Caudate Lobe | |
|---|---|---|---|---|---|---|
| Functional/ surgical term** | Right (part of) liver<br>[Right portal lobe*] | | Left (part of) liver<br>[Left portal lobe+] | | Posterior (part of) liver | |
| | Right lateral division | Right medial division | Left medial division | Left lateral division | [Right caudate lobe*] | [Left caudate lobe+] |
| | Posterior lateral segment<br>**Segment VII**<br>[Posterior superior area] | Posterior medial segment<br>**Segment VIII**<br>[Anterior superior area] | [Medial superior area]<br><br>Left medial segment<br>**Segment IV** | Lateral segment<br>**Segment II**<br>[Lateral superior area] | Posterior segment<br>**Segment I** | |
| | Right anterior lateral segment<br>**Segment VI**<br>[Posterior inferior area] | Anterior medial segment<br>**Segment V**<br>[Anterior inferior area] | [Medial inferior area = quadrate lobe] | Left anterior lateral segment<br>**Segment III**<br>[Lateral inferior area] | | |

** The labels in the table and figure above reflect the new Terminologia Anatomica: International Anatomical Terminology Previous terminology is in brackets.

*+ Under the schema of the previous terminology, the caudate lobe was divided into right and left halves, and *the right half of the caudate lobe was considered a subdivision of the right portal lobe; + the left half of the caudate lobe was considered a subdivision of the left portal lobe.

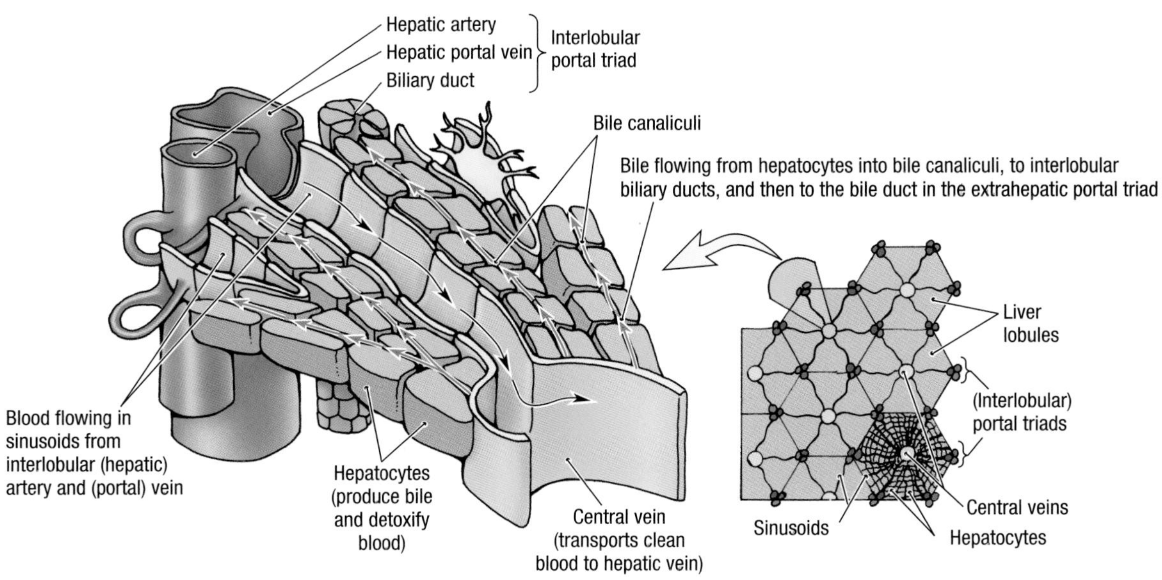
Hepatic artery
Hepatic portal vein
Biliary duct
Interlobular portal triad
Bile canaliculi
Bile flowing from hepatocytes into bile canaliculi, to interlobular biliary ducts, and then to the bile duct in the extrahepatic portal triad
Liver lobules
(Interlobular) portal triads
Central veins
Hepatocytes
Sinusoids
Blood flowing in sinusoids from interlobular (hepatic) artery and (portal) vein
Hepatocytes (produce bile and detoxify blood)
Central vein (transports clean blood to hepatic vein)

## 2.50 Flow of blood and bile in the liver

This small part of a liver lobule shows the components of the interlobular portal triad and the positioning of the sinusoids and bile canaliculi. Right: The cut surface of the liver shows the hexagonal pattern of the lobules.

- With the exception of lipids, every substance absorbed by the alimentary tract is received first by the liver, via the hepatic portal vein. In addition to its many metabolic activities, the liver stores glycogen and secretes bile.
- There is progressive destruction of hepatocytes in cirrhosis of the liver and replacement of them by fibrous tissue. This tissue surrounds the intrahepatic blood vessels and biliary ducts, making the liver firm and impeding circulation of blood through it.

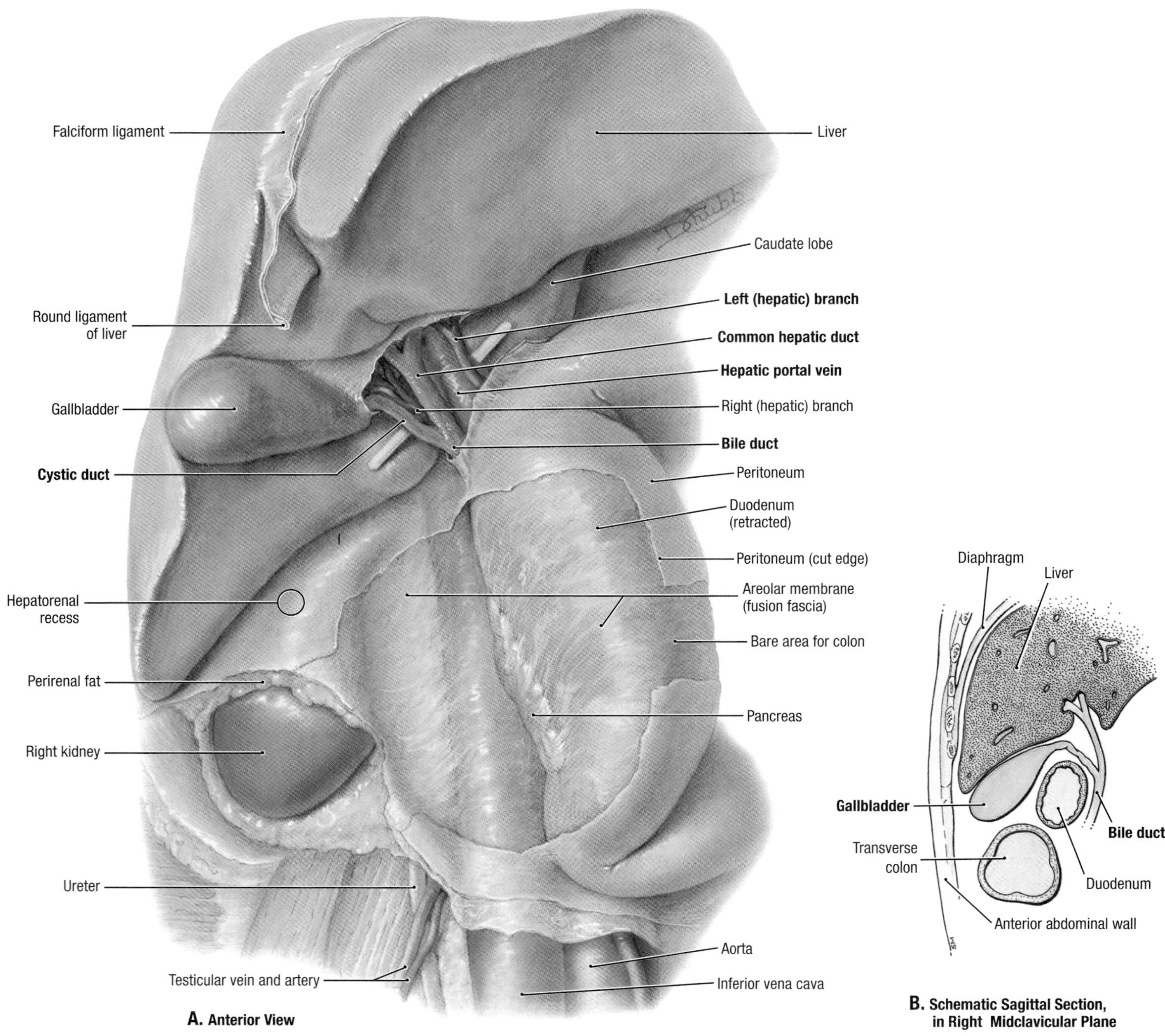
Falciform ligament
Liver
Caudate lobe
Left (hepatic) branch
Round ligament of liver
Common hepatic duct
Hepatic portal vein
Gallbladder
Right (hepatic) branch
Bile duct
Cystic duct
Peritoneum
Duodenum (retracted)
Peritoneum (cut edge)
Hepatorenal recess
Areolar membrane (fusion fascia)
Bare area for colon
Perirenal fat
Pancreas
Right kidney
Ureter
Aorta
Testicular vein and artery
Inferior vena cava
A. Anterior View
Diaphragm
Liver
Gallbladder
Bile duct
Transverse colon
Duodenum
Anterior abdominal wall
B. Schematic Sagittal Section, in Right Midclavicular Plane

## 2.51 Exposure of the portal triad

**A.** The portal triad typically consists of the hepatic portal vein (posteriorly), the hepatic artery proper (ascending from the left), and the bile passages (descending to the right). Here, the hepatic artery proper is replaced by a left hepatic branch, arising directly from the common hepatic artery, and a right hepatic branch, arising from the superior mesenteric artery (a common variation). A rod traverses the omental (epiploic) foramen. The lesser omentum and transverse colon are removed, and the peritoneum is cut along the right border of the duodenum; this part of the duodenum is retracted anteriorly. The space opened up reveals two smooth areolar membranes (fusion fascia) normally applied to each other that are vestiges of the embryonic peritoneum originally covering these surfaces **B.** Typical relations of gallbladder, cystic duct, and bile duct to the duodenum.

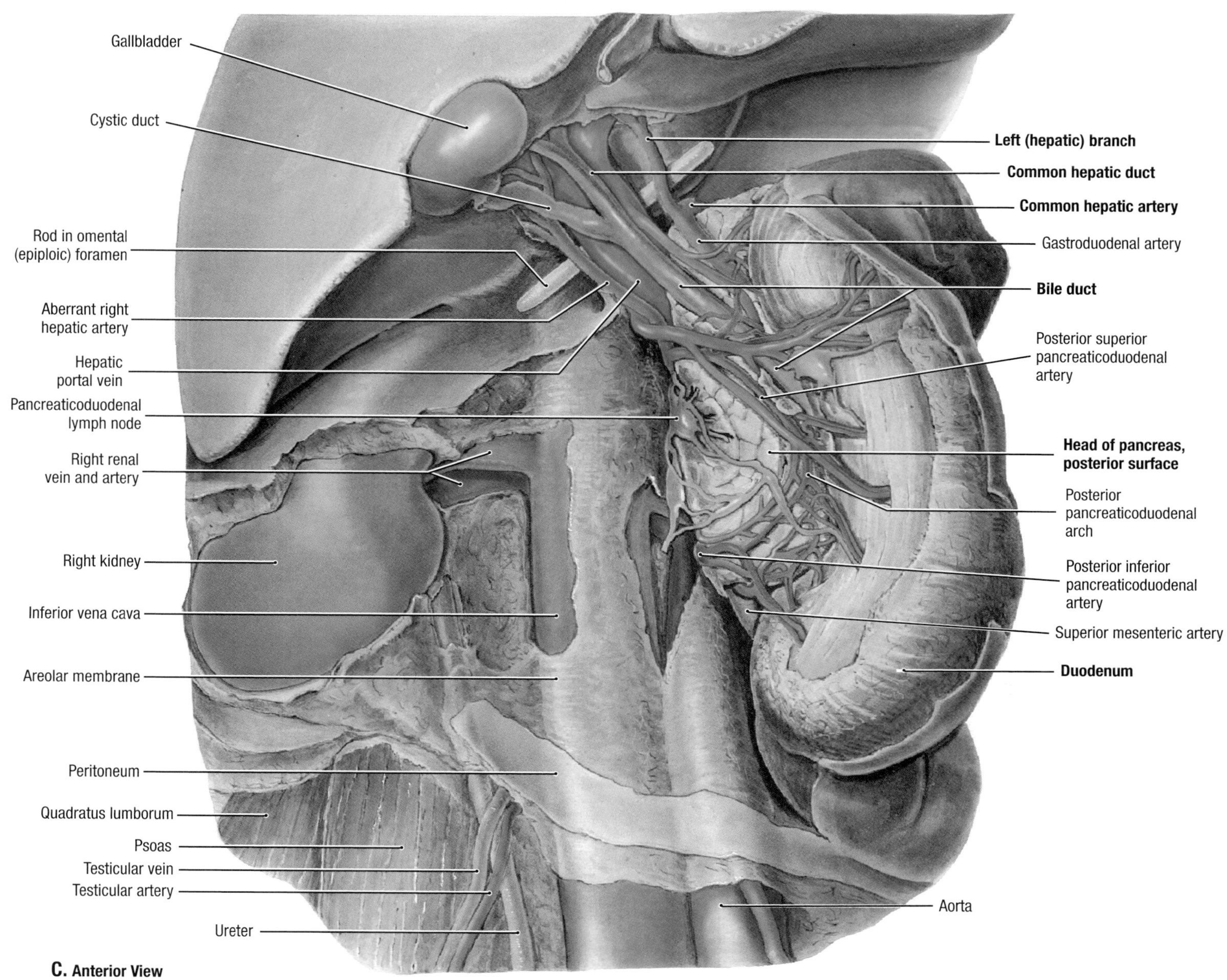
Gallbladder
Cystic duct
Rod in omental (epiploic) foramen
Aberrant right hepatic artery
Hepatic portal vein
Pancreaticoduodenal lymph node
Right renal vein and artery
Right kidney
Inferior vena cava
Areolar membrane
Peritoneum
Quadratus lumborum
Psoas
Testicular vein
Testicular artery
Ureter
Left (hepatic) branch
Common hepatic duct
Common hepatic artery
Gastroduodenal artery
Bile duct
Posterior superior pancreaticoduodenal artery
Head of pancreas, posterior surface
Posterior pancreaticoduodenal arch
Posterior inferior pancreaticoduodenal artery
Superior mesenteric artery
Duodenum
Aorta

**C. Anterior View**

## 2.51 Exposure of the portal triad *(continued)*

**C.** Continuing the dissection in **A**, the secondarily retroperitoneal viscera (duodenum and head of the pancreas) are retracted anteriorly and to the left. The areolar membrane (fusion fascia) covering the posterior aspect of the pancreas and duodenum is largely removed, and that covering the anterior aspect of the great vessels is partly removed. A common method for reducing portal hypertension is to divert blood from the portal venous system to the systemic venous system by creating a communication between the portal vein and the IVC. This portacaval anastomosis of portosystemic shunt may be created where these vessels lie close to each other posterior to the liver.

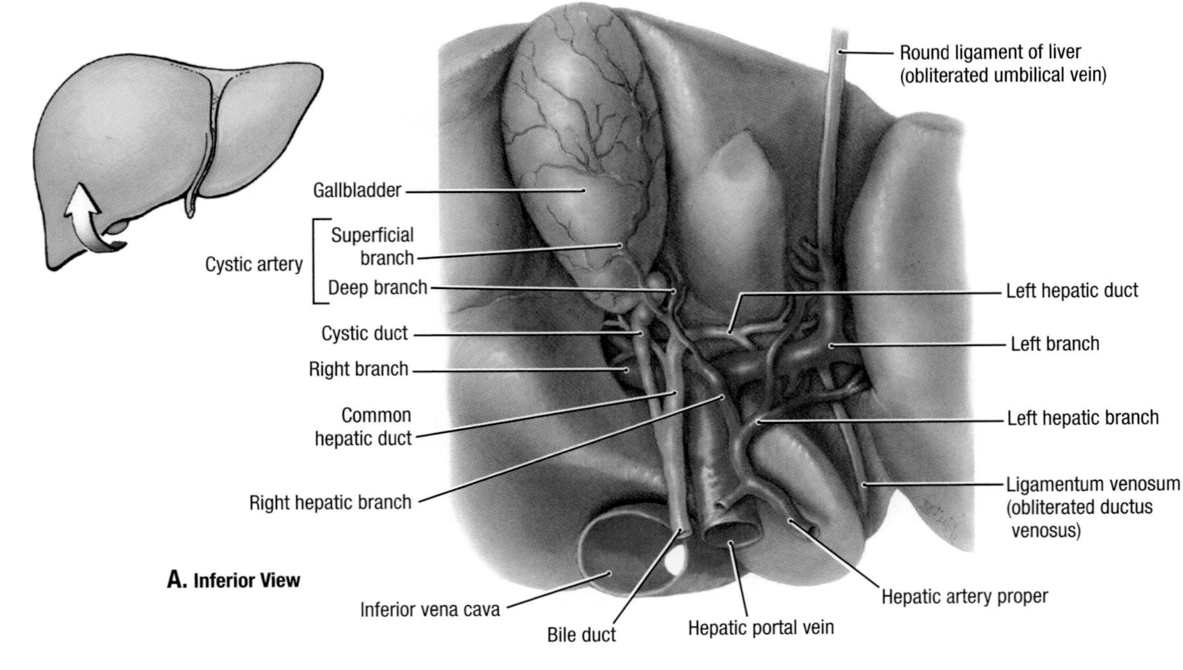
Round ligament of liver
(obliterated umbilical vein)
Gallbladder
Cystic artery
Superficial branch
Deep branch
Cystic duct
Right branch
Common hepatic duct
Right hepatic branch
Left hepatic duct
Left branch
Left hepatic branch
Ligamentum venosum
(obliterated ductus venosus)
Hepatic artery proper
Inferior vena cava
Bile duct
Hepatic portal vein
A. Inferior View

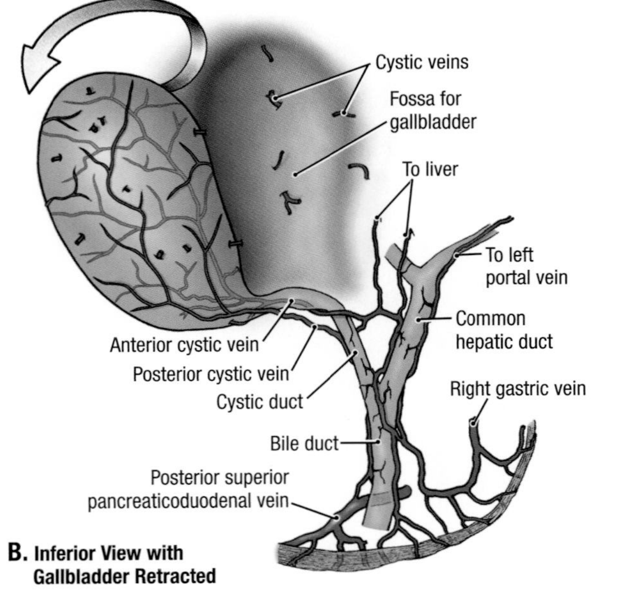
Cystic veins
Fossa for gallbladder
To liver
To left portal vein
Common hepatic duct
Anterior cystic vein
Posterior cystic vein
Cystic duct
Right gastric vein
Bile duct
Posterior superior pancreaticoduodenal vein
B. Inferior View with Gallbladder Retracted

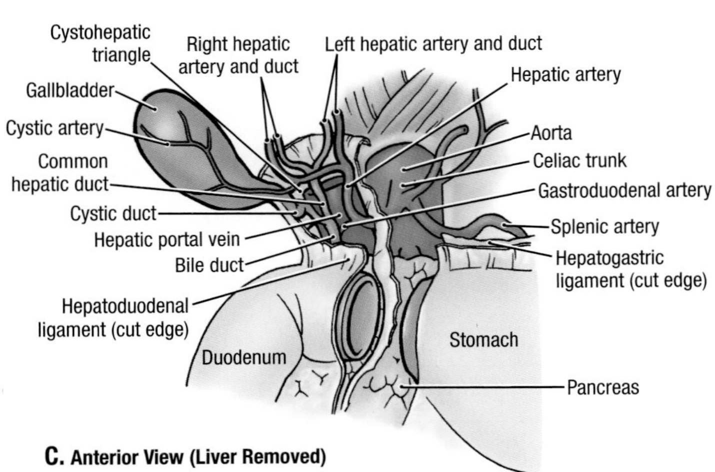
Cystohepatic triangle
Right hepatic artery and duct
Left hepatic artery and duct
Hepatic artery
Gallbladder
Cystic artery
Common hepatic duct
Cystic duct
Hepatic portal vein
Bile duct
Aorta
Celiac trunk
Gastroduodenal artery
Splenic artery
Hepatogastric ligament (cut edge)
Hepatoduodenal ligament (cut edge)
Duodenum
Stomach
Pancreas
C. Anterior View (Liver Removed)

## 2.52 Gallbladder and structures of porta hepatis

**A.** Gallbladder, cystic artery and extrahepatic bile ducts. The inferior border of the liver is elevated to demonstrate its visceral surface (as in orientation figure). **B.** Venous drainage of the gall bladder and extrahepatic ducts. Most veins are tributaries of the hepatic portal vein, but some drain directly to the liver. **C.** Portal triad within the hepatoduodenal ligament (free edge of lesser omentum).

Gallstones are concretions, pebble(s), in the gallbladder or extrahepatic biliary ducts. The cystohepatic triangle (Calot), between the common hepatic duct, cystic duct, and liver is an important endoscopic landmark for locating the cystic artery.

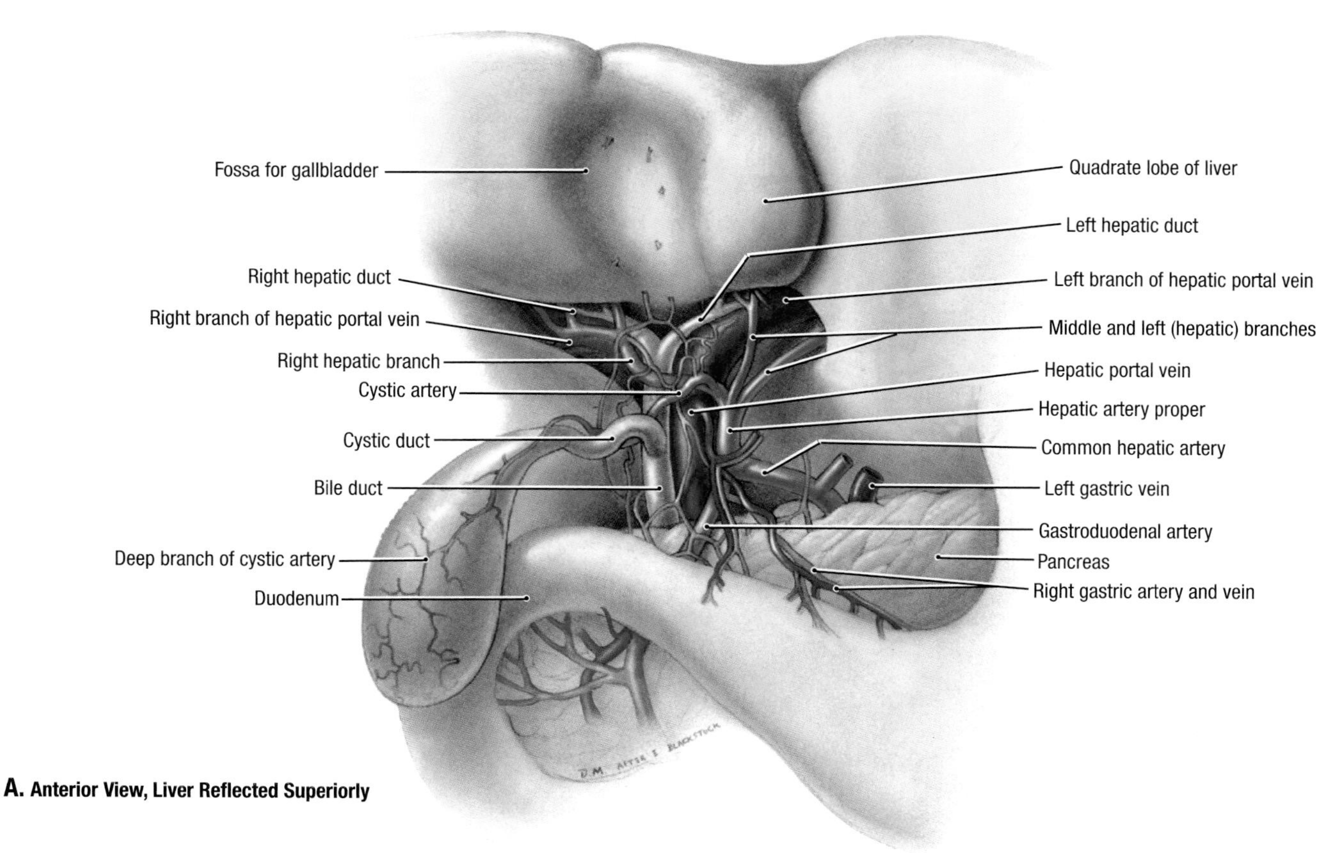
Fossa for gallbladder
Right hepatic duct
Right branch of hepatic portal vein
Right hepatic branch
Cystic artery
Cystic duct
Bile duct
Deep branch of cystic artery
Duodenum
Quadrate lobe of liver
Left hepatic duct
Left branch of hepatic portal vein
Middle and left (hepatic) branches
Hepatic portal vein
Hepatic artery proper
Common hepatic artery
Left gastric vein
Gastroduodenal artery
Pancreas
Right gastric artery and vein

**A.** **Anterior View, Liver Reflected Superiorly**

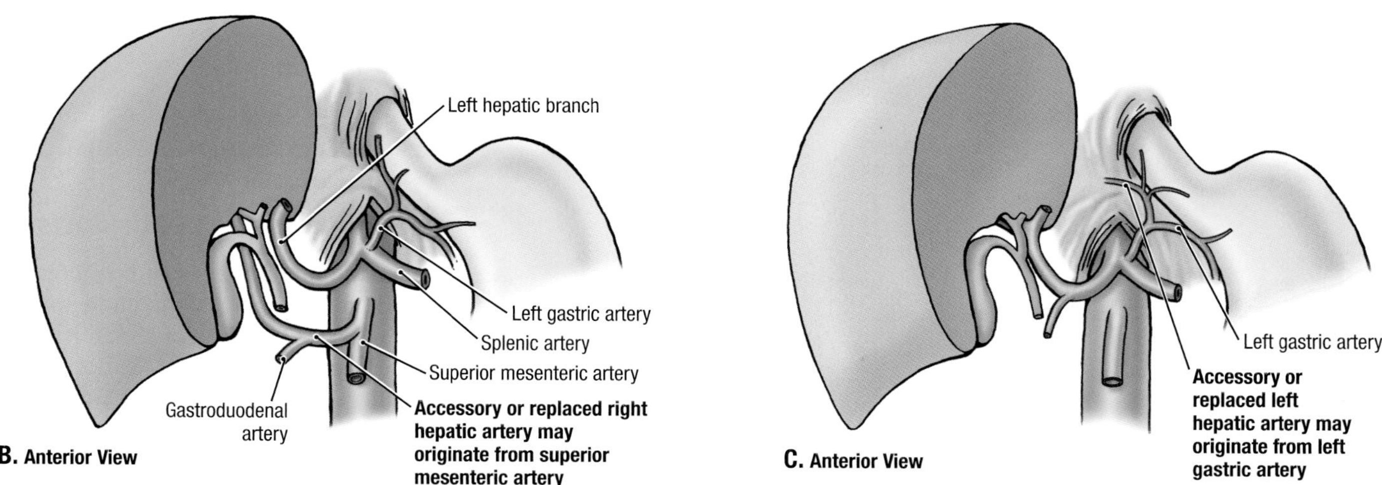
Left hepatic branch
Left gastric artery
Splenic artery
Superior mesenteric artery
Gastroduodenal artery
Accessory or replaced right hepatic artery may originate from superior mesenteric artery
Left gastric artery
Accessory or replaced left hepatic artery may originate from left gastric artery

**B.** **Anterior View**

**C.** **Anterior View**

## 2.53 Vessels in porta hepatis

**A.** Hepatic and cystic vessels. The liver is reflected superiorly. The gallbladder, freed from its bed, or fossa, has remained nearly in its anatomical position, pulled slightly to the right. The deep branch of the cystic artery on the deep, or attached, surface of the gallbladder anastomoses with branches of the superficial branch of the cystic artery and sends twigs into the bed of the gallbladder. Veins (not all shown) accompany most arteries. **B.** Aberrant (accessory or replaced) right hepatic artery. **C.** Aberrant left hepatic artery.

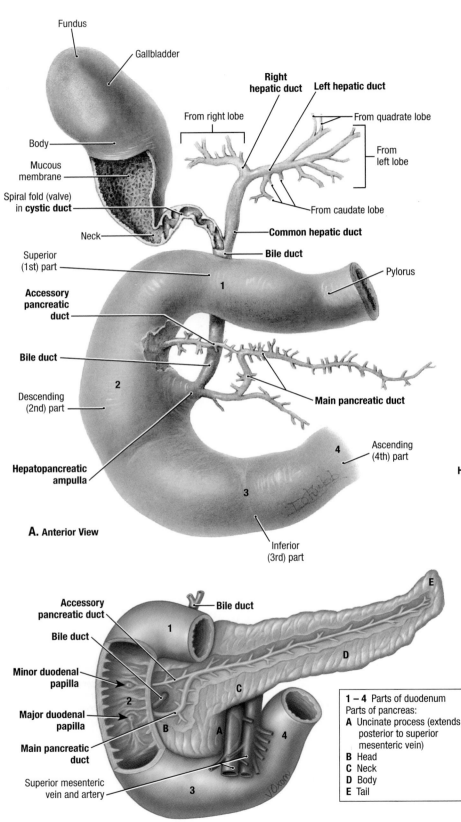

Fundus
Gallbladder
Body
Mucous membrane
Spiral fold (valve) in **cystic duct**
Neck
**Right hepatic duct**
**Left hepatic duct**
From right lobe
From quadrate lobe
From left lobe
From caudate lobe
**Common hepatic duct**
**Bile duct**
Superior (1st) part
Pylorus
**Accessory pancreatic duct**
**Bile duct**
Descending (2nd) part
**Main pancreatic duct**
Ascending (4th) part
**Hepatopancreatic ampulla**
Inferior (3rd) part
1
2
3
4

**A.** Anterior View

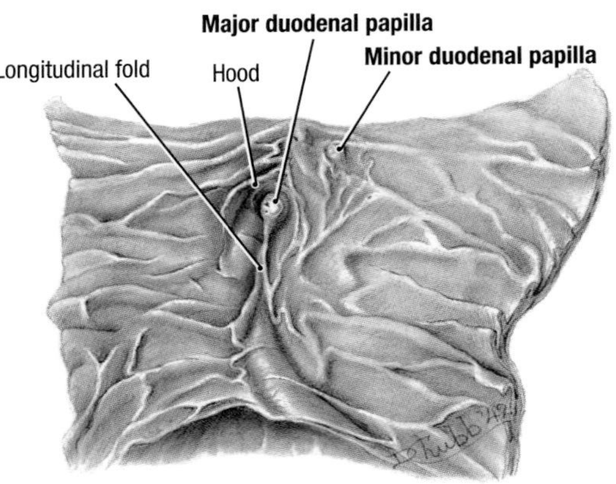
Major duodenal papilla
Minor duodenal papilla
Longitudinal fold
Hood

**C.** Internal View

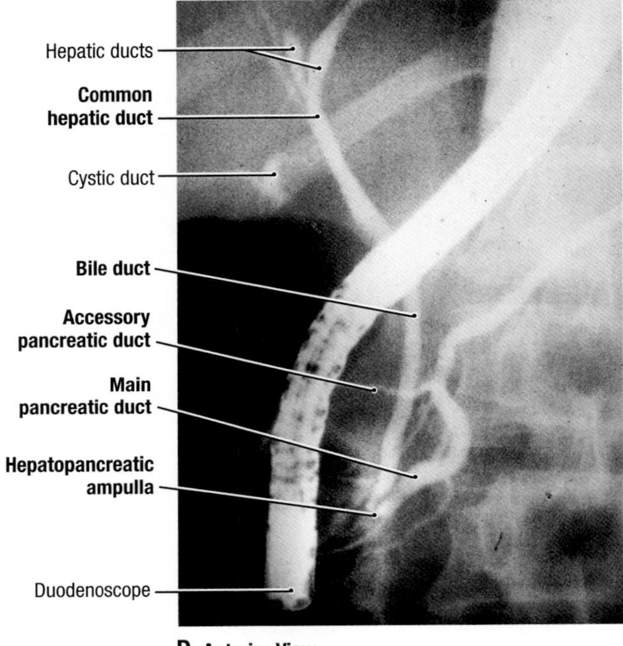
Hepatic ducts
Common hepatic duct
Cystic duct
Bile duct
Accessory pancreatic duct
Main pancreatic duct
Hepatopancreatic ampulla
Duodenoscope

**D.** Anterior View

**Accessory pancreatic duct**
**Bile duct**
**Minor duodenal papilla**
**Major duodenal papilla**
**Main pancreatic duct**
Superior mesenteric vein and artery
1
2
3
4
A
B
C
D
E

**1 – 4** Parts of duodenum
Parts of pancreas:
**A** Uncinate process (extends posterior to superior mesenteric vein)
**B** Head
**C** Neck
**D** Body
**E** Tail

**B.** Anterior View

## 2.54 Bile and pancreatic ducts

**A.** Extrahepatic bile passages and pancreatic ducts. **B.** Descending (2nd) part of the duodenum (interior). **C.** Endoscopic retrograde cholangiography and pancreatography (ERCP) demonstrating the bile and pancreatic ducts. The right and left hepatic ducts collect bile from the liver; the common hepatic duct unites with the cystic duct superior to the duodenum to form the bile duct which descends posterior to the superior (1st) part of the duodenum. The bile duct joins the main pancreatic duct, forming the hepatopancreatic ampulla, which opens on the major duodenal papilla. This opening is the narrowest part of the biliary passages and is the common site for impaction of a gallstone. Gallstones may produce biliary colic (pain in the epigastric region). The accessory pancreatic duct opens on the minor duodenal papilla.

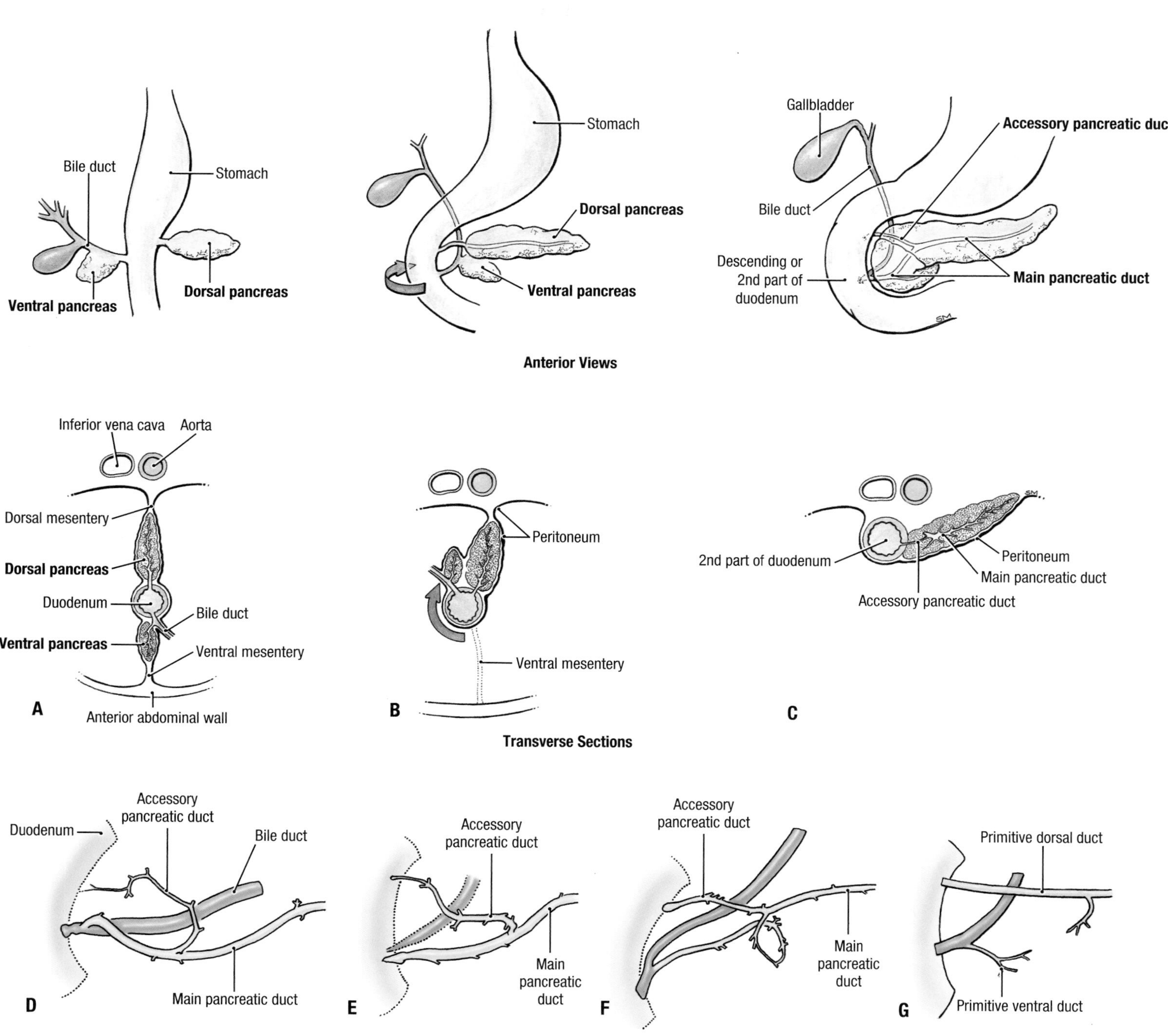
Bile duct
Stomach
Ventral pancreas
Dorsal pancreas
Stomach
Dorsal pancreas
Ventral pancreas
Gallbladder
Accessory pancreatic duct
Bile duct
Descending or 2nd part of duodenum
Main pancreatic duct
Anterior Views
Inferior vena cava
Aorta
Dorsal mesentery
Dorsal pancreas
Duodenum
Bile duct
Ventral pancreas
Ventral mesentery
A
Anterior abdominal wall
Peritoneum
Ventral mesentery
B
2nd part of duodenum
Peritoneum
Main pancreatic duct
Accessory pancreatic duct
C
Transverse Sections
Duodenum
Accessory pancreatic duct
Bile duct
Main pancreatic duct
D
Accessory pancreatic duct
Main pancreatic duct
E
Accessory pancreatic duct
Main pancreatic duct
F
Primitive dorsal duct
Primitive ventral duct
G
Anterior Views

## 2.55 Development and variability of the pancreatic ducts

**A–C.** Anterior views (top) and transverse sections (bottom) of the stages in the development of the pancreas. **A.** The small, primitive ventral bud arises in common with the bile duct, and a larger, primitive dorsal bud arises independently from the duodenum. **B.** The 2nd, or descending, part of the duodenum rotates on its long axis, which brings the ventral bud and bile duct posterior to the dorsal bud. **C.** A connecting segment unites the dorsal duct to the ventral duct, whereupon the duodenal end of the dorsal duct atrophies, and the direction of flow within it is reversed. **D–G.** Common variations of the pancreatic duct. **D.** An accessory duct that has lost its connection with the duodenum. **E.** An accessory duct that is large enough to relieve an obstructed main duct. **F.** An accessory duct that could probably substitute for the main duct. **G.** A persisting primitive dorsal duct unconnected to the primitive ventral duct.

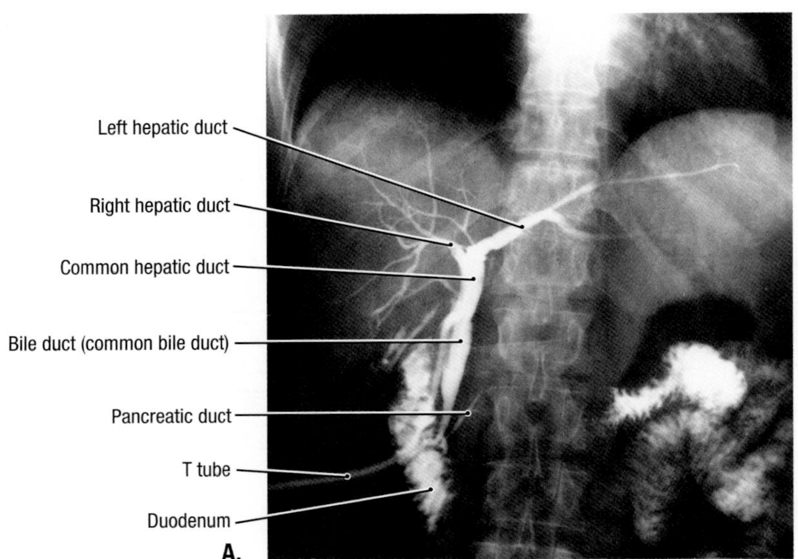
Left hepatic duct
Right hepatic duct
Common hepatic duct
Bile duct (common bile duct)
Pancreatic duct
T tube
Duodenum
A.

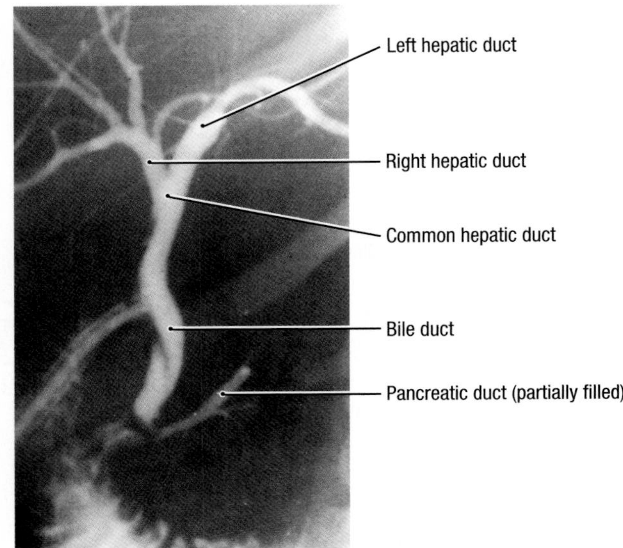
Left hepatic duct
Right hepatic duct
Common hepatic duct
Bile duct
Pancreatic duct (partially filled)
B.

## 2.56 Radiographs of biliary passages

After a cholecystectomy (removal of the gallbladder), contrast medium was injected with a T tube inserted into the bile passages. The biliary passages are visualized in the superior abdomen in **A** and are more localized in **B**.

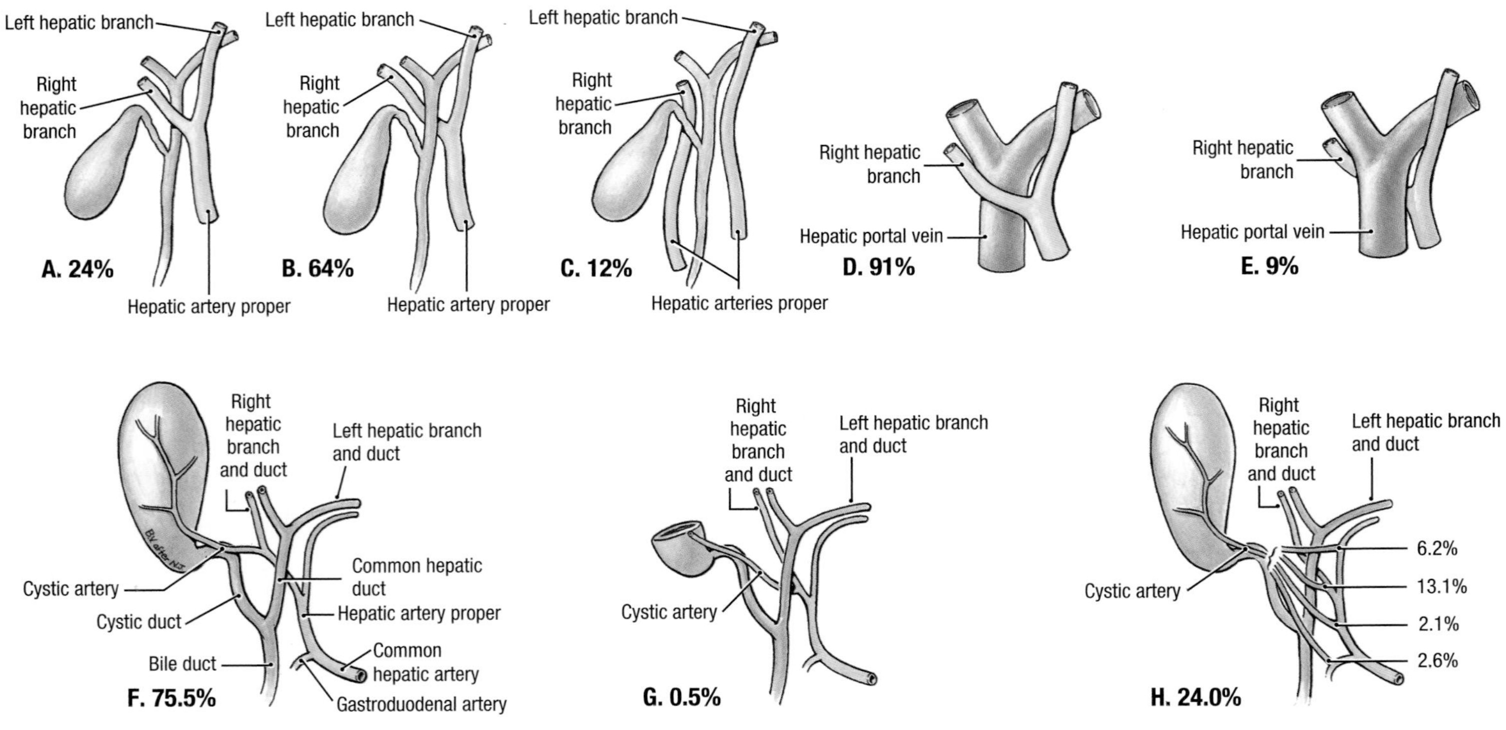
Left hepatic branch
Right hepatic branch
A. 24%
Hepatic artery proper
Left hepatic branch
Right hepatic branch
B. 64%
Hepatic artery proper
Left hepatic branch
Right hepatic branch
C. 12%
Hepatic arteries proper
Right hepatic branch
Hepatic portal vein
D. 91%
Right hepatic branch
Hepatic portal vein
E. 9%
Right hepatic branch and duct
Left hepatic branch and duct
Cystic artery
Cystic duct
Bile duct
Common hepatic duct
Hepatic artery proper
Common hepatic artery
Gastroduodenal artery
F. 75.5%
Right hepatic branch and duct
Left hepatic branch and duct
Cystic artery
G. 0.5%
Right hepatic branch and duct
Left hepatic branch and duct
Cystic artery
6.2%
13.1%
2.1%
2.6%
H. 24.0%
Anterior Views

## 2.57 Variations in hepatic and cystic arteries

In a study of 165 cadavers, five patterns were observed. **A.** Right hepatic artery crossing anterior to bile passages, 24%. **B.** Right hepatic artery crossing posterior to bile passages, 64%. **C.** Aberrant artery arising from the superior mesenteric artery, 12%. The artery crossed anterior **(D)** to the portal vein in 91%, and posterior **(E)** in 9%. The cystic artery usually arises from the right hepatic artery in the angle between the common hepatic duct and cystic duct, without crossing the common hepatic duct **(F** and **G)**. However, when it arises on the left of the bile passages, it almost always crosses anterior to the passages **(H)**.

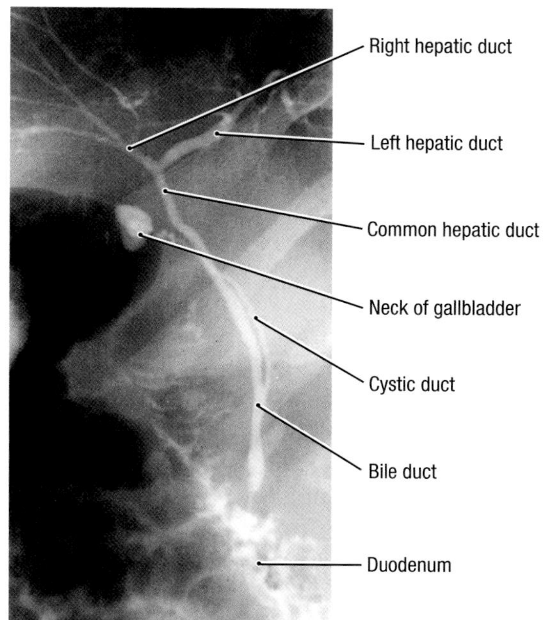
Right hepatic duct
Left hepatic duct
Common hepatic duct
Neck of gallbladder
Cystic duct
Bile duct
Duodenum

**A. Anterior View**

Parts of gallbladder:

Neck

Body

Fundus

**B. Anterior View**

## 2.58 Endoscopic retrograde cholangiography of gallbladder and biliary passages

**A.** Cystic duct. **B.** Parts of gallbladder.

Endoscopic retrograde cholangiography (ERCP) is done by first passing a fiberoptic endoscope through the mouth, esophagus, and stomach. Then the duodenum is entered and a cannula is inserted into the major duodenal papilla and advanced under fluoroscopic control into the duct of choice (bile duct or pancreatic duct) for injection of radiographic contrast medium.

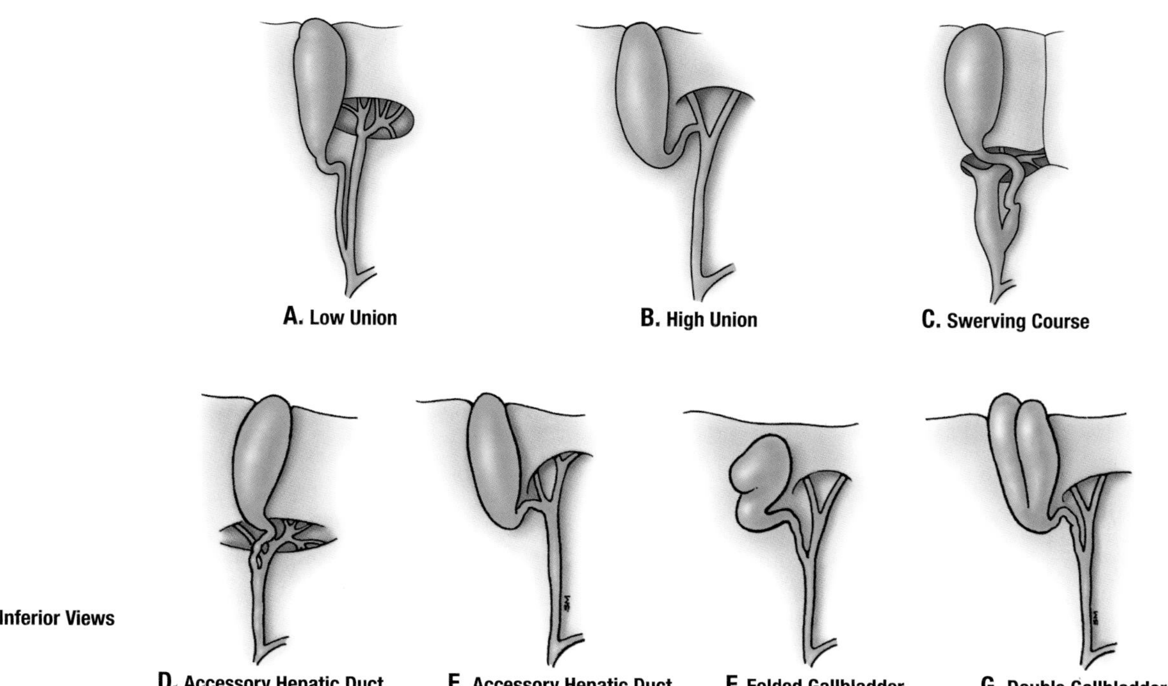
A. Low Union
B. High Union
C. Swerving Course
Inferior Views
D. Accessory Hepatic Duct
E. Accessory Hepatic Duct
F. Folded Gallbladder
G. Double Gallbladder

## 2.59 Variations of cystic and hepatic ducts and gallbladder

The cystic duct usually lies on the right side of the common hepatic duct, joining it just above the superior (1st) part of the duodenum, but this varies as in **A–C**. Of 95 gallbladders and bile passages studied, 7 had accessory ducts. Of these, 4 joined the common hepatic duct near the cystic duct **(D)**, 2 joined the cystic duct **(E)**, and 1 was an anastomosing duct connecting the cystic with the common hepatic duct. **F.** Folded gallbladder. **G.** Double gallbladder.

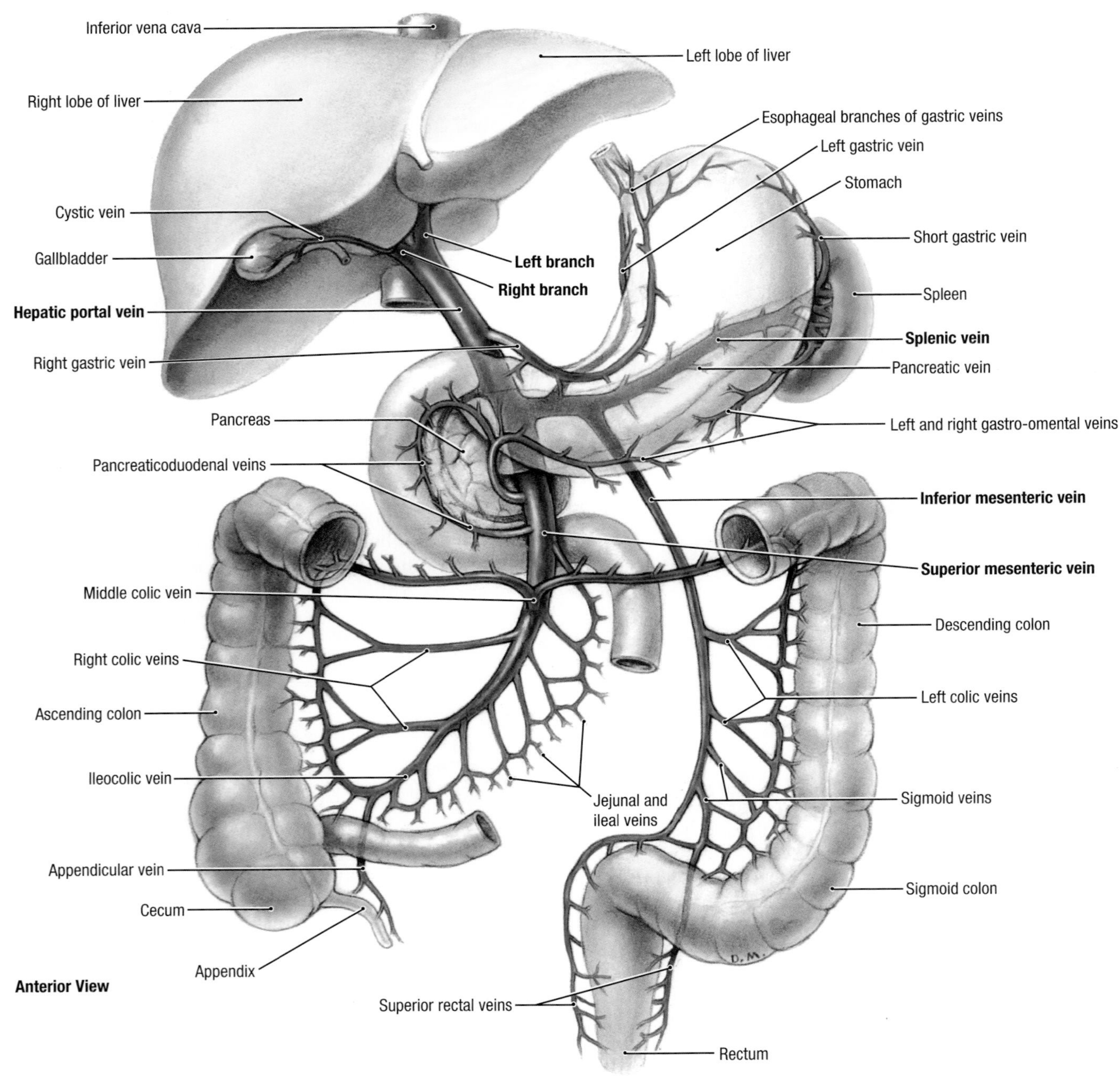
Inferior vena cava
Left lobe of liver
Right lobe of liver
Esophageal branches of gastric veins
Left gastric vein
Stomach
Cystic vein
Short gastric vein
Gallbladder
Left branch
Right branch
Spleen
Hepatic portal vein
Splenic vein
Right gastric vein
Pancreatic vein
Left and right gastro-omental veins
Pancreas
Pancreaticoduodenal veins
Inferior mesenteric vein
Superior mesenteric vein
Middle colic vein
Descending colon
Right colic veins
Left colic veins
Ascending colon
Ileocolic vein
Jejunal and ileal veins
Sigmoid veins
Appendicular vein
Sigmoid colon
Cecum
Appendix
Anterior View
Superior rectal veins
Rectum

## 2.60 Portal venous system

- The hepatic portal vein drains venous blood from the gastrointestinal tract, spleen, pancreas, and gallbladder to the sinusoids of the liver; from here, the blood is conveyed to the systemic venous system by the hepatic veins that drain directly to the inferior vena cava.
- The hepatic portal vein forms posterior to the neck of the pancreas by the union of the superior mesenteric and splenic veins, with the inferior mesenteric vein joining at or near the angle of union.
- The splenic vein drains blood from the inferior mesenteric, left gastro-omental (epiploic), short gastric, and pancreatic veins.
- The right gastro-omental, pancreaticoduodenal, jejunal, ileal, right, and middle colic veins drain into the superior mesenteric vein.
- The inferior mesenteric vein commences in the rectal plexus as the superior rectal vein and, after crossing the common iliac vessels, becomes the inferior mesenteric vein; branches include the sigmoid and left colic veins.
- The hepatic portal vein divides into right and left branches at the porta hepatis. The left branch carries mainly, but not exclusively, blood from the inferior mesenteric, gastric, and splenic veins, and the right branch carries blood mainly from the superior mesenteric vein.

Azygos vein
Esophageal vein
Inferior vena cava
(1)
Stomach
Liver
Left gastric vein
Hepatic portal vein
Splenic vein
Superior mesenteric vein
Inferior mesenteric vein
Paraumbilical vein
(3)
Umbilicus
Colic vein
(4)
Colon
Epigastric veins
Retroperitoneal veins
Superior rectal vein
Middle rectal veins
Inferior rectal vein
(2)
Anus
SM AFTER NJ

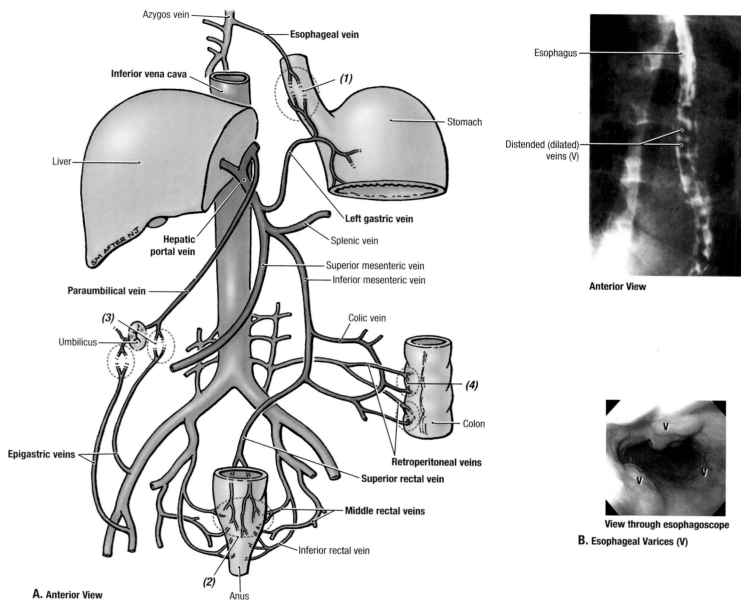

**A. Anterior View**

Esophagus
Distended (dilated) veins (V)

**Anterior View**

V
V
V

**View through esophagoscope**

**B. Esophageal Varices (V)**

## 2.61 Portacaval system

**A.** Portacaval system. In this diagram, portal tributaries are dark blue, and systemic tributaries and communicating veins are light blue. In portal hypertension (as in hepatic cirrhosis), the portal blood cannot pass freely through the liver, and the portocaval anastomoses become engorged, dilated, or even varicose; as a consequence, these veins may rupture. The sites of the portocaval anastomosis shown are between *(1)* esophageal veins draining into the azygos vein (systemic) and left gastric vein (portal), which when dilated are esophageal varices, also shown in **B**; *(2)* the inferior and middle rectal veins, draining into the inferior vena cava (systemic) and the superior rectal vein continuing as the inferior mesenteric vein (portal) (hemorrhoids result if the vessels are dilated); *(3)* paraumbilical veins (portal) and small epigastric veins of the anterior abdominal wall (systemic), which when varicose form "caput medusae" (so named because of the resemblance of the radiating veins to the serpents on the head of Medusa, a character in Greek mythology); and *(4)* twigs of colic veins (portal) anastomosing with systemic retroperitoneal veins. **B.** Esophageal varices. **C.** Caput medusae.

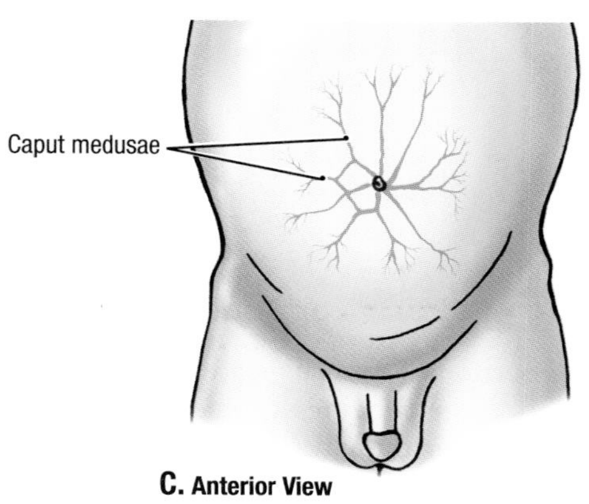
Caput medusae

**C. Anterior View**

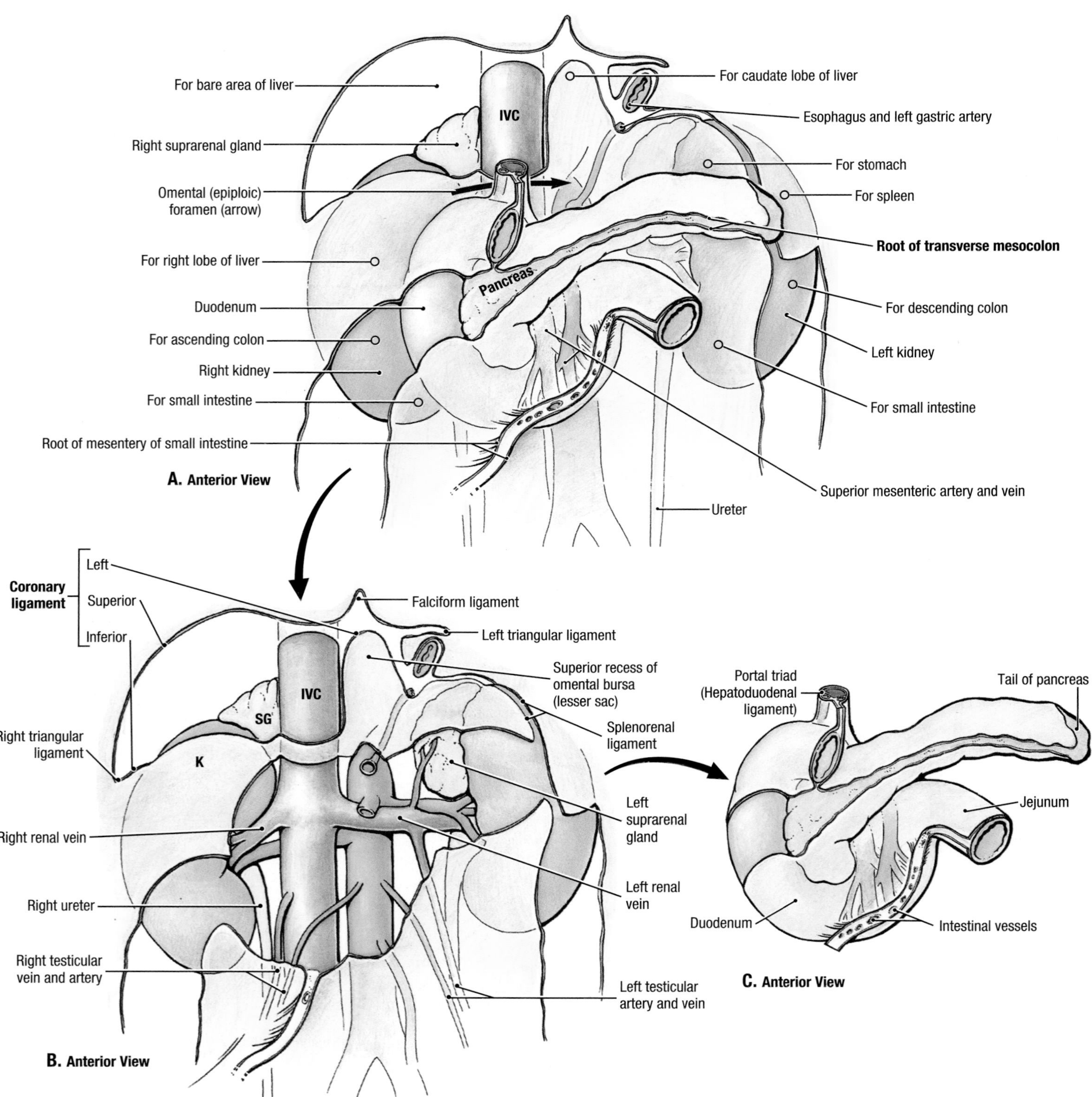
For bare area of liver
IVC
For caudate lobe of liver
Esophagus and left gastric artery
Right suprarenal gland
For stomach
Omental (epiploic) foramen (arrow)
For spleen
Root of transverse mesocolon
For right lobe of liver
Pancreas
For descending colon
Duodenum
For ascending colon
Left kidney
Right kidney
For small intestine
For small intestine
Root of mesentery of small intestine
Superior mesenteric artery and vein
A. Anterior View
Ureter
Coronary ligament
Left
Superior
Inferior
Falciform ligament
Left triangular ligament
Superior recess of omental bursa (lesser sac)
IVC
SG
Splenorenal ligament
Right triangular ligament
K
Right renal vein
Left suprarenal gland
Left renal vein
Right ureter
Right testicular vein and artery
Left testicular artery and vein
B. Anterior View
Portal triad (Hepatoduodenal ligament)
Tail of pancreas
Jejunum
Duodenum
Intestinal vessels
C. Anterior View

## 2.62 Posterior abdominal viscera and their anterior relations

The peritoneal coverings are yellow. **A.** Duodenum and pancreas in situ. Note the line of attachment of the root of the transverse mesocolon is to the body and tail of the pancreas. The viscera contacting specific regions are indicated by the term “for.” The omental (epiploic) foramen is traversed by an arrow. **B.** After removal of duodenum and pancreas. The three parts of the coronary ligament are attached to the diaphragm, except where the inferior vena cava (IVC), suprarenal gland (SG), and kidney (K) intervene. **C.** Pancreas and duodenum removed from **A.**

Celiac ganglion
**Celiac trunk**
Posterior vagal trunk in esophageal hiatus
Inferior phrenic artery and plexus
Hepatic veins
Spleen
Inferior phrenic artery
Costodiaphragmatic recess
**Right suprarenal gland**
10th rib
**Inferior vena cava**
**Left suprarenal gland**
Diaphragm
**Abdominal aorta**
**Superior mesenteric artery**
Subcostal artery
Descending colon
Subcostal nerve
Sympathetic trunk
Transversus abdominis
Quadratus lumborum
External oblique
Iliohypogastric and ilioinguinal nerves
Internal oblique
Transversus abdominis
**Left common iliac artery and vein**
Inferior mesenteric artery and vein
Iliacus
Lateral cutaneous nerve of thigh
**Testicular artery and vein**
Psoas
Femoral nerve
**Ureter**
Sigmoid colon
Psoas fascia
Right internal iliac artery
Genitofemoral nerve
Testicular artery and vein
**External iliac artery and vein**
Ductus deferens

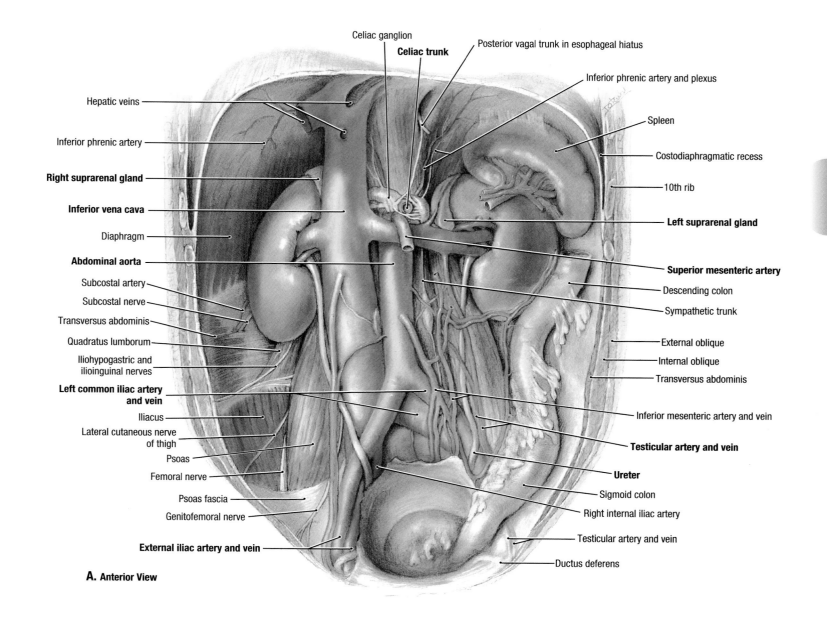

**A. Anterior View**

## 2.63 Viscera and vessels of posterior abdominal wall

**A.** Great vessels, kidneys, and suprarenal glands. **B.** Relationships of left renal vein and inferior (3rd) part of duodenum to aorta and superior mesenteric artery.

- The abdominal aorta is shorter and smaller in caliber than the inferior vena cava.
- The inferior mesenteric artery arises about 4 cm superior to the aortic bifurcation and crosses the left common iliac vessels to become the superior rectal artery.
- The left renal vein drains the left testis, left suprarenal gland, and left kidney; the renal arteries are posterior to the renal veins.
- The ureter crosses the external iliac artery just beyond the common iliac bifurcation.
- The testicular vessels cross anterior to the ureter and join the ductus deferens at the deep inguinal ring.
- In **B**, the left renal vein and duodenum (and uncinate process of pancreas—not shown) pass between the aorta posteriorly and the superior mesenteric artery, anteriorly; they may be compressed like nuts in a nutcracker.

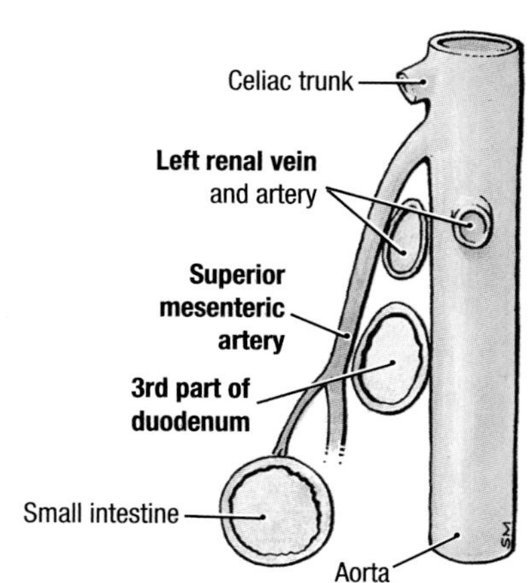
Celiac trunk
Left renal vein
and artery
Superior
mesenteric
artery
3rd part of
duodenum
Small intestine
Aorta

**B. Lateral View (from left)**

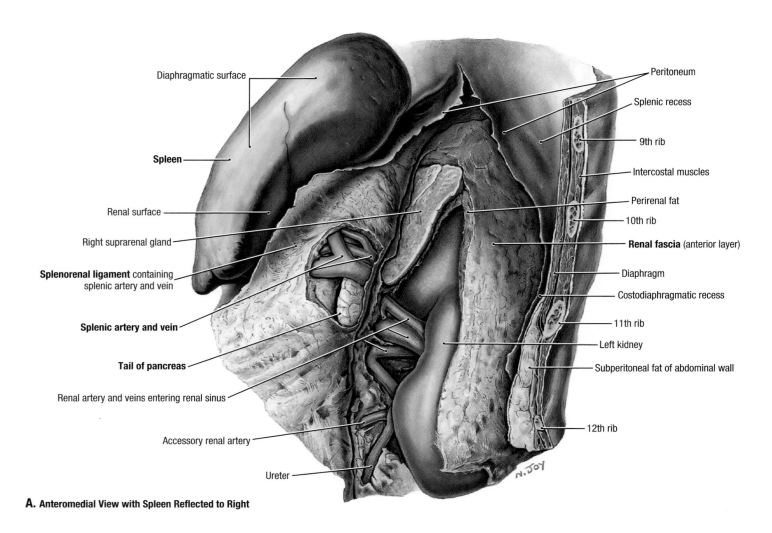

Diaphragmatic surface
Spleen
Renal surface
Right suprarenal gland
**Splenorenal ligament** containing splenic artery and vein
**Splenic artery and vein**
**Tail of pancreas**
Renal artery and veins entering renal sinus
Accessory renal artery
Ureter
Peritoneum
Splenic recess
9th rib
Intercostal muscles
Perirenal fat
10th rib
**Renal fascia** (anterior layer)
Diaphragm
Costodiaphragmatic recess
11th rib
Left kidney
Subperitoneal fat of abdominal wall
12th rib
N. JOY

**A. Anteromedial View with Spleen Reflected to Right**

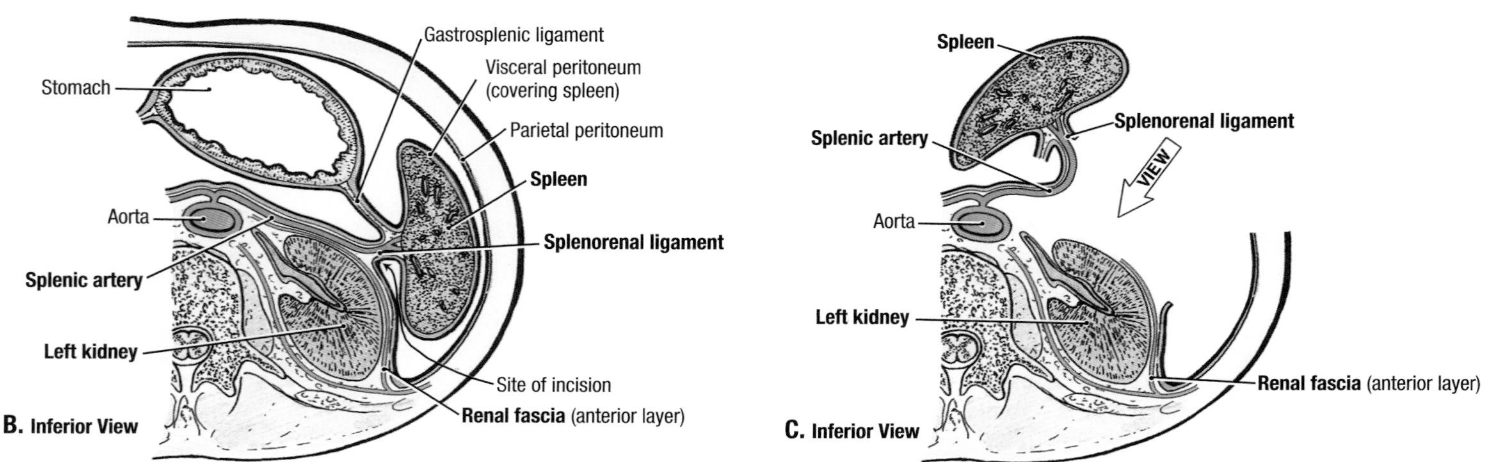
Gastrosplenic ligament
Stomach
Visceral peritoneum (covering spleen)
Parietal peritoneum
**Spleen**
Aorta
**Splenorenal ligament**
**Splenic artery**
**Left kidney**
Site of incision
**Renal fascia** (anterior layer)
**Spleen**
**Splenic artery**
**Splenorenal ligament**
VIEW
Aorta
**Left kidney**
**Renal fascia** (anterior layer)

**B. Inferior View**

**C. Inferior View**

## 2.64 Exposure of the left kidney and suprarenal gland

**A.** Dissection. **B.** Schematic section with spleen and splenorenal ligament intact. **C.** Procedure used in **A** to expose the kidney. The spleen and splenorenal ligament are reflected anteriorly, with the splenic vessels and tail of the pancreas. Part of the renal fascia of the kidney is removed. Note the proximity of the splenic vein and left renal vein, enabling a splenorenal shunt to be established surgically to relieve portal hypertension.

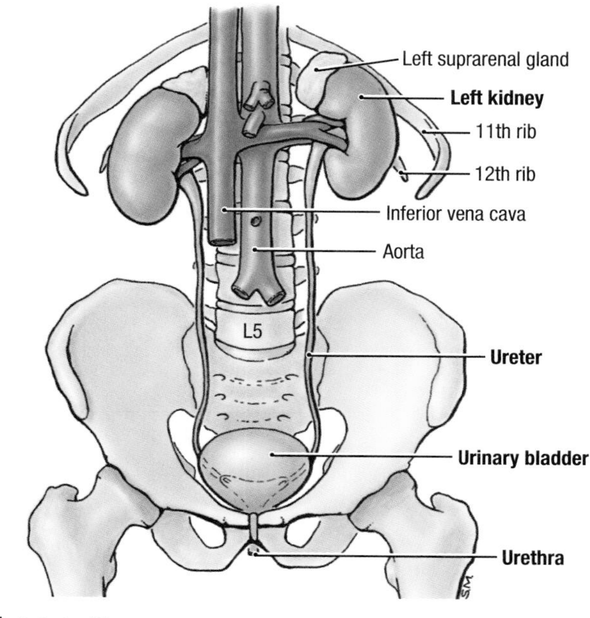
Left suprarenal gland
Left kidney
11th rib
12th rib
Inferior vena cava
Aorta
L5
Ureter
Urinary bladder
Urethra

**A.** Anterior View

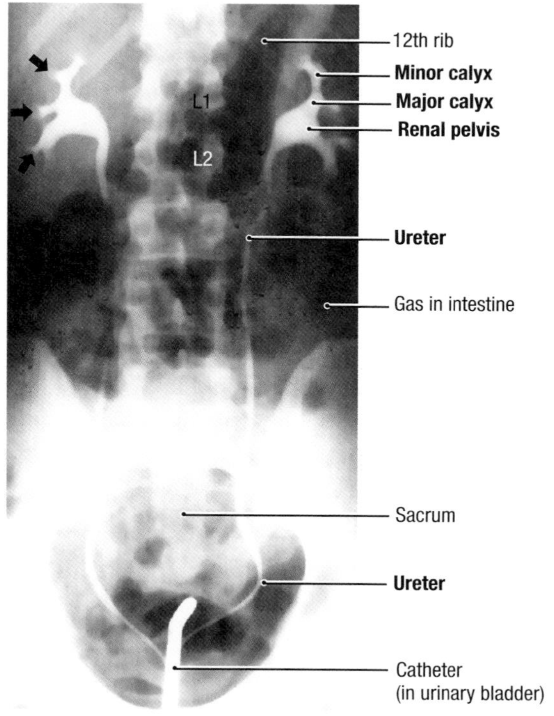
12th rib
Minor calyx
Major calyx
Renal pelvis
L1
L2
Ureter
Gas in intestine
Sacrum
Ureter
Catheter
(in urinary bladder)

**B.** Anteroposterior Pyelogram

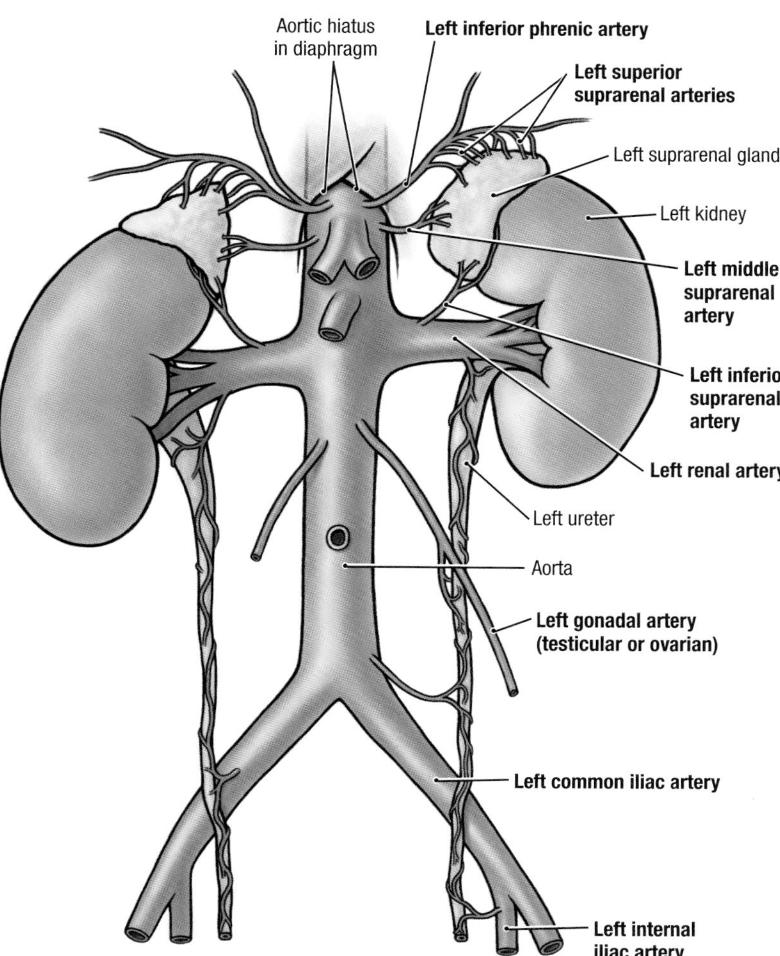
Aortic hiatus
in diaphragm
Left inferior phrenic artery
Left superior
suprarenal arteries
Left suprarenal gland
Left kidney
Left middle
suprarenal
artery
Left inferior
suprarenal
artery
Left renal artery
Left ureter
Aorta
Left gonadal artery
(testicular or ovarian)
Left common iliac artery
Left internal
iliac artery

**C.** Anterior View

## 2.65 Kidneys and suprarenal glands

**A.** Overview of urinary system. **B.** Pyelogram. Radiopaque material occupies the cavities that normally conduct urine. Note the papillae (indicated with arrows) bulging into the minor calices, which empty into a major calyx that opens, in turn, into the renal pelvis drained by the ureter. **C.** Arterial supply of the suprarenal glands, kidneys and ureters.

Renal transplantation is now an established operation for the treatment of selected cases of chronic renal failure. The kidney can be removed from the donor without damaging the suprarenal gland because of the weak septum of renal fascia that separates the kidney from this gland. The site for transplanting a kidney is in the iliac fossa of the greater pelvis. The renal artery and vein are joined to the external iliac artery and vein, respectively, and the ureter is sutured into the urinary bladder.

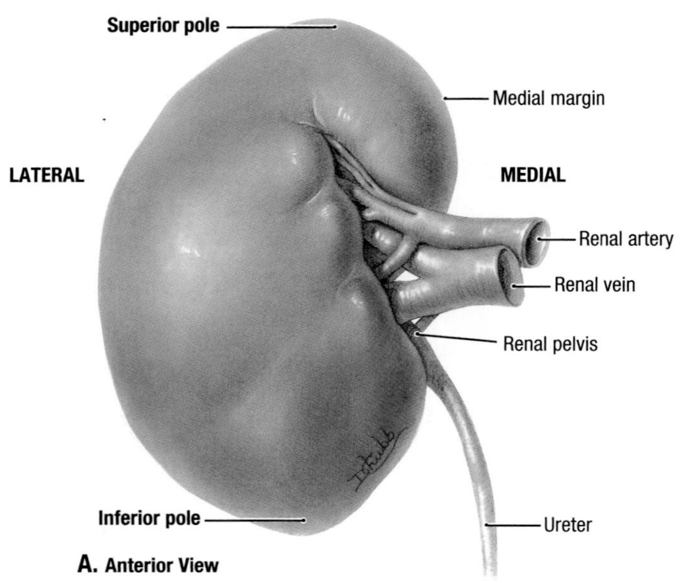
Superior pole
Medial margin
LATERAL
MEDIAL
Renal artery
Renal vein
Renal pelvis
Inferior pole
Ureter
A. Anterior View

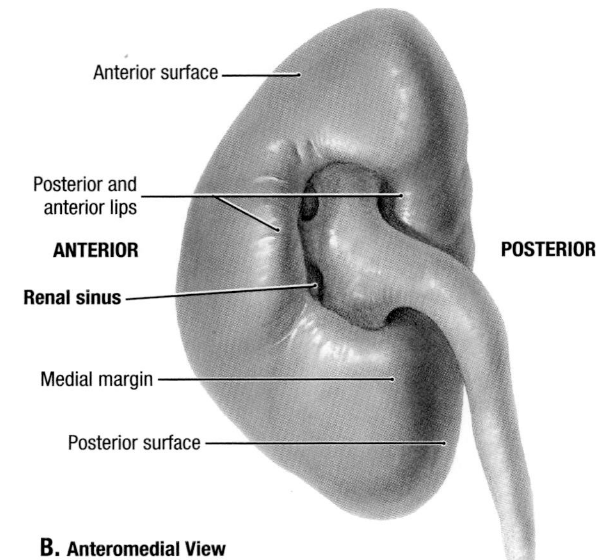
Anterior surface
Posterior and anterior lips
ANTERIOR
POSTERIOR
Renal sinus
Medial margin
Posterior surface
B. Anteromedial View

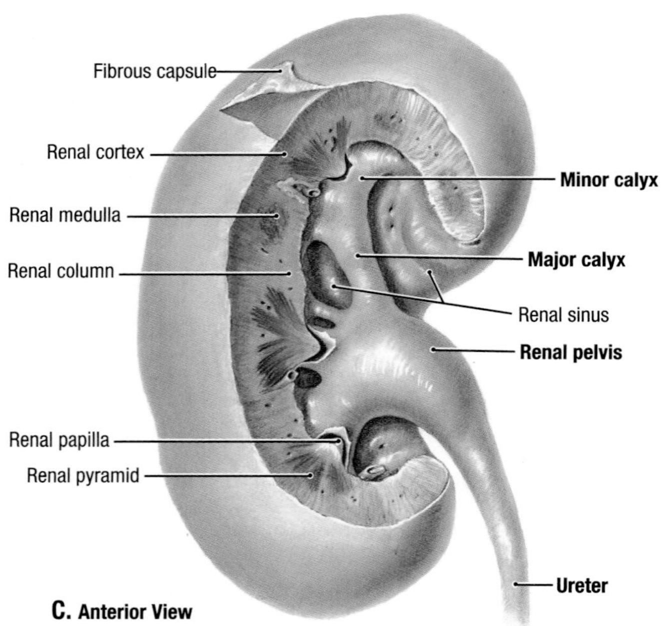
Fibrous capsule
Renal cortex
Renal medulla
Renal column
Minor calyx
Major calyx
Renal sinus
Renal pelvis
Renal papilla
Renal pyramid
Ureter
C. Anterior View

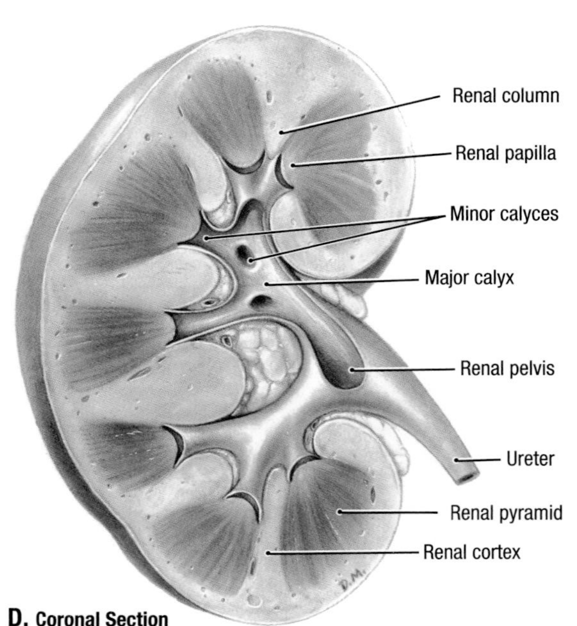
Renal column
Renal papilla
Minor calyces
Major calyx
Renal pelvis
Ureter
Renal pyramid
Renal cortex
D. Coronal Section

## 2.66 Structure of kidney

**A.** External features. The superior pole of the kidney is closer to the median plane than the inferior pole. Approximately 25% of kidneys may have a 2nd, 3rd, and even 4th accessory renal artery branching from the aorta. These multiple vessels enter through the renal sinus or at the superior or inferior pole. **B.** Renal sinus. The renal sinus is a vertical "pocket" opening on the medial side of the kidney. Tucked into the pocket are the renal pelvis and renal vessels in a matrix of perirenal fat. **C.** Renal calices. The anterior wall of the renal sinus has been cut away to expose the renal pelvis and the calices. **D.** Internal features. Cysts in the kidney, multiple or solitary, are common and usually benign findings during ultrasound examinations and dissection of cadavers. Adult polycystic disease of the kidneys, however, is an important cause of renal failure.

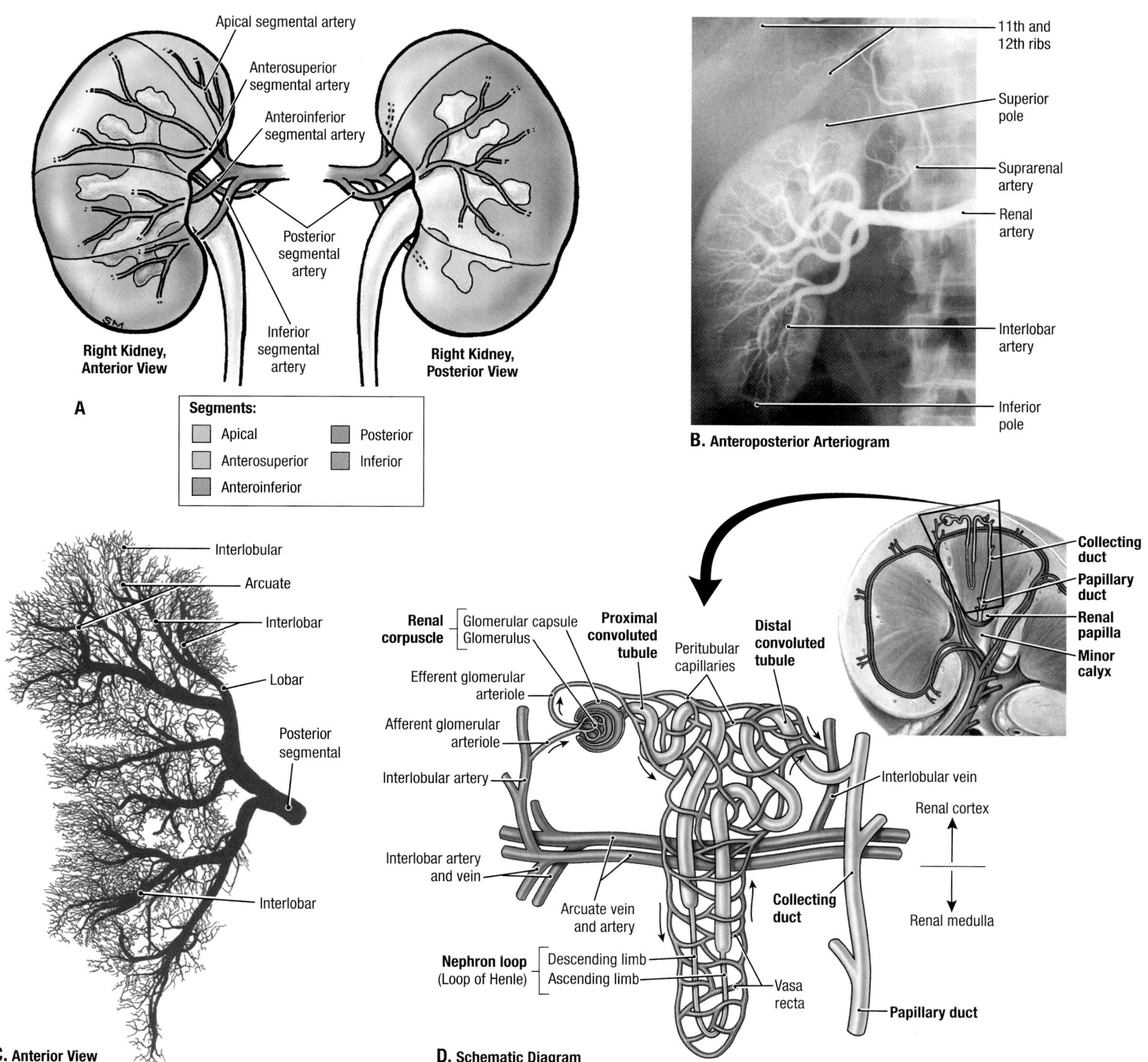
Apical segmental artery
Anterosuperior segmental artery
Anteroinferior segmental artery
Posterior segmental artery
Inferior segmental artery
Right Kidney, Anterior View
Right Kidney, Posterior View
A
Segments:
Apical
Anterosuperior
Anteroinferior
Posterior
Inferior
11th and 12th ribs
Superior pole
Suprarenal artery
Renal artery
Interlobar artery
Inferior pole
B. Anteroposterior Arteriogram
Interlobular
Arcuate
Interlobar
Lobar
Posterior segmental
Interlobar
C. Anterior View
Renal corpuscle
Glomerular capsule
Glomerulus
Proximal convoluted tubule
Peritubular capillaries
Distal convoluted tubule
Efferent glomerular arteriole
Afferent glomerular arteriole
Interlobular artery
Interlobular vein
Renal cortex
Renal medulla
Interlobar artery and vein
Arcuate vein and artery
Collecting duct
Nephron loop (Loop of Henle)
Descending limb
Ascending limb
Vasa recta
Papillary duct
Collecting duct
Papillary duct
Renal papilla
Minor calyx
D. Schematic Diagram

## 2.67 Segments of the kidneys

**A.** Segmental arteries. Segmental arteries do not anastomose significantly with other segmental arteries; they are end arteries. The area supplied by each segmented artery is an independent, surgically respectable unit or renal segment. **B.** Renal arteriogram. **C.** Corrosion cast of posterior segmental artery of kidney. **D.** The nephron is the functional unit of the kidney consisting of a renal corpuscle, proximal tubule, nephron loop and distal tubule. Papillary ducts open onto renal papillae, emptying into minor calices.

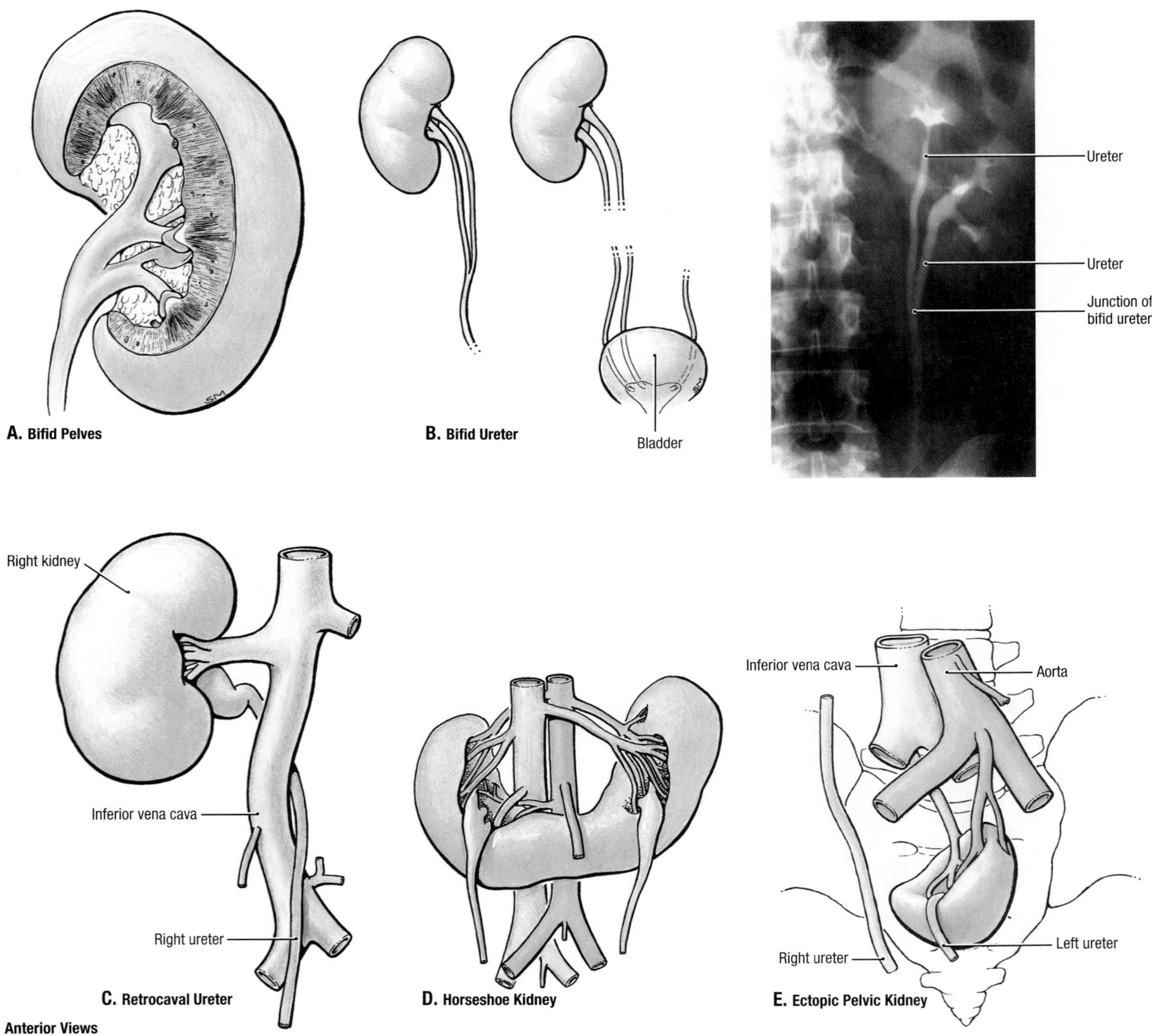
Ureter
Ureter
Junction of bifid ureter
Bladder
A. Bifid Pelves
B. Bifid Ureter
Right kidney
Inferior vena cava
Right ureter
C. Retrocaval Ureter
D. Horseshoe Kidney
Inferior vena cava
Aorta
Left ureter
Right ureter
E. Ectopic Pelvic Kidney
Anterior Views

## 2.68 Anomalies of kidney and ureter

**A.** Bifid pelves. The pelves are almost replaced by two long major calices, which extend outside the sinus. **B.** Duplicated, or bifid, ureters. These can be unilateral or bilateral, and complete or incomplete. **C.** Retrocaval ureter. The ureter courses posterior and then anterior to the inferior vena cava. **D.** Horseshoe kidney. The right and left kidneys are fused in the midline. **E.** Ectopic pelvic kidney. Pelvic kidneys have no fatty capsule and can be unilateral or bilateral. During childbirth, they may cause obstruction and suffer injury.

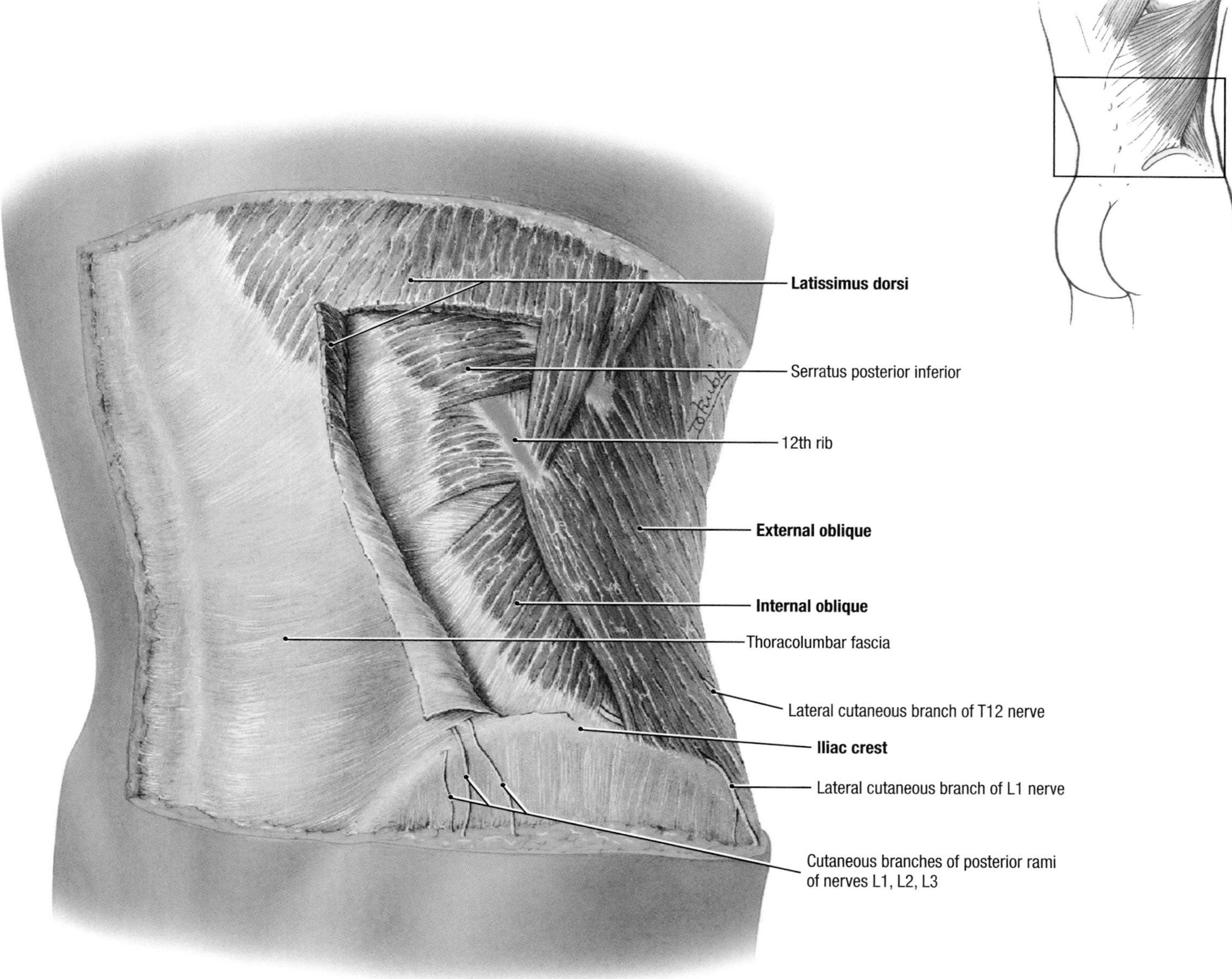
Latissimus dorsi
Serratus posterior inferior
12th rib
External oblique
Internal oblique
Thoracolumbar fascia
Lateral cutaneous branch of T12 nerve
Iliac crest
Lateral cutaneous branch of L1 nerve
Cutaneous branches of posterior rami of nerves L1, L2, L3
Posterolateral View

## 2.69 Exposure of kidney

The latissimus dorsi is partially reflected.

- The external oblique muscle has an oblique, free posterior border that extends from the tip of the 12th rib to the midpoint of the iliac crest.
- The internal oblique muscle extends posteriorly beyond the border of the external oblique muscle.

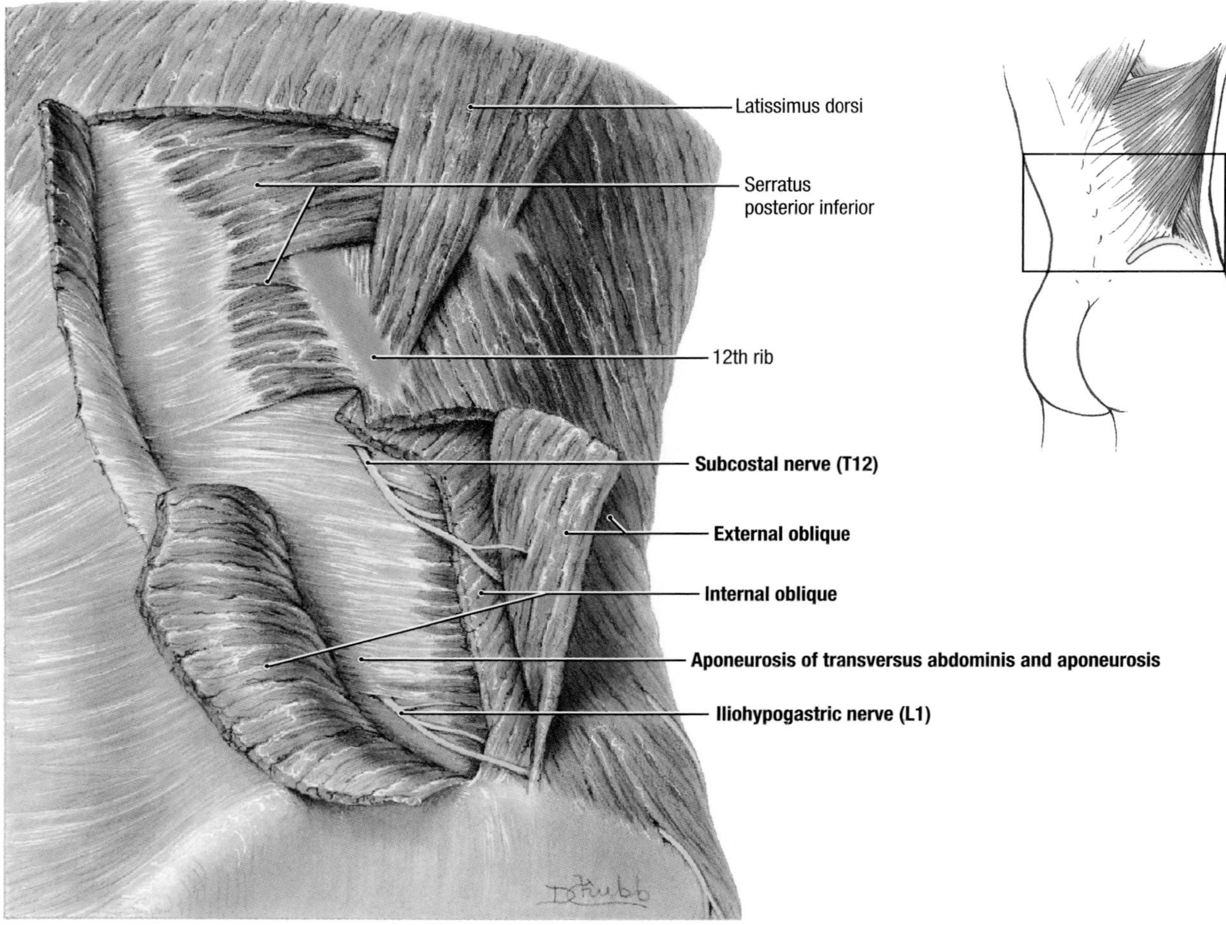
Latissimus dorsi
Serratus posterior inferior
12th rib
Subcostal nerve (T12)
External oblique
Internal oblique
Aponeurosis of transversus abdominis and aponeurosis
Iliohypogastric nerve (L1)
Posterolateral View

## 2.70 Exposure of kidney—II

The external oblique muscle is incised and reflected laterally, and the internal oblique muscle is incised and reflected medially; the transversus abdominis muscle and its posterior aponeurosis are exposed where pierced by the subcostal (T12) and iliohypogastric (L1) nerves. These nerves give off motor twigs and lateral cutaneous branches and continue anteriorly between the internal oblique and transversus abdominis muscles.

## 2.71 Exposure of kidney—III and renal fascia

**A.** Dissection. The posterior aponeurosis of the transversus abdominis muscle is divided between the subcostal and iliohypogastric nerves and lateral to the oblique lateral border of the quadratus lumborum muscle; the retroperitoneal fat surrounding the kidney is exposed. **B.** Renal fascia and retroperitoneal fat, schematic transverse section. The renal fascia is within this fat; the portion of fat internal to the renal fascia is termed perinephric fat (perirenal fat capsule), and the fat immediately external is paranephric fat (pararenal fat body).

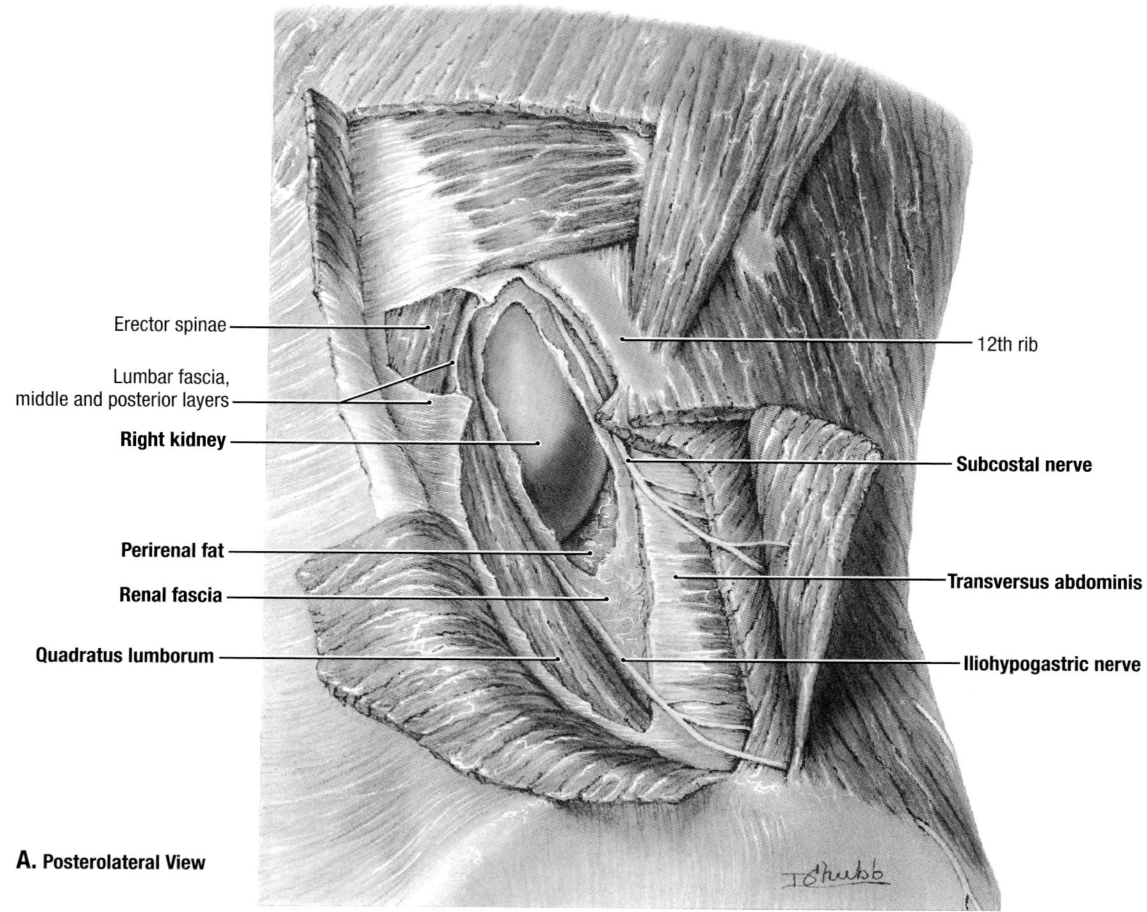
Erector spinae
Lumbar fascia, middle and posterior layers
Right kidney
Perirenal fat
Renal fascia
Quadratus lumborum
12th rib
Subcostal nerve
Transversus abdominis
Iliohypogastric nerve

**A.** **Posterolateral View**

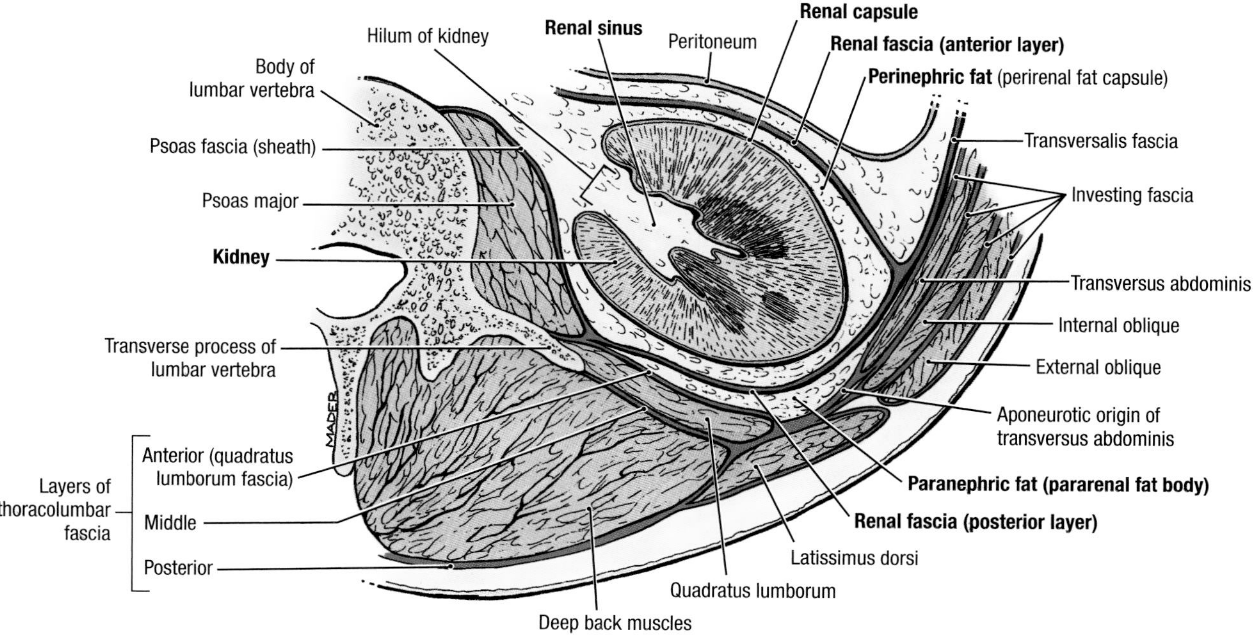
Hilum of kidney
Renal sinus
Peritoneum
Renal capsule
Renal fascia (anterior layer)
Perinephric fat (perirenal fat capsule)
Body of lumbar vertebra
Psoas fascia (sheath)
Psoas major
Kidney
Transverse process of lumbar vertebra
Transversalis fascia
Investing fascia
Transversus abdominis
Internal oblique
External oblique
Aponeurotic origin of transversus abdominis
Paranephric fat (pararenal fat body)
Renal fascia (posterior layer)
Latissimus dorsi
Quadratus lumborum
Deep back muscles
Layers of thoracolumbar fascia
Anterior (quadratus lumborum fascia)
Middle
Posterior
MADER

**B.** **Transverse Section**

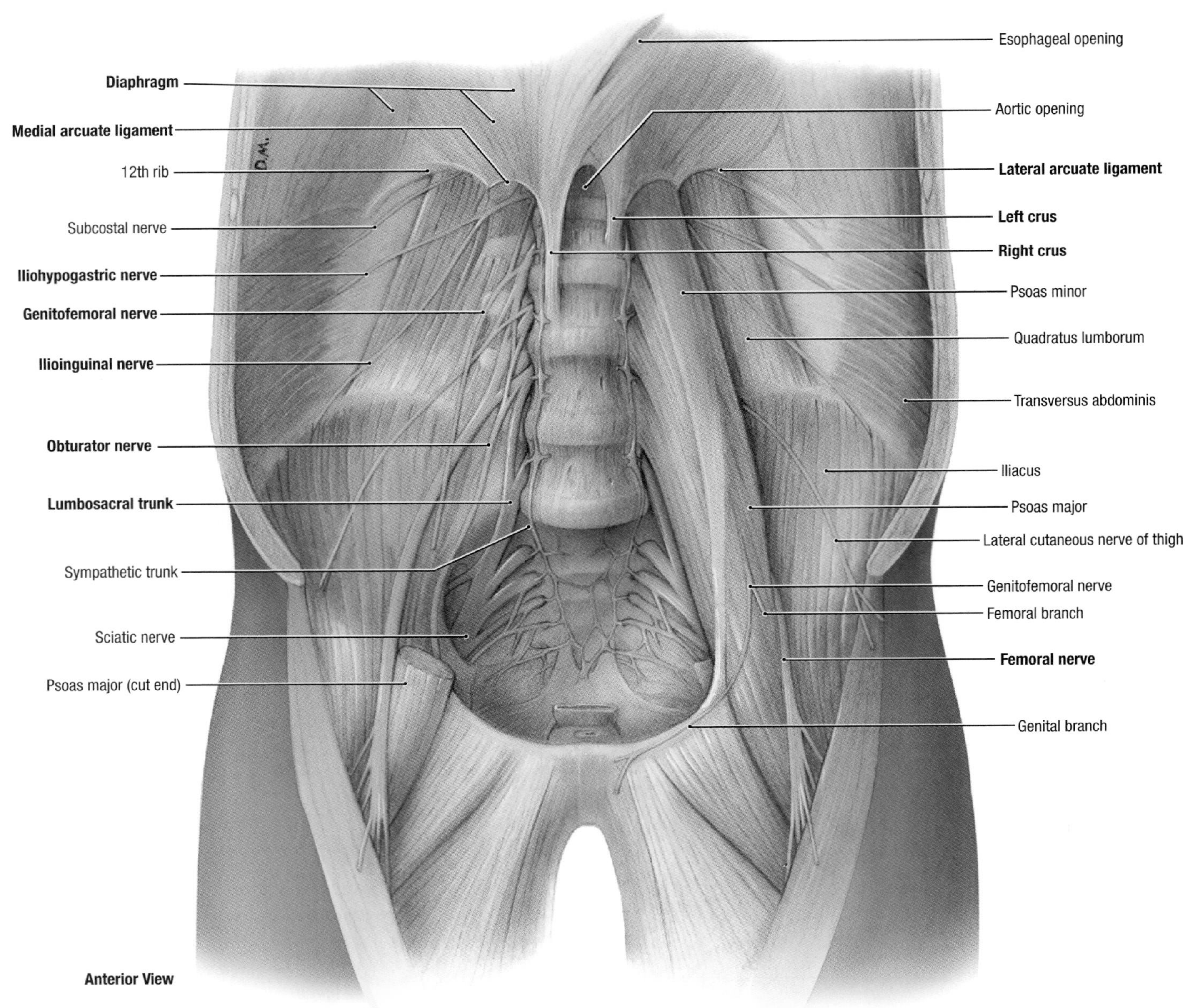
Esophageal opening
Diaphragm
Aortic opening
Medial arcuate ligament
12th rib
Lateral arcuate ligament
Subcostal nerve
Left crus
Right crus
Iliohypogastric nerve
Psoas minor
Genitofemoral nerve
Quadratus lumborum
Ilioinguinal nerve
Transversus abdominis
Obturator nerve
Iliacus
Lumbosacral trunk
Psoas major
Lateral cutaneous nerve of thigh
Sympathetic trunk
Genitofemoral nerve
Femoral branch
Sciatic nerve
Femoral nerve
Psoas major (cut end)
Genital branch
Anterior View

**2.72 Lumbar plexus and vertebral attachment of diaphragm**

**TABLE 2.5 PRINCIPAL MUSCLES OF POSTERIOR ABDOMINAL WALL**

| Muscle | Superior Attachments | Inferior Attachments | Innervation | Actions |
|---|---|---|---|---|
| **Psoas major,**[a b] | Transverse processes of lumbar vertebrae; sides of bodies of T12–L5 vertebrae and intervening invertebral discs | By a strong tendon to lesser trochanter of femur | Anterior rami of lumbar nerves (**L1, L2,** L3) | Acting inferiorly with iliacus, it flexes thigh at hip; acting superiorly, it flexes vertebral column laterally; it is used to balance the trunk; during sitting it acts inferiorly with iliacus to flex trunk |
| **Iliacus**[a] | Superior two thirds of iliac fossa, ala of sacrum; and anterior sacroiliac ligaments | Lesser trochanter of femur and shaft inferior to it, and to psoas major tendon | Femoral nerve (**L2,** L3) | Flexes thigh and stabilizes hip joint; acts with psoas major |
| **Quadratus lumborum** | Medial half of inferior border of 12th rib and tips of lumbar transverse processes | Iliolumbar ligament and internal lip of iliac crest | Anterior rami of T12 and L1-L4 nerves | Extends and laterally flexes vertebral column; fixes 12th rib during inspiration |

[a] Psoas major and iliacus muscles are often described together as the iliopsoas muscle when flexion of the thigh is discussed.

[b] Psoas minor attaches proximally to the sides of bodies of T12–L1 vertebrae and intervertebral disc and distally to the pectineal line and iliopectineal eminence via the iliopectineal arch; it does not cross the hip joint. It is used to balance the trunk, in conjunction with psoas major. Innervation is from the anterior rami of lumbar nerves (L1, L2).

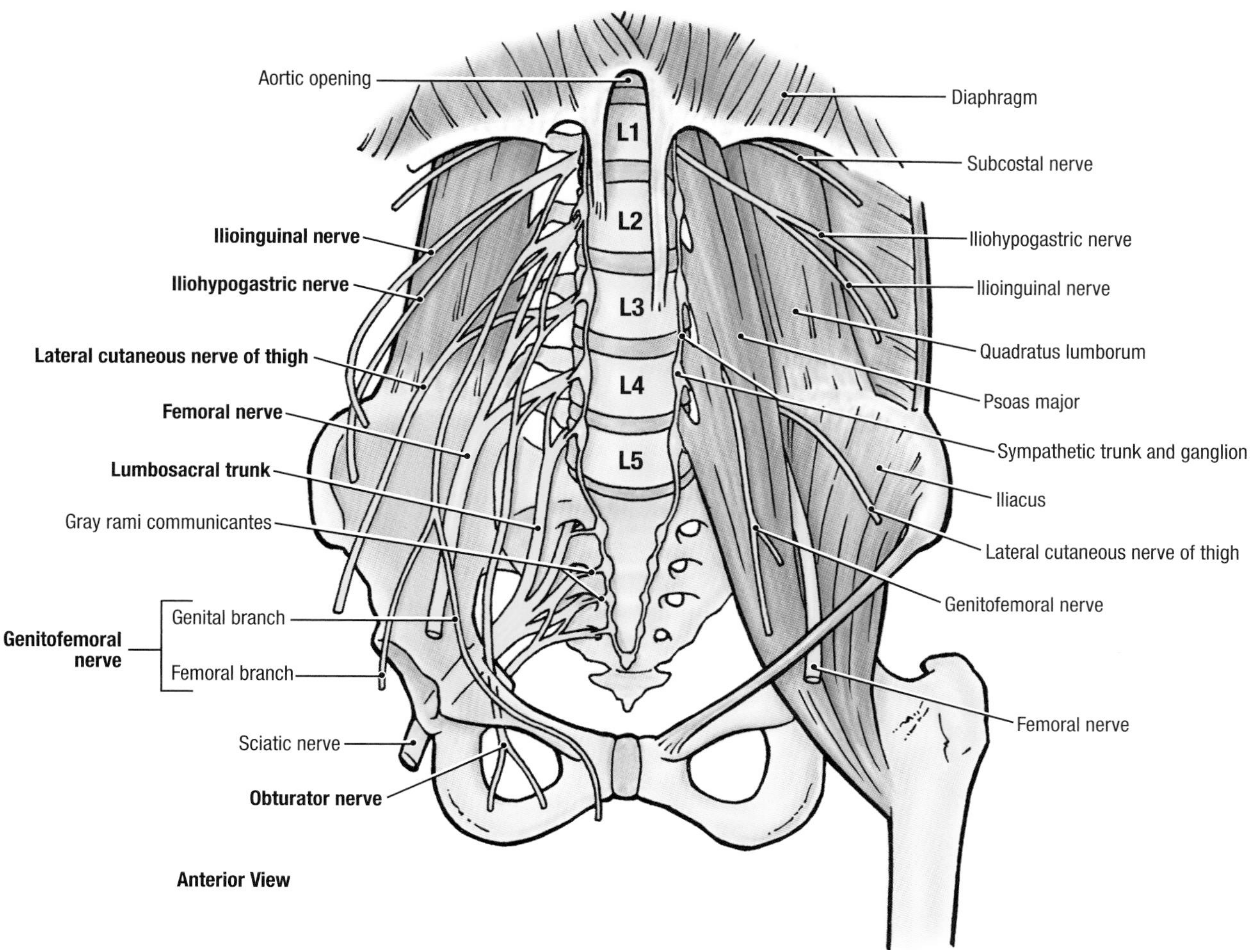
Aortic opening
Diaphragm
L1
L2
L3
L4
L5
Subcostal nerve
Ilioinguinal nerve
Iliohypogastric nerve
Iliohypogastric nerve
Ilioinguinal nerve
Quadratus lumborum
Lateral cutaneous nerve of thigh
Psoas major
Femoral nerve
Sympathetic trunk and ganglion
Lumbosacral trunk
Iliacus
Gray rami communicantes
Lateral cutaneous nerve of thigh
Genitofemoral nerve
Genital branch
Genitofemoral nerve
Femoral branch
Femoral nerve
Sciatic nerve
Obturator nerve
Anterior View

## 2.73 Nerves of the lumbar plexus

The lumbar plexus of nerves is in the posterior part of the psoas major, anterior to the lumbar transverse processes. This nerve network is composed of the anterior rami of L1-L4 nerves. All rami receive gray rami communicates from the sympathetic trunks. The following nerves are branches of the lumbar plexus:

- Ilioinguinal and iliohypogastric nerves (L1) arise from the anterior ramus of L1 and enter the abdomen posterior to the medial arcuate ligaments and pass inferolaterally, anterior to the quadratus lumborum muscle; they pierce the transversus abdominis muscle near the anterior superior iliac spine and pass through the internal and external oblique muscles to supply the skin of the suprapubic and inguinal regions.
- Lateral cutaneous nerve of thigh (L2, L3) runs inferolaterally on the iliacus muscle and enters the thigh posterior to the inguinal ligament, just medial to the anterior superior iliac spine; it supplies the skin on the anterolateral surface of the thigh.
- Femoral nerve (L2-L4) emerges from the lateral border of the psoas and innervates the iliacus muscle and the extensor muscles of the knee.
- Genitofemoral nerve (L1, L2) pierces the anterior surface of the psoas major muscle and runs inferiorly on it deep to the psoas fascia; it divides lateral to the common and external iliac arteries into femoral and genital branches.
- Obturator nerve (L2-L4) emerges from the medial border of the psoas to supply the adductor muscles of the thigh.
- Lumbosacral trunk (L4, L5) passes over the ala (wing) of the sacrum and descends into the pelvis to take part in the formation of the sacral plexus along with the anterior rami of S1-S4 nerves.

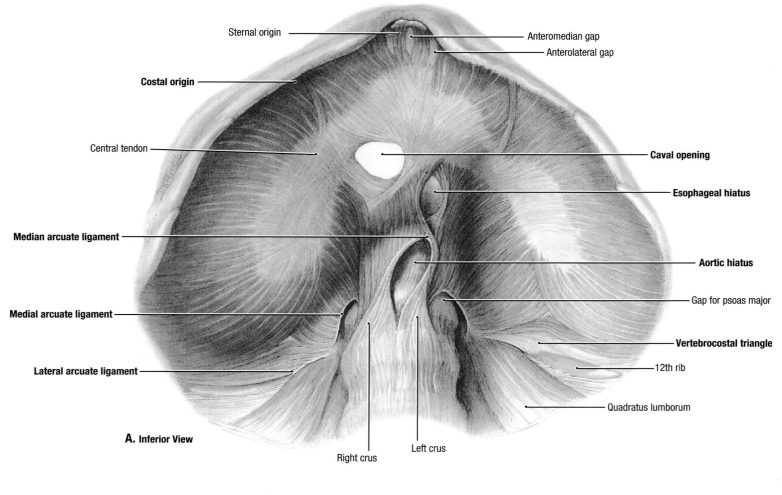

Sternal origin
Anteromedian gap
Anterolateral gap
Costal origin
Central tendon
Caval opening
Esophageal hiatus
Median arcuate ligament
Aortic hiatus
Gap for psoas major
Medial arcuate ligament
Vertebrocostal triangle
Lateral arcuate ligament
12th rib
Quadratus lumborum
A. Inferior View
Right crus
Left crus

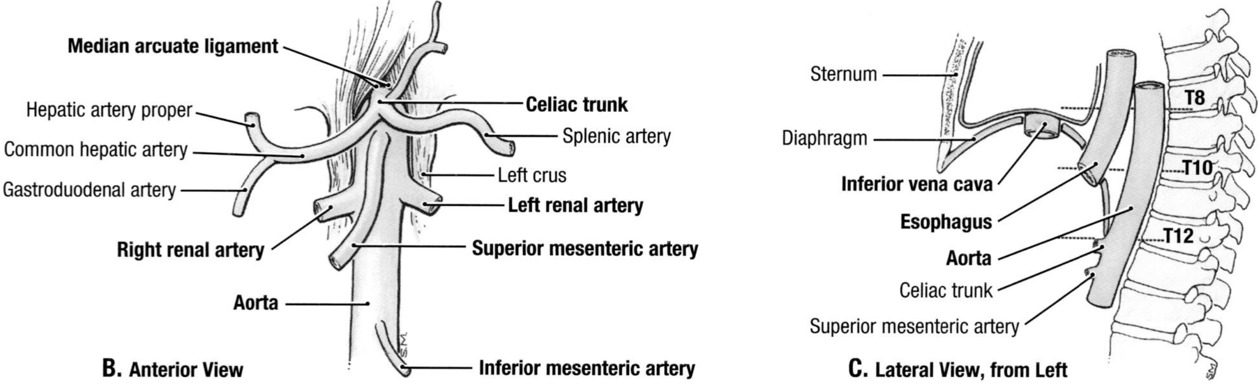
Median arcuate ligament
Hepatic artery proper
Celiac trunk
Splenic artery
Common hepatic artery
Left crus
Gastroduodenal artery
Left renal artery
Right renal artery
Superior mesenteric artery
Aorta
Inferior mesenteric artery
B. Anterior View
Sternum
T8
Diaphragm
T10
Inferior vena cava
Esophagus
T12
Aorta
Celiac trunk
Superior mesenteric artery
C. Lateral View, from Left

## 2.74 Diaphragm

**A.** Dissection. The clover-shaped central tendon is the aponeurotic insertion of the muscle. The diaphragm in this specimen fails to arise from the left lateral arcuate ligament, leaving a potential opening, the vertebrocostal triangle, through which abdominal contents may be herniated into the thoracic cavity. **B.** Median arcuate ligament and branches of the aorta. **C.** Openings of the diaphragm. There are three major openings through which major structures pass from the thorax into the abdomen: the caval opening for the inferior vena cava, most anterior, at the T8 vertebral level to the right of the midline; the esophageal hiatus, intermediate, at T10 level and to the left; and the aortic hiatus, which allows the aorta to pass posterior to the vertebral attachment of the diaphragm in the midline at T12.

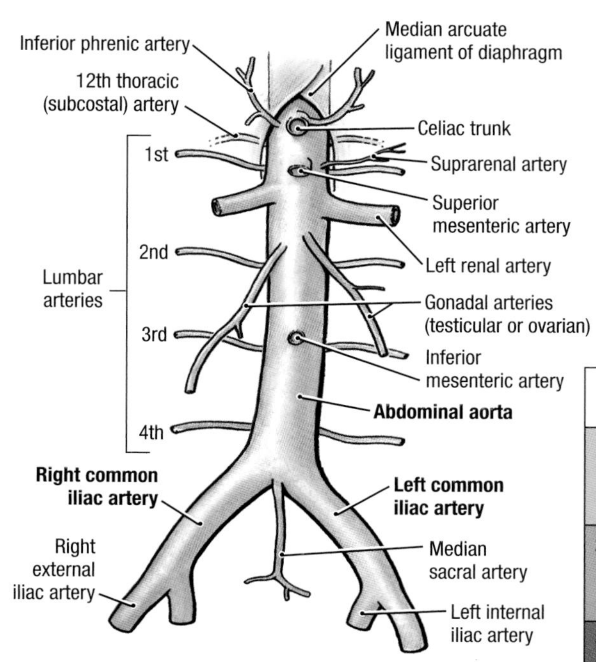
Inferior phrenic artery
12th thoracic (subcostal) artery
Median arcuate ligament of diaphragm
Celiac trunk
Suprarenal artery
Superior mesenteric artery
Left renal artery
Gonadal arteries (testicular or ovarian)
Inferior mesenteric artery
Abdominal aorta
1st
2nd
3rd
4th
Lumbar arteries
Right common iliac artery
Left common iliac artery
Median sacral artery
Right external iliac artery
Left internal iliac artery

A. Anterior View

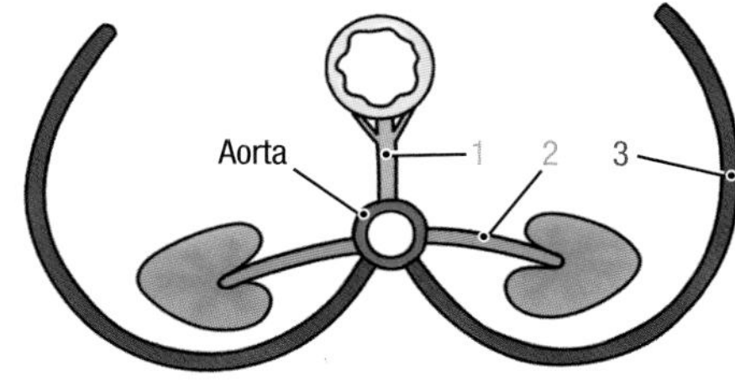
Aorta
1
2
3

Three Vascular Planes

| | Vascular plane | Class | Distribution | Abdominal Branches (Arteries) | Vertebral Level |
|---|---|---|---|---|---|
| 1 | Anterior midline | Unpaired visceral | Alimentary tract | Celiac | T12 |
| | | | | Superior mesenteric (SMA) | L1 |
| | | | | Inferior mesenteric (IMA) | L3 |
| 2 | Lateral | Paired visceral | Urogenital and endocrine organs | Suprarenal | L1 |
| | | | | Renal | L1 |
| | | | | Gonadal (testicular or ovarian) | L2 |
| 3 | Postero-lateral | Paired parietal (segmental) | Diaphragm Body Wall | Subcostal | T12 |
| | | | | Inferior phrenic | T12 |
| | | | | Lumbar | L1–L4 |

Right
Intermediate (middle)
Left
Hepatic veins
Azygos vein
Right inferior phrenic vein
Hemiazygos vein
Left inferior phrenic vein
Inferior vena cava
Right suprarenal vein
Right renal vein
Posterior intercostal veins
1st
2nd
3rd
4th
5th
Lumbar veins
Left renal vein
Left gonadal vein (testicular or ovarian)
Right gonadal vein (testicular or ovarian)
Ascending lumbar vein
Left common iliac vein
Left external iliac vein
Left internal iliac vein
Median sacral vein
Right common iliac vein

B. Anterior View

## 2.75 Abdominal aorta and inferior vena cava and their branches

**A.** Branches of abdominal aorta. **B.** Tributaries of the inferior vena cava (IVC). The asymmetry in the renal and common iliac veins reflects the placement of the IVC to the right of the midline.

Rupture of an aneurysm (localized enlargement) of the abdominal aorta causes severe pain in the abdomen or back. If unrecognized, a ruptured aneurysm has a mortality of nearly 90% because of heavy blood loss. Surgeons can repair an aneurysm by opening it, inserting a prosthetic graft (such as one made of Dacron), and sewing the wall of the aneurysmal aorta over the graft to protect it. Aneurysms may also be treated by endovascular catheterization procedures.

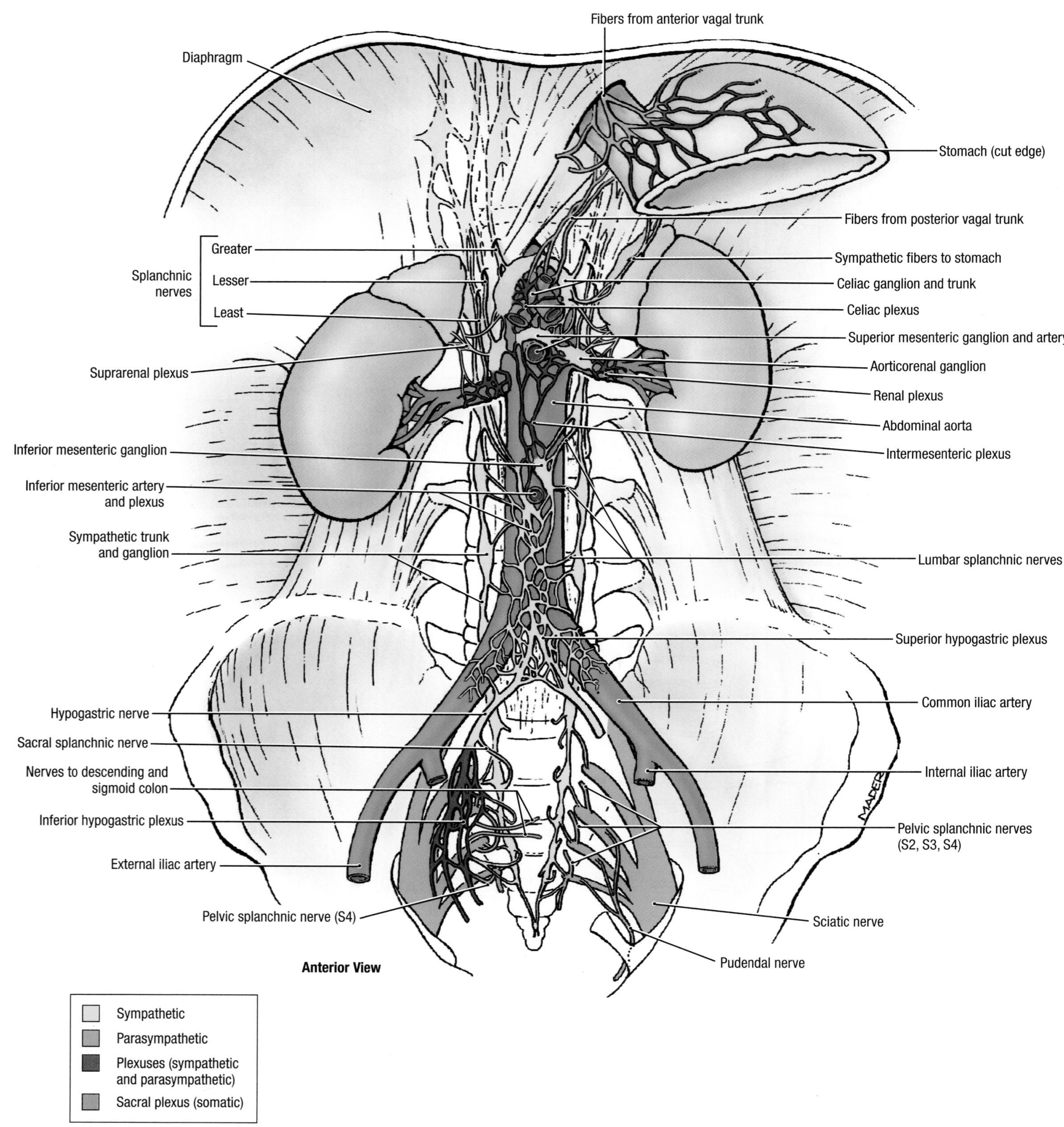
Fibers from anterior vagal trunk
Diaphragm
Stomach (cut edge)
Fibers from posterior vagal trunk
Splanchnic nerves
Greater
Lesser
Least
Sympathetic fibers to stomach
Celiac ganglion and trunk
Celiac plexus
Superior mesenteric ganglion and artery
Suprarenal plexus
Aorticorenal ganglion
Renal plexus
Abdominal aorta
Intermesenteric plexus
Inferior mesenteric ganglion
Inferior mesenteric artery and plexus
Sympathetic trunk and ganglion
Lumbar splanchnic nerves
Superior hypogastric plexus
Common iliac artery
Hypogastric nerve
Sacral splanchnic nerve
Internal iliac artery
Nerves to descending and sigmoid colon
Inferior hypogastric plexus
Pelvic splanchnic nerves (S2, S3, S4)
External iliac artery
MADER
Pelvic splanchnic nerve (S4)
Sciatic nerve
Pudendal nerve
Anterior View
Sympathetic
Parasympathetic
Plexuses (sympathetic and parasympathetic)
Sacral plexus (somatic)

**2.76 Abdominopelvic nerve plexuses and ganglia**

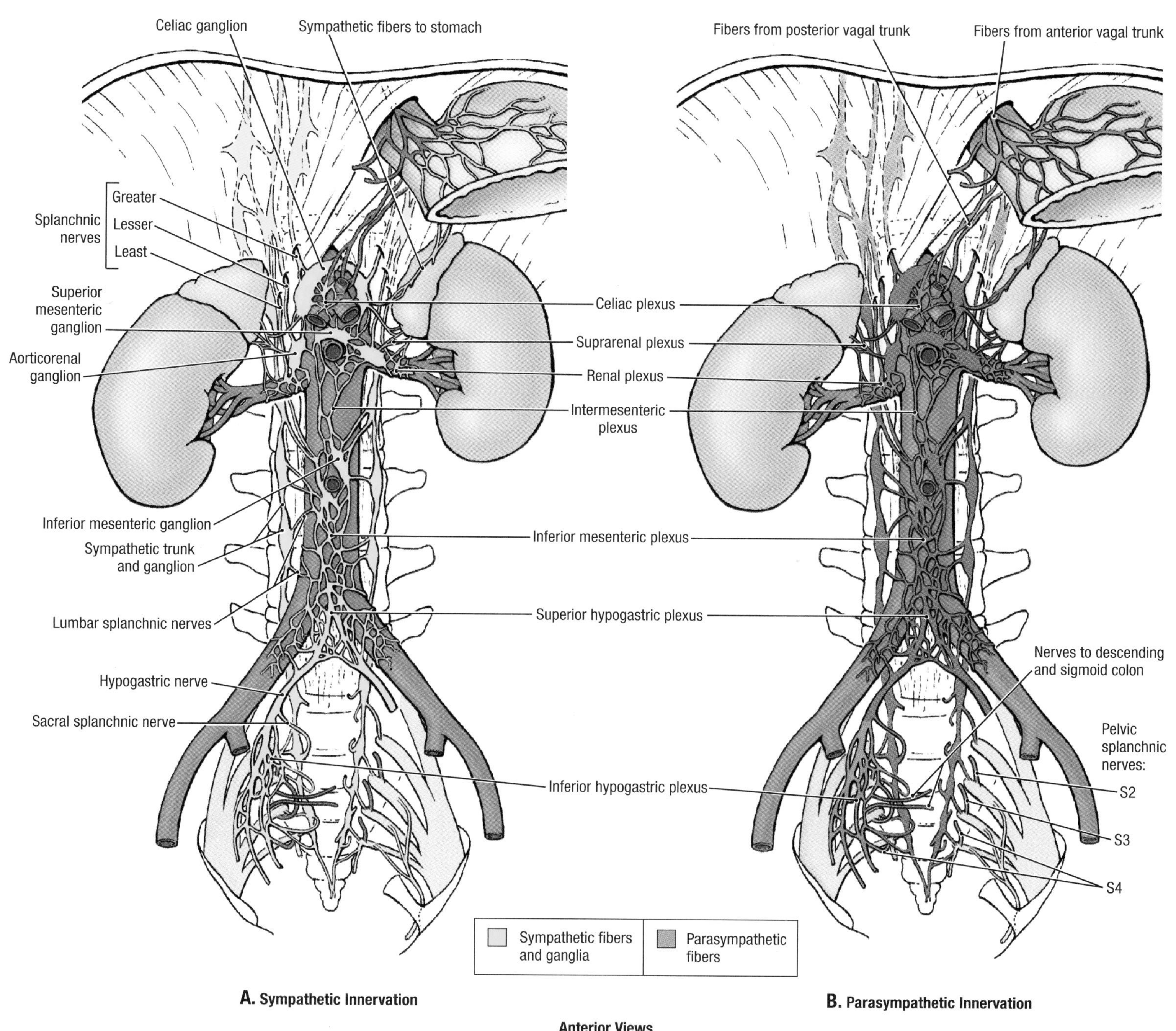
Celiac ganglion
Sympathetic fibers to stomach
Splanchnic nerves
Greater
Lesser
Least
Superior mesenteric ganglion
Aorticorenal ganglion
Inferior mesenteric ganglion
Sympathetic trunk and ganglion
Lumbar splanchnic nerves
Hypogastric nerve
Sacral splanchnic nerve
Celiac plexus
Suprarenal plexus
Renal plexus
Intermesenteric plexus
Inferior mesenteric plexus
Superior hypogastric plexus
Inferior hypogastric plexus
Fibers from posterior vagal trunk
Fibers from anterior vagal trunk
Nerves to descending and sigmoid colon
Pelvic splanchnic nerves:
S2
S3
S4
Sympathetic fibers and ganglia
Parasympathetic fibers
A. Sympathetic Innervation
B. Parasympathetic Innervation
Anterior Views

**2.77 Overview of autonomic nervous system**

**A.** Sympathetic. **B.** Parasympathetic.

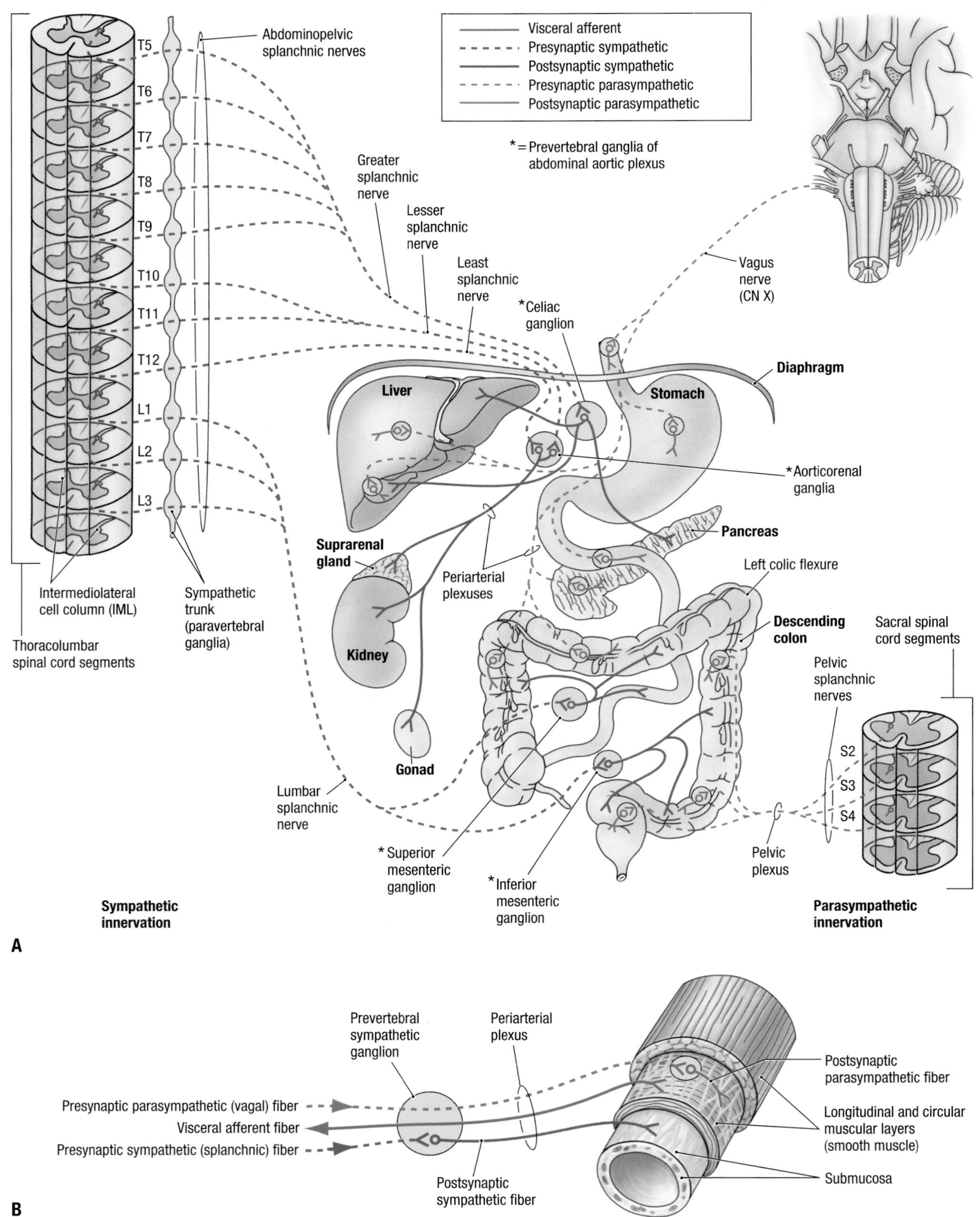

Visceral afferent
Presynaptic sympathetic
Postsynaptic sympathetic
Presynaptic parasympathetic
Postsynaptic parasympathetic
*= Prevertebral ganglia of abdominal aortic plexus
T5
T6
T7
T8
T9
T10
T11
T12
L1
L2
L3
Abdominopelvic splanchnic nerves
Greater splanchnic nerve
Lesser splanchnic nerve
Least splanchnic nerve
*Celiac ganglion
Vagus nerve (CN X)
Diaphragm
Liver
Stomach
*Aorticorenal ganglia
Pancreas
Suprarenal gland
Periarterial plexuses
Left colic flexure
Descending colon
Sacral spinal cord segments
Pelvic splanchnic nerves
Kidney
Intermediolateral cell column (IML)
Sympathetic trunk (paravertebral ganglia)
Thoracolumbar spinal cord segments
Gonad
S2
S3
S4
Lumbar splanchnic nerve
*Superior mesenteric ganglion
*Inferior mesenteric ganglion
Pelvic plexus
Sympathetic innervation
Parasympathetic innervation
A
Prevertebral sympathetic ganglion
Periarterial plexus
Presynaptic parasympathetic (vagal) fiber
Visceral afferent fiber
Presynaptic sympathetic (splanchnic) fiber
Postsynaptic sympathetic fiber
Postsynaptic parasympathetic fiber
Longitudinal and circular muscular layers (smooth muscle)
Submucosa
B


**2.78 Origin and distribution of presynaptic and postsynaptic sympathetic and parasympathetic fibers, and the ganglia involved in supplying abdominal viscera**

**A.** Overview. **B.** Fibers supplying the intrinsic plexuses of abdominal viscera.

**TABLE 2.6 AUTONOMIC INNERVATION OF THE ABDOMINAL VISCERA (SPLANCHNIC NERVES)**

| Splanchnic Nerves | Autonomic Fiber Type[a] | System | Origin | Destination |
|---|---|---|---|---|
| A. **Cardiopulmonary** (Cervical and upper thoracic) | Postsynaptic | Sympathetic | Cervical and upper thoracic sympathetic trunk | Thoracic cavity (viscera superior to level of diaphragm) |
| B. **Abdominopelvic**<br>1. Lower thoracic<br>a. Greater<br>b. Lesser<br>c. Least<br>2. Lumbar<br>3. Sacral | Presynaptic | Sympathetic | Lower thoracic and abdominopelvic sympathetic trunk:<br>1. Thoracic sympathetic trunk:<br>a. T5–T9 or T10 level<br>b. T10–T11 level<br>c. T12 level<br>2. Abdominal sympathetic trunk<br>3. Pelvic (sacral) sympathetic trunk | Abdominopelvic cavity (prevertebral ganglia serving viscera and suprarenal glands inferior to level of diaphragm)<br>1. Abdominal prevertebral ganglia:<br>a. Celiac ganglia<br>b. Aorticorenal ganglia<br>c. & 2. Other abdominal prevertebral ganglia (superior and inferior mesenteric, and of inter-mesenteric/hypogastric plexuses<br>3. Pelvic prevertebral ganglia |
| C. **Pelvic** | Presynaptic | Parasympathetic | Anterior rami of S2–S4 spinal nerves | Intrinsic ganglia of descending and sigmoid colon, rectum, and pelvic viscera |

[a]Splanchnic nerves also convey visceral afferent fibers, which are not part of the autonomic nervous system.

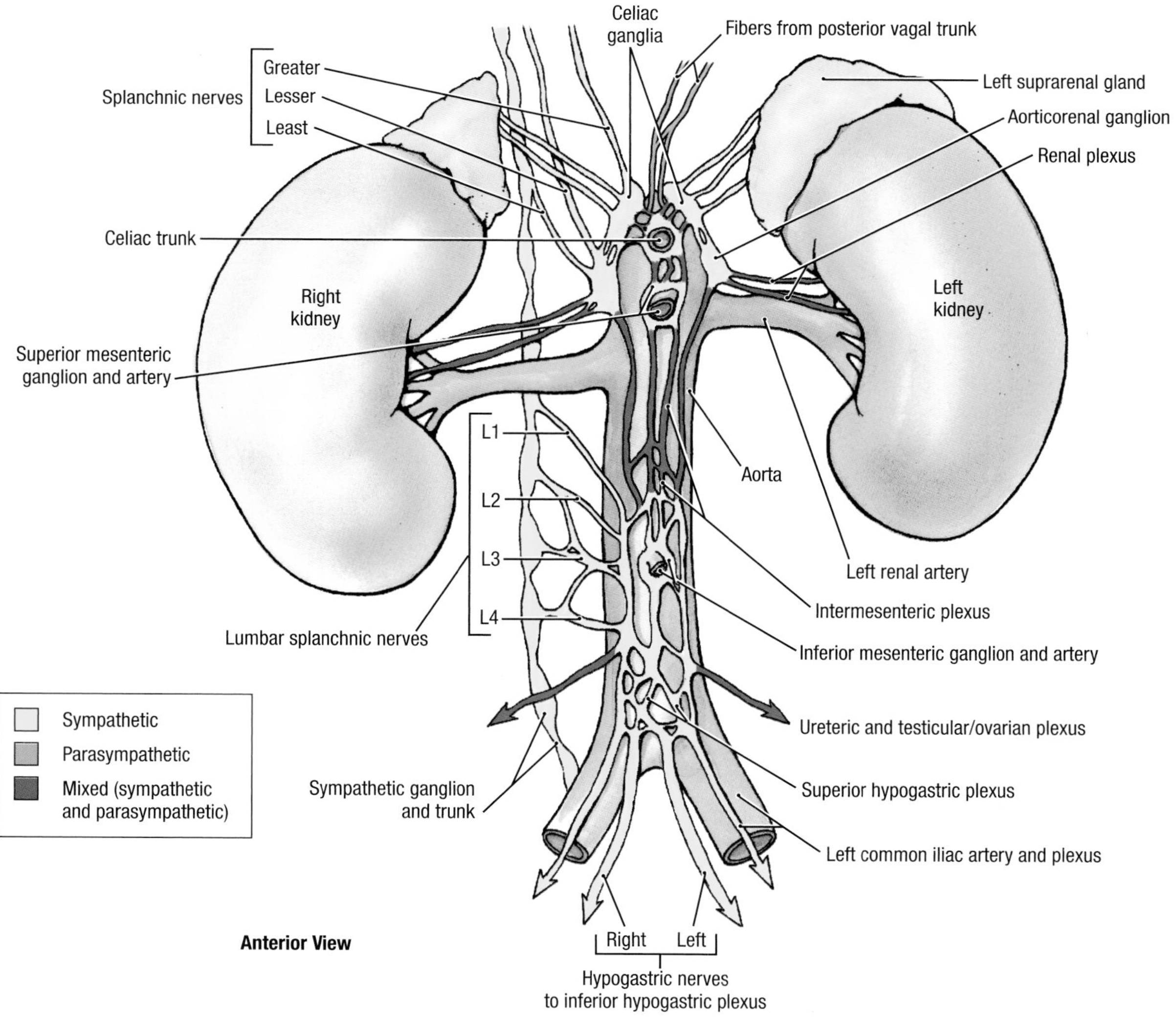
Celiac ganglia
Fibers from posterior vagal trunk
Splanchnic nerves
Greater
Lesser
Least
Left suprarenal gland
Aorticorenal ganglion
Renal plexus
Celiac trunk
Right kidney
Left kidney
Superior mesenteric ganglion and artery
L1
L2
L3
L4
Aorta
Left renal artery
Intermesenteric plexus
Inferior mesenteric ganglion and artery
Lumbar splanchnic nerves
Sympathetic
Parasympathetic
Mixed (sympathetic and parasympathetic)
Ureteric and testicular/ovarian plexus
Sympathetic ganglion and trunk
Superior hypogastric plexus
Left common iliac artery and plexus
Anterior View
Right
Left
Hypogastric nerves to inferior hypogastric plexus

**2.79 Abdominal nerve plexuses and ganglia**

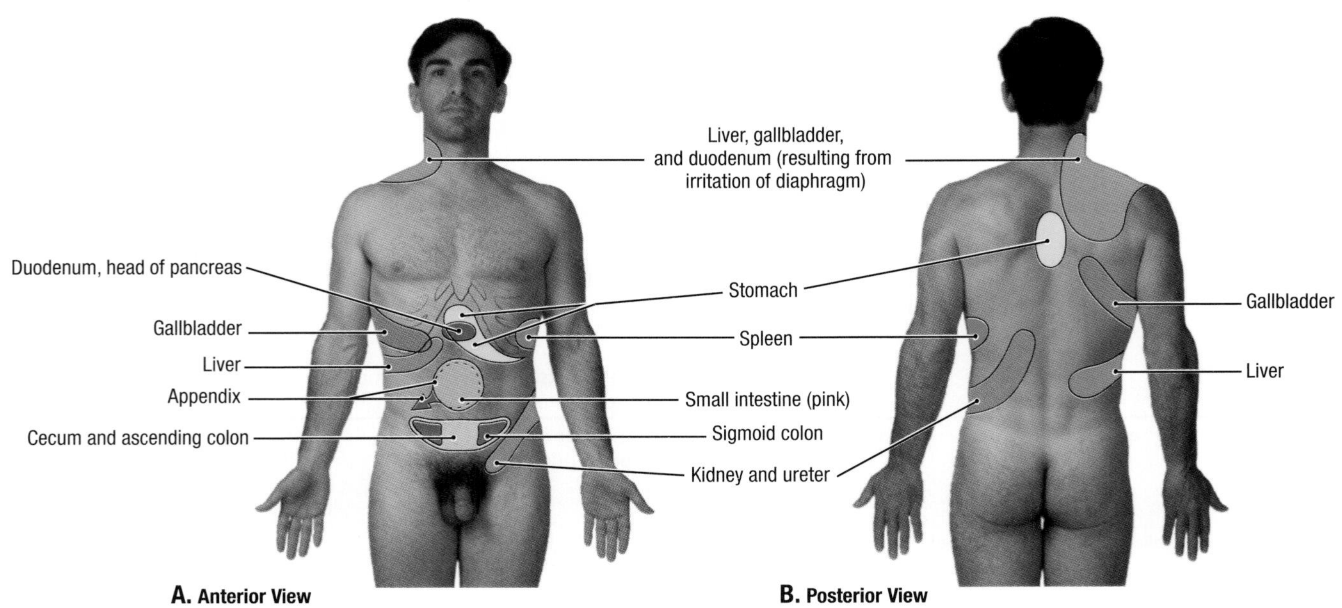
Liver, gallbladder, and duodenum (resulting from irritation of diaphragm)
Duodenum, head of pancreas
Gallbladder
Liver
Appendix
Cecum and ascending colon
Stomach
Spleen
Small intestine (pink)
Sigmoid colon
Kidney and ureter
Gallbladder
Liver
A. Anterior View
B. Posterior View

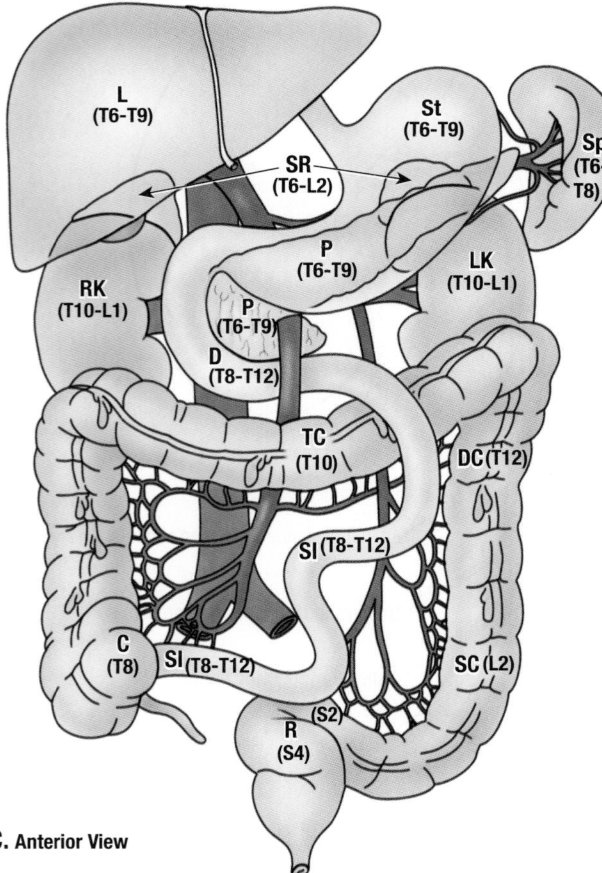
L (T6-T9)
St (T6-T9)
Sp (T6-T8)
SR (T6-L2)
P (T6-T9)
RK (T10-L1)
LK (T10-L1)
P (T6-T9)
D (T8-T12)
TC (T10)
DC (T12)
SI (T8-T12)
C (T8)
SI (T8-T12)
SC (L2)
(S2)
R (S4)

C. Anterior View

| | | | |
|---|---|---|---|
| C | Cecum | RK | Right kidney |
| D | Duodenum | SC | Sigmoid colon |
| DC | Descending colon | SI | Small intestine |
| L | Liver | Sp | Spleen |
| LK | Left kidney | SR | Suprarenal glands |
| P | Pancreas | St | Stomach |
| R | Rectum | TC | Transverse colon |

## 2.80 Surface projections of visceral pain

**A.** and **B.** Pain arising from a viscus (organ) varies from dull to severe but is poorly localized. It radiates to the part of the body supplied by somatic sensory fibers associated with the same spinal ganglion and segment of the spinal cord that receive visceral sensory (autonomic) fibers from the viscus concerned. The pain is interpreted by the brain as though the irritation occurred in the area of skin supplied by the posterior roots of the affected segments. This is called visceral referred pain. **C.** Approximate spinal cord segments and spinal sensory ganglia involved in sympathetic and visceral afferent (pain) innervation of abdominal viscera.

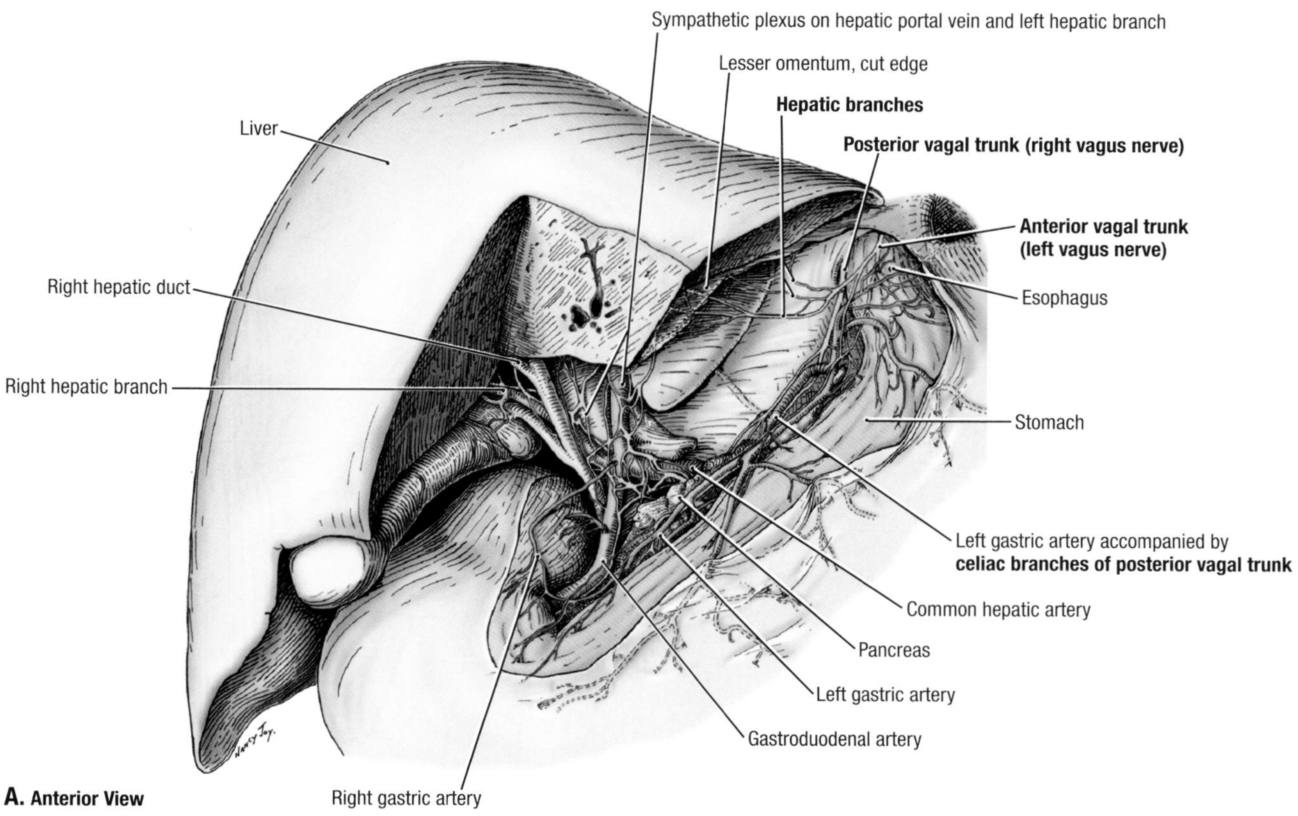
Sympathetic plexus on hepatic portal vein and left hepatic branch
Lesser omentum, cut edge
Hepatic branches
Posterior vagal trunk (right vagus nerve)
Liver
Anterior vagal trunk
(left vagus nerve)
Esophagus
Right hepatic duct
Right hepatic branch
Stomach
Left gastric artery accompanied by
celiac branches of posterior vagal trunk
Common hepatic artery
Pancreas
Left gastric artery
Gastroduodenal artery
Right gastric artery

**A. Anterior View**

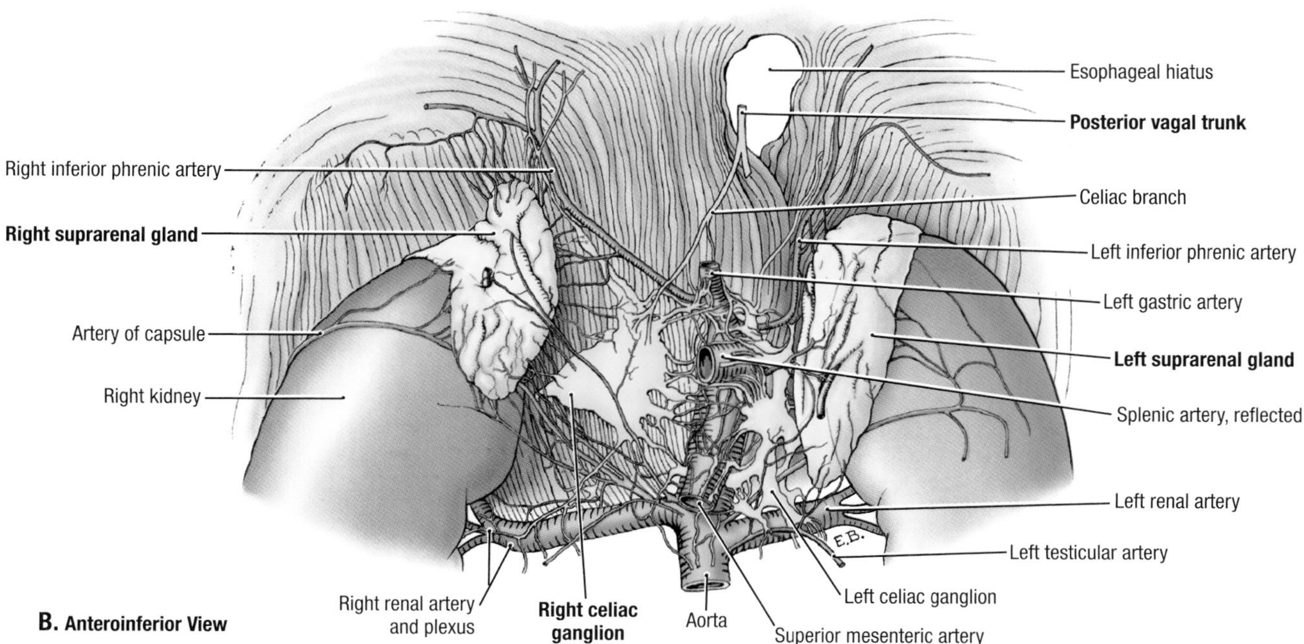
Esophageal hiatus
Posterior vagal trunk
Right inferior phrenic artery
Celiac branch
Right suprarenal gland
Left inferior phrenic artery
Left gastric artery
Artery of capsule
Left suprarenal gland
Right kidney
Splenic artery, reflected
Left renal artery
Left testicular artery
Right renal artery
and plexus
Right celiac
ganglion
Aorta
Left celiac ganglion
Superior mesenteric artery

**B. Anteroinferior View**

## 2.81 Vagus nerves in abdomen

**A.** Anterior and posterior vagal trunks. **B.** Celiac plexus and ganglia and suprarenal glands.

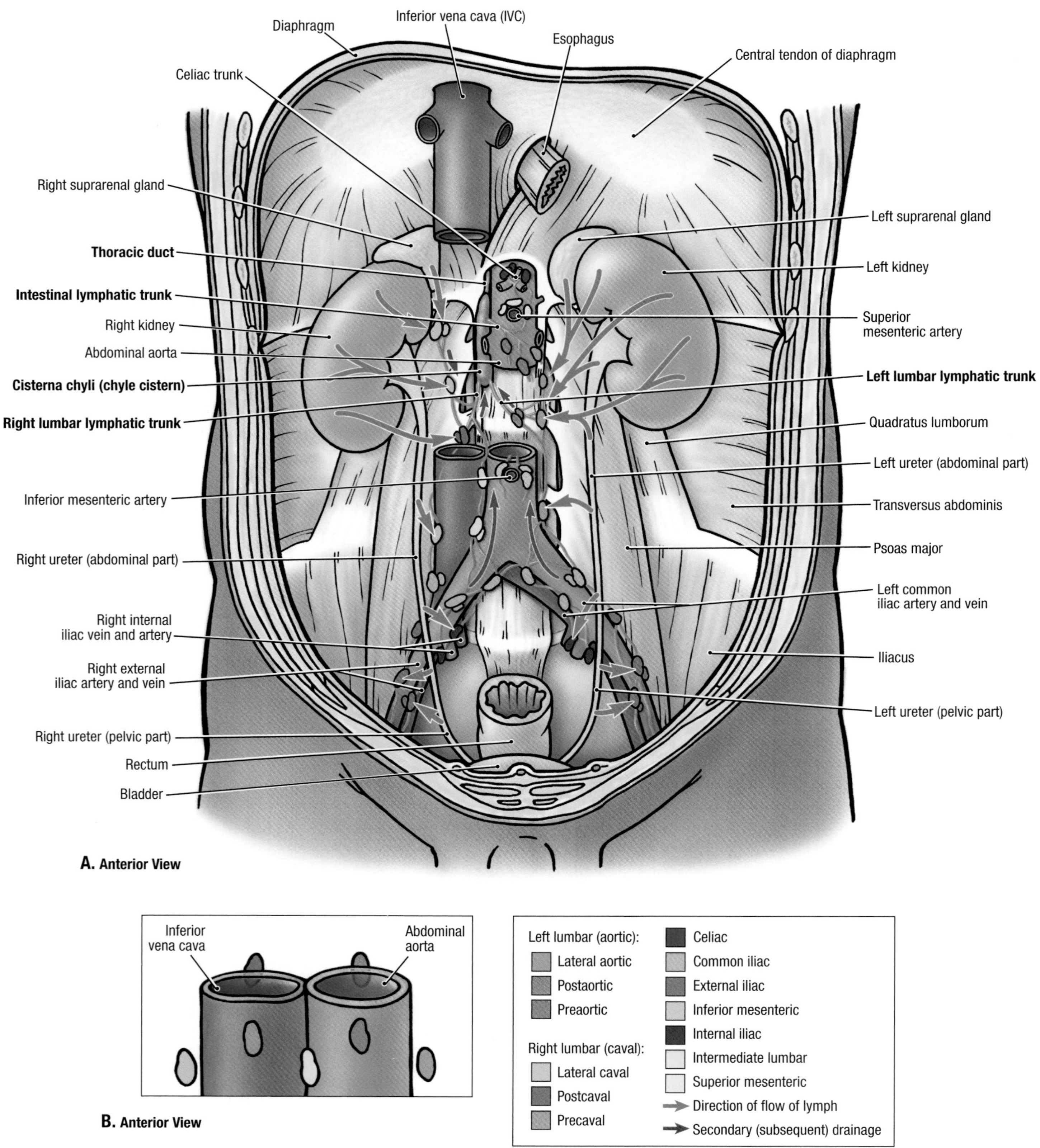
Diaphragm
Inferior vena cava (IVC)
Esophagus
Central tendon of diaphragm
Celiac trunk
Right suprarenal gland
Thoracic duct
Intestinal lymphatic trunk
Right kidney
Abdominal aorta
Cisterna chyli (chyle cistern)
Right lumbar lymphatic trunk
Inferior mesenteric artery
Right ureter (abdominal part)
Right internal iliac vein and artery
Right external iliac artery and vein
Right ureter (pelvic part)
Rectum
Bladder
Left suprarenal gland
Left kidney
Superior mesenteric artery
Left lumbar lymphatic trunk
Quadratus lumborum
Left ureter (abdominal part)
Transversus abdominis
Psoas major
Left common iliac artery and vein
Iliacus
Left ureter (pelvic part)
A. Anterior View
Inferior vena cava
Abdominal aorta
B. Anterior View
Left lumbar (aortic):
Lateral aortic
Postaortic
Preaortic
Right lumbar (caval):
Lateral caval
Postcaval
Precaval
Celiac
Common iliac
External iliac
Inferior mesenteric
Internal iliac
Intermediate lumbar
Superior mesenteric
Direction of flow of lymph
Secondary (subsequent) drainage

**2.82 Lymphatic drainage of suprarenal glands, kidneys, and ureters**

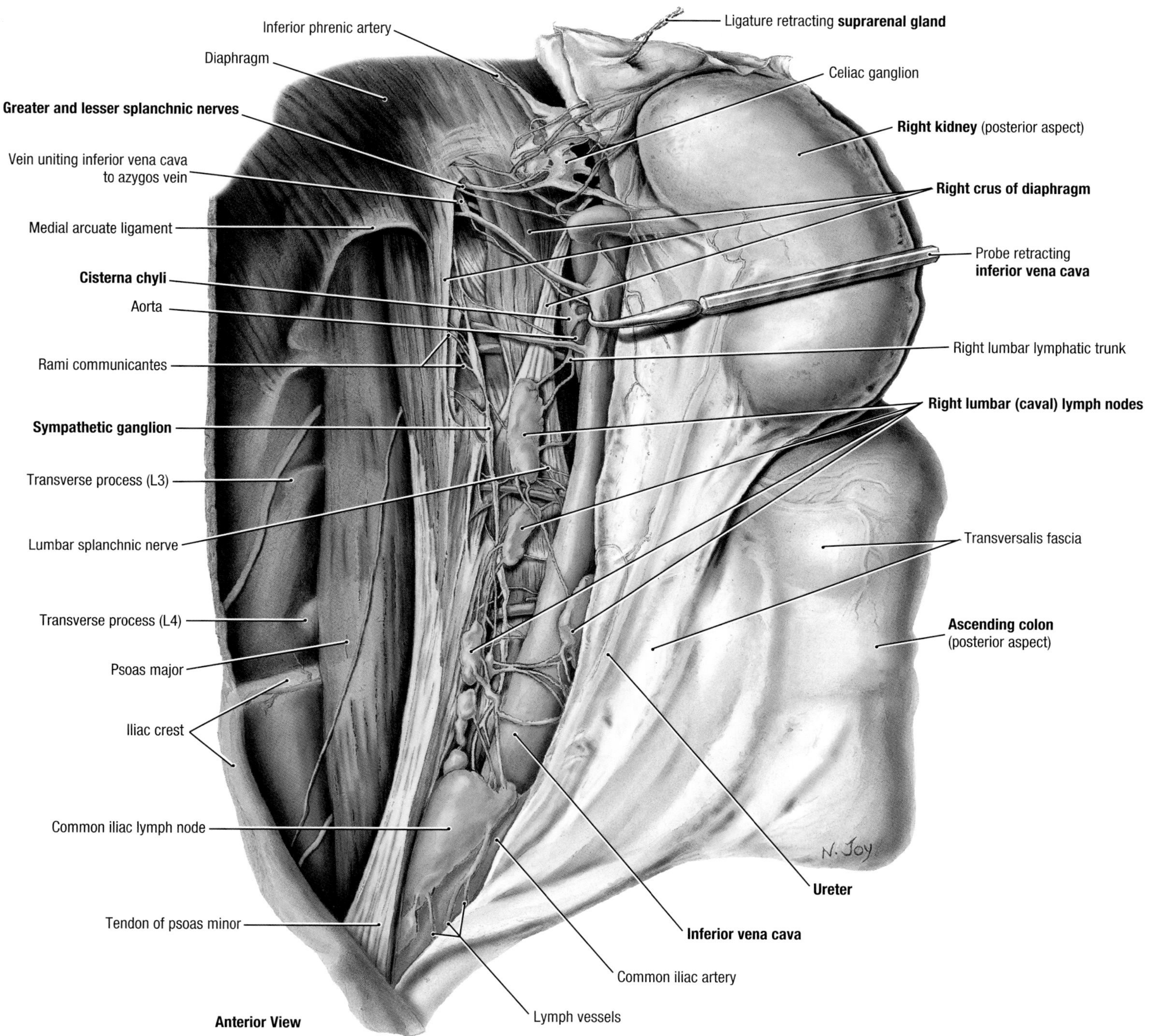
Inferior phrenic artery
Ligature retracting suprarenal gland
Diaphragm
Celiac ganglion
Greater and lesser splanchnic nerves
Right kidney (posterior aspect)
Vein uniting inferior vena cava to azygos vein
Right crus of diaphragm
Medial arcuate ligament
Probe retracting inferior vena cava
Cisterna chyli
Aorta
Right lumbar lymphatic trunk
Rami communicantes
Right lumbar (caval) lymph nodes
Sympathetic ganglion
Transverse process (L3)
Transversalis fascia
Lumbar splanchnic nerve
Transverse process (L4)
Ascending colon (posterior aspect)
Psoas major
Iliac crest
Common iliac lymph node
N. Joy
Ureter
Tendon of psoas minor
Inferior vena cava
Common iliac artery
Anterior View
Lymph vessels

## 2.83 Lumbar lymph nodes, sympathetic trunk, nerves, and ganglia

The right suprarenal gland, kidney, ureter, and colon are reflected to the left; the inferior vena cava is pulled medially, and the third and fourth lumbar veins are removed. In this specimen, the greater and lesser splanchnic nerves, the sympathetic trunk, and a communicating vein pass through an unusually wide cleft in the right crus. The splanchnic nerves convey preganglionic fibers arising from the cell bodies in the (thoracolumbar) sympathetic trunk. The greater splanchnic nerve is from thoracic ganglia 5 to 9, and the lesser from thoracic ganglia 10 to 11.

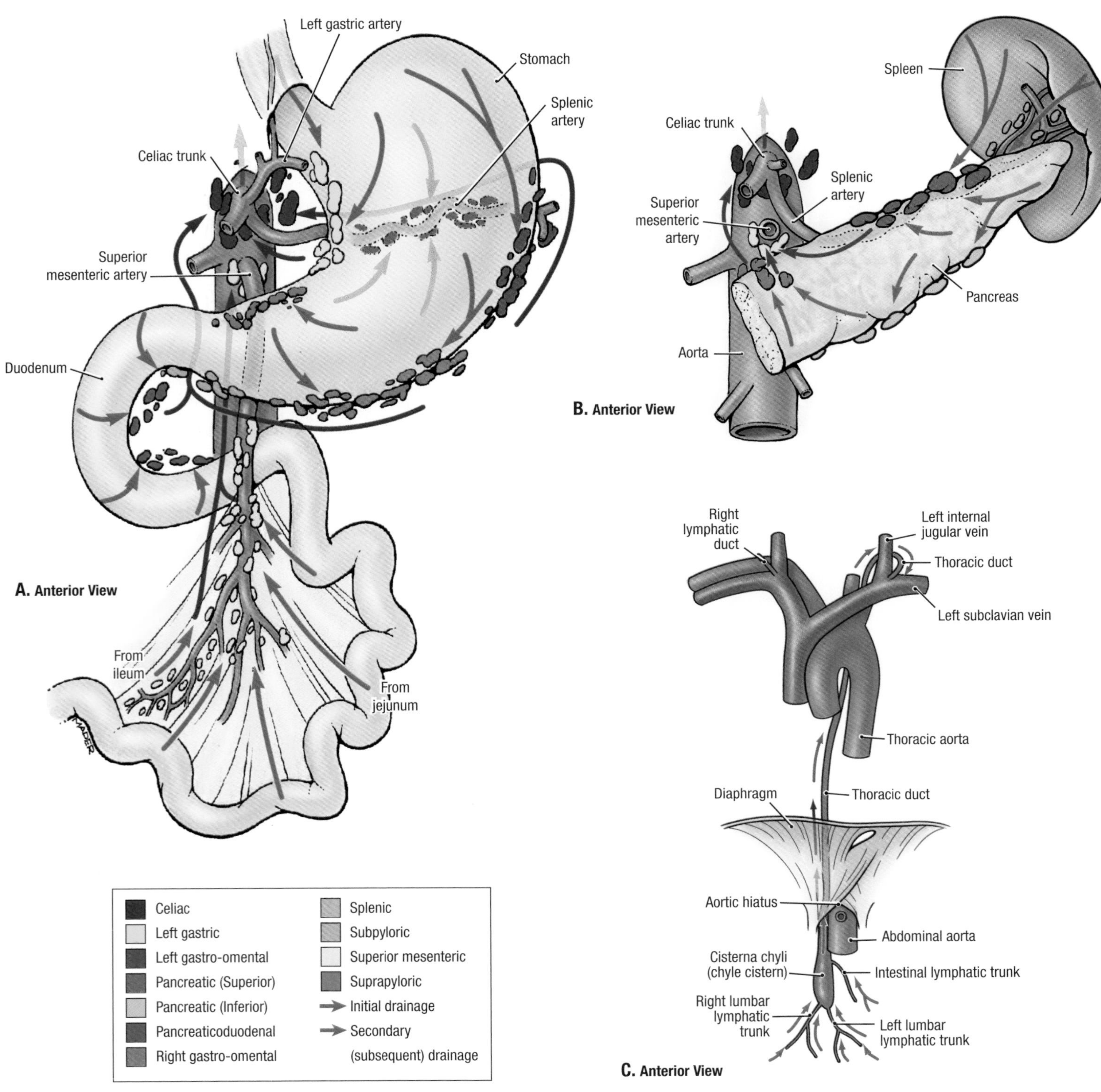

Left gastric artery
Stomach
Splenic artery
Celiac trunk
Superior mesenteric artery
Duodenum
A. Anterior View
From ileum
From jejunum
Spleen
Celiac trunk
Splenic artery
Superior mesenteric artery
Pancreas
Aorta
B. Anterior View
Right lymphatic duct
Left internal jugular vein
Thoracic duct
Left subclavian vein
Thoracic aorta
Diaphragm
Thoracic duct
Aortic hiatus
Abdominal aorta
Cisterna chyli (chyle cistern)
Intestinal lymphatic trunk
Right lumbar lymphatic trunk
Left lumbar lymphatic trunk
C. Anterior View
Celiac
Left gastric
Left gastro-omental
Pancreatic (Superior)
Pancreatic (Inferior)
Pancreaticoduodenal
Right gastro-omental
Splenic
Subpyloric
Superior mesenteric
Suprapyloric
Initial drainage
Secondary (subsequent) drainage


## 2.84 Lymphatic drainage

**A.** Stomach and small intestine. **B.** Spleen and pancreas. **C.** Drainage from lumbar and intestinal lymphatic trunks. The *arrows* indicate the direction of lymph flow; each group of lymph nodes is color coded. Lymph from the abdominal nodes drains into the cisterna chyli, origin of the inferior end of the thoracic duct. The thoracic duct receives all lymph that forms inferior to the diaphragm and left upper quadrant (thorax and left upper limb) and empties into the junction of the left subclavian and left internal jugular veins.

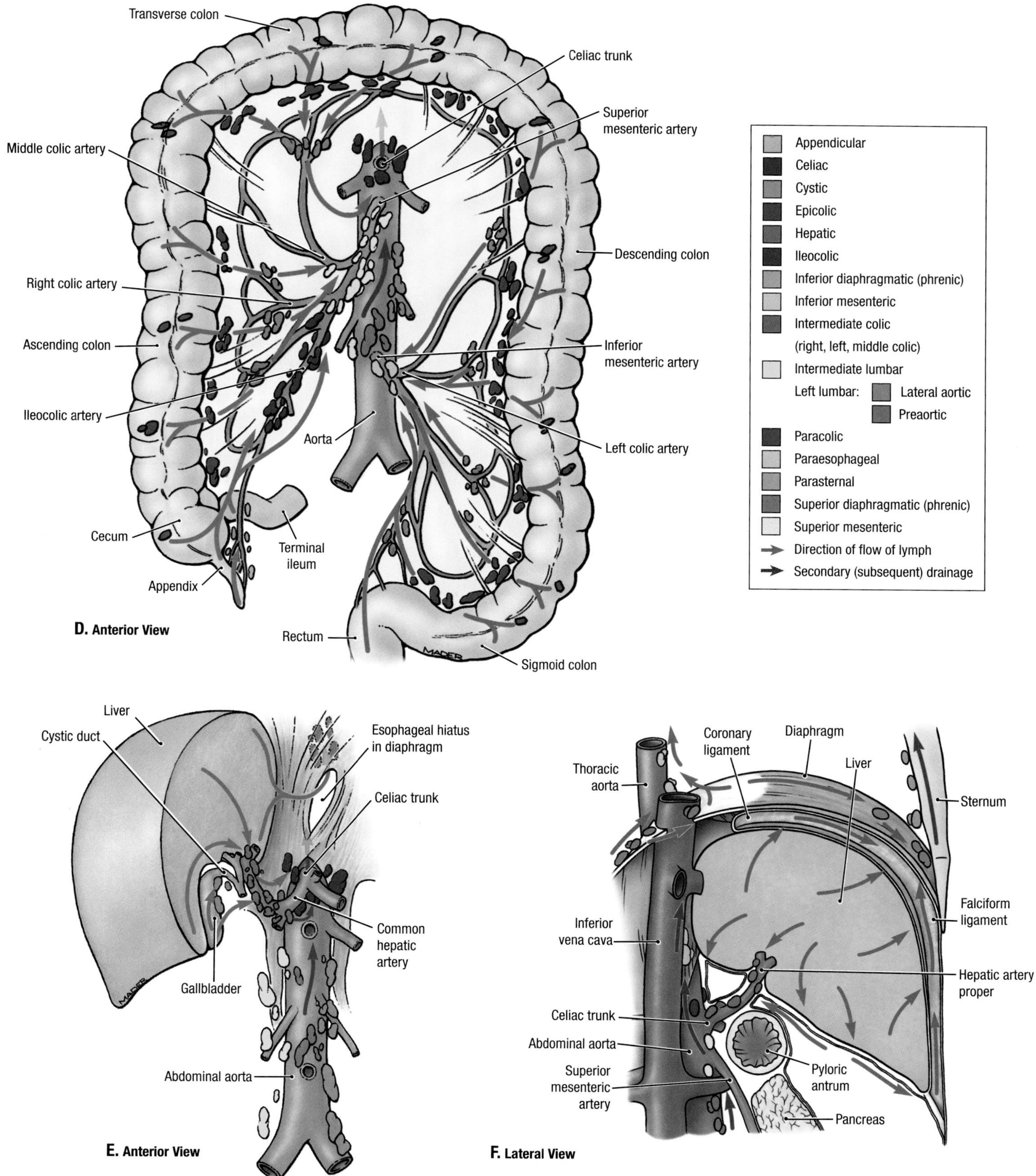
Transverse colon
Celiac trunk
Superior mesenteric artery
Middle colic artery
Descending colon
Right colic artery
Ascending colon
Inferior mesenteric artery
Ileocolic artery
Aorta
Left colic artery
Cecum
Terminal ileum
Appendix
Rectum
Sigmoid colon
D. Anterior View
Appendicular
Celiac
Cystic
Epicolic
Hepatic
Ileocolic
Inferior diaphragmatic (phrenic)
Inferior mesenteric
Intermediate colic
(right, left, middle colic)
Intermediate lumbar
Left lumbar:
Lateral aortic
Preaortic
Paracolic
Paraesophageal
Parasternal
Superior diaphragmatic (phrenic)
Superior mesenteric
Direction of flow of lymph
Secondary (subsequent) drainage
Liver
Cystic duct
Esophageal hiatus in diaphragm
Celiac trunk
Common hepatic artery
Gallbladder
Abdominal aorta
E. Anterior View
Thoracic aorta
Coronary ligament
Diaphragm
Liver
Sternum
Falciform ligament
Inferior vena cava
Hepatic artery proper
Celiac trunk
Abdominal aorta
Superior mesenteric artery
Pyloric antrum
Pancreas
F. Lateral View

**2.84 Lymphatic drainage *(continued)***

**D.** Large intestine. **E.** Liver and gallbladder. **F.** Liver.

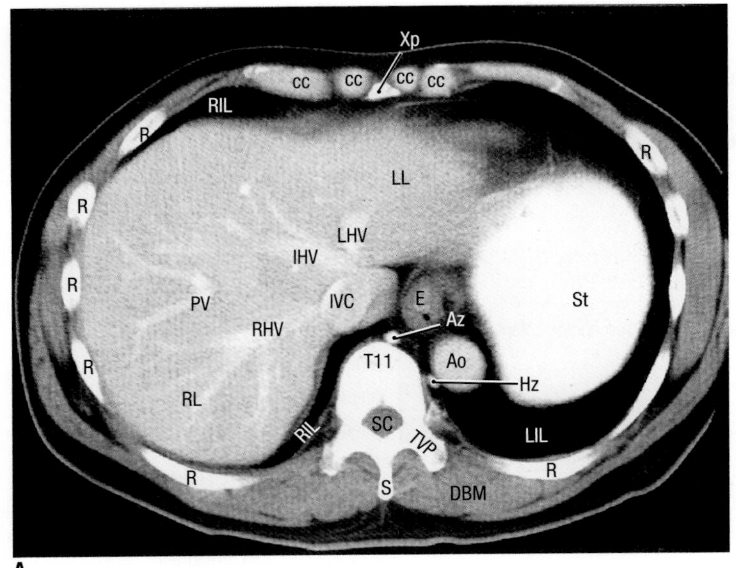
Xp
cc
cc
cc
cc
RIL
R
LL
LHV
IHV
PV
IVC
E
Az
St
RHV
T11
Ao
Hz
RL
RIL
SC
TVP
LIL
S
DBM

A

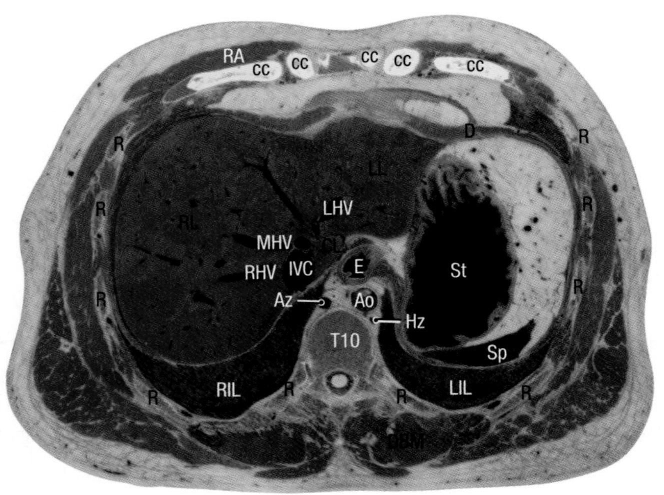
RA
cc
cc
cc
cc
cc
D
R
LL
LHV
RL
MHV
CL
RHV
IVC
E
St
Az
Ao
Hz
T10
Sp
RIL
LIL
DBM

B

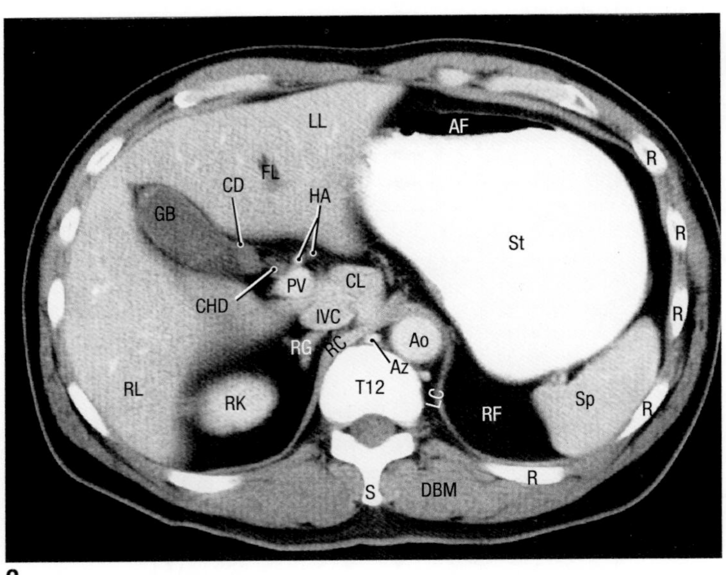
LL
AF
FL
CD
HA
GB
St
R
CHD
PV
CL
IVC
Ao
RG
RC
Az
T12
LC
RL
RK
RF
Sp
S
DBM

C

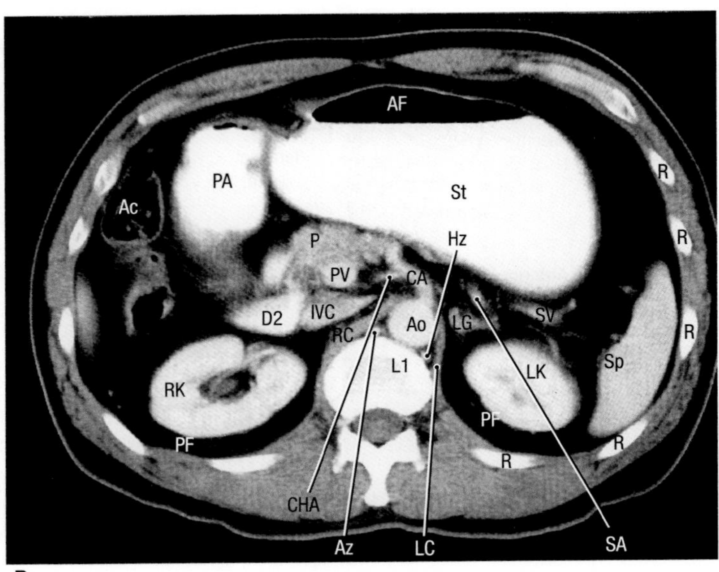
AF
PA
St
Ac
P
Hz
PV
CA
D2
IVC
RC
Ao
LG
SV
L1
RK
LK
Sp
PF
PF
R
CHA
Az
LC
SA

D

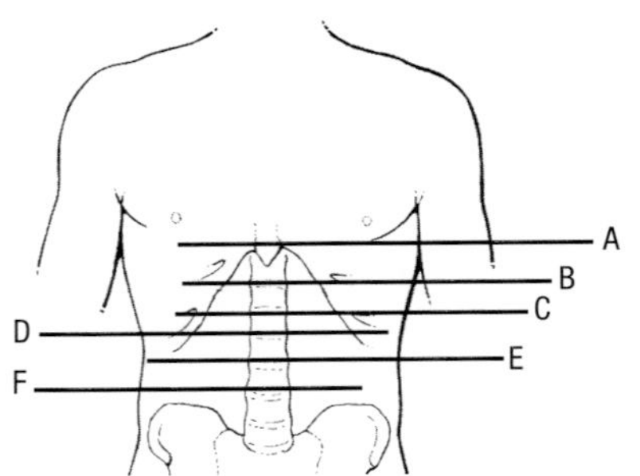
A
B
C
D
E
F

| | | | | | |
|---|---|---|---|---|---|
| Ac | Ascending colon | DBM | Deep back muscles | LC | Left crus of diaphragm |
| AF | Air-fluid level of stomach | Dc | Descending colon | LG | Left suprarenal gland |
| Ao | Aorta | D2 | Descending part of duodenum | LHV | Left hepatic vein |
| Az | Azygos vein | D3 | Inferior part of duodenum | LIL | Left inferior lobe of lung |
| CA | Celiac artery | E | Esophagus | LK | Left kidney |
| cc | Costal cartilage | FL | Falciform ligament | LL | Left lobe of liver |
| CD | Cystic duct | GB | Gallbladder | LRV | Left renal vein |
| CHA | Common hepatic artery | HA | Hepatic artery | LU | Left ureter |
| CHD | Common hepatic duct | Hz | Hemiazygos vein | IHV | Intermediate hepatic vein |
| CL | Caudate lobe of liver | IMV | Inferior mesenteric vein | P | Pancreas |
| D | Diaphragm | IVC | Inferior vena cava | PA | Pyloric antrum of stomach |

**2.85 Transverse or horizontal (axial) MRIs of the abdomen**

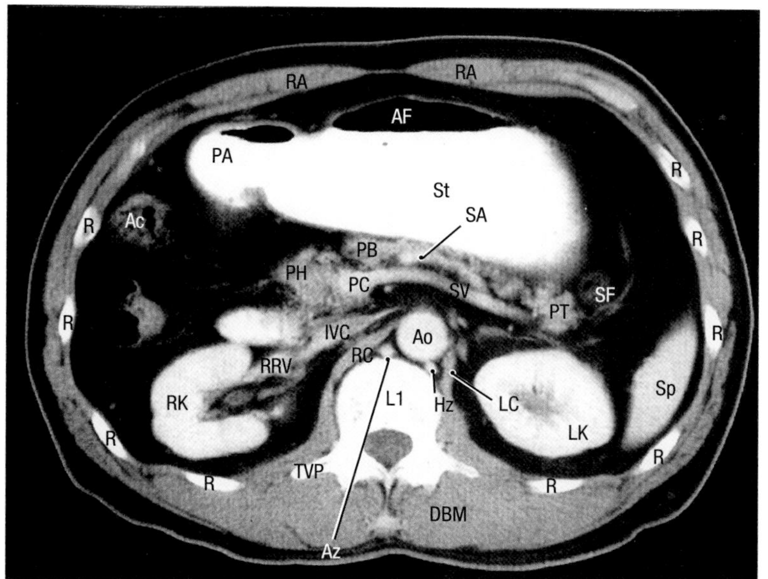
RA
RA
AF
PA
St
SA
R
Ac
PB
PH
PC
SV
PT
SF
IVC
Ao
RC
RRV
L1
Hz
LC
RK
LK
Sp
TVP
DBM
Az

E

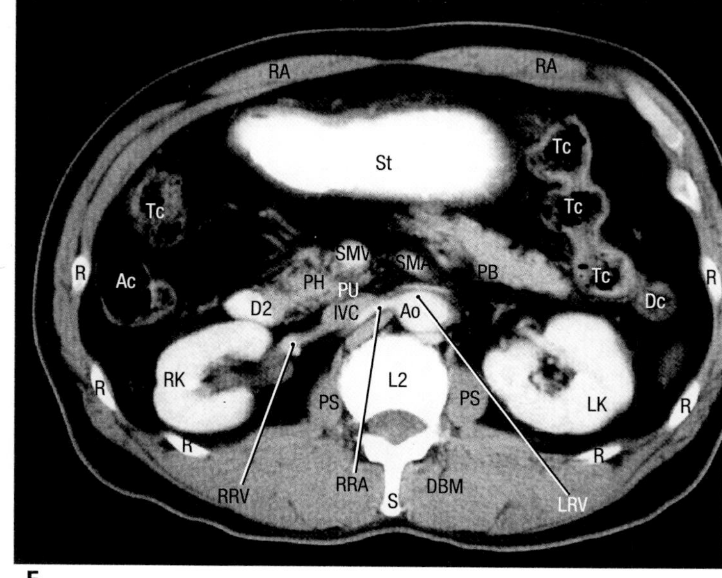
RA
RA
St
Tc
Ac
SMV
SMA
PB
PH
PU
D2
IVC
Ao
Dc
RK
L2
PS
PS
LK
RRV
RRA
S
DBM
LRV

F

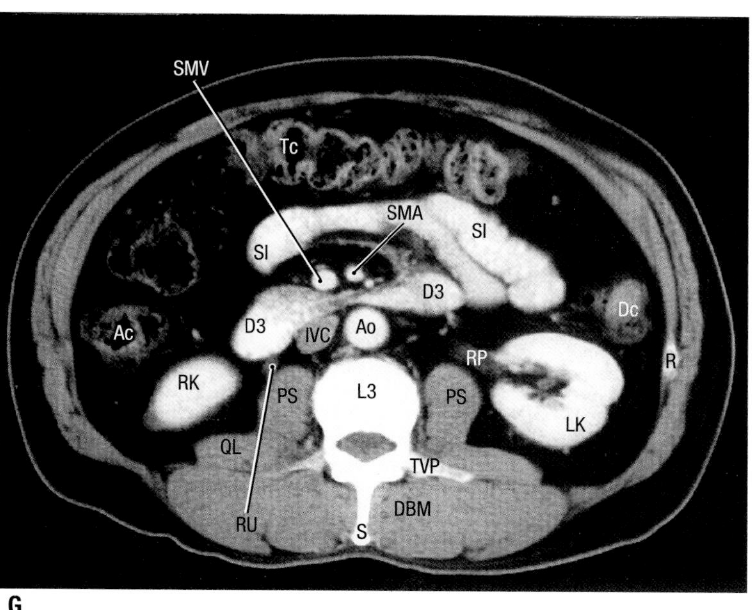
SMV
Tc
SMA
SI
SI
D3
D3
Dc
Ac
IVC
Ao
RP
RK
PS
L3
PS
LK
QL
TVP
RU
DBM
S

G

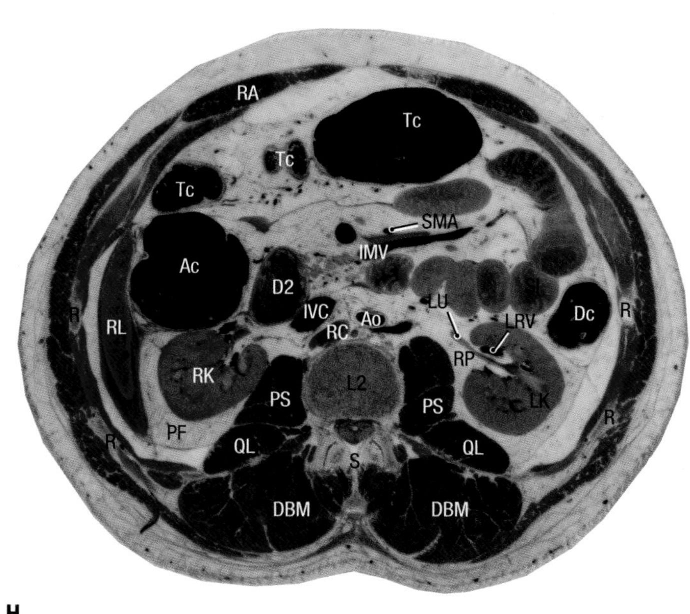
RA
Tc
Tc
Tc
SMA
IMV
Ac
D2
IVC
Ao
LU
LRV
Dc
RL
RC
RP
RK
L2
PS
PS
LK
PF
QL
QL
S
DBM
DBM

H

| | | | | | | | |
|---|---|---|---|---|---|---|---|
| PB | Body of pancreas | R | Rib | RP | Renal pelvis | SMA | Superior mesenteric artery |
| PC | Portal confluence | RA | Rectus abdominis | RRA | Right renal artery | SMV | Superior mesenteric vein |
| PF | Perinephric fat | RC | Right crus of diaphragm | RRV | Right renal vein | Sp | Spleen |
| PH | Head of pancreas | RF | Retroperitoneal fat | RU | Right ureter | St | Stomach |
| PS | Psoas muscle | RG | Right suprarenal gland | S | Spinous process | SV | Splenic vein |
| PT | Tail of pancreas | RHV | Right hepatic vein | SA | Splenic artery | Tc | Transverse colon |
| PU | Uncinate process of pancreas | RIL | Right inferior lobe of lung | SC | Spinal cord | TVP | Transverse process |
| PV | Hepatic portal vein | RK | Right kidney | SF | Splenic flexure | Xp | Xiphoid process |
| QL | Quadratus lumborum | RL | Right lobe of liver | SI | Small intestine | | |

**2.85** **Transverse or horizontal (axial) MRIs of the abdomen *(continued)***

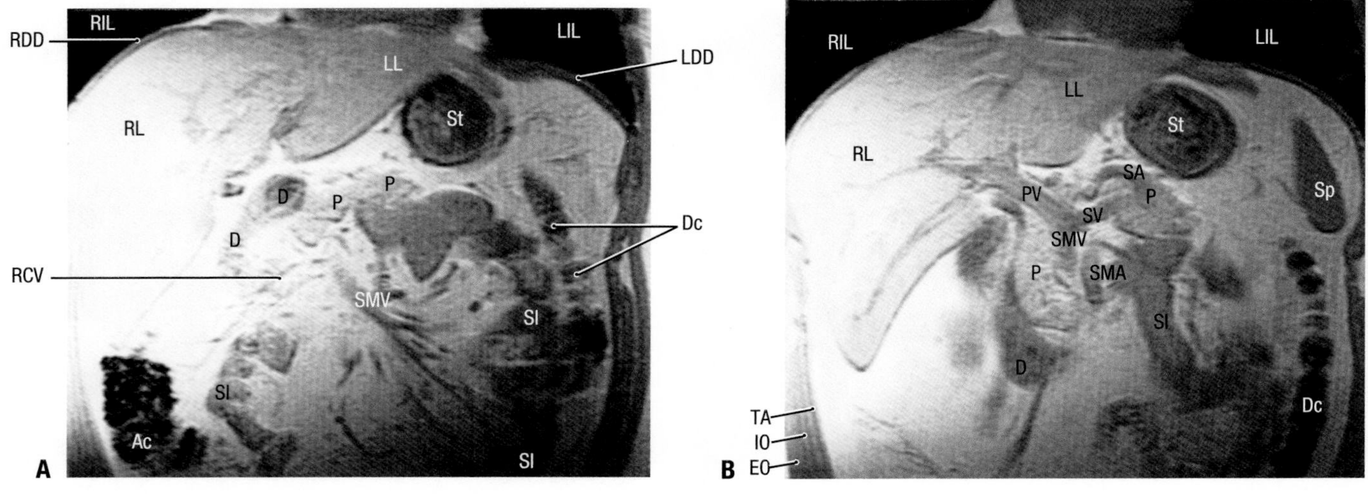
RIL
RDD
LIL
LL
LDD
RL
St
P
D
P
Dc
D
RCV
SMV
SI
SI
Ac
SI
A
RIL
LIL
LL
St
RL
SA
PV
P
Sp
SV
SMV
P
SMA
SI
D
TA
IO
EO
Dc
B

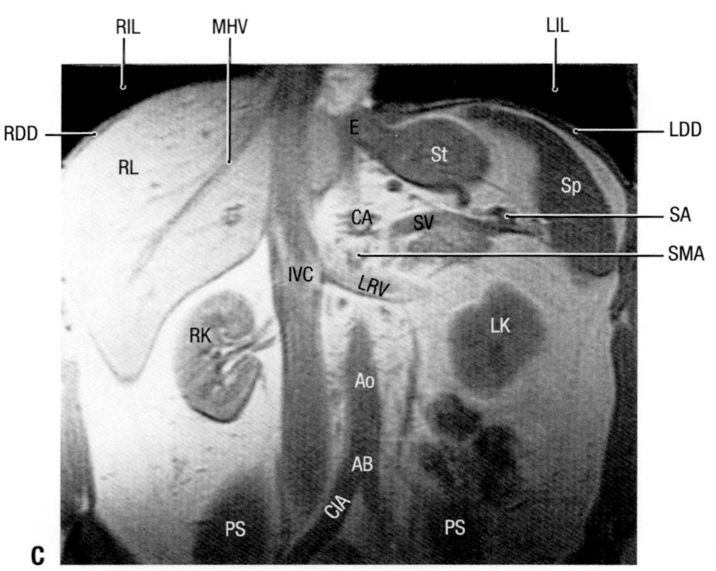
RIL
MHV
LIL
RDD
E
LDD
St
RL
Sp
CA
SV
SA
SMA
IVC
LRV
RK
LK
Ao
AB
CIA
PS
PS
C

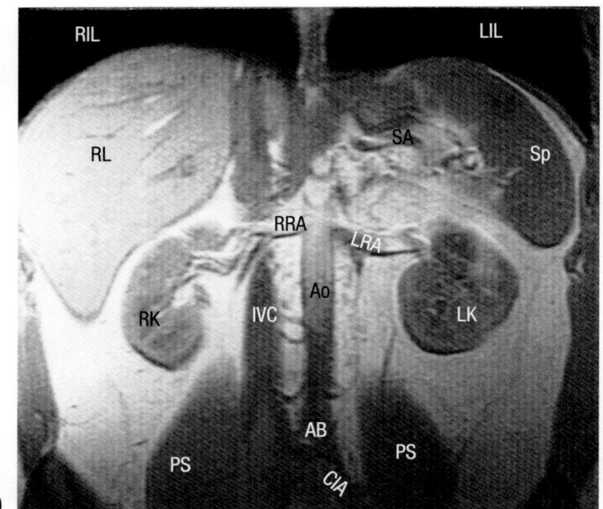
RIL
LIL
SA
RL
Sp
RRA
LRA
Ao
RK
IVC
LK
AB
PS
PS
CIA
D

| | | | | | |
|---|---|---|---|---|---|
| AB | Aortic bifurcation | LIL | Left lung (inferior lobe) | RK | Right kidney |
| Ac | Ascending colon | LK | Left kidney | RL | Right lobe of liver |
| Ao | Aorta | LL | Left lobe of liver | RRA | Right renal artery |
| CA | Celiac artery | LRA | Left renal artery | SA | Splenic artery |
| CIA | Common iliac artery | LRV | Left renal vein | SI | Small intestine |
| D | Duodenum | MHV | Middle hepatic vein | SMA | Superior mesenteric artery |
| Dc | Descending colon | P | Pancreas | SMV | Superior mesenteric vein |
| E | Esophagus | PV | Portal vein | Sp | Spleen |
| EO | External oblique | PS | Psoas | St | Stomach |
| IO | Internal oblique | RCV | Right colic vein | SV | Splenic vein |
| IVC | Inferior vena cava | RDD | Right dome of diaphragm | TA | Transversus abdominis |
| LDD | Left dome of diaphragm | RIL | Right lung (inferior lobe) | | |

**2.86 Coronal MRIs of the abdomen**

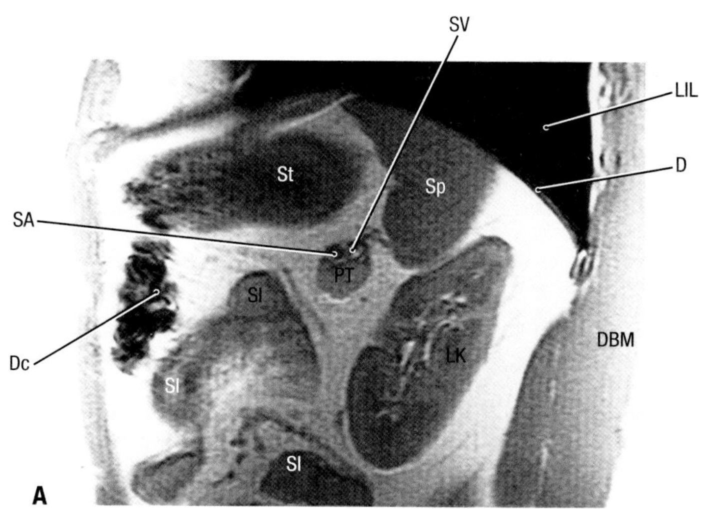
SV
LIL
D
St
Sp
SA
PT
SI
Dc
SI
LK
DBM
SI
A

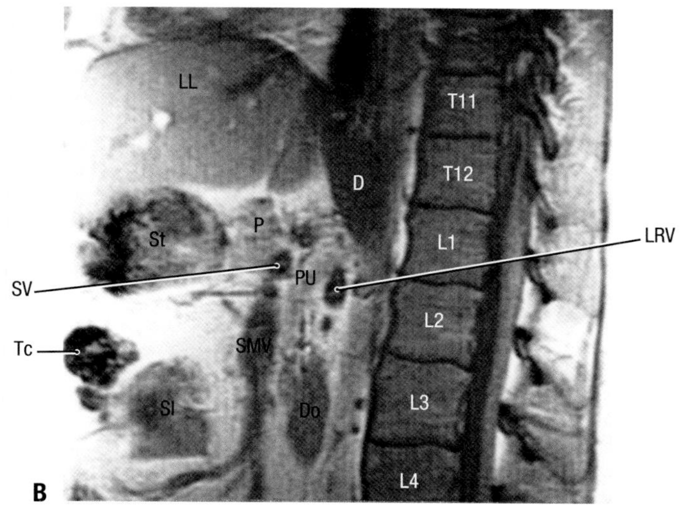
LL
T11
T12
D
P
St
L1
LRV
SV
PU
L2
Tc
SMV
SI
Do
L3
L4
B

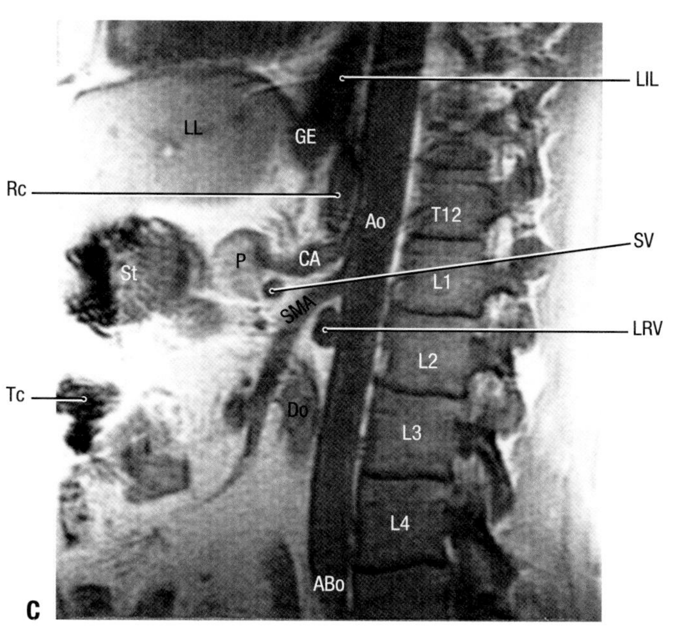
LIL
LL
GE
Rc
Ao
T12
SV
P
CA
St
L1
SMA
LRV
L2
Tc
Do
L3
L4
ABo
C

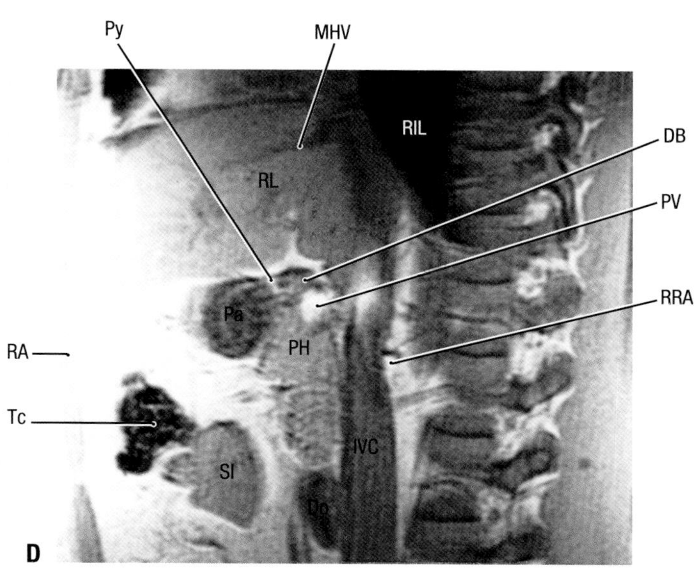
Py
MHV
RIL
DB
RL
PV
RRA
Pa
PH
RA
Tc
SI
IVC
Do
D

| | | | | | |
|---|---|---|---|---|---|
| Ao | Aorta | LL | Left lobe of liver | RC | Right crus |
| ABo | Bifurcation of aorta | LRV | Left renal vein | RIL | Inferior lobe of right lung |
| CA | Celiac artery | MHV | Middle hepatic vein | RL | Right lobe of right liver |
| D | Diaphragm | P | Pancreas | RRA | Right renal artery |
| DB | Bulb of duodenum | Pa | Pyloric antrum | SA | Splenic artery |
| Dc | Descending colon | PC | Portal confluence | SI | Small intestine |
| Do | Duodenum | PH | Head of pancreas | SMA | Superior mesenteric artery |
| DBM | Deep back muscles | PT | Tail of pancreas | SMV | Superior mesenteric vein |
| GE | Gastroesophageal junction | PV | Portal vein | Sp | Spleen |
| IVC | Inferior vena cava | PU | Uncinate process of pancreas | St | Stomach |
| LIL | Inferior lobe of left lung | Py | Pylorus of stomach | SV | Splenic vein |
| LK | Left kidney | RA | Rectus abdominus | Tc | Transverse colon |

**2.87 Sagittal MRIs of the abdomen**

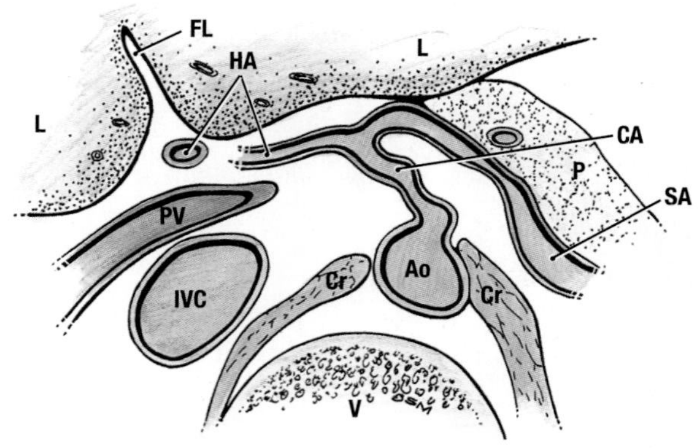
FL
HA
L
L
CA
P
SA
PV
IVC
Cr
Ao
Cr
V

A. Transverse Section, Inferior View

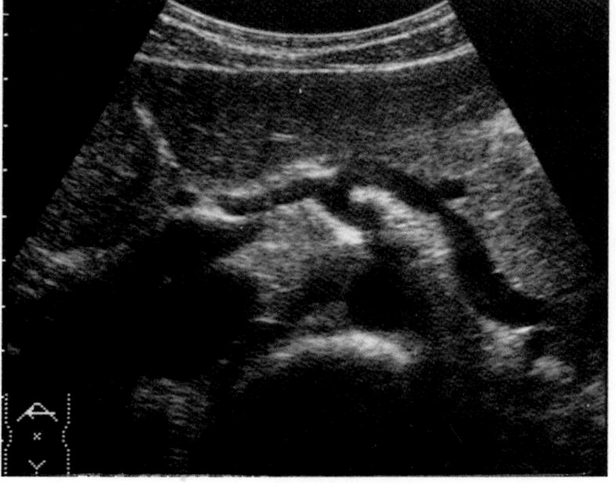

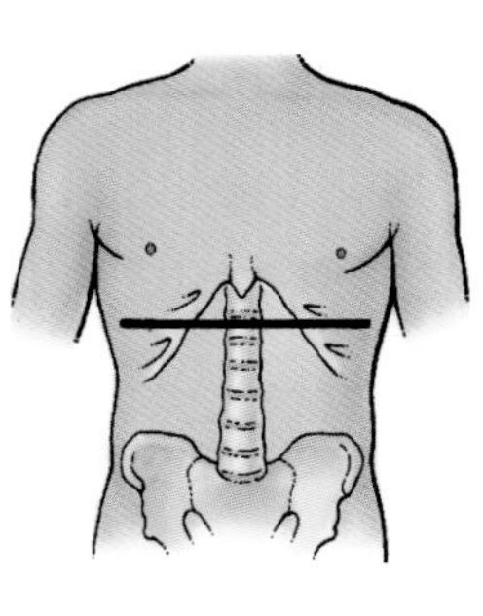

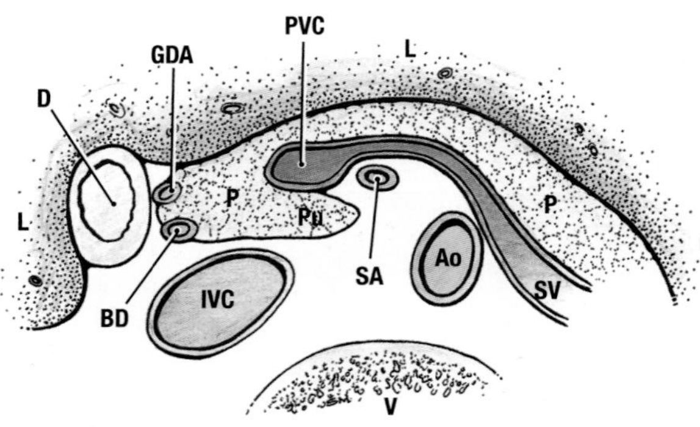
PVC
GDA
L
D
P
Pu
P
L
SA
Ao
SV
BD
IVC
V

B. Transverse Section, Inferior View

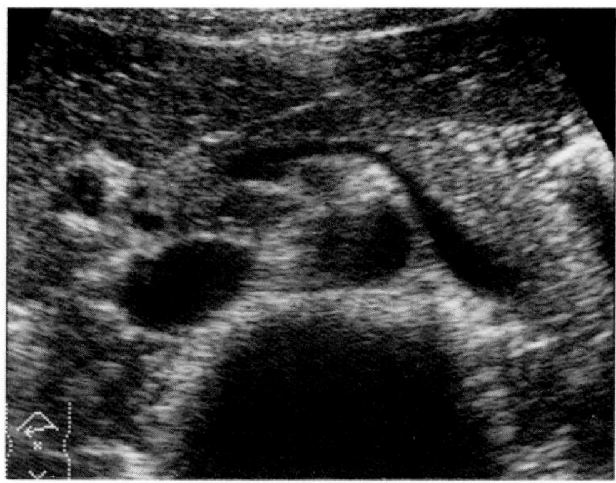

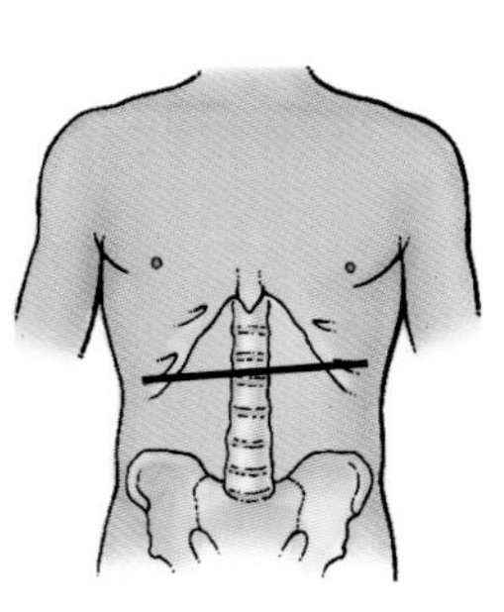

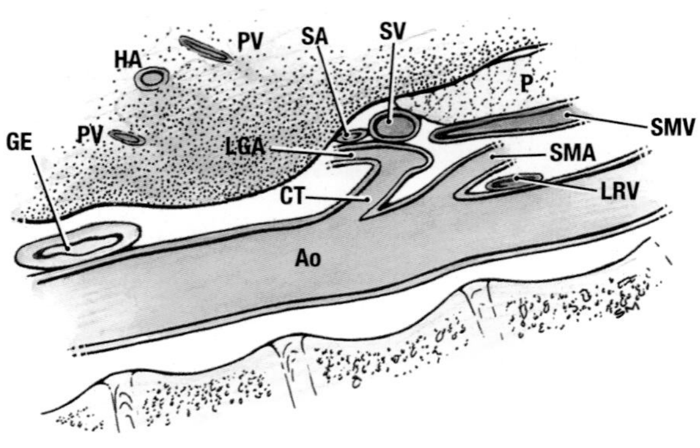
PV
SA
SV
HA
P
GE
PV
LGA
SMV
SMA
CT
LRV
Ao

C. Median Section, Right Lateral View

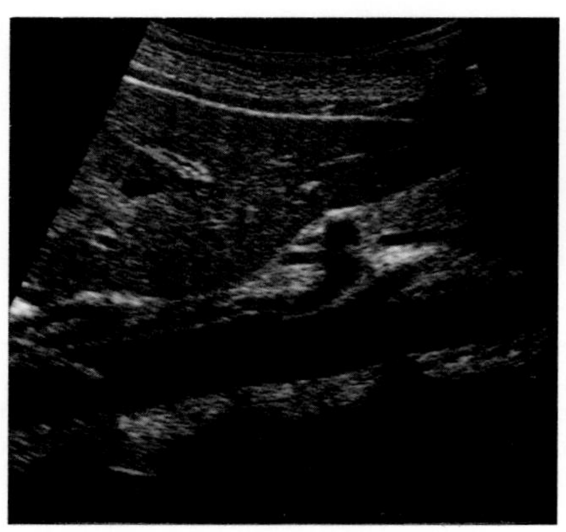

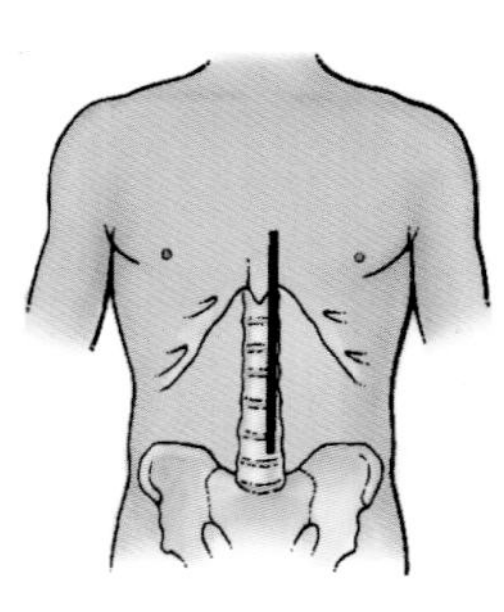

## 2.88 Ultrasound scans and MR angiogram of the abdomen

**A.** Transverse ultrasound scan through celiac trunk. **B.** Transverse ultrasound scan through pancreas. **C** and **D.** Sagittal ultrasound scans through the aorta, celiac trunk, and superior mesenteric artery. (**D.** With Doppler.) **E.** MR angiogram of abdominal aorta and branches. **F.** Transverse ultrasound scan at hilum of left kidney with the left renal artery and vein (with Doppler). **G.** Sagittal ultrasound scan of the right kidney.

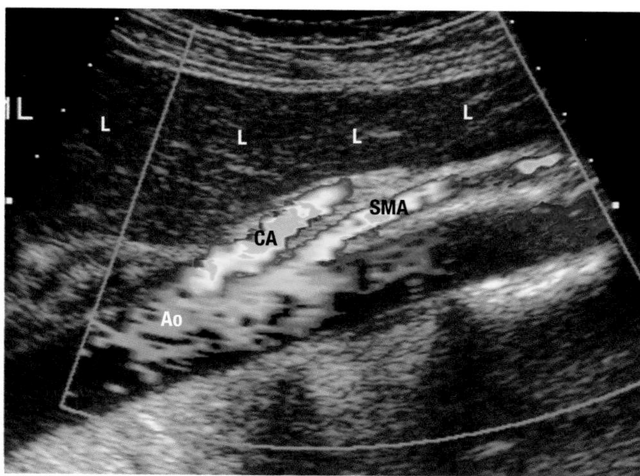
L
L
L
L
L
SMA
CA
Ao

**D. Median Section, Right Lateral View**

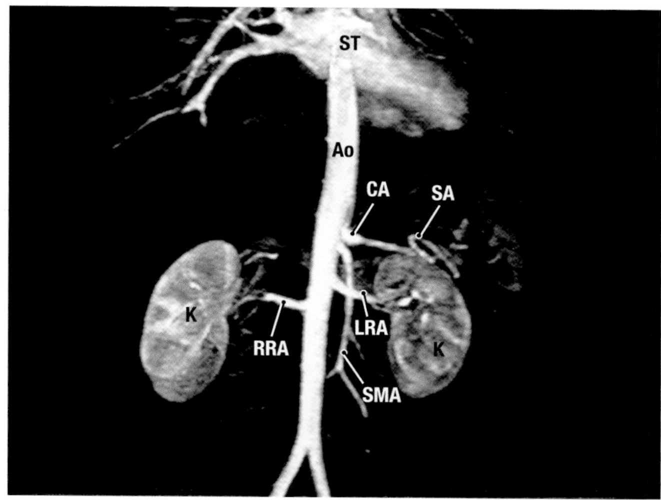
ST
Ao
CA
SA
K
RRA
LRA
K
SMA

**E. Anterior View**

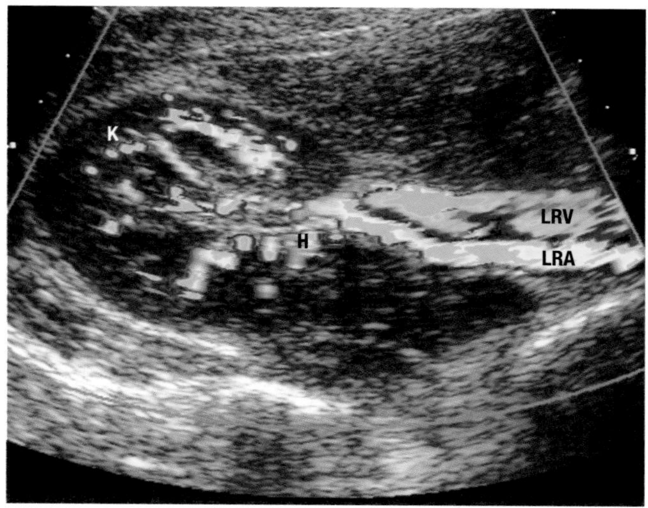
K
H
LRV
LRA

**F. Transverse Section**

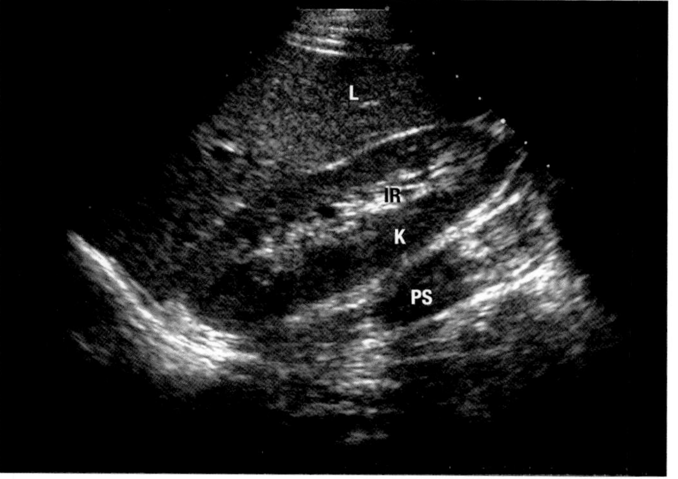
L
IR
K
PS

**G. Sagittal Section, Right Lateral View**

A major advantage of ultrasonography is its ability to produce real-time images, demonstrating motion of structures and flow within blood vessels. In Doppler ultrasonography (**D** and **F**) the shifts in frequency between emitted ultrasonic waves and their echoes are used to measure the velocities of moving objects. This technique is based on the principle of the Doppler effect. Blood flow through vessels is displayed in color, superimposed on the two-dimensional cross-sectional image. (slow flow: blue, fast flow: orange)

| | | | | | |
|---|---|---|---|---|---|
| Ao | Aorta | IR | Intrarenal fat | PV | Portal vein |
| BD | Bile duct | IVC | Inferior vena cava | PVC | Portal venous confluence |
| CA | Celiac artery | K | Cortex of kidney | RRA | Right renal artery |
| Cr | Crus of diaphragm | L | Liver | SA | Splenic artery |
| D | Duodenum | LGA | Left gastric artery | SMA | Superior mesenteric artery |
| FL | Falciform ligament | LRA | Left renal artery | SMV | Superior mesenteric vein |
| GDA | Gastroduodenal artery | LRV | Left renal vein | ST | Stomach |
| GE | Gastroesophageal junction | P | Pancreas | SV | Splenic vein |
| H | Hilum of kidney | PS | Psoas | V | Vertebra |
| HA | Hepatic artery | Pu | Uncinate process of pancreas | | |

**2.88 Ultrasound scans and MR angiogram of the abdomen *(continued)***

CHAPTER 3

# PELVIS AND PERINEUM

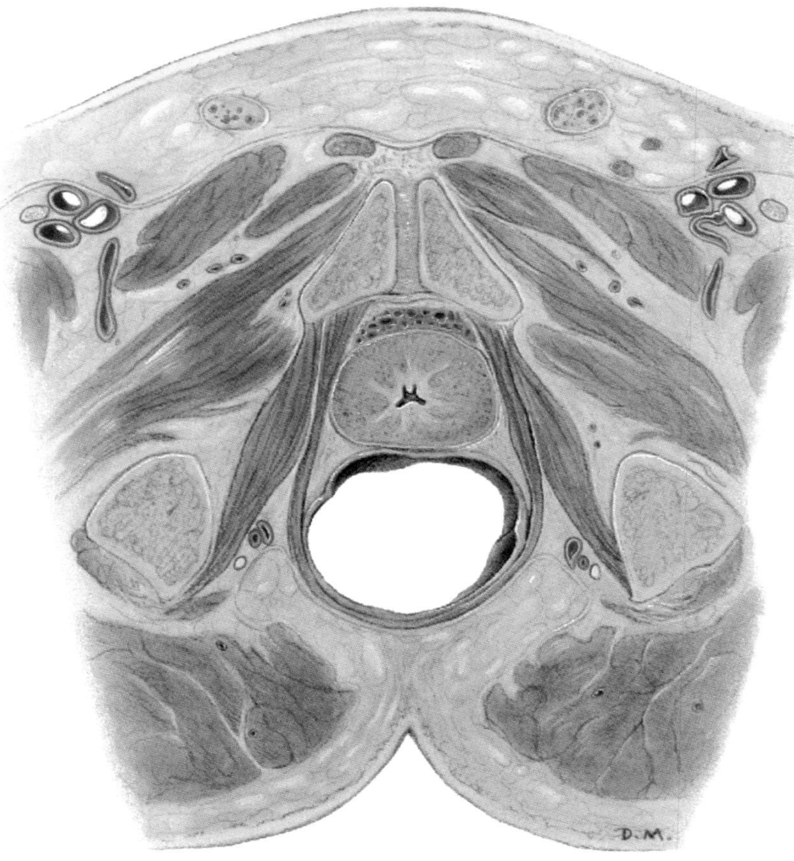

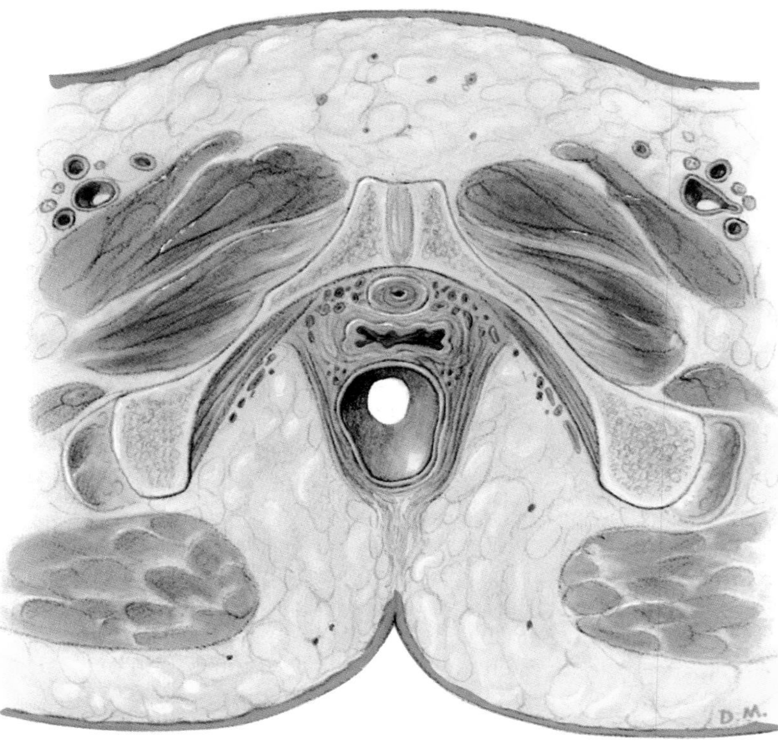


- Pelvic Girdle 194
- Ligaments of Pelvic Girdle 200
- Floor and Walls of Pelvis 202
- Sacral and Coccygeal Plexuses 206
- Peritoneal Reflections in Pelvis 208
- Rectum and Anal Canal 210
- Organs of Male Pelvis 216
- Vessels of Male Pelvis 224
- Lymphatic Drainage of Male Pelvis and Perineum 228
- Innervation of Male Pelvic Organs 230
- Organs of Female Pelvis 232
- Vessels of Female Pelvis 240
- Lymphatic Drainage of Female Pelvis and Perineum 244
- Innervation of Female Pelvic Organs 246
- Subperitoneal Region of Pelvis 250
- Surface Anatomy of Perineum 252
- Overview of Male and Female Perineum 254
- Male Perineum 261
- Female Perineum 269
- Imaging of Pelvis and Perineum 276

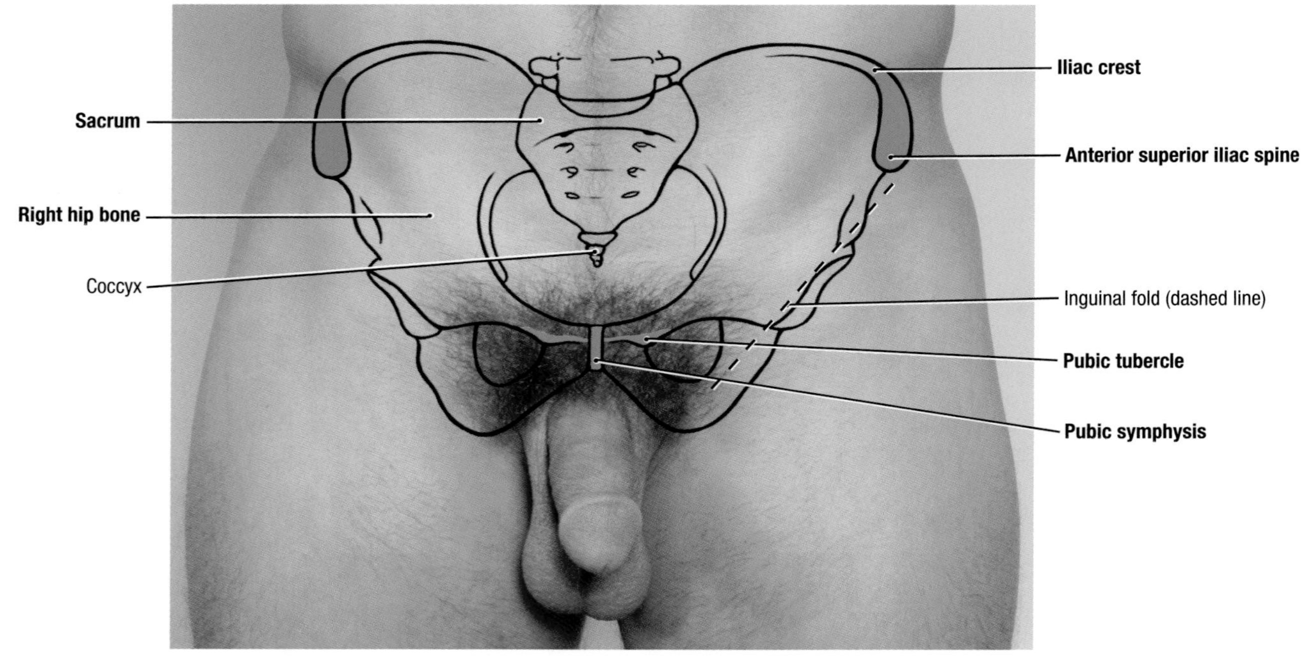
Sacrum
Right hip bone
Coccyx
Iliac crest
Anterior superior iliac spine
Inguinal fold (dashed line)
Pubic tubercle
Pubic symphysis

**A.** Anterior View

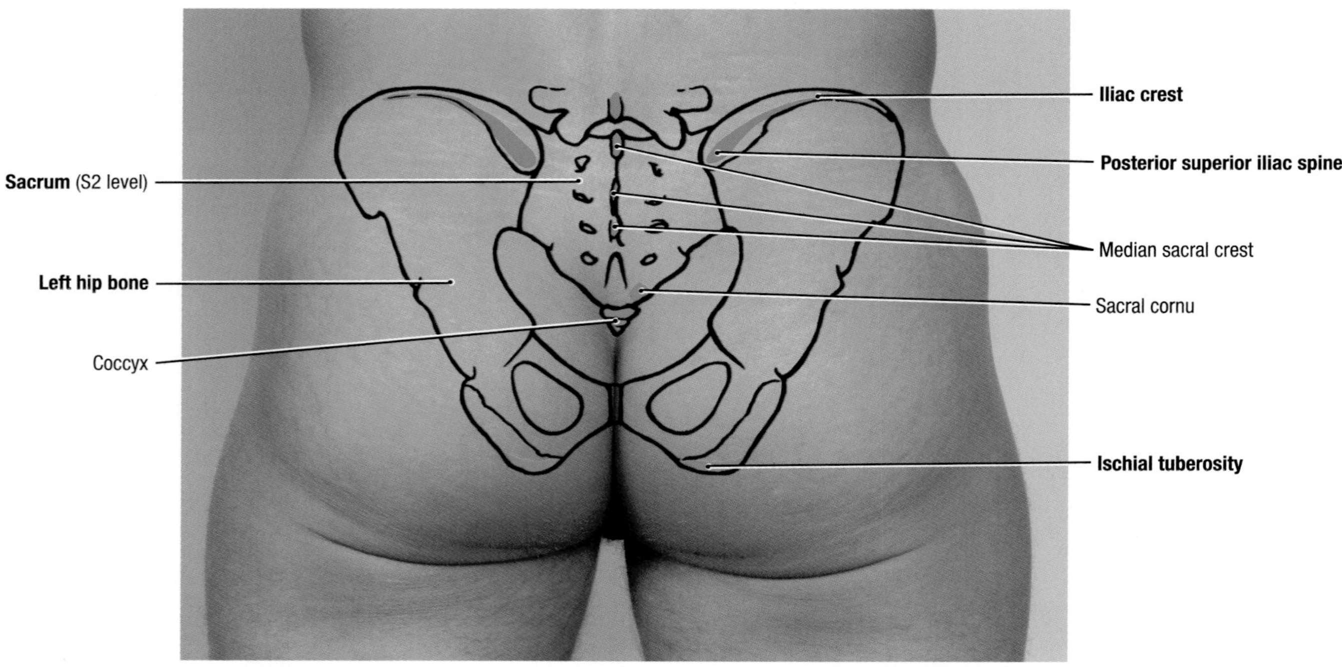
Sacrum (S2 level)
Left hip bone
Coccyx
Iliac crest
Posterior superior iliac spine
Median sacral crest
Sacral cornu
Ischial tuberosity

**B.** Posterior View

## 3.1 Surface anatomy of the male pelvic girdle

The pelvic girdle (bony pelvis) is a basin-shaped ring of three bones (right and left hip bones and sacrum) that connects the vertebral column to the femora. Palpable features *(green)* should be symmetrical across the midline. **A.** The anterior third of the iliac crests are subcutaneous and usually easily palpable. The remainder of the crests may also be palpable, depending on the thickness of the overlying subcutaneous tissue (fat). The inguinal ligament spans between the palpable anterior superior iliac spine (ASIS) and pubic tubercle, located superior to the lateral and medial ends of the inguinal fold. **B.** The posterior superior iliac spine is usually palpable and often lies deep to a visible dimple, indicating the S-2 vertebral level. The ischial tuberosities may be palpated when the thigh is flexed at the hip joint.

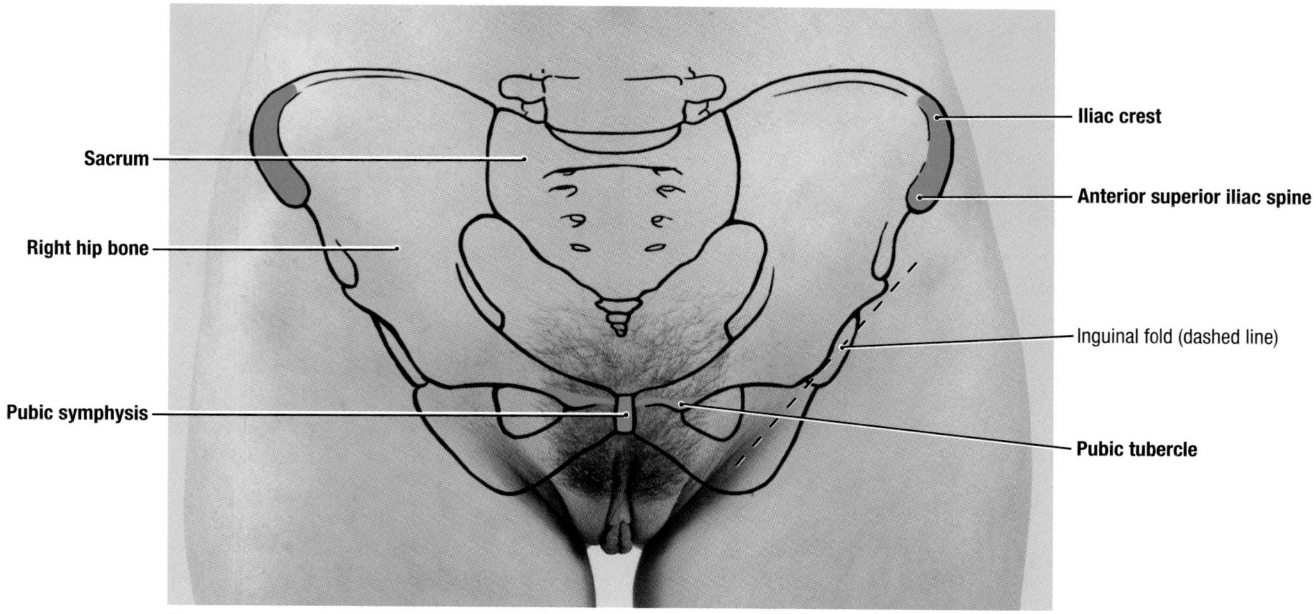
Sacrum
Right hip bone
Pubic symphysis
Iliac crest
Anterior superior iliac spine
Inguinal fold (dashed line)
Pubic tubercle

**A.** Anterior View

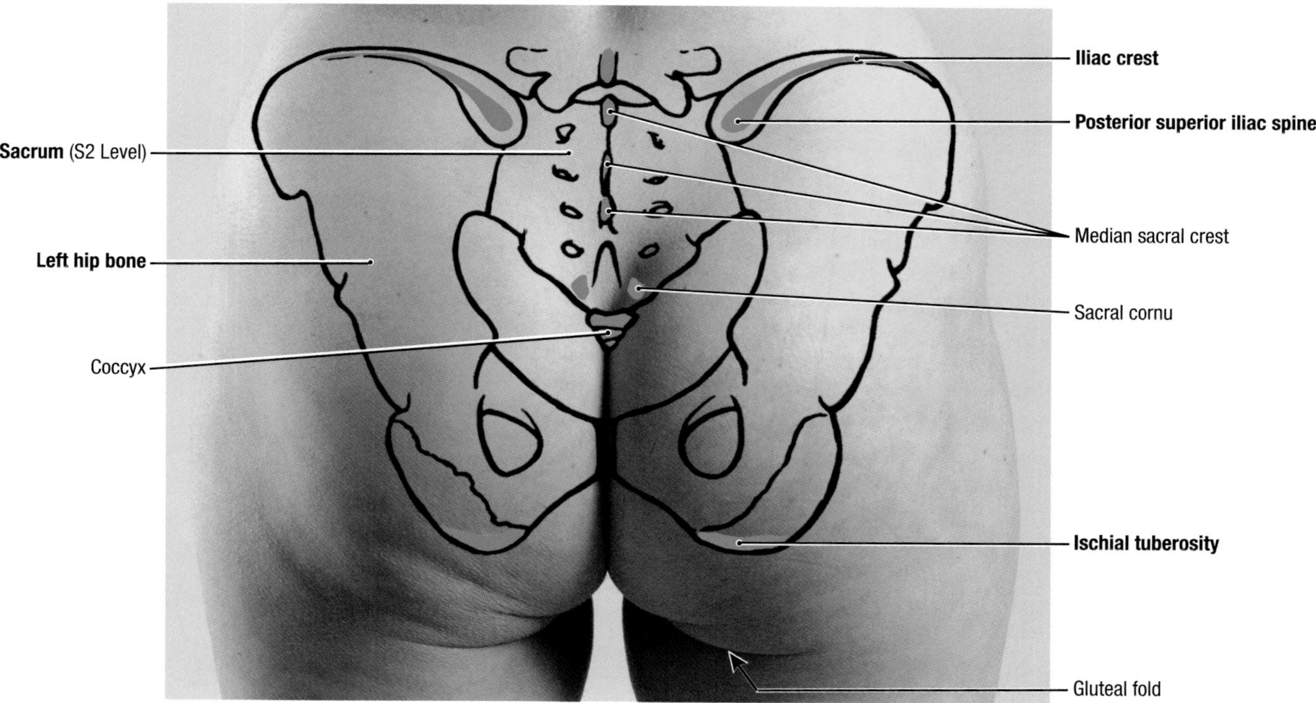
Sacrum (S2 Level)
Left hip bone
Coccyx
Iliac crest
Posterior superior iliac spine
Median sacral crest
Sacral cornu
Ischial tuberosity
Gluteal fold

**B.** Posterior View

## 3.2 Surface anatomy of the female pelvic girdle

The female pelvic girdle is relatively wider and shallower than that of the male, related to its additional roles of bearing the weight of the gravid uterus in late pregnancy, and allowing passage of the fetus through the pelvic outlet during childbirth (parturition). (*Green:* palpable features) **A.** The hip bones are joined anteriorly at the pubic symphysis. The presence of a thick overlying pubic fat-pad forming the mons pubis may interfere with palpation of the pubic tubercles and symphysis. **B.** Posteriorly the hip bones are joined to the sacrum at the sacroiliac joints.

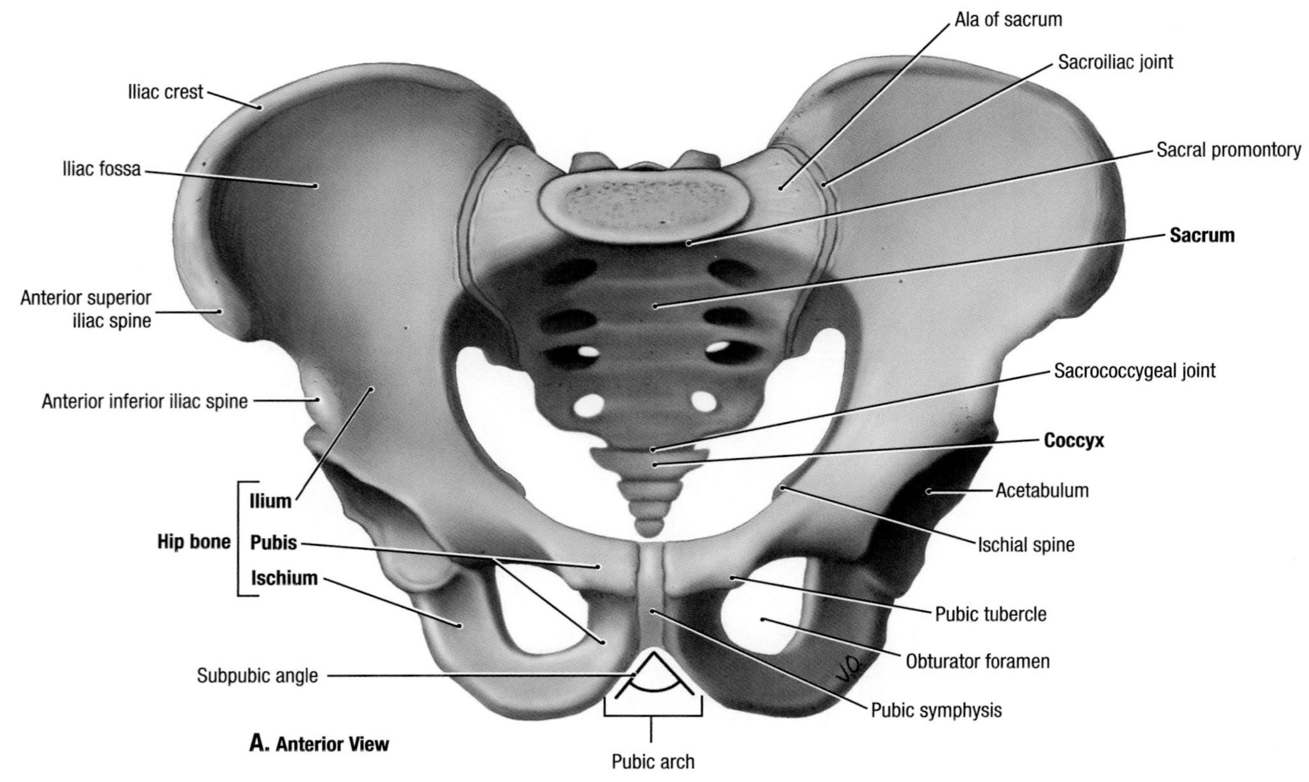
Ala of sacrum
Sacroiliac joint
Iliac crest
Iliac fossa
Sacral promontory
Sacrum
Anterior superior iliac spine
Anterior inferior iliac spine
Sacrococcygeal joint
Coccyx
Acetabulum
Hip bone
Ilium
Pubis
Ischium
Ischial spine
Pubic tubercle
Obturator foramen
Subpubic angle
Pubic symphysis
Pubic arch

A. Anterior View

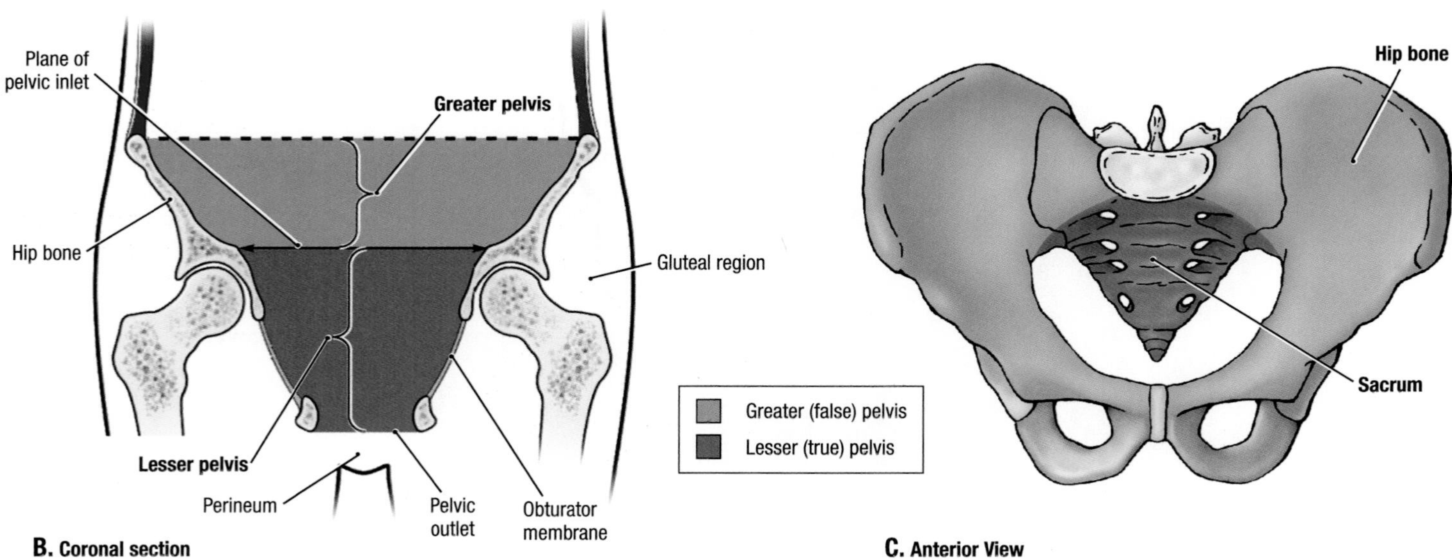
Plane of pelvic inlet
Greater pelvis
Hip bone
Gluteal region
Lesser pelvis
Perineum
Pelvic outlet
Obturator membrane
Greater (false) pelvis
Lesser (true) pelvis
Hip bone
Sacrum

B. Coronal section

C. Anterior View

## 3.3 Bones and divisions of pelvis

**A.** Bones of pelvis. The three bones composing the pelvis are the pubis, ischium, and ilium. **B** and **C.** Lesser and greater pelvis, schematic illustrations. The plane of the pelvic inlet (*double-headed arrow* in **B**) separates the greater pelvis (part of the abdominal cavity) from the lesser pelvis (pelvic cavity).

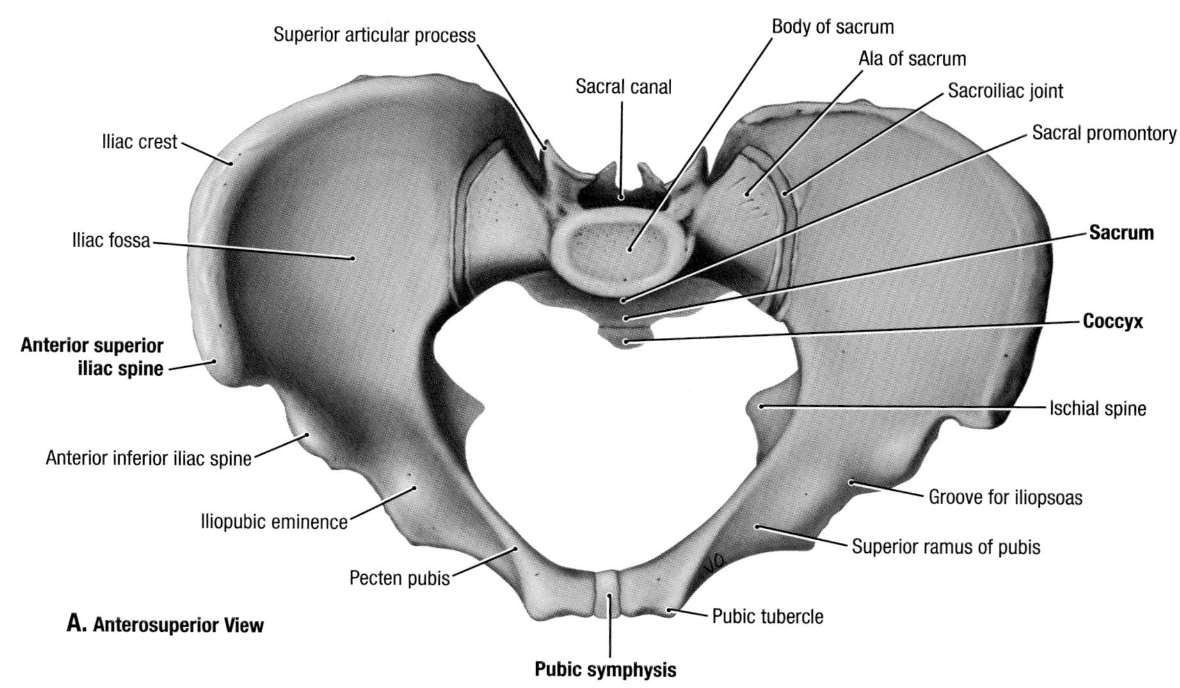
Superior articular process
Body of sacrum
Ala of sacrum
Sacral canal
Sacroiliac joint
Sacral promontory
Iliac crest
Iliac fossa
Sacrum
Coccyx
Anterior superior iliac spine
Ischial spine
Anterior inferior iliac spine
Groove for iliopsoas
Iliopubic eminence
Superior ramus of pubis
Pecten pubis
Pubic tubercle
Pubic symphysis
A. Anterosuperior View

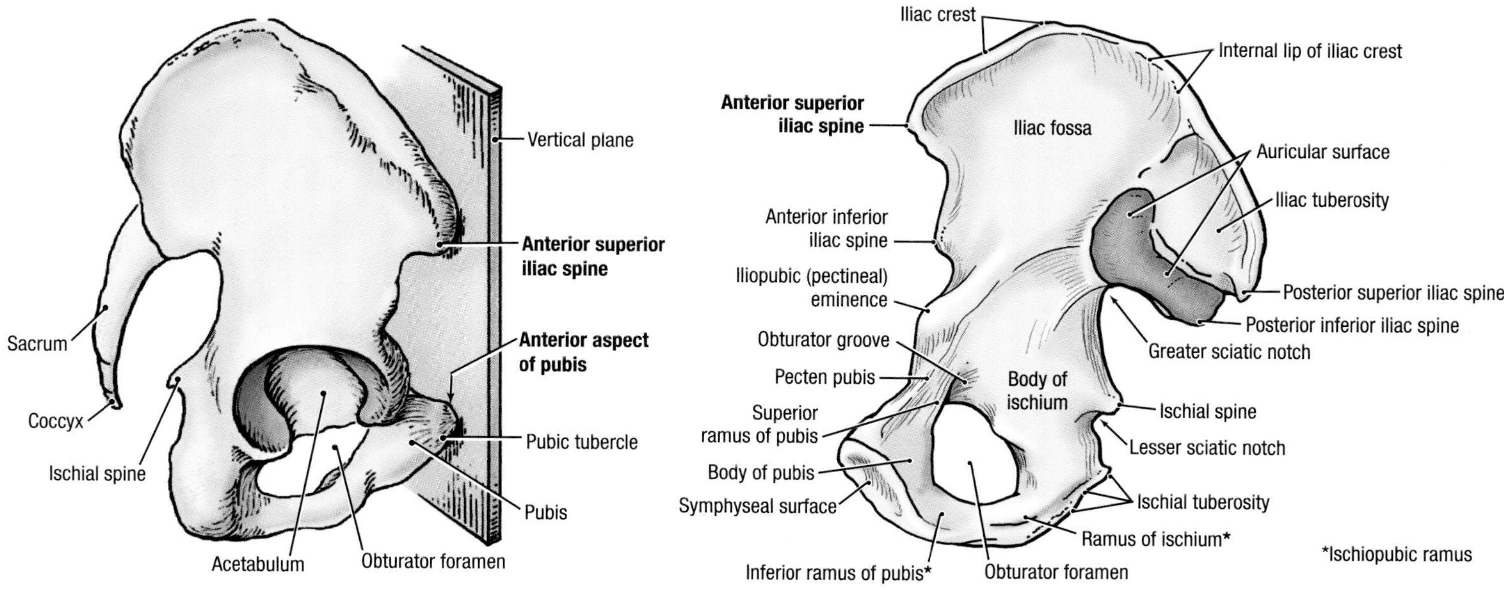
Vertical plane
Anterior superior iliac spine
Anterior aspect of pubis
Sacrum
Coccyx
Ischial spine
Pubic tubercle
Pubis
Acetabulum
Obturator foramen
Iliac crest
Internal lip of iliac crest
Anterior superior iliac spine
Iliac fossa
Auricular surface
Iliac tuberosity
Anterior inferior iliac spine
Iliopubic (pectineal) eminence
Posterior superior iliac spine
Posterior inferior iliac spine
Greater sciatic notch
Obturator groove
Pecten pubis
Body of ischium
Superior ramus of pubis
Ischial spine
Lesser sciatic notch
Body of pubis
Symphyseal surface
Ischial tuberosity
Ramus of ischium*
Inferior ramus of pubis*
Obturator foramen
*Ischiopubic ramus
B. Lateral View

C. Medial Aspect

## 3.4 Pelvis, anatomical position

**A.** Pelvic girdle. **B.** Placement of hip bone in anatomical position. In the anatomical position: (1) the anterior superior iliac spine and the anterior aspect of the pubis lie in the same vertical plane; (2) the sacrum is located superiorly, the coccyx posteriorly and the pubic symphysis anteroinferiorly. **C.** Features of hip bone.

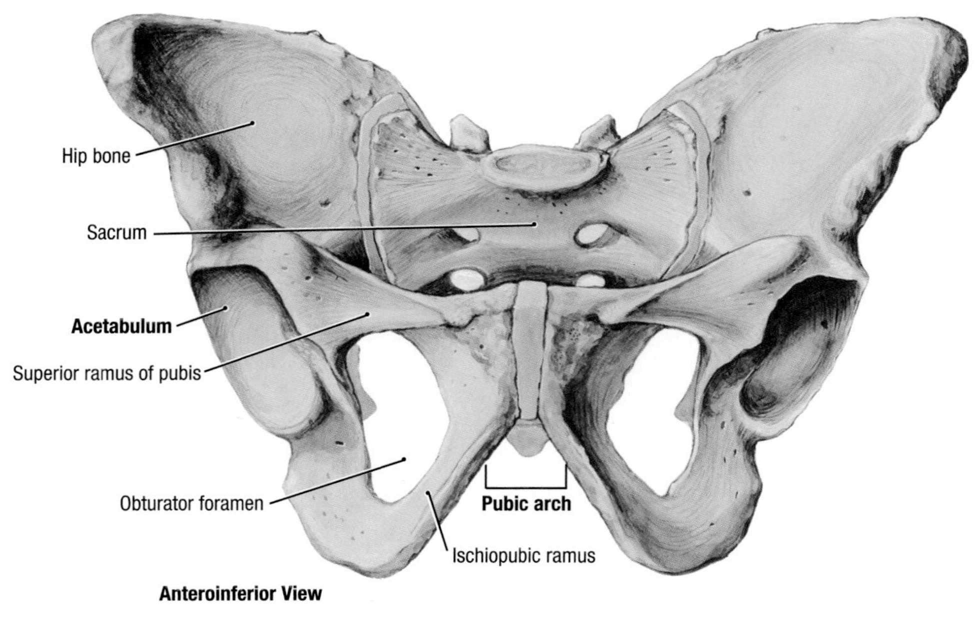
Hip bone
Sacrum
Acetabulum
Superior ramus of pubis
Obturator foramen
Pubic arch
Ischiopubic ramus
Anteroinferior View

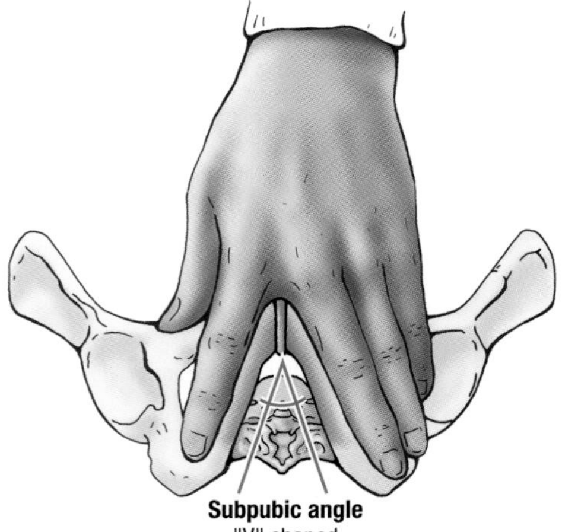
Subpubic angle
"V" shaped

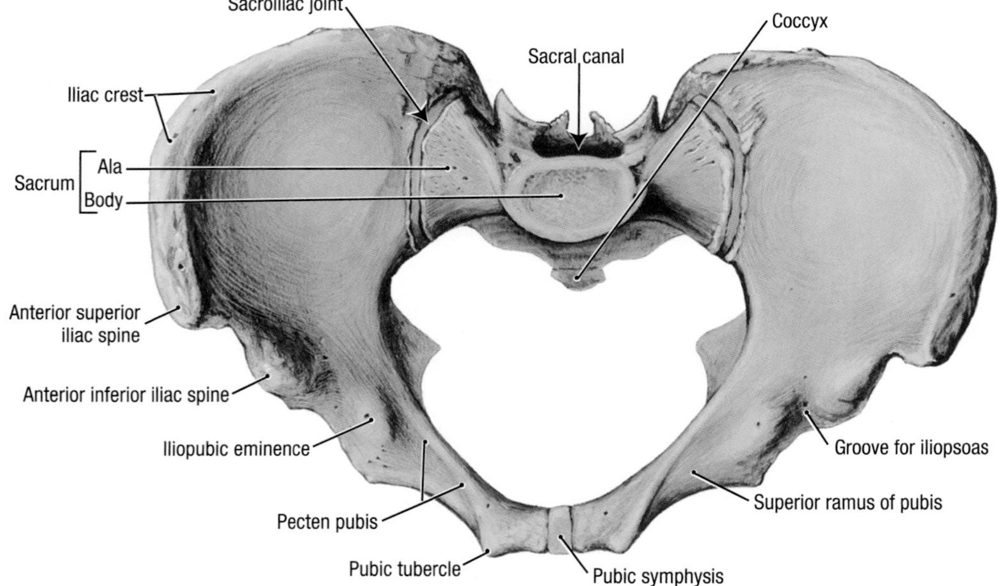
Sacroiliac joint
Coccyx
Sacral canal
Iliac crest
Sacrum
Ala
Body
Anterior superior iliac spine
Anterior inferior iliac spine
Iliopubic eminence
Groove for iliopsoas
Superior ramus of pubis
Pecten pubis
Pubic tubercle
Pubic symphysis
Anterosuperior View

## 3.5 Male pelvic girdle

**TABLE 3.1 DIFFERENCES BETWEEN MALE AND FEMALE PELVES** (continued on next page)

| Bony pelvis | Male | Female |
|---|---|---|
| General structure | Thick and heavy | Thin and light |
| Greater pelvis (pelvis major) | Deep | Shallow |
| Lesser pelvis (pelvis minor) | Narrow and deep, tapering | Wide and shallow, cylindrical |
| Pelvic inlet (superior pelvic aperture) | Heart shaped, narrow | Oval or rounded, wide |

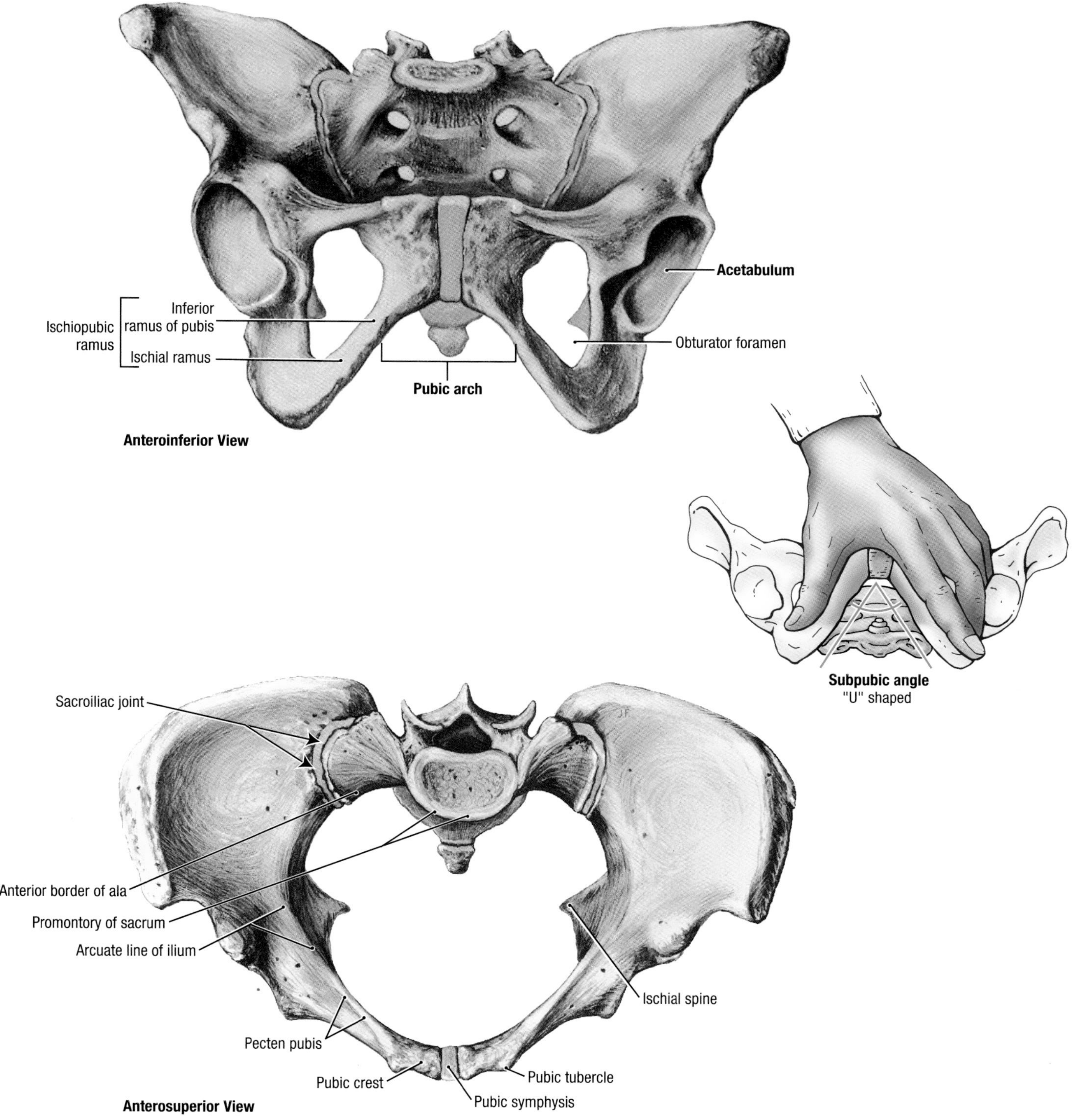
Acetabulum
Ischiopubic ramus
Inferior ramus of pubis
Ischial ramus
Obturator foramen
Pubic arch
Anteroinferior View
Subpubic angle
"U" shaped
Sacroiliac joint
Anterior border of ala
Promontory of sacrum
Arcuate line of ilium
Ischial spine
Pecten pubis
Pubic crest
Pubic tubercle
Pubic symphysis
Anterosuperior View

## 3.6 Female pelvic girdle

**TABLE 3.1 DIFFERENCES BETWEEN MALE AND FEMALE PELVES *(continued)***

| Bony pelvis | Male | Female |
|---|---|---|
| Pelvic outlet (inferior pelvic aperture) | Comparatively small | Comparatively large |
| Pubic arch and subpubic angle | Narrow | Wide |
| Obturator foramen | Round | Oval |
| Acetabulum | Large | Small |

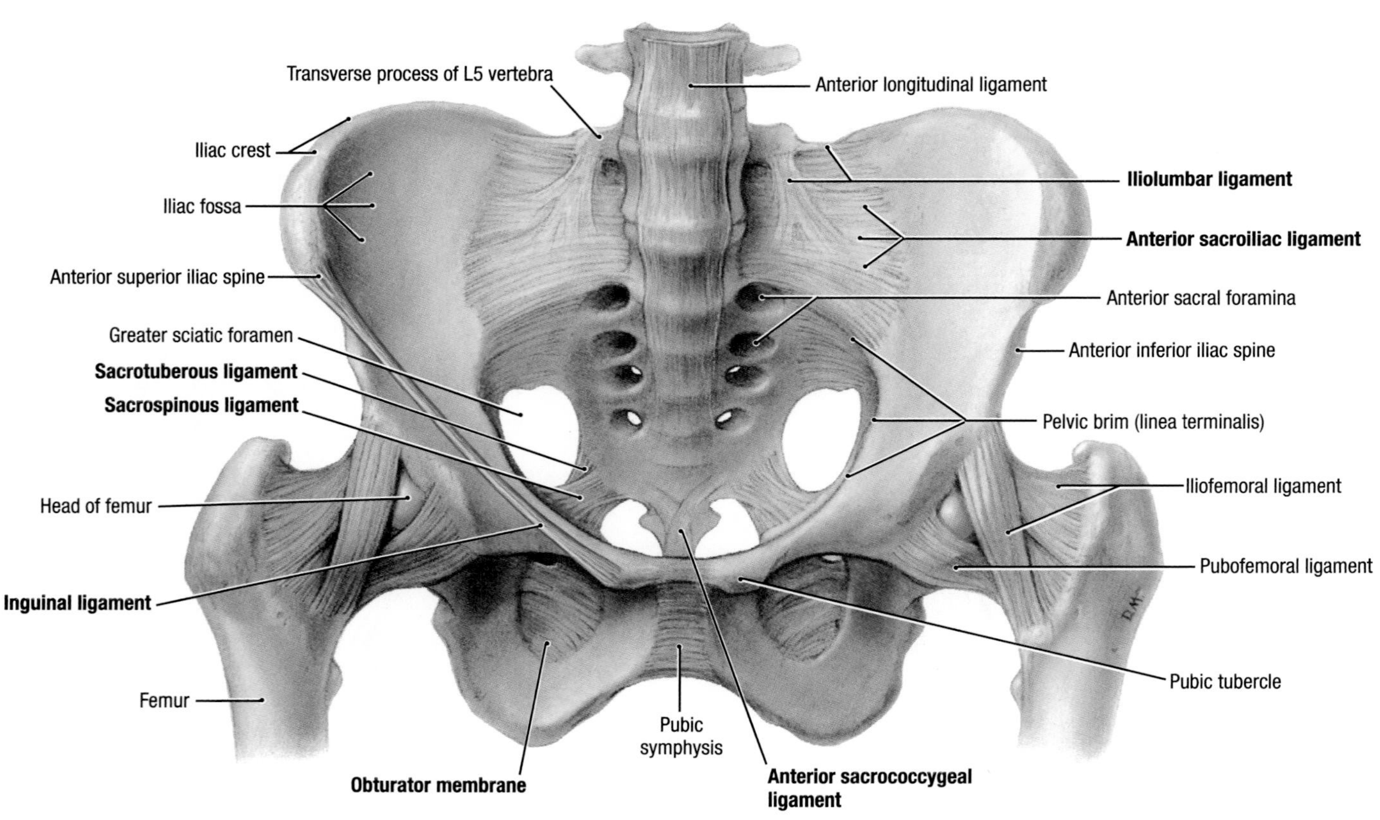
Transverse process of L5 vertebra
Anterior longitudinal ligament
Iliac crest
Iliolumbar ligament
Iliac fossa
Anterior sacroiliac ligament
Anterior superior iliac spine
Anterior sacral foramina
Greater sciatic foramen
Anterior inferior iliac spine
Sacrotuberous ligament
Sacrospinous ligament
Pelvic brim (linea terminalis)
Iliofemoral ligament
Head of femur
Pubofemoral ligament
Inguinal ligament
Pubic tubercle
Femur
Pubic symphysis
Obturator membrane
Anterior sacrococcygeal ligament
A. Anterior View

## 3.7 Pelvis and pelvic ligaments

**A.** Ligaments of pelvis, anterior aspect of pelvis.

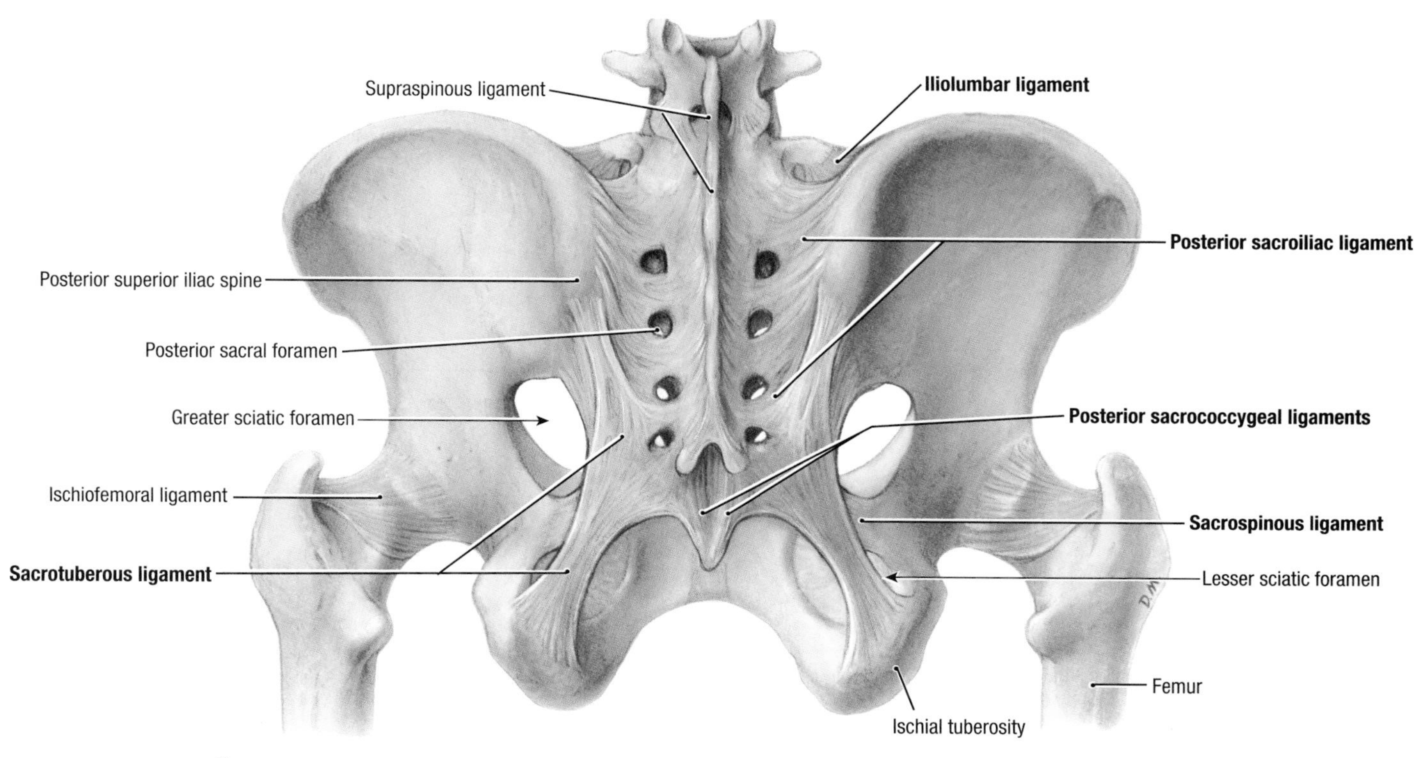
Supraspinous ligament
Iliolumbar ligament
Posterior sacroiliac ligament
Posterior superior iliac spine
Posterior sacral foramen
Greater sciatic foramen
Posterior sacrococcygeal ligaments
Ischiofemoral ligament
Sacrospinous ligament
Sacrotuberous ligament
Lesser sciatic foramen
Femur
Ischial tuberosity

**B.** **Posterior View**

## 3.7 Pelvis and pelvic ligaments *(continued)*

**B.** Ligaments of pelvis, posterior aspect of pelvis.

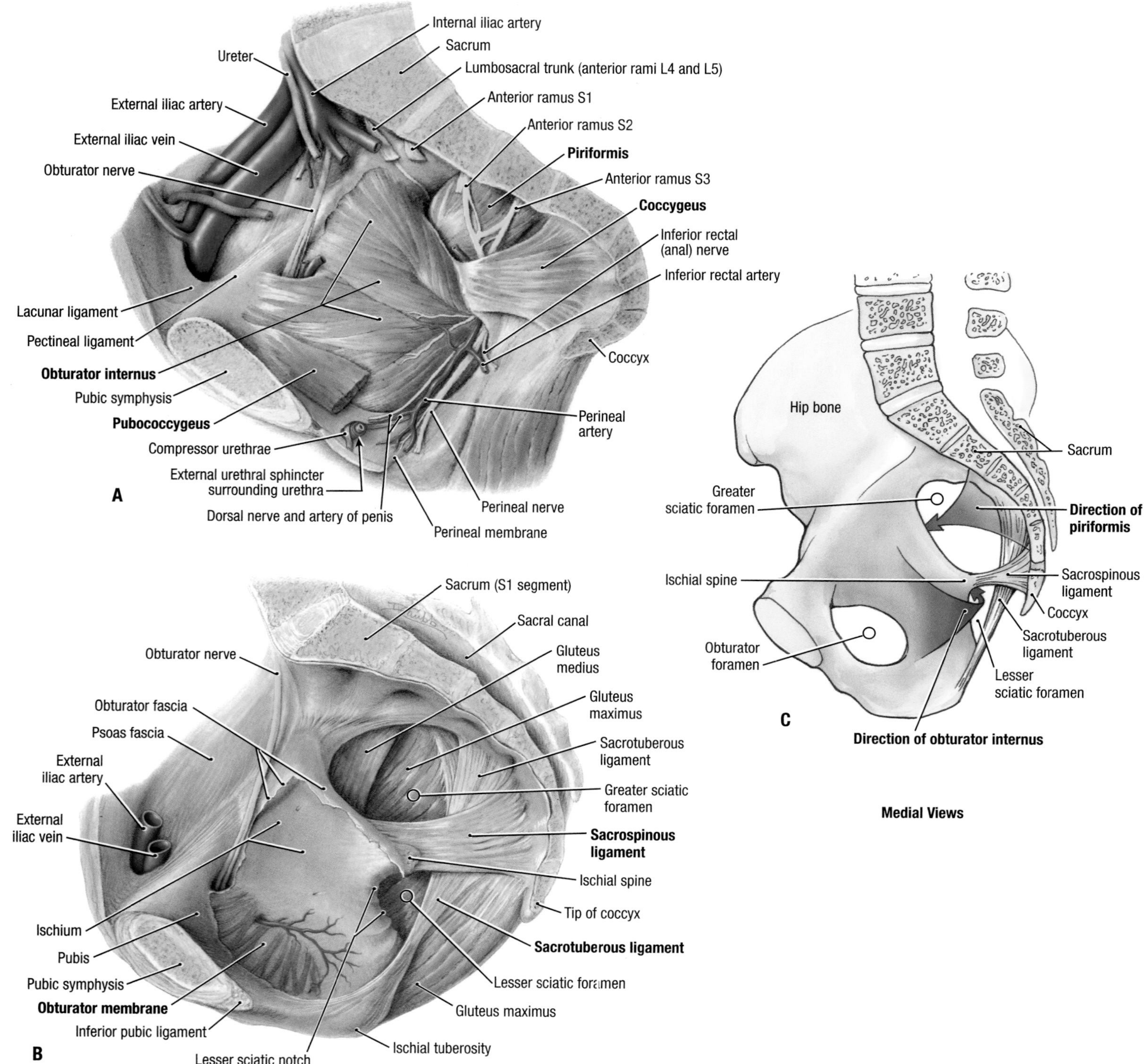

Internal iliac artery
Sacrum
Ureter
Lumbosacral trunk (anterior rami L4 and L5)
External iliac artery
Anterior ramus S1
Anterior ramus S2
External iliac vein
Piriformis
Obturator nerve
Anterior ramus S3
Coccygeus
Inferior rectal (anal) nerve
Inferior rectal artery
Lacunar ligament
Pectineal ligament
Obturator internus
Coccyx
Pubic symphysis
Pubococcygeus
Perineal artery
Compressor urethrae
External urethral sphincter surrounding urethra
A
Perineal nerve
Dorsal nerve and artery of penis
Perineal membrane
Sacrum (S1 segment)
Sacral canal
Obturator nerve
Gluteus medius
Obturator fascia
Gluteus maximus
Psoas fascia
Sacrotuberous ligament
External iliac artery
Greater sciatic foramen
External iliac vein
Sacrospinous ligament
Ischial spine
Ischium
Tip of coccyx
Sacrotuberous ligament
Pubis
Lesser sciatic foramen
Pubic symphysis
Obturator membrane
Gluteus maximus
Inferior pubic ligament
Ischial tuberosity
B
Lesser sciatic notch
Hip bone
Sacrum
Greater sciatic foramen
Direction of piriformis
Ischial spine
Sacrospinous ligament
Coccyx
Obturator foramen
Sacrotuberous ligament
Lesser sciatic foramen
C
Direction of obturator internus
Medial Views


## 3.8 Obturator internus and piriformis

- On the lateral pelvic wall the obturator foramen is closed by the obturator membrane; the obturator internus muscle attaches mainly to the obturator membrane and exits the lesser pelvis through the lesser sciatic foramen; obturator fascia lies on the medial surface of the muscle.
- Piriformis lies on the posterolateral pelvic wall and leaves the lesser pelvis through the greater sciatic foramen.

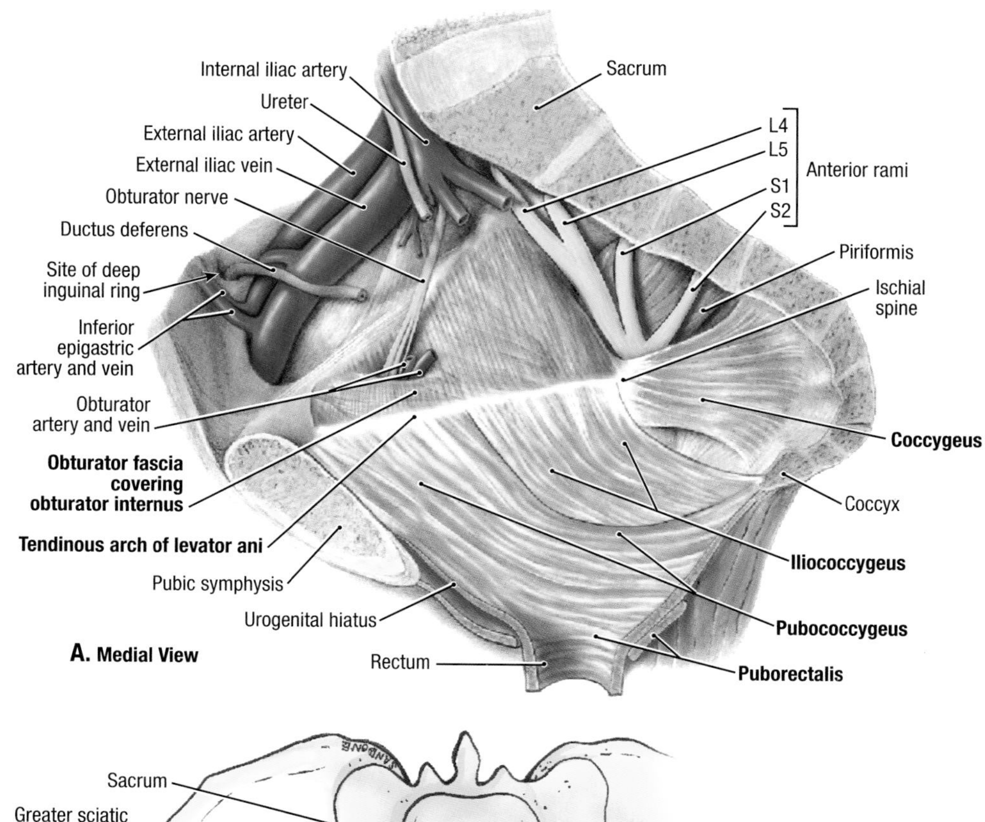
Internal iliac artery
Ureter
External iliac artery
External iliac vein
Obturator nerve
Ductus deferens
Site of deep inguinal ring
Inferior epigastric artery and vein
Obturator artery and vein
Obturator fascia covering obturator internus
Tendinous arch of levator ani
Pubic symphysis
Urogenital hiatus
A. Medial View
Rectum
Sacrum
L4
L5
S1
S2
Anterior rami
Piriformis
Ischial spine
Coccygeus
Coccyx
Iliococcygeus
Pubococcygeus
Puborectalis

**Muscles of floor of pelvis*:**

Pelvic diaphragm (PD) = Levator ani (LA) + Coccygeus (C)
(PD = LA + C)

Levator ani (LA) = Pubococcygeus (PC) + Iliococcygeus (IC)
(LA = PC + IC)

Pubococcygeus (PC ♀) = Puborectalis (PR) + Pubovaginalis (PV)
(PC = PR + PV ♀)

Pubococcygeus (PC ♂) = Puborectalis (PR) + Puboprostaticus
(PC = PR + LP ♂) (Levator prostatae [LP])

*Formulas: Dr. Larry M. Ross.
The University of Texas Medical School at Houston

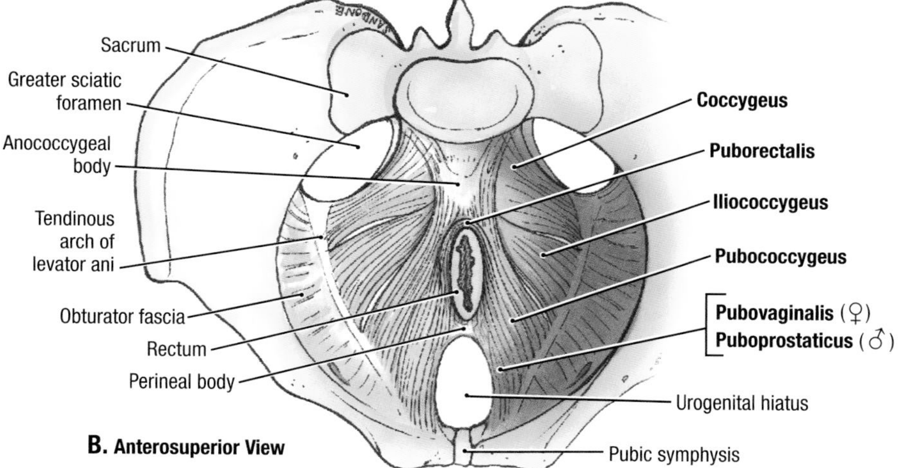
Sacrum
Greater sciatic foramen
Anococcygeal body
Tendinous arch of levator ani
Obturator fascia
Rectum
Perineal body
B. Anterosuperior View
Coccygeus
Puborectalis
Iliococcygeus
Pubococcygeus
Pubovaginalis (♀)
Puboprostaticus (♂)
Urogenital hiatus
Pubic symphysis

## 3.9 Muscles of the pelvic diaphragm

**A.** The pelvic floor is formed by the funnel- or bowl-shaped pelvic diaphragm. The funnel shape can be seen in a medial view of a median section. **B.** The bowl shape from a superior view.

**TABLE 3.2 MUSCLES OF PELVIC WALLS AND FLOOR**

| Boundary | Muscle | Proximal attachment | Distal attachment | Innervation | Main Action |
|---|---|---|---|---|---|
| Lateral wall | Obturator internus | Pelvic surfaces of ilium and ischium, obturator membrane | Greater trochanter of femur | Nerve to obturator internus (L5, S1, S2) | Rotates thigh laterally; assists in holding head of femur in acetabulum |
| Posterolateral wall | Piriformis | Pelvic surface of S2–S4 segments, superior margin of greater sciatic notch, sacrotuberous ligament | | Anterior rami of S1 and S2 | Rotates thigh laterally; abducts thigh; assists in holding head of femur in acetabulum |
| Floor | Levator ani (pubococcygeus, puborectalis, and iliococcygeus) | Body of pubis, tendinous arch of obturator fascia, ischial spine | Perineal body, coccyx, anococcygeal ligament, walls of prostate or vagina, rectum, and anal canal | Nerve to levator ani (branches of S4), inferior anal (rectal) nerve, and coccygeal plexus | Forms most of pelvic diaphragm that helps support pelvic viscera and resists increases in intra-abdominal pressure |
| | Coccygeus (ischiococcygeus) | Ischial spine | Inferior end of sacrum and coccyx | Branches of S4 and S5 spinal nerves | Forms small part of pelvic diaphragm that supports pelvic viscera; flexes coccyx |

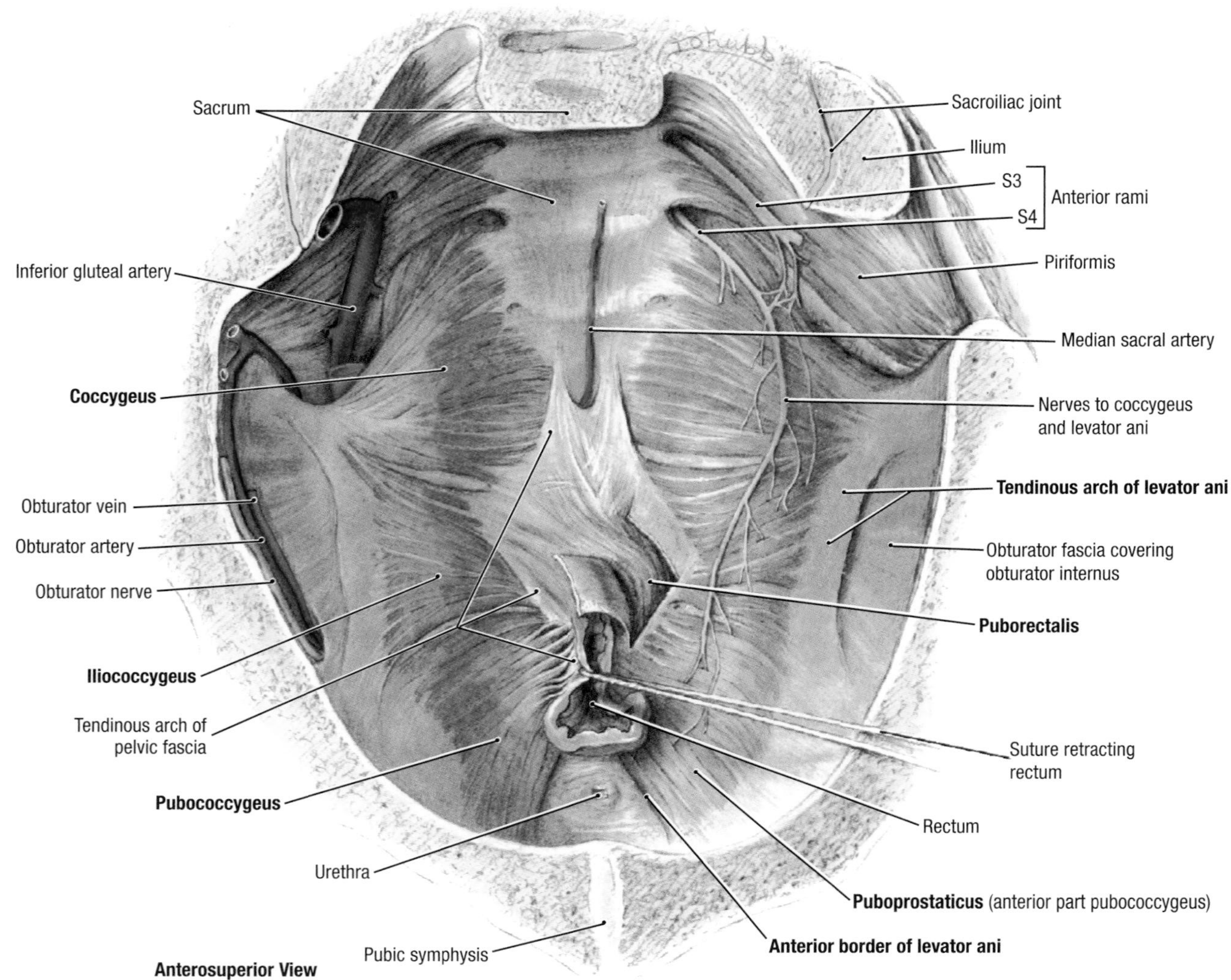
Sacrum
Sacroiliac joint
Ilium
S3
S4
Anterior rami
Piriformis
Inferior gluteal artery
Median sacral artery
Coccygeus
Nerves to coccygeus and levator ani
Tendinous arch of levator ani
Obturator vein
Obturator artery
Obturator fascia covering obturator internus
Obturator nerve
Puborectalis
Iliococcygeus
Tendinous arch of pelvic fascia
Suture retracting rectum
Pubococcygeus
Rectum
Urethra
Puboprostaticus (anterior part pubococcygeus)
Anterior border of levator ani
Pubic symphysis
Anterosuperior View

## 3.10 Floor and walls of male pelvis, pelvic diaphragm

The pelvic viscera are removed, and the bony pelvis has been cut to show the levator ani and coccygeus muscles.

- The pubococcygeus muscle arises mainly from the pubic bone, the iliococcygeus muscle from the tendinous arch, and the coccygeus muscle from the ischial spine.
- In the male, the anterior part of the pubococcygeus muscle that lies adjacent to the prostate is the puboprostaticus.
- Although not part of the pelvic diaphragm, the piriformis assists in closure of the pelvic outlet, largely occluding the greater sciatic foramen.

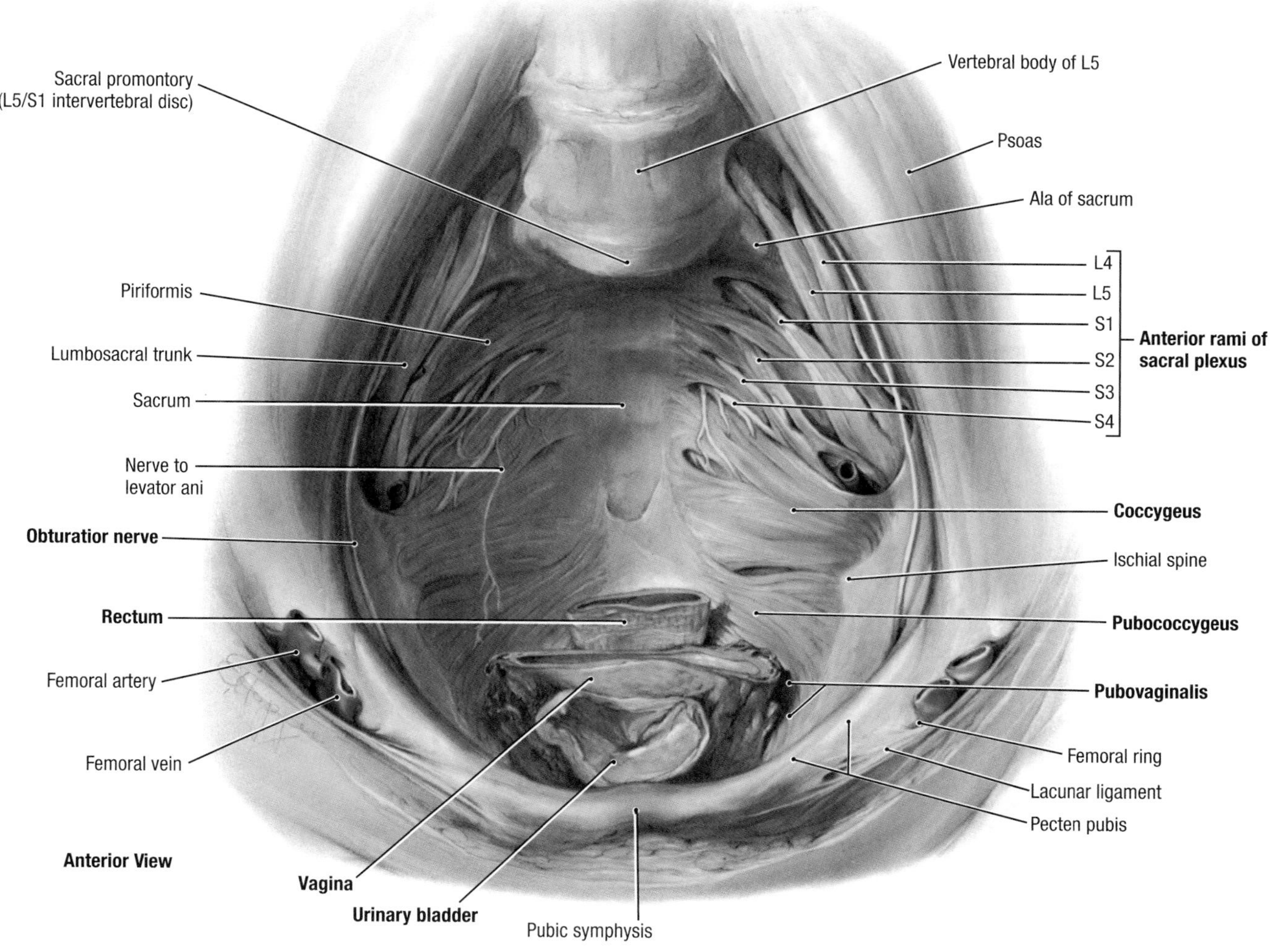
Sacral promontory (L5/S1 intervertebral disc)
Vertebral body of L5
Psoas
Ala of sacrum
L4
L5
S1
S2
S3
S4
Anterior rami of sacral plexus
Piriformis
Lumbosacral trunk
Sacrum
Nerve to levator ani
Obturatior nerve
Coccygeus
Ischial spine
Rectum
Pubococcygeus
Femoral artery
Pubovaginalis
Femoral vein
Femoral ring
Lacunar ligament
Pecten pubis
Anterior View
Vagina
Urinary bladder
Pubic symphysis

## 3.11 Floor and walls of female pelvis

The pelvic viscera are removed to reveal the levator ani and coccygeus muscles.

- Note the relative positions of the bladder, vagina, and rectum as they penetrate the pelvic floor.
- Branches of S3 and S4 nerves supply the levator ani and coccygeus muscles; the pudendal nerve, through its perineal branch, also supplies the levator ani muscle (see Table 3.2).
- The obturator nerve runs along the lateral wall of the pelvis and enters the thigh by passing through the obturator canal.
- The anterior rami of L4–S4 are part of the sacral plexus, almost all of which exits the pelvis via the greater sciatic foramen with the piriformis.

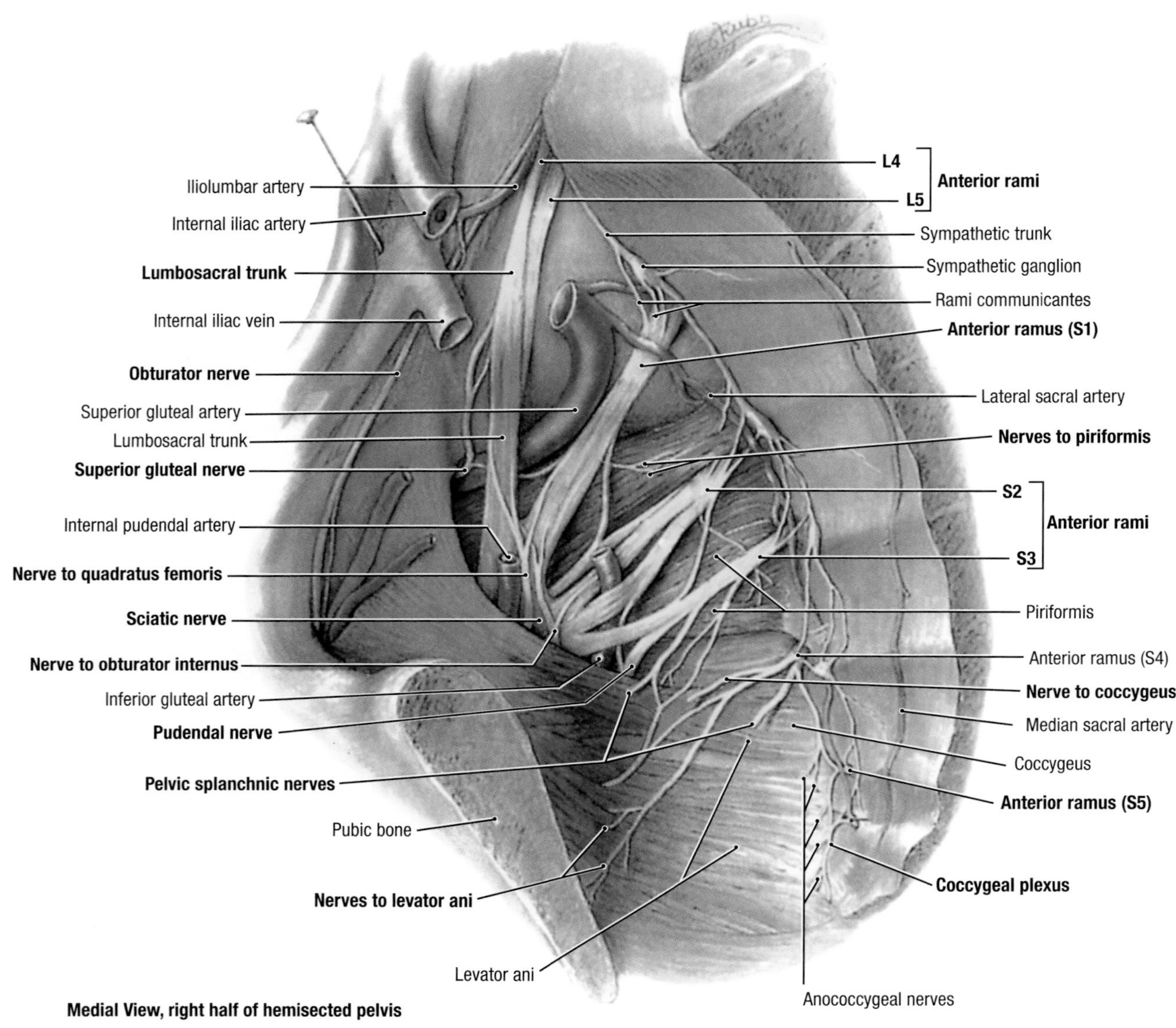
Iliolumbar artery
Internal iliac artery
Lumbosacral trunk
Internal iliac vein
Obturator nerve
Superior gluteal artery
Lumbosacral trunk
Superior gluteal nerve
Internal pudendal artery
Nerve to quadratus femoris
Sciatic nerve
Nerve to obturator internus
Inferior gluteal artery
Pudendal nerve
Pelvic splanchnic nerves
Pubic bone
Nerves to levator ani
Levator ani
L4
L5
Anterior rami
Sympathetic trunk
Sympathetic ganglion
Rami communicantes
Anterior ramus (S1)
Lateral sacral artery
Nerves to piriformis
S2
S3
Anterior rami
Piriformis
Anterior ramus (S4)
Nerve to coccygeus
Median sacral artery
Coccygeus
Anterior ramus (S5)
Coccygeal plexus
Anococcygeal nerves

**Medial View, right half of hemisected pelvis**

## 3.12 Sacral and coccygeal nerve plexuses

- The sympathetic trunk or its ganglia send rami communicantes to each sacral and coccygeal nerve.
- The anterior ramus from L4 joins that of L5 to form the lumbosacral trunk.
- The anterior rami of S1 and S2 supply the piriformis muscle; S3 and S4 supply the coccygeus and levator ani muscles.
- The sciatic nerve arises from anterior rami of L4, L5, S1, S2, and S3; the pudendal nerve from S2, S3, and S4; and the coccygeal plexus from S4, S5, and coccygeal segments.

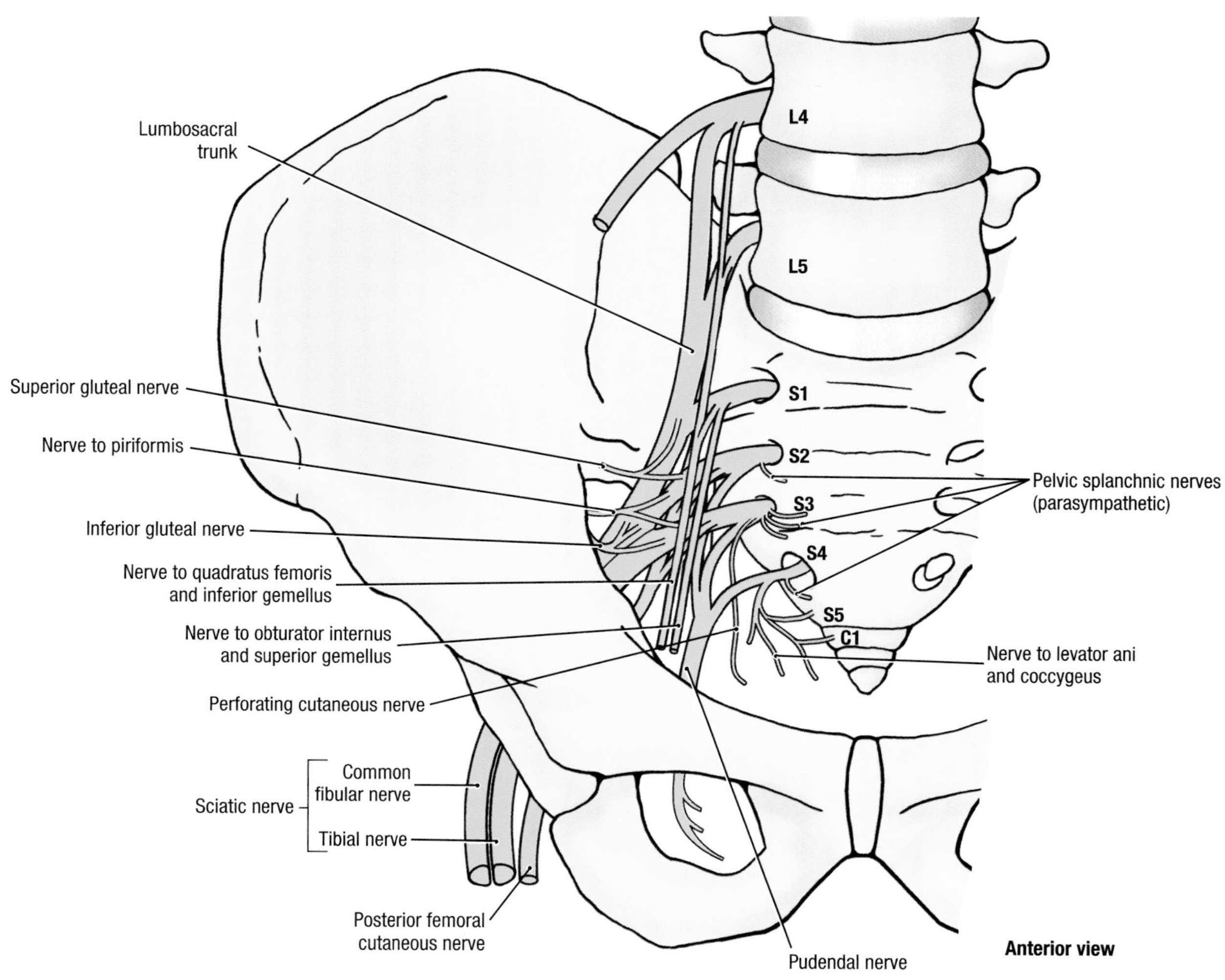
L4
L5
S1
S2
S3
S4
S5
C1
Lumbosacral trunk
Superior gluteal nerve
Nerve to piriformis
Inferior gluteal nerve
Nerve to quadratus femoris and inferior gemellus
Nerve to obturator internus and superior gemellus
Perforating cutaneous nerve
Sciatic nerve
Common fibular nerve
Tibial nerve
Posterior femoral cutaneous nerve
Pudendal nerve
Pelvic splanchnic nerves (parasympathetic)
Nerve to levator ani and coccygeus
Anterior view

**TABLE 3.3 NERVES OF SACRAL AND COCCYGEAL PLEXUSES**

| Nerve | Origin | Distribution |
|---|---|---|
| **Sciatic** | L4, L5, S1, S2, S3 | Articular branches to hip joint and muscular branches to flexors of knee in thigh and all muscles in leg and foot |
| **Superior gluteal** | L4, L5, S1 | Gluteus medius and gluteus minimus muscles |
| **Nerve to quadratus femoris and inferior gemellus** | L4, L5, S1 | Quadratus femoris and inferior gemellus muscles |
| **Inferior gluteal** | L5, S1, S2 | Gluteus maximus muscle |
| **Nerve to obturator internus and superior gemellus** | L5, S1, S2 | Obturator internus and superior gemellus muscles |
| **Nerve to piriformis** | S1, S2 | Piriformis muscle |
| **Posterior femoral cutaneous** | S2, S3 | Cutaneous branches to buttock and uppermost medial and posterior surfaces of thigh |
| **Perforating cutaneous** | S2, S3 | Cutaneous branches to medial part of buttock |
| **Pudendal** | S2, S3, S4 | Structures in perineum, sensory to genitalia, muscular branches to perineal muscles, external urethral sphincter, and external anal sphincter |
| **Pelvic splanchnic** | S2, S3, S4 | Pelvic viscera via inferior hypogastric and pelvic plexuses |
| **Nerves to levator ani and coccygeus** | S3, S4 | Levator ani and coccygeus muscles |

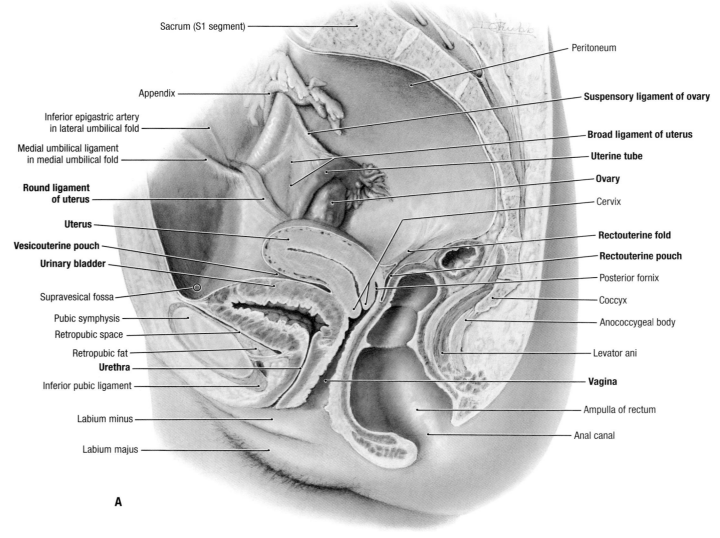

Sacrum (S1 segment)
Appendix
Inferior epigastric artery in lateral umbilical fold
Medial umbilical ligament in medial umbilical fold
**Round ligament of uterus**
**Uterus**
**Vesicouterine pouch**
**Urinary bladder**
Supravesical fossa
Pubic symphysis
Retropubic space
Retropubic fat
**Urethra**
Inferior pubic ligament
Labium minus
Labium majus
Peritoneum
**Suspensory ligament of ovary**
**Broad ligament of uterus**
**Uterine tube**
**Ovary**
Cervix
**Rectouterine fold**
**Rectouterine pouch**
Posterior fornix
Coccyx
Anococcygeal body
Levator ani
**Vagina**
Ampulla of rectum
Anal canal

**A**

**Medial Views**

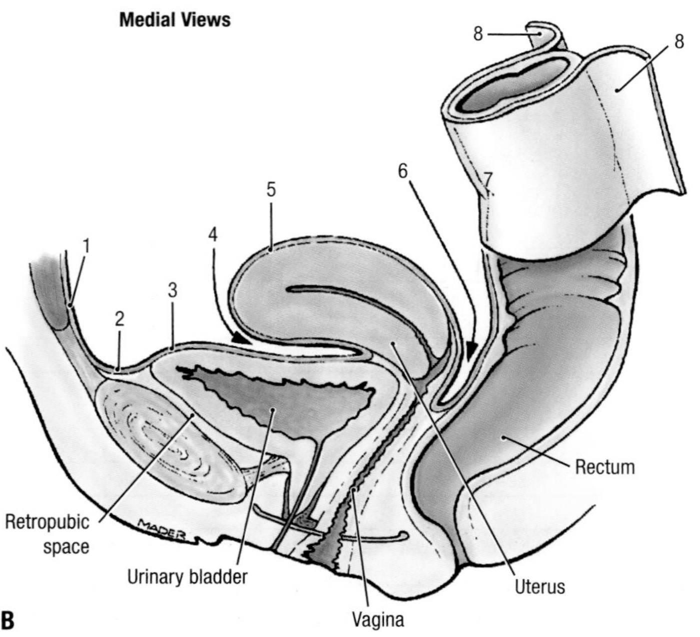
1
2
3
4
5
6
7
8
8
Rectum
Retropubic space
Urinary bladder
Vagina
Uterus
MADER

**B**

**Female:**
Peritoneum passes:
- From the anterior abdominal wall *(1)*
- Superior to the pubic bone *(2)*
- On the superior surface of the urnary bladder *(3)*
- From the bladder to the uterus, forming the vesicouterine pouch *(4)*
- On the fundus and body of the uterus, posterior formix. and all of the vagina *(5)*
- Between the rectum and uterus, forming the rectouterine pouch *(6)*
- On the anterior and lateral sides of the rectum *(7)*
- Posteriorly to become the sigmoid mesocolon *(8)*

## 3.13 Right half of hemisected female pelvis

**A.** Organs in situ.

- The urethra, the vagina, and the rectum are parallel to one another; the uterus is nearly at right angles to these structures when the bladder is empty.

**B.** Peritoneum covering female pelvic organs.

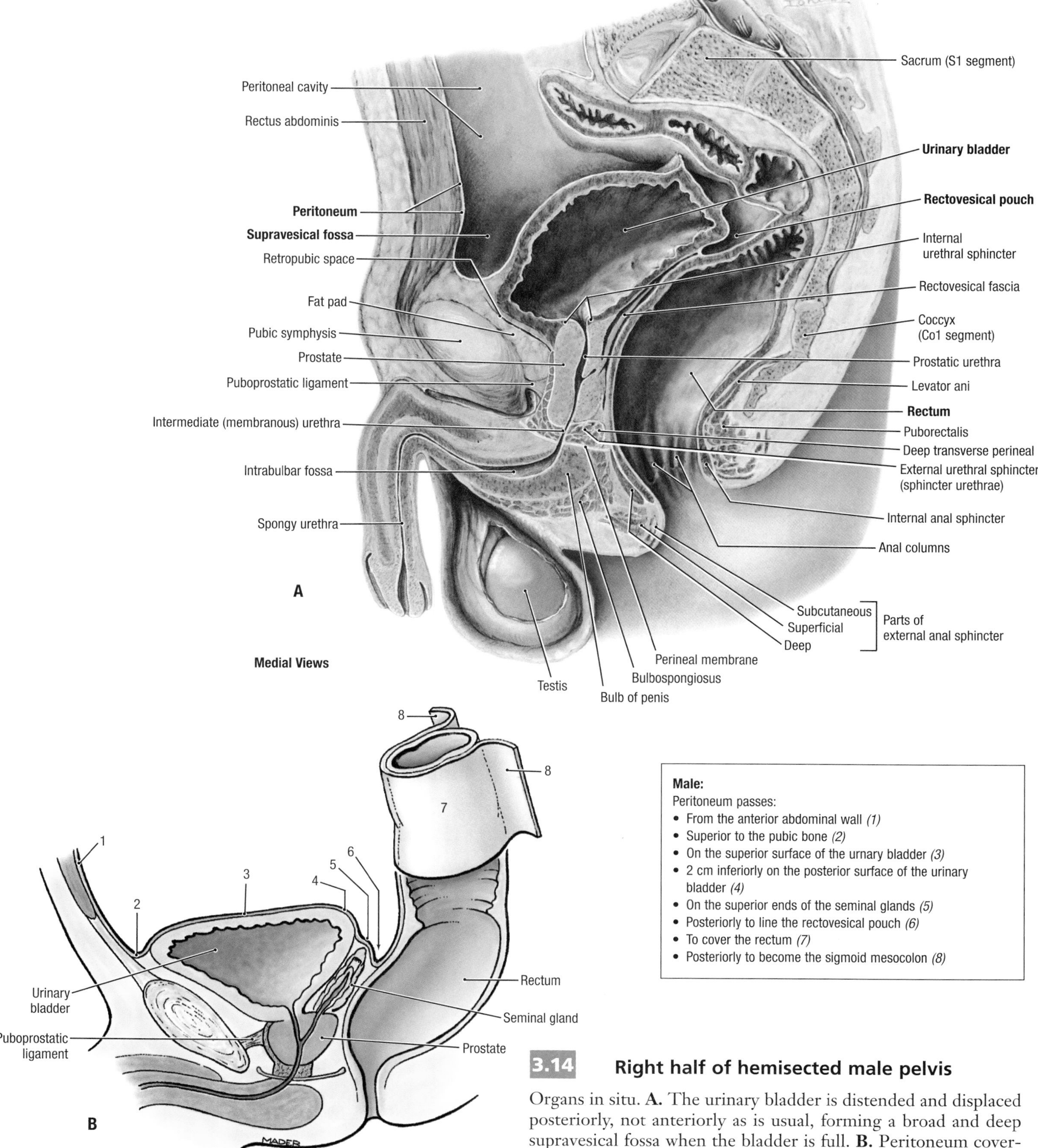
Peritoneal cavity
Rectus abdominis
Peritoneum
Supravesical fossa
Retropubic space
Fat pad
Pubic symphysis
Prostate
Puboprostatic ligament
Intermediate (membranous) urethra
Intrabulbar fossa
Spongy urethra
A
Medial Views
Sacrum (S1 segment)
Urinary bladder
Rectovesical pouch
Internal urethral sphincter
Rectovesical fascia
Coccyx (Co1 segment)
Prostatic urethra
Levator ani
Rectum
Puborectalis
Deep transverse perineal
External urethral sphincter (sphincter urethrae)
Internal anal sphincter
Anal columns
Subcutaneous
Superficial
Deep
Parts of external anal sphincter
Perineal membrane
Bulbospongiosus
Testis
Bulb of penis
8
8
7
1
2
3
4
5
6
Urinary bladder
Puboprostatic ligament
Rectum
Seminal gland
Prostate
B

**Male:**

Peritoneum passes:

- From the anterior abdominal wall *(1)*
- Superior to the pubic bone *(2)*
- On the superior surface of the urnary bladder *(3)*
- 2 cm inferiorly on the posterior surface of the urinary bladder *(4)*
- On the superior ends of the seminal glands *(5)*
- Posteriorly to line the rectovesical pouch *(6)*
- To cover the rectum *(7)*
- Posteriorly to become the sigmoid mesocolon *(8)*

## 3.14 Right half of hemisected male pelvis

Organs in situ. **A.** The urinary bladder is distended and displaced posteriorly, not anteriorly as is usual, forming a broad and deep supravesical fossa when the bladder is full. **B.** Peritoneum covering male pelvic organs.

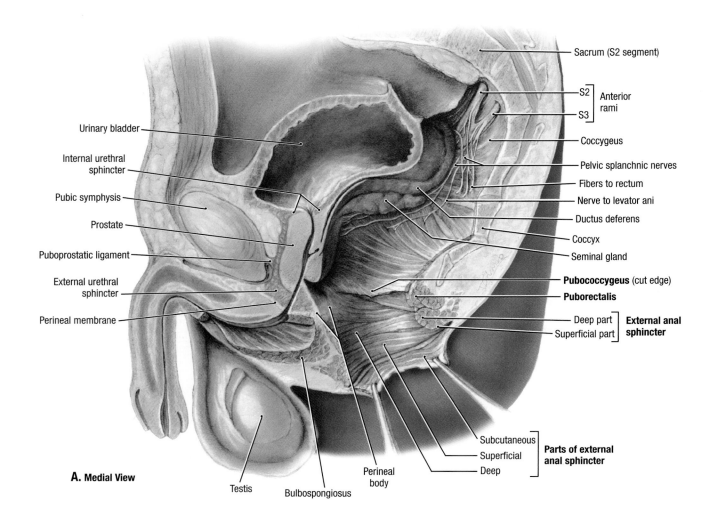

Sacrum (S2 segment)
S2
S3
Anterior rami
Coccygeus
Pelvic splanchnic nerves
Fibers to rectum
Nerve to levator ani
Ductus deferens
Coccyx
Seminal gland
**Pubococcygeus** (cut edge)
**Puborectalis**
Deep part
Superficial part
**External anal sphincter**
Urinary bladder
Internal urethral sphincter
Pubic symphysis
Prostate
Puboprostatic ligament
External urethral sphincter
Perineal membrane
Subcutaneous
Superficial
Deep
**Parts of external anal sphincter**
Testis
Bulbospongiosus
Perineal body

**A. Medial View**

## 3.15 Anal sphincters and anal canal

**A.** Levator ani, in right half of hemisected pelvis.

- The subcutaneous fibers of the external anal sphincter are reflected with forceps. The pubococcygeus muscle is cut to reveal the anal canal, to which it is, in part, attached.

**B.** Puborectalis.

- The innermost part of the pubococcygeus muscle, the puborectalis, forms a U-shaped muscular "sling" around the anorectal junction, which maintains the anorectal (perineal) flexure.

**C.** External and internal anal sphincters.

- The internal anal sphincter is a thickening of the inner, circular muscular coat of the anal canal.
- The external anal sphincter has three continuous zones: deep, superficial, and subcutaneous; the deep part intermingles with the puborectalis muscle posteriorly.
- The longitudinal muscle layer of the rectum separates the internal and external anal sphincters and terminates in the subcutaneous tissue and skin around the anus.

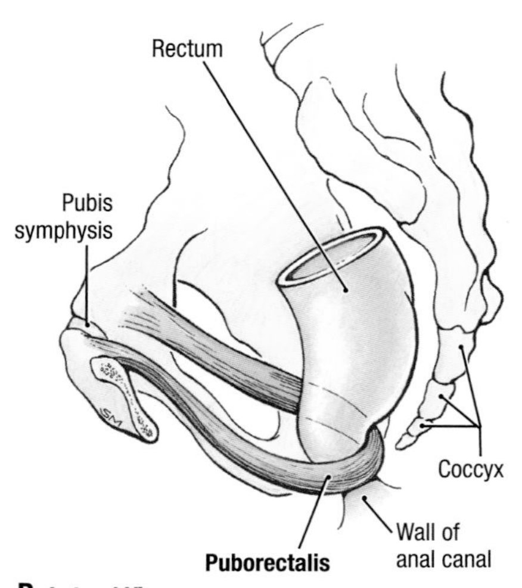
Rectum
Pubis symphysis
Coccyx
Wall of anal canal
Puborectalis

**B. Lateral View**

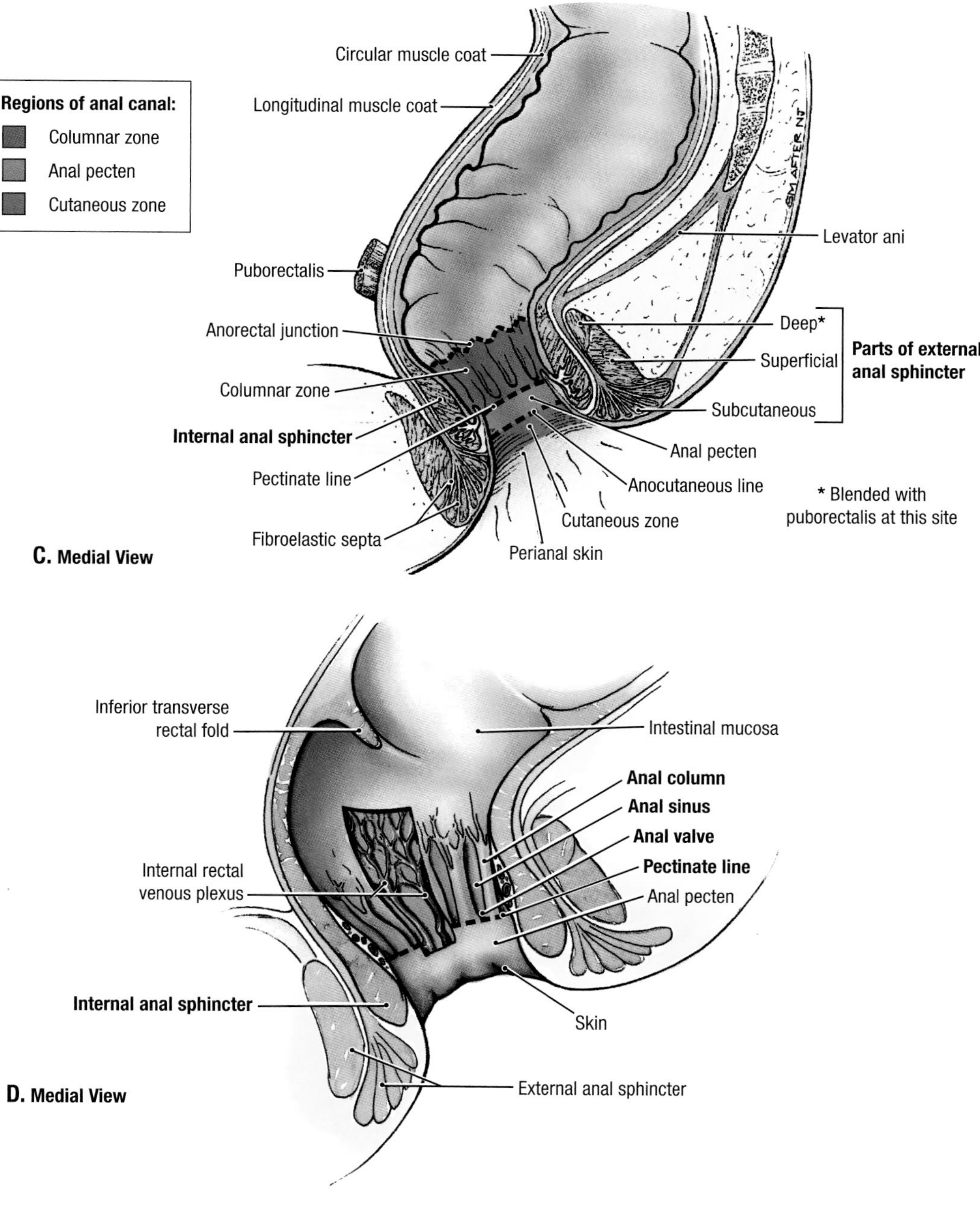
Regions of anal canal:
Columnar zone
Anal pecten
Cutaneous zone
Circular muscle coat
Longitudinal muscle coat
Puborectalis
Anorectal junction
Columnar zone
Internal anal sphincter
Pectinate line
Fibroelastic septa
Levator ani
Deep*
Superficial
Subcutaneous
Parts of external anal sphincter
Anal pecten
Anocutaneous line
Cutaneous zone
Perianal skin
* Blended with puborectalis at this site
C. Medial View
Inferior transverse rectal fold
Intestinal mucosa
Anal column
Anal sinus
Anal valve
Pectinate line
Anal pecten
Internal rectal venous plexus
Internal anal sphincter
Skin
External anal sphincter
D. Medial View

## 3.15 Anal sphincters and anal canal *(continued)*

**D.** Features of the anal canal.

- The anal columns are 5 to 10 vertical folds of mucosa separated by anal valves; they contain portions of the rectal venous plexus.
- The pecten is a smooth area of hairless stratified epithelium that lies between the anal valves superiorly and the inferior border of the internal anal sphincter inferiorly.
- The pectinate line is an irregular line at the base of the anal valves where the intestinal mucosa is continuous with the pecten; this indicates the junction of the *superior part of the anal canal (derived from embryonic hindgut)* and the inferior part of the *anal canal (derived from the anal pit [proctodeum])*. Innervation is visceral proximal to the line and somatic distally; lymphatic drainage is to the pararectal nodes proximally and to the superficial inguinal nodes distally.

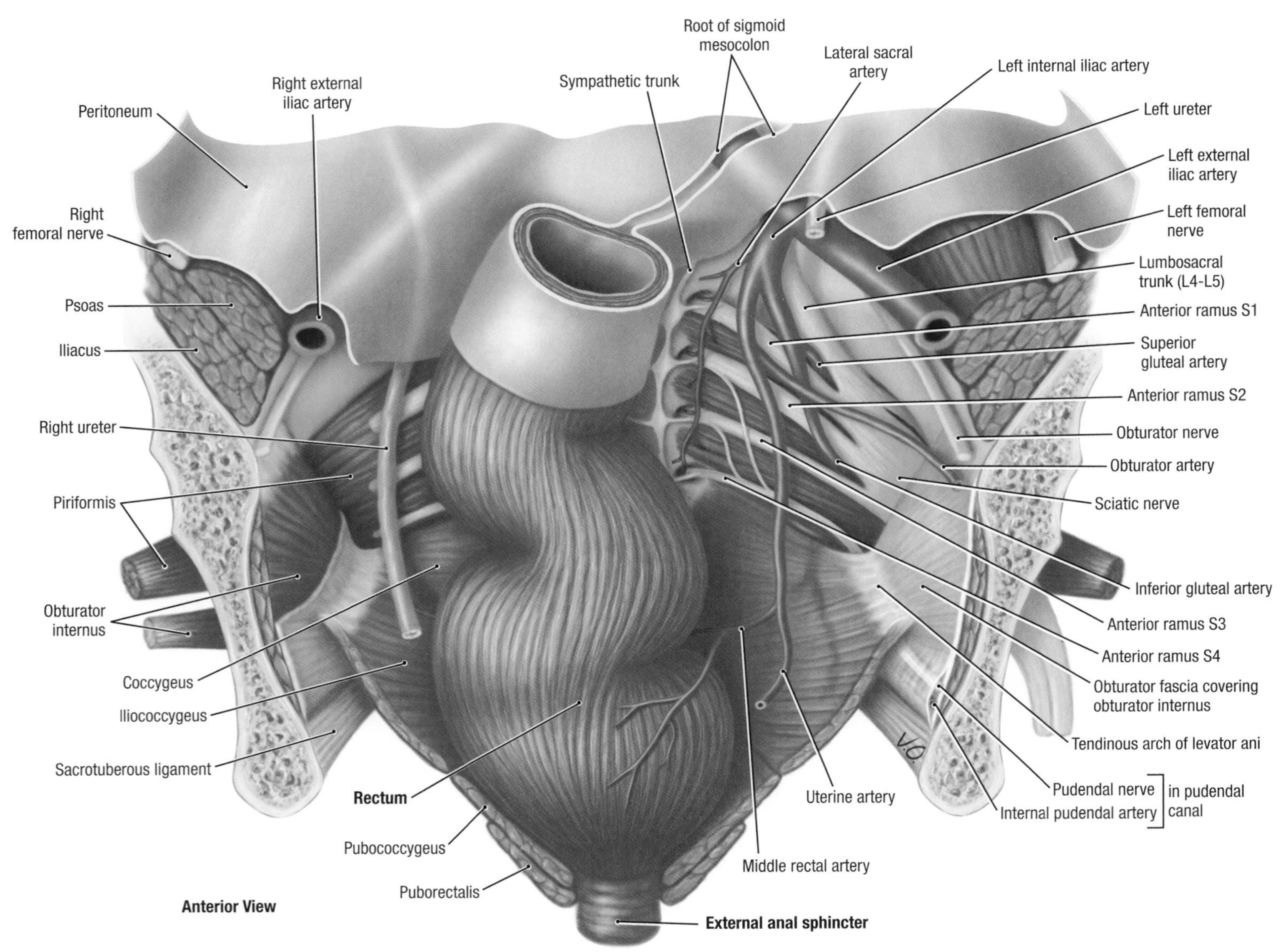
Root of sigmoid mesocolon
Lateral sacral artery
Left internal iliac artery
Sympathetic trunk
Right external iliac artery
Peritoneum
Left ureter
Left external iliac artery
Left femoral nerve
Right femoral nerve
Lumbosacral trunk (L4-L5)
Psoas
Anterior ramus S1
Iliacus
Superior gluteal artery
Anterior ramus S2
Right ureter
Obturator nerve
Obturator artery
Piriformis
Sciatic nerve
Inferior gluteal artery
Obturator internus
Anterior ramus S3
Anterior ramus S4
Coccygeus
Obturator fascia covering obturator internus
Iliococcygeus
Tendinous arch of levator ani
Sacrotuberous ligament
Pudendal nerve
Internal pudendal artery
in pudendal canal
Rectum
Uterine artery
Pubococcygeus
Middle rectal artery
Puborectalis
Anterior View
External anal sphincter

## 3.16 Rectum, anal canal, and neurovascular structures of the posterior pelvis

The pelvis is coronally bisected anterior to the rectum and anal canal. The superior gluteal artery often passes posteriorly between the anterior rami of L5 and S1, and the inferior gluteal artery between S2 and S3.

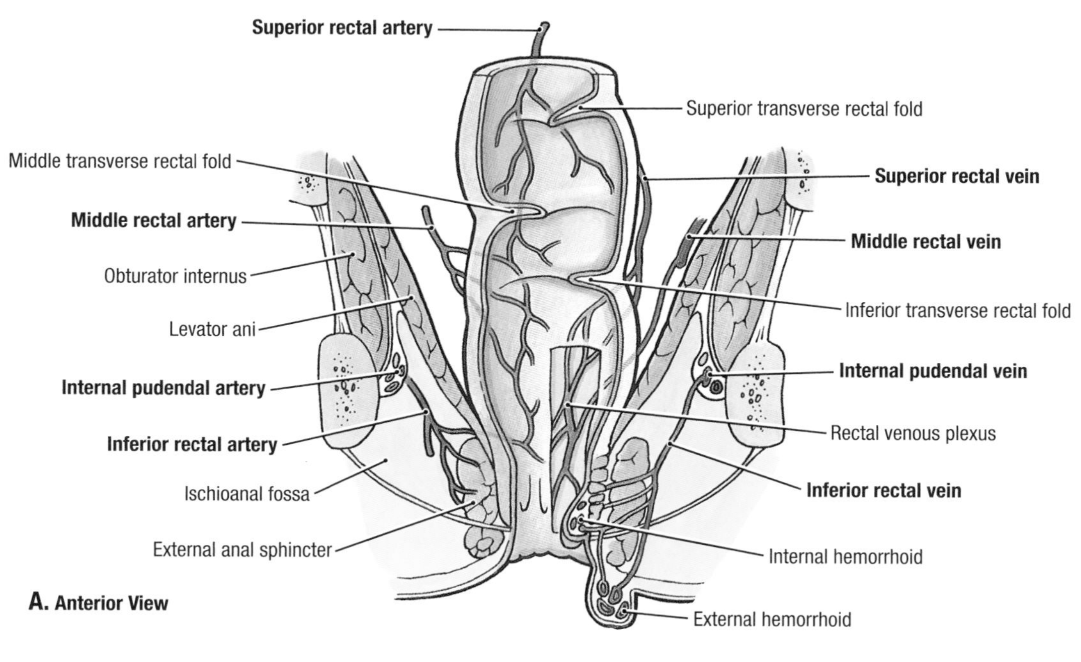
Superior rectal artery
Superior transverse rectal fold
Middle transverse rectal fold
Superior rectal vein
Middle rectal artery
Middle rectal vein
Obturator internus
Inferior transverse rectal fold
Levator ani
Internal pudendal artery
Internal pudendal vein
Inferior rectal artery
Rectal venous plexus
Ischioanal fossa
Inferior rectal vein
External anal sphincter
Internal hemorrhoid
External hemorrhoid
A. Anterior View

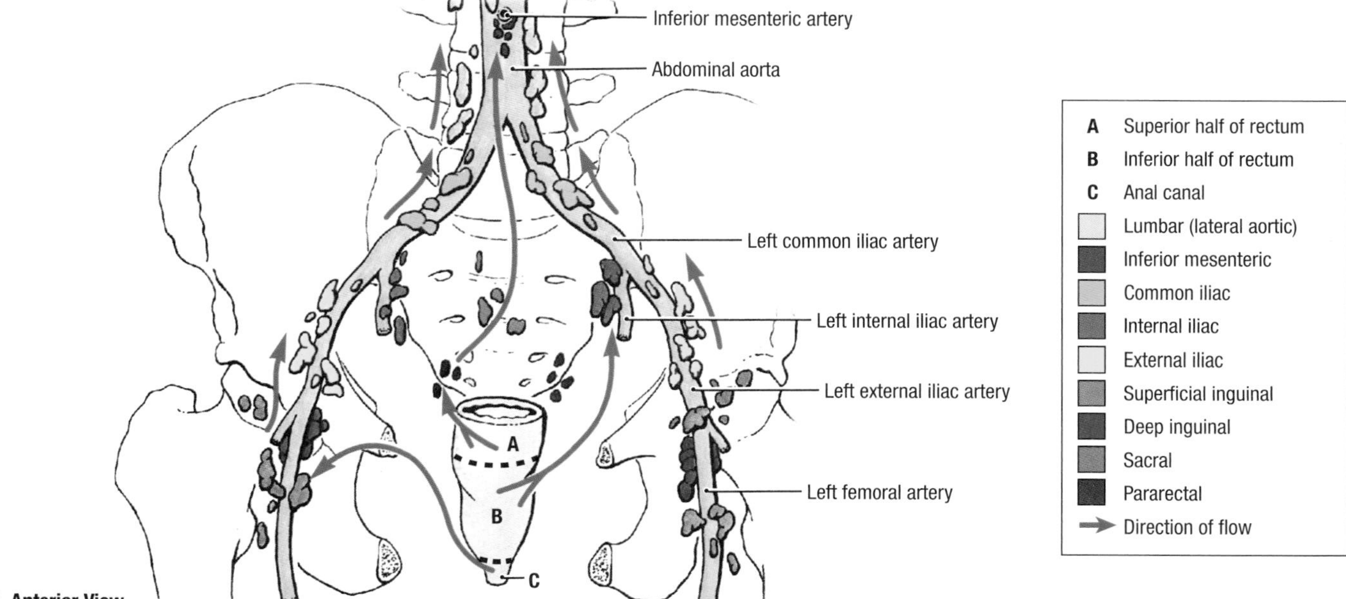
Inferior mesenteric artery
Abdominal aorta
A Superior half of rectum
B Inferior half of rectum
C Anal canal
Lumbar (lateral aortic)
Inferior mesenteric
Common iliac
Internal iliac
External iliac
Superficial inguinal
Deep inguinal
Sacral
Pararectal
Direction of flow
Left common iliac artery
Left internal iliac artery
Left external iliac artery
Left femoral artery
A
B
C
B. Anterior View

## 3.17 Vasculature of rectum

**A.** Arterial and venous drainage.

- The continuation of the inferior mesenteric artery, the superior rectal artery, supplies the proximal part of rectum.
- Right and left middle rectal arteries, usually arising from the inferior vesical (male) or uterine (female) arteries, supply the middle and inferior parts of the rectum.
- Inferior rectal arteries, arising from the internal pudendal arteries, supply the anorectal junction and the anal canal.

**B.** Lymphatic drainage.

- The superior, middle, and inferior rectal veins drain the rectum and anal canal; there are anastomoses between the plexuses formed by all three veins.
- The rectal venous plexus surrounds the distal rectum and anal canal and consists of an internal rectal plexus deep to the epithelium of the anal canal and an external rectal plexus external to the muscular coats of the wall of the anal canal.
- The superior rectal vein drains into the portal system, and the middle and inferior veins drain into the systemic system; thus, this is an important area of portacaval anastomosis.

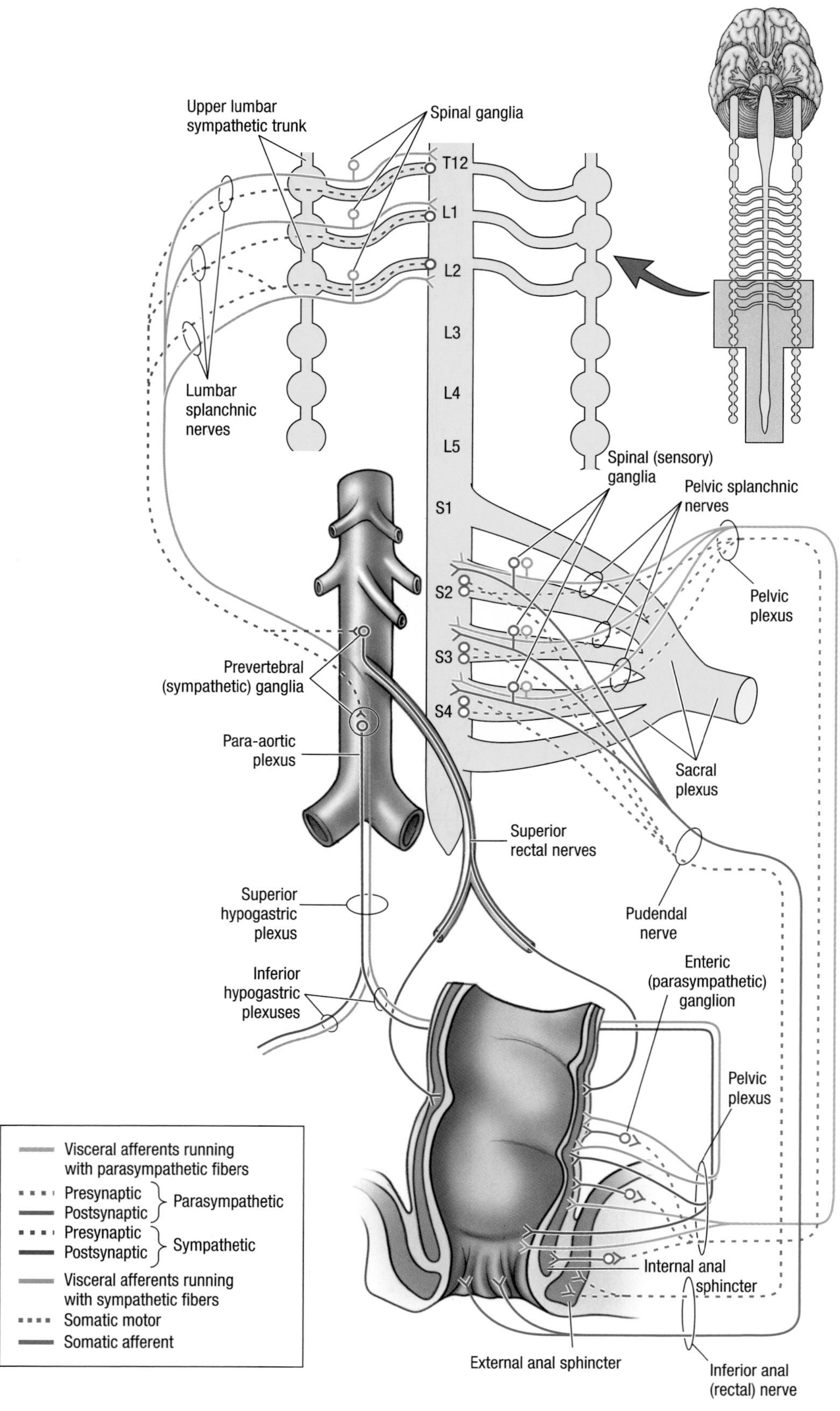
Upper lumbar sympathetic trunk
Spinal ganglia
T12
L1
L2
L3
L4
L5
S1
S2
S3
S4
Lumbar splanchnic nerves
Spinal (sensory) ganglia
Pelvic splanchnic nerves
Pelvic plexus
Prevertebral (sympathetic) ganglia
Para-aortic plexus
Sacral plexus
Superior rectal nerves
Superior hypogastric plexus
Pudendal nerve
Inferior hypogastric plexuses
Enteric (parasympathetic) ganglion
Pelvic plexus
Internal anal sphincter
External anal sphincter
Inferior anal (rectal) nerve
Visceral afferents running with parasympathetic fibers
Presynaptic
Postsynaptic
Parasympathetic
Presynaptic
Postsynaptic
Sympathetic
Visceral afferents running with sympathetic fibers
Somatic motor
Somatic afferent

## 3.18 Innervation of rectum and anal canal

The lumbar and pelvic spinal nerves and hypogastric plexuses have been retracted laterally for clarity.

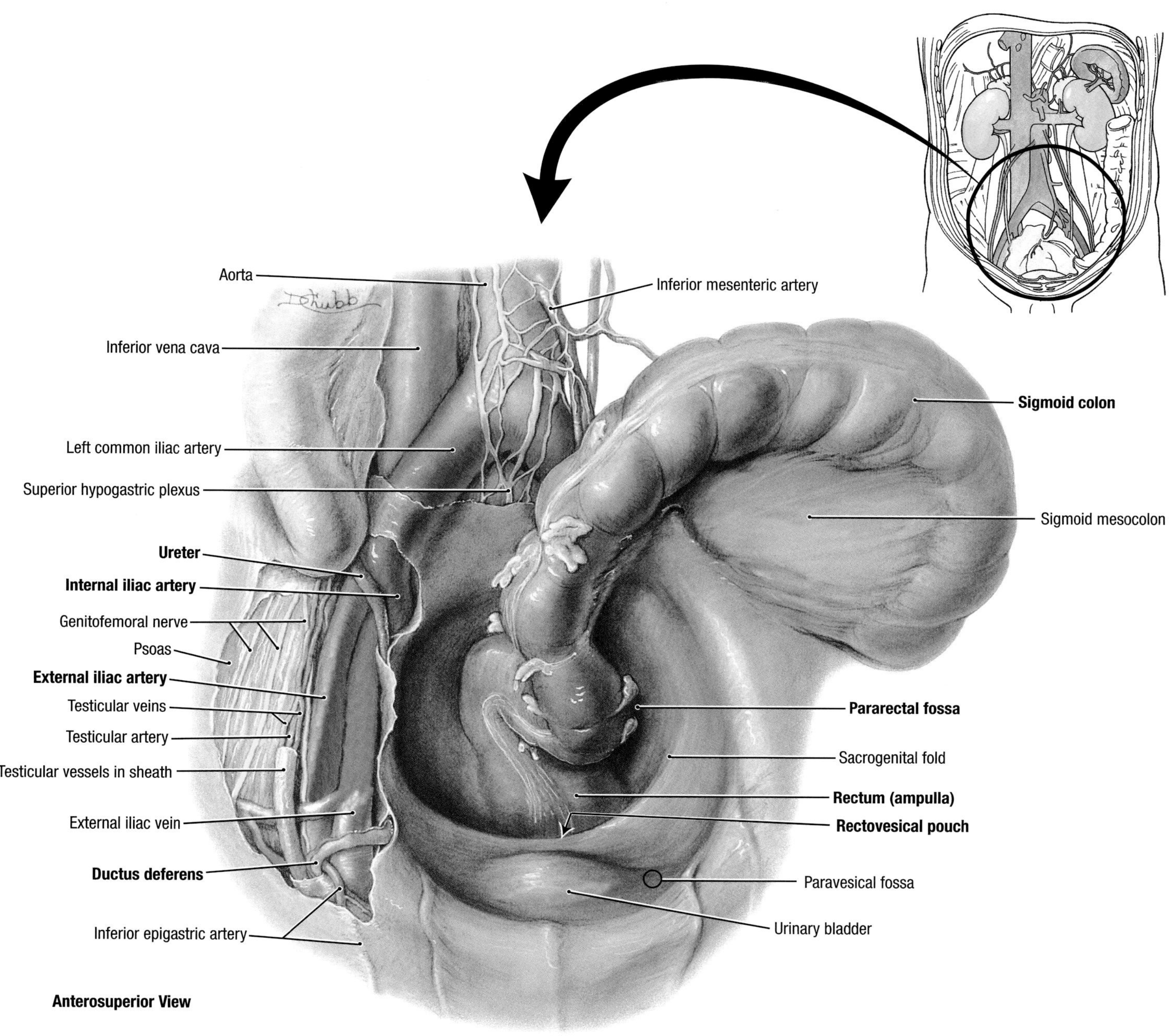
Aorta
Inferior mesenteric artery
Inferior vena cava
Sigmoid colon
Left common iliac artery
Superior hypogastric plexus
Sigmoid mesocolon
Ureter
Internal iliac artery
Genitofemoral nerve
Psoas
External iliac artery
Testicular veins
Testicular artery
Testicular vessels in sheath
Pararectal fossa
Sacrogenital fold
Rectum (ampulla)
Rectovesical pouch
External iliac vein
Ductus deferens
Paravesical fossa
Inferior epigastric artery
Urinary bladder
Anterosuperior View

## 3.19 Rectum in situ

- The sigmoid colon begins at the left pelvic brim and becomes the rectum anterior to the third sacral segment in the midline.
- The superior hypogastric plexus lies inferior to the bifurcation of the aorta and anterior to the left common iliac vein.
- The ureter adheres to the external aspect of the peritoneum, crosses the external iliac vessels, and descends anterior to the internal iliac artery. The ductus deferens and its artery also adhere to the peritoneum, cross the external iliac vessels, and then hook around the inferior epigastric artery to join the other components of the spermatic cord.
- The genitofemoral nerve lies on the psoas.

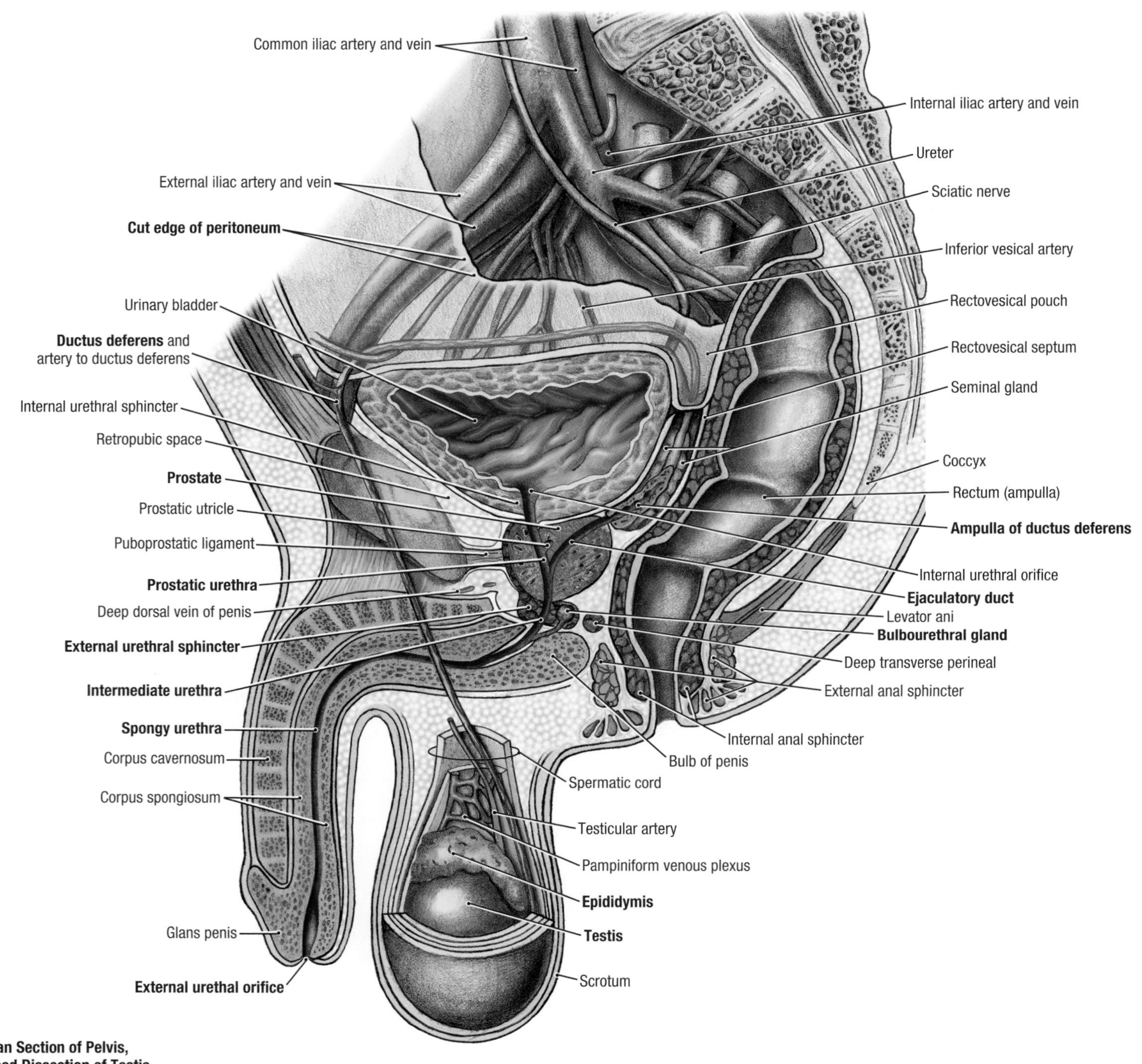
Common iliac artery and vein
Internal iliac artery and vein
Ureter
Sciatic nerve
External iliac artery and vein
Cut edge of peritoneum
Inferior vesical artery
Urinary bladder
Rectovesical pouch
Ductus deferens and artery to ductus deferens
Rectovesical septum
Internal urethral sphincter
Seminal gland
Retropubic space
Coccyx
Prostate
Rectum (ampulla)
Prostatic utricle
Ampulla of ductus deferens
Puboprostatic ligament
Internal urethral orifice
Prostatic urethra
Ejaculatory duct
Deep dorsal vein of penis
Levator ani
External urethral sphincter
Bulbourethral gland
Deep transverse perineal
Intermediate urethra
External anal sphincter
Spongy urethra
Internal anal sphincter
Corpus cavernosum
Bulb of penis
Spermatic cord
Corpus spongiosum
Testicular artery
Pampiniform venous plexus
Epididymis
Glans penis
Testis
Scrotum
External urethal orifice

**Median Section of Pelvis, Stepped Dissection of Testis**

## 3.20 Male pelvic organs and external genitalia

- Most of the pelvic viscera are subperitoneal, embedded in a matrix of fatty endopelvic fascia.
- The genital tract is demonstrated in its entirety; it merges with the urinary tract in the prostatic urethra.

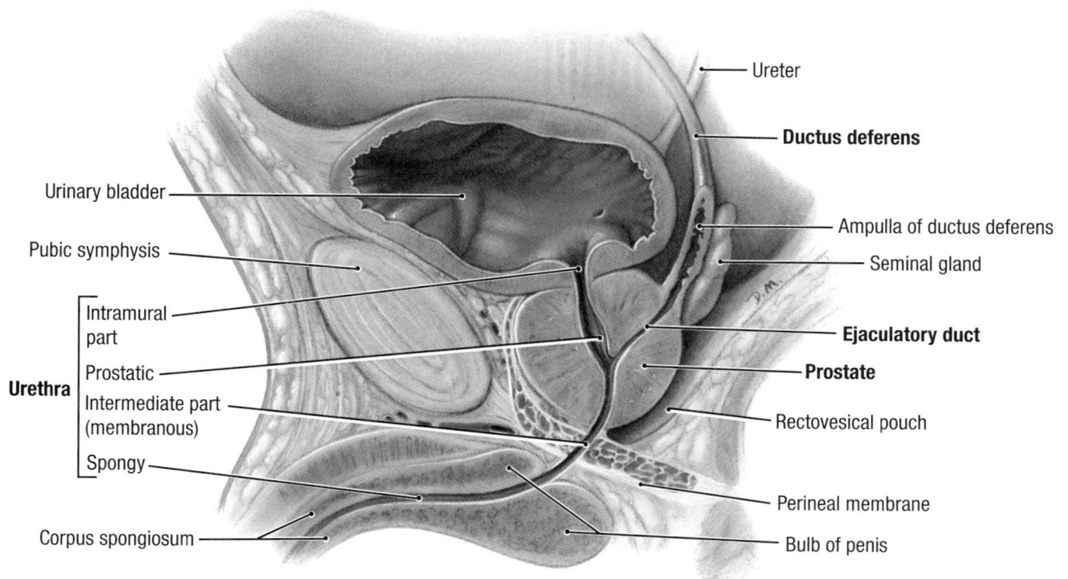
Ureter
Ductus deferens
Urinary bladder
Ampulla of ductus deferens
Pubic symphysis
Seminal gland
Urethra
Intramural part
Prostatic
Intermediate part (membranous)
Spongy
Ejaculatory duct
Prostate
Rectovesical pouch
Perineal membrane
Corpus spongiosum
Bulb of penis

**A. Median Section**

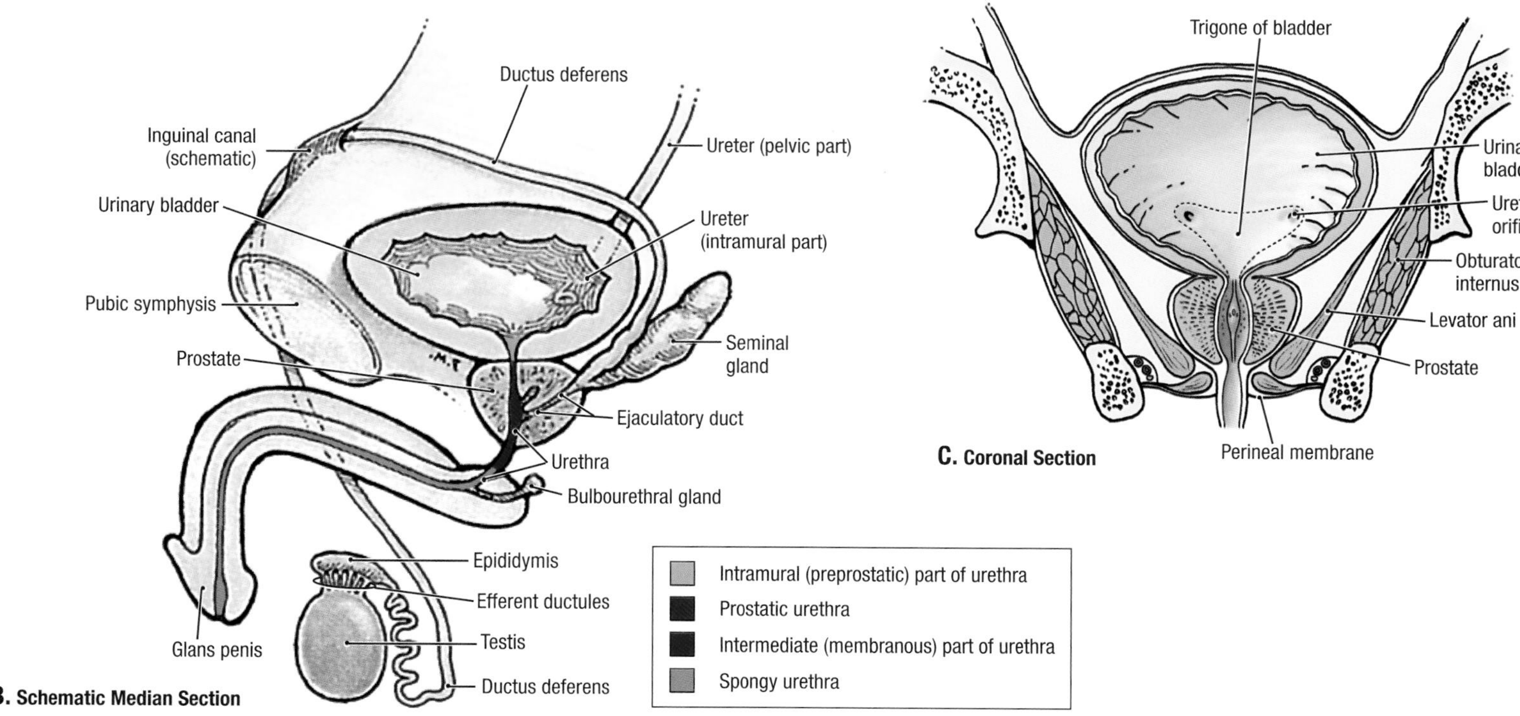
Ductus deferens
Inguinal canal (schematic)
Ureter (pelvic part)
Urinary bladder
Ureter (intramural part)
Pubic symphysis
Seminal gland
Prostate
Ejaculatory duct
Urethra
Bulbourethral gland
Epididymis
Efferent ductules
Testis
Glans penis
Ductus deferens
Intramural (preprostatic) part of urethra
Prostatic urethra
Intermediate (membranous) part of urethra
Spongy urethra
Trigone of bladder
Urinary bladder
Uretic orifice
Obturator internus
Levator ani
Prostate
Perineal membrane

**B. Schematic Median Section**

**C. Coronal Section**

## 3.21 Urinary bladder, prostate, and ductus deferens

**A.** Dissection. The ejaculatory duct (approximately 2 cm in length) is formed by the union of the ductus deferens and duct of the seminal gland; it passes anteriorly and inferiorly through the substance of the prostate to enter the prostatic urethra on the seminal colliculus. **B.** Overview of urogenital system, schematic illustration. **C.** Coronal section through urinary bladder and prostate.

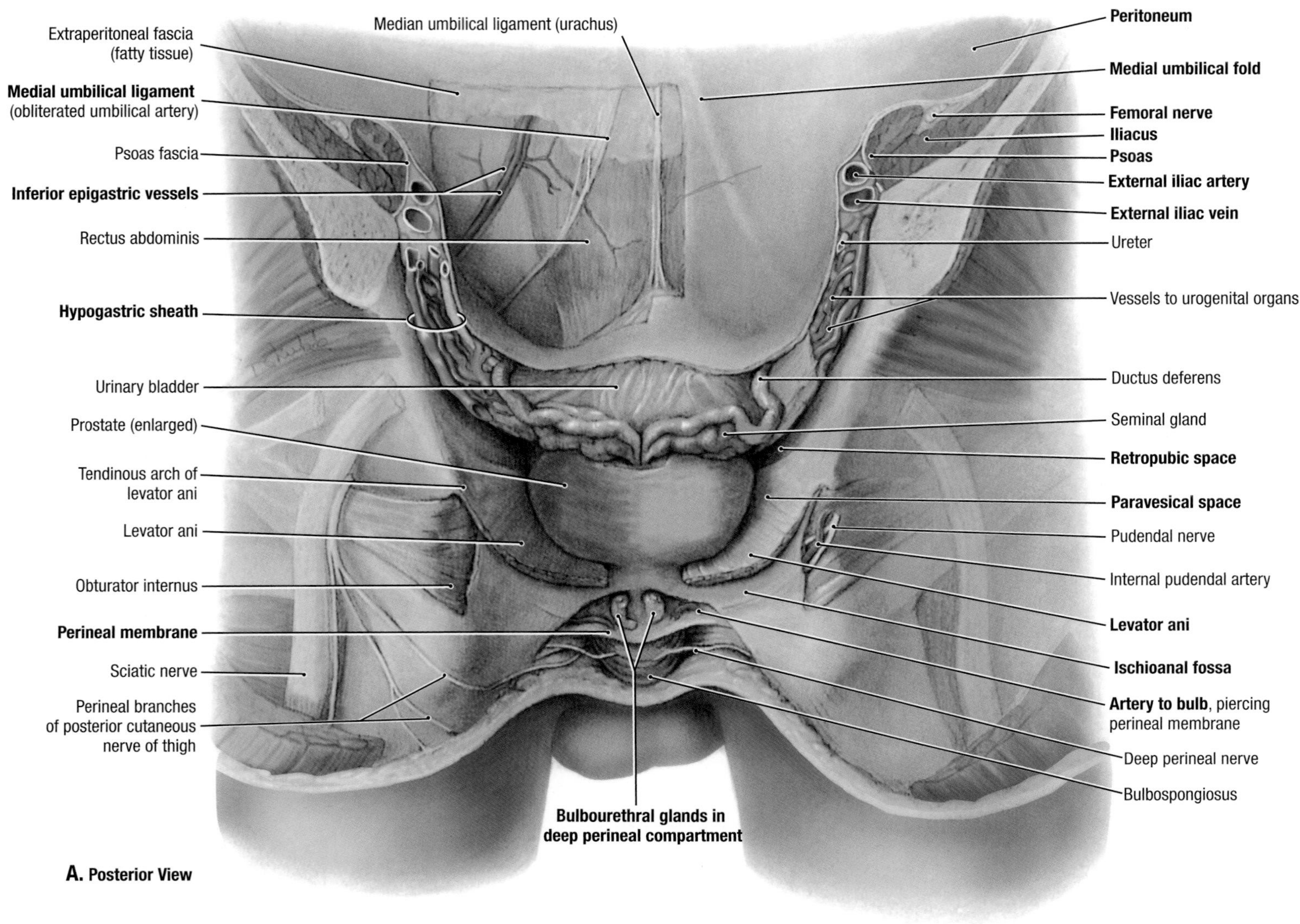
Extraperitoneal fascia (fatty tissue)
Median umbilical ligament (urachus)
Peritoneum
Medial umbilical fold
Medial umbilical ligament (obliterated umbilical artery)
Psoas fascia
Femoral nerve
Iliacus
Psoas
Inferior epigastric vessels
External iliac artery
External iliac vein
Rectus abdominis
Ureter
Hypogastric sheath
Vessels to urogenital organs
Urinary bladder
Ductus deferens
Prostate (enlarged)
Seminal gland
Retropubic space
Tendinous arch of levator ani
Paravesical space
Levator ani
Pudendal nerve
Obturator internus
Internal pudendal artery
Levator ani
Perineal membrane
Ischioanal fossa
Sciatic nerve
Artery to bulb, piercing perineal membrane
Perineal branches of posterior cutaneous nerve of thigh
Deep perineal nerve
Bulbospongiosus
Bulbourethral glands in deep perineal compartment

**A.** Posterior View

## 3.22 Posterior approach to anterior pelvic and perineal structures and spaces

**A.** Dissection. The rectovesical septum and all pelvic and perineal structures posterior to it have been removed. **B.** Posterior surface of inferior part of anterior abdominal wall with umbilical folds and ligaments and anterior pelvic viscera. **C.** Schematic coronal section through the anterior pelvis (plane of urinary bladder and prostate) demonstrating pelvic fascia.

- In **A** and **B**, the inferior epigastric artery and accompanying veins enter the rectus sheath, covered posteriorly with peritoneum to form the lateral umbilical fold. The medial umbilical fold is formed by peritoneum overlying the medial umbilical ligament (obliterated umbilical artery), and the median umbilical fold is formed by the median umbilical ligament (urachus).
- In **A**, the femoral nerve lies between the psoas and iliacus muscles, covered on their internal aspects with psoas (membranous parietal) fascia; the external iliac artery and vein lie within the areolar extraperitoneal fascia.
- The pelvic genitourinary organs are subperitoneal. Near the bladder, the ureter accompanies a "leash" of internal iliac vessels and derivatives within the fibroareolar hypogastric sheath.
- The levator ani and its fascial coverings separate the retropubic and paravesical spaces of the pelvis from the ischioanal fossae of the perineum. The fat that occupies these spaces has been removed.
- The bulbourethral glands and the initial part of the artery to the bulb lie superior to the perineal membrane in the deep perineal compartment.

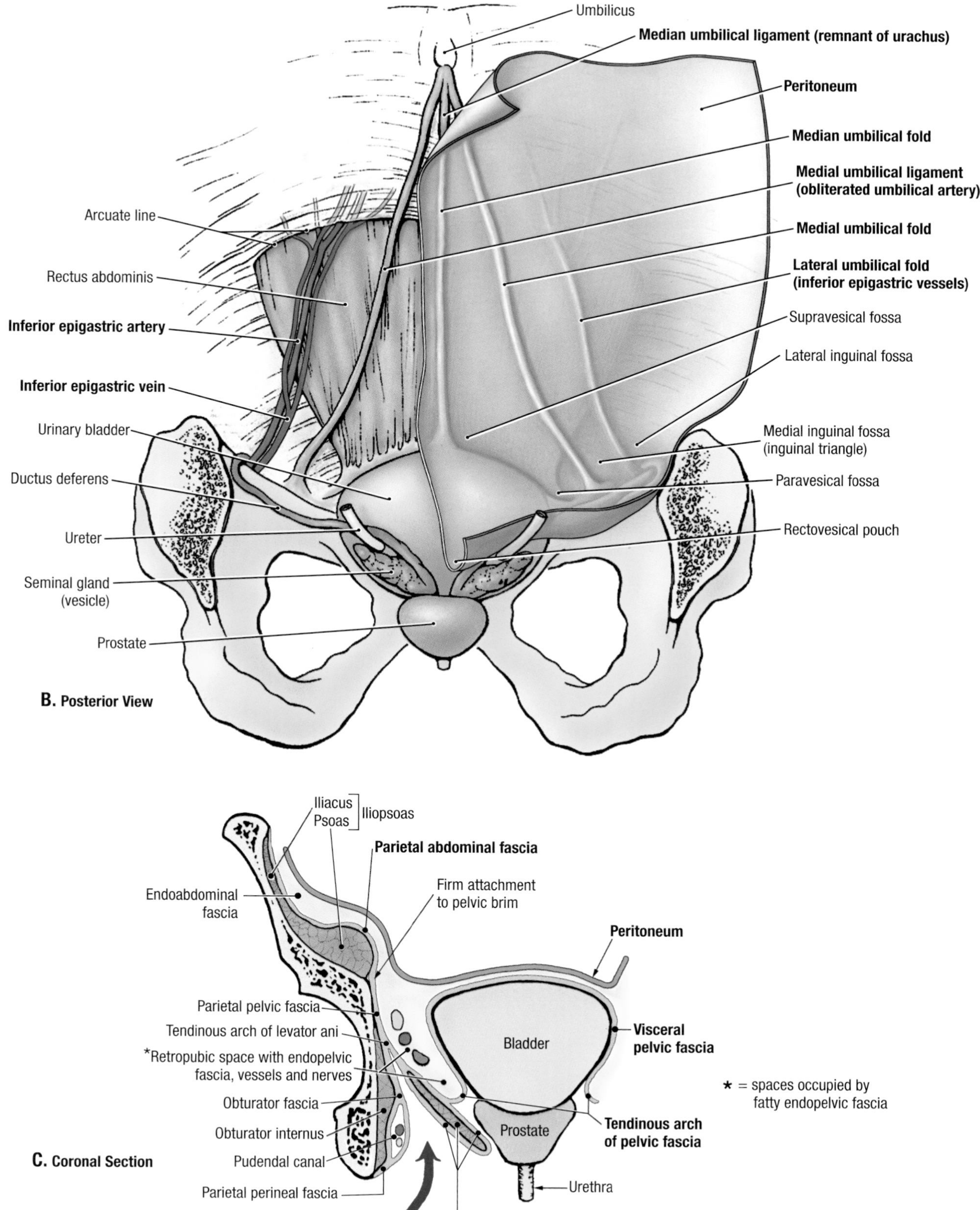
Umbilicus
Median umbilical ligament (remnant of urachus)
Peritoneum
Median umbilical fold
Medial umbilical ligament (obliterated umbilical artery)
Medial umbilical fold
Lateral umbilical fold (inferior epigastric vessels)
Supravesical fossa
Lateral inguinal fossa
Medial inguinal fossa (inguinal triangle)
Paravesical fossa
Rectovesical pouch
Arcuate line
Rectus abdominis
Inferior epigastric artery
Inferior epigastric vein
Urinary bladder
Ductus deferens
Ureter
Seminal gland (vesicle)
Prostate
B. Posterior View
Iliacus
Psoas
Iliopsoas
Parietal abdominal fascia
Endoabdominal fascia
Firm attachment to pelvic brim
Peritoneum
Parietal pelvic fascia
Tendinous arch of levator ani
*Retropubic space with endopelvic fascia, vessels and nerves
Obturator fascia
Obturator internus
Pudendal canal
Parietal perineal fascia
*Ischioanal (ischiorectal) fossa
Bladder
Prostate
Visceral pelvic fascia
* = spaces occupied by fatty endopelvic fascia
Tendinous arch of pelvic fascia
Urethra
Levator ani with superior and inferior parietal fascia
C. Coronal Section

**3.22 Posterior approach to anterior pelvic and perineal structures and spaces *(continued)***

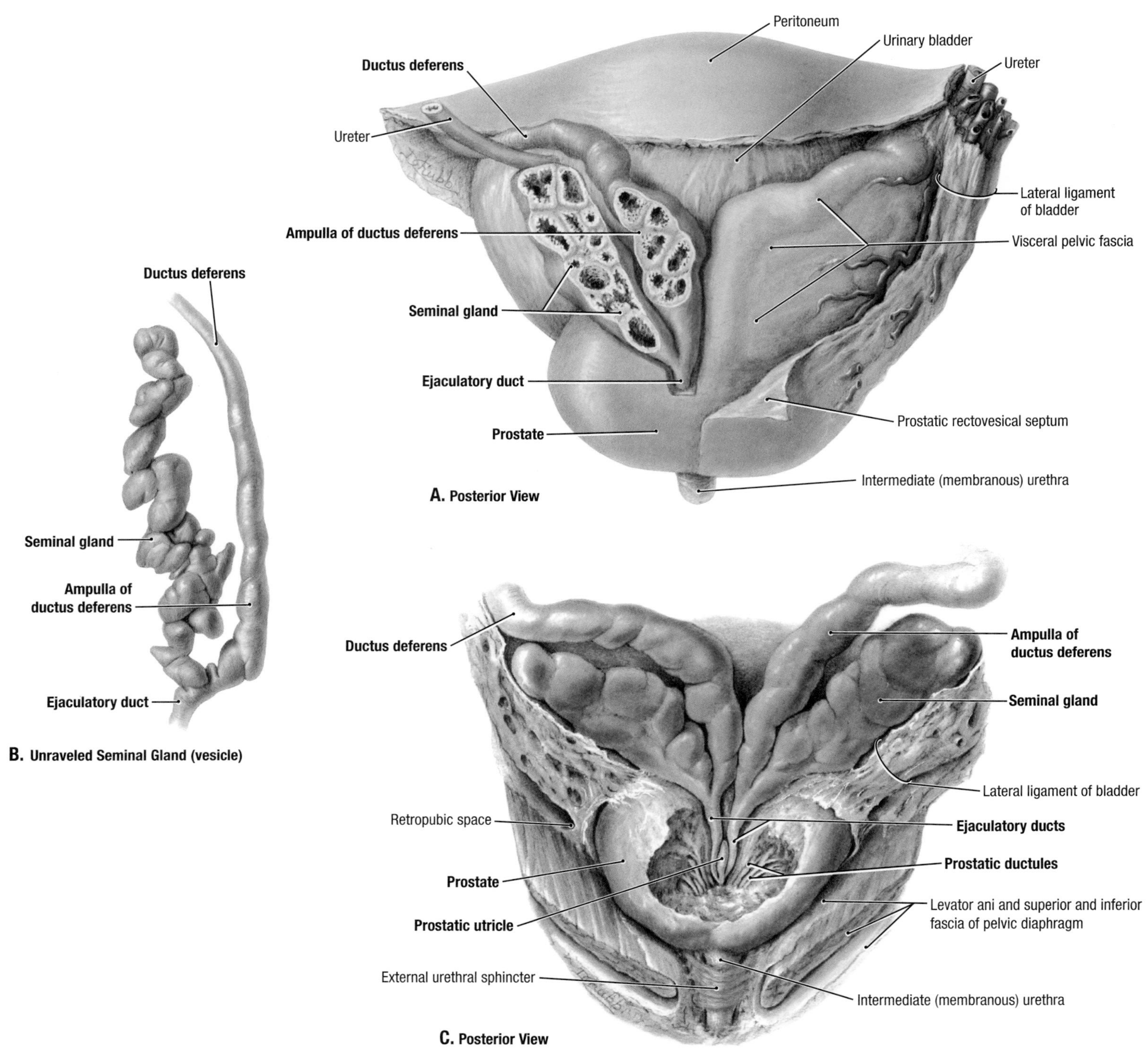

Peritoneum
Urinary bladder
Ductus deferens
Ureter
Ureter
Lateral ligament of bladder
Ampulla of ductus deferens
Visceral pelvic fascia
Seminal gland
Ejaculatory duct
Prostatic rectovesical septum
Prostate
Intermediate (membranous) urethra
A. Posterior View
Ductus deferens
Seminal gland
Ampulla of ductus deferens
Ejaculatory duct
B. Unraveled Seminal Gland (vesicle)
Ductus deferens
Ampulla of ductus deferens
Seminal gland
Lateral ligament of bladder
Retropubic space
Ejaculatory ducts
Prostatic ductules
Prostate
Levator ani and superior and inferior fascia of pelvic diaphragm
Prostatic utricle
External urethral sphincter
Intermediate (membranous) urethra
C. Posterior View


## 3.23 Seminal glands and prostate

**A.** Bladder, ductus deferens, seminal glands (vesicles), and prostate. The left seminal gland and ampulla of the ductus deferens are dissected and opened; part of the prostate is cut away to expose the ejaculatory duct. **B.** Seminal vesicle, unraveled. The vesicle is a tortuous tube with numerous dilatations. The ampulla of the ductus deferens has similar dilatations. **C.** Prostate, dissected posteriorly. The ejaculatory duct (approximately 2 cm in length) is formed by the union of the ductus deferens and the duct of the seminal gland; it passes anteriorly and inferiorly through the substance of the prostate to enter the prostatic urethra on the seminal colliculus. The prostatic utricle lies between the ends of the two ejaculatory ducts. The prostatic ductules mostly open onto the prostatic sinus.

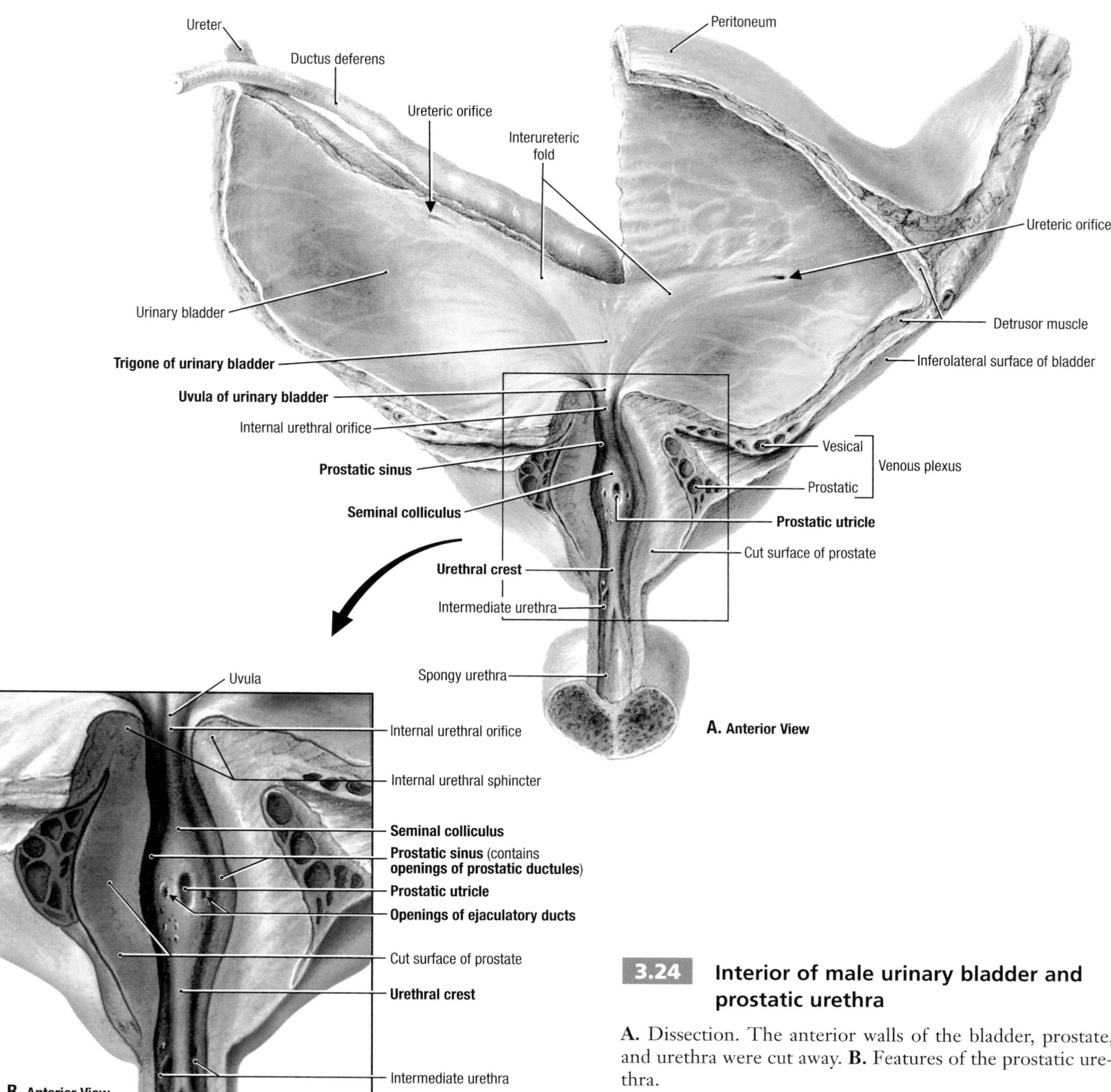
Ureter
Ductus deferens
Peritoneum
Ureteric orifice
Interureteric fold
Ureteric orifice
Urinary bladder
Detrusor muscle
Inferolateral surface of bladder
Trigone of urinary bladder
Uvula of urinary bladder
Internal urethral orifice
Vesical
Venous plexus
Prostatic
Prostatic sinus
Seminal colliculus
Prostatic utricle
Cut surface of prostate
Urethral crest
Intermediate urethra
Spongy urethra
A. Anterior View
Uvula
Internal urethral orifice
Internal urethral sphincter
Seminal colliculus
Prostatic sinus (contains openings of prostatic ductules)
Prostatic utricle
Openings of ejaculatory ducts
Cut surface of prostate
Urethral crest
Intermediate urethra
B. Anterior View

## 3.24 Interior of male urinary bladder and prostatic urethra

**A.** Dissection. The anterior walls of the bladder, prostate, and urethra were cut away. **B.** Features of the prostatic urethra.

- The mucous membrane is smooth over the trigone of the urinary bladder (triangular region demarcated by ureteric and internal urethral orifices) but folded elsewhere, especially when the bladder is empty.
- The opening of the prostatic utricle is in the seminal colliculus on the urethral crest; there is an orifice of an ejaculatory duct on each side of the prostatic utricle. The prostatic fascia encloses a venous plexus..

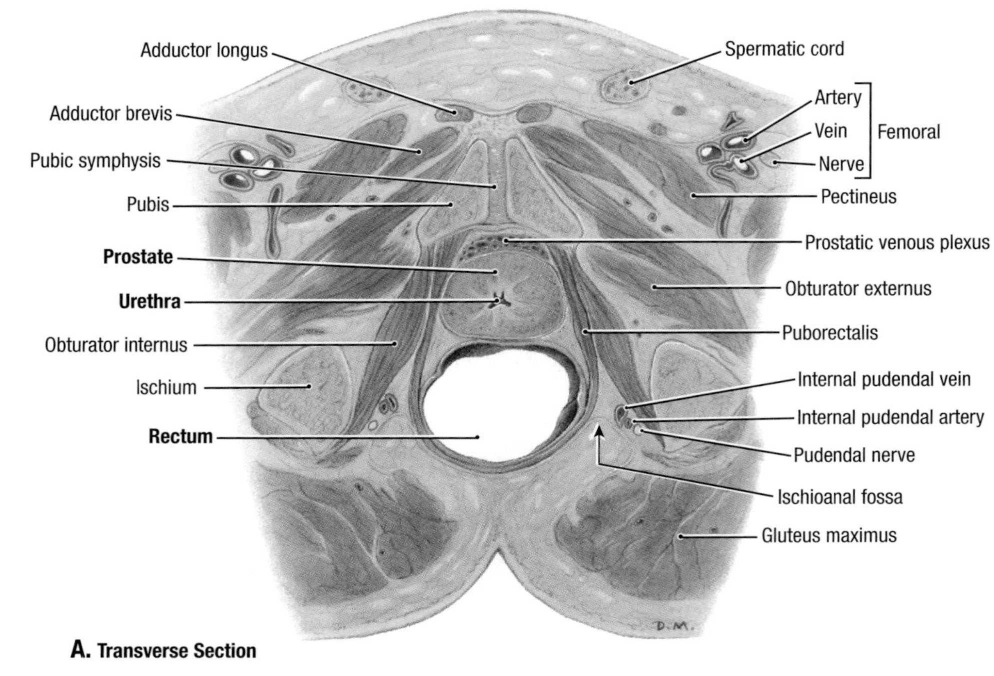
Adductor longus
Adductor brevis
Pubic symphysis
Pubis
Prostate
Urethra
Obturator internus
Ischium
Rectum
Spermatic cord
Artery
Vein
Nerve
Femoral
Pectineus
Prostatic venous plexus
Obturator externus
Puborectalis
Internal pudendal vein
Internal pudendal artery
Pudendal nerve
Ischioanal fossa
Gluteus maximus
D.M.

**A. Transverse Section**

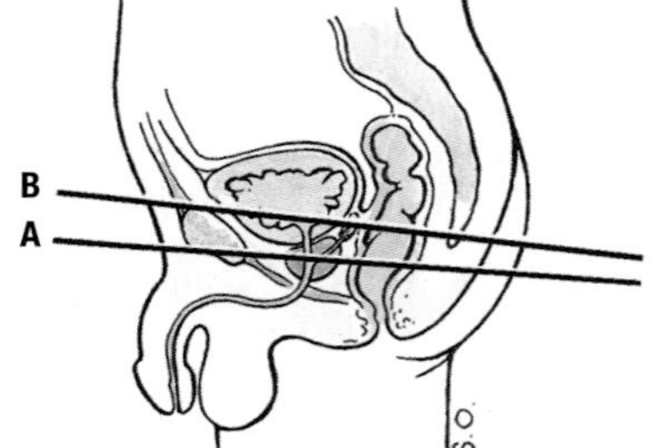
B
A
S.O.

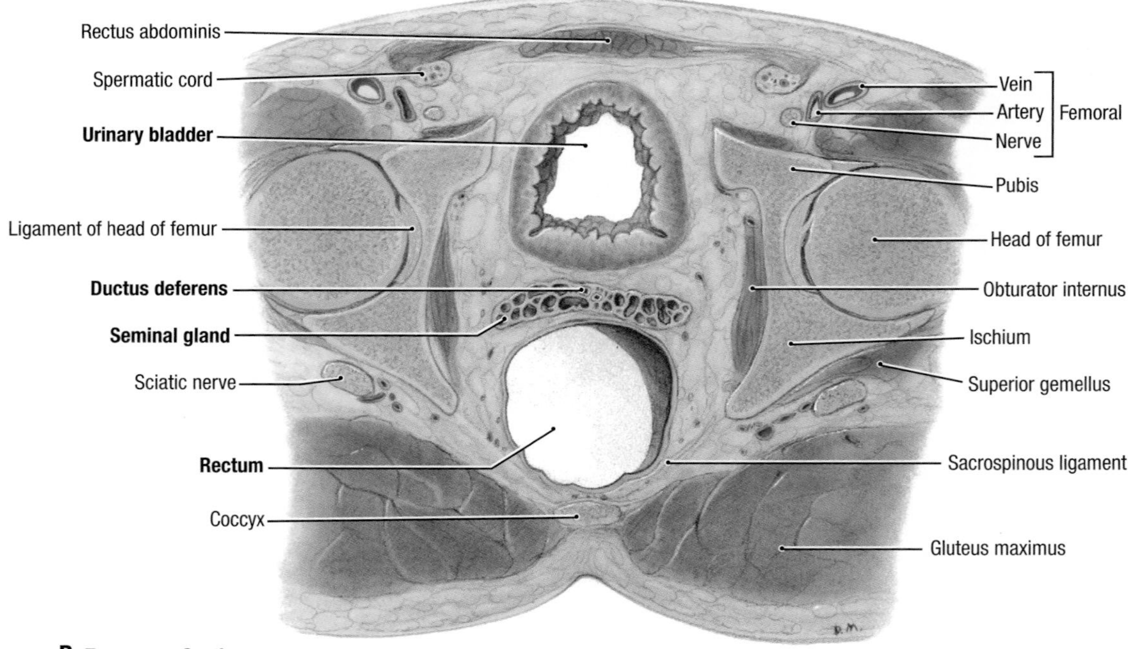
Rectus abdominis
Spermatic cord
Urinary bladder
Ligament of head of femur
Ductus deferens
Seminal gland
Sciatic nerve
Rectum
Coccyx
Vein
Artery
Nerve
Femoral
Pubis
Head of femur
Obturator internus
Ischium
Superior gemellus
Sacrospinous ligament
Gluteus maximus
D.M.

**B. Transverse Section**

## 3.25 Male pelvis, transverse sections

**A.** Section through prostate and puborectalis. **B.** Section through urinary bladder and seminal gland.

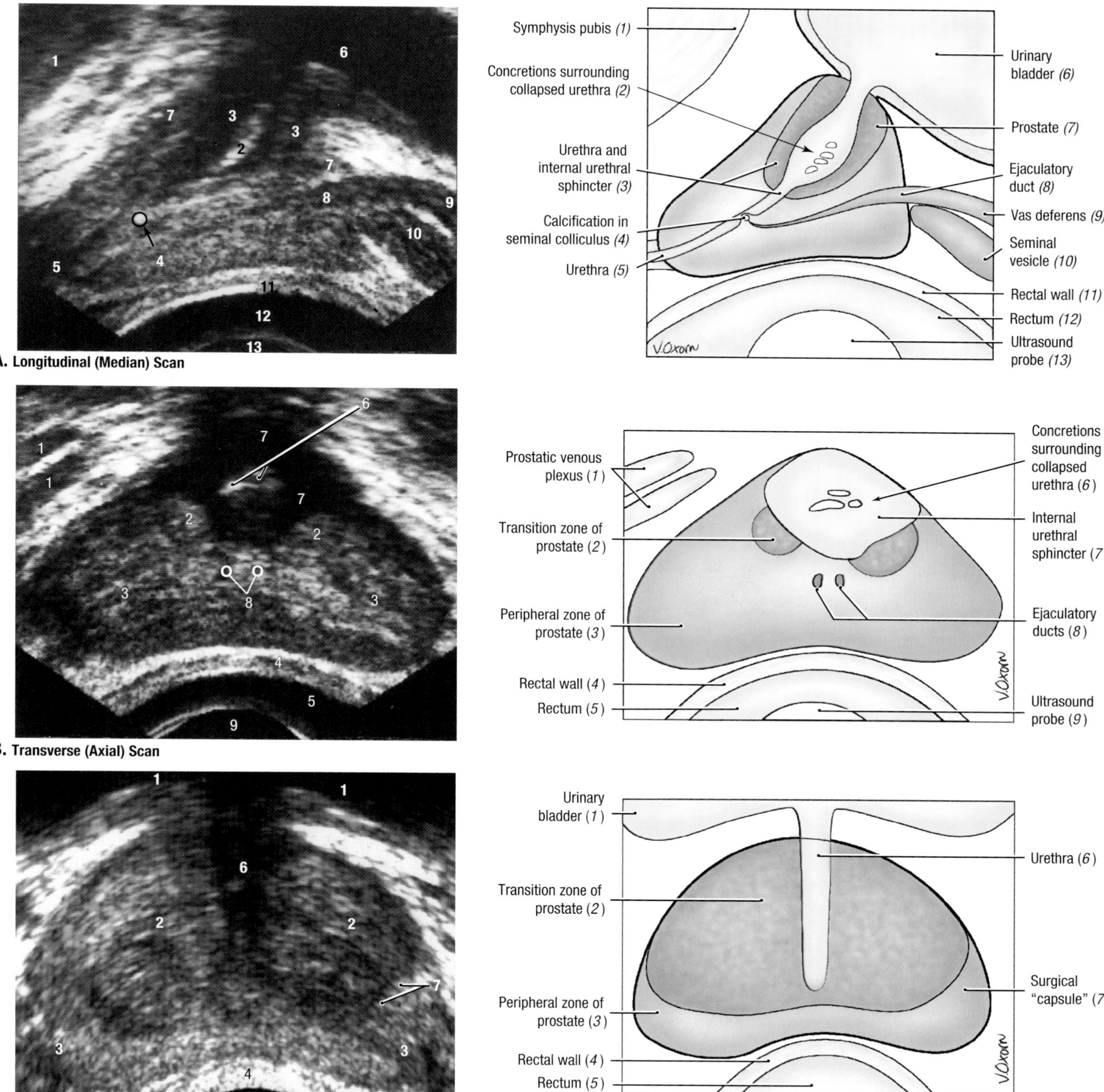
Symphysis pubis (1)
Concretions surrounding collapsed urethra (2)
Urethra and internal urethral sphincter (3)
Calcification in seminal colliculus (4)
Urethra (5)
Urinary bladder (6)
Prostate (7)
Ejaculatory duct (8)
Vas deferens (9)
Seminal vesicle (10)
Rectal wall (11)
Rectum (12)
Ultrasound probe (13)
V.Oxorn
Prostatic venous plexus (1)
Transition zone of prostate (2)
Peripheral zone of prostate (3)
Rectal wall (4)
Rectum (5)
Concretions surrounding collapsed urethra (6)
Internal urethral sphincter (7)
Ejaculatory ducts (8)
Ultrasound probe (9)
V.Oxorn
Urinary bladder (1)
Transition zone of prostate (2)
Peripheral zone of prostate (3)
Rectal wall (4)
Rectum (5)
Urethra (6)
Surgical "capsule" (7)
V.Oxorn

**A. Longitudinal (Median) Scan**

**B. Transverse (Axial) Scan**

**C. Transverse (Axial) Scan**

## 3.26 Transrectal ultrasound scans of male pelvis

**A.** In this longitudinal ultrasound scan, the probe was inserted into the rectum to scan the anteriorly located prostate. The ducts of the glands in the peripheral zone open into the prostatic sinuses, whereas the ducts of the glands in the central (internal) zone open into the prostatic sinuses and onto the seminal colliculus. The large peripheral zone (3) is the common site for carcinomas. **B.** Normal prostate of young male. **C.** Benign prostatic hyperplasia. Note the enlarged transition zone (2). The transition zone of the prostate normally starts becoming hyperplastic after age 30. The numbers in parentheses correspond to labels on the ultrasound scan.

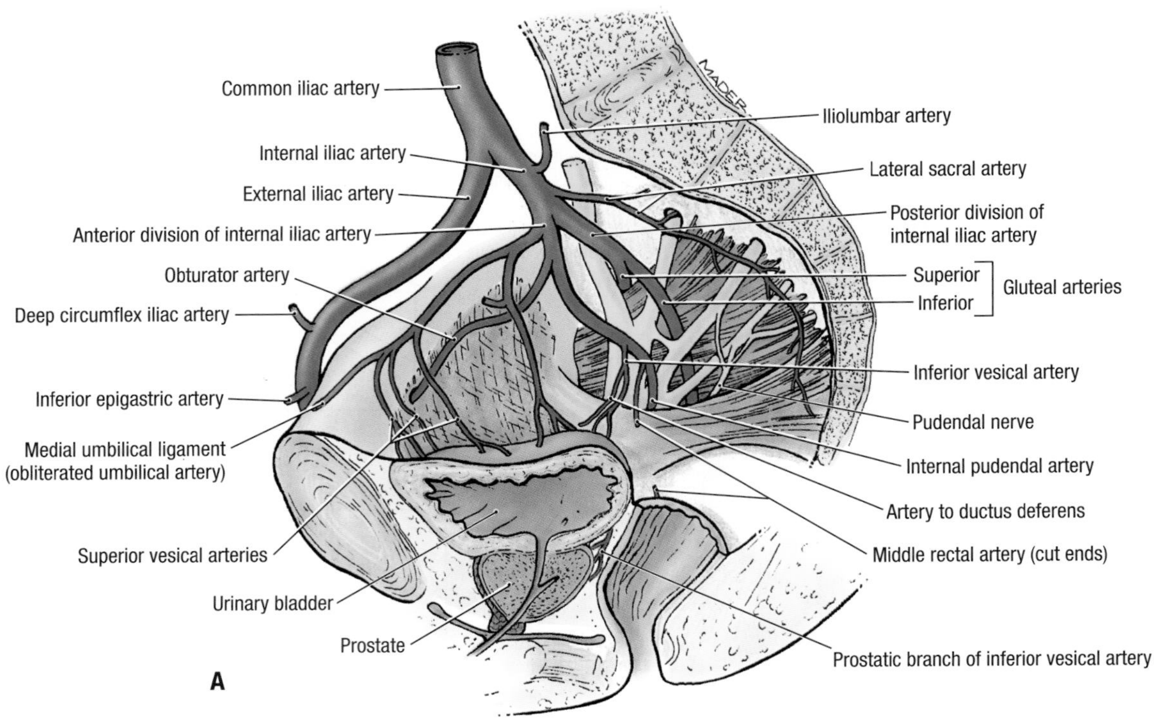
Common iliac artery
Internal iliac artery
External iliac artery
Anterior division of internal iliac artery
Obturator artery
Deep circumflex iliac artery
Inferior epigastric artery
Medial umbilical ligament (obliterated umbilical artery)
Superior vesical arteries
Urinary bladder
Prostate
A
Iliolumbar artery
Lateral sacral artery
Posterior division of internal iliac artery
Superior
Inferior
Gluteal arteries
Inferior vesical artery
Pudendal nerve
Internal pudendal artery
Artery to ductus deferens
Middle rectal artery (cut ends)
Prostatic branch of inferior vesical artery

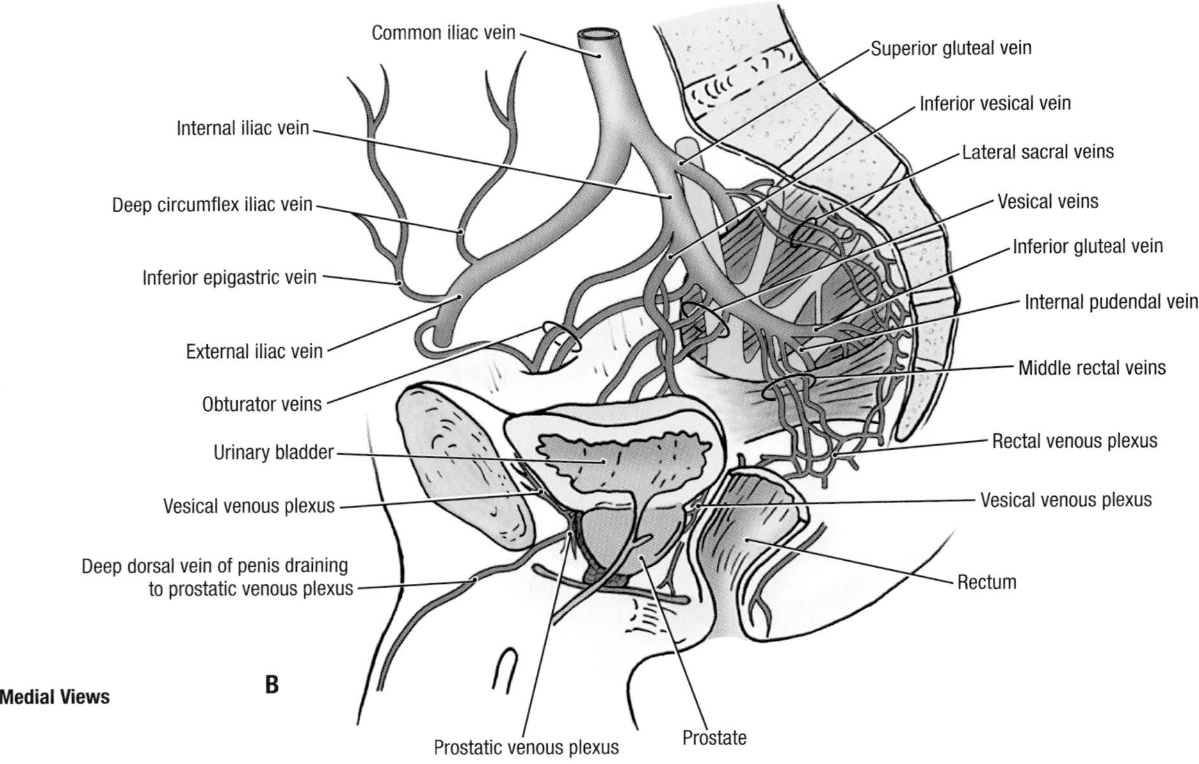
Common iliac vein
Internal iliac vein
Deep circumflex iliac vein
Inferior epigastric vein
External iliac vein
Obturator veins
Urinary bladder
Vesical venous plexus
Deep dorsal vein of penis draining to prostatic venous plexus
Medial Views
B
Prostatic venous plexus
Prostate
Superior gluteal vein
Inferior vesical vein
Lateral sacral veins
Vesical veins
Inferior gluteal vein
Internal pudendal vein
Middle rectal veins
Rectal venous plexus
Vesical venous plexus
Rectum

**3.27 Arteries and veins of male pelvis**

**A.** Arteries. **B.** Pelvic veins and venous plexuses.

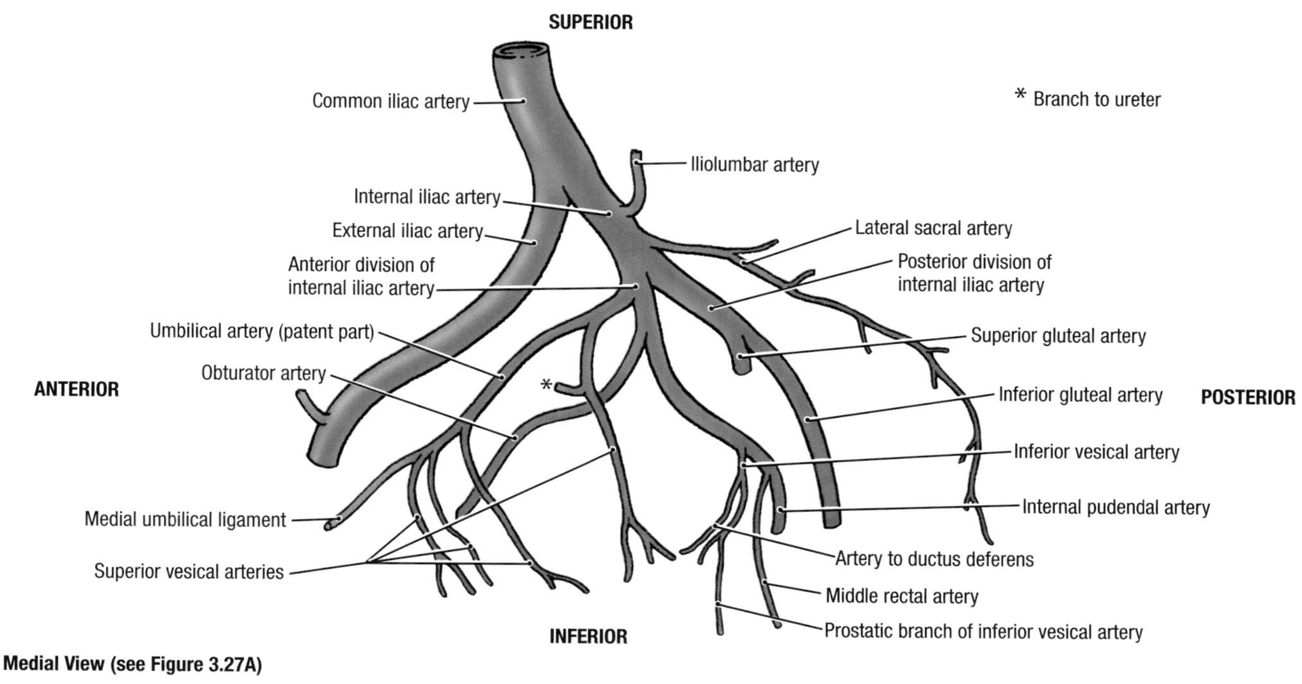
SUPERIOR
Common iliac artery
* Branch to ureter
Iliolumbar artery
Internal iliac artery
External iliac artery
Lateral sacral artery
Anterior division of internal iliac artery
Posterior division of internal iliac artery
Umbilical artery (patent part)
Superior gluteal artery
Obturator artery
ANTERIOR
Inferior gluteal artery
POSTERIOR
Inferior vesical artery
Medial umbilical ligament
Internal pudendal artery
Superior vesical arteries
Artery to ductus deferens
Middle rectal artery
INFERIOR
Prostatic branch of inferior vesical artery
Medial View (see Figure 3.27A)

## TABLE 3.4 ARTERIES OF MALE PELVIS

| Artery | Origin | Course | Distribution |
|---|---|---|---|
| Internal iliac | Common iliac artery | Passes medially over pelvic brim and descends into pelvic cavity; often forms anterior and posterior divisions | Main blood supply to pelvic organs, gluteal muscles, and perineum |
| Anterior division of internal iliac | Internal iliac artery | Passes laterally along lateral wall of pelvis, dividing into visceral, obturator, and internal pudendal arteries | Pelvic viscera, perineum, and muscles of superior medial thigh |
| Umbilical | Anterior division of internal iliac artery | Short pelvic course; gives off superior vesical arteries, then obliterates, becoming medial umbilical ligament | Urinary bladder and, in some males, ductus deferens |
| Superior vesical | Patent part of umbilical artery | Usually multiple; pass to superior aspect of urinary bladder | Superior aspect of urinary bladder and distal ureter |
| Artery to ductus deferens | Superior or inferior vesical artery | Runs subperitoneally to ductus deferens | Ductus deferens |
| Obturator | Anterior division of internal iliac artery | Runs anteroinferiorly on lateral pelvic wall | Pelvic muscles, nutrient artery to ilium, head of femur and medial compartment of thigh |
| Inferior vesical | | Passes subperitoneally giving rise to prostatic artery and occasionally the artery to the ductus deferens | Inferior aspect of urinary bladder, pelvic ureter, seminal glands, and prostate |
| Middle rectal | | Descends in pelvis to rectum | Seminal glands, prostate, and inferior part of rectum |
| Internal pudendal | | Exits pelvis through greater sciatic foramen and enters perineum via lesser sciatic foramen | Main artery to perineum, including muscles and skin of anal and urogenital triangles; erectile bodies |
| Posterior division of internal iliac artery | Internal iliac artery | Passes posteriorly and gives rise to parietal branches | Pelvic wall and gluteal region |
| Iliolumbar | Posterior division of internal iliac artery | Ascends anterior to sacroiliac joint and posterior to common iliac vessels and psoas major | Iliacus, psoas major, quadratus lumborum muscles, and cauda equina in vertebral canal |
| Lateral sacral (superior and inferior) | | Run on anteromedial aspect of piriformis to send branches into pelvic sacral foramina | Piriformis muscle, structures in sacral canal and erector spinae muscles |
| Testicular (gonadal) [see Fig. 3.28A ] | Abdominal aorta | Descends retroperitoneally; traverses inguinal canal and enters scrotum | Abdominal ureter, testis and epididymis |

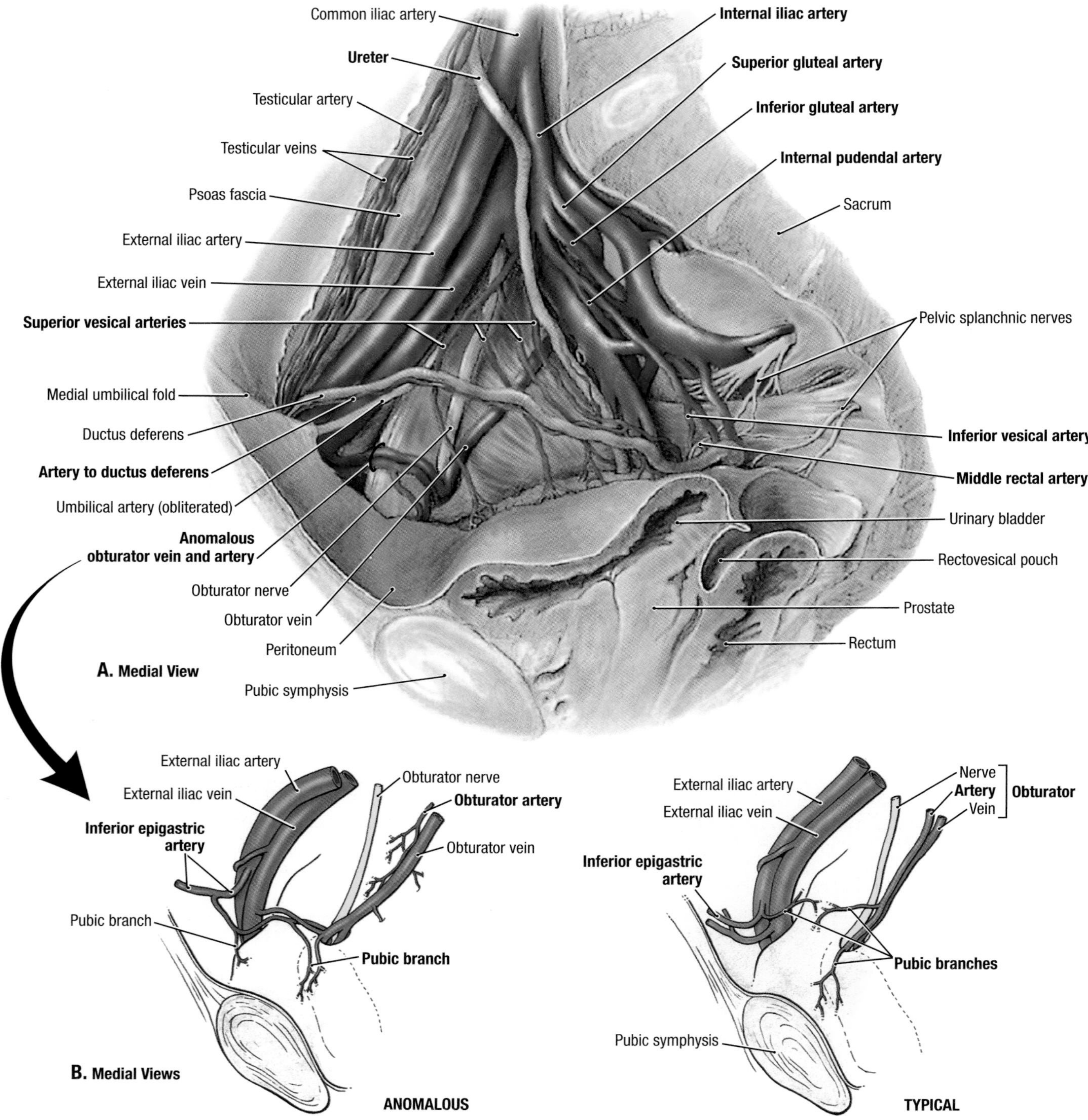
Common iliac artery
Ureter
Testicular artery
Testicular veins
Psoas fascia
External iliac artery
External iliac vein
Superior vesical arteries
Medial umbilical fold
Ductus deferens
Artery to ductus deferens
Umbilical artery (obliterated)
Anomalous obturator vein and artery
Obturator nerve
Obturator vein
Peritoneum
A. Medial View
Pubic symphysis
Internal iliac artery
Superior gluteal artery
Inferior gluteal artery
Internal pudendal artery
Sacrum
Pelvic splanchnic nerves
Inferior vesical artery
Middle rectal artery
Urinary bladder
Rectovesical pouch
Prostate
Rectum
External iliac artery
External iliac vein
Inferior epigastric artery
Pubic branch
Obturator nerve
Obturator artery
Obturator vein
Pubic branch
B. Medial Views
ANOMALOUS
External iliac artery
External iliac vein
Inferior epigastric artery
Nerve
Artery
Vein
Obturator
Pubic branches
Pubic symphysis
TYPICAL

## 3.28 Pelvic vessels in situ; lateral pelvic wall

**A.** Dissection. **B.** Usual and anomalous obturator arteries.

- The ureter crosses the external iliac artery at its origin (common iliac bifurcation), and the ductus deferens crosses the external iliac artery at its termination (deep inguinal ring).
- In this specimen, an anomalous (replaced) obturator artery branches from the inferior epigastric artery **(B)**.

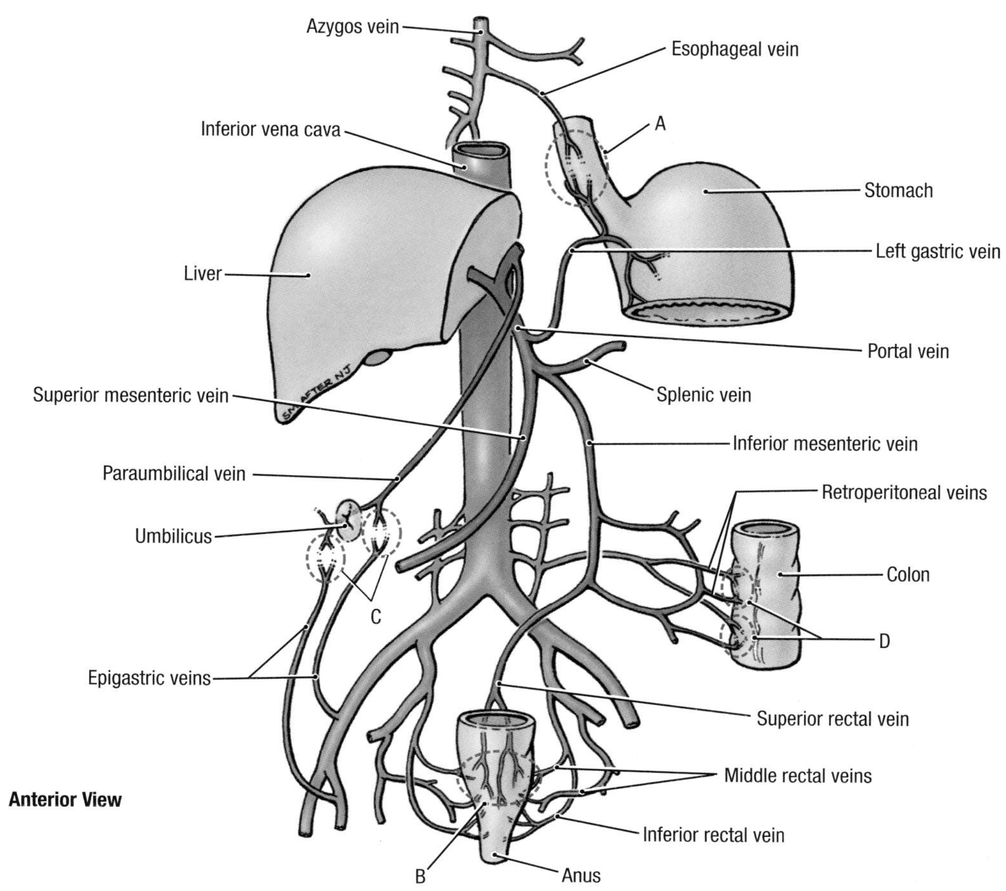
Azygos vein
Esophageal vein
Inferior vena cava
A
Stomach
Left gastric vein
Liver
Portal vein
Superior mesenteric vein
Splenic vein
Inferior mesenteric vein
Paraumbilical vein
Retroperitoneal veins
Umbilicus
Colon
C
D
Epigastric veins
Superior rectal vein
Middle rectal veins
Anterior View
Inferior rectal vein
B
Anus

## 3.29 Portal–systemic anastomoses

The portal tributaries are *purple*, and systemic tributaries are *blue*. *A–D* indicate sites of portal systemic anastomoses. *A*, between portal and systemic esophageal veins; *B*, between portal and systemic rectal veins; *C*, paraumbilical veins (portal) anastomosing with small epigastric veins of the anterior abdominal wall (systemic); *D*, twigs of colic veins (portal) anastomosing with retroperitoneal veins (systemic).

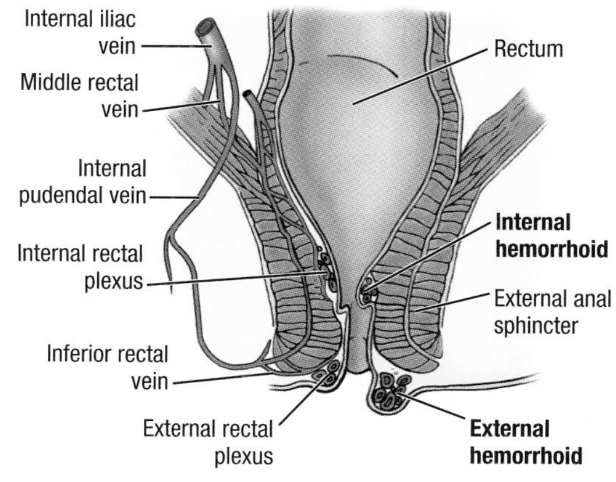
Internal iliac vein
Rectum
Middle rectal vein
Internal pudendal vein
Internal hemorrhoid
Internal rectal plexus
External anal sphincter
Inferior rectal vein
External rectal plexus
External hemorrhoid
Anterior view of coronal section

**Internal hemorrhoids** (piles) are prolapses of rectal mucosa containing the normally dilated veins of the *internal rectal venous plexus*. Internal hemorrhoids are thought to result from a breakdown of the muscularis mucosae, a smooth muscle layer deep to the mucosa (see figure at right). Internal hemorrhoids that prolapse through the anal canal are often compressed by the contracted sphincters, impeding blood flow. As a result, they tend to strangulate, ulcerate, and bleed.

**External hemorrhoids** are thromboses (blood clots) in the veins of the *external rectal venous plexus* and are covered by skin. Predisposing factors for hemorrhoids include pregnancy, chronic constipation, and any disorder that impedes venous return. The superior rectal vein drains into the inferior mesenteric vein, whereas the middle and inferior rectal veins drain through the systemic system into the inferior vena cava. Any abnormal increase in pressure in the valveless portal system or veins of the trunk may cause enlargement of the superior rectal veins, resulting in an increase in blood flow or stasis in the internal rectal venous plexus. In *portal hypertension* that occurs in relation to *hepatic cirrhosis*, the portocaval anastomosis (e.g., esophageal) may become varicose and rupture.

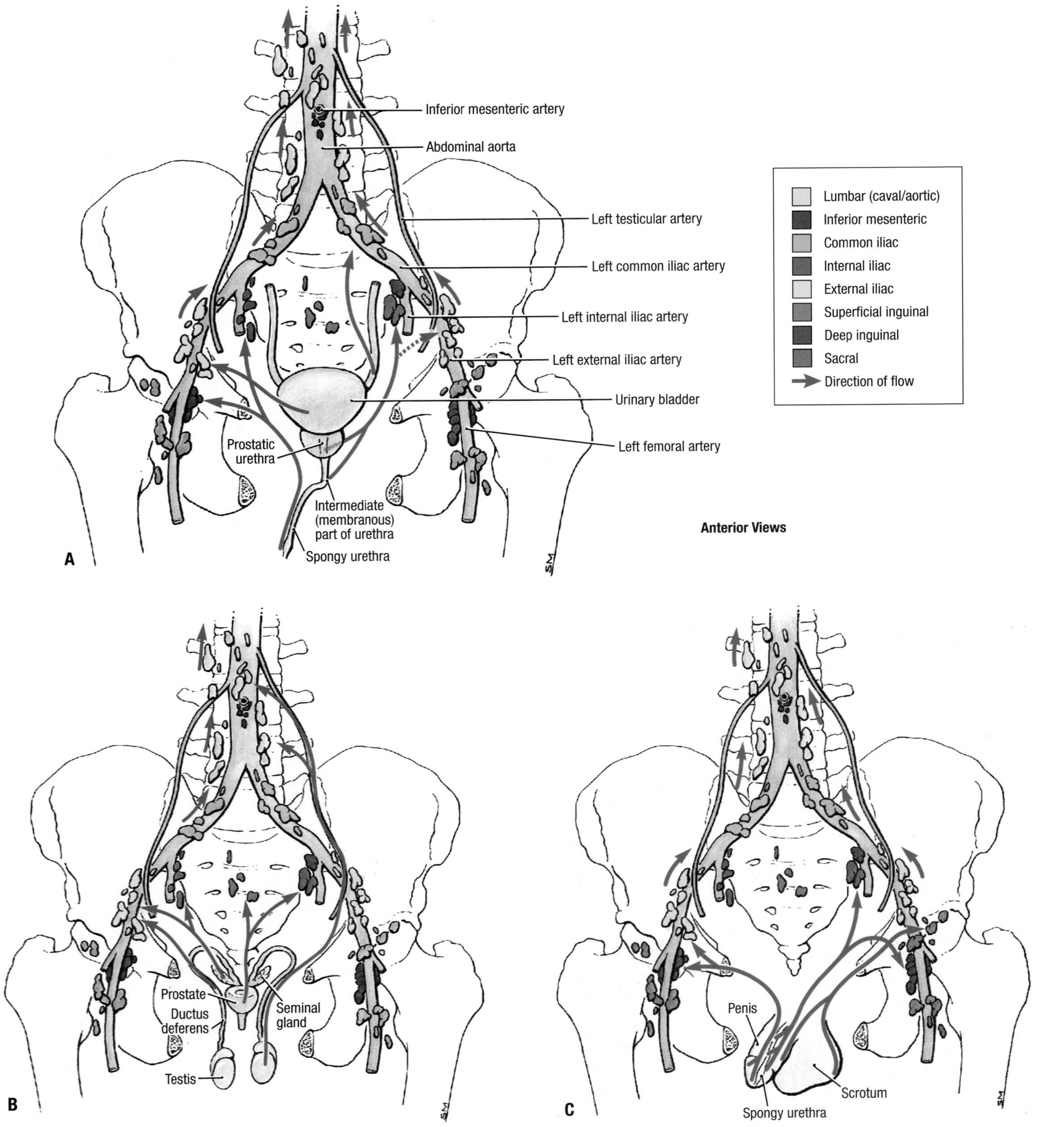

Inferior mesenteric artery
Abdominal aorta
Left testicular artery
Left common iliac artery
Left internal iliac artery
Left external iliac artery
Urinary bladder
Left femoral artery
Prostatic urethra
Intermediate (membranous) part of urethra
Spongy urethra
A
Lumbar (caval/aortic)
Inferior mesenteric
Common iliac
Internal iliac
External iliac
Superficial inguinal
Deep inguinal
Sacral
Direction of flow
Anterior Views
Prostate
Ductus deferens
Seminal gland
Testis
B
Penis
Scrotum
Spongy urethra
C

**3.30 Lymphatic drainage of male pelvis and perineum**

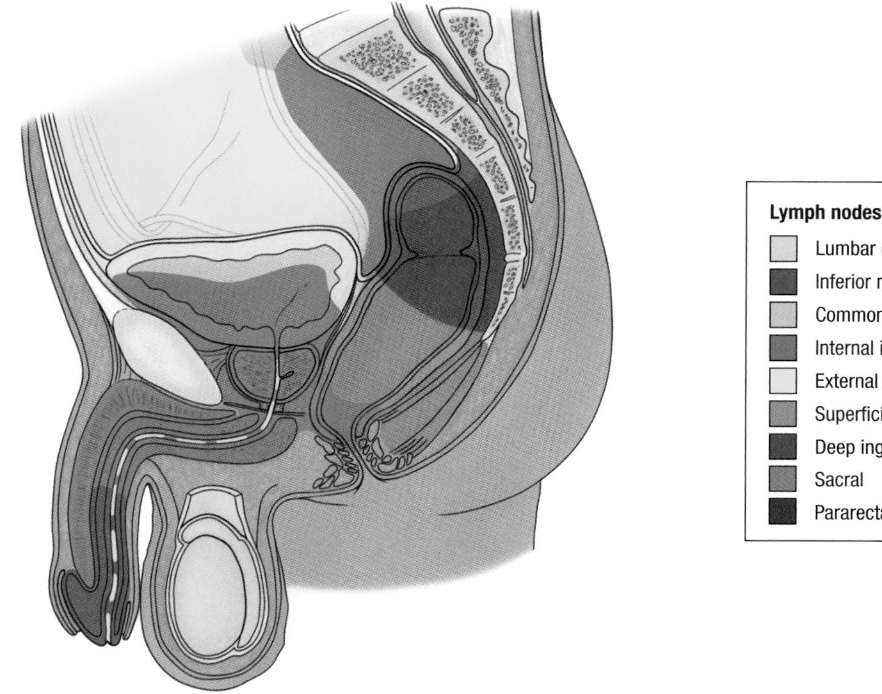
Lymph nodes:
Lumbar (caval/aortic)
Inferior mesenteric
Common iliac
Internal iliac
External iliac
Superficial inguinal
Deep inguinal
Sacral
Pararectal

**TABLE 3.5 LYMPHATIC DRAINAGE OF THE MALE PELVIS AND PERINEUM**

| Lymph Node Group | Structures Typically Draining to Lymph Node Group |
|---|---|
| Lumbar | Gonads and associated structures (including testicular vessels), urethra, testis, epididymis, common iliac nodes |
| Inferior mesenteric nodes | Superiormost rectum, sigmoid colon, descending colon, pararectal nodes |
| Common iliac nodes | External and internal iliac lymph nodes |
| Internal iliac nodes | Inferior pelvic structures, deep perineal structures, sacral nodes, prostatic urethra, prostate, base of bladder, inferior part of pelvic ureter, inferior part of seminal glands, cavernous bodies, anal canal (above pectinate line), inferior rectum |
| External iliac nodes | Anterosuperior pelvic structures, deep inguinal nodes, superior aspect of bladder, superior part of pelvic ureter, upper part of seminal gland, pelvic part of ductus deferens, intermediate and spongy urethra |
| Superficial inguinal nodes | Lower limb, superficial drainage of inferolateral quadrant of trunk, including anterior abdominal wall inferior to umbilicus, gluteal region, superficial perineal structures, skin of perineum including skin and prepuce of penis, scrotum, perianal skin, anal canal inferior to pectinate line |
| Deep inguinal nodes | Glans of penis, distal spongy urethra, superficial inguinal nodes |
| Sacral nodes | Posteroinferior pelvic structures, inferior rectum |
| Pararectal nodes | Superior rectum |

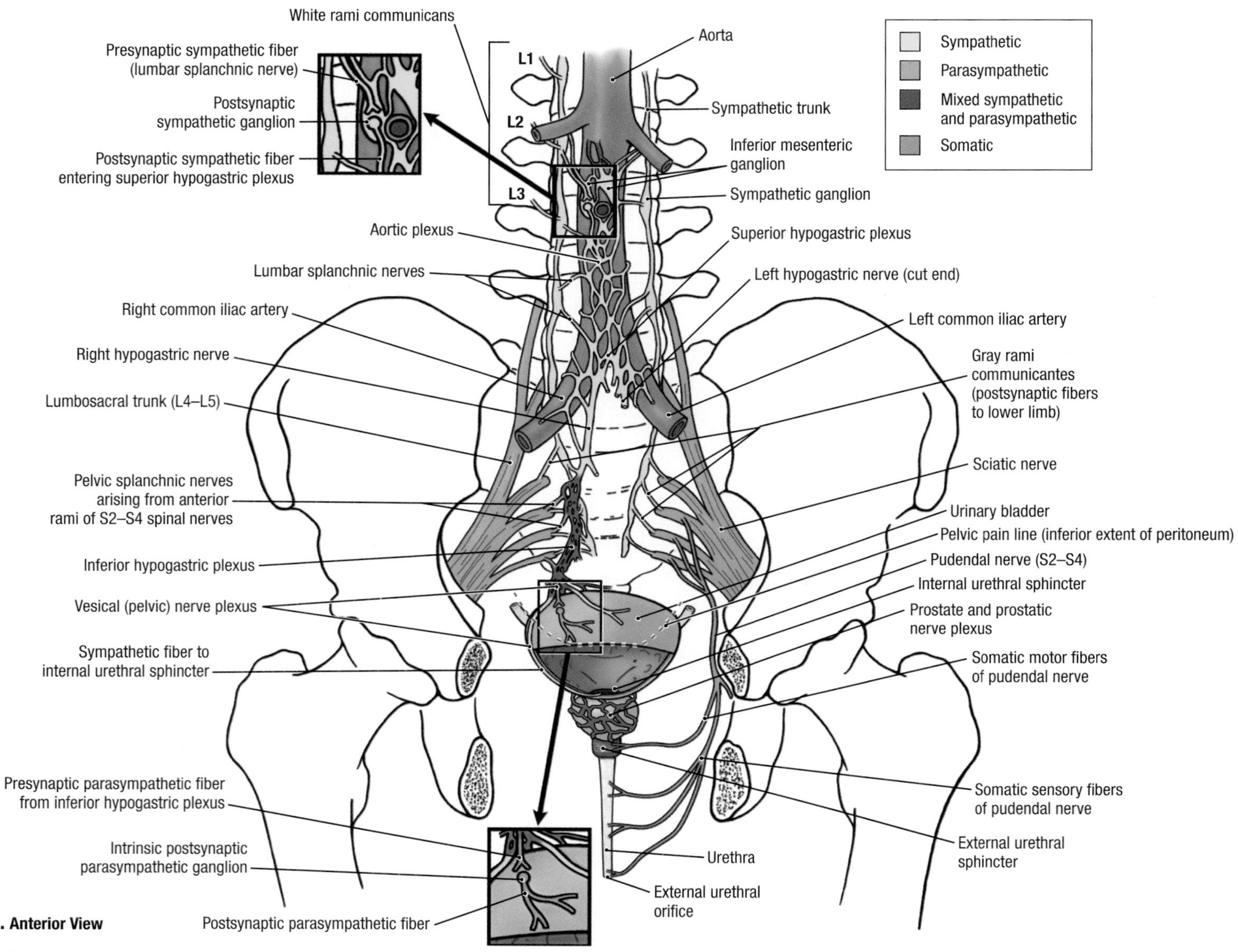
White rami communicans
Presynaptic sympathetic fiber (lumbar splanchnic nerve)
Postsynaptic sympathetic ganglion
Postsynaptic sympathetic fiber entering superior hypogastric plexus
L1
L2
L3
Aorta
Sympathetic trunk
Inferior mesenteric ganglion
Sympathetic ganglion
Sympathetic
Parasympathetic
Mixed sympathetic and parasympathetic
Somatic
Aortic plexus
Superior hypogastric plexus
Lumbar splanchnic nerves
Left hypogastric nerve (cut end)
Right common iliac artery
Left common iliac artery
Right hypogastric nerve
Gray rami communicantes (postsynaptic fibers to lower limb)
Lumbosacral trunk (L4–L5)
Sciatic nerve
Pelvic splanchnic nerves arising from anterior rami of S2–S4 spinal nerves
Urinary bladder
Pelvic pain line (inferior extent of peritoneum)
Pudendal nerve (S2–S4)
Inferior hypogastric plexus
Internal urethral sphincter
Vesical (pelvic) nerve plexus
Prostate and prostatic nerve plexus
Sympathetic fiber to internal urethral sphincter
Somatic motor fibers of pudendal nerve
Presynaptic parasympathetic fiber from inferior hypogastric plexus
Somatic sensory fibers of pudendal nerve
Intrinsic postsynaptic parasympathetic ganglion
External urethral sphincter
Urethra
External urethral orifice
Postsynaptic parasympathetic fiber

**A. Anterior View**

### TABLE 3.6 EFFECT OF SYMPATHETIC AND PARASYMPATHETIC STIMULATION ON THE URINARY TRACT, GENITAL SYSTEM, AND RECTUM

| Organ, Tract, or System | Effect of Sympathetic Stimulation | Effect of Parasympathetic Stimulation |
|---|---|---|
| Urinary tract | Vasoconstriction of renal vessels slows urine formation; internal sphincter of male bladder contracted to prevent retrograde ejaculation and maintain urinary continence | Inhibits contraction of internal sphincter of bladder in males; contracts detrusor muscle of the bladder wall causing urination |
| Genital system | Causes ejaculation and vasoconstriction resulting in remission of erection | Produces engorgement (erection) of erectile tissues of the external genitals |
| Rectum | Maintains tonus of internal anal sphincter; inhibits peristalsis of rectum | Rectal contraction (peristalsis) for defecation; inhibition of contraction of internal anal sphincter |

The parasympathetic system is restricted in its distribution to the head, neck, and body cavities (except for erectile tissues of genitalia); otherwise, parasympathetic fibers are never found in the body wall and limbs. Sympathetic fibers, by comparison, are distributed to all vascularized portions of the body.

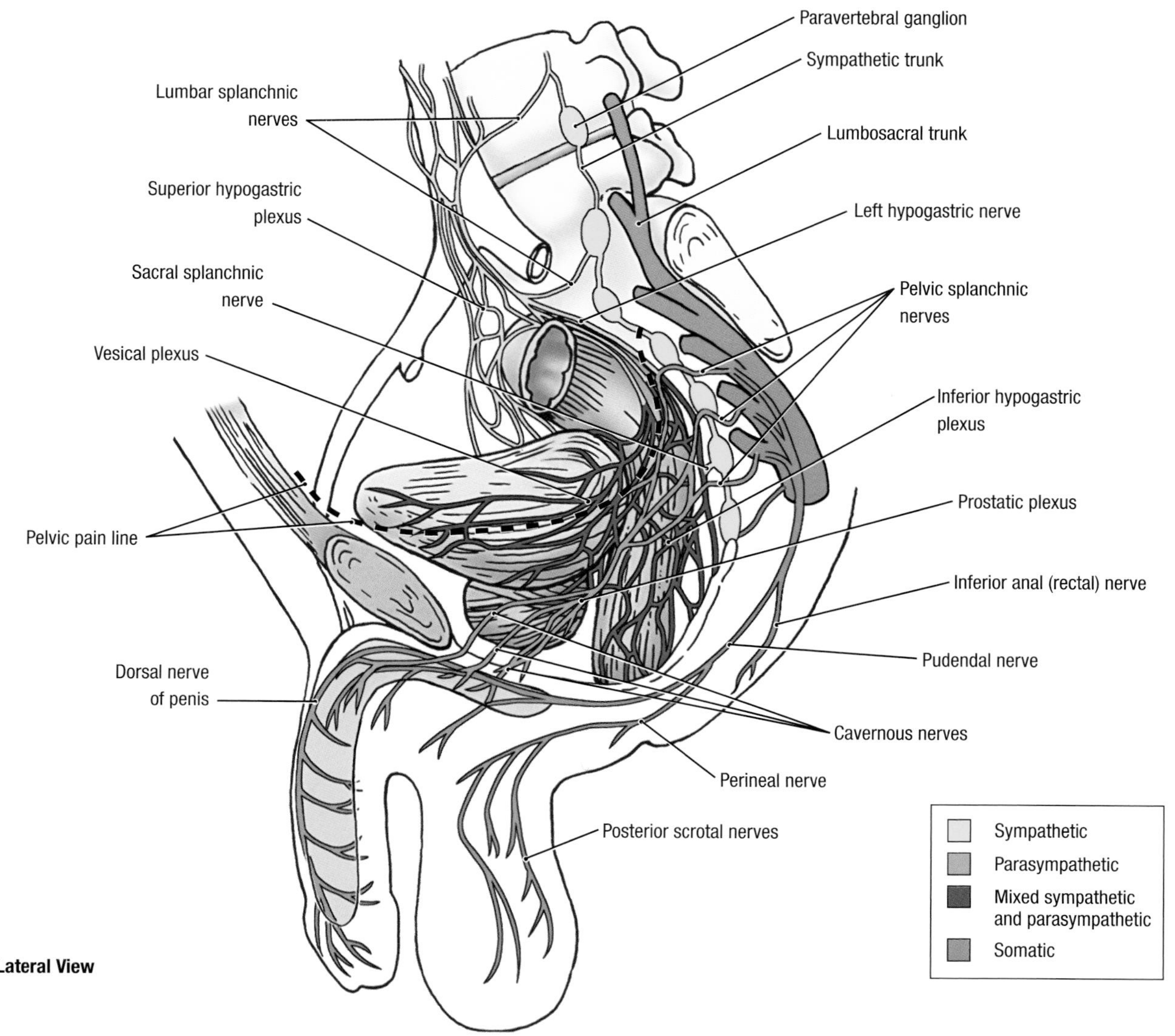
Paravertebral ganglion
Sympathetic trunk
Lumbar splanchnic nerves
Lumbosacral trunk
Superior hypogastric plexus
Left hypogastric nerve
Sacral splanchnic nerve
Pelvic splanchnic nerves
Vesical plexus
Inferior hypogastric plexus
Prostatic plexus
Pelvic pain line
Inferior anal (rectal) nerve
Pudendal nerve
Dorsal nerve of penis
Cavernous nerves
Perineal nerve
Posterior scrotal nerves
Sympathetic
Parasympathetic
Mixed sympathetic and parasympathetic
Somatic
B. Lateral View

## 3.31 Innervation of male pelvis and perineum

**A.** Overview. **B.** Innervation of prostate and external genitalia.

- The primary function of the sacral sympathetic trunks is to provide postsynaptic fibers to the sacral plexus for sympathetic innervation of the lower limb.
- The periarterial plexuses of the ovarian, superior rectal, and internal iliac arteries are minor routes by which sympathetic fibers enter the pelvis. Their primary function is vasomotion of the arteries they accompany.
- The hypogastric plexuses (superior and inferior) are networks of sympathetic and visceral afferent nerve fibers.
- The superior hypogastric plexus carries fibers conveyed to and from the aortic (intermesenteric) plexus by the L3 and L4 splanchnic nerves. The superior hypogastric plexus divides into right and left hypogastric nerves that merge with the parasympathetic pelvic splanchnic nerves to form the inferior hypogastric plexuses.
- The fibers of the inferior hypogastric plexuses continue to the pelvic viscera upon which they form pelvic plexuses, e.g., prostatic nerve plexus.
- The pelvic splanchnic nerves convey presynaptic parasympathetic fibers from the S2–S4 spinal cord segments, which make up the sacral outflow of the parasympathetic system.
- Visceral afferents conveying unconscious reflex sensation follow the course of the parasympathetic fibers retrogradely to the spinal sensory ganglia of S2–S4, as do those transmitting pain sensations from the viscera inferior to the pelvic pain line (structures that do not contact the peritoneum plus the distal sigmoid colon and rectum). Visceral afferent fibers conducting pain from structures superior to the pelvic pain line (structures in contact with the peritoneum, except for the distal sigmoid colon and rectum) follow the sympathetic fibers retrogradely to inferior thoracic and superior lumbar spinal ganglia.

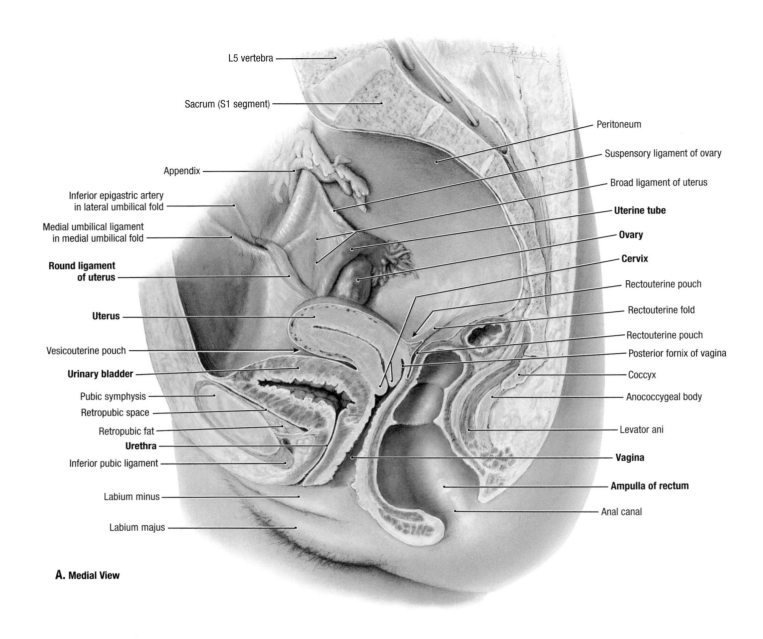

L5 vertebra
Sacrum (S1 segment)
Appendix
Inferior epigastric artery in lateral umbilical fold
Medial umbilical ligament in medial umbilical fold
**Round ligament of uterus**
**Uterus**
Vesicouterine pouch
**Urinary bladder**
Pubic symphysis
Retropubic space
Retropubic fat
**Urethra**
Inferior pubic ligament
Labium minus
Labium majus
Peritoneum
Suspensory ligament of ovary
Broad ligament of uterus
**Uterine tube**
**Ovary**
**Cervix**
Rectouterine pouch
Rectouterine fold
Rectouterine pouch
Posterior fornix of vagina
Coccyx
Anococcygeal body
Levator ani
**Vagina**
**Ampulla of rectum**
Anal canal

**A. Medial View**

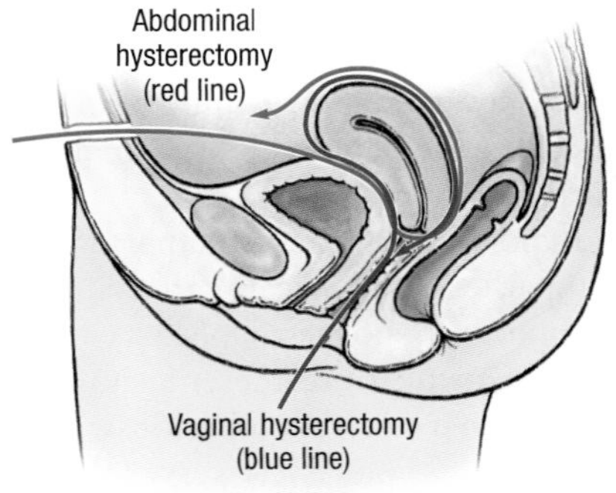
Abdominal hysterectomy (red line)
Vaginal hysterectomy (blue line)

**B. Medial View**

## 3.32 Female pelvic organs in situ

**A.** Median section. The uterus is bent on itself (anteflexed) at the junction of its body and the cervix; the cervix, opening on the anterior wall of the vagina, has a short, round, anterior lip and a long, thin, posterior lip. **B.** Hysterectomy (excision of the uterus) is performed through the lower anterior abdominal wall or through the vagina. Because the uterine artery crosses superior to the ureter near the lateral fornix of the vagina, the ureter is in danger of being inadvertently clamped or severed when the uterine artery is tied off during a hysterectomy.

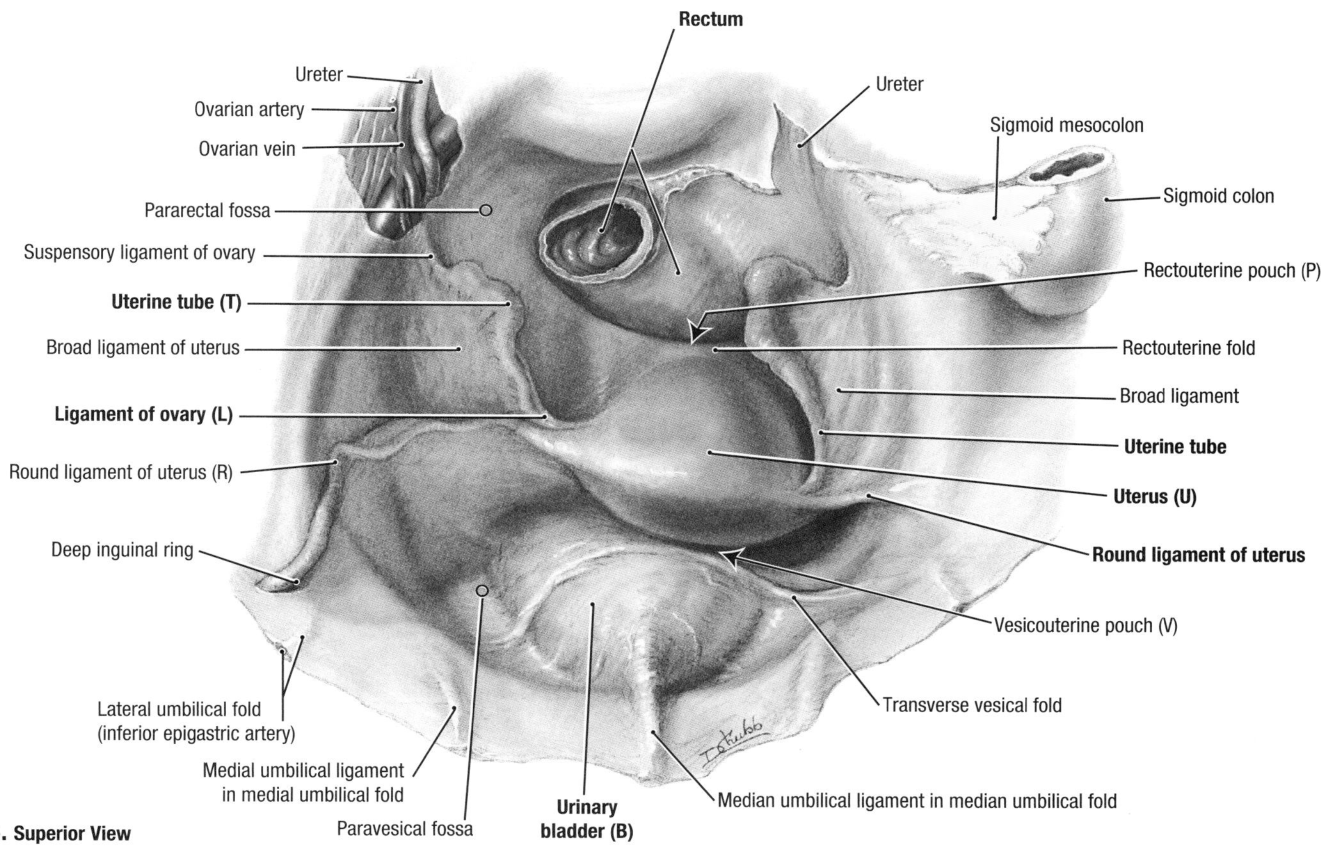
Rectum
Ureter
Ovarian artery
Ovarian vein
Pararectal fossa
Suspensory ligament of ovary
Uterine tube (T)
Broad ligament of uterus
Ligament of ovary (L)
Round ligament of uterus (R)
Deep inguinal ring
Lateral umbilical fold
(inferior epigastric artery)
Medial umbilical ligament
in medial umbilical fold
Paravesical fossa
Urinary
bladder (B)
Ureter
Sigmoid mesocolon
Sigmoid colon
Rectouterine pouch (P)
Rectouterine fold
Broad ligament
Uterine tube
Uterus (U)
Round ligament of uterus
Vesicouterine pouch (V)
Transverse vesical fold
Median umbilical ligament in median umbilical fold

**C.** **Superior View**

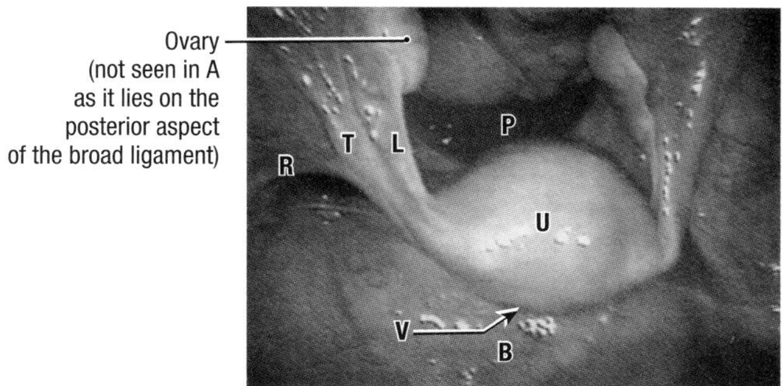
Ovary
(not seen in A
as it lies on the
posterior aspect
of the broad ligament)
R
T
L
P
U
V
B

**D.** **Laparoscopic View of Normal Pelvis**

## 3.32 Female pelvic organs in situ *(continued)*

**C.** True pelvis with peritoneum intact, viewed from above. The uterus is usually asymmetrically placed. The round ligament of the female takes the same subperitoneal course as the ductus deferens of the male.

**D.** Laparoscopy involves inserting a laparoscope into the peritoneal cavity through a small incision below the umbilicus. Insufflation of inert gas creates a pneumoperitoneum to provide space to visualize the pelvic organs. Additional openings (ports) can be made to introduce other instruments for manipulation or to enable therapeutic procedures (e.g., ligation of the uterine tubes).

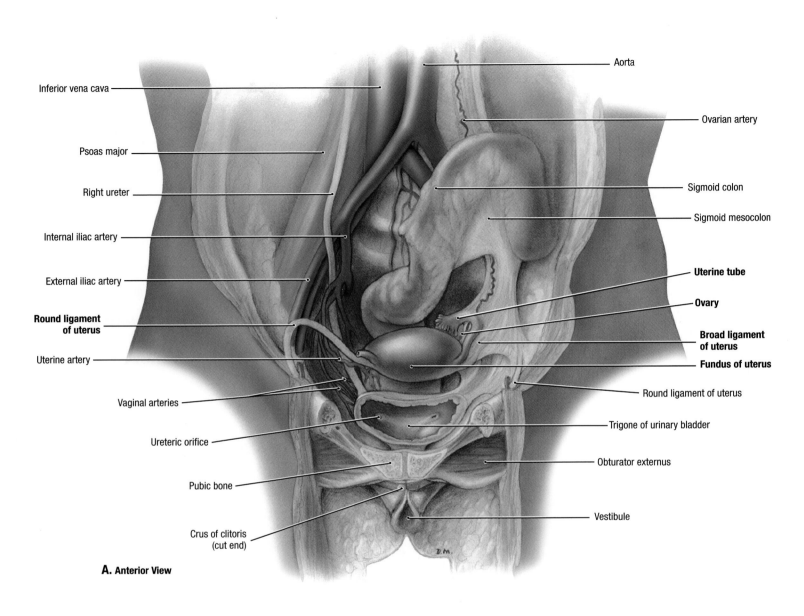

Aorta
Inferior vena cava
Ovarian artery
Psoas major
Right ureter
Sigmoid colon
Sigmoid mesocolon
Internal iliac artery
External iliac artery
**Uterine tube**
**Ovary**
**Round ligament of uterus**
**Broad ligament of uterus**
Uterine artery
**Fundus of uterus**
Round ligament of uterus
Vaginal arteries
Trigone of urinary bladder
Ureteric orifice
Obturator externus
Pubic bone
Vestibule
Crus of clitoris (cut end)

**A. Anterior View**

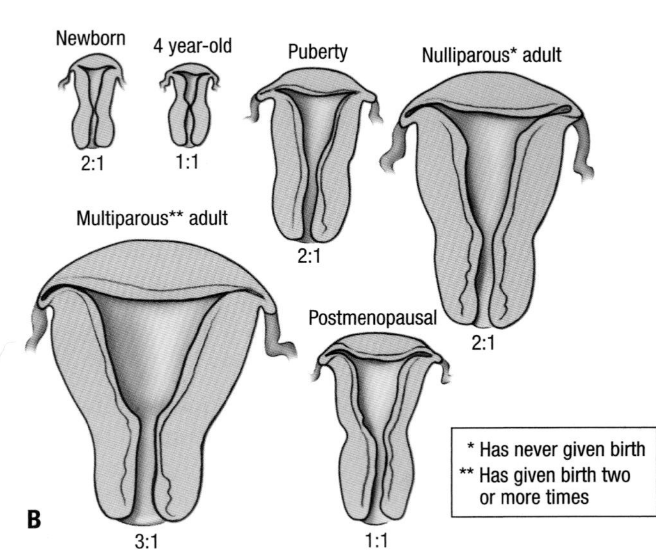

Newborn
2:1
4 year-old
1:1
Puberty
2:1
Nulliparous* adult
2:1
Multiparous** adult
3:1
Postmenopausal
1:1
* Has never given birth
** Has given birth two or more times
B


## 3.33 Female genital organs

**A.** Dissection. Part of the pubic bones, the anterior aspect of the bladder, and—on the specimen's right side—the uterine tube, ovary, broad ligament, and peritoneum covering the lateral wall of the pelvis have been removed. **B.** Lifetime changes in uterine size and proportion (body to cervical ratio, e.g., 2:1). All these stages represent normal anatomy for the particular age and reproductive status of the woman.

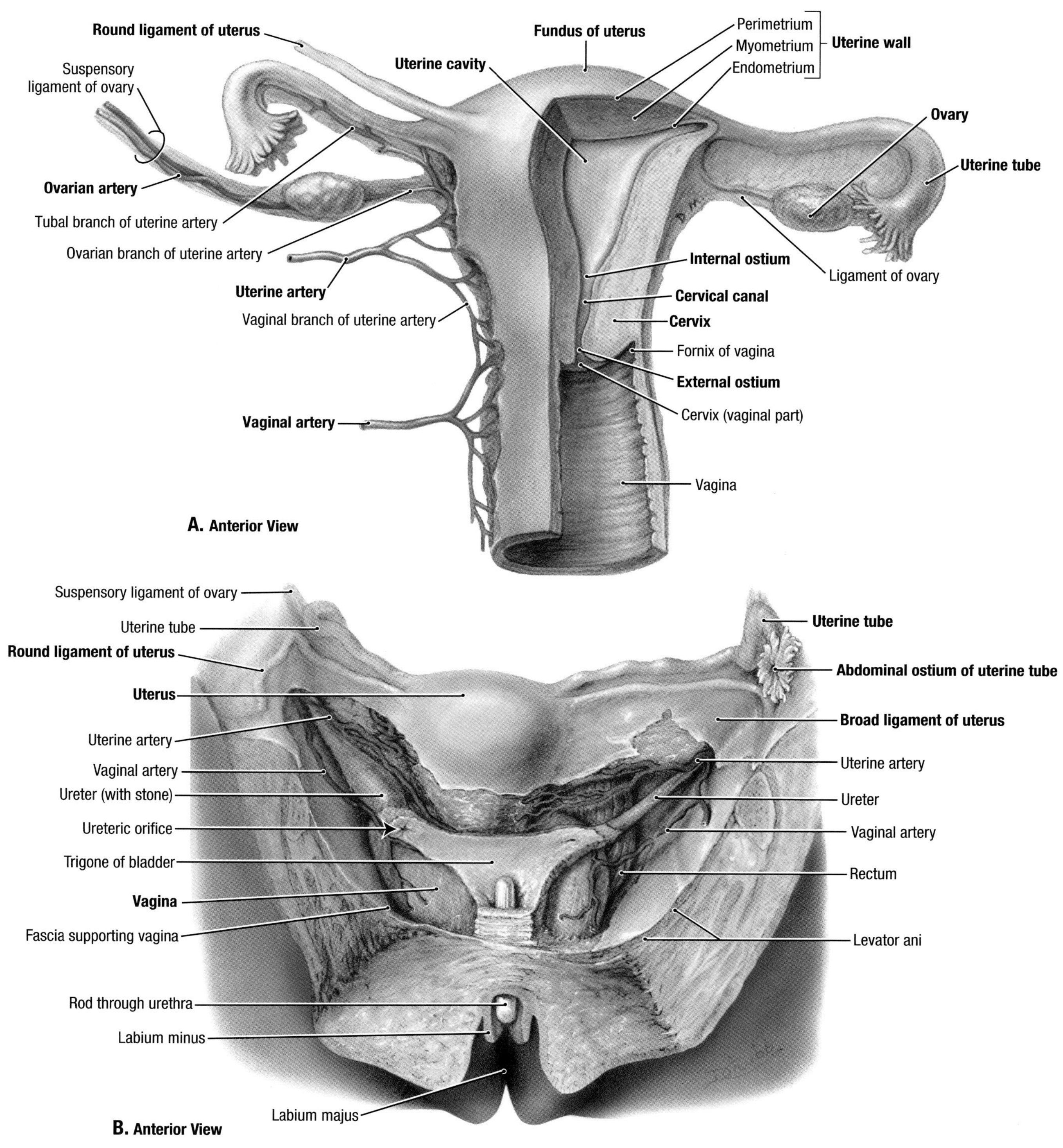
Round ligament of uterus
Suspensory ligament of ovary
Ovarian artery
Tubal branch of uterine artery
Ovarian branch of uterine artery
Uterine artery
Vaginal branch of uterine artery
Vaginal artery
Uterine cavity
Fundus of uterus
Perimetrium
Myometrium
Endometrium
Uterine wall
Ovary
Uterine tube
Ligament of ovary
Internal ostium
Cervical canal
Cervix
Fornix of vagina
External ostium
Cervix (vaginal part)
Vagina
A. Anterior View
Suspensory ligament of ovary
Uterine tube
Round ligament of uterus
Uterus
Uterine artery
Vaginal artery
Ureter (with stone)
Ureteric orifice
Trigone of bladder
Vagina
Fascia supporting vagina
Rod through urethra
Labium minus
Labium majus
B. Anterior View
Uterine tube
Abdominal ostium of uterine tube
Broad ligament of uterus
Uterine artery
Ureter
Vaginal artery
Rectum
Levator ani

## 3.34 Uterus and its adnexa

**A.** Blood supply. On the specimen's left side, part of the uterine wall with the round ligament and the vaginal wall have been cut away to expose the cervix, uterine cavity, and thick muscular wall of the uterus, the myometrium. On the specimen's right side, the ovarian artery (from the aorta) and uterine artery (from the internal iliac) supply the ovary, uterine tube, and uterus and anastomose in the broad ligament along the lateral aspect of the uterus. The uterine artery sends a uterine branch to supply the uterine body and fundus and a vaginal branch to supply the cervix and vagina. **B.** Uterus and broad ligament. The pubic bones and bladder, trigone excepted, are removed, as a continued dissection from Figure 3.33.

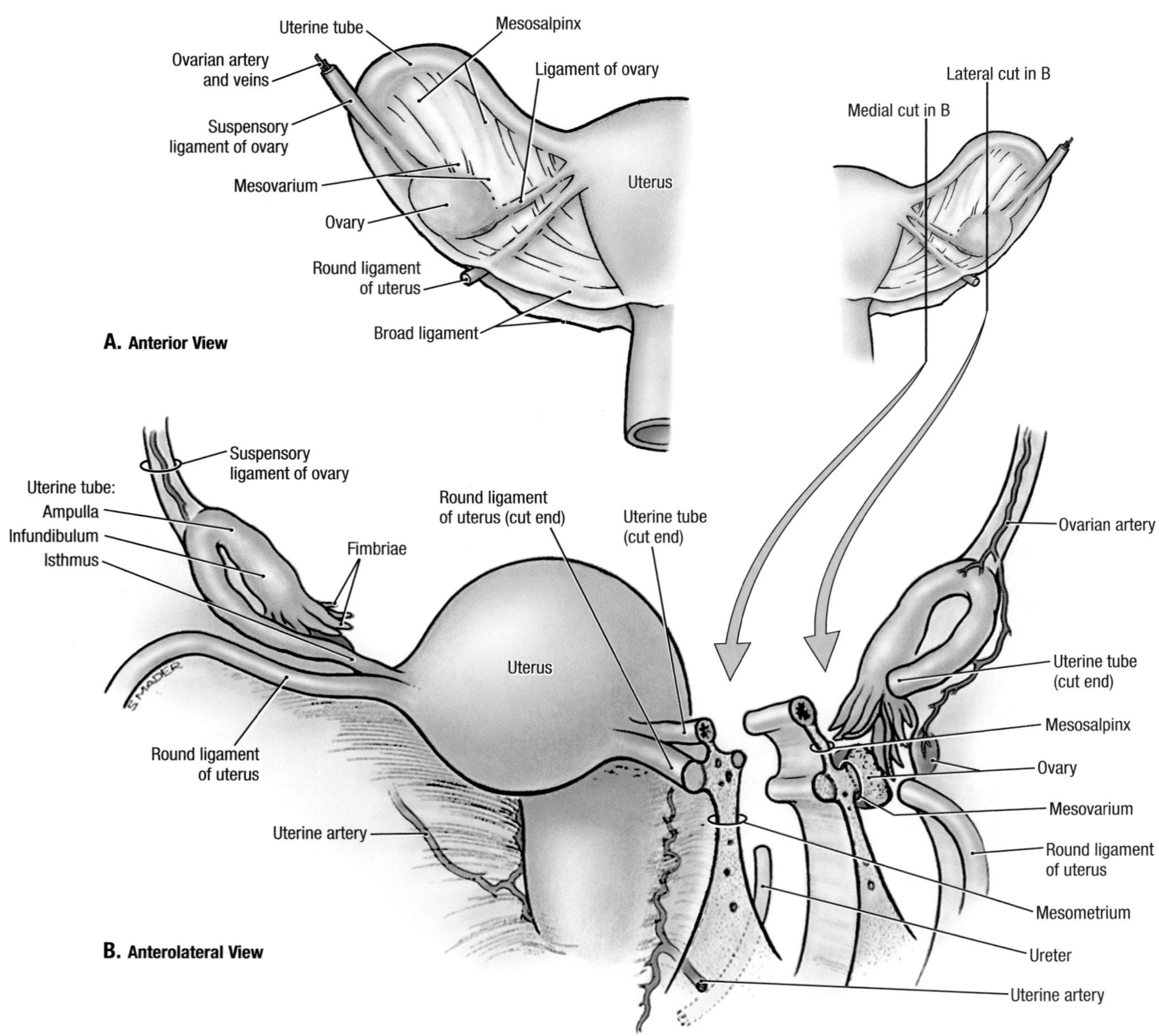
Uterine tube
Mesosalpinx
Ovarian artery and veins
Ligament of ovary
Lateral cut in B
Medial cut in B
Suspensory ligament of ovary
Mesovarium
Uterus
Ovary
Round ligament of uterus
Broad ligament
A. Anterior View
Suspensory ligament of ovary
Uterine tube:
Ampulla
Infundibulum
Isthmus
Round ligament of uterus (cut end)
Uterine tube (cut end)
Ovarian artery
Fimbriae
Uterus
Uterine tube (cut end)
Mesosalpinx
Ovary
Round ligament of uterus
Mesovarium
Uterine artery
Round ligament of uterus
Mesometrium
Ureter
B. Anterolateral View
Uterine artery

## 3.35 Uterus and broad ligament

**A** and **B.** Two paramedian sections show "mesenteries" with the prefix meso-. "Salpinx" is the Greek word for trumpet or tube, "metro" for uterus. The mesentery of the uterus and uterine tube is called the broad ligament. The major part of the broad ligament, the *mesometrium*, is attached to the uterus. The ovary is attached: to the broad ligament by a mesentery of its own, called the *mesovarium*; to the uterus by the ligament of the ovary; and near the pelvic brim, by the suspensory ligament of the ovary containing the ovarian vessels. The part of the broad ligament superior to the level of the mesovarium is called the *mesosalpinx*. **C.** Uterus in situ. **D.** Uterus and adnexa, removed from cadaver.

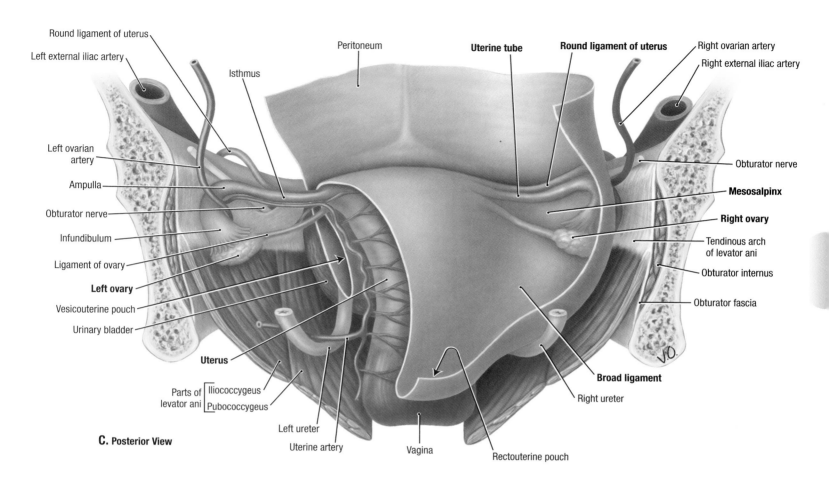

Round ligament of uterus
Left external iliac artery
Isthmus
Peritoneum
Uterine tube
Round ligament of uterus
Right ovarian artery
Right external iliac artery
Left ovarian artery
Ampulla
Obturator nerve
Infundibulum
Ligament of ovary
Left ovary
Vesicouterine pouch
Urinary bladder
Uterus
Obturator nerve
Mesosalpinx
Right ovary
Tendinous arch of levator ani
Obturator internus
Obturator fascia
Broad ligament
Right ureter
Parts of levator ani
Iliococcygeus
Pubococcygeus
Left ureter
Uterine artery
Vagina
Rectouterine pouch

**C.** Posterior View

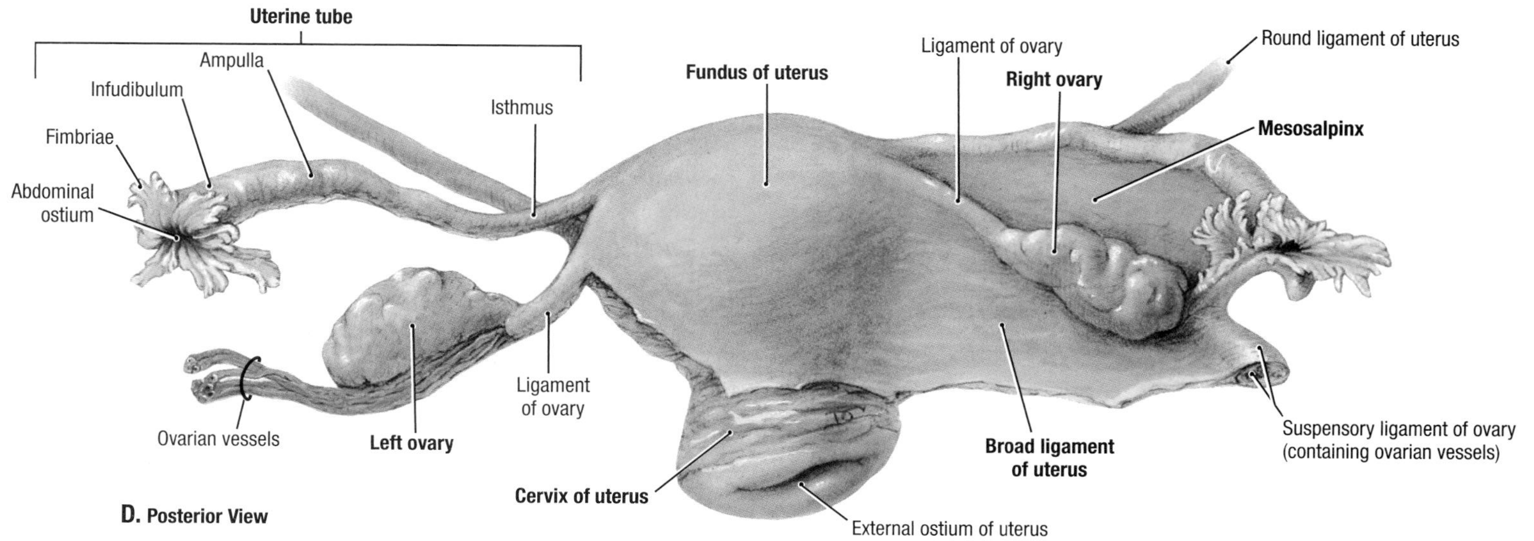
Uterine tube
Ampulla
Infudibulum
Fimbriae
Abdominal ostium
Isthmus
Fundus of uterus
Ligament of ovary
Right ovary
Round ligament of uterus
Mesosalpinx
Ovarian vessels
Left ovary
Ligament of ovary
Cervix of uterus
Broad ligament of uterus
External ostium of uterus
Suspensory ligament of ovary (containing ovarian vessels)

**D.** Posterior View

**3.35 Uterus and broad ligament *(continued)***

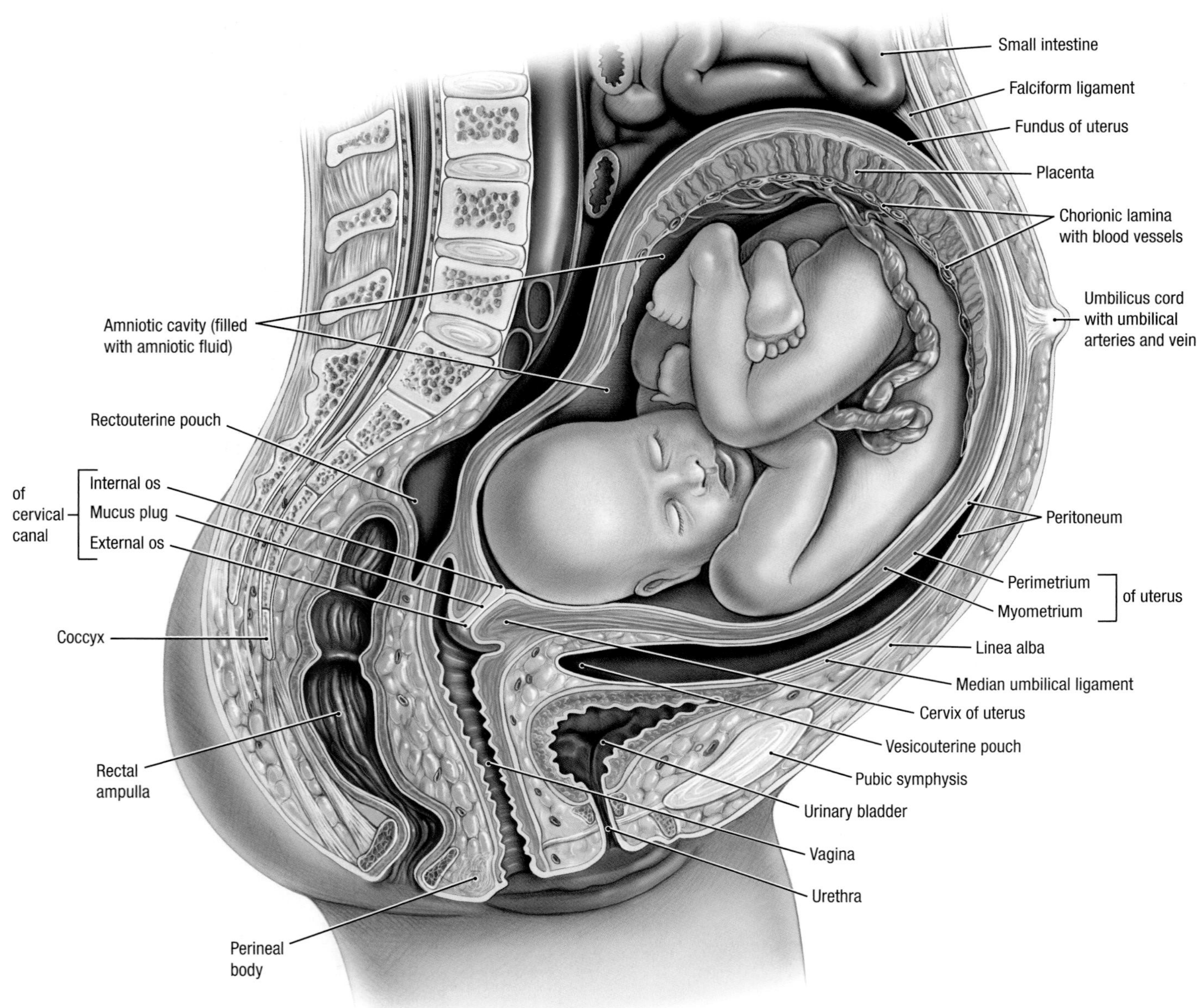
Small intestine
Falciform ligament
Fundus of uterus
Placenta
Chorionic lamina with blood vessels
Umbilicus cord with umbilical arteries and vein
Amniotic cavity (filled with amniotic fluid)
Rectouterine pouch
of cervical canal
Internal os
Mucus plug
External os
Peritoneum
Perimetrium
Myometrium
of uterus
Coccyx
Linea alba
Median umbilical ligament
Cervix of uterus
Vesicouterine pouch
Pubic symphysis
Rectal ampulla
Urinary bladder
Vagina
Urethra
Perineal body

**3.36 Pregnant uterus**

**A.** Median section; fetus is intact.

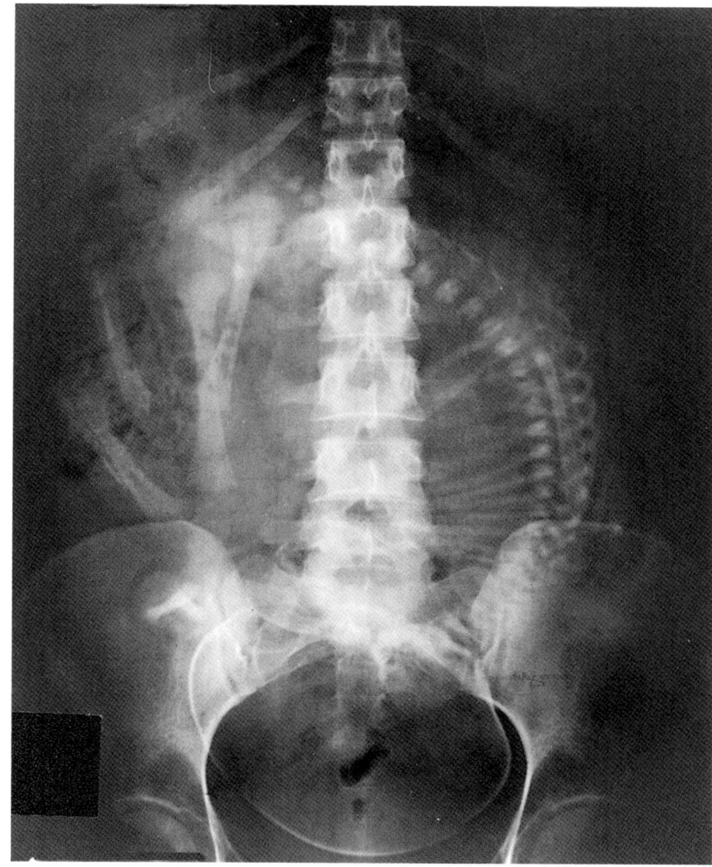

**B.** Anteroposterior View

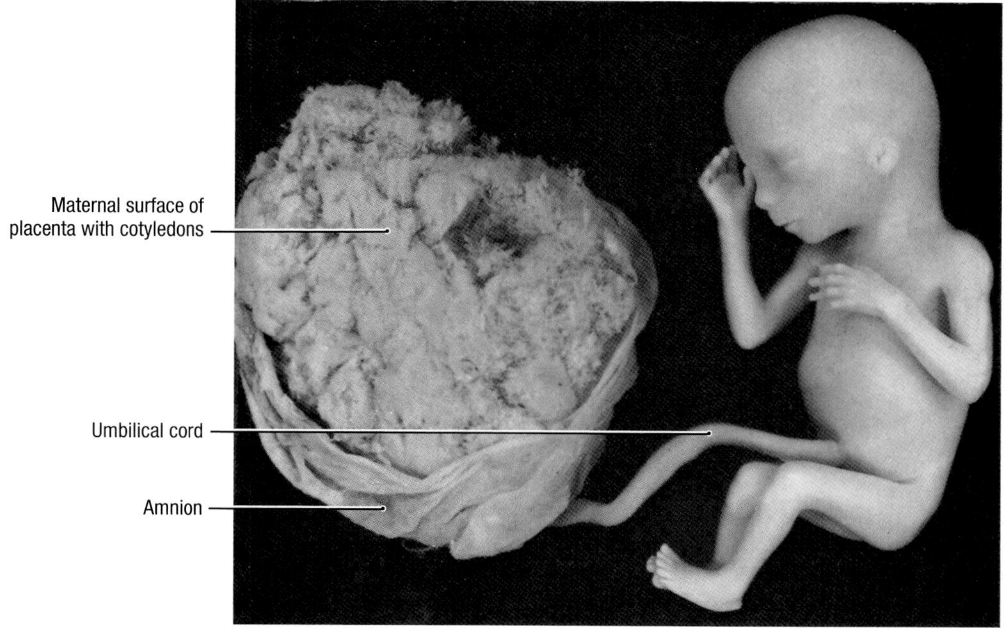
Maternal surface of placenta with cotyledons
Umbilical cord
Amnion

**C.** Maternal Surface of Placenta

## 3.36 Pregnant uterus *(continued)*

**B.** Radiograph of fetus. **C.** Photograph of an 18-week-old fetus connected to the placenta by the umbilical cord.

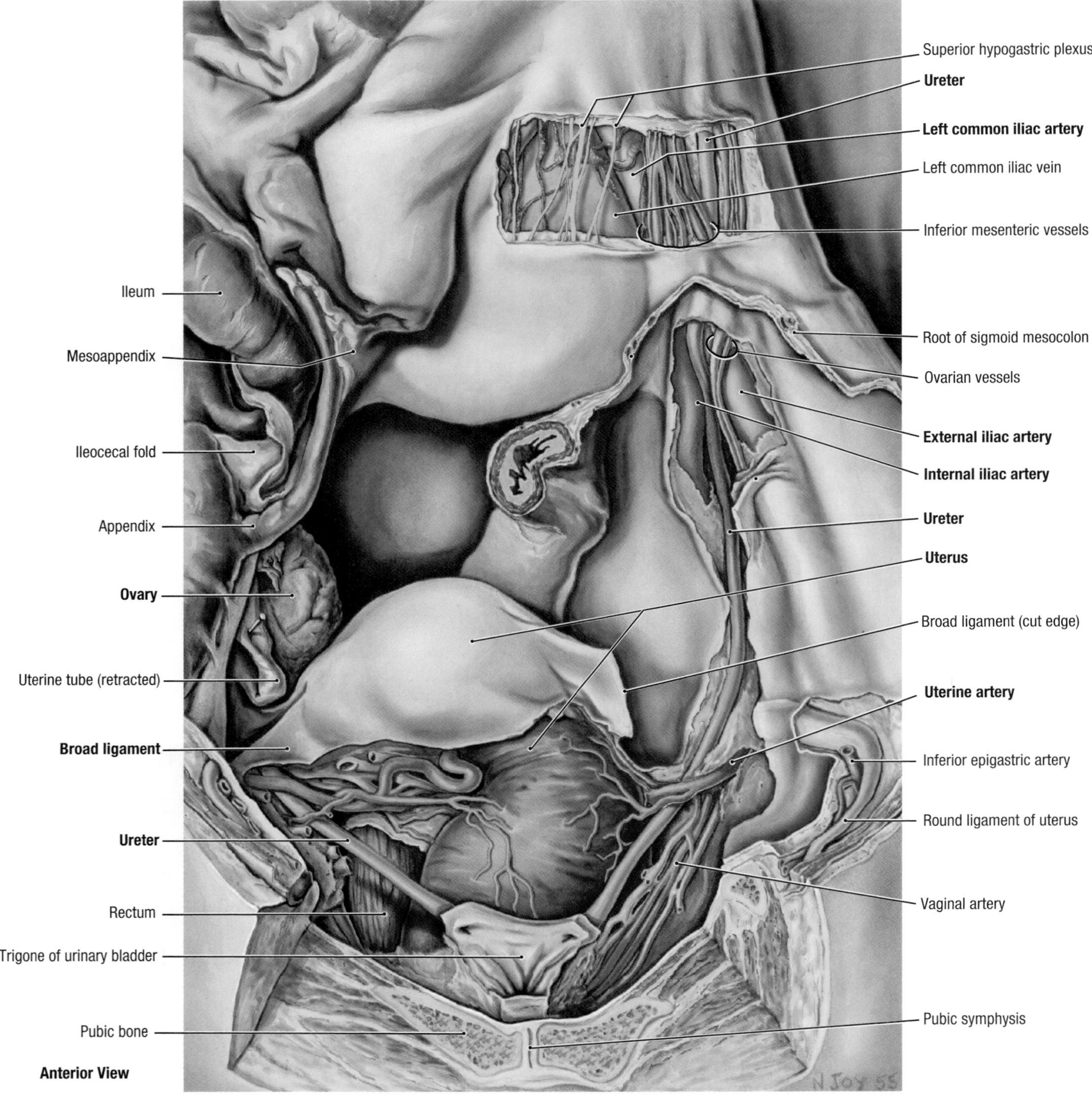
Superior hypogastric plexus
Ureter
Left common iliac artery
Left common iliac vein
Inferior mesenteric vessels
Ileum
Mesoappendix
Root of sigmoid mesocolon
Ovarian vessels
External iliac artery
Internal iliac artery
Ileocecal fold
Appendix
Ureter
Uterus
Ovary
Broad ligament (cut edge)
Uterine tube (retracted)
Uterine artery
Broad ligament
Inferior epigastric artery
Round ligament of uterus
Ureter
Rectum
Vaginal artery
Trigone of urinary bladder
Pubic bone
Pubic symphysis
Anterior View
N. JOY 55

## 3.37 Ureter and relationship to uterine artery

- Most of the pubic symphysis and most of the bladder (except the trigone) have been removed as in Figure 3.34B.
- The left ureter is crossed by the ovarian vessels and nerves; the apex of the inverted V-shaped root of the sigmoid mesocolon is situated anterior to the left ureter.
- The left ureter crosses the external iliac artery at the bifurcation of the common iliac artery and then descends anterior to the internal iliac artery; its course is subperitoneal from where it enters the pelvis to where it passes deep to the broad ligament and is crossed by the uterine artery.

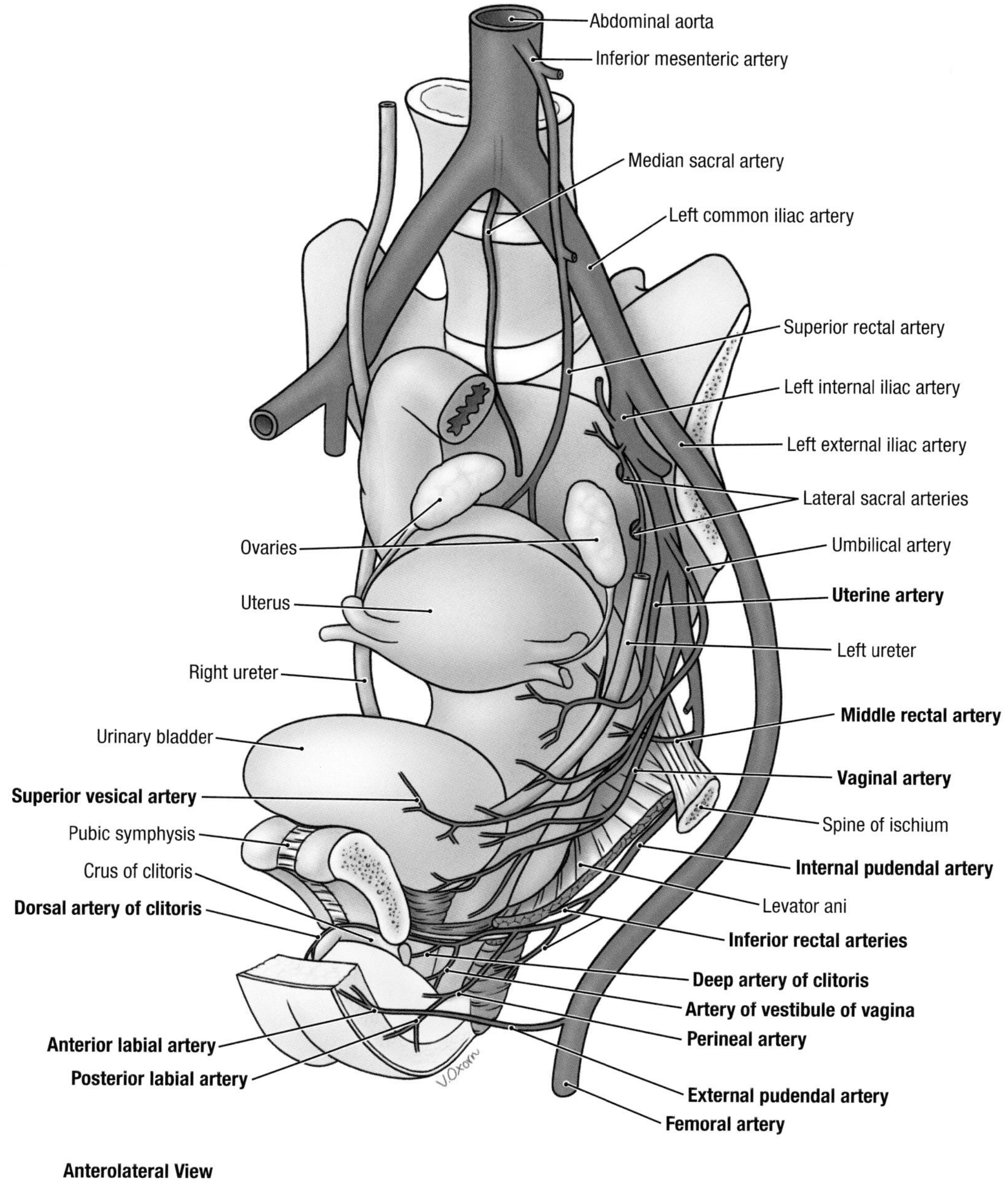
Abdominal aorta
Inferior mesenteric artery
Median sacral artery
Left common iliac artery
Superior rectal artery
Left internal iliac artery
Left external iliac artery
Lateral sacral arteries
Umbilical artery
Uterine artery
Left ureter
Middle rectal artery
Vaginal artery
Spine of ischium
Internal pudendal artery
Levator ani
Inferior rectal arteries
Deep artery of clitoris
Artery of vestibule of vagina
Perineal artery
External pudendal artery
Femoral artery
Ovaries
Uterus
Right ureter
Urinary bladder
Superior vesical artery
Pubic symphysis
Crus of clitoris
Dorsal artery of clitoris
Anterior labial artery
Posterior labial artery
Anterolateral View

## 3.38 Arterial supply of female pelvis and perineum

- The blood supply of the uterus is mainly from the *uterine arteries*, with potential collateral supply from the ovarian arteries.
- The arteries supplying the superior part of the vagina derive from the *uterine arteries*; the arteries supplying the middle and inferior parts of the vagina derive from the *vaginal* and *internal pudendal arteries*.
- The superior vesical arteries supply the anterosuperior parts of the bladder; the vaginal arteries supply the posteroinferior parts of the bladder.

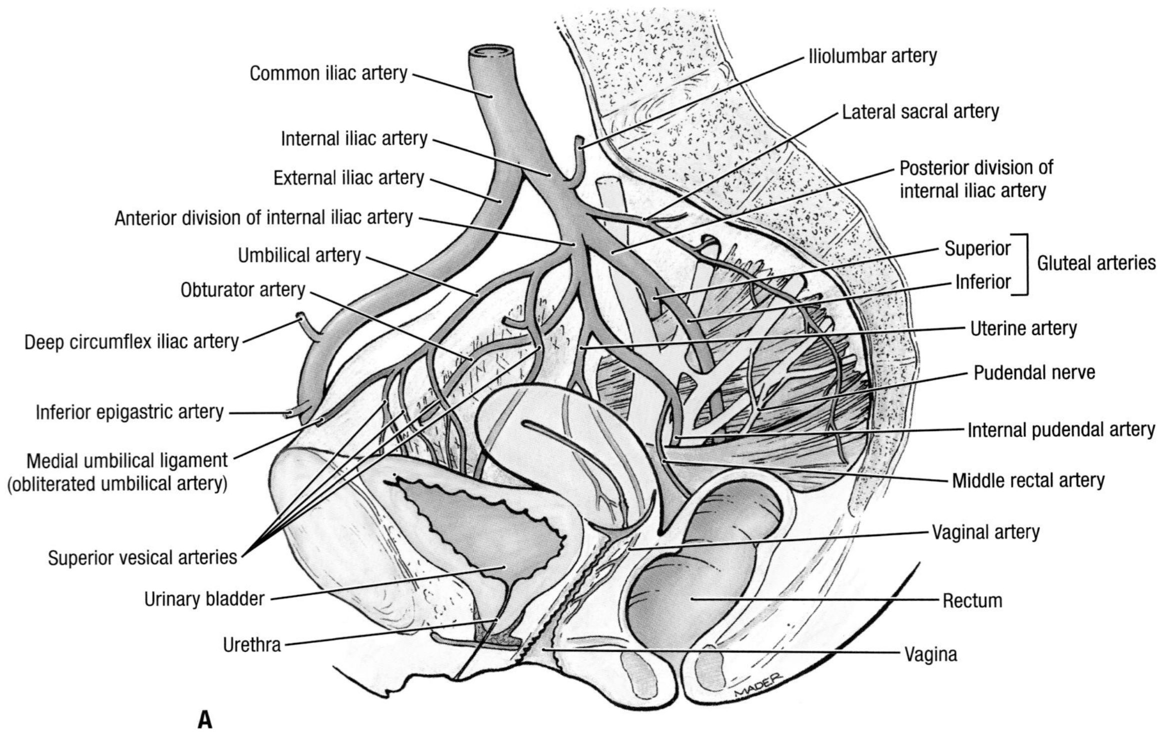
Common iliac artery
Internal iliac artery
External iliac artery
Anterior division of internal iliac artery
Umbilical artery
Obturator artery
Deep circumflex iliac artery
Inferior epigastric artery
Medial umbilical ligament (obliterated umbilical artery)
Superior vesical arteries
Urinary bladder
Urethra
Iliolumbar artery
Lateral sacral artery
Posterior division of internal iliac artery
Superior
Inferior
Gluteal arteries
Uterine artery
Pudendal nerve
Internal pudendal artery
Middle rectal artery
Vaginal artery
Rectum
Vagina
A

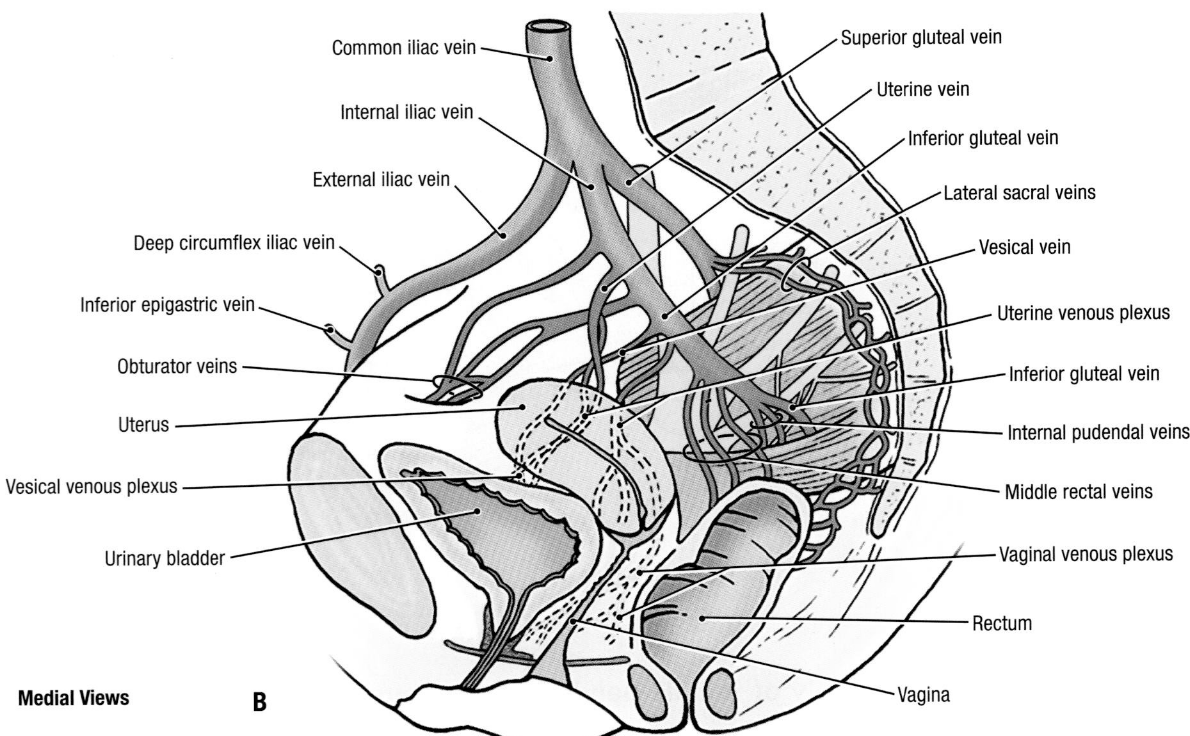
Common iliac vein
Internal iliac vein
External iliac vein
Deep circumflex iliac vein
Inferior epigastric vein
Obturator veins
Uterus
Vesical venous plexus
Urinary bladder
Superior gluteal vein
Uterine vein
Inferior gluteal vein
Lateral sacral veins
Vesical vein
Uterine venous plexus
Inferior gluteal vein
Internal pudendal veins
Middle rectal veins
Vaginal venous plexus
Rectum
Vagina
Medial Views
B

**3.39 Arteries and veins of female pelvis**

**A.** Arteries. **B.** Pelvic veins and venous plexuses.

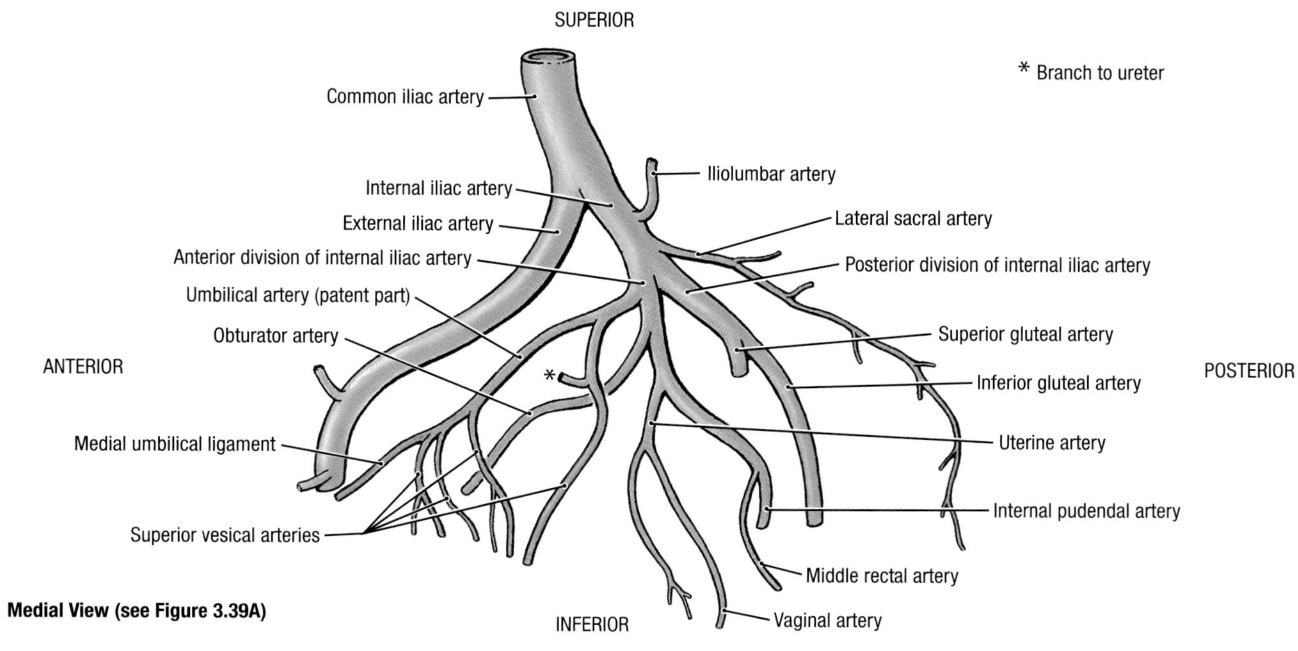
SUPERIOR
* Branch to ureter
Common iliac artery
Iliolumbar artery
Internal iliac artery
Lateral sacral artery
External iliac artery
Anterior division of internal iliac artery
Posterior division of internal iliac artery
Umbilical artery (patent part)
Obturator artery
Superior gluteal artery
ANTERIOR
Inferior gluteal artery
POSTERIOR
Medial umbilical ligament
Uterine artery
Internal pudendal artery
Superior vesical arteries
Middle rectal artery
INFERIOR
Vaginal artery

**Medial View (see Figure 3.39A)**

**TABLE 3.7 ARTERIES OF FEMALE PELVIS**

| Artery | Origin | Course | Distribution |
|---|---|---|---|
| Internal iliac | Common iliac artery | Passes over pelvic brim and descends into pelvic cavity | Main blood supply to pelvic organs, gluteal muscles, and perineum |
| Anterior division of internal iliac artery | Internal iliac artery | Passes anteriorly along lateral wall of pelvis, dividing into visceral, obturator, and internal pudendal arteries | Pelvic viscera and muscles of superior medial thigh, and perineum |
| Umbilical | Anterior division of internal iliac artery | Short pelvic course, gives off superior vesical arteries | Superior aspect of urinary bladder |
| Superior vesical artery | Patent proximal part of umbilical artery | Usually multiple, pass to superior aspect of urinary bladder | Superior aspect of urinary bladder |
| Obturator | Anterior division of internal iliac artery | Runs anteroinferiorly on lateral pelvic wall | Pelvic muscles, nutrient artery to ilium, head of femur, and muscles of medial compartment of thigh |
| Uterine | | Runs anteromedially in base of broad ligament/superior cardinal ligament; gives rise to vaginal branch, then crosses ureter superiorly to reach lateral aspect of uterine cervix | Uterus, ligaments of uterus, medial parts of uterine tube and ovary, and superior vagina |
| Vaginal | | Divides into vaginal and inferior vesical branches | Vaginal branch: lower vagina, vestibular bulb, and adjacent rectum; inferior vesical branch: fundus of urinary bladder |
| Middle rectal | | Descends in pelvis to inferior part of rectum | Inferior part of rectum |
| Internal pudendal | | Exits pelvis via greater sciatic foramen and enters perineum (ischioanal fossa) via lesser sciatic foramen | Main artery to perineum including muscles of anal canal and perineum, skin and urogenital triangle, and erectile bodies |
| Posterior division of internal iliac artery | Internal iliac artery | Passes posteriorly and gives rise to parietal branches | Pelvic wall and gluteal region |
| Iliolumbar | Posterior division of internal iliac artery | Ascends anterior to sacroiliac joint and posterior to common iliac vessels and psoas major | Iliacus, psoas major, quadratus lumborum muscles, and cauda equina in vertebral canal |
| Lateral sacral (superior and inferior) | | Run on anteromedial aspect of piriformis | Piriformis muscle, structures in sacral canal and erector spinae muscles |
| Ovarian | Abdominal aorta | Crosses pelvic brim and descends in suspensory ligament to ovary | Abdominal and/or pelvic ureter, ovary, and ampullary end of uterine tube |

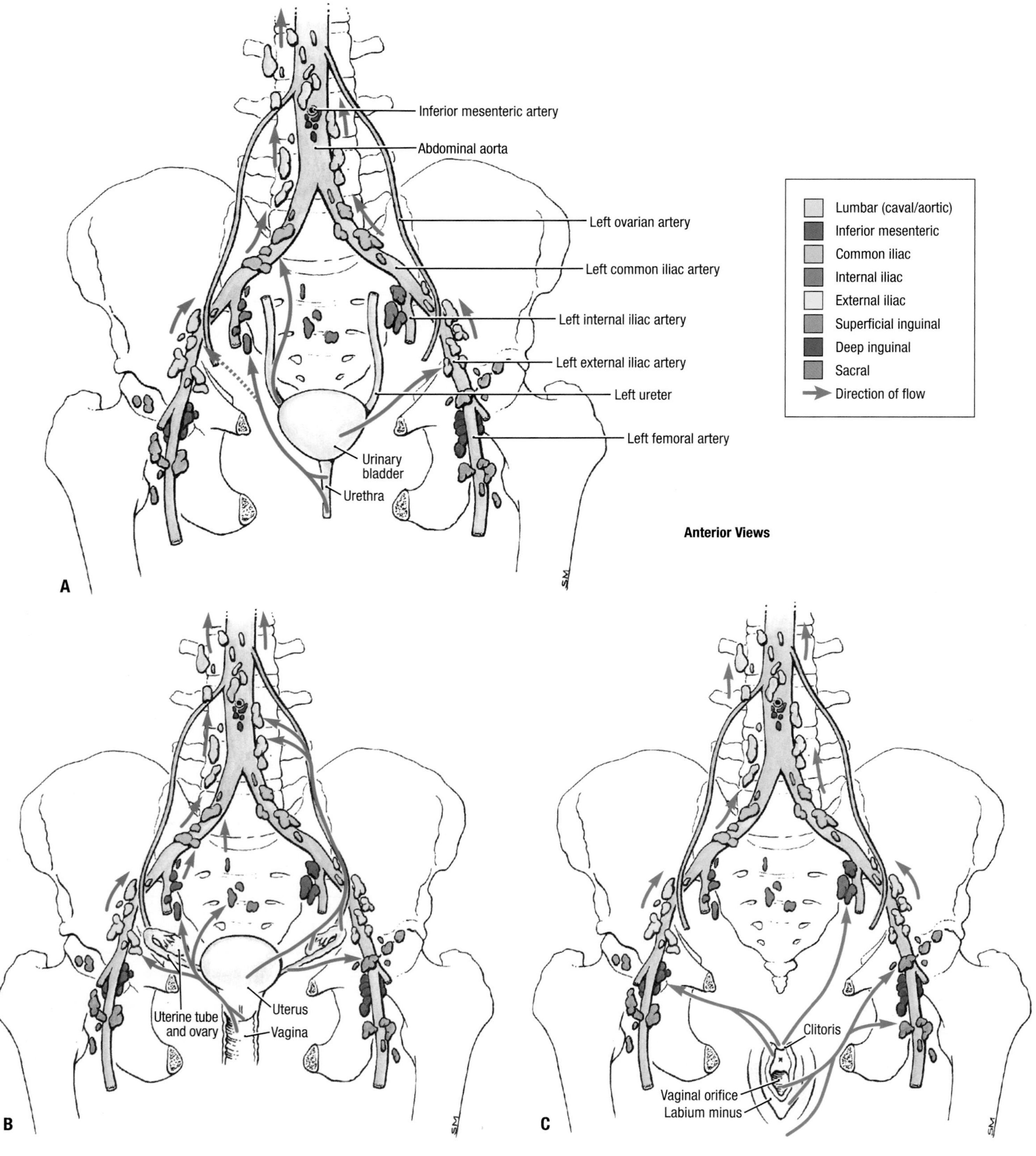
Inferior mesenteric artery
Abdominal aorta
Left ovarian artery
Left common iliac artery
Left internal iliac artery
Left external iliac artery
Left ureter
Left femoral artery
Urinary bladder
Urethra
Lumbar (caval/aortic)
Inferior mesenteric
Common iliac
Internal iliac
External iliac
Superficial inguinal
Deep inguinal
Sacral
Direction of flow
Anterior Views
A
Uterine tube and ovary
Uterus
Vagina
B
Clitoris
Vaginal orifice
Labium minus
C

**3.40 Lymphatic drainage of female pelvis and perineum**

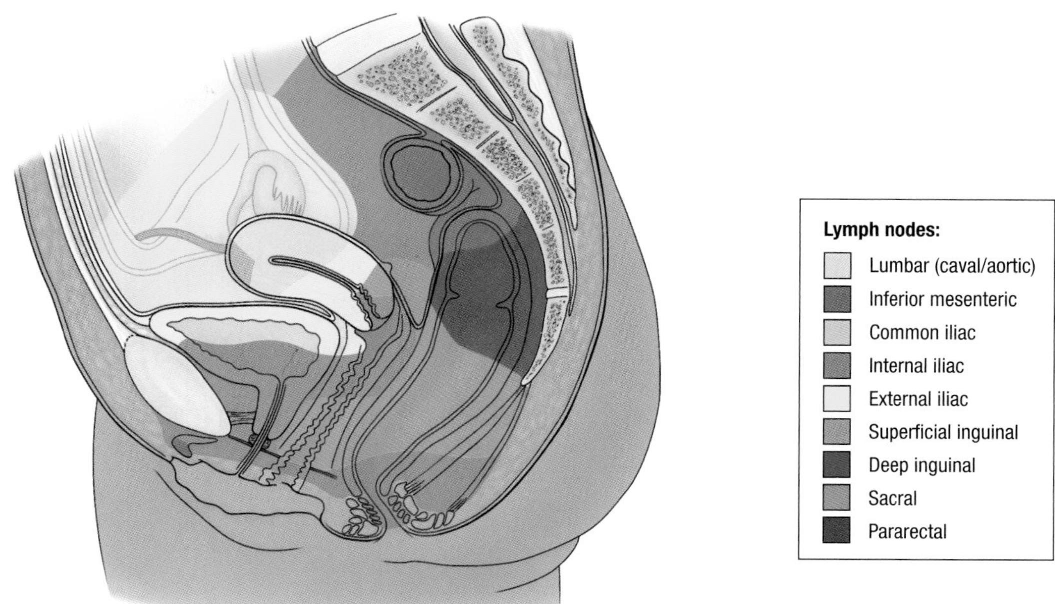
Lymph nodes:
Lumbar (caval/aortic)
Inferior mesenteric
Common iliac
Internal iliac
External iliac
Superficial inguinal
Deep inguinal
Sacral
Pararectal

**TABLE 3.8 LYMPHATIC DRAINAGE OF THE STRUCTURES OF THE FEMALE PELVIS AND PERINEUM**

| Lymph Node Group | Structures Typically Draining to Lymph Node Group |
|---|---|
| Lumbar | Gonads and associated structures (along ovarian vessels), ovary, uterine tube (except isthmus and intrauterine parts), fundus of uterus, common iliac nodes |
| Inferior mesenteric | Superiormost rectum, sigmoid colon, descending colon, pararectal nodes |
| Common iliac | External and internal iliac lymph nodes |
| Internal iliac | Inferior pelvic structures, deep perineal structures, sacral nodes, base of bladder, inferior pelvic ureter, anal canal (above pectinate line), inferior rectum, middle and upper vagina, cervix, body of uterus , sacral nodes |
| External iliac | Anterosuperior pelvic structures, deep inguinal nodes, superior bladder, superior pelvic ureter, upper vagina, cervix, lower body of uterus |
| Superficial inguinal | Lower limb, superficial drainage of inferolateral quadrant of trunk, including anterior abdominal wall inferior to umbilicus, gluteal region, superolateral uterus (near attachment of round ligament), skin of perineum including vulva, ostium of vagina (inferior to hymen), prepuce of clitoris, perianal skin, anal canal inferior to pectinate line |
| Deep inguinal | Glans of clitoris, superficial inguinal nodes |
| Sacral | Posteroinferior pelvic structures, inferior rectum, inferior vagina |
| Pararectal | Superior rectum |

## 3.41 Innervation of female pelvic viscera

- Pelvic splanchnic nerves (S2–S4) supply parasympathetic motor fibers to the uterus and vagina (and vasodilator fibers to the erectile tissue of the clitoris and bulb of the vestibule; not shown).
- Presynaptic sympathetic fibers pass through the lumbar splanchnic nerves to synapse in prevertebral ganglia; the postsynaptic fibers travel through the superior and inferior hypogastric plexuses to reach the pelvic viscera.
- Visceral afferent fibers conducting pain from intraperitoneal viscera travel with the sympathetic fibers to the T12–L2 spinal ganglia. Visceral afferent fibers conducting pain from subperitoneal viscera travel with parasympathetic fibers to the S2–S4 spinal ganglia.
- Somatic sensation from the opening of the vagina also passes to the S2–S4 spinal ganglia via the pudendal nerve.
- Muscular contractions of the uterus are hormonally induced.

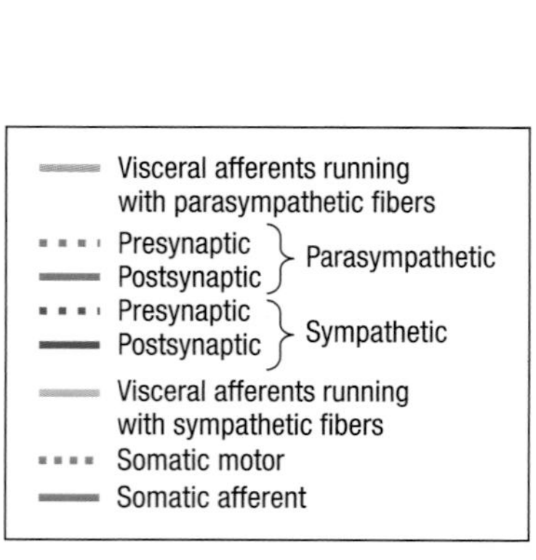
Visceral afferents running with parasympathetic fibers
Presynaptic
Postsynaptic
Parasympathetic
Presynaptic
Postsynaptic
Sympathetic
Visceral afferents running with sympathetic fibers
Somatic motor
Somatic afferent

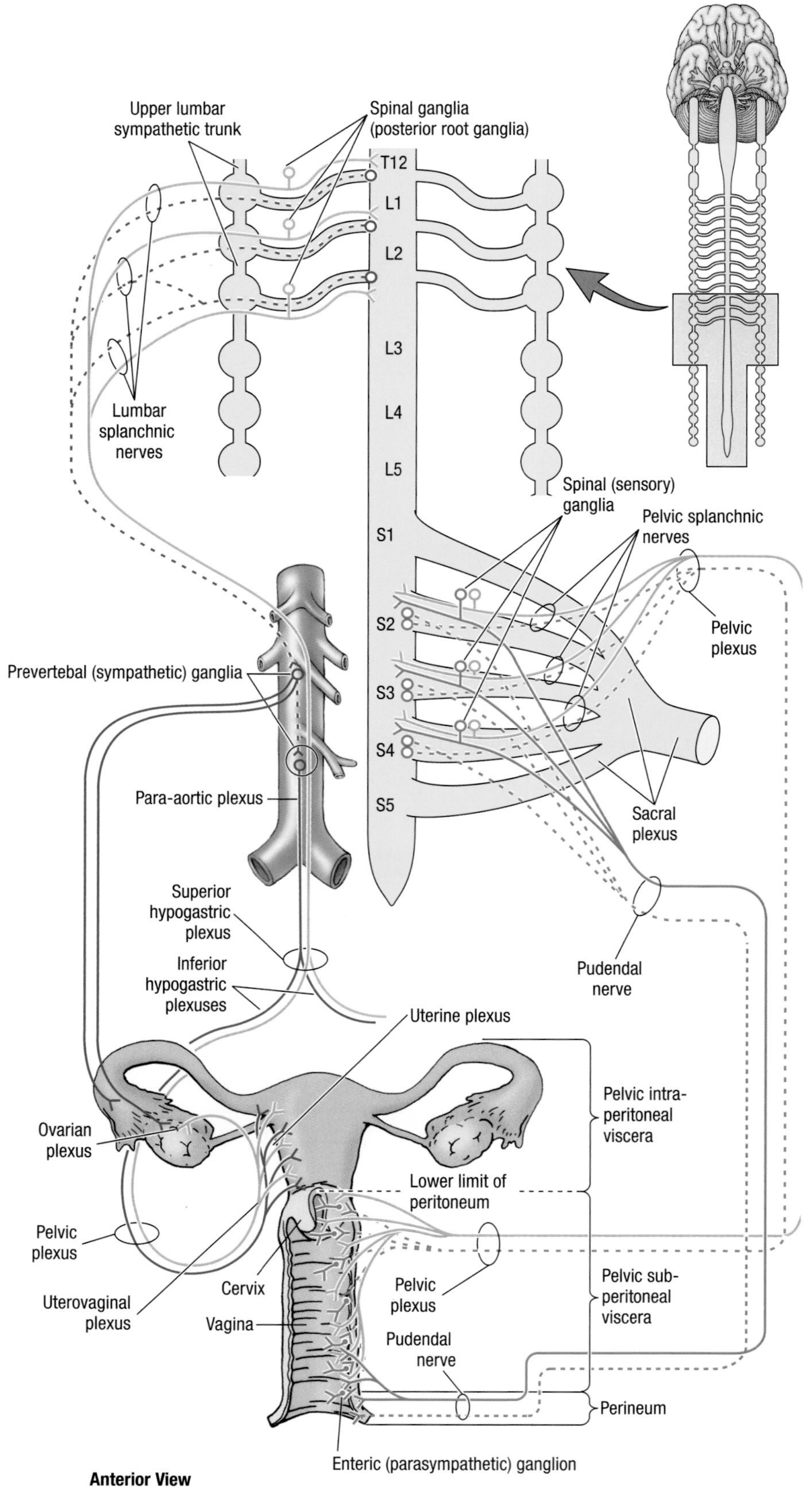

**Anterior View**

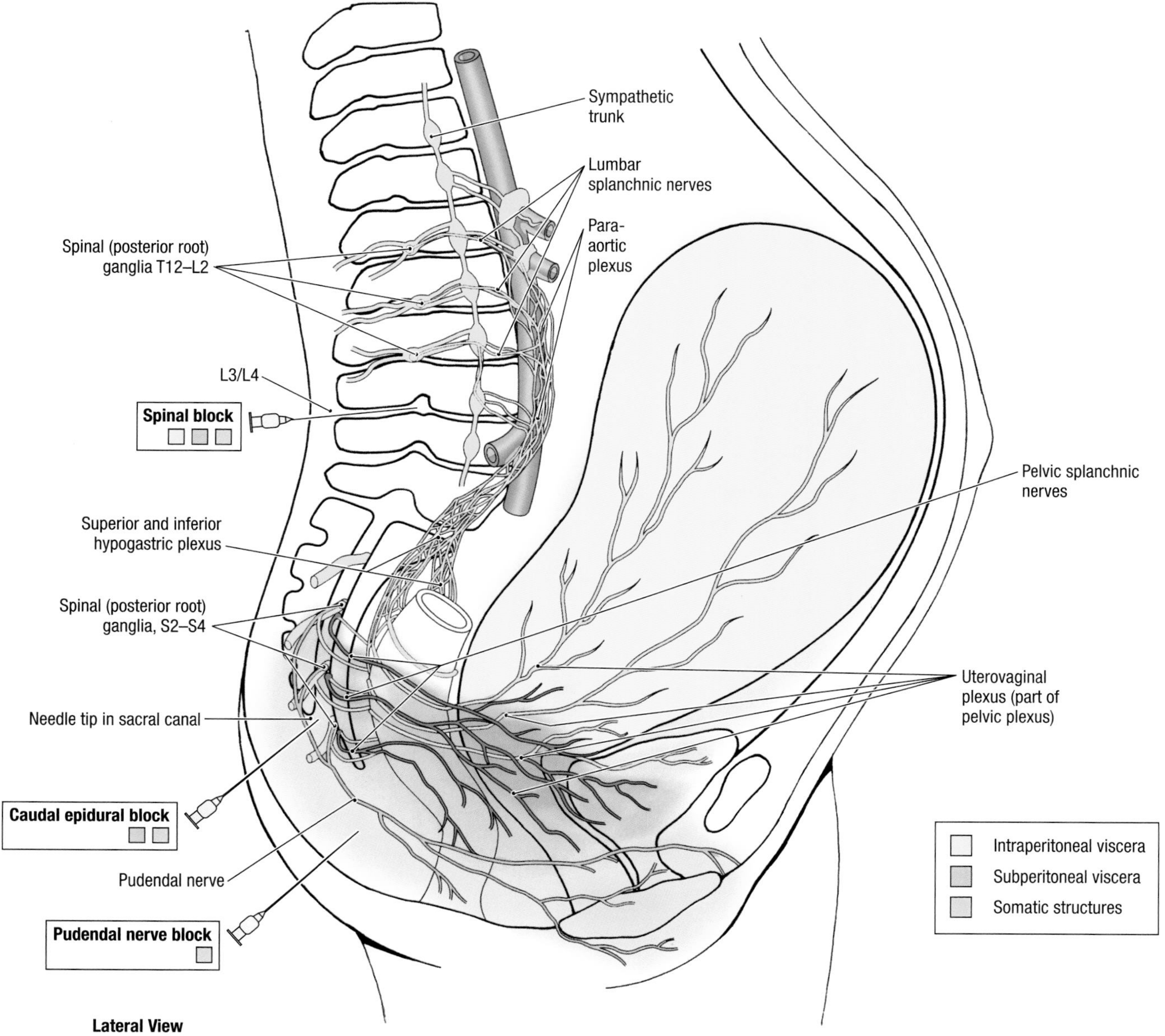
Sympathetic trunk
Lumbar splanchnic nerves
Para-aortic plexus
Spinal (posterior root) ganglia T12–L2
L3/L4
Spinal block
Superior and inferior hypogastric plexus
Spinal (posterior root) ganglia, S2–S4
Needle tip in sacral canal
Caudal epidural block
Pudendal nerve
Pudendal nerve block
Pelvic splanchnic nerves
Uterovaginal plexus (part of pelvic plexus)
Intraperitoneal viscera
Subperitoneal viscera
Somatic structures
Lateral View

## 3.42 Innervation of pelvic viscera during pregnancy; nerve blocks

- A spinal block, in which the anesthetic agent is introduced with a needle into the spinal subarachnoid space at the L3–L4 vertebral level produces complete anesthesia inferior to approximately the waist level. The perineum, pelvic floor, and birth canal are anesthetized, and motor and sensory functions of the entire lower limbs, as well as sensation of uterine contractions, are temporarily eliminated.
- With the caudal epidural block, the anesthetic agent is administered using an in-dwelling catheter in the sacral canal. The entire birth canal, pelvic floor, and most of the perineum are anesthetized, but the lower limbs are not usually affected. The mother is aware of her uterine contractions.
- A pudendal nerve block is a peripheral nerve block that provides local anesthesia over the S2–S4 dermatomes (most of the perineum) and the inferior quarter of the vagina. It does not block pain from the superior birth canal (uterine cervix and superior vagina, so the mother is able to feel uterine contractions.

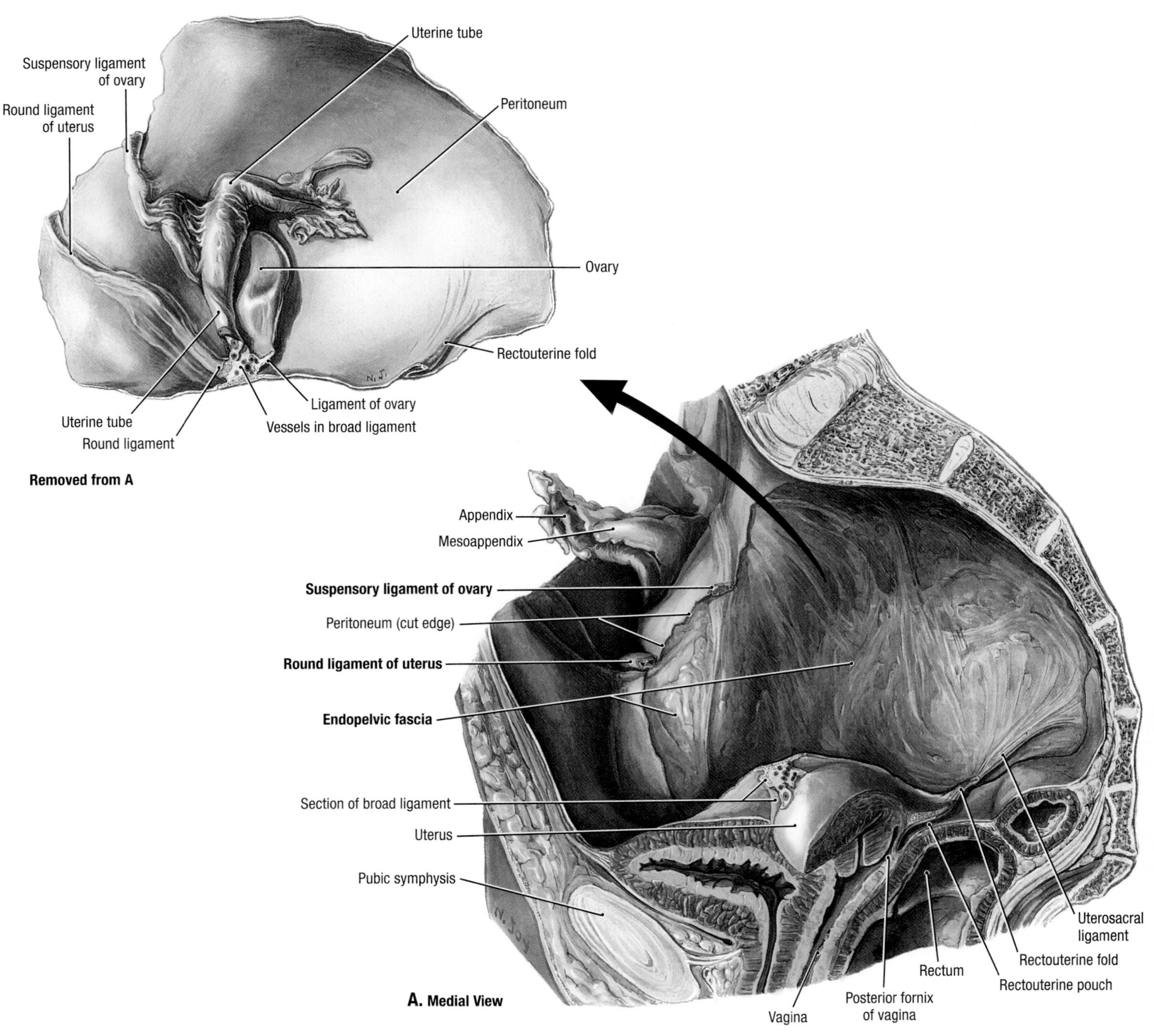
Uterine tube
Suspensory ligament of ovary
Round ligament of uterus
Peritoneum
Ovary
Rectouterine fold
Ligament of ovary
Vessels in broad ligament
Uterine tube
Round ligament
Removed from A
Appendix
Mesoappendix
Suspensory ligament of ovary
Peritoneum (cut edge)
Round ligament of uterus
Endopelvic fascia
Section of broad ligament
Uterus
Pubic symphysis
A. Medial View
Uterosacral ligament
Rectouterine fold
Rectum
Rectouterine pouch
Posterior fornix of vagina
Vagina

## 3.43 Serial dissection of autonomic nerves of female pelvis

**A.** Broad ligament and peritoneum of the lateral wall of the pelvic cavity have been removed to expose the endopelvic fascia.

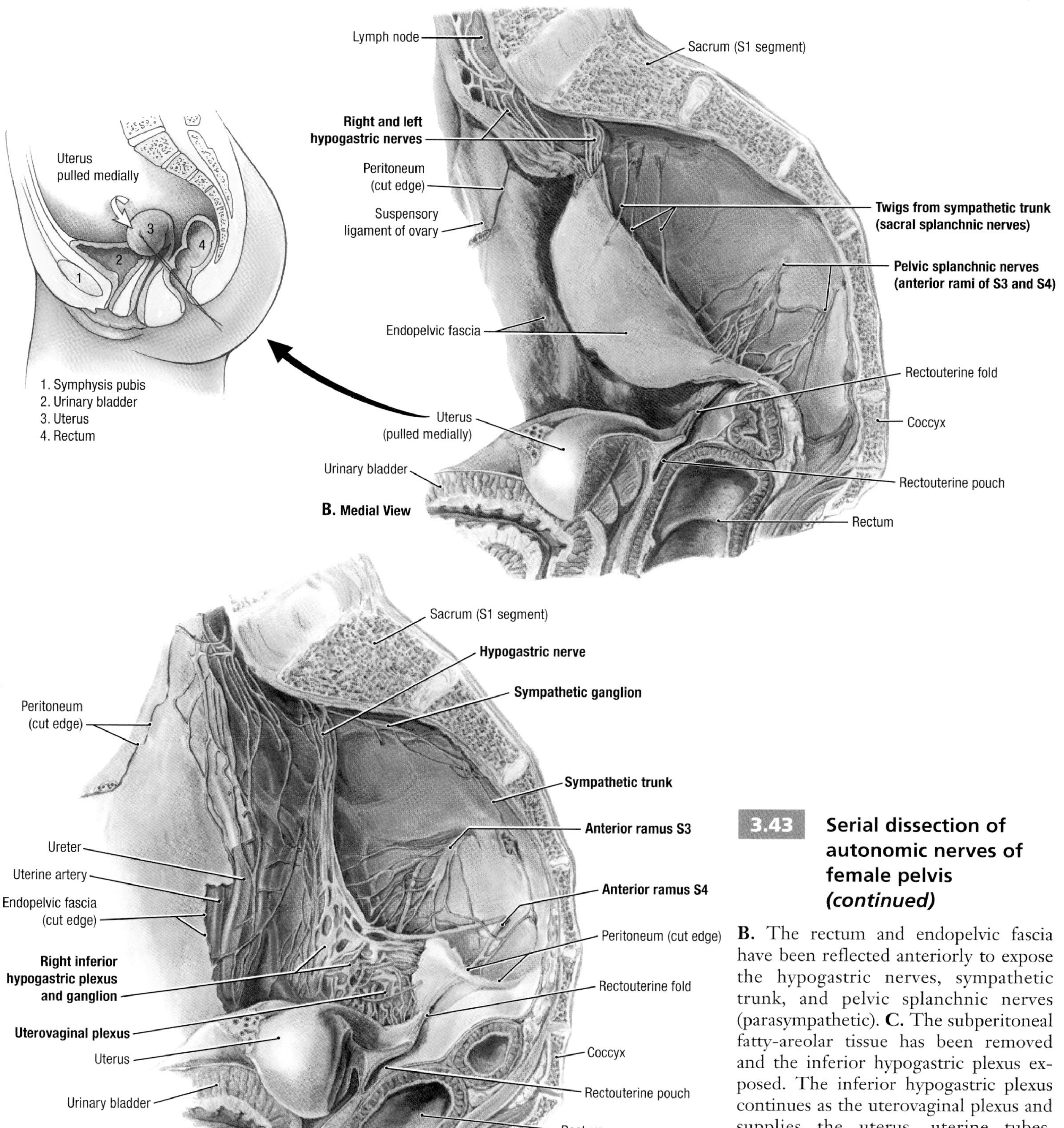
Uterus
pulled medially
1. Symphysis pubis
2. Urinary bladder
3. Uterus
4. Rectum
Lymph node
Sacrum (S1 segment)
Right and left
hypogastric nerves
Peritoneum
(cut edge)
Suspensory
ligament of ovary
Twigs from sympathetic trunk
(sacral splanchnic nerves)
Pelvic splanchnic nerves
(anterior rami of S3 and S4)
Endopelvic fascia
Rectouterine fold
Uterus
(pulled medially)
Coccyx
Urinary bladder
Rectouterine pouch
B. Medial View
Rectum
Sacrum (S1 segment)
Hypogastric nerve
Sympathetic ganglion
Peritoneum
(cut edge)
Sympathetic trunk
Anterior ramus S3
Ureter
Uterine artery
Anterior ramus S4
Endopelvic fascia
(cut edge)
Peritoneum (cut edge)
Right inferior
hypogastric plexus
and ganglion
Rectouterine fold
Uterovaginal plexus
Uterus
Coccyx
Urinary bladder
Rectouterine pouch
Rectum
C. Medial View

## 3.43 Serial dissection of autonomic nerves of female pelvis *(continued)*

**B.** The rectum and endopelvic fascia have been reflected anteriorly to expose the hypogastric nerves, sympathetic trunk, and pelvic splanchnic nerves (parasympathetic). **C.** The subperitoneal fatty-areolar tissue has been removed and the inferior hypogastric plexus exposed. The inferior hypogastric plexus continues as the uterovaginal plexus and supplies the uterus, uterine tubes, vagina, urethra, greater vestibular glands, erectile tissue of the clitoris, and bulb of the vestibule.

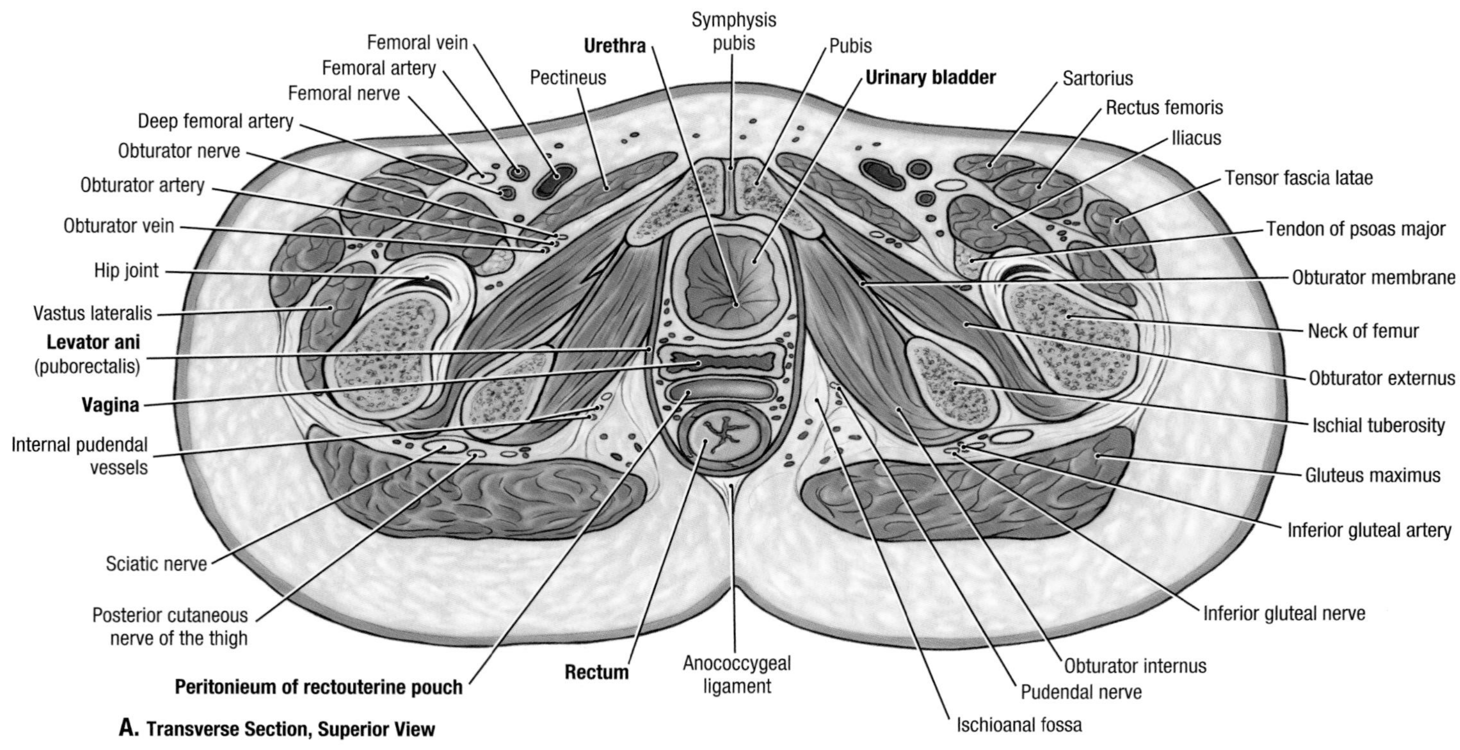

Femoral vein
Femoral artery
Femoral nerve
Deep femoral artery
Obturator nerve
Obturator artery
Obturator vein
Hip joint
Vastus lateralis
Levator ani (puborectalis)
Vagina
Internal pudendal vessels
Sciatic nerve
Posterior cutaneous nerve of the thigh
Peritonieum of rectouterine pouch
Rectum
Anococcygeal ligament
Urethra
Pectineus
Symphysis pubis
Pubis
Urinary bladder
Sartorius
Rectus femoris
Iliacus
Tensor fascia latae
Tendon of psoas major
Obturator membrane
Neck of femur
Obturator externus
Ischial tuberosity
Gluteus maximus
Inferior gluteal artery
Inferior gluteal nerve
Obturator internus
Pudendal nerve
Ischioanal fossa


**A. Transverse Section, Superior View**

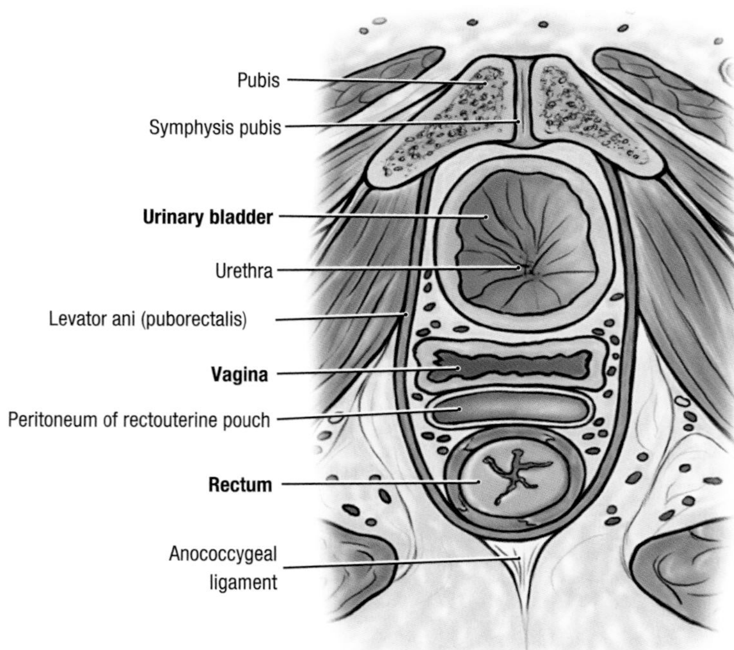

Pubis
Symphysis pubis
Urinary bladder
Urethra
Levator ani (puborectalis)
Vagina
Peritoneum of rectouterine pouch
Rectum
Anococcygeal ligament


**B. Transverse Section**

## 3.44 Transverse section through female pelvis

**A.** Transverse section through the ischial tuberosities. **B.** Enlargement of central part of section including the bladder, vagina, rectum, and rectouterine pouch.

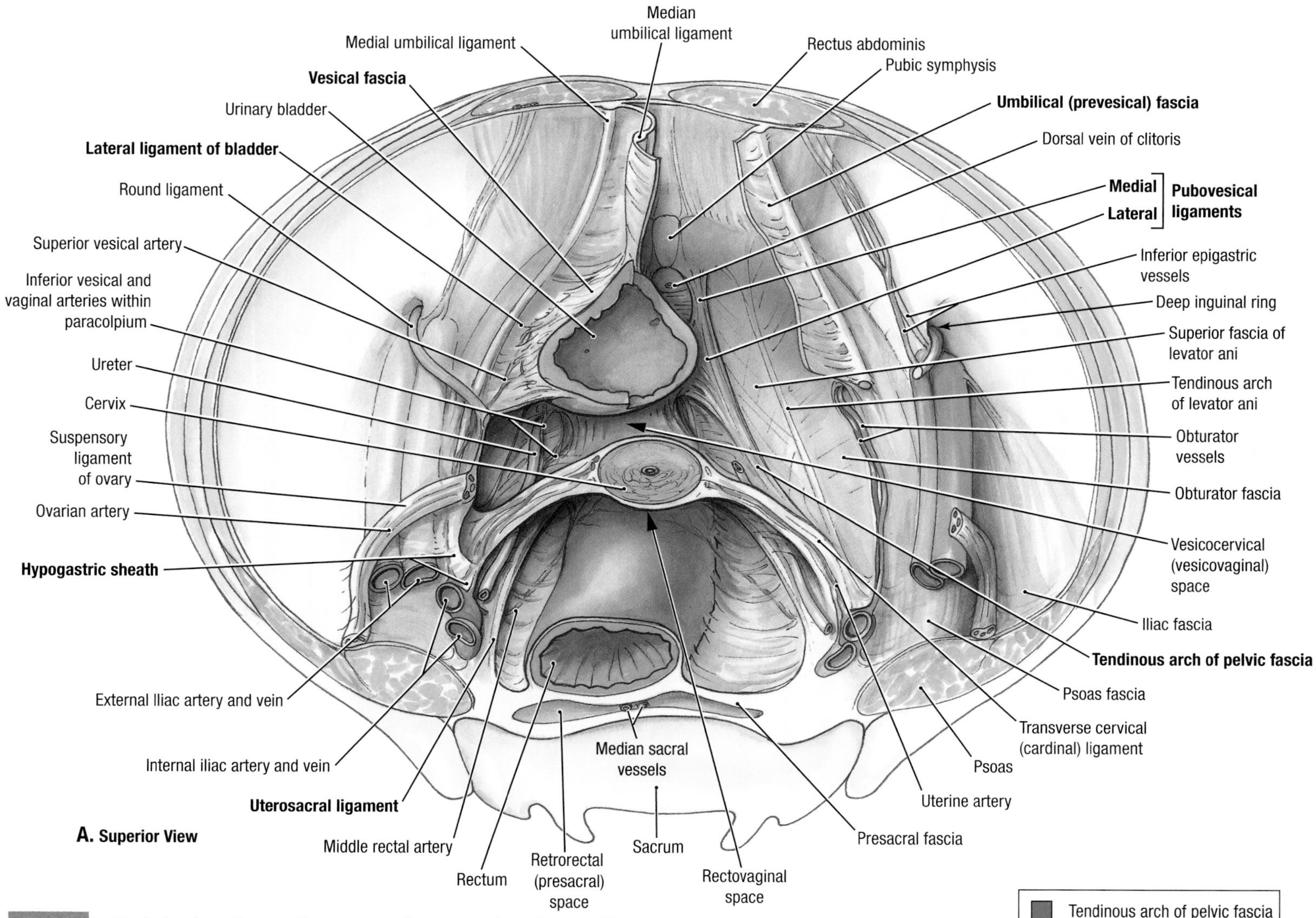

Median umbilical ligament
Medial umbilical ligament
Vesical fascia
Urinary bladder
Lateral ligament of bladder
Round ligament
Superior vesical artery
Inferior vesical and vaginal arteries within paracolpium
Ureter
Cervix
Suspensory ligament of ovary
Ovarian artery
Hypogastric sheath
External iliac artery and vein
Internal iliac artery and vein
Uterosacral ligament
Middle rectal artery
Rectum
Retrorectal (presacral) space
Median sacral vessels
Sacrum
Rectovaginal space
Presacral fascia
Uterine artery
Psoas
Transverse cervical (cardinal) ligament
Psoas fascia
Tendinous arch of pelvic fascia
Iliac fascia
Vesicocervical (vesicovaginal) space
Obturator fascia
Obturator vessels
Tendinous arch of levator ani
Superior fascia of levator ani
Deep inguinal ring
Inferior epigastric vessels
Medial / Lateral Pubovesical ligaments
Dorsal vein of clitoris
Umbilical (prevesical) fascia
Pubic symphysis
Rectus abdominis

**A.** Superior View

## 3.45 Pelvic fascia and supporting mechanism of cervix and upper vagina

**A.** Greater and lesser pelvis demonstrating pelvic viscera and endopelvic fascia. **B.** Schematic illustration of fascial ligaments and areolar spaces at level of tendinous arch of pelvic fascia.

- Note the parietal pelvic fascia covering the obturator internus and levator ani muscles and the visceral pelvic fascia surrounding the pelvic organs. These membranous fasciae are continuous where the organs penetrate the pelvic floor, forming a tendinous arch of pelvic fascia bilaterally.
- The endopelvic fascia lies between, and is continuous with, both visceral and parietal layers of pelvic fascia. The loose, areolar portions of the endopelvic fascia have been removed; the fibrous, condensed portions remain. Note the condensation of this fascia into the hypogastric sheath, containing the vessels to the pelvic viscera, the ureters, and (in the male) the ductus deferens.
- Observe the ligamentous extensions of the hypogastric sheath: the lateral ligament of the urinary bladder, the transverse cervical ligament at the base of the broad ligament, and a less prominent lamina posteriorly containing the middle rectal vessels.

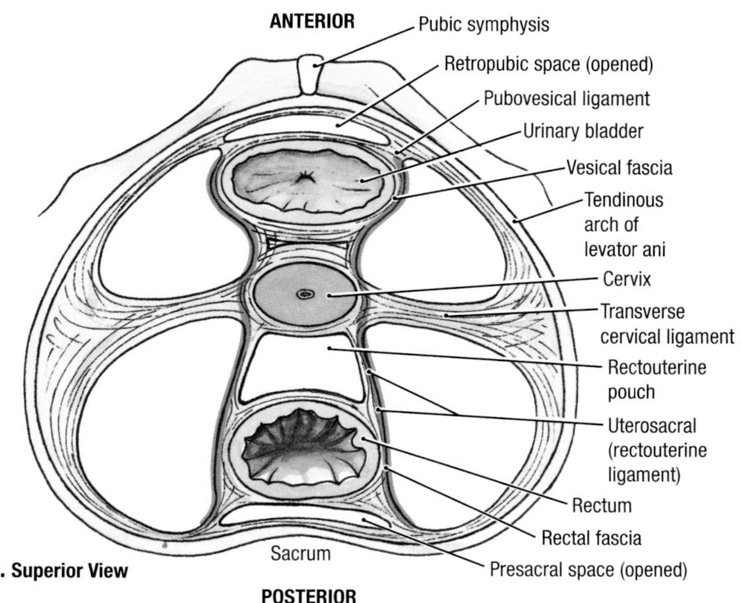
Tendinous arch of pelvic fascia
ANTERIOR
Pubic symphysis
Retropubic space (opened)
Pubovesical ligament
Urinary bladder
Vesical fascia
Tendinous arch of levator ani
Cervix
Transverse cervical ligament
Rectouterine pouch
Uterosacral (rectouterine ligament)
Rectum
Rectal fascia
Presacral space (opened)
Sacrum
POSTERIOR

**B.** Superior View

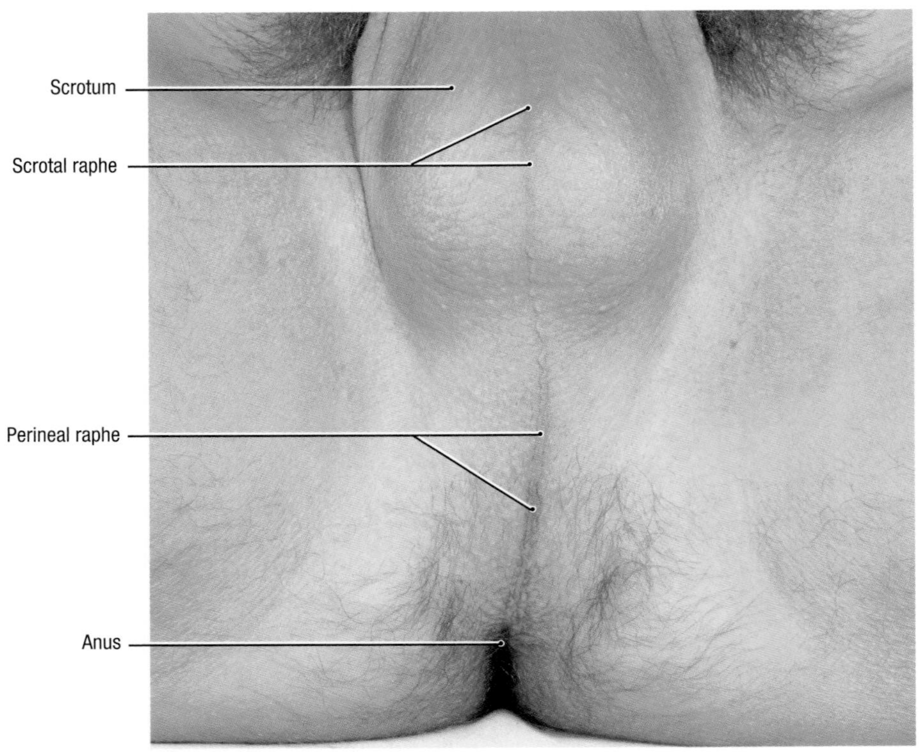
Scrotum
Scrotal raphe
Perineal raphe
Anus

A. Inferior View

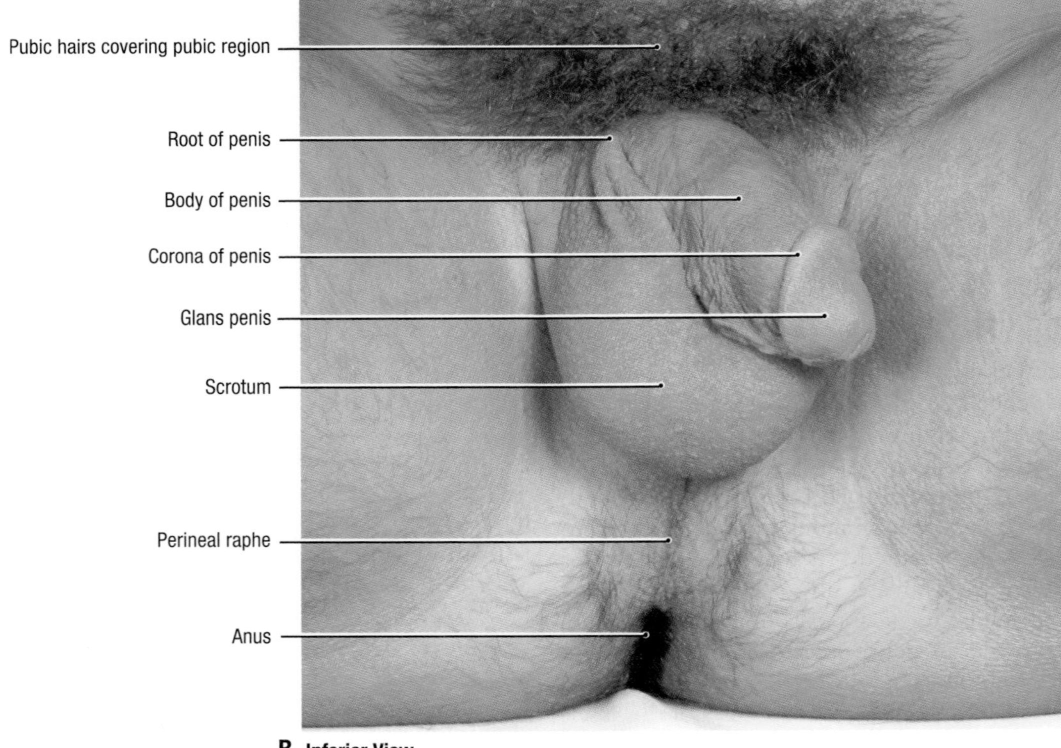
Pubic hairs covering pubic region
Root of penis
Body of penis
Corona of penis
Glans penis
Scrotum
Perineal raphe
Anus

B. Inferior View

## 3.46 Surface anatomy of male perineum

**A.** Scrotum and anal region. **B.** Penis, scrotum, and anal region.

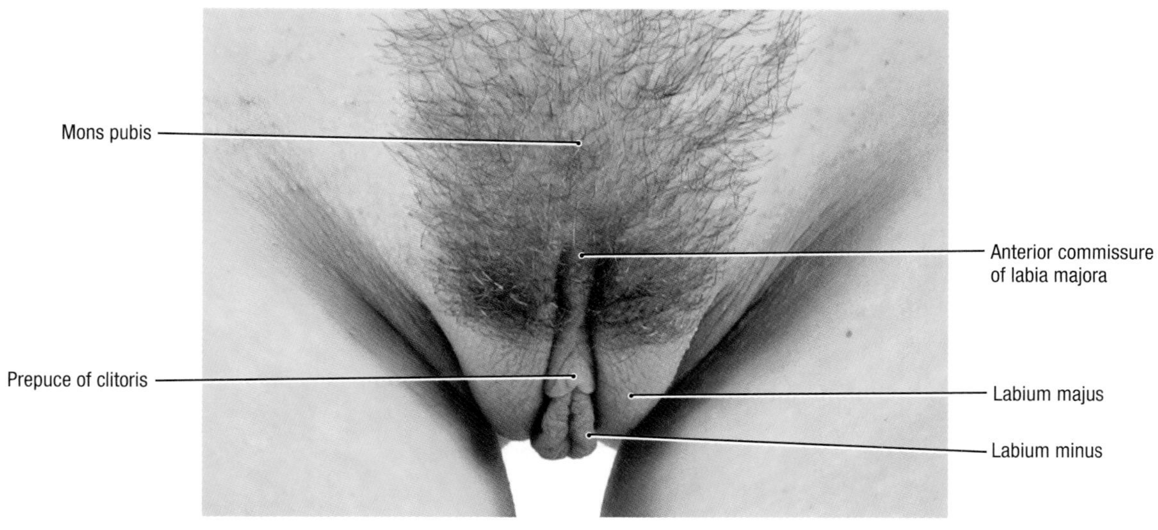
Mons pubis
Anterior commissure of labia majora
Prepuce of clitoris
Labium majus
Labium minus

**A. Anterior View**

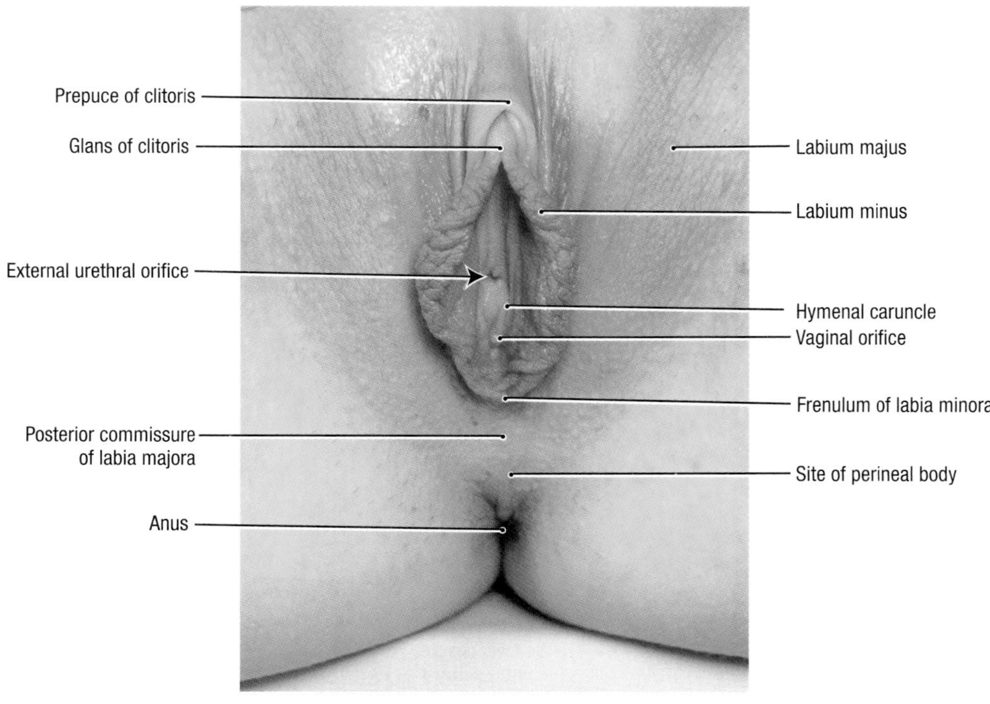
Prepuce of clitoris
Glans of clitoris
Labium majus
Labium minus
External urethral orifice
Hymenal caruncle
Vaginal orifice
Frenulum of labia minora
Posterior commissure of labia majora
Site of perineal body
Anus

**B. Antero-inferior View (Lithotomy Position)**

## 3.47 Surface anatomy of the female perineum

**A.** External genitalia (pudendum; vulva), standing position. **B.** Vestibule of vagina and the external urethral and vaginal orifices opening into it (recumbent position).

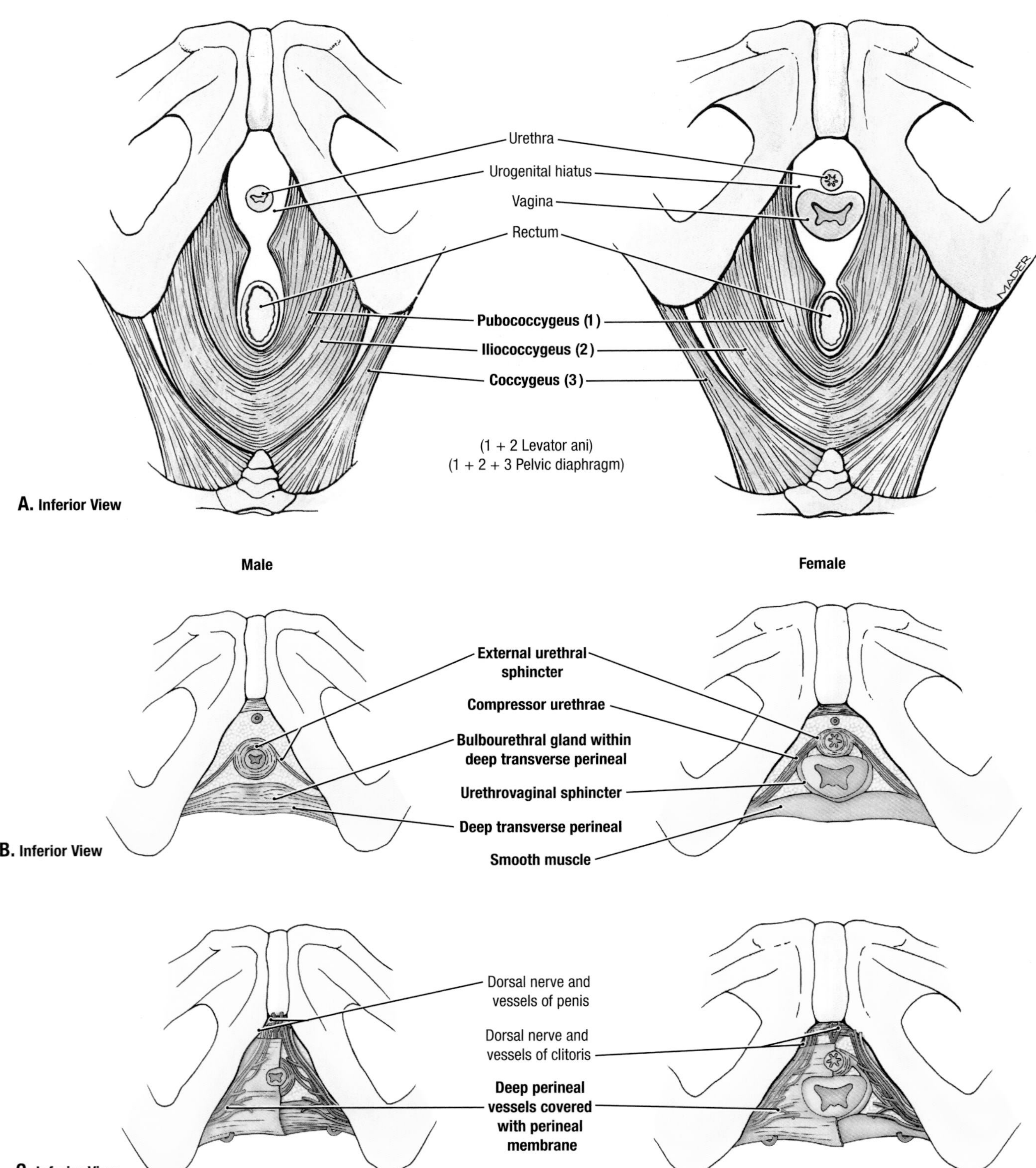
Urethra
Urogenital hiatus
Vagina
Rectum
Pubococcygeus (1)
Iliococcygeus (2)
Coccygeus (3)
(1 + 2 Levator ani)
(1 + 2 + 3 Pelvic diaphragm)
MADER
A. Inferior View
Male
Female
External urethral sphincter
Compressor urethrae
Bulbourethral gland within deep transverse perineal
Urethrovaginal sphincter
Deep transverse perineal
Smooth muscle
B. Inferior View
Dorsal nerve and vessels of penis
Dorsal nerve and vessels of clitoris
Deep perineal vessels covered with perineal membrane
C. Inferior View

## 3.48 Male and female perineal compartments

**A–F.** Sequential demonstration of structures of the perineal compartments, from deep to superficial. **A–C.** Deep perineal compartment (superior to perineal membrane). **A.** Pelvic diaphragm. **B.** Muscles of deep perineal compartment. **C.** Deep perineal vessels and nerves, covered by perineal membrane on right side.

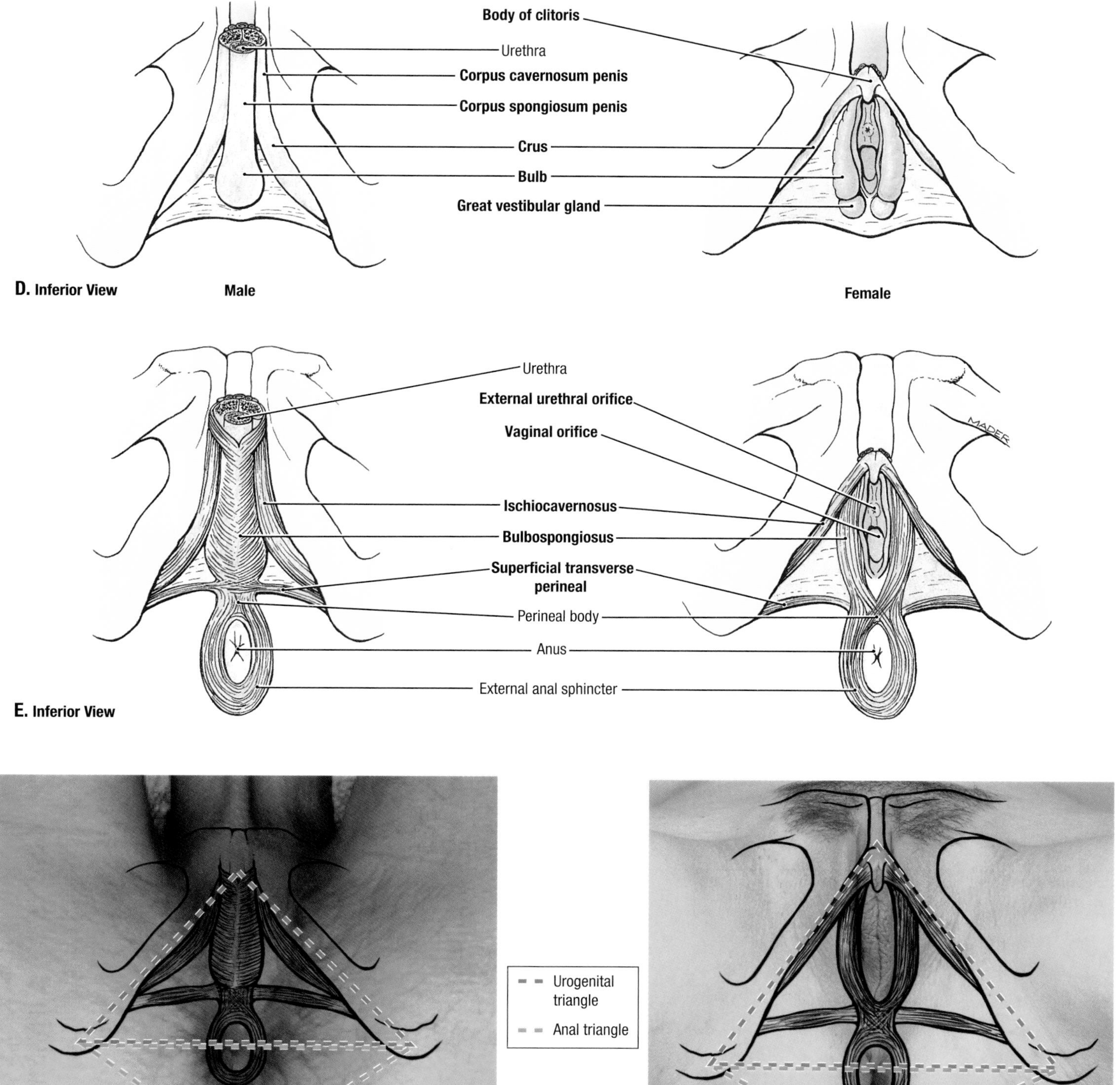
Body of clitoris
Urethra
Corpus cavernosum penis
Corpus spongiosum penis
Crus
Bulb
Great vestibular gland
D. Inferior View
Male
Female
Urethra
External urethral orifice
Vaginal orifice
Ischiocavernosus
Bulbospongiosus
Superficial transverse perineal
Perineal body
Anus
External anal sphincter
E. Inferior View
MADER
Urogenital triangle
Anal triangle
F. Inferior View

**3.48 Male and female perineal compartments *(continued)***

**D–F.** Superficial perineal compartment (inferior to perineal membrane). **D.** Erectile bodies. **E.** Muscles of superficial perineal compartment. F. Superficial muscles imposed on surface anatomy of perineum.

## TABLE 3.9 MUSCLES OF PERINEUM

| Muscle | Origin | Course and Insertion | Innervation | Main Action |
|---|---|---|---|---|
| **External anal sphincter** | Skin and fascia surrounding anus; coccyx via anococcygeal ligament | Passes around lateral aspects of anal canal; insertion into perineal body | Inferior anal (rectal) nerve, a branch of pudendal nerve (S2–S4) | Constricts anal canal during peristalsis, resisting defecation; supports and fixes perineal body and pelvic floor |
| **Bulbospongiosus** | *Male:* median raphe on ventral surface of bulb of penis; perineal body | *Male:* surrounds lateral aspects of bulb of penis and most proximal part of body of penis, inserting into perineal membrane, dorsal aspect of corpora spongiosum and cavernosa, and fascia of bulb of penis | Muscular (deep) branch of perineal nerve, a branch of thepudendal nerve (S2–S4) | *Male:* supports and fixes perineal body/pelvic floor; compresses bulb of penis to expel last drops of urine/semen; assists erection by compressing outflow via deep perineal vein and by pushing blood from bulb into body of penis |
| | *Female:* perineal body | *Female:* passes on each side of lower vagina, enclosing bulb and greater vestibular gland; inserts onto pubic arch and fascia of corpora cavernosa of clitoris | | *Female:* supports and fixes perineal body/pelvic floor; "sphincter" of vagina; assists in erection of clitoris (and perhaps bulb of vestibule); compresses greater vestibular gland |
| **Ischiocavernosus** | Internal surface of ischiopubic ramus and ischial tuberosity | Embraces crus of penis or clitoris, inserting onto the inferior and medial aspects of the crus and to the perineal membrane medial to the crus | | Maintains erection of penis or clitoris by compressing outflow veins and pushing blood from the root of penis or clitoris into the body of penis or clitoris |
| **Superficial transverse perineal** | Internal surface of ischiopubic ramus and ischial tuberosity | Passes along inferior aspect of posterior border of perineal membrane to perineal body | | Supports and fixes perineal body (pelvic floor) to support abdominopelvic viscera and resist increased intraabdominal pressure |
| **Deep transverse perineal (male only)** | | Passes along superior aspect of posterior border of perineal membrane to perineal body, and external anal sphincter | Muscular (deep) branch of perineal nerve | |
| **Smooth muscle (female only)** | Ischiopubic rami | Passes to lateral wall of urethra and vagina | Autonomic nerves | Quantity of smooth muscle increases with age; function uncertain |
| **External urethral sphincter** | | Surrounds urethra superior to perineal membrane; in males, also ascends anterior aspect of prostate | Dorsal nerve of penis or clitoris, the terminal branch of the pudendal nerve (S2–S4) | Compresses urethra to maintain urinary continence |
| **Compressor urethrae (females only)** | Internal surface of ischiopubic ramus | Continuous with external urethral sphincter | | Compresses urethra; with pelvic diaphragm; assists in elongation of urethra |
| **Urethrovaginal sphincter (females only)** | Anterior side of urethra | Continuous with compressor urethrae; extends posteriorly on lateral wall of urethra and vagina to interdigitate with fibers from opposite side of perineal body | | Compresses urethra and vagina |

Oelrich TM. The urethral sphincter muscle in the male. Am J Anat 1980;158:229–246.
Oelrich TM. The striated urogenital sphincter muscle in the female. Anat Rec 1983;205:223–232.
Mirilas P, Skandalakis JE. Urogenital diaphragm: an erroneous concept casting its shadow over the sphincter urethrae and deep perineal space. J Am Coll Surg 2004;198:279–290.
DeLancey JO. Correlative study of paraurethral anatomy. Obstet Gynecol 1986;68:91–97.

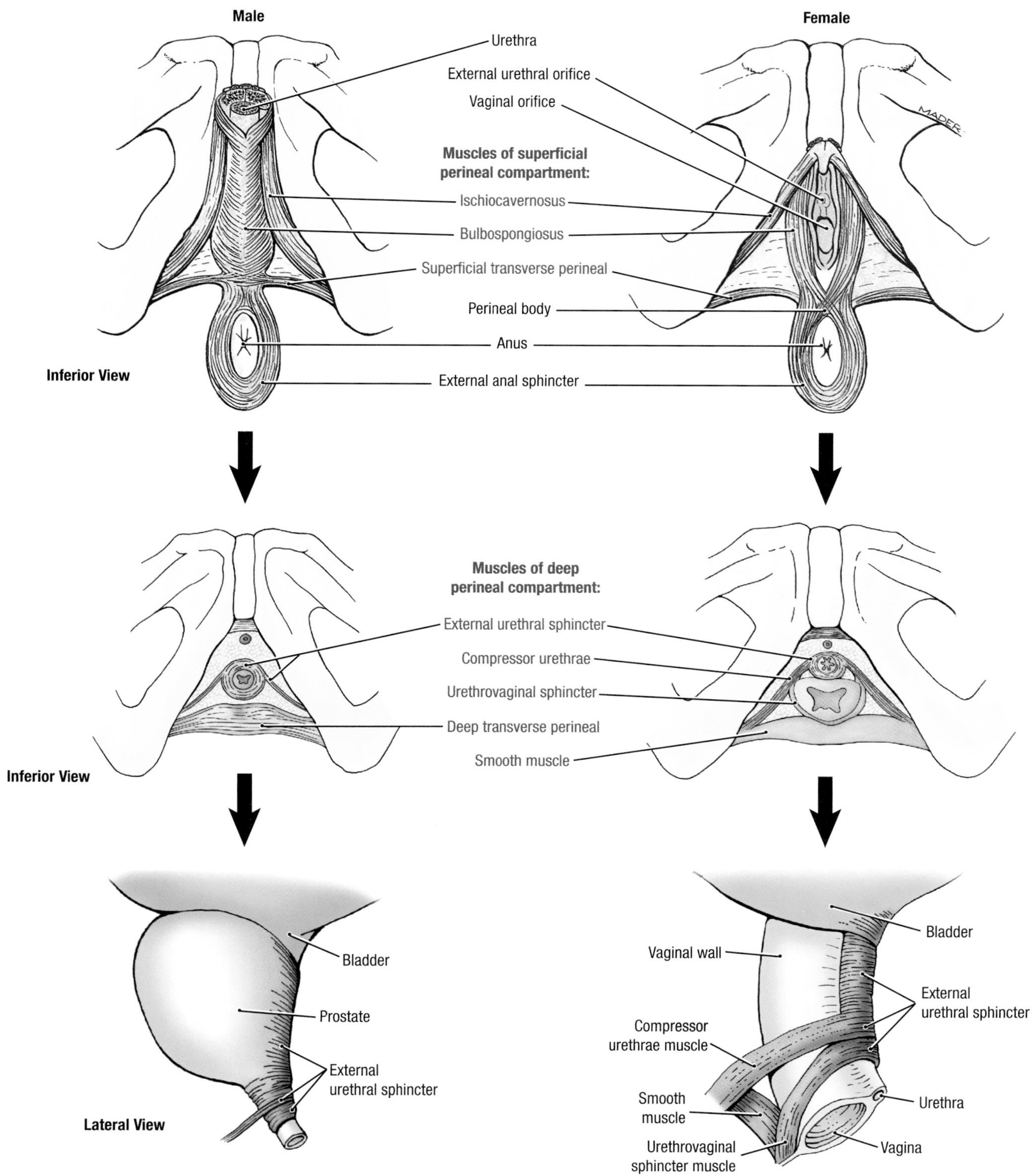
Male
Female
Urethra
External urethral orifice
Vaginal orifice
Muscles of superficial perineal compartment:
Ischiocavernosus
Bulbospongiosus
Superficial transverse perineal
Perineal body
Anus
External anal sphincter
Inferior View
MADER
Muscles of deep perineal compartment:
External urethral sphincter
Compressor urethrae
Urethrovaginal sphincter
Deep transverse perineal
Smooth muscle
Inferior View
Bladder
Prostate
External urethral sphincter
Lateral View
Bladder
Vaginal wall
External urethral sphincter
Compressor urethrae muscle
Smooth muscle
Urethra
Urethrovaginal sphincter muscle
Vagina

**TABLE 3.9 MUSCLES OF PERINEUM *(continued)***

A potential subcutaneous perineal space (pouch) lies between the membranous layer of the subcutaneous tissue of the perineum and the perineal fascia (investing fascia of the superficial perineal muscles). The superficial perineal compartment (pouch) is an enclosed compartment bounded inferiorly by the perineal fascia and superiorly by the perineal membrane. The deep compartment is bounded inferiorly by the perineal membrane and continues superiorly to the (inferior investing fascia of the) pelvic diaphragm. (Oelich, 1980, 1983; DeLancy 1986; Mirilus, 2004).

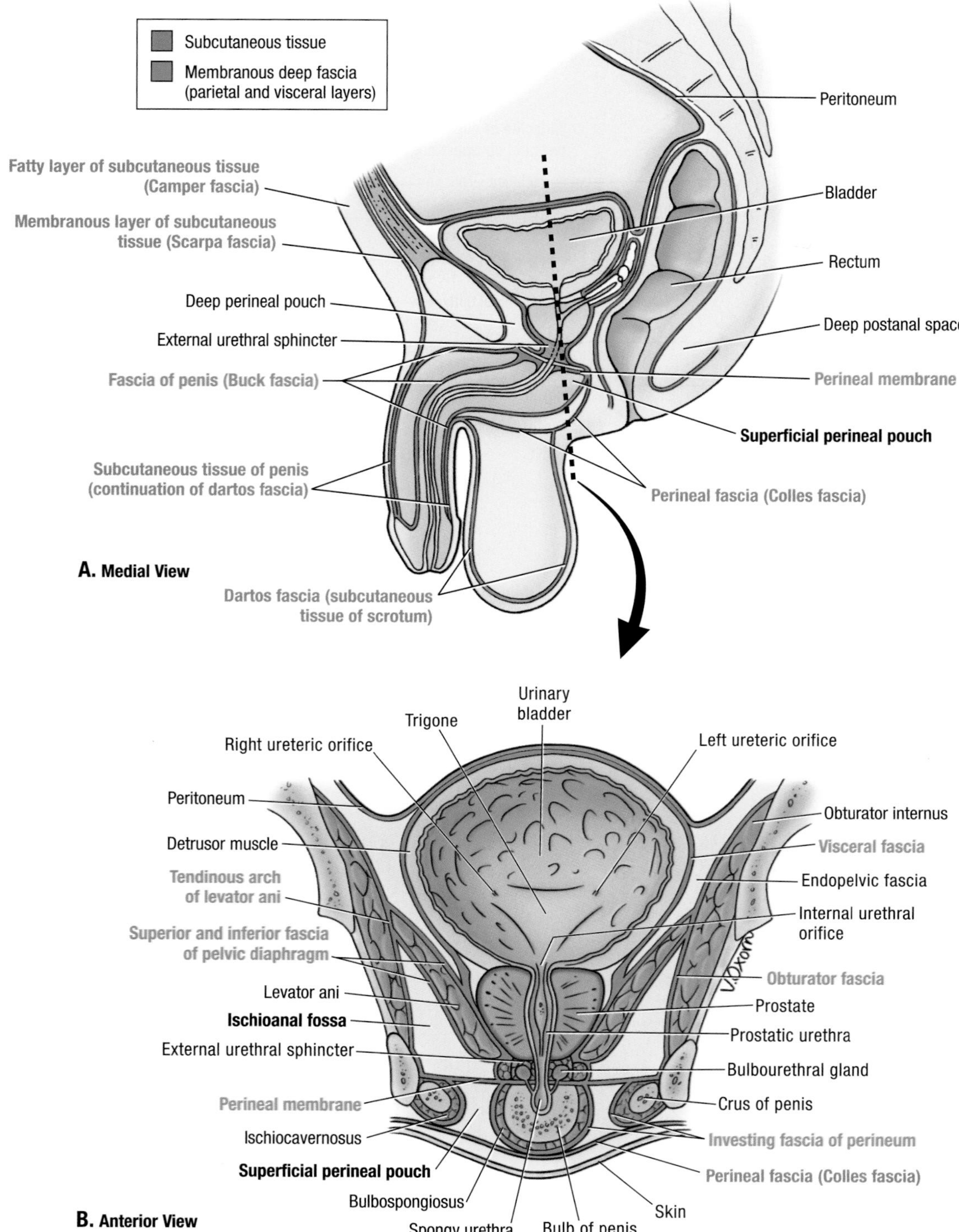

Subcutaneous tissue
Membranous deep fascia (parietal and visceral layers)
Peritoneum
Fatty layer of subcutaneous tissue (Camper fascia)
Bladder
Membranous layer of subcutaneous tissue (Scarpa fascia)
Rectum
Deep perineal pouch
Deep postanal space
External urethral sphincter
Fascia of penis (Buck fascia)
Perineal membrane
Superficial perineal pouch
Subcutaneous tissue of penis (continuation of dartos fascia)
Perineal fascia (Colles fascia)
A. Medial View
Dartos fascia (subcutaneous tissue of scrotum)
Urinary bladder
Trigone
Right ureteric orifice
Left ureteric orifice
Peritoneum
Obturator internus
Detrusor muscle
Visceral fascia
Tendinous arch of levator ani
Endopelvic fascia
Internal urethral orifice
Superior and inferior fascia of pelvic diaphragm
Obturator fascia
Levator ani
Prostate
Ischioanal fossa
Prostatic urethra
External urethral sphincter
Bulbourethral gland
Perineal membrane
Crus of penis
Ischiocavernosus
Investing fascia of perineum
Superficial perineal pouch
Perineal fascia (Colles fascia)
Bulbospongiosus
Skin
B. Anterior View
Spongy urethra
Bulb of penis


## 3.49 Perineal fascia and perineal compartments

**A.** Fascia of male perineum, median section. **B.** Compartments of male perineum, coronal section.

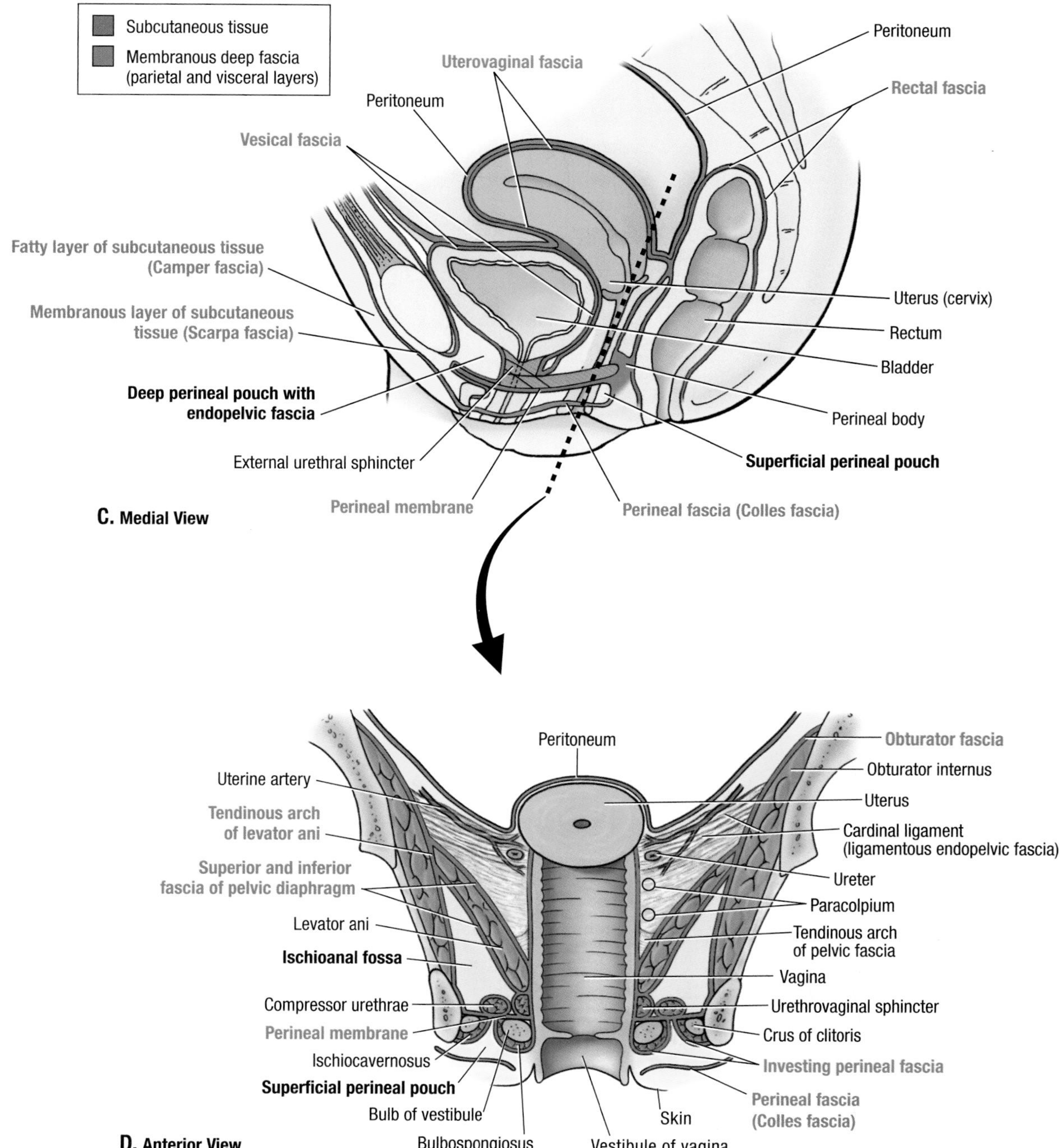
Subcutaneous tissue
Membranous deep fascia (parietal and visceral layers)
Peritoneum
Uterovaginal fascia
Peritoneum
Rectal fascia
Vesical fascia
Fatty layer of subcutaneous tissue (Camper fascia)
Membranous layer of subcutaneous tissue (Scarpa fascia)
Deep perineal pouch with endopelvic fascia
External urethral sphincter
Perineal membrane
Perineal fascia (Colles fascia)
Superficial perineal pouch
Perineal body
Bladder
Rectum
Uterus (cervix)
C. Medial View
Peritoneum
Obturator fascia
Obturator internus
Uterus
Cardinal ligament (ligamentous endopelvic fascia)
Ureter
Paracolpium
Tendinous arch of pelvic fascia
Vagina
Urethrovaginal sphincter
Crus of clitoris
Investing perineal fascia
Perineal fascia (Colles fascia)
Skin
Vestibule of vagina
Uterine artery
Tendinous arch of levator ani
Superior and inferior fascia of pelvic diaphragm
Levator ani
Ischioanal fossa
Compressor urethrae
Perineal membrane
Ischiocavernosus
Superficial perineal pouch
Bulb of vestibule
Bulbospongiosus
D. Anterior View

## 3.49 Perineal fascia and perineal compartments *(continued)*

**C.** Fascia of female perineum, median section. **D.** Compartments of female perineum, coronal section.

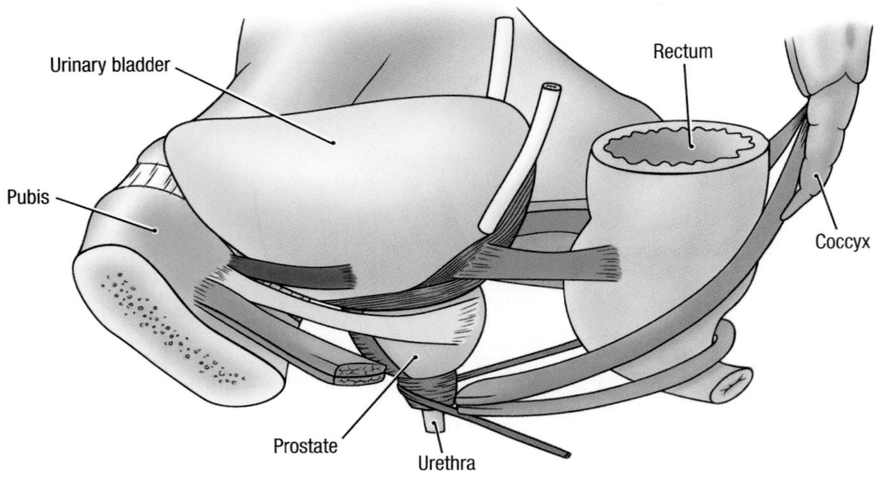
Urinary bladder
Rectum
Pubis
Coccyx
Prostate
Urethra

MALE:
- Puboprostaticus
- Pubococcygeus
- Puborectalis
- Muscle of uvula
- Rectovesicalis

Muscles compressing urethra:
- Internal urethral sphincter
- Pubovesicalis
- External urethral sphincter

**A.** **Left Lateral View, Male**

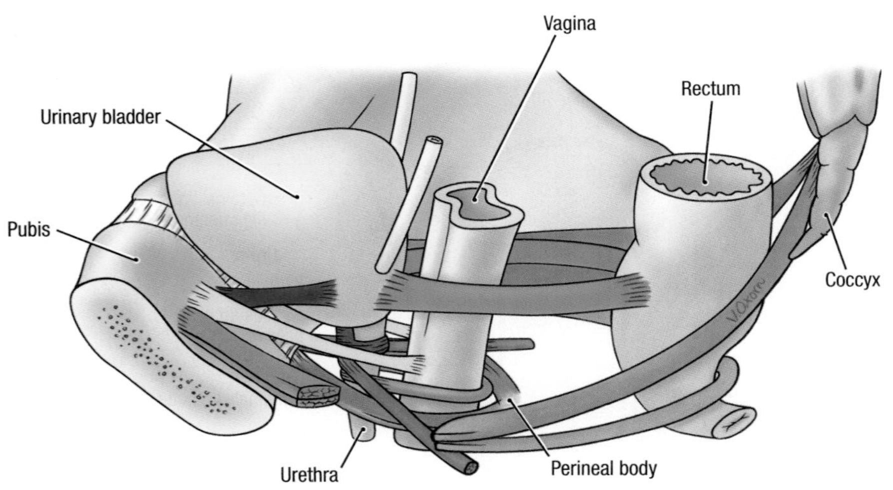
Vagina
Urinary bladder
Rectum
Pubis
Coccyx
Urethra
Perineal body

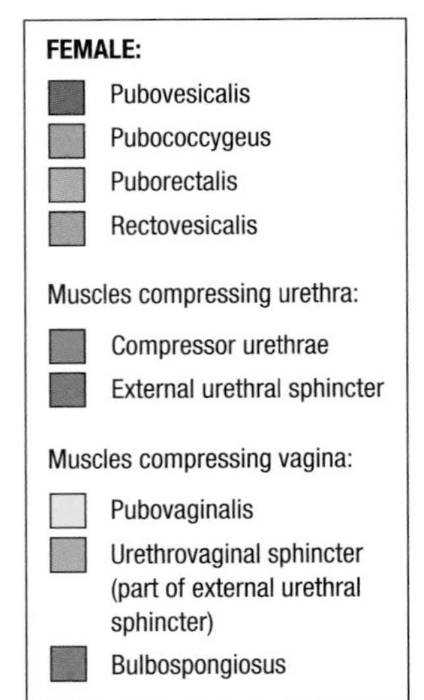
FEMALE:
Pubovesicalis
Pubococcygeus
Puborectalis
Rectovesicalis
Muscles compressing urethra:
Compressor urethrae
External urethral sphincter
Muscles compressing vagina:
Pubovaginalis
Urethrovaginal sphincter (part of external urethral sphincter)
Bulbospongiosus

**B.** **Left Lateral View, Female**

**3.50 Supporting and compressor/sphincteric muscles of pelvis**

**A.** Male. **B.** Female.

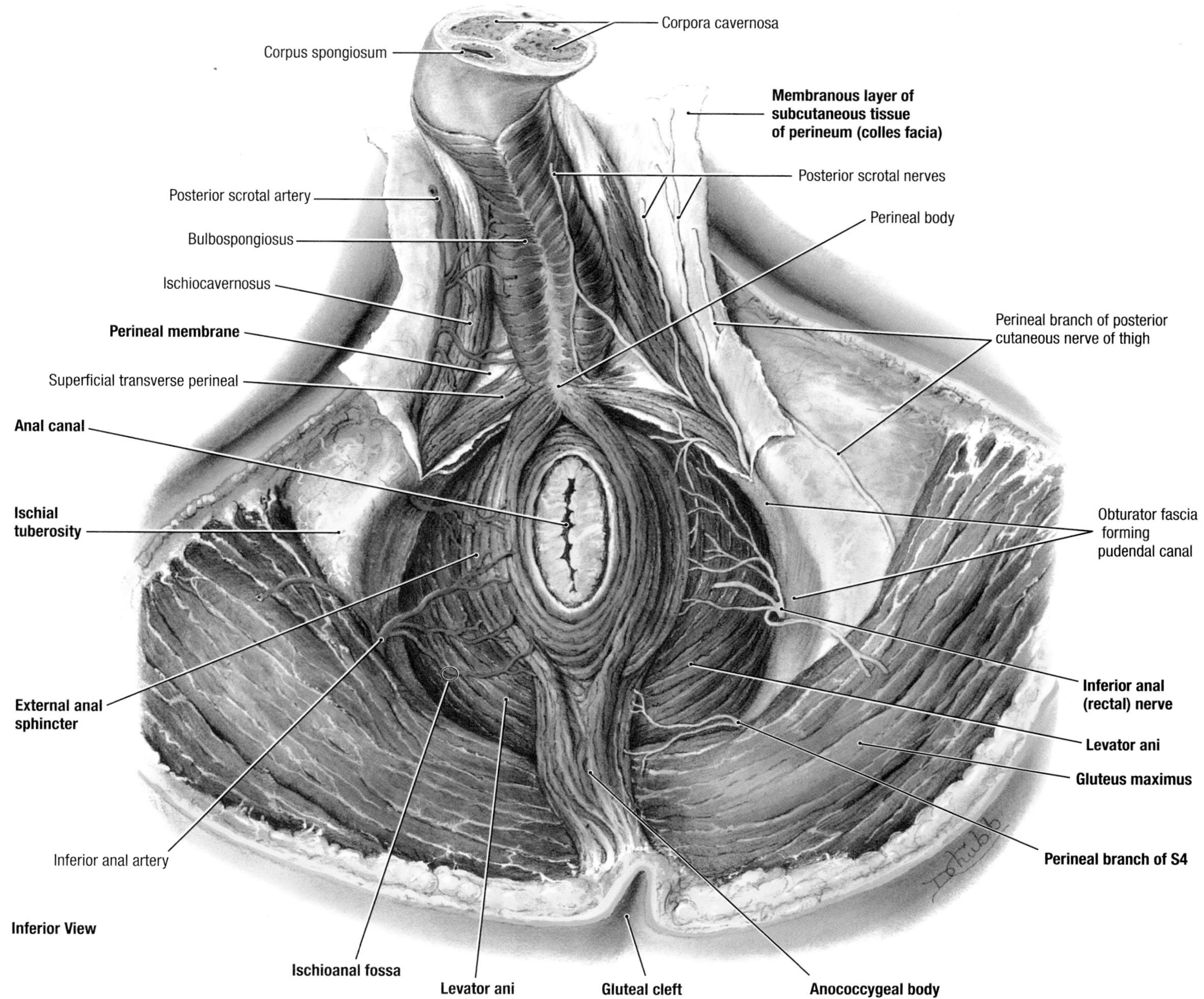
Corpora cavernosa
Corpus spongiosum
Membranous layer of subcutaneous tissue of perineum (colles facia)
Posterior scrotal nerves
Posterior scrotal artery
Perineal body
Bulbospongiosus
Ischiocavernosus
Perineal branch of posterior cutaneous nerve of thigh
Perineal membrane
Superficial transverse perineal
Anal canal
Ischial tuberosity
Obturator fascia forming pudendal canal
Inferior anal (rectal) nerve
External anal sphincter
Levator ani
Gluteus maximus
Perineal branch of S4
Inferior anal artery
Inferior View
Ischioanal fossa
Levator ani
Gluteal cleft
Anococcygeal body

## 3.51 Dissection of male perineum—I

Superficial dissection.

- The membranous layer of subcutaneous tissue of the perineum was incised and reflected, opening the subcutaneous perineal compartment (pouch) in which the cutaneous nerves course.
- The perineal membrane is exposed between the three paired muscles of the superficial compartment; although not evident here, the muscles are individually ensheathed with investing fascia.
- The anal canal is surrounded by the external anal sphincter. The superficial fibers of the sphincter anchor the anal canal anteriorly to the perineal body and posteriorly, via the anococcygeal body (ligament), to the coccyx and skin of the gluteal cleft.
- Ischioanal (ischiorectal) fossae, from which fat bodies have been removed, lie on each side of the external anal sphincter. The fossae are also bound medially and superiorly by the levator ani; laterally by the ischial tuberosities and obturator internus fascia; and posteriorly by the gluteus maximus overlying the sacrotuberous ligaments. An anterior recess of each ischioanal fossa extends superior to the perineal membrane.
- In the lateral wall of the fossa, the inferior anal (rectal) nerve emerges from the pudendal canal and, with the perineal branch of S4, supplies the voluntary external anal sphincter and peri-anal skin; most cutaneous twigs have been removed.

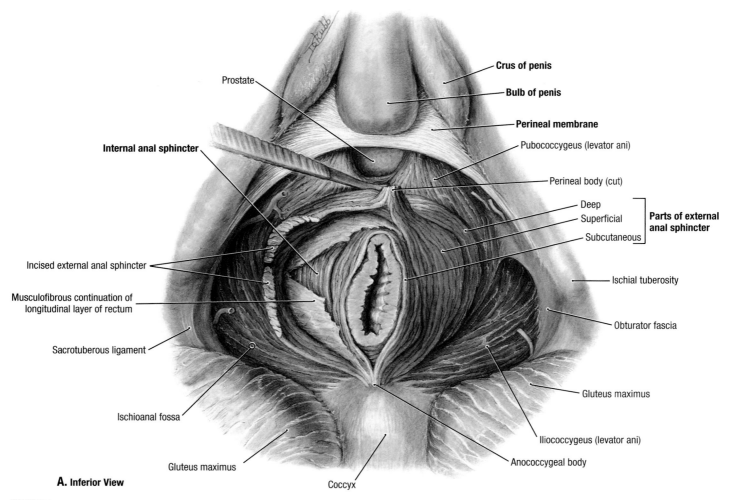

Crus of penis
Bulb of penis
Perineal membrane
Prostate
Pubococcygeus (levator ani)
Internal anal sphincter
Perineal body (cut)
Deep
Superficial
Subcutaneous
Parts of external anal sphincter
Incised external anal sphincter
Ischial tuberosity
Musculofibrous continuation of longitudinal layer of rectum
Obturator fascia
Sacrotuberous ligament
Gluteus maximus
Ischioanal fossa
Iliococcygeus (levator ani)
Gluteus maximus
Anococcygeal body
Coccyx

**A.** Inferior View

## 3.52 Dissection of the male perineum—II

**A.** The superficial perineal muscles have been removed, revealing the roots of the erectile bodies (crura and bulb) of the penis, attached to the ischiopubic rami and perineal membrane. On the left side the superficial and deep parts of the external anal sphincter were incised and reflected; the underlying musculofibrous continuation of the outer longitudinal layer of the muscular layer of the rectum is cut to reveal thickening of the inner circular layer that comprises the internal anal sphincter. **B.** Rupture of the spongy urethra in the bulb of the penis results in urine passing (extravasating) into the subcutaneous perineal compartment. The attachments of the membranous layer of subcutaneous tissue determine the direction and restrictions of flow of the extravasated urine. Urine and blood may pass deep to the continuations of the membranous layer in the scrotum, penis, and inferior abdominal wall. The urine cannot pass laterally and inferiorly into the thighs because the membranous layer fuses with the fascia lata (deep fascia of the thigh), nor posteriorly into the anal triangle due to continuity with the perineal membrane and perineal body.

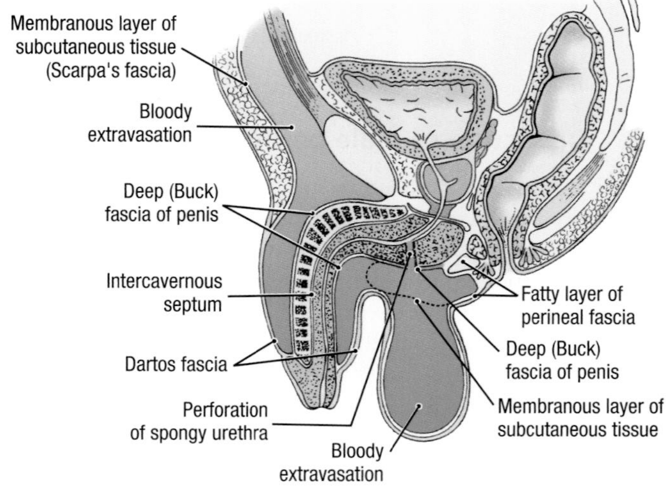
Membranous layer of subcutaneous tissue (Scarpa's fascia)
Bloody extravasation
Deep (Buck) fascia of penis
Intercavernous septum
Dartos fascia
Perforation of spongy urethra
Bloody extravasation
Fatty layer of perineal fascia
Deep (Buck) fascia of penis
Membranous layer of subcutaneous tissue

**B.** Medial view (from left)

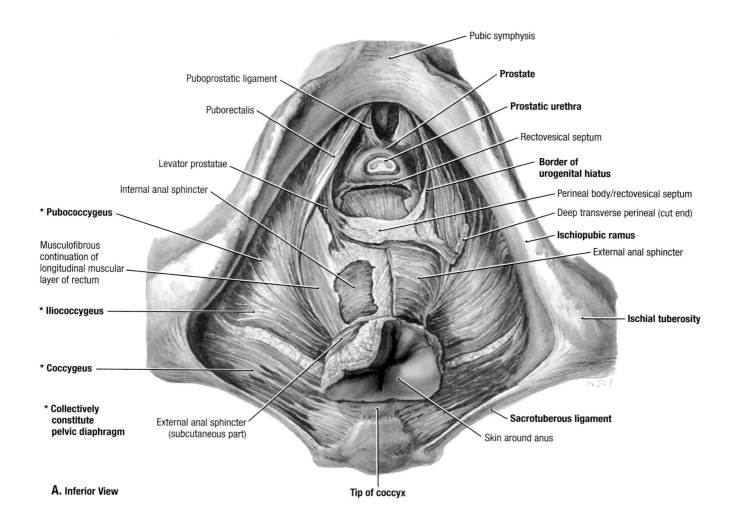

Pubic symphysis
Puboprostatic ligament
Prostate
Puborectalis
Prostatic urethra
Rectovesical septum
Levator prostatae
Border of urogenital hiatus
Internal anal sphincter
Perineal body/rectovesical septum
* Pubococcygeus
Deep transverse perineal (cut end)
Ischiopubic ramus
Musculofibrous continuation of longitudinal muscular layer of rectum
External anal sphincter
* Iliococcygeus
Ischial tuberosity
* Coccygeus
* Collectively constitute pelvic diaphragm
External anal sphincter (subcutaneous part)
Sacrotuberous ligament
Skin around anus

A. Inferior View

Tip of coccyx

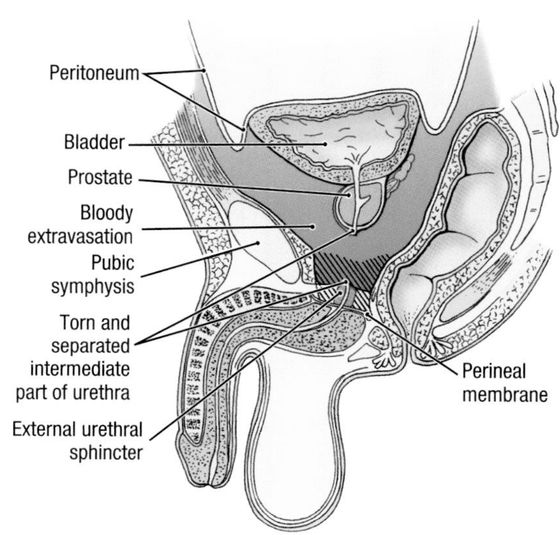
Peritoneum
Bladder
Prostate
Bloody extravasation
Pubic symphysis
Torn and separated intermediate part of urethra
External urethral sphincter
Perineal membrane

B. Medial View (from left)

## 3.53 Dissection of the male perineum—III

**A.** The perineal membrane and structures superficial to it have been removed. The prostatic urethra, base of the prostate, and rectum are visible through the urogenital hiatus of the pelvic diaphragm. The osseofibrous boundaries are demonstrated. **B.** Rupture of the intermediate part of the urethra results in extravasation of urine and blood into the deep perineal compartment. The fluid may pass superiorly through the urogenital hiatus and distribute extraperitoneally around the prostate and bladder.

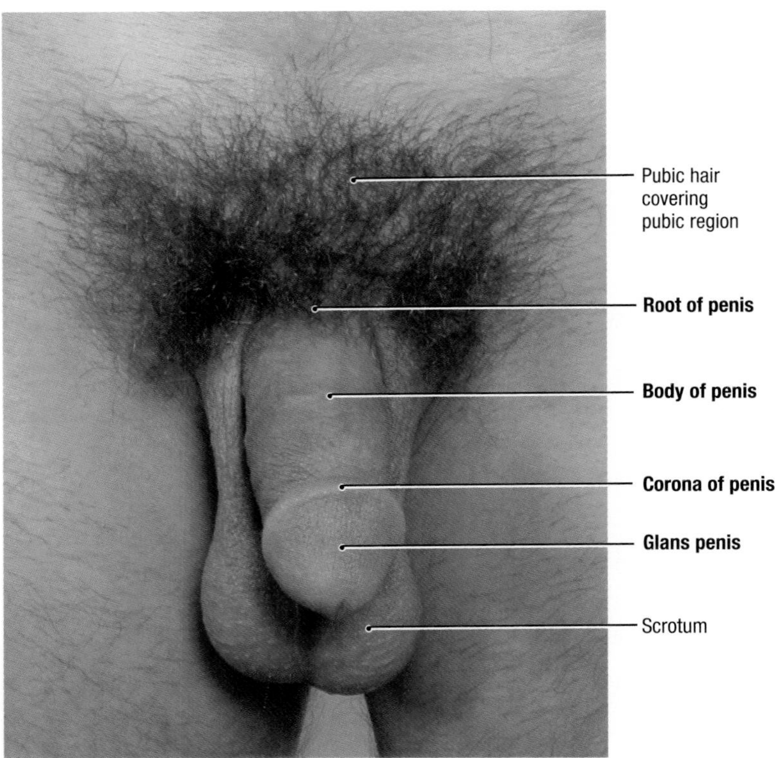
Pubic hair covering pubic region
Root of penis
Body of penis
Corona of penis
Glans penis
Scrotum

**A.** Anterior View

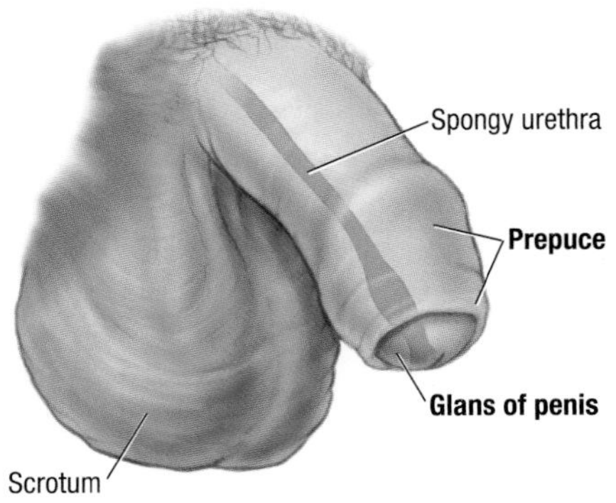
Spongy urethra
Prepuce
Glans of penis
Scrotum

**B.** Right Anterolateral View

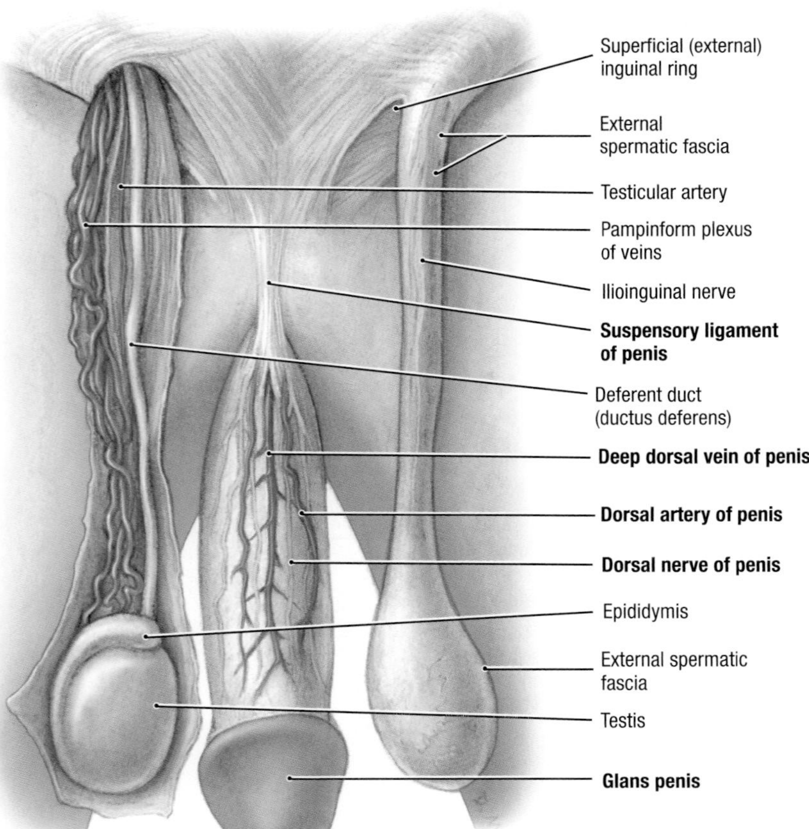
Superficial (external) inguinal ring
External spermatic fascia
Testicular artery
Pampinform plexus of veins
Ilioinguinal nerve
Suspensory ligament of penis
Deferent duct (ductus deferens)
Deep dorsal vein of penis
Dorsal artery of penis
Dorsal nerve of penis
Epididymis
External spermatic fascia
Testis
Glans penis

**C.** Anterior View

## 3.54 Glans, prepuce, and neurovascular bundle of penis

**A.** Surface anatomy, penis circumcised. **B.** Uncircumcised penis. **C.** Vessels and nerves of penis and contents of spermatic cord.

In **C:**

- The superficial and deep fasciae covering the penis are removed to expose the midline deep dorsal vein and the bilateral dorsal arteries and nerves of the penis. The triangular suspensory ligament of the penis attaches to the region of the pubic symphysis and blends with the deep fascia of the penis.
- On the specimen's left, the spermatic cord passes through the external inguinal ring and picks up a covering of external spermatic fascia from the margins of the superficial inguinal ring.
- On the specimen's right, the coverings of the spermatic cord and testis are incised and reflected, and the contents of the cord are separated.

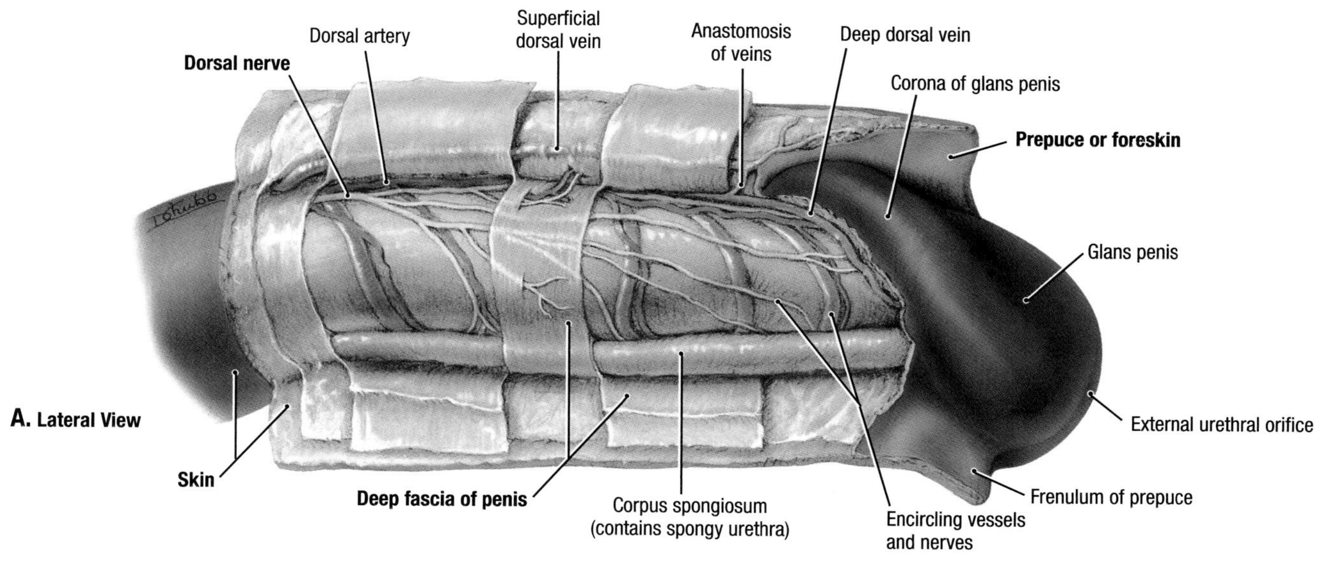
Dorsal nerve
Dorsal artery
Superficial dorsal vein
Anastomosis of veins
Deep dorsal vein
Corona of glans penis
Prepuce or foreskin
Glans penis
External urethral orifice
Frenulum of prepuce
Encircling vessels and nerves
Corpus spongiosum (contains spongy urethra)
Deep fascia of penis
Skin
A. Lateral View

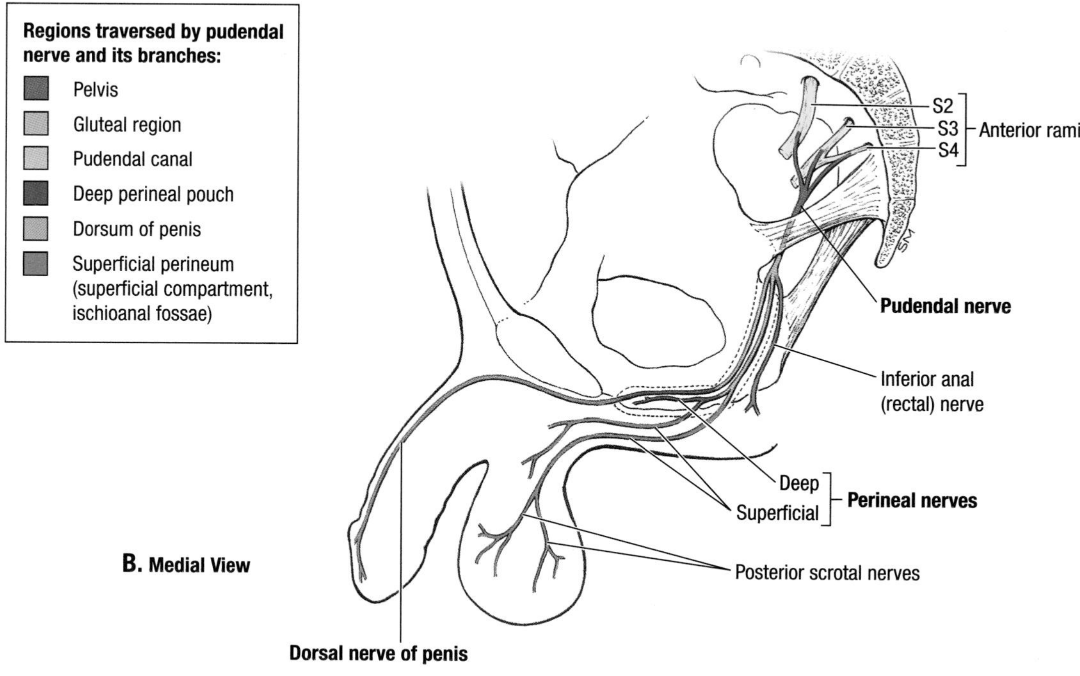
Regions traversed by pudendal nerve and its branches:
Pelvis
Gluteal region
Pudendal canal
Deep perineal pouch
Dorsum of penis
Superficial perineum (superficial compartment, ischioanal fossae)
S2
S3
S4
Anterior rami
Pudendal nerve
Inferior anal (rectal) nerve
Deep
Superficial
Perineal nerves
Posterior scrotal nerves
B. Medial View
Dorsal nerve of penis

## 3.55 Layers and nerves of penis

**A.** Dissection. The skin, subcutaneous tissue, and deep fascia of the penis and prepuce are reflected separately. **B.** Distribution of pudendal nerve, right hemipelvis. Five regions transversed by the nerve are demonstrated.

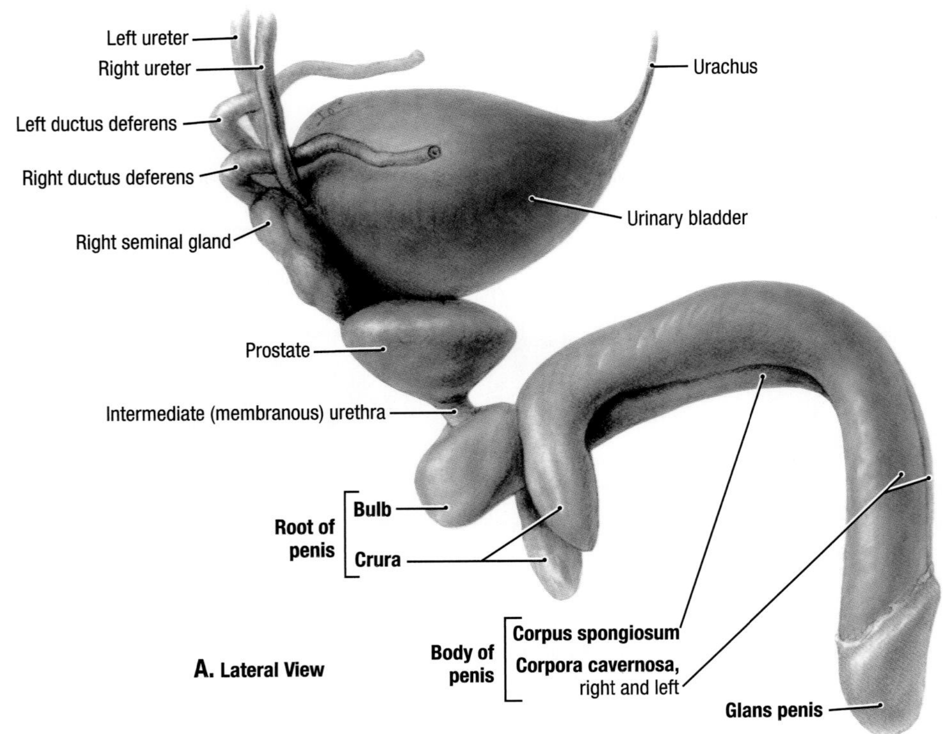
Left ureter
Right ureter
Left ductus deferens
Right ductus deferens
Right seminal gland
Urachus
Urinary bladder
Prostate
Intermediate (membranous) urethra
Root of penis
Bulb
Crura
Body of penis
Corpus spongiosum
Corpora cavernosa, right and left
Glans penis
A. Lateral View

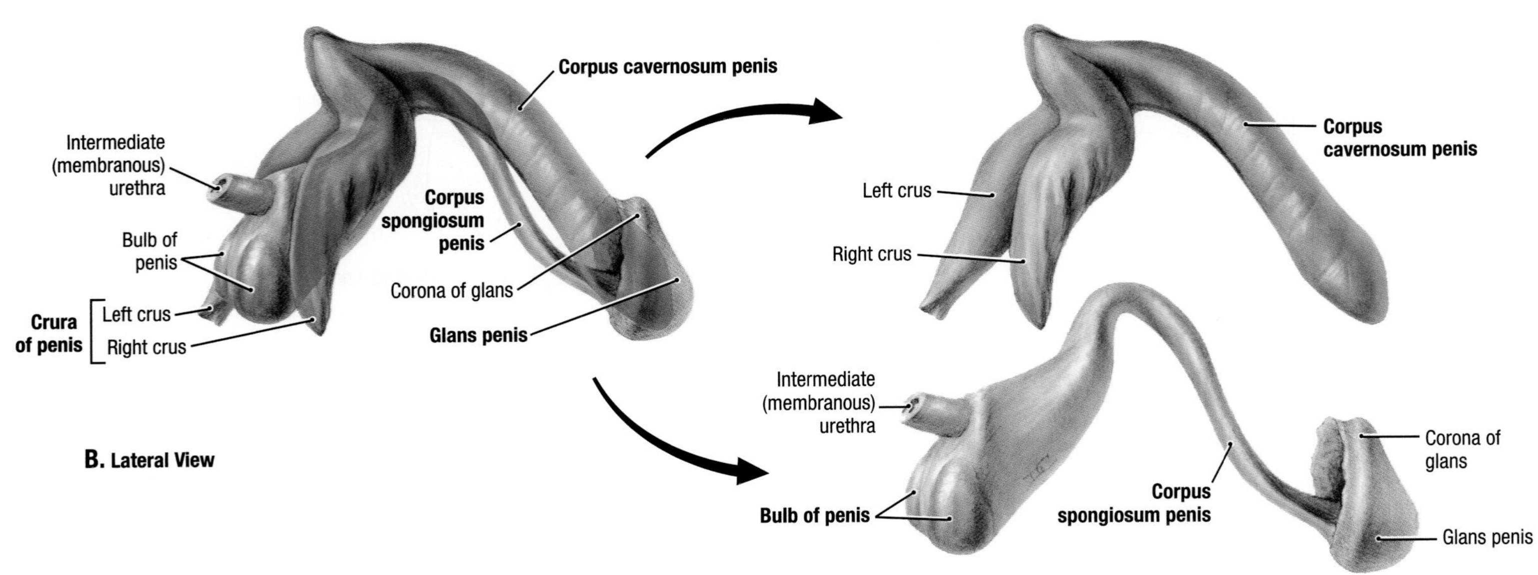
Intermediate (membranous) urethra
Bulb of penis
Crura of penis
Left crus
Right crus
Corpus cavernosum penis
Corpus spongiosum penis
Corona of glans
Glans penis
B. Lateral View
Corpus cavernosum penis
Left crus
Right crus
Intermediate (membranous) urethra
Bulb of penis
Corpus spongiosum penis
Corona of glans
Glans penis
C. Lateral View

## 3.56 Male urogenital system, erectile bodies

**A.** Pelvic components of genital and urinary tracts and erectile bodies of perineum. **B.** Dissection of male erectile bodies (corpora cavernosa and corpus spongiosum). **C.** Corpus spongiosum and corpora cavernosa, separated. The corpora cavernosa is bent where the penis is suspended by the suspensory ligament of the penis from the pubic symphysis. The corpus spongiosum extends posteriorly as the bulb of the penis and terminates anteriorly as the glans.

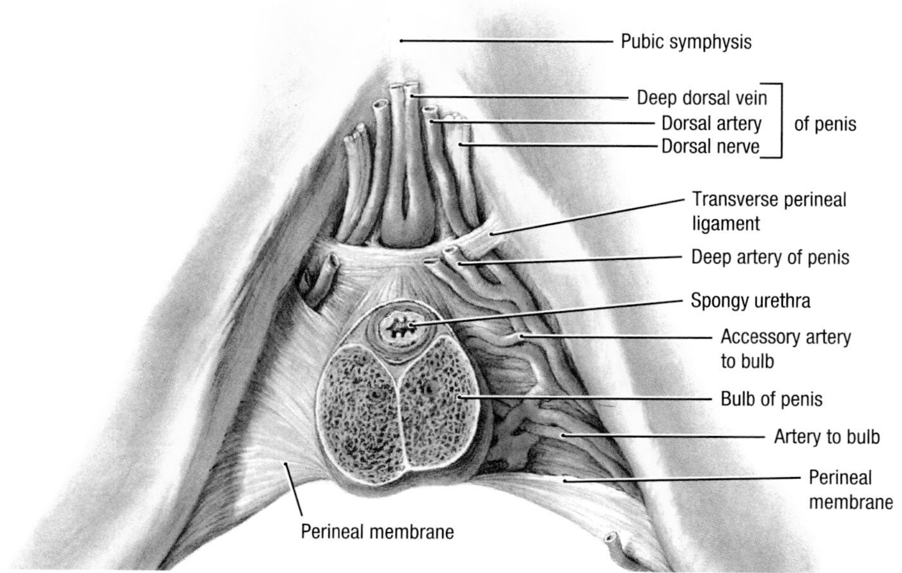
Pubic symphysis
Deep dorsal vein
Dorsal artery
Dorsal nerve
of penis
Transverse perineal ligament
Deep artery of penis
Spongy urethra
Accessory artery to bulb
Bulb of penis
Artery to bulb
Perineal membrane
Perineal membrane

**A.** **Anterior/Inferior View**

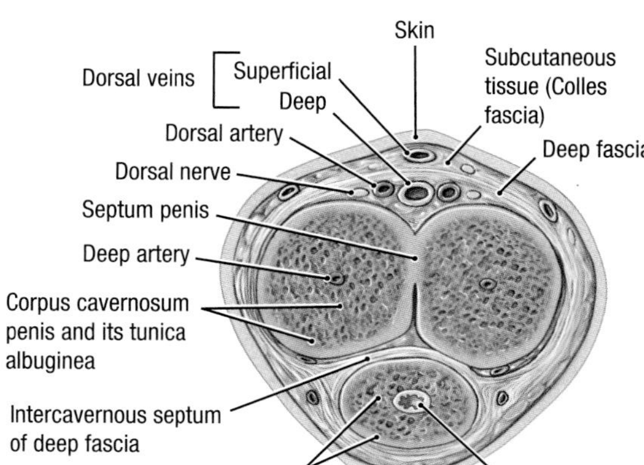
DORSUM
Skin
Subcutaneous tissue (Colles fascia)
Deep fascia
Dorsal veins
Superficial
Deep
Dorsal artery
Dorsal nerve
Septum penis
Deep artery
Corpus cavernosum penis and its tunica albuginea
Intercavernous septum of deep fascia
Corpus spongiosum penis and its tunica albuginea
Spongy urethra
URETHRAL SURFACE

**C.** **Transverse Section**

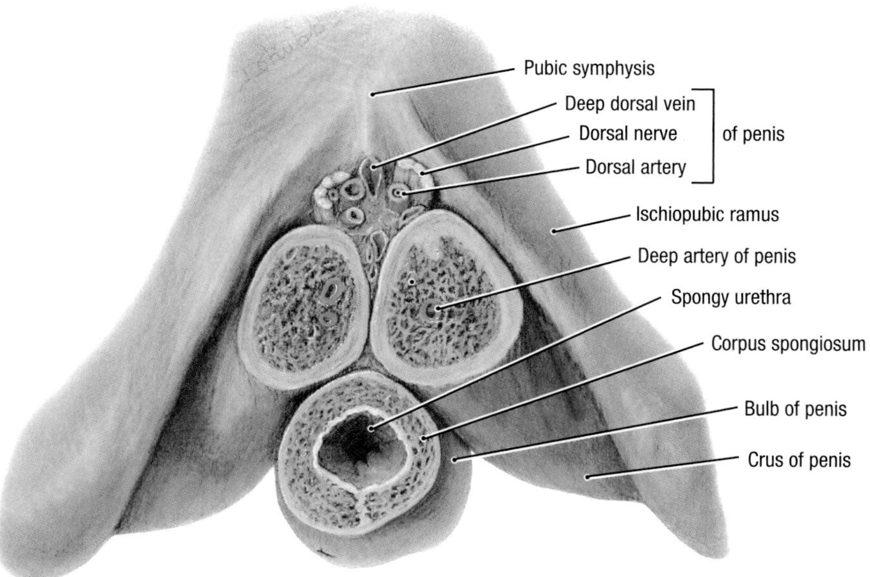
Pubic symphysis
Deep dorsal vein
Dorsal nerve
Dorsal artery
of penis
Ischiopubic ramus
Deep artery of penis
Spongy urethra
Corpus spongiosum
Bulb of penis
Crus of penis

**B.** **Anterior View**

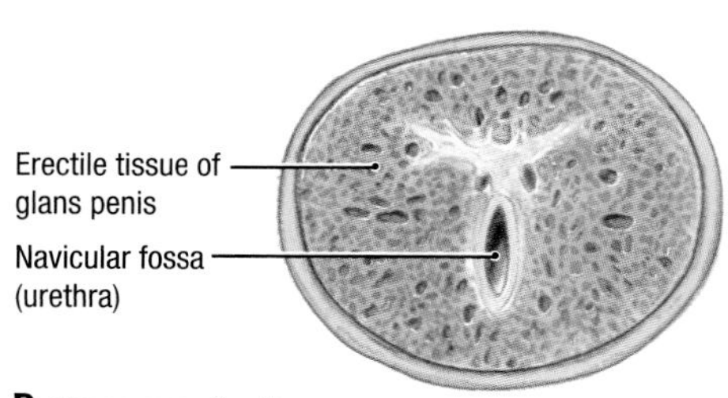
Erectile tissue of glans penis
Navicular fossa (urethra)

**D.** **Transverse Section**

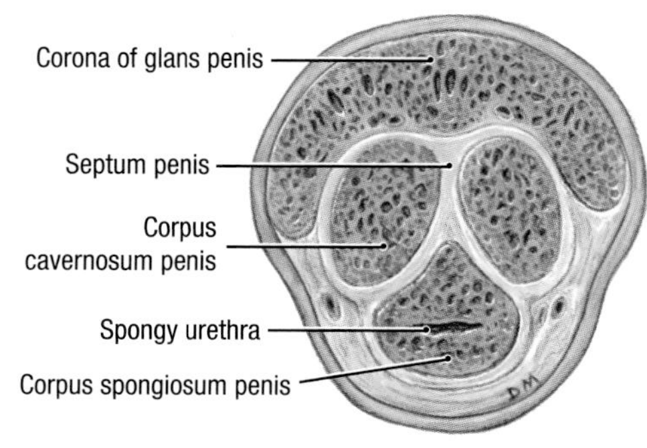
Corona of glans penis
Septum penis
Corpus cavernosum penis
Spongy urethra
Corpus spongiosum penis

**E.** **Transverse Section**

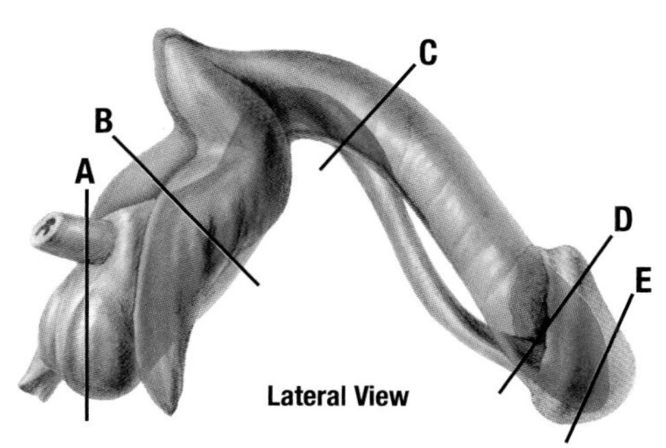
A
B
C
D
E
Lateral View

## 3.57 Cross sections of penis

**A.** Transverse section through bulb of penis with crura removed. The bulb is cut posterior to the entry of the intermediate urethra. On the left side, the perineal membrane is partially removed, opening the deep perineal compartment. **B.** The crura and bulb of penis have been sectioned obliquely. The spongy urethra is dilated within the bulb of the penis. **C.** Transverse section through body of penis. **D.** Transverse section through the proximal part of the glans penis. **E.** Transverse section through the distal part of the glans penis.

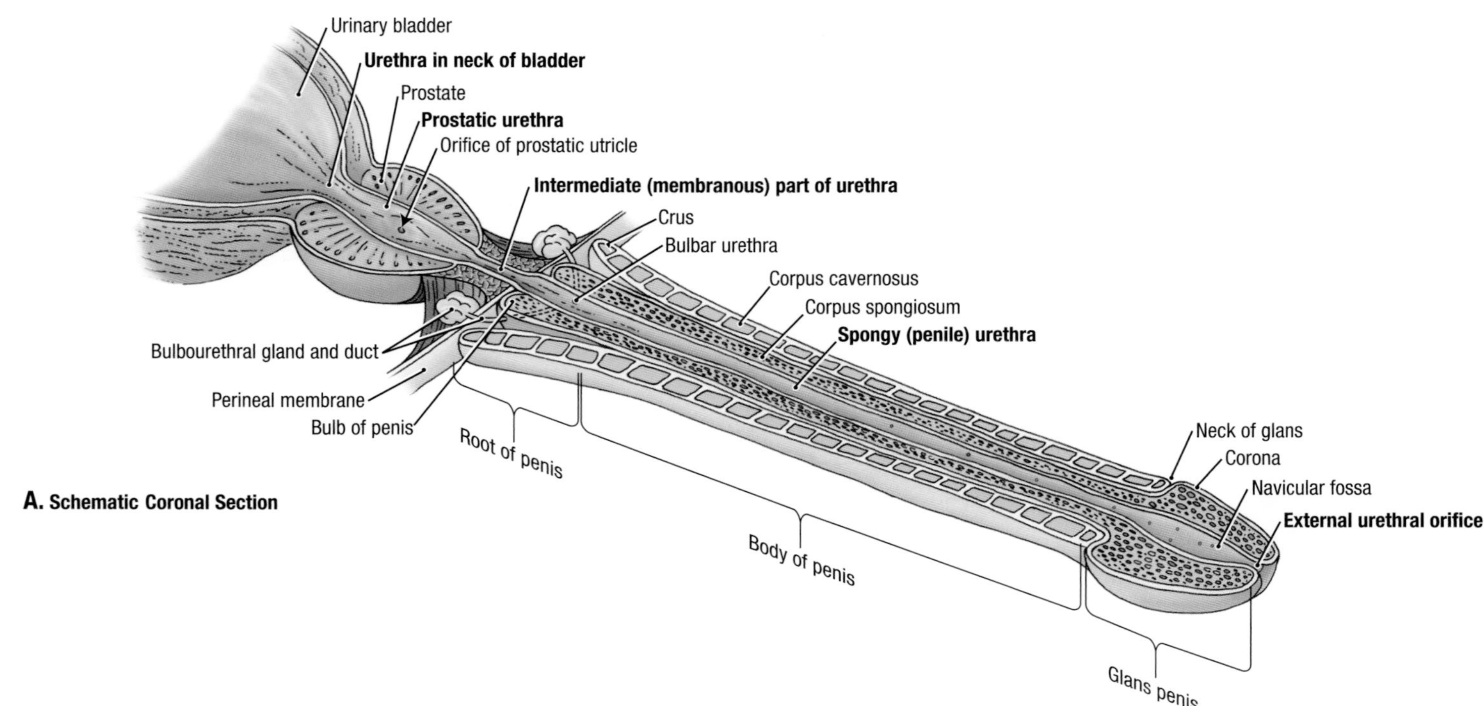
Urinary bladder
Urethra in neck of bladder
Prostate
Prostatic urethra
Orifice of prostatic utricle
Intermediate (membranous) part of urethra
Crus
Bulbar urethra
Corpus cavernosus
Corpus spongiosum
Spongy (penile) urethra
Bulbourethral gland and duct
Perineal membrane
Bulb of penis
Root of penis
Body of penis
Neck of glans
Corona
Navicular fossa
External urethral orifice
Glans penis

**A.** Schematic Coronal Section

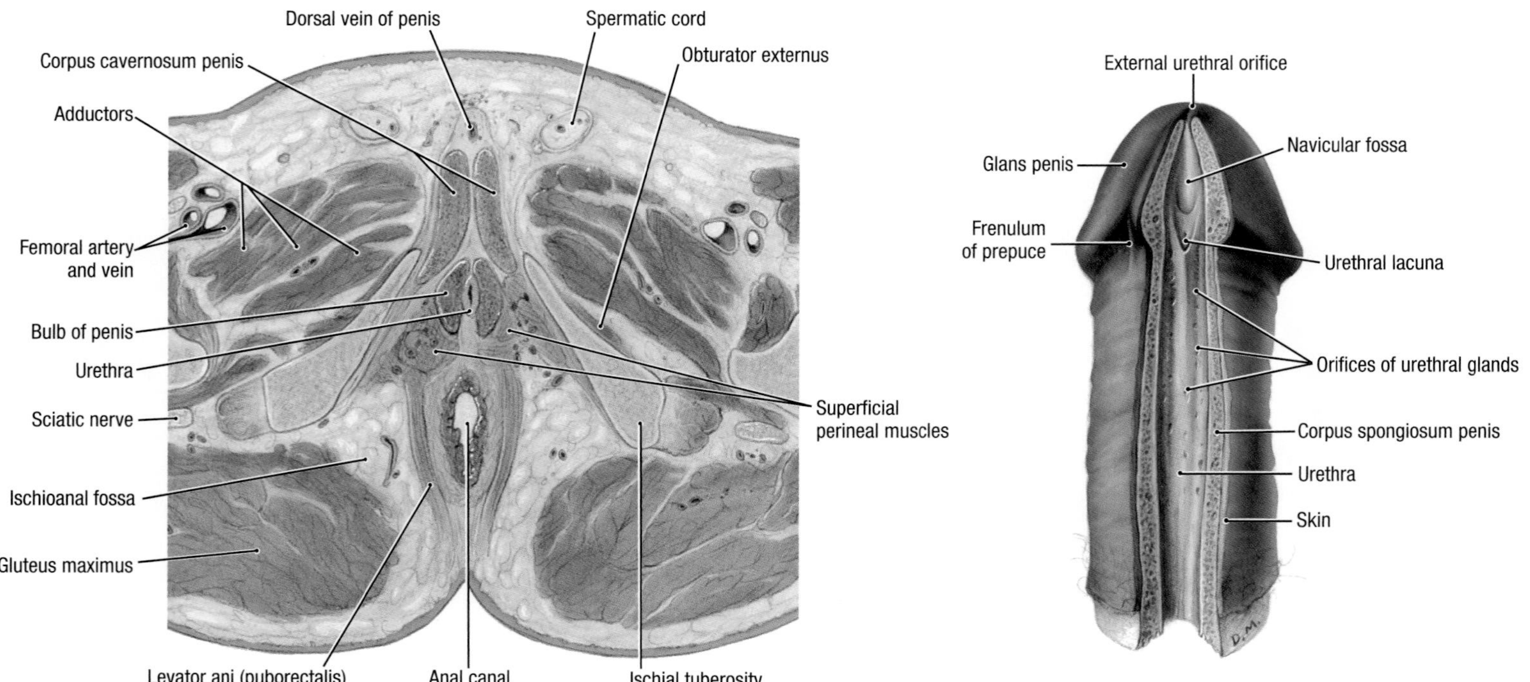
Dorsal vein of penis
Spermatic cord
Corpus cavernosum penis
Obturator externus
Adductors
Femoral artery and vein
Bulb of penis
Urethra
Sciatic nerve
Superficial perineal muscles
Ischioanal fossa
Gluteus maximus
Levator ani (puborectalis)
Anal canal
Ischial tuberosity
External urethral orifice
Glans penis
Navicular fossa
Frenulum of prepuce
Urethral lacuna
Orifices of urethral glands
Corpus spongiosum penis
Urethra
Skin

**B.** Transverse Section, Inferior View

**C.** Urethal Aspect of Distal Penis

## 3.58 Urethra

**A.** Urethra and related structures. B. Transverse section of body passing through the bulb of the penis. **C.** Spongy urethra, interior. A longitudinal incision was made on the urethral surface of the penis and carried through the floor of the urethra, allowing a view of the dorsal surface of the interior of the urethra.

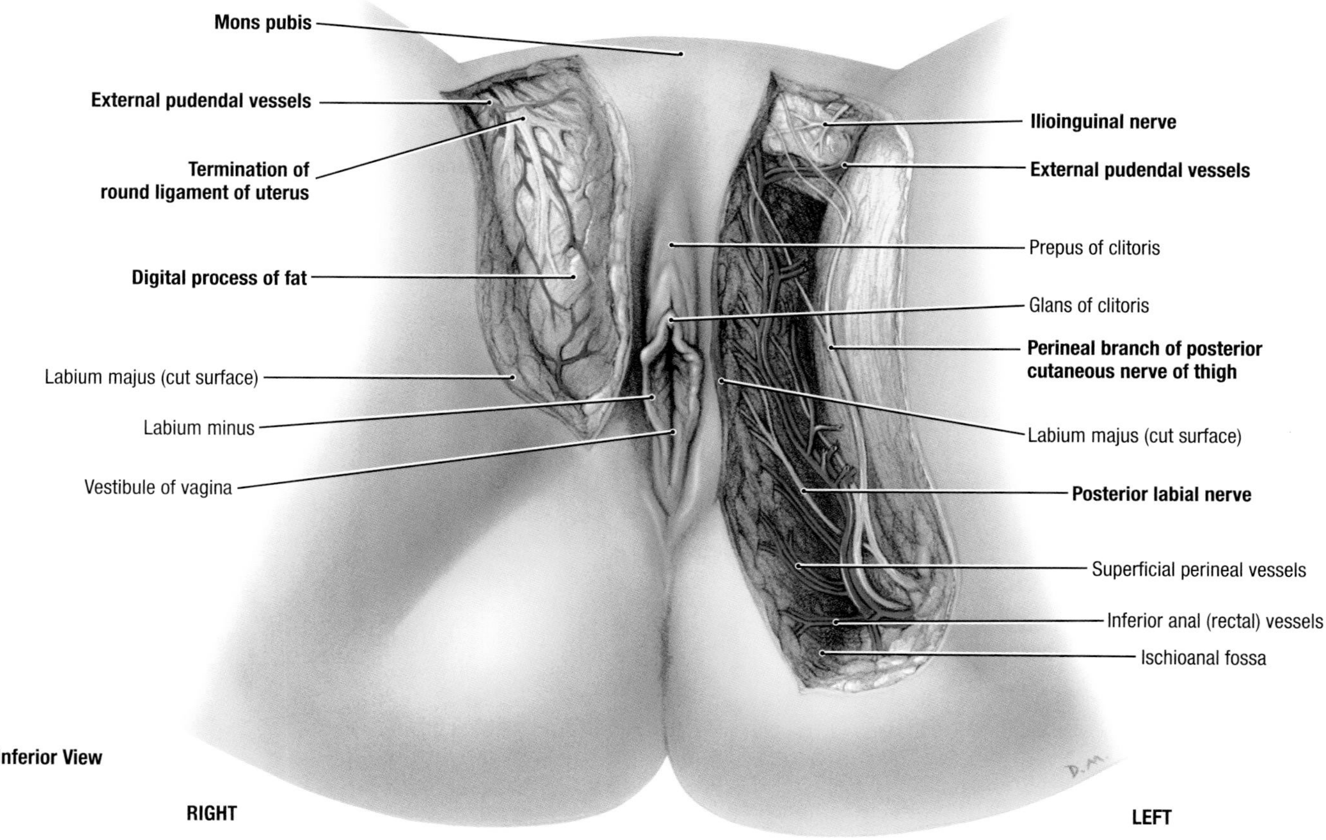
Mons pubis
External pudendal vessels
Termination of round ligament of uterus
Digital process of fat
Labium majus (cut surface)
Labium minus
Vestibule of vagina
Ilioinguinal nerve
External pudendal vessels
Prepus of clitoris
Glans of clitoris
Perineal branch of posterior cutaneous nerve of thigh
Labium majus (cut surface)
Posterior labial nerve
Superficial perineal vessels
Inferior anal (rectal) vessels
Ischioanal fossa
Inferior View
RIGHT
LEFT

## 3.59 Female perineum—I

Superficial dissection. On the right side of the specimen:

- A long digital process of fat lies deep to the subcutaneous fatty tissue and descends into the labium majus.
- The round ligament of the uterus ends as a branching band of fascia that spreads out superficial to the fatty digital process.

On the left side of the specimen:

- Most of the fatty digital process is removed.
- The mons pubis is the rounded fatty prominence anterior to the pubic symphysis and bodies of the pubic bones.
- The posterior labial vessels and nerves (S2, S3) are joined by the perineal branch of the posterior cutaneous nerve of thigh (S1, S2, S3) and run anteriorly to the mons pubis. At the mons pubis the vessels anastomose with the external pudendal vessels, and the nerves overlap in supply with the ilioinguinal nerve (L1).

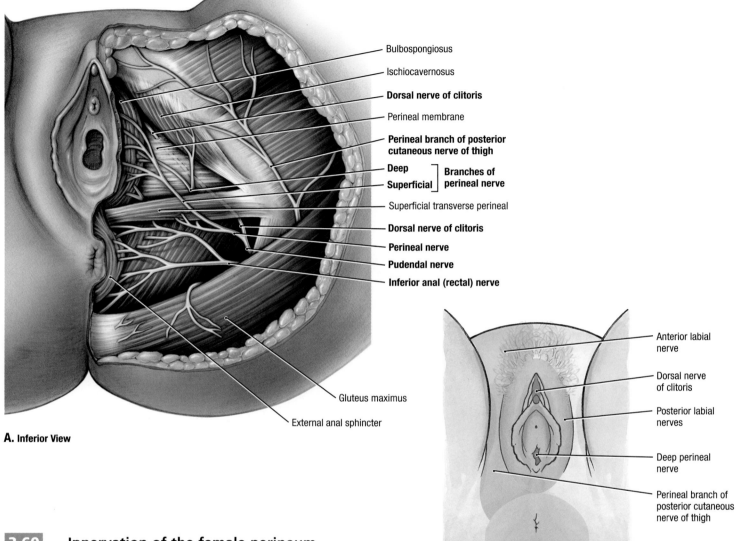

Bulbospongiosus
Ischiocavernosus
**Dorsal nerve of clitoris**
Perineal membrane
**Perineal branch of posterior cutaneous nerve of thigh**
**Deep** / **Superficial** — **Branches of perineal nerve**
Superficial transverse perineal
**Dorsal nerve of clitoris**
**Perineal nerve**
**Pudendal nerve**
**Inferior anal (rectal) nerve**
Gluteus maximus
External anal sphincter

**A. Inferior View**

Anterior labial nerve
Dorsal nerve of clitoris
Posterior labial nerves
Deep perineal nerve
Perineal branch of posterior cutaneous nerve of thigh
Inferior rectal (anal) nerve
Inferior clunial nerves

**B. Inferior View**

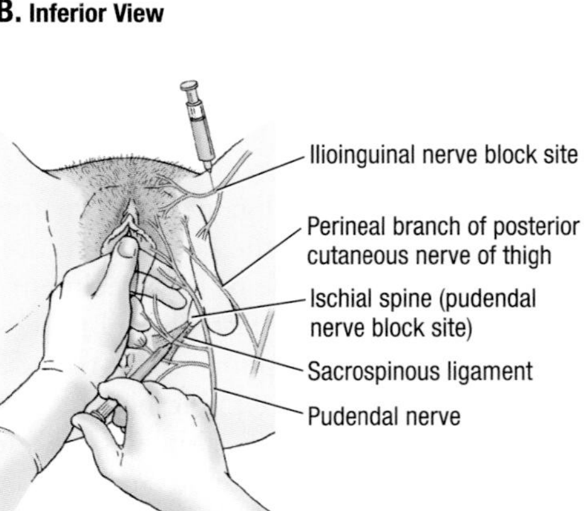
Ilioinguinal nerve block site
Perineal branch of posterior cutaneous nerve of thigh
Ischial spine (pudendal nerve block site)
Sacrospinous ligament
Pudendal nerve

**C. Inferior View**

## 3.60 Innervation of the female perineum

**A** and **B.** The anterior aspect of the perineum is supplied by anterior labial nerves, derived from the ilioinguinal nerve and genital branch of the genitofemoral nerve. The pudendal nerve is the main nerve of the perineum. Posterior labial nerves, derived from the superficial perineal nerve, supply most of the vulva. The deep perineal nerve supplies the orifice of the vagina and superficial perineal muscles; and the dorsal nerve of the clitoris supplies deep perineal muscles and sensations to the clitoris. The inferior anal (rectal) nerve, also from the pudendal nerve, innervates the external anal sphincter and the perianal skin. The lateral perineum is supplied by the perineal branch of the posterior cutaneous nerve of the thigh. **C.** To relieve the pain experienced during childbirth, pudendal nerve block anesthesia may be performed by injecting a local anesthetic agent into the tissue surrounding the pudendal nerve, near the ischial spine. A pudendal nerve block does not abolish sensations from the anterior and lateral parts of the perineum. Therefore, a block of the ilioinguinal and/or perineal branch of the posterior cutaneous nerve of the thigh may also need to be performed.

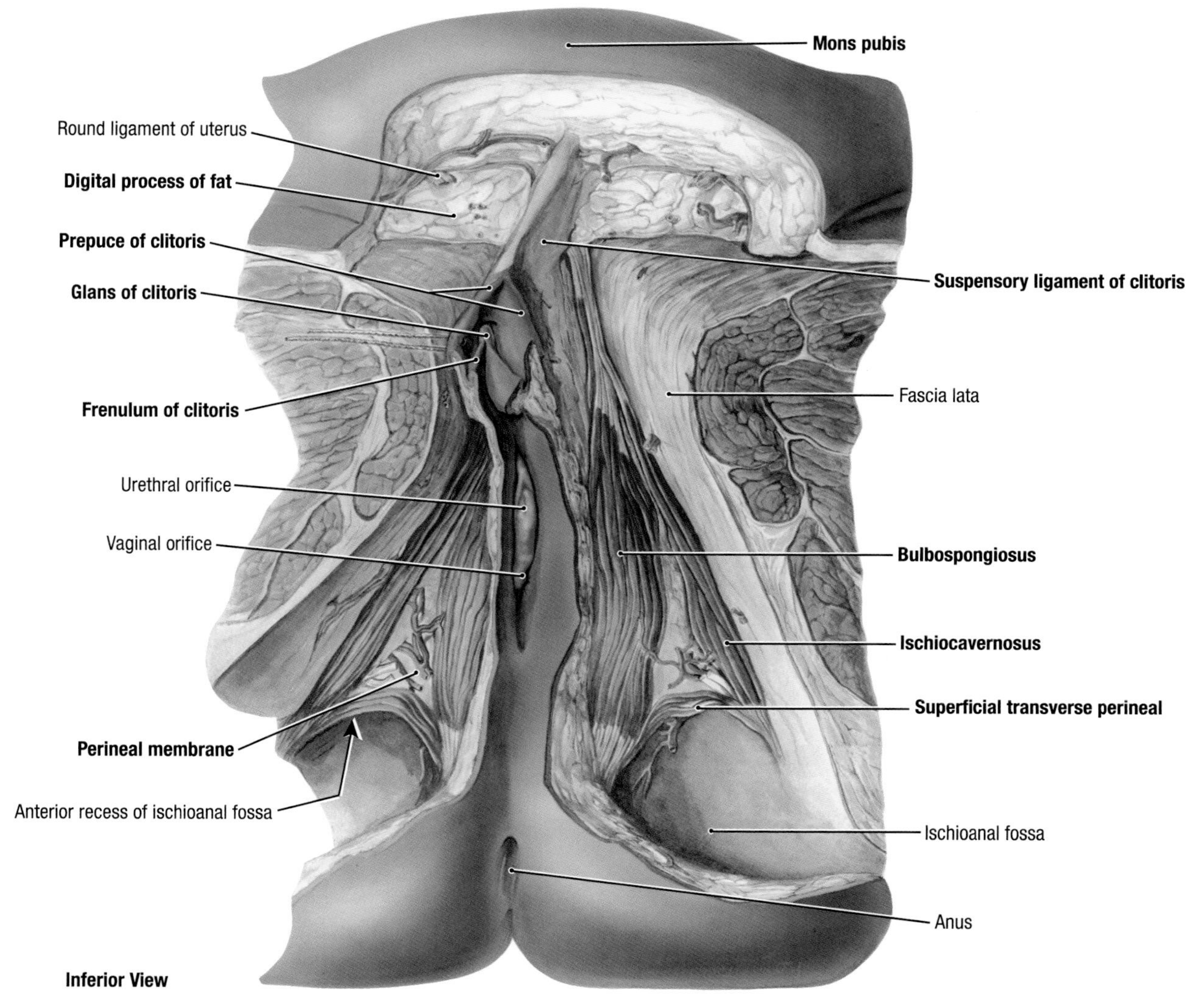
Mons pubis
Round ligament of uterus
Digital process of fat
Prepuce of clitoris
Glans of clitoris
Suspensory ligament of clitoris
Fascia lata
Frenulum of clitoris
Urethral orifice
Vaginal orifice
Bulbospongiosus
Ischiocavernosus
Superficial transverse perineal
Perineal membrane
Anterior recess of ischioanal fossa
Ischioanal fossa
Anus
Inferior View

## 3.61 Female perineum—II

- Note the thickness of the subcutaneous fatty tissue of the mons pubis and the encapsulated digital process of fat deep to this. The suspensory ligament of the clitoris descends from the linea alba.
- Anteriorly, each labium minus forms two laminae or folds: the lateral laminae of the labia pass on each side of the glans clitoris and unite, forming a hood that partially or completely covers the glans, the prepuce (foreskin) of the clitoris. The medial laminae of the labia merge posterior to the glans, forming the frenulum of the clitoris.
- There are three muscles on each side: bulbospongiosus, ischiocavernosus, and superficial transverse perineal; the perineal membrane is visible between them.
- The bulbospongiosus muscle overlies the bulb of the vestibule and the great vestibular gland. In the male, the muscles of the two sides are united by a median raphe; in the female, the orifice of the vagina separates the right from the left.

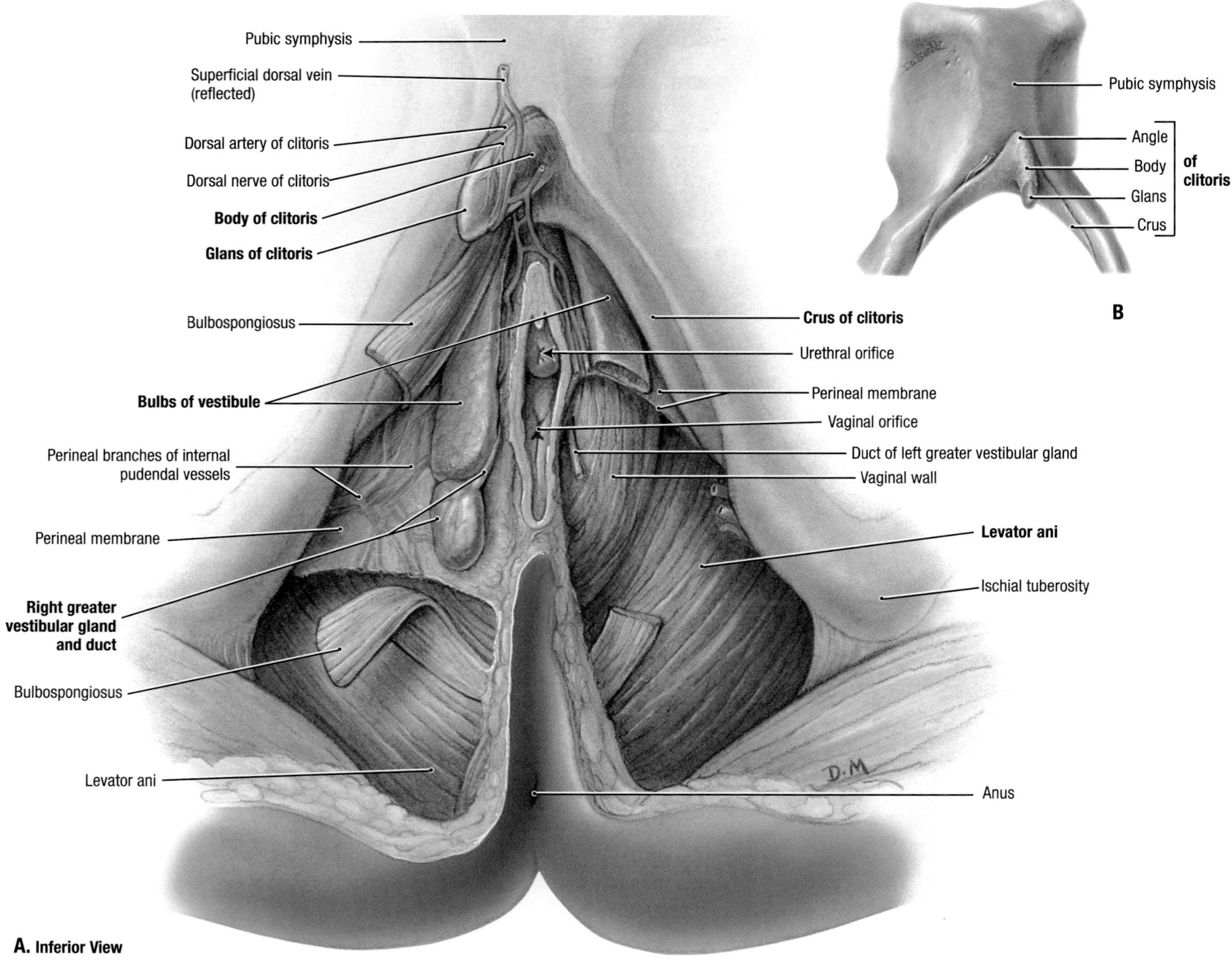
Pubic symphysis
Superficial dorsal vein (reflected)
Dorsal artery of clitoris
Dorsal nerve of clitoris
Body of clitoris
Glans of clitoris
Bulbospongiosus
Bulbs of vestibule
Perineal branches of internal pudendal vessels
Perineal membrane
Right greater vestibular gland and duct
Bulbospongiosus
Levator ani
Crus of clitoris
Urethral orifice
Perineal membrane
Vaginal orifice
Duct of left greater vestibular gland
Vaginal wall
Levator ani
Ischial tuberosity
Anus
D.M.
A. Inferior View
Pubic symphysis
Angle
Body
Glans
Crus
of clitoris
B

## 3.62 Female perineum—III

**A.** Deeper dissection. **B.** Clitoris.

In **A:**

- The bulbospongiosus muscle is reflected on the right side and mostly removed on the left side; the posterior portion of the bulb of the vestibule and the greater vestibular gland have been removed on the left side.
- The glans and body of the clitoris is displaced to the right so that the distribution of the dorsal vessels and nerve of the clitoris can be seen.
- Homologues of the bulb of the penis, the bulbs of the vestibule exist as two masses of elongated erectile tissue that lie along the sides of the vaginal orifice; veins connect the bulbs of the vestibule to the glans of the clitoris.
- On the specimen's right side, the greater vestibular gland is situated at the posterior end of the bulb; both structures are covered by bulbospongiosus muscle.
- On the specimen's left side, the bulb, gland, and perineal membrane are cut away, thereby revealing the external aspect of the vaginal wall.

In **B:**

- The body of the clitoris, composed of two crura (corpora cavernosa), is capped by the glans.

Pubic symphysis
Obturator externus
Clitoris (cut surface)
Urethral orifice
Urethrovaginal sphincter
Ischiopubic ramus
Labium minus (cut surface)
Vaginal orifice with hymenal carunculae
Vestibule of vagina
Pubovaginalis
Vaginal wall
Levator ani
Internal pudendal vessels
Ischial tuberosity
Coccygeus
Perineal body
Sacrotuberous ligament
External anal sphincter
Ishioanal fossa
Anus
Gluteus maximus
Anococcygeal body
D.M.
Coccyx

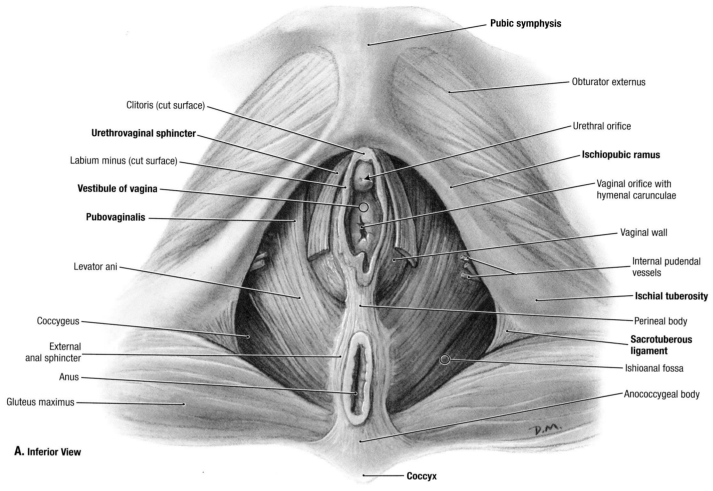

**A. Inferior View**

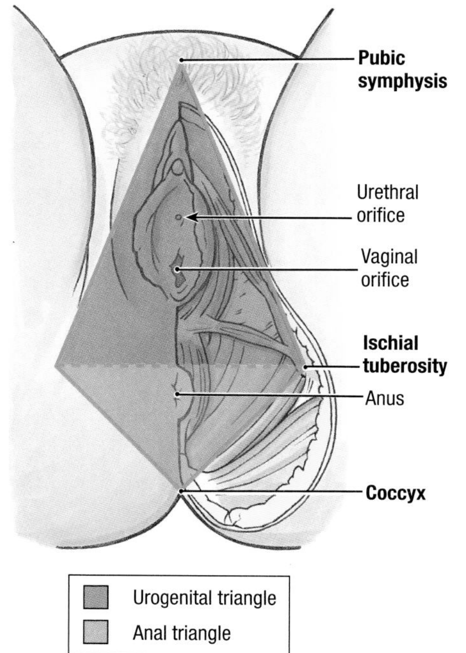
Pubic symphysis
Urethral orifice
Vaginal orifice
Ischial tuberosity
Anus
Coccyx
Urogenital triangle
Anal triangle

**B. Inferior View**

## 3.63 Female perineum—IV

**A.** Deep perineal compartment. The perineal membrane and smooth muscle corresponding in position to the deep transverse perineal muscle in the male have been removed.

- The most anterior and medial part of the levator ani muscle, the pubovaginalis, passes posterior to the vaginal orifice.
- The urethrovaginal sphincter, part of the external urethral sphincter of the female, rests on the urethra and straddles the vagina.
- The labia minora (cut short here) bound the vestibule of the vagina.

**A** and **B.** The osseoligamentous boundaries of the diamond-shaped perineum are the pubic symphysis, ischiopubic rami, ischial tuberosities, sacrotuberous ligaments, and coccyx. For descriptive purposes, a transverse line connecting the ischial tuberosities subdivides the diamond into urogenital and anal triangles.

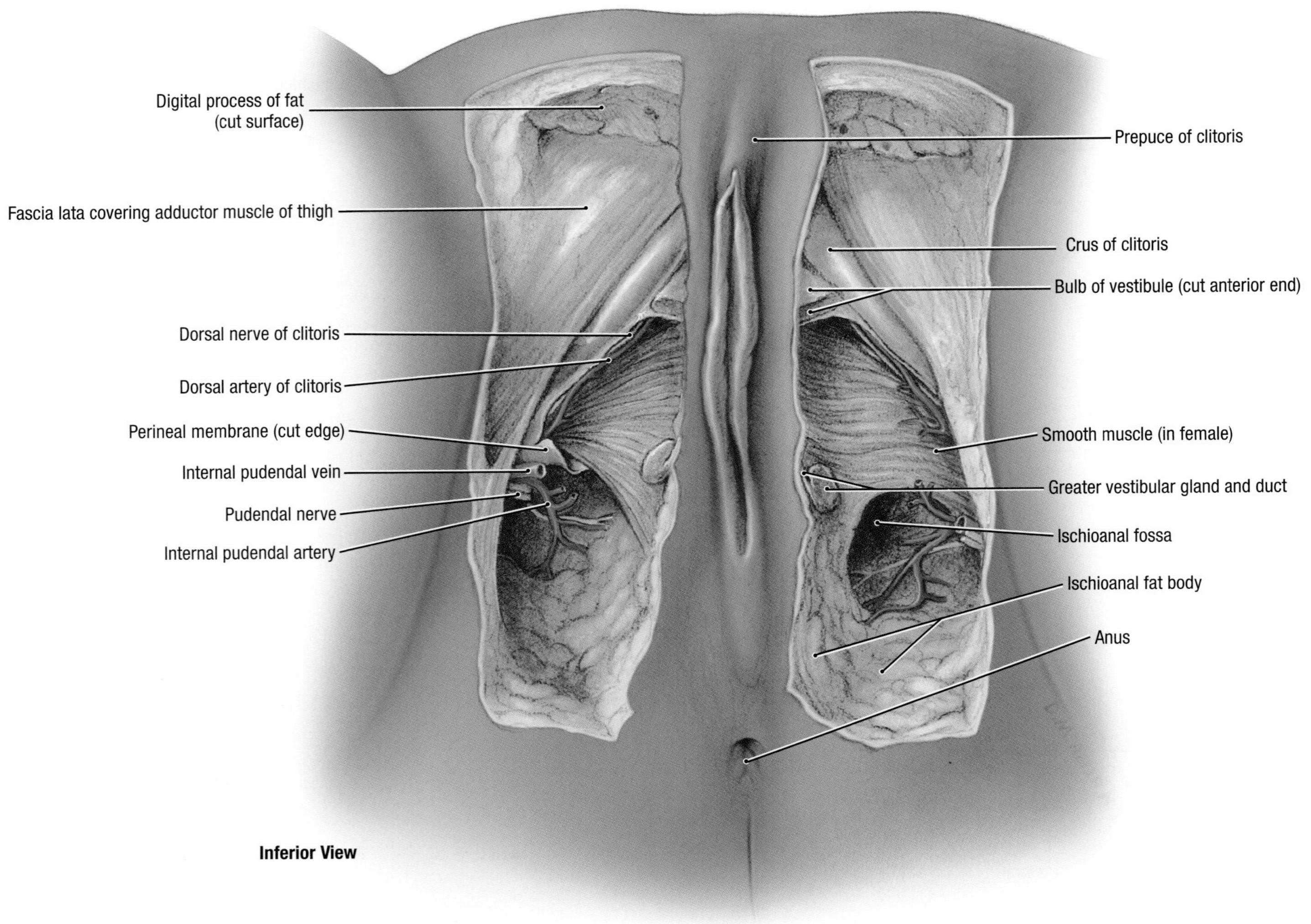
Digital process of fat (cut surface)
Fascia lata covering adductor muscle of thigh
Dorsal nerve of clitoris
Dorsal artery of clitoris
Perineal membrane (cut edge)
Internal pudendal vein
Pudendal nerve
Internal pudendal artery
Prepuce of clitoris
Crus of clitoris
Bulb of vestibule (cut anterior end)
Smooth muscle (in female)
Greater vestibular gland and duct
Ischioanal fossa
Ischioanal fat body
Anus
Inferior View

## 3.64 Female perineum—V

This is a different dissection than the previous series, with the vulva undissected centrally but the perineum dissected deeply on each side. Although most of the perineal membrane and bulbs of the vestibule have been removed, the greater vestibular glands (structures of the superficial perineal compartment) have been left in place. The development and extent of the smooth muscle layer corresponding in position to the voluntary deep transverse perineal muscles of the male is highly variable, being relatively extensive in this case, blending centrally with voluntary fibers of the external urethral sphincter and the perineal body.

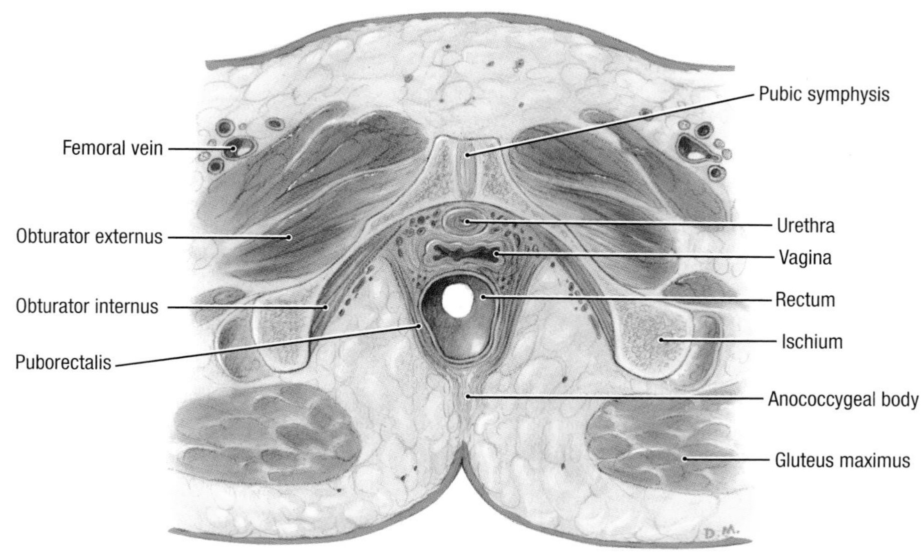
Pubic symphysis
Femoral vein
Obturator externus
Urethra
Vagina
Obturator internus
Rectum
Ischium
Puborectalis
Anococcygeal body
Gluteus maximus

**A.** Transverse Section

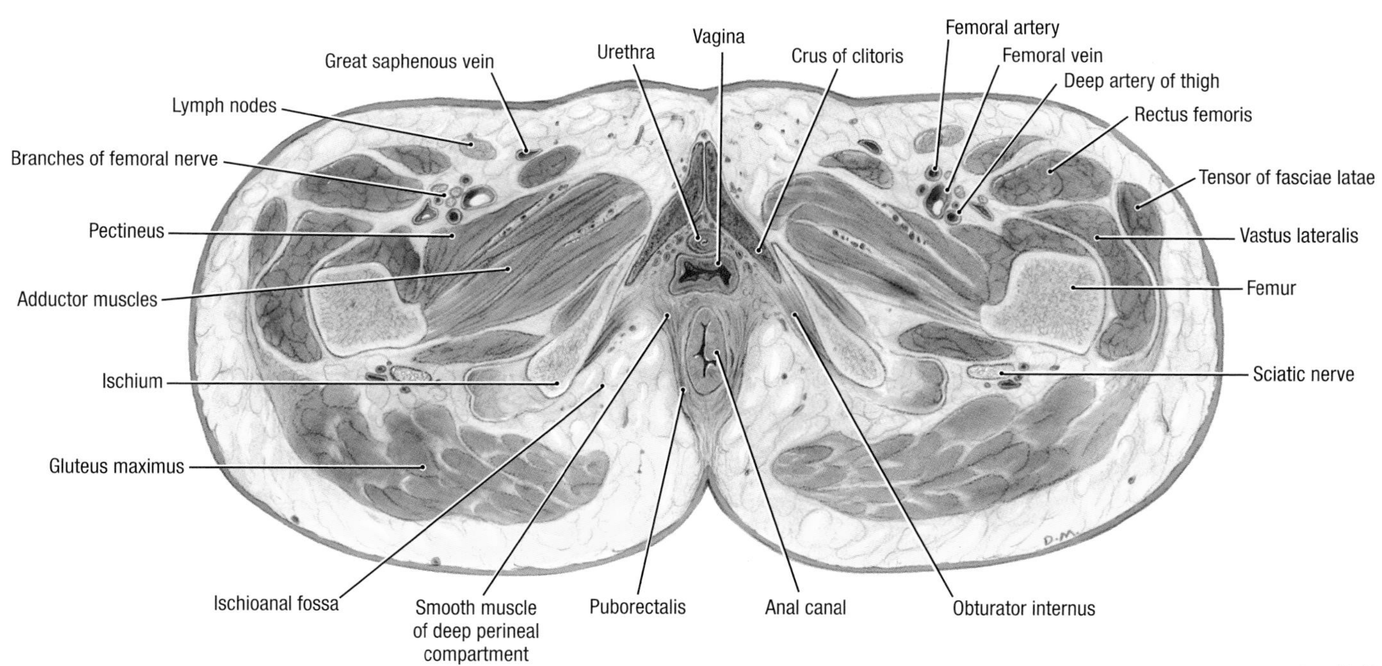
Vagina
Femoral artery
Urethra
Crus of clitoris
Femoral vein
Great saphenous vein
Deep artery of thigh
Lymph nodes
Rectus femoris
Branches of femoral nerve
Tensor of fasciae latae
Pectineus
Vastus lateralis
Femur
Adductor muscles
Ischium
Sciatic nerve
Gluteus maximus
Ischioanal fossa
Smooth muscle of deep perineal compartment
Puborectalis
Anal canal
Obturator internus

**B.** Transverse Section

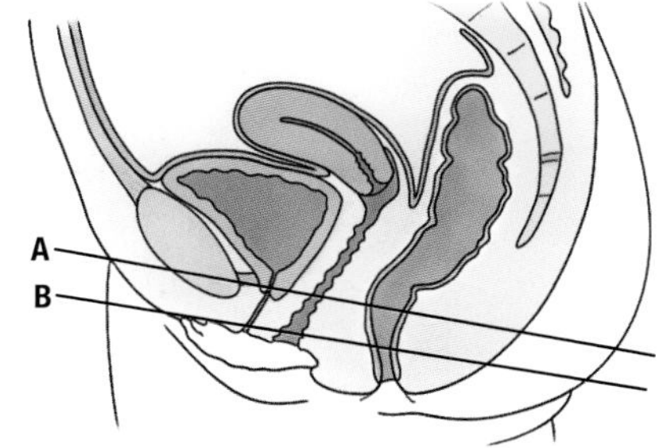
A
B

## 3.65 Female perineum—V

**A.** Section through vagina and urethra at base of urinary bladder. **B.** Section through vagina, urethra, and crura of clitoris.

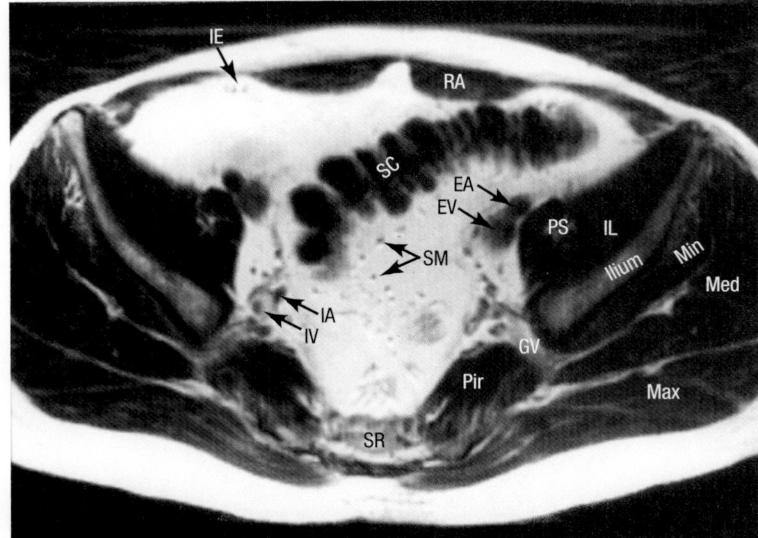
IE
RA
SC
EA
EV
SM
PS
IL
Ilium
Min
Med
IA
IV
GV
Pir
Max
SR

A

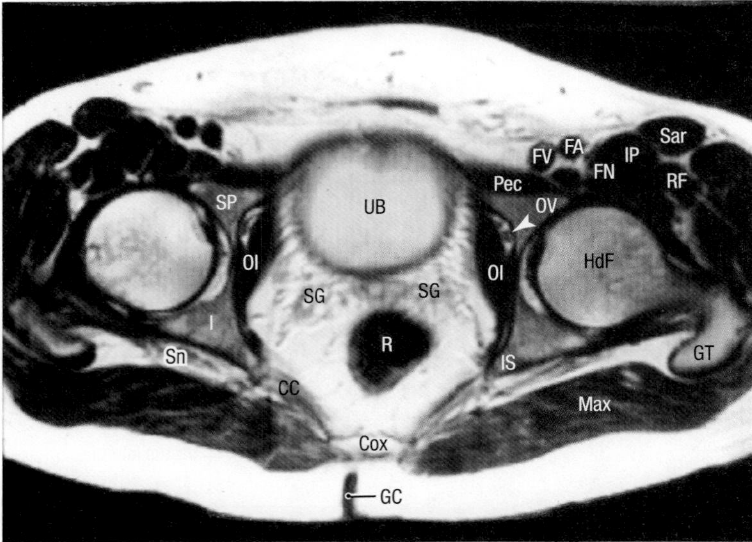
FV
FA
IP
Sar
FN
Pec
RF
SP
UB
OV
OI
HdF
OI
SG
SG
I
R
Sn
GT
IS
CC
Max
Cox
GC

B

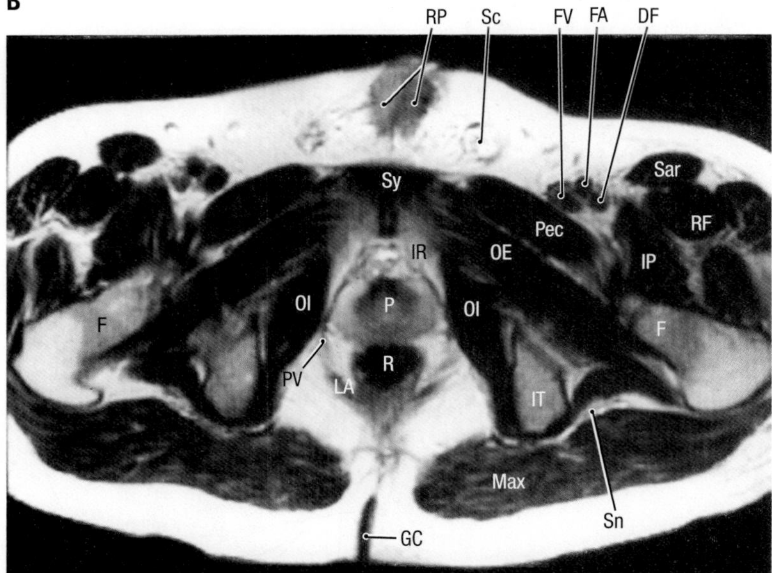
RP
Sc
FV
FA
DF
Sar
Sy
RF
Pec
IR
OE
IP
OI
P
OI
F
F
PV
LA
R
IT
Max
Sn
GC

C

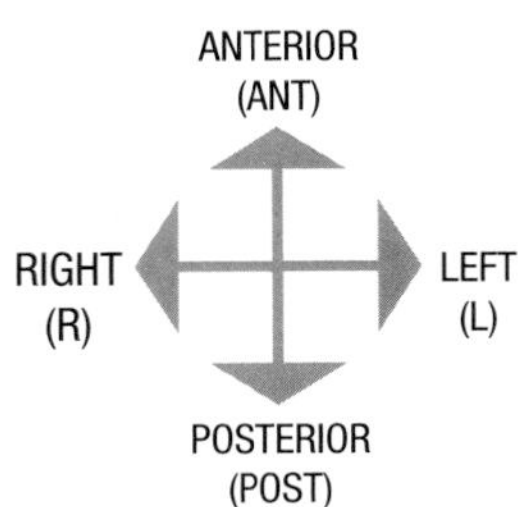
ANTERIOR
(ANT)
RIGHT
(R)
LEFT
(L)
POSTERIOR
(POST)

| | |
|---|---|
| **A** | **Anus** |
| Ad | Adductor muscles |
| Bi | Biceps femoris tendon |
| **Bu** | **Bulb of penis** |
| **Cav** | **Corpus cavernosum penis** |
| CC | Coccygeus |
| Cox | Coccyx |
| **Cr** | **Crus of penis** |
| DD | Ductus deferens |
| DF | Deep femoral artery |
| DVP | Dorsal vein of penis |
| EA | External iliac artery |
| EAS | External anal sphincter |
| EV | External iliac vein |
| F | Femur |
| FA | Femoral artery |
| FN | Femoral nerve |
| FV | Femoral vein |
| GC | Gluteal cleft |
| GSV | Great saphenous vein |
| GT | Greater trochanter |
| GV | Superior gluteal vein |
| HdF | Head of femur |
| I | Body of ischium |
| IA | Internal iliac artery |
| **IAF** | **Ischioanal fossa (pararectal fat)** |
| **IC** | **Ischiocavernosus** |
| IE | Inferior epigastric vessels |
| IL | Iliacus |
| IP | Iliopsoas |
| IPR | Ischiopubic ramus |
| IR | Inferior pubic ramus |
| IS | Ischial spine |
| IT | Ischial tuberosity |
| IV | Internal iliac vein |
| **LA** | **Levator ani** |
| Max | Gluteus maximus |
| Med | Gluteus medius |
| Min | Gluteus minimus |
| OE | Obturator externus |
| OI | Obturator internus |
| OV | Obturator vessels and nerve |
| **P** | **Prostate** |
| **PB** | **Perineal body** |
| Pec | Pectineus |
| Pir | Piriformis |
| **PR** | **Puborectalis** |
| PS | Psoas |
| PV | Pudenal vessels and nerves |
| QF | Quadratus femoris |
| **R** | **Rectum** |
| RA | Rectus abdominis |
| RF | Rectus femoris |
| **RP** | **Root of penis** |
| Sar | Sartorius |
| Sc | Spermatic cord |
| SC | Sigmoid colon |
| **SG** | **Seminal gland** |
| SM | Sigmoidal vessels in mesentery of sigmoid colon |
| Sn | Sciatic nerve |
| SP | Superior ramus of pubis |
| SR | Sacrum |
| Sy | Pubic symphysis |
| **U** | **Urethra** |
| **UB** | **Urinary bladder** |
| VI | Vastus intermedius |

**(Organs/structures of male pelvis and perineum are in boldface)**

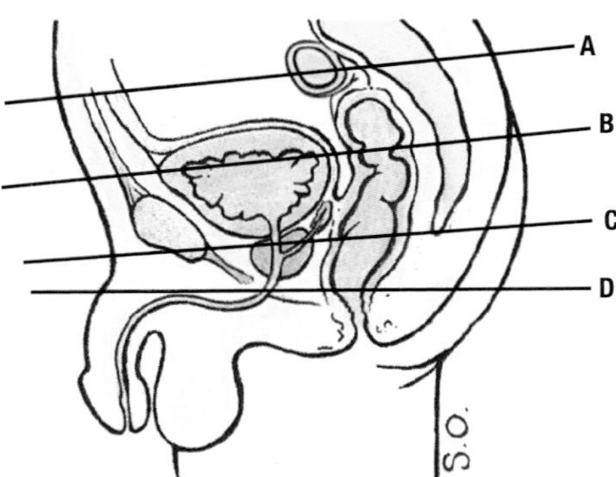
A
B
C
D
S.O.

**3.66 Transverse (axial) MRIs and sectional specimen of the male pelvis and perineum, inferior views**

**A–D.** MRIs. **E.** Anatomical section.

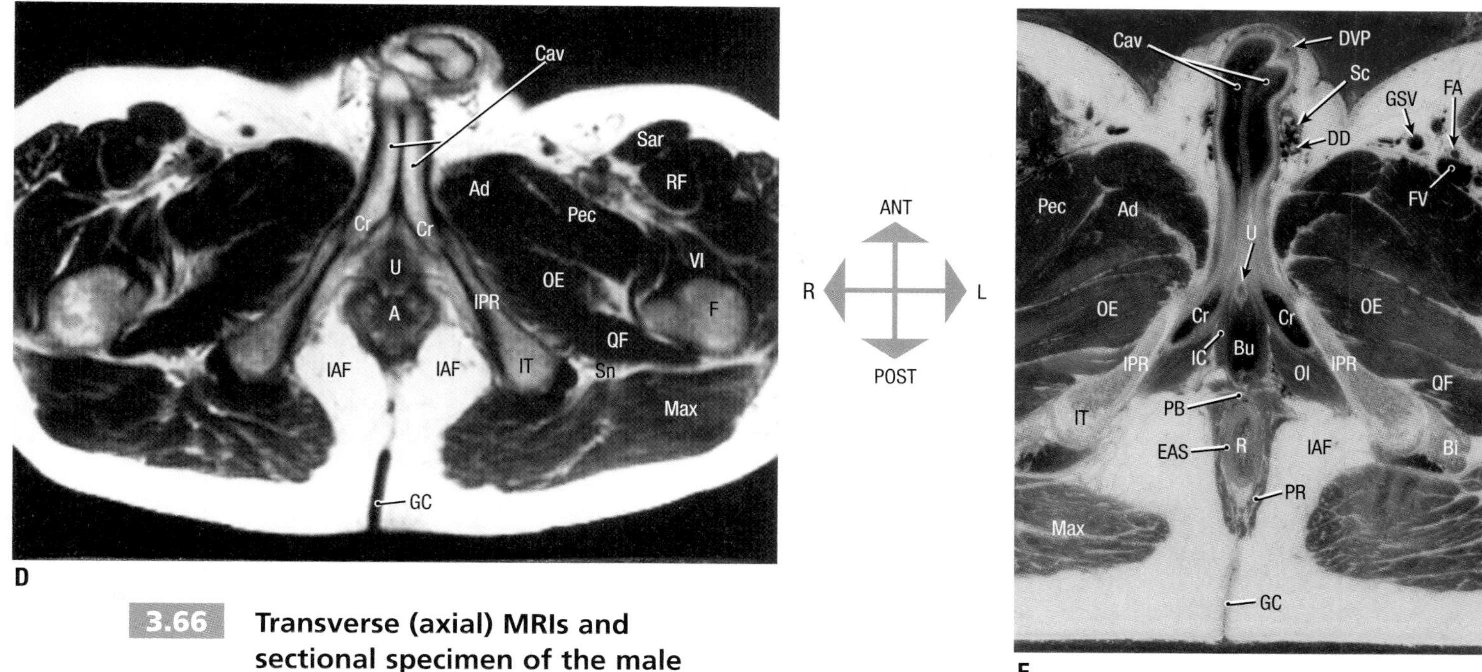
Cav
Sar
Ad
RF
Pec
Cr
Cr
U
VI
OE
A
IPR
F
QF
IAF
IAF
IT
Sn
Max
GC
D
ANT
R
L
POST
Cav
DVP
Sc
GSV
FA
DD
FV
Pec
Ad
U
OE
OE
Cr
Cr
IC
Bu
IPR
OI
IPR
QF
IT
PB
IAF
EAS
R
Bi
PR
Max
GC
E

**3.66 Transverse (axial) MRIs and sectional specimen of the male pelvis and perineum, inferior views *(continued)***

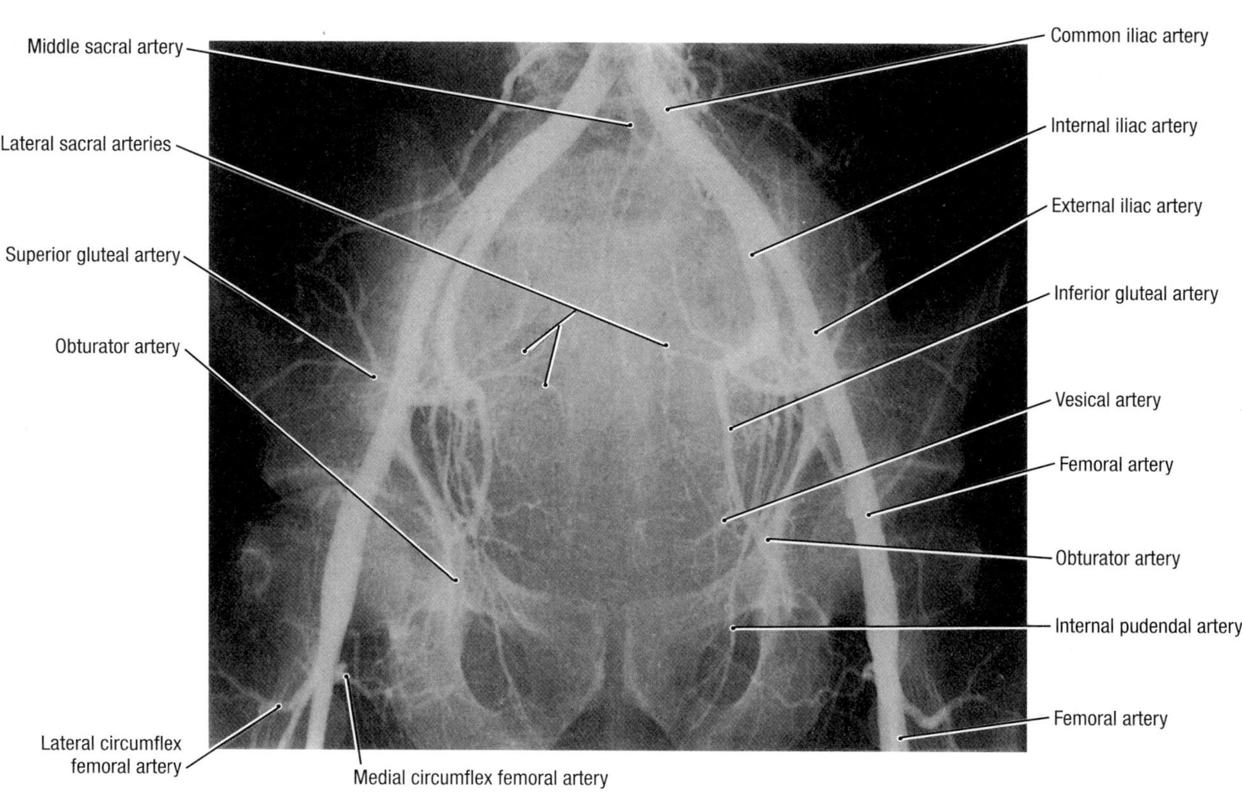
Middle sacral artery
Lateral sacral arteries
Superior gluteal artery
Obturator artery
Lateral circumflex femoral artery
Medial circumflex femoral artery
Common iliac artery
Internal iliac artery
External iliac artery
Inferior gluteal artery
Vesical artery
Femoral artery
Obturator artery
Internal pudendal artery
Femoral artery
Anteroposterior View

**3.67 Pelvic angiography**

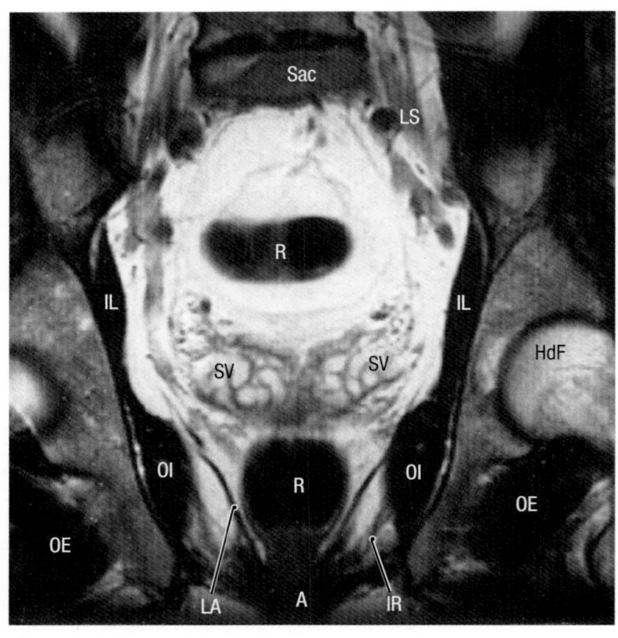
Sac
LS
R
IL
IL
HdF
SV
SV
OI
OI
R
OE
OE
LA
A
IR

A

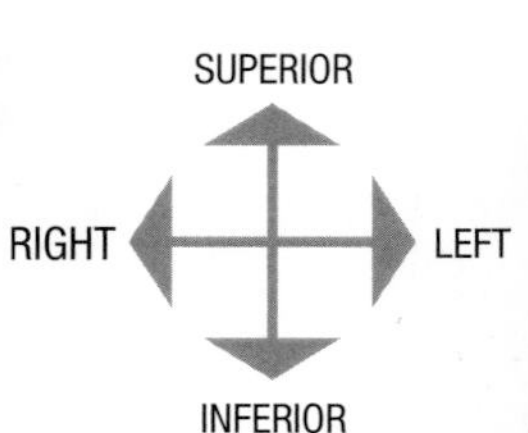
SUPERIOR
RIGHT
LEFT
INFERIOR

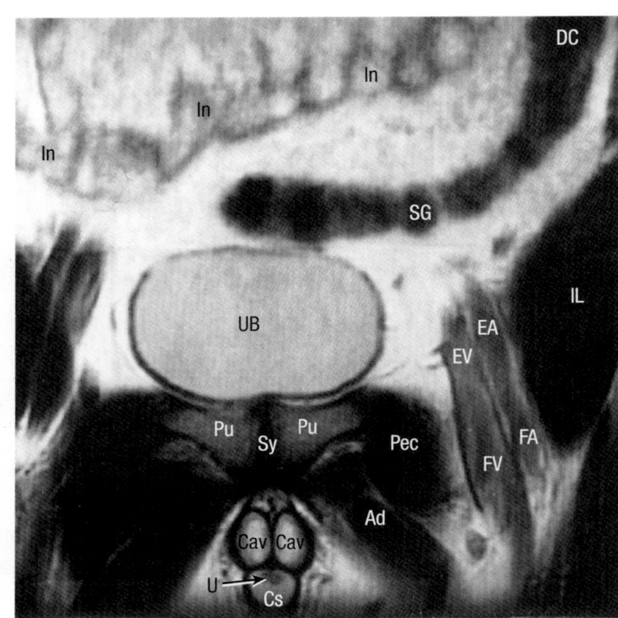
DC
In
In
In
SG
UB
IL
EA
EV
Pu
Pu
Sy
Pec
FA
FV
Ad
Cav
Cav
U
Cs

B

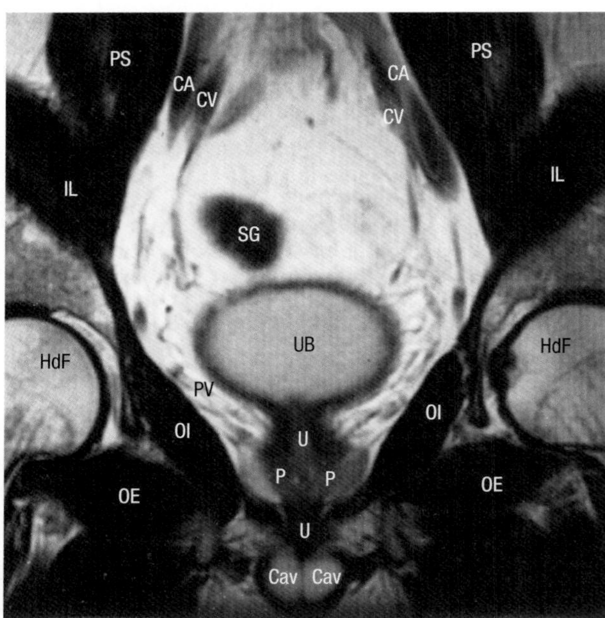
PS
PS
CA
CV
CA
CV
IL
IL
SG
UB
HdF
HdF
PV
OI
OI
U
P
P
OE
OE
U
Cav
Cav

C

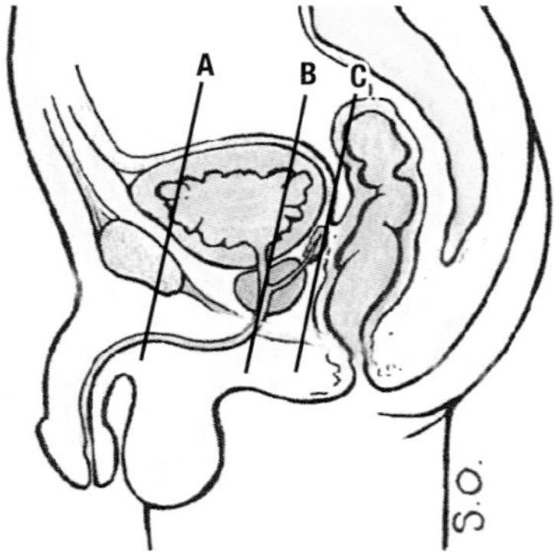
A
B
C
S.O.

| | |
|---|---|
| **A** | **Anus** |
| Ad | Adductors |
| CA | Common iliac artery |
| **Cav** | **Corpus cavernosum penis** |
| **Cs** | **Corpus spongiosum penis** |
| CV | Common iliac vein |
| DC | Descending colon |
| EA | External iliac artery |
| EV | External iliac vein |
| FA | Femoral artery |
| FV | Femoral vein |
| HdF | Head of femur |
| IL | Iliacus |
| In | Small intestine |
| **IR** | **Inferior rectal nerve and vessels** |
| **LA** | **Levator ani** |
| LS | Lumbosacral trunk |
| OE | Obturator externus |
| **OI** | **Obturator internus** |
| **P** | **Prostate** |
| Pec | Pectineus |
| PS | Psoas |
| Pu | Pubic bone |
| **PV** | **Pelvic vessels and nerves** |
| **R** | **Rectum** |
| **Sac** | **Sacrum** |
| SC | Sigmoid colon |
| **SG** | **Seminal vesicle** |
| **Sy** | **Pubic symphysis** |
| **U** | **Urethra** |
| **UB** | **Urinary bladder** |

## 3.68 Coronal MRIs of the male pelvis and perineum, anterior views

**MALE**

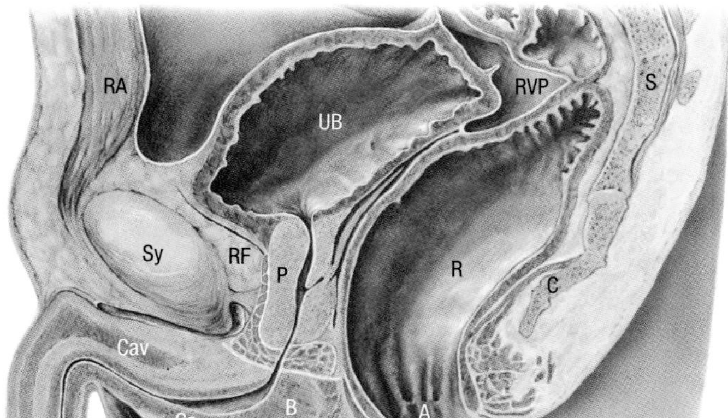
RA
UB
RVP
S
Sy
RF
P
R
C
Cav
Cs
B
A

Median Section

**FEMALE**

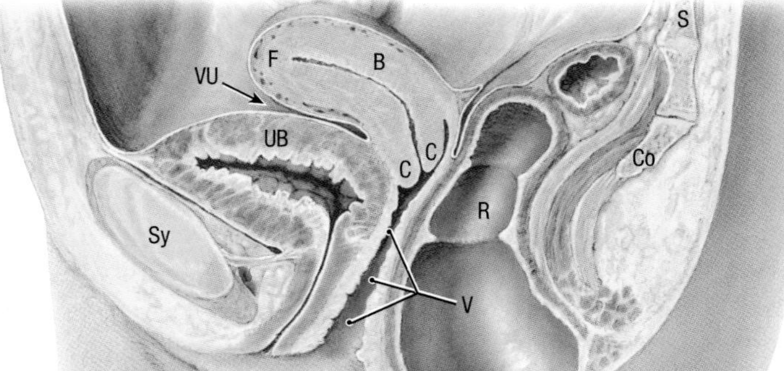
S
F
B
VU
UB
C
C
Co
R
Sy
V

Median Section

| | |
|---|---|
| A | Anus |
| B | Bulb of penis |
| Co | Coccyx |
| Cav | Corpus cavernosum penis |
| Cs | Corpus spongiosum penis |
| P | Prostate |
| PP | Prostatic venous plexus |
| R | Rectum |
| RA | Rectus abdominis |
| RF | Retropubic fat |
| RVP | Rectovesical pouch |
| S | Sacrum |
| SG | Seminal gland |
| SN | Sacral nerves |
| Sy | Pubic symphysis |
| UB | Urinary bladder |

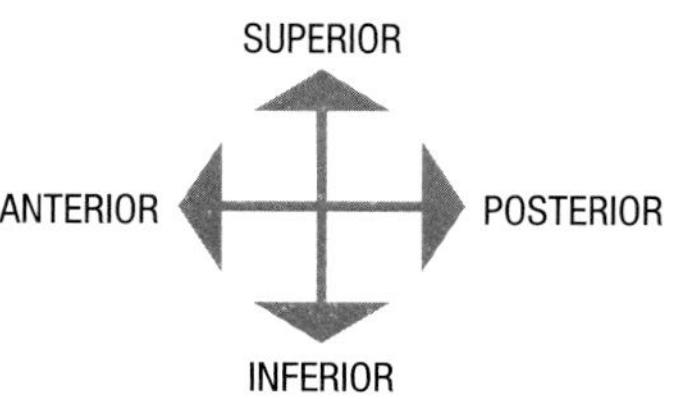
SUPERIOR
ANTERIOR
POSTERIOR
INFERIOR

| | |
|---|---|
| B | Body of uterus |
| C | Cervix of uterus |
| Co | Coccyx |
| E | Endometrium |
| EF | Endopelvic fascia |
| F | Fundus of uterus |
| M | Myometrium |
| R | Rectum |
| RA | Rectus abdominis |
| S | Sacrum |
| Sy | Pubis symphysis |
| UB | Urinary bladder |
| V | Vagina |
| VU | Vesicouterine pouch |

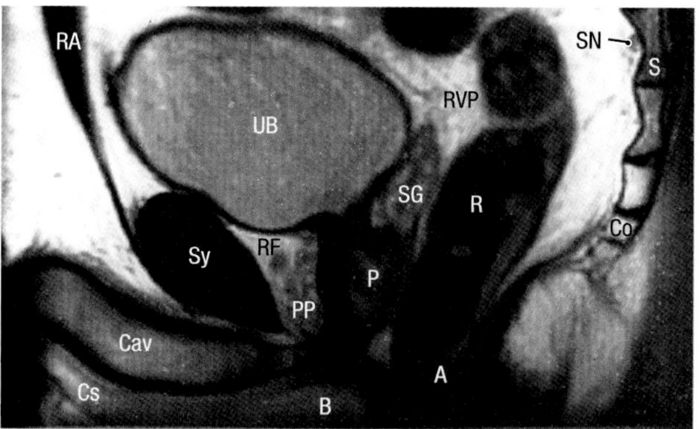
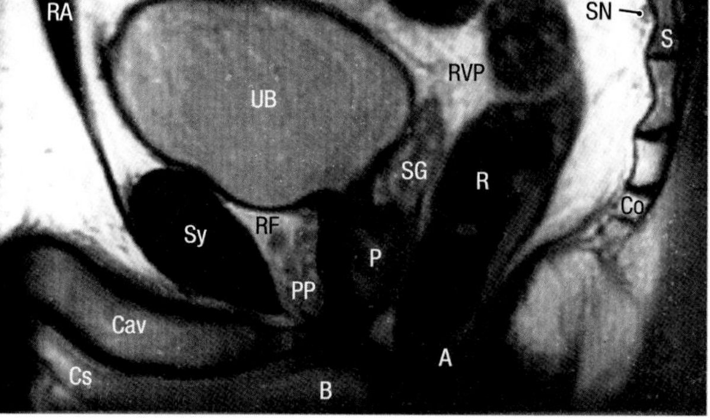
RA
SN
S
UB
RVP
SG
R
Co
Sy
RF
P
PP
Cav
Cs
B
A

Median MRI Scan

Median MRI Scan

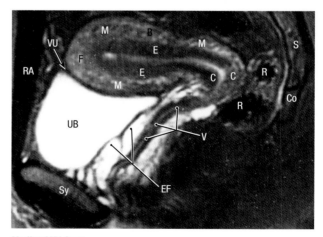

**3.69 Median MRIs of the male and female pelvis and perineum**

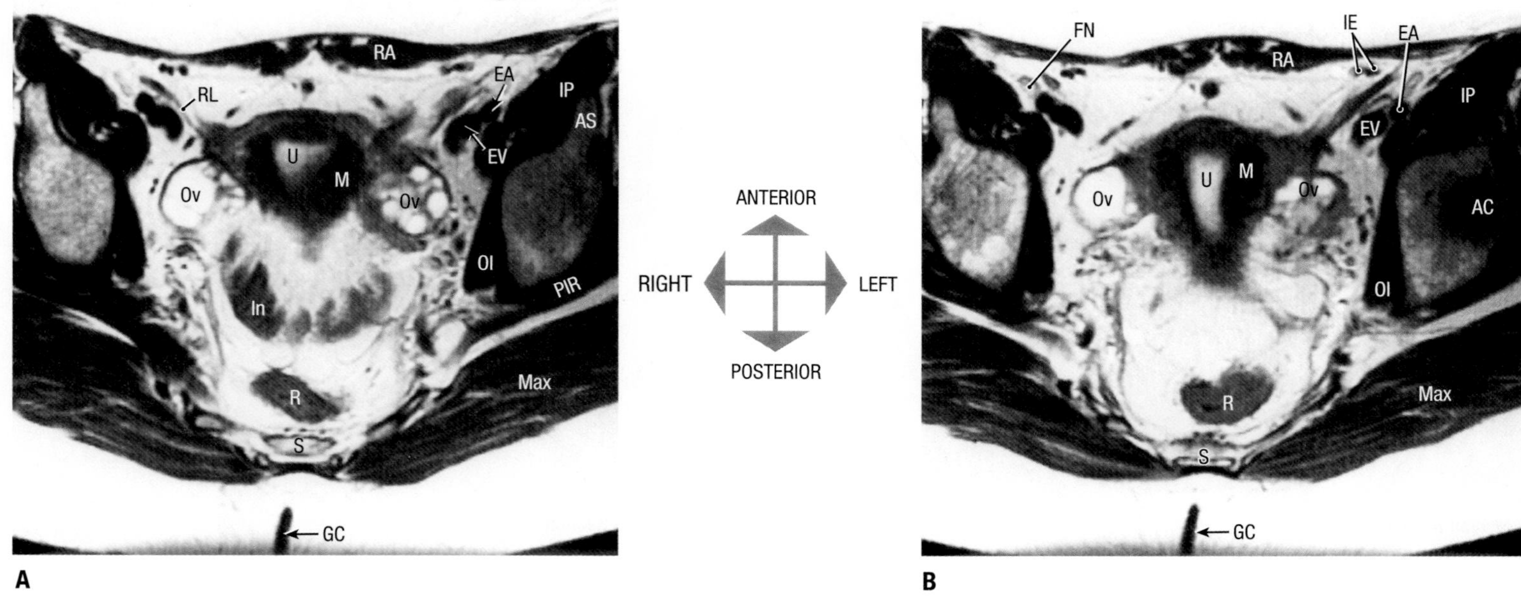
RA
RL
EA
IP
AS
U
M
EV
Ov
Ov
OI
PIR
In
Max
R
S
GC
A
ANTERIOR
RIGHT
LEFT
POSTERIOR
FN
IE
EA
RA
IP
EV
U
M
Ov
Ov
AC
OI
Max
R
S
GC
B

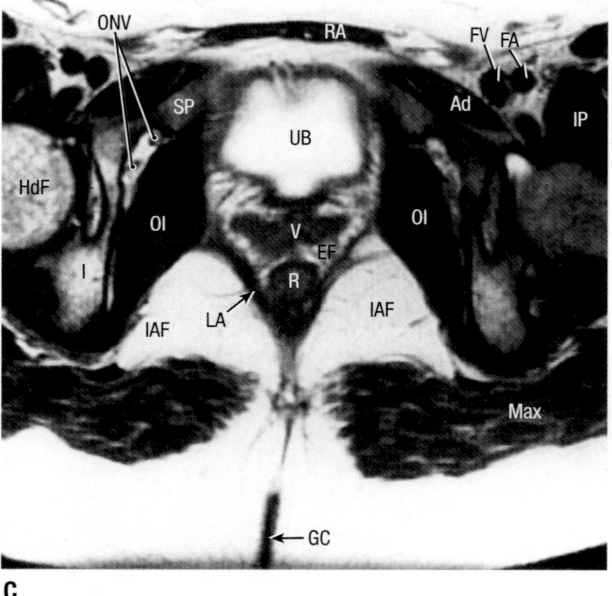
ONV
RA
FV
FA
SP
Ad
IP
UB
HdF
OI
OI
V
EF
I
R
LA
IAF
IAF
Max
GC
C

| | | | |
|---|---|---|---|
| **A** | **Anus** | **M** | **Myometrium** |
| AC | Acetabulum | Max | Gluteus maximus |
| Ad | Adductor muscles | OE | Obturator externus |
| AS | Anterior superior iliac spine | **OI** | **Obturator internus** |
| BC | Body of clitoris | **Ov** | **Ovary** |
| CC | Crus of clitoris | OV | Obturator vessels |
| EA | External iliac artery | Pd | Pudendal nerve and vessels |
| EF | Endopelvic fascia | Pec | Pectineus |
| EV | External iliac vein | PIR | Piriformis |
| FA | Femoral artery | **Pm** | **Perineal membrane** |
| FN | Femoral nerve | **Pu** | **Pubic bone** |
| FV | Femoral vein | QF | Quadratus femoris |
| GC | Gluteal cleft | **R** | **Rectum** |
| HdF | Head of femur | RA | Rectus abdominis |
| I | Ilium | **RF** | **Recto-uterine fold** |
| **IAF** | **Ischioanal fossa** | **RL** | **Round ligament** |
| IE | Inferior epigastric vessels | **S** | **Sacrum** |
| In | Intestine | SP | Superior ramus of pubis |
| IP | Iliopsoas | Sy | Pubic symphysis |
| IPR | Ischiopubic ramus | **U** | **Uterus** |
| IT | Ischial tuberosity | **UB** | **Urinary bladder** |
| **LA** | **Levator ani** | **Ur** | **Urethra** |
| Lin | Linea alba | **V** | **Vagina** |
| **LM** | **Labia majus** | **Ve** | **Vestibule** |

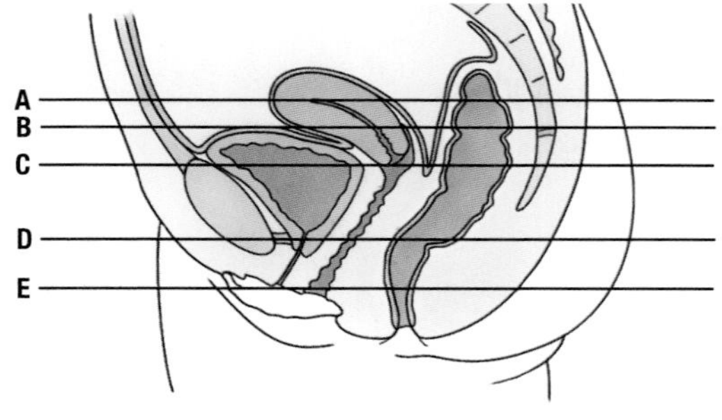
A
B
C
D
E

**3.70 Transverse (axial) MRIs and sectional specimens of the female pelvis and perineum, inferior views**

**A–C.** MRIs.

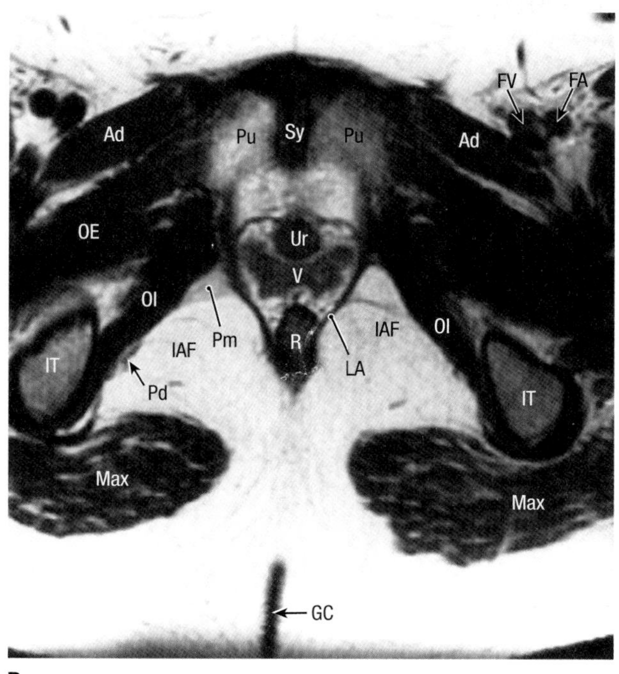
FV
FA
Ad
Pu
Sy
Pu
Ad
OE
Ur
V
OI
Pm
IAF
R
IAF
OI
IT
Pd
LA
IT
Max
Max
GC
D

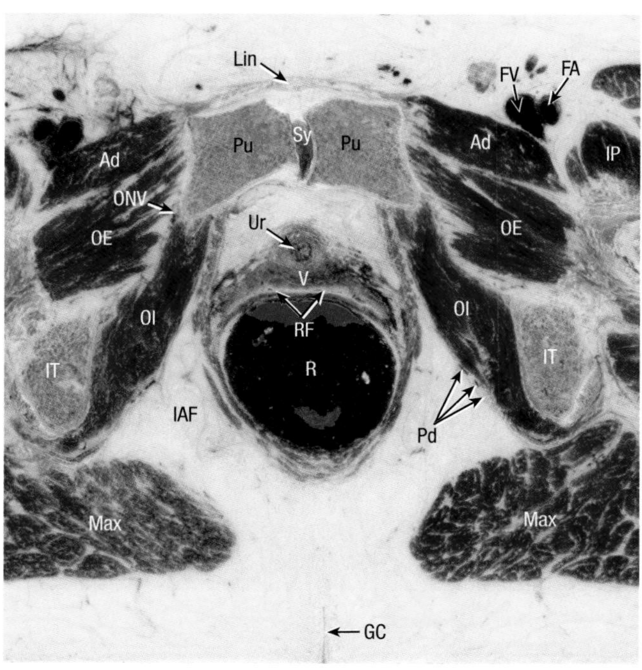
Lin
FV
FA
Ad
Pu
Sy
Pu
Ad
IP
ONV
OE
Ur
OE
V
OI
RF
OI
IT
R
IT
IAF
Pd
Max
Max
GC
E

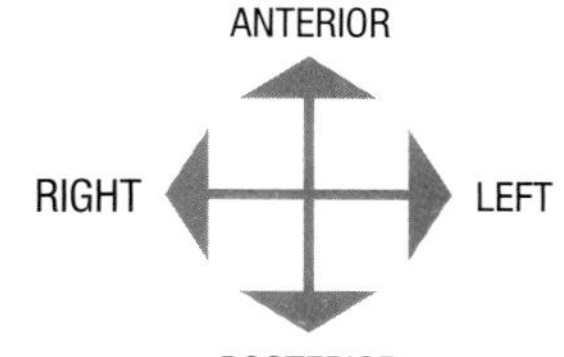
ANTERIOR
RIGHT
LEFT
POSTERIOR

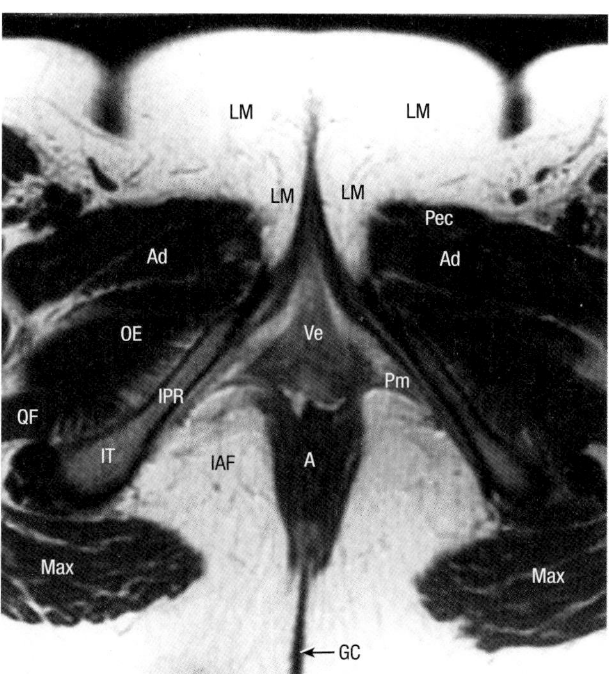
LM
LM
LM
LM
Pec
Ad
Ad
OE
Ve
Pm
IPR
QF
IT
IAF
A
Max
Max
GC
F

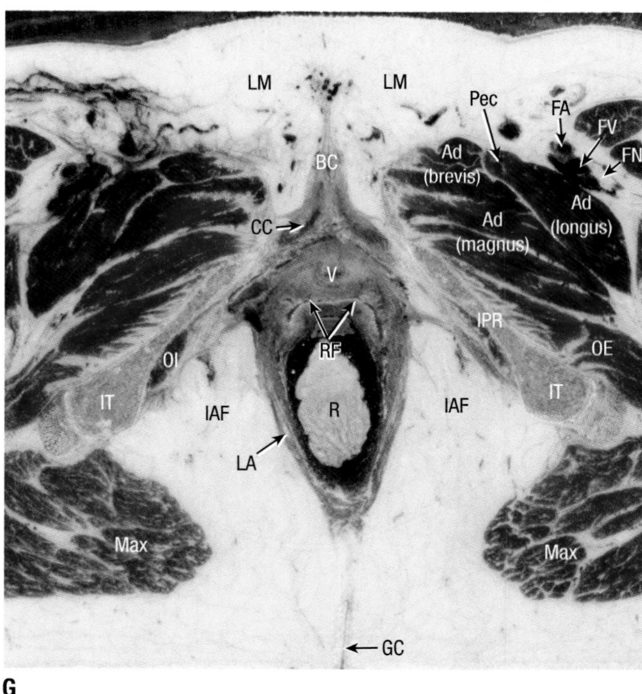
LM
LM
Pec
FA
FV
FN
BC
Ad
(brevis)
Ad
(magnus)
Ad
(longus)
CC
V
RF
IPR
OE
OI
IT
IAF
R
IAF
IT
LA
Max
Max
GC
G

**3.70** **Transverse (axial) MRIs and sectional specimens of the female pelvis and perineum, inferior views *(continued)***

**D and F.** MRIs. **E and G.** Anatomical sections.

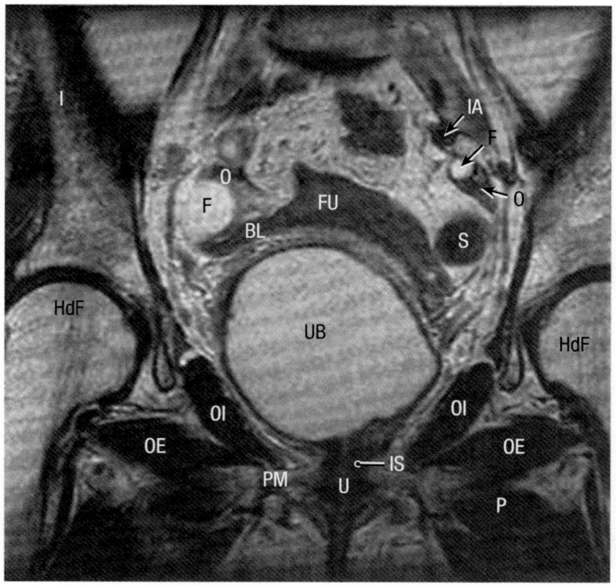

A

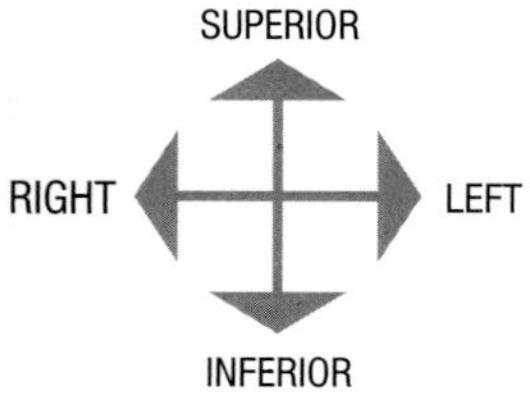

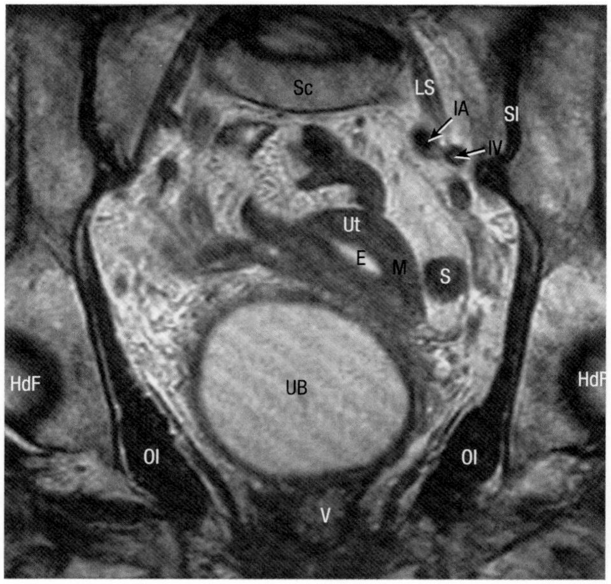

B

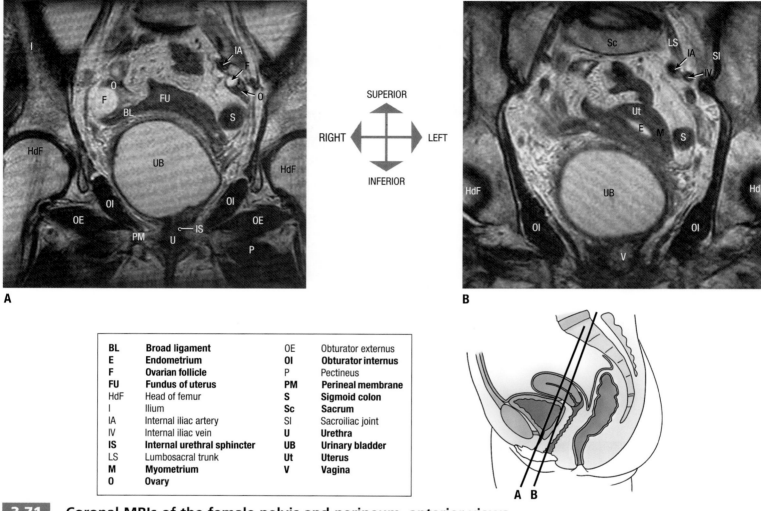

| | | | |
|---|---|---|---|
| **BL** | **Broad ligament** | OE | Obturator externus |
| **E** | **Endometrium** | **OI** | **Obturator internus** |
| **F** | **Ovarian follicle** | P | Pectineus |
| **FU** | **Fundus of uterus** | **PM** | **Perineal membrane** |
| HdF | Head of femur | **S** | **Sigmoid colon** |
| I | Ilium | **Sc** | **Sacrum** |
| IA | Internal iliac artery | SI | Sacroiliac joint |
| IV | Internal iliac vein | **U** | **Urethra** |
| **IS** | **Internal urethral sphincter** | **UB** | **Urinary bladder** |
| LS | Lumbosacral trunk | **Ut** | **Uterus** |
| **M** | **Myometrium** | **V** | **Vagina** |
| **O** | **Ovary** | | |

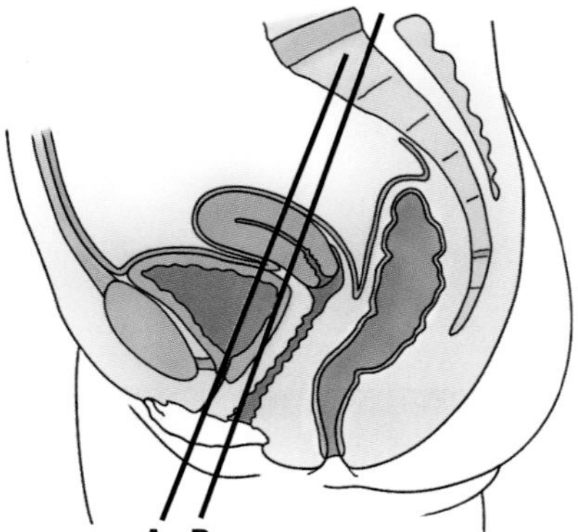

**3.71 Coronal MRIs of the female pelvis and perineum, anterior views**

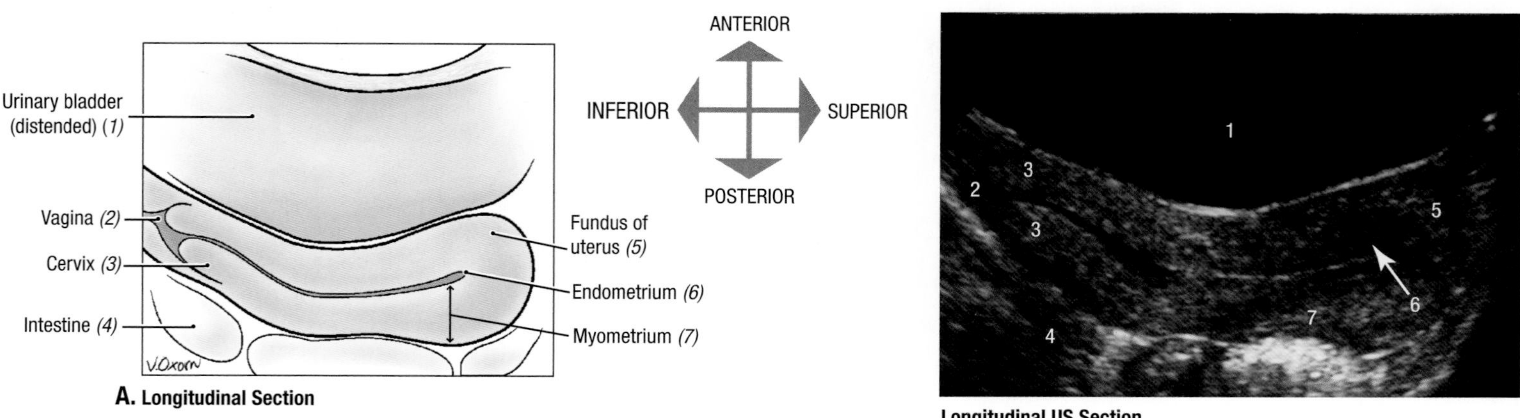
Urinary bladder (distended) (1)
Vagina (2)
Cervix (3)
Intestine (4)
Fundus of uterus (5)
Endometrium (6)
Myometrium (7)
V.Oxorn
ANTERIOR
INFERIOR
SUPERIOR
POSTERIOR
1
2
3
3
4
5
6
7

**A.** Longitudinal Section

Longitudinal US Section

**3.72 Ultrasound scans of female pelvis**

**A.** Median (transabdominal) ultrasound scan and orientation drawing (numbers in parentheses correspond to labels on the ultrasound scan).

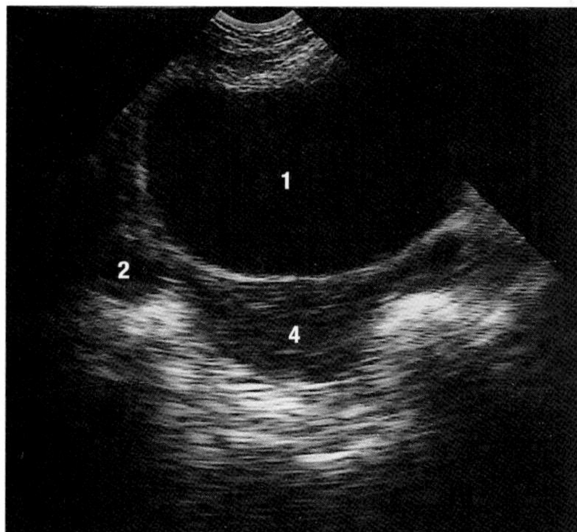
1
2
4

B. Transverse (Axial) Scan

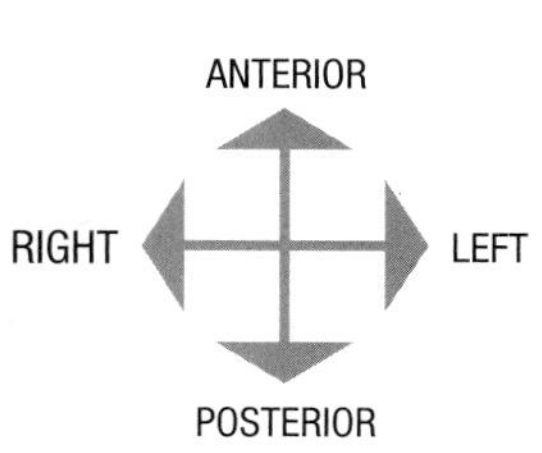
ANTERIOR
RIGHT
LEFT
POSTERIOR

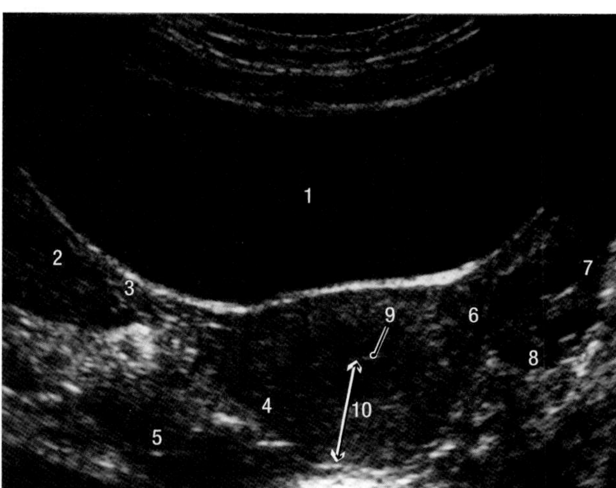
1
2
3
4
5
6
7
8
9
10

C. Transverse (Axial) Scan

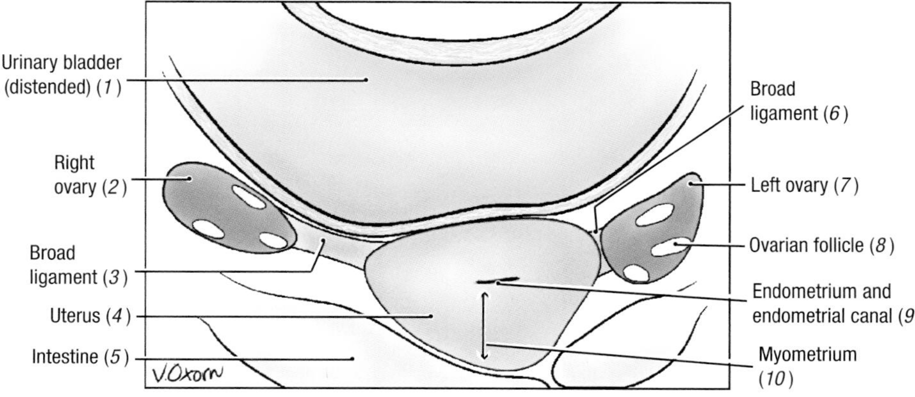
Urinary bladder (distended) (1)
Right ovary (2)
Broad ligament (3)
Uterus (4)
Intestine (5)
Broad ligament (6)
Left ovary (7)
Ovarian follicle (8)
Endometrium and endometrial canal (9)
Myometrium (10)

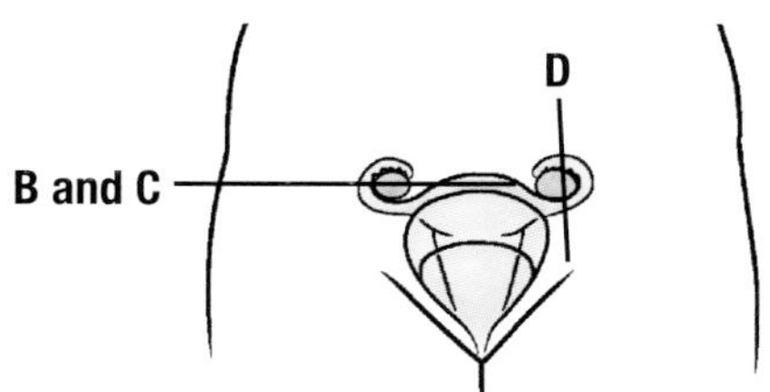
D
B and C

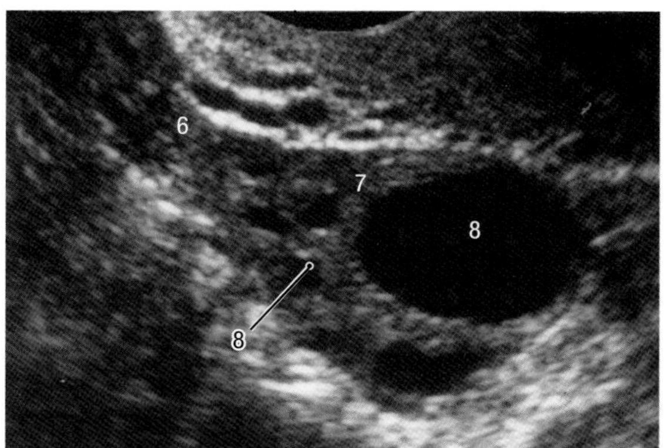
6
7
8
8

D. Sagittal Scan

## 3.72 Ultrasound scans of female pelvis *(continued)*

**B** and **C.** Transabdominal axial (transverse) scan through uterus and ovaries. Transabdominal US scanning requires a fully distended urinary bladder to displace the bowel loops from the pelvis and to provide an acoustical window through which to observe pelvic anatomy.

**D.** Transvaginal sagittal scan of left ovary (numbers in parentheses correspond to labels on the ultrasound scans). Transvaginal and transrectal ultrasonography enables the placing of the probe closer to the structures of interest, allowing increased resolution.

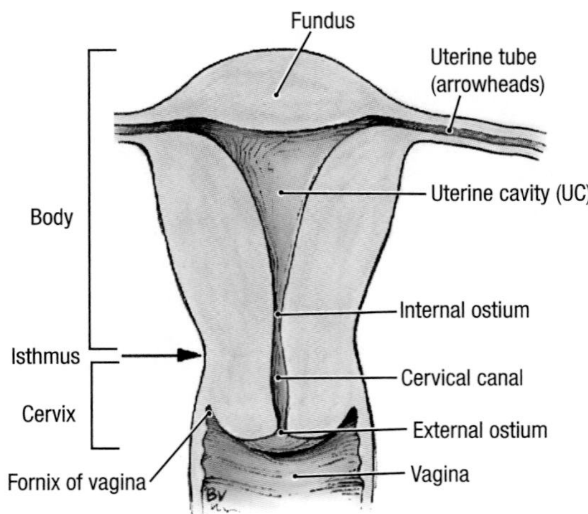
Fundus
Uterine tube
(arrowheads)
Uterine cavity (UC)
Body
Internal ostium
Isthmus
Cervical canal
Cervix
External ostium
Fornix of vagina
Vagina

**A.** Coronal Section

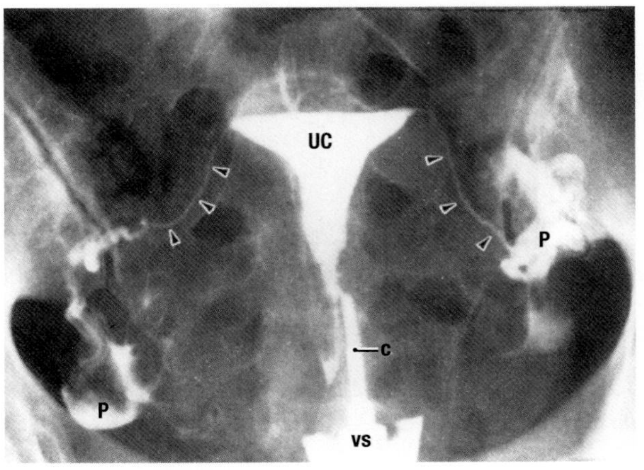
UC
P
c
P
VS

**B.** Hysterosalpingogram of Normal Uterus, Anteroposterior View

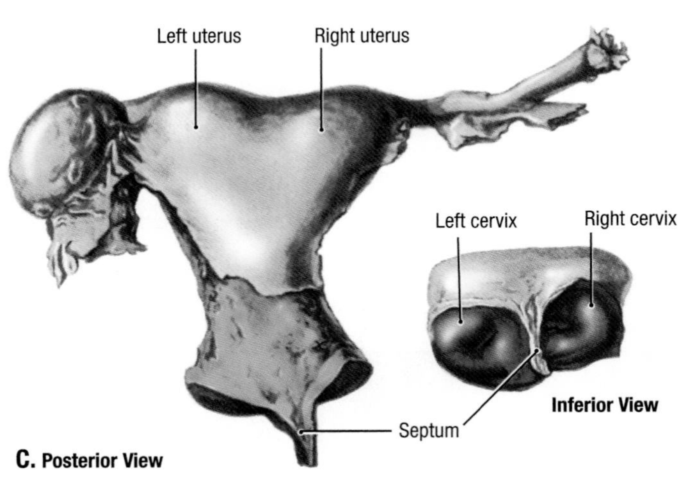
Left uterus
Right uterus
Left cervix
Right cervix
Inferior View
Septum

**C.** Posterior View

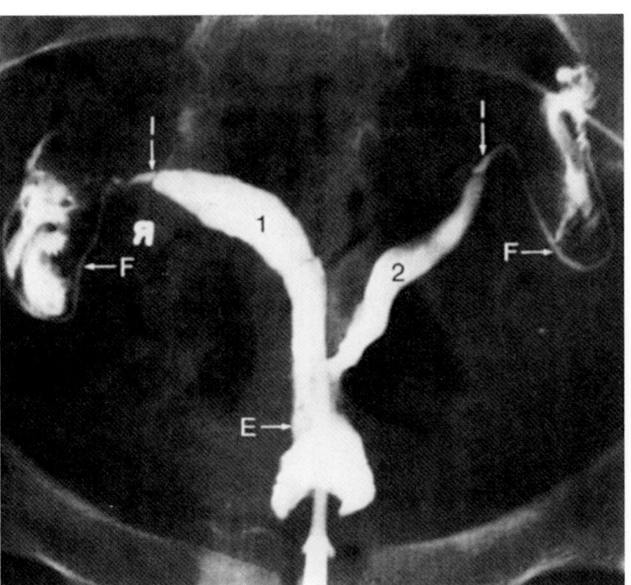
1
F
2
F
E

**D.** Hysterosalpingogram of Bicornate Uterus, Anteroposterior View

## 3.73 Radiograph of uterus and uterine tubes (hysterosalpingogram)

**A.** Coronal section of uterus. **B.** Radiopaque material was injected into the uterus through external os of the uterus. The contrast medium traveled through the triangular uterine cavity (UC) and uterine tubes (arrowheads) and passed into the pararectal fossae (P) of the peritoneal cavity. c, catheter in the cervical canal; vs, vaginal speculum. The female genital tract is in direct communication with the peritoneal cavity and is, therefore, a potential pathway for the spread of an infection from the vagina and uterus. **C.** Illustration of duplicated uterus. **D.** Hysterosalpingogram of a bicornate ("two horned") uterus. 1 and 2, uterine cavities; E, cervical canal; F, uterine tubes; I, isthmus of tubes.

CHAPTER 4

# BACK

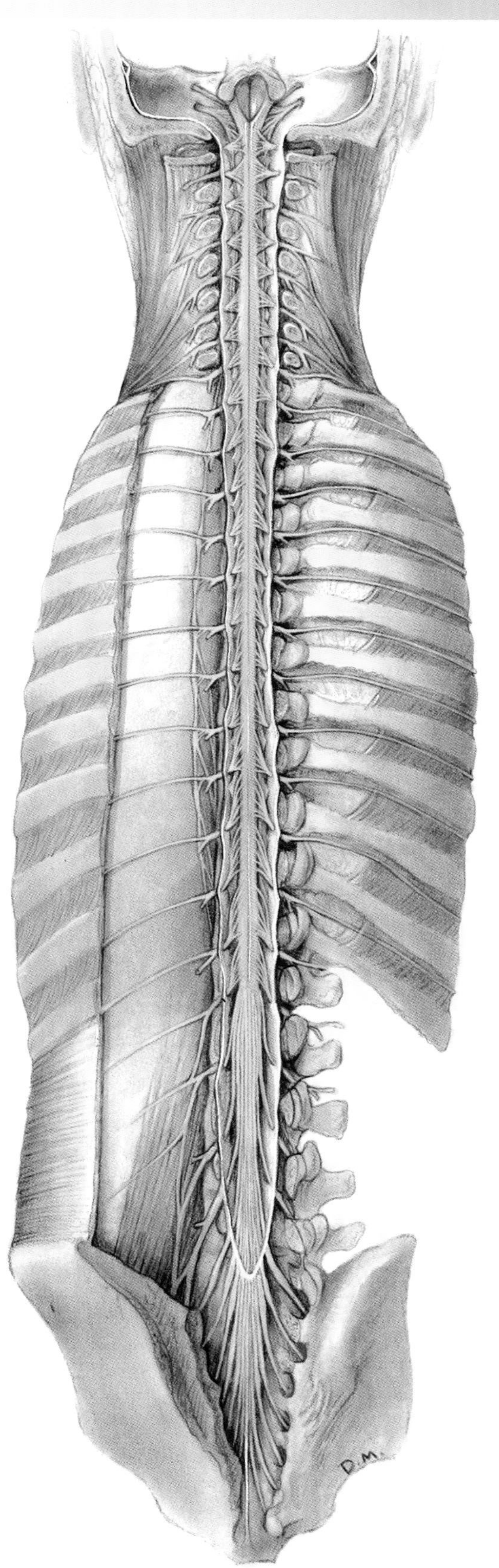
D.M.

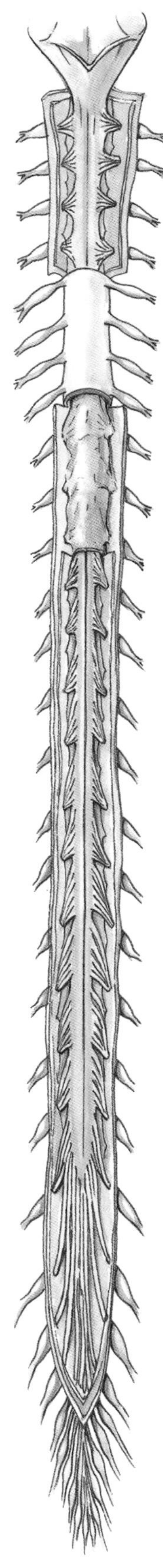


- Overview of Vertebral Column **286**
- Cervical Spine **294**
- Craniovertebral Joints **298**
- Thoracic Spine **300**
- Lumbar Spine **302**
- Ligaments and Intervertebral Discs **304**
- Vertebral Venous Plexuses **309**
- Bones, Joints, and Ligaments of Pelvic Girdle **310**
- Anomalies of Vertebrae **318**
- Muscles of Back **320**
- Suboccipital Region **330**
- Spinal Cord and Meninges **334**
- Components of Spinal Nerves **343**
- Dermatomes and Myotomes **348**
- Imaging of Vertebral Column **350**

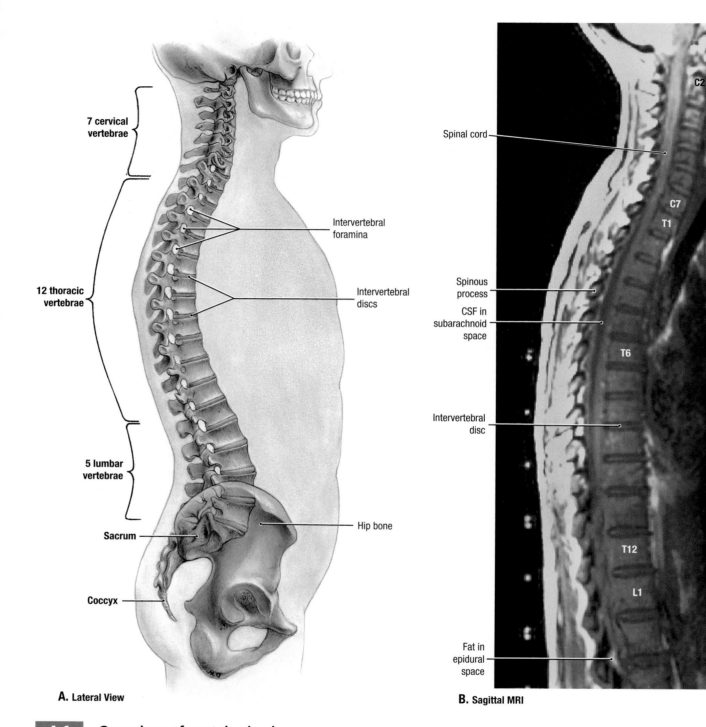

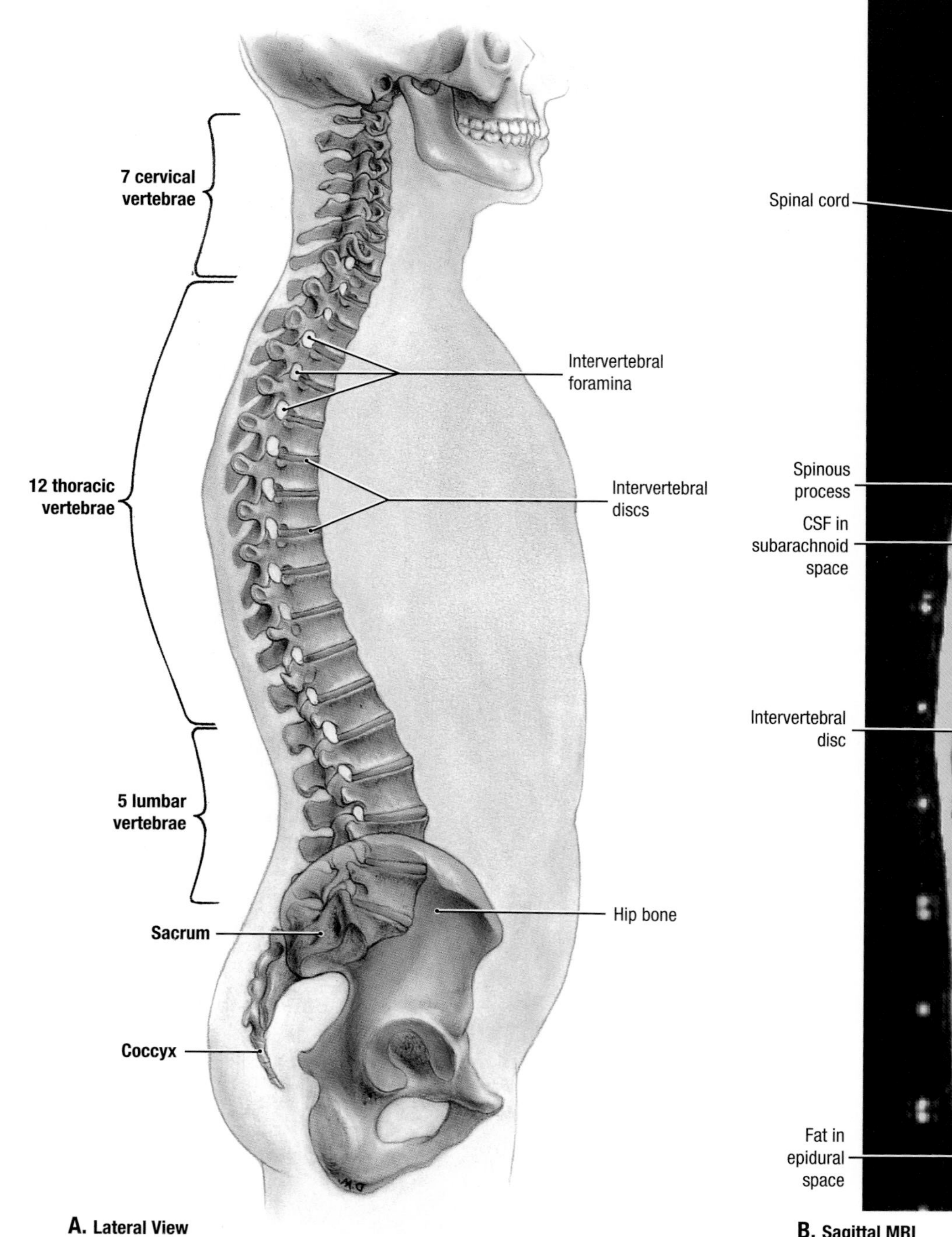
7 cervical vertebrae
12 thoracic vertebrae
5 lumbar vertebrae
Sacrum
Coccyx
Intervertebral foramina
Intervertebral discs
Hip bone
A. Lateral View
C2
Spinal cord
C7
T1
Spinous process
CSF in subarachnoid space
T6
Intervertebral disc
T12
L1
Fat in epidural space
B. Sagittal MRI

## 4.1 Overview of vertebral column

**A.** Vertebral column showing articulation with skull and hip bone.
**B.** Sagittal MRI, lateral view.

- The vertebral column usually consists of 24 separate (presacral) vertebrae, 5 fused vertebrae in the sacrum, and variably 4 fused or separate coccygeal vertebrae. Of the 24 separate vertebrae, 12 support ribs (thoracic), 7 are in the neck (cervical), and 5 are in the lumbar region (lumbar).
- Vertebrae contributing to the posterior walls of the thoracic and pelvic cavities are concave anteriorly; elsewhere (in the cervical and lumbar regions) they are convex anteriorly.
- The spinal nerves exit the vertebral (spinal) canal via the intervertebral foramina. There are 8 cervical, 12 thoracic, 5 lumbar, 5 sacral, and 1 to 2 coccygeal spinal nerves.
- Note the size and shape of the vertebral bodies, the direction of the spinous processes, and the spinal cord in the vertebral canal (in **B**).

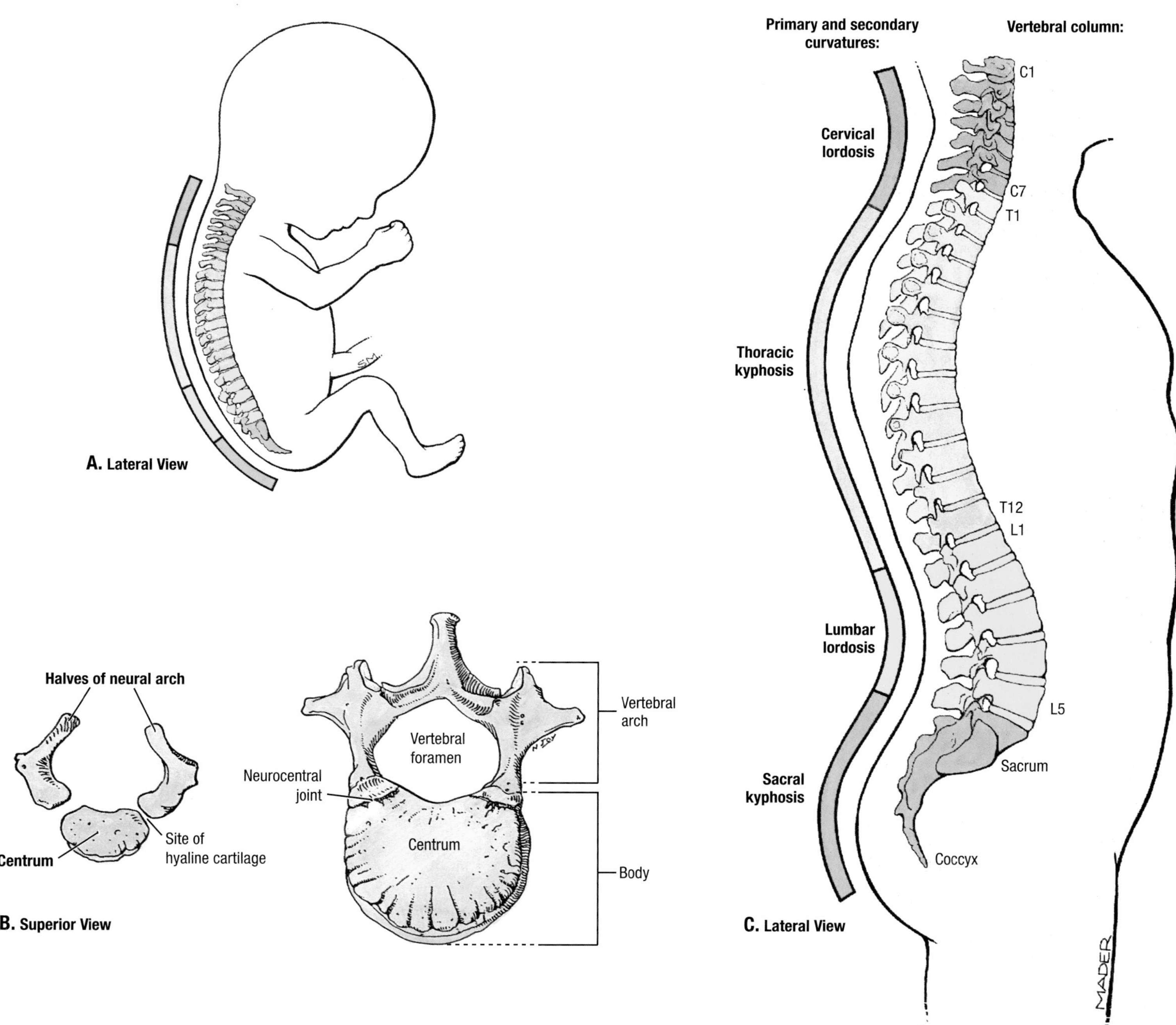
A. Lateral View
Halves of neural arch
Centrum
Site of
hyaline cartilage
Neurocentral
joint
Vertebral
foramen
Centrum
Vertebral
arch
Body
B. Superior View
Primary and secondary
curvatures:
Vertebral column:
Cervical
lordosis
Thoracic
kyphosis
Lumbar
lordosis
Sacral
kyphosis
C1
C7
T1
T12
L1
L5
Sacrum
Coccyx
C. Lateral View
MADER

## 4.2 Curvatures of vertebral column

**A.** Fetus. Note the C-shaped curvature of the fetal spine, which is concave anteriorly over its entire length. **B.** Development of the vertebrae. At birth, a vertebra consists of three bony parts (two halves of the neural arch and the centrum) united by hyaline cartilage. At age 2, the halves of each neural arch begin to fuse, proceeding from the lumbar to the cervical region; at approximately age 7, the arches begin to fuse to the centrum, proceeding from the cervical to lumbar regions. **C.** Adult. The four curvatures of the adult vertebral column include the cervical lordosis, which is convex anteriorly and lies between vertebrae C1 and T2; the thoracic kyphosis, which is concave anteriorly, between vertebrae T2 and T12; the lumbar lordosis, convex anteriorly and lying between T12 and the lumbosacral joint; and the sacral kyphosis, concave anteriorly and spanning from the lumbosacral joint to the tip of the coccyx. The anteriorly concave thoracic kyphosis and sacrococcygeal kyphosis are primary curves, and the anteriorly convex cervical lordosis and lumbar lordosis are secondary curves that develop after birth. The cervical lordosis develops when the child begins to hold the head up, and the lumbar kyphosis develops when the child begins to walk.

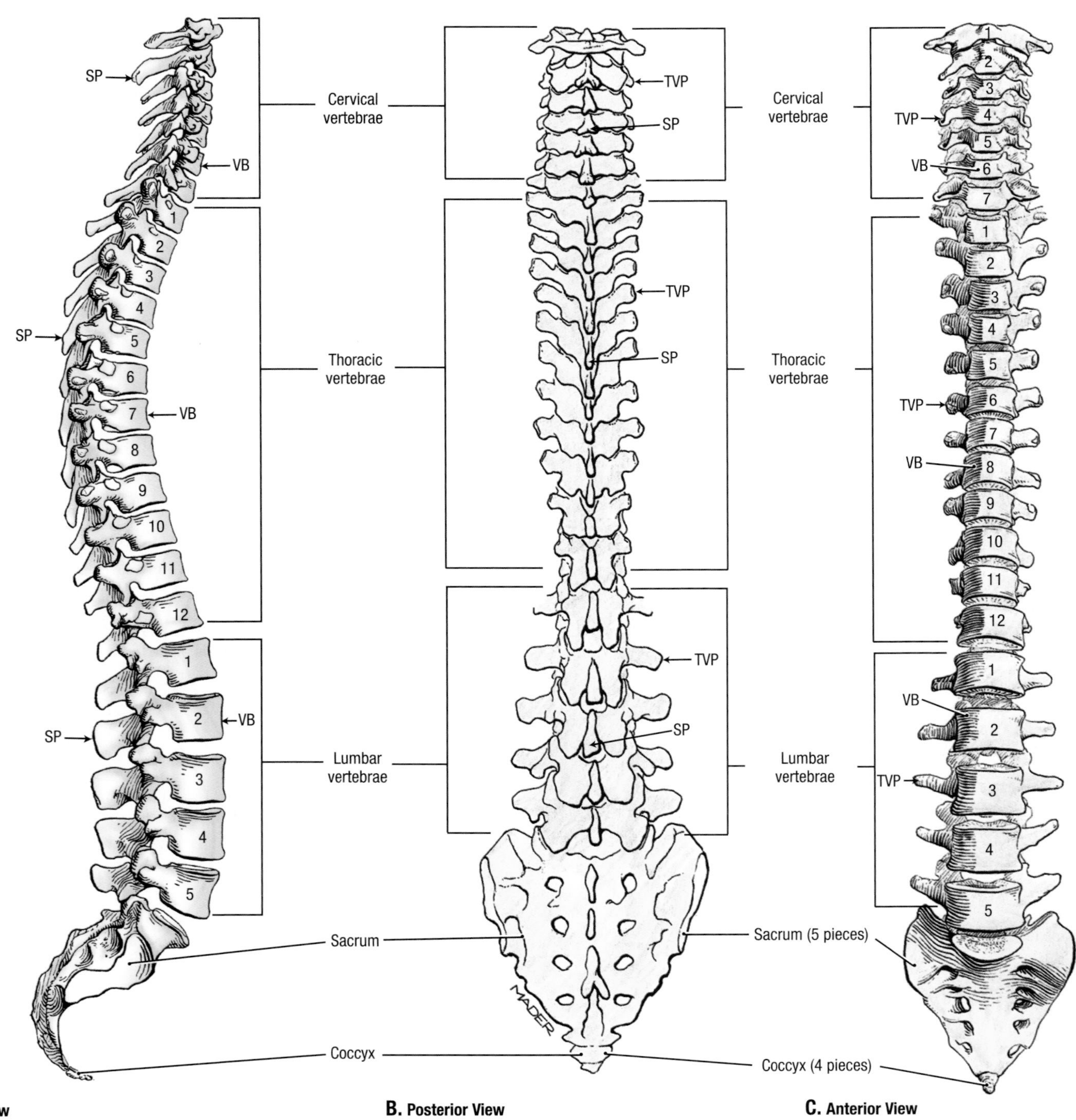
SP
VB
SP
VB
SP
VB
Cervical vertebrae
Thoracic vertebrae
Lumbar vertebrae
Sacrum
Coccyx
TVP
SP
TVP
SP
TVP
SP
MADER
Cervical vertebrae
Thoracic vertebrae
Lumbar vertebrae
Sacrum (5 pieces)
Coccyx (4 pieces)
TVP
VB
TVP
VB
VB
TVP

**A.** Lateral View **B.** Posterior View **C.** Anterior View

## 4.3 Three views of the vertebral column

- The vertebral bodies (VB) vary in size and shape.
- Transverse processes (TVP) in the cervical region are directed laterally, inferiorly and anteriorly. In the thoracic region, they are directed laterally posteriorly, and superiorly, have a facet for the tubercle of the rib, and are stout. In the lumbar region, the TVPs point laterally and are long and slender.
- Generally, spinous processes (SP) are bifid in caucasians in the cervical region, long and spinelike in the thoracic region, and stout and oblong in the lumbar region. The cervical and thoracic SPs often overlap the adjacent, inferior vertebrae.

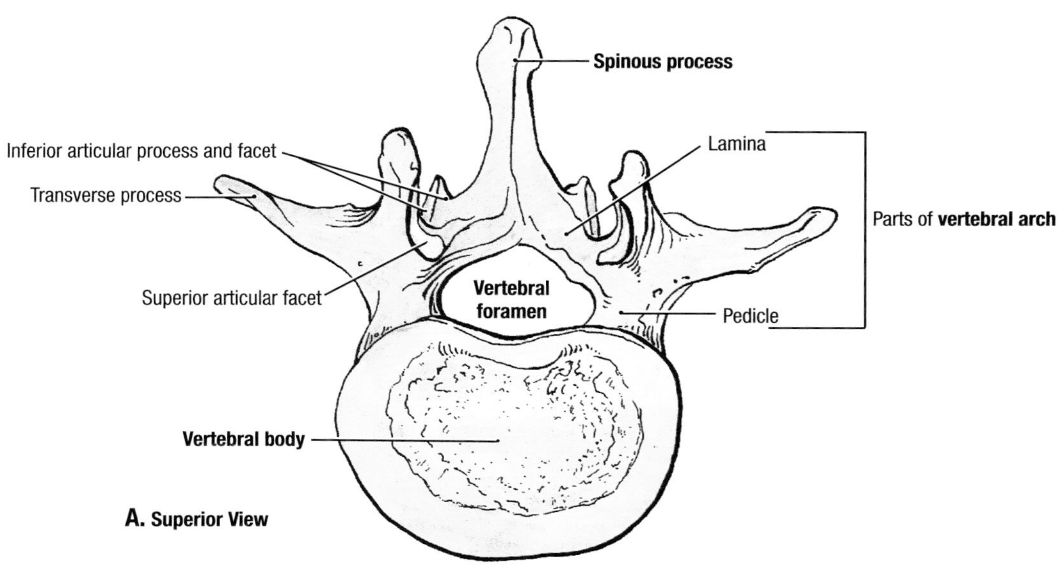
Spinous process
Inferior articular process and facet
Lamina
Transverse process
Parts of vertebral arch
Superior articular facet
Vertebral foramen
Pedicle
Vertebral body
A. Superior View

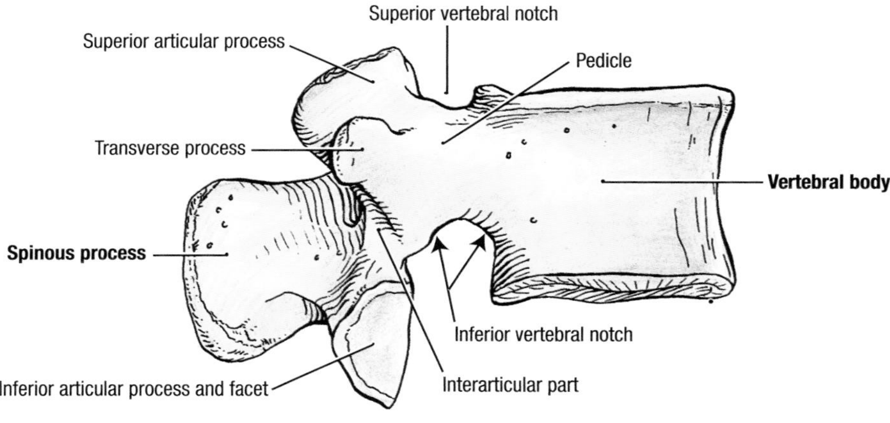
Superior vertebral notch
Superior articular process
Pedicle
Transverse process
Vertebral body
Spinous process
Inferior vertebral notch
Inferior articular process and facet
Interarticular part
B. Lateral View

## 4.4 Typical vertebra

A typical vertebra (e.g., the 2nd lumbar vertebra) consists of the following parts:

- A vertebral body, situated anteriorly, functions to support weight.
- A vertebral arch, posterior to the body, with the body, encloses the vertebral foramen. Collectively, the vertebral foramina constitute the vertebral canal, in which the spinal cord lies. The function of a vertebral arch is to protect the spinal cord. The vertebral arch consists of two rounded pedicles, one on each side, which arise from the body, and two flat plates called laminae that unite posteriorly in the midline.
- Three processes, two transverse and one spinous, provide attachment for muscles and are the levers that help move the vertebrae.
- Four articular processes, two superior and two inferior, each have an articular facet. The articular processes project superiorly and inferiorly from the vertebral arch and come into apposition with the articular facet of the corresponding processes of the vertebrae above and below. The direction of the articular facets determines the nature of the movement between adjacent vertebrae and prevents the vertebrae from slipping anteriorly.

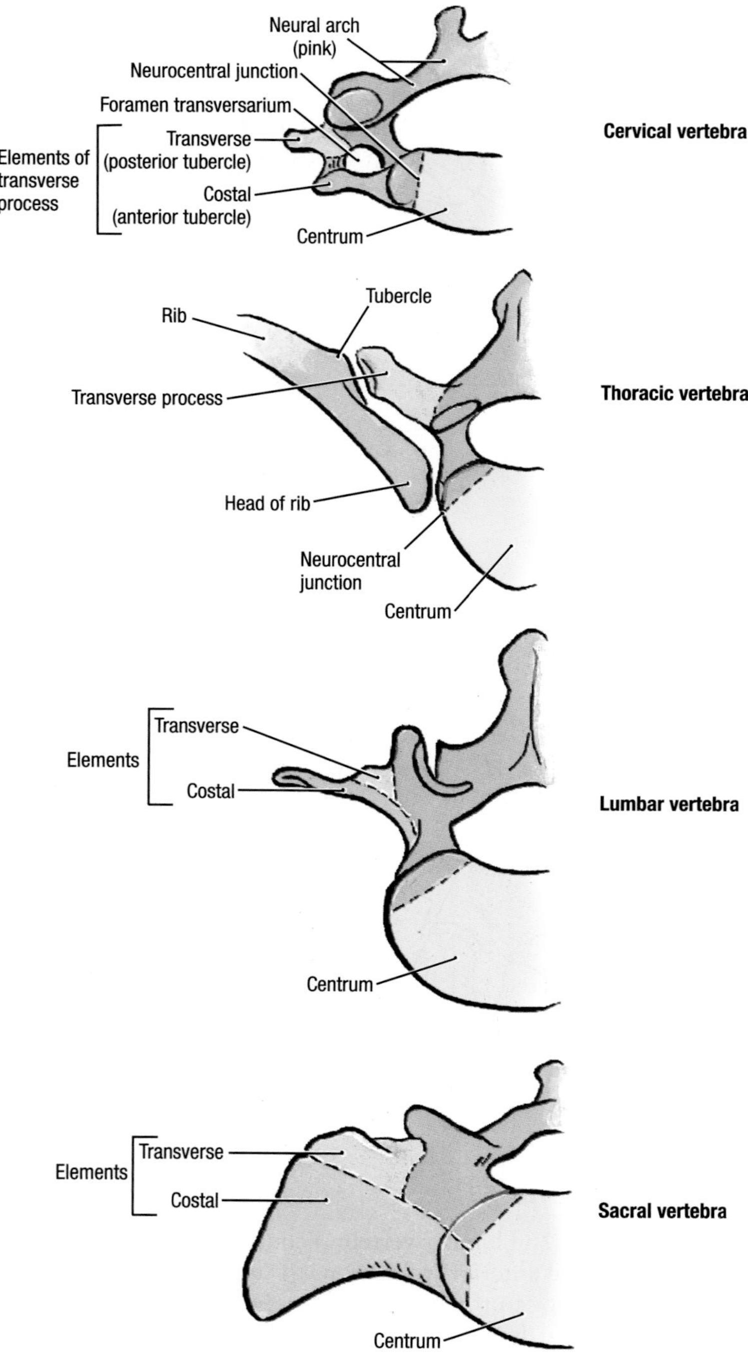
Neural arch
(pink)
Neurocentral junction
Foramen transversarium
Elements of transverse process
Transverse
(posterior tubercle)
Costal
(anterior tubercle)
Centrum
Cervical vertebra
Tubercle
Rib
Transverse process
Head of rib
Neurocentral junction
Centrum
Thoracic vertebra
Elements
Transverse
Costal
Centrum
Lumbar vertebra
Elements
Transverse
Costal
Centrum
Sacral vertebra
Superior Views

## 4.5 Homologous parts of vertebrae

A rib is a free costal element in the thoracic region; in the cervical and lumbar regions, it is represented by the anterior part of a transverse process, and in the sacrum, by the anterior part of the lateral mass. The heads of the ribs (thoracic region) articulate with the sides of the vertebral bodies posterior to the neurocentral junctions.

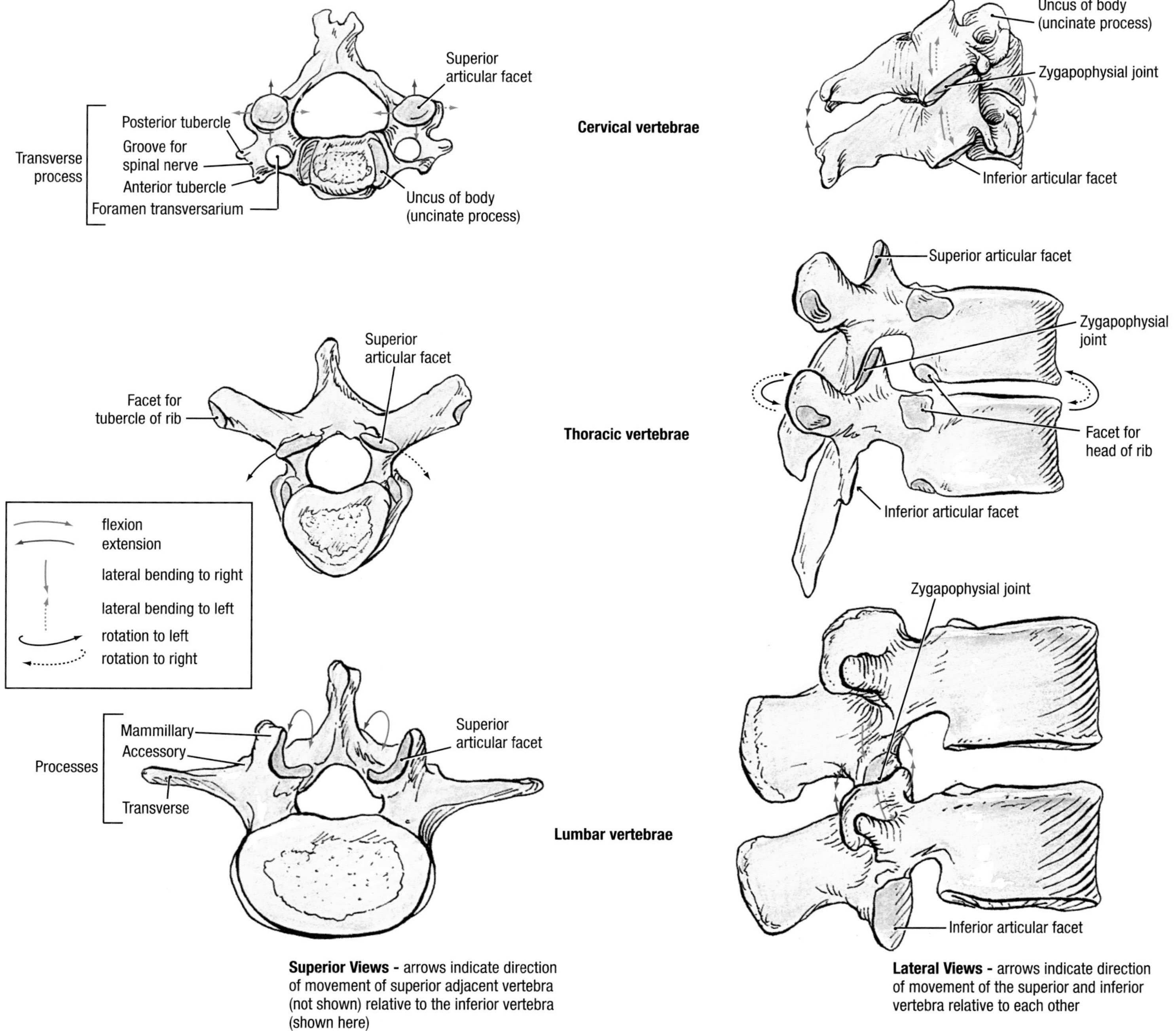
Superior
articular facet
Posterior tubercle
Transverse process
Groove for
spinal nerve
Anterior tubercle
Foramen transversarium
Uncus of body
(uncinate process)
Cervical vertebrae
Uncus of body
(uncinate process)
Zygapophysial joint
Inferior articular facet
Superior
articular facet
Facet for
tubercle of rib
Thoracic vertebrae
Superior articular facet
Zygapophysial
joint
Facet for
head of rib
Inferior articular facet
flexion
extension
lateral bending to right
lateral bending to left
rotation to left
rotation to right
Processes
Mammillary
Accessory
Transverse
Superior
articular facet
Lumbar vertebrae
Zygapophysial joint
Inferior articular facet

**Superior Views -** arrows indicate direction of movement of superior adjacent vertebra (not shown) relative to the inferior vertebra (shown here)

**Lateral Views -** arrows indicate direction of movement of the superior and inferior vertebra relative to each other

## 4.6 Vertebral features and movements

Direction of movement is indicated by *arrows*.

- In the thoracic and lumbar regions, the superior articular facets lie posterior to the pedicles, and the inferior facets are anterior to the laminae. Superior articular facets in the cervical region face mainly superiorly, in the thoracic region, mainly posteriorly, and in the lumbar region, mainly medially. The change in direction is gradual from cervical to thoracic but abrupt from thoracic to lumbar.
- Although movements between adjacent vertebrae are relatively small, especially in the thoracic region, the summation of all the small movements produces a considerable range of movement of the vertebral column as a whole.
- Movements of the vertebral column are freer in the cervical and lumbar regions than in the thoracic region. Lateral bending is freest in the cervical and lumbar regions; flexion of the vertebral column is greatest in the cervical region; extension is most marked in the lumbar region, but the interlocking articular processes prevent rotation.
- The thoracic region is most stable because of the external support gained from the articulations of the ribs and costal cartilages with the sternum. The direction of the articular facets permits rotation, but flexion, extension, and lateral bending is severely restricted.

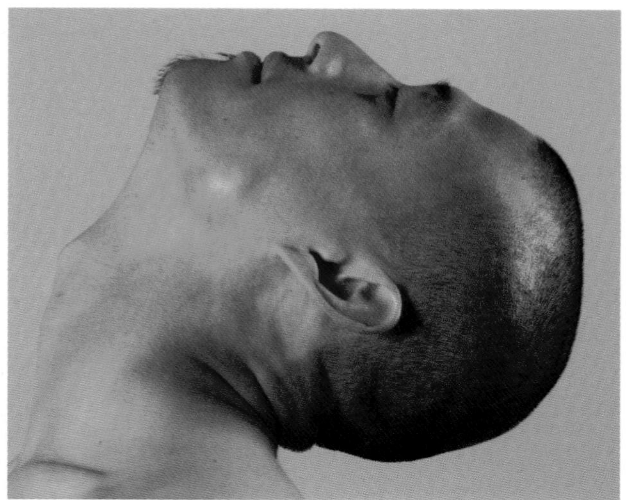
A. Lateral View

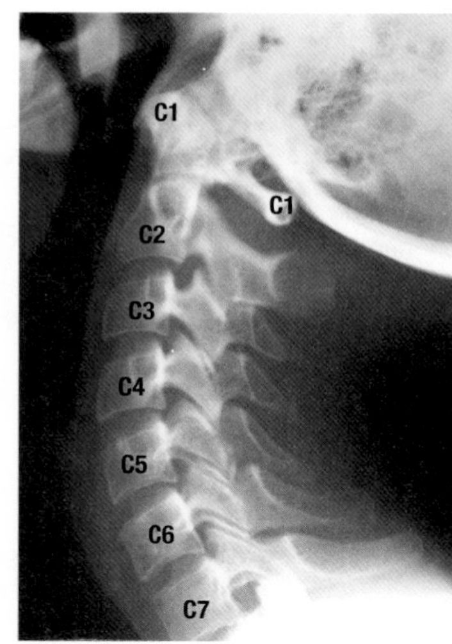
C1
C1
C2
C3
C4
C5
C6
C7
B. Lateral View

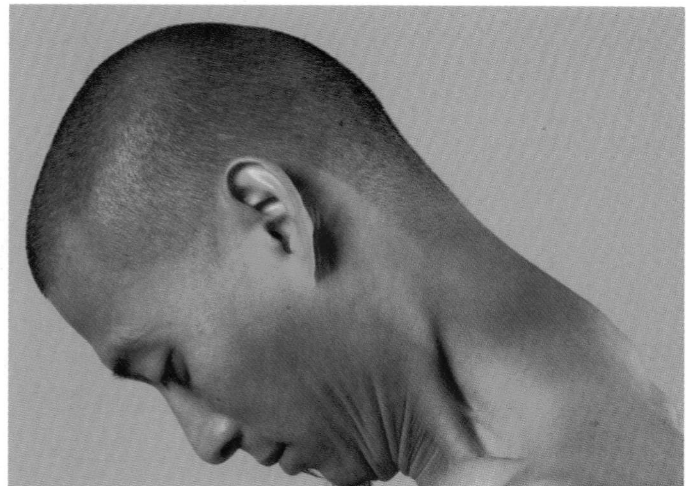
C. Lateral View

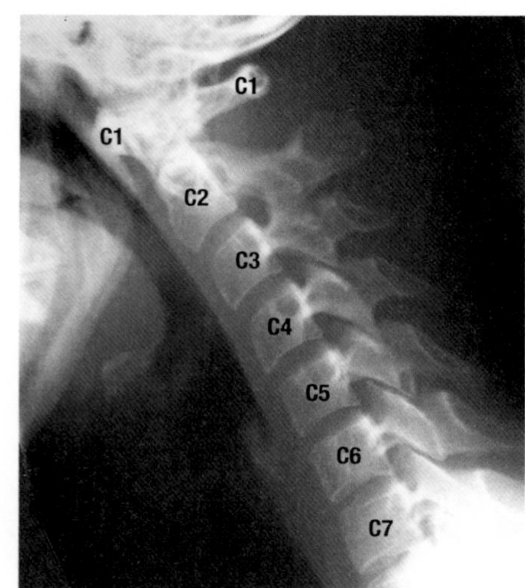
C1
C1
C2
C3
C4
C5
C6
C7
D. Lateral View

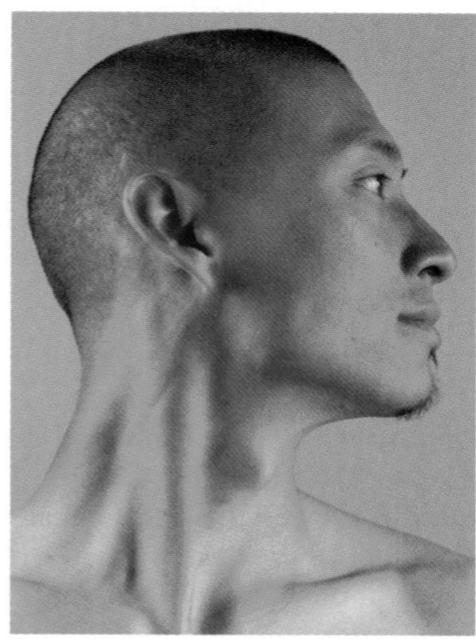
E. Anterior View

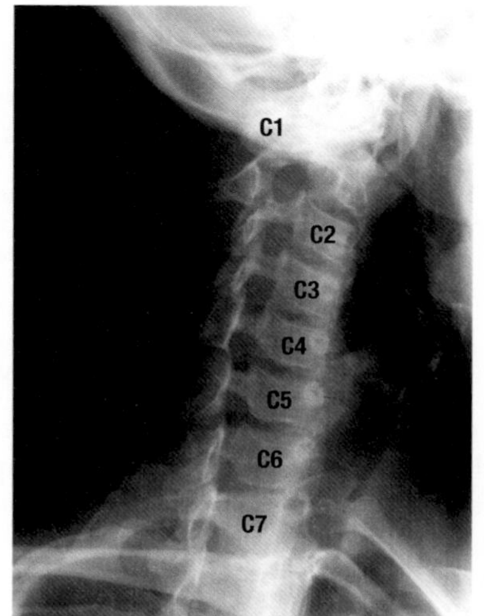
C1
C2
C3
C4
C5
C6
C7
F. Oblique View

## 4.7 Surface anatomy with radiographic correlation of selected movements of the cervical spine

**A.** Extension of the neck. **B.** Radiograph of the extended cervical spine. **C.** Flexion of the neck. **D.** Radiograph of the flexed cervical spine. **E.** Head turned (rotated) to left. **F.** Radiograph of cervical spine rotated to left.

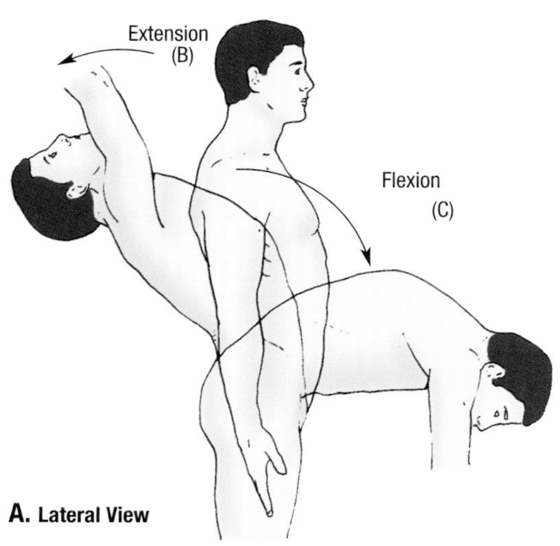
Extension
(B)
Flexion
(C)

**A.** Lateral View

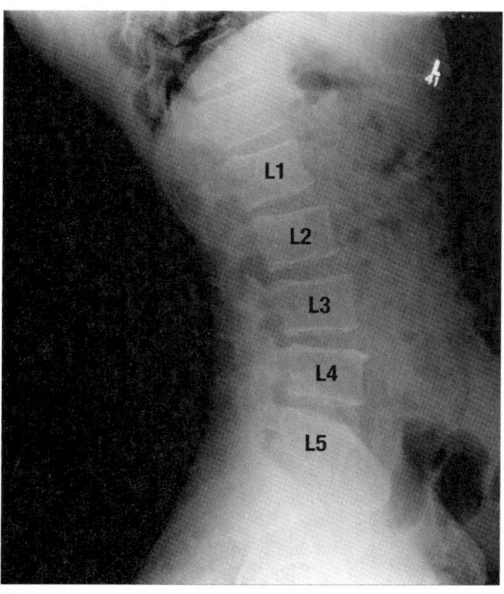
L1
L2
L3
L4
L5

**B.** Lateral View

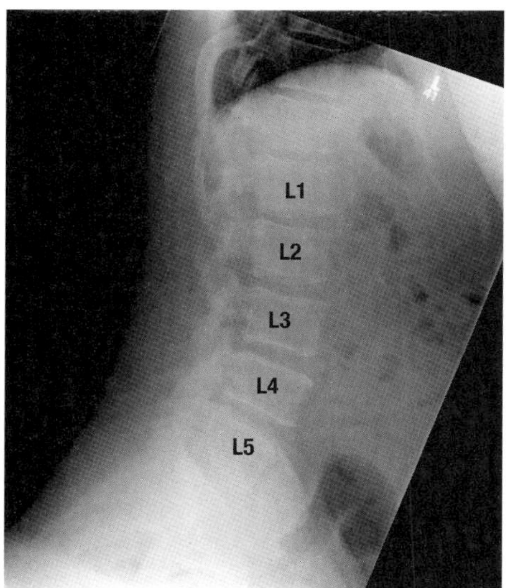
L1
L2
L3
L4
L5

**C.** Lateral View

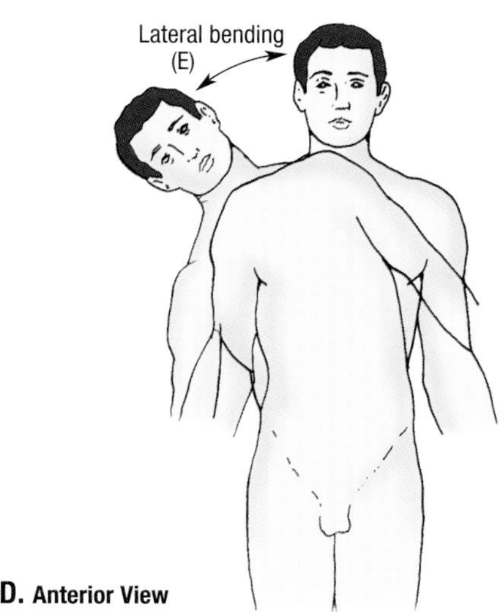
Lateral bending
(E)

**D.** Anterior View

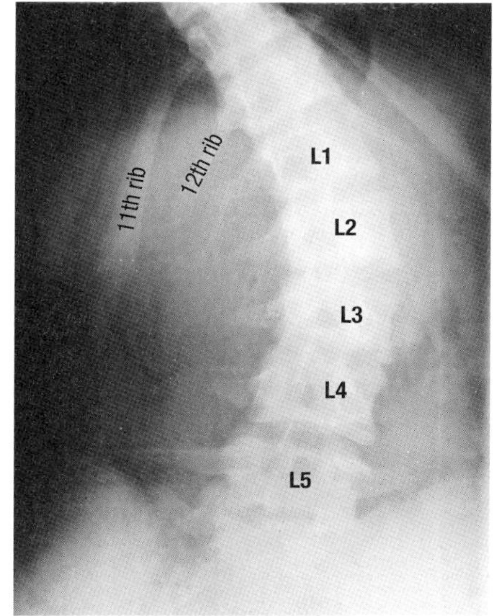
11th rib
12th rib
L1
L2
L3
L4
L5

**E.** Anteroposterior View

## 4.8 Surface anatomy with radiographic correlation of selected movements of the lumbar spine

**A.** Flexion and extension of the trunk. **B.** Radiograph of the extended lumbar spine. **C.** Radiograph of the flexed lumbar spine. **D.** Lateral bending of the trunk. **E.** Radiograph of the lumbar spine during lateral bending.

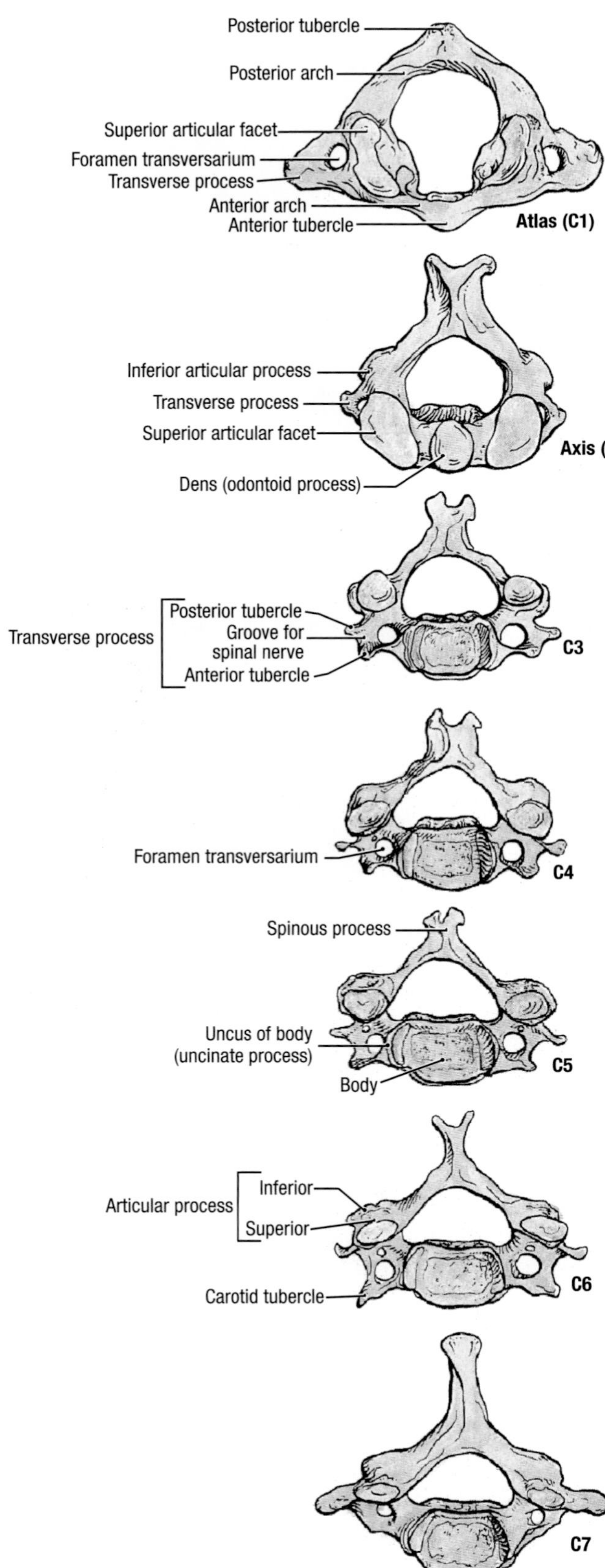
Posterior tubercle
Posterior arch
Superior articular facet
Foramen transversarium
Transverse process
Anterior arch
Anterior tubercle
Atlas (C1)
Inferior articular process
Transverse process
Superior articular facet
Axis (C2)
Dens (odontoid process)
Transverse process
Posterior tubercle
Groove for spinal nerve
Anterior tubercle
C3
Foramen transversarium
C4
Spinous process
Uncus of body (uncinate process)
Body
C5
Articular process
Inferior
Superior
Carotid tubercle
C6
C7
Superior Views

**TABLE 4.1 TYPICAL CERVICAL VERTEBRAE (C3-C7)[a]**

| Part | Distinctive Characteristics |
|---|---|
| Body | Small and wider from side to side than anteroposteriorly; superior surface is concave with uncus of body (uncinate process); inferior surface is convex |
| Vertebral foramen | Large and triangular |
| Transverse processes | Foramina transversaria small or absent in C7; vertebral arteries and accompanying venous and sympathetic plexuses pass through foramina, except C7, which transmits only small accessory vertebral veins; anterior and posterior tubercles separated by groove for spinal nerve |
| Articular processes | Superior articular facets directed superoposteriorly; inferior articular facets directed inferoanteriorly; obliquely placed facets are most nearly horizontal in this region |
| Spinous process | Short (C3–C5) and bifid, only in Caucasians (C3–C5); process of C6 is long but that of C7 is longer; C7 is called "vertebra prominens" |

[a]C1 and C2 vertebrae are atypical.

## 4.9 Cervical vertebrae

The bodies of the cervical vertebrae can be dislocated in neck injuries with less force than is required to fracture them. Because of the large vertebral canal in the cervical region, slight dislocation can occur without damaging the spinal cord. When a cervical vertebra is severely dislocated, it injures the spinal cord. If the dislocation does not result in "facet jumping" with locking of the displaced articular processes, the cervical vertebrae may self-reduce ("slip back into place") so that a radiograph may not indicate that the cord has been injured. MRI may reveal the resulting soft tissue damage.

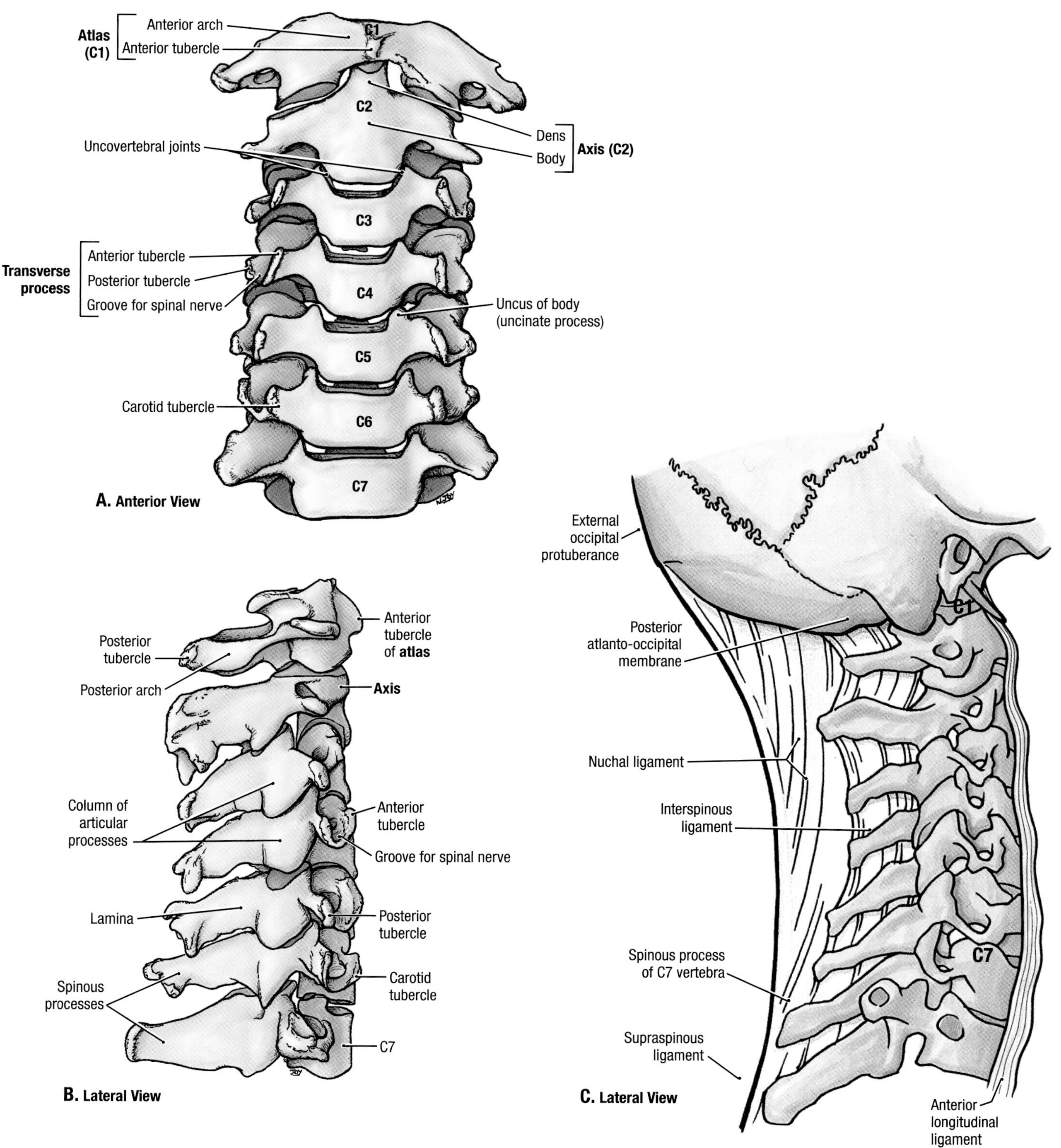
Atlas (C1)
Anterior arch
Anterior tubercle
C1
C2
Dens
Body
Axis (C2)
Uncovertebral joints
C3
Transverse process
Anterior tubercle
Posterior tubercle
Groove for spinal nerve
C4
Uncus of body (uncinate process)
C5
Carotid tubercle
C6
C7
A. Anterior View
Posterior tubercle
Posterior arch
Anterior tubercle of atlas
Axis
Column of articular processes
Anterior tubercle
Groove for spinal nerve
Lamina
Posterior tubercle
Spinous processes
Carotid tubercle
C7
B. Lateral View
External occipital protuberance
Posterior atlanto-occipital membrane
C1
Nuchal ligament
Interspinous ligament
Spinous process of C7 vertebra
C7
Supraspinous ligament
Anterior longitudinal ligament
C. Lateral View

**4.10 Cervical spine**

**A** and **B.** Articulated cervical vertebrae. **C.** Ligaments.

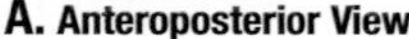
Uncovertebral joint
Uncal process of body of C5
Pedicle
1st rib
Transverse process of T2
Clavicle
Spinous process of T2
C3
C7

**A. Anteroposterior View**

D
FJ
AT
C1
FJ
C2
TVP
C3
A
P
UV
C4
C5
C6

**C. Anterior View**

| | | | |
|---|---|---|---|
| A | Anterior tubercle of transverse process | PA | Posterior arch of C1 |
| AA | Anterior arch of C1 | PT | Posterior tubercle of C1 |
| AT | Anterior tubercle of C1 | SF | Superior articular facet of C1 |
| C1-C7 | Vertebrae | SP | Spinous process |
| D | Dens (odontoid) process of C2 | T | Foramen transversarium |
| FJ | Zygapophysial (facet) joint | TVP | Transverse process |
| La | Lamina | UV | Uncovertebral joint |
| P | Posterior tubercle of transverse process | VC | Vertebral canal |

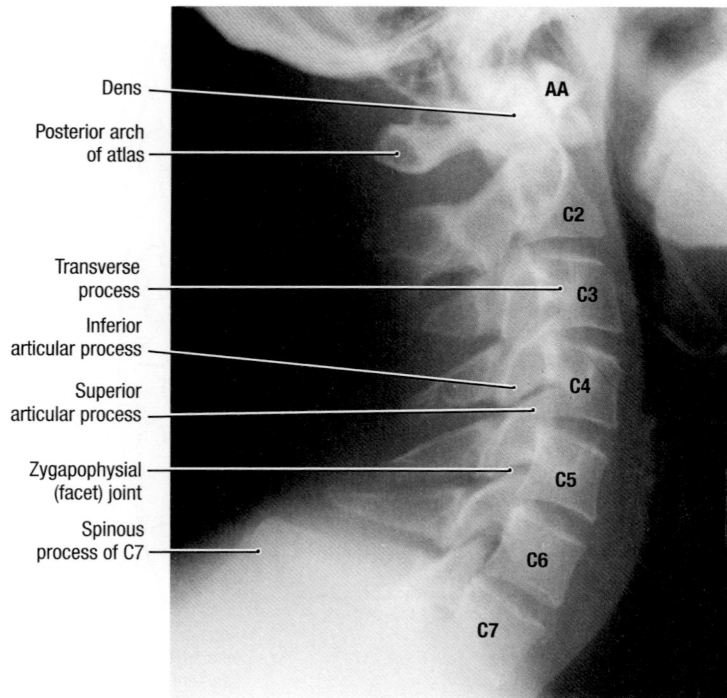
Dens
Posterior arch of atlas
Transverse process
Inferior articular process
Superior articular process
Zygapophysial (facet) joint
Spinous process of C7
AA
C2
C3
C4
C5
C6
C7

**B. Lateral View**

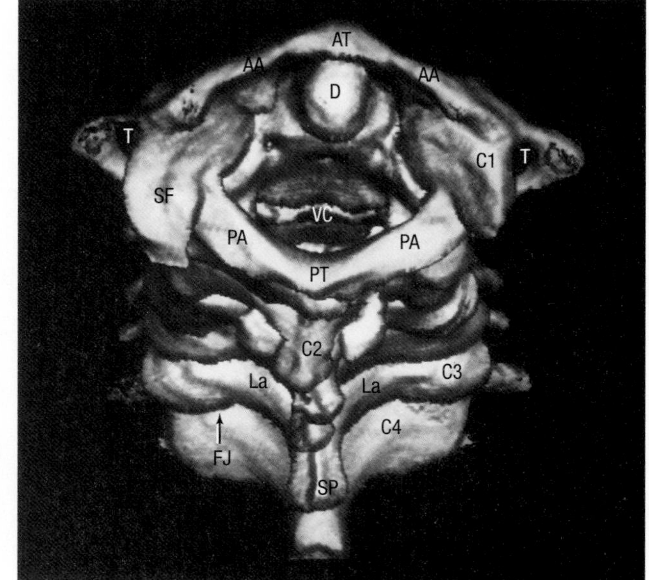
AT
AA
AA
D
T
T
C1
SF
VC
PA
PA
PT
C2
C3
La
La
C4
FJ
SP

**D. Posterior View**

## 4.11 Imaging of the cervical spine

**A and B.** Radiographs. The arrowheads demarcate the margins of the *(black)* column of air in the trachea. **C and D.** Three-dimensional (3D) reconstructed computed tomographic (CT) images.

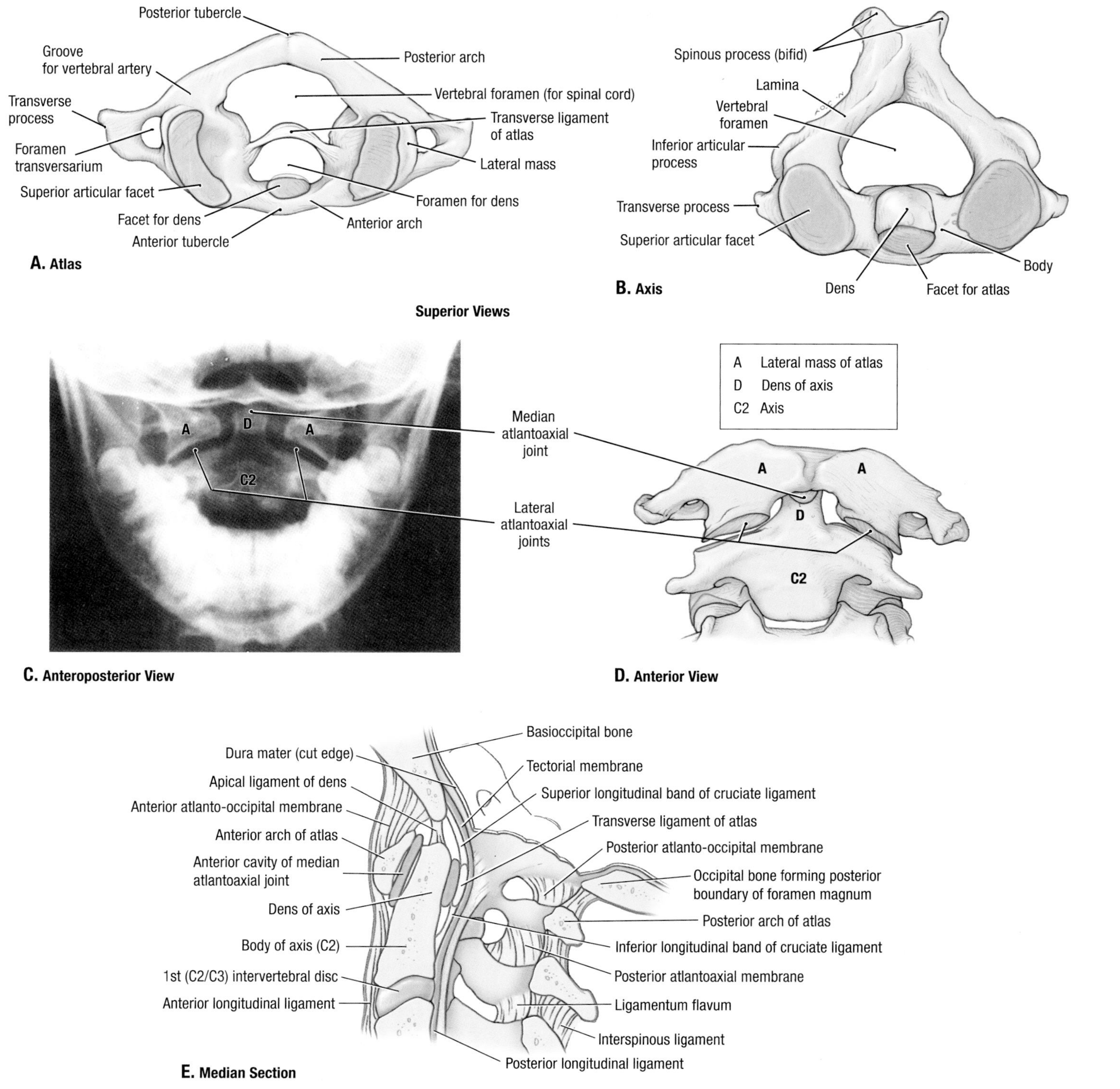

Posterior tubercle
Groove for vertebral artery
Transverse process
Foramen transversarium
Superior articular facet
Facet for dens
Anterior tubercle
Posterior arch
Vertebral foramen (for spinal cord)
Transverse ligament of atlas
Lateral mass
Foramen for dens
Anterior arch

**A. Atlas**

Spinous process (bifid)
Lamina
Vertebral foramen
Inferior articular process
Transverse process
Superior articular facet
Dens
Facet for atlas
Body

**B. Axis**

**Superior Views**

A D A C2
Median atlantoaxial joint
Lateral atlantoaxial joints

**C. Anteroposterior View**

| | |
|---|---|
| A | Lateral mass of atlas |
| D | Dens of axis |
| C2 | Axis |

A A D C2

**D. Anterior View**

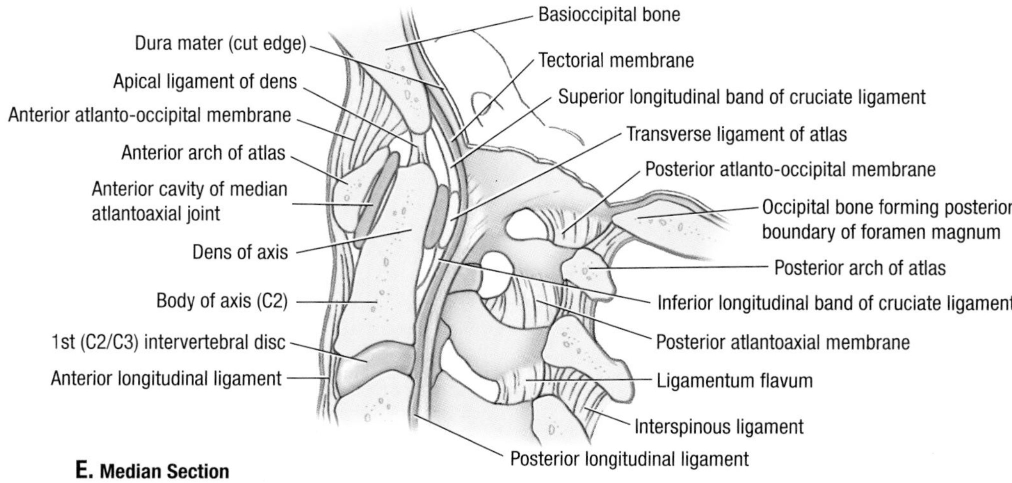
Dura mater (cut edge)
Apical ligament of dens
Anterior atlanto-occipital membrane
Anterior arch of atlas
Anterior cavity of median atlantoaxial joint
Dens of axis
Body of axis (C2)
1st (C2/C3) intervertebral disc
Anterior longitudinal ligament
Basioccipital bone
Tectorial membrane
Superior longitudinal band of cruciate ligament
Transverse ligament of atlas
Posterior atlanto-occipital membrane
Occipital bone forming posterior boundary of foramen magnum
Posterior arch of atlas
Inferior longitudinal band of cruciate ligament
Posterior atlantoaxial membrane
Ligamentum flavum
Interspinous ligament
Posterior longitudinal ligament

**E. Median Section**

## 4.12 Atlas and axis and the atlantoaxial joint

**A.** Atlas. **B.** Axis. **C.** Radiograph taken through the open mouth. **D.** Articulated atlas and axis. **E.** Median section with ligaments.

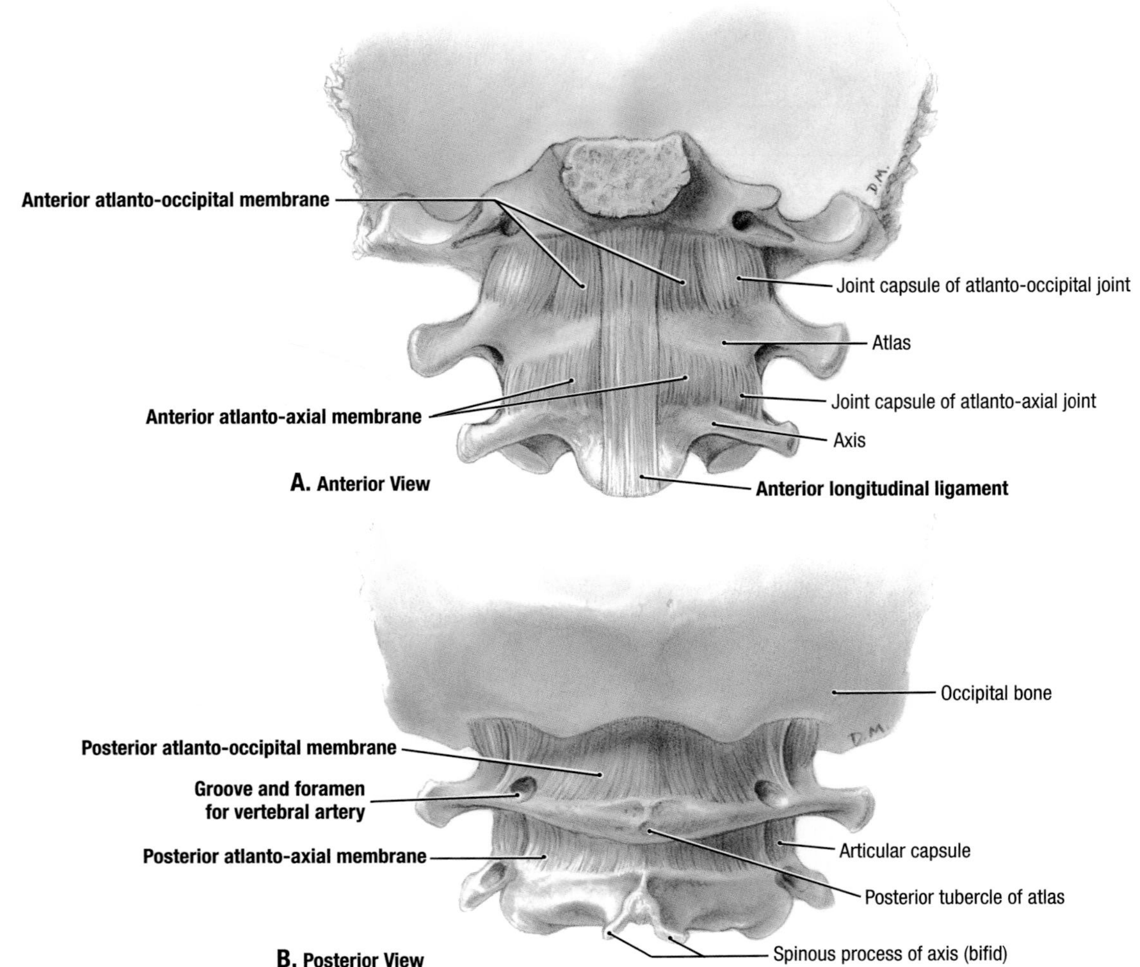
Anterior atlanto-occipital membrane
Joint capsule of atlanto-occipital joint
Atlas
Anterior atlanto-axial membrane
Joint capsule of atlanto-axial joint
Axis
A. Anterior View
Anterior longitudinal ligament
Occipital bone
Posterior atlanto-occipital membrane
Groove and foramen for vertebral artery
Posterior atlanto-axial membrane
Articular capsule
Posterior tubercle of atlas
Spinous process of axis (bifid)
B. Posterior View

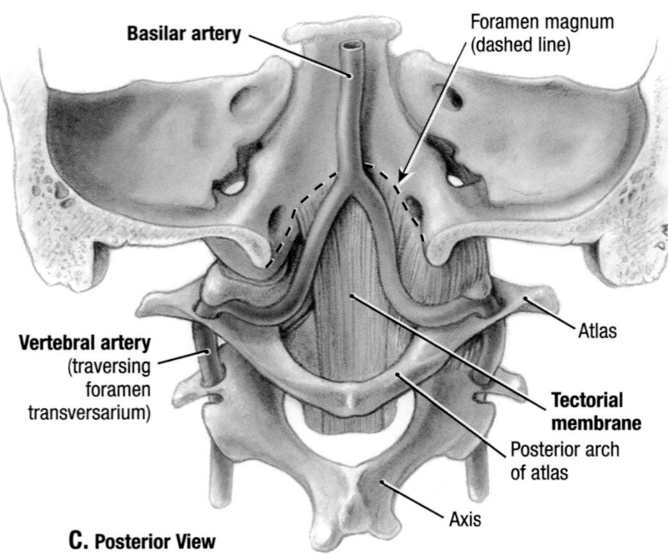
Basilar artery
Foramen magnum (dashed line)
Atlas
Vertebral artery (traversing foramen transversarium)
Tectorial membrane
Posterior arch of atlas
Axis
C. Posterior View

## 4.13 Craniovertebral joints and vertebral artery

**A.** Anterior atlanto-axial and atlanto-occipital membranes. The anterior longitudinal ligament ascends to blend with, and form a central thickening in, the anterior atlanto-axial and atlanto-occipital membranes. **B.** Posterior atlanto-axial and atlanto-occipital membranes. Inferior to the axis (C2 vertebra), ligamenta flava occur in this position. **C.** Tectorial membrane and vertebral artery. The tectorial membrane is a superior continuation of the posterior longitudinal ligament superior to the axis. After coursing through the foramina transversaria of vertebrae C6–C1, the arteries turning medially, grooving the superior aspect of the posterior arch of the atlas and piercing the posterior atlanto-occipital membrane **(B).** The right and left vertebral arteries traverse the foramen magnum and merge to form the intracranial basilar artery.

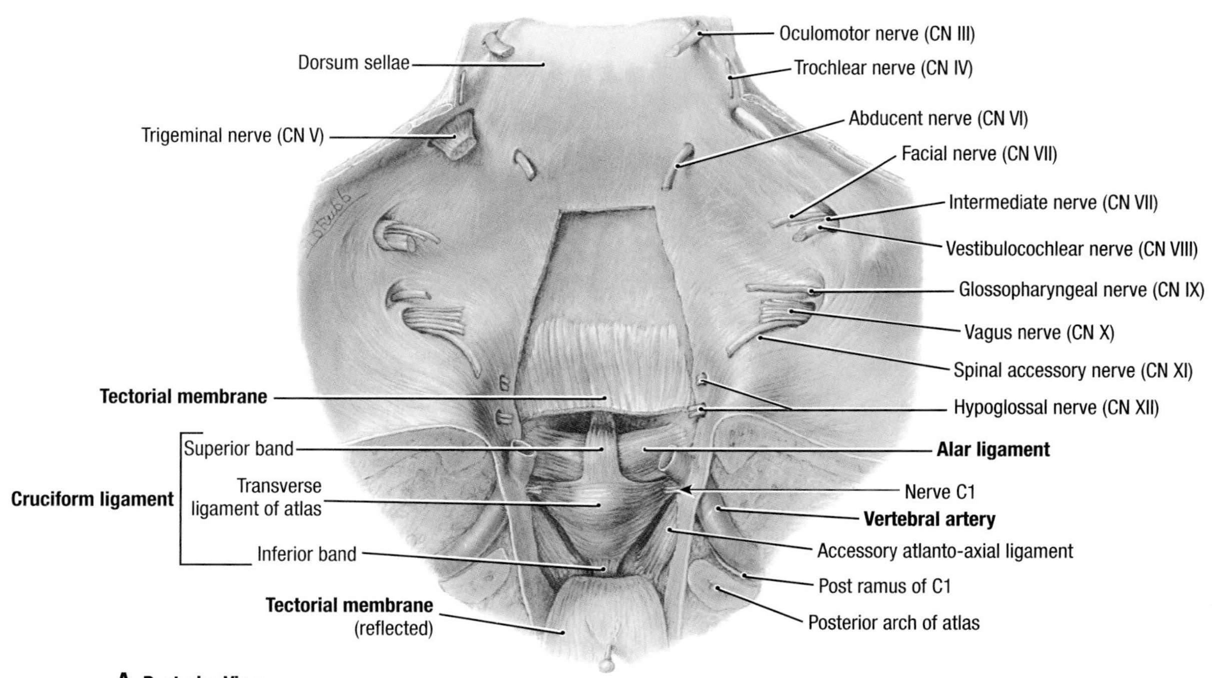
Dorsum sellae
Oculomotor nerve (CN III)
Trochlear nerve (CN IV)
Trigeminal nerve (CN V)
Abducent nerve (CN VI)
Facial nerve (CN VII)
Intermediate nerve (CN VII)
Vestibulocochlear nerve (CN VIII)
Glossopharyngeal nerve (CN IX)
Vagus nerve (CN X)
Spinal accessory nerve (CN XI)
Tectorial membrane
Hypoglossal nerve (CN XII)
Cruciform ligament
Superior band
Alar ligament
Transverse ligament of atlas
Nerve C1
Vertebral artery
Accessory atlanto-axial ligament
Inferior band
Post ramus of C1
Tectorial membrane (reflected)
Posterior arch of atlas

**A.** Posterior View

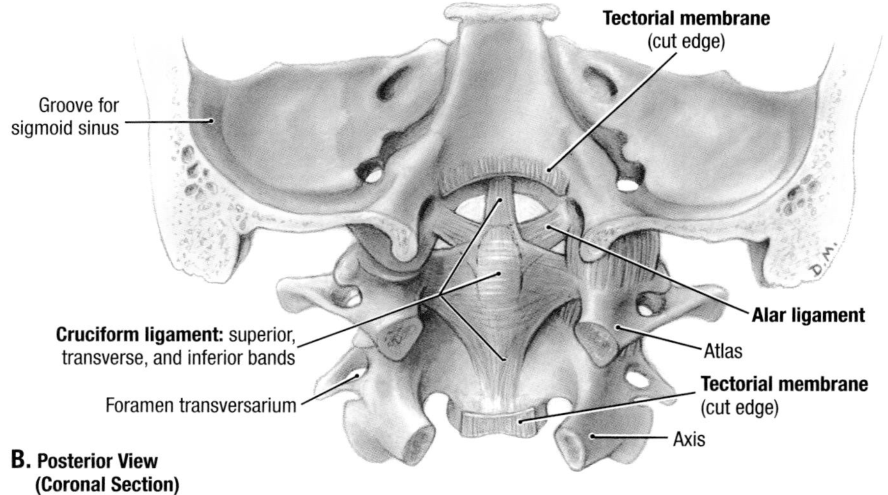
Tectorial membrane (cut edge)
Groove for sigmoid sinus
Alar ligament
Cruciform ligament: superior, transverse, and inferior bands
Atlas
Tectorial membrane (cut edge)
Foramen transversarium
Axis

**B.** Posterior View (Coronal Section)

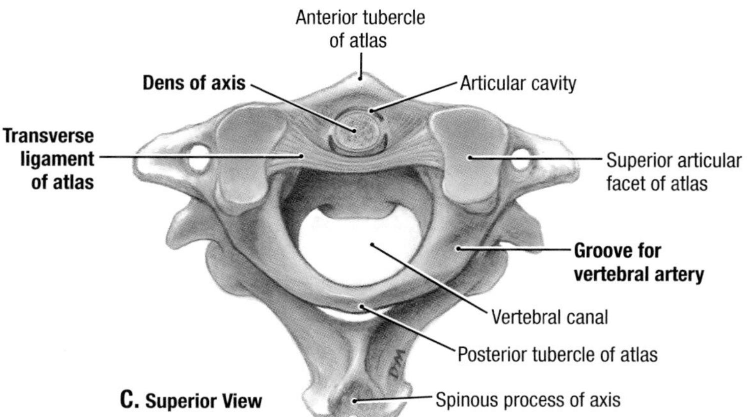
Anterior tubercle of atlas
Dens of axis
Articular cavity
Transverse ligament of atlas
Superior articular facet of atlas
Groove for vertebral artery
Vertebral canal
Posterior tubercle of atlas
Spinous process of axis

**C.** Superior View

## 4.14 Ligaments of atlanto-occipital and atlantoaxial joints

**A.** Cranial nerves and dura mater of posterior cranial fossa with dura mater and tentorial membrane incised and removed to reveal the medial atlanto-axial joint. **B.** The alar ligaments serve as check ligaments for the rotary movements of the atlanto-axial joints. **B** and **C.** The transverse ligament (band) of the cruciform ligament provides the posterior wall of a socket that receives the dens of the axis, forming a pivot joint.

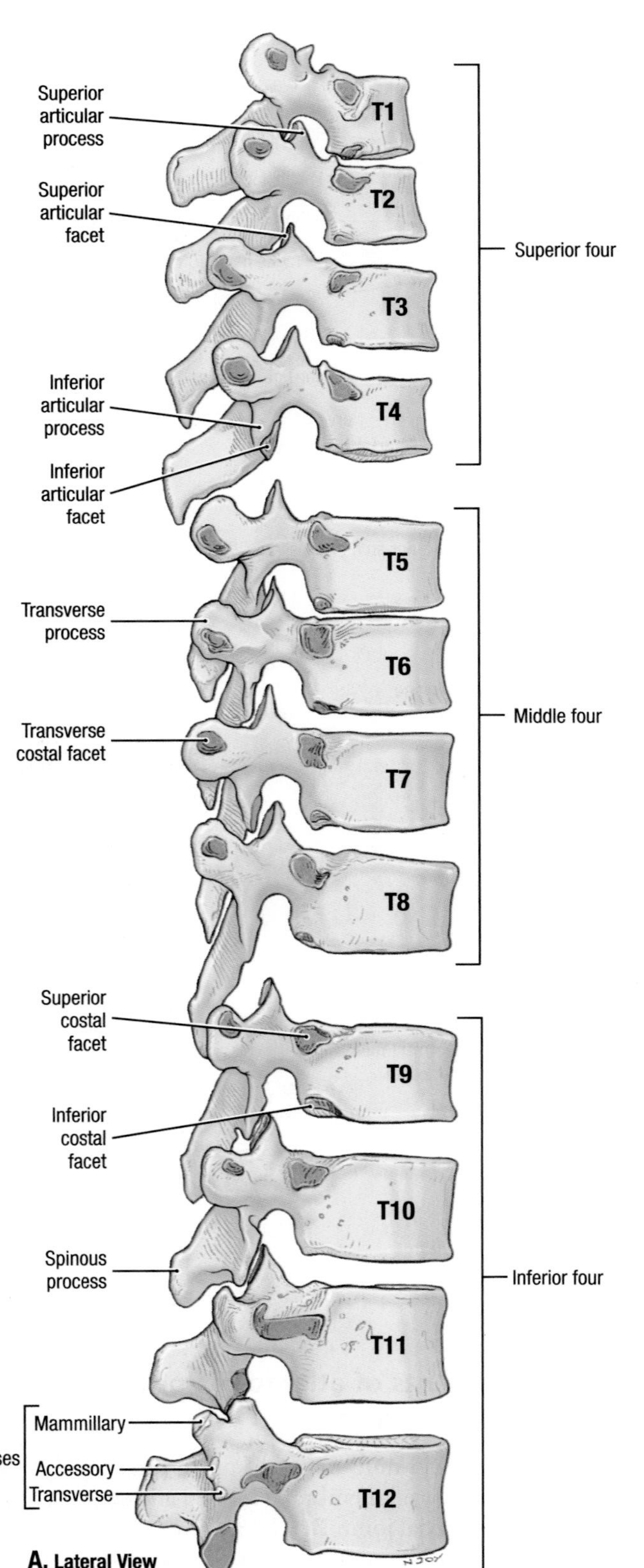
Superior articular process
Superior articular facet
Inferior articular process
Inferior articular facet
Transverse process
Transverse costal facet
Superior costal facet
Inferior costal facet
Spinous process
Processes
Mammillary
Accessory
Transverse
T1
T2
T3
T4
T5
T6
T7
T8
T9
T10
T11
T12
Superior four
Middle four
Inferior four

A. Lateral View

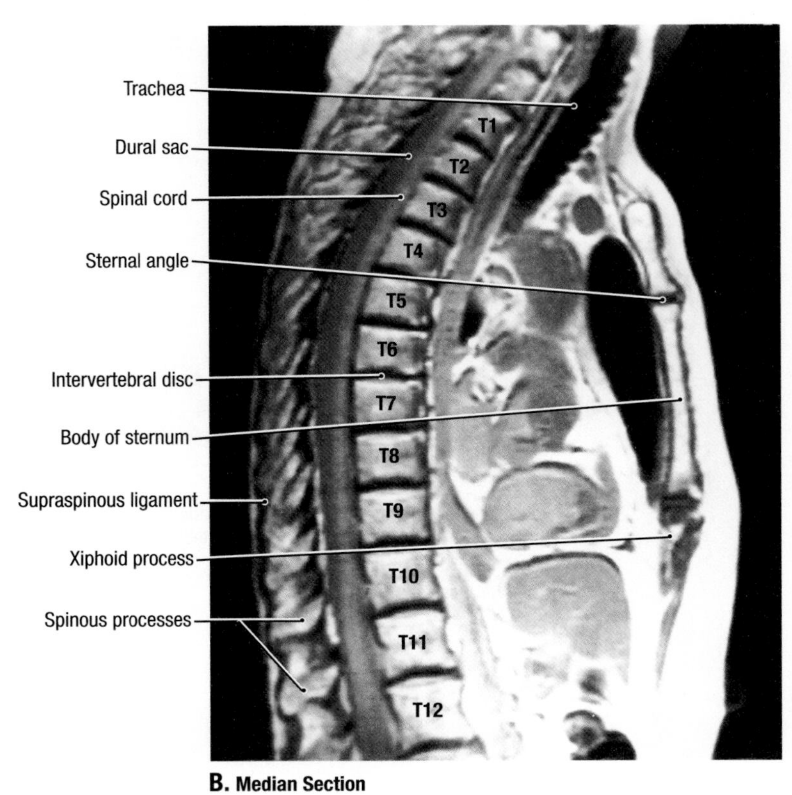
Trachea
Dural sac
Spinal cord
Sternal angle
Intervertebral disc
Body of sternum
Supraspinous ligament
Xiphoid process
Spinous processes
T1
T2
T3
T4
T5
T6
T7
T8
T9
T10
T11
T12

B. Median Section

**TABLE 4.2 THORACIC VERTEBRAE**

| Part | Distinctive Characteristics |
|---|---|
| **Body** | Heart-shaped; has one or two costal facets for articulation with head of rib |
| **Vertebral foramen** | Circular and smaller than those of cervical and lumbar vertebrae |
| **Transverse processes** | Long and strong and extend posterolaterally; length diminishes from T1 to T12; T1–T10 have transverse costal facets for articulation with tubercle of a rib |
| **Articular processes** | Superior articular facets directed posteriorly and slightly laterally; inferior articular facets directed anteriorly and slightly medially |
| **Spinous process** | Long and slopes posteroinferiorly; tip extends to level of vertebral body below |

**4.15 Thoracic vertebrae**

**A.** Features. **B.** MRI scan of thoracic spine, median section.

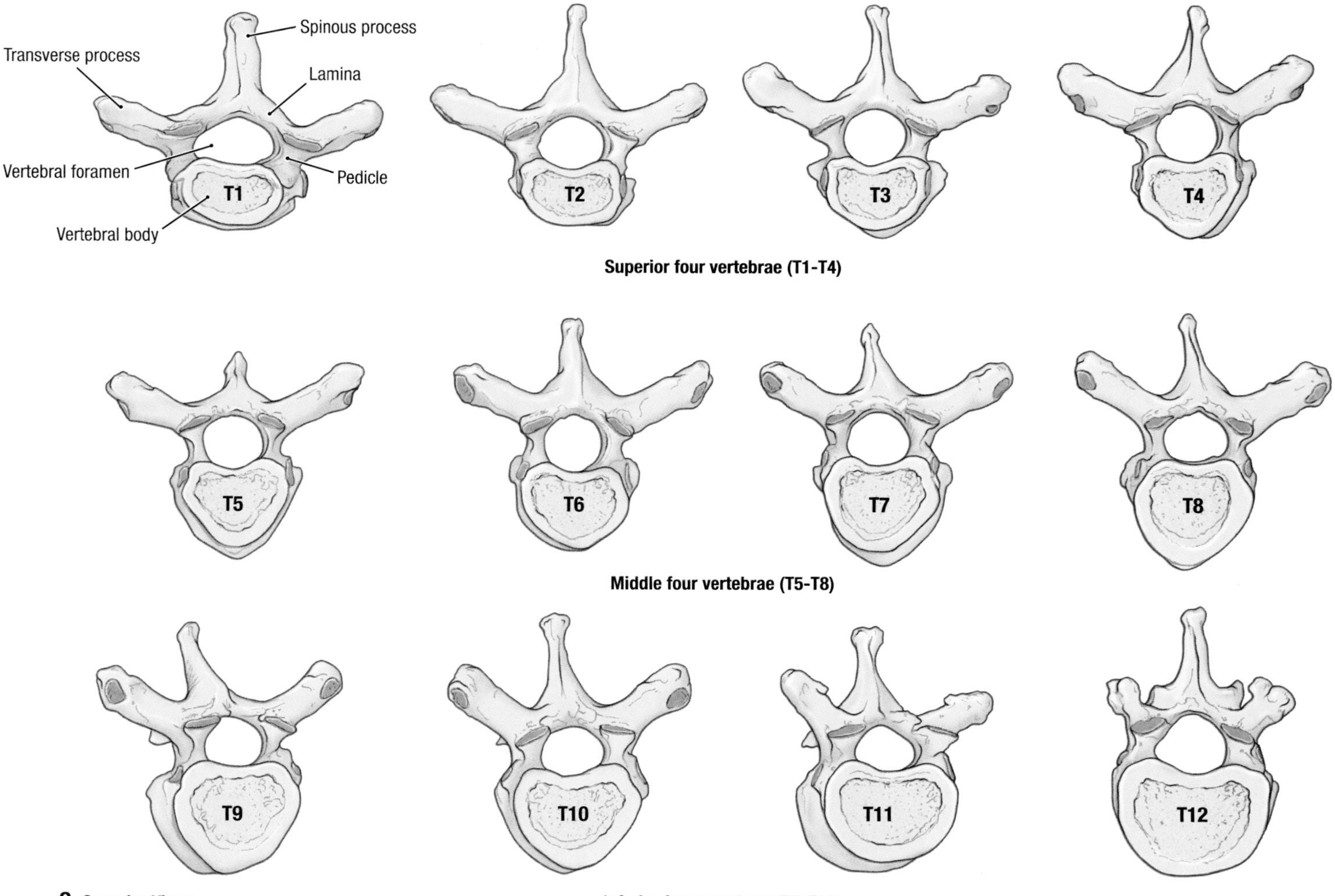

Spinous process
Transverse process
Lamina
Vertebral foramen
Pedicle
Vertebral body
T1 T2 T3 T4

**Superior four vertebrae (T1-T4)**

T5 T6 T7 T8

**Middle four vertebrae (T5-T8)**

T9 T10 T11 T12

**C. Superior Views**

**Inferior four vertebrae (T9-T12)**

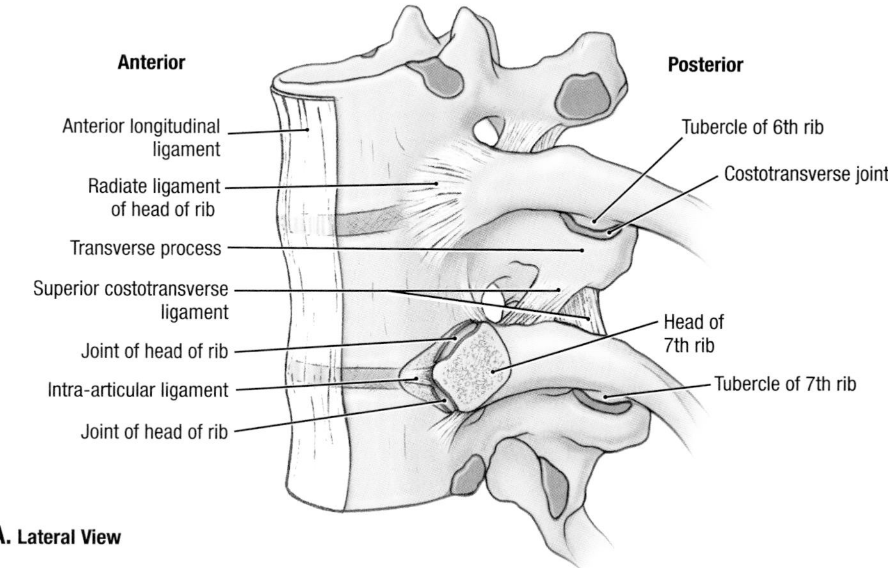
Anterior
Posterior
Anterior longitudinal ligament
Radiate ligament of head of rib
Transverse process
Superior costotransverse ligament
Joint of head of rib
Intra-articular ligament
Joint of head of rib
Tubercle of 6th rib
Costotransverse joint
Head of 7th rib
Tubercle of 7th rib

**A. Lateral View**

## 4.15 Thoracic vertebrae *(continued)*

**C.** Comparative anatomy. The vertebral bodies increase in size as the vertebral column descends, each bearing an increasing amount of weight transferred by the vertebra above. Although the characteristics of the superior aspect of vertebra T12 are distinctly thoracic, its inferior aspect has lumbar characteristics for articulation with vertebra L1. The abrupt transition allowing primarily rotational movements with vertebra T11 while disallowing rotational movements with vertebral L1 makes vertebra T12 especially susceptible to fracture. **D.** Intra- and extra-articular ligaments of the costovertebral articulations. Typically, the head of each rib articulates with the bodies of two adjacent vertebrae and the invertebral disc between them, and the tubercle of the rib articulates with the transverse process of the inferior vertebra.

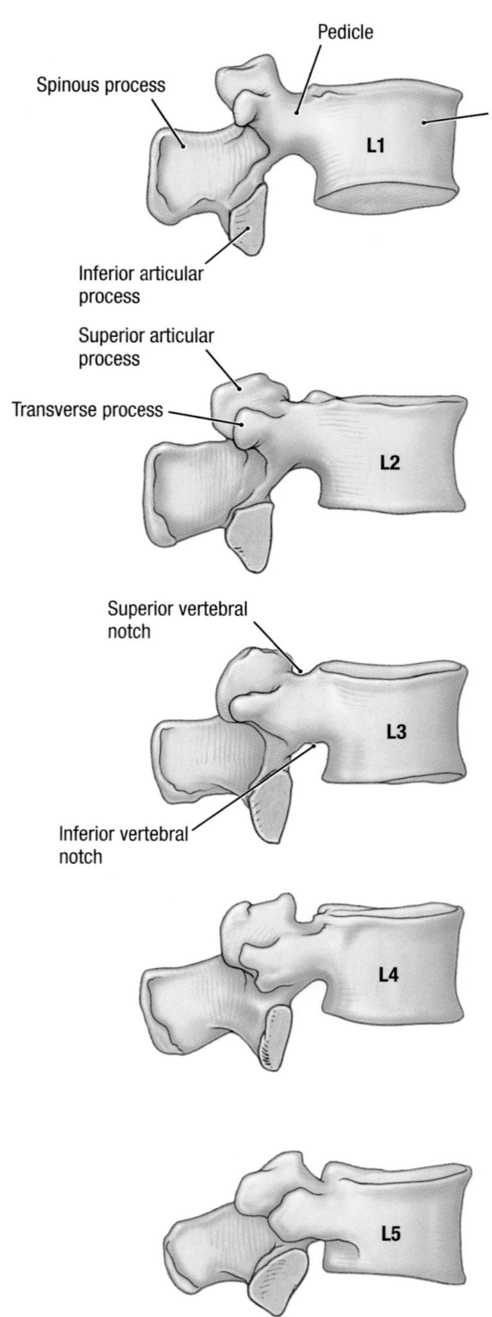
Pedicle
Spinous process
Vertebral body
L1
Inferior articular process
Superior articular process
Transverse process
L2
Superior vertebral notch
L3
Inferior vertebral notch
L4
L5

**A.** Lateral Views

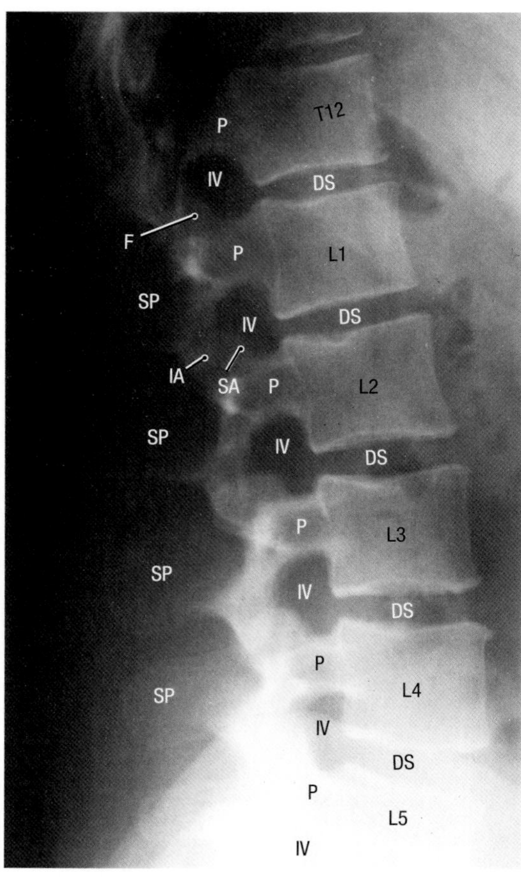
T12
P
IV
DS
F
P
L1
SP
IV
DS
IA
SA
P
L2
SP
IV
DS
P
L3
SP
IV
DS
P
SP
L4
IV
DS
P
L5
IV

**B.** Lateral View

| Key for B | |
|---|---|
| F | Zygapophysial (facet) joint |
| DS | Intervertebral disc space |
| IA | Inferior articular process |
| IV | Intervertebral foramen |
| P | Pedicle |
| SA | Superior articular process |
| SP | Spinous process |
| T12–L5 | Vertebral bodies |

**TABLE 4.3 LUMBAR VERTEBRAE**

| Part | Distinctive Characteristics |
|---|---|
| Body | Massive; kidney-shaped when viewed superiorly |
| Vertebral foramen | Triangular; larger than in thoracic vertebrae and smaller than in cervical vertebrae |
| Transverse processes | Long and slender; accessory process on posterior surface of base of each transverse process |
| Articular processes | Superior articular facets directed posteromedially (or medially); inferior articular facets directed anterolaterally (or laterally); mamillary process on posterior surface of each superior articular process |
| Spinous process | Short and sturdy; thick, broad, and rectangular |

## 4.16 Lumbar vertebrae

**A, C,** and **D.** Features. **B.** Radiograph. A laminectomy is the surgical excision of one or more spinous processes and their supporting laminae in a particular region of the vertebral column i.e., removal of most of the vertebral arch by transecting the pedicles. Laminectomies provide access to the vertebral canal to relieve pressure on the spinal cord or nerve roots, commonly caused by a tumor, herniated IV disc, or bony hypertrophy (excess growth). Laminectomies are most commonly performed in the lumbar region.

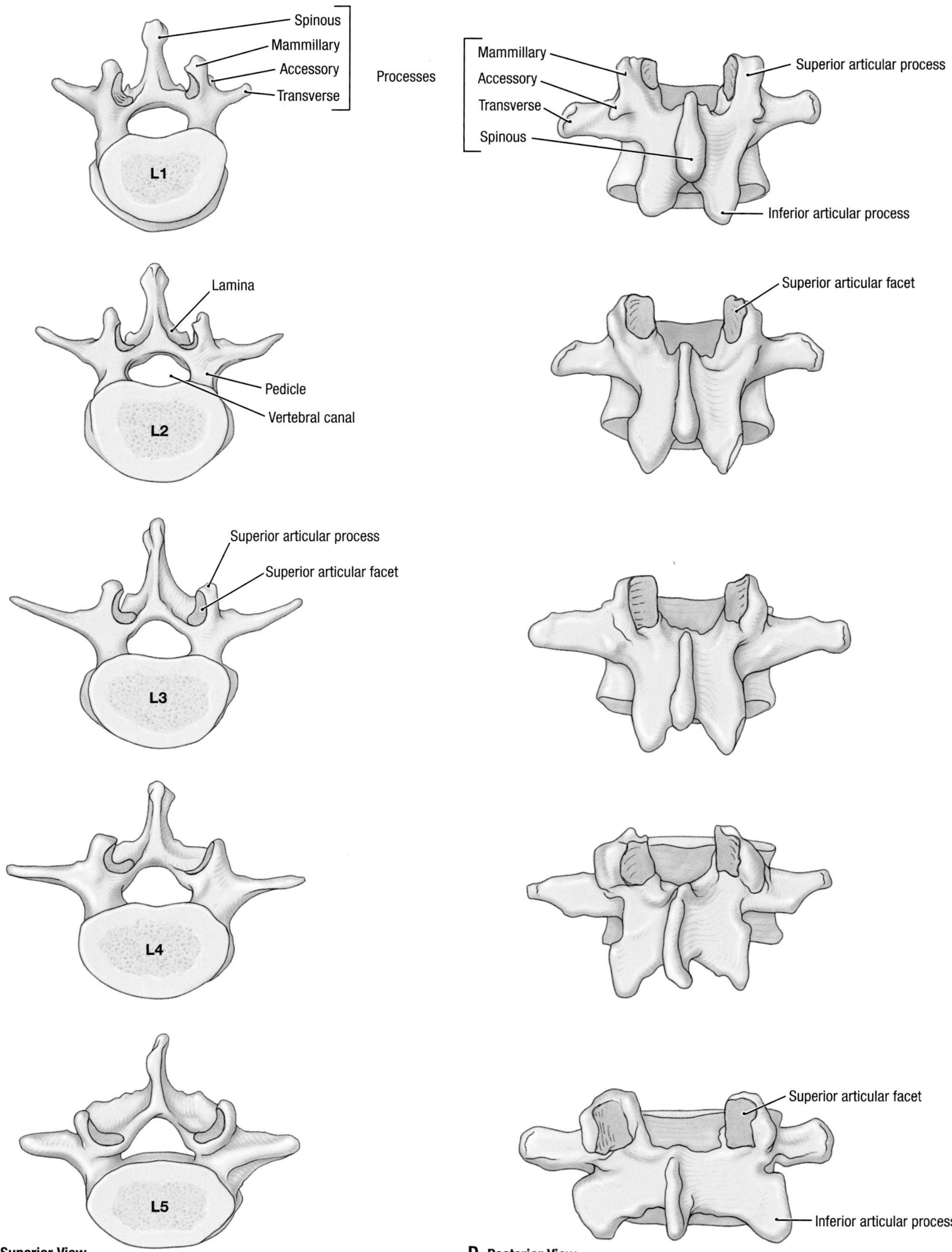
Spinous
Mammillary
Accessory
Transverse
Processes
L1
Lamina
Pedicle
Vertebral canal
L2
Superior articular process
Superior articular facet
L3
L4
L5
Mammillary
Accessory
Transverse
Spinous
Superior articular process
Inferior articular process
Superior articular facet
Superior articular facet
Inferior articular process

**C.** **Superior View**

**D.** **Posterior View**

**4.16 Lumbar vertebrae *(continued)***

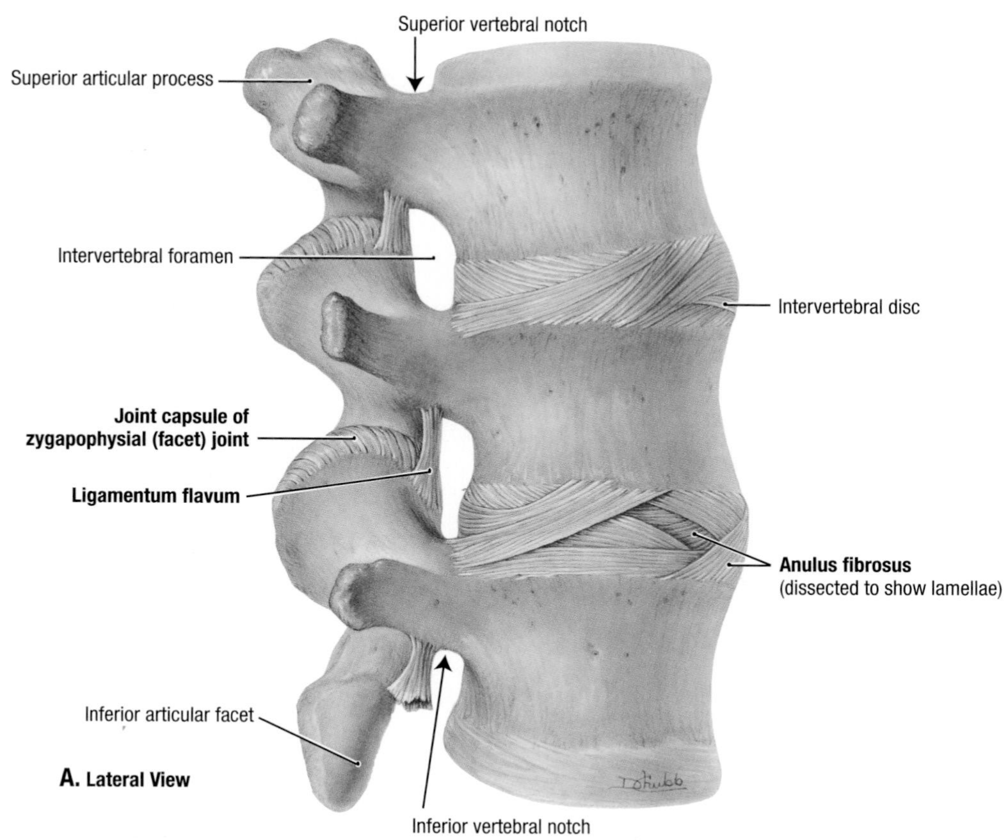
Superior vertebral notch
Superior articular process
Intervertebral foramen
Intervertebral disc
Joint capsule of zygapophysial (facet) joint
Ligamentum flavum
Anulus fibrosus
(dissected to show lamellae)
Inferior articular facet
A. Lateral View
Inferior vertebral notch

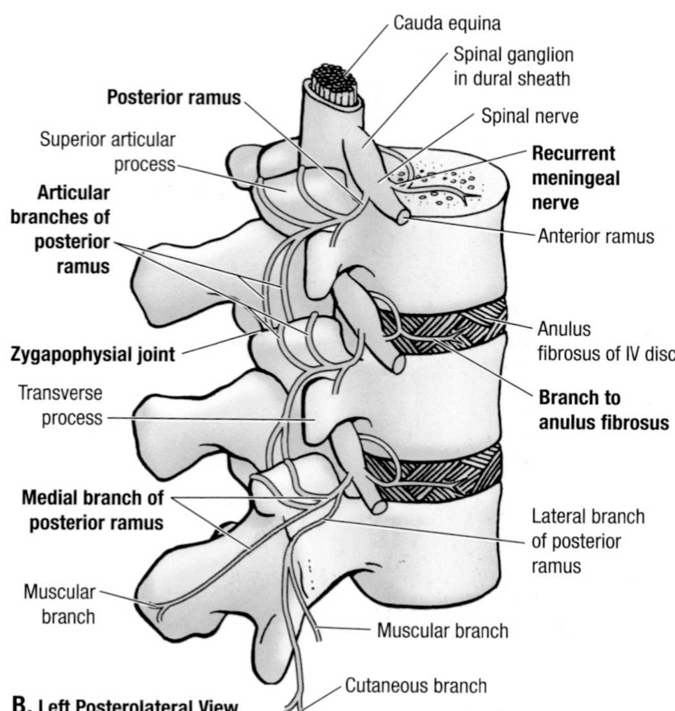
Cauda equina
Spinal ganglion in dural sheath
Posterior ramus
Spinal nerve
Superior articular process
Recurrent meningeal nerve
Articular branches of posterior ramus
Anterior ramus
Anulus fibrosus of IV disc
Zygapophysial joint
Transverse process
Branch to anulus fibrosus
Medial branch of posterior ramus
Lateral branch of posterior ramus
Muscular branch
Muscular branch
Cutaneous branch
B. Left Posterolateral View

When the zygapophyseal joints are injured or develop osteophytes during aging (osteoarthritis), the related spinal nerves are affected. This causes pain along the distribution pattern of the dermatomes and spasm in the muscles derived from the associated myotomes (a myotome consists of all the muscles or parts of muscles receiving innervation from one spinal nerve). Denervation of lumbar zygapophysial joints is a procedure that may be used for treatment of back pain caused by disease of these joints. The nerves are sectioned near the joints or are destroyed by radiofrequency percutaneous rhizolysis (root dissolution). The denervation process is directed at the articular branches of two adjacent posterior rami of the spinal nerves because each joint receives innervation from both the nerve exiting that level and the superadjacent nerve.

## 4.17 Structure and innervation of intervertebral discs and zygapophysial joints

**A.** Anulus fibrosus and intervertebral foramen. Sections have been removed from the superficial layers of the inferior intervertebral disc to show the change in direction of the fibers in the concentric layers of the anulus fibrosus. **B.** Innervation of zygapophysial joint and intervertebral disc.

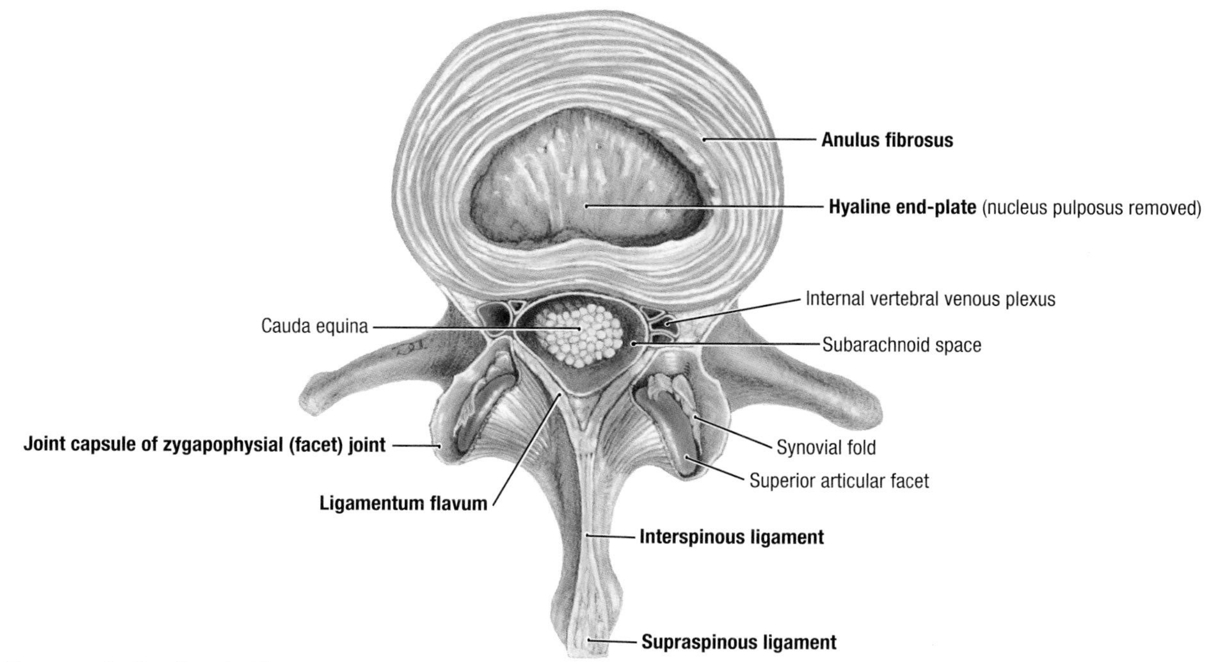
Anulus fibrosus
Hyaline end-plate (nucleus pulposus removed)
Internal vertebral venous plexus
Cauda equina
Subarachnoid space
Joint capsule of zygapophysial (facet) joint
Synovial fold
Superior articular facet
Ligamentum flavum
Interspinous ligament
Supraspinous ligament

C. Transverse Section, Superior View

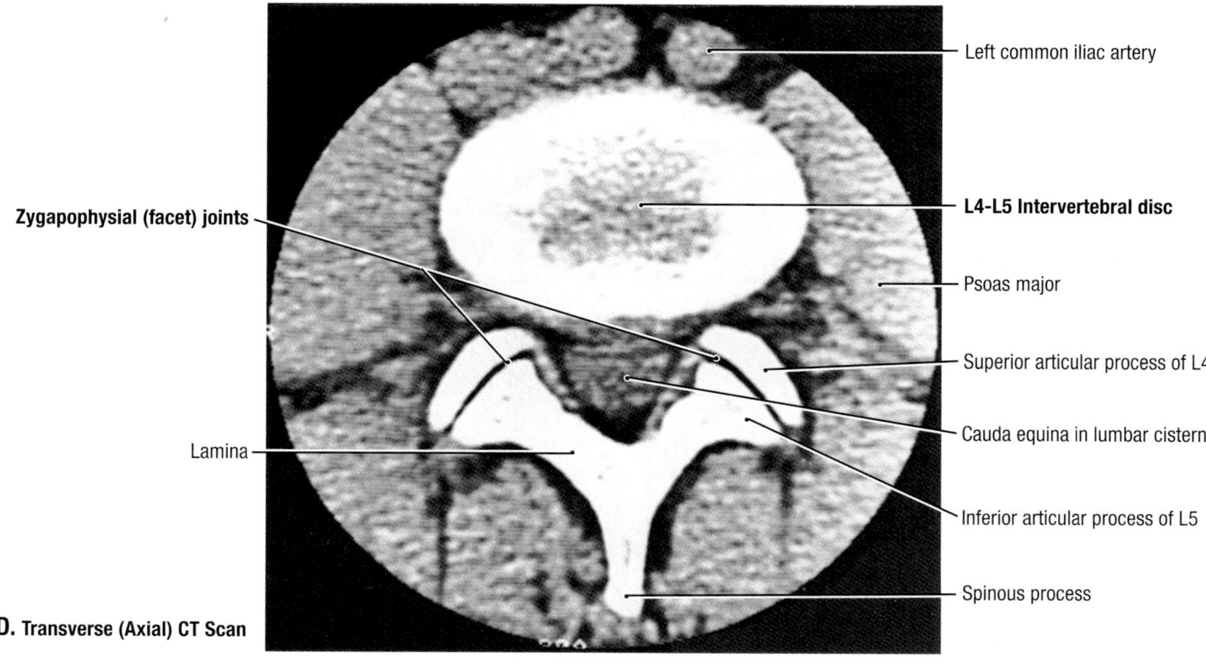
Left common iliac artery
L4-L5 Intervertebral disc
Zygapophysial (facet) joints
Psoas major
Superior articular process of L4
Cauda equina in lumbar cistern
Lamina
Inferior articular process of L5
Spinous process

D. Transverse (Axial) CT Scan

## 4.17 Structure and innervation of intervertebral discs and zygapophysial joints *(continued)*

**C.** Transverse section. The nucleus pulposus has been removed, and the cartilaginous epiphyseal plate exposed. There are fewer rings of the anulus fibrosus posteriorly, and consequently, this portion of the annulus fibrosus is thinner. The ligamentum flavum, interspinous, and supraspinous ligaments are continuous. **D.** CT image of L4/L5 intervertebral disc.

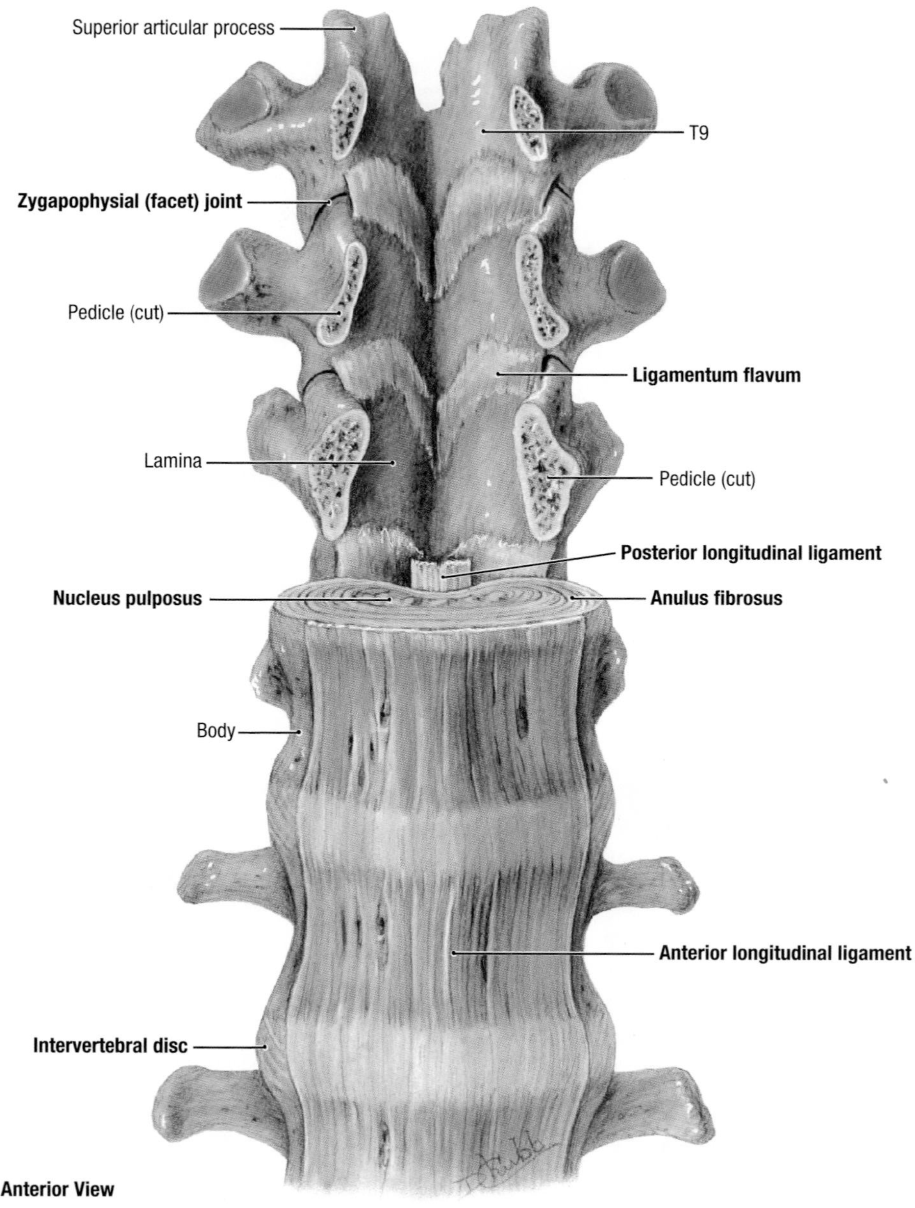
Superior articular process
T9
Zygapophysial (facet) joint
Pedicle (cut)
Ligamentum flavum
Lamina
Pedicle (cut)
Posterior longitudinal ligament
Nucleus pulposus
Anulus fibrosus
Body
Anterior longitudinal ligament
Intervertebral disc

A. Anterior View

## 4.18 Intervertebral discs: ligaments and movements

**A.** Anterior longitudinal ligament and ligamenta flava. The pedicles of T9 to T11 were sawed through, and the posterior aspect of the bodies is shown in **B.**
**B.** Posterior longitudinal ligament. **C.** Intervertebral disc during loading and movement.

- The anterior and posterior longitudinal ligaments are ligaments of the vertebral bodies; the ligamenta flava are ligaments of the vertebral arches.
- The anterior longitudinal ligament consists of broad, strong, fibrous bands that are attached to the intervertebral discs and vertebral bodies anteriorly and are perforated by the foramina for arteries and veins passing to and from the vertebral bodies.
- The ligamenta flava, composed of elastic fibers, extend between adjacent laminae; right and left ligaments converge in the median plane. They extend laterally to the articular processes, where they blend with the joint capsule of the zygapophysial joint.

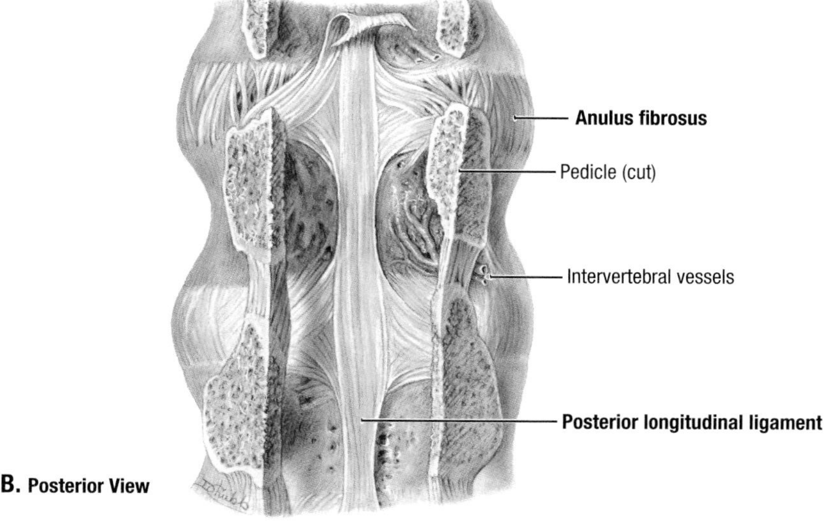
Anulus fibrosus
Pedicle (cut)
Intervertebral vessels
Posterior longitudinal ligament

**B.** Posterior View

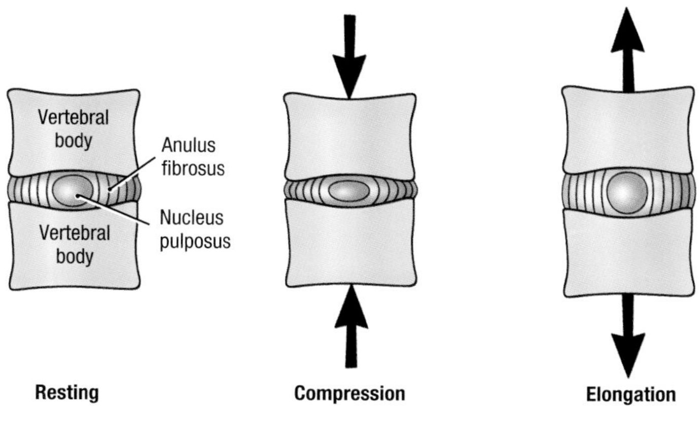
Vertebral body
Anulus fibrosus
Nucleus pulposus
Vertebral body
Resting
Compression
Elongation
Anterior Views

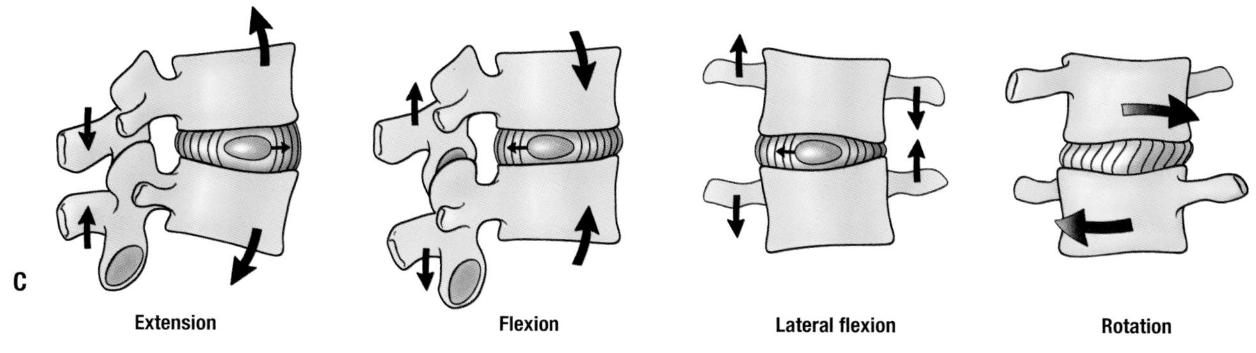
C
Extension
Flexion
Lateral flexion
Rotation
Lateral Views
Anterior Views

## 4.18 Intervertebral discs: ligaments and movements *(continued)*

- The posterior longitudinal ligament is a narrow band passing from disc to disc, spanning the posterior surfaces of the vertebral bodies (in **B**). The ligament is diamond shaped posterior to each intervertebral disc, where it exchanges fibers with the anulus fibrosus; the ligament extends to the sacrum inferiorly and becomes the tectorial membrane cranially.
- The movement or loading of the intervertebral disc changes its shape and the position of the nucleus pulposus. Flexion and extension movements cause compression and elongation simultaneously.

Anterior longitudinal ligament
Posterior longitudinal ligament
L1
Ligamentum flavum
Nucleus pulposus protruding posteriorly
L2
Interspinous ligament
Cavity for nucleus pulposus
Intervertebral foramen
Anulus fibrosus
Hyaline plate
L3
Supraspinous ligament
Spinal nerve
Nucleus pulposus protruding into vertebral bodies
Anterior and posterior nerve roots
Bursa
Canal for basivertebral vein
Dura mater
L4
Median Section

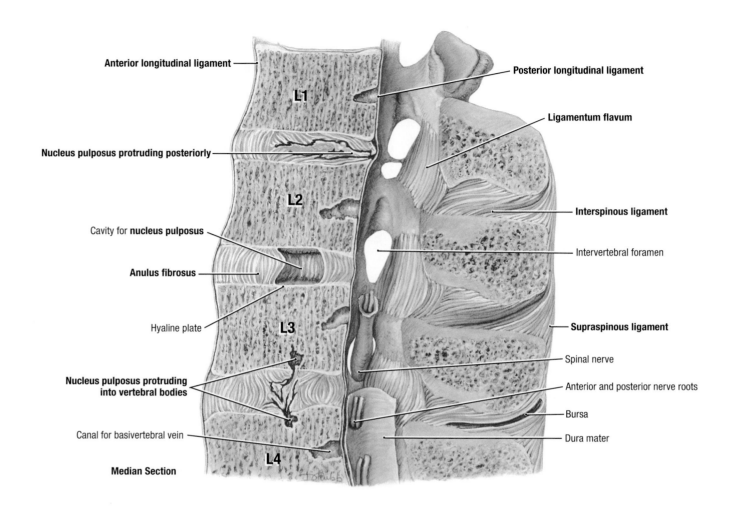

## 4.19 Lumbar region of vertebral column

The nucleus pulposus of the normal disc between L2 and L3 has been removed from the enclosing anulus fibrosus.

- The ligamentum flavum extends from the superior border and adjacent part of the posterior aspect of one lamina to the inferior border and adjacent part of the anterior aspect of the lamina above and extends laterally to become continuous with the fibrous capsule of the zygapophysial joint.
- The obliquely placed interspinous ligament unites the superior and inferior borders of two adjacent spines.
- The bursa between L3 and L4 spines is presumably the result of habitual hyperextension, which brings the lumbar spines into contact.

The nucleus pulposus of the disc between L1 and L2 has herniated posteriorly through the anulus. Herniation or protrusion of the gelatinous nucleus pulposus into or through the anulus fibrosus is a well-recognized cause of low back and lower limb pain. If degeneration of the posterior longitudinal ligament and wearing of the anulus fibrosus has occurred, the nucleus pulposus may herniate into the vertebral canal and compress the spinal cord or nerve roots of spinal nerves in the cauda equina. Herniations usually occur posterolaterally, where the anulus is relatively thin and does not receive support from the posterior or anterior longitudinal ligaments.

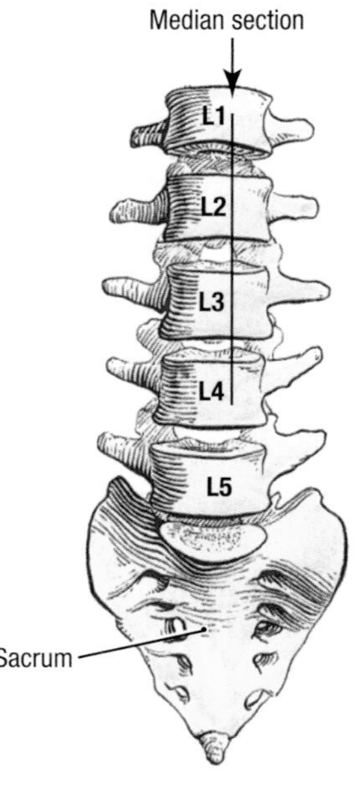
Median section
L1
L2
L3
L4
L5
Sacrum

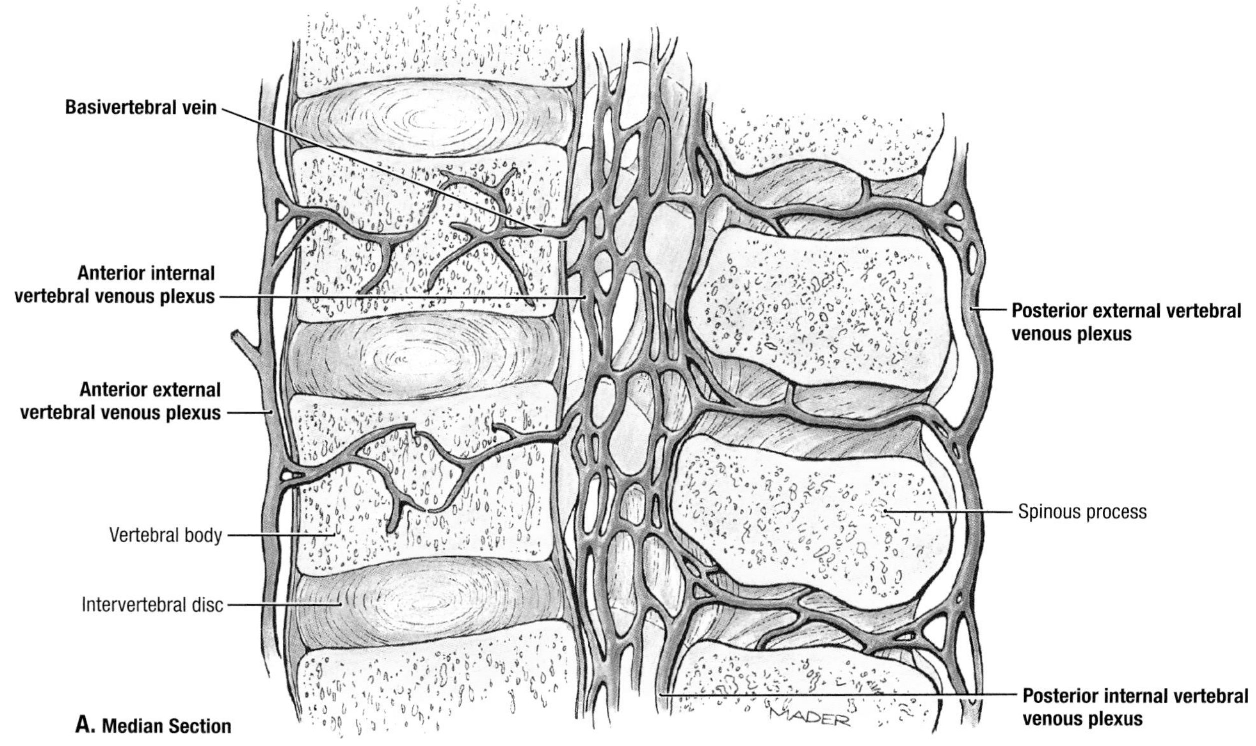
Basivertebral vein
Anterior internal vertebral venous plexus
Anterior external vertebral venous plexus
Vertebral body
Intervertebral disc
Posterior external vertebral venous plexus
Spinous process
Posterior internal vertebral venous plexus
MADER

**A.** Median Section

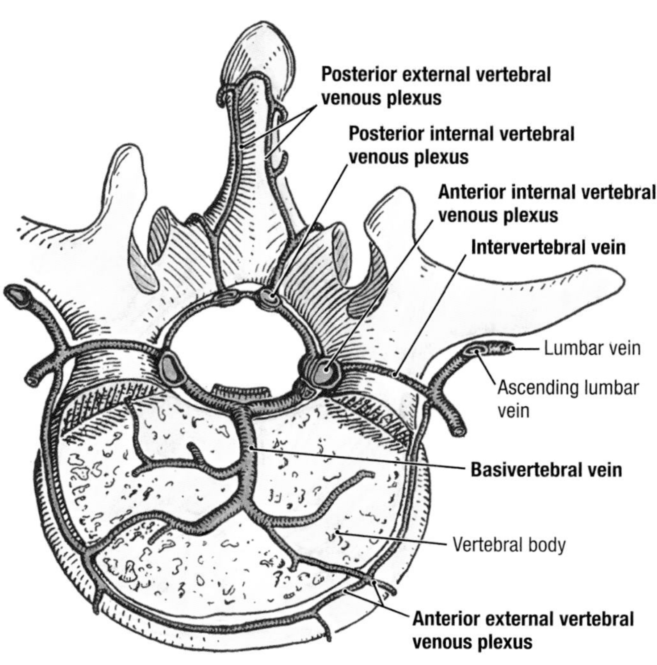
Posterior external vertebral venous plexus
Posterior internal vertebral venous plexus
Anterior internal vertebral venous plexus
Intervertebral vein
Lumbar vein
Ascending lumbar vein
Basivertebral vein
Vertebral body
Anterior external vertebral venous plexus

**B.** Superior View

## 4.20 Vertebral venous plexuses

**A.** Median section of lumbar spine. **B.** Superior view of lumbar vertebra with the vertebral body sectioned transversely.

- There are internal and external vertebral venous plexuses, communicating with each other and with both systemic veins and the portal system. Infection and tumors can spread from the areas drained by the systemic and portal veins to the vertebral venous system and lodge in the vertebrae, spinal cord, brain, or skull.
- The internal vertebral venous plexus, located in the vertebral canal, consists of a plexus of thin-walled, valveless veins that surround the dura mater. Cranially, the internal venous plexus communicates through the foramen magnum with the occipital and basilar sinuses; at each spinal segment, the plexus receives veins from the spinal cord and a basivertebral vein from the vertebral body. The plexus is drained by intervertebral veins that pass through the intervertebral and sacral foramina to the vertebral, intercostal, lumbar, and lateral sacral veins.
- The anterior external vertebral venous plexus is formed by veins that course through the body of each vertebra. Veins that pass through the ligamenta flava form the posterior external vertebral venous plexus. In the cervical region, these plexuses communicate with the occipital and deep cervical veins. In the thoracic, lumbar, and pelvic regions, the azygos (or hemiazygos), ascending lumbar, and lateral sacral veins, respectively, further link segment to segment.

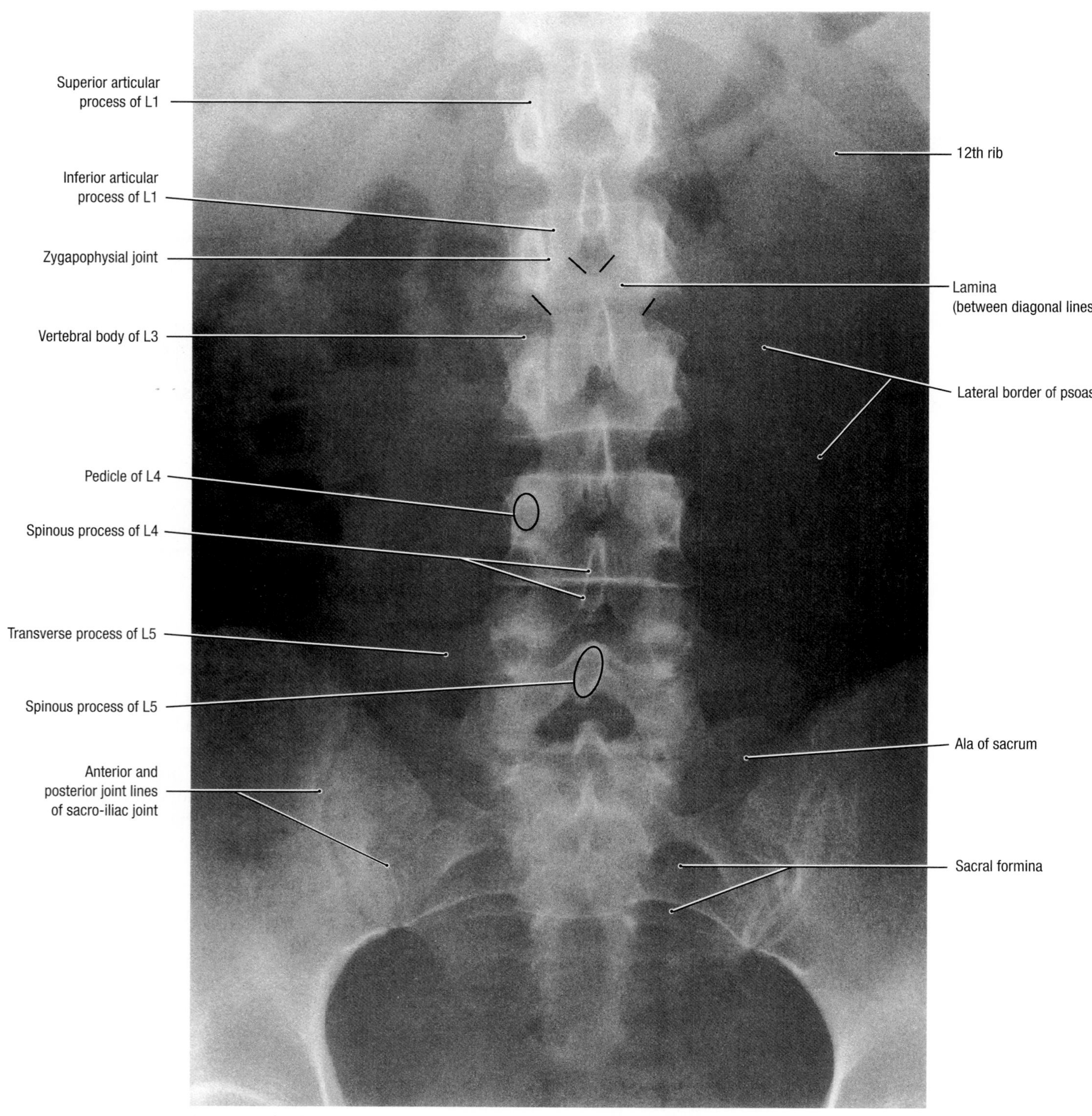
Superior articular process of L1
Inferior articular process of L1
Zygapophysial joint
Vertebral body of L3
Pedicle of L4
Spinous process of L4
Transverse process of L5
Spinous process of L5
Anterior and posterior joint lines of sacro-iliac joint
12th rib
Lamina (between diagonal lines)
Lateral border of psoas
Ala of sacrum
Sacral formina

**Anteroposterior View**

## 4.21 Radiograph of inferior thoracic and lumbosacral spine

Note the bodies and processes of the five lumbar vertebrae, the labeled spinous and transverse processes of L5, the sinuous sacro-iliac joint, the lateral margin of the right and left psoas muscles, and the 12th rib.

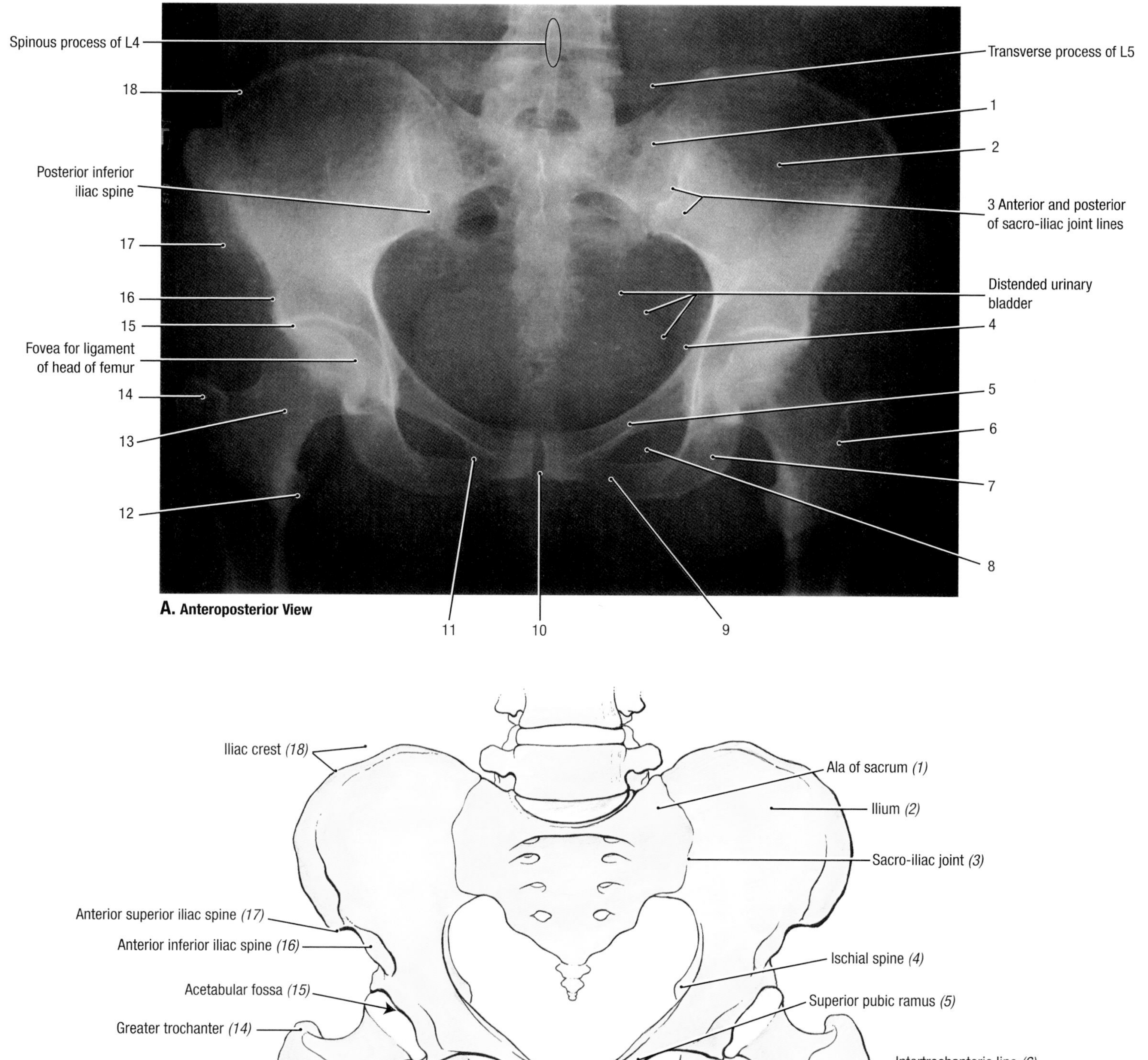
Spinous process of L4
18
Posterior inferior iliac spine
17
16
15
Fovea for ligament of head of femur
14
13
12
Transverse process of L5
1
2
3 Anterior and posterior of sacro-iliac joint lines
Distended urinary bladder
4
5
6
7
8
A. Anteroposterior View
11
10
9
Iliac crest (18)
Ala of sacrum (1)
Ilium (2)
Sacro-iliac joint (3)
Anterior superior iliac spine (17)
Anterior inferior iliac spine (16)
Acetabular fossa (15)
Greater trochanter (14)
Neck of femur (13)
Lesser trochanter (12)
Ischial spine (4)
Superior pubic ramus (5)
Intertrochanteric line (6)
Ischial tuberosity (7)
Obturator foramen (8)
Pubic tubercle (11)
Body of pubis
Ischiopubic ramus (9)
Pubic symphysis (10)
B. Anterior View
MADER

**4.22 Pelvis**

**A.** Radiograph of pelvis. **B.** Bony pelvis with articulated femora.

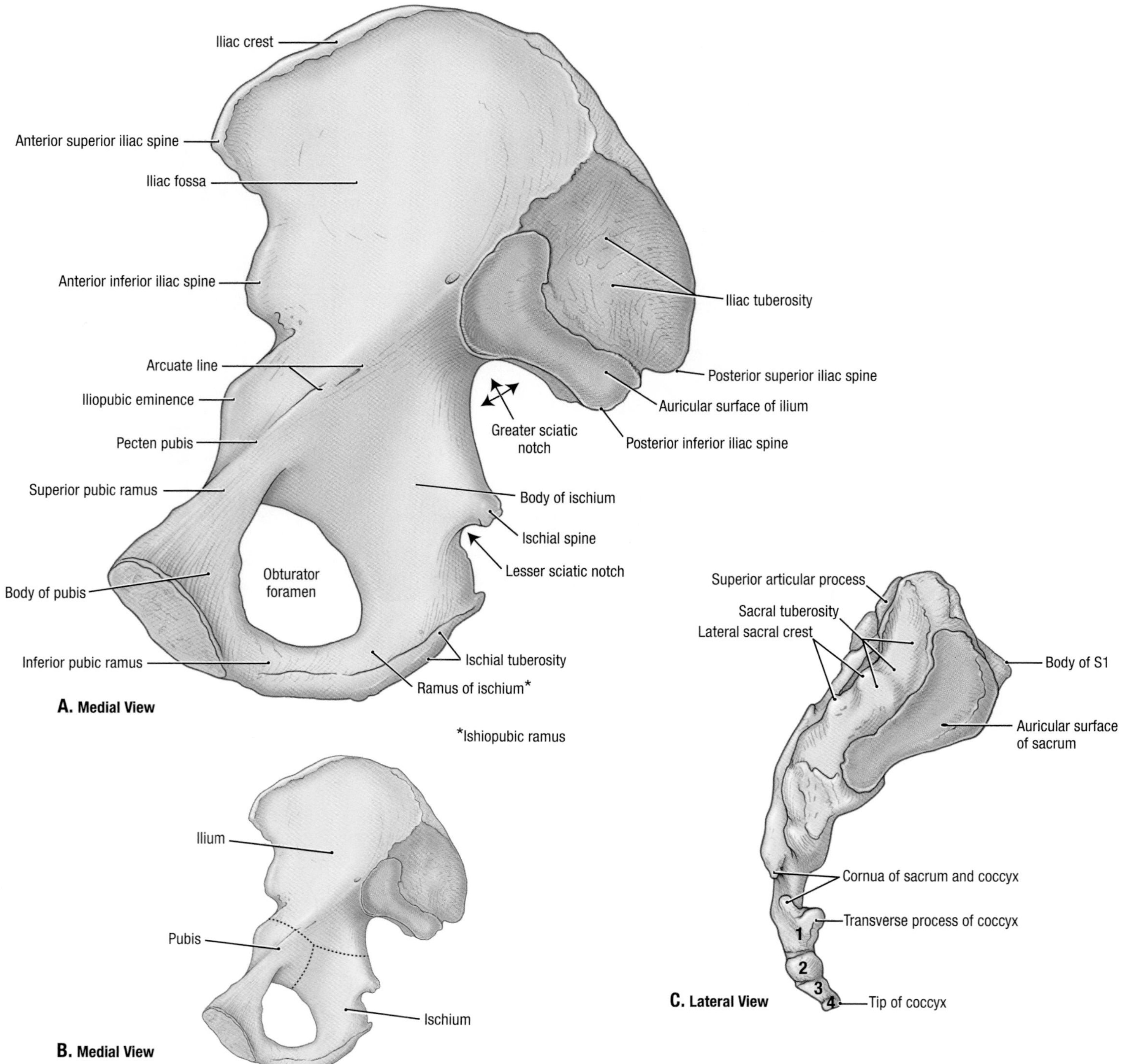
Iliac crest
Anterior superior iliac spine
Iliac fossa
Anterior inferior iliac spine
Arcuate line
Iliopubic eminence
Pecten pubis
Superior pubic ramus
Body of pubis
Inferior pubic ramus
Obturator foramen
Iliac tuberosity
Posterior superior iliac spine
Auricular surface of ilium
Posterior inferior iliac spine
Greater sciatic notch
Body of ischium
Ischial spine
Lesser sciatic notch
Ischial tuberosity
Ramus of ischium*
A. Medial View
*Ishiopubic ramus
Ilium
Pubis
Ischium
B. Medial View
Superior articular process
Sacral tuberosity
Lateral sacral crest
Body of S1
Auricular surface of sacrum
Cornua of sacrum and coccyx
Transverse process of coccyx
1
2
3
4
Tip of coccyx
C. Lateral View

## 4.23 Hip bone, sacrum, and coccyx

**A.** Features of hip bone. **B.** Ilium, ischium, and pubis. **C.** Sacrum and coccyx.

- Each hip bone consists of three bones: ilium, ischium, and pubis. The ilium is the superior, larger part of the hip bone, forming the superior part of the acetabulum, the deep socket on the lateral aspect of the hip bone that articulates with the head of the femur. The ischium forms the posteroinferior part of the acetabulum and hip bone. The pubis forms the anterior part of the acetabulum and anteromedial part of the hip bone.
- Anterosuperiorly, the auricular, ear-shaped surface of the sacrum articulates with the auricular surface of the ilium; the sacral and iliac tuberosities are for the attachment of the posterior sacro-iliac and interosseous sacro-iliac ligaments.

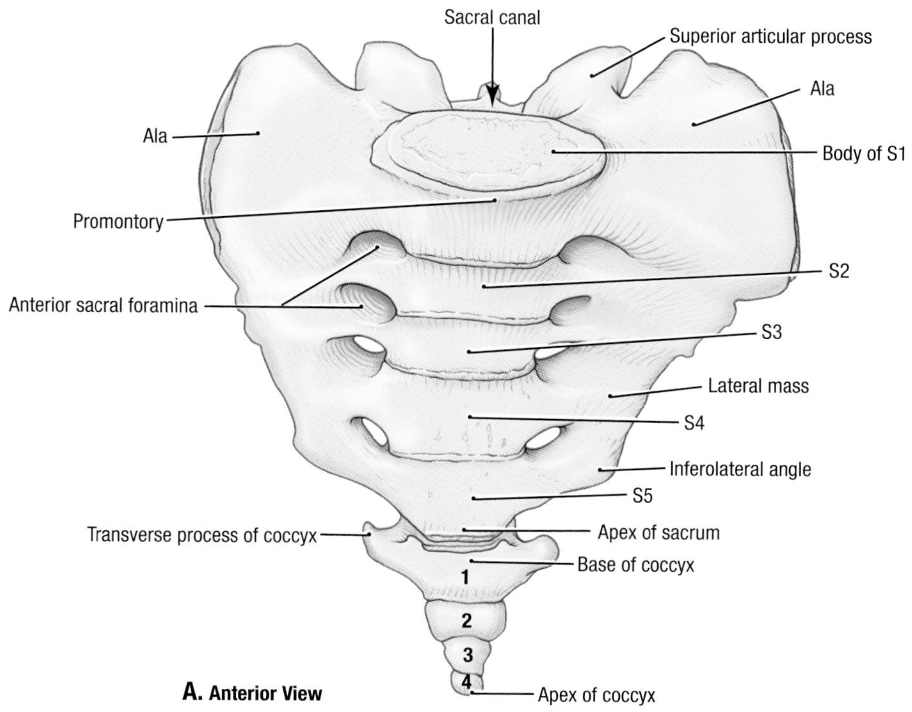
Sacral canal
Superior articular process
Ala
Ala
Body of S1
Promontory
S2
Anterior sacral foramina
S3
Lateral mass
S4
Inferolateral angle
S5
Transverse process of coccyx
Apex of sacrum
Base of coccyx
1
2
3
4
Apex of coccyx

**A. Anterior View**

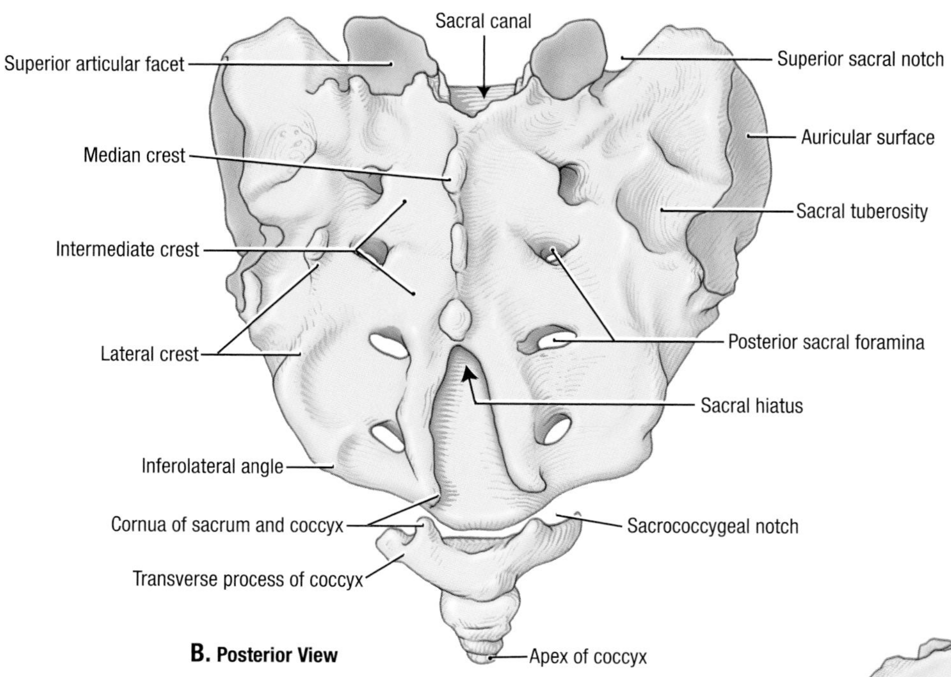
Sacral canal
Superior articular facet
Superior sacral notch
Auricular surface
Median crest
Sacral tuberosity
Intermediate crest
Posterior sacral foramina
Lateral crest
Sacral hiatus
Inferolateral angle
Cornua of sacrum and coccyx
Sacrococcygeal notch
Transverse process of coccyx
Apex of coccyx

**B. Posterior View**

1

2

3

4

5

**C. Anterior View**

## 4.24 Sacrum and coccyx

**A.** Pelvic (anterior) surface. **B.** Dorsal (posterior surface). **C.** Sacrum in youth.

- In **A** the five sacral bodies are demarcated in the mature sacrum by four transverse lines ending laterally in four pairs of anterior sacral foramina. The coccyx has four pieces—the first having a pair of transverse processes and a pair of cornua (horns).
- The costal (lateral) elements begin to fuse around puberty. The bodies begin to fuse from inferior to superior at about the 17th to 18th year, with fusion usually completed by the 23rd year.

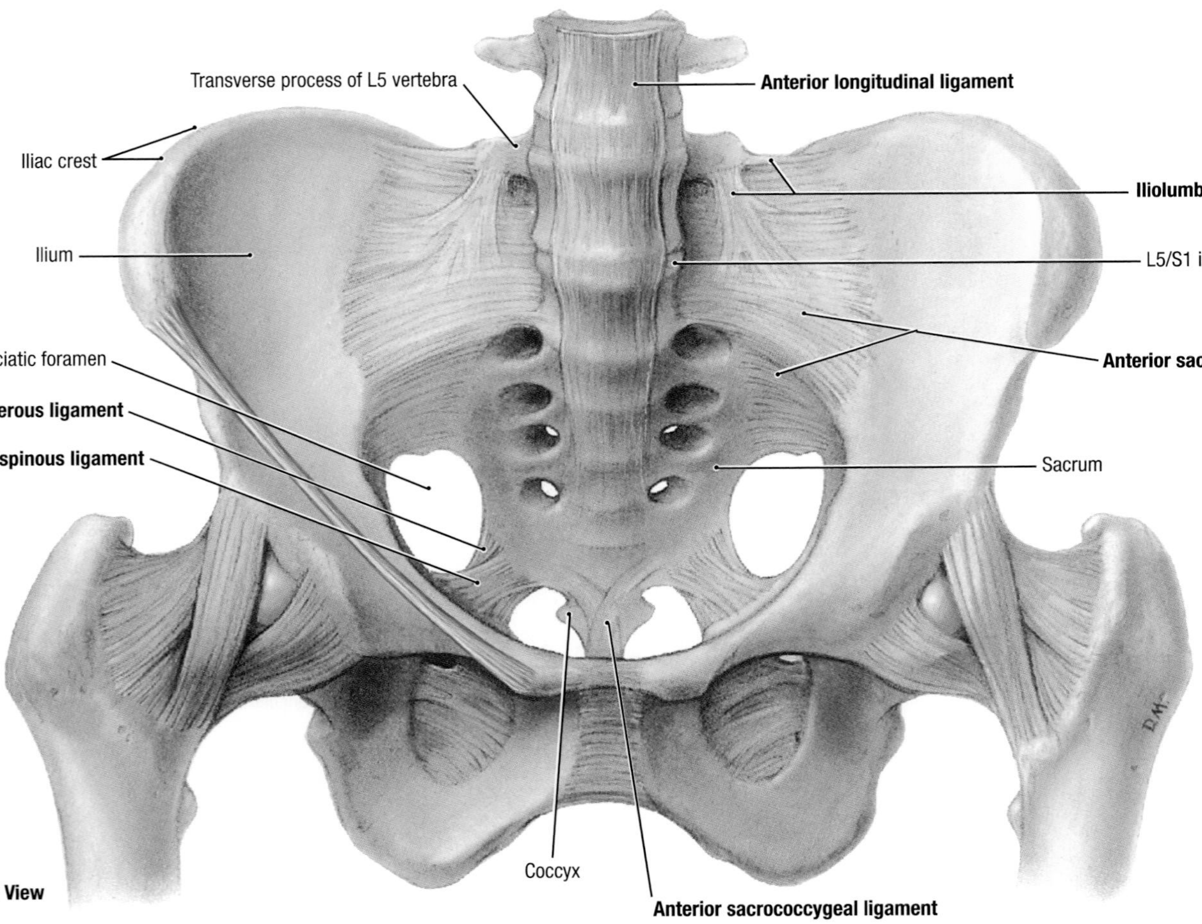

Transverse process of L5 vertebra
Anterior longitudinal ligament
Iliac crest
Iliolumbar ligament
Ilium
L5/S1 intervertebral disc
Greater sciatic foramen
Anterior sacro-iliac ligament
Sacrotuberous ligament
Sacrospinous ligament
Sacrum
Coccyx
Anterior sacrococcygeal ligament

**A. Anterior View**

## 4.25 Lumbar and pelvic ligaments

- The anterior sacro-iliac ligament is part of the fibrous capsule anteriorly and spans between the lateral aspect of the sacrum and the ilium, anterior to the auricular surfaces.

During pregnancy, the pelvic joint and ligaments relax, and pelvic movements increase. The sacro-iliac interlocking mechanism is less effective because the relaxation permits greater rotation of the pelvis and contributes to the lordotic posture often assumed during pregnancy with the change in the center of gravity. Relaxation of the sacro-iliac joints and pubic symphysis permits as much as 10–15% increase in diameters (mostly transverse), facilitating passage of the fetus through the pelvic canal. The coccyx is also allowed to move posteriorly.

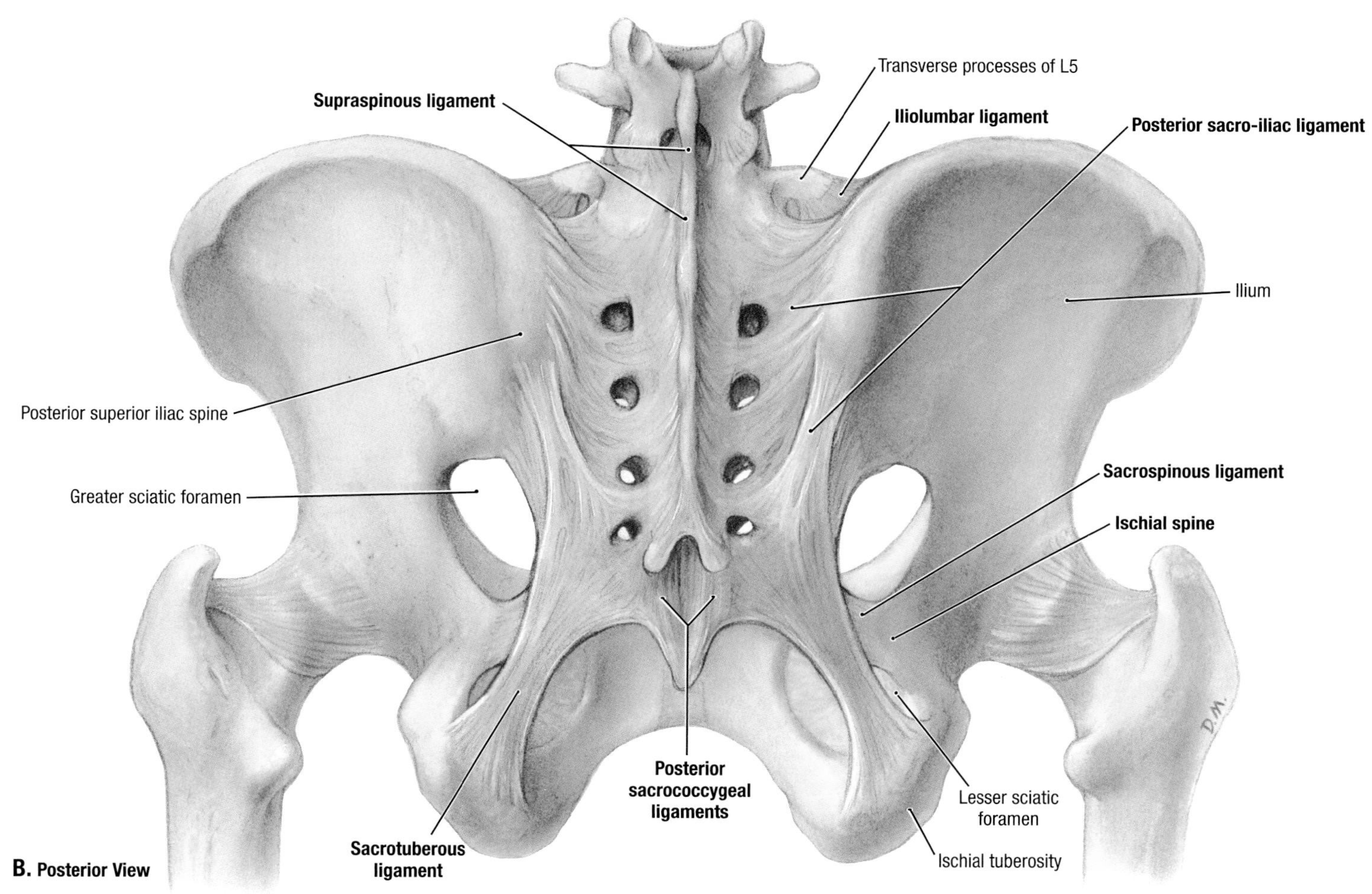
Transverse processes of L5
Supraspinous ligament
Iliolumbar ligament
Posterior sacro-iliac ligament
Ilium
Posterior superior iliac spine
Greater sciatic foramen
Sacrospinous ligament
Ischial spine
Posterior sacrococcygeal ligaments
Lesser sciatic foramen
Sacrotuberous ligament
Ischial tuberosity
B. Posterior View

## 4.25 Lumbar and pelvic ligaments *(continued)*

- The sacrotuberous ligaments attach the sacrum, ilium, and coccyx to the ischial tuberosity; the sacrospinous ligaments unite the sacrum and coccyx to the ischial spine. The sacrotuberous and sacrospinous ligaments convert the sciatic notches of the hip bones into greater and lesser sciatic foramina.
- The fibers of the posterior sacro-iliac ligament vary in obliquity; the superior fibers are shorter and lie between the ilium and superior part of the sacrum; the longer, obliquely oriented inferior fibers span between the posterior superior iliac spine and the inferior part of the sacrum, also blending with the sacrotuberous ligament.
- The interosseous sacro-iliac ligament lies deep to the posterior sacro-iliac ligament (see Fig. 4.26).
- The iliolumbar ligaments unite the ilia and transverse processes of L5; the lumbosacral portions of the ligaments descend to the alae of the sacrum and blend with the anterior sacro-iliac ligaments.

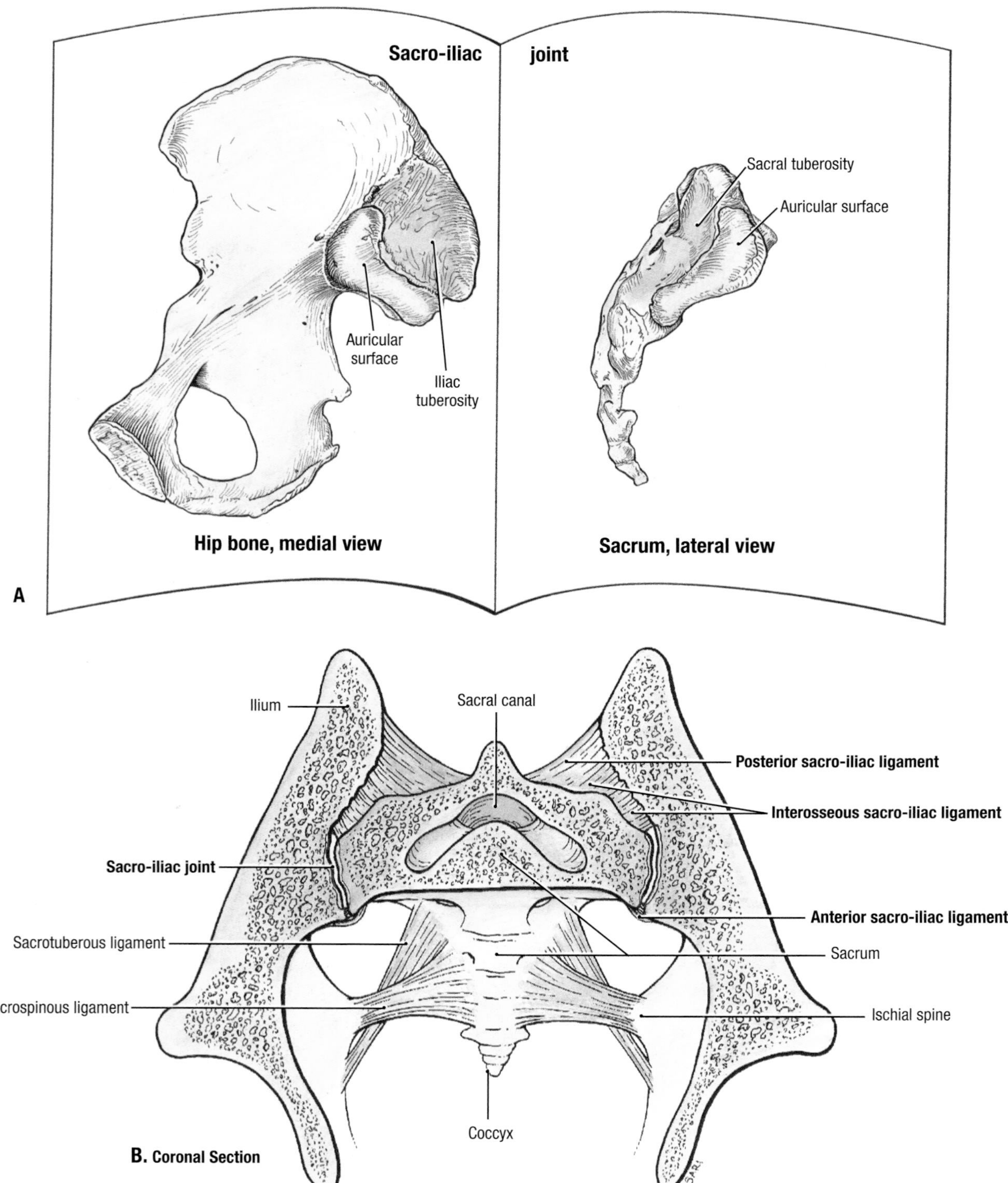
Sacro-iliac
joint
Auricular surface
Iliac tuberosity
Sacral tuberosity
Auricular surface
Hip bone, medial view
Sacrum, lateral view
A
Ilium
Sacral canal
Posterior sacro-iliac ligament
Interosseous sacro-iliac ligament
Sacro-iliac joint
Anterior sacro-iliac ligament
Sacrotuberous ligament
Sacrum
Sacrospinous ligament
Ischial spine
Coccyx
B. Coronal Section

## 4.26 Articular surfaces of sacro-iliac joint and ligaments

**A.** Articular surfaces. Note the auricular surface (articular area, *blue*) of the sacrum and hip bone and the roughened areas superior and posterior to the auricular areas *(orange)* for the attachment of the interosseous sacro-iliac ligament. **B.** Sacro-iliac ligaments. Note the sacro-iliac joints and the strong interosseous sacro-iliac ligament that lies inferior and anterior to the posterior sacro-iliac ligament. The interosseous sacro-iliac ligament consists of short fibers connecting the sacral tuberosity to the iliac tuberosity. The sacrum is suspended from the ilia by the sacro-iliac ligaments.

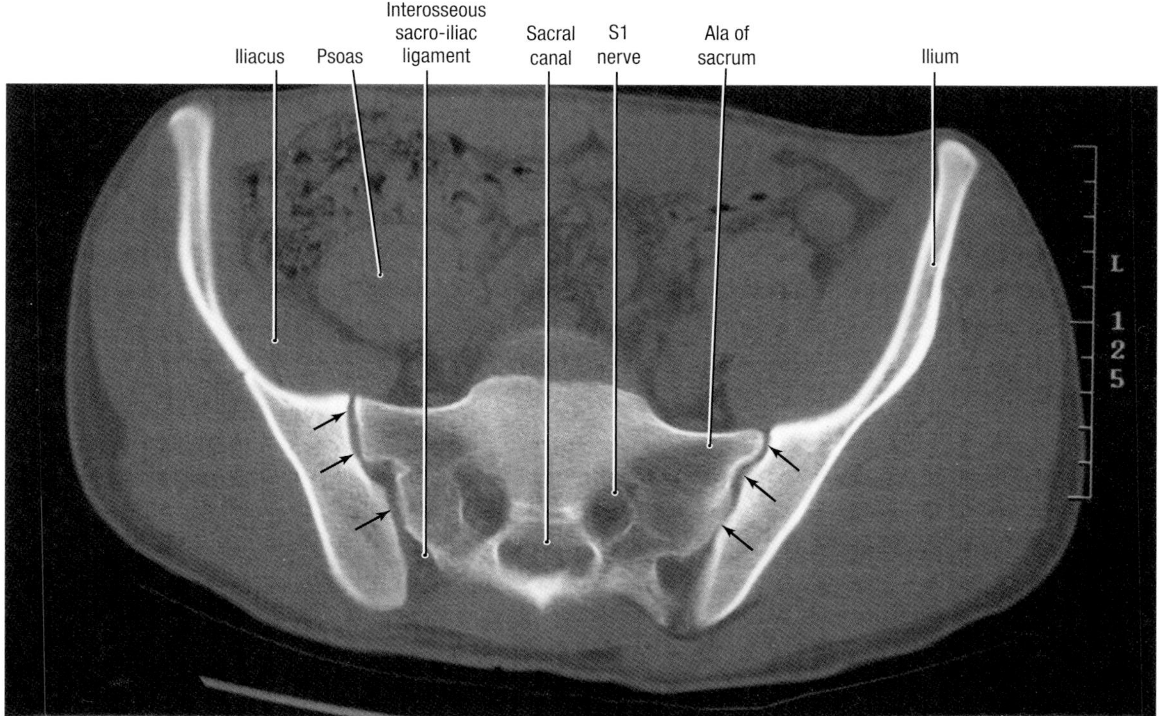
Iliacus
Psoas
Interosseous sacro-iliac ligament
Sacral canal
S1 nerve
Ala of sacrum
Ilium
L
1
2
5

**A.** Transverse (axial) CT Scan

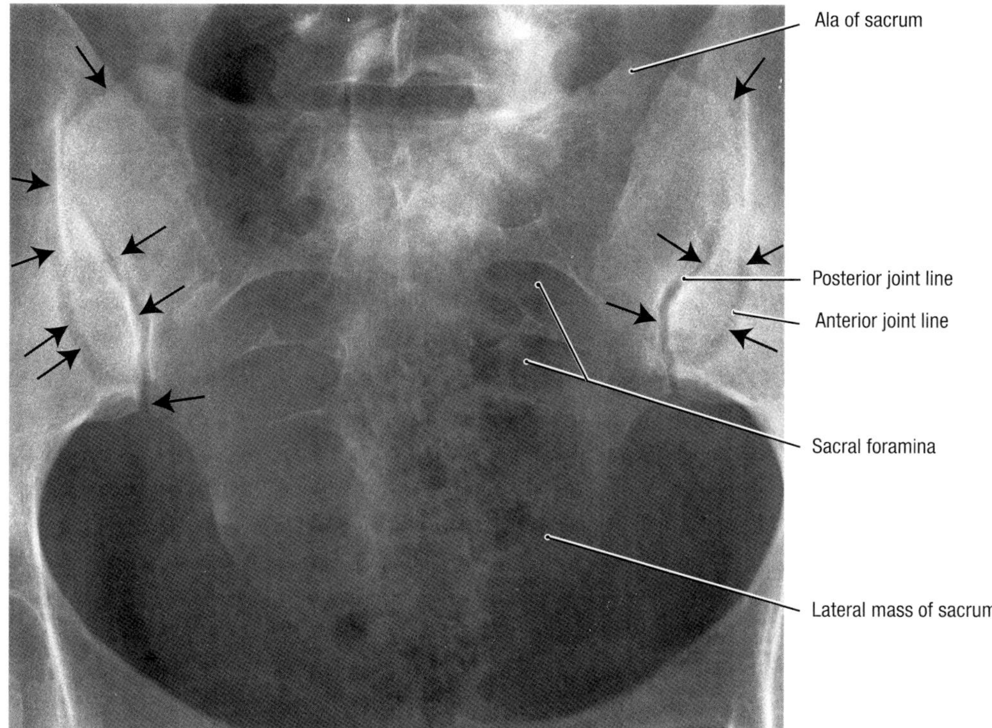
Ala of sacrum
Posterior joint line
Anterior joint line
Sacral foramina
Lateral mass of sacrum

**B.** Anteroposterior View

## 4.27 Imaging of the sacro-iliac joint

**A.** CT scan. The sacro-iliac joint is indicated by *arrows*. Note that the articular surfaces of the ilium and sacrum have irregular shapes that result in partial interlocking of the bones. The sacro-iliac joint is oblique, with the anterior aspect of the joint situated lateral to the posterior aspect of the joint. **B.** Radiograph. Due to the oblique placement of the sacro-iliac joints, the anterior and posterior joint lines appear separately.

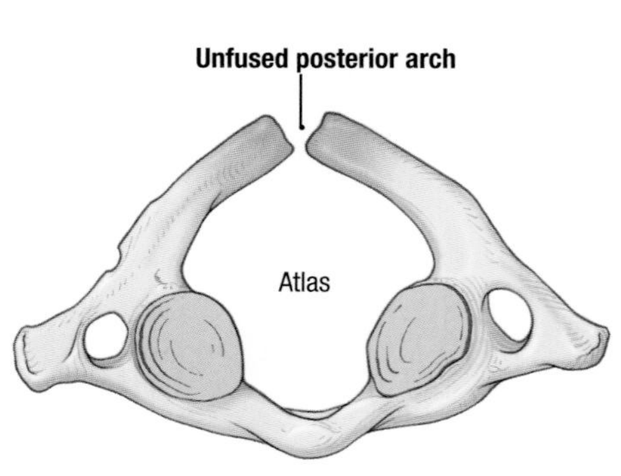
Unfused posterior arch
Atlas

A. Inferior View

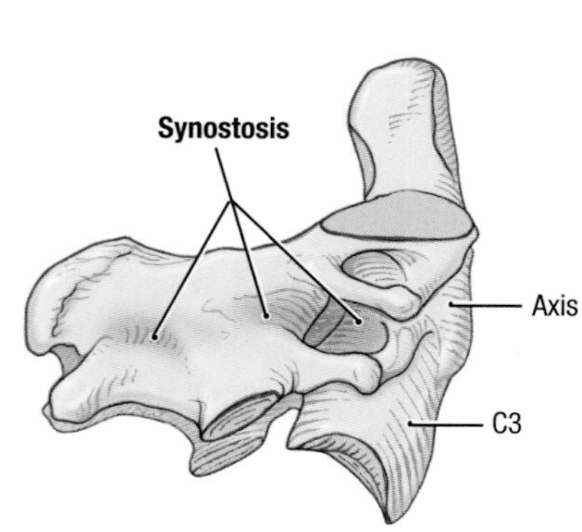
Synostosis
Axis
C3

B. Lateral View

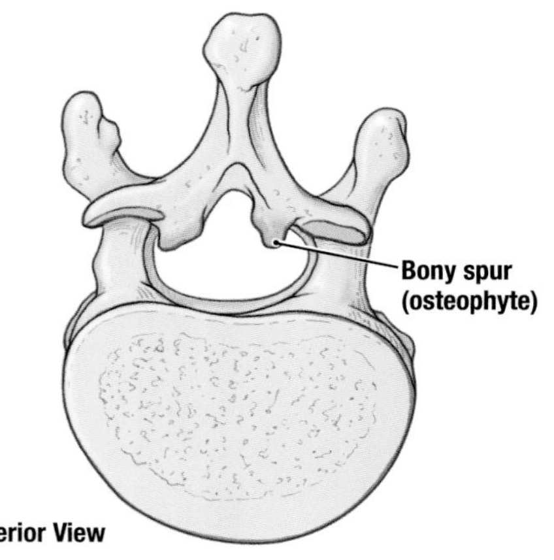
Bony spur
(osteophyte)

C. Superior View

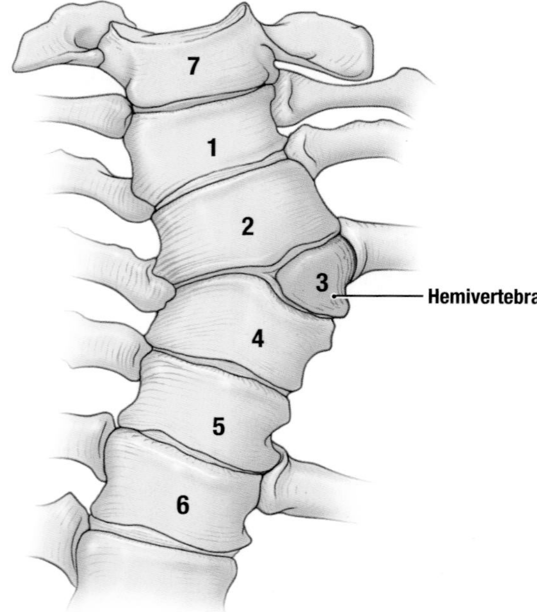
7
1
2
3
Hemivertebra
4
5
6

D. Anterior View

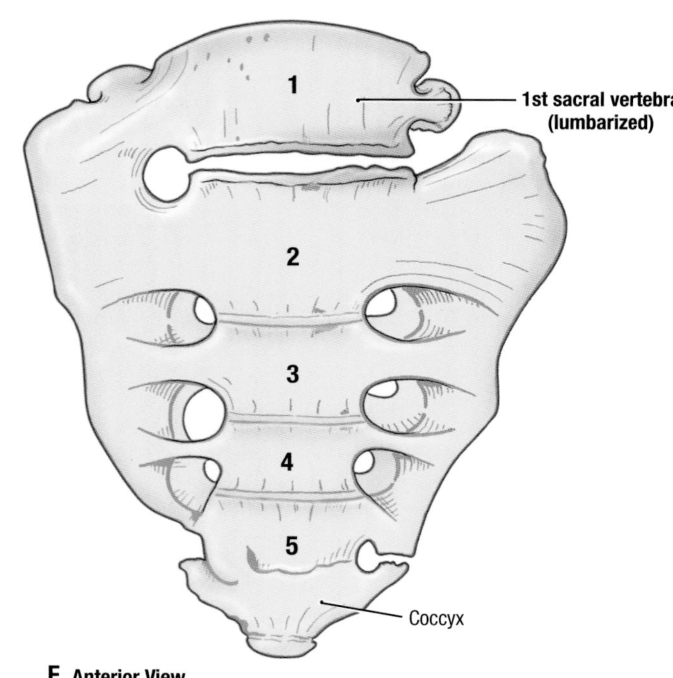
1
1st sacral vertebra
(lumbarized)
2
3
4
5
Coccyx

E. Anterior View

## 4.28 Anomalies of the vertebrae

**A.** Unfused posterior arch of the atlas. The centrum fused to the right and left halves of the neural arch, but the arch did not fuse in the midline posteriorly. **B.** Synostosis (fusion) of vertebrae C2 (axis) and C3. **C.** Bony spurs. Sharp bony spurs may grow from the laminae inferiorly into the ligamenta flava, thereby reducing the lengths of the functional portions of these ligaments. When the vertebral column is flexed, the ligaments may be torn. **D.** Hemivertebra. The entire right half of T3 and the corresponding rib are absent. The left lamina and the spine are fused with those of T4, and the left intervertebral foramen is reduced in size. Observe the associated scoliosis (lateral curvature of the spine). **E.** Transitional lumbosacral vertebra. Here, the 1st sacral vertebra is partly free (lumbarized). Not uncommonly, the 5th lumbar vertebra may be partly fused to the sacrum (sacralized).

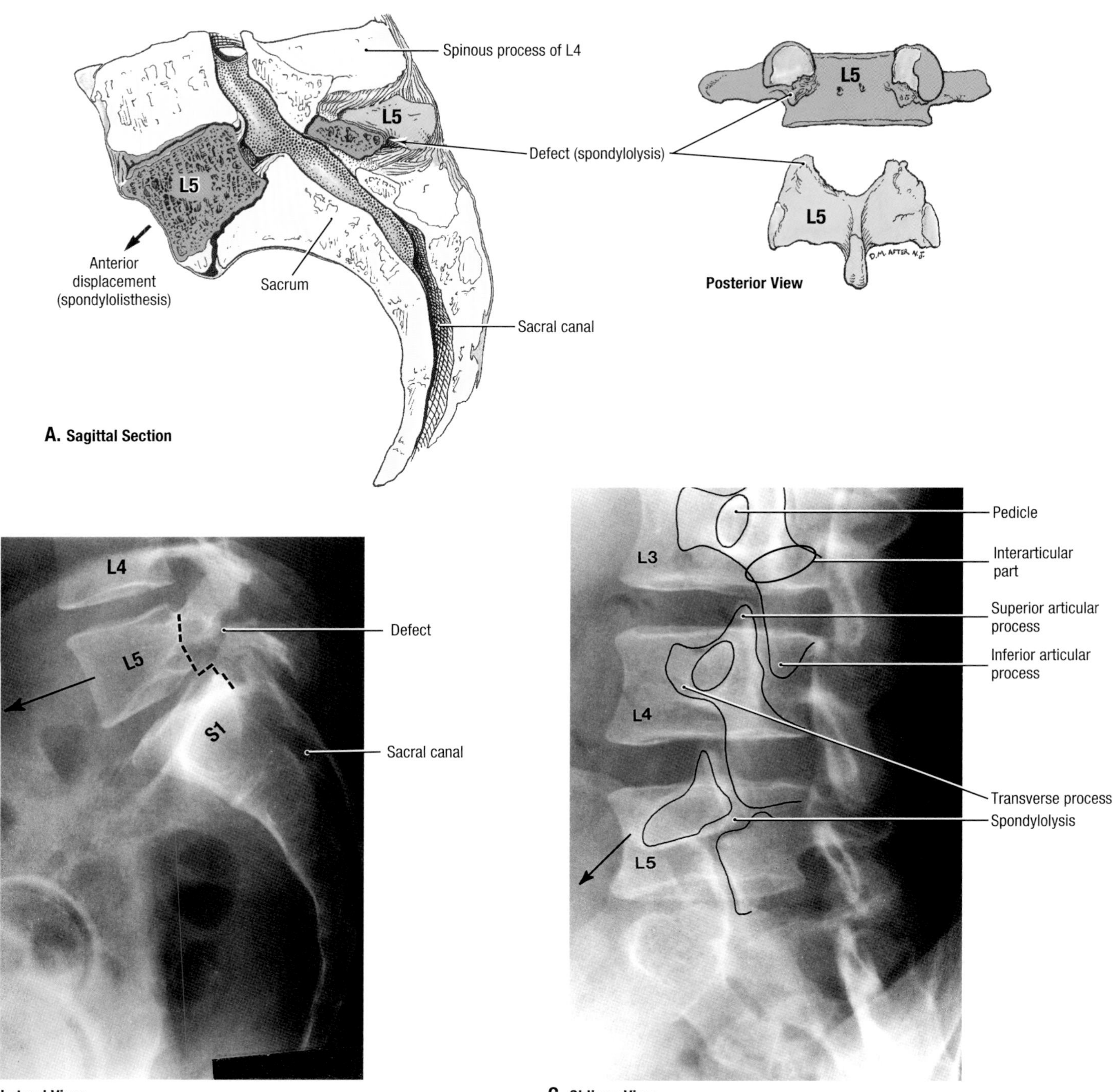
Spinous process of L4
L5
L5
Defect (spondylolysis)
Anterior displacement (spondylolisthesis)
Sacrum
Sacral canal
L5
L5
Posterior View
A. Sagittal Section
L4
L5
S1
Defect
Sacral canal
B. Lateral View
L3
L4
L5
Pedicle
Interarticular part
Superior articular process
Inferior articular process
Transverse process
Spondylolysis
C. Oblique View

## 4.29 Spondylolysis and spondylolisthesis

**A.** Articulated and isolated spondylolytic L5 vertebra. The vertebra has an oblique defect (spondylolysis) through the interarticular part (pars interarticularis). The defect may be traumatic or congenital in origin. The interarticular part is the region of the lamina of a lumbar vertebra between the superior and inferior articular processes. Also, the vertebral body of L5 has slipped anteriorly (spondylolisthesis). **B** and **C.** Radiographs. In **B,** the *dotted line* following the posterior vertebral margins of L5 and the sacrum shows the anterior displacement of L5 *(arrow)*. In **C,** note the superimposed outline of a dog: the head is the transverse process, the eye is the pedicle, and the ear is the superior articular process. The lucent (dark) cleft across the "neck" of the dog is the spondylolysis; the anterior displacement *(arrow)* is the spondylolisthesis.

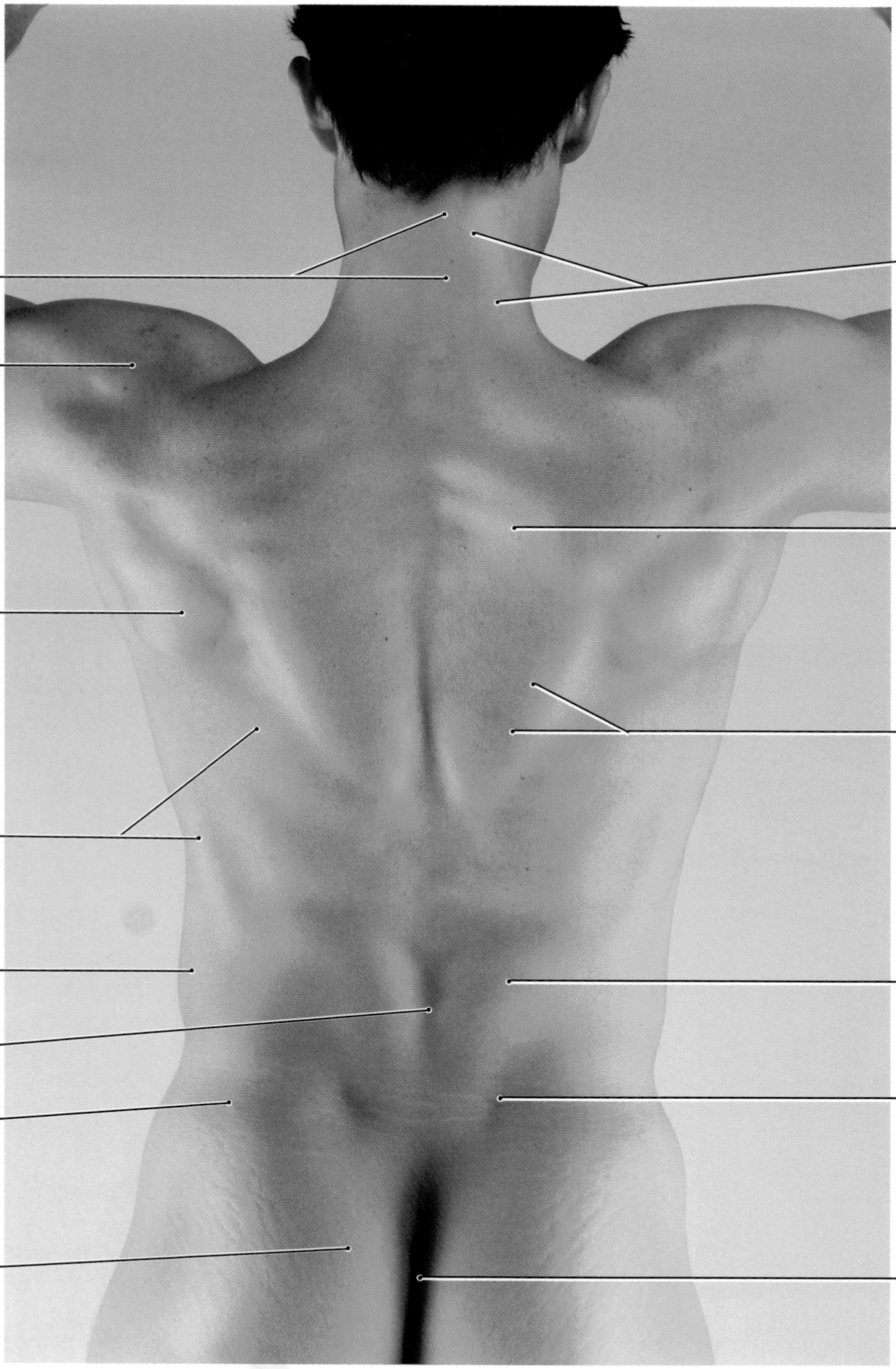

Site of nuchal ligament
Spinal (posterior) part of deltoid
Teres major
Latissimus dorsi
External oblique
Posterior median furrow
Gluteus medius
Gluteus maximus
Posterior View
Descending (superior) part of trapezius
Transverse (middle) part of trapezius
Ascending (inferior) part of trapezius
Erector spine
Site of posterior superior iliac spine
Intergluteal cleft

## 4.30 Surface anatomy of back

- The arms are abducted, so the scapulae have rotated superiorly on the thoracic wall.
- The latissimus dorsi and teres major muscles form the posterior axillary fold.
- The trapezius muscle has three parts: descending, transverse, and ascending.
- Note the deep median furrow that separates the longitudinal bulges formed by the contracted erector spinae group of muscles;
- Dimples (depressions) indicate the site of the posterior superior iliac spines, which usually lie at the level of the sacro-iliac joint.

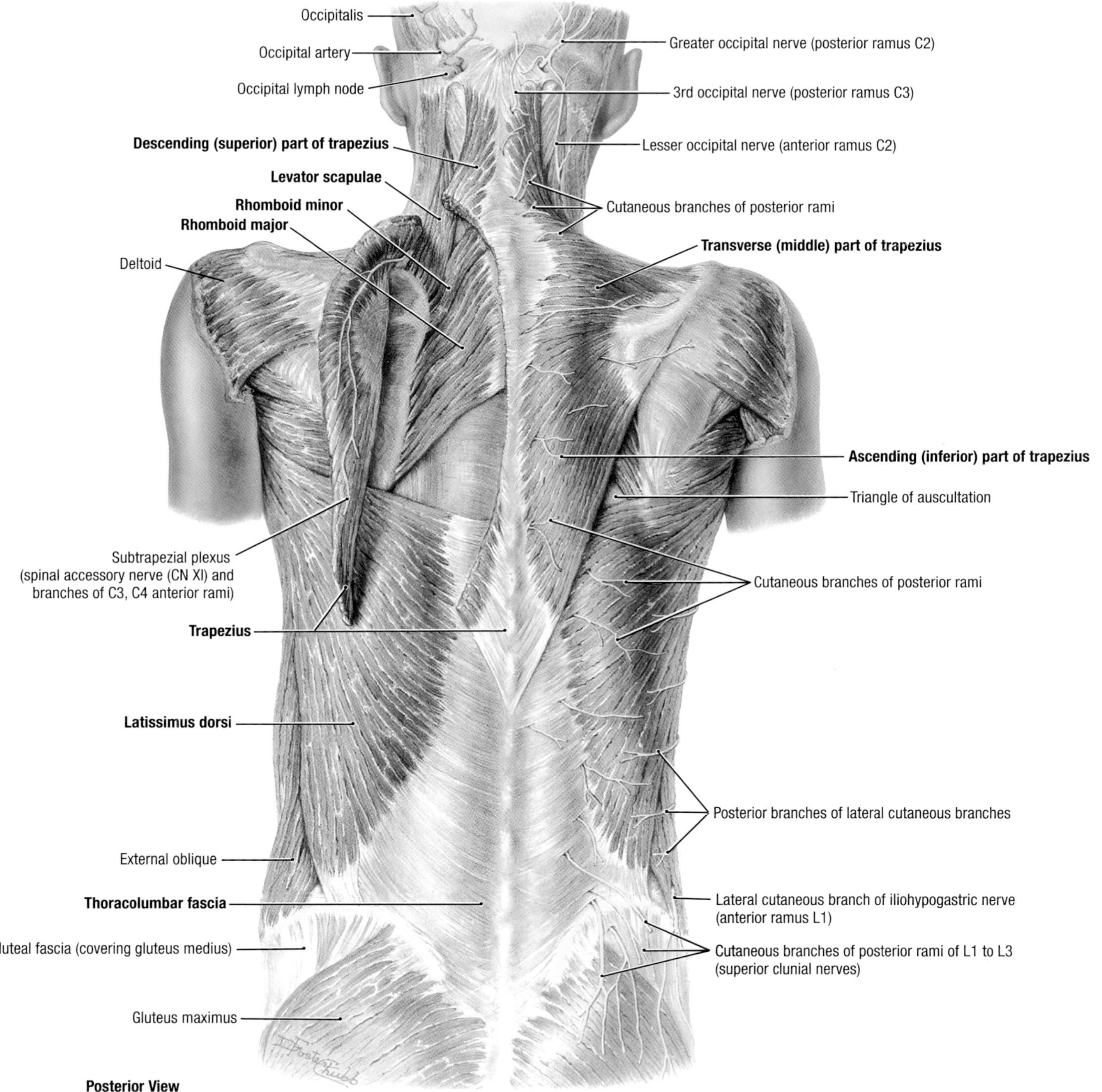
Occipitalis
Occipital artery
Occipital lymph node
Descending (superior) part of trapezius
Levator scapulae
Rhomboid minor
Rhomboid major
Deltoid
Greater occipital nerve (posterior ramus C2)
3rd occipital nerve (posterior ramus C3)
Lesser occipital nerve (anterior ramus C2)
Cutaneous branches of posterior rami
Transverse (middle) part of trapezius
Ascending (inferior) part of trapezius
Triangle of auscultation
Subtrapezial plexus (spinal accessory nerve (CN XI) and branches of C3, C4 anterior rami)
Cutaneous branches of posterior rami
Trapezius
Latissimus dorsi
Posterior branches of lateral cutaneous branches
External oblique
Thoracolumbar fascia
Lateral cutaneous branch of iliohypogastric nerve (anterior ramus L1)
Gluteal fascia (covering gluteus medius)
Cutaneous branches of posterior rami of L1 to L3 (superior clunial nerves)
Gluteus maximus
Posterior View

## 4.31 Superficial muscles of back

On the *left*, the trapezius muscle is reflected. Observe two layers: the trapezius and latissimus dorsi muscles, and the levator scapulae and rhomboids minor and major. These axial appendicular muscles help attach the upper limb to the trunk.

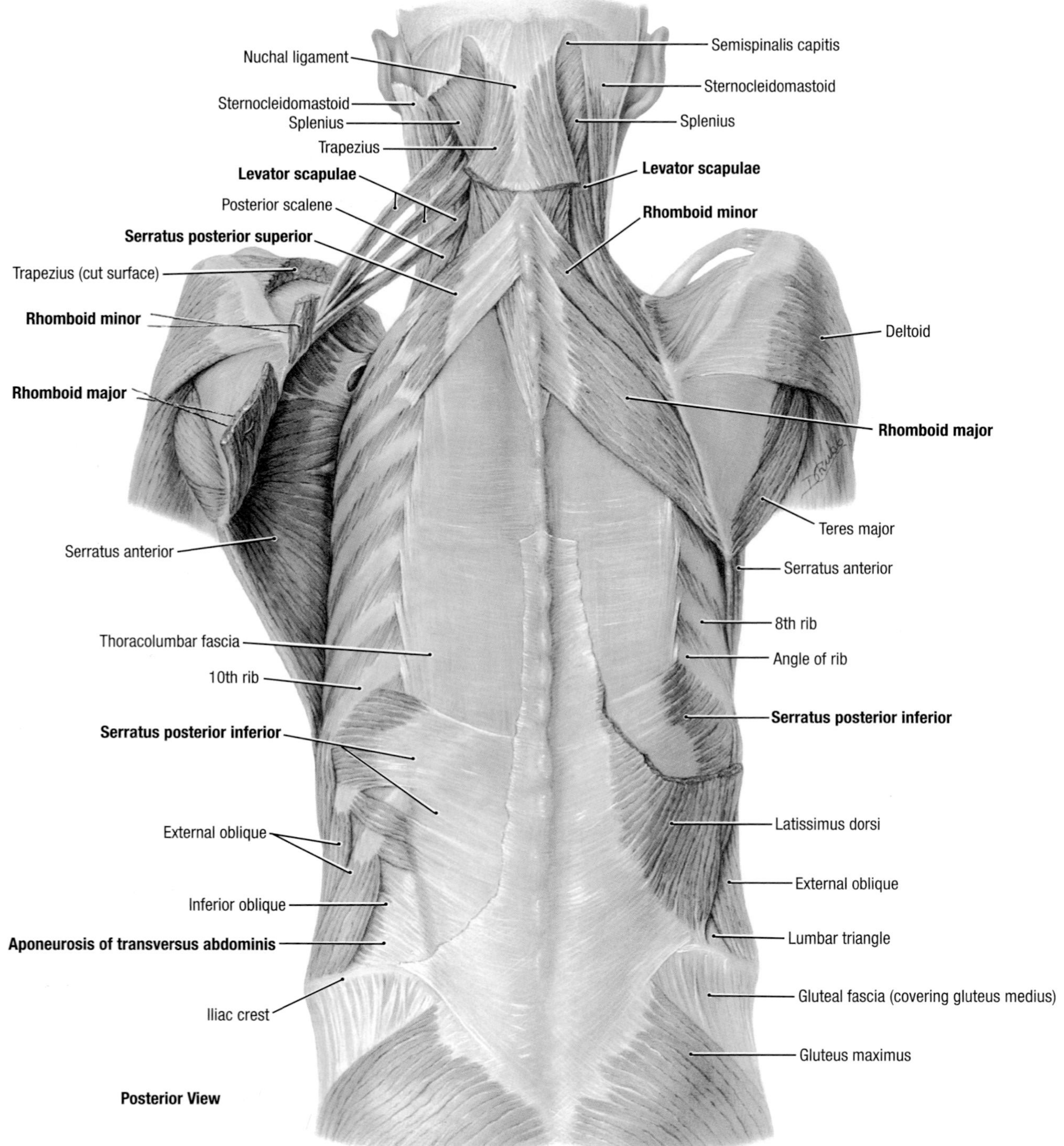
Nuchal ligament
Semispinalis capitis
Sternocleidomastoid
Sternocleidomastoid
Splenius
Splenius
Trapezius
Levator scapulae
Levator scapulae
Posterior scalene
Rhomboid minor
Serratus posterior superior
Trapezius (cut surface)
Rhomboid minor
Deltoid
Rhomboid major
Rhomboid major
Teres major
Serratus anterior
Serratus anterior
8th rib
Thoracolumbar fascia
Angle of rib
10th rib
Serratus posterior inferior
Serratus posterior inferior
Latissimus dorsi
External oblique
External oblique
Inferior oblique
Lumbar triangle
Aponeurosis of transversus abdominis
Gluteal fascia (covering gluteus medius)
Iliac crest
Gluteus maximus
Posterior View

## 4.32 Intermediate muscles of back

The trapezius and latissimus dorsi muscles are largely cut away on both sides. On the *left*, the rhomboid muscles have been severed, allowing the vertebral border of the scapula to be raised from the thoracic wall. The serratus posterior superior and inferior form the intermediate layer of muscles, passing from the vertebral spines to the ribs; the two muscles slope in opposite directions and are muscles of respiration. The thoracolumbar fascia extends laterally to the angles of the ribs, becoming thin superiorly and passing deep to the serratus posterior superior muscle. The fascia gives attachment to the latissimus dorsi and serratus posterior inferior muscles (see Fig. 4.34).

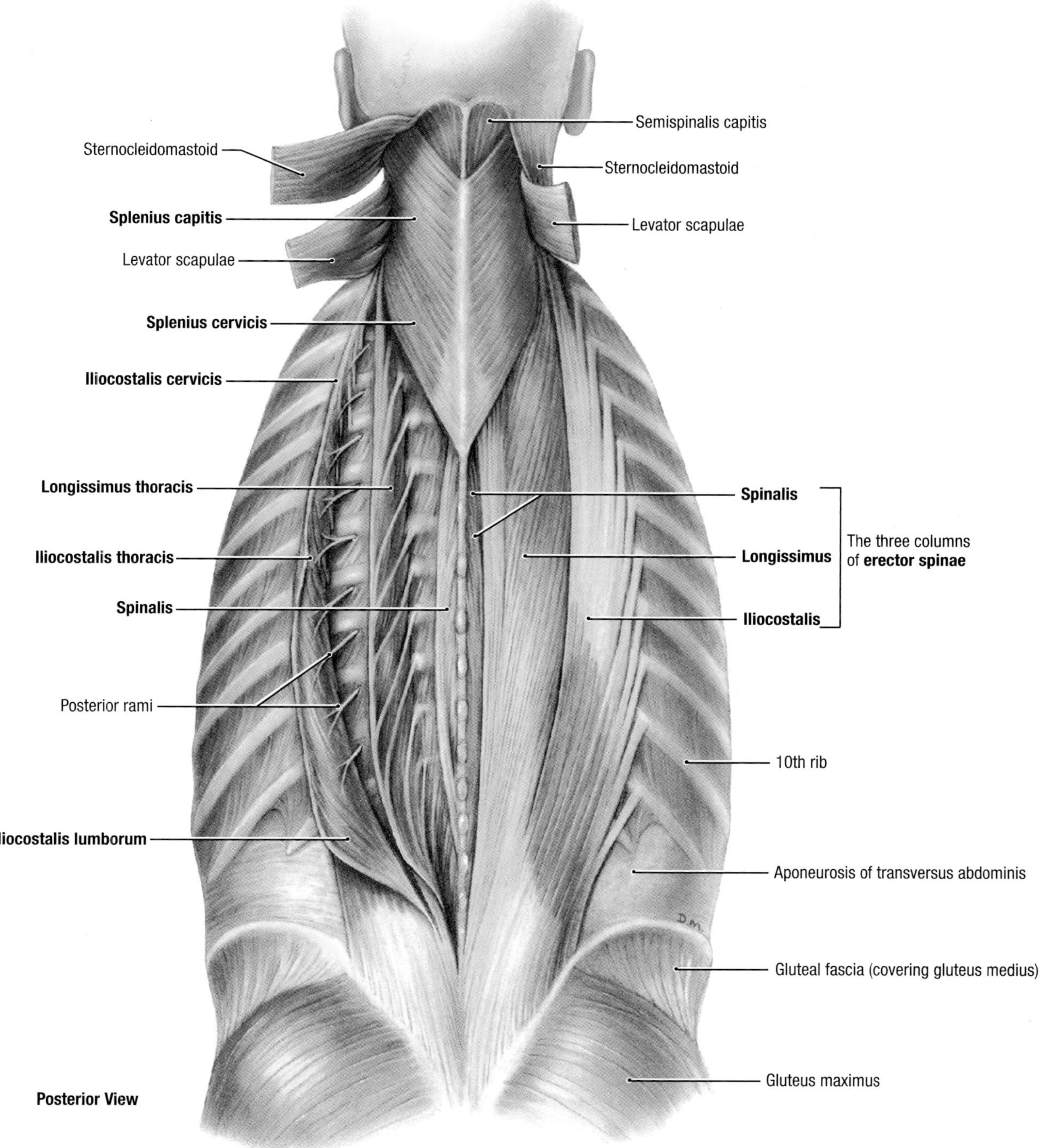
Sternocleidomastoid
Splenius capitis
Levator scapulae
Splenius cervicis
Iliocostalis cervicis
Longissimus thoracis
Iliocostalis thoracis
Spinalis
Posterior rami
Iliocostalis lumborum
Posterior View
Semispinalis capitis
Sternocleidomastoid
Levator scapulae
Spinalis
Longissimus
Iliocostalis
The three columns of erector spinae
10th rib
Aponeurosis of transversus abdominis
Gluteal fascia (covering gluteus medius)
Gluteus maximus

## 4.33 Deep muscles of back: splenius and erector spinae

On the *right* of the body, the erector spinae muscles are in situ, lying between the spinous processes medially and the angles of the ribs laterally. The eretor spinae split into three longitudinal columns: iliocostalis laterally, longissimus in the middle, and spinalis medially. On the *left*, the longissimus muscle is pulled laterally to show the insertion into the transverse processes and ribs; not shown here are its extensions to the neck and head, longissimus cervicis and capitis.

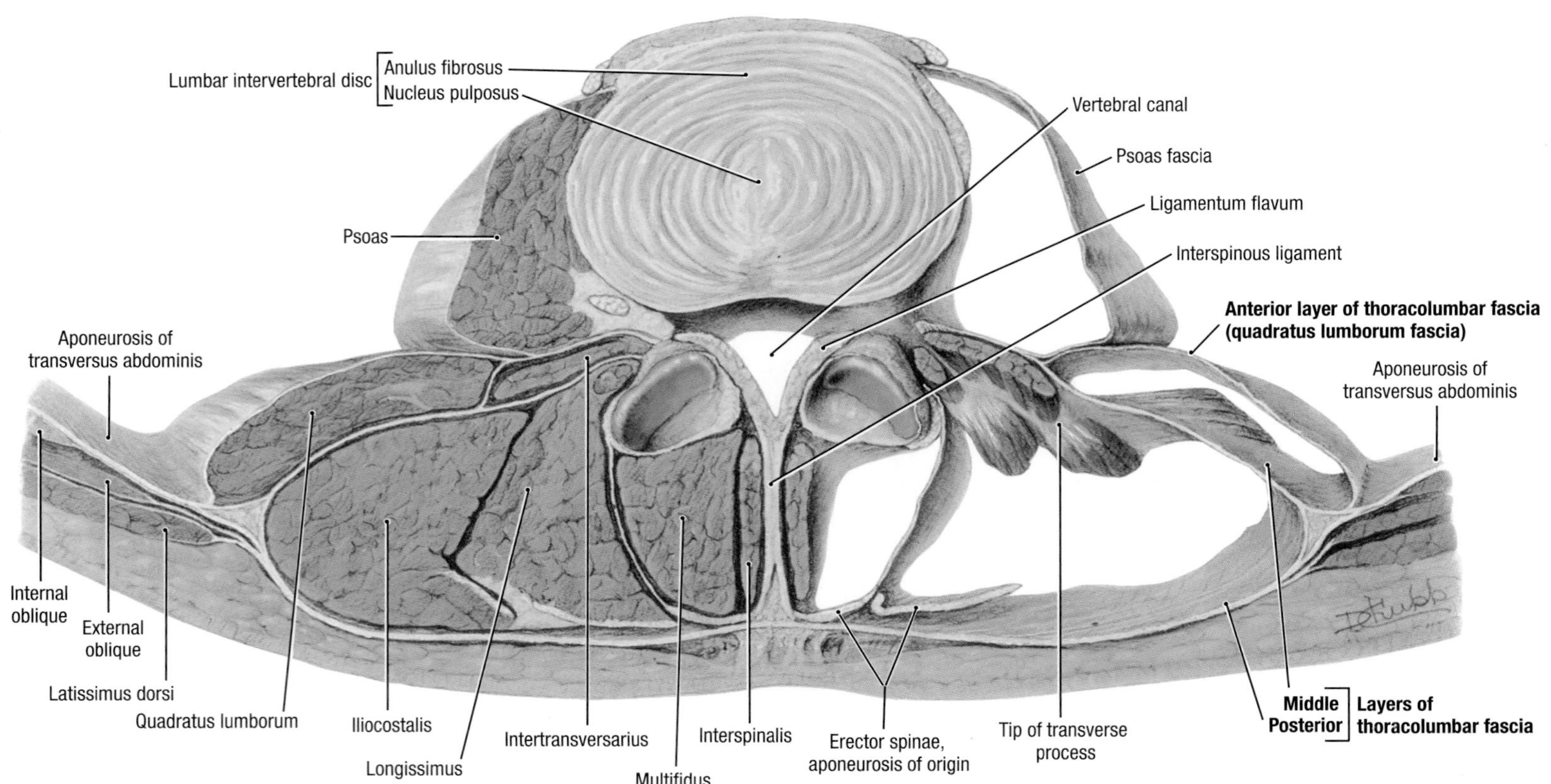
Lumbar intervertebral disc
Anulus fibrosus
Nucleus pulposus
Vertebral canal
Psoas fascia
Ligamentum flavum
Interspinous ligament
Psoas
Anterior layer of thoracolumbar fascia (quadratus lumborum fascia)
Aponeurosis of transversus abdominis
Aponeurosis of transversus abdominis
Internal oblique
External oblique
Latissimus dorsi
Quadratus lumborum
Iliocostalis
Longissimus
Intertransversarius
Multifidus
Interspinalis
Erector spinae, aponeurosis of origin
Tip of transverse process
Middle
Posterior
Layers of thoracolumbar fascia

**Transverse Section (Dissected), Superior View**

## 4.34 Transverse section of back muscles and thoracolumbar fascia

- On the *left*, the muscles are seen in their fascial sheaths or compartments; on the *right*, the muscles have been removed from their sheaths.
- The deep back muscles extend from the pelvis to the cranium and are enclosed in fascia. This fascia attaches medially to the nuchal ligament, the tips of the spinous processes, the supraspinous ligament, and the median crest of the sacrum. The lateral attachment of the fascia is to the cervical transverse processes, the angles of the ribs and to the aponeurosis of transversus abdominis. The thoracic and lumbar parts of the fascia are named thoracolumbar fascia.
- The aponeurosis of transversus abdominis and posterior aponeurosis of internal oblique muscles split into two strong sheets, the middle and posterior layers of the thoracolumbar fascia. The anterior layer of thoracolumbar fascia is the deep fascia of the quadratus lumborum (quadratus lumborum fascia). The posterior layer of the thoracolumbar fascia provides proximal attachment for the latissimus dorsi muscle and, at a higher level, the serratus posterior inferior muscle.

Back strain is a common back problem that usually results from extreme movements of the vertebral column, such as extension or rotation. Back strain refers to some stretching or microscopic tearing of muscle fibers and/or ligaments of the back. The muscles usually involved are those producing movements of the lumbar IV joints.

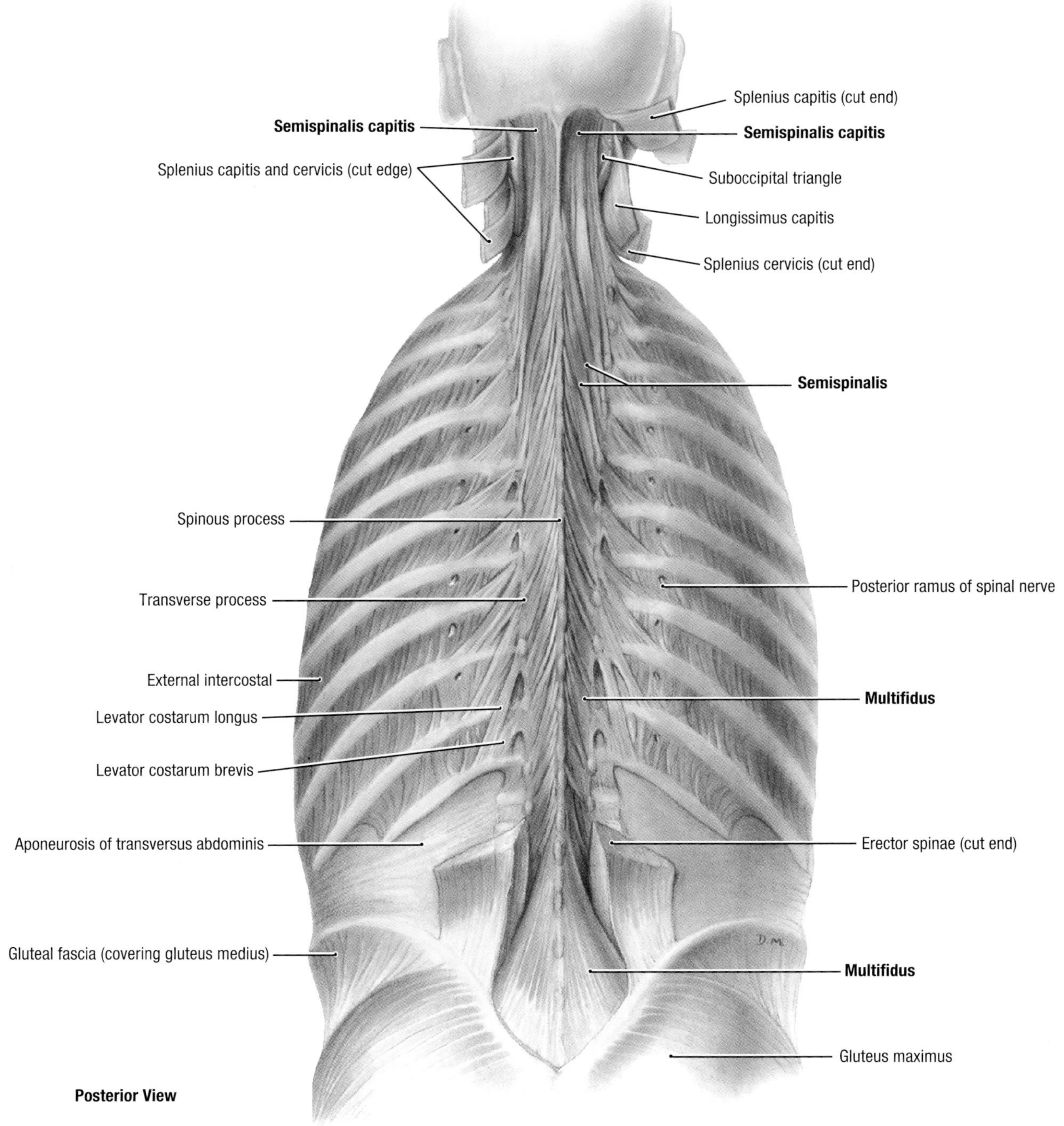
Splenius capitis (cut end)
Semispinalis capitis
Semispinalis capitis
Splenius capitis and cervicis (cut edge)
Suboccipital triangle
Longissimus capitis
Splenius cervicis (cut end)
Semispinalis
Spinous process
Transverse process
Posterior ramus of spinal nerve
External intercostal
Multifidus
Levator costarum longus
Levator costarum brevis
Aponeurosis of transversus abdominis
Erector spinae (cut end)
Gluteal fascia (covering gluteus medius)
Multifidus
Gluteus maximus
Posterior View

## 4.35 Deep muscles of back: semispinalis and multifidus

- The semispinalis, multifidus, and rotatores muscles constitute the transversospinalis group of deep muscles. In general, their bundles pass obliquely in a superomedial direction, from transverse processes to spinous processes in successively deeper layers. The bundles of semispinalis span approximately five interspaces, those of multifidus approximately three, and those of rotatores, one or two.
- The semispinalis (thoracis, cervicis, and capitis) muscles extend from the lower thoracic region to the skull; the semispinalis capitis, a powerful extensor muscle, originates from the lower cervical and upper thoracic vertebrae and inserts into the occipital bone between the superior and inferior nuchal lines.
- The multifidus muscle extends from the sacrum to the spine of the axis. In the lumbosacral region it emerges from the aponeurosis of the erector spinae, and extends from the sacrum, and mammillary processes of the lumbar vertebrae, to insert into spinous processes approximately three segments higher.

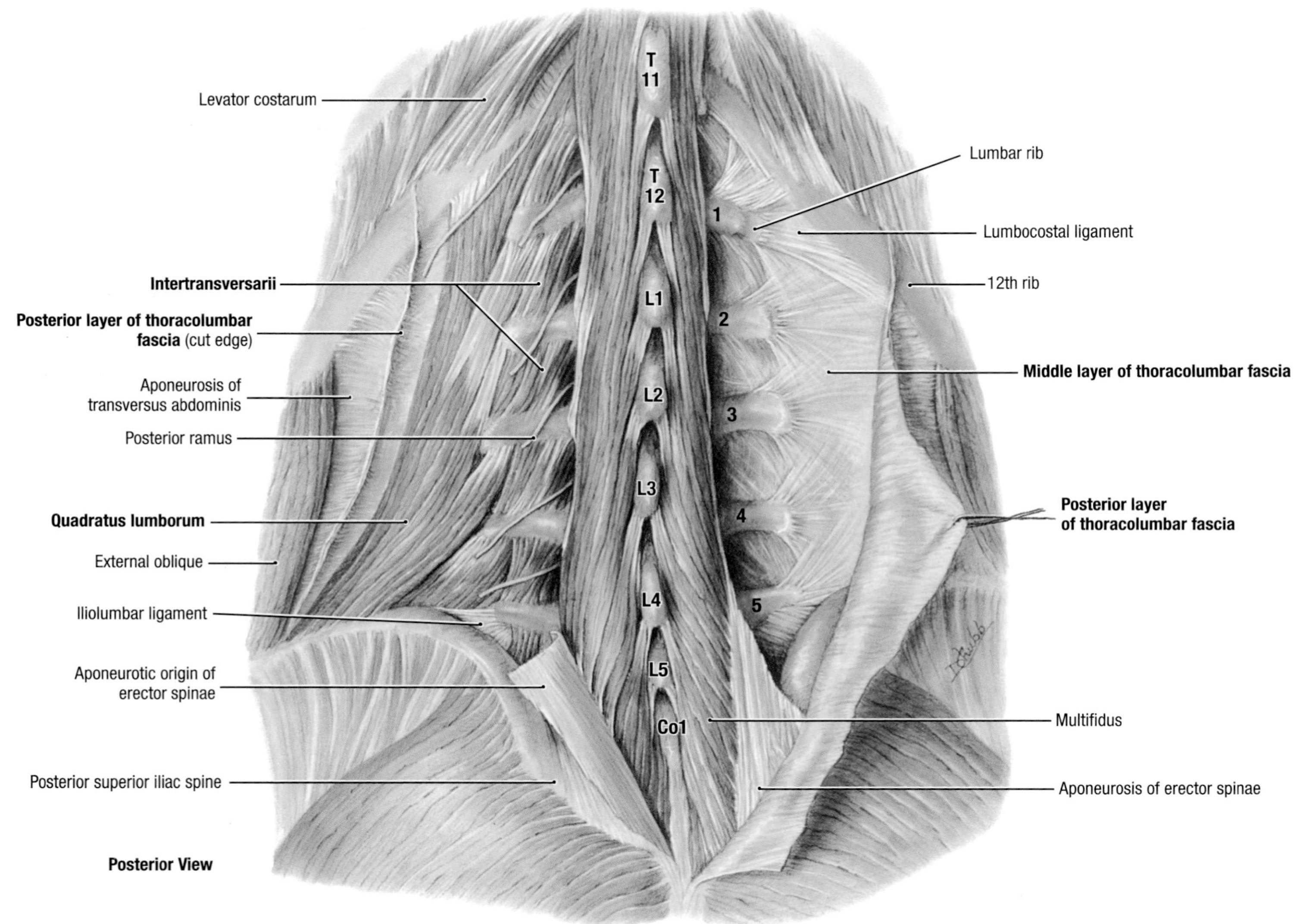
T 11
T 12
L1
L2
L3
L4
L5
Co1
1
2
3
4
5
Levator costarum
Intertransversarii
Posterior layer of thoracolumbar fascia (cut edge)
Aponeurosis of transversus abdominis
Posterior ramus
Quadratus lumborum
External oblique
Iliolumbar ligament
Aponeurotic origin of erector spinae
Posterior superior iliac spine
Posterior View
Lumbar rib
Lumbocostal ligament
12th rib
Middle layer of thoracolumbar fascia
Posterior layer of thoracolumbar fascia
Multifidus
Aponeurosis of erector spinae

## 4.36 Back: multifidus, quadratus lumborum, and thoracolumbar fascia

*Right:* After removal of erector spinae at the L1 level, the middle layer of thoracolumbar fascia extends from the tip of each lumbar transverse process in a fan-shaped manner. A short lumbar rib is present at the level of L1. *Left:* After removal of the posterior and middle layers of thoracolumbar fascia, the lateral border of the quadratus lumborum muscle is oblique, and the medial border is in continuity with the intertransversarii.

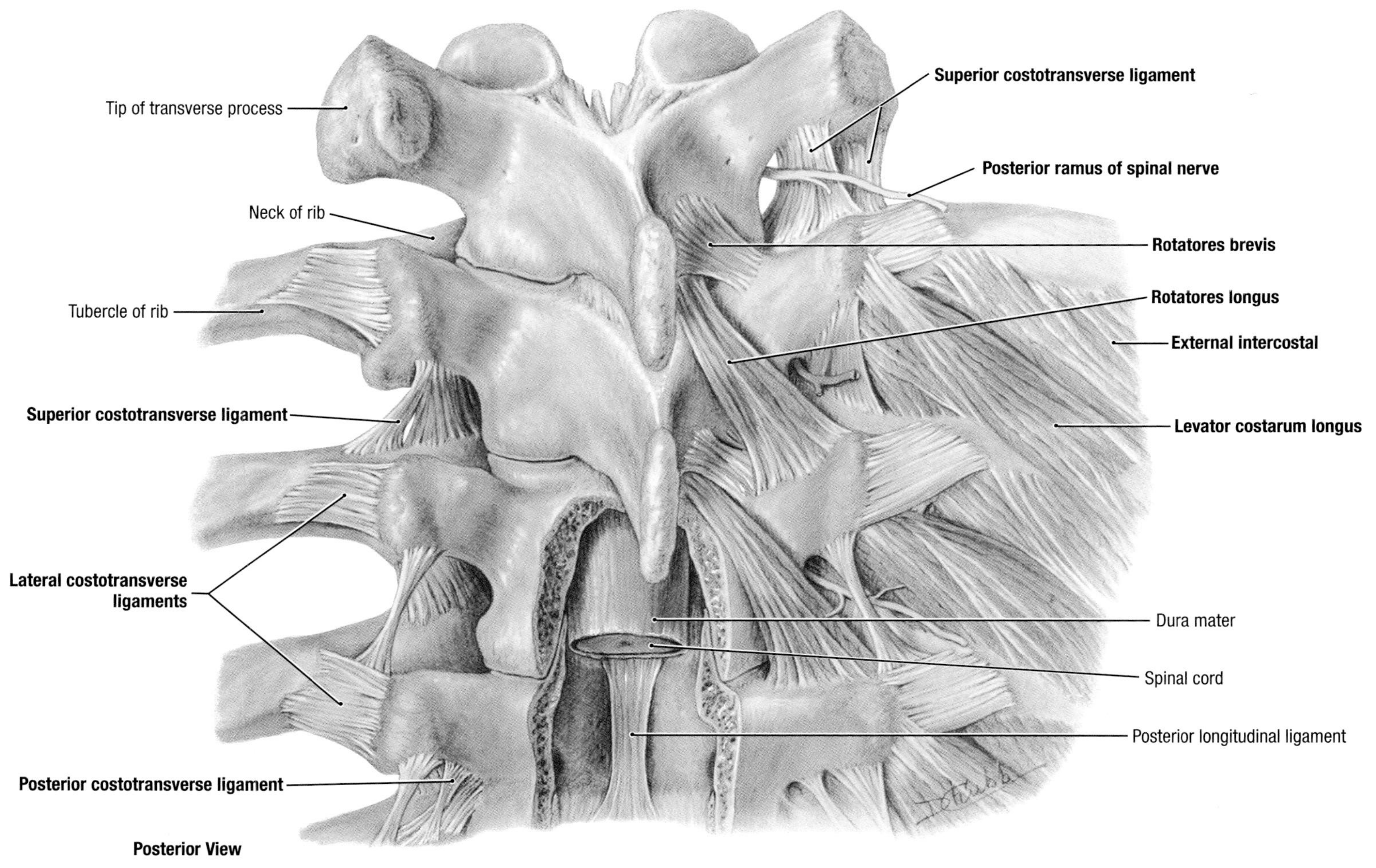
Tip of transverse process
Neck of rib
Tubercle of rib
Superior costotransverse ligament
Lateral costotransverse ligaments
Posterior costotransverse ligament
Posterior View
Superior costotransverse ligament
Posterior ramus of spinal nerve
Rotatores brevis
Rotatores longus
External intercostal
Levator costarum longus
Dura mater
Spinal cord
Posterior longitudinal ligament

## 4.37 Rotatores and costotransverse ligaments

- Of the three layers of transversospinalis, or oblique muscles of the back (semispinalis, multifidus, rotatores), the rotatores are the deepest and shortest. They pass from the root of one transverse process superomedially to the junction of the transverse process and lamina of the vertebra above. Rotatores longus span two vertebrae.
- The levatores costarum pass from the tip of one transverse process inferiorly to the rib below; some span two ribs.
- The superior costotransverse ligament splits laterally into two sheets, between which lie the levatores costarum and external intercostal muscles; the posterior ramus passes posterior to this ligament.
- The lateral costotransverse ligament is strong and joins the tubercle of the rib to the tip of the transverse process. It forms the posterior aspect of the joint capsule of the costotransverse joint.

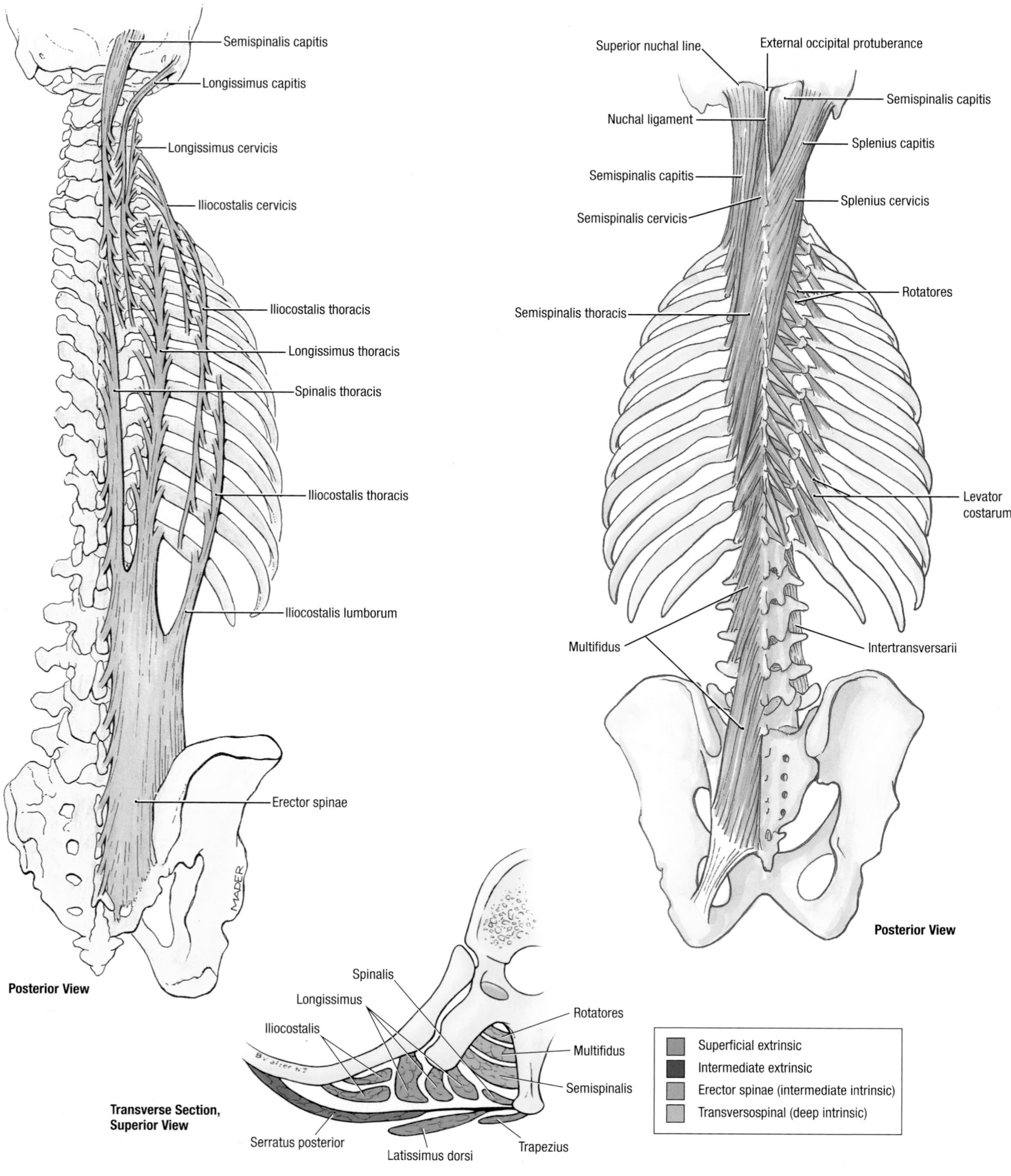
Semispinalis capitis
Longissimus capitis
Longissimus cervicis
Iliocostalis cervicis
Iliocostalis thoracis
Longissimus thoracis
Spinalis thoracis
Iliocostalis thoracis
Iliocostalis lumborum
Erector spinae
MADER
Superior nuchal line
External occipital protuberance
Semispinalis capitis
Nuchal ligament
Splenius capitis
Semispinalis capitis
Splenius cervicis
Semispinalis cervicis
Rotatores
Semispinalis thoracis
Levator costarum
Multifidus
Intertransversarii
Spinalis
Longissimus
Iliocostalis
Rotatores
Multifidus
Semispinalis
Serratus posterior
Latissimus dorsi
Trapezius
Superficial extrinsic
Intermediate extrinsic
Erector spinae (intermediate intrinsic)
Transversospinal (deep intrinsic)

**Posterior View**

**Posterior View**

**Transverse Section, Superior View**

TABLE 4.4 INTRINSIC BACK MUSCLES[a]

| MUSCLES | ORIGIN | INSERTION | NERVE SUPPLY[b] | MAIN ACTIONS |
|---|---|---|---|---|
| **Superficial layer**<br>Splenius | Arises from nuchal ligament and spinous processes of C7–T3 or T4 vertebrae | *Splenius capitis:* fibers run superolaterally to mastoid process of temporal bone and lateral third of superior nuchal line of occipital bone<br>*Splenius cervicis:* posterior tubercles of transverse processes of C1–C3 or C4 vertebrae | Posterior rami of spinal nerves | *Acting unilaterally*: laterally bend to side of active muscles; *Acting bilaterally*: extend head and neck |
| **Intermediate layer**<br>Erector spinae | Arises by a broad tendon from posterior part of iliac crest, posterior surface of sacrum, sacral and inferior lumbar spinous processes, and supraspinous ligament | *Iliocostalis (lumborum, thoracis, and cervicis):* fibers run superiorly to angles of lower ribs and cervical transverse processes<br>*Longissimus (thoracis, cervicis, and capitis):* fibers run superiorly to ribs between tubercles and angles to transverse processes in thoracic and cervical regions, and to mastoid process of temporal bone<br>*Spinalis (thoracis, cervicis, and capitis):* fibers run superiorly to spinous processes in the upper thoracic region and to skull | | *Acting unilaterally:* laterally bend vertebral column to side of active muscles; *Acting bilaterally:* extend vertebral column and head; as back is flexed, control movement by gradually lengthening their fibers |
| **Deep layer**<br>Transversospinalis | *Semispinalis:* arises from thoracic and cervical transverse processes | *Semispinalis: thoracis, cervicis, and capitis;* fibers run superomedially and attach to occipital bone and spinous processes in thoracic and cervical regions, spanning four to six segments | | *Acting unilaterally:* rotate head and neck contralaterally; *Acting bilaterally:* extend head and thoracic cervical regions |
| | *Multifidus:* arises from sacrum and ilium, transverse processes of T1–L5, and articular processes of C4–C7 | *Multifidus (lumborum, thoracis, and cervicis):* fibers pass superomedially to spinous processes, spanning two to four segments | | Stabilizes vertebrae during local movements of vertebral column |
| | *Rotatores:* arise from transverse processes of vertebrae; best developed in thoracic region | *Rotatores (thoracis and cervicis):* Pass superomedially and attach to junction of lamina and transverse process of vertebra of origin or into spinous process above their origin, spanning one to two segments | | Stabilize vertebrae and assist with local extension and rotary movements |
| **Minor deep layer**<br>Interspinales | Superior surfaces of spinous processes of cervical and lumbar vertebrae | Inferior surfaces of spinous processes of vertebrae superior to vertebrae of origin | Posterior rami of spinal nerves | Aid in extension and rotation of vertebral column |
| Intertransversarii | Transverse processes of cervical and lumbar vertebrae | Transverse processes of adjacent vertebrae | Posterior and anterior rami of spinal nerves | Aid in lateral bending of vertebral column; *Acting bilaterally:* stabilize vertebral column |
| Levatores costarum | Tips of transverse processes of C7 and T1–T11 vertebrae | Pass inferolaterally and insert on rib between its tubercle and angle | Posterior rami of C8–T11 spinal nerves | Elevate ribs, assisting inspiration<br>Assist with lateral bending of vertebral column |

[a]See figures on opposite page.
[b]Most back muscles are innervated by dorsal rami of spinal nerves, but a few are innervated by anterior rami. Intertransversarii of cervical region are supplied by anterior rami.

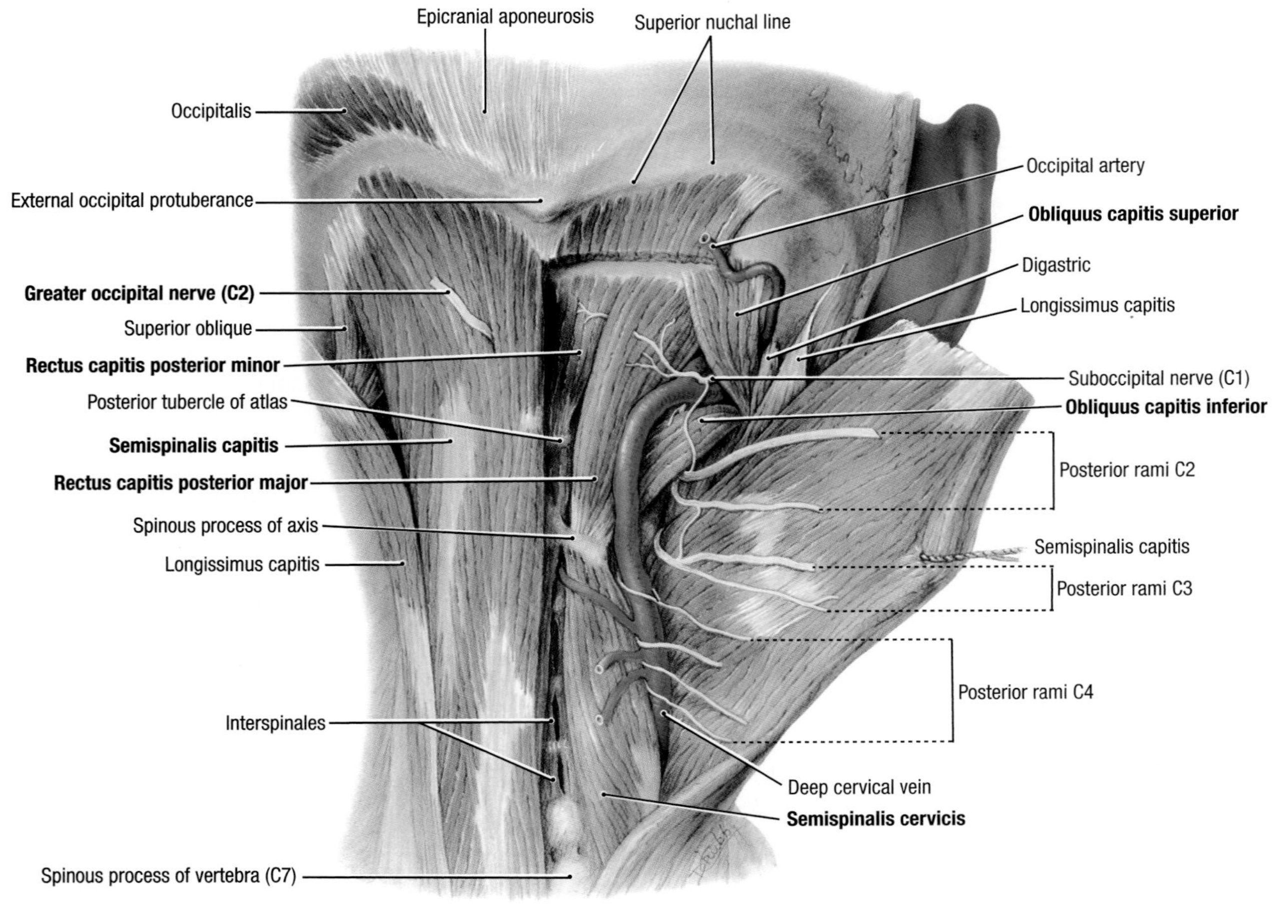
Epicranial aponeurosis
Superior nuchal line
Occipitalis
External occipital protuberance
Occipital artery
Obliquus capitis superior
Digastric
Longissimus capitis
Greater occipital nerve (C2)
Superior oblique
Rectus capitis posterior minor
Suboccipital nerve (C1)
Obliquus capitis inferior
Posterior tubercle of atlas
Semispinalis capitis
Rectus capitis posterior major
Posterior rami C2
Spinous process of axis
Longissimus capitis
Semispinalis capitis
Posterior rami C3
Posterior rami C4
Interspinales
Deep cervical vein
Semispinalis cervicis
Spinous process of vertebra (C7)
Posterior View

## 4.38 Suboccipital region—I

The trapezius, sternocleidomastoid, and splenius muscles are removed. The right semispinalis capitis muscle is cut and turned laterally.

- The semispinalis capitis, the great extensor muscle of the head and neck, forms the posterior wall of the suboccipital region. It is pierced by the greater occipital nerve (posterior ramus of C2) and has free medial and lateral borders at this level.
- The greater occipital nerve, when followed caudally, leads to the inferior border of the obliquus capitis inferior muscle, around which it turns. Following the inferior border of the obliquus capitis inferior muscle medially from the nerve leads to the spinous process of the axis; followed laterally, this leads to the transverse process of the atlas.
- Five muscles (all paired) are attached to the spinous process of the axis: obliquus capitis inferior, rectus capitis posterior major, semispinalis cervicis, multifidus, and interspinalis; the latter two are largely concealed by the semispinalis cervicis.

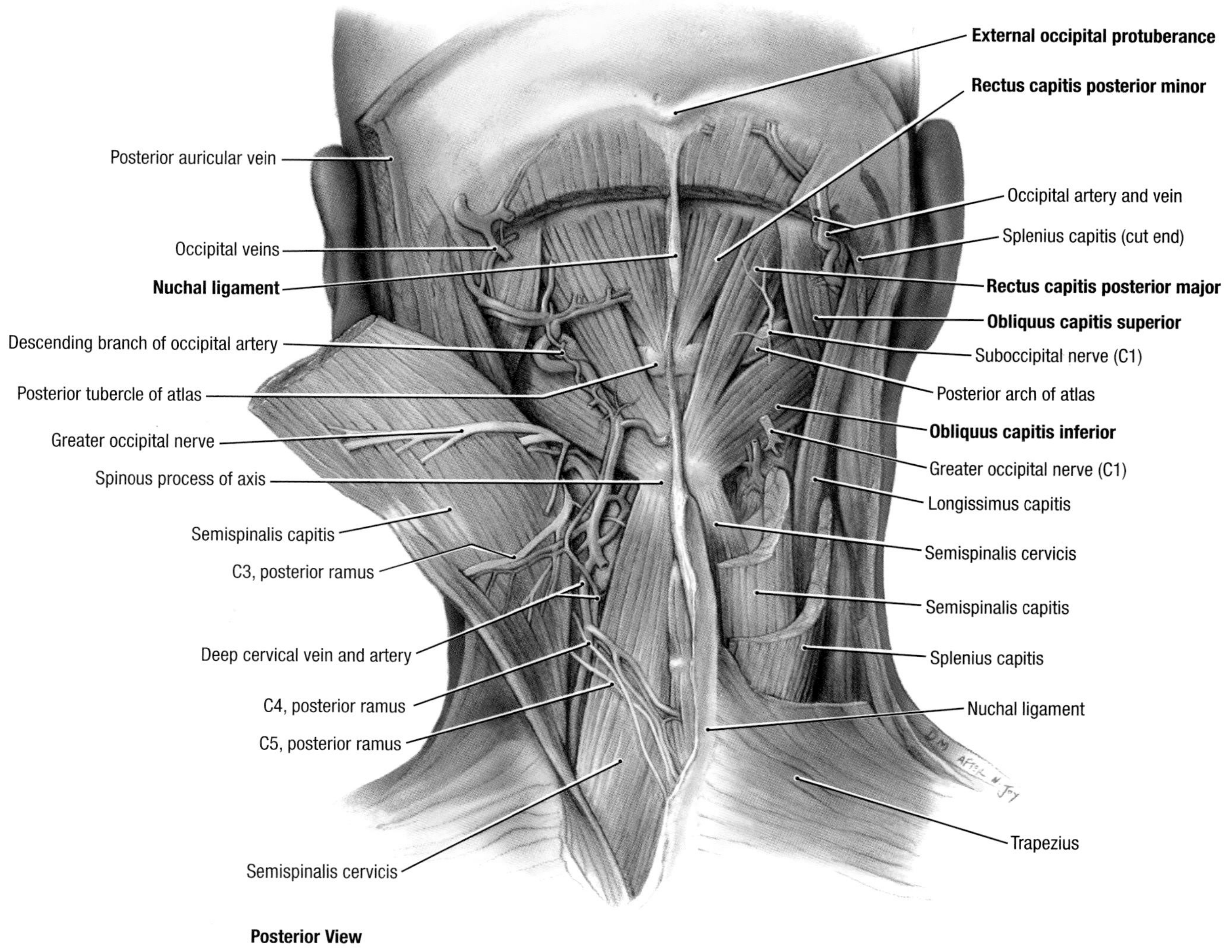
External occipital protuberance
Rectus capitis posterior minor
Posterior auricular vein
Occipital artery and vein
Splenius capitis (cut end)
Occipital veins
Nuchal ligament
Rectus capitis posterior major
Obliquus capitis superior
Descending branch of occipital artery
Suboccipital nerve (C1)
Posterior tubercle of atlas
Posterior arch of atlas
Obliquus capitis inferior
Greater occipital nerve
Greater occipital nerve (C1)
Spinous process of axis
Longissimus capitis
Semispinalis capitis
Semispinalis cervicis
C3, posterior ramus
Semispinalis capitis
Deep cervical vein and artery
Splenius capitis
C4, posterior ramus
Nuchal ligament
C5, posterior ramus
Trapezius
Semispinalis cervicis
Posterior View

## 4.39 Suboccipital region—II

The semispinalis capitis is reflected on the *left* and removed on the *right* side of the body.

- The suboccipital region contains four pairs of structures: two straight muscles, the rectus capitis posterior major and minor; two oblique muscles, the obliquus capitis superior and obliquus capitis inferior; two nerves (posterior rami), C1 suboccipital (motor) and C2 greater occipital (sensory); and two arteries, the occipital and vertebral.
- The nuchal ligament, which represents the cervical part of the supraspinous ligament, is a median, thin, fibrous partition attached to the spinous processes of cervical vertebrae and the external occipital crest; its posterior border gives origin to the trapezius muscle and extends superiorly to the external occipital protuberance.
- The suboccipital triangle is bounded by three muscles: obliquus capitis superior and inferior, and rectus capitis posterior major.
- The suboccipital nerve (posterior ramus of C1) supplies the three muscles bounding the suboccipital triangle and also the rectus capitis minor muscle and communicates with the greater occipital nerve.
- The occipital veins along with the suboccipital nerve (posterior ramus of C1) emerge through the suboccipital triangle to join the deep cervical vein.
- The posterior arch of the atlas forms the floor of the suboccipital triangle.

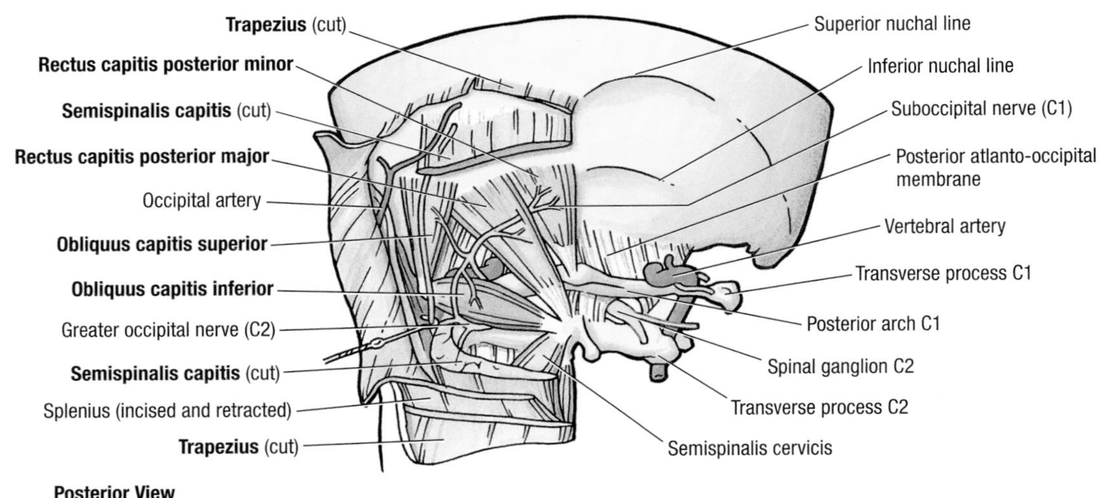
Trapezius (cut)
Rectus capitis posterior minor
Semispinalis capitis (cut)
Rectus capitis posterior major
Occipital artery
Obliquus capitis superior
Obliquus capitis inferior
Greater occipital nerve (C2)
Semispinalis capitis (cut)
Splenius (incised and retracted)
Trapezius (cut)
Superior nuchal line
Inferior nuchal line
Suboccipital nerve (C1)
Posterior atlanto-occipital membrane
Vertebral artery
Transverse process C1
Posterior arch C1
Spinal ganglion C2
Transverse process C2
Semispinalis cervicis
Posterior View

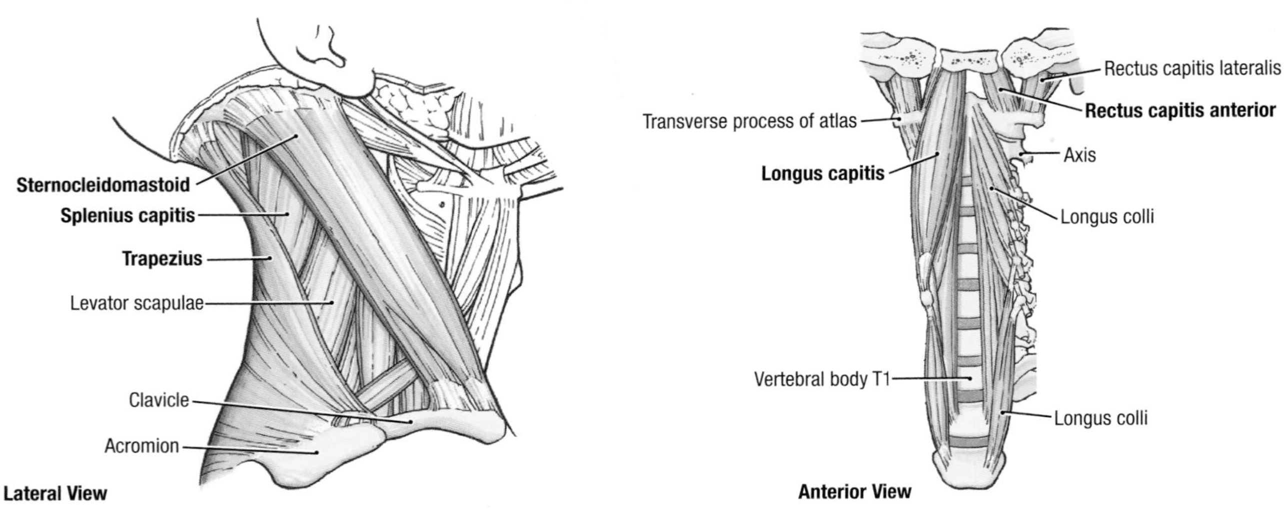
Sternocleidomastoid
Splenius capitis
Trapezius
Levator scapulae
Clavicle
Acromion
Lateral View
Rectus capitis lateralis
Rectus capitis anterior
Transverse process of atlas
Axis
Longus capitis
Longus colli
Vertebral body T1
Longus colli
Anterior View

## TABLE 4.5 MUSCLES OF THE ATLANTO-OCCIPITAL AND ATLANTOAXIAL JOINTS

**MOVEMENTS OF ATLANTO-OCCIPITAL JOINTS**

| *FLEXION* | *EXTENSION* | *LATERAL BENDING* |
|---|---|---|
| Longus capitis<br>Rectus capitis anterior<br>Anterior fibers of sternocleidomastoid | Rectus capitis posterior major and minor<br>Obliquus capitis superior<br>Semispinalis capitis<br>Splenius capitis<br>Longissimus capitis<br>Trapezius | Sternocleidomastoid<br>Obliquus capitis superior and inferior<br>Rectus capitis lateralis<br>Splenius capitis |

**ROTATION OF ATLANTOAXIAL JOINTS**[a]

| *IPSILATERAL*[b] | *CONTRALATERAL* |
|---|---|
| Obliquus capitis inferior<br>Rectus capitis posterior, major and minor<br>Longissimus capitis<br>Splenius capitis | Sternocleidomastoid<br>Semispinalis capitis |

[a]Rotation is the specialized movement at these joints. Movement of one joint involves the other.
[b]Same side to which head is rotated.

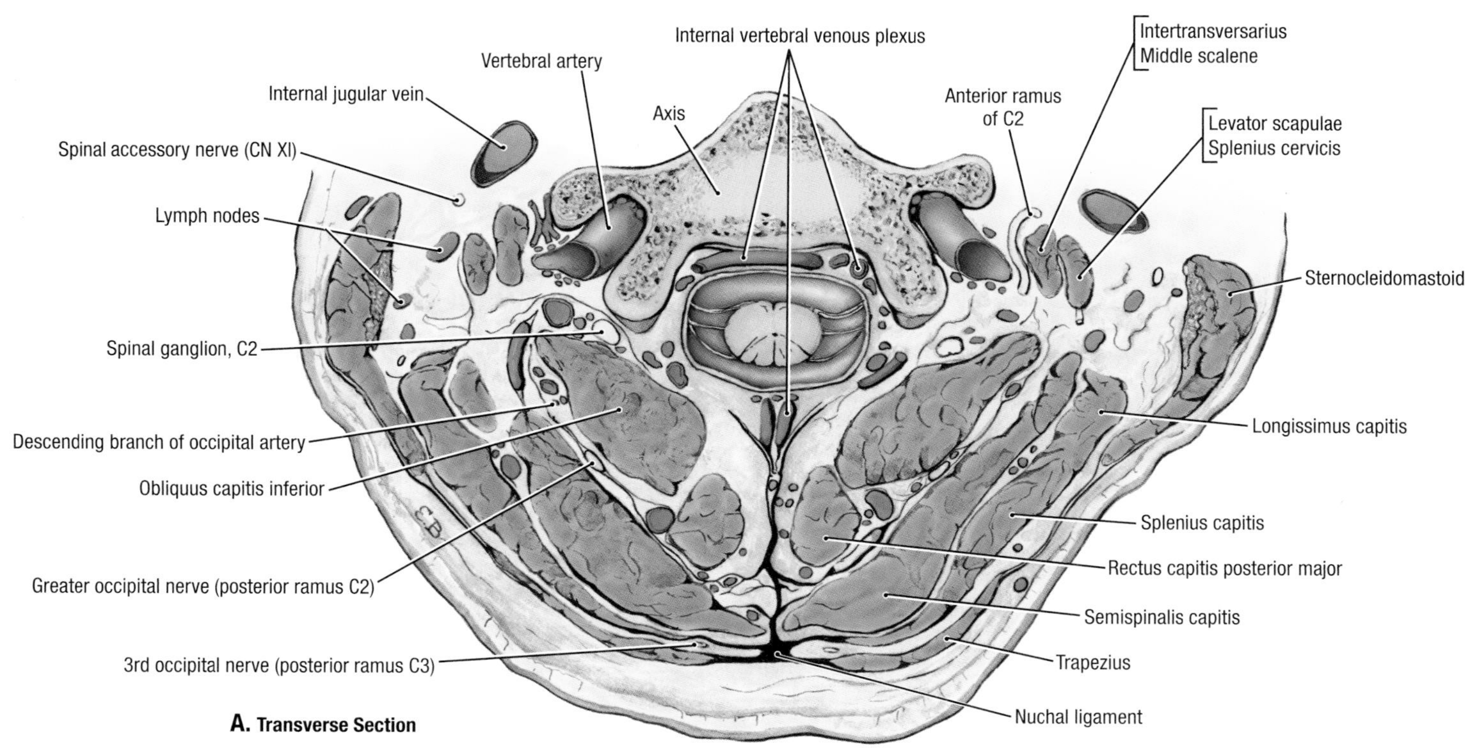
Internal vertebral venous plexus
Vertebral artery
Intertransversarius
Middle scalene
Internal jugular vein
Axis
Anterior ramus of C2
Levator scapulae
Splenius cervicis
Spinal accessory nerve (CN XI)
Lymph nodes
Sternocleidomastoid
Spinal ganglion, C2
Longissimus capitis
Descending branch of occipital artery
Obliquus capitis inferior
Splenius capitis
Rectus capitis posterior major
Greater occipital nerve (posterior ramus C2)
Semispinalis capitis
Trapezius
3rd occipital nerve (posterior ramus C3)
Nuchal ligament

**A. Transverse Section**

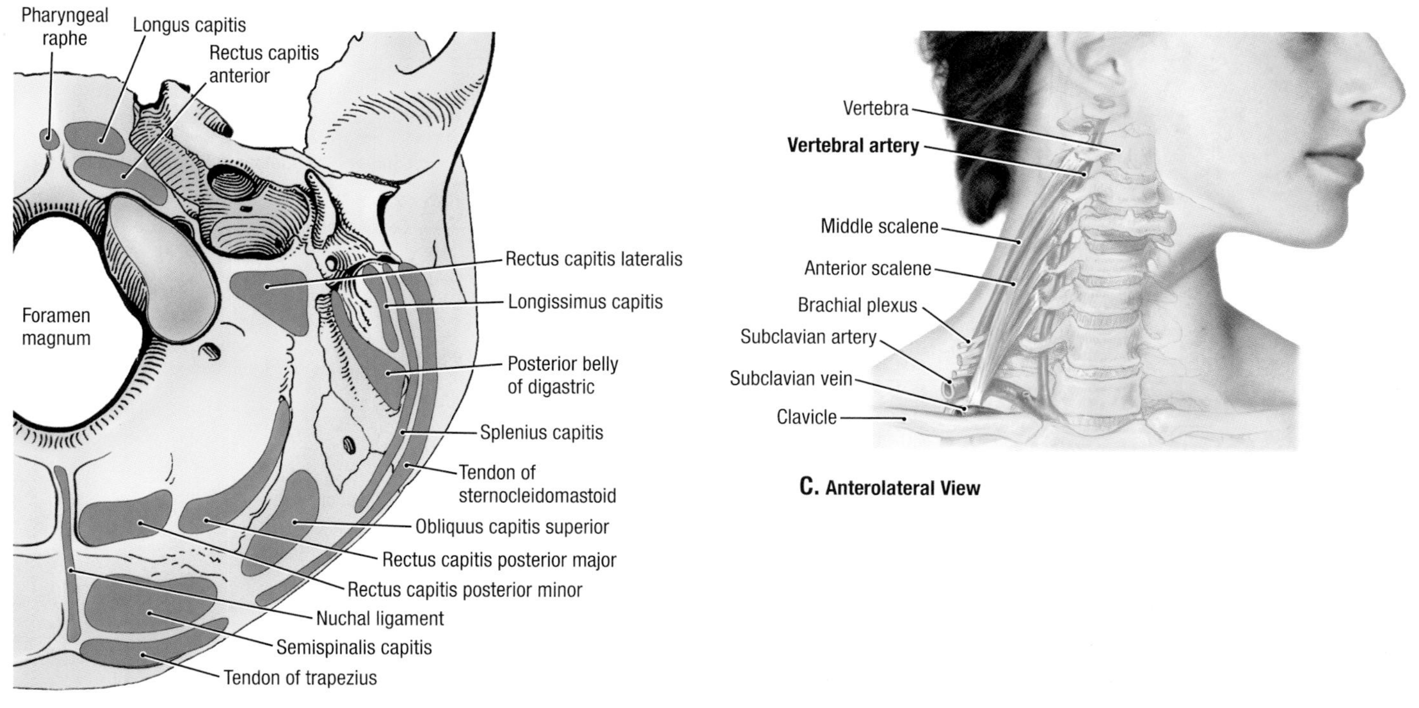
Pharyngeal raphe
Longus capitis
Rectus capitis anterior
Rectus capitis lateralis
Longissimus capitis
Foramen magnum
Posterior belly of digastric
Splenius capitis
Tendon of sternocleidomastoid
Obliquus capitis superior
Rectus capitis posterior major
Rectus capitis posterior minor
Nuchal ligament
Semispinalis capitis
Tendon of trapezius
Vertebra
Vertebral artery
Middle scalene
Anterior scalene
Brachial plexus
Subclavian artery
Subclavian vein
Clavicle

**B. Inferior View**

**C. Anterolateral View**

## 4.40 Nuchal Region

**A.** Transverse section at the level of the axis. **B.** Muscle attachments to inferior aspect of skull. **C.** Vertebral artery.

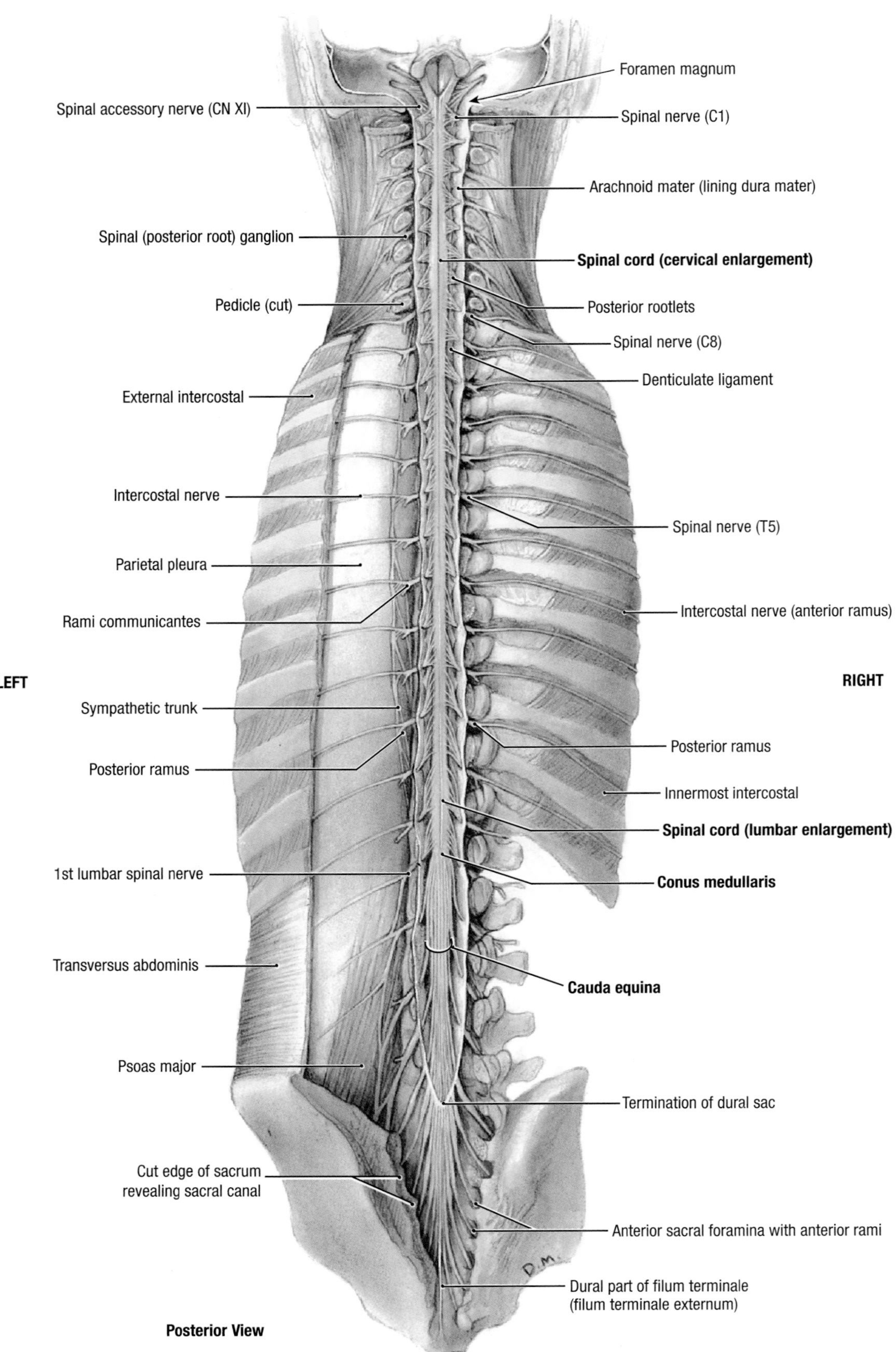
Foramen magnum
Spinal accessory nerve (CN XI)
Spinal nerve (C1)
Arachnoid mater (lining dura mater)
Spinal (posterior root) ganglion
Spinal cord (cervical enlargement)
Pedicle (cut)
Posterior rootlets
Spinal nerve (C8)
Denticulate ligament
External intercostal
Intercostal nerve
Spinal nerve (T5)
Parietal pleura
Rami communicantes
Intercostal nerve (anterior ramus)
LEFT
RIGHT
Sympathetic trunk
Posterior ramus
Posterior ramus
Innermost intercostal
Spinal cord (lumbar enlargement)
1st lumbar spinal nerve
Conus medullaris
Transversus abdominis
Cauda equina
Psoas major
Termination of dural sac
Cut edge of sacrum
revealing sacral canal
Anterior sacral foramina with anterior rami
Dural part of filum terminale
(filum terminale externum)
Posterior View

**4.41 Spinal cord in situ**

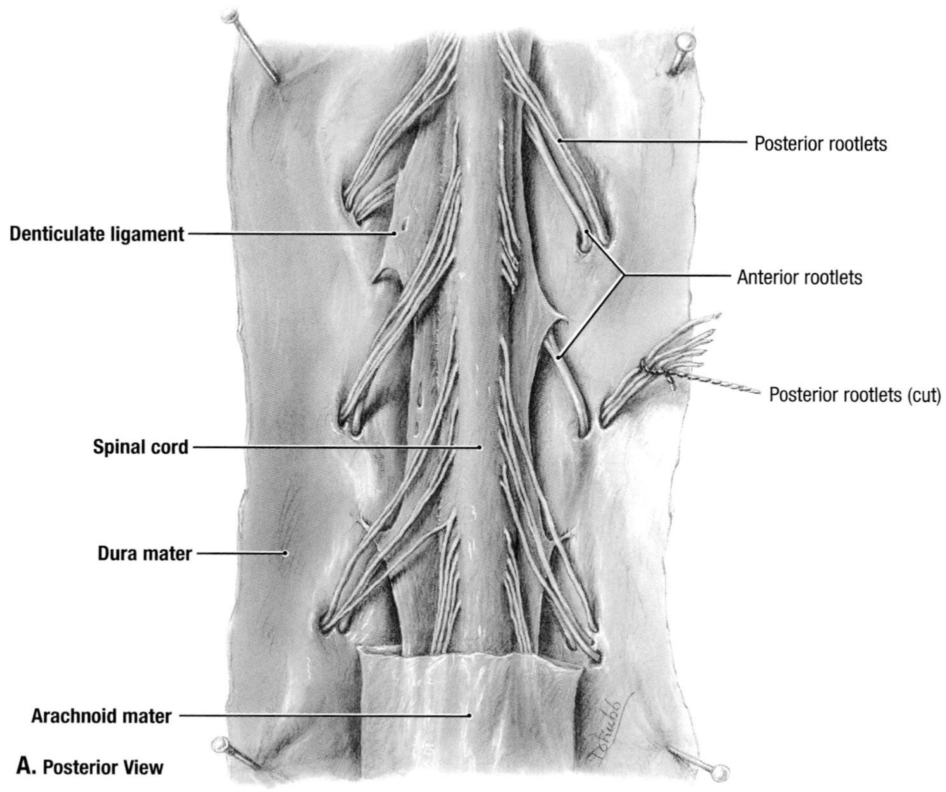
Posterior rootlets
Denticulate ligament
Anterior rootlets
Posterior rootlets (cut)
Spinal cord
Dura mater
Arachnoid mater
A. Posterior View

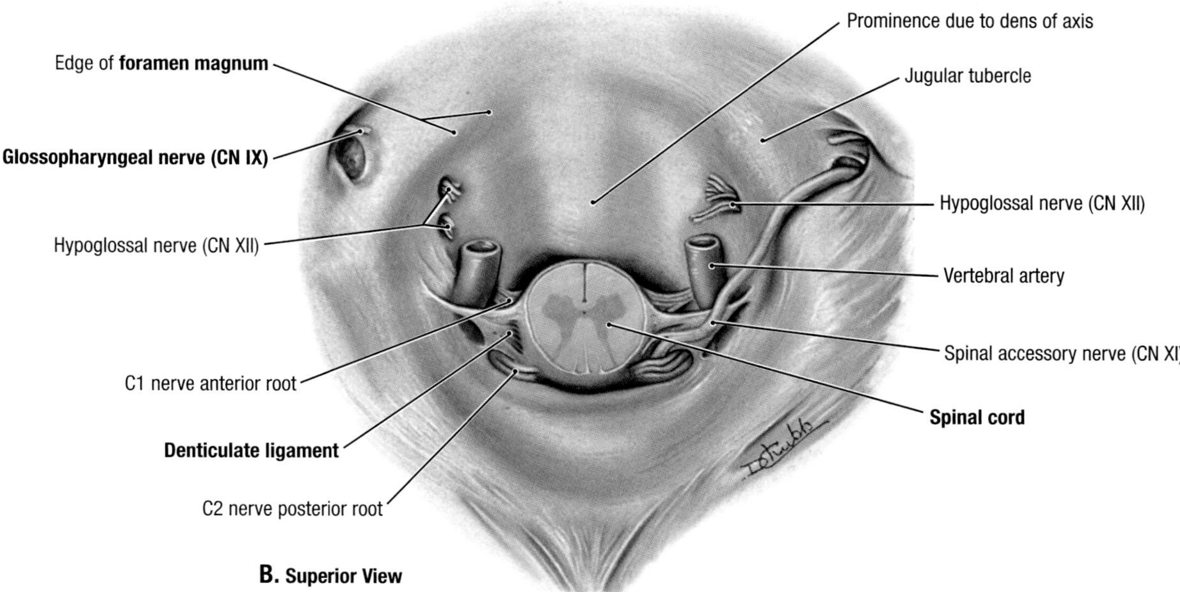
Prominence due to dens of axis
Edge of foramen magnum
Jugular tubercle
Glossopharyngeal nerve (CN IX)
Hypoglossal nerve (CN XII)
Hypoglossal nerve (CN XII)
Vertebral artery
Spinal accessory nerve (CN XI)
C1 nerve anterior root
Spinal cord
Denticulate ligament
C2 nerve posterior root
B. Superior View

## 4.42 Spinal cord and meninges

**A.** Dural sac cut open. The denticulate ligament anchors the cord to the dural sac between successive nerve roots by means of strong, toothlike processes. The anterior nerve roots lie anterior to the denticulate ligament, and the posterior nerve roots lie posterior to the ligament. **B.** Structures of vertebral canal seen through foramen magnum. The spinal cord, vertebral arteries, spinal accessory nerve (CN XI), and most superior part of the denticulate ligament pass through the foramen magnum within the meninges.

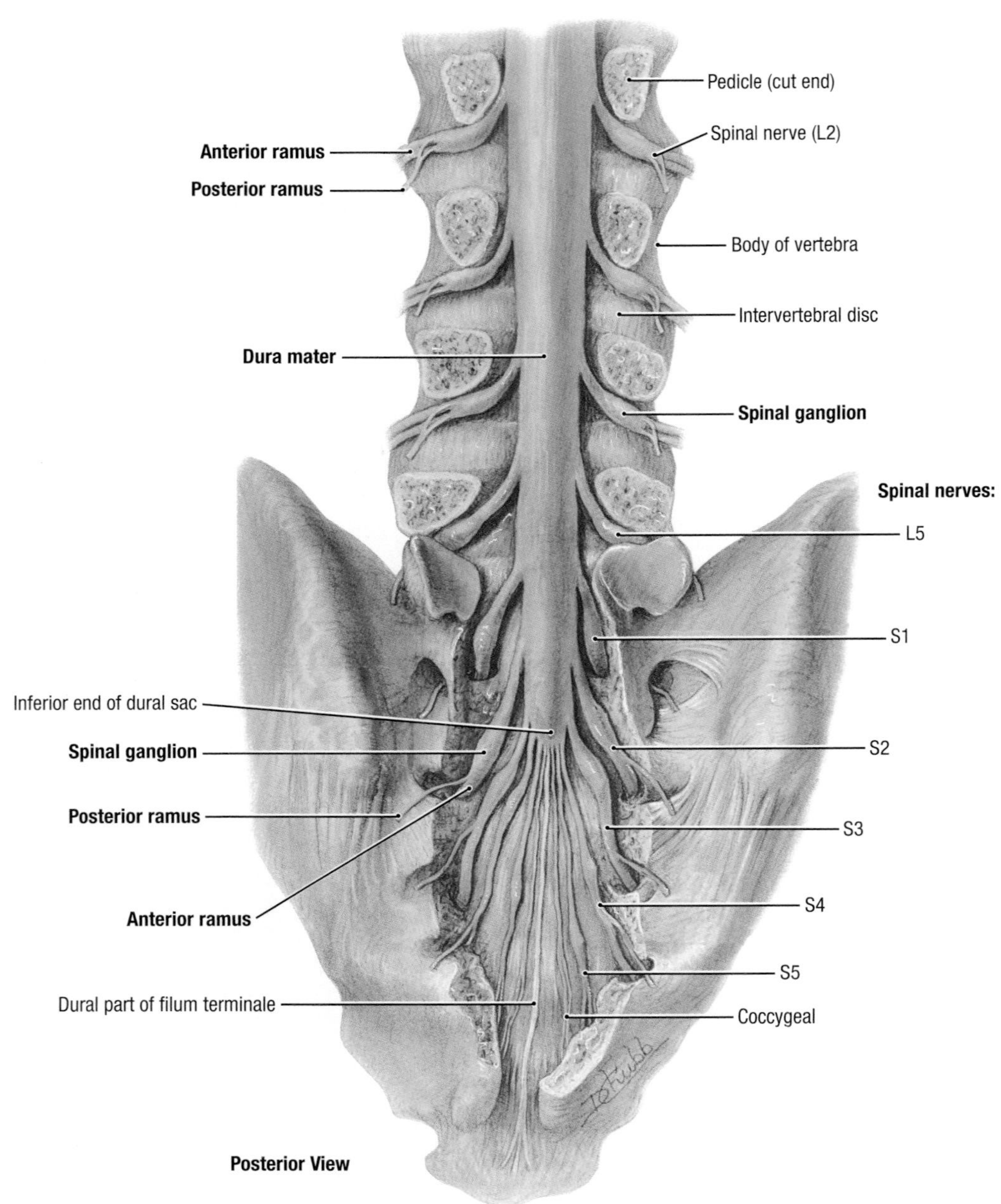
Pedicle (cut end)
Spinal nerve (L2)
Anterior ramus
Posterior ramus
Body of vertebra
Intervertebral disc
Dura mater
Spinal ganglion
Spinal nerves:
L5
S1
Inferior end of dural sac
Spinal ganglion
S2
Posterior ramus
S3
Anterior ramus
S4
S5
Dural part of filum terminale
Coccygeal
Posterior View

## 4.43 Inferior end of dural sac—I

The posterior parts of the lumbar vertebrae and sacrum were removed.

- The inferior limit of the dural sac is at the level of the posterior superior iliac spine (body of 2nd sacral vertebra); the dura continues as the dural part of the filum terminale (filum terminale externum).
- The lumbar spinal ganglia are in the intervertebral foramina, and the sacral spinal ganglia are somewhat asymmetrically placed within the sacral canal.
- The posterior rami are smaller than the anterior rami.

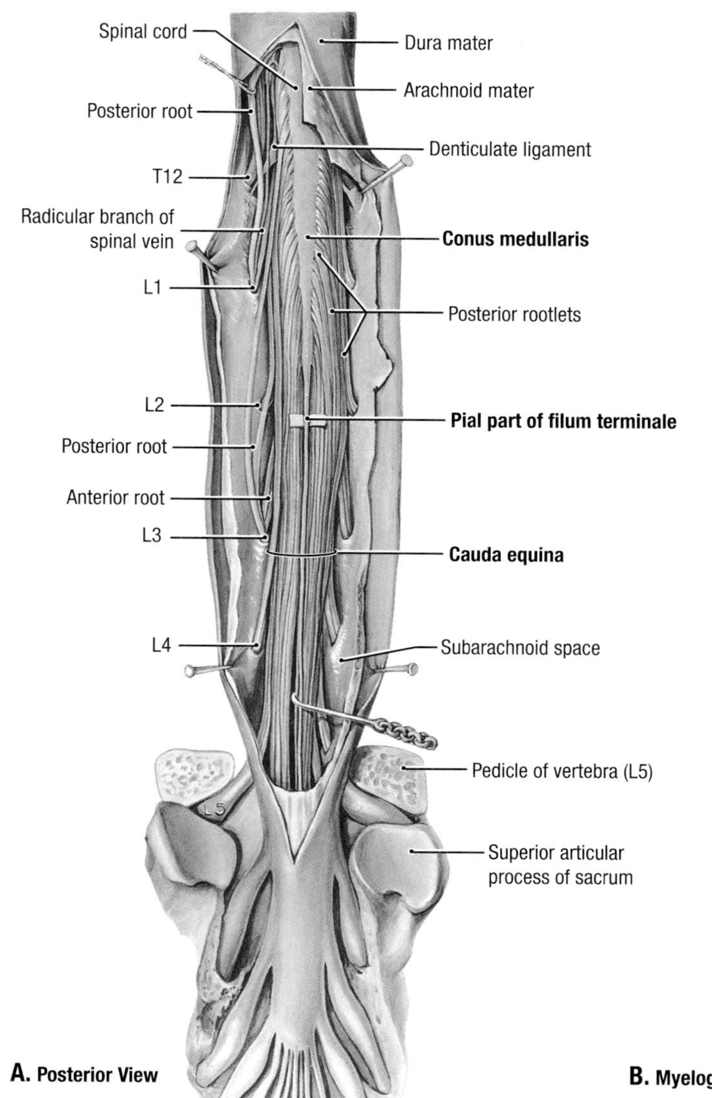
Spinal cord
Dura mater
Arachnoid mater
Posterior root
Denticulate ligament
T12
Radicular branch of spinal vein
Conus medullaris
L1
Posterior rootlets
L2
Pial part of filum terminale
Posterior root
Anterior root
L3
Cauda equina
L4
Subarachnoid space
Pedicle of vertebra (L5)
L5
Superior articular process of sacrum

A. Posterior View

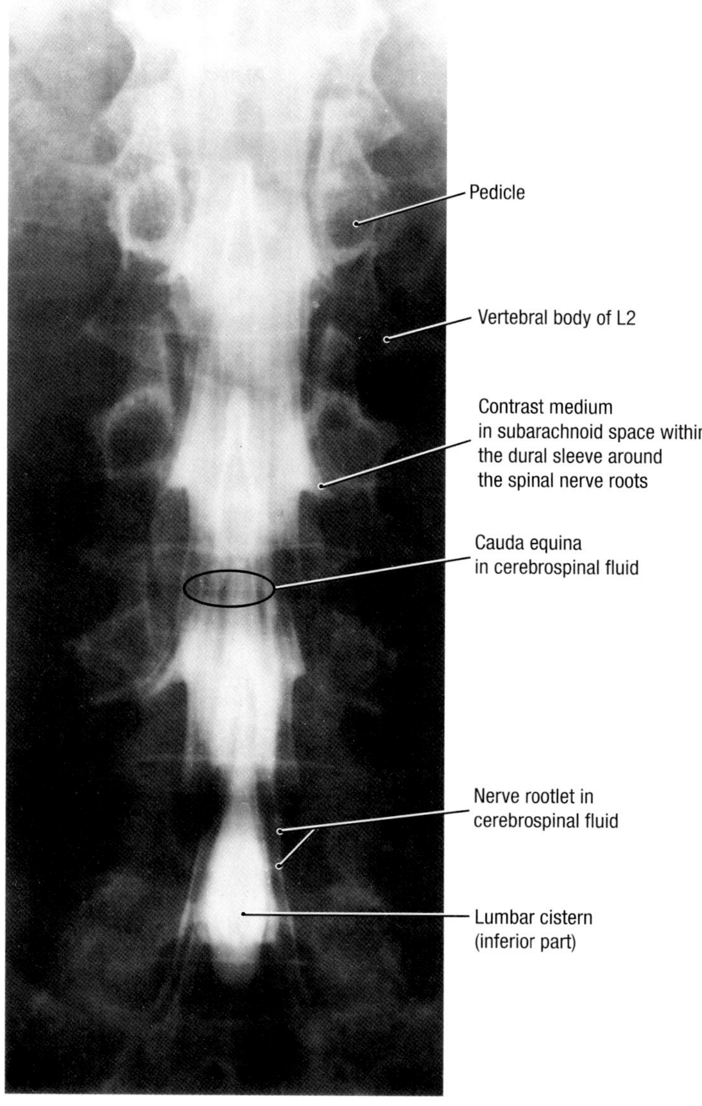
Pedicle
Vertebral body of L2
Contrast medium in subarachnoid space within the dural sleeve around the spinal nerve roots
Cauda equina in cerebrospinal fluid
Nerve rootlet in cerebrospinal fluid
Lumbar cistern (inferior part)

B. Myelogram

## 4.44 Inferior end of dural sac—II

**A.** Inferior dural sac and lumbar cistern of subarachnoid space, opened. **B.** Myelogram of the lumbar region of the vertebral column. Contrast medium was injected into the subarachnoid space. **C.** Termination of spinal cord, in situ, sagittal section.

- The conus medullaris, or conical lower end of the spinal cord, continues as a glistening thread, the plial part of the filum terminale (filum terminale internum), which descends with the posterior and anterior nerve roots; these constitute the cauda equina.
- In the adult, the spinal cord usually ends at the level of the disc between L1 and L2. Variations: 95% of cords end within the limits of the bodies of L1 and L2, whereas 3% end posterior to the inferior half of T12, and 2% posterior to L3.
- The subarachnoid space usually ends at the level of the disc between S1 and S2, but it can be more inferior.

To obtain a sample of CSF from the lumbar cistern, a lumbar puncture needle, fitted with a stylet, is inserted into the subarachnoid space. Flexion of the vertebral column facilitates insertion of the needle by stretching the ligamenta flava and spreading the laminae and spinous processes apart. The needle is inserted in the midline between the spinous processes of the L3 and L4 (or the L4 and L5) vertebrae. At these levels in adults, there is little danger of damaging the spinal cord.

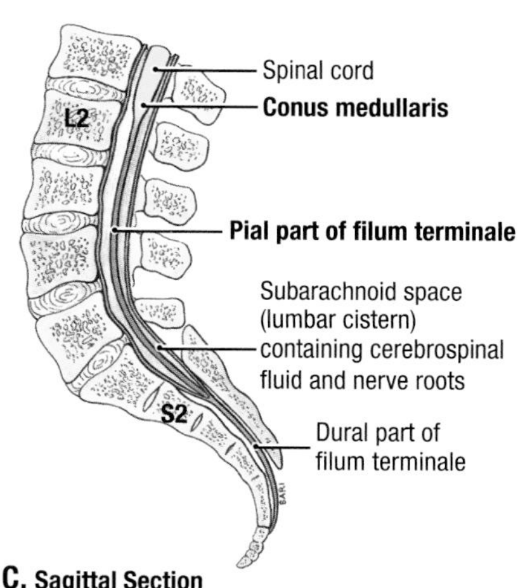
L2
Spinal cord
Conus medullaris
Pial part of filum terminale
Subarachnoid space (lumbar cistern) containing cerebrospinal fluid and nerve roots
S2
Dural part of filum terminale

C. Sagittal Section

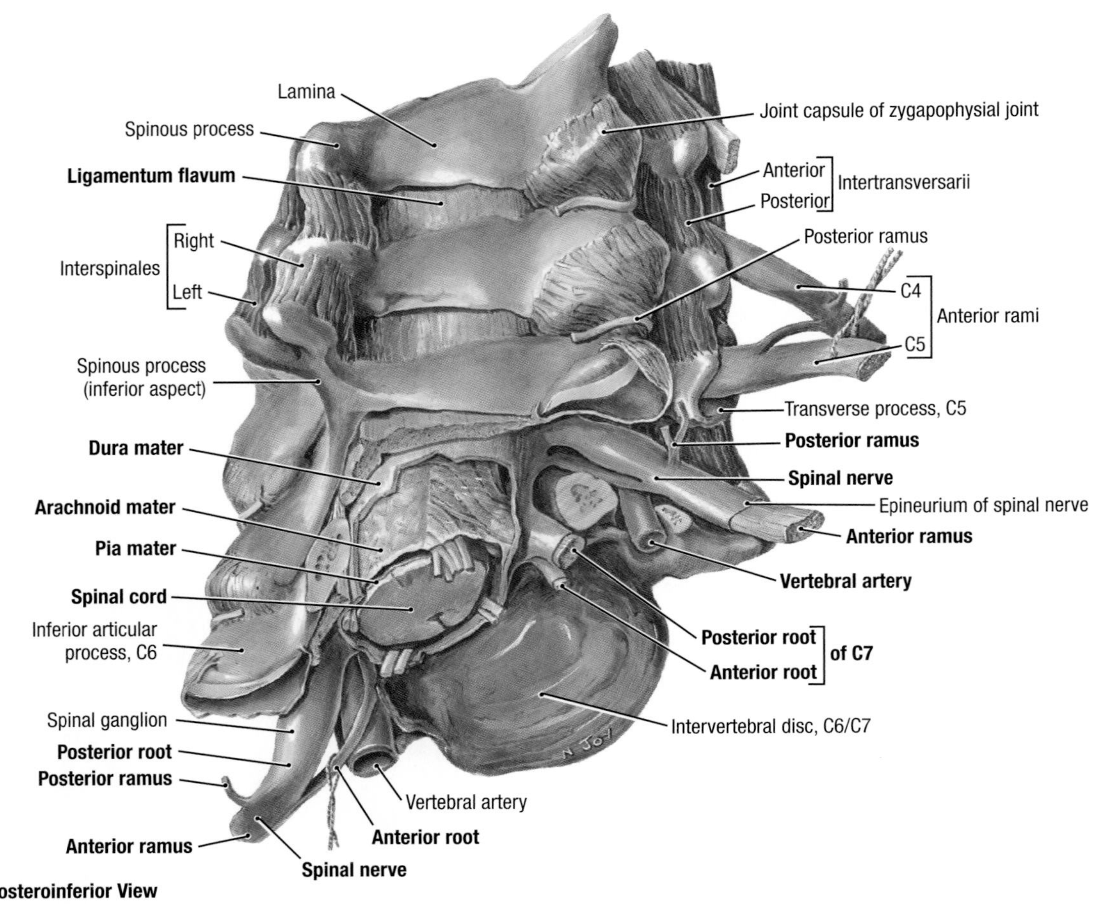
Lamina
Spinous process
Ligamentum flavum
Interspinales
Right
Left
Spinous process (inferior aspect)
Dura mater
Arachnoid mater
Pia mater
Spinal cord
Inferior articular process, C6
Spinal ganglion
Posterior root
Posterior ramus
Anterior ramus
Spinal nerve
Anterior root
Vertebral artery
Joint capsule of zygapophysial joint
Anterior
Posterior
Intertransversarii
Posterior ramus
C4
C5
Anterior rami
Transverse process, C5
Posterior ramus
Spinal nerve
Epineurium of spinal nerve
Anterior ramus
Vertebral artery
Posterior root
Anterior root
of C7
Intervertebral disc, C6/C7

A. Posteroinferior View

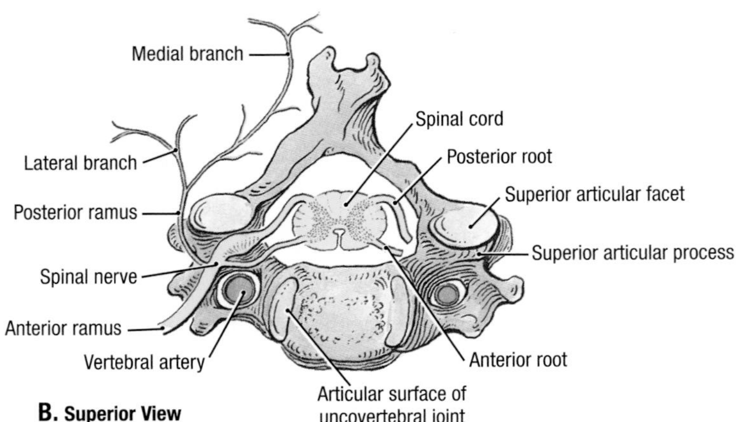
Medial branch
Lateral branch
Posterior ramus
Spinal nerve
Anterior ramus
Vertebral artery
Spinal cord
Posterior root
Superior articular facet
Superior articular process
Anterior root
Articular surface of uncovertebral joint

B. Superior View

## 4.45 Lower cervical vertebrae and associated structures and nerves

**A.** Relationship of cervical spinal cord, spinal nerves, and coverings. The anterior and posterior roots, in a common or separate dural sleeve, unite beyond the spinal ganglion to form a spinal nerve that immediately divides into a small posterior and large anterior ramus. The roots pass anterior to the zygapophysial joints and unite as they exit the intervertebral foramina and pass posterior to the vertebral artery. The posterior ramus curves dorsally around the superior articular process, and the anterior ramus rests on the transverse process, which is grooved to support it. **B.** Transverse section of spinal cord in situ. Note the vulnerability of the vertebral artery, spinal cord, and nerve roots to arthritic expansion from articular processes and the vertebral body, particularly the lateral edge of the superior surface of the body, the uncovertebral joint (joint of Luschka).

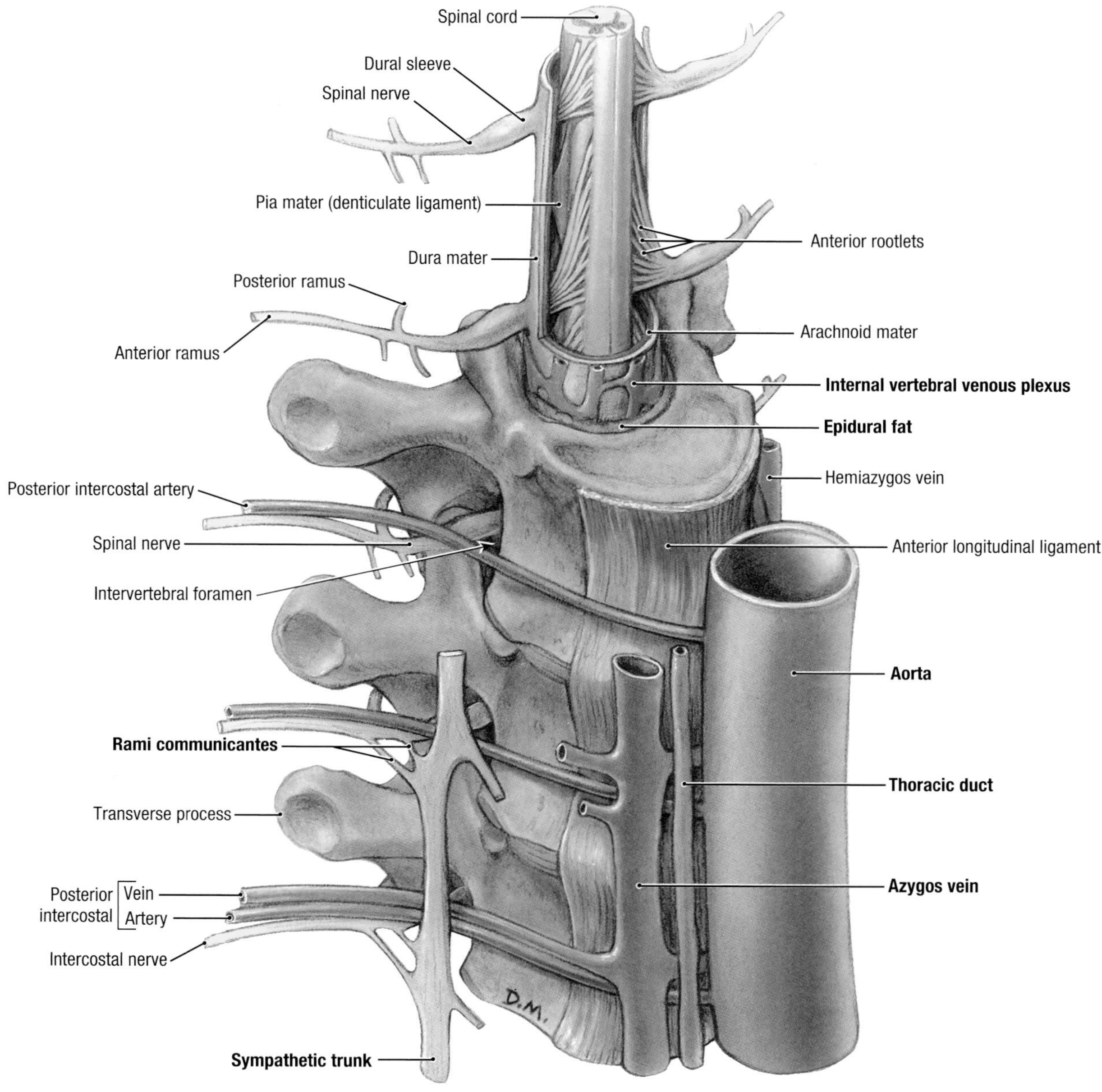
Spinal cord
Dural sleeve
Spinal nerve
Pia mater (denticulate ligament)
Anterior rootlets
Dura mater
Posterior ramus
Arachnoid mater
Anterior ramus
Internal vertebral venous plexus
Epidural fat
Hemiazygos vein
Posterior intercostal artery
Spinal nerve
Anterior longitudinal ligament
Intervertebral foramen
Aorta
Rami communicantes
Thoracic duct
Transverse process
Azygos vein
Posterior intercostal
Vein
Artery
Intercostal nerve
Sympathetic trunk
D.M.

**Right Anterolateral View**

## 4.46 Spinal cord and prevertebral structures

The vertebrae have been removed superiorly to expose the spinal cord and meninges.

- The aorta descends to the left of the midline, with the thoracic duct and azygos vein to its right.
- Typically, the azygos vein is on the right side of the vertebral bodies, and the hemiazygous vein is on the left.
- The thoracic sympathetic trunk and ganglia lie lateral to the thoracic vertebrae; the rami communicantes connect the sympathetic ganglia with the spinal nerve.
- A sleeve of dura mater surrounds the spinal nerves and blends with the sheath (epineurium) of the spinal nerve.
- The dura mater is separated from the walls of the vertebral canal by epidural fat and the internal vertebral venous plexus.

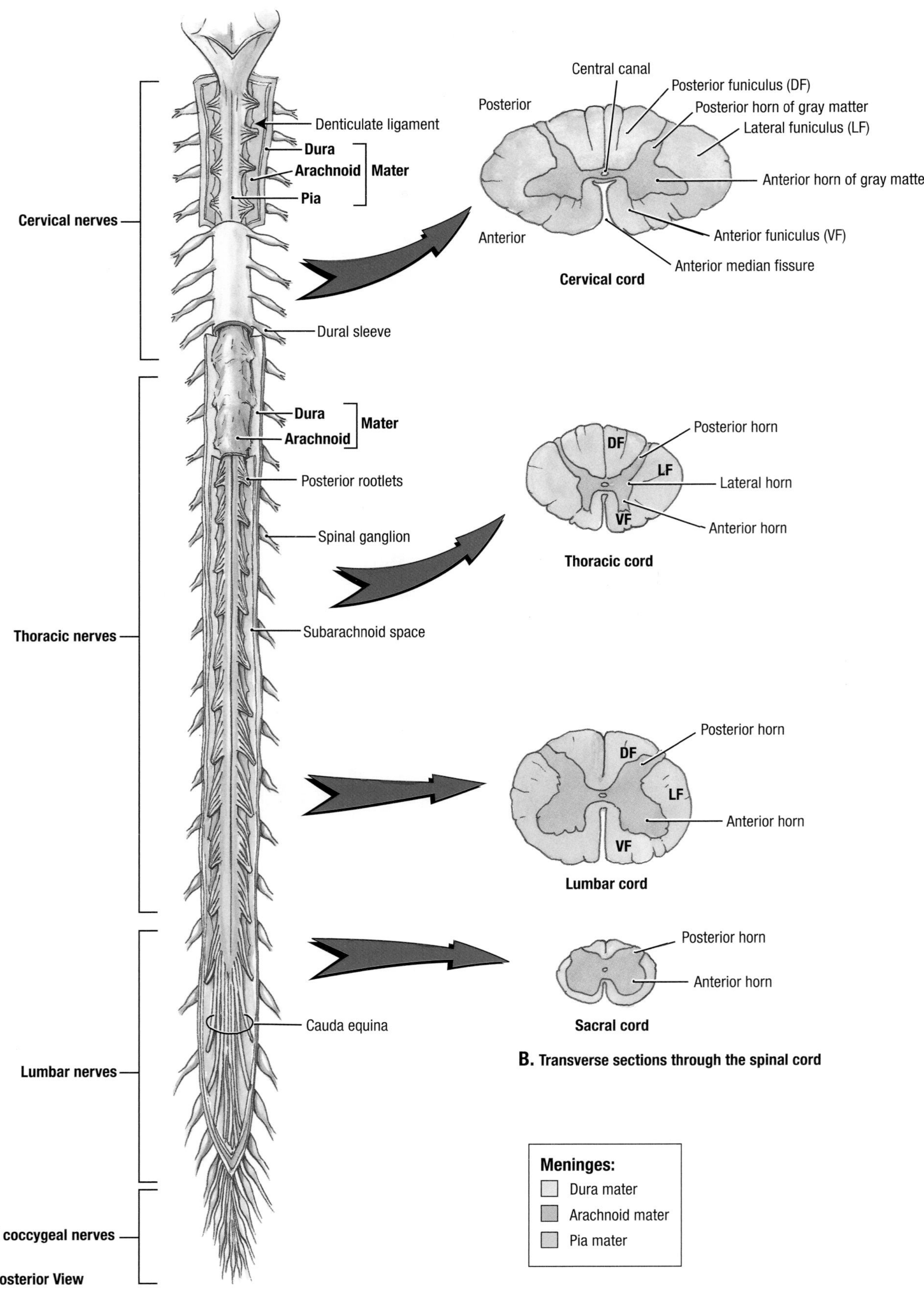
Cervical nerves
Thoracic nerves
Lumbar nerves
Sacral and coccygeal nerves
Denticulate ligament
Dura
Arachnoid
Pia
Mater
Dural sleeve
Dura
Arachnoid
Mater
Posterior rootlets
Spinal ganglion
Subarachnoid space
Cauda equina
A. Posterior View
Central canal
Posterior funiculus (DF)
Posterior horn of gray matter
Lateral funiculus (LF)
Posterior
Anterior horn of gray matter
Anterior
Anterior funiculus (VF)
Anterior median fissure
Cervical cord
Posterior horn
DF
LF
Lateral horn
VF
Anterior horn
Thoracic cord
Posterior horn
DF
LF
Anterior horn
VF
Lumbar cord
Posterior horn
Anterior horn
Sacral cord
B. Transverse sections through the spinal cord
Meninges:
Dura mater
Arachnoid mater
Pia mater

**4.47 Isolated spinal cord and spinal nerve roots with coverings and regional sections**

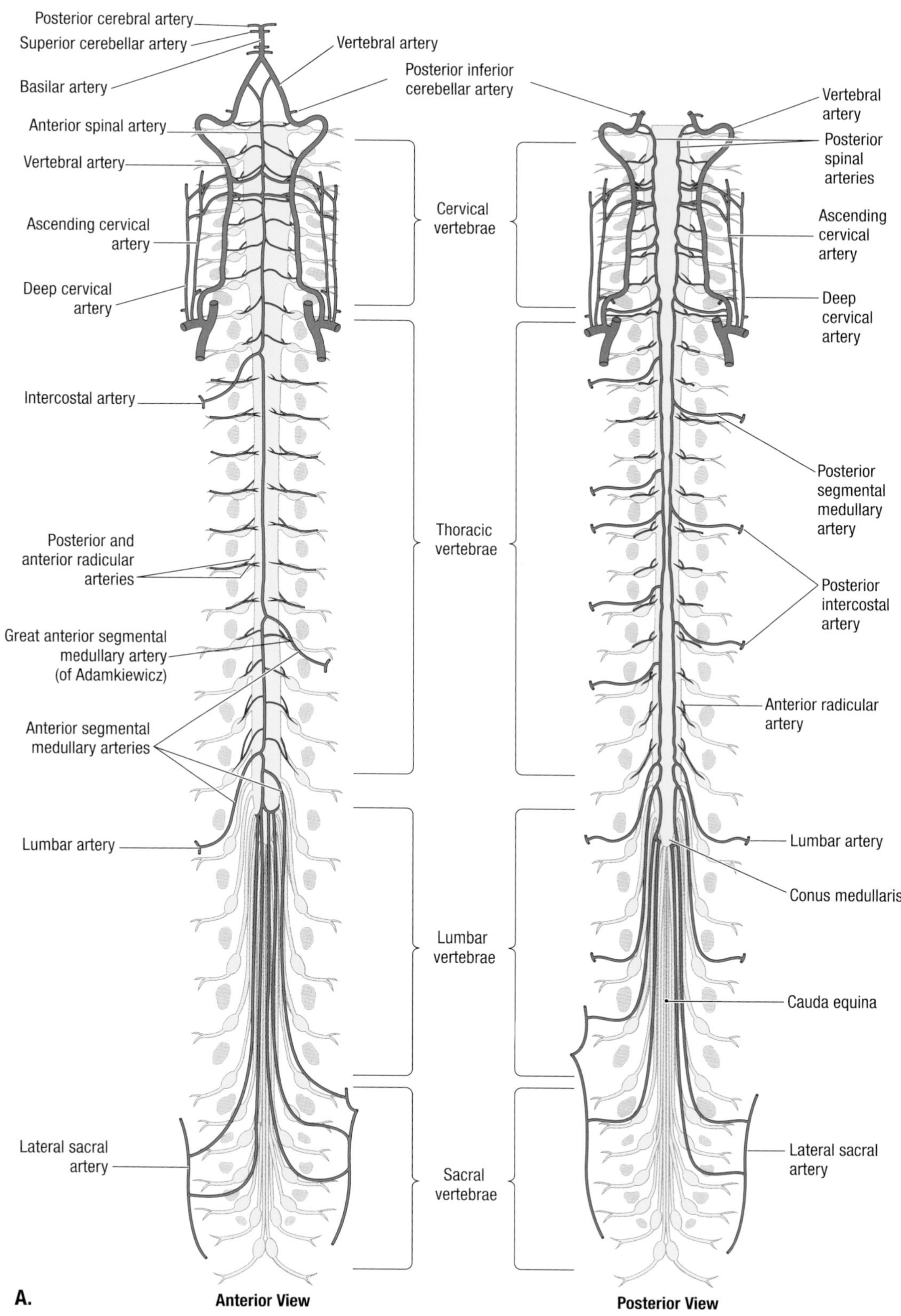
Posterior cerebral artery
Superior cerebellar artery
Basilar artery
Anterior spinal artery
Vertebral artery
Ascending cervical artery
Deep cervical artery
Intercostal artery
Posterior and anterior radicular arteries
Great anterior segmental medullary artery (of Adamkiewicz)
Anterior segmental medullary arteries
Lumbar artery
Lateral sacral artery
Vertebral artery
Posterior inferior cerebellar artery
Cervical vertebrae
Thoracic vertebrae
Lumbar vertebrae
Sacral vertebrae
Vertebral artery
Posterior spinal arteries
Ascending cervical artery
Deep cervical artery
Posterior segmental medullary artery
Posterior intercostal artery
Anterior radicular artery
Lumbar artery
Conus medullaris
Cauda equina
Lateral sacral artery
A.
Anterior View
Posterior View

## 4.48 Blood supply of spinal cord

**A.** Arteries of spinal cord. The segmental reinforcements of blood supply from the segmental medullary arteries are important in supplying blood to the anterior and posterior spinal arteries. Fractures, dislocations, and fracture-dislocations may interfere with the blood supply to the spinal cord from the spinal and medullary arteries. Deficiency of blood supply (ischemia) of the spinal cord affects its function and can lead to muscle weakness and paralysis. The spinal cord may also suffer circulatory impairment if the segmental medullary arteries, particularly the great anterior segmental medullary artery (of Adamkiewicz), are narrowed by obstructive arterial disease.

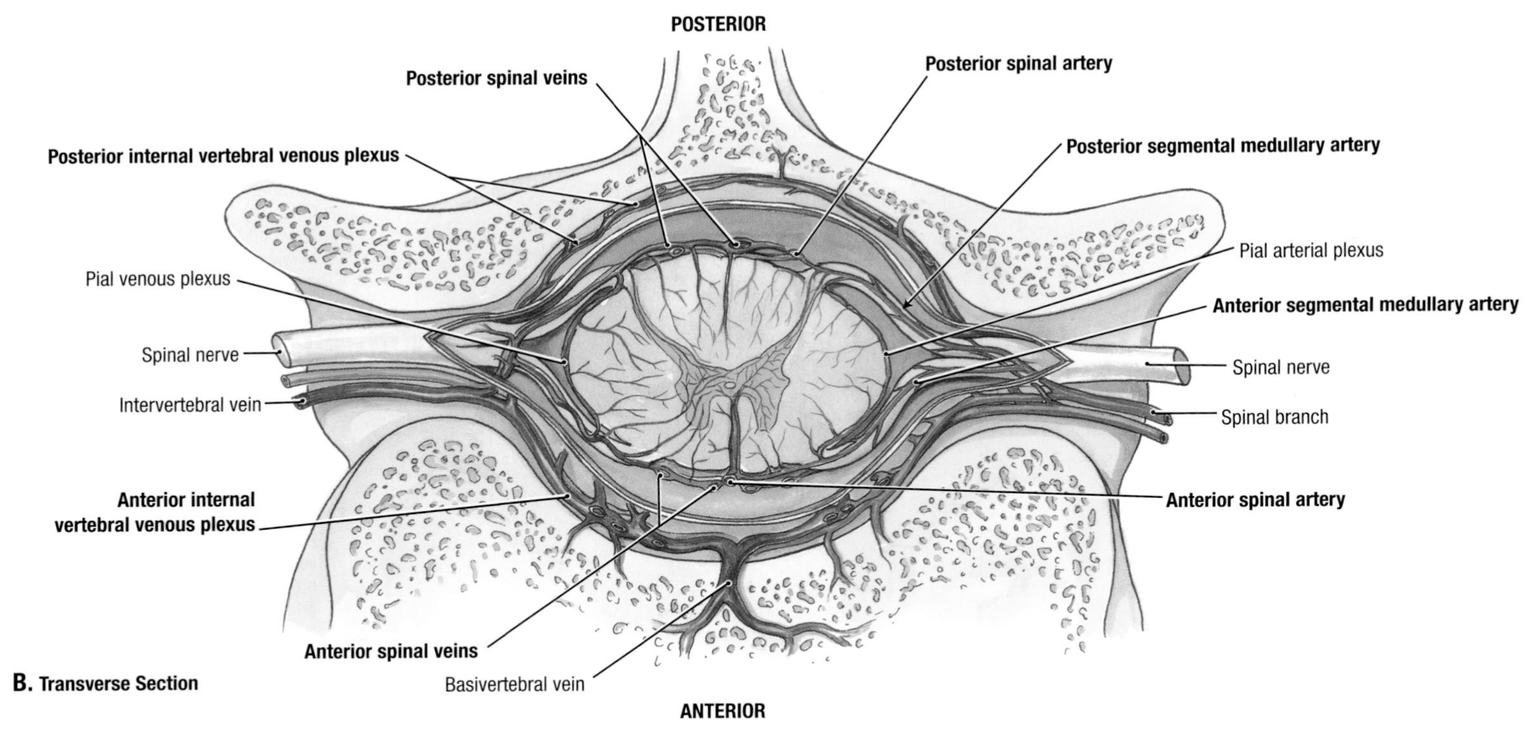
POSTERIOR
Posterior spinal veins
Posterior spinal artery
Posterior internal vertebral venous plexus
Posterior segmental medullary artery
Pial arterial plexus
Pial venous plexus
Anterior segmental medullary artery
Spinal nerve
Spinal nerve
Intervertebral vein
Spinal branch
Anterior internal vertebral venous plexus
Anterior spinal artery
Anterior spinal veins
Basivertebral vein
ANTERIOR

**B.** **Transverse Section**

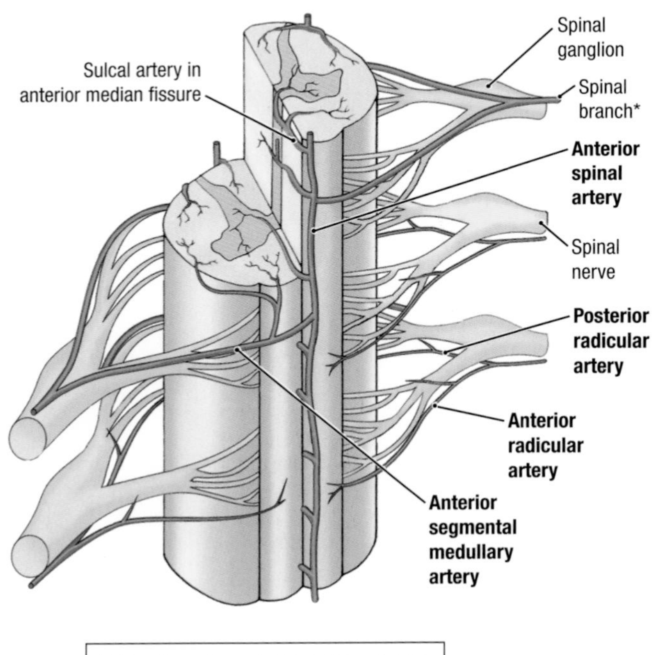
Spinal ganglion
Sulcal artery in anterior median fissure
Spinal branch*
Anterior spinal artery
Spinal nerve
Posterior radicular artery
Anterior radicular artery
Anterior segmental medullary artery
* Spinal branches arise from the vertebral, intercostal, lumbar, or sacral artery, depending on level of spinal cord.

**C.** **Anterolateral View**

## 4.48 Blood supply of spinal cord *(continued)*

B. Arterial supply and venous drainage. C. Segmental medullary and radicular arteries. Three longitudinal arteries supply the spinal cord: an anterior spinal artery, formed by the union of branches of vertebral arteries, and paired posterior spinal arteries, each of which is a branch of either the vertebral artery or the posterior inferior cerebellar artery.

- The spinal arteries run longitudinally from the medulla oblongata of the brainstem to the conus medullaris of the spinal cord. By themselves, the anterior and posterior spinal arteries supply only the short superior part of the spinal cord. The circulation to much of the spinal cord depends on segmental medullary and radicular arteries.
- The anterior and posterior segmental medullary arteries enter the intervertebral foramen to unite with the spinal arteries to supply blood to the spinal cord. The great anterior segmented medullary artery (Adamkiewicz artery) occurs on the left side in 65% of people. It reinforces the circulation to two thirds of the spinal cord.
- Posterior and anterior roots of the spinal nerves and their coverings are supplied by posterior and anterior radicular arteries, which run along the nerve roots. These vessels do not reach the posterior or anterior spinal arteries.
- The 3 anterior and 3 posterior spinal veins are arranged longitudinally; they communicate freely with each other and are drained by up to 12 anterior and posterior medullary and radicular veins. The veins draining the spinal cord join the internal vertebral plexus in the epidural space.

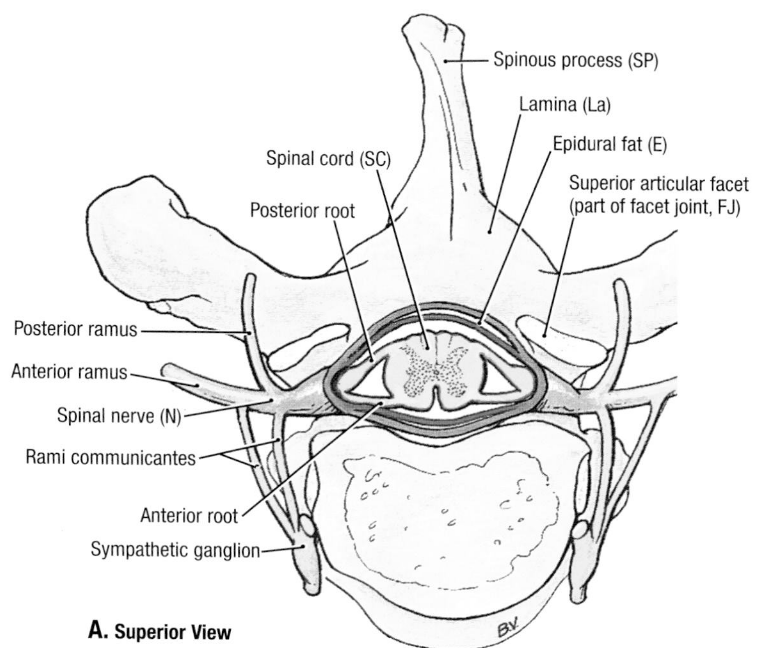
Spinous process (SP)
Lamina (La)
Epidural fat (E)
Spinal cord (SC)
Superior articular facet
(part of facet joint, FJ)
Posterior root
Posterior ramus
Anterior ramus
Spinal nerve (N)
Rami communicantes
Anterior root
Sympathetic ganglion

**A. Superior View**

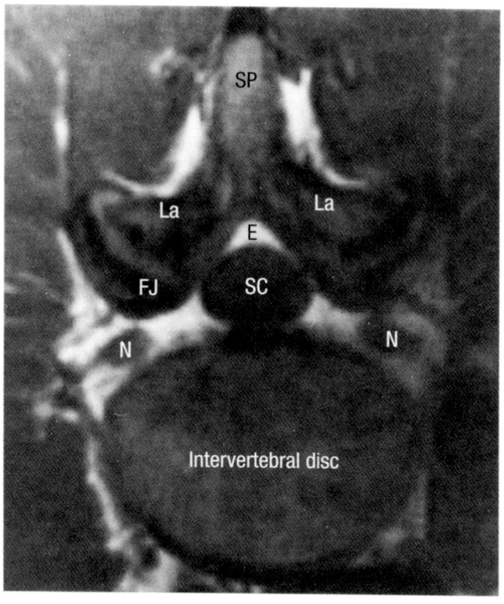
SP
La
La
E
FJ
SC
N
N
Intervertebral disc

**B. Transverse (axial) MRI**

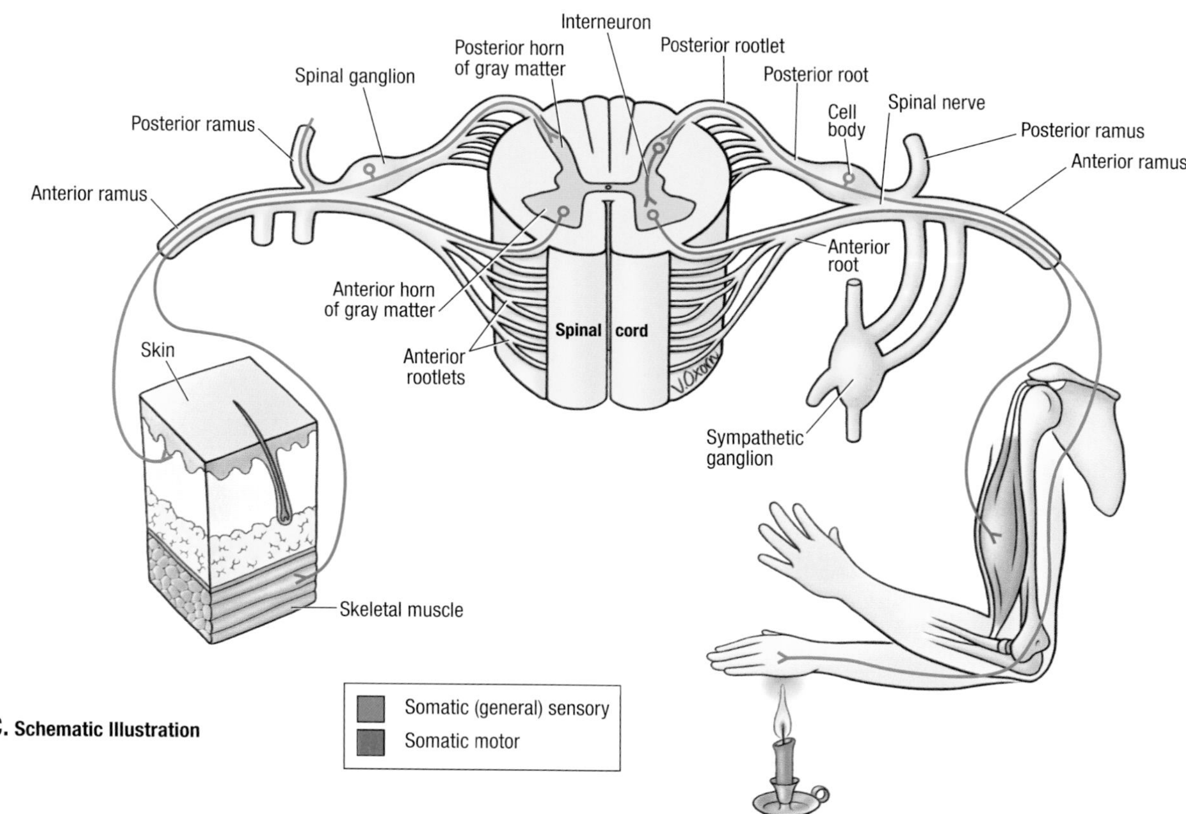
Interneuron
Posterior horn
of gray matter
Posterior rootlet
Spinal ganglion
Posterior root
Cell
body
Spinal nerve
Posterior ramus
Posterior ramus
Anterior ramus
Anterior ramus
Anterior
root
Anterior horn
of gray matter
Spinal cord
Skin
Anterior
rootlets
Sympathetic
ganglion
Skeletal muscle
Somatic (general) sensory
Somatic motor

**C. Schematic Illustration**

## 4.49 Overview of somatic nervous system

**A.** Spinal cord in situ in vertebral canal. **B.** T1 axial (transverse) MRI of lumbar spine. **C.** Components of typical spinal nerve. The somatic nervous system, or voluntary nervous system, composed of somatic parts of the CNS and PNS, provides general sensory and motor innervation to all parts of the body (G. *soma*), except the viscera in the body cavities, smooth muscle, and glands. The somatic (general) sensory fibers transmit sensations of touch, pain, temperature, and position from sensory receptors. The somatic motor fibers permit voluntary and reflexive movement by causing contraction of skeletal muscles, such as occurs when one touches a candle flame.

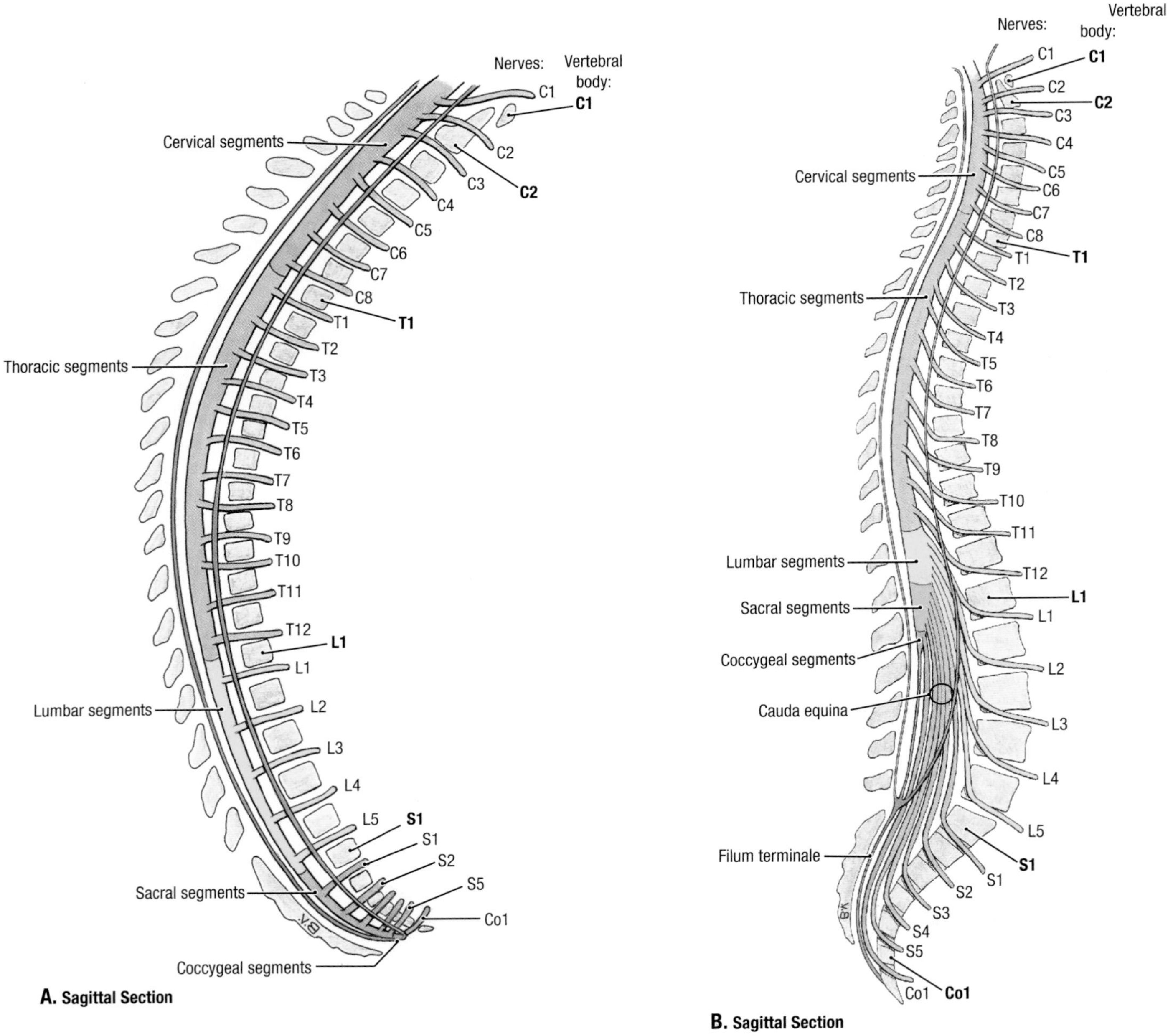

A. Sagittal Section

B. Sagittal Section

## 4.50 Spinal cord and spinal nerves

**A.** Spinal cord at 12 weeks gestation. **B.** Spinal cord of an adult.

- Early in development, the spinal cord and vertebral (spinal) canal are nearly equal in length. The canal grows longer, so spinal nerves have an increasingly longer course to reach the intervertebral foramen at the correct level for their exit. The spinal cord of adults terminates between vertebral bodies L1–L2. The remaining spinal nerves, seeking their intervertebral foramen of exit, form the cauda equina.
- All 31 pairs of spinal nerves—8 cervical (C), 12 thoracic (T), 5 lumbar (L), 5 sacral (S), and 1 coccygeal (Co)—arise from the spinal cord and exit through the intervertebral foramina in the vertebral column.

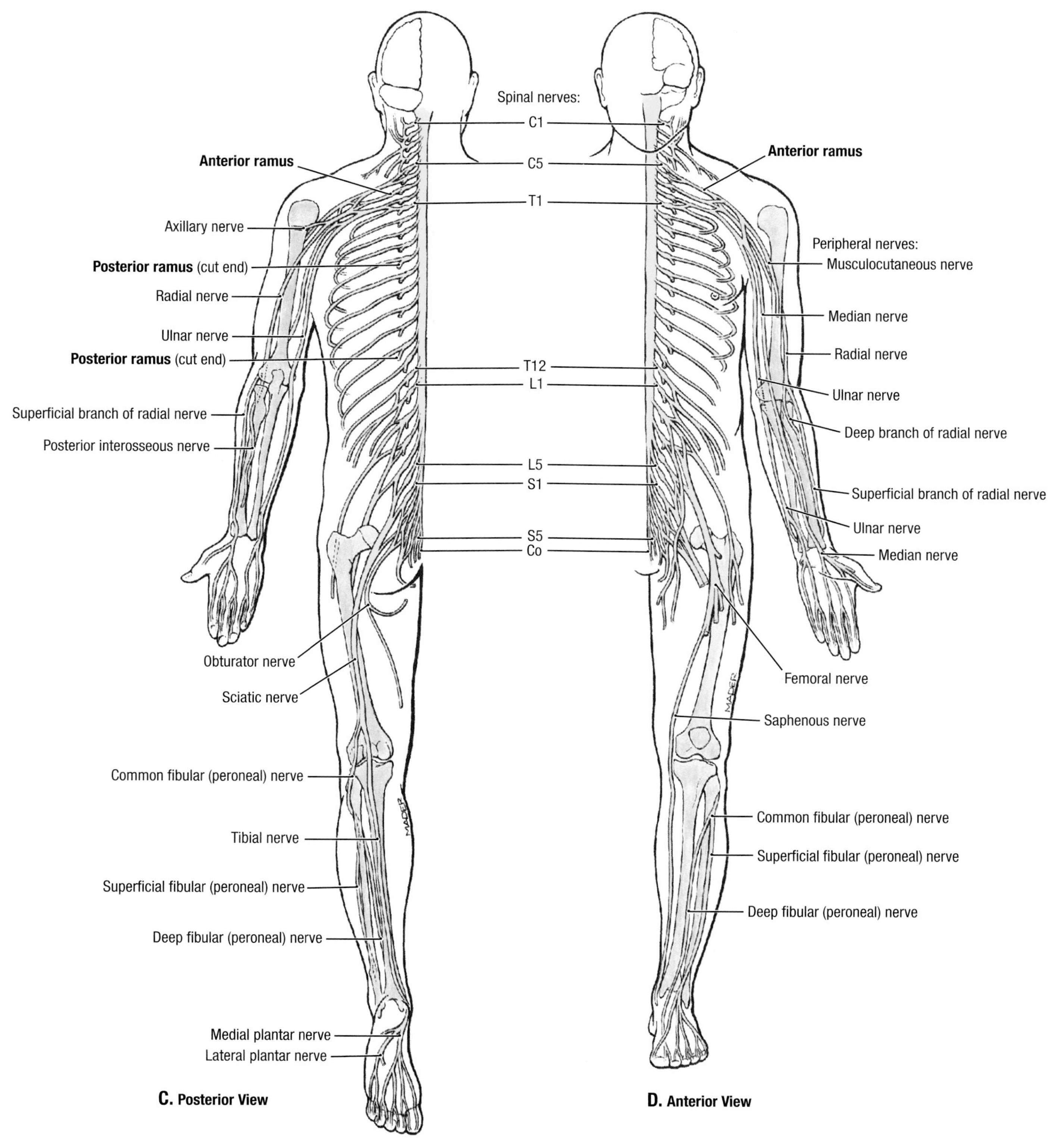
Spinal nerves:
C1
C5
T1
T12
L1
L5
S1
S5
Co
Anterior ramus
Axillary nerve
Posterior ramus (cut end)
Radial nerve
Ulnar nerve
Posterior ramus (cut end)
Superficial branch of radial nerve
Posterior interosseous nerve
Obturator nerve
Sciatic nerve
Common fibular (peroneal) nerve
Tibial nerve
Superficial fibular (peroneal) nerve
Deep fibular (peroneal) nerve
Medial plantar nerve
Lateral plantar nerve
C. Posterior View
Anterior ramus
Peripheral nerves:
Musculocutaneous nerve
Median nerve
Radial nerve
Ulnar nerve
Deep branch of radial nerve
Superficial branch of radial nerve
Ulnar nerve
Median nerve
Femoral nerve
Saphenous nerve
Common fibular (peroneal) nerve
Superficial fibular (peroneal) nerve
Deep fibular (peroneal) nerve
D. Anterior View

## 4.50 Spinal cord and spinal nerves *(continued)*

**C** and **D.** Peripheral nerves.

- The anterior rami supply nerve fibers to the anterior and lateral regions of the trunk and upper and lower limbs.
- The posterior rami supply nerve fibers to synovial joints of the vertebral column, deep muscles of the back, and overlying skin.

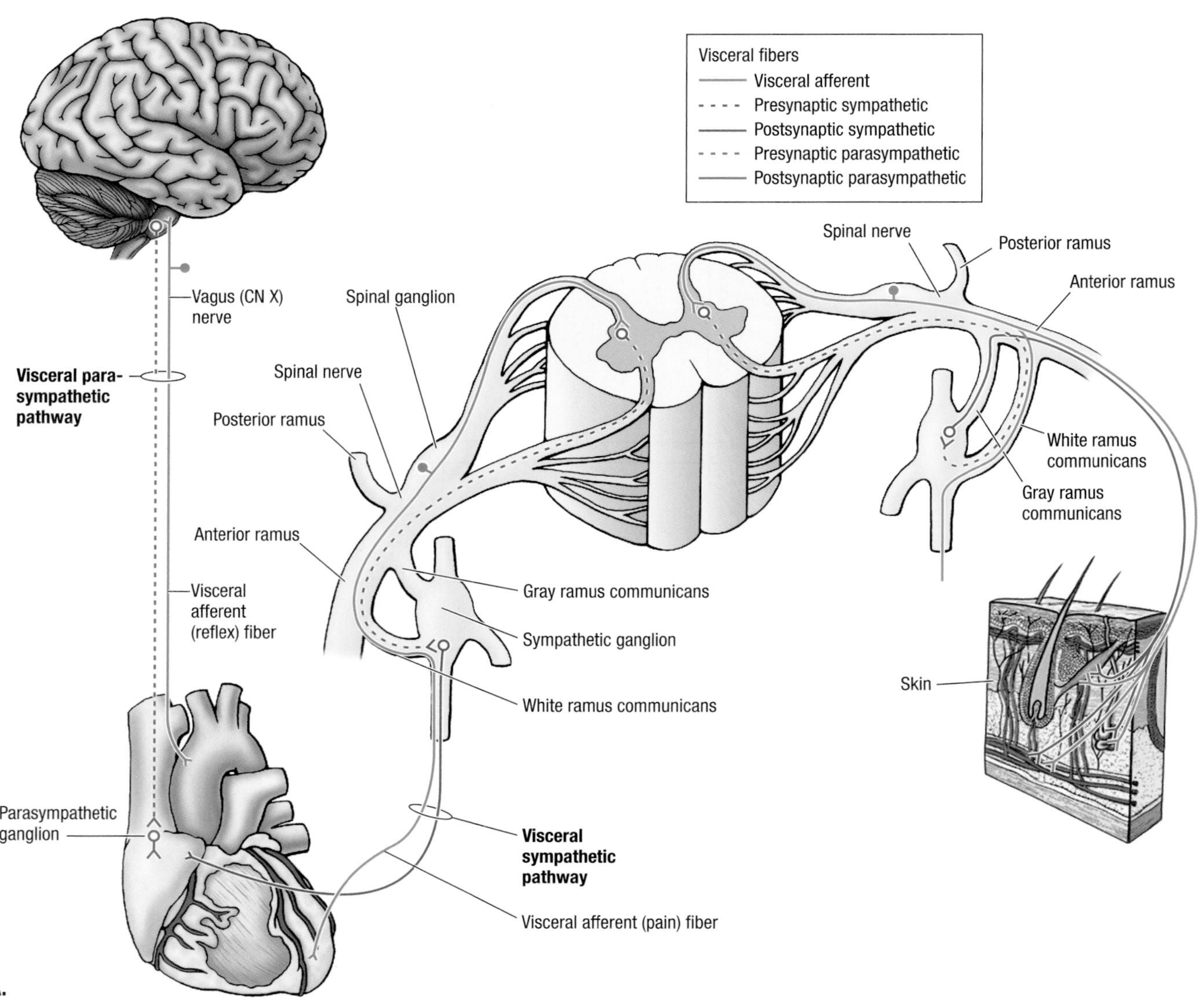
Visceral fibers
Visceral afferent
Presynaptic sympathetic
Postsynaptic sympathetic
Presynaptic parasympathetic
Postsynaptic parasympathetic
Vagus (CN X) nerve
Visceral parasympathetic pathway
Spinal ganglion
Spinal nerve
Posterior ramus
Anterior ramus
Visceral afferent (reflex) fiber
Gray ramus communicans
Sympathetic ganglion
White ramus communicans
Parasympathetic ganglion
Visceral sympathetic pathway
Visceral afferent (pain) fiber
Spinal nerve
Posterior ramus
Anterior ramus
White ramus communicans
Gray ramus communicans
Skin
A.

## 4.51 Visceral afferent and visceral efferent (motor) innervation

**A.** Schematic illustration. Visceral afferent fibers have important relationships to the CNS, both anatomically and functionally. We are usually unaware of the sensory input of these fibers, which provides information about the condition of the body's internal environment. This information is integrated in the CNS, often triggering visceral or somatic reflexes or both. Visceral reflexes regulate blood pressure and chemistry by altering such functions as heart and respiratory rates and vascular resistance. Visceral sensation that reaches a conscious level is generally categorized as pain that is usually poorly localized and may be perceived as hunger or nausea. However, adequate stimulation may elicit true pain. Most visceral/reflex (unconscious) sensation and some pain travel in visceral afferent fibers that accompany the parasympathetic fibers retrograde. Most visceral pain impulses (from the heart and most organs of the peritoneal cavity) travel along visceral afferent fibers accompanying sympathetic fibers.

Visceral efferent (motor) innervation. The efferent nerve fibers and ganglia of the ANS are organized into two systems or divisions.

1. Sympathetic (thoracolumbar) division. In general, the effects of sympathetic stimulation are catabolic (preparing the body for "flight or fight").
2. Parasympathetic (craniosacral) division. In general, the effects of parasympathetic stimulation are anabolic (promoting normal function and conserving energy).

Conduction of impulses from the CNS to the effector organ involves a series of two neurons in both sympathetic and parasympathetic systems. The cell body of the presynaptic (preganglionic) neuron (first neuron) is located in the gray matter of the CNS. Its fiber (axon) synapses on the cell body of a postsynaptic (postganglionic) neuron, the second neuron in the series. The cell bodies of such second neurons are located in autonomic ganglia outside the CNS, and the postsynaptic fibers terminate on the effector organ (smooth muscle, modified cardiac muscle, or glands).

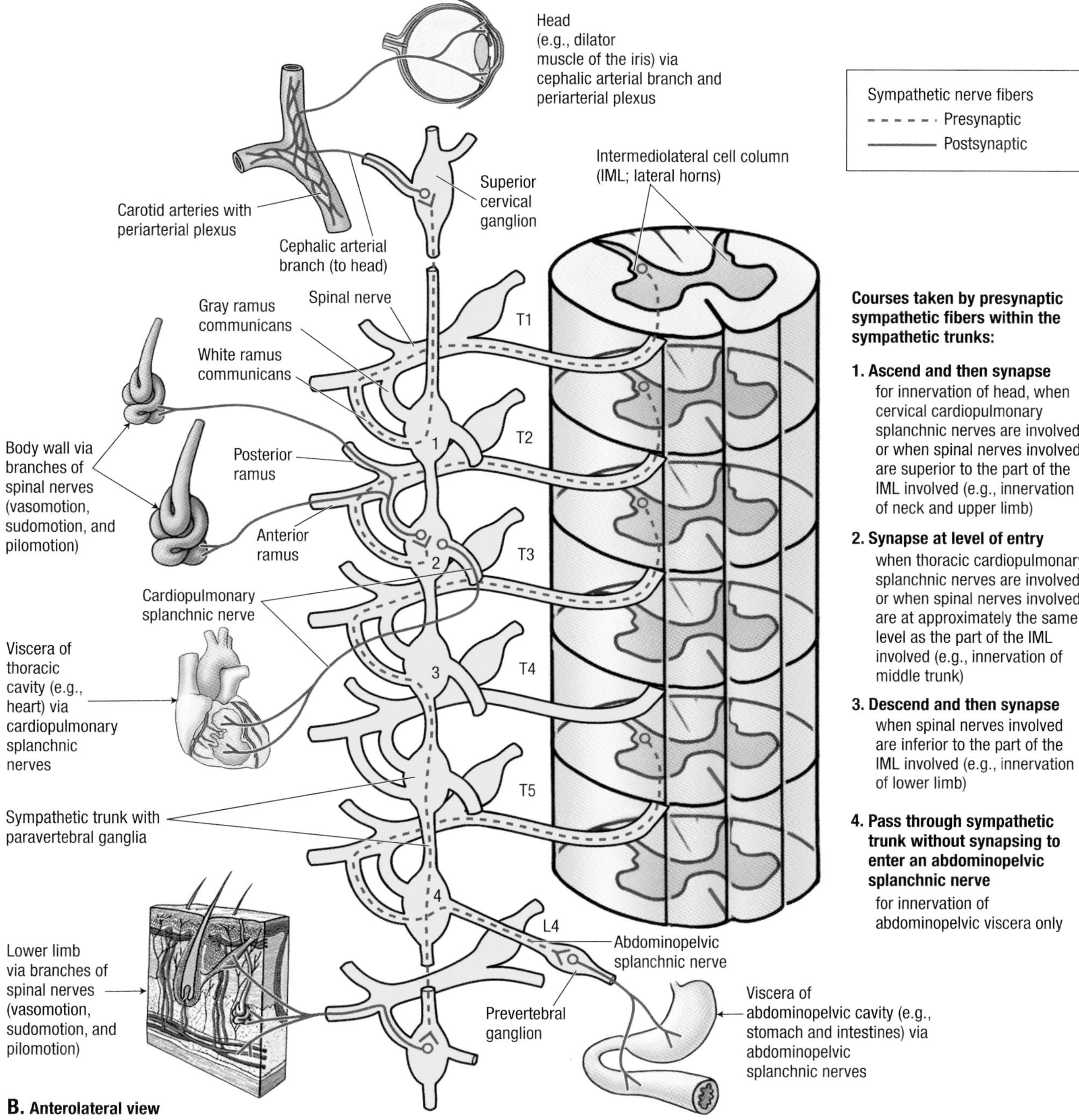
Head
(e.g., dilator
muscle of the iris) via
cephalic arterial branch and
periarterial plexus
Sympathetic nerve fibers
Presynaptic
Postsynaptic
Intermediolateral cell column
(IML; lateral horns)
Superior
cervical
ganglion
Carotid arteries with
periarterial plexus
Cephalic arterial
branch (to head)
Spinal nerve
Gray ramus
communicans
White ramus
communicans
T1
T2
T3
T4
T5
L4
Body wall via
branches of
spinal nerves
(vasomotion,
sudomotion, and
pilomotion)
Posterior
ramus
Anterior
ramus
Cardiopulmonary
splanchnic nerve
Viscera of
thoracic
cavity (e.g.,
heart) via
cardiopulmonary
splanchnic
nerves
Sympathetic trunk with
paravertebral ganglia
Lower limb
via branches of
spinal nerves
(vasomotion,
sudomotion, and
pilomotion)
Abdominopelvic
splanchnic nerve
Prevertebral
ganglion
Viscera of
abdominopelvic cavity (e.g.,
stomach and intestines) via
abdominopelvic
splanchnic nerves
Courses taken by presynaptic
sympathetic fibers within the
sympathetic trunks:
1. Ascend and then synapse
for innervation of head, when
cervical cardiopulmonary
splanchnic nerves are involved,
or when spinal nerves involved
are superior to the part of the
IML involved (e.g., innervation
of neck and upper limb)
2. Synapse at level of entry
when thoracic cardiopulmonary
splanchnic nerves are involved,
or when spinal nerves involved
are at approximately the same
level as the part of the IML
involved (e.g., innervation of
middle trunk)
3. Descend and then synapse
when spinal nerves involved
are inferior to the part of the
IML involved (e.g., innervation
of lower limb)
4. Pass through sympathetic
trunk without synapsing to
enter an abdominopelvic
splanchnic nerve
for innervation of
abdominopelvic viscera only
B. Anterolateral view

## 4.51 Visceral afferent and visceral efferent (motor) innervation *(continued)*

**B. Courses taken by sympathetic motor fibers.** Presynaptic fibers all follow the same course until they reach the sympathetic trunks. In the sympathetic trunks, they follow one of four possible courses. Fibers involved in providing sympathetic innervation to the body wall and limbs or viscera above the level of the diaphragm follow paths 1–3. They synapse in the paravertebral ganglia of the sympathetic trunks. Fibers involved in innervating abdominopelvic viscera follow path 4 to prevertebral ganglion via abdominopelvic splanchnic nerves.

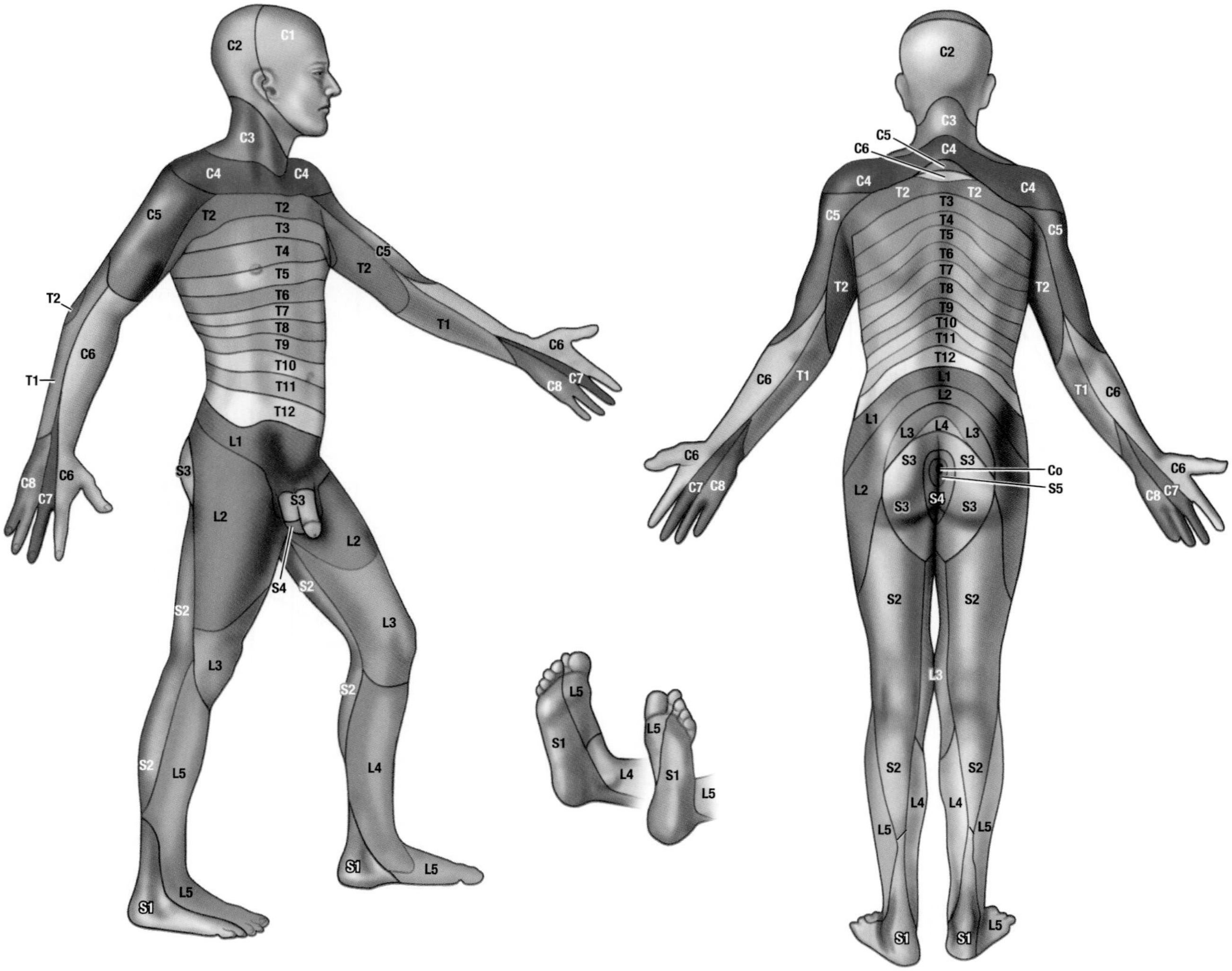

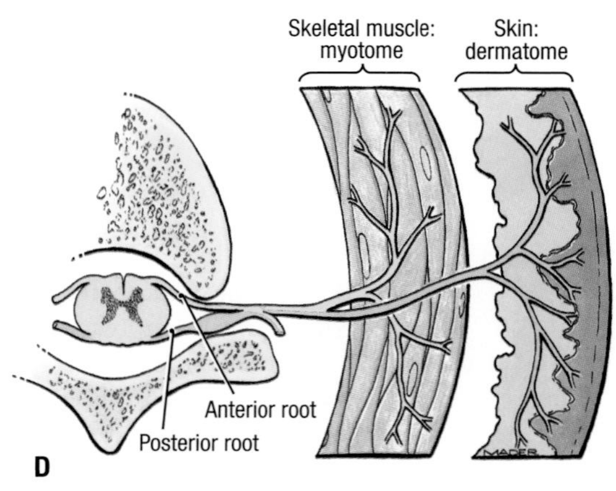
Skeletal muscle: myotome
Skin: dermatome
Anterior root
Posterior root
D

## 4.52 Dermatomes

**A–C.** Dermatome map (Foerster, 1933). The Keegan and Garrett (1948) dermatome map is not included here. The two schemes are similar in the trunk but differ in the limbs, where both are presented. **D.** Schematic illustration of a dermatome and myotome. The unilateral area of skin innervated by the general sensory fibers of a single spinal nerve is called a dermatome. From clinical studies of lesions in the posterior roots or spinal nerves, dermatome maps have been devised that indicate the typical pattens of innervation of the skin by specific spinal nerves.

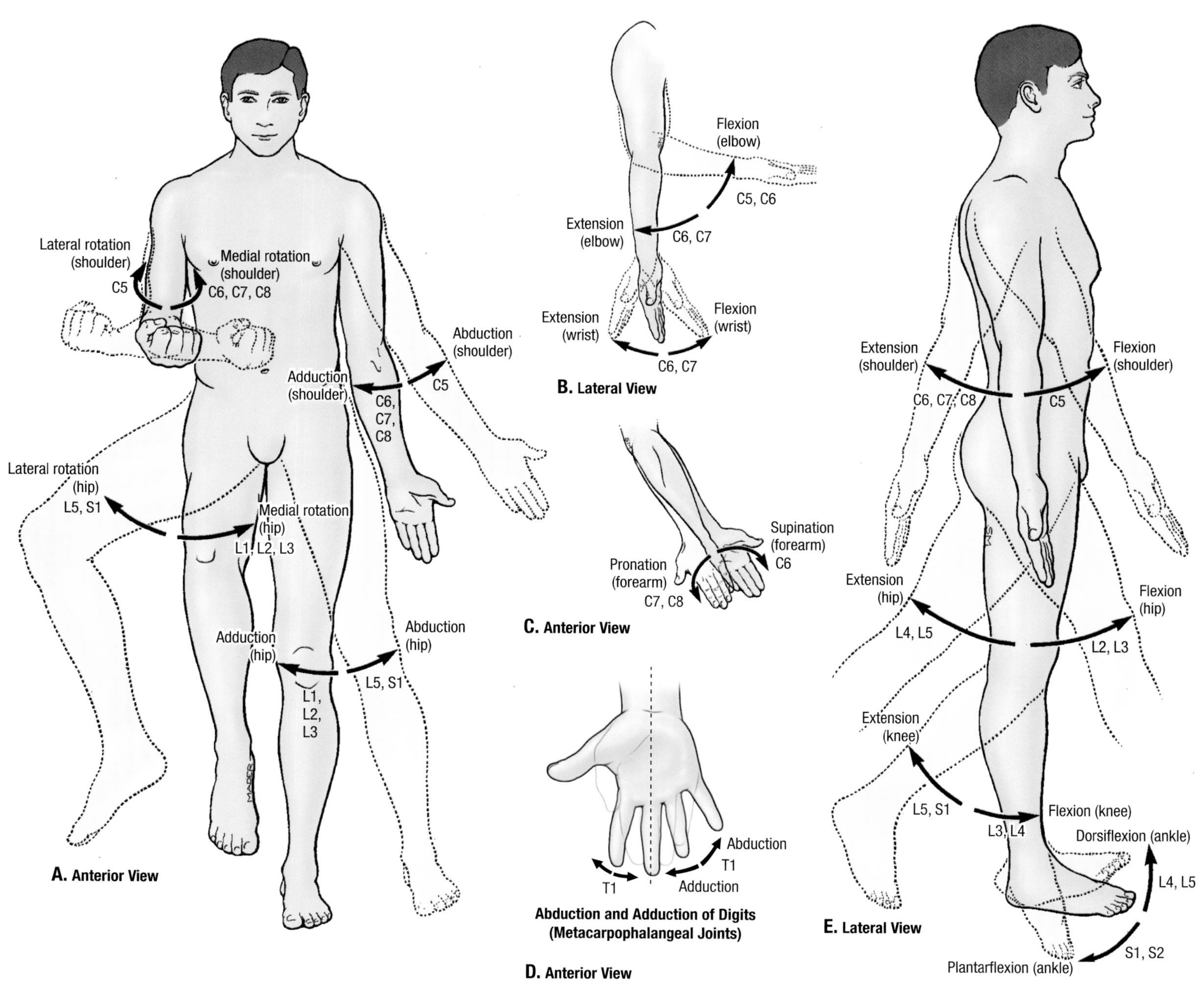
Lateral rotation
(shoulder)
C5
Medial rotation
(shoulder)
C6, C7, C8
Abduction
(shoulder)
C5
Adduction
(shoulder)
C6,
C7,
C8
Lateral rotation
(hip)
L5, S1
Medial rotation
(hip)
L1, L2, L3
Abduction
(hip)
Adduction
(hip)
L5, S1
L1,
L2,
L3
A. Anterior View
Flexion
(elbow)
C5, C6
Extension
(elbow)
C6, C7
Extension
(wrist)
Flexion
(wrist)
C6, C7
B. Lateral View
Supination
(forearm)
C6
Pronation
(forearm)
C7, C8
C. Anterior View
Abduction
T1
T1
Adduction
Abduction and Adduction of Digits
(Metacarpophalangeal Joints)
D. Anterior View
Extension
(shoulder)
Flexion
(shoulder)
C6, C7, C8
C5
Extension
(hip)
Flexion
(hip)
L4, L5
L2, L3
Extension
(knee)
L5, S1
Flexion (knee)
L3, L4
Dorsiflexion (ankle)
L4, L5
S1, S2
Plantarflexion (ankle)
E. Lateral View

## 4.53 Myotomes

Somatic motor (general somatic efferent) fibers transmit impulses to skeletal (voluntary) muscles. The unilateral muscle mass receiving innervation from the somatic motor fibers conveyed by a single spinal nerve is a myotome. Each skeletal muscle is innervated by the somatic motor fibers of several spinal nerves; therefore, the muscle myotome will consist of several segments. The muscle myotomes have been grouped by joint movement to facilitate clinical testing. The intrinsic muscles of the hand constitute a single myotome—T1.

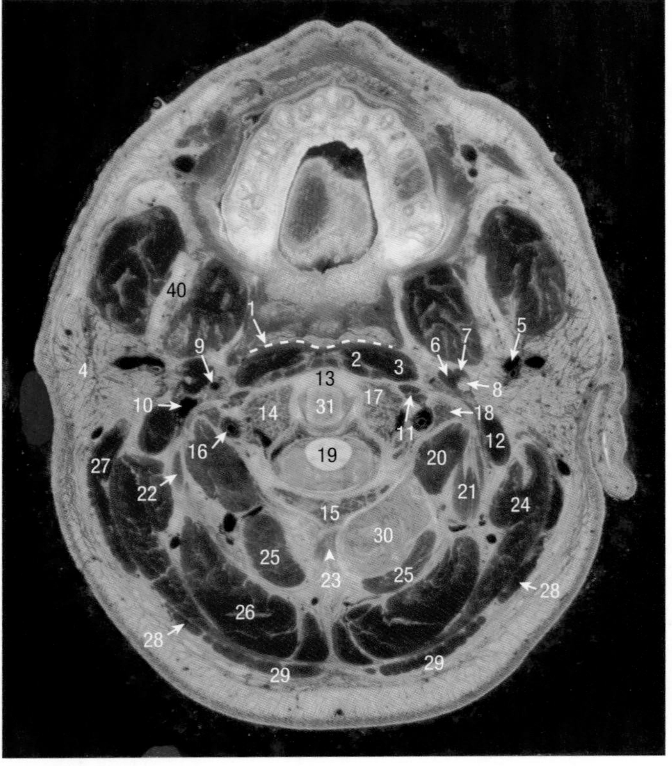

40
1
9
2
3
6
7
5
4
13
8
10
14
31
17
18
11
16
19
20
12
27
22
21
24
15
30
25
23
25
28
26
28
29
29


**A. Inferior View**

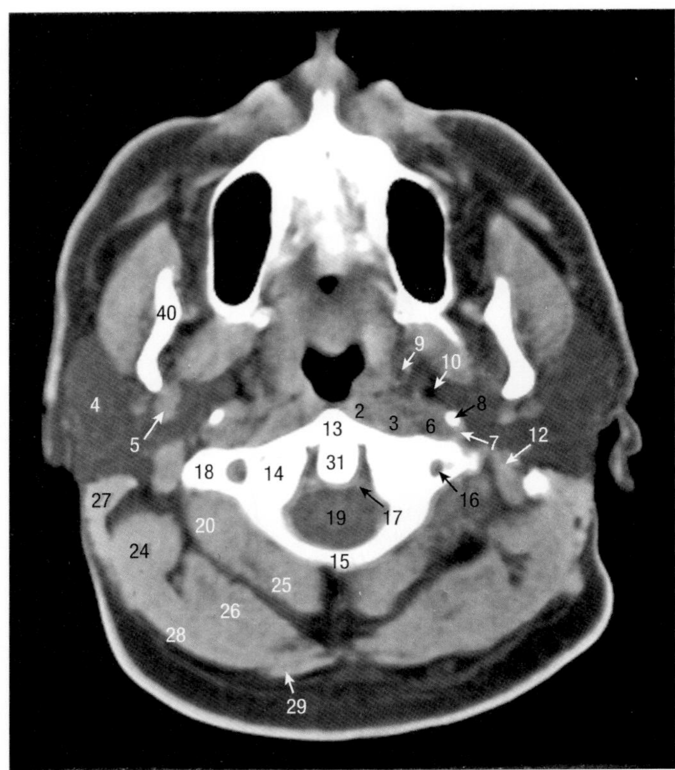

40
9
10
8
2
3
4
13
6
7
12
5
18
14
31
16
27
17
20
19
24
15
25
26
28
29


**B. Inferior View**

| | |
|---|---|
| 1 | Site of retropharyngeal space |
| 2 | Longus colli |
| 3 | Longus capitis |
| 4 | Parotid gland |
| 5 | Retromandibular vein |
| 6 | Stylopharyngeus |
| 7 | Styloglossus |
| 8 | Stylohyoid muscle and ligament/process |
| 9 | Internal carotid artery |
| 10 | Internal jugular vein |
| 11 | Rectus capitis lateralis |
| 12 | Posterior belly of digastric |
| 13 | Anterior arch of atlas (C1) |
| 14 | Lateral mass of atlas (C1) |
| 15 | Posterior arch of atlas (C1) |
| 16 | Vertebral artery |
| 17 | Transverse ligament of atlas (C1) |
| 18 | Transverse process of atlas (C1) |
| 19 | Spinal cord |
| 20 | Rectus capitis posterior major |
| 21 | Obliquus capitis inferior |
| 22 | Obliquus capitis superior |
| 23 | Spinous process of atlas (C1) |
| 24 | Longissimus capitis |
| 25 | Rectus capitis posterior minor |
| 26 | Semispinalis capitis |
| 27 | Sternocleidomastoid |
| 28 | Splenius capitis |
| 29 | Trapezius |
| 30 | Fatty mass |
| 31 | Dens of axis (C2) |
| 32 | Anterior tubercle of atlas (C1) |
| 33 | Inferior articular facet of atlas (C1) |
| 34 | Foramen magnum |
| 35 | Foramen transversarium |
| 36 | Posterior tubercle of atlas (C1) |
| 37 | Mastoid process |
| 38 | Occipital bone of skull |
| 39 | External occipital protuberance |
| 40 | Ramus of mandible |

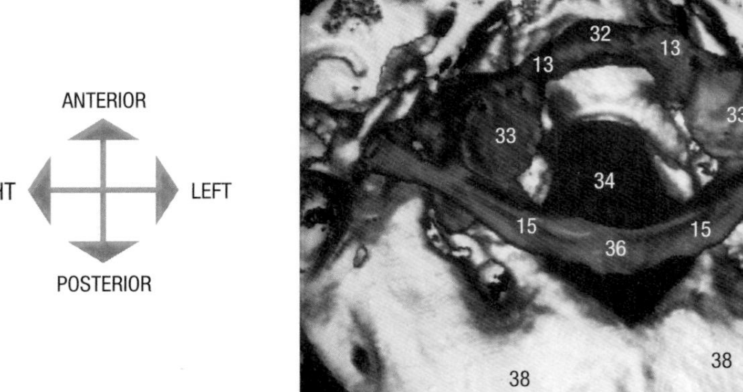

ANTERIOR
RIGHT
LEFT
POSTERIOR
32
13
13
37
35
33
33
34
15
15
36
38
38
39


**C. Posteroinferior View**

## 4.54 Imaging of superior nuchal region at the level of the atlas

**A.** Transverse section of specimen. **B.** Transverse computed tomographic (CT) scan. **C.** Three-dimensional (3D) CT of the base of the skull and atlas.

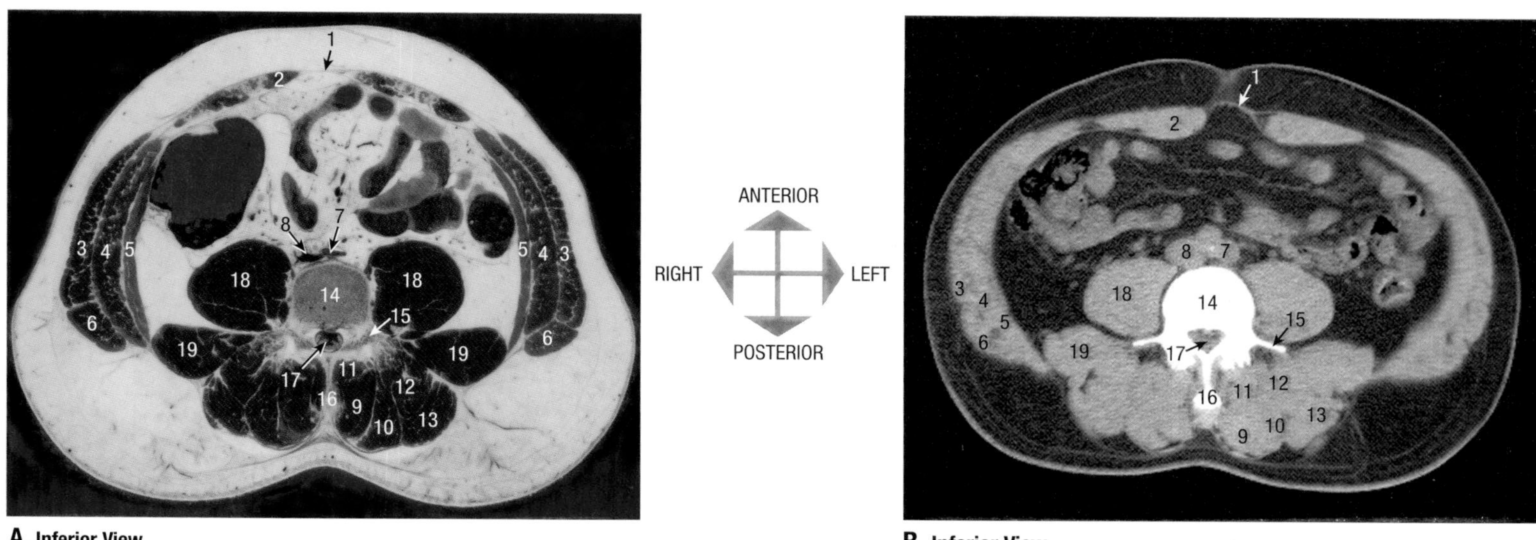
ANTERIOR
RIGHT
LEFT
POSTERIOR

**A.** Inferior View

**B.** Inferior View

| 1 | Linea alba | 6 | Latissimus dorsi | 11 | Multifidus | 16 | Spinous process |
|---|---|---|---|---|---|---|---|
| 2 | Rectus abdominis | 7 | Descending aorta | 12 | Rotatores | 17 | Cauda equina |
| 3 | External oblique | 8 | Inferior vena cava | 13 | Iliocostalis | 18 | Psoas major |
| 4 | Internal oblique | 9 | Spinalis | 14 | 4th lumbar vertebra | 19 | Quadratus lumborum |
| 5 | Transversus abdominis | 10 | Longissimus | 15 | Transverse process | | |

**4.55 Imaging of lumbar spine at L4**

**A.** Transverse section of specimen. **B.** Transverse computed tomographic (CT) scan.

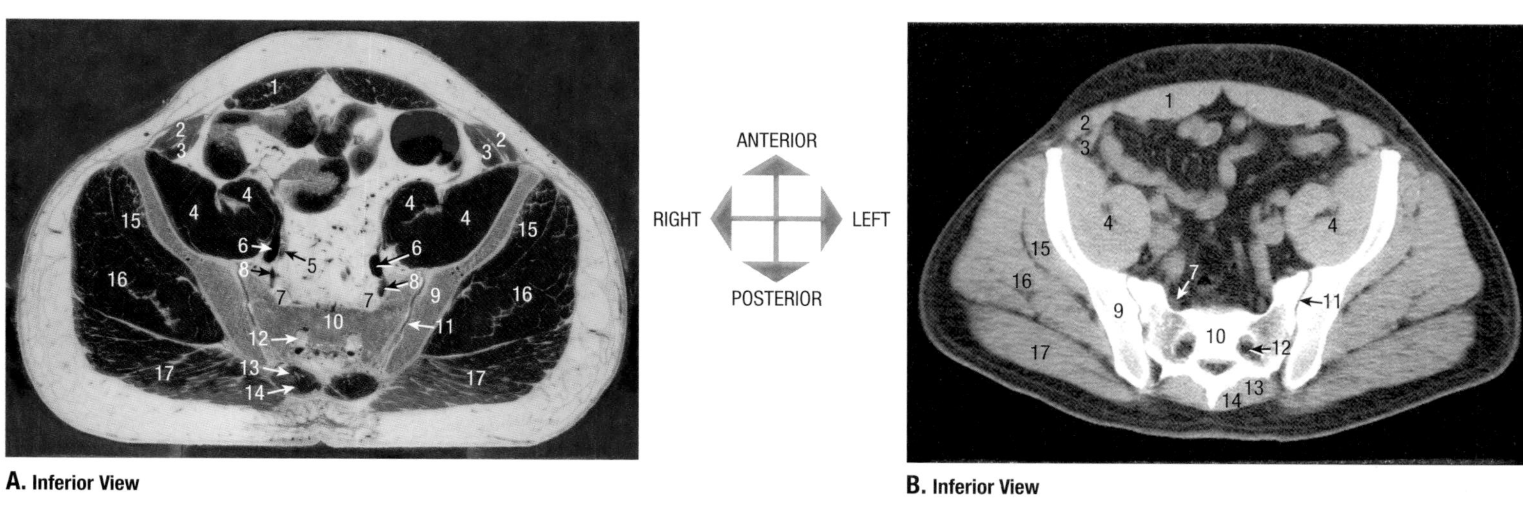
ANTERIOR
RIGHT
LEFT
POSTERIOR

**A.** Inferior View

**B.** Inferior View

| 1 | Rectus abdominis | 6 | Internal iliac vein | 10 | 2nd sacral vertebra | 14 | Erector spinae |
|---|---|---|---|---|---|---|---|
| 2 | External oblique | 7 | Anterior rami | 11 | Sacro-iliac joint | 15 | Gluteus minimis |
| 3 | Internal oblique | 8 | Superior gluteal vessels | 12 | Sacral nerve root | 16 | Gluteus medius |
| 4 | Iliopsoas | 9 | Body of ilium | 13 | Multifidus | 17 | Gluteus maximus |
| 5 | Internal iliac artery | | | | | | |

**4.56 Imaging of sacro-iliac joint**

**A.** Transverse section of specimen. **B.** Transverse computed tomographic (CT) scan.

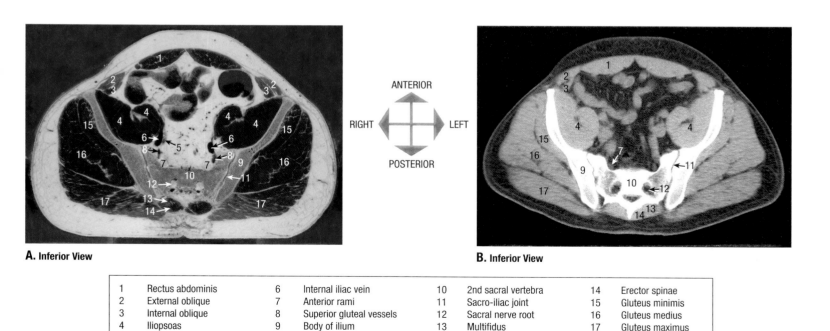

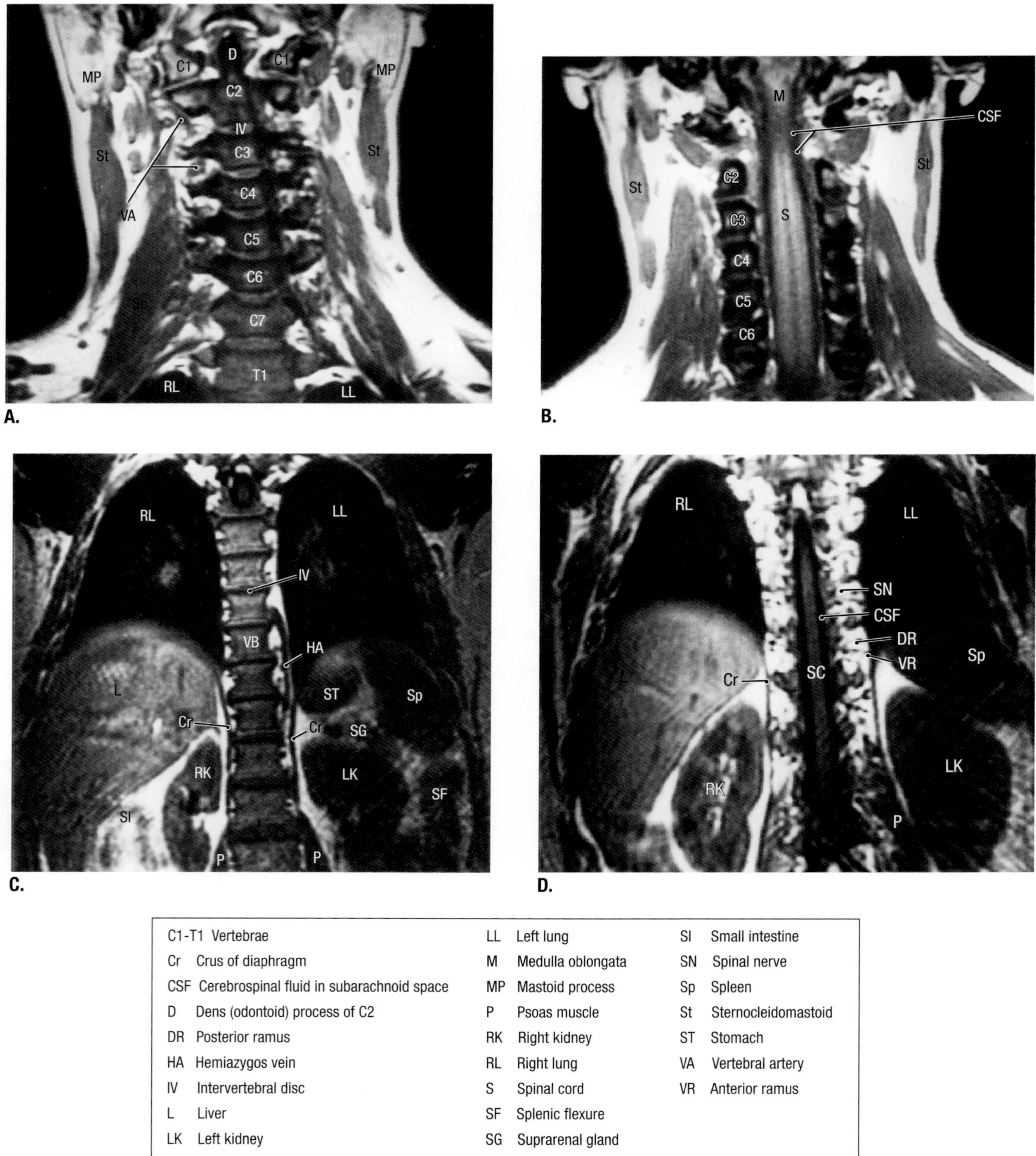
A.
MP
C1
D
C1
MP
C2
IV
C3
St
St
VA
C4
C5
C6
Sc
C7
T1
RL
LL
B.
M
CSF
St
St
C2
S
C3
C4
C5
C6
C.
RL
LL
IV
VB
HA
L
ST
Sp
Cr
Cr
SG
RK
LK
SF
SI
P
P
D.
RL
LL
SN
CSF
DR
Sp
VR
Cr
SC
LK
RK
P
C1-T1 Vertebrae
Cr Crus of diaphragm
CSF Cerebrospinal fluid in subarachnoid space
D Dens (odontoid) process of C2
DR Posterior ramus
HA Hemiazygos vein
IV Intervertebral disc
L Liver
LK Left kidney
LL Left lung
M Medulla oblongata
MP Mastoid process
P Psoas muscle
RK Right kidney
RL Right lung
S Spinal cord
SF Splenic flexure
SG Suprarenal gland
SI Small intestine
SN Spinal nerve
Sp Spleen
St Sternocleidomastoid
ST Stomach
VA Vertebral artery
VR Anterior ramus

## 4.57 Coronal MRI scans of cervical and thoracic spine

**A** and **B.** Cervical spine. **C** and **D.** Thoracic spine.

CHAPTER 5

# LOWER LIMB

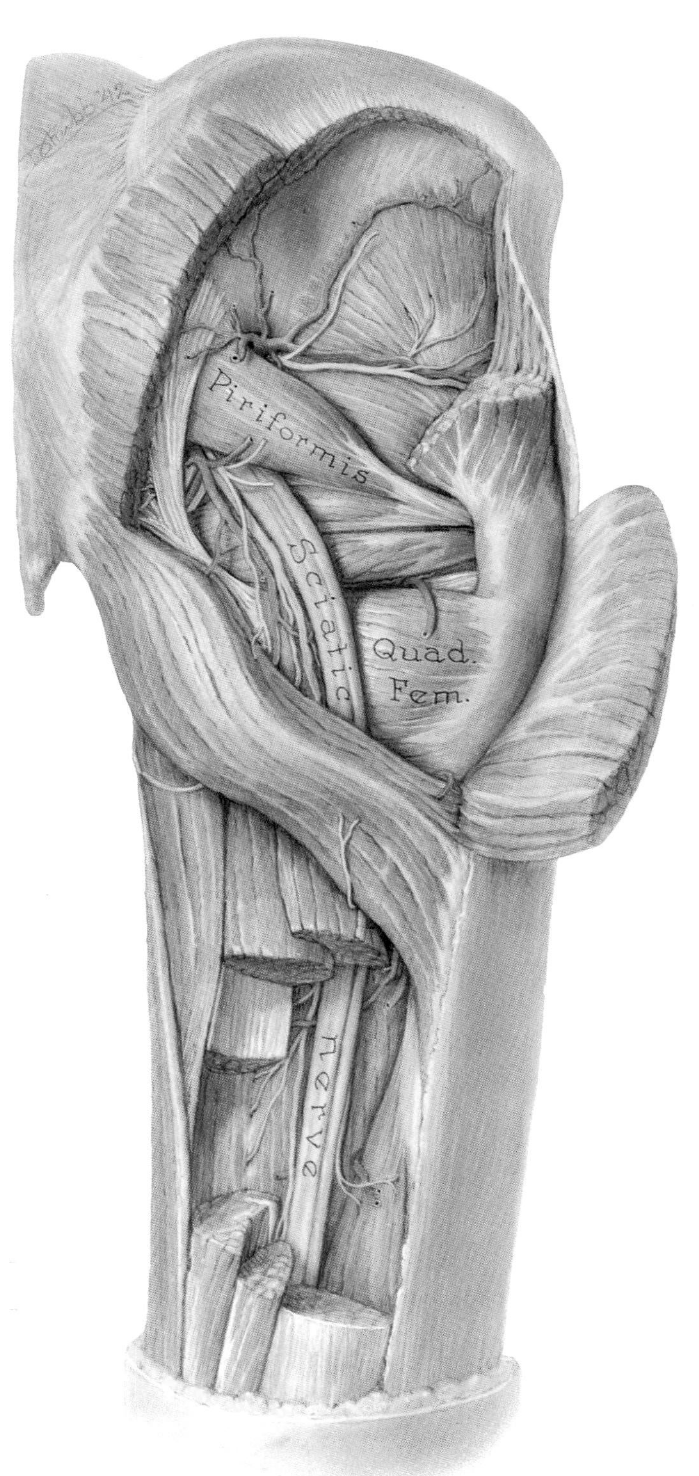

Piriformis
Sciatic
Quad.
Fem.
Nerve



- Systemic Overview of Lower Limb **354**
  - Bones **355**
  - Nerves **356**
  - Blood Vessels **362**
  - Lymphatics **366**
  - Musculofascial Compartments **368**
- Retroinguinal Passage and Femoral Triangle **370**
- Anterior and Medial Compartments of Thigh **374**
- Lateral Thigh **383**
- Gluteal Region and Posterior Compartment of Thigh **384**
- Hip Joint **394**
- Knee Region **402**
- Knee Joint **408**
- Anterior and Lateral Compartments of Leg, Dorsum of Foot **422**
- Posterior Compartment of Leg **432**
- Tibiofibular Joints **442**
- Sole of Foot **443**
- Ankle, Subtalar, and Foot Joints **448**
- Arches of Foot **466**
- Bony Anomalies **467**
- Imaging and Sectional Anatomy **468**

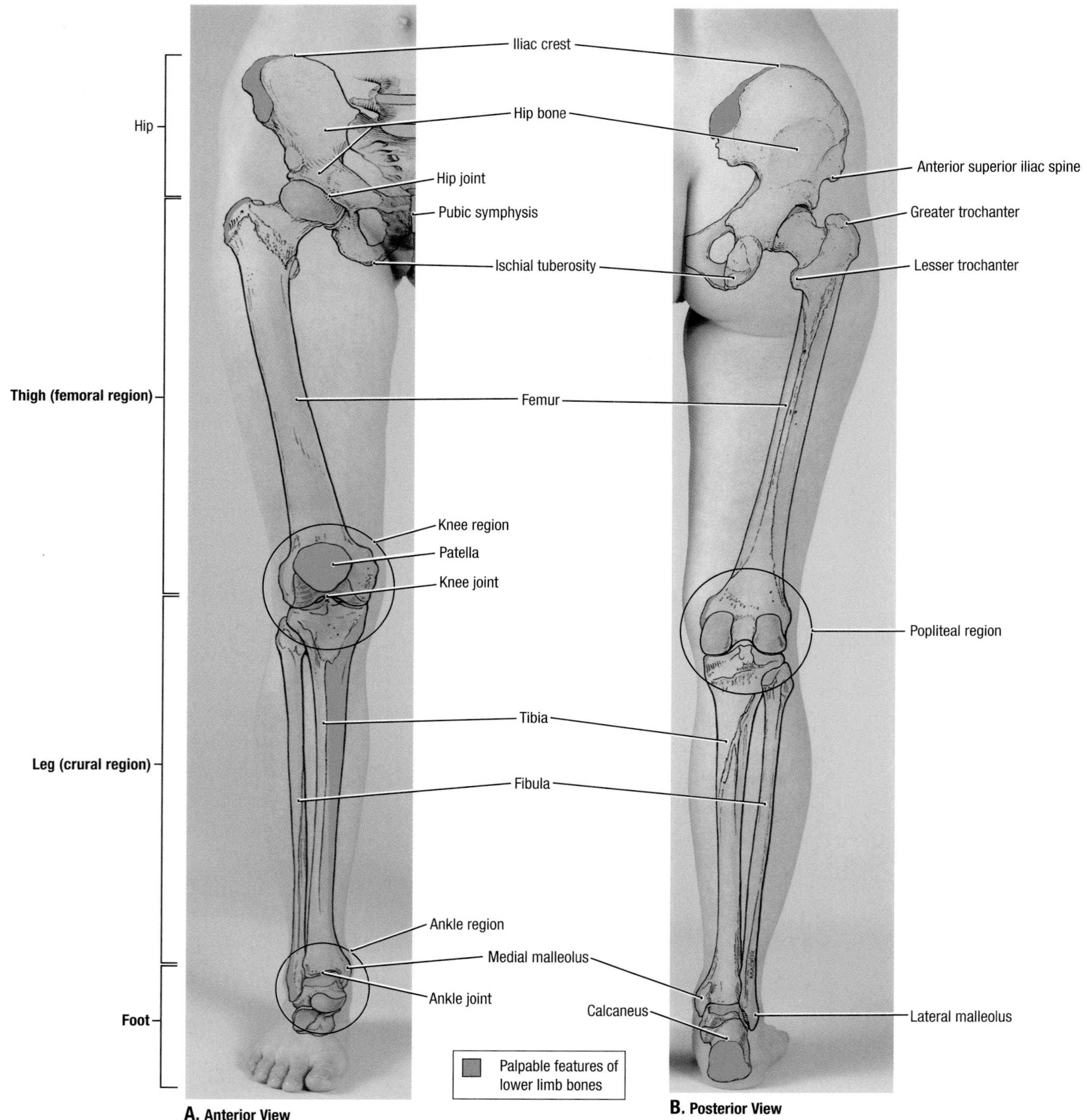
Hip
Thigh (femoral region)
Leg (crural region)
Foot
Iliac crest
Hip bone
Hip joint
Pubic symphysis
Ischial tuberosity
Anterior superior iliac spine
Greater trochanter
Lesser trochanter
Femur
Knee region
Patella
Knee joint
Popliteal region
Tibia
Fibula
Ankle region
Medial malleolus
Ankle joint
Calcaneus
Lateral malleolus
Palpable features of lower limb bones
A. Anterior View
B. Posterior View

## 5.1 Regions, bones, and major joints of lower limb

The hip bones meet anteriorly at the symphysis pubis and articulate with the sacrum posteriorly. The femur articulates with the hip bone proximally and the tibia distally. The tibia and fibula are the bones of the leg that join the foot at the ankle.

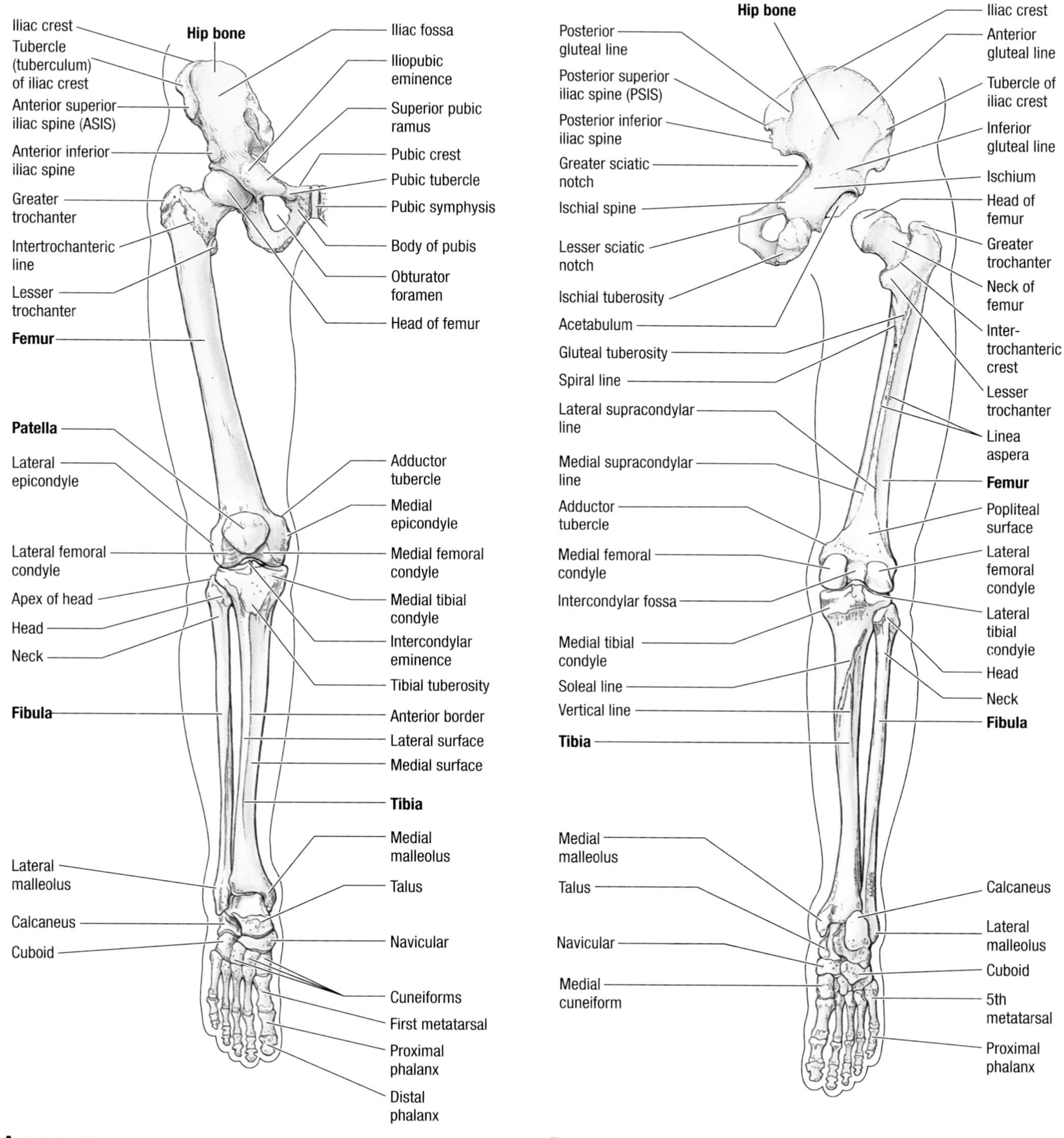
Iliac crest
Hip bone
Iliac fossa
Tubercle (tuberculum) of iliac crest
Iliopubic eminence
Anterior superior iliac spine (ASIS)
Superior pubic ramus
Anterior inferior iliac spine
Pubic crest
Pubic tubercle
Greater trochanter
Pubic symphysis
Intertrochanteric line
Body of pubis
Obturator foramen
Lesser trochanter
Head of femur
Femur
Patella
Lateral epicondyle
Adductor tubercle
Medial epicondyle
Lateral femoral condyle
Medial femoral condyle
Apex of head
Medial tibial condyle
Head
Intercondylar eminence
Neck
Tibial tuberosity
Fibula
Anterior border
Lateral surface
Medial surface
Tibia
Medial malleolus
Lateral malleolus
Talus
Calcaneus
Navicular
Cuboid
Cuneiforms
First metatarsal
Proximal phalanx
Distal phalanx
A. Anterior View
Hip bone
Iliac crest
Posterior gluteal line
Anterior gluteal line
Posterior superior iliac spine (PSIS)
Tubercle of iliac crest
Posterior inferior iliac spine
Inferior gluteal line
Greater sciatic notch
Ischium
Ischial spine
Head of femur
Lesser sciatic notch
Greater trochanter
Neck of femur
Ischial tuberosity
Acetabulum
Inter-trochanteric crest
Gluteal tuberosity
Spiral line
Lesser trochanter
Lateral supracondylar line
Linea aspera
Medial supracondylar line
Femur
Adductor tubercle
Popliteal surface
Medial femoral condyle
Lateral femoral condyle
Intercondylar fossa
Lateral tibial condyle
Medial tibial condyle
Head
Soleal line
Neck
Vertical line
Fibula
Tibia
Medial malleolus
Talus
Calcaneus
Lateral malleolus
Navicular
Cuboid
Medial cuneiform
5th metatarsal
Proximal phalanx
B. Posterior View

## 5.2 Features of bones of lower limb

The foot is in full plantarflexion. The hip joint is disarticulated in **B** to demonstrate the acetabulum of the hip bone and the entire head of the femur.

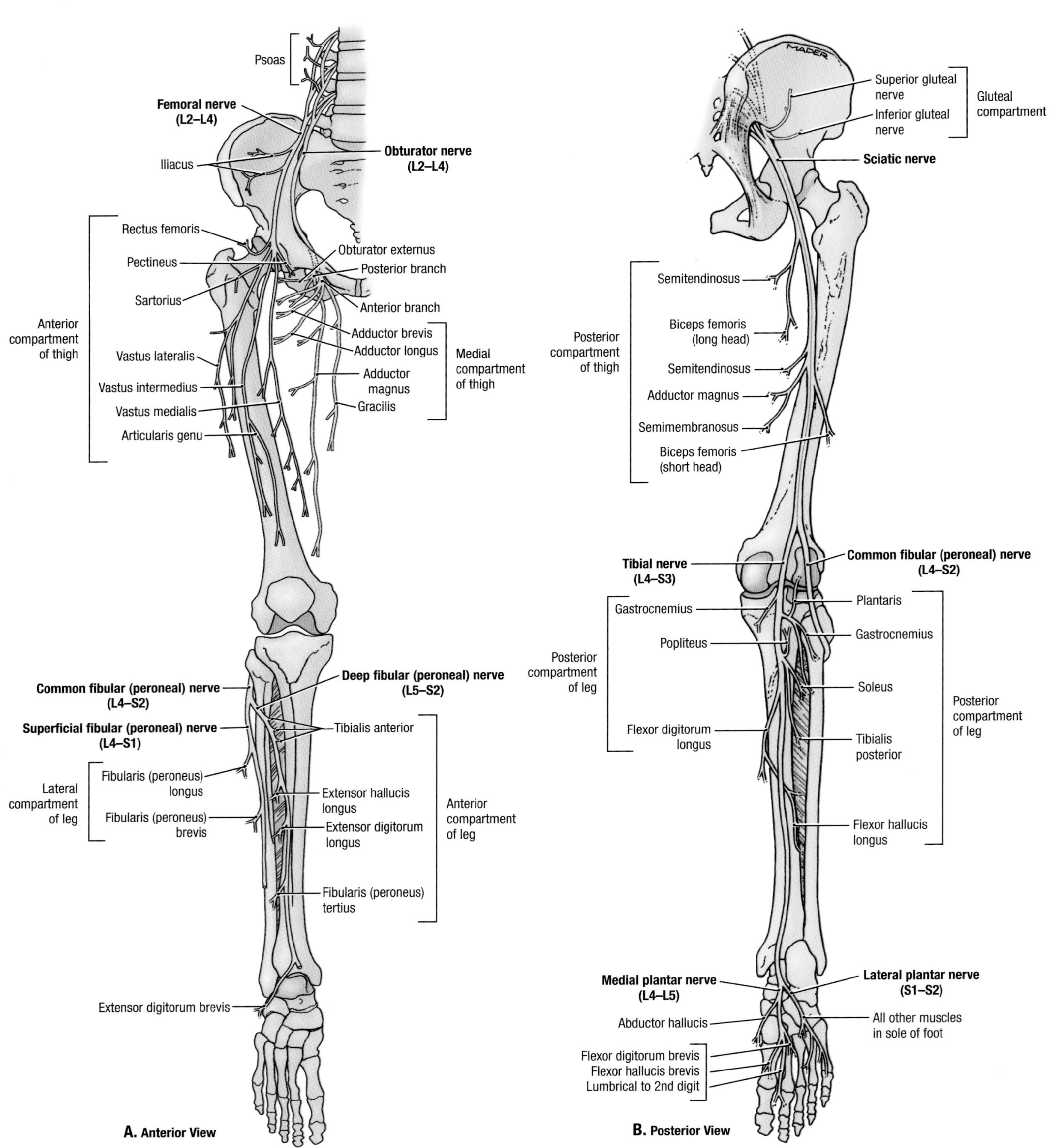
Psoas
Femoral nerve (L2–L4)
Iliacus
Obturator nerve (L2–L4)
Anterior compartment of thigh
Rectus femoris
Pectineus
Sartorius
Vastus lateralis
Vastus intermedius
Vastus medialis
Articularis genu
Obturator externus
Posterior branch
Anterior branch
Adductor brevis
Adductor longus
Adductor magnus
Gracilis
Medial compartment of thigh
Common fibular (peroneal) nerve (L4–S2)
Superficial fibular (peroneal) nerve (L4–S1)
Deep fibular (peroneal) nerve (L5–S2)
Tibialis anterior
Lateral compartment of leg
Fibularis (peroneus) longus
Fibularis (peroneus) brevis
Extensor hallucis longus
Extensor digitorum longus
Fibularis (peroneus) tertius
Anterior compartment of leg
Extensor digitorum brevis
A. Anterior View
MADER
Superior gluteal nerve
Inferior gluteal nerve
Gluteal compartment
Sciatic nerve
Posterior compartment of thigh
Semitendinosus
Biceps femoris (long head)
Semitendinosus
Adductor magnus
Semimembranosus
Biceps femoris (short head)
Tibial nerve (L4–S3)
Common fibular (peroneal) nerve (L4–S2)
Posterior compartment of leg
Gastrocnemius
Popliteus
Flexor digitorum longus
Plantaris
Gastrocnemius
Soleus
Tibialis posterior
Flexor hallucis longus
Posterior compartment of leg
Medial plantar nerve (L4–L5)
Lateral plantar nerve (S1–S2)
Abductor hallucis
All other muscles in sole of foot
Flexor digitorum brevis
Flexor hallucis brevis
Lumbrical to 2nd digit
B. Posterior View

**5.3 Overview of motor innervation of lower limb**

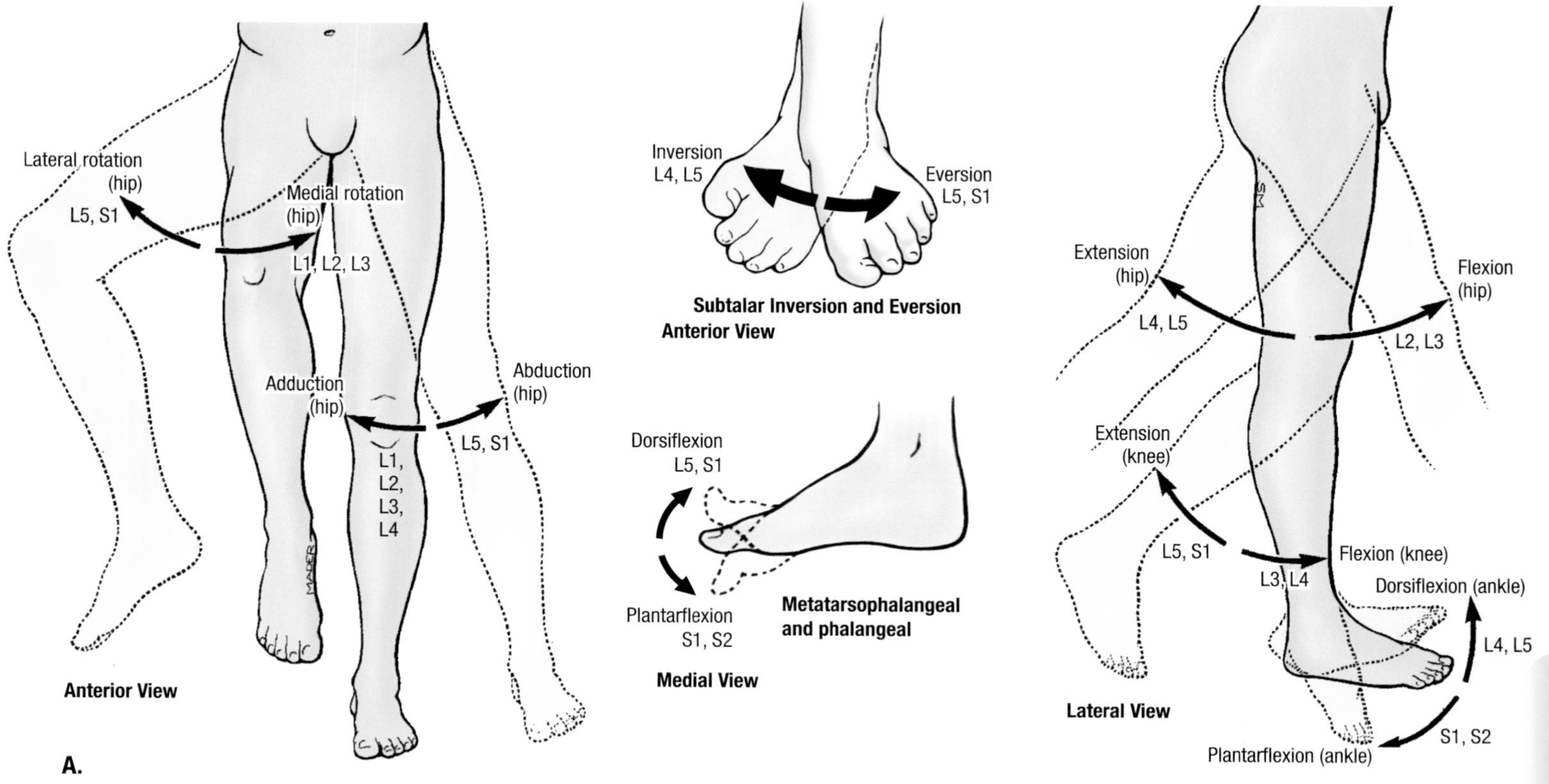
Lateral rotation (hip)
L5, S1
Medial rotation (hip)
L1, L2, L3
Adduction (hip)
L1, L2, L3, L4
Abduction (hip)
L5, S1
Anterior View
A.
Inversion L4, L5
Eversion L5, S1
Subtalar Inversion and Eversion
Anterior View
Dorsiflexion L5, S1
Plantarflexion S1, S2
Metatarsophalangeal and phalangeal
Medial View
Extension (hip)
L4, L5
Flexion (hip)
L2, L3
Extension (knee)
L5, S1
Flexion (knee)
L3, L4
Dorsiflexion (ankle)
L4, L5
S1, S2
Plantarflexion (ankle)
Lateral View

| Myotatic (Deep Tendon) Reflex | Spinal Cord Segments |
|---|---|
| Quadriceps | L3/L4 |
| Calcaneal (Achilles) | S1/S2 |

## 5.4 Myotomes and deep tendon reflexes

**A.** Myotomes. Somatic motor (general somatic efferent) fibers transmit impulses to skeletal (voluntary) muscles. The unilateral muscle mass receiving innervation from the somatic motor fibers conveyed by a single spinal nerve is a myotome. Each skeletal muscle is usually innervated by the somatic motor fibers of several spinal nerves; therefore, the muscle myotome will consist of several segments. The muscle myotomes have been grouped by joint movement to facilitate clinical testing.

**B.** Myotactic (deep tendon) reflexes. A myotatic (stretch) reflex is an involuntary contraction of a muscle in response to being stretched. Deep tendon reflexes (e.g., "knee jerk") are monosynaptic stretch reflexes that are elicited by briskly tapping the tendon with a reflex hammer. Each tendon reflex is mediated by specific spinal nerves. Stretch reflexes control muscle tone (e.g., in antigravity, muscles that keep the body upright against gravity).

**TABLE 5.1 MOTOR NERVES OF LOWER LIMB**

| Nerve | Origin | Course | Distribution in Leg |
|---|---|---|---|
| **Femoral** | Lumbar plexus (L2–L4) | Passes deep to midpoint of inguinal ligament, lateral to femoral vessels, dividing into muscular and cutaneous branches in femoral triangle | Anterior thigh muscles, hip and knee joints |
| **Obturator** | Lumbar plexus (L2–L4) | Enters thigh via obturator foramen and divides; its anterior branch descends between adductor longus and adductor brevis; its posterior branch descends between adductor brevis and adductor magnus | *Anterior branch:* adductor longus, adductor brevis, gracilis, and pectineus; *posterior branch:* obturator externus, and adductor magnus |
| **Sciatic** | Sacral plexus (L4–S3) | Enters gluteal region through greater sciatic foramen, usually passing inferior to piriformis, descends in posterior compartment of thigh, bifurcating at apex of popliteal fossa into tibial and common fibular (peroneal) nerves | Muscles of posterior thigh, leg and foot; skin of posterolateral leg and foot |
| **Tibial** | Sciatic nerve | Terminal branch of sciatic nerve arising at apex of popliteal fossa; descends through popliteal fossa with popliteal vessels, continuing in deep posterior compartment of leg with posterior tibial vessels; bifurcates into medial and lateral plantar nerves | Hamstring muscles of posterior compartment of thigh, muscles of posterior compartment of leg, and sole of foot |
| **Common fibular** | Sciatic nerve | Terminal branch of sciatic nerve arising at apex of popliteal fossa; follows medial border of biceps femoris and its tendon to wind around neck of fibula deep to fibularis longus, where it bifurcates into superficial and deep fibular nerves | Short head of biceps femoris, muscles of anterior and lateral leg, and dorsum of foot |
| **Superficial fibular** | Common fibular nerve | Arises deep to fibularis longus on neck of fibula and descends in lateral compartment of the leg; pierces crural fascia in distal third of leg to become cutaneous | Fibularis longus and brevis muscles |
| **Deep fibular** | Common fibular nerve | Arises deep to fibularis longus on neck of fibula; passes through extensor digitorum longus into anterior compartment, descending on interosseous membrane; crosses ankle joint and enters dorsum of foot | Muscles of anterior compartment of leg and dorsum of foot |

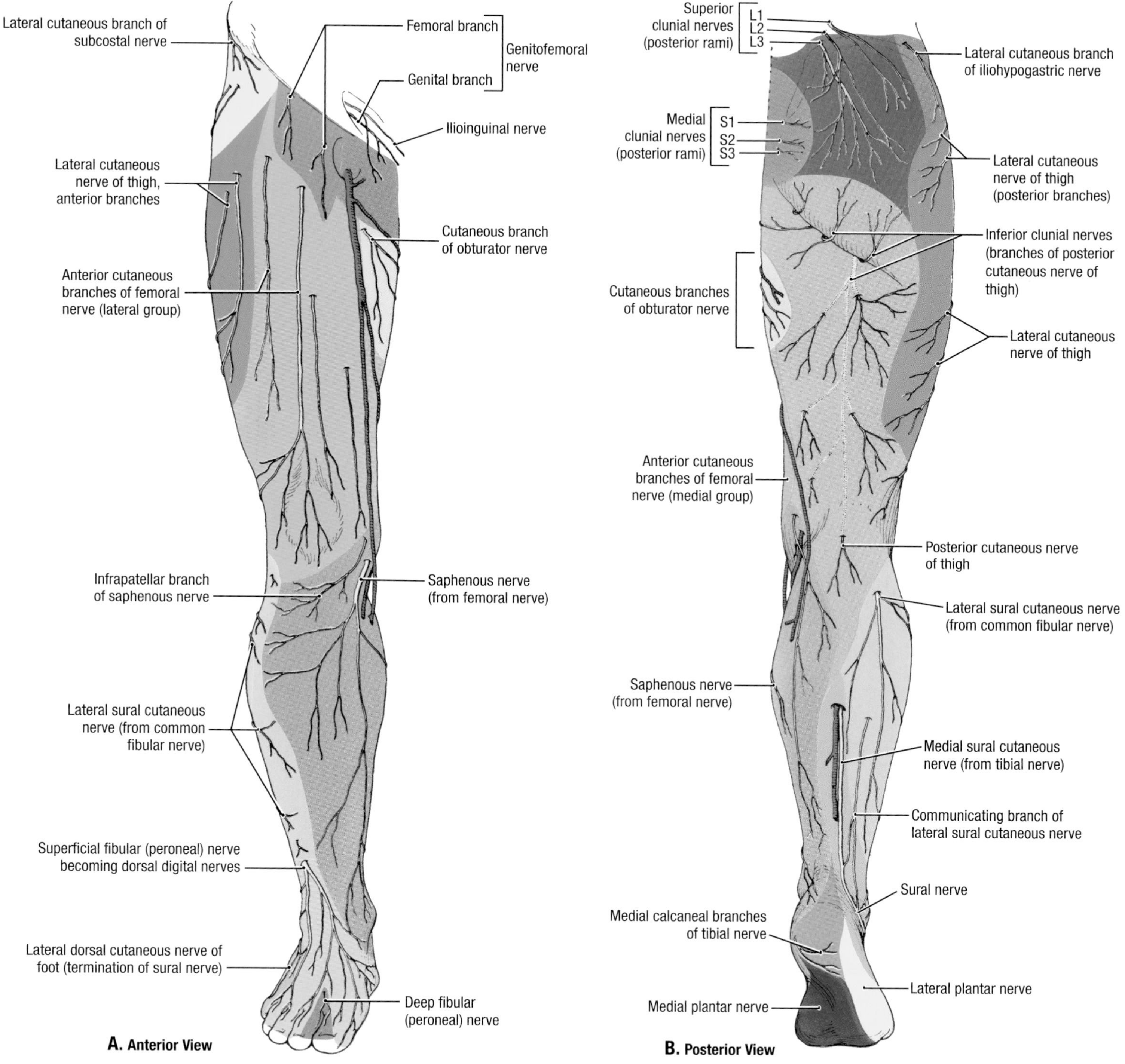
Lateral cutaneous branch of subcostal nerve
Femoral branch
Genital branch
Genitofemoral nerve
Ilioinguinal nerve
Lateral cutaneous nerve of thigh, anterior branches
Cutaneous branch of obturator nerve
Anterior cutaneous branches of femoral nerve (lateral group)
Infrapatellar branch of saphenous nerve
Saphenous nerve (from femoral nerve)
Lateral sural cutaneous nerve (from common fibular nerve)
Superficial fibular (peroneal) nerve becoming dorsal digital nerves
Lateral dorsal cutaneous nerve of foot (termination of sural nerve)
Deep fibular (peroneal) nerve
A. Anterior View
Superior clunial nerves (posterior rami)
L1
L2
L3
Lateral cutaneous branch of iliohypogastric nerve
Medial clunial nerves (posterior rami)
S1
S2
S3
Lateral cutaneous nerve of thigh (posterior branches)
Inferior clunial nerves (branches of posterior cutaneous nerve of thigh)
Cutaneous branches of obturator nerve
Lateral cutaneous nerve of thigh
Anterior cutaneous branches of femoral nerve (medial group)
Posterior cutaneous nerve of thigh
Lateral sural cutaneous nerve (from common fibular nerve)
Saphenous nerve (from femoral nerve)
Medial sural cutaneous nerve (from tibial nerve)
Communicating branch of lateral sural cutaneous nerve
Sural nerve
Medial calcaneal branches of tibial nerve
Lateral plantar nerve
Medial plantar nerve
B. Posterior View

## 5.5 Cutaneous nerves of lower limb

Cutaneous nerves in the subcutaneous tissue supply the skin of the lower limb. The cutaneous innervation of the lower limb reflects both the original segmental innervation of the skin via separate spinal nerves in its dermatomal pattern (Fig. 5.7) and the result of plexus formation of segmental peripheral nerves. In **B,** the medial sural cutaneous nerve (*sural* is Latin for calf) is joined between the popliteal fossa and posterior aspect of the ankle by a communicating branch of the lateral sural cutaneous nerve to form the sural nerve. The level of the junction is variable and is low in this specimen.

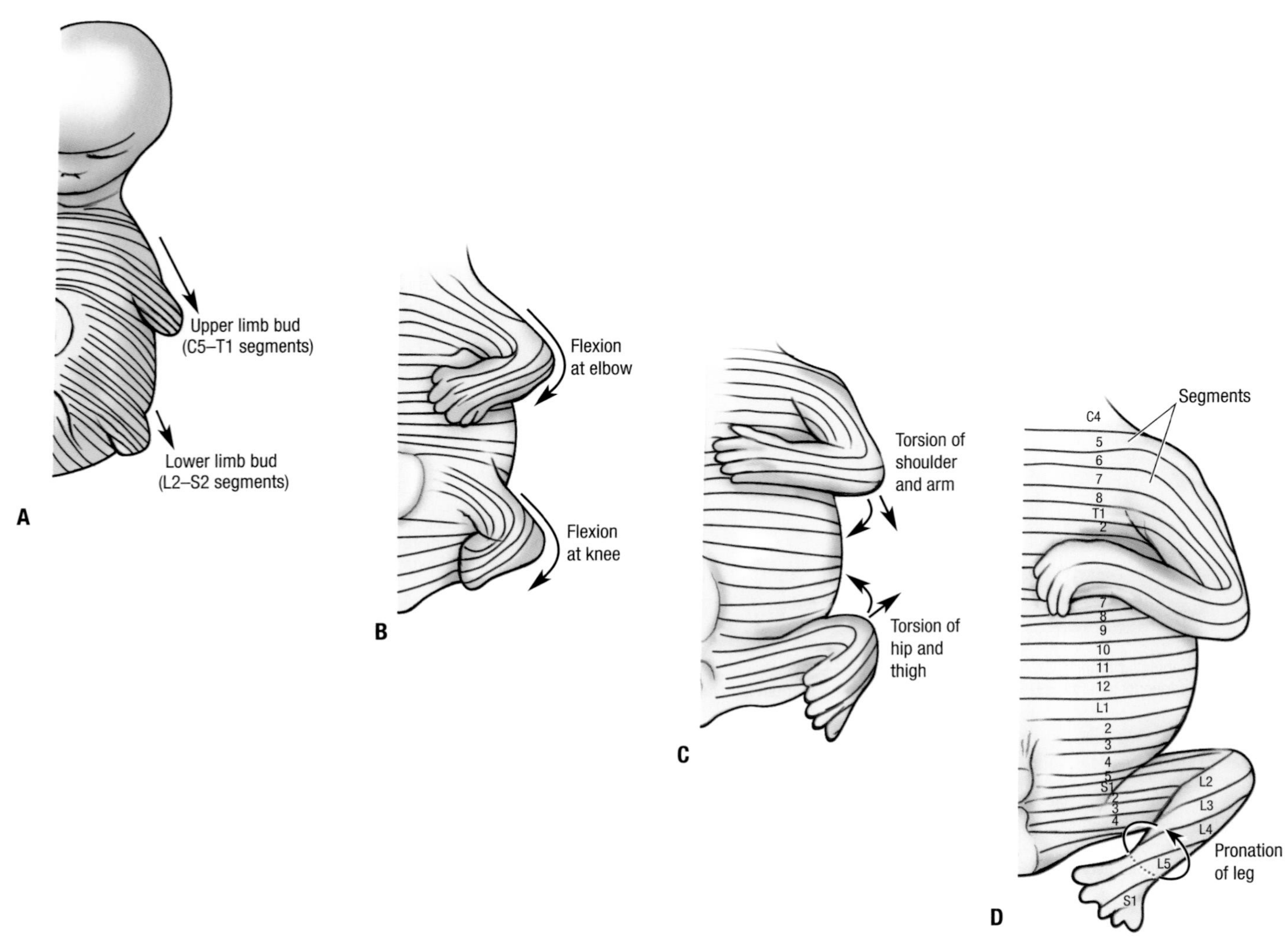
Upper limb bud
(C5–T1 segments)
Lower limb bud
(L2–S2 segments)
A
Flexion
at elbow
Flexion
at knee
B
Torsion of
shoulder
and arm
Torsion of
hip and
thigh
C
Segments
C4
5
6
7
8
T1
2
7
8
9
10
11
12
L1
2
3
4
5
S1
2
3
4
L2
L3
L4
L5
S1
Pronation
of leg
D
Anterior (Ventral) Views

## 5.6 Rotation of limbs during development; effect on lower limb dermatome pattern

**A.** During early development, the trunk is divided into segments (metameres) that correspond to, and receive innervation from, the corresponding spinal cord segments. During the 4th week of development, the upper limb buds appear as elevations of the C5 to T1 segments of the ventrolateral body wall. Following the cranial-to-caudal pattern of development the lower limb buds appear about a week later (5th week). The lower limb buds grow laterally from broader bases formed by the L2 to S2 segments.

**B.** The distal ends of the limb buds flatten into paddlelike hand plates and foot plates that are elongated in the craniocaudal axis. Initially, both the thumb and the great toe are on the cranial sides of the developing hand and foot, directed superiorly, with the palms and soles directed anteriorly. Where gaps develop between the precursors of the long bones (future elbow and knee joints), flexures occur. At first, the limbs bend anteriorly, so that the elbow and knee are directed laterally, causing the palm and sole to be directed medially (toward the trunk).

**C.** By the end of the 7th week, the proximal parts of the upper and lower limbs undergo a 90-degree torsion around their long axes, but in opposite directions, so that the elbow becomes directed caudally and the knee cranially.

**D.** In the lower limb, the torsion of the proximal limb is accompanied by a permanent pronation (twisting) of the leg, so that the foot becomes oriented with the great toe on the medial side.

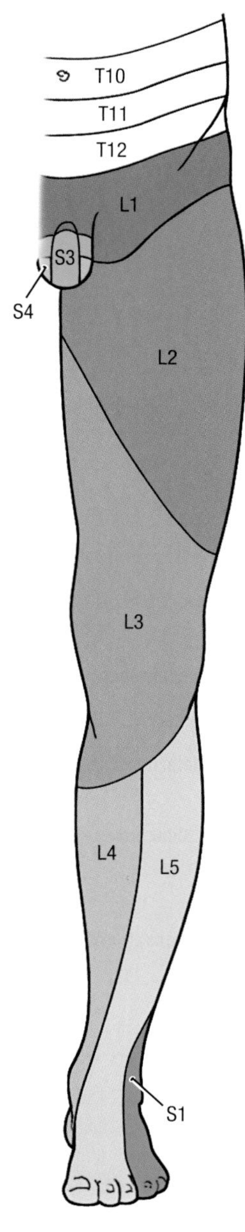
T10
T11
T12
L1
S3
S4
L2
L3
L4
L5
S1
A. Anterior View

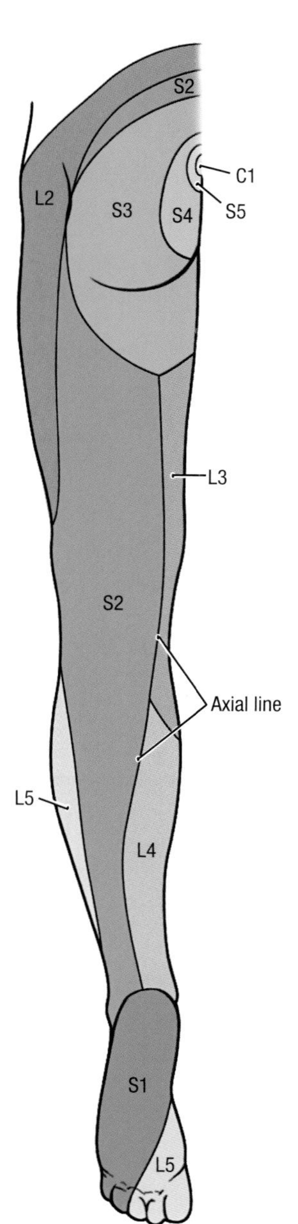
S2
C1
S5
L2
S3
S4
L3
S2
Axial line
L5
L4
S1
L5
B. Posterior View

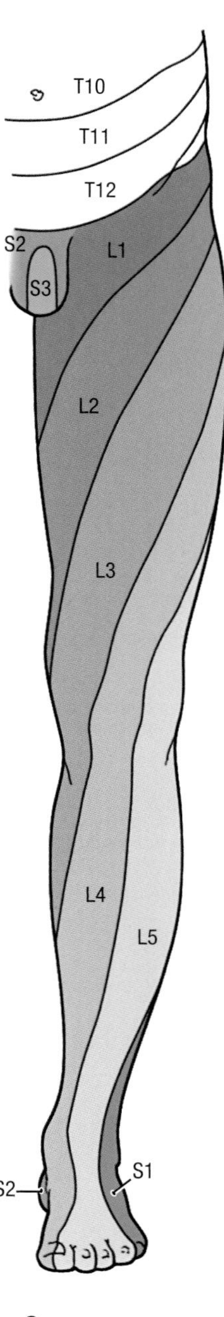
T10
T11
T12
S2
L1
S3
L2
L3
L4
L5
S2
S1
C. Anterior View

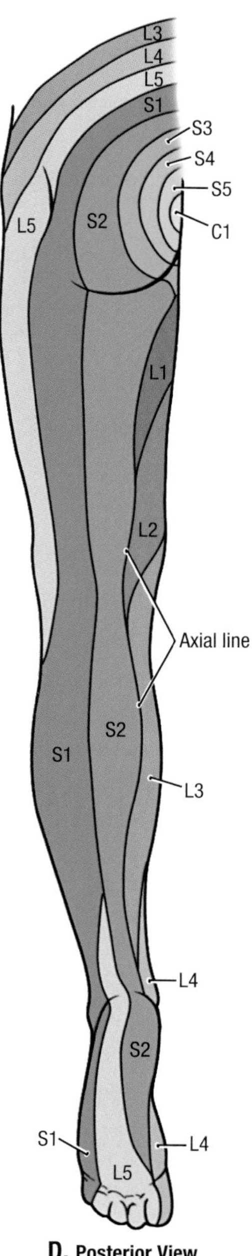
L3
L4
L5
S1
S3
S4
S5
C1
L5
S2
L1
L2
Axial line
S2
S1
L3
L4
S2
S1
L4
L5
D. Posterior View

## 5.7 Dermatomes of lower limb

The dermatomal, or segmental, pattern of distribution of sensory nerve fibers persists despite the merging of spinal nerves in plexus formation during development. Two different dermatome maps are commonly used. **A** and **B.** The dermatome pattern of the lower limb according to Foerster (1933) is preferred by many because of its correlation with clinical findings. **C** and **D.** The dermatome pattern of the lower limb according to Keegan and Garrett (1948) is preferred by others for its aesthetic uniformity and obvious correlation with development. Although depicted as distinct zones, adjacent dermatomes overlap considerably, except along the axial line.

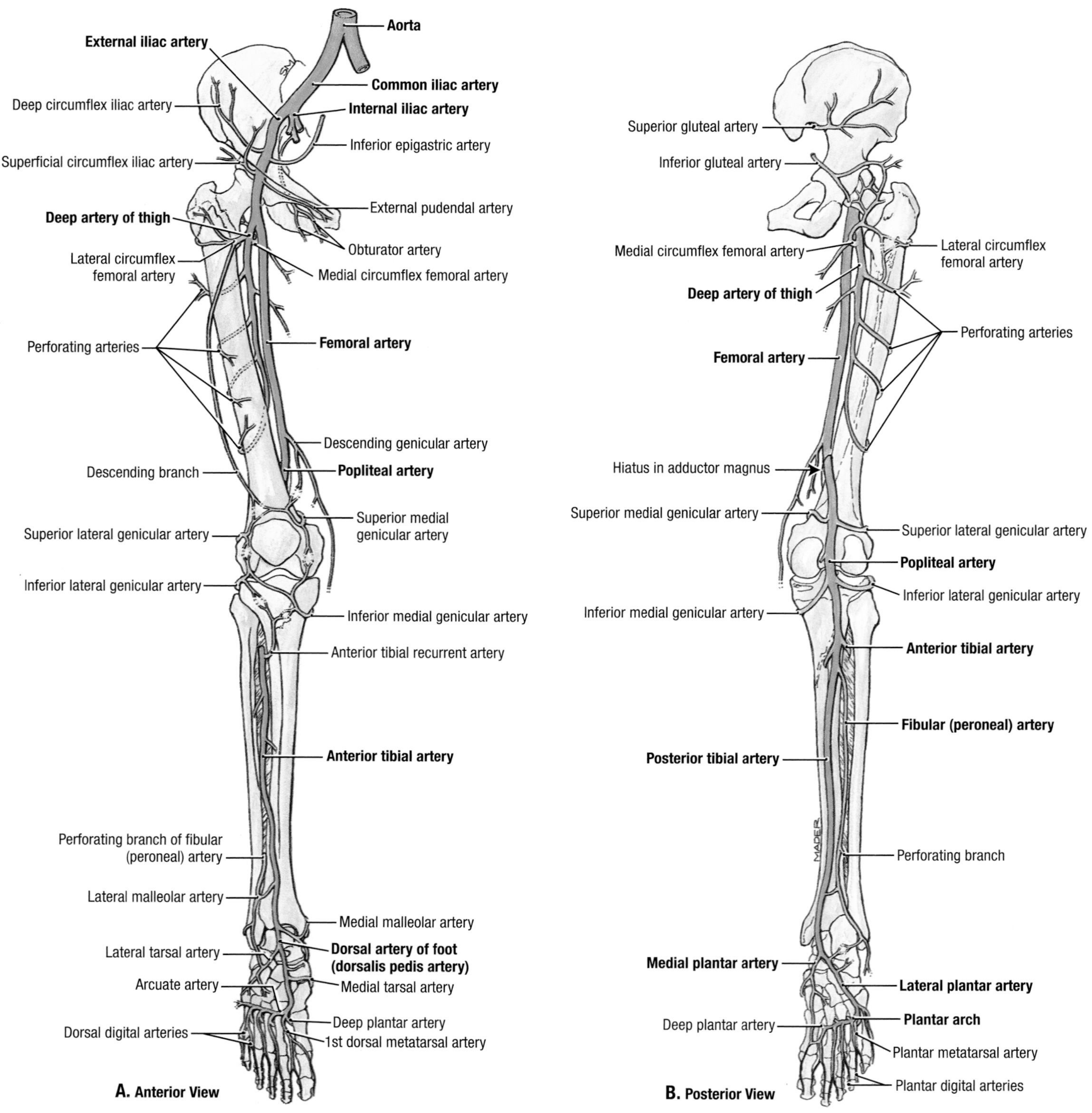
Aorta
External iliac artery
Common iliac artery
Internal iliac artery
Deep circumflex iliac artery
Inferior epigastric artery
Superficial circumflex iliac artery
External pudendal artery
Deep artery of thigh
Obturator artery
Lateral circumflex femoral artery
Medial circumflex femoral artery
Perforating arteries
Femoral artery
Descending genicular artery
Descending branch
Popliteal artery
Superior medial genicular artery
Superior lateral genicular artery
Inferior lateral genicular artery
Inferior medial genicular artery
Anterior tibial recurrent artery
Anterior tibial artery
Perforating branch of fibular (peroneal) artery
Lateral malleolar artery
Medial malleolar artery
Lateral tarsal artery
Dorsal artery of foot (dorsalis pedis artery)
Arcuate artery
Medial tarsal artery
Deep plantar artery
Dorsal digital arteries
1st dorsal metatarsal artery
A. Anterior View
Superior gluteal artery
Inferior gluteal artery
Medial circumflex femoral artery
Lateral circumflex femoral artery
Deep artery of thigh
Perforating arteries
Femoral artery
Hiatus in adductor magnus
Superior medial genicular artery
Superior lateral genicular artery
Popliteal artery
Inferior lateral genicular artery
Inferior medial genicular artery
Anterior tibial artery
Fibular (peroneal) artery
Posterior tibial artery
MADER
Perforating branch
Medial plantar artery
Lateral plantar artery
Plantar arch
Deep plantar artery
Plantar metatarsal artery
Plantar digital arteries
B. Posterior View

## 5.8 Overview of arteries of lower limb

The arteries often anastomose or communicate to form networks to ensure blood supply distal to the joint throughout the range of movement. If a main channel is slowly occluded, the smaller alternate channels can usually increase in size, providing a collateral circulation that ensures the blood supply to structures distal to the blockage.

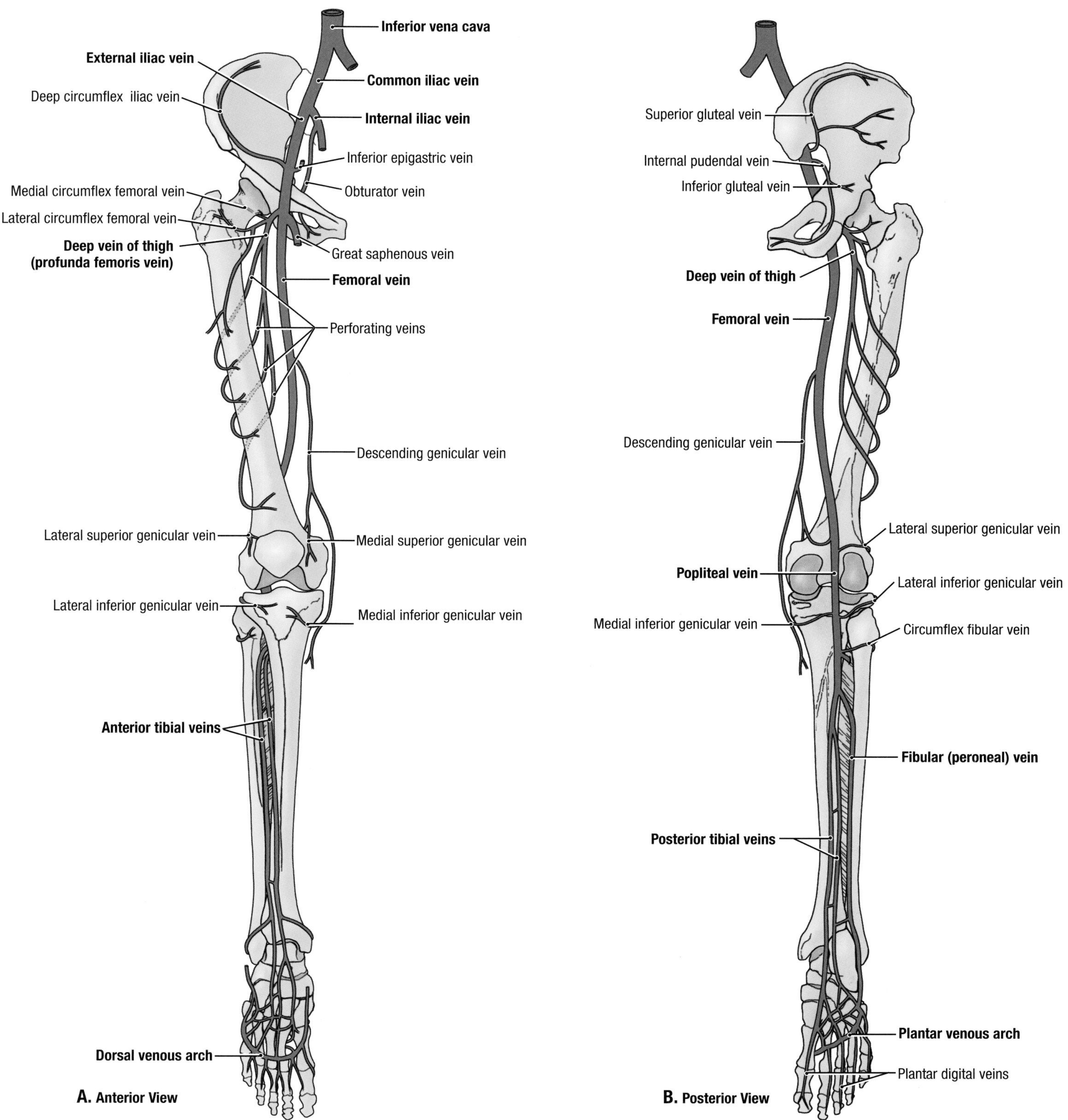
Inferior vena cava
External iliac vein
Common iliac vein
Deep circumflex iliac vein
Internal iliac vein
Inferior epigastric vein
Medial circumflex femoral vein
Obturator vein
Lateral circumflex femoral vein
Deep vein of thigh (profunda femoris vein)
Great saphenous vein
Femoral vein
Perforating veins
Descending genicular vein
Lateral superior genicular vein
Medial superior genicular vein
Lateral inferior genicular vein
Medial inferior genicular vein
Anterior tibial veins
Dorsal venous arch
A. Anterior View
Superior gluteal vein
Internal pudendal vein
Inferior gluteal vein
Deep vein of thigh
Femoral vein
Descending genicular vein
Lateral superior genicular vein
Popliteal vein
Lateral inferior genicular vein
Medial inferior genicular vein
Circumflex fibular vein
Fibular (peroneal) vein
Posterior tibial veins
Plantar venous arch
Plantar digital veins
B. Posterior View

## 5.9 Deep veins of lower limb

Deep veins lie internal to the deep fascia. Although only the anterior and posterior tibial veins are depicted as paired structures in this schematic illustration, typically in the limbs deep veins occur as paired, continually interanastomosing accompanying veins (L., venae comitantes) surrounding and sharing the name of the artery they accompany.

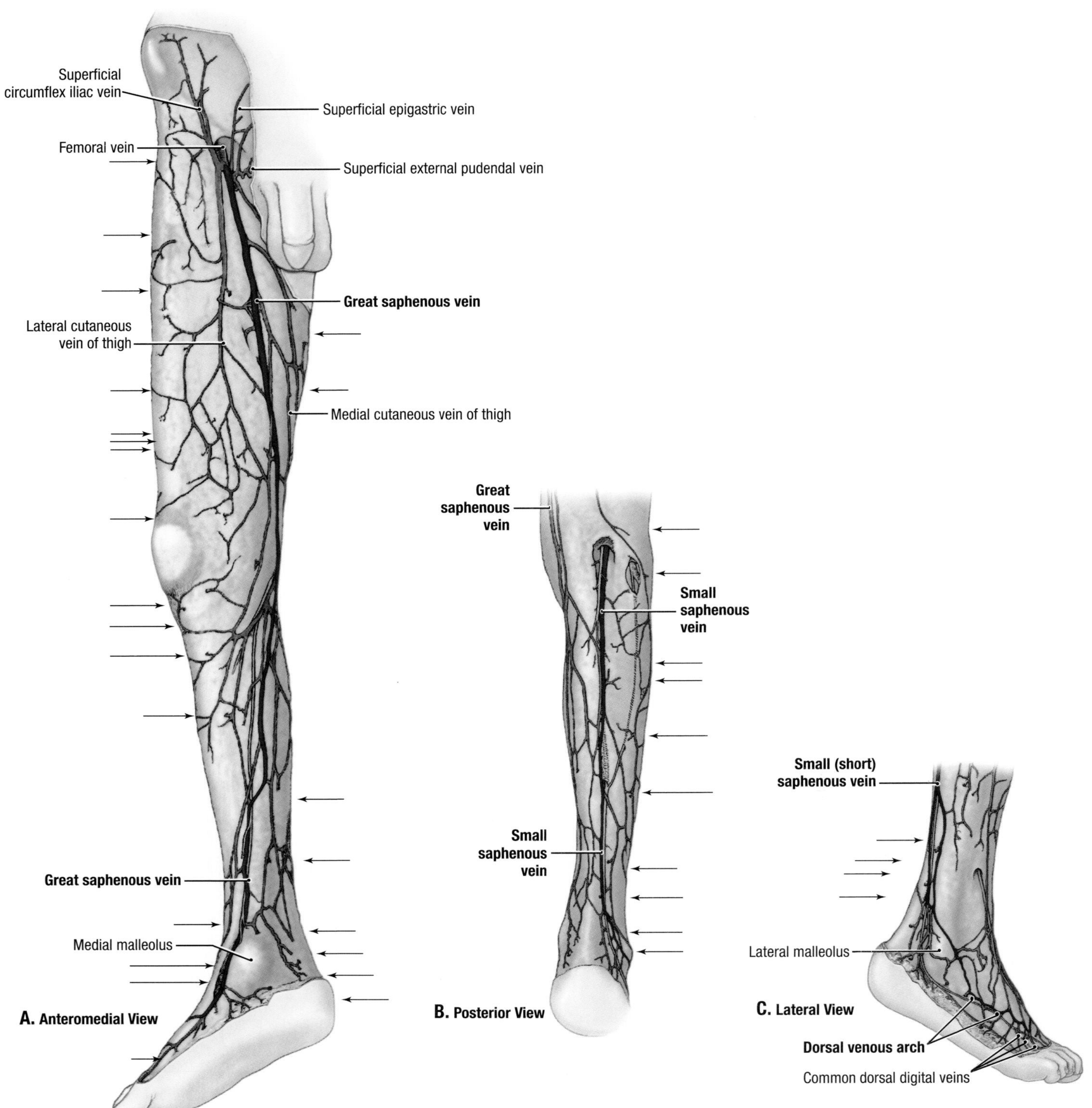
Superficial circumflex iliac vein
Superficial epigastric vein
Femoral vein
Superficial external pudendal vein
Great saphenous vein
Lateral cutaneous vein of thigh
Medial cutaneous vein of thigh
Great saphenous vein
Medial malleolus
A. Anteromedial View
Great saphenous vein
Small saphenous vein
Small saphenous vein
B. Posterior View
Small (short) saphenous vein
Lateral malleolus
C. Lateral View
Dorsal venous arch
Common dorsal digital veins

## 5.10 Superficial veins of lower limb

The *arrows* indicate where perforating veins penetrate the deep fascia. Blood is continuously shunted from these superficial veins in the subcutaneous tissue to deep veins via the perforating veins. Vein grafts obtained by surgically harvesting parts of the great saphenous vein are used to bypass obstructions in blood vessels (e.g., an occlusion of a coronary artery or its branches). When part of the vein is used as a bypass, it is reversed so that the valves do not obstruct blood flow. Because there are so many anastomosing leg veins, removal of the great saphenous vein rarely affects circulation seriously, provided the deep veins are intact.

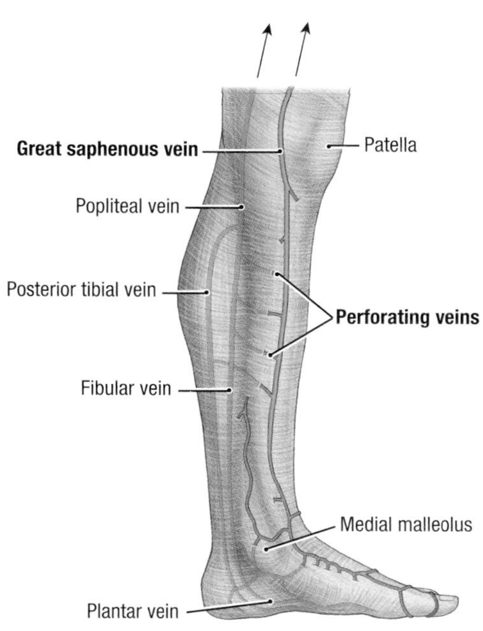
Great saphenous vein
Patella
Popliteal vein
Posterior tibial vein
Perforating veins
Fibular vein
Medial malleolus
Plantar vein

**A. Medial View**

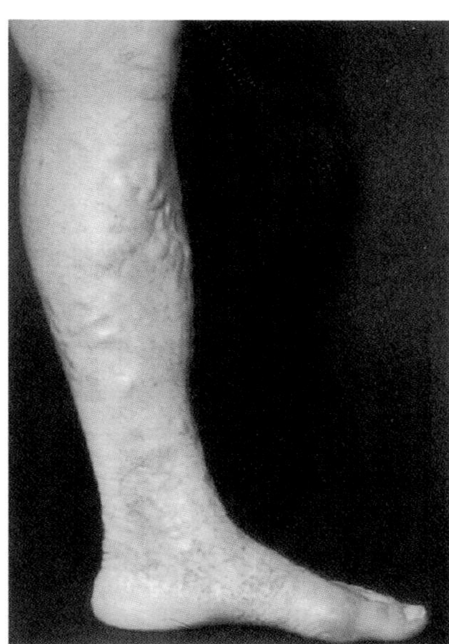

**B. Medial View, Varicose Veins**

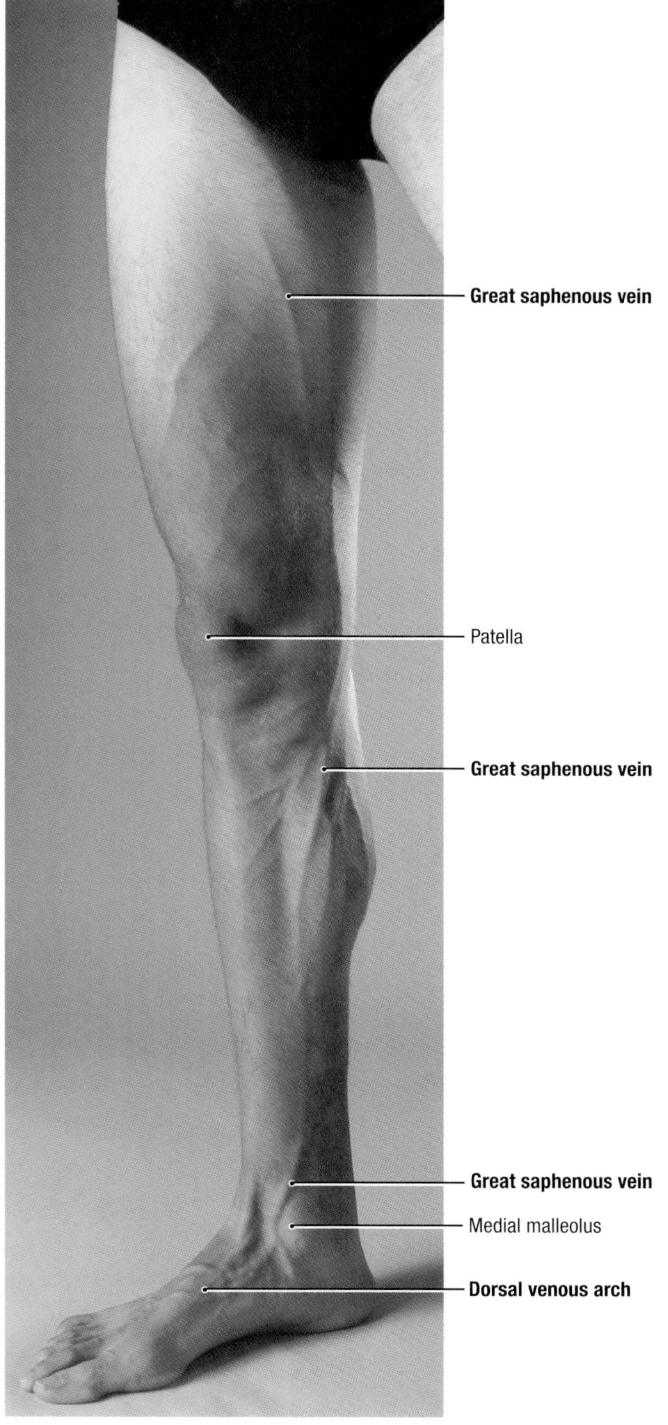
Great saphenous vein
Patella
Great saphenous vein
Great saphenous vein
Medial malleolus
Dorsal venous arch

**C. Anteromedial View, Normal Veins (distended following exercise)**

## 5.11 Drainage and surface anatomy of superficial veins of lower limb

**A.** Schematic diagram of drainage of superficial veins. Blood is repeatedly shunted from the superficial veins (e.g., great saphenous vein) to the deep veins (e.g., fibular and posterior tibial veins) via perforating veins that penetrate the deep fascia. Muscular compression of deep veins assists return of blood to the heart against gravity.

**B.** Varicose veins form when either the deep fascia or the valves of the perforating veins are incompetent. This allows the muscular compression that normally propels blood toward the heart to push blood from the deep to the superficial veins. Consequently, superficial veins become enlarged and tortuous. **C.** Normal veins, distended following exercise.

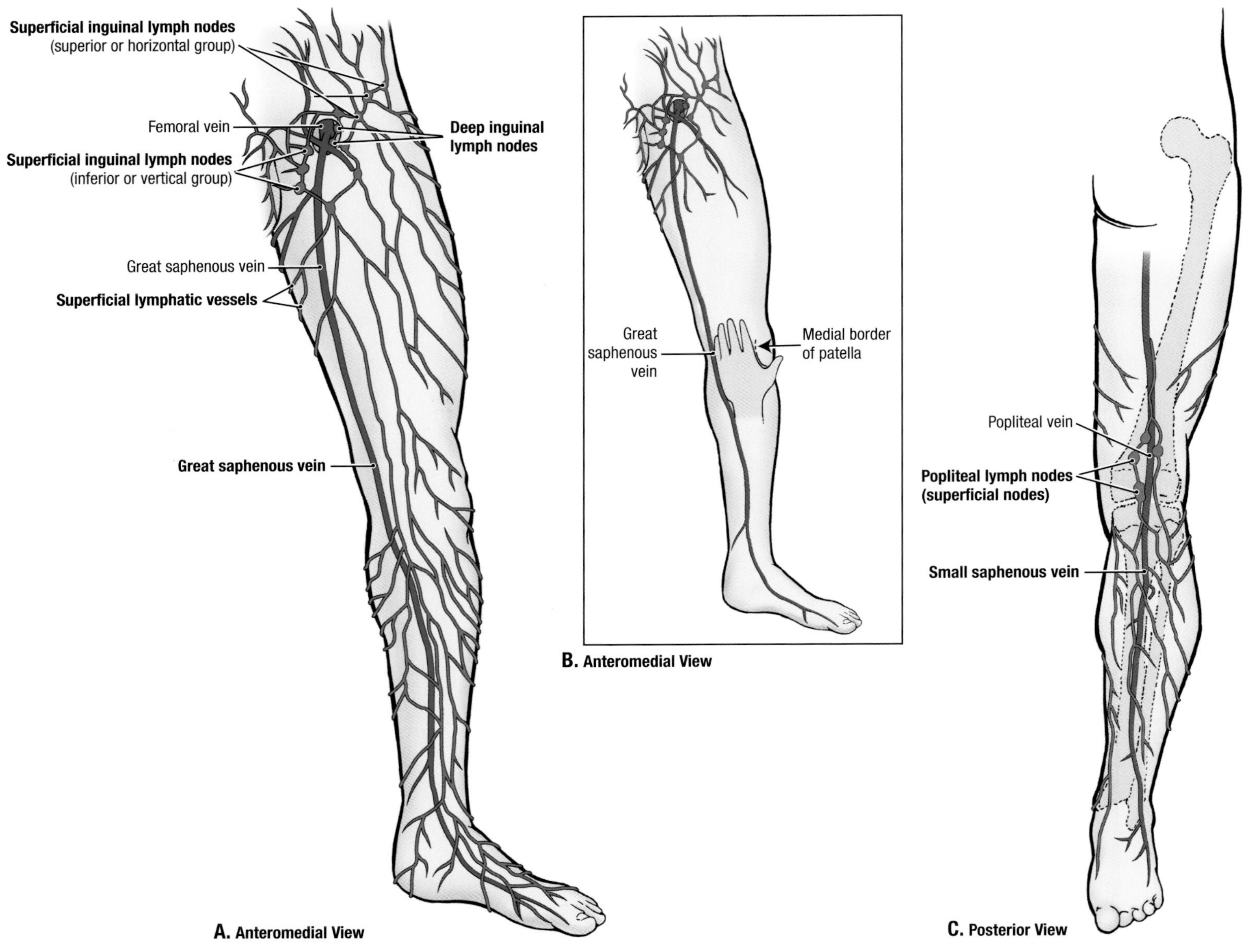
Superficial inguinal lymph nodes
(superior or horizontal group)
Femoral vein
Deep inguinal lymph nodes
Superficial inguinal lymph nodes
(inferior or vertical group)
Great saphenous vein
Superficial lymphatic vessels
Great saphenous vein
A. Anteromedial View
Great saphenous vein
Medial border of patella
B. Anteromedial View
Popliteal vein
Popliteal lymph nodes
(superficial nodes)
Small saphenous vein
C. Posterior View

## 5.12 Superficial lymphatic drainage of lower limb

The superficial lymphatic vessels converge on and accompany the saphenous veins and their tributaries in the superficial fascia. The lymphatic vessels along the great saphenous vein drain into the superficial inguinal lymph nodes; those along the small saphenous vein drain into the popliteal lymph nodes. Lymph from the superficial inguinal nodes drains to the deep inguinal and external iliac nodes. Lymph from the popliteal nodes ascends through deep lymphatic vessels accompanying the deep blood vessels to the deep inguinal nodes. In **B,** note that the great saphenous vein lies anterior to the medial malleolus and a hand's breadth posterior to the medial aspect of the patella. Lymph nodes enlarge when diseased. Abrasions and minor sepsis, caused by pathogenic microorganisms or their toxins in the blood or other tissues, may produce slight enlargement of the superficial inguinal nodes (lymphadenopathy) in otherwise healthy people. Malignancies (e.g., of the external genitalia and uterus) and perineal abscesses also result in enlargement of these nodes.

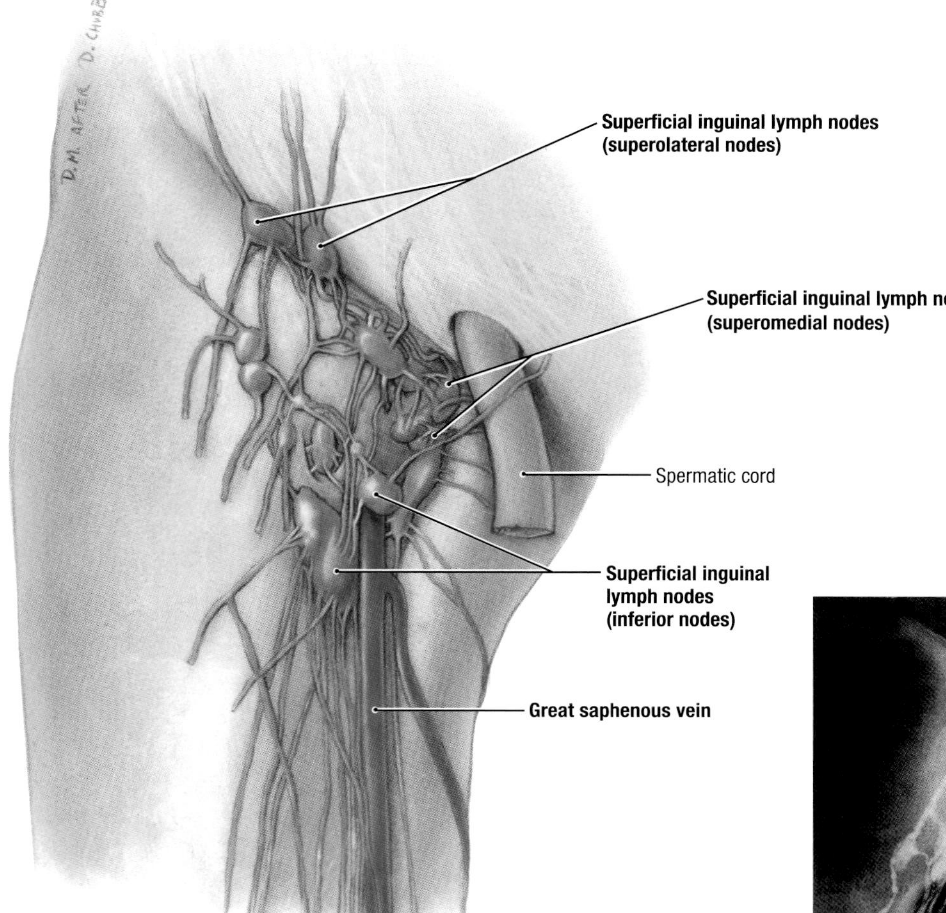
Superficial inguinal lymph nodes (superolateral nodes)
Superficial inguinal lymph nodes (superomedial nodes)
Spermatic cord
Superficial inguinal lymph nodes (inferior nodes)
Great saphenous vein
D.M. AFTER D. CHUBB

**A.** Anterior View

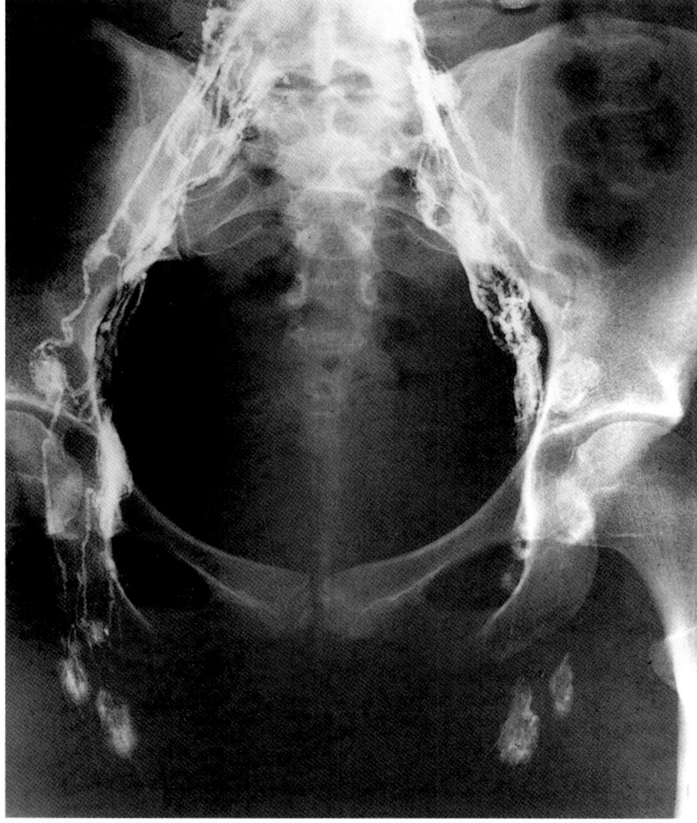

**B.** Anteroposterior View

## 5.13 Inguinal lymph nodes

**A.** Dissection. **B.** Lymphangiogram.

- Observe the arrangement of the nodes: a proximal chain parallel to the inguinal ligament (superolateral and superomedial superficial inguinal lymph nodes) and a distal chain on the sides of the great saphenous vein (inferior superficial inguinal lymph nodes). Efferent vessels leave these nodes and pass deep to the inguinal ligament to enter the external iliac nodes. Some of the lymphatic vessels traverse the femoral canal, and others ascend alongside the femoral artery and vein, some inside the femoral sheath, and some outside it.
- Note the anastomosis between the lymph vessels.

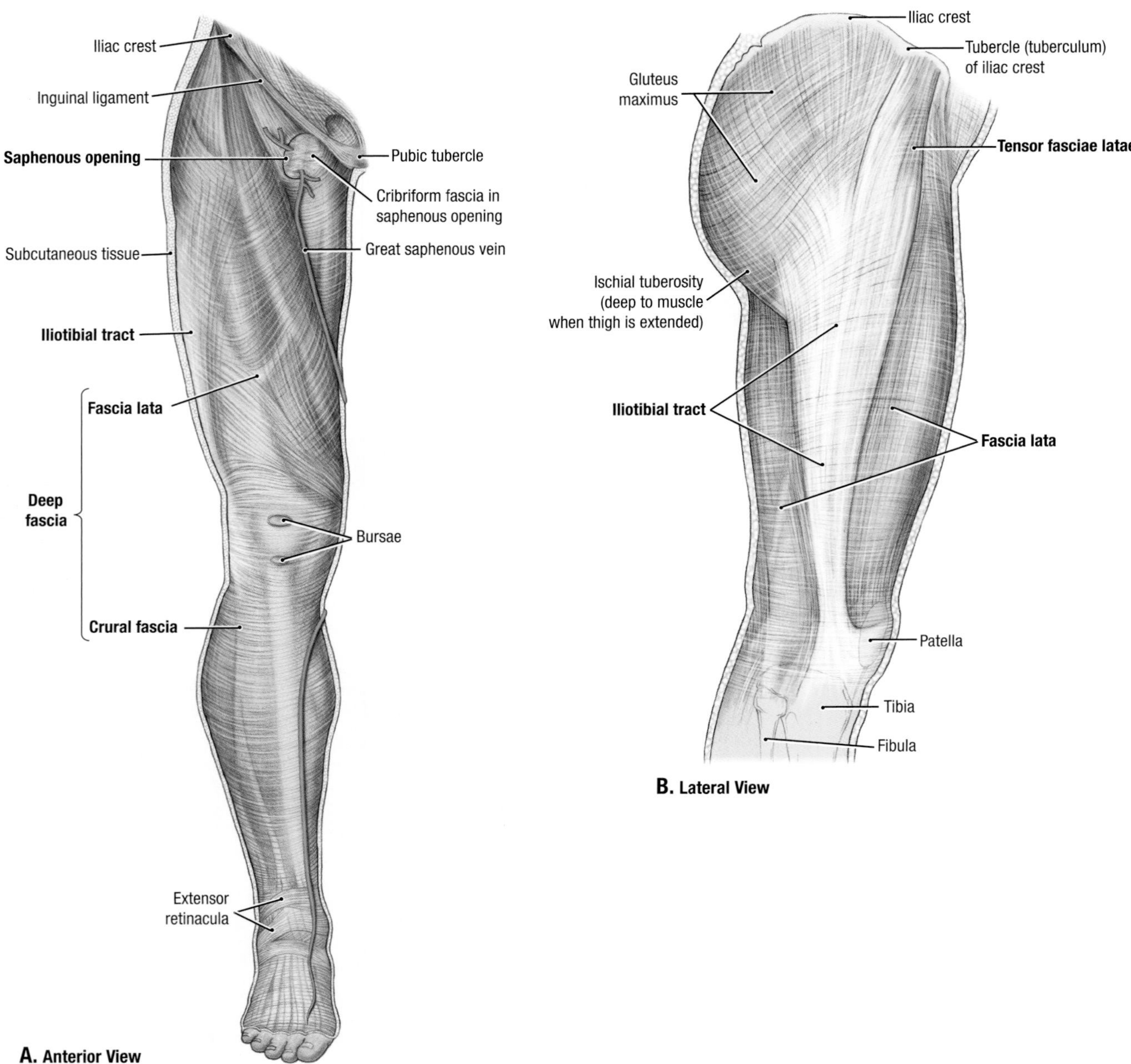
Iliac crest
Inguinal ligament
Saphenous opening
Pubic tubercle
Cribriform fascia in saphenous opening
Subcutaneous tissue
Great saphenous vein
Iliotibial tract
Fascia lata
Deep fascia
Bursae
Crural fascia
Extensor retinacula
A. Anterior View
Iliac crest
Tubercle (tuberculum) of iliac crest
Gluteus maximus
Tensor fasciae latae
Ischial tuberosity (deep to muscle when thigh is extended)
Iliotibial tract
Fascia lata
Patella
Tibia
Fibula
B. Lateral View

## 5.14 Fascia and musculofascial compartments of lower limb

**A.** Anterior skin and subcutaneous tissue have been removed to reveal the deep fascia of the thigh (fascia lata) and leg (crural fascia). **B.** Lateral skin and subcutaneous tissue have been removed to reveal the fascia lata. The fascia lata is thick laterally and forms the iliotibial tract. The iliotibial tract serves as a common aponeurosis for the gluteus maximus and tensor fasciae latae muscles.

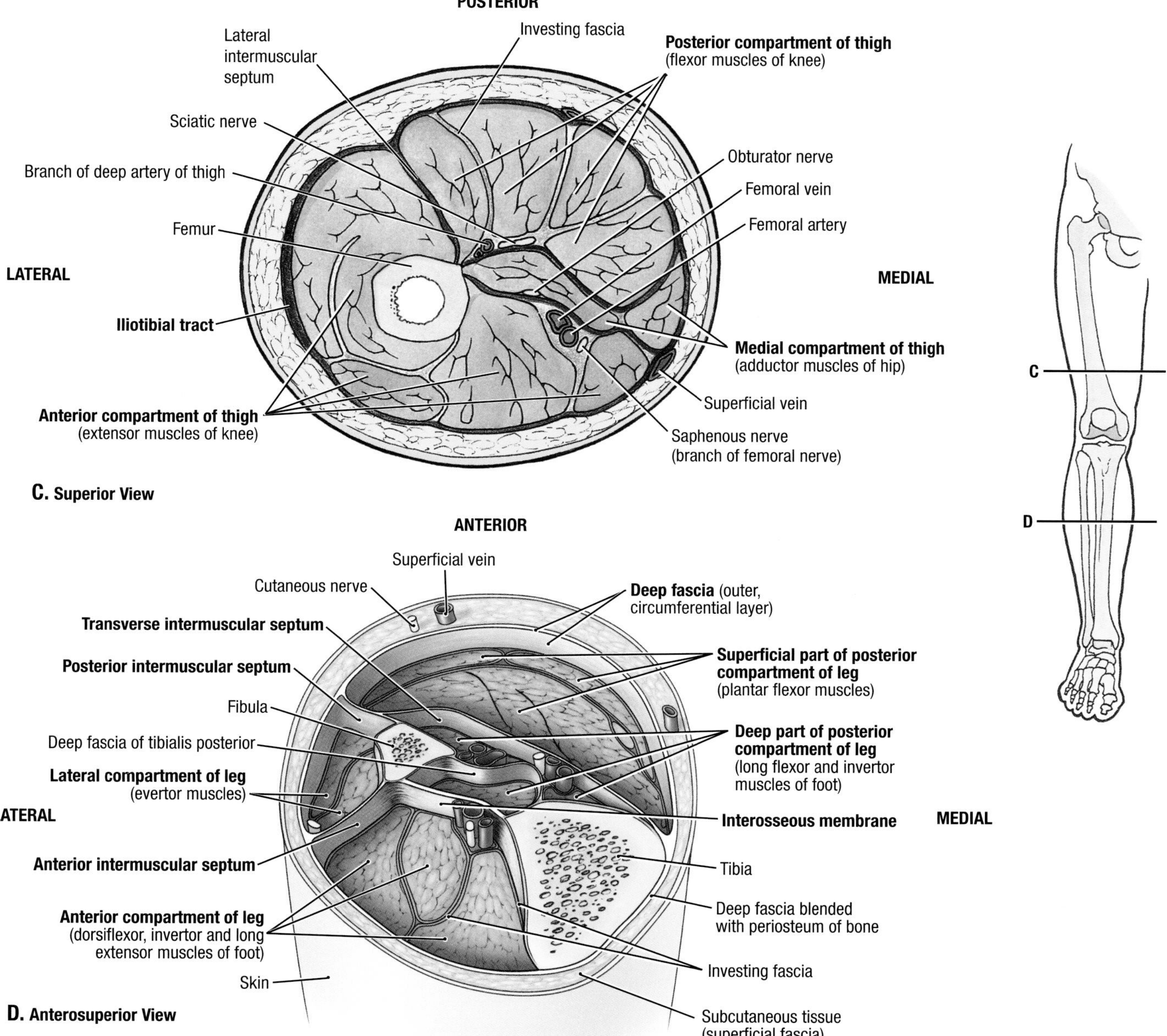
POSTERIOR
Lateral intermuscular septum
Investing fascia
Posterior compartment of thigh (flexor muscles of knee)
Sciatic nerve
Obturator nerve
Branch of deep artery of thigh
Femoral vein
Femur
Femoral artery
LATERAL
MEDIAL
Iliotibial tract
Medial compartment of thigh (adductor muscles of hip)
Superficial vein
Anterior compartment of thigh (extensor muscles of knee)
Saphenous nerve (branch of femoral nerve)
C. Superior View
ANTERIOR
C
D
Superficial vein
Cutaneous nerve
Deep fascia (outer, circumferential layer)
Transverse intermuscular septum
Posterior intermuscular septum
Superficial part of posterior compartment of leg (plantar flexor muscles)
Fibula
Deep fascia of tibialis posterior
Deep part of posterior compartment of leg (long flexor and invertor muscles of foot)
Lateral compartment of leg (evertor muscles)
LATERAL
Interosseous membrane
MEDIAL
Anterior intermuscular septum
Tibia
Deep fascia blended with periosteum of bone
Anterior compartment of leg (dorsiflexor, invertor and long extensor muscles of foot)
Investing fascia
Skin
D. Anterosuperior View
Subcutaneous tissue (superficial fascia)

## 5.14 Fascia and musculofascial compartments of lower limb *(continued)*

**C** and **D.** The fascial compartments of the thigh **(C)** and leg **(D)** are demonstrated in transverse section. The fascial compartments contain muscles that generally perform common functions and share common innervation, and contain the spread of infection. While both thigh and leg have anterior and posterior compartments, the thigh also includes a medial compartment and the leg a lateral compartment. Trauma to muscles and/or vessels in the compartments may product hemorrhage, edema, and inflammation of the muscles. Because the septa, deep fascia, and bony attachments firmly bound the compartments, increased volume resulting from these processes raises intracompartmental pressure. In compartment syndromes, structures within or distal to the compressed area become ischemic and may become permanently injured (e.g., compression of capillary beds results in denervation and consequent paralysis of muscles). A fasciotomy (incision of bounding fascia or septum) may be performed to relieve the pressure in the compartment and restore circulation.

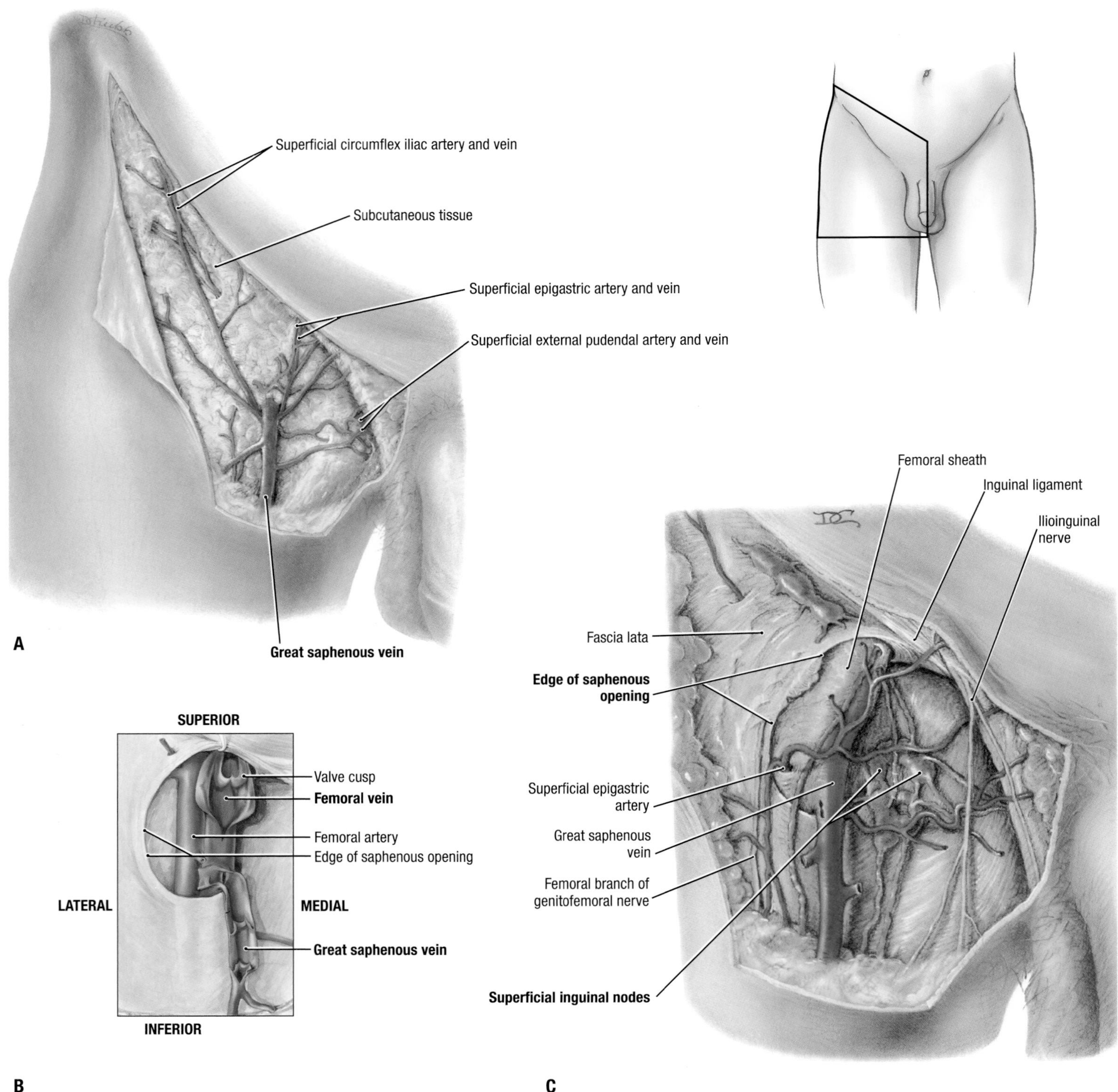
Superficial circumflex iliac artery and vein
Subcutaneous tissue
Superficial epigastric artery and vein
Superficial external pudendal artery and vein
A
Great saphenous vein
SUPERIOR
Valve cusp
Femoral vein
Femoral artery
Edge of saphenous opening
LATERAL
MEDIAL
Great saphenous vein
INFERIOR
B
Femoral sheath
Inguinal ligament
Ilioinguinal nerve
Fascia lata
Edge of saphenous opening
Superficial epigastric artery
Great saphenous vein
Femoral branch of genitofemoral nerve
Superficial inguinal nodes
C

## 5.15 Superficial inguinal vessels and saphenous opening

**A.** Superficial inguinal vessels. The arteries are branches of the femoral artery, and the veins are tributaries of the great saphenous vein. **B.** Valves of the proximal part of femoral and great saphenous veins. **C.** Saphenous opening.

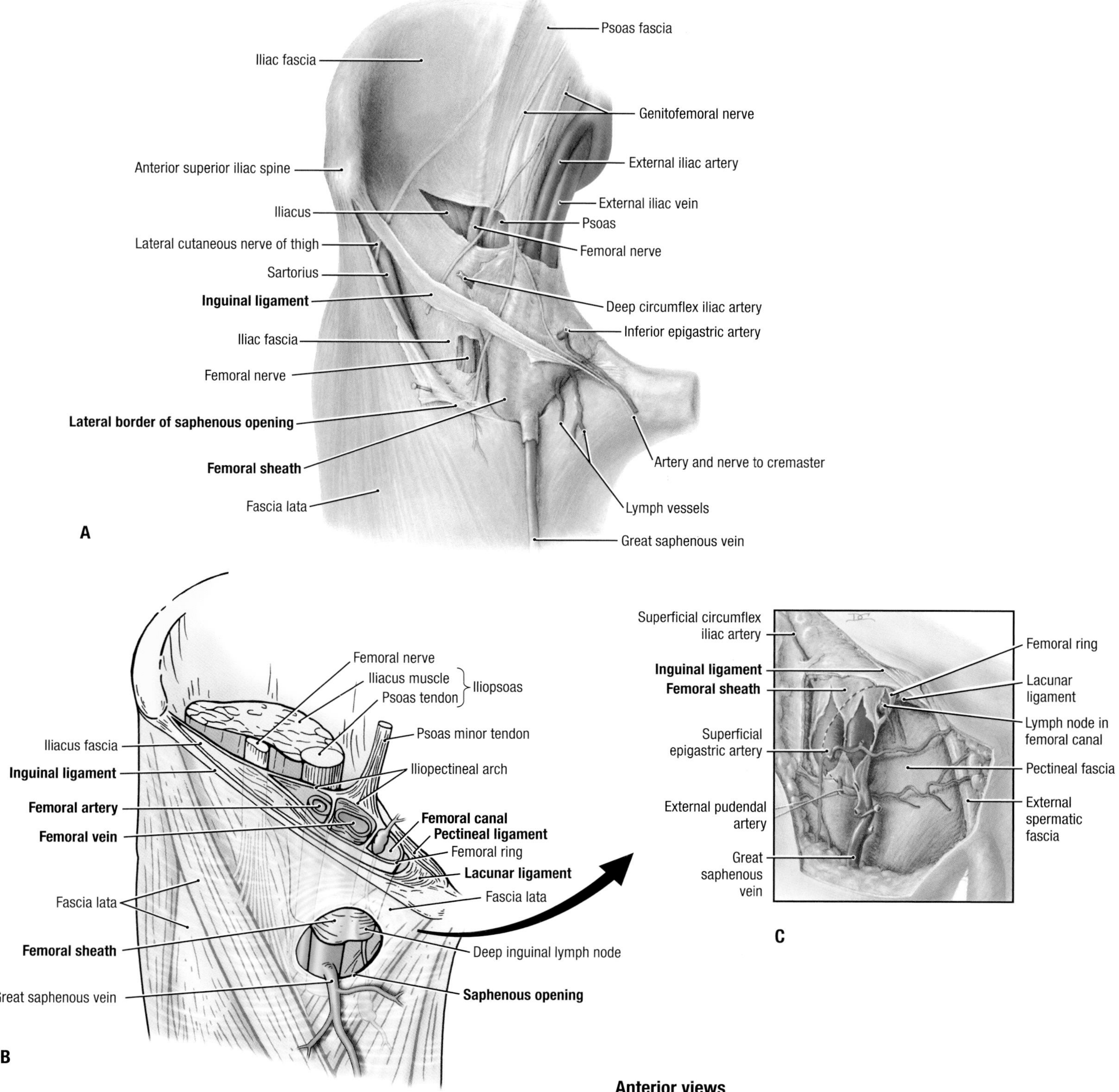
Psoas fascia
Iliac fascia
Genitofemoral nerve
Anterior superior iliac spine
External iliac artery
External iliac vein
Iliacus
Psoas
Lateral cutaneous nerve of thigh
Femoral nerve
Sartorius
Inguinal ligament
Deep circumflex iliac artery
Inferior epigastric artery
Iliac fascia
Femoral nerve
Lateral border of saphenous opening
Artery and nerve to cremaster
Femoral sheath
Fascia lata
Lymph vessels
A
Great saphenous vein
Femoral nerve
Iliacus muscle
Psoas tendon
Iliopsoas
Psoas minor tendon
Iliacus fascia
Inguinal ligament
Iliopectineal arch
Femoral artery
Femoral canal
Femoral vein
Pectineal ligament
Femoral ring
Lacunar ligament
Fascia lata
Fascia lata
Femoral sheath
Deep inguinal lymph node
Great saphenous vein
Saphenous opening
B
Superficial circumflex iliac artery
Inguinal ligament
Femoral sheath
Superficial epigastric artery
External pudendal artery
Great saphenous vein
Femoral ring
Lacunar ligament
Lymph node in femoral canal
Pectineal fascia
External spermatic fascia
C
Anterior views

## 5.16 Femoral sheath and inguinal ligament

**A.** Dissection. **B.** Schematic illustration. The femoral sheath contains the femoral artery, vein, and lymph vessels, but the femoral nerve, lying posterior to the iliacus fascia, is outside the femoral sheath. **C.** Femoral sheath and femoral ring.

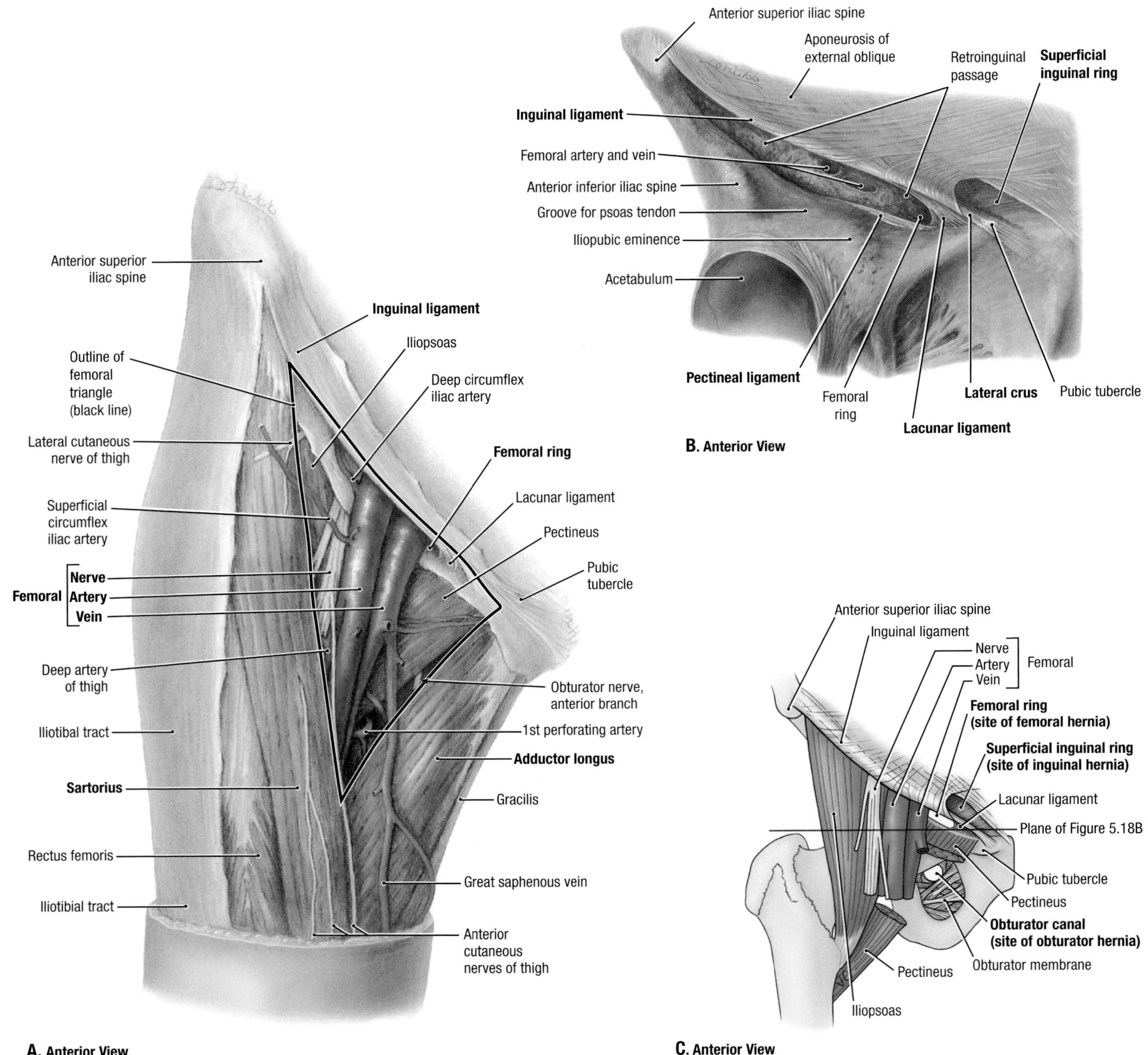
Anterior superior iliac spine
Inguinal ligament
Outline of femoral triangle (black line)
Iliopsoas
Deep circumflex iliac artery
Lateral cutaneous nerve of thigh
Femoral ring
Superficial circumflex iliac artery
Lacunar ligament
Pectineus
Femoral
Nerve
Artery
Vein
Pubic tubercle
Deep artery of thigh
Obturator nerve, anterior branch
Iliotibal tract
1st perforating artery
Adductor longus
Sartorius
Gracilis
Rectus femoris
Great saphenous vein
Iliotibial tract
Anterior cutaneous nerves of thigh
A. Anterior View
Anterior superior iliac spine
Aponeurosis of external oblique
Retroinguinal passage
Superficial inguinal ring
Inguinal ligament
Femoral artery and vein
Anterior inferior iliac spine
Groove for psoas tendon
Iliopubic eminence
Acetabulum
Pectineal ligament
Femoral ring
Lateral crus
Pubic tubercle
Lacunar ligament
B. Anterior View
Anterior superior iliac spine
Inguinal ligament
Nerve
Artery
Vein
Femoral
Femoral ring (site of femoral hernia)
Superficial inguinal ring (site of inguinal hernia)
Lacunar ligament
Plane of Figure 5.18B
Pubic tubercle
Pectineus
Obturator canal (site of obturator hernia)
Obturator membrane
Pectineus
Iliopsoas
C. Anterior View

**5.17 Structures passing to/from femoral triangle via retroinguinal passage**

**A.** Dissection. The boundaries of the femoral triangle are the inguinal ligament superiorly (base of triangle), the medial border of the sartorius (lateral side), and the lateral border of the adductor longus (medial side). The point at which the lateral and medial sides converge inferiorly forms the apex. The femoral triangle is bisected by the femoral vessels. **B.** Retroinguinal passage between the inguinal ligament anteriorly and the bony pelvis posteriorly. **C.** The iliopsoas muscle, the femoral nerve, artery, and vein, and the lymphatic vessels draining the inguinal nodes pass deep to the inguinal ligament to enter the anterior thigh or return to the trunk. Three potential sites for hernia formation are indicated. Pulsations of the femoral artery can be felt distal to the inguinal ligament, midway between the anterior superior iliac spine and the pubic tubercle.

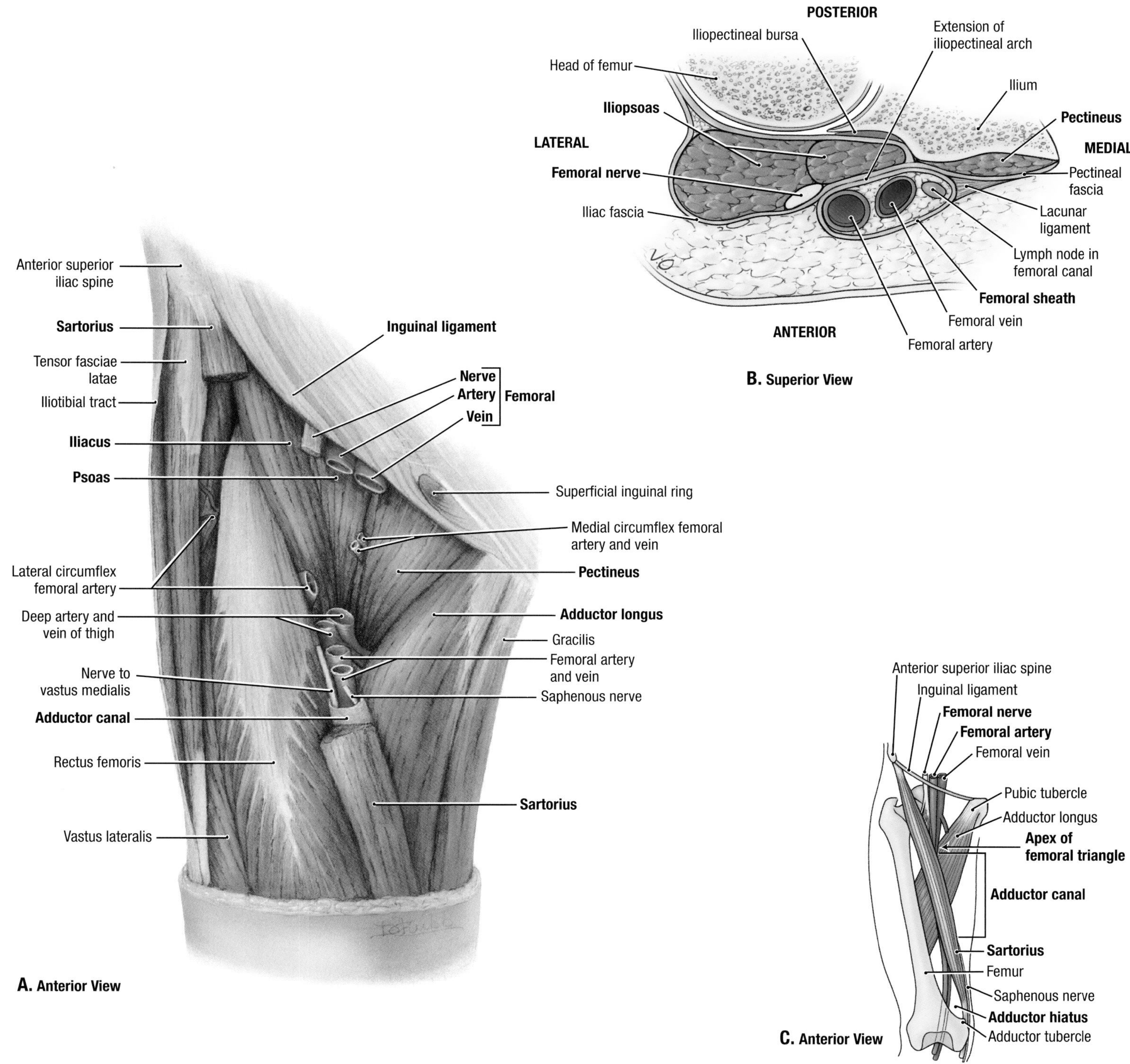
Anterior superior iliac spine
Sartorius
Tensor fasciae latae
Iliotibial tract
Iliacus
Psoas
Lateral circumflex femoral artery
Deep artery and vein of thigh
Nerve to vastus medialis
Adductor canal
Rectus femoris
Vastus lateralis
Inguinal ligament
Nerve
Artery
Vein
Femoral
Superficial inguinal ring
Medial circumflex femoral artery and vein
Pectineus
Adductor longus
Gracilis
Femoral artery and vein
Saphenous nerve
Sartorius
A. Anterior View
POSTERIOR
Iliopectineal bursa
Extension of iliopectineal arch
Head of femur
Ilium
Iliopsoas
Pectineus
LATERAL
MEDIAL
Femoral nerve
Pectineal fascia
Iliac fascia
Lacunar ligament
Lymph node in femoral canal
Femoral sheath
Femoral vein
ANTERIOR
Femoral artery
B. Superior View
Anterior superior iliac spine
Inguinal ligament
Femoral nerve
Femoral artery
Femoral vein
Pubic tubercle
Adductor longus
Apex of femoral triangle
Adductor canal
Sartorius
Femur
Saphenous nerve
Adductor hiatus
Adductor tubercle
C. Anterior View

## 5.18 Floor of femoral canal and retroinguinal passage

**A.** Dissection. Portions of the sartorius muscle, femoral vessels, and femoral nerve have been removed revealing the floor of the femoral triangle, formed by the iliopsoas laterally and the pectineus medially. At the apex of the triangle the femoral vessels, saphenous nerve, and the nerve to the vastus medialis pass deep to the sartorius into the adductor (subsartorial) canal. **B.** Transverse section of the femoral triangle at the level of head of femur. (Level of section is indicated in Fig. 5.17**C.**) The iliopsoas and femoral nerve traverse the retroinguinal passage and femoral triangle in a fascial sheath separate from the femoral vessels, which are contained within the femoral sheath. **C.** Schematic illustration of course of femoral vessels. The adductor canal extends from the triangle's apex to the adductor hiatus, by which the vessels enter and leave the popliteal fossa.

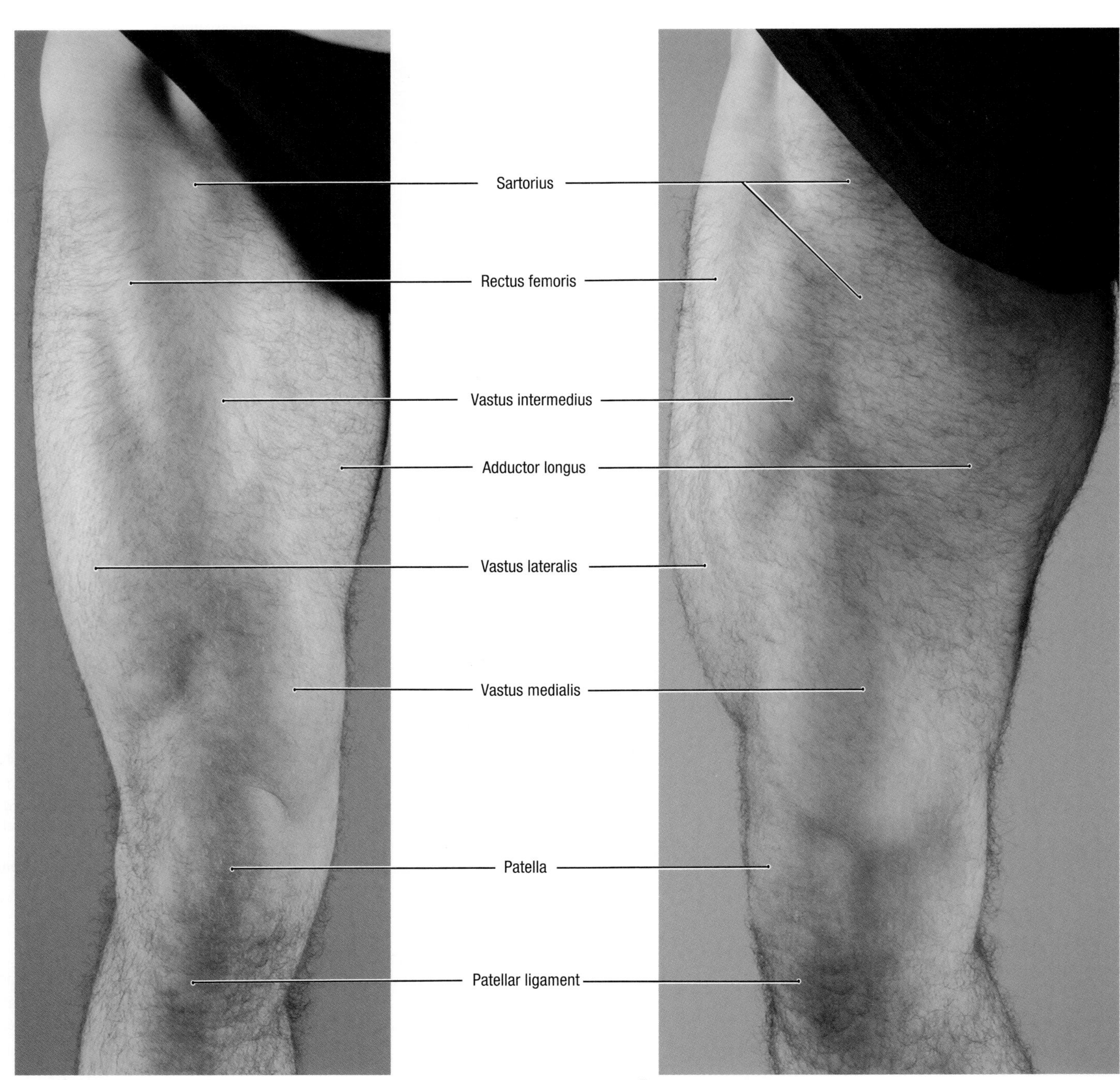
Sartorius
Rectus femoris
Vastus intermedius
Adductor longus
Vastus lateralis
Vastus medialis
Patella
Patellar ligament
A. Anterior View
B. Anteromedial View

**5.19 Surface anatomy of anterior and medial aspects of thigh**

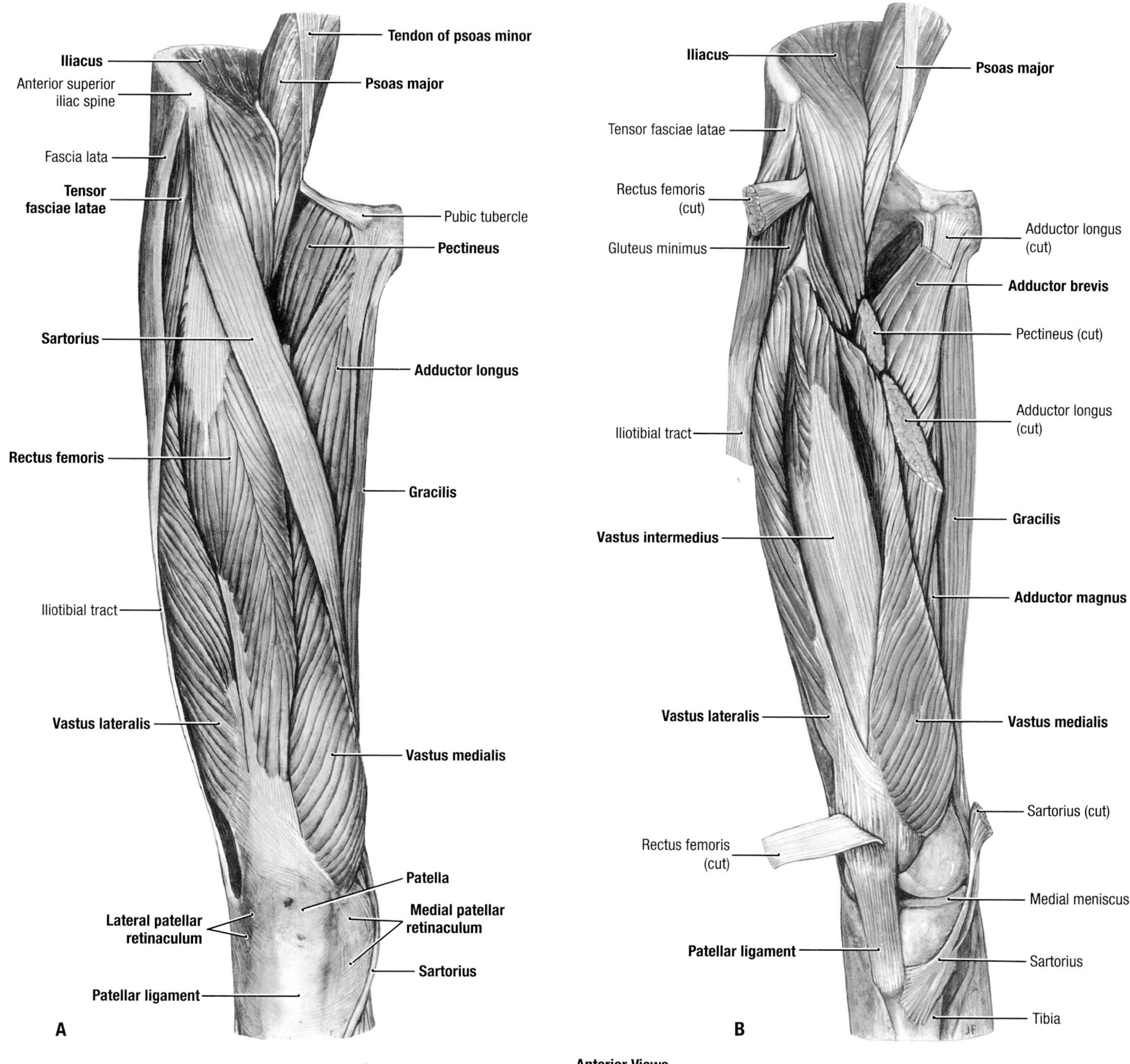
Tendon of psoas minor
Iliacus
Anterior superior iliac spine
Psoas major
Fascia lata
Tensor fasciae latae
Pubic tubercle
Pectineus
Sartorius
Adductor longus
Rectus femoris
Gracilis
Iliotibial tract
Vastus lateralis
Vastus medialis
Patella
Lateral patellar retinaculum
Medial patellar retinaculum
Sartorius
Patellar ligament
A
Iliacus
Psoas major
Tensor fasciae latae
Rectus femoris (cut)
Adductor longus (cut)
Gluteus minimus
Adductor brevis
Pectineus (cut)
Adductor longus (cut)
Iliotibial tract
Gracilis
Vastus intermedius
Adductor magnus
Vastus lateralis
Vastus medialis
Sartorius (cut)
Rectus femoris (cut)
Medial meniscus
Patellar ligament
Sartorius
Tibia
B
Anterior Views

## 5.20 Anterior and medial thigh muscles

**A.** Superficial dissection. **B.** Deep dissection. The central portions of the muscle bellies of the sartorius, rectus femoris, pectineus, and adductor longus muscles have been removed. Weakness of the vastus medialis or vastus lateralis, resulting from arthritis or trauma to the knee joint, for example, can result in abnormal patellar movement and loss of joint stability.

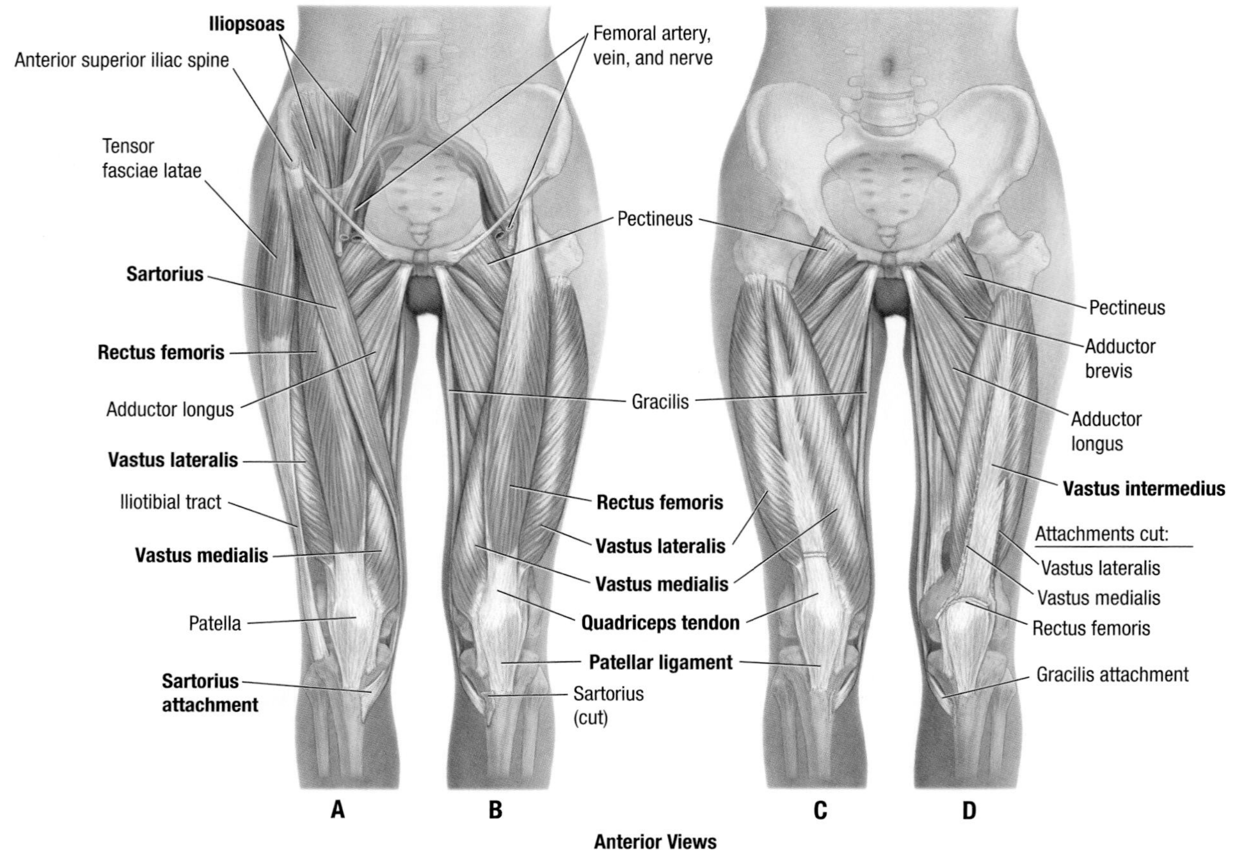
Iliopsoas
Anterior superior iliac spine
Tensor fasciae latae
Sartorius
Rectus femoris
Adductor longus
Vastus lateralis
Iliotibial tract
Vastus medialis
Patella
Sartorius attachment
Femoral artery, vein, and nerve
Pectineus
Gracilis
Rectus femoris
Vastus lateralis
Vastus medialis
Quadriceps tendon
Patellar ligament
Sartorius (cut)
Pectineus
Adductor brevis
Adductor longus
Vastus intermedius
Attachments cut:
Vastus lateralis
Vastus medialis
Rectus femoris
Gracilis attachment
A
B
C
D
Anterior Views

**Table 5.2 Anterior and medial thigh muscles, in situ.**

**A** to **D.** Sequential dissection from superficial to deep.

A "hip pointer," which is a contusion of the iliac crest, usually occurs at its anterior part (e.g., where the sartorius attaches to the anterior superior iliac spine). This is one of the most common injuries to the hip region, usually occurring in association with collision sports. Contusions cause bleeding from ruptured capillaries and infiltration of blood into the muscles, tendons, and other soft tissues. The term hip pointer may also refer to avulsion of bony muscle attachments, for example, of the sartorius or rectus femoris from the anterior iliac spines or of the iliopsoas from the lesser trochanter of the femur. However, these injuries should be called avulsion fractures.

A person with a paralyzed quadriceps cannot extend the leg against resistance and usually presses on the distal end of the thigh during walking to prevent inadvertent flexion of the knee joint.

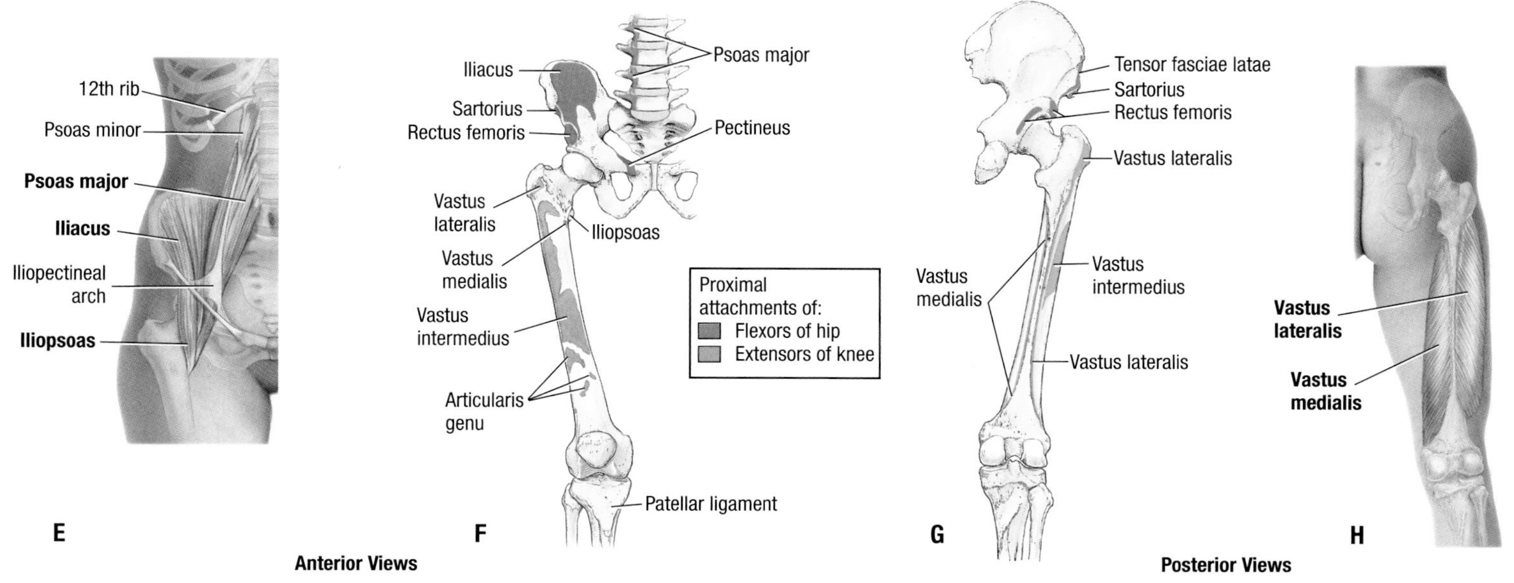
12th rib
Psoas minor
Psoas major
Iliacus
Iliopectineal arch
Iliopsoas
E
Iliacus
Sartorius
Rectus femoris
Psoas major
Pectineus
Vastus lateralis
Iliopsoas
Vastus medialis
Vastus intermedius
Articularis genu
Patellar ligament
Proximal attachments of:
Flexors of hip
Extensors of knee
F
Anterior Views
Tensor fasciae latae
Sartorius
Rectus femoris
Vastus lateralis
Vastus medialis
Vastus intermedius
Vastus lateralis
G
Vastus lateralis
Vastus medialis
H
Posterior Views

**TABLE 5.2 MUSCLES OF ANTERIOR THIGH**

| Muscle | Proximal Attachment[d] | Distal Attachment[d] | Innervation[a] | Main Actions |
|---|---|---|---|---|
| **Iliopsoas** | | | | |
| Psoas major | Lateral aspects of T12–L5 vertebrae and IV discs; transverse processes of all lumbar vertebrae | Lesser trochanter of femur | Anterior rami of lumbar nerves (**L1, L2,** and L3) | Flexes thigh at hip joint and stabilizes this joint[b] |
| Iliacus | Iliac crest, iliac fossa, ala of sacrum and anterior sacro-iliac ligaments | Tendon of psoas major, lesser trochanter, and femur distal to it | Femoral nerve (L2 and L3) | |
| Tensor fasciae latae | Anterior superior iliac spine and anterior part of iliac crest | Iliotibial tract that attaches to lateral condyle of tibia | Superior gluteal (L4 and L5) | Abducts, medially rotates, and flexes thigh; helps to keep knee extended; steadies trunk on thigh |
| Sartorius | Anterior superior iliac spine and superior part of notch inferior to it | Superior part of medial surface of tibia | Femoral nerve (L2 and L3) | Flexes, abducts, and laterally rotates thigh at hip joint; flexes leg at knee joint[c] |
| **Quadriceps femoris** | | | | |
| Rectus femoris | Anterior inferior iliac spine and ilium superior to acetabulum | Base of patella and by patellar ligament to tibial tuberosity; medial and lateral vasti also attach to tibia and patella via aponeuroses (medial and lateral patellar | Femoral nerve (L2, **L3**, and **L4**) | Extends leg at knee joint; rectus femoris also steadies hip joint and helps iliopsoas to flex thigh |
| Vastus lateralis | Greater trochanter and lateral lip of linea aspera of femur | | | |
| Vastus medialis | Intertrochanteric line and medial lip of linea aspera of femur | | | |
| Vastus intermedius | Anterior and lateral surfaces of body of femur | | | |

[a]Numbers indicate spinal cord segmental innervation of nerves (e.g., L1, L2, and L3 indicate that nerves supplying psoas major are derived from first three lumbar segments of the spinal cord; boldface type [**L1**, **L2**] indicates main segmental innervation). Damage to one or more of these spinal cord segments or to motor nerve roots arising from these segments results in paralysis of the muscles concerned.
[b]Psoas major is also a postural muscle that helps control deviation of trunk and is active during standing.
[c]Four actions of sartorius (L. *sartor*, tailor) produce the once common cross-legged sitting position used by tailors—hence the name.
[d]See also Figure 5.22 for muscle attachments.

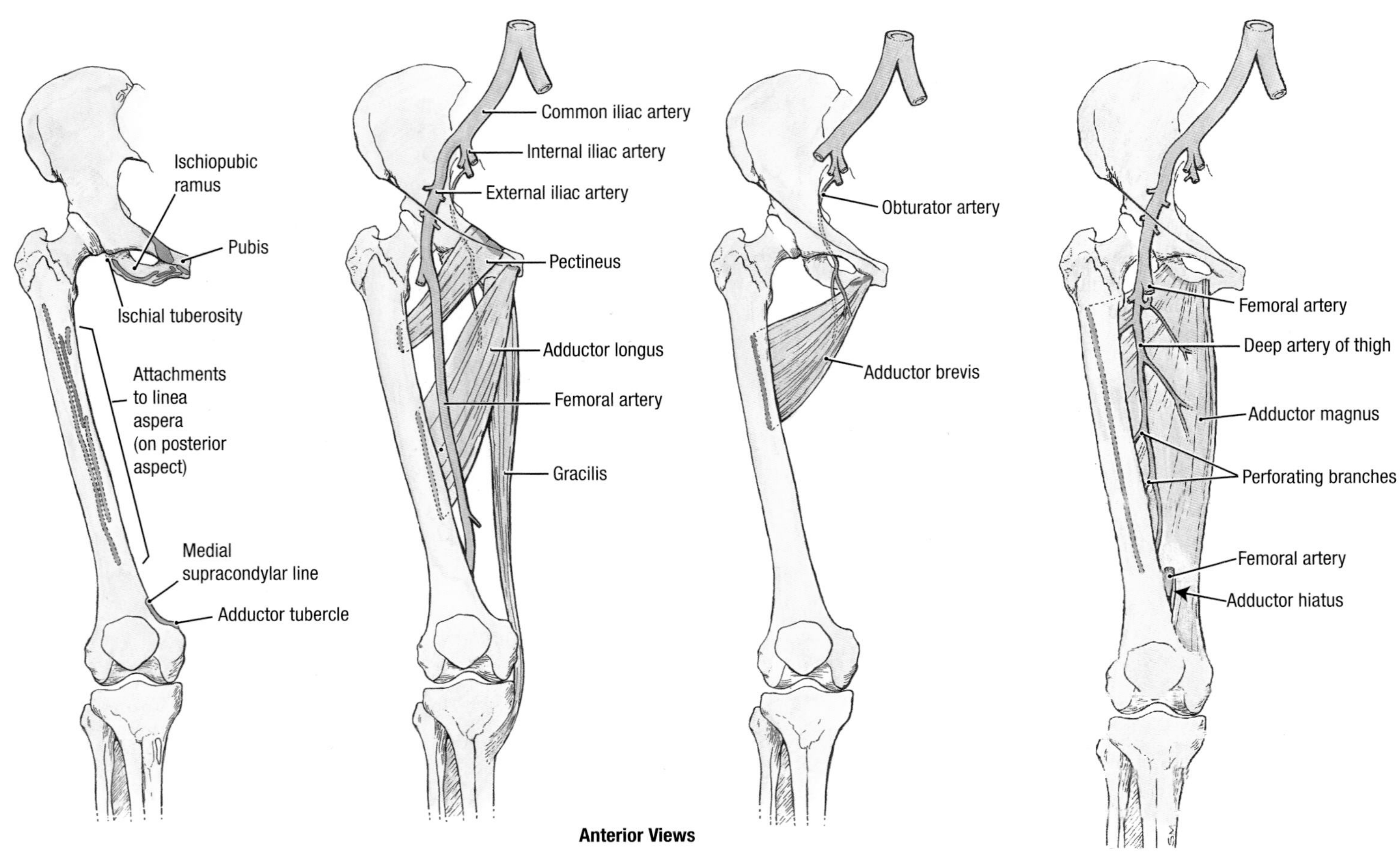

Ischiopubic ramus
Pubis
Ischial tuberosity
Attachments to linea aspera (on posterior aspect)
Medial supracondylar line
Adductor tubercle
Common iliac artery
Internal iliac artery
External iliac artery
Pectineus
Adductor longus
Femoral artery
Gracilis
Obturator artery
Adductor brevis
Femoral artery
Deep artery of thigh
Adductor magnus
Perforating branches
Femoral artery
Adductor hiatus
Anterior Views


## TABLE 5.3 MUSCLES OF MEDIAL THIGH

| Muscle | Proximal Attachment | Distal Attachment[a] | Innervation[b] | Main Actions |
|---|---|---|---|---|
| Pectineus | Superior pubic ramus | Pectineal line of femur, just inferior to lesser trochanter | Femoral nerve (**L2** and L3) may receive a branch from obturator nerve | Adducts and flexes thigh; assists with medial rotation of thigh |
| Adductor longus | Body of pubis inferior to pubic crest | Middle third of linea aspera of femur | Obturator nerve, anterior branch (L2, **L3**, and L4) | Adducts thigh |
| Adductor brevis | Body of pubis and inferior pubic ramus | Pectineal line and proximal part of linea aspera of femur | Obturator nerve (L2, **L3**, and L4) | Adducts thigh and, to some extent, flexes it |
| Adductor magnus | Inferior pubic ramus, ramus of ischium (adductor part), and ischial tuberosity | Gluteal tuberosity, linea aspera, medial supracondylar line (adductor part), and adductor tubercle of femur (hamstring part) | *Adductor part:* obturator nerve (L2, **L3**, and **L4**) *Hamstring part:* tibial part of sciatic nerve **(L4)** | Adducts thigh; its adductor part also flexes thigh, and its hamstring part extends it |
| Gracilis | Body of pubis and inferior pubic ramus | Superior part of medial surface of tibia | Obturator nerve (**L2** and L3) | Adducts thigh, flexes leg, and helps rotate it medially |
| Obturator externus | Margins of obturator foramen and obturator membrane | Trochanteric fossa of femur | Obturator nerve (L3 and **L4)** | Laterally rotates thigh; steadies head of femur in acetabulum |

Collectively, the first five muscles listed are the adductors of the thigh, but their actions are more complex (e.g., they act as flexors of the hip joint during flexion of the knee joint and are active during walking).

[a]See Figure 5.22 for muscle attachments.

[b]See Table 5.1 for explanation of segmental innervation.

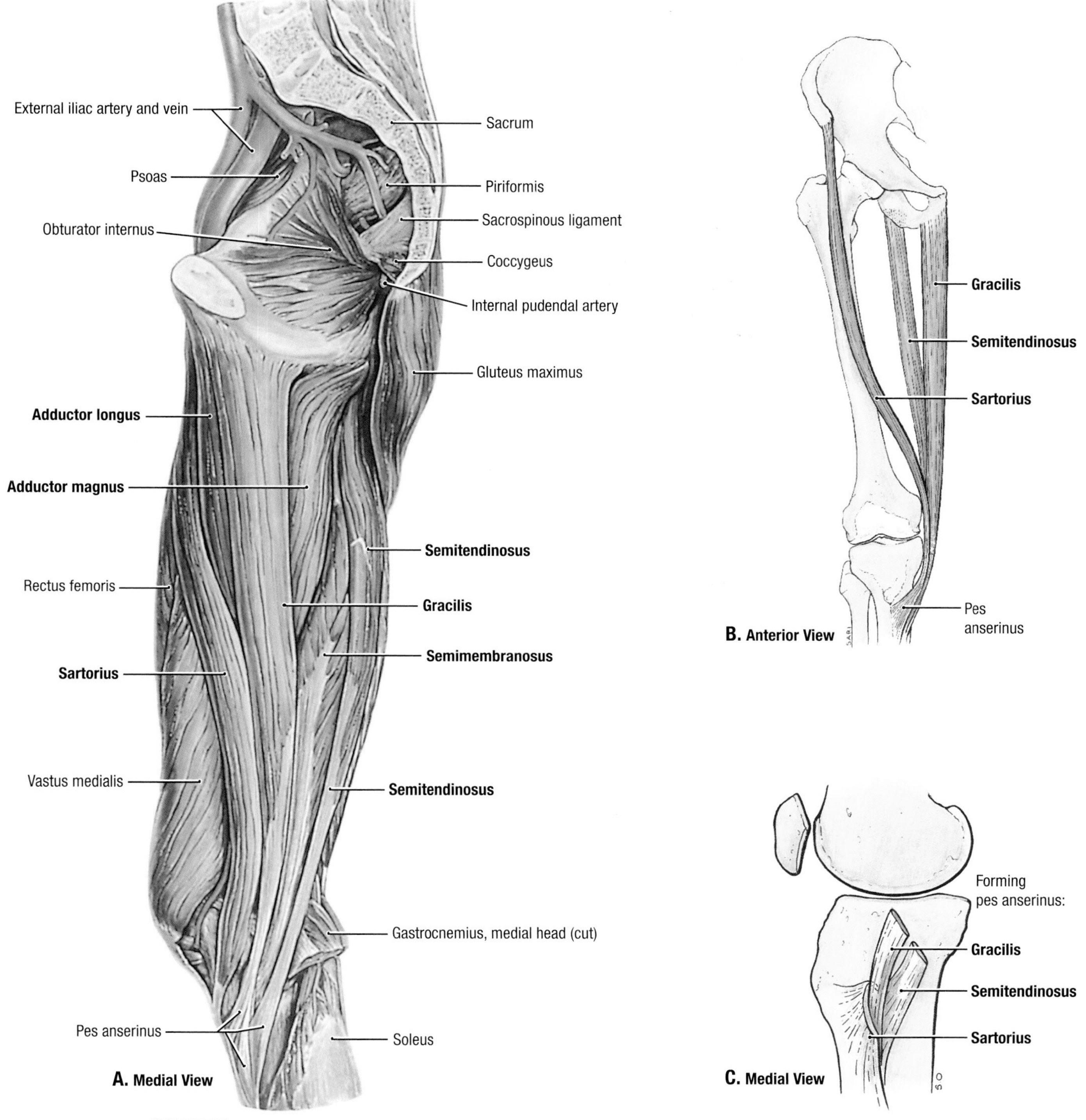
External iliac artery and vein
Psoas
Obturator internus
Sacrum
Piriformis
Sacrospinous ligament
Coccygeus
Internal pudendal artery
Gluteus maximus
Adductor longus
Adductor magnus
Semitendinosus
Rectus femoris
Gracilis
Semimembranosus
Sartorius
Vastus medialis
Semitendinosus
Gastrocnemius, medial head (cut)
Pes anserinus
Soleus
A. Medial View
Gracilis
Semitendinosus
Sartorius
Pes anserinus
B. Anterior View
Forming pes anserinus:
Gracilis
Semitendinosus
Sartorius
C. Medial View

## 5.21 Muscles of medial aspect of thigh

**A.** Dissection. **B.** Muscular tripod. The sartorius, gracilis, and semitendinosus muscles form an inverted tripod arising from three different components of the hip bone. These muscles course within three different compartments, perform three different functions, and are innervated by three different nerves yet share a common distal attachment. **C.** Distal attachment of sartorius, gracilis, and semitendinosus muscles. All three tendons become thin and aponeurotic and are collectively referred to as the pes anserinus. The gracilis is a relatively weak member of the adductor group and hence can be removed without noticeable loss of its actions on the leg. Surgeons often transplant the gracilis, or part of it, with its nerve and blood vessels to replace a damaged muscle in the hand, for example.

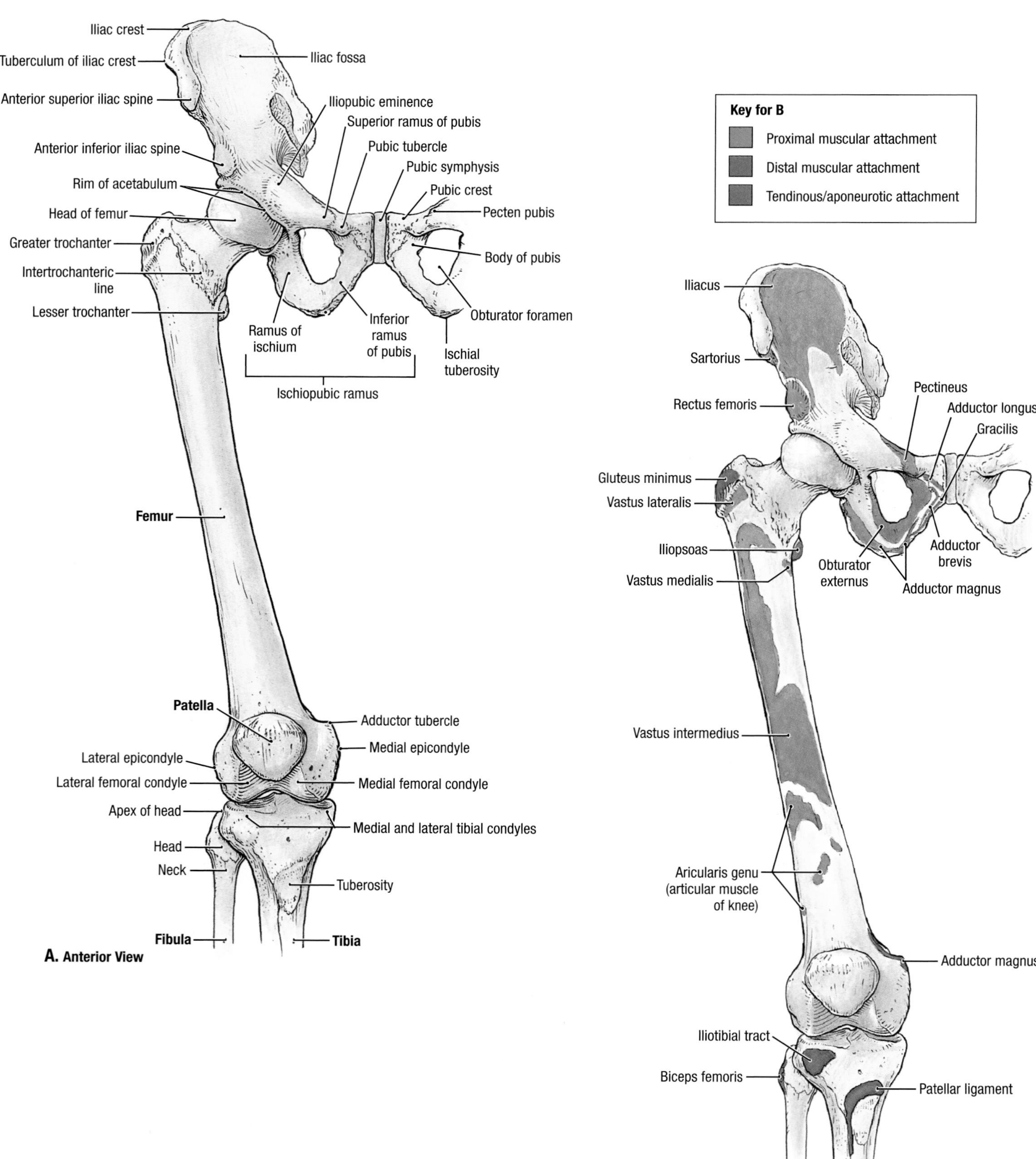
Iliac crest
Tuberculum of iliac crest
Iliac fossa
Anterior superior iliac spine
Iliopubic eminence
Superior ramus of pubis
Anterior inferior iliac spine
Pubic tubercle
Pubic symphysis
Rim of acetabulum
Pubic crest
Head of femur
Pecten pubis
Greater trochanter
Body of pubis
Intertrochanteric line
Lesser trochanter
Obturator foramen
Ramus of ischium
Inferior ramus of pubis
Ischial tuberosity
Ischiopubic ramus
Femur
Patella
Adductor tubercle
Medial epicondyle
Lateral epicondyle
Lateral femoral condyle
Medial femoral condyle
Apex of head
Medial and lateral tibial condyles
Head
Neck
Tuberosity
Fibula
Tibia
A. Anterior View
Key for B
Proximal muscular attachment
Distal muscular attachment
Tendinous/aponeurotic attachment
Iliacus
Sartorius
Rectus femoris
Pectineus
Adductor longus
Gracilis
Gluteus minimus
Vastus lateralis
Iliopsoas
Obturator externus
Adductor brevis
Vastus medialis
Adductor magnus
Vastus intermedius
Aricularis genu (articular muscle of knee)
Adductor magnus
Iliotibial tract
Biceps femoris
Patellar ligament
B. Anterior View

**5.22 Bones of the thigh and proximal leg**

**A.** Bony features. **B.** Muscle attachment sites.

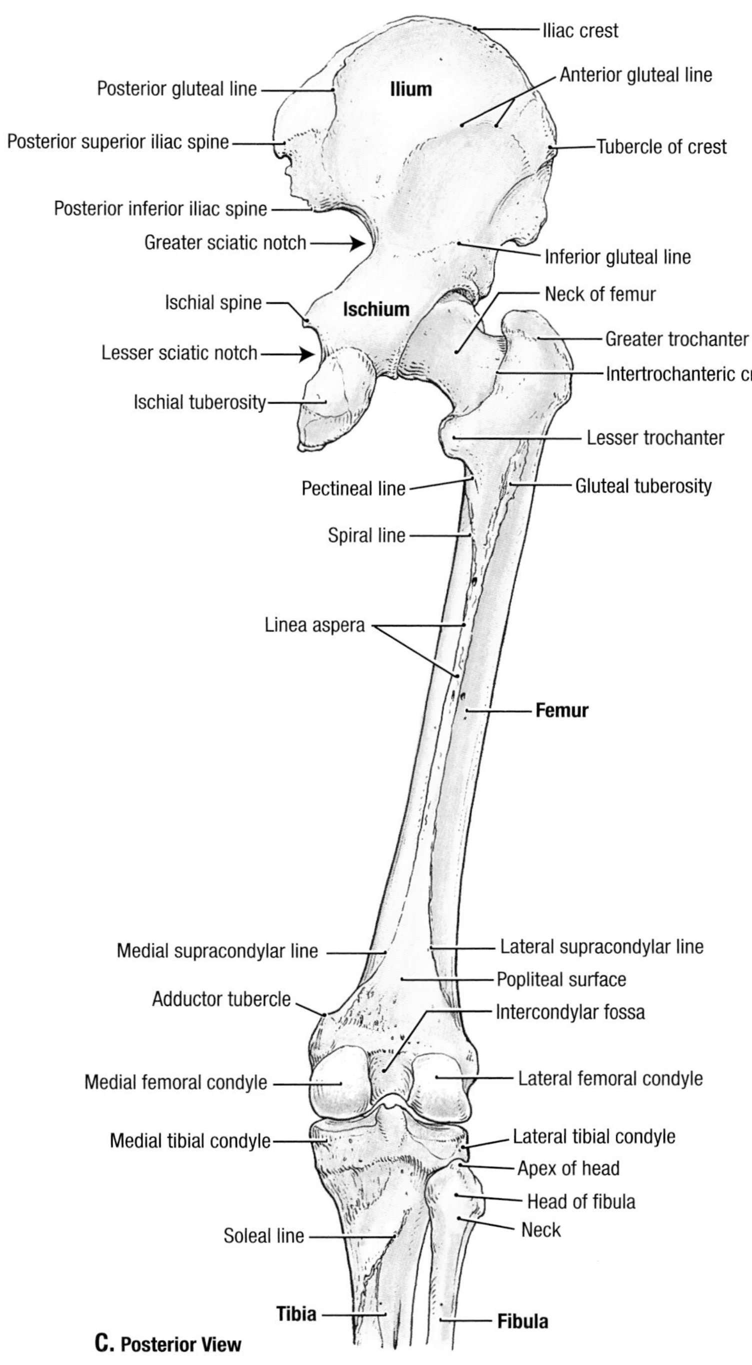
Iliac crest
Posterior gluteal line
Ilium
Anterior gluteal line
Posterior superior iliac spine
Tubercle of crest
Posterior inferior iliac spine
Greater sciatic notch
Inferior gluteal line
Ischial spine
Ischium
Neck of femur
Lesser sciatic notch
Greater trochanter
Intertrochanteric crest
Ischial tuberosity
Lesser trochanter
Pectineal line
Gluteal tuberosity
Spiral line
Linea aspera
Femur
Medial supracondylar line
Lateral supracondylar line
Popliteal surface
Adductor tubercle
Intercondylar fossa
Medial femoral condyle
Lateral femoral condyle
Medial tibial condyle
Lateral tibial condyle
Apex of head
Head of fibula
Soleal line
Neck
Tibia
Fibula

**C.** Posterior View

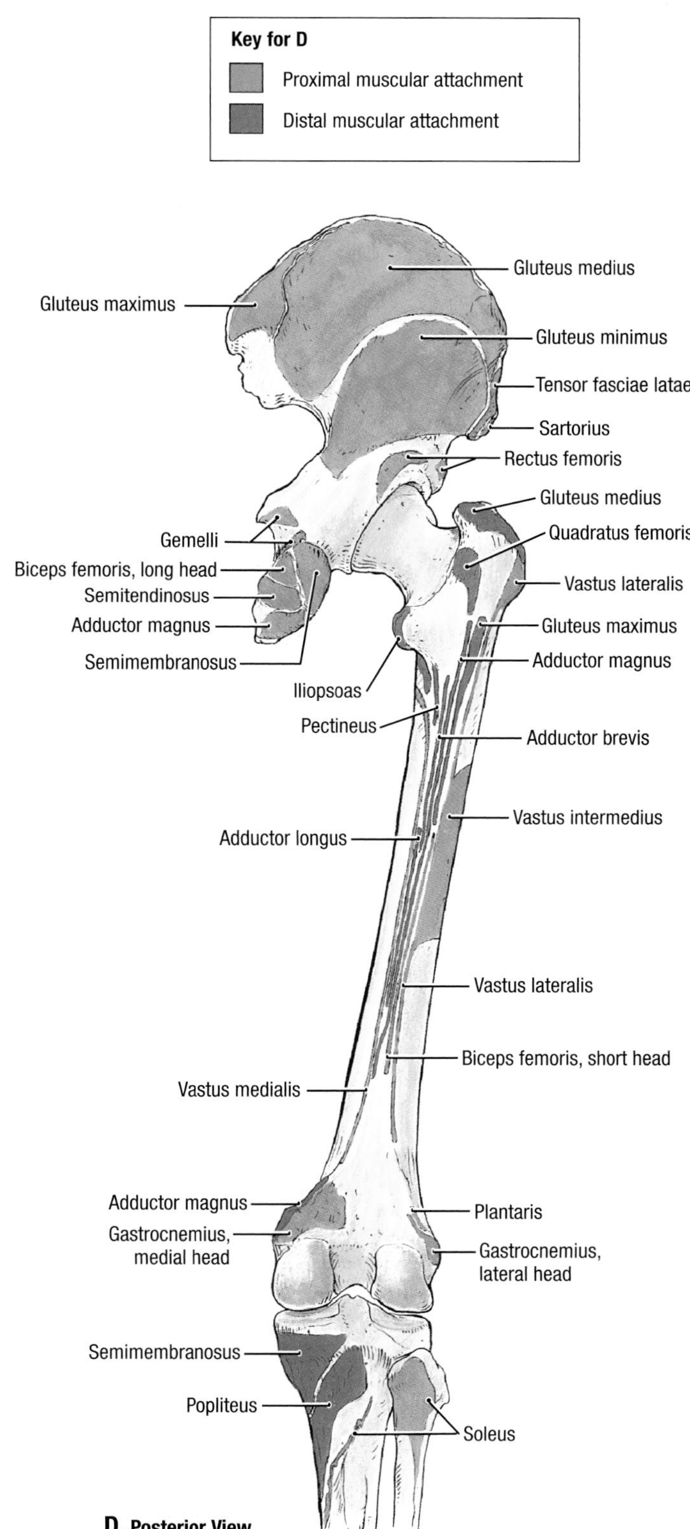
Key for D
Proximal muscular attachment
Distal muscular attachment
Gluteus medius
Gluteus maximus
Gluteus minimus
Tensor fasciae latae
Sartorius
Rectus femoris
Gluteus medius
Quadratus femoris
Gemelli
Biceps femoris, long head
Vastus lateralis
Semitendinosus
Adductor magnus
Gluteus maximus
Adductor magnus
Semimembranosus
Iliopsoas
Pectineus
Adductor brevis
Vastus intermedius
Adductor longus
Vastus lateralis
Biceps femoris, short head
Vastus medialis
Adductor magnus
Plantaris
Gastrocnemius, medial head
Gastrocnemius, lateral head
Semimembranosus
Popliteus
Soleus

**D.** Posterior View

**5.22 Bones of the thigh and proximal leg *(continued)***

**C.** Bony features. **D.** Muscle attachment sites.

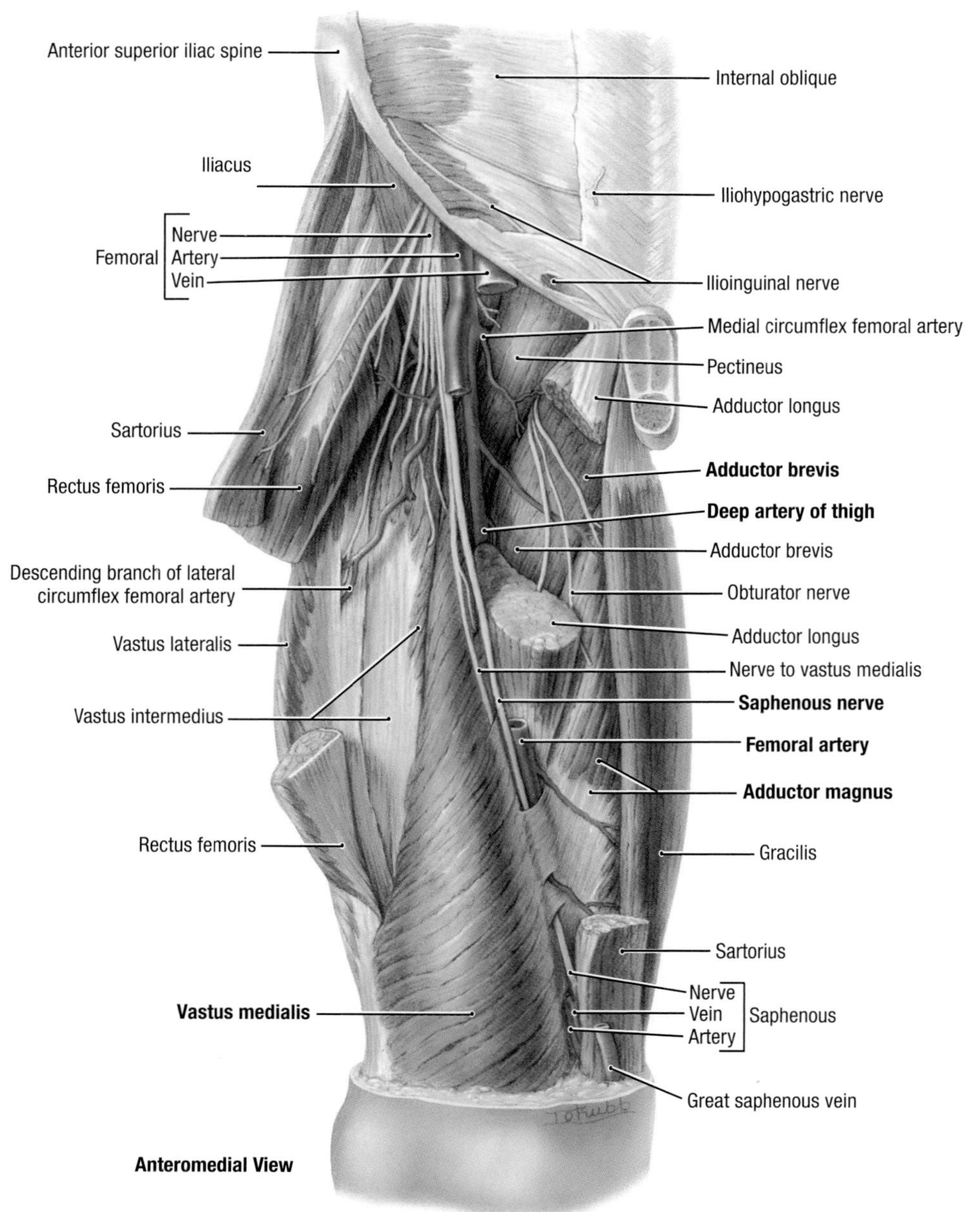
Anterior superior iliac spine
Internal oblique
Iliacus
Iliohypogastric nerve
Femoral
Nerve
Artery
Vein
Ilioinguinal nerve
Medial circumflex femoral artery
Pectineus
Adductor longus
Sartorius
Adductor brevis
Rectus femoris
Deep artery of thigh
Adductor brevis
Descending branch of lateral circumflex femoral artery
Obturator nerve
Vastus lateralis
Adductor longus
Nerve to vastus medialis
Saphenous nerve
Vastus intermedius
Femoral artery
Adductor magnus
Rectus femoris
Gracilis
Sartorius
Vastus medialis
Nerve
Vein
Artery
Saphenous
Great saphenous vein
Anteromedial View

## 5.23 Anteromedial aspect of thigh

- The limb is rotated laterally.
- The femoral nerve breaks up into several nerves on entering the thigh.
- The femoral artery lies between two motor territories: that of the obturator nerve, which is medial, and that of the femoral nerve, which is lateral. No motor nerve crosses anterior to the femoral artery, but the twig to the pectineus muscle crosses posterior to the femoral artery.
- The nerve to the vastus medialis muscle and the saphenous nerve accompany the femoral artery into the adductor canal. The saphenous nerve and artery and their anastomotic accompanying vein emerge from the canal distally between the sartorius and gracilis muscles.
- The deep artery of the thigh arises approximately 4 cm distal to the inguinal ligament, lies posterior to the femoral artery, and disappears posterior to the adductor longus muscle. It supplies the thigh through the medial and lateral circumflex femoral branches and the perforating arteries that pass through the adductor magnus muscle on their way to the posterior aspect of the thigh.

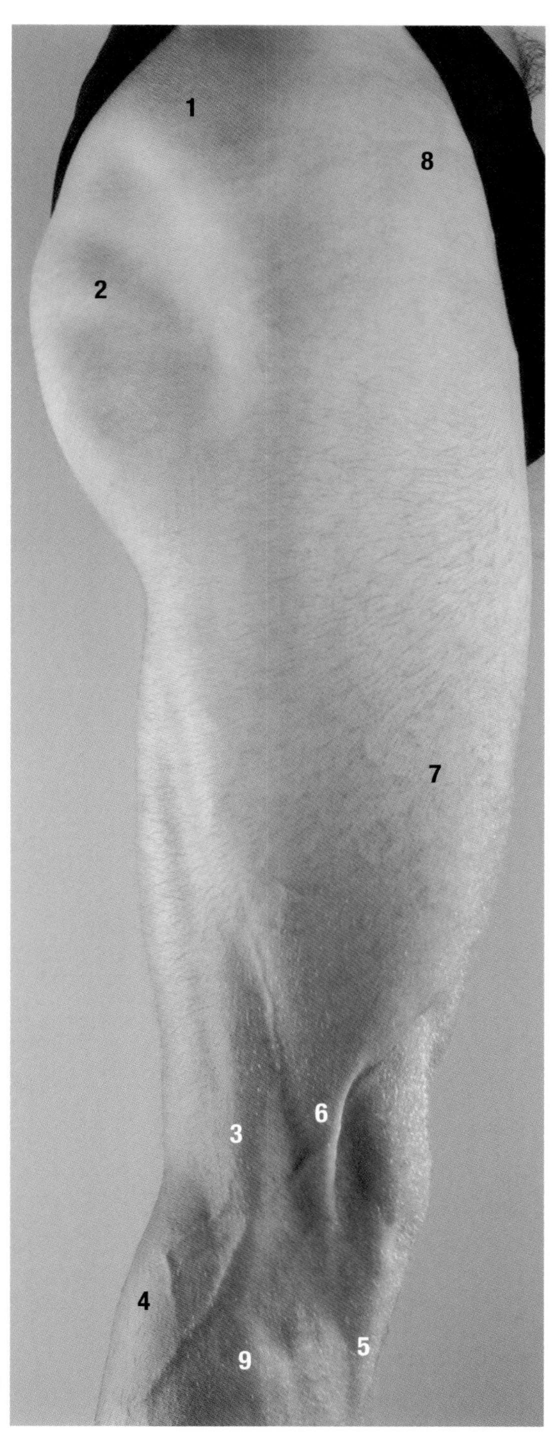
1
8
2
7
6
3
4
9
5

A. Lateral View

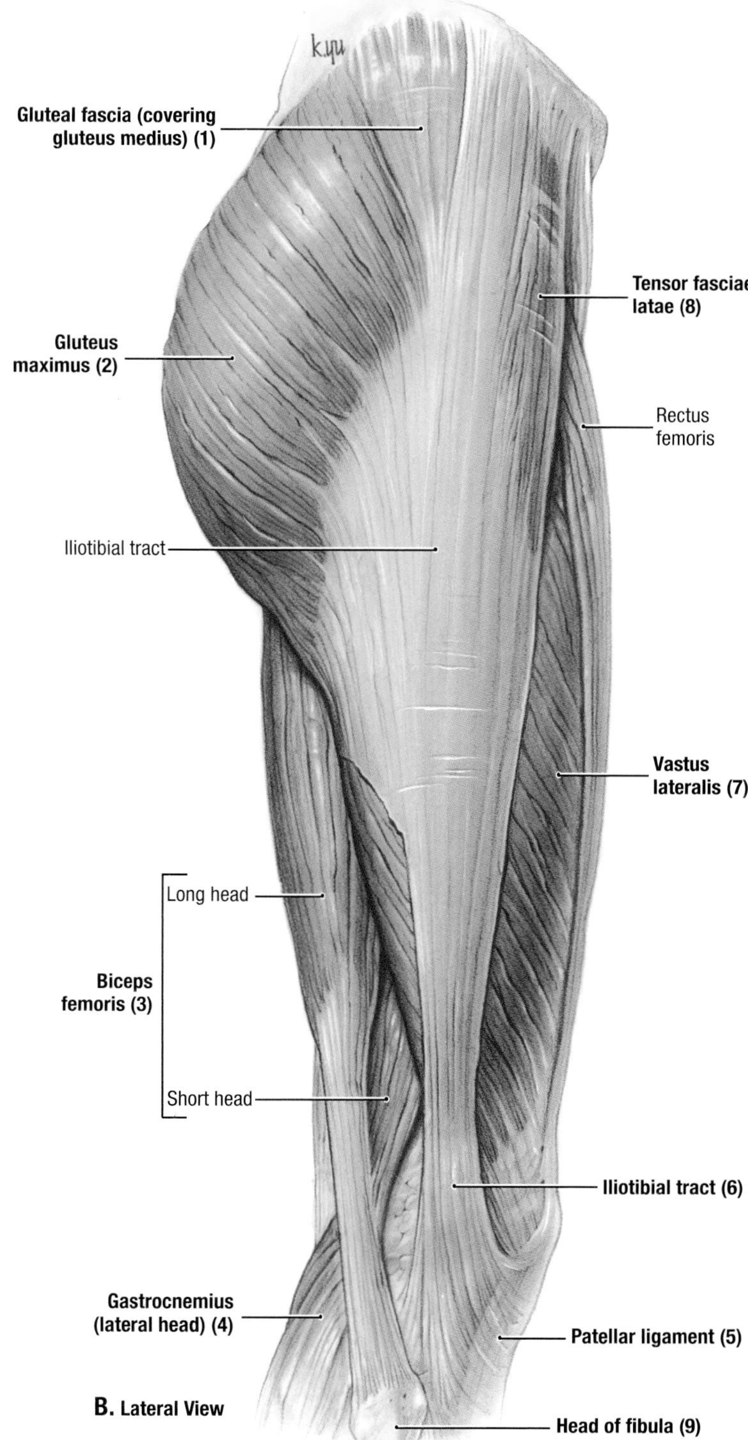
Gluteal fascia (covering gluteus medius) (1)
Tensor fasciae latae (8)
Gluteus maximus (2)
Rectus femoris
Iliotibial tract
Vastus lateralis (7)
Long head
Biceps femoris (3)
Short head
Iliotibial tract (6)
Gastrocnemius (lateral head) (4)
Patellar ligament (5)
Head of fibula (9)

B. Lateral View

## 5.24 Lateral aspect of thigh

**A.** Surface anatomy (*numbers* refer to structures in **B**). **B.** Dissection showing the iliotibial tract, a thickening of the fascia lata, which serves as a tendon for the gluteus maximus and tensor fasciae latae. The iliotibial tract attaches to the anterolateral (Gerdy) tubercle of the lateral condyle of the tibia. The biceps femoris tendon attaches on the head of the fibula.

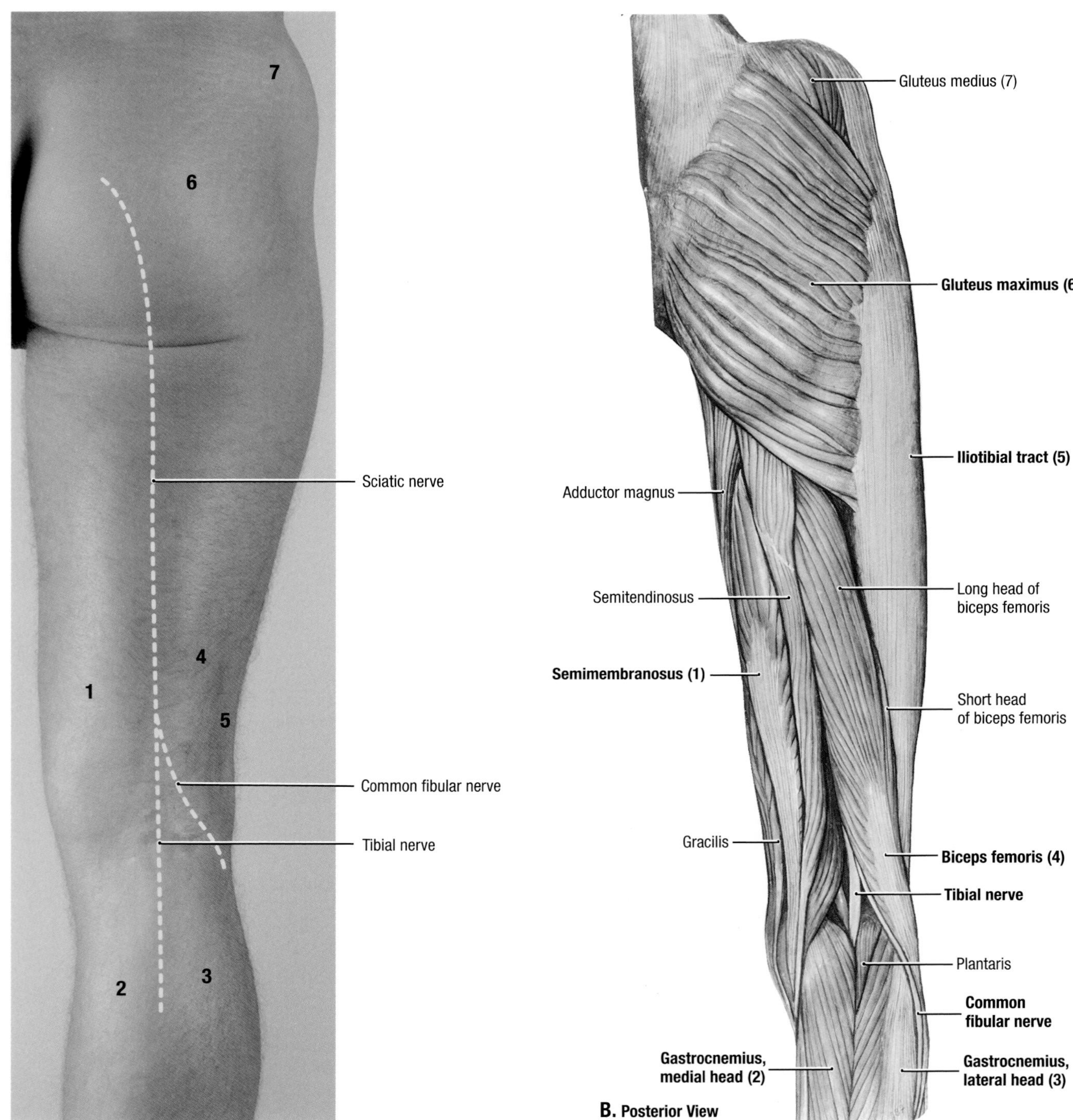
7
6
Sciatic nerve
4
1
5
Common fibular nerve
Tibial nerve
2
3
A. Posterior View
Gluteus medius (7)
Gluteus maximus (6)
Iliotibial tract (5)
Adductor magnus
Semitendinosus
Long head of biceps femoris
Semimembranosus (1)
Short head of biceps femoris
Gracilis
Biceps femoris (4)
Tibial nerve
Plantaris
Common fibular nerve
Gastrocnemius, medial head (2)
Gastrocnemius, lateral head (3)
B. Posterior View

## 5.25 Muscles of the gluteal region and posterior aspect of thigh—I

**A.** Surface anatomy (*numbers* refer to structures in **B**). **B.** Superficial dissection of muscles of gluteal region and posterior thigh (hamstring muscles consisting of semimembranosus, semitendinosus, and biceps femoris). Hamstring strains (pulled and/or torn hamstrings) are common in running, jumping, and quick-start sports. The muscular exertion required to excel in these sports may tear part of the proximal attachments of the hamstrings from the ischial tuberosity.

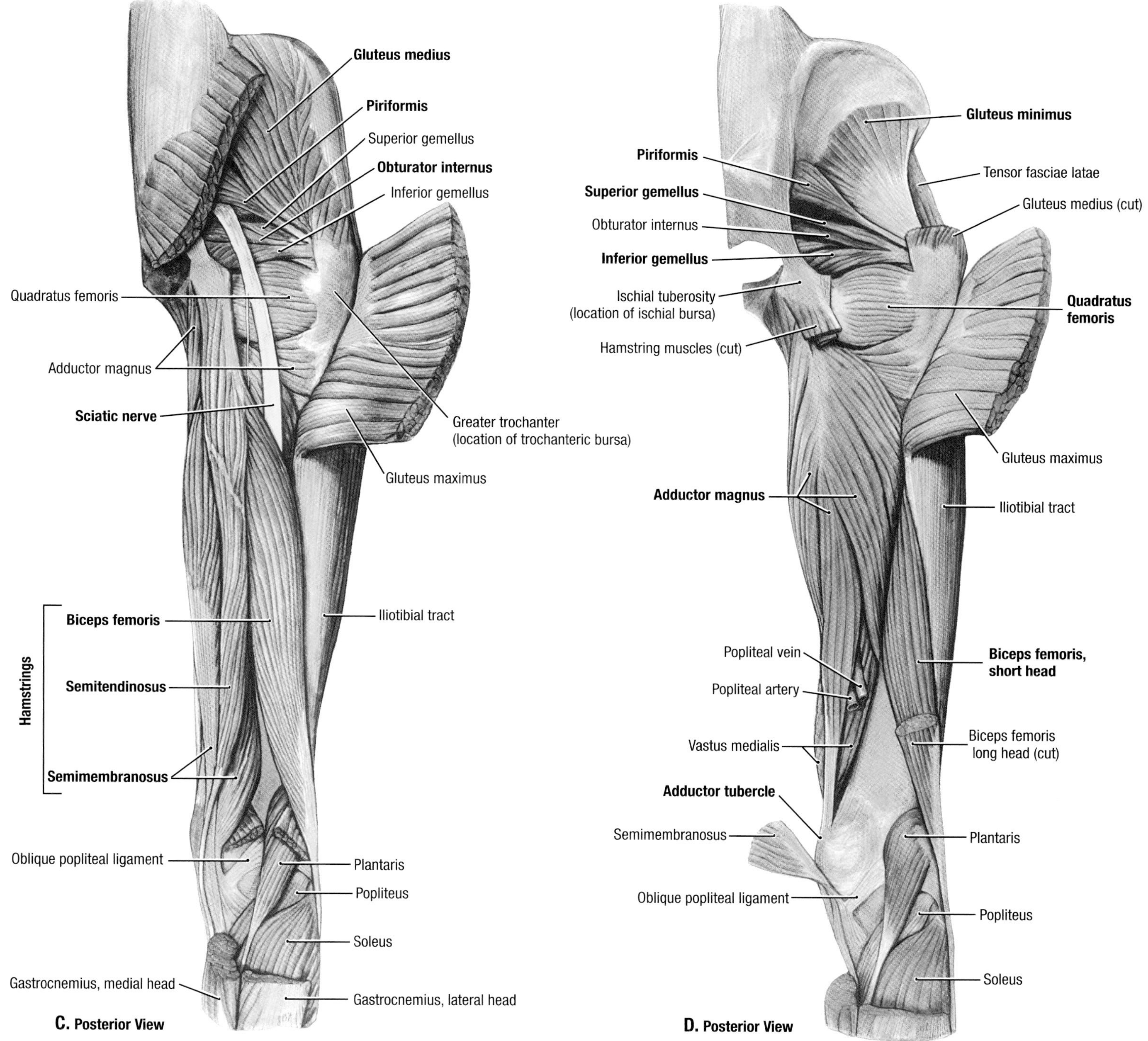
Gluteus medius
Piriformis
Superior gemellus
Obturator internus
Inferior gemellus
Quadratus femoris
Adductor magnus
Sciatic nerve
Greater trochanter
(location of trochanteric bursa)
Gluteus maximus
Biceps femoris
Iliotibial tract
Hamstrings
Semitendinosus
Semimembranosus
Oblique popliteal ligament
Plantaris
Popliteus
Soleus
Gastrocnemius, medial head
Gastrocnemius, lateral head
C. Posterior View
Gluteus minimus
Piriformis
Tensor fasciae latae
Superior gemellus
Gluteus medius (cut)
Obturator internus
Inferior gemellus
Ischial tuberosity
(location of ischial bursa)
Quadratus femoris
Hamstring muscles (cut)
Gluteus maximus
Adductor magnus
Iliotibial tract
Popliteal vein
Biceps femoris, short head
Popliteal artery
Vastus medialis
Biceps femoris long head (cut)
Adductor tubercle
Semimembranosus
Plantaris
Oblique popliteal ligament
Popliteus
Soleus
D. Posterior View

## 5.25 Muscles of gluteal region and posterior aspect of thigh—*(continued)*—II and III

**C.** Muscles of gluteal region and posterior thigh with gluteus maximus reflected. **D.** Adductor magnus muscle. The adductor magnus is a large muscle with two parts: one belongs to the adductor group and the other to the hamstring group. The adductor part is innervated by the obturator nerve and the hamstring part by the tibial portion of the sciatic nerve. The trochanteric bursa separates the superior fibers of the gluteus maximus from the greater trochanter of the femur.

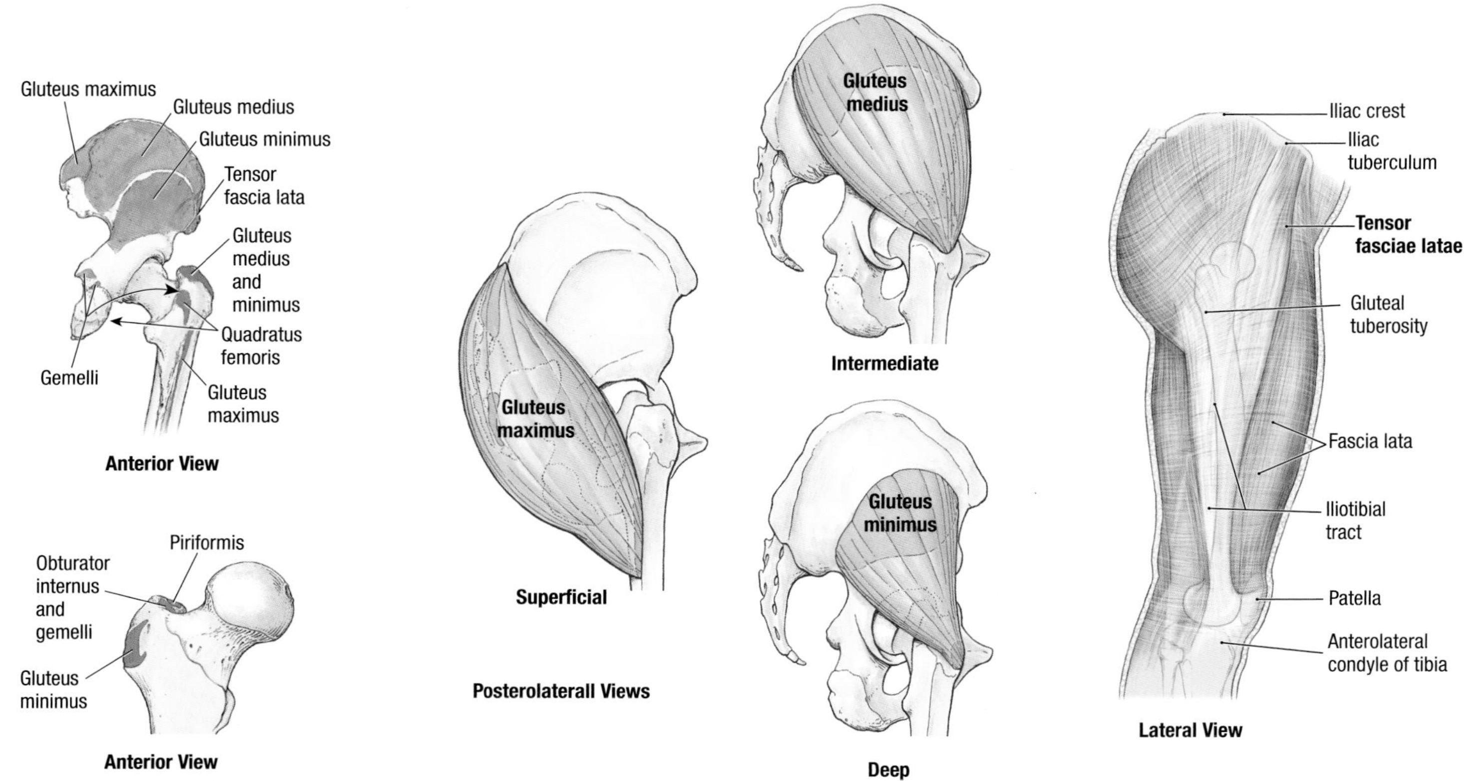
Gluteus maximus
Gluteus medius
Gluteus minimus
Tensor fascia lata
Gluteus medius and minimus
Quadratus femoris
Gemelli
Gluteus maximus
Anterior View
Piriformis
Obturator internus and gemelli
Gluteus minimus
Anterior View
Gluteus maximus
Superficial
Posterolaterall Views
Gluteus medius
Intermediate
Gluteus minimus
Deep
Iliac crest
Iliac tuberculum
Tensor fasciae latae
Gluteal tuberosity
Fascia lata
Iliotibial tract
Patella
Anterolateral condyle of tibia
Lateral View

## TABLE 5.4 MUSCLES OF GLUTEAL REGION

| Muscle | Proximal Attachment[a] *(red)* | Distal Attachment[a] *(blue)* | Innervation[b] | Main Actions |
|---|---|---|---|---|
| Gluteus maximus | Ilium posterior to posterior gluteal line, dorsal surface of sacrum and coccyx, sacrotuberous ligament | Iliotibial tract that inserts into lateral condyle of tibia; some fibers to gluteal tuberosity | Inferior gluteal nerve (L5, **S1**, **S2**) | Extends thigh and assists in lateral rotation; steadies thigh and assists in raising trunk from flexed position |
| Gluteus medius | External surface of ilium between anterior and posterior gluteal lines; gluteal fascia | Lateral surface of greater trochanter of femur | Superior gluteal nerve (**L5,** S1) | Abducts and medially rotates thigh; keeps pelvis level when opposite leg is off ground and advances pelvis during swing phase of gait; TFL also contributes to stability of extended knee |
| Gluteus minimus | External surface of ilium between anterior and inferior gluteal lines | Anterior surface of greater trochanter of femur | | |
| Tensor fasciae latae (TFL) | Anterior superior iliac spine and iliac crest | Iliotibial tract that attaches to lateral condyle (Gerdy tubercle) of tibia | | |
| Piriformis | Anterior surface of sacrum and sacrotuberous ligament | Superior border of greater trochanter of femur | Anterior rami of S1 and S2 | Laterally rotate extended thigh and abduct flexed thigh; steady femoral head in acetabulum |
| Obturator internus | Pelvic surface of obturator membrane and surrounding bones | Medial surface of greater trochanter of femur by common tendons | Nerve to obturator internus (L5, S1) Nerve to quadratus femoris (L5, S1) | |
| Superior gemellus | Ischial spine | | | |
| Inferior gemellus | Ischial tuberosity | | | |
| Quadratus femoris | Lateral border of ischial tuberosity | Quadrate tubercle on intertrochanteric crest of femur | | Laterally rotates thigh,[c] steadies femoral head in acetabulum |

[a]See Figure 5.22 for muscle attachments.

[b]See Table 5.1 for explanation of segmental innervation.

[c]There are six lateral rotators of the thigh: piriformis, obturator internus, gemelli (superior and inferior), quadratus femoris, and obturator externus. These muscles also stabilize the hip joint.

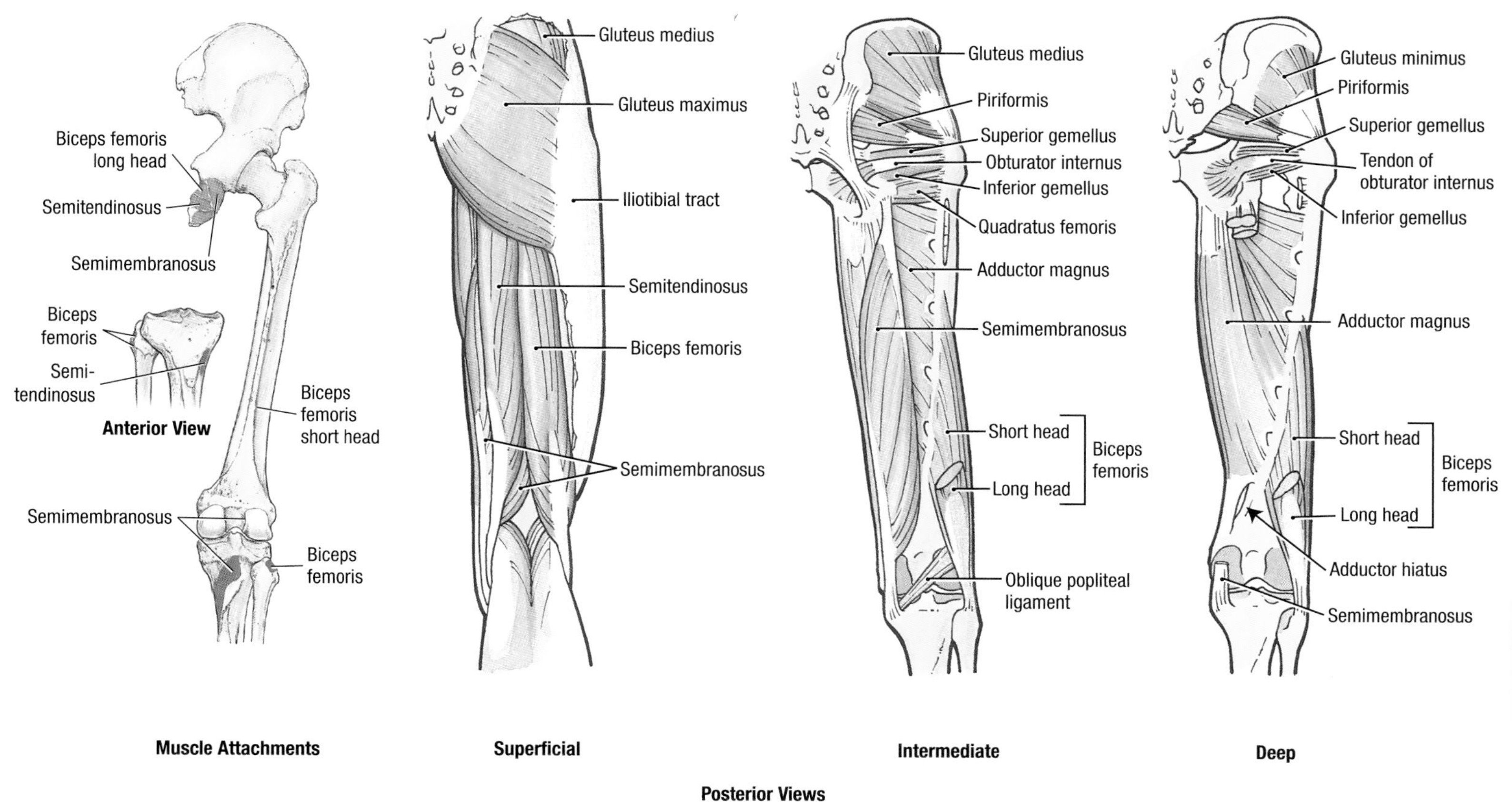
Biceps femoris long head
Semitendinosus
Semimembranosus
Biceps femoris
Semi-tendinosus
Anterior View
Biceps femoris short head
Semimembranosus
Biceps femoris
Gluteus medius
Gluteus maximus
Iliotibial tract
Semitendinosus
Biceps femoris
Semimembranosus
Gluteus medius
Piriformis
Superior gemellus
Obturator internus
Inferior gemellus
Quadratus femoris
Adductor magnus
Semimembranosus
Short head
Long head
Biceps femoris
Oblique popliteal ligament
Gluteus minimus
Piriformis
Superior gemellus
Tendon of obturator internus
Inferior gemellus
Adductor magnus
Short head
Long head
Biceps femoris
Adductor hiatus
Semimembranosus
Muscle Attachments
Superficial
Intermediate
Deep
Posterior Views

## TABLE 5.5 MUSCLES OF POSTERIOR THIGH (HAMSTRING)

| Muscle[a] | Proximal Attachment[a] *(red)* | Distal Attachment[a] *(blue)* | Innervation[b] | Main Actions |
|---|---|---|---|---|
| **Semitendinosus** | Ischial tuberosity | Medial surface of superior part of tibia | Tibial division of sciatic nerve (**L5**, **S1**, and S2) | Extend thigh; flex leg and rotate it medially; when thigh and leg are flexed, can extend trunk |
| **Semimembranosus** | | Posterior part of medial condyle of tibia; reflected attachment forms oblique popliteal ligament to lateral femoral condyle | | |
| **Biceps femoris** | *Long head:* ischial tuberosity; *Short head:* linea aspera and lateral supracondylar line of femur | Lateral side of head of fibula; tendon is split at this site by fibular collateral ligament of knee | *Long head:* tibial division of sciatic nerve (L5, **S1**, and S2); *Short head:* common fibular (peroneal) division of sciatic nerve (L5, **S1**, and S2) | Flexes leg and rotates it laterally; extends thigh (e.g., when initiating a walking gait) |

[a]See Figure 5.22 for muscle attachments.
[b]See Table 5.1 for explanation of segmental innervation.

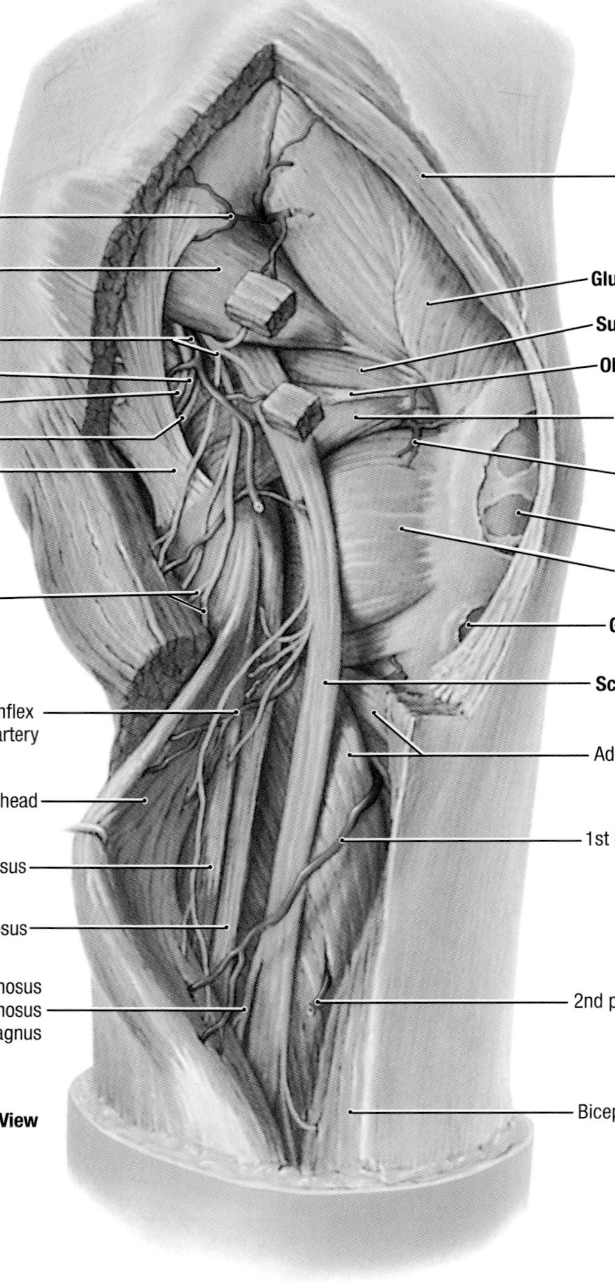

Superior gluteal artery
Piriformis
Inferior gluteal artery and nerve
Internal pudendal artery
Pudendal nerve
Nerve to obturator internus
Sacrotuberous ligament
Posterior cutaneous nerve of thigh
Branch of medial circumflex femoral artery
Biceps femoris, long head
Semitendinosus
Semimembranosus
Nerve to Semimembranosus, Semitendinosus, Adductor magnus
Gluteus maximus
Gluteus medius
Superior gemellus
Obturator internus
Inferior gemellus
Branch of medial circumflex femoral artery
Trochanteric bursa
Quadratus femoris
Gluteofemoral bursa
Sciatic nerve
Adductor magnus
1st perforating artery
2nd perforating artery
Biceps femoris, short head

**A. Posterior View**

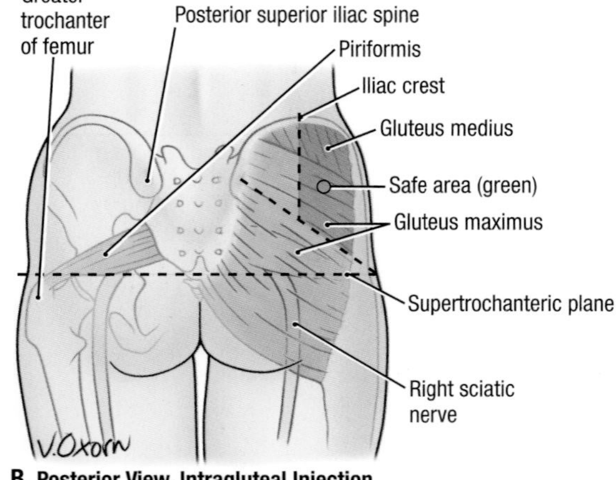

Greater trochanter of femur
Posterior superior iliac spine
Piriformis
Iliac crest
Gluteus medius
Safe area (green)
Gluteus maximus
Supertrochanteric plane
Right sciatic nerve
V.Oxorn


**B. Posterior View, Intragluteal Injection**

## 5.26 Muscles of gluteal region and posterior aspect of thigh—IV

**A.** Dissection. The gluteus maximus muscle is split superiorly and inferiorly, and the middle part is excised; two cubes remain to identify its nerve. The gluteus maximus is the only muscle to cover the greater trochanter; it is aponeurotic and has underlying bursae where it glides on the trochanter (trochanteric bursa) and the aponeurosis of the vastus lateralis muscle (gluteofemoral bursa). Diffuse deep pain in the lateral thigh region, especially during stair climbing or rising from a seated position, may be caused by trochanteric bursitis. This type of friction bursitis is characterized by point tenderness over the greater trochanter; however, the pain radiates along the iliotibial tract. **B.** Intragluteal injection. Injections can be made safely only into the superolateral part of the buttock, avoiding injury to the sciatic and gluteal nerves.

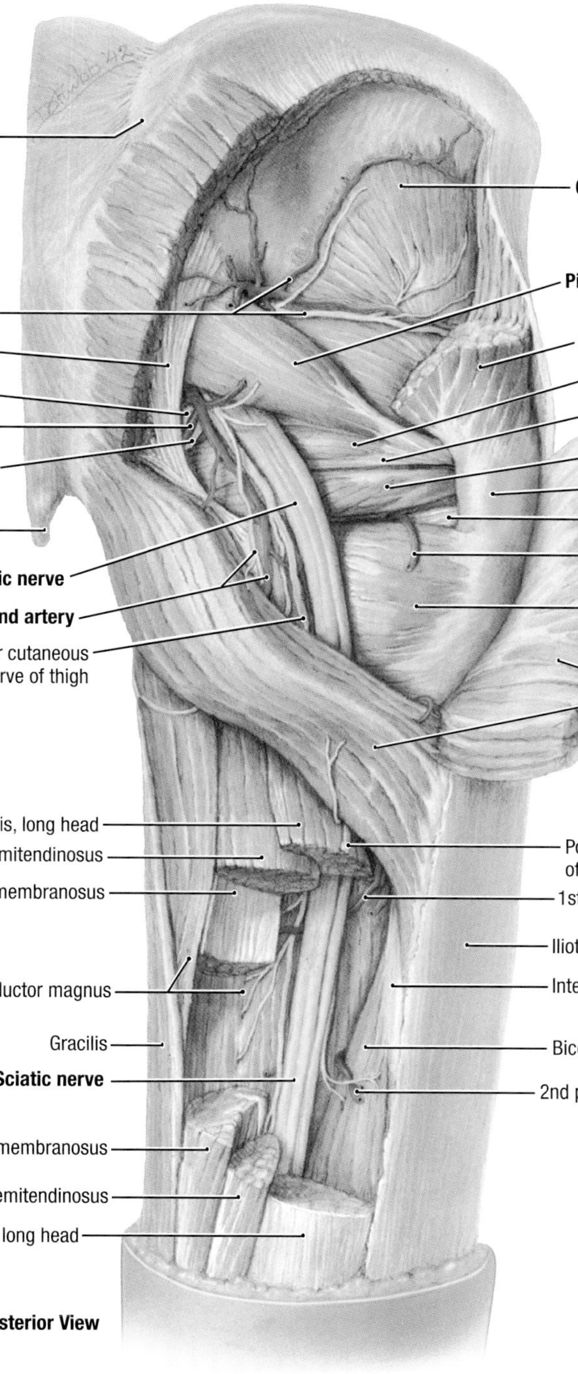

Posterior superior iliac spine
Gluteus minimus
Piriformis
Superior gluteal artery and nerve
Sacrotuberous ligament
Gluteus medius
Superior gemellus
Pudendal nerve
Obturator internus tendon
Internal pudendal artery
Inferior gemellus
Nerve to obturator internus
Greater trochanter
Tip of coccyx
Obturator externus tendon
Medial circumflex femoral artery
Sciatic nerve
Inferior gluteal nerve and artery
Quadratus femoris
Posterior cutaneous nerve of thigh
Gluteus maximus
Biceps femoris, long head
Semitendinosus
Posterior cutaneous nerve of thigh
Semimembranosus
1st perforating artery
Iliotibial tract
Adductor magnus
Intermuscular septum
Gracilis
Biceps femoris, short head
Sciatic nerve
2nd perforating artery
Semimembranosus
Semitendinosus
Biceps femoris, long head
A. Posterior View

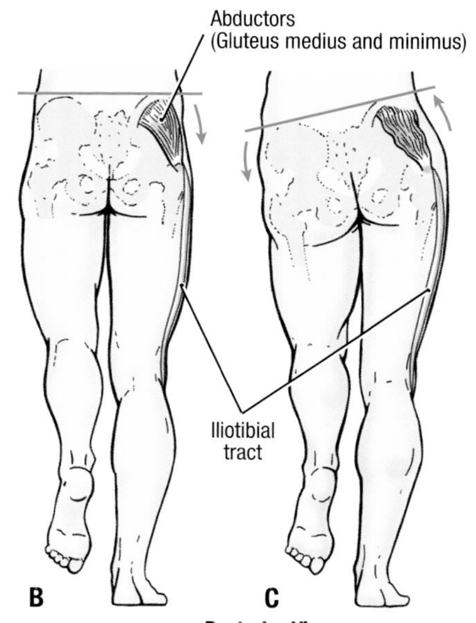
Abductors (Gluteus medius and minimus)
Iliotibial tract
B
C
Posterior Views

## 5.27 Muscles of gluteal region and posterior aspect of thigh—V

**A.** The proximal three quarters of the gluteus maximus muscle is reflected, and parts of the gluteus medius and the three hamstring muscles are excised. The superior gluteal vessels and nerves emerge superior to the piriformis muscle; all other vessels and nerves emerge inferior to it. **B.** When the weight is borne by one limb, the muscles on the supported side fix the pelvis so that it does not sag to the unsupported side, keeping the pelvis level. **C.** When the right abductors are paralyzed, owing to a lesion of the right superior gluteal nerve, fixation by these muscles is lost and the pelvis tilts to the unsupported left side (positive Trendelenburg sign).

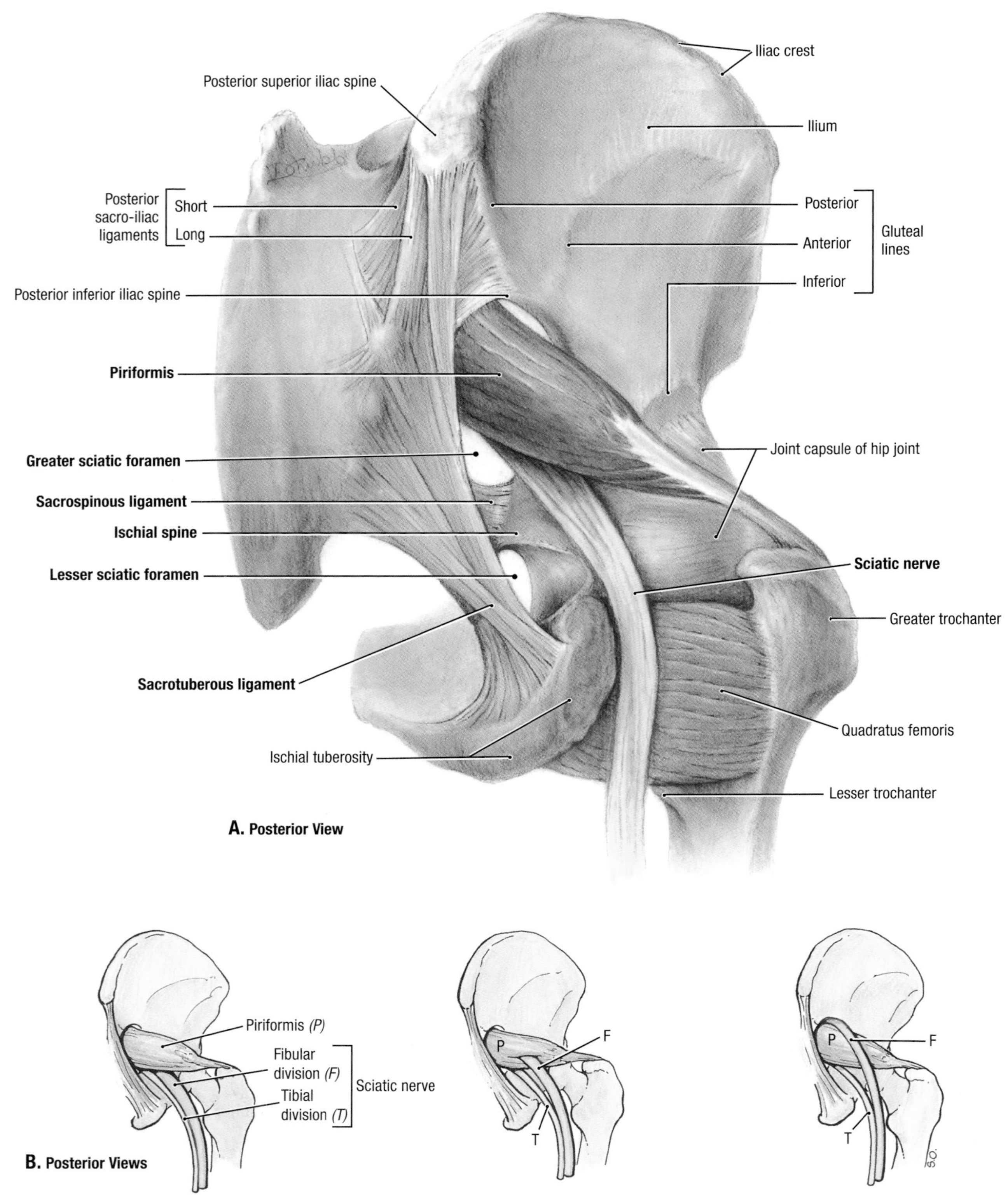
Iliac crest
Posterior superior iliac spine
Ilium
Posterior sacro-iliac ligaments
Short
Long
Posterior
Anterior
Inferior
Gluteal lines
Posterior inferior iliac spine
Piriformis
Greater sciatic foramen
Joint capsule of hip joint
Sacrospinous ligament
Ischial spine
Lesser sciatic foramen
Sciatic nerve
Greater trochanter
Sacrotuberous ligament
Quadratus femoris
Ischial tuberosity
Lesser trochanter
A. Posterior View
Piriformis (P)
Fibular division (F)
Tibial division (T)
Sciatic nerve
P
F
T
P
F
T
B. Posterior Views

## 5.28 Lateral rotators of hip, sciatic nerve, and ligaments of gluteal region

**A.** Piriformis and quadratus femoris. In the anatomical position the tip of the coccyx lies superior to the level of the ischial tuberosity and inferior to that of the ischial spine. The lateral border of the sciatic nerve lies midway between the lateral surface of the greater trochanter and the medial surface of the ischial tuberosity.

**B.** Relationship of sciatic nerve to piriformis muscle. Of 640 limbs studied in Dr. Grant's laboratory, in 87%, the tibial and fibular (peroneal) divisions passed inferior to the piriformis *(left);* in 12.2%, the fibular (peroneal) division passed through the piriformis *(center);* and in 0.5% the fibular (peroneal) division passed superior to the piriformis *(right)*.

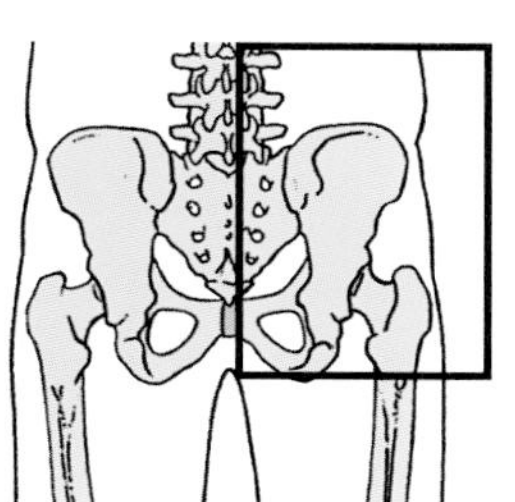

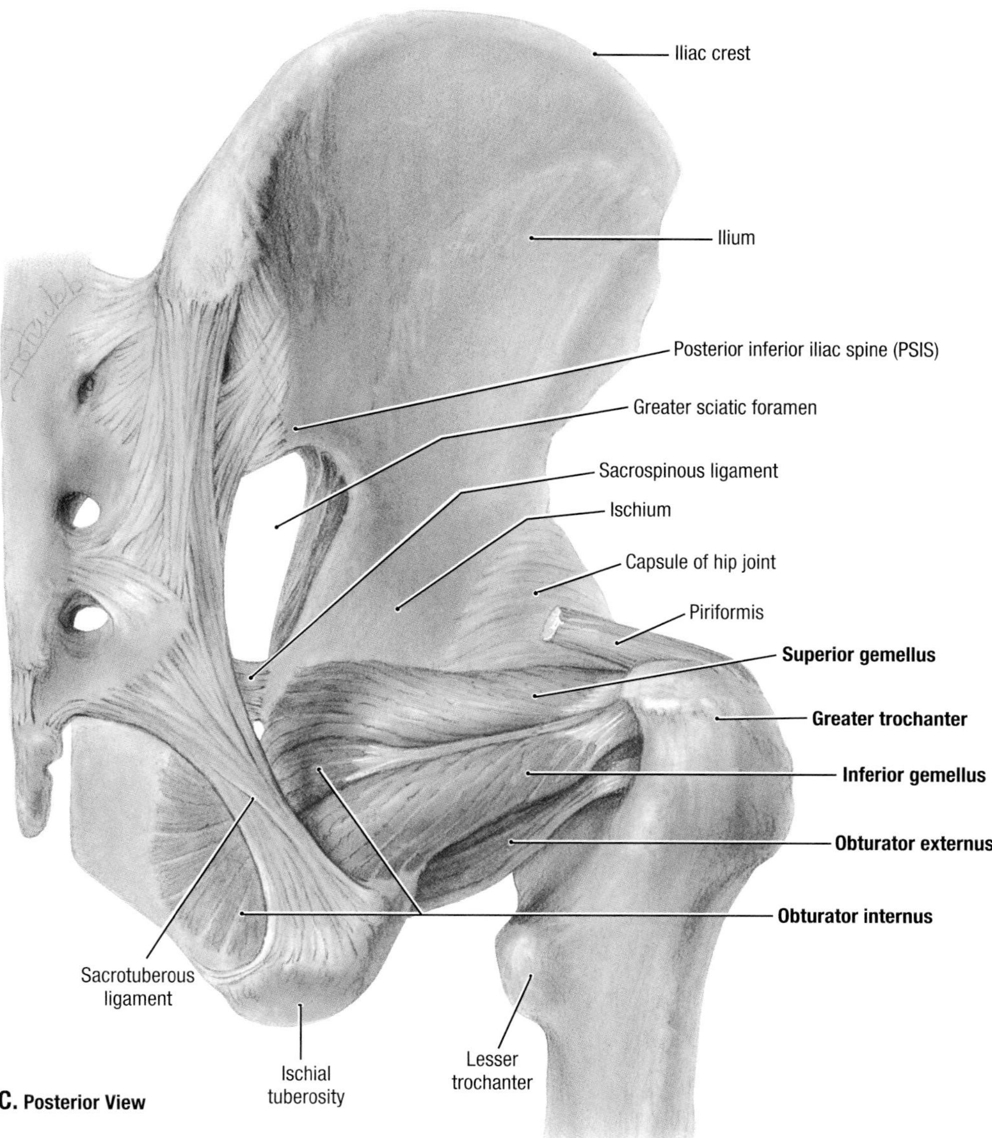
Iliac crest
Ilium
Posterior inferior iliac spine (PSIS)
Greater sciatic foramen
Sacrospinous ligament
Ischium
Capsule of hip joint
Piriformis
Superior gemellus
Greater trochanter
Inferior gemellus
Obturator externus
Obturator internus
Sacrotuberous ligament
Ischial tuberosity
Lesser trochanter

**C. Posterior View**

## 5.28 Lateral rotators of hip, sciatic nerve, and ligaments of gluteal region *(continued)*

**C.** Obturator internus, obturator externus, and superior and inferior gemelli.

- The obturator internus is located partly in the pelvis, where it covers most of the lateral wall of the lesser pelvis. It leaves the pelvis through the lesser sciatic foramen, makes a right-angle turn, becomes tendinous, and receives the distal attachments of the gemelli before attaching to the medial surface of the greater trochanter (trochanteric fossa).
- The obturator externus extends from the external surface of the obturator membrane and surrounding bone of the pelvis to the posterior aspect of the greater trochanter, passing directly under the acetabulum and neck of the femur.
- Sensation conveyed by the sciatic nerve can be blocked by injecting an anesthetic agent a few centimeters inferior to the midpoint of the line joining the PSIS and the superior border of the greater trochanter. Paresthesia radiates to the foot because of anesthesia of the plantar nerves, which are terminal branches of the tibial nerve derived from the sciatic nerve.
- In the approximately 12% of people in whom the common fibular division of the sciatic nerve passes through the piriformis, this muscle may compress the nerve.

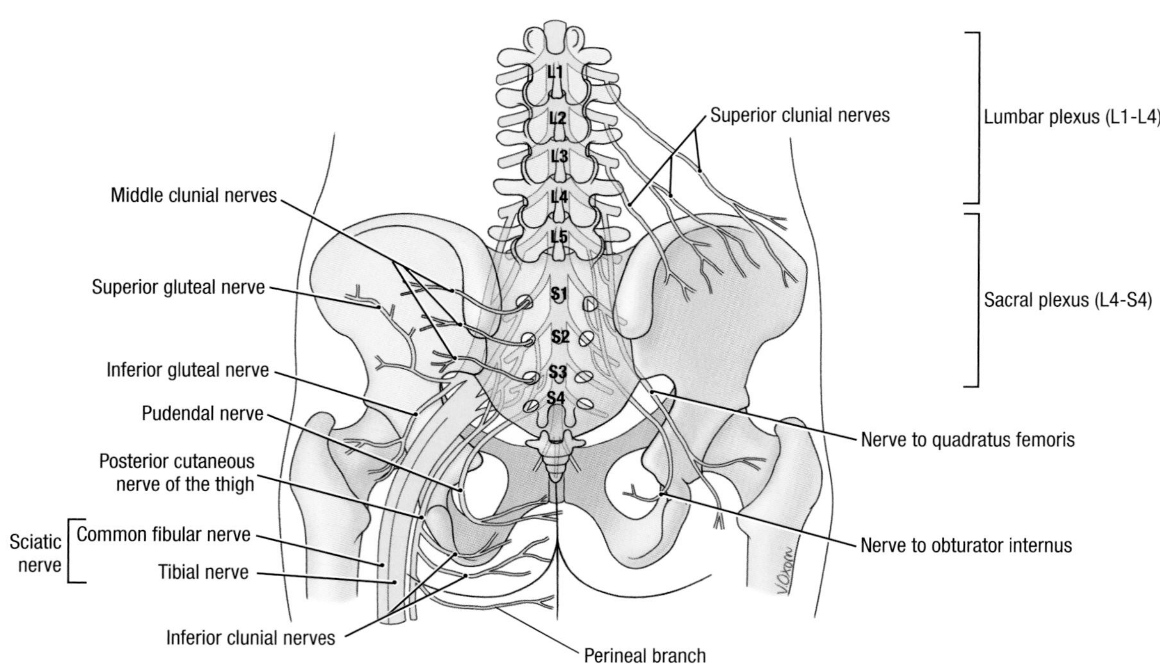
L1
L2
L3
L4
L5
S1
S2
S3
S4
Superior clunial nerves
Lumbar plexus (L1-L4)
Middle clunial nerves
Superior gluteal nerve
Sacral plexus (L4-S4)
Inferior gluteal nerve
Pudendal nerve
Nerve to quadratus femoris
Posterior cutaneous nerve of the thigh
Sciatic nerve
Common fibular nerve
Tibial nerve
Nerve to obturator internus
Inferior clunial nerves
Perineal branch

**TABLE 5.6 NERVES OF GLUTEAL REGION**

| Nerve | Origin | Course | Distribution in Gluteal Region |
|---|---|---|---|
| **Clunial (superior, middle, and inferior)** | *Superior:* posterior rami of L1–L3 nerves *Middle:* posterior rami of S1–S3 nerves *Inferior:* posterior cutaneous nerve of thigh | *Superior nerves* cross iliac crest; *middle nerves* exit through posterior sacral foramina and enter gluteal region; *inferior nerves* curve around inferior border of gluteal maximus | Gluteal region as far laterally as greater trochanter |
| **Sciatic** | Sacral plexus (L4–S3) | Exits pelvis via greater sciatic foramen inferior to piriformis to enter gluteal region | No muscles in gluteal region |
| **Posterior cutaneous nerve of thigh** | Sacral plexus (S1–S3) | Exits pelvis via greater sciatic foramen inferior to piriformis, emerges from inferior border of gluteus maximus coursing deept to fascia lata | Skin of buttock via inferior cluneal branches, skin over posterior thigh and popliteal fossa; skin of lateral perineum and upper medial thigh via perineal branch |
| **Superior gluteal** | Anterior rami of L4–S1 nerves | Exits pelvis via greater sciatic foramen superior to piriformis; courses between gluteus medius and minimus | Gluteus medius, gluteus minimus, and tensor fasciae latae |
| **Inferior gluteal** | Anterior rami of L5–S2 nerves | Exits pelvis via greater sciatic foramen inferior to piriformis, dividing into mutliple branches | Gluteus maximus |
| **Nerve to quadratus femoris** | Anterior rami of L4–S1 nerves | Exits pelvis via greater sciatic foramen deep to sciatic nerve | Posterior hip joint, inferior gemellus, and quadratus femoris |
| **Pudendal** | Anterior rami of S2–S4 nerves | Exits pelvis via greater sciatic foramen inferior to piriformis; descends posterior to sacrospinous ligament; enters perineum (pudenal canal) through lesser sciatic foramen | No structures in gluteal region (supplies most of perineum) |
| **Nerve to obturator internus** | Anterior rami of L5–S2 nerves | Exits pelvis via greater sciatic foramen inferior to piriformis; descends posterior to ischial spine; enters lesser sciatic foramen and passes to obturator internus | Superior gemellus and obturator internus |

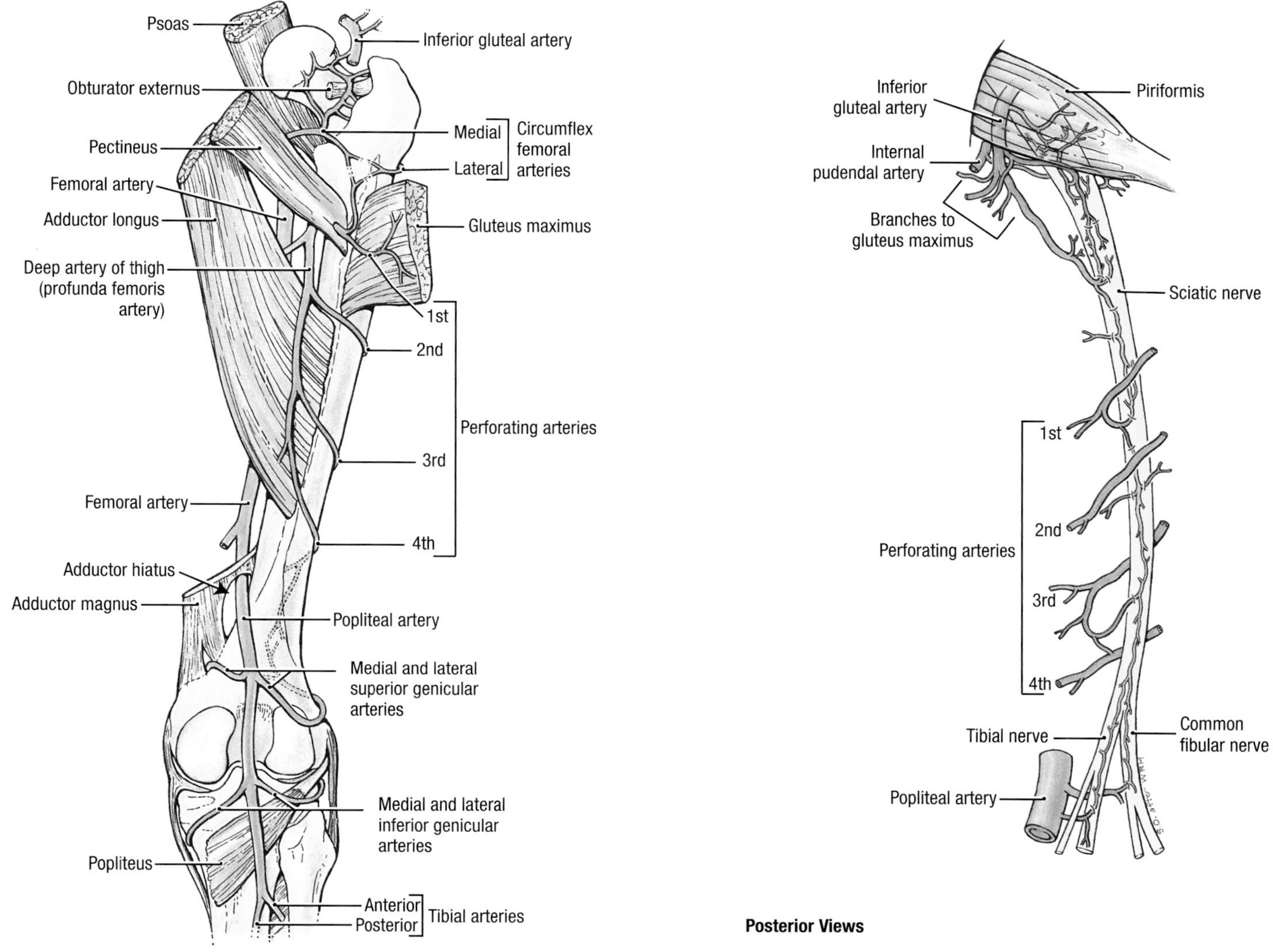
Psoas
Inferior gluteal artery
Obturator externus
Pectineus
Medial
Lateral
Circumflex femoral arteries
Femoral artery
Adductor longus
Gluteus maximus
Deep artery of thigh (profunda femoris artery)
1st
2nd
Perforating arteries
3rd
Femoral artery
4th
Adductor hiatus
Adductor magnus
Popliteal artery
Medial and lateral superior genicular arteries
Medial and lateral inferior genicular arteries
Popliteus
Anterior
Posterior
Tibial arteries
Inferior gluteal artery
Piriformis
Internal pudendal artery
Branches to gluteus maximus
Sciatic nerve
1st
2nd
Perforating arteries
3rd
4th
Tibial nerve
Common fibular nerve
Popliteal artery

Posterior Views

**TABLE 5.7 ARTERIES OF GLUTEAL REGION AND POSTERIOR THIGH**

| Artery | Course | Distribution/Structures Supplied |
|---|---|---|
| **Superior gluteal** | Enters gluteal region through greater sciatic foramen superior to piriformis; divides into superficial and deep branches; anastomoses with inferior gluteal and medial circumflex femoral arteries | *Superficial branch:* superior gluteus maximus<br>*Deep branch:* runs between gluteus medius and minimus, supplying both and tensor fasciae latae |
| **Inferior gluteal** | Enters gluteal region through greater sciatic foramen inferior to piriformis; descends on medial side of sciatic nerve; anastomoses with superior gluteal artery and participates in cruciate anastomosis of thigh | Inferior gluteus maximus, obturator internus, quadratus femoris, and superior parts of hamstring muscles |
| **Internal pudendal** | Enters gluteal region through greater sciatic foramen; descends posterior to ischial spine; exits gluteal region via lesser sciatic foramen to perineum | No structures in gluteal region (supplies external genitalia and muscles in perineal region) |
| **Perforating arteries (from deep femoral artery)** | Perforate aponeurotic portion of adductor magnus attachment and medial intermuscular septum to enter and supply muscular branches to posterior compartment; then pierce lateral intermuscular septum to enter posterolateral aspect of anterior compartment | Majority (central portions) of hamstring muscles in posterior compartment; posterior portion of vastus lateralis in anterior compartment; femur (via femoral nutrient arteries); reinforce arterial supply of sciatic nerve |

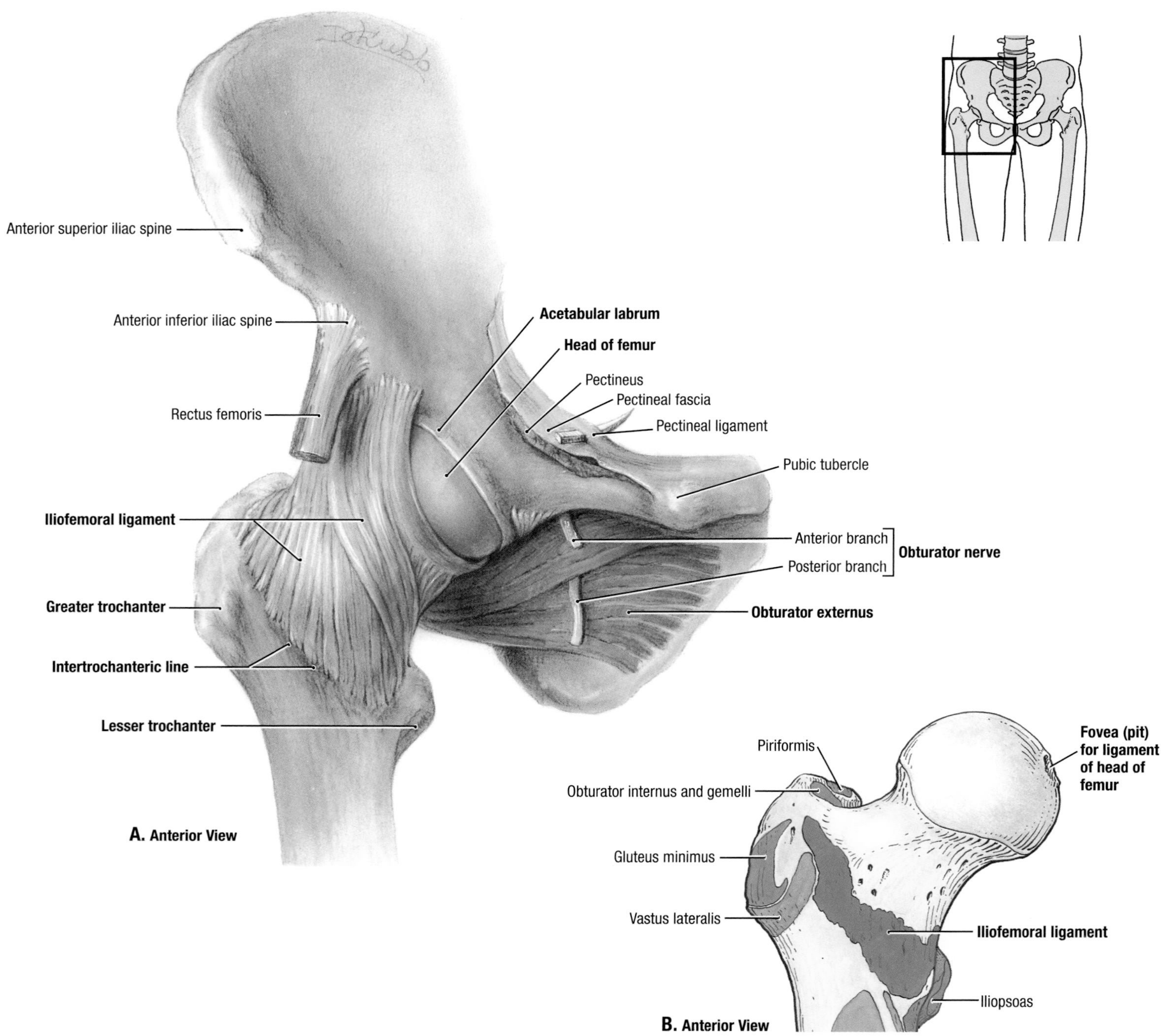
Anterior superior iliac spine
Anterior inferior iliac spine
Rectus femoris
Iliofemoral ligament
Greater trochanter
Intertrochanteric line
Lesser trochanter
A. Anterior View
Acetabular labrum
Head of femur
Pectineus
Pectineal fascia
Pectineal ligament
Pubic tubercle
Anterior branch
Posterior branch
Obturator nerve
Obturator externus
Piriformis
Obturator internus and gemelli
Gluteus minimus
Vastus lateralis
Fovea (pit) for ligament of head of femur
Iliofemoral ligament
Iliopsoas
B. Anterior View

## 5.29 Hip joint

**A.** Iliofemoral ligament. **B.** Muscle attachments of anterior aspect of the proximal femur.

In **A**:

- The head of the femur is exposed just medial to the iliofemoral ligament and faces superiorly, medially, and anteriorly. At the site of the subtendinous bursa of psoas, the capsule is weak or (as in this specimen) partially deficient, but it is guarded by the psoas tendon.
- The iliofemoral ligament, shaped like an inverted "Y." Superiorly it is attached deep to the rectus femoris muscle; the ligament becomes tight on medial rotation of the femur.
- The pectineus muscle is thin, and its fascia blends with the pectineal ligament.

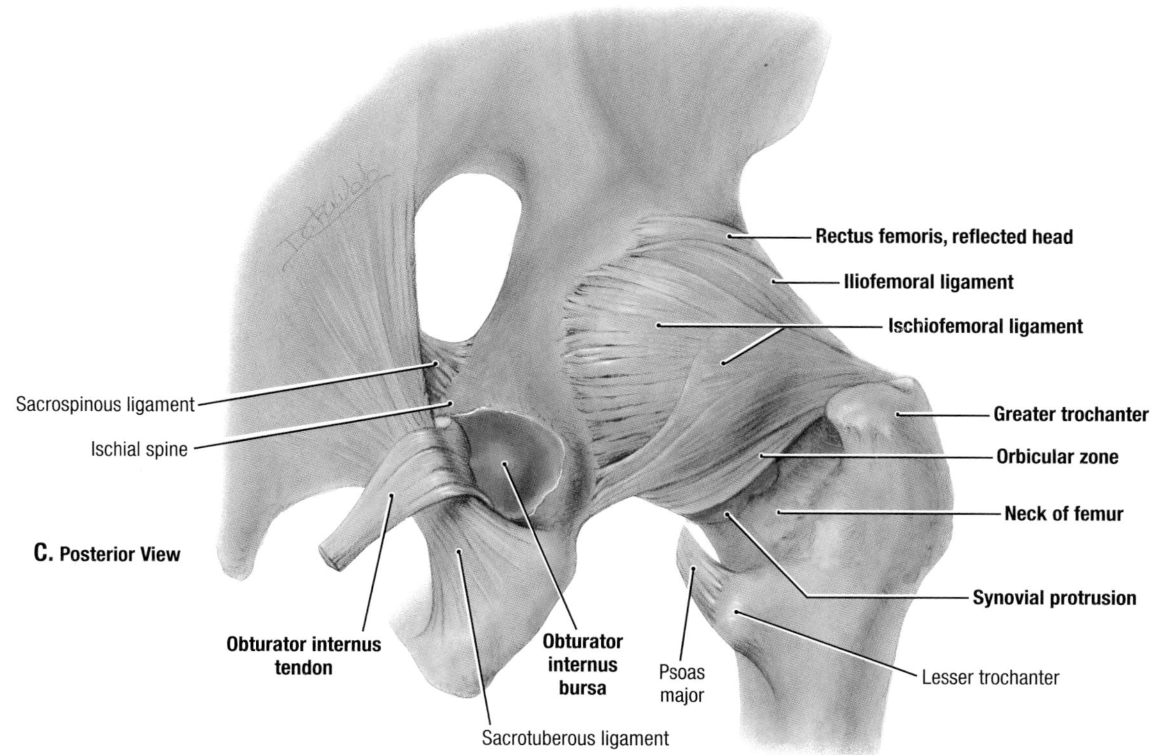
Rectus femoris, reflected head
Iliofemoral ligament
Ischiofemoral ligament
Sacrospinous ligament
Ischial spine
Greater trochanter
Orbicular zone
Neck of femur
C. Posterior View
Synovial protrusion
Obturator internus tendon
Obturator internus bursa
Psoas major
Lesser trochanter
Sacrotuberous ligament

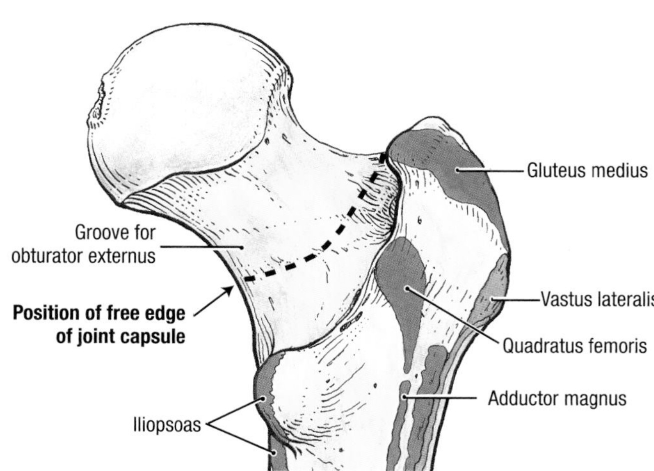
Gluteus medius
Groove for obturator externus
Vastus lateralis
Position of free edge of joint capsule
Quadratus femoris
Adductor magnus
Iliopsoas
D. Posterior View

## 5.29 Hip joint *(continued)*

**C.** Ischiofemoral ligament. **D.** Muscle attachments onto the posterior aspect of proximal femur. In **C**:

- The fibers of the capsule spiral to become taut during extension and medial rotation of the femur.
- The synovial membrane protrudes inferior to the fibrous capsule and forms a bursa for the tendon of the obturator externus muscle. Note the large subtendinous bursa of the obturator internus at the lesser sciatic notch, where the tendon turns 90° to attach to the greater trochanter.

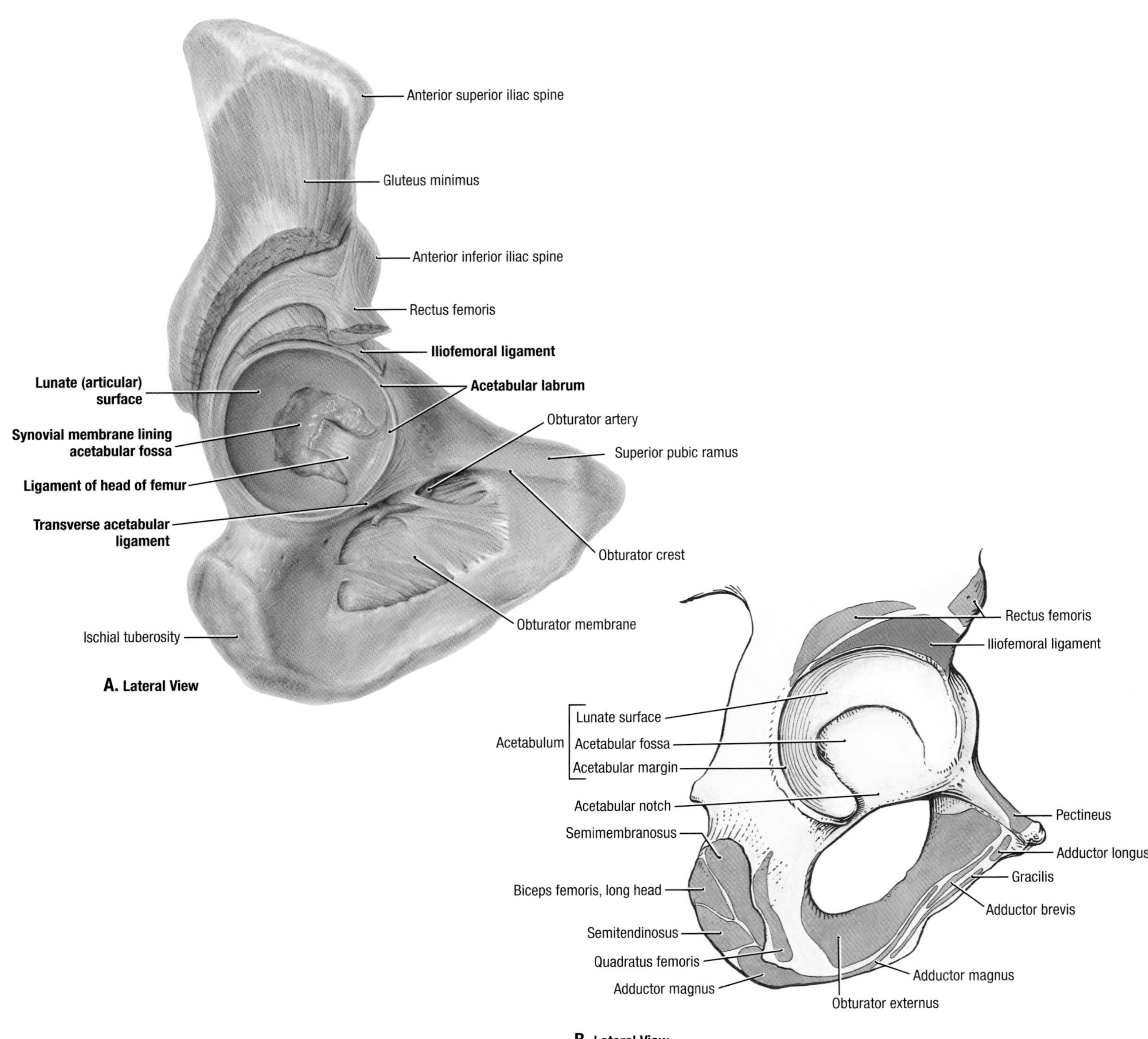
Anterior superior iliac spine
Gluteus minimus
Anterior inferior iliac spine
Rectus femoris
Iliofemoral ligament
Lunate (articular) surface
Acetabular labrum
Obturator artery
Synovial membrane lining acetabular fossa
Superior pubic ramus
Ligament of head of femur
Transverse acetabular ligament
Obturator crest
Obturator membrane
Ischial tuberosity
A. Lateral View
Rectus femoris
Iliofemoral ligament
Acetabulum
Lunate surface
Acetabular fossa
Acetabular margin
Acetabular notch
Pectineus
Semimembranosus
Adductor longus
Gracilis
Biceps femoris, long head
Adductor brevis
Semitendinosus
Quadratus femoris
Adductor magnus
Adductor magnus
Obturator externus
B. Lateral View

## 5.30 Acetabular region

**A.** Dissection of acetabulum. **B.** Muscle attachments of acetabular region.

In **A**:

- The transverse acetabular ligament bridges the acetabular notch.
- The acetabular labrum is attached to the acetabular rim and transverse acetabular ligament and forms a complete ring around the head of the femur.
- The ligament of the head of the femur lies between the head of the femur and the acetabulum. These fibers are attached superiorly to the pit (fovea) on the head of the femur and inferiorly to the transverse acetabular ligament and the margins of the acetabular notch. The artery of the ligament of the head of the femur passes through the acetabular notch and into the ligament of the head of the femur.

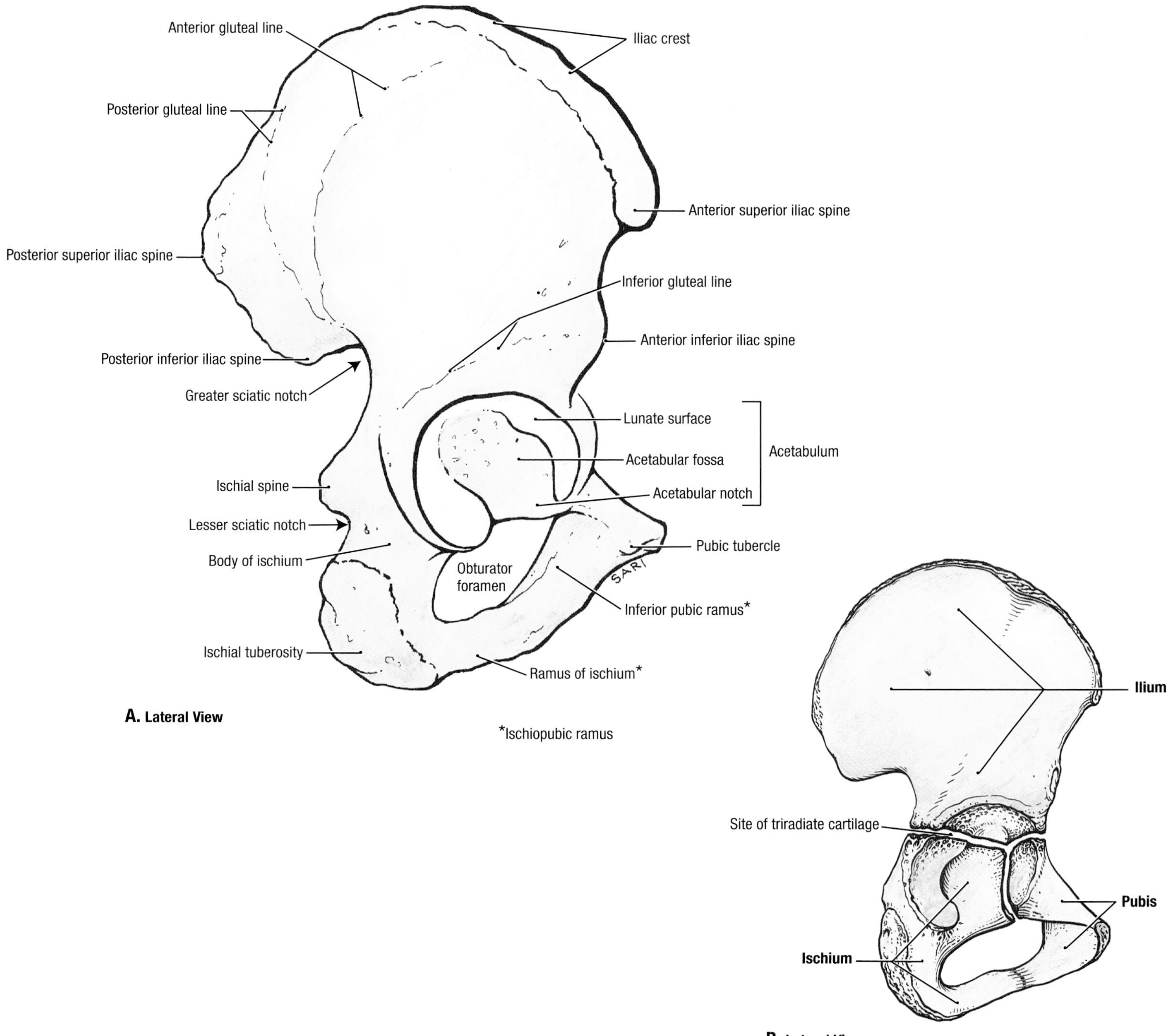
Anterior gluteal line
Iliac crest
Posterior gluteal line
Anterior superior iliac spine
Posterior superior iliac spine
Inferior gluteal line
Anterior inferior iliac spine
Posterior inferior iliac spine
Greater sciatic notch
Lunate surface
Acetabular fossa
Acetabulum
Acetabular notch
Ischial spine
Lesser sciatic notch
Pubic tubercle
Body of ischium
Obturator foramen
Inferior pubic ramus*
Ischial tuberosity
Ramus of ischium*
A. Lateral View
*Ischiopubic ramus
Ilium
Site of triradiate cartilage
Pubis
Ischium
B. Lateral View

## 5.31 Hip bone

**A.** Features of the lateral aspect. In the anatomical position, the anterior superior iliac spine and pubic tubercle are in the same coronal plane, and the ischial spine and superior end of the pubic symphysis are in the same horizontal plane; the internal aspect of the body of the pubis faces superiorly, and the acetabulum faces inferolaterally. **B.** Hip bone in youth. The three parts of the hip bone (ilium, ischium, and pubis) meet in the acetabulum at the triradiate synchondrosis. One or more primary centers of ossification appear in the triradiate cartilage at approximately the 12th year. Secondary centers of ossification appear along the length of the iliac crest, at the anterior inferior iliac spine, the ischial tuberosity, and the symphysis pubis at about puberty; fusion is usually complete by age 23.

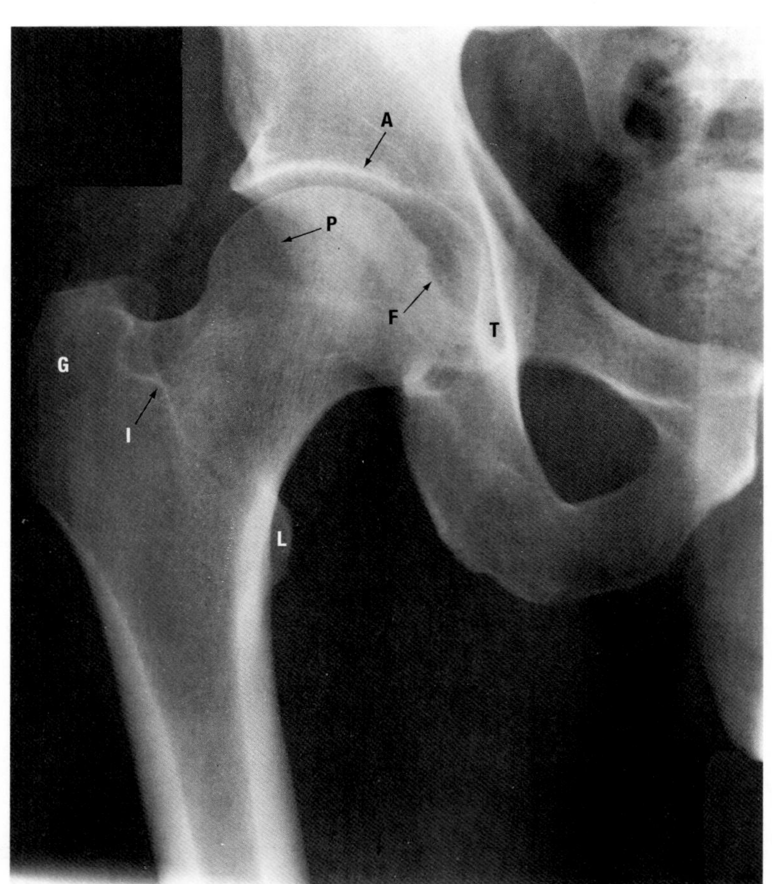
A
P
F
T
G
I
L

A. Anteroposterior View

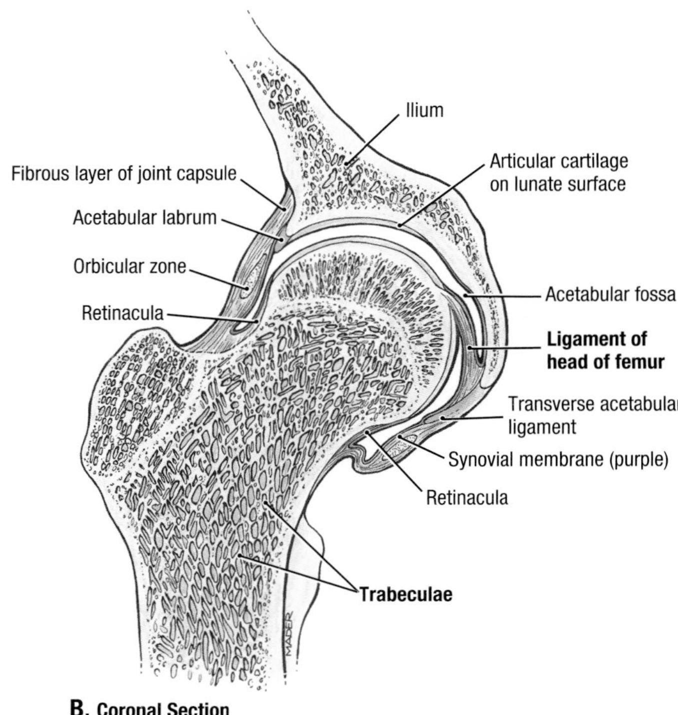
Ilium
Fibrous layer of joint capsule
Articular cartilage on lunate surface
Acetabular labrum
Orbicular zone
Acetabular fossa
Retinacula
Ligament of head of femur
Transverse acetabular ligament
Synovial membrane (purple)
Retinacula
Trabeculae
MADER

B. Coronal Section

## 5.32 Radiograph and coronal section of hip joint

**A.** Radiograph. On the femur, note the greater *(G)* and lesser *(L)* trochanters, the intertrochanteric crest *(I)*, and the pit or fovea *(F)* for the ligament of the head. On the pelvis, note the roof *(A)* and posterior rim *(P)* of the acetabulum and the "teardrop" appearance *(T)* caused by the superimposition of structures at the inferior margin of the acetabulum. **B.** Coronal section. Observe the bony trabeculae projecting into the head of the femur. The ligament of the head of the femur becomes taut during adduction of the hip joint, such as when crossing the legs. **C.** Hip replacement. The hip joint is subject to severe traumatic injury and degenerative disease. Osteoarthritis of the hip joint, characterized by pain, edema, limitation of motion, and erosion of articular cartilage, is a common cause of disability. During hip replacement, a metal prosthesis anchored to the person's femur by bone cement replaces the femoral head and neck. A plastic socket is cemented to the hip bone to replace the acetabulum. See Figure 5.34 blue box.

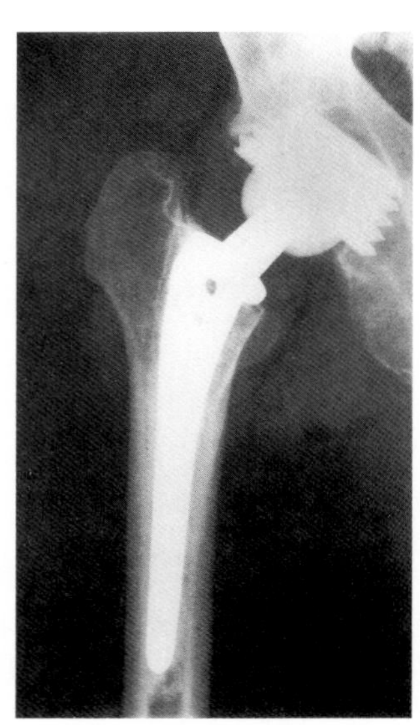

C. Hip Prosthesis

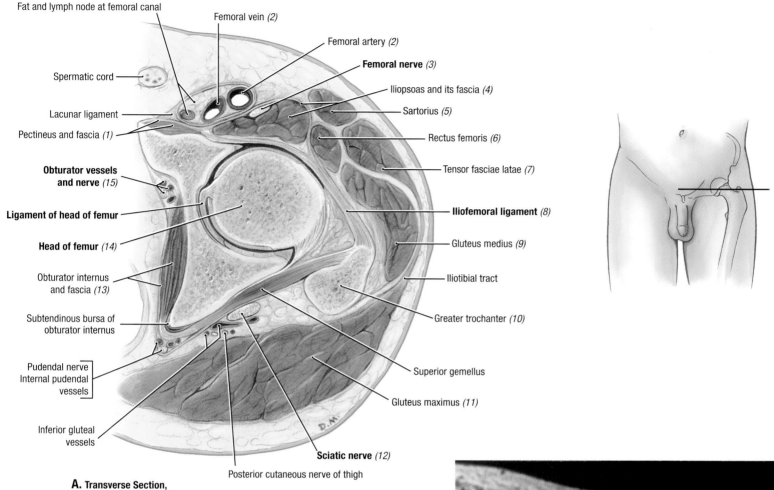

Fat and lymph node at femoral canal
Femoral vein *(2)*
Femoral artery *(2)*
**Femoral nerve** *(3)*
Spermatic cord
Iliopsoas and its fascia *(4)*
Lacunar ligament
Sartorius *(5)*
Pectineus and fascia *(1)*
Rectus femoris *(6)*
**Obturator vessels and nerve** *(15)*
Tensor fasciae latae *(7)*
**Ligament of head of femur**
**Iliofemoral ligament** *(8)*
**Head of femur** *(14)*
Gluteus medius *(9)*
Obturator internus and fascia *(13)*
Iliotibial tract
Subtendinous bursa of obturator internus
Greater trochanter *(10)*
Pudendal nerve
Internal pudendal vessels
Superior gemellus
Gluteus maximus *(11)*
Inferior gluteal vessels
**Sciatic nerve** *(12)*
Posterior cutaneous nerve of thigh

**A. Transverse Section, Inferior View**

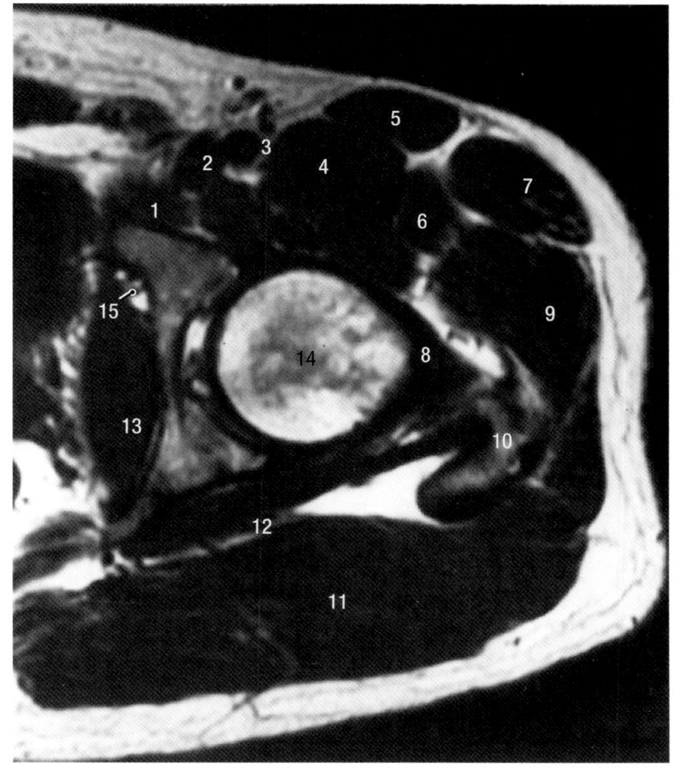
1
2
3
4
5
6
7
8
9
10
11
12
13
14
15

**B. Transverse MRI**

## 5.33 Transverse section through thigh at level of hip joint

**A.** Transverse section. **B.** MRI (*numbers* refer to structures in A).

In **A**:

- The fibrous capsule of the joint is thick where it forms the iliofemoral ligament and thin posterior to the subtendinous bursa of psoas and tendon.
- The femoral sheath, enclosing the femoral artery, vein, lymph node, lymph vessels, and fat, is free, except posteriorly where, between the psoas and pectineus muscles, it is attached to the capsule of the hip joint.
- The femoral vein is located at the interval between the psoas and pectineus muscles. The femoral nerve lies between the iliacus muscle and fascia.

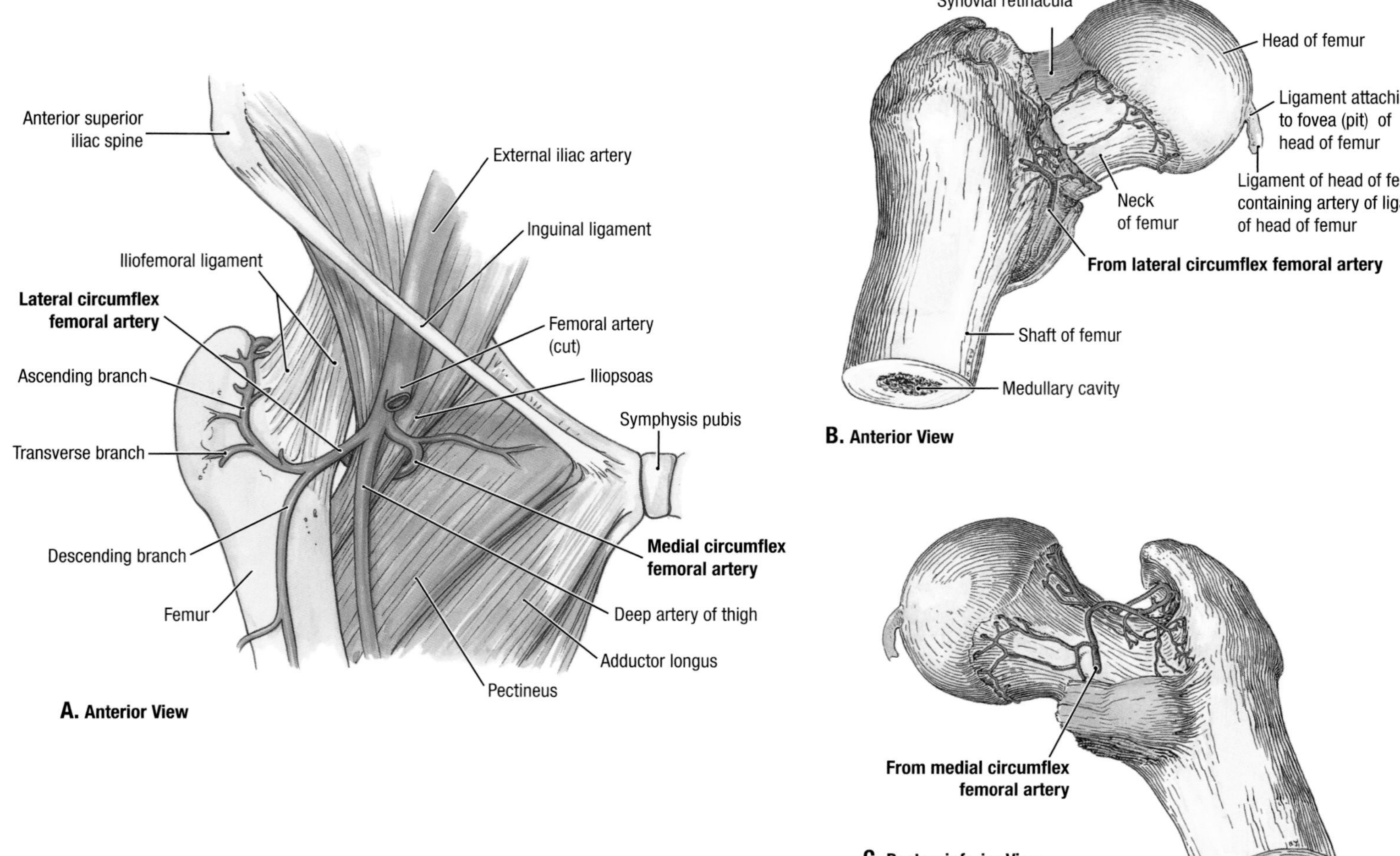
Anterior superior iliac spine
External iliac artery
Inguinal ligament
Iliofemoral ligament
Lateral circumflex femoral artery
Femoral artery (cut)
Ascending branch
Iliopsoas
Symphysis pubis
Transverse branch
Medial circumflex femoral artery
Descending branch
Deep artery of thigh
Femur
Adductor longus
Pectineus
A. Anterior View
Synovial retinacula
Head of femur
Ligament attaching to fovea (pit) of head of femur
Ligament of head of femur containing artery of ligament of head of femur
Neck of femur
From lateral circumflex femoral artery
Shaft of femur
Medullary cavity
B. Anterior View
From medial circumflex femoral artery
C. Posteroinferior View

## 5.34 Blood supply to head of femur

**A.** Medial and lateral circumflex femoral arteries in femoral triangle. **B.** Branches of lateral circumflex femoral artery. **C.** Branches of medial circumflex femoral artery.

- Branches of the medial and lateral circumflex femoral arteries ascend on the posterosuperior and posteroinferior parts of the neck of the femur. The vessels ascend in synovial retinacula—reflections of synovial membrane along the neck of the femur. The retinacula (in **B** and **C**) have been mostly removed; thus, the vessels can be clearly visualized.
- The branches of the medial and lateral circumflex femoral arteries perforate the bone just distal to the head of the femur, where they anastomose with branches from the artery of the ligament of the head of the femur and with medullary branches located within the shaft of the femur.
- The ligament of the head of the femur usually contains the artery of the ligament of the head of the femur, a branch of the obturator artery. The artery enters the head of the femur only when the center of the ossification has extended to the pit (fovea) for the ligament of the head (12th to 14th year). When present, this anastomosis persists even in advanced age; however, in 20% of persons, it is never established.

Fractures of the femoral neck often disrupt the blood supply to the head of the femur. The medial circumflex femoral artery supplies most of the blood to the head and neck of the femur and is often torn when the femoral neck is fractured. In some cases, the blood supplied by the artery of the ligament of the head may be the only blood received by the proximal fragment of the femoral head, which may be inadequate. If the blood vessels are ruptured, the fragment of bone may receive no blood and undergo aseptic necrosis.

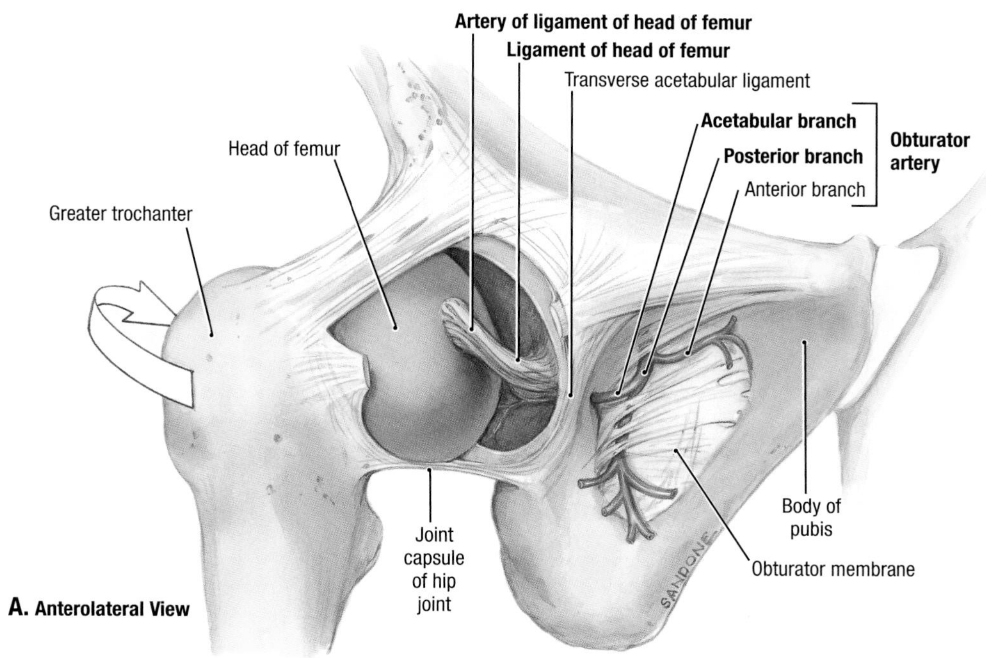
Artery of ligament of head of femur
Ligament of head of femur
Transverse acetabular ligament
Acetabular branch
Posterior branch
Anterior branch
Obturator artery
Head of femur
Greater trochanter
Joint capsule of hip joint
Body of pubis
Obturator membrane
A. Anterolateral View

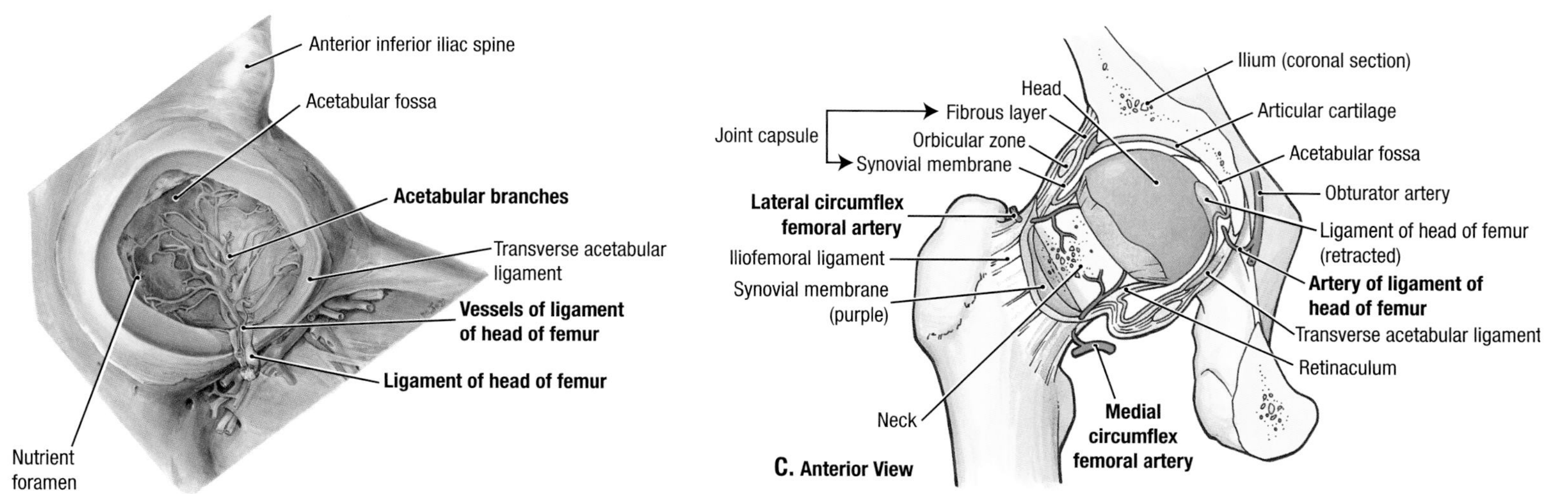
Anterior inferior iliac spine
Acetabular fossa
Acetabular branches
Transverse acetabular ligament
Vessels of ligament of head of femur
Ligament of head of femur
Nutrient foramen
B. Lateral View
Ilium (coronal section)
Head
Fibrous layer
Joint capsule
Orbicular zone
Synovial membrane
Articular cartilage
Acetabular fossa
Obturator artery
Lateral circumflex femoral artery
Iliofemoral ligament
Synovial membrane (purple)
Ligament of head of femur (retracted)
Artery of ligament of head of femur
Transverse acetabular ligament
Retinaculum
Neck
Medial circumflex femoral artery
C. Anterior View

## 5.35 Blood vessels of acetabular fossa and ligament of head of femur

**A.** Obturator artery. The hip joint has been dislocated to reveal the ligament of the head of the femur. The obturator artery divides into anterior and posterior branches, and the acetabular branch arises from the posterior branch. The artery of the ligament of the head of the femur is a branch of the acetabular artery and can be seen traveling in the ligament to the head of the femur. **B.** Acetabular artery and vein. The acetabular branches (artery and vein) pass through the acetabular foramen and enter the acetabular fossa, where they diverge in the fatty areolar tissue. The branches radiate to the margin of the fossa, where they enter nutrient foramina. **C.** Blood supply of the head and neck of the femur. A section of bone has been removed from the femoral neck.

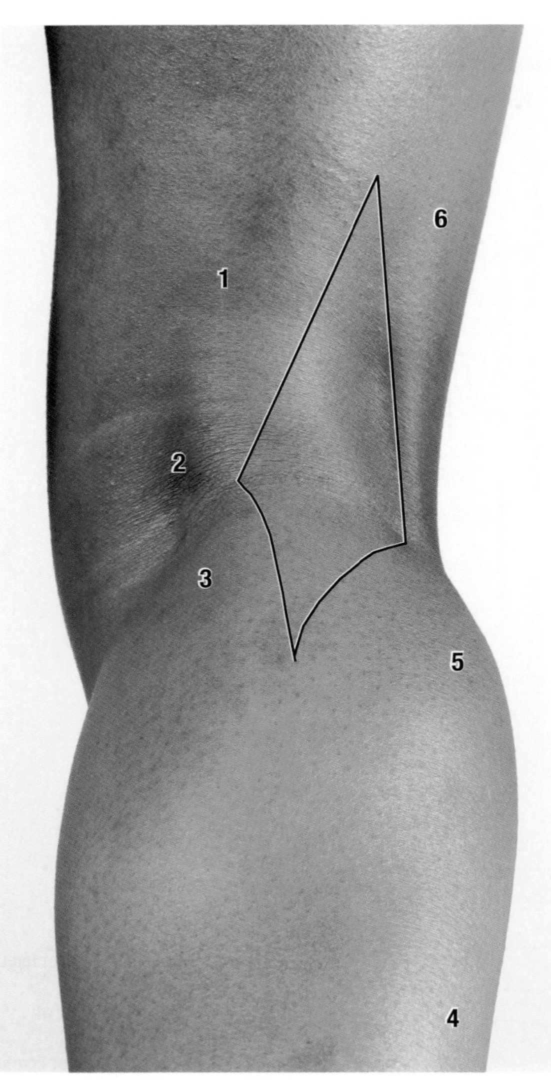
6
1
2
3
5
4

A. Posterior View

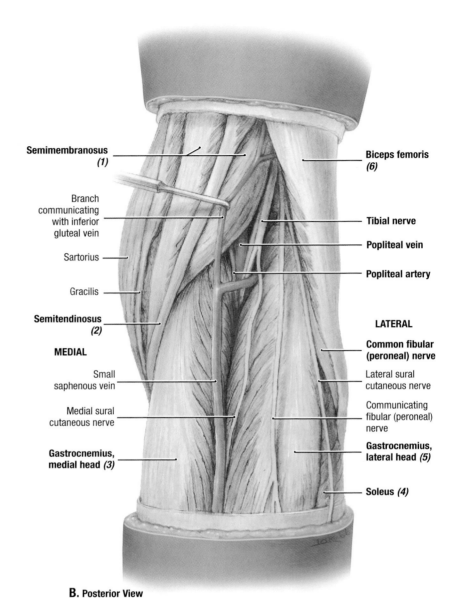

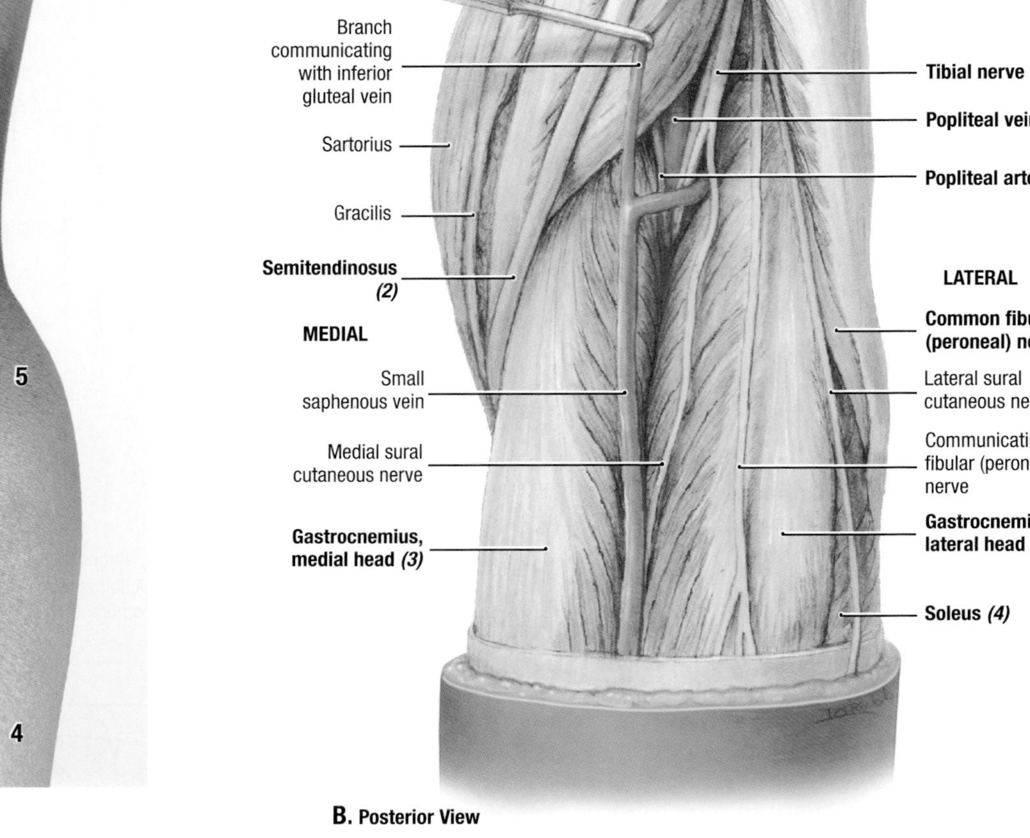
Semimembranosus (1)
Branch communicating with inferior gluteal vein
Sartorius
Gracilis
Semitendinosus (2)
MEDIAL
Small saphenous vein
Medial sural cutaneous nerve
Gastrocnemius, medial head (3)
Biceps femoris (6)
Tibial nerve
Popliteal vein
Popliteal artery
LATERAL
Common fibular (peroneal) nerve
Lateral sural cutaneous nerve
Communicating fibular (peroneal) nerve
Gastrocnemius, lateral head (5)
Soleus (4)

B. Posterior View

## 5.36 Popliteal fossa

**A.** Surface anatomy (*numbers* refer to structures in B). **B.** Superficial dissection.

- The two heads of the gastrocnemius muscle are embraced on the medial side by the semimembranosus muscle, which is overlaid by the semitendinosus muscle, and on the lateral side by the biceps femoris muscle.
- The small saphenous vein runs between the two heads of the gastrocnemius muscle. Deep to this vein is the medial sural cutaneous nerve, which, followed proximally, leads to the tibial nerve. The tibial nerve is superficial to the popliteal vein, which, in turn, is superficial to the popliteal artery.

Because the popliteal artery is deep in the popliteal fossa, it may be difficult to feel the popliteal pulse. Palpation of this pulse is commonly performed by placing the person in the prone position with the knee flexed to relax the popliteal fascia and hamstrings. The pulsations are best felt in the inferior part of the fossa. Weakening or loss of the popliteal pulse is a sign of femoral artery obstruction.

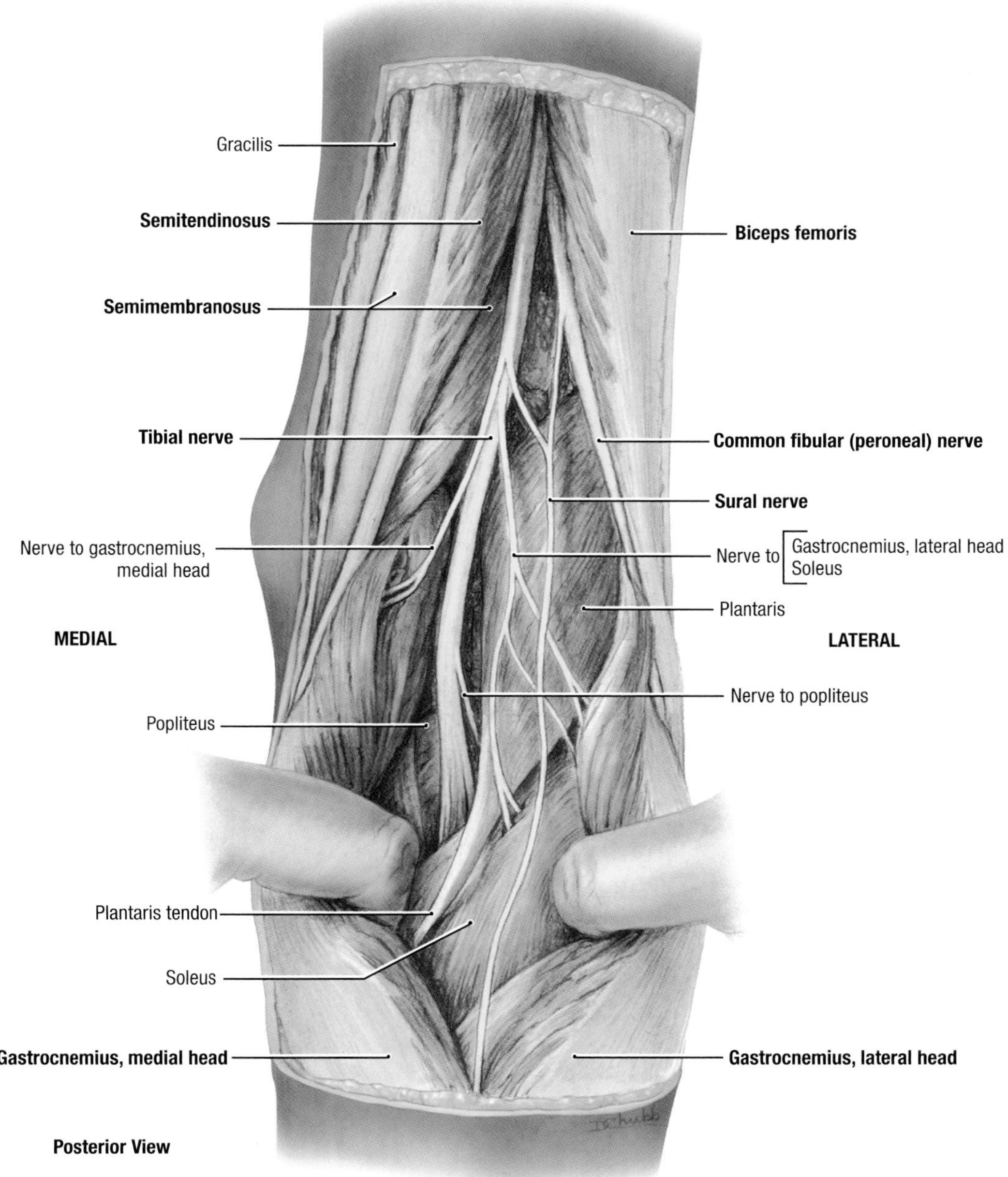
Gracilis
Semitendinosus
Semimembranosus
Tibial nerve
Nerve to gastrocnemius, medial head
MEDIAL
Popliteus
Plantaris tendon
Soleus
Gastrocnemius, medial head
Posterior View
Biceps femoris
Common fibular (peroneal) nerve
Sural nerve
Nerve to Gastrocnemius, lateral head
Soleus
Plantaris
LATERAL
Nerve to popliteus
Gastrocnemius, lateral head

## 5.37 Nerves of popliteal fossa

The two heads of the gastrocnemius muscle are separated.

- A cutaneous branch of the tibial nerve joins a cutaneous branch of the common fibular (peroneal) nerve to form the sural nerve. In this specimen, the junction is high; usually it is 5 to 8 cm proximal to the ankle.

All motor branches in this region emerge from the tibial nerve, one branch from its medial side and the others from its lateral side; hence, it is safer to dissect on the medial side.

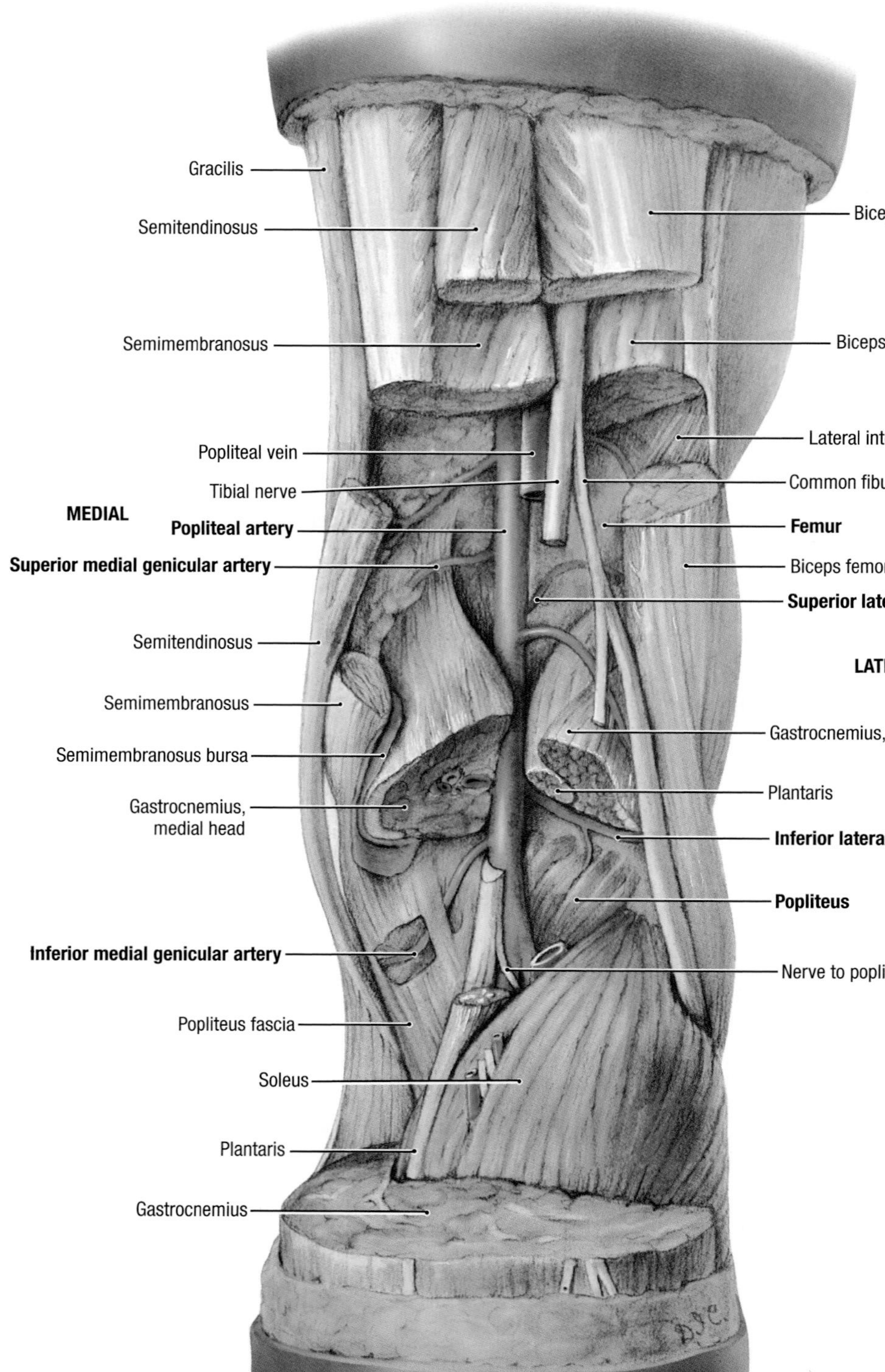
Gracilis
Semitendinosus
Semimembranosus
Popliteal vein
Tibial nerve
MEDIAL
Popliteal artery
Superior medial genicular artery
Semitendinosus
Semimembranosus
Semimembranosus bursa
Gastrocnemius, medial head
Inferior medial genicular artery
Popliteus fascia
Soleus
Plantaris
Gastrocnemius
Posterior View
Biceps femoris, long head
Biceps femoris, short head
Lateral intermuscular septum
Common fibular (peroneal) nerve
Femur
Biceps femoris
Superior lateral genicular artery
LATERAL
Gastrocnemius, lateral head
Plantaris
Inferior lateral genicular artery
Popliteus
Nerve to popliteus

## 5.38 Deep dissection of popliteal fossa

The common fibular (peroneal) nerve follows the posterior border of the biceps femoris muscle and, in this specimen, gives off two cutaneous branches. The popliteal artery lies on the floor of the popliteal fossa. The floor is formed by the femur, capsule of the knee joint, and popliteus muscle and fascia. The popliteal artery gives off genicular branches that also lie on the floor of the fossa. A popliteal aneurysm (abnormal dilation of all or part of the popliteal artery) usually causes edema (swelling) and pain in the popliteal fossa. If the femoral artery has to be ligated, blood can bypass the occlusion through the genicular anastomosis and reach the popliteal artery distal to the ligation.

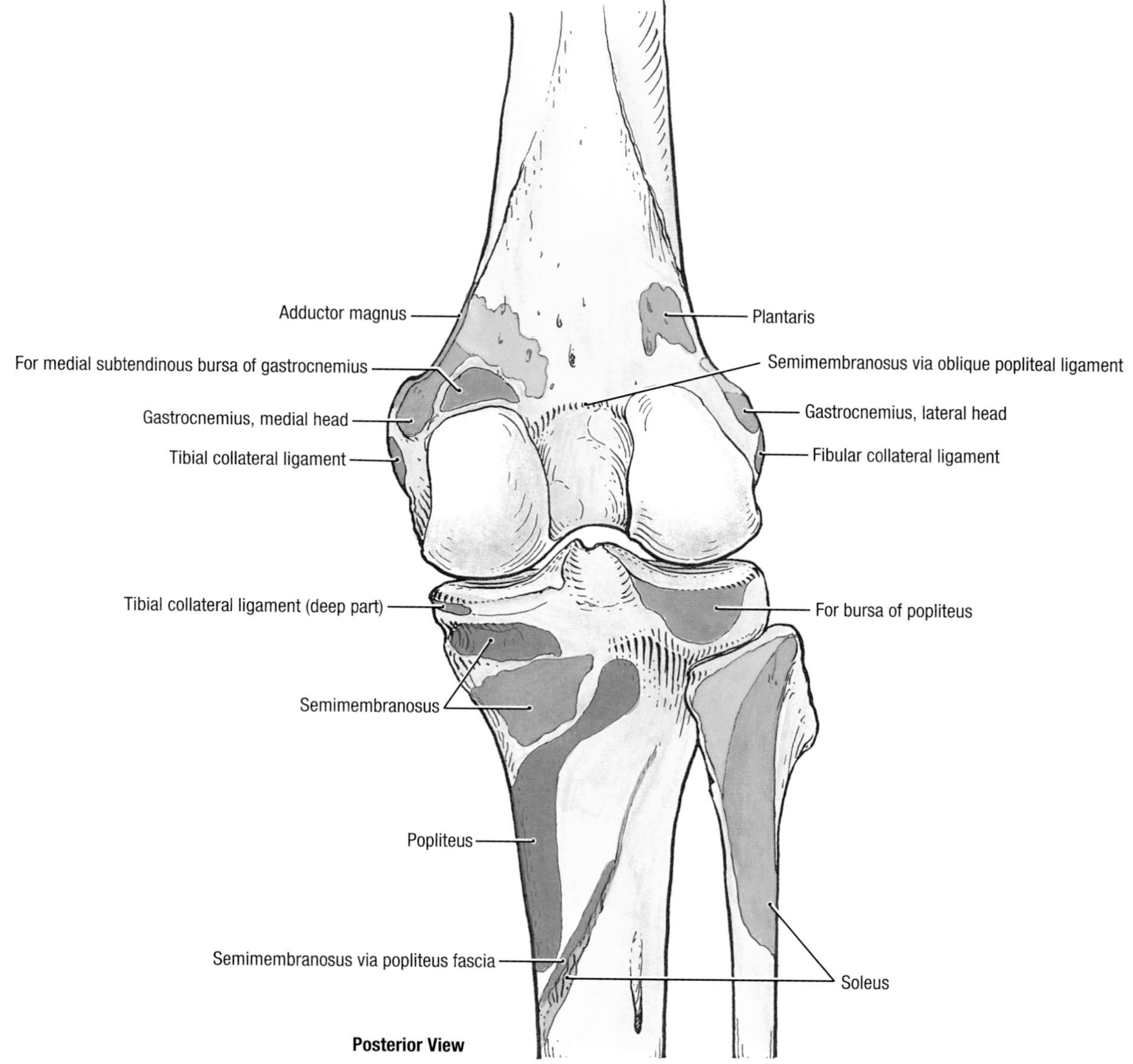
Adductor magnus
Plantaris
For medial subtendinous bursa of gastrocnemius
Semimembranosus via oblique popliteal ligament
Gastrocnemius, medial head
Gastrocnemius, lateral head
Tibial collateral ligament
Fibular collateral ligament
Tibial collateral ligament (deep part)
For bursa of popliteus
Semimembranosus
Popliteus
Semimembranosus via popliteus fascia
Soleus
Posterior View

**5.39 Attachment of muscles of popliteal region**

Lighter tones are secondary attachments.

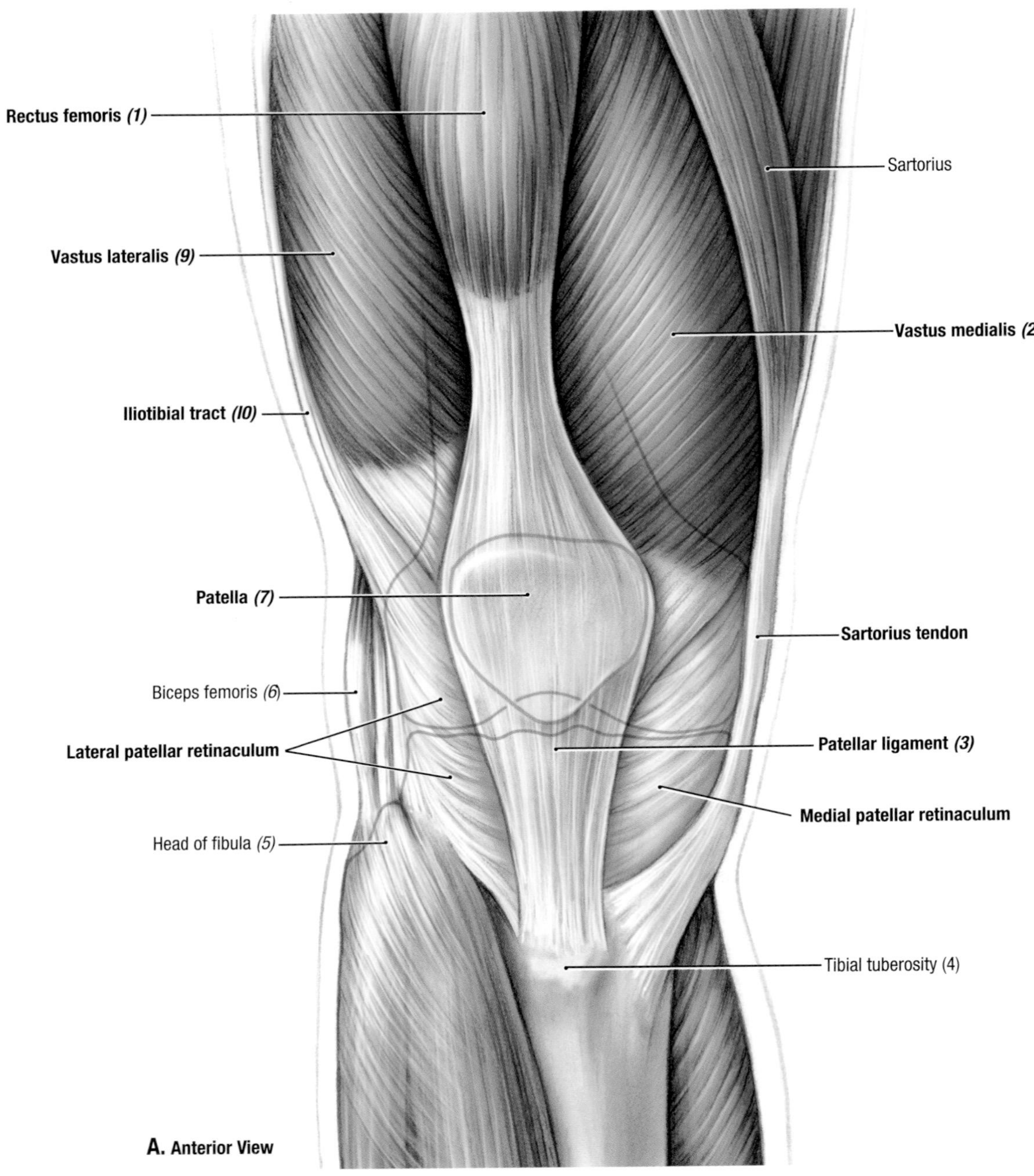
Rectus femoris (1)
Sartorius
Vastus lateralis (9)
Vastus medialis (2)
Iliotibial tract (10)
Patella (7)
Sartorius tendon
Biceps femoris (6)
Lateral patellar retinaculum
Patellar ligament (3)
Medial patellar retinaculum
Head of fibula (5)
Tibial tuberosity (4)
A. Anterior View

## 5.40 Anterior aspect of knee

**A.** Distal thigh and knee regions.

Note that the tendons of the four parts of the quadriceps unite to form the quadriceps tendon, a broad band that attaches to the patella. The patellar ligament, a continuation of the quadriceps tendon, attaches the patella to the tibial tuberosity. The lateral and medial patellar retinacula, formed largely by continuation of the iliotibial tract, and investing fascia of the vasti muscles, maintains alignment of the patella and patellar ligament. The retinacula also form the anterolateral and anteromedial portions of the fibrous layer of the joint capsule of the knee.

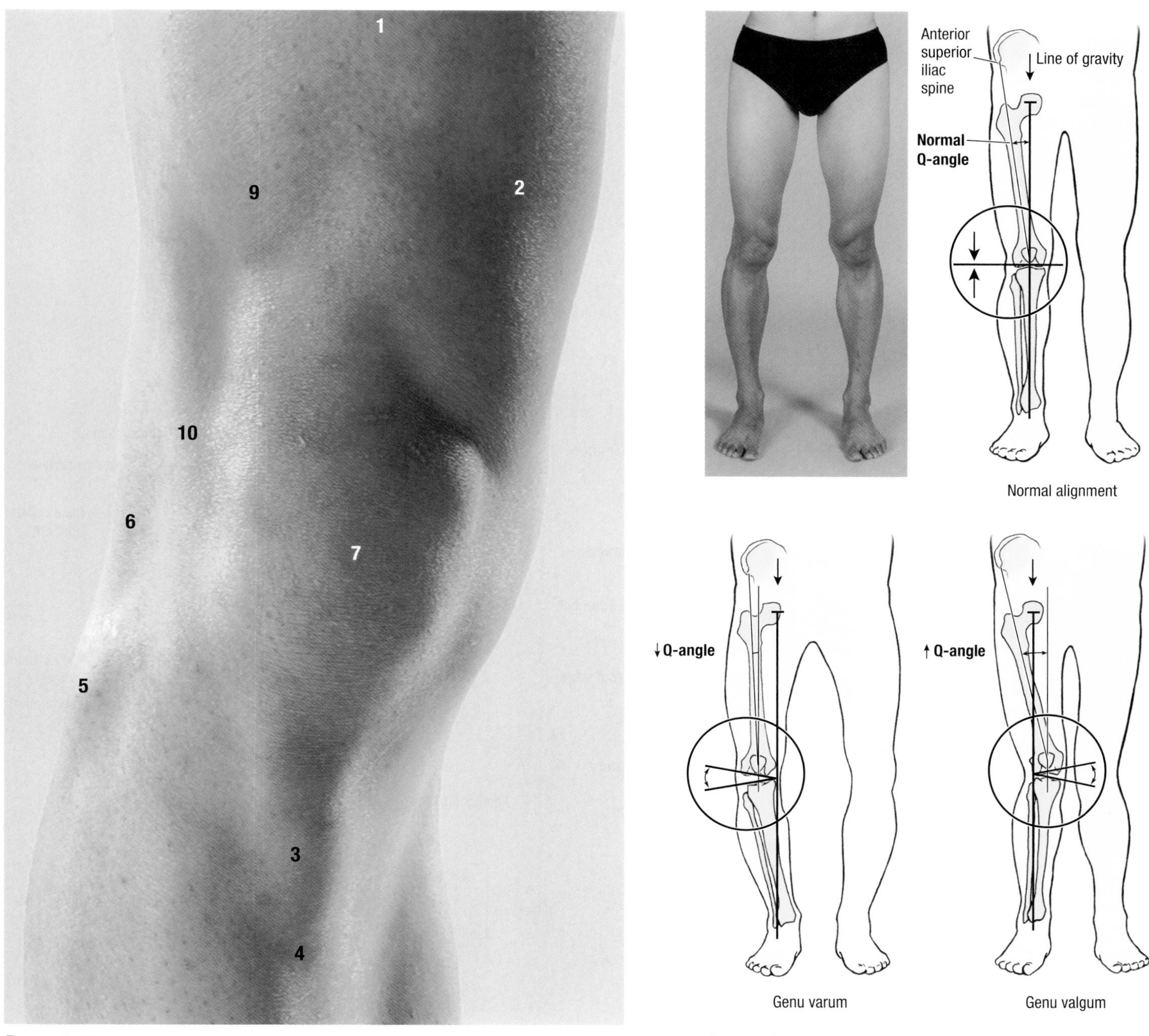
1
2
9
10
6
7
5
3
4
Anterior superior iliac spine
Line of gravity
Normal Q-angle
Normal alignment
↓Q-angle
↑Q-angle
Genu varum
Genu valgum

**B.** Anterior Views

**C.** Anterior Views

## 5.40 Anterior aspect of knee *(continued)*

**B.** Surface anatomy (numbers refer to structures in **A**). The femur is placed diagonally within the thigh, whereas the tibia is almost vertical within the leg, creating an angle at the knee between the long axes of the bones. The angle between the two bones, referred to clinically as the Q-angle, is assessed by drawing a line from the anterior superior iliac spine to the middle of the patella and extrapolating a second (vertical) line passing through the middle of the patella and tibial tuberosity. The Q-angle is typically greater in adult females, owing to their wider pelves. **C.** Genu valgum and genu varum. A medial angulation of the leg in relation to the thigh, in which the femur is abnormally vertical and the Q-angle is small, is a deformity called genu varum (bowleg) that causes unequal weight bearing resulting in arthrosis (destruction of knee cartilages), and an overstressed fibular collateral ligament. A lateral angulation of the leg (large Q-angle, >17°) in relation to the thigh is called genu valgum (knock-knee). This results in excess stress and degeneration of the lateral structures of the knee joint.

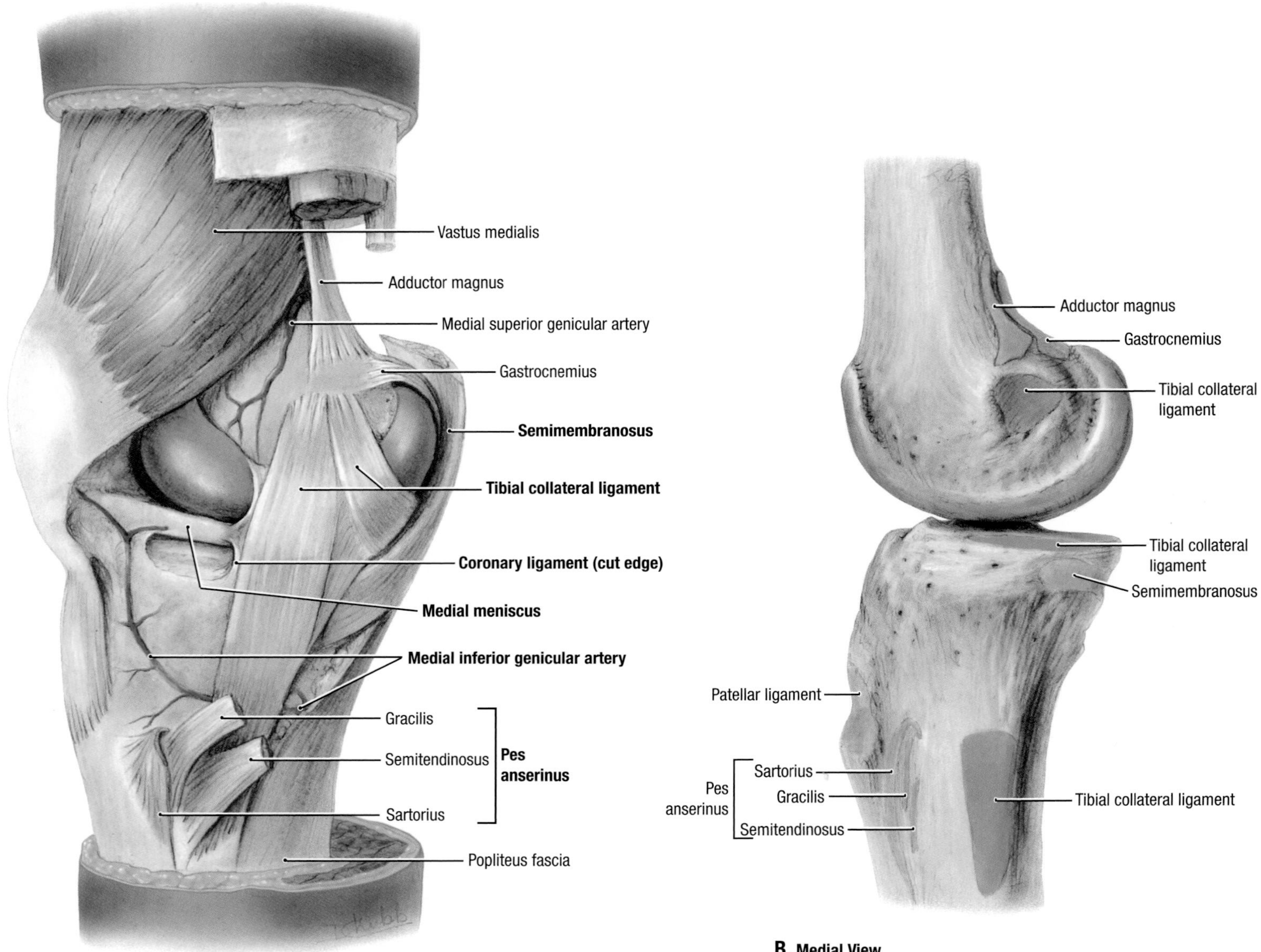
Vastus medialis
Adductor magnus
Medial superior genicular artery
Gastrocnemius
Semimembranosus
Tibial collateral ligament
Coronary ligament (cut edge)
Medial meniscus
Medial inferior genicular artery
Gracilis
Semitendinosus
Pes anserinus
Sartorius
Popliteus fascia
A. Medial View
Adductor magnus
Gastrocnemius
Tibial collateral ligament
Tibial collateral ligament
Semimembranosus
Patellar ligament
Pes anserinus
Sartorius
Gracilis
Semitendinosus
Tibial collateral ligament
B. Medial View

## 5.41 Medial aspect of knee

**A.** Dissection. The bandlike part of the tibial collateral ligament attaches to the medial epicondyle of the femur, bridges superficial to the insertion of the semimembranosus muscle, and crosses the medial inferior genicular artery. Distally, the ligament is crossed by the three tendons forming the pes anserinus (sartorius, gracilis, and semitendinosus). **B.** Bones, showing muscle and ligament attachment sites.

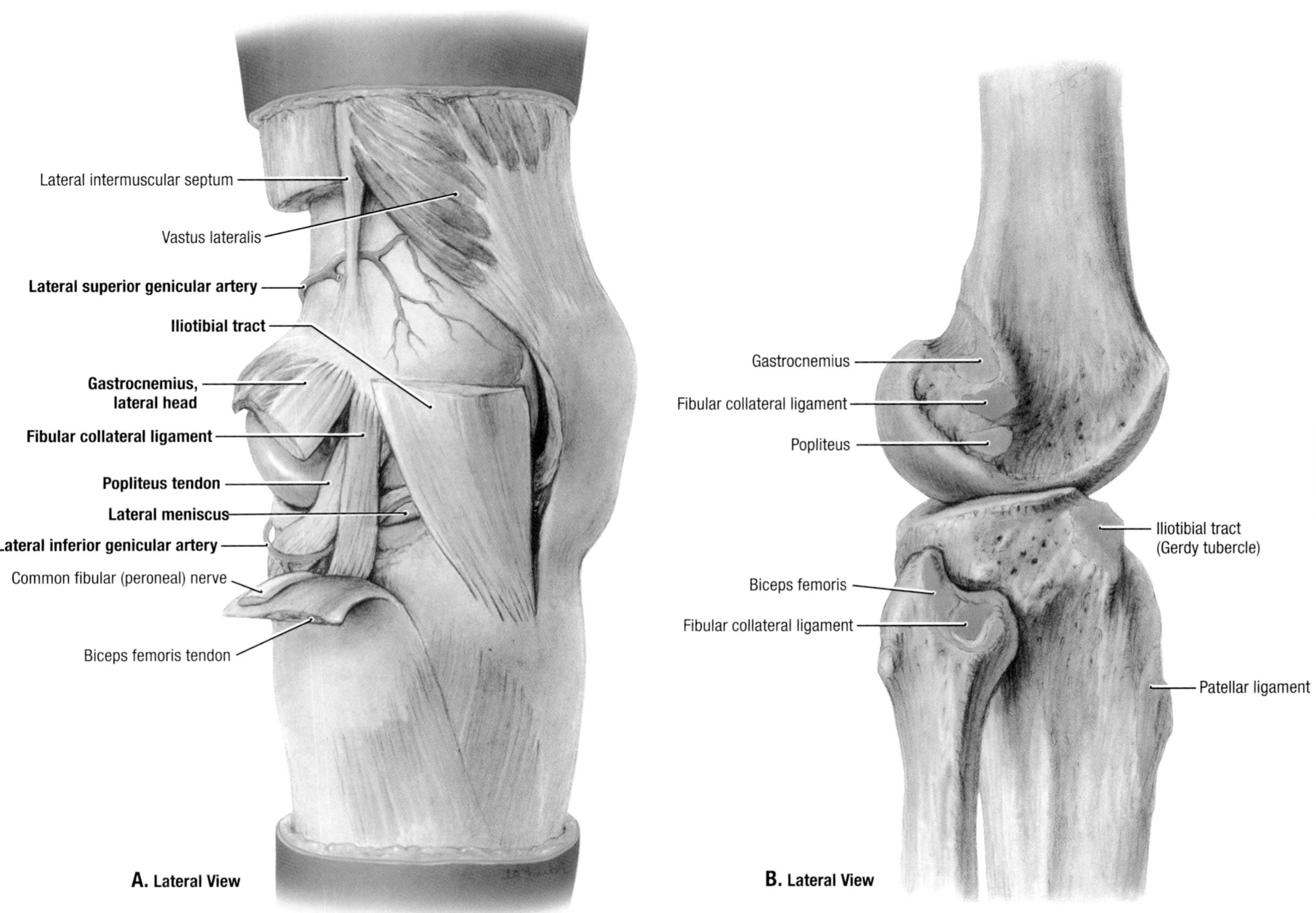
Lateral intermuscular septum
Vastus lateralis
Lateral superior genicular artery
Iliotibial tract
Gastrocnemius, lateral head
Fibular collateral ligament
Popliteus tendon
Lateral meniscus
Lateral inferior genicular artery
Common fibular (peroneal) nerve
Biceps femoris tendon
A. Lateral View
Gastrocnemius
Fibular collateral ligament
Popliteus
Iliotibial tract (Gerdy tubercle)
Biceps femoris
Fibular collateral ligament
Patellar ligament
B. Lateral View

## 5.42 Lateral aspect of knee

**A.** Dissection. **B.** Bones, showing muscle and ligament attachments.

Three structures arise from the lateral epicondyle and are uncovered by reflecting the biceps muscle: the gastrocnemius muscle is posterosuperior; the popliteus muscle is anteroinferior; and the fibular collateral ligament is in between, crossing superficial to the popliteus muscle. The lateral inferior genicular artery courses along the lateral meniscus.

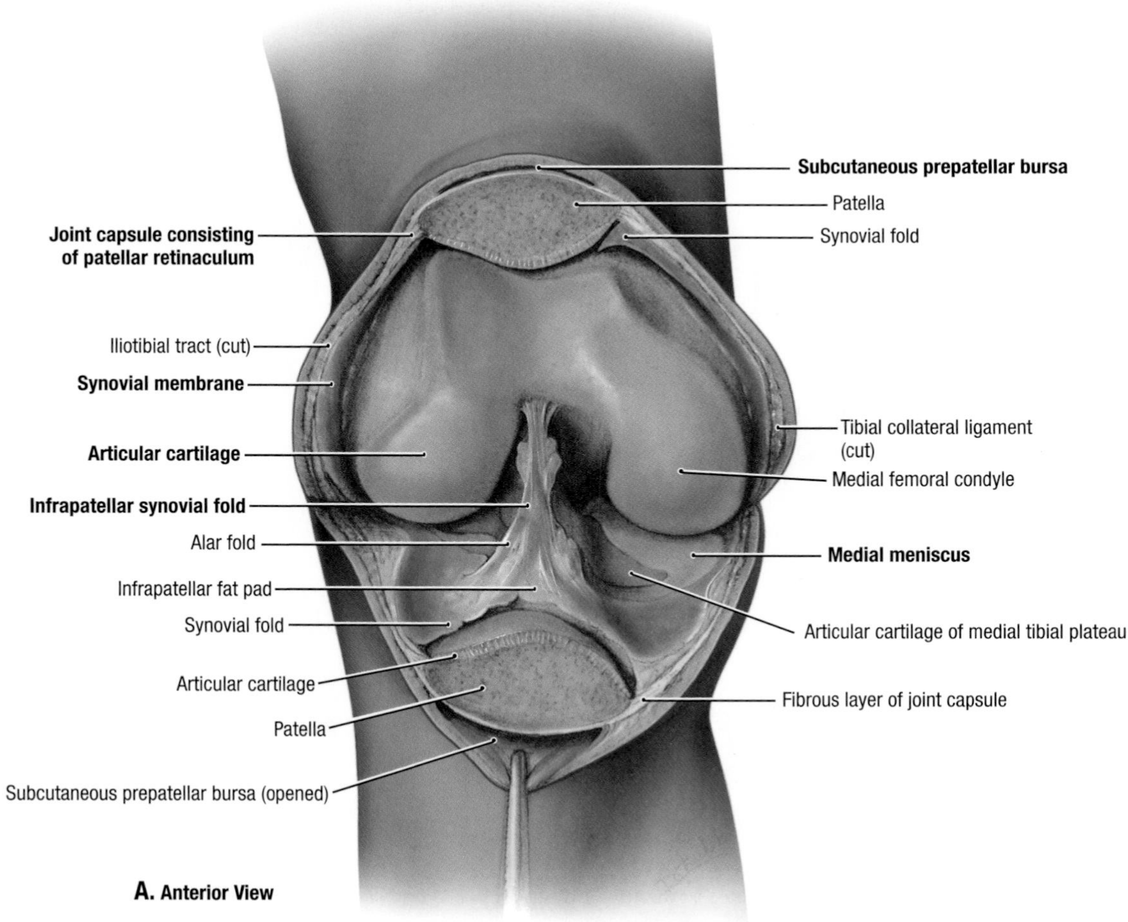
Subcutaneous prepatellar bursa
Patella
Synovial fold
Joint capsule consisting of patellar retinaculum
Iliotibial tract (cut)
Synovial membrane
Articular cartilage
Infrapatellar synovial fold
Alar fold
Infrapatellar fat pad
Synovial fold
Articular cartilage
Patella
Subcutaneous prepatellar bursa (opened)
Tibial collateral ligament (cut)
Medial femoral condyle
Medial meniscus
Articular cartilage of medial tibial plateau
Fibrous layer of joint capsule
A. Anterior View

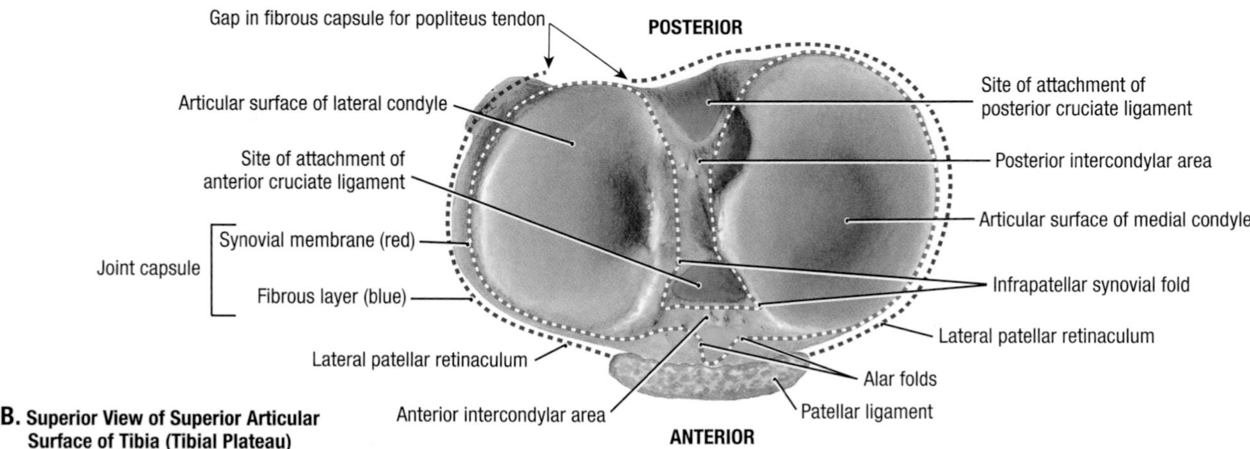
Gap in fibrous capsule for popliteus tendon
POSTERIOR
Articular surface of lateral condyle
Site of attachment of anterior cruciate ligament
Joint capsule
Synovial membrane (red)
Fibrous layer (blue)
Lateral patellar retinaculum
Anterior intercondylar area
ANTERIOR
Site of attachment of posterior cruciate ligament
Posterior intercondylar area
Articular surface of medial condyle
Infrapatellar synovial fold
Lateral patellar retinaculum
Alar folds
Patellar ligament
B. Superior View of Superior Articular Surface of Tibia (Tibial Plateau)

## 5.43 Fibrous layer and synovial membrane of joint capsule

**A.** Dissection. **B.** Attachment of the layers of the joint capsule to the tibia. The fibrous layer (blue dotted line) and synovial membrane (red dotted line) are adjacent on each side, but they part company centrally to accommodate intercondylar and infrapatellar structures that are intracapsular (inside the fibrous layer) but extra-articular (excluded from the articular cavity by synovial membrane).

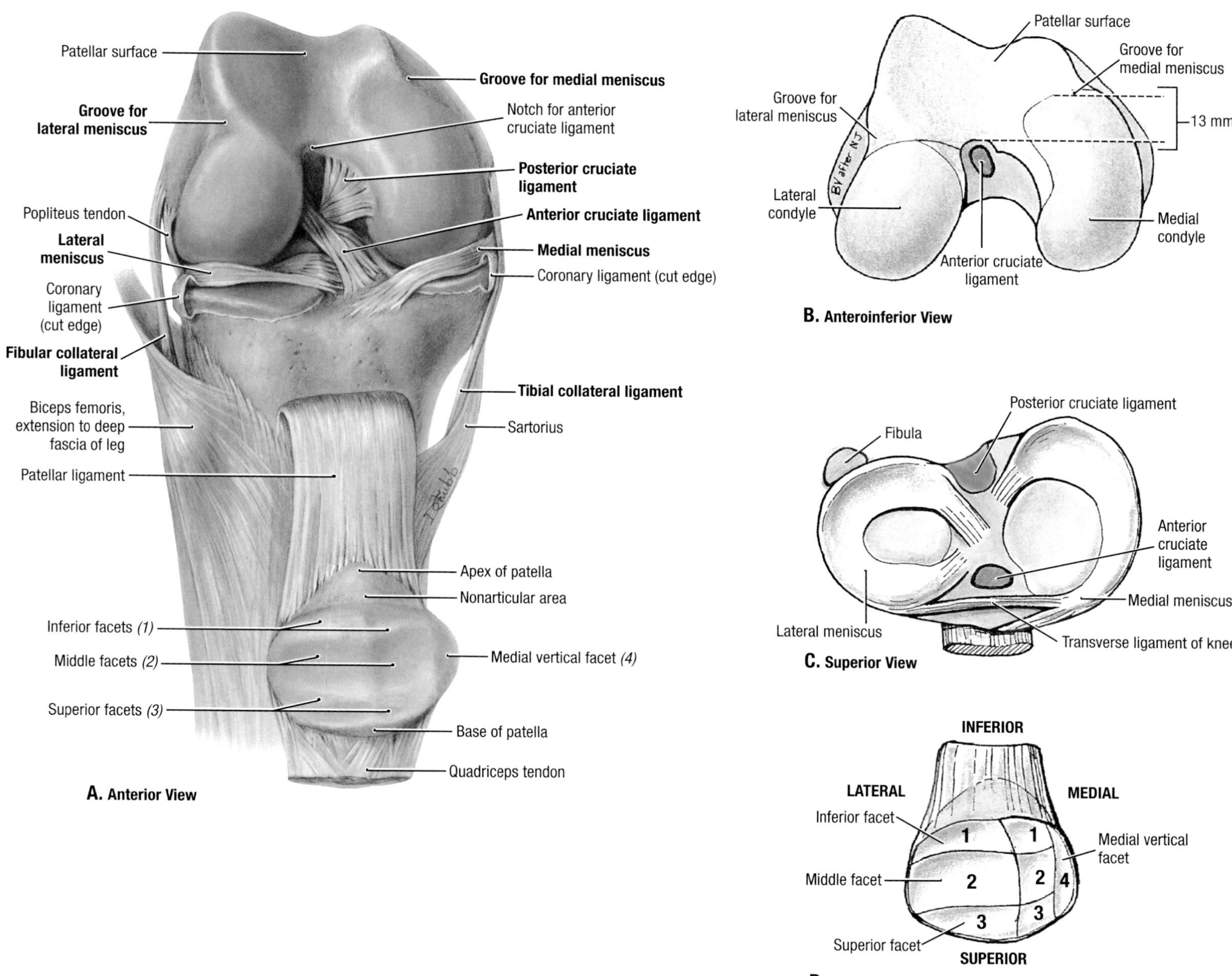
Patellar surface
Groove for medial meniscus
Groove for lateral meniscus
Notch for anterior cruciate ligament
Posterior cruciate ligament
Popliteus tendon
Anterior cruciate ligament
Lateral meniscus
Medial meniscus
Coronary ligament (cut edge)
Coronary ligament (cut edge)
Fibular collateral ligament
Tibial collateral ligament
Biceps femoris, extension to deep fascia of leg
Sartorius
Patellar ligament
Apex of patella
Nonarticular area
Inferior facets (1)
Middle facets (2)
Medial vertical facet (4)
Superior facets (3)
Base of patella
Quadriceps tendon
A. Anterior View
Patellar surface
Groove for medial meniscus
Groove for lateral meniscus
13 mm
Lateral condyle
Medial condyle
Anterior cruciate ligament
B. Anteroinferior View
Posterior cruciate ligament
Fibula
Anterior cruciate ligament
Medial meniscus
Lateral meniscus
Transverse ligament of knee
C. Superior View
INFERIOR
LATERAL
MEDIAL
Inferior facet
Medial vertical facet
Middle facet
Superior facet
SUPERIOR
D. Posterior View

## 5.44 Articular surfaces and ligaments of knee joint

**A.** Flexed knee joint with patella reflected. There are indentations on the sides of the femoral condyles at the junction of the patellar and tibial articular areas. The lateral tibial articular area is shorter than the medial one. The notch at the anterolateral part of the intercondylar notch is for the anterior cruciate ligament on full extension. **B.** Distal femur. **C.** Tibial plateaus. **D.** Articular surfaces of patella. The three paired facets (superior, middle, and inferior) on the posterior surface of the patella articulate with the patellar surface of the femur successively during *(1)* extension, *(2)* slight flexion, *(3)* flexion, and the most medial vertical facet on the patella *(4)* articulates during full flexion with the cresenteric facet on the medial margin of the intercondylar notch of the femur.

When the patella is dislocated, it nearly always dislocates laterally. The tendency toward lateral dislocation is normally counterbalanced by the medial, more horizontal pull of the powerful vastus medialis. In addition, the more anterior projection of the lateral femoral condyle and deeper slope for the large lateral patellar facet provides a mechanical deterrent to lateral dislocation. An imbalance of the lateral pull and the mechanisms resisting it result in abnormal tracking of the patella within the patellar groove and chronic patellar pain, even if actual dislocation does not occur. See Figure 5.49 blue box.

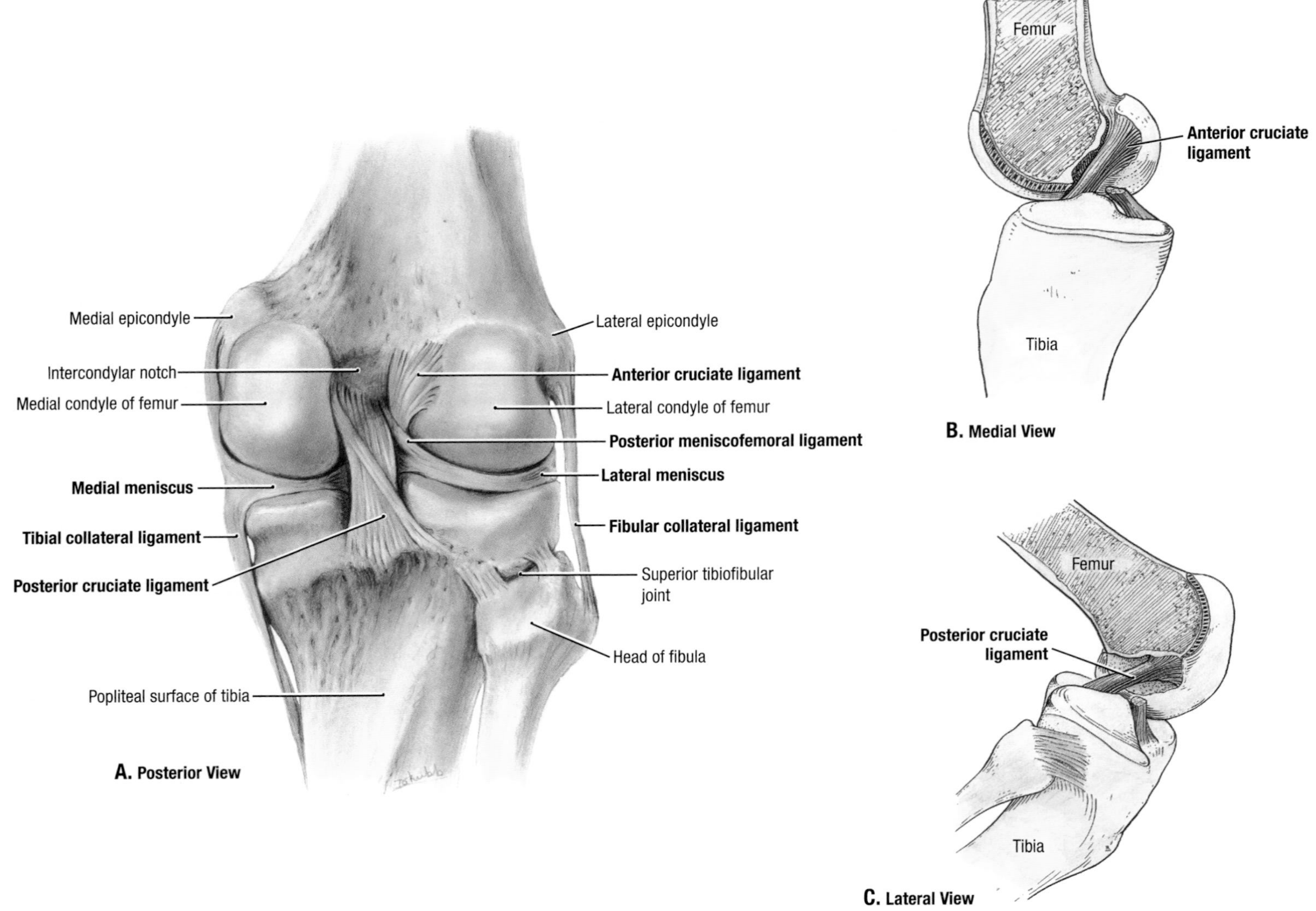
Medial epicondyle
Intercondylar notch
Medial condyle of femur
Medial meniscus
Tibial collateral ligament
Posterior cruciate ligament
Popliteal surface of tibia
Lateral epicondyle
Anterior cruciate ligament
Lateral condyle of femur
Posterior meniscofemoral ligament
Lateral meniscus
Fibular collateral ligament
Superior tibiofibular joint
Head of fibula
A. Posterior View
Femur
Anterior cruciate ligament
Tibia
B. Medial View
Femur
Posterior cruciate ligament
Tibia
C. Lateral View

## 5.45 Ligaments of knee joint

**A.** Posterior aspect of joint. The bandlike tibial (medial) collateral ligament is attached to the medial meniscus, and the cordlike fibular (lateral) collateral ligament is separated from the lateral meniscus by the width of the popliteus tendon (removed). The posterior cruciate ligament is joined by a cord from the lateral meniscus called the posterior meniscofemoral ligament. The posterior meniscofemoral ligament attaches to the medial condyle of the femur just posterior to the attachment of the posterior cruciate ligament. **B.** Anterior cruciate ligament. **C.** Posterior cruciate ligament. In each illustration, half the femur is sagittally sectioned and removed with the proximal part of the corresponding cruciate ligament. Note that the posterior cruciate ligament prevents the femur from sliding anteriorly on the tibia, particularly when the knee is flexed. The anterior cruciate ligament prevents the femur from sliding posteriorly on the tibia, preventing hyperextension of the knee, and limits medial rotation of the femur when the foot is on the ground (i.e., when the leg is fixed). Injury to the knee joint is frequently caused by a blow to the lateral side of the extended knee or excessive lateral twisting of the flexed knee, which disrupts the tibial collateral ligament and concomitantly tears and/or detaches the medial meniscus from the joint capsule. This injury is common in athletes who twist their flexed knees while running (e.g., in football and soccer). The anterior cruciate ligament, which serves as a pivot for rotary movements of the knee, is taut during flexion and may also tear subsequent to the rupture of the tibial collateral ligament, creating an "unhappy triad" of knee injuries.

Anterior intercondylar area
Articular surface of lateral condyle
Medial intercondylar tubercle
Lateral intercondylar tubercle
Posterior intercondylar area
Articular surface of medial condyle

**A. Superior View**

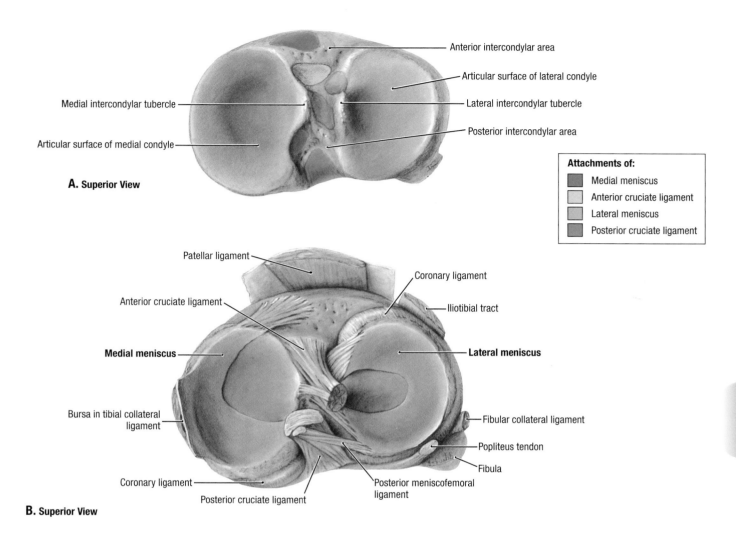

**Attachments of:**
Medial meniscus
Anterior cruciate ligament
Lateral meniscus
Posterior cruciate ligament

Patellar ligament
Coronary ligament
Anterior cruciate ligament
Iliotibial tract
**Medial meniscus**
**Lateral meniscus**
Bursa in tibial collateral ligament
Fibular collateral ligament
Popliteus tendon
Fibula
Coronary ligament
Posterior meniscofemoral ligament
Posterior cruciate ligament

**B. Superior View**

## 5.46 Cruciate ligaments and menisci

**A.** Attachments sites on tibia. **B.** Menisci in situ.

- The lateral tibial condyle is flatter, shorter from anterior to posterior, and more circular. The medial condyle is concave, longer from anterior to posterior, and more oval.
- The menisci conform to the shapes of the surfaces on which they rest. Because the horns of the lateral meniscus are attached close together and its coronary ligament is slack, this meniscus can slide anteriorly and posteriorly on the (flat) condyle; because the horns of the medial meniscus are attached further apart, its movements on the (concave) condyle are restricted.

Arthroscopy is an endoscopic examination that allows visualization of the interior of the knee joint cavity with minimal disruption of tissue. The arthroscope and one (or more) additional canula(e) are inserted through tiny incisions, known as portals. The second canula is for passage of specialized tools (e.g., manipulative probes or forceps) or equipment for trimming, shaping, or removing damaged tissue. This technique allows removal of torn menisci, loose bodies in the joint such as bone chips, and debridement (the excision of devitalized articular cartilaginous material in advanced cases of arthritis). Ligament repair or replacement may also be performed using an arthroscope.

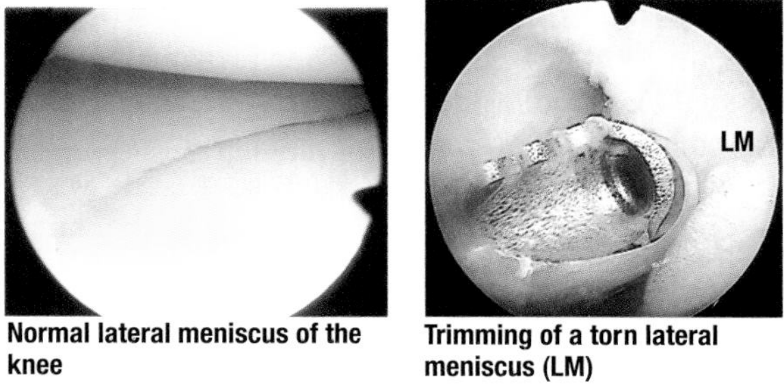
LM

**Normal lateral meniscus of the knee** **Trimming of a torn lateral meniscus (LM)**

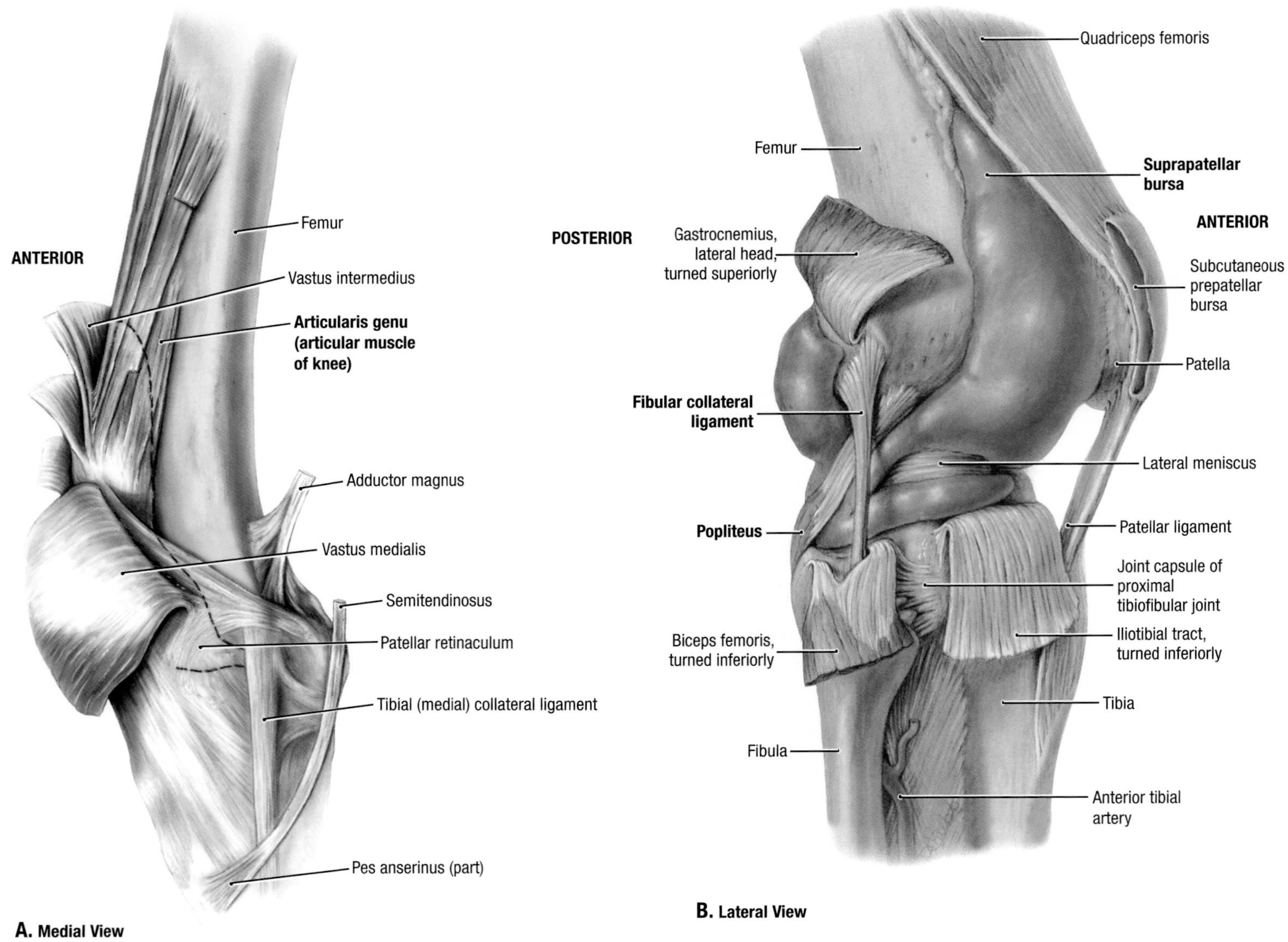
ANTERIOR
Femur
Vastus intermedius
Articularis genu (articular muscle of knee)
Adductor magnus
Vastus medialis
Semitendinosus
Patellar retinaculum
Tibial (medial) collateral ligament
Pes anserinus (part)
POSTERIOR
Quadriceps femoris
Femur
Suprapatellar bursa
ANTERIOR
Gastrocnemius, lateral head, turned superiorly
Subcutaneous prepatellar bursa
Patella
Fibular collateral ligament
Lateral meniscus
Popliteus
Patellar ligament
Joint capsule of proximal tibiofibular joint
Biceps femoris, turned inferiorly
Iliotibial tract, turned inferiorly
Tibia
Fibula
Anterior tibial artery

**A.** Medial View

**B.** Lateral View

## 5.47 Articularis genu and suprapatellar bursa

**A.** Articularis genu (articular muscle of the knee). This muscle lies deep to the vastus intermedius muscle and consists of fibers arising from the anterior surface of the femur proximally and attaching into the synovial membrane distally. The articularis genu pulls the synovial membrane of the suprapatellar bursa *(dotted line)* superiorly during extension of the knee so that it will not be caught between the patella and femur within the knee joint. **B.** Lateral aspect of knee. Latex was injected into the articular cavity and fixed with acetic acid. The distended synovial membrane was exposed and cleaned. The gastrocnemius muscle was reflected proximally, and the biceps femoris muscle and the iliotibial tract were reflected distally. The extent of the synovial capsule: superiorly, it rises superior to the patella, where it rests on a layer of fat that allows it to glide freely with movements of the joint; this superior part is called the suprapatellar bursa; posteriorly, it rises as high as the origin of the gastrocnemius muscle; laterally, it curves inferior to the lateral femoral epicondyle, where the popliteus tendon and fibular collateral ligament are attached; and inferiorly, it bulges inferior to the lateral meniscus, overlapping the tibia (the coronary ligament is removed to show this). Prepatellar bursitis (housemaid's knee) is usually a friction bursitis caused by friction between the skin and the patella. The suprapatellar bursa communicates with the articular cavity of the knee joint; consequently, abrasions or penetrating wounds superior to the patella may result in suprapatellar bursitis caused by bacteria entering the bursa from the torn skin. The infection may spread to the knee joint.

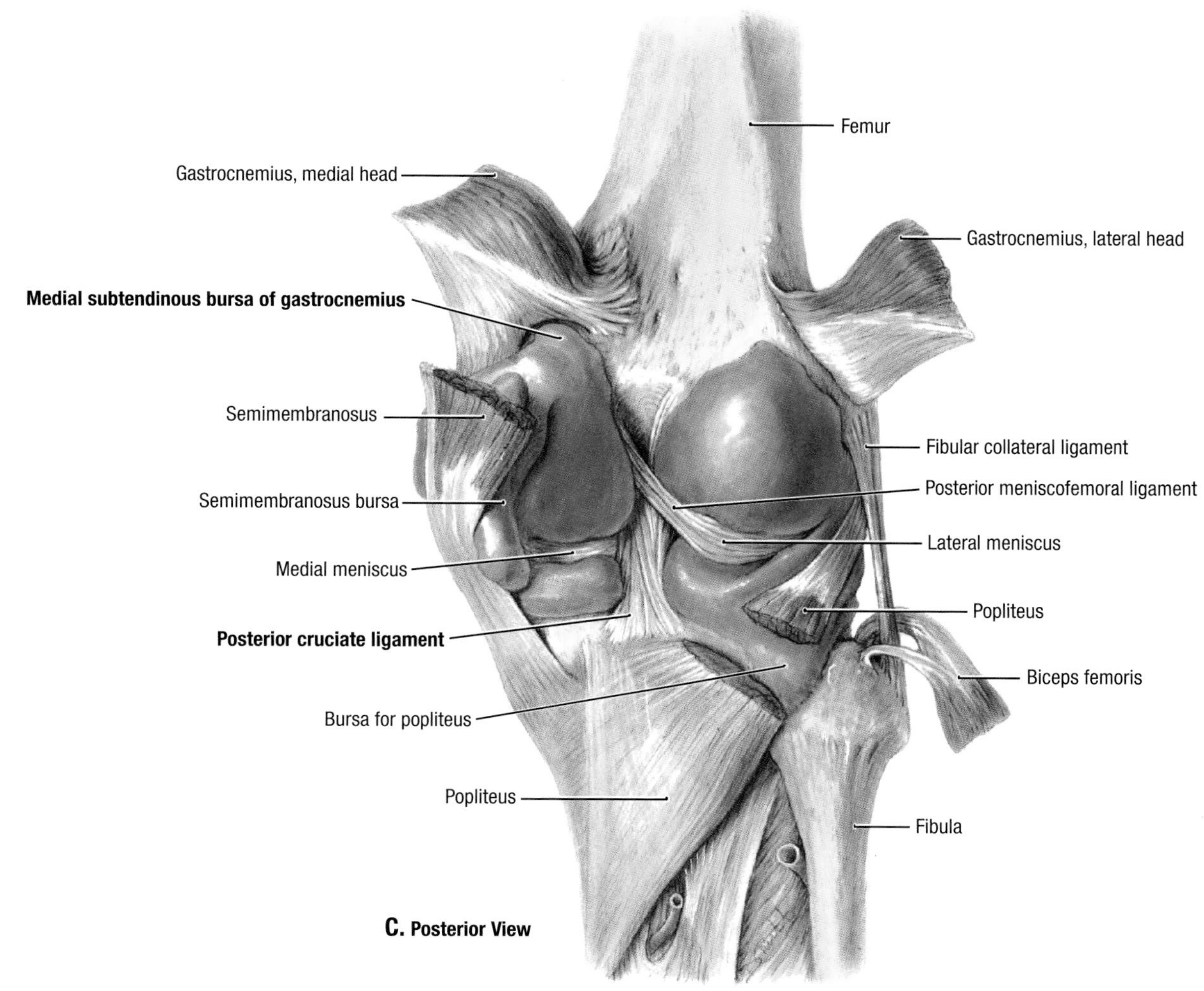
Femur
Gastrocnemius, medial head
Gastrocnemius, lateral head
Medial subtendinous bursa of gastrocnemius
Semimembranosus
Fibular collateral ligament
Posterior meniscofemoral ligament
Semimembranosus bursa
Lateral meniscus
Medial meniscus
Popliteus
Posterior cruciate ligament
Biceps femoris
Bursa for popliteus
Popliteus
Fibula

**C. Posterior View**

## 5.47 Distended knee joint *(continued)*

**TABLE 5.8 BURSAE AROUND KNEE**

| Bursa | Location | Structural Features or Functions |
|---|---|---|
| **Suprapatellar** | Between femur and tendon of quadriceps femoris | Held in position by articular muscle of knee; communicates freely with synovial cavity of knee joint |
| **Popliteus** | Between tendon of popliteus and lateral condyle of tibia | Opens into synovial cavity of knee joint, inferior to lateral meniscus |
| **Anserine** | Separates tendons of sartorius, gracilis, and semitendinosus from tibia and tibial collateral ligament | Area where tendons of these muscles attach to tibia resembles the foot of a goose (L. *pes,* foot; L. *anser,* goose) |
| **Medial subtendinous bursa of gastrocnemius** | Lies deep to proximal attachment of tendon of medial head of gastrocnemius | This bursa is an extension of synovial cavity of knee joint |
| **Semimembranosus** | Located between medial head of gastrocnemius and semimembranosus tendon | Related to the distal attachment of semimembranosus |
| **Subcutaneous prepatellar** | Lies between skin and anterior surface of patella | Allows free movement of skin over patella during movements of leg |
| **Subcutaneous infrapatellar** | Located between skin and tibial tuberosity | Helps knee to withstand pressure when kneeling |
| **Deep infrapatellar** | Lies between patellar ligament and anterior surface of tibia | Separated from knee joint by infrapatellar fat-pad |

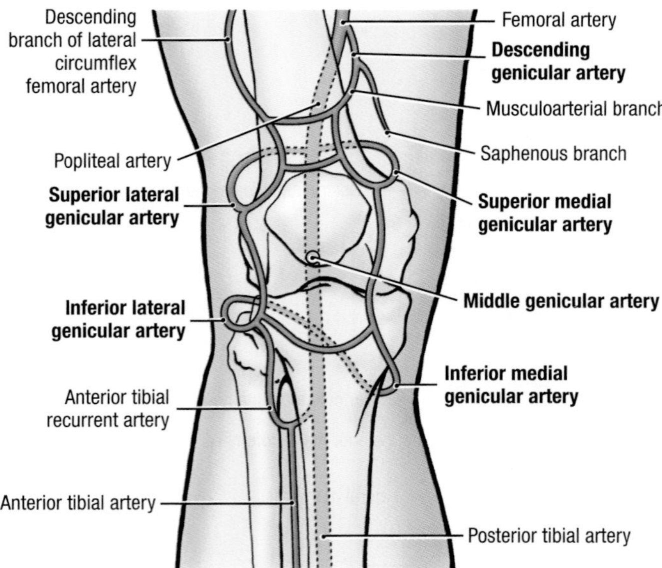
Descending branch of lateral circumflex femoral artery
Femoral artery
Descending genicular artery
Musculoarterial branch
Saphenous branch
Popliteal artery
Superior lateral genicular artery
Superior medial genicular artery
Middle genicular artery
Inferior lateral genicular artery
Inferior medial genicular artery
Anterior tibial recurrent artery
Anterior tibial artery
Posterior tibial artery

**A.** **Anterior View**

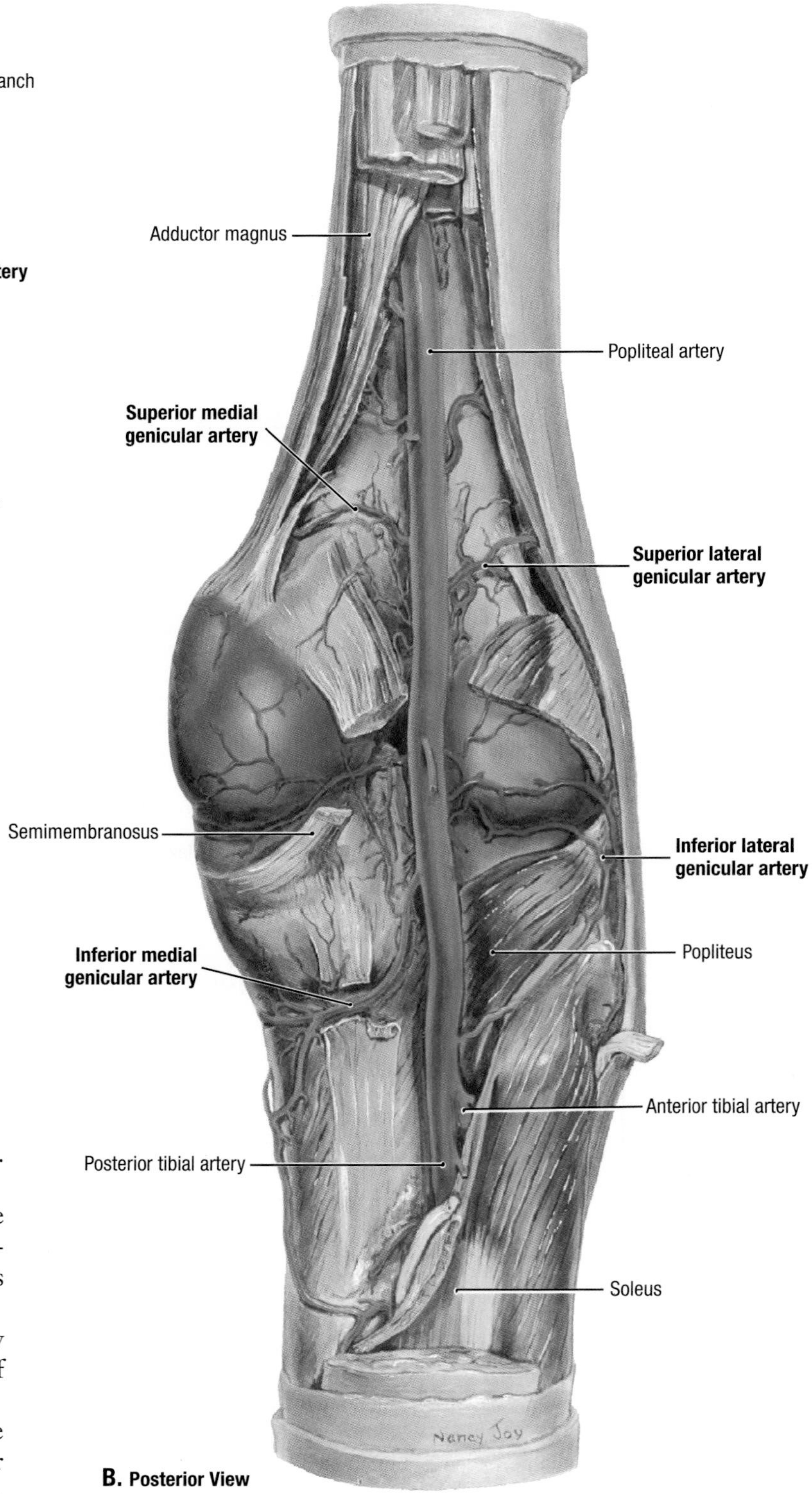

Adductor magnus
Popliteal artery
Superior medial genicular artery
Superior lateral genicular artery
Semimembranosus
Inferior lateral genicular artery
Inferior medial genicular artery
Popliteus
Anterior tibial artery
Posterior tibial artery
Soleus
Nancy Joy

**B.** **Posterior View**

## 5.48 Anastomoses around knee

**A.** Genicular anastomosis on the anterior aspect of the knee.
**B.** Popliteal artery in popliteal fossa.

- The popliteal artery runs from the adductor hiatus (in the adductor magnus muscle) proximally to the inferior border of the popliteus muscle distally, where it bifurcates into the anterior and posterior tibial arteries.
- The three anterior relations of the popliteal artery include the femur (fat intervening), the joint capsule of the knee; and the popliteus muscle.
- Five genicular branches of the popliteal artery supply the capsule and ligaments of the knee joint. The genicular arteries are the superior lateral, superior medial, middle, inferior lateral, and inferior medial genicular arteries.

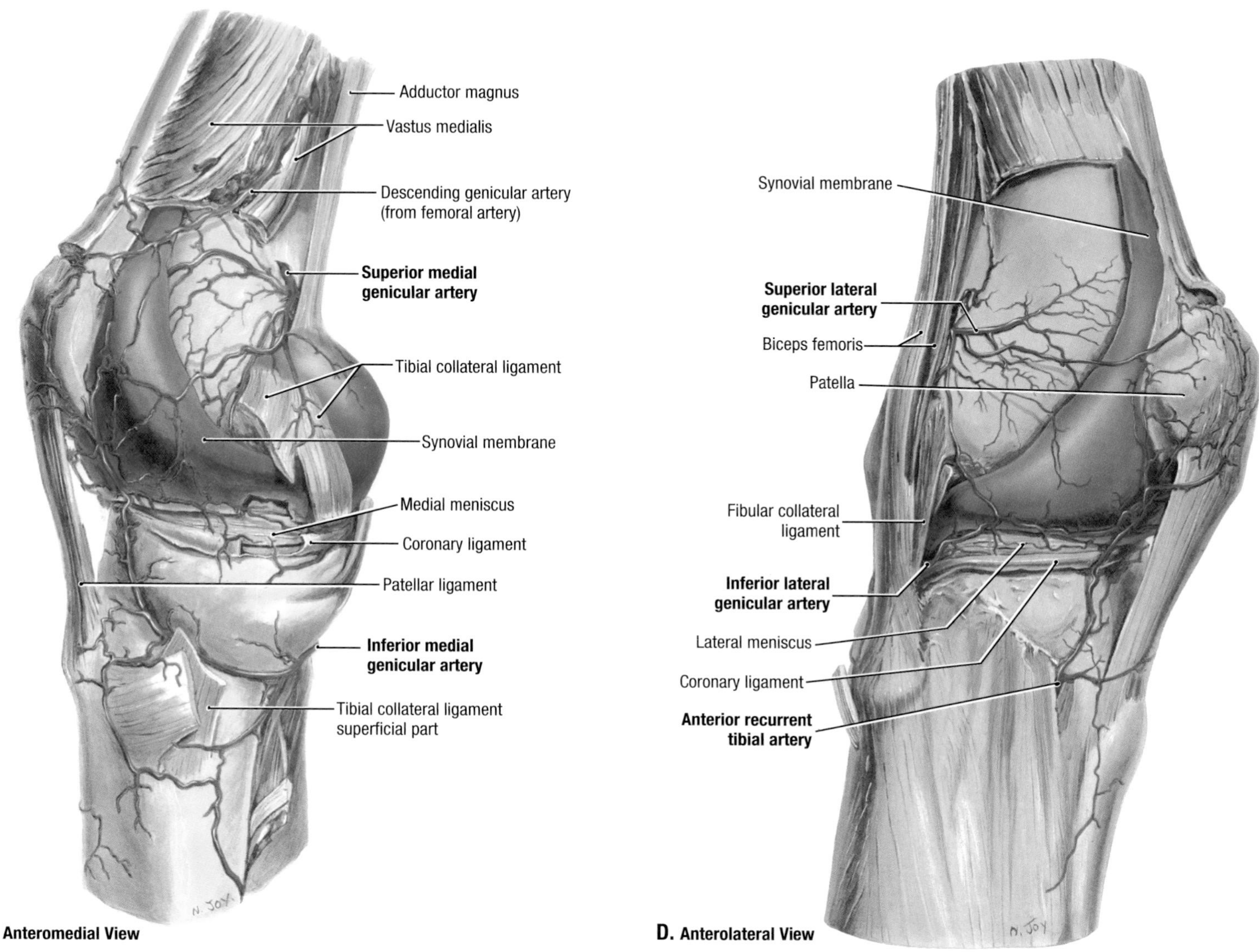
Adductor magnus
Vastus medialis
Descending genicular artery (from femoral artery)
Superior medial genicular artery
Tibial collateral ligament
Synovial membrane
Medial meniscus
Coronary ligament
Patellar ligament
Inferior medial genicular artery
Tibial collateral ligament superficial part
C. Anteromedial View
Synovial membrane
Superior lateral genicular artery
Biceps femoris
Patella
Fibular collateral ligament
Inferior lateral genicular artery
Lateral meniscus
Coronary ligament
Anterior recurrent tibial artery
D. Anterolateral View

## 5.48 Anastomoses around knee *(continued)*

**C.** Medial aspect of the knee showing superior and inferior medial genicular arteries. **D.** Lateral aspect of the knee showing superior and inferior lateral genicular arteries.

The genicular arteries participate in the formation of the periarticular genicular anastomosis, a network of vessels surrounding the knee that provides collateral circulation capable of maintaining blood supply to the leg during full knee flexion, which may kink the popliteal artery. Other contributors to this important anastomosis are the descending genicular artery, a branch of the femoral artery, superomedially; descending branch of the lateral circumflex femoral artery, superolaterally; and anterior tibial recurrent artery, a branch of the anterior tibial artery, inferolaterally.

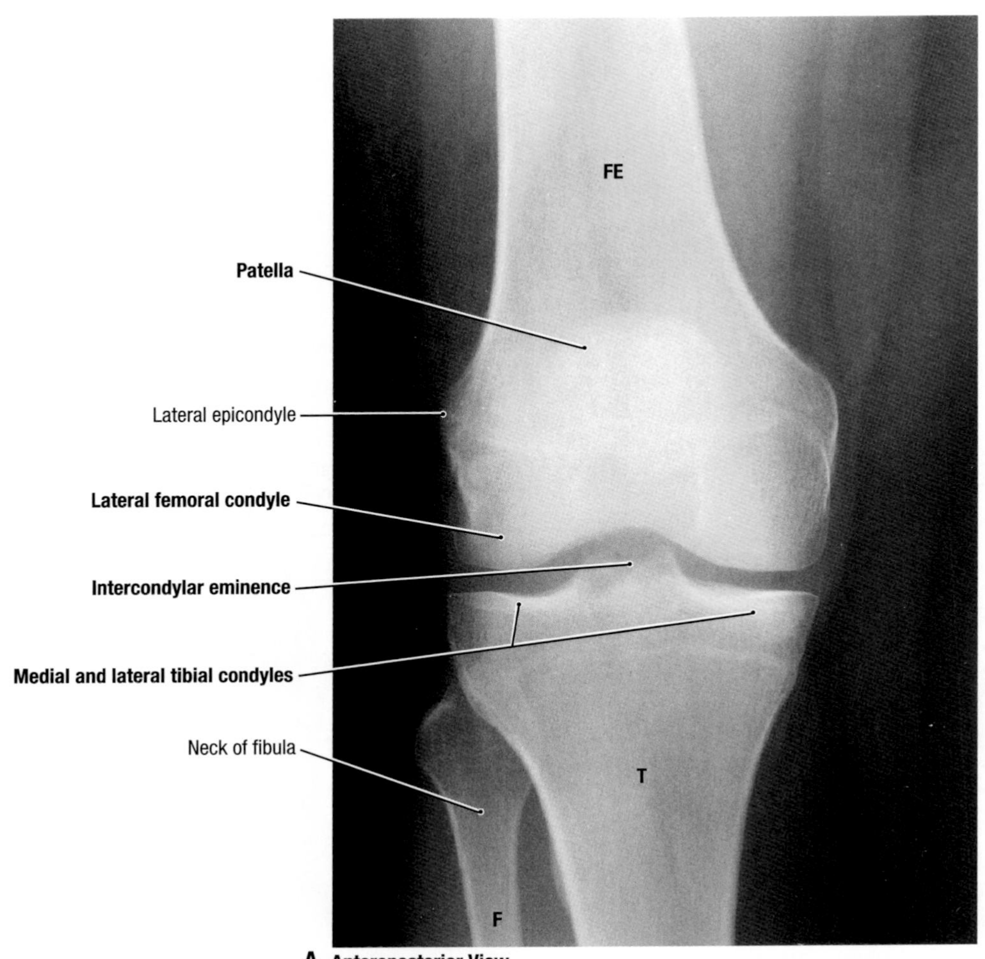
FE
Patella
Lateral epicondyle
Lateral femoral condyle
Intercondylar eminence
Medial and lateral tibial condyles
Neck of fibula
T
F

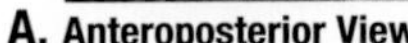
**A.** Anteroposterior View

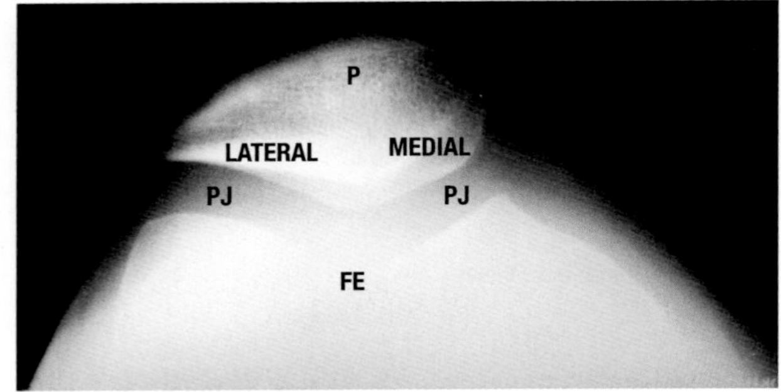
P
LATERAL
MEDIAL
PJ
PJ
FE

**B.** Skyline View (Knee in Flexion)

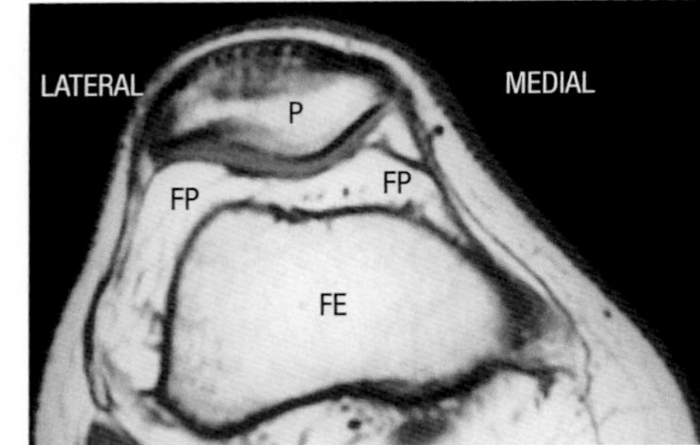
LATERAL
MEDIAL
P
FP
FP
FE

**C.** Transverse MRI

## 5.49 Imaging of the knee and patellofemoral articulation

**A.** Anteroposterior radiograph of knee. **B.** Radiograph of patella (knee joint flexed). *FE,* femur; *FP,* fat pad; *P,* patella; *PJ,* patellofemoral joint. **C.** Transverse MRI showing the patellofemoral joint.

Pain deep to the patella often results from excessive running, especially downhill; hence, this type of pain is often called "runner's knee." The pain results from repetitive microtrauma caused by abnormal tracking of the patella relative to the patellar surface of the femur, a condition known as the patellofemoral syndrome. This syndrome may also result from a direct blow to the patella and from osteoarthritis of the patellofemoral compartment (degenerative wear and tear of articular cartilages). In some cases, strengthening of the vastus medialis corrects patellofemoral dysfunction. This muscle tends to prevent lateral dislocation of the patella resulting from the Q-angle because the vastus medialis attaches to and pulls on the medial border of the patella. Hence, weakness of the vastus medialis predisposes the individual to patellofemoral dysfunction and patellar dislocation.

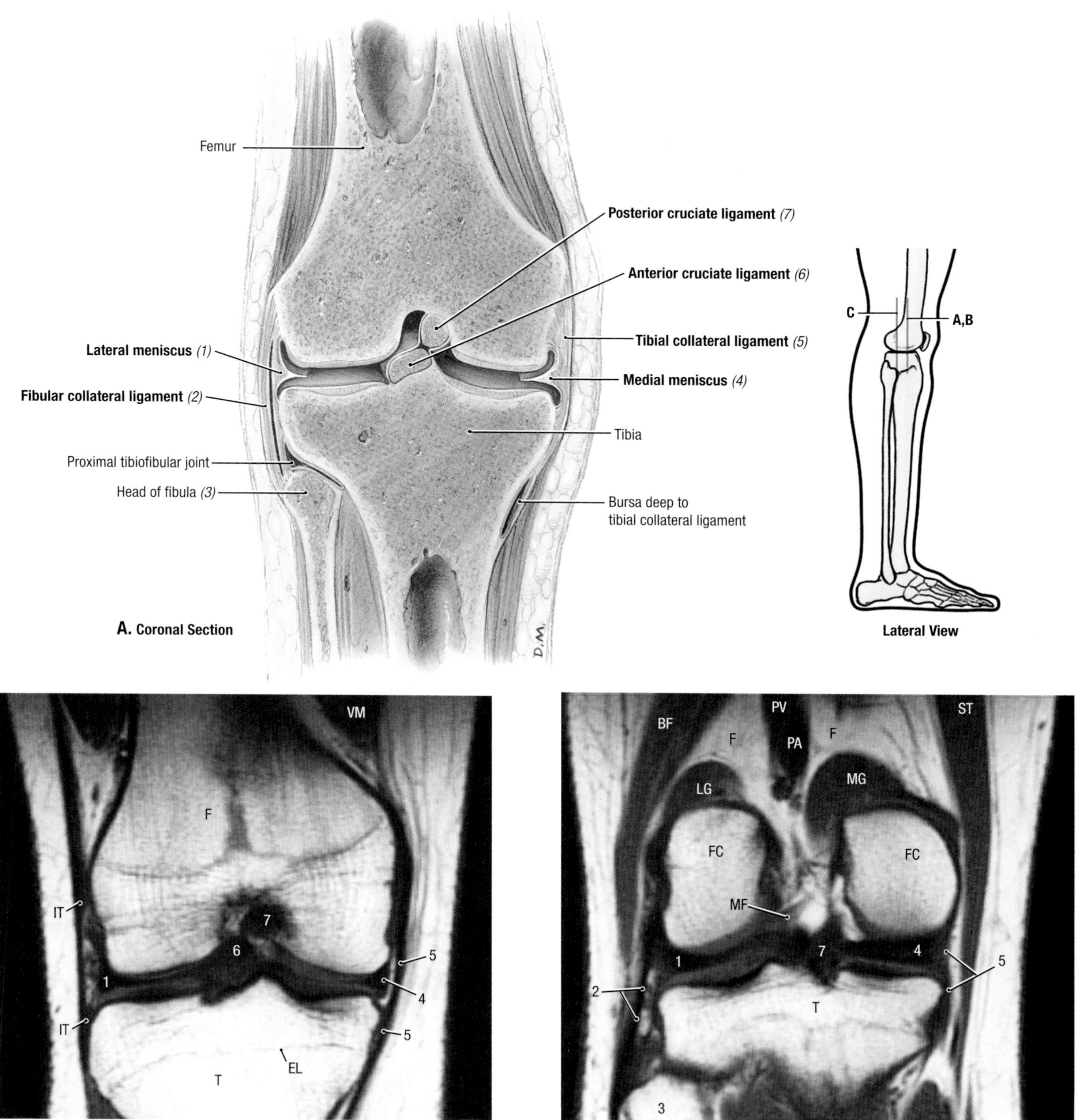
Femur
Posterior cruciate ligament (7)
Anterior cruciate ligament (6)
Tibial collateral ligament (5)
Lateral meniscus (1)
Medial meniscus (4)
Fibular collateral ligament (2)
Tibia
Proximal tibiofibular joint
Head of fibula (3)
Bursa deep to
tibial collateral ligament
A. Coronal Section
C
A,B
Lateral View
VM
F
IT
7
6
5
1
4
IT
5
EL
T
B. Coronal MRI
BF
PV
ST
F
PA
F
LG
MG
FC
FC
MF
1
7
4
5
2
T
3
C. Coronal MRI

## 5.50 Coronal section and MRIs of knee

**A.** Section through intercondylar notch of femur, tibia, and fibula. **B.** MRI through intercondylar notch of femur and tibia. **C.** MRI through femoral condyles tibia and fibula. *Numbers* in MRIs refer to structures in **A.** *VM*, vastus medialis; *EL*, epiphyseal line; *IT*, iliotibial tract; *FC*, femoral condyle; *BF*, biceps femoris; *ST*, semitendinosus; *LG*, lateral head of gastrocnemius; *MG*, medial head of gastrocnemius; *PV*, popliteal vein; *PA*, popliteal artery; *F*, fat in popliteal fossa; *MF*, meniscofemoral ligament.

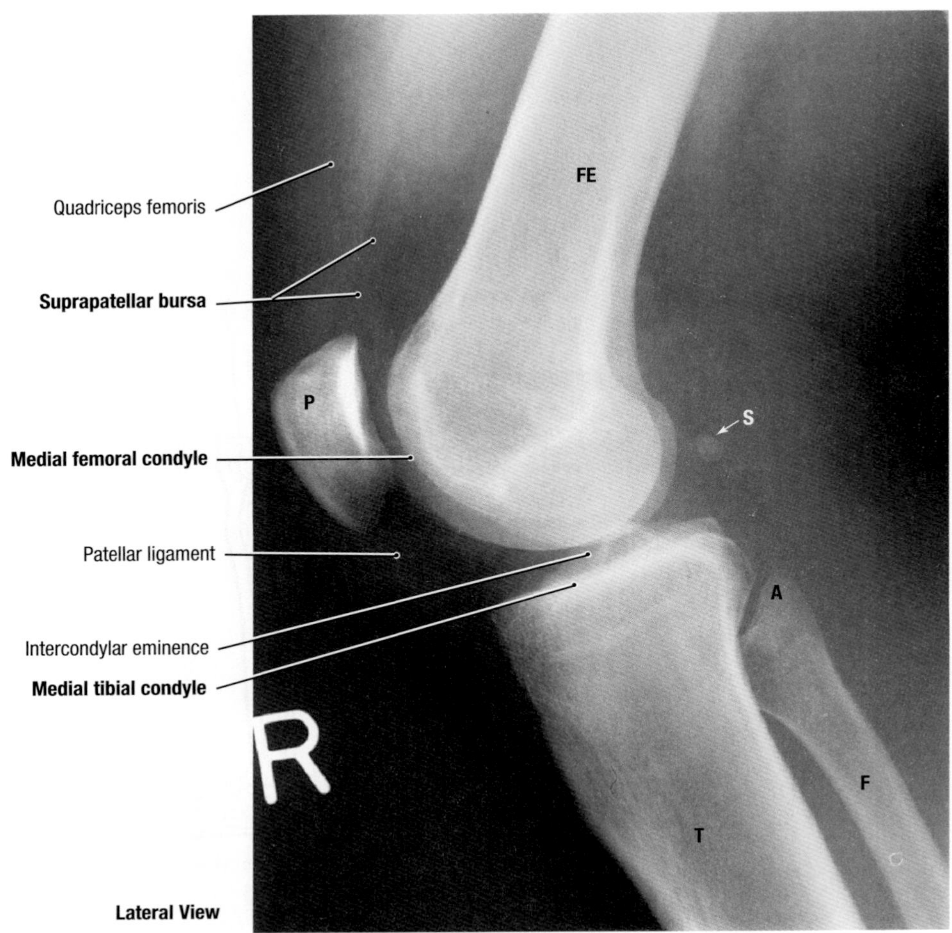

Quadriceps femoris
Suprapatellar bursa
Medial femoral condyle
Patellar ligament
Intercondylar eminence
Medial tibial condyle
FE
P
S
A
F
T
R
Lateral View


## 5.51 Radiograph of knee

Lateral radiograph of flexed knee. *FE*, femur; *T*, tibia; *F*, fibula; *A*, apex of fibula; *S*, fabella; *P*, patella. The fabella is a sesamoid bone in the lateral head of gastrocnemius muscle.

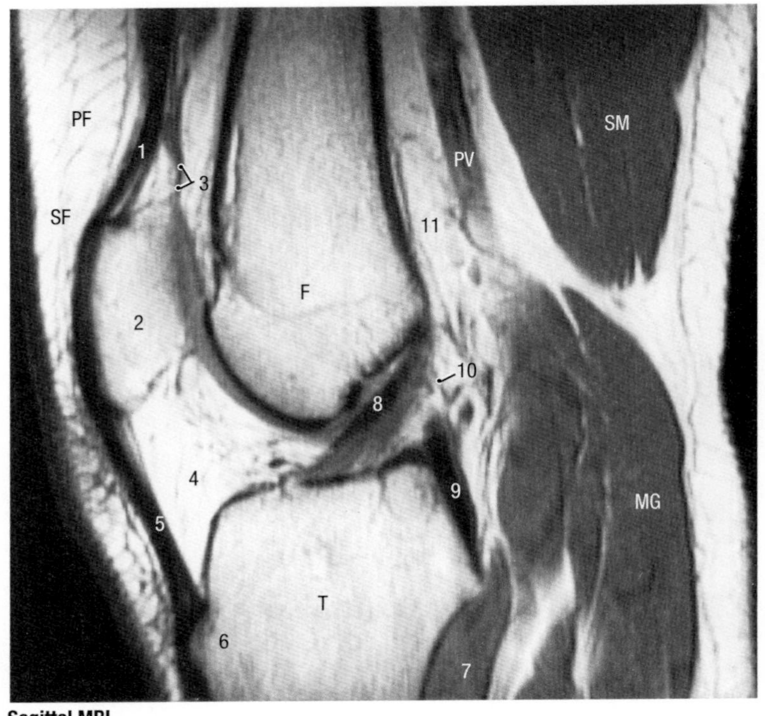

PF
SM
1
3
PV
SF
11
F
2
10
8
4
9
MG
5
T
6
7


**B.** Sagittal MRI

## 5.52 Sagittal section and MRIs of knee

**A.** *(Opposite page)*. Section through lateral aspect of intercondylar notch of femur. **B.** MRI through medial aspect of intercondylar notch of femur showing cruciate ligaments. **C.** MRI through medial femoral and tibial condyles. *Numbers* in MRIs refer to structures in **A.** *SM*, semimembranosus; *ST*, semitendinosus; *MG*, medial head of gastrocnemius; *VM*, vastus medialis; *PF*, prefemoral fat; *SF*, suprapatellar fat; *AM*, anterior horn of medial meniscus; *PM*, posterior horn of medial meniscus; *PV*, popliteal vessels.

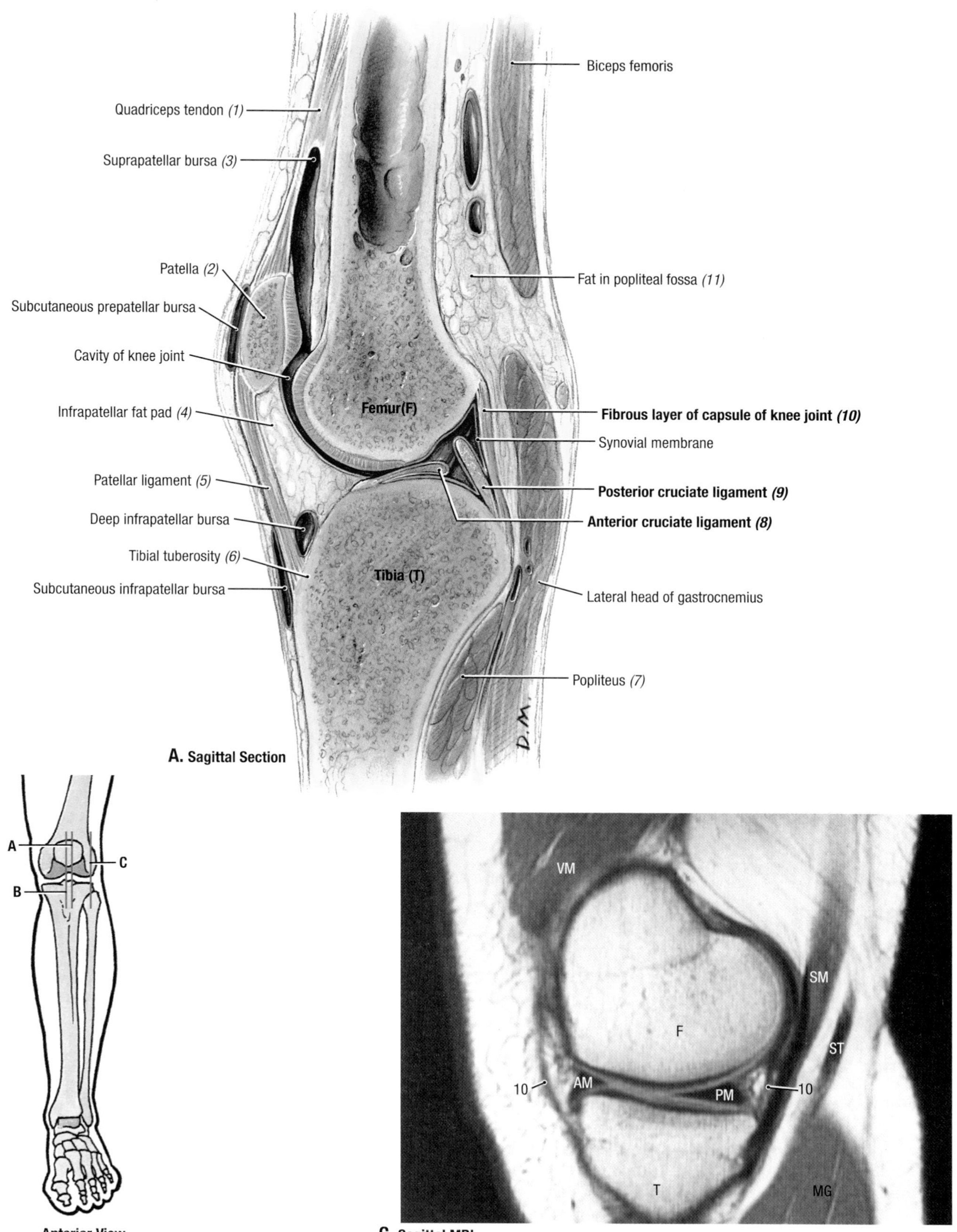
Quadriceps tendon (1)
Suprapatellar bursa (3)
Patella (2)
Subcutaneous prepatellar bursa
Cavity of knee joint
Infrapatellar fat pad (4)
Patellar ligament (5)
Deep infrapatellar bursa
Tibial tuberosity (6)
Subcutaneous infrapatellar bursa
Biceps femoris
Fat in popliteal fossa (11)
Fibrous layer of capsule of knee joint (10)
Synovial membrane
Posterior cruciate ligament (9)
Anterior cruciate ligament (8)
Lateral head of gastrocnemius
Popliteus (7)
Femur(F)
Tibia (T)
D.M.
A. Sagittal Section
A
B
C
Anterior View
VM
SM
F
ST
10
AM
PM
10
T
MG
C. Sagittal MRI

**5.52 Sagittal section and MRIs of knee *(continued)***

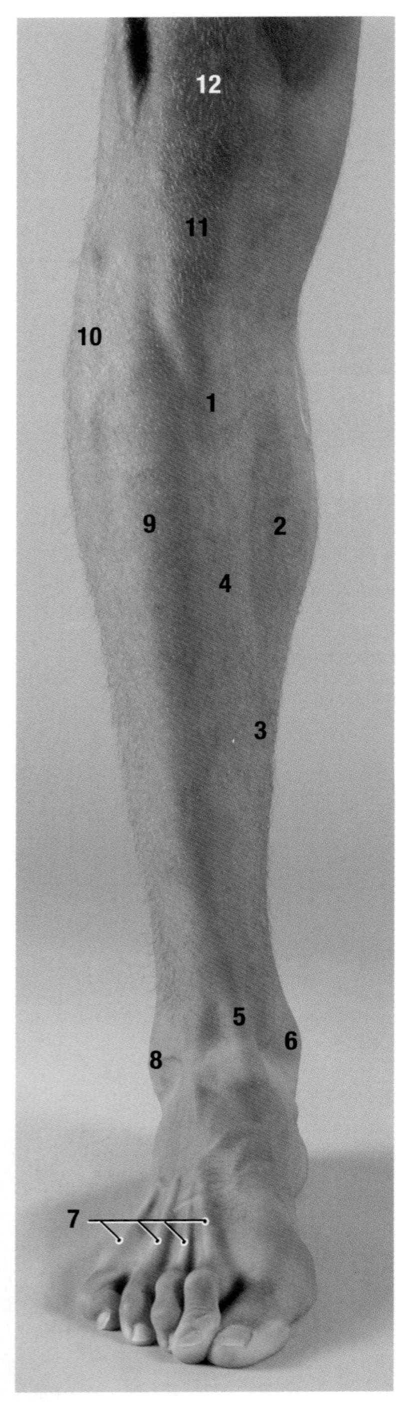
12
11
10
1
9
2
4
3
5
6
8
7

A. Anterior View

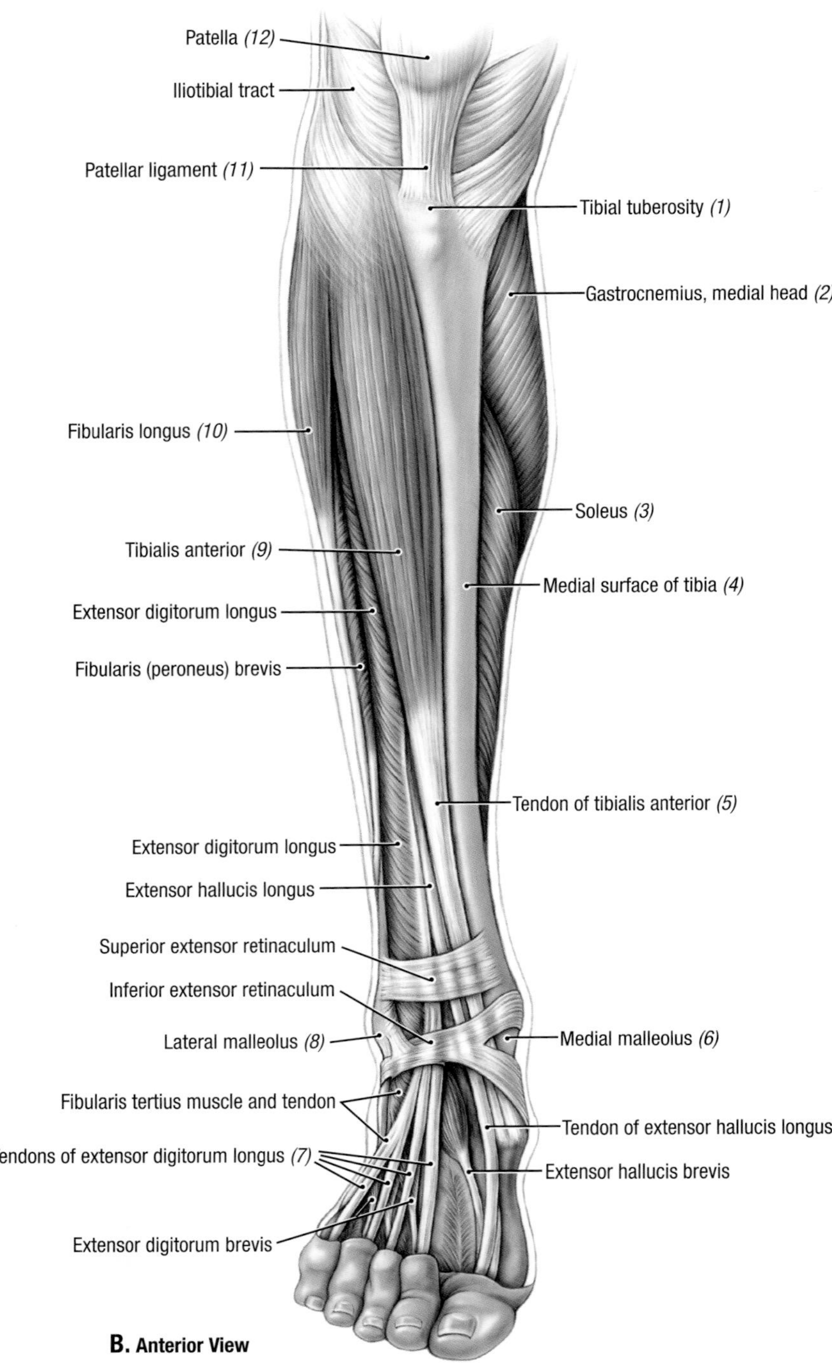
Patella (12)
Iliotibial tract
Patellar ligament (11)
Tibial tuberosity (1)
Gastrocnemius, medial head (2)
Fibularis longus (10)
Soleus (3)
Tibialis anterior (9)
Medial surface of tibia (4)
Extensor digitorum longus
Fibularis (peroneus) brevis
Tendon of tibialis anterior (5)
Extensor digitorum longus
Extensor hallucis longus
Superior extensor retinaculum
Inferior extensor retinaculum
Lateral malleolus (8)
Medial malleolus (6)
Fibularis tertius muscle and tendon
Tendon of extensor hallucis longus
Tendons of extensor digitorum longus (7)
Extensor hallucis brevis
Extensor digitorum brevis

B. Anterior View

## 5.53 Anterior leg—superficial muscles

**A.** Surface anatomy (*numbers* refer to structures labeled in **B**). **B.** Dissection.

The muscles of the anterior compartment are ankle dorsiflexors/toe extensors. They are active in walking as they concentrically contract to raise the forefoot to clear the ground during the swing phase of the gait cycle and eccentrically contract to lower the forefoot to the ground after the heel strike of the stance phase.

Shin splints, edema, and pain in the area of the distal third of the tibia, result from repetitive microtrauma of the anterior compartment muscles, especially the tibialis anterior. This produces a mild form of anterior compartment syndrome. The pain commonly occurs during traumatic injury or athletic overexertion of the muscles. Edema and muscle-tendon inflammation causes swelling that reduces blood flow to the muscles. The swollen ischemic muscles are painful and tender to pressure.

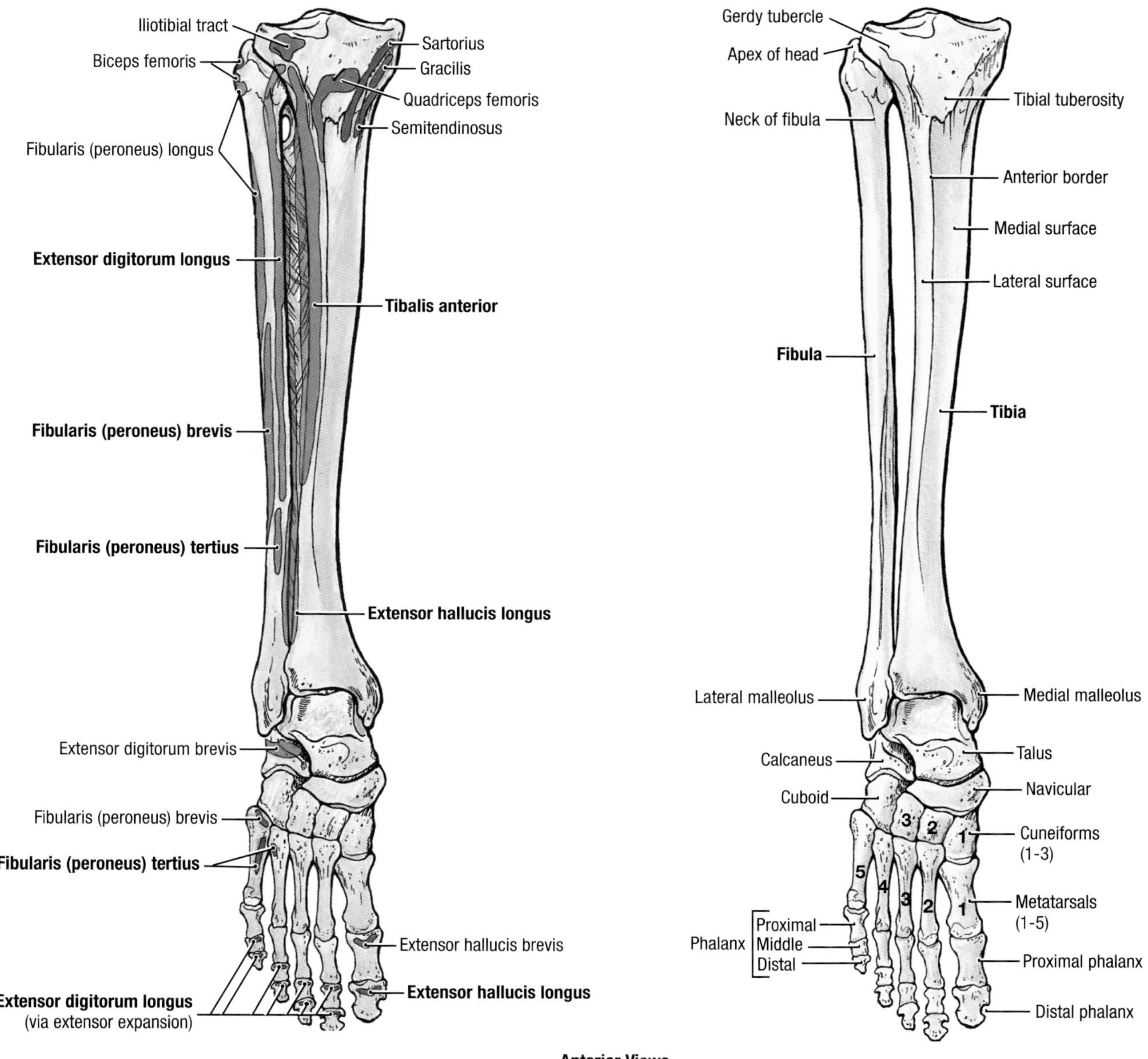
Iliotibial tract
Biceps femoris
Fibularis (peroneus) longus
Sartorius
Gracilis
Quadriceps femoris
Semitendinosus
Extensor digitorum longus
Tibalis anterior
Fibularis (peroneus) brevis
Fibularis (peroneus) tertius
Extensor hallucis longus
Extensor digitorum brevis
Fibularis (peroneus) brevis
Fibularis (peroneus) tertius
Extensor hallucis brevis
Extensor hallucis longus
Extensor digitorum longus
(via extensor expansion)
Gerdy tubercle
Apex of head
Neck of fibula
Tibial tuberosity
Anterior border
Medial surface
Lateral surface
Fibula
Tibia
Lateral malleolus
Medial malleolus
Calcaneus
Talus
Cuboid
Navicular
Cuneiforms
(1-3)
Metatarsals
(1-5)
Phalanx
Proximal
Middle
Distal
Proximal phalanx
Distal phalanx

Anterior Views

## TABLE 5.9 MUSCLES OF THE ANTERIOR COMPARTMENT OF LEG

| Muscle | Proximal Attachment | Distal Attachment | Innervation[a] | Main Actions |
|---|---|---|---|---|
| **Tibialis anterior** | Lateral condyle and superior half of lateral surface of tibia | Medial and inferior surfaces of medial cuneiform and base of first metatarsal | Deep fibular (peroneal) nerve (**L4**–L5) | Dorsiflexes ankle and inverts foot |
| **Extensor hallucis longus** | Middle part of anterior surface of fibula and interosseous membrane | Dorsal aspect of base of distal phalanx of great toe (hallux) | Deep fibular (peroneal) nerve (L5–S1) | Extends great toe and dorsiflexes ankle |
| **Extensor digitorum longus** | Lateral condyle of tibia and superior three fourths of anterior surface of interosseous membrane | Middle and distal phalanges of lateral four digits | | Extends lateral four digits and dorsiflexes ankle |
| **Fibularis (peroneus) tertius** | Inferior third of anterior surface of fibula and interosseus membrane | Dorsum of base of fifth metatarsal | | Dorsiflexes ankle and aids in eversion of foot |

[a]See Table 5.1 for explanation of segmental innervation.

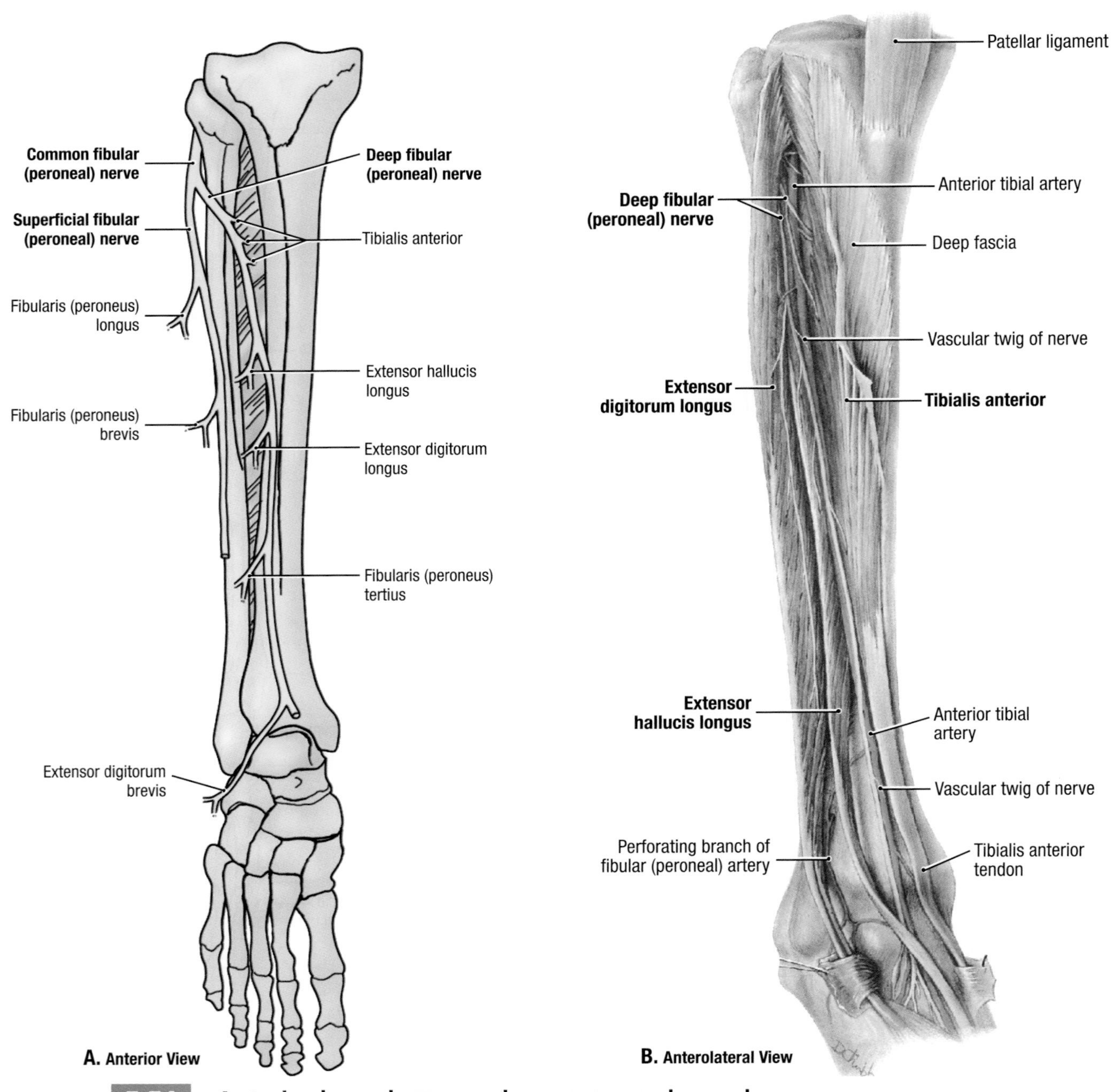
Common fibular (peroneal) nerve
Superficial fibular (peroneal) nerve
Fibularis (peroneus) longus
Fibularis (peroneus) brevis
Extensor digitorum brevis
Deep fibular (peroneal) nerve
Tibialis anterior
Extensor hallucis longus
Extensor digitorum longus
Fibularis (peroneus) tertius
A. Anterior View
Patellar ligament
Anterior tibial artery
Deep fibular (peroneal) nerve
Deep fascia
Vascular twig of nerve
Extensor digitorum longus
Tibialis anterior
Extensor hallucis longus
Anterior tibial artery
Vascular twig of nerve
Perforating branch of fibular (peroneal) artery
Tibialis anterior tendon
B. Anterolateral View

**5.54 Anterior leg—deep muscles, nerves and vessels**

**TABLE 5.10 COMMON, SUPERFICIAL, AND DEEP FIBULAR NERVES**

| Nerve | Origin | Course | Distribution/Structure(s) Supplied |
|---|---|---|---|
| **Common fibular** | Sciatic nerve | Forms as sciatic nerve bifurcates at apex of popliteal fossa and follows medial border of biceps femoris; winds around neck of fibula, dividing into superficial and deep fibular nerves | Skin on lateral part of posterior aspect of leg via the lateral sural nerve; lateral aspect of knee joint via its articular branch |
| **Superficial fibular** | Common fibular nerve | Arises deep to fibularis longus and descends in lateral compartment of leg; pierces crural fascia at distal third of leg to become cutaneous | Fibularis longus and brevis and skin on distal third of anterolateral surface of leg and dorsum of foot |
| **Deep fibular** | Common fibular nerve | Arises deep to fibularis longus; passes through extensor digitorum longus, descends on interosseous membrane, and enters dorsum of foot | Anterior muscles of leg, dorsum of foot, and skin of first interdigital cleft; dorsal aspect of joints crossed via articular branches |

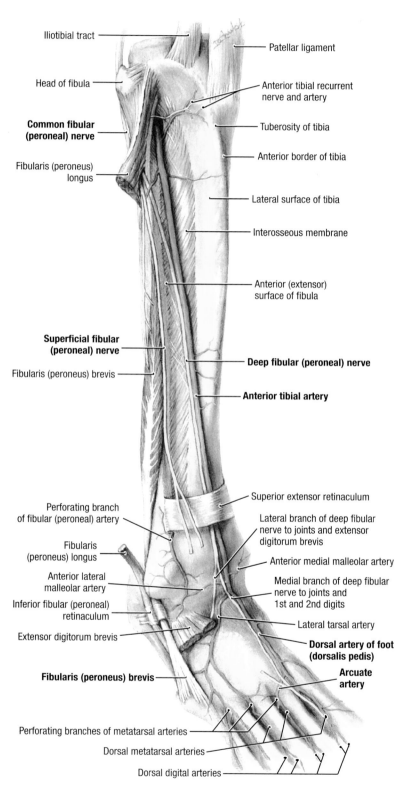

Iliotibial tract
Patellar ligament
Head of fibula
Anterior tibial recurrent nerve and artery
Common fibular (peroneal) nerve
Tuberosity of tibia
Anterior border of tibia
Fibularis (peroneus) longus
Lateral surface of tibia
Interosseous membrane
Anterior (extensor) surface of fibula
Superficial fibular (peroneal) nerve
Deep fibular (peroneal) nerve
Fibularis (peroneus) brevis
Anterior tibial artery
Superior extensor retinaculum
Perforating branch of fibular (peroneal) artery
Lateral branch of deep fibular nerve to joints and extensor digitorum brevis
Fibularis (peroneus) longus
Anterior medial malleolar artery
Anterior lateral malleolar artery
Medial branch of deep fibular nerve to joints and 1st and 2nd digits
Inferior fibular (peroneal) retinaculum
Lateral tarsal artery
Extensor digitorum brevis
Dorsal artery of foot (dorsalis pedis)
Fibularis (peroneus) brevis
Arcuate artery
Perforating branches of metatarsal arteries
Dorsal metatarsal arteries
Dorsal digital arteries

**C. Anterolateral View**

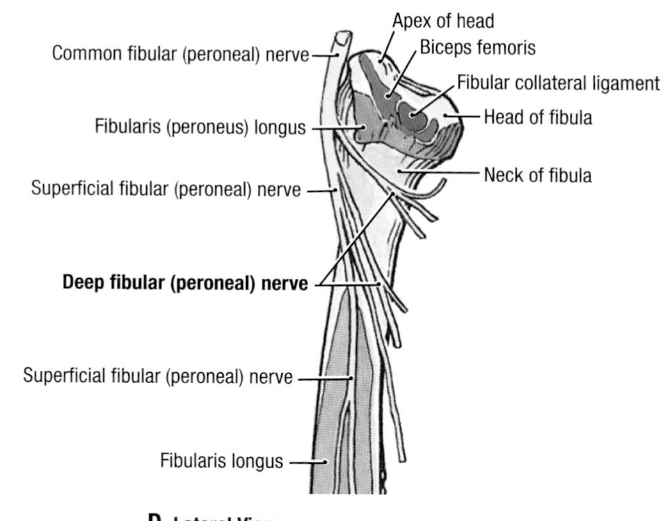
Apex of head
Biceps femoris
Common fibular (peroneal) nerve
Fibular collateral ligament
Head of fibula
Fibularis (peroneus) longus
Neck of fibula
Superficial fibular (peroneal) nerve
Deep fibular (peroneal) nerve
Superficial fibular (peroneal) nerve
Fibularis longus

**D. Lateral View**

## 5.54 Anterior leg—deep muscles, nerves and vessels *(continued)*

**A.** Overview of motor innervation. **B.** Deep dissection of the anterior compartment of the leg. The muscles are separated to display the anterior tibial artery and deep fibular nerve. **C.** Neurovascular structures. **D.** Relations of common fibular nerve and branches to the proximal fibula.

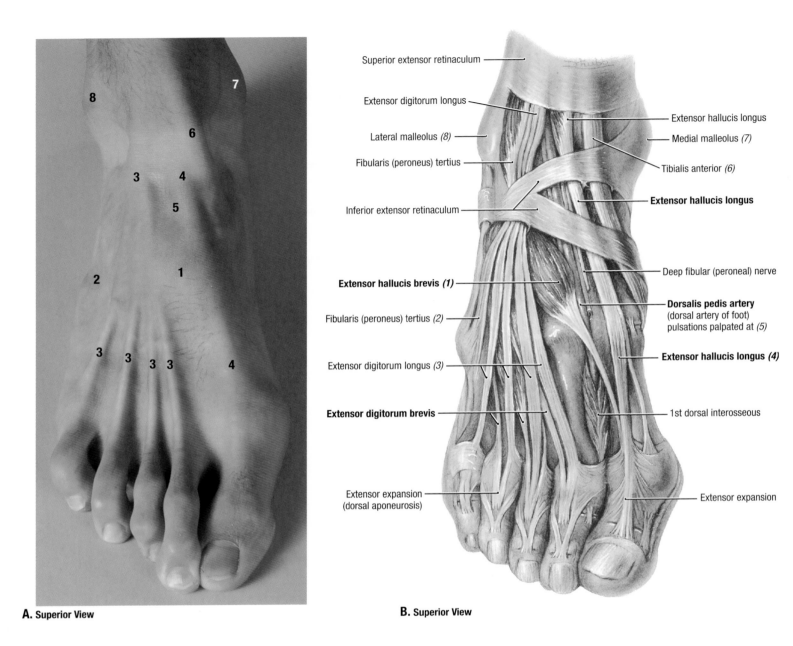

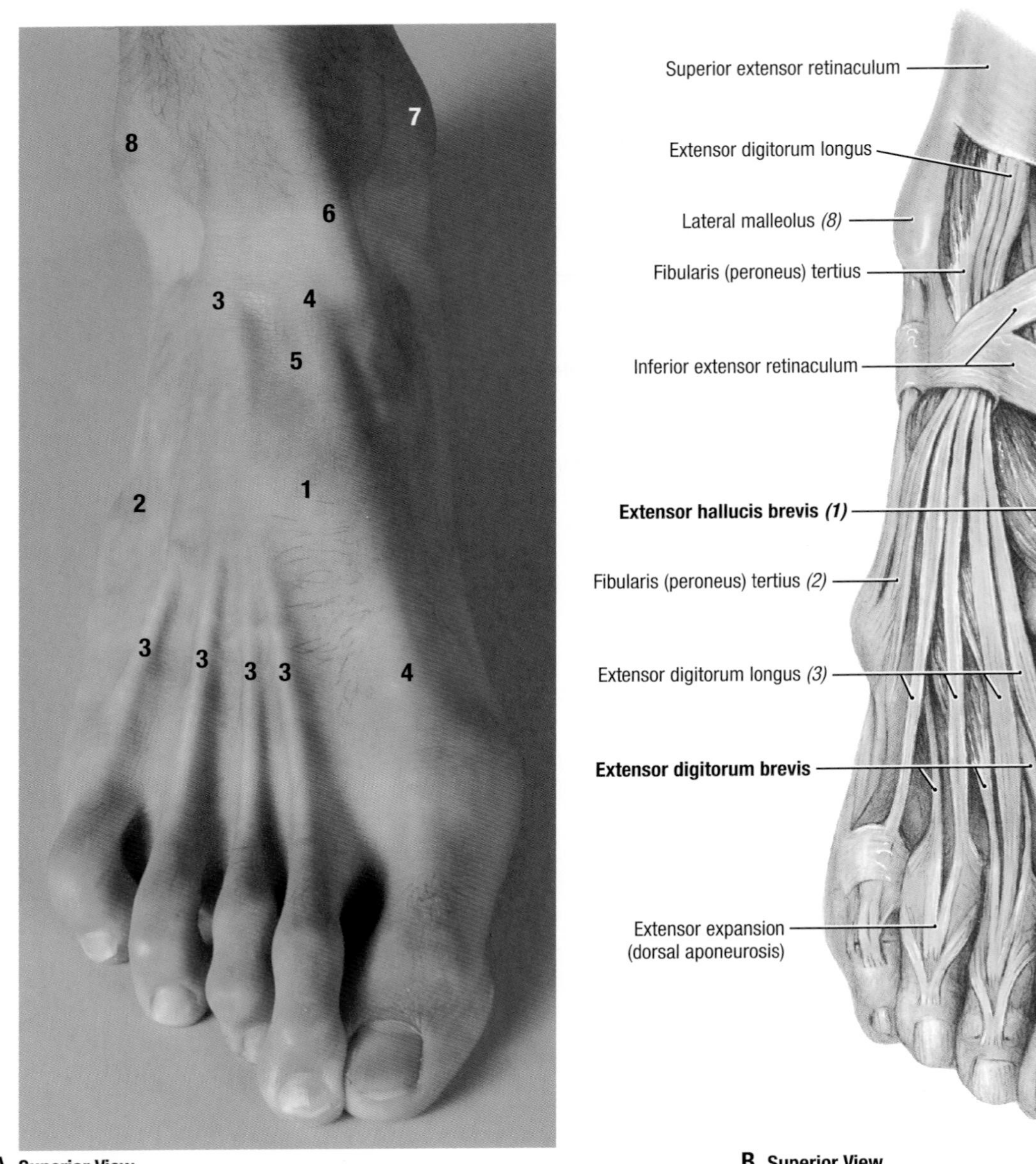
8
7
6
3
4
5
2
1
3
3
3 3
4
Superior extensor retinaculum
Extensor digitorum longus
Lateral malleolus (8)
Fibularis (peroneus) tertius
Inferior extensor retinaculum
Extensor hallucis brevis (1)
Fibularis (peroneus) tertius (2)
Extensor digitorum longus (3)
Extensor digitorum brevis
Extensor expansion
(dorsal aponeurosis)
Extensor hallucis longus
Medial malleolus (7)
Tibialis anterior (6)
Extensor hallucis longus
Deep fibular (peroneal) nerve
Dorsalis pedis artery
(dorsal artery of foot)
pulsations palpated at (5)
Extensor hallucis longus (4)
1st dorsal interosseous
Extensor expansion

**A.** Superior View

**B.** Superior View

## 5.55 Dorsum of foot

**A.** Surface anatomy (*numbers* refer to structures labeled in **B**). **B.** Dissection. The dorsal vein of foot and deep fibular nerve are cut. At the ankle, the dorsalis pedis artery (dorsal artery of foot) and deep fibular nerve lie midway between the malleoli. On the dorsum of the foot, the dorsal artery of foot is crossed by the extensor hallucis brevis muscle and disappears between the two heads of the first dorsal interosseous muscle.

Clinically, knowing the location of the belly of the extensor digitorum brevis is important for distinguishing this muscle from abnormal edema. Contusion and tearing of the muscle fibers and associated blood vessels result in a hematoma, producing edema anteromedial to the lateral malleolus. Most people who have not seen this inflamed muscle assume they have a severely sprained ankle.

Dorsalis pedis pulses may be palpated with the feet slightly dorsiflexed. The pulses are usually easy to palpate because the dorsal arteries of the foot are subcutaneous and pass along a line from the extensor retinaculum to a point just lateral to the extensor hallucis longus tendon. A diminished or absent dorsalis pedis pulse usually suggests vascular insufficiency resulting from arterial disease.

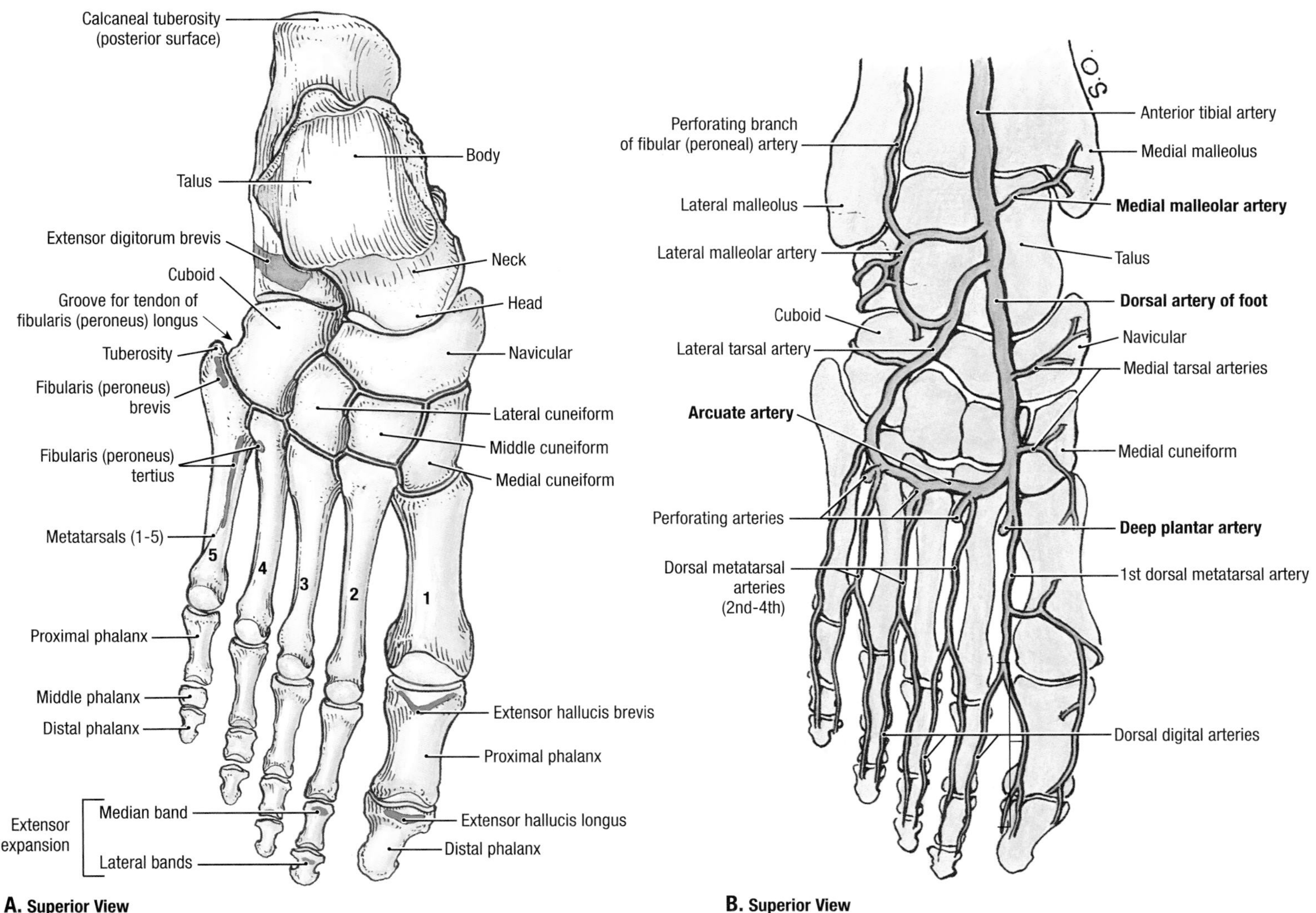
Calcaneal tuberosity (posterior surface)
Talus
Body
Extensor digitorum brevis
Cuboid
Neck
Groove for tendon of fibularis (peroneus) longus
Head
Tuberosity
Navicular
Fibularis (peroneus) brevis
Lateral cuneiform
Middle cuneiform
Fibularis (peroneus) tertius
Medial cuneiform
Metatarsals (1-5)
5
4
3
2
1
Proximal phalanx
Middle phalanx
Distal phalanx
Extensor hallucis brevis
Proximal phalanx
Extensor expansion
Median band
Lateral bands
Extensor hallucis longus
Distal phalanx
A. Superior View
Perforating branch of fibular (peroneal) artery
Anterior tibial artery
Medial malleolus
Lateral malleolus
Medial malleolar artery
Lateral malleolar artery
Talus
Dorsal artery of foot
Cuboid
Navicular
Lateral tarsal artery
Medial tarsal arteries
Arcuate artery
Medial cuneiform
Perforating arteries
Deep plantar artery
Dorsal metatarsal arteries (2nd-4th)
1st dorsal metatarsal artery
Dorsal digital arteries
B. Superior View

**5.56 Attachments of muscles and arteries of the dorsum of foot**

**A.** Attachments. **B.** Arterial supply.

**TABLE 5.11 ARTERIAL SUPPLY TO DORSUM OF FOOT**

| Artery | Origin | Course and Distribution |
|---|---|---|
| **(L. *dorsalis pedis*) Dorsal artery of foot** | Continuation of anterior tibial artery distal to talocrural joint | Descends anteromedially to 1st interosseous space and divides into plantar and arcuate arteries |
| **Lateral tarsal artery** | Dorsal artery of foot | Runs an arched course laterally beneath extensor digitorum brevis to anastomose with branches of arcuate artery |
| **Arcuate artery** | | Runs laterally from 1st interosseous space across bases of lateral four metatarsals, deep to extensor tendons |
| **Deep plantar artery** | | Passes to sole of foot and joins plantar arch |
| **Metatarsal arteries** 1st | Deep plantar artery | Run between metatarsals to clefts of toes where each vessel divides into two dorsal digital arteries. |
| 2nd to 4th | Arcuate artery | Perforating arteries connect to plantar arch and plantar metatarsal arteries. |
| **Dorsal digital arteries** | Metatarsal arteries | Pass to sides of adjoining toes |

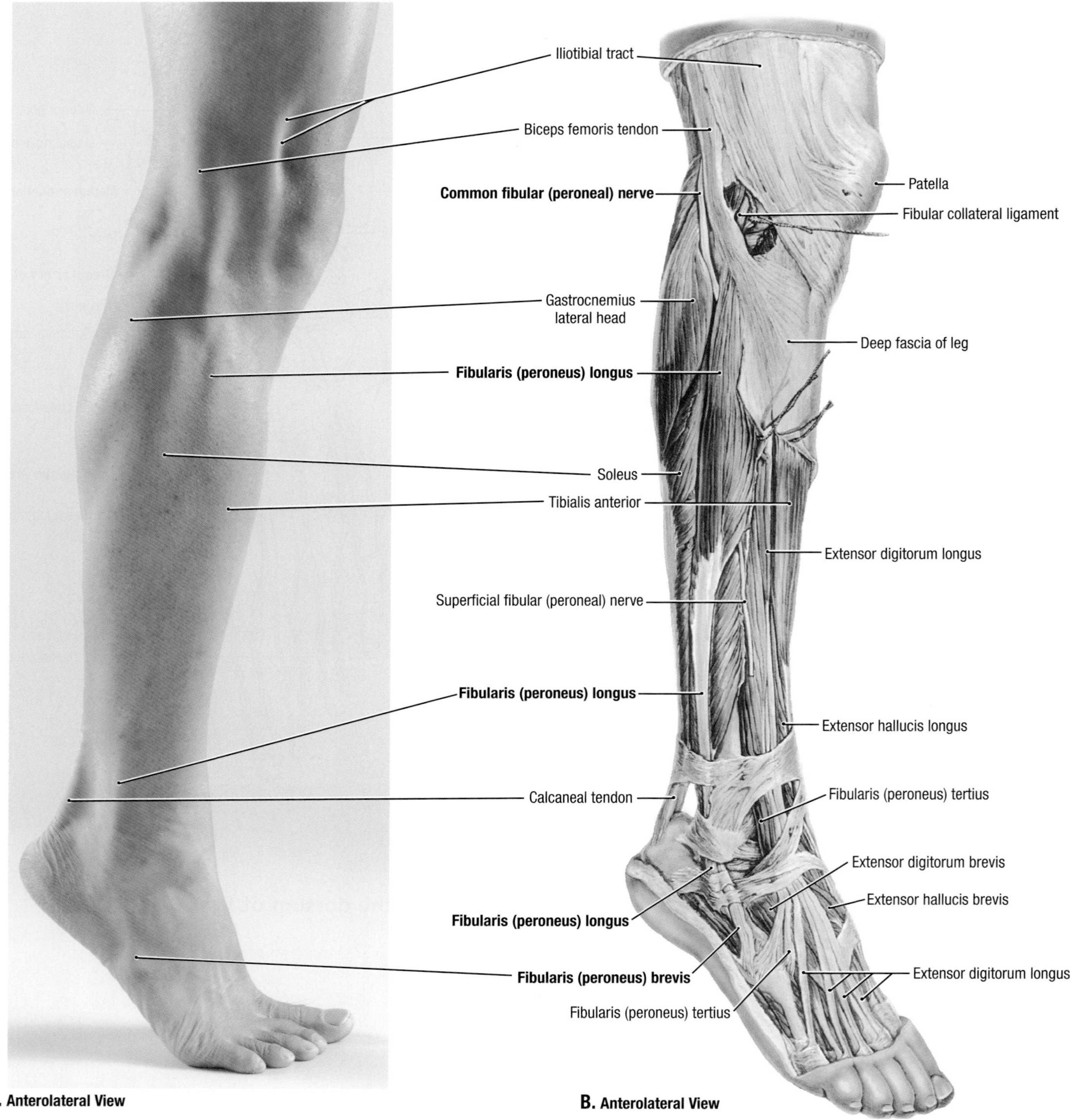
Iliotibial tract
Biceps femoris tendon
Common fibular (peroneal) nerve
Patella
Fibular collateral ligament
Gastrocnemius lateral head
Deep fascia of leg
Fibularis (peroneus) longus
Soleus
Tibialis anterior
Extensor digitorum longus
Superficial fibular (peroneal) nerve
Fibularis (peroneus) longus
Extensor hallucis longus
Calcaneal tendon
Fibularis (peroneus) tertius
Extensor digitorum brevis
Extensor hallucis brevis
Fibularis (peroneus) longus
Fibularis (peroneus) brevis
Extensor digitorum longus
Fibularis (peroneus) tertius
A. Anterolateral View
B. Anterolateral View

## 5.57 Muscles of lateral aspect of leg and foot

**A.** Surface anatomy. **B.** Dissection

- The two fibular (peroneal) muscles both attach to two thirds of the fibula, the fibularis (peroneus) longus muscle to the proximal two thirds, and the fibularis (peroneus) brevis muscle to the distal two thirds. Where they overlap, the fibularis brevis muscle lies anteriorly.
- The fibularis (peroneus) longus muscle enters the foot by hooking around the cuboid and traveling medially to the base of the first metatarsal and medial cuneiform.

The common fibular (peroneal) nerve is in contact with the neck of the fibula deep to the fibularis longus muscle. Here it is vulnerable to injury with serious implications; because it supplies the extensor and everter muscle groups, loss of function results in foot-drop (inability to dorsiflex the ankle) and difficulty in everting the foot.

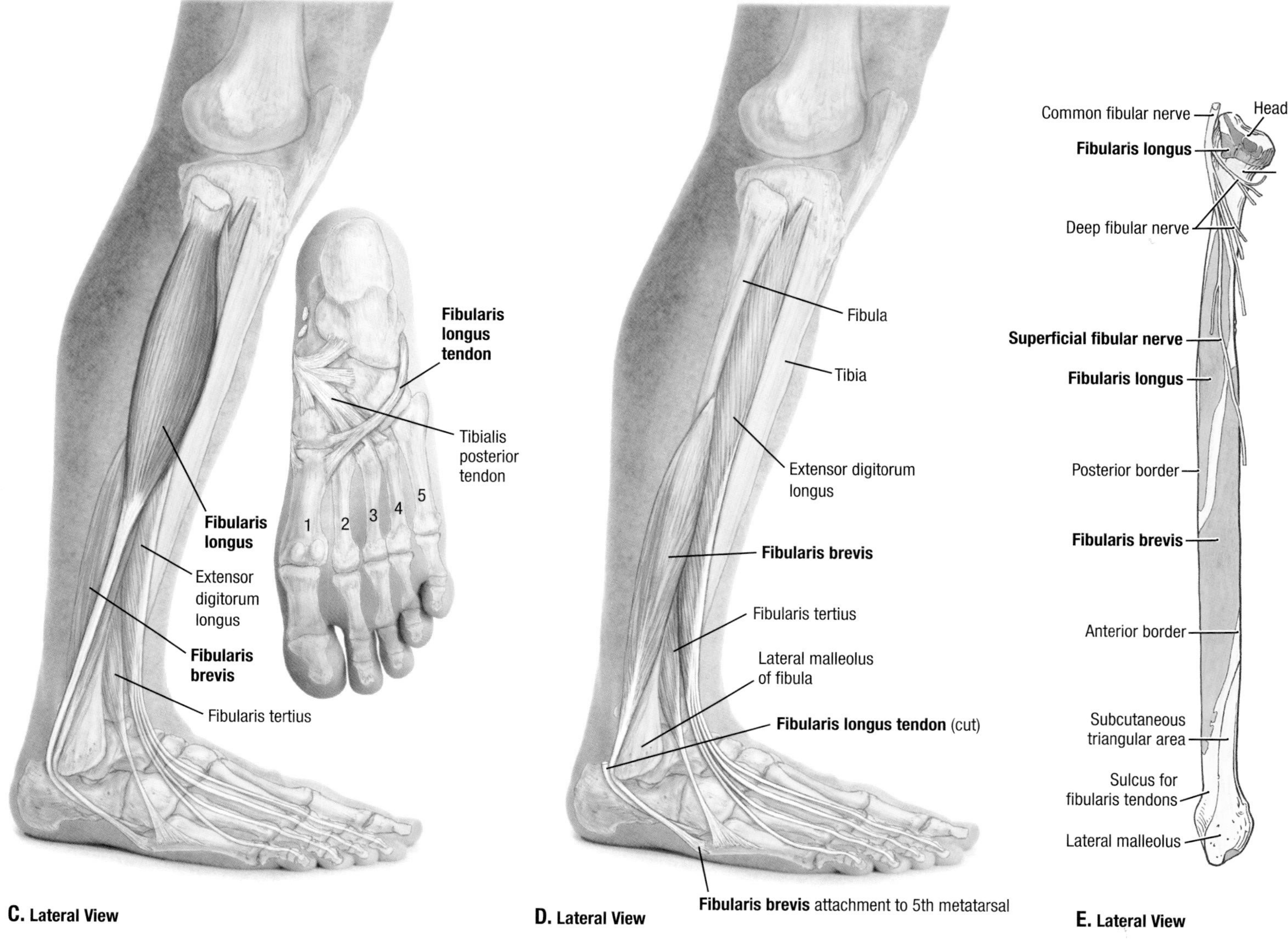
Fibularis longus tendon
Tibialis posterior tendon
1
2
3
4
5
Fibularis longus
Extensor digitorum longus
Fibularis brevis
Fibularis tertius
C. Lateral View
Fibula
Tibia
Extensor digitorum longus
Fibularis brevis
Fibularis tertius
Lateral malleolus of fibula
Fibularis longus tendon (cut)
Fibularis brevis attachment to 5th metatarsal
D. Lateral View
Common fibular nerve
Head
Fibularis longus
Deep fibular nerve
Superficial fibular nerve
Fibularis longus
Posterior border
Fibularis brevis
Anterior border
Subcutaneous triangular area
Sulcus for fibularis tendons
Lateral malleolus
E. Lateral View

**5.57 Muscles of lateral aspect of leg and foot *(continued)***

**C.** Fibularis (peroneus) longus. **D.** Fibularis (peroneus) brevis. **E.** Attachments sites on fibula.

**TABLE 5.12 MUSCLES OF THE LATERAL COMPARTMENT OF LEG**

| Muscle | Proximal Attachment | Distal Attachment | Innervation[a] | Main Actions |
|---|---|---|---|---|
| **Fibularis (peroneus) longus** | Head and superior two thirds of lateral surface of fibula | Base of first metatarsal and medial cuneiform | Superficial fibular (peroneal) nerve (**L5, S1,** and **S2**) | Evert foot and weakly plantarflex ankle |
| **Fibularis (peroneus) brevis** | Inferior two thirds of lateral surface of fibula | Dorsal surface of tuberosity on lateral side of base of fifth metatarsal | | |

[a]See Table 5.1 for explanation of segmental innervation

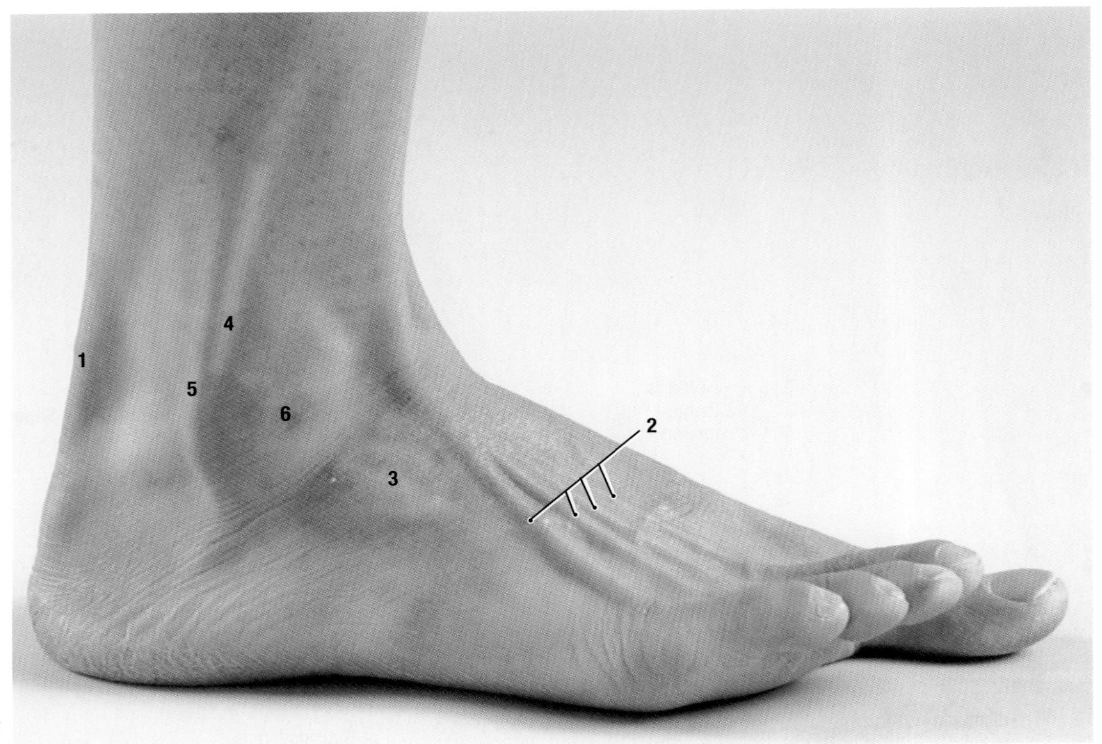
4
1
5
6
2
3

**A.** Lateral View

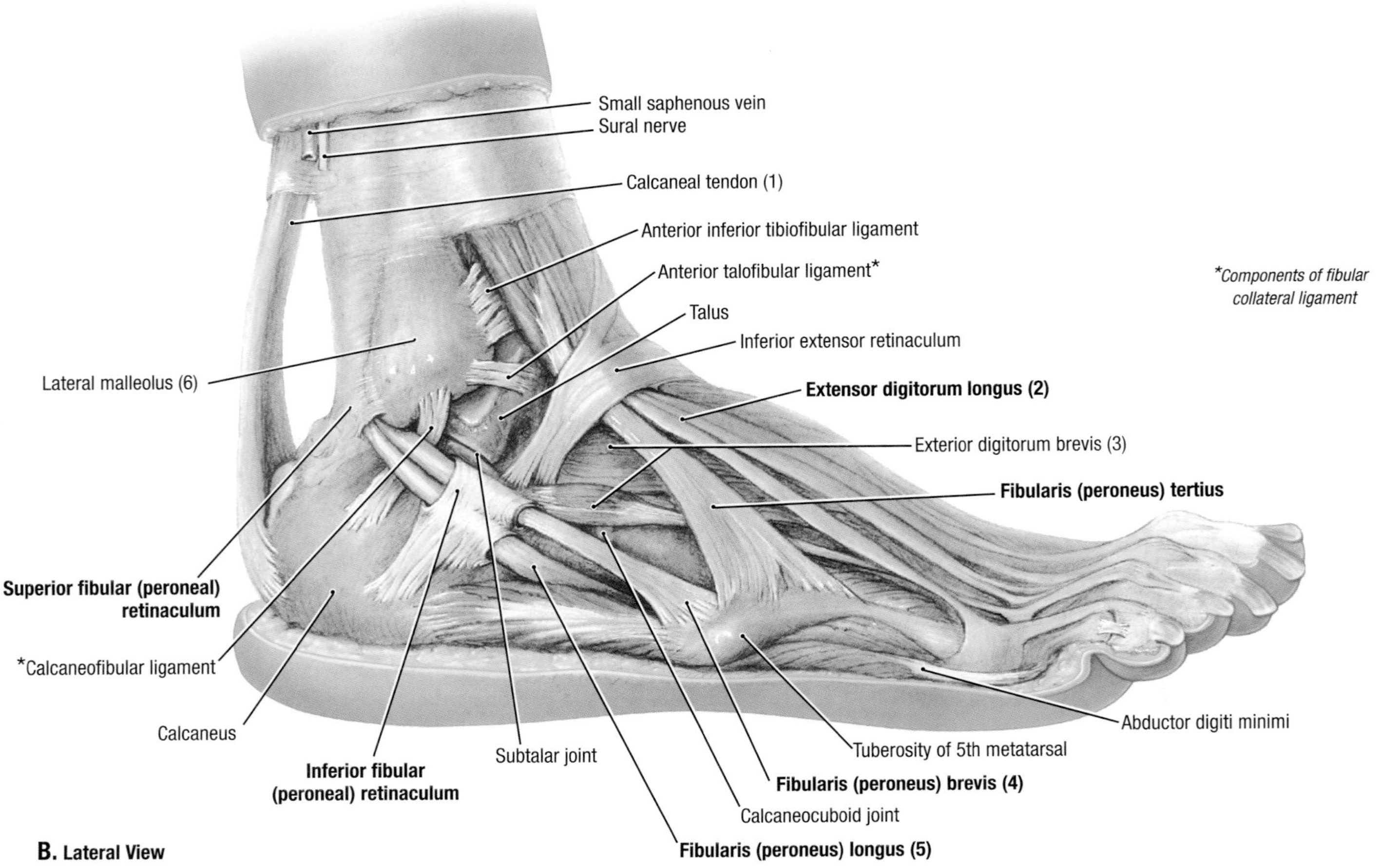

Small saphenous vein
Sural nerve
Calcaneal tendon (1)
Anterior inferior tibiofibular ligament
Anterior talofibular ligament*
Talus
Inferior extensor retinaculum
Lateral malleolus (6)
**Extensor digitorum longus (2)**
Exterior digitorum brevis (3)
**Fibularis (peroneus) tertius**
**Superior fibular (peroneal) retinaculum**
*Calcaneofibular ligament
Calcaneus
Abductor digiti minimi
Tuberosity of 5th metatarsal
Subtalar joint
**Inferior fibular (peroneal) retinaculum**
**Fibularis (peroneus) brevis (4)**
Calcaneocuboid joint
**Fibularis (peroneus) longus (5)**

**Components of fibular collateral ligament*

**B.** Lateral View

## 5.58 Synovial sheaths and tendons at ankle

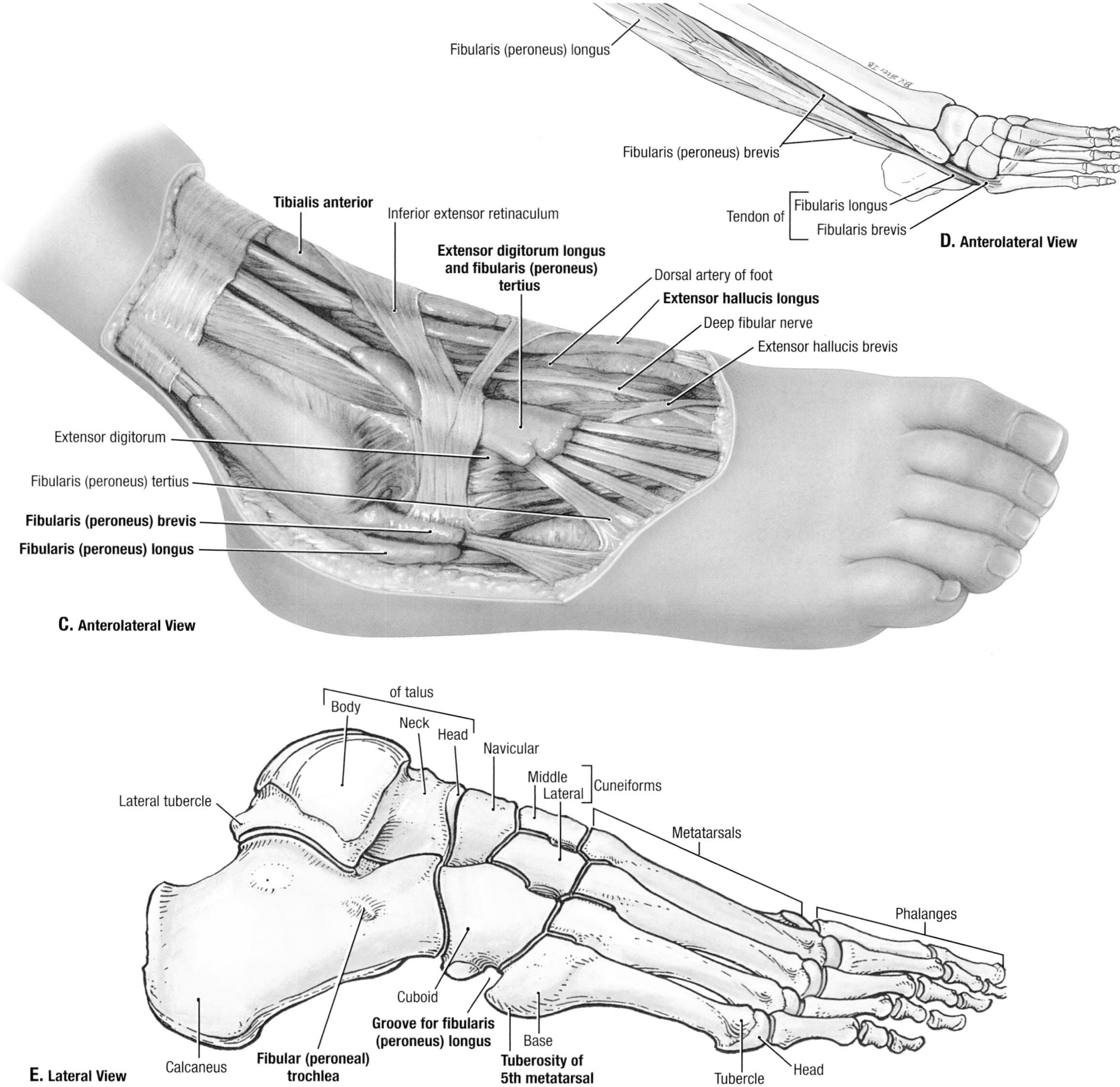
Fibularis (peroneus) longus
Fibularis (peroneus) brevis
Tendon of
Fibularis longus
Fibularis brevis
D. Anterolateral View
Tibialis anterior
Inferior extensor retinaculum
Extensor digitorum longus and fibularis (peroneus) tertius
Dorsal artery of foot
Extensor hallucis longus
Deep fibular nerve
Extensor hallucis brevis
Extensor digitorum
Fibularis (peroneus) tertius
Fibularis (peroneus) brevis
Fibularis (peroneus) longus
C. Anterolateral View
of talus
Body
Neck
Head
Navicular
Middle
Lateral
Cuneiforms
Lateral tubercle
Metatarsals
Phalanges
Cuboid
Groove for fibularis (peroneus) longus
Base
Tuberosity of 5th metatarsal
Calcaneus
Fibular (peroneal) trochlea
Tubercle
Head
E. Lateral View

## 5.58 Synovial sheaths and tendons at ankle *(continued)*

**A.** Surface anatomy (*numbers* refer to structures labeled in **B**). **B.** Tendons at the lateral aspect of the ankle. **C.** Synovial sheaths of tendons on the anterolateral aspect of the ankle. The tendons of the fibularis (peroneus) longus and fibularis (peroneus) brevis muscles are enclosed in a common synovial sheath posterior to the lateral malleolus. This sheath splits into two, one for each tendon, posterior to the fibular (peroneal) trochlea. **D.** Schematic illustration of fibularis longus and brevis. **E.** Lateral aspect of bones of foot.

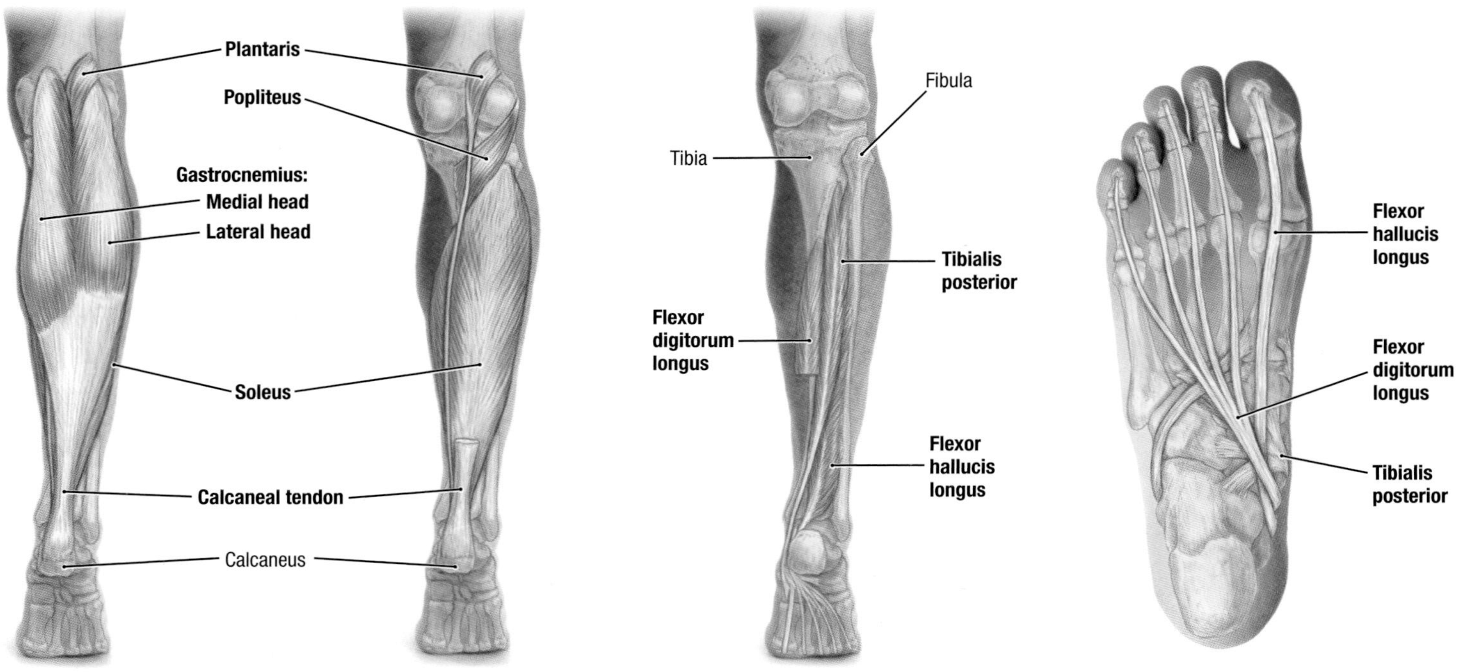
Plantaris
Popliteus
Gastrocnemius:
Medial head
Lateral head
Soleus
Calcaneal tendon
Calcaneus
Fibula
Tibia
Tibialis posterior
Flexor digitorum longus
Flexor hallucis longus
Flexor hallucis longus
Flexor digitorum longus
Tibialis posterior

## TABLE 5.13 MUSCLES OF THE POSTERIOR COMPARTMENT OF LEG

| Muscle | Proximal Attachment | Distal Attachment | Innervation[a] | Main Actions |
|---|---|---|---|---|
| **Superficial muscles** | | | | |
| Gastrocnemius | *Lateral head:* lateral aspect of lateral condyle of femur<br>*Medial head:* popliteal surface of femur, superior to medial condyle to medial condyle | | | Plantarflexes ankle when knee is extended; raises heel during walking, and flexes leg at knee joint |
| Soleus | Posterior aspect of head of fibula, superior fourth of posterior surface of fibula, soleal lne and medial border of tibia | Posterior surface of calcaneus with calcaneal tendon (tendocalcaneus) | Tibial nerve (S1 and S2) | Plantarflexes ankle (independent of knee position) and steadies leg on foot |
| Plantaris | Inferior end of lateral supracondylar supracondylar line of femur and oblique popliteal ligament | | | Weakly assists gastrocnemius in plantarflexing ankle and flexing knee |
| **Deep muscles** | | | | |
| Popliteus | Lateral surface of lateral condyle of femur and lateral meniscus | Posterior surface of tibia, superior to soleal line | Tibial nerve (**L4,** L5, and S1) | Unlocks fully extended knee (laterally rotates femur 5° on planted tibia); weakly flexes knee |
| Flexor hallucis longus | Inferior two thirds of posterior surface of fibula and inferior part of interosseous membrane | Base of distal phalanx of great toe (hallux) | | Flexes great toe at all joints and plantarflexes ankle; supports medial longitudinal arch of foot |
| Flexor digitorum longus | Medial part of posterior surface of tibia inferior to soleal line, and by a broad tendon to fibula | Bases of distal phalanges of lateral four digits | Tibial nerve (**S2** and S3) | Flexes lateral four digits and plantarflexes ankle; supports longitudinal arches of foot |
| Tibialis posterior | Interosseous membrane, posterior surface of tibia inferior to soleal line and posterior surface of fibula | Tuberosity of navicular, cuneiform, and cuboid and bases of metatarsals 2–4 | Tibial nerve (L4 and L5) | Plantarflexes ankle and inverts foot |

[a]See Table 5.1 for explanation of segmental innervation.

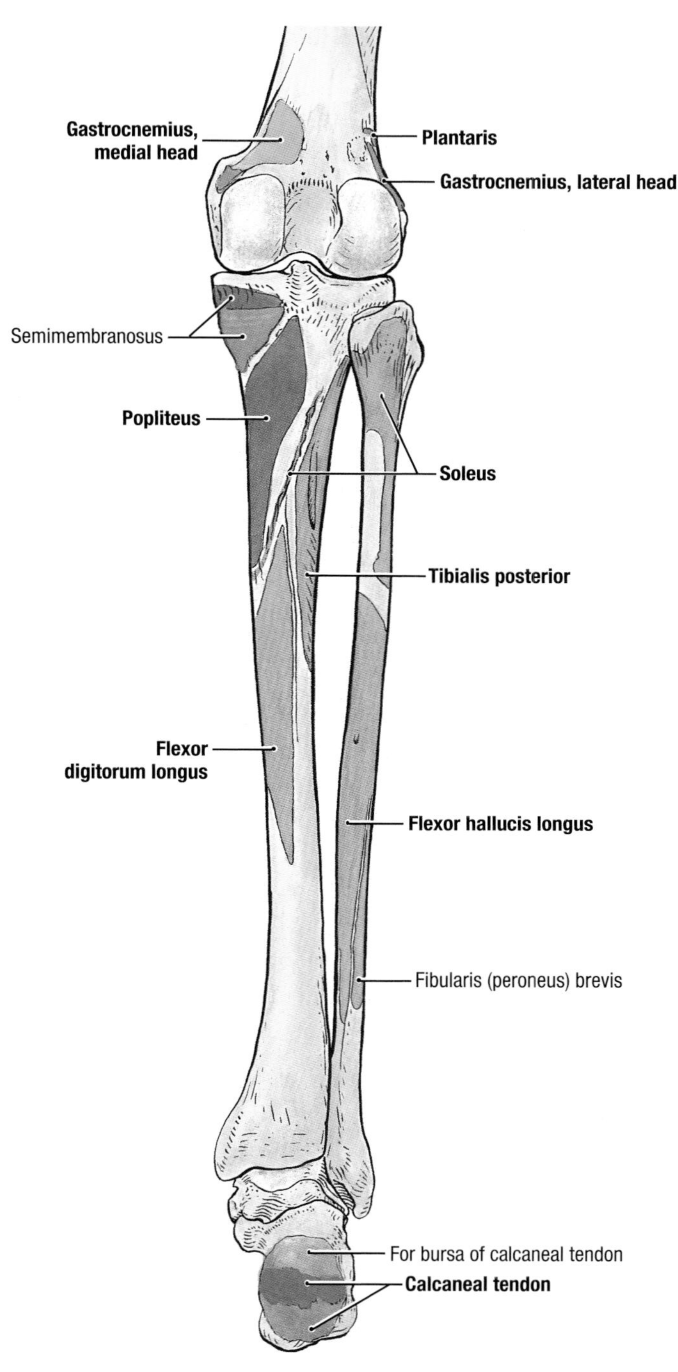
Gastrocnemius, medial head
Plantaris
Gastrocnemius, lateral head
Semimembranosus
Popliteus
Soleus
Tibialis posterior
Flexor digitorum longus
Flexor hallucis longus
Fibularis (peroneus) brevis
For bursa of calcaneal tendon
Calcaneal tendon

**A.** Posterior View

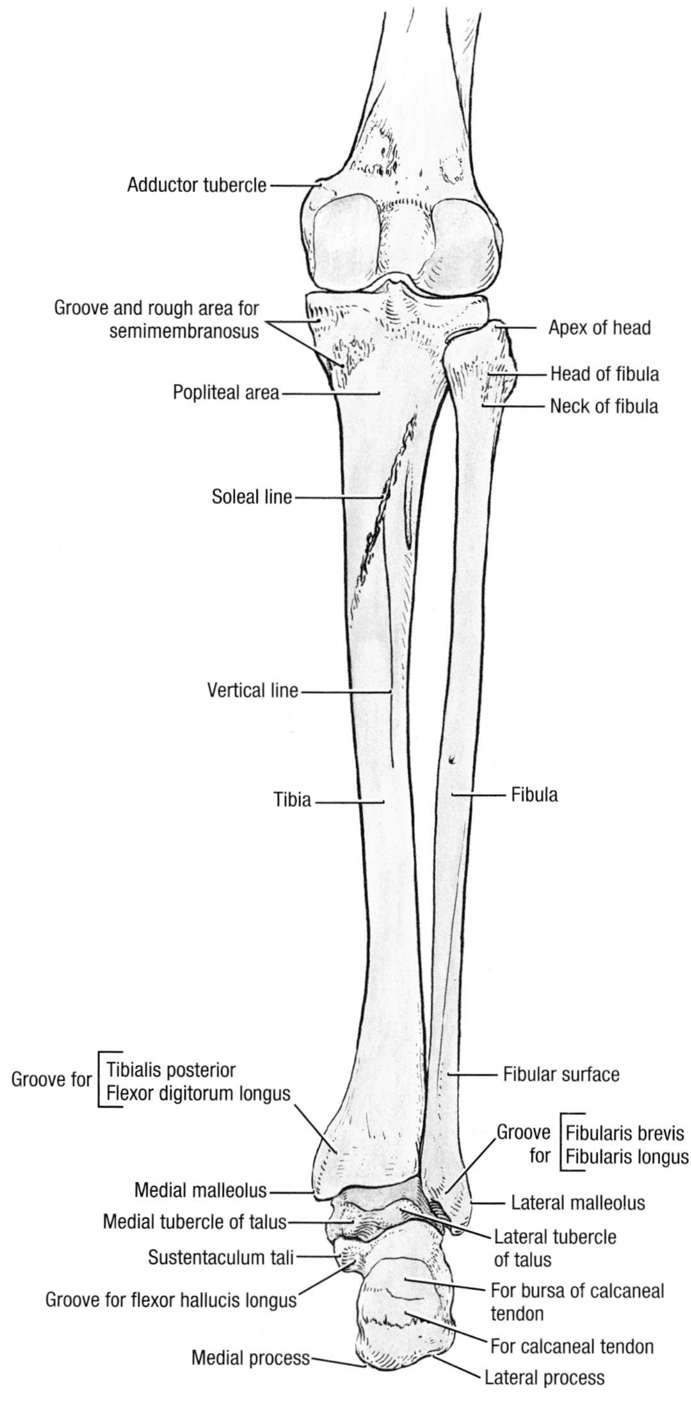
Adductor tubercle
Groove and rough area for semimembranosus
Apex of head
Head of fibula
Neck of fibula
Popliteal area
Soleal line
Vertical line
Tibia
Fibula
Groove for
Tibialis posterior
Flexor digitorum longus
Fibular surface
Groove for
Fibularis brevis
Fibularis longus
Medial malleolus
Lateral malleolus
Medial tubercle of talus
Lateral tubercle of talus
Sustentaculum tali
Groove for flexor hallucis longus
For bursa of calcaneal tendon
For calcaneal tendon
Medial process
Lateral process

**B.** Posterior View

## 5.59 Bones of the posterior aspect of leg

**A.** Muscle attachments. **B.** Features of bones.

The tibial shaft is narrowest at the junction of its middle and inferior thirds, which is the most frequent site of fracture. Unfortunately, this area of the bone also has the poorest blood supply.

Fibular fractures commonly occur 2–6 cm proximal to the distal end of the lateral malleolus and are often associated with fracture/dislocations of the ankle joint, which are combined with tibial fractures. When a person slips and the foot is forced into an excessively inverted position, the ankle ligaments tear, forcibly tilting the talus against the lateral malleolus and shearing it off.

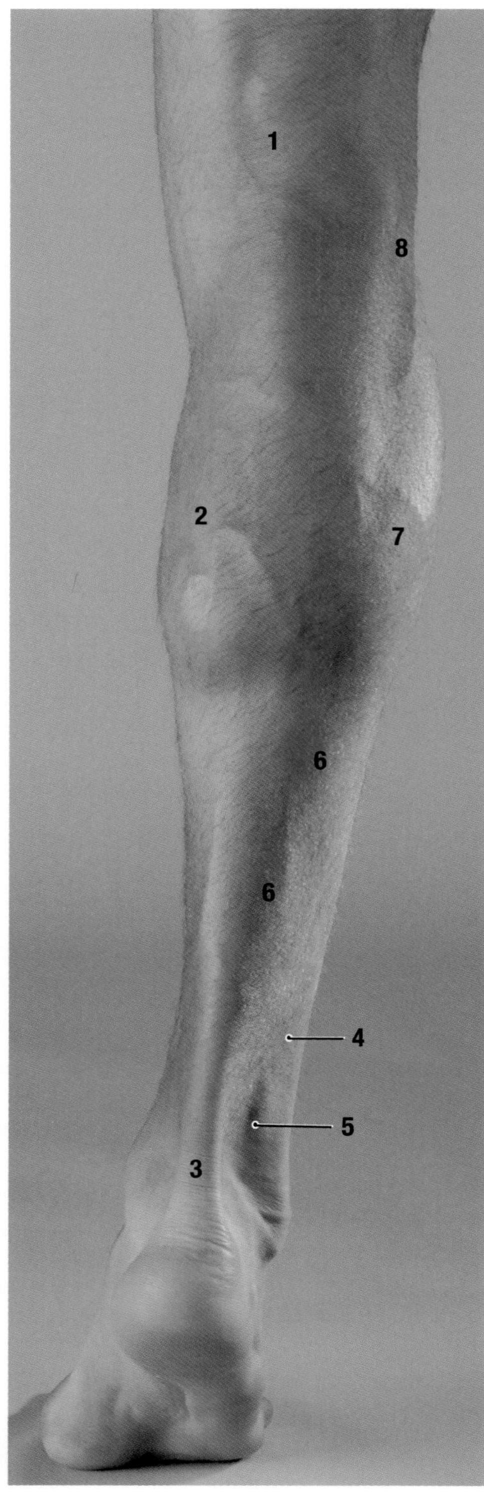
1
8
2
7
6
6
4
5
3

**A.** Posterior View

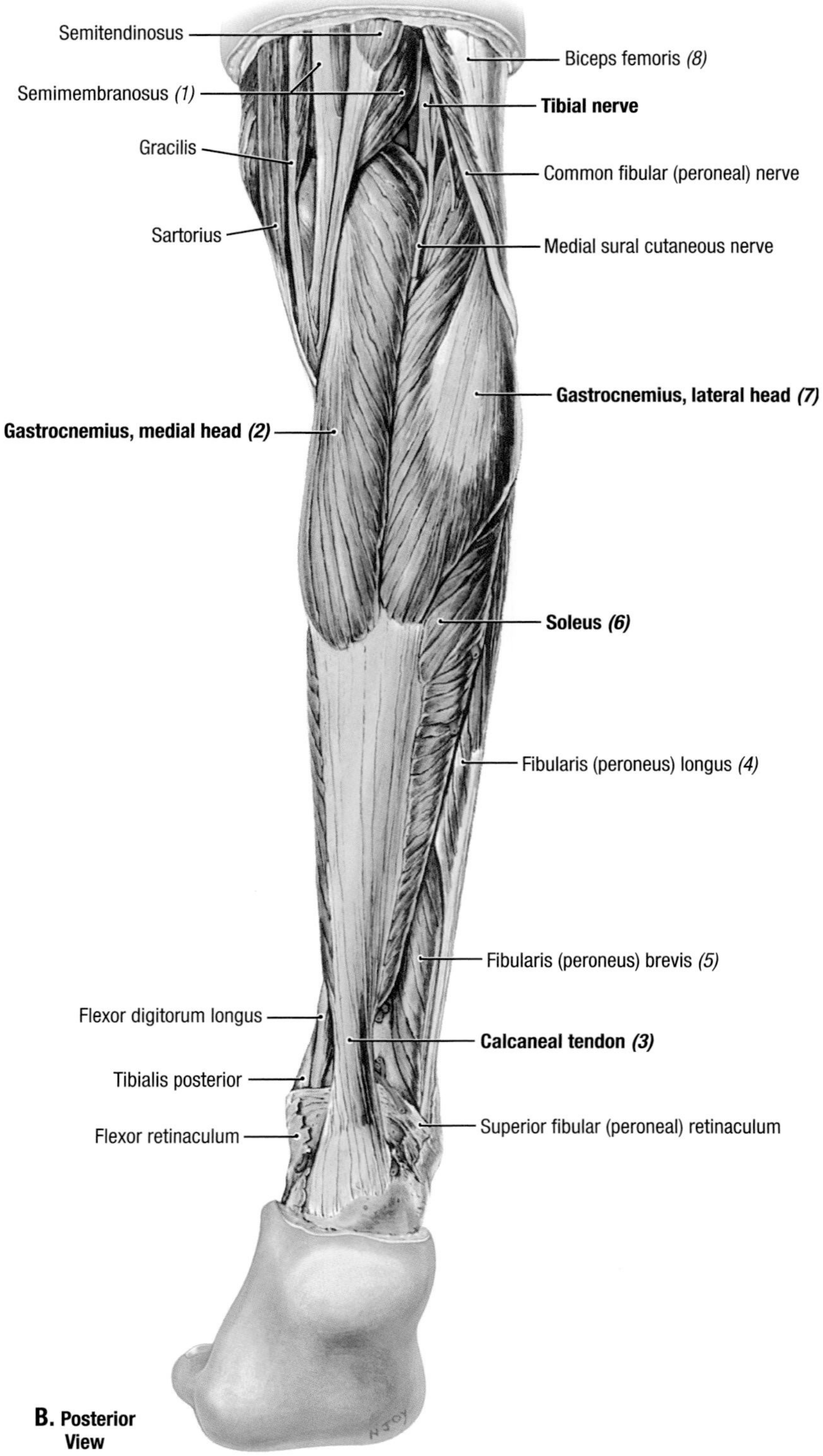

Semitendinosus
Biceps femoris *(8)*
Semimembranosus *(1)*
**Tibial nerve**
Gracilis
Common fibular (peroneal) nerve
Sartorius
Medial sural cutaneous nerve
**Gastrocnemius, lateral head *(7)***
**Gastrocnemius, medial head *(2)***
**Soleus *(6)***
Fibularis (peroneus) longus *(4)*
Fibularis (peroneus) brevis *(5)*
Flexor digitorum longus
**Calcaneal tendon *(3)***
Tibialis posterior
Flexor retinaculum
Superior fibular (peroneal) retinaculum
N JOY

**B.** Posterior View

## 5.60 Posterior leg, superficial muscles of posterior compartment

**A.** Surface anatomy (*numbers* refer to structures labeled in **B**). **B.** Dissection. Gastrocnemius strain (tennis leg) is a painful calf injury resulting from partial tearing of the medial belly of the muscle at or near its musculotendinous junction. It is caused by overstretching the muscle during simultaneous full extension of the knee and dorsiflexion of the ankle.

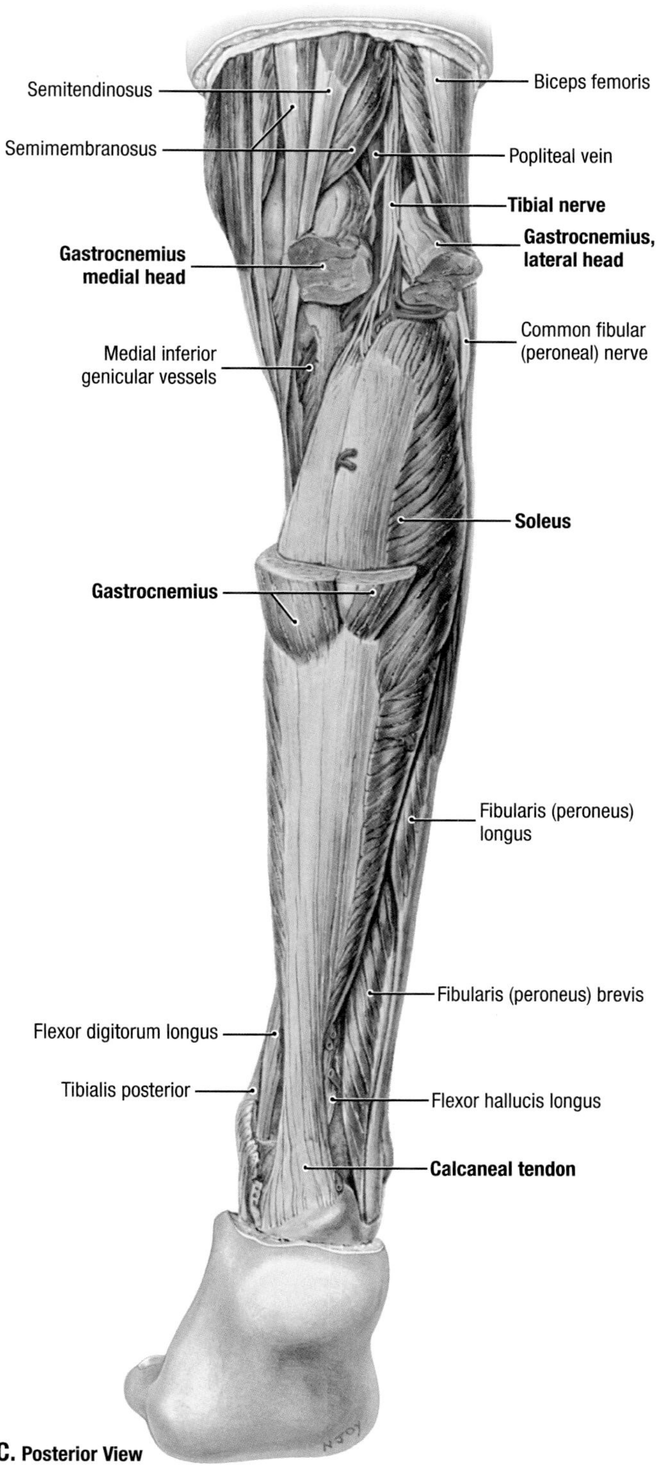
Semitendinosus
Biceps femoris
Semimembranosus
Popliteal vein
Tibial nerve
Gastrocnemius medial head
Gastrocnemius, lateral head
Common fibular (peroneal) nerve
Medial inferior genicular vessels
Soleus
Gastrocnemius
Fibularis (peroneus) longus
Fibularis (peroneus) brevis
Flexor digitorum longus
Tibialis posterior
Flexor hallucis longus
Calcaneal tendon

C. Posterior View

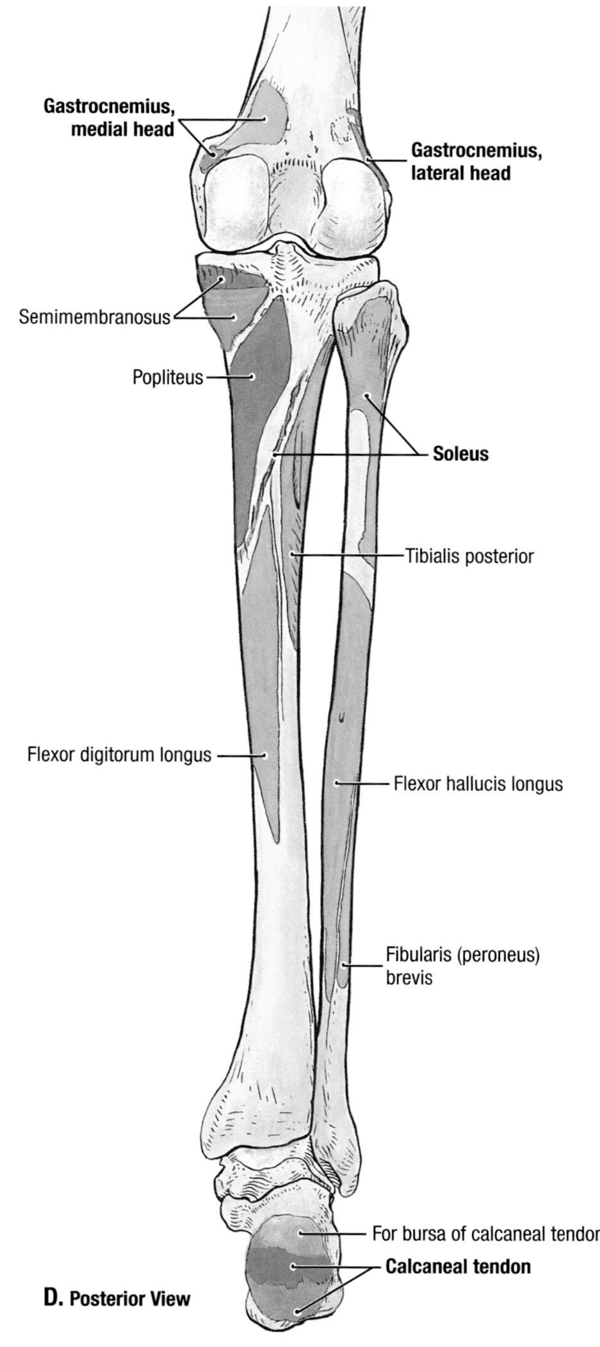
Gastrocnemius, medial head
Gastrocnemius, lateral head
Semimembranosus
Popliteus
Soleus
Tibialis posterior
Flexor digitorum longus
Flexor hallucis longus
Fibularis (peroneus) brevis
For bursa of calcaneal tendon
Calcaneal tendon

D. Posterior View

**5.60 Posterior leg, superficial muscles of posterior compartment *(continued)***

**C.** Dissection revealing soleus. **D.** Bones of leg showing muscle attachments. Inflammation of the calcaneal tendon due to microscopic tears of collagen fibers in the tendon, particularly just superior to its attachment to the calcaneus, results in tendinitis, which causes pain during walking. Calcaneal tendon rupture is probably the most severe acute muscular problem of the leg. Following complete rupture of the tendon, passive dorsiflexion is excessive, and the person cannot plantarflex against resistance.

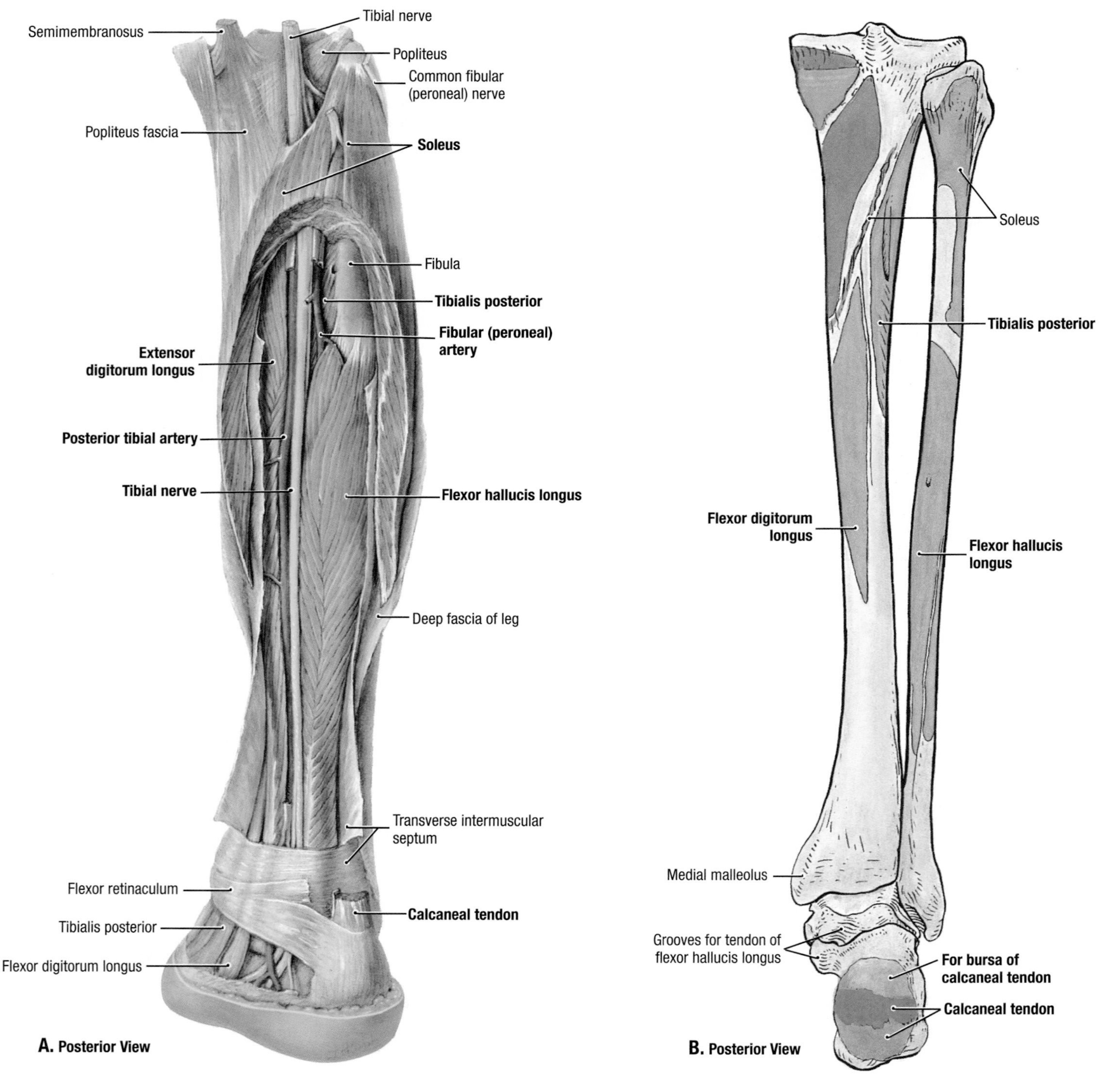
Semimembranosus
Tibial nerve
Popliteus
Common fibular (peroneal) nerve
Popliteus fascia
Soleus
Fibula
Tibialis posterior
Fibular (peroneal) artery
Extensor digitorum longus
Posterior tibial artery
Tibial nerve
Flexor hallucis longus
Deep fascia of leg
Transverse intermuscular septum
Flexor retinaculum
Calcaneal tendon
Tibialis posterior
Flexor digitorum longus
A. Posterior View
Soleus
Tibialis posterior
Flexor digitorum longus
Flexor hallucis longus
Medial malleolus
Grooves for tendon of flexor hallucis longus
For bursa of calcaneal tendon
Calcaneal tendon
B. Posterior View

## 5.61 Posterior leg, deep muscles of posterior compartment

**A.** Superficial dissection. The calcaneal tendon (Achilles tendon) is cut, the gastrocnemius muscle is removed, and only a horseshoe-shaped proximal part of the soleus muscle remains in place. **B.** Bones of leg showing muscle attachments. Calcaneal bursitis results from inflammation of the bursa of the calcaneal tendon located between the calcaneal tendon and the superior part of the posterior surface of the calcaneus. Calcaneal bursitis causes pain posterior to the heel and occurs commonly during long-distance running, basketball, and tennis. It is caused by excessive friction on the bursa as the calcaneal tendon continuously slides over it.

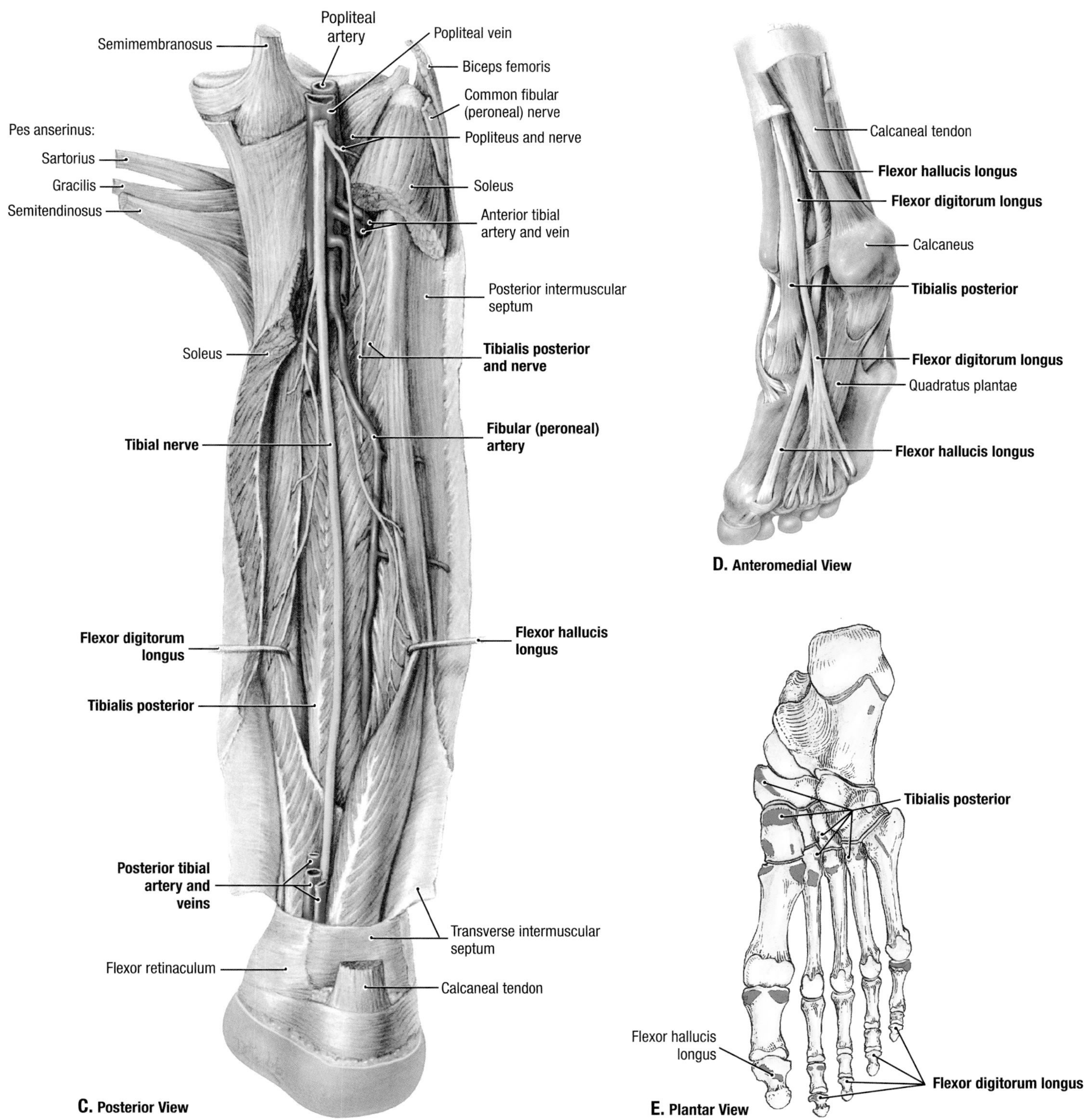
Semimembranosus
Popliteal artery
Popliteal vein
Biceps femoris
Common fibular (peroneal) nerve
Pes anserinus:
Sartorius
Gracilis
Semitendinosus
Popliteus and nerve
Soleus
Anterior tibial artery and vein
Posterior intermuscular septum
Soleus
Tibialis posterior and nerve
Tibial nerve
Fibular (peroneal) artery
Flexor digitorum longus
Flexor hallucis longus
Tibialis posterior
Posterior tibial artery and veins
Transverse intermuscular septum
Flexor retinaculum
Calcaneal tendon
C. Posterior View
Calcaneal tendon
Flexor hallucis longus
Flexor digitorum longus
Calcaneus
Tibialis posterior
Flexor digitorum longus
Quadratus plantae
Flexor hallucis longus
D. Anteromedial View
Tibialis posterior
Flexor hallucis longus
Flexor digitorum longus
E. Plantar View

## 5.61 Posterior leg, deep muscles of posterior compartment *(continued)*

**C.** Deeper dissection. The flexor hallucis longus and flexor digitorum longus are pulled apart, and the posterior tibial artery is partly excised. The tibialis posterior lies deep to the two long digital flexors. **D.** Crossing of muscles (tendons) of the deep compartment superoposterior to the medial malleolus and into the sole of the foot. **E.** Bones of foot showing muscle attachments.

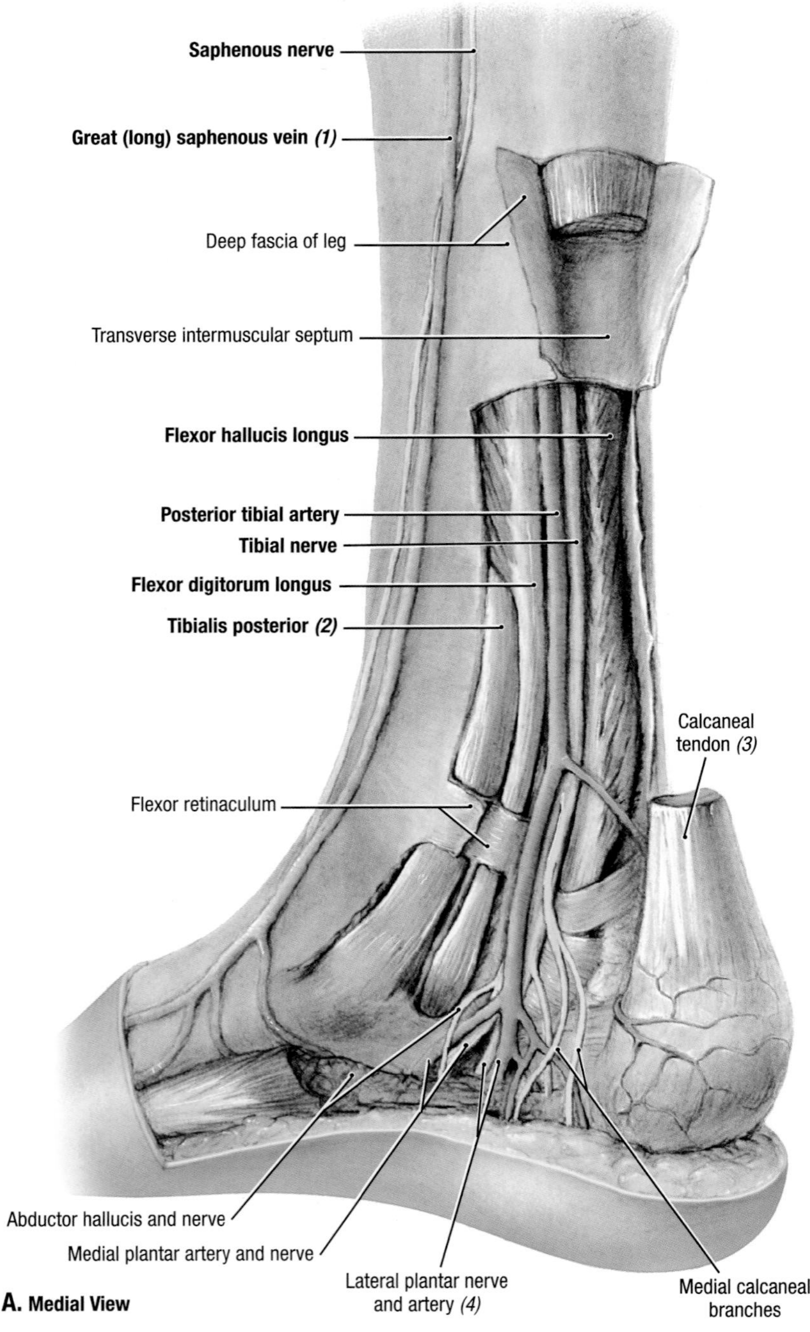
Saphenous nerve
Great (long) saphenous vein (1)
Deep fascia of leg
Transverse intermuscular septum
Flexor hallucis longus
Posterior tibial artery
Tibial nerve
Flexor digitorum longus
Tibialis posterior (2)
Calcaneal tendon (3)
Flexor retinaculum
Abductor hallucis and nerve
Medial plantar artery and nerve
Lateral plantar nerve and artery (4)
Medial calcaneal branches

A. Medial View

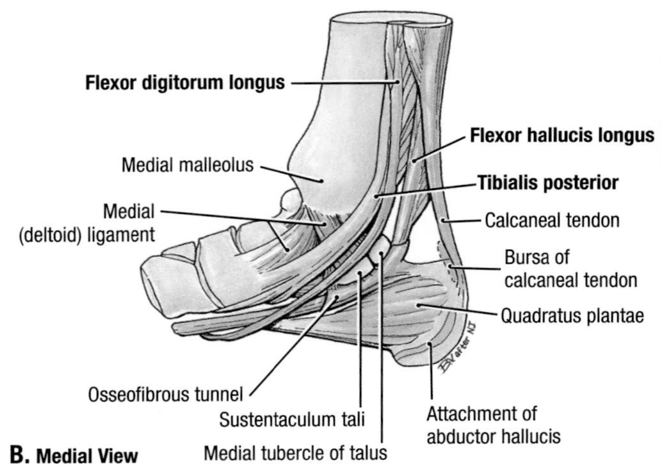
Flexor digitorum longus
Flexor hallucis longus
Medial malleolus
Tibialis posterior
Medial (deltoid) ligament
Calcaneal tendon
Bursa of calcaneal tendon
Quadratus plantae
Osseofibrous tunnel
Sustentaculum tali
Attachment of abductor hallucis
Medial tubercle of talus

B. Medial View

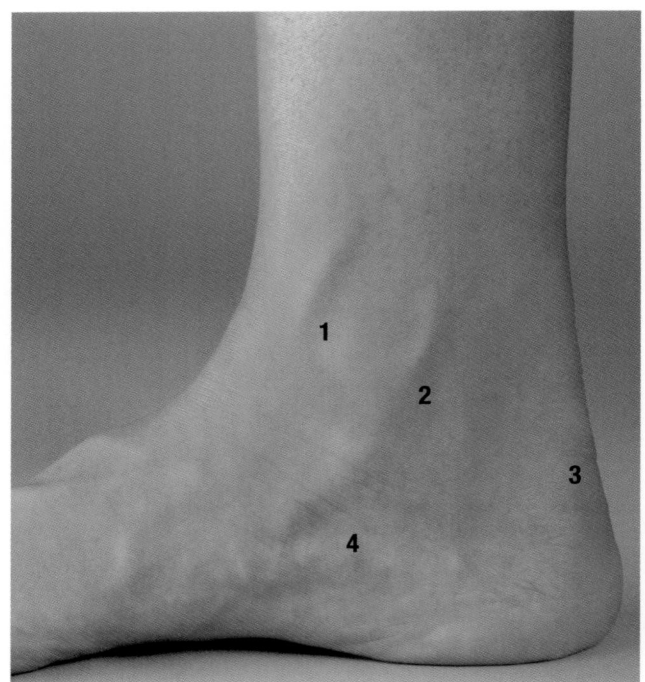
1
2
3
4

C. Medial View

## 5.62 Medial ankle region

**A.** Dissection. The calcaneal tendon and posterior part of the abductor hallucis were excised. **B.** Schematic illustration of the tendons passing posterior to medial malleolus. **C.** Surface anatomy (*numbers* refer to structures labeled in **A**).

- The posterior tibial artery and the tibial nerve lie between the flexor digitorum longus and flexor hallucis longus muscles and divide into medial and lateral plantar branches.
- The tibialis posterior and flexor digitorum longus tendons occupy separate osseofibrous tunnels posterior to the medial malleolus.
- The posterior tibial pulse can usually be palpated between the posterior surface of the medial malleolus and the medial border of the calcaneal tendon.

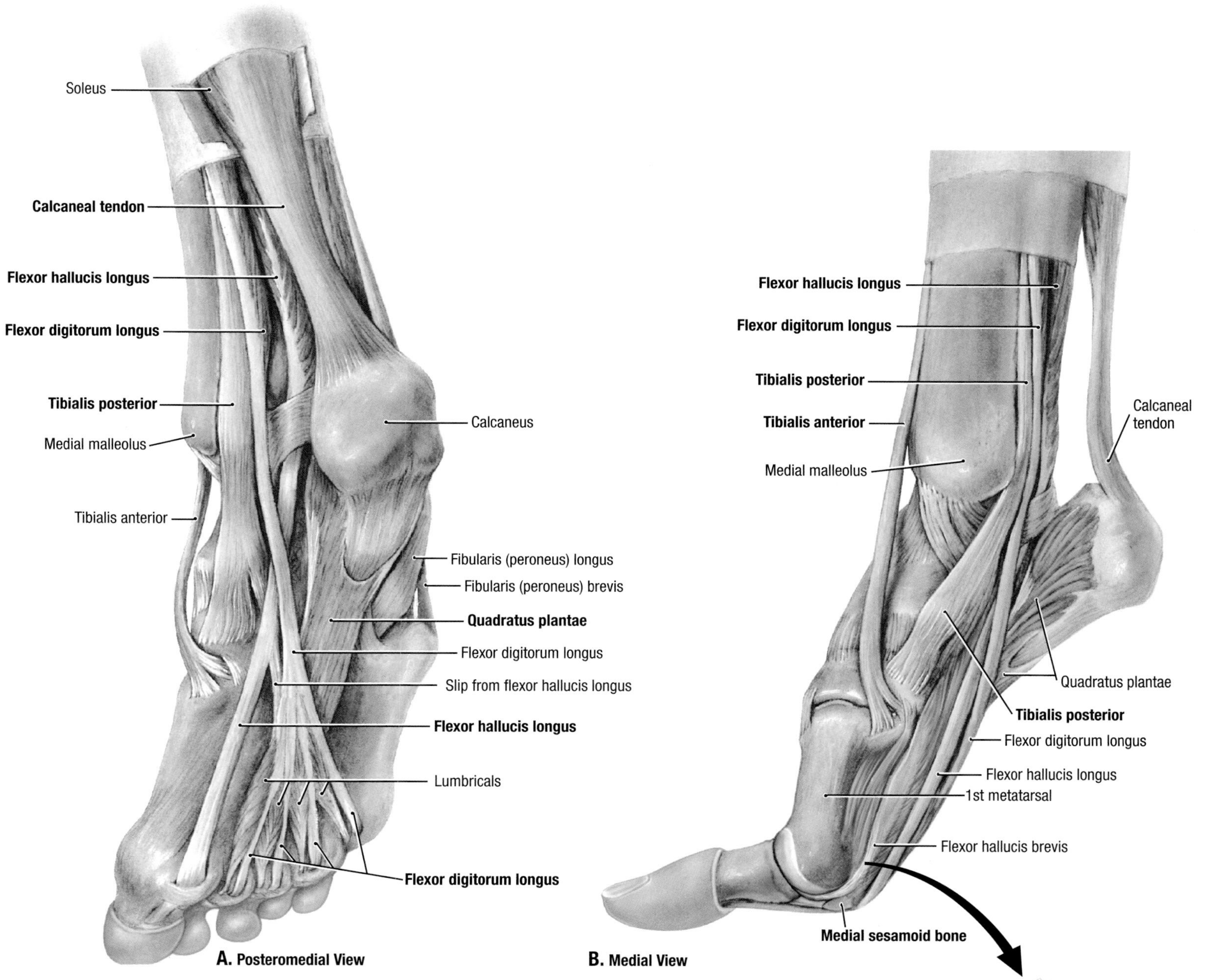

Soleus
Calcaneal tendon
Flexor hallucis longus
Flexor digitorum longus
Tibialis posterior
Medial malleolus
Tibialis anterior
Calcaneus
Fibularis (peroneus) longus
Fibularis (peroneus) brevis
Quadratus plantae
Flexor digitorum longus
Slip from flexor hallucis longus
Flexor hallucis longus
Lumbricals
Flexor digitorum longus

A. Posteromedial View

Flexor hallucis longus
Flexor digitorum longus
Tibialis posterior
Tibialis anterior
Medial malleolus
Calcaneal tendon
Quadratus plantae
Tibialis posterior
Flexor digitorum longus
Flexor hallucis longus
1st metatarsal
Flexor hallucis brevis
Medial sesamoid bone

B. Medial View

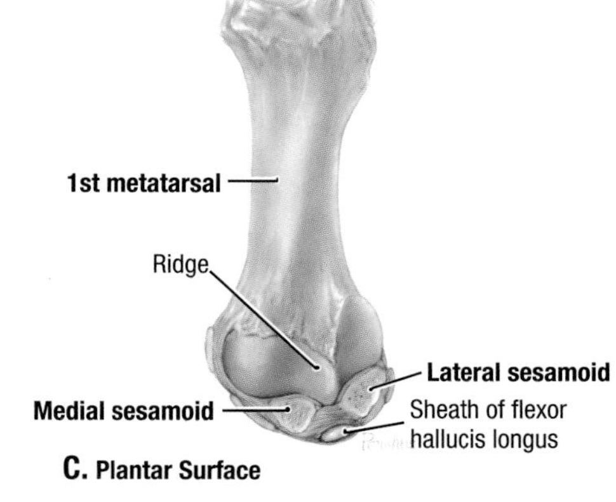
1st metatarsal
Ridge
Lateral sesamoid
Medial sesamoid
Sheath of flexor hallucis longus

C. Plantar Surface

## 5.63 Medial ankle and foot

**A.** Tendons of deep compartment of the leg traced to their distal attachments in the sole of the foot. **B.** Foot raised as in walking and sesamoid bones of the great toe. The sesamoid bones of the great toe are located on each side of a bony ridge on the 1st metatarsal.

- The sesamoid bones are a "footstool" for the first metatarsal, giving it increased height.
- By inserting into the flexor digitorum longus muscle, the quadratus plantae muscle modifies the oblique pull of the flexor tendons.
- The flexor hallucis longus muscle uses three pulleys: a groove on the posterior aspect of the distal end of the tibia, a groove on the posterior aspect of the talus, and a groove inferior to the sustentaculum tali.
- The flexor digitorum longus muscle crosses superficial to the tibialis posterior, superoposterior to the medial malleolus.

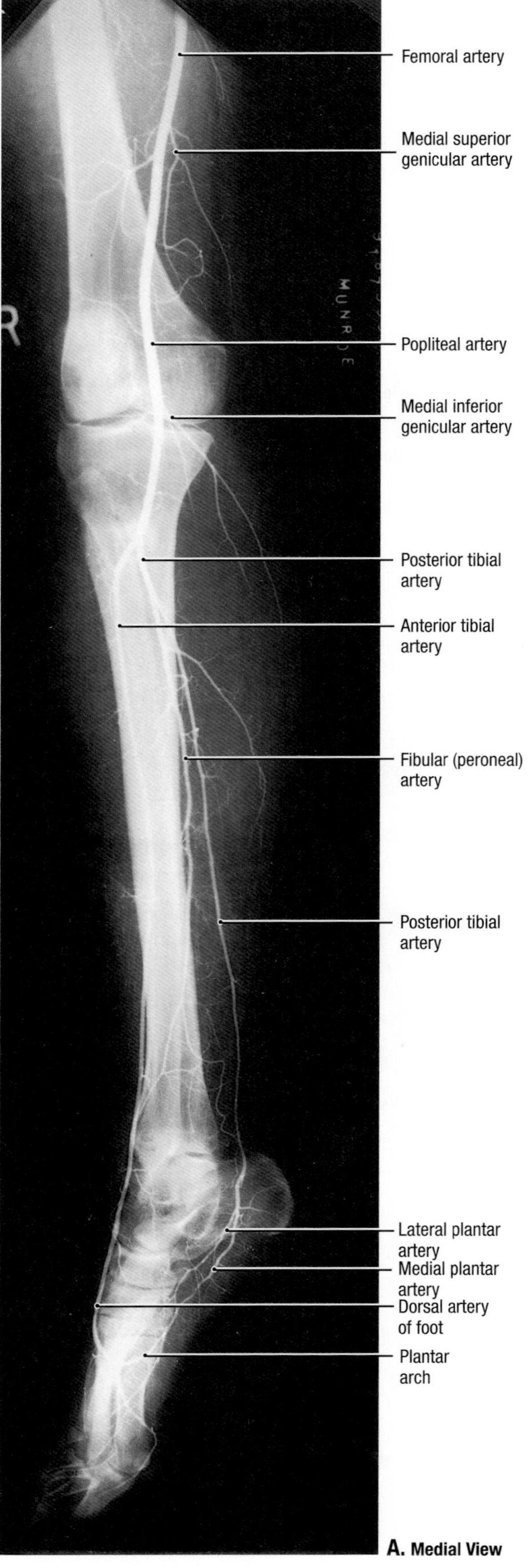
Femoral artery
Medial superior genicular artery
Popliteal artery
Medial inferior genicular artery
Posterior tibial artery
Anterior tibial artery
Fibular (peroneal) artery
Posterior tibial artery
Lateral plantar artery
Medial plantar artery
Dorsal artery of foot
Plantar arch

**A. Medial View**

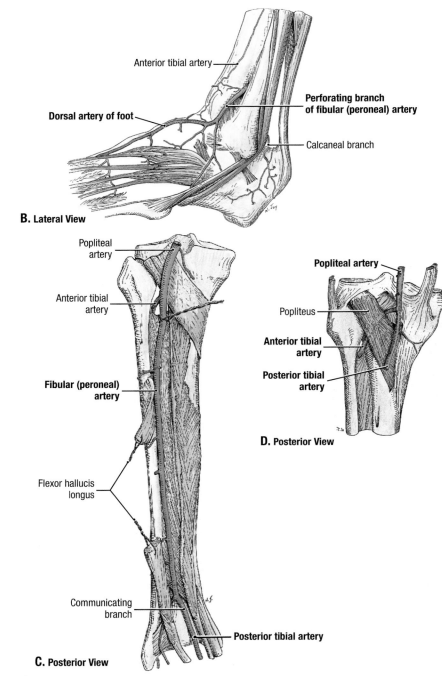

Anterior tibial artery
**Perforating branch of fibular (peroneal) artery**
**Dorsal artery of foot**
Calcaneal branch

**B. Lateral View**

Popliteal artery
Anterior tibial artery
**Fibular (peroneal) artery**
Flexor hallucis longus
Communicating branch
**Posterior tibial artery**

**C. Posterior View**

**Popliteal artery**
Popliteus
**Anterior tibial artery**
**Posterior tibial artery**

**D. Posterior View**

## 5.64 Popliteal arteriogram and arterial anomalies

**A.** Popliteal arteriogram. The femoral artery becomes the popliteal artery at the adductor hiatus. The anterior tibial artery continues as the dorsalis pedis (dorsal artery of the foot). The posterior tibial artery terminates as the medial and lateral plantar arteries; its major branch is the fibular artery. **B.** Anomalous dorsal artery of the foot. The perforating branch of the fibular artery rarely continues as the dorsal artery of the foot, but when it does, the anterior tibial artery ends proximal to the ankle or is a slender vessel. **C.** Absence of posterior tibial artery. Compensatory enlargement of the fibular artery was found to occur in approximately 5% of limbs. **D.** High division of popliteal artery. Along with the anterior tibial artery descending anterior to the popliteus muscle; this anomaly was found to occur in approximately 2% of limbs.

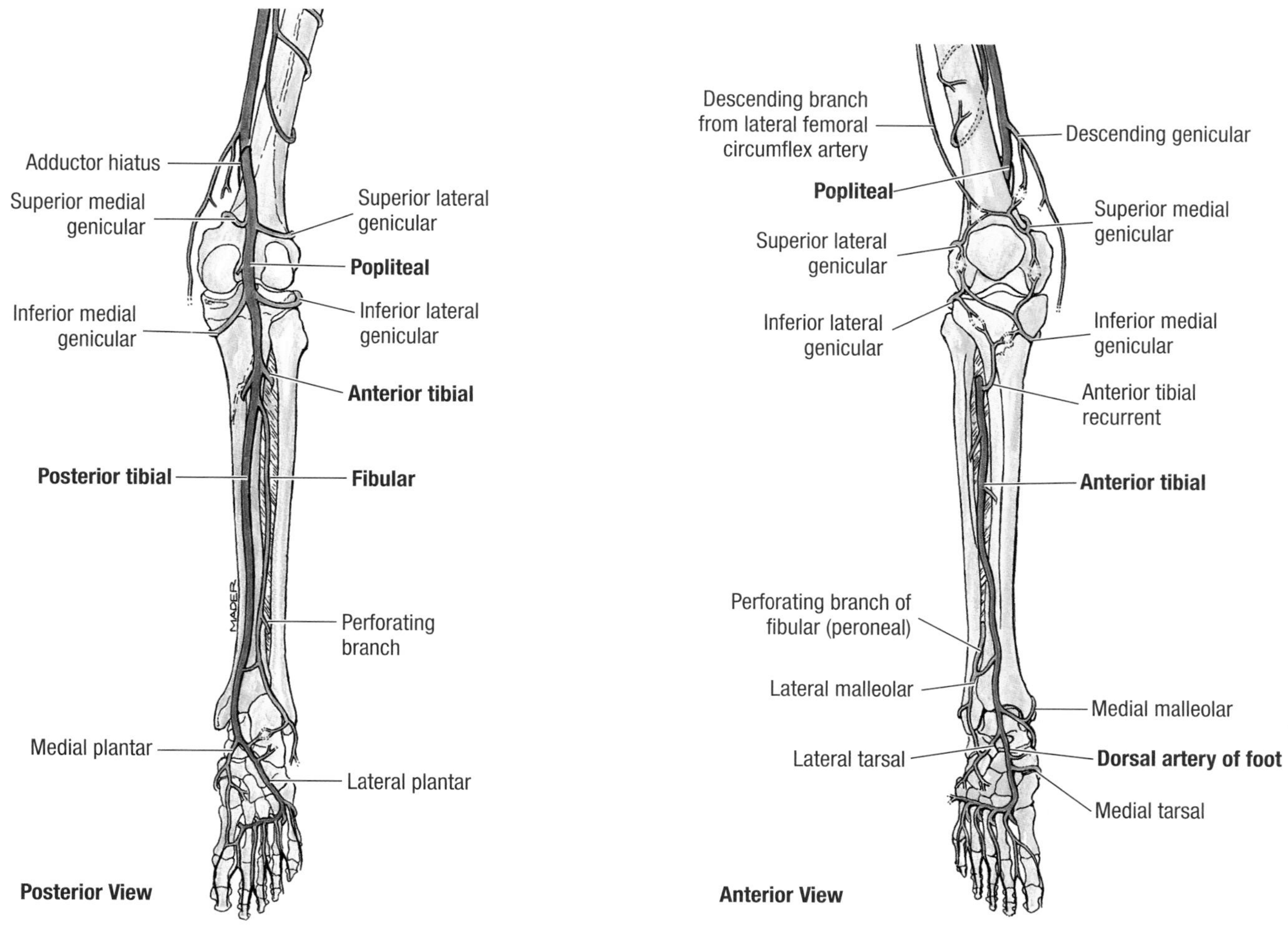
Adductor hiatus
Superior medial genicular
Superior lateral genicular
Popliteal
Inferior medial genicular
Inferior lateral genicular
Anterior tibial
Posterior tibial
Fibular
MADER
Perforating branch
Medial plantar
Lateral plantar
Posterior View
Descending branch from lateral femoral circumflex artery
Descending genicular
Popliteal
Superior medial genicular
Superior lateral genicular
Inferior lateral genicular
Inferior medial genicular
Anterior tibial recurrent
Anterior tibial
Perforating branch of fibular (peroneal)
Lateral malleolar
Medial malleolar
Lateral tarsal
Dorsal artery of foot
Medial tarsal
Anterior View

**TABLE 5.14 ARTERIAL SUPPLY OF LEG AND FOOT**

| Artery | Origin | Course | Distribution in Leg |
|---|---|---|---|
| **Popliteal** | Continuation of femoral artery at adductor hiatus | Passes through popliteal fossa to leg; divides into anterior and posterior tibial arteries at lower border of popliteus | Lateral and medial aspects of knee via genicular arteries |
| **Anterior tibial** | Popliteal | Passes between tibia and fibula into anterior compartment through gap superior to interosseous membrane; descends between tibialis anterior and extensor digitorum longus muscles | Anterior compartment |
| **Dorsal artery of foot (dorsalis pedis)** | Continuation of anterior tibial artery distal to talocrural joint | Descends to first interosseous space; divides into plantar and arcuate arteries | Muscles on dorsum of foot; pierces first dorsal interosseous muscle as deep plantar artery; joins deep plantar arch |
| **Posterior tibial** | Popliteal | Passes through posterior compartment; divides into medial and lateral plantar arteries posterior to medial malleolus | Posterior and lateral compartments, nutrient artery passes to tibia |
| **Fibular (peroneal)** | Posterior tibial | Descends in posterior compartment adjacent to posterior intermuscular septum | Posterior compartment: perforating branches supply lateral compartment |
| **Medial plantar** | | In foot between abductor hallucis and flexor digitorum brevis muscles | Supplies mainly muscles of great toe and skin on medial side of sole of foot |
| **Lateral plantar** | Posterior tibial | Runs anterolaterally deep to abductor hallucis and flexor digitorum brevis, then arches medially to form deep plantar arch | Supplies remainder (lateral aspect) of sole of foot |

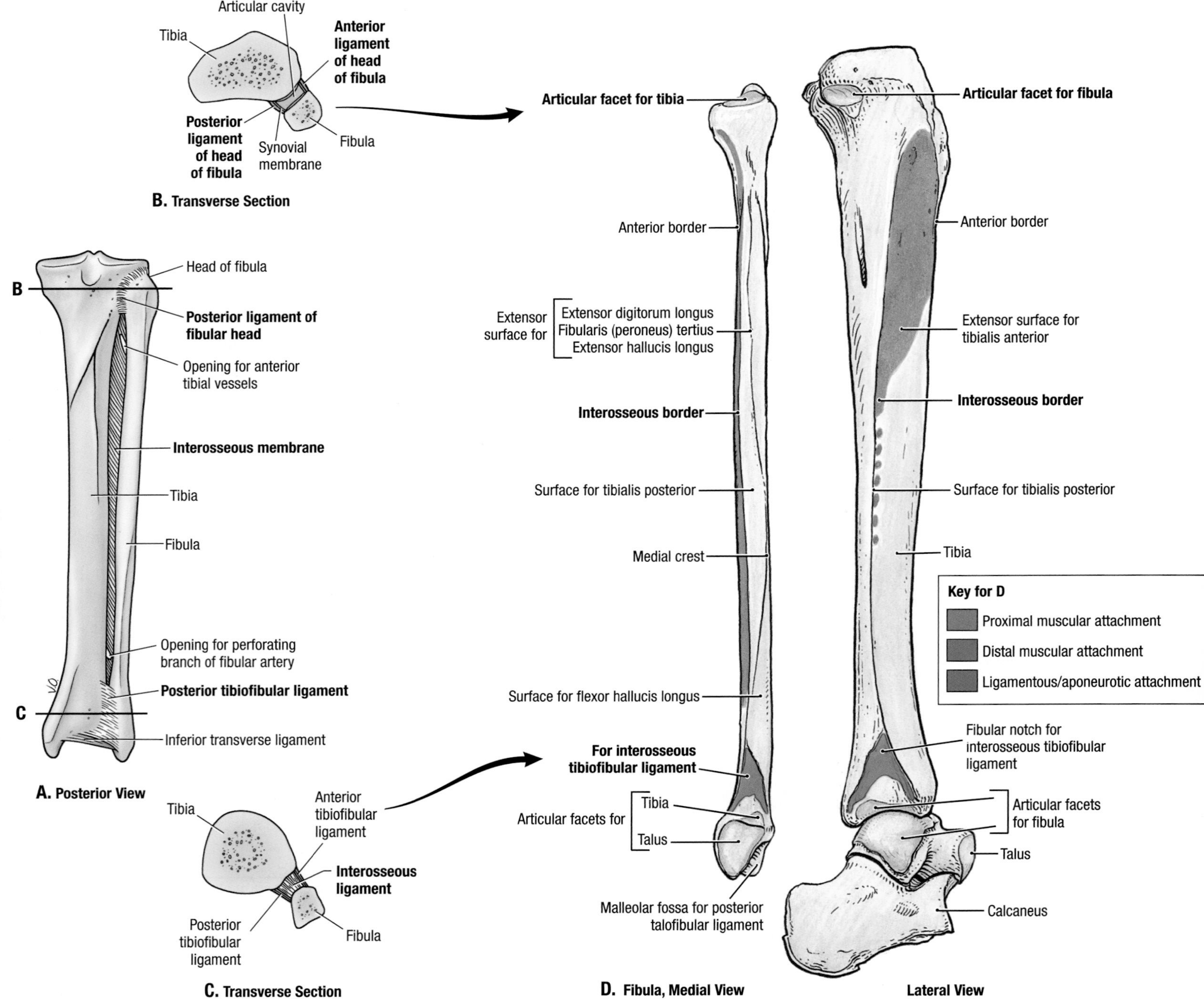
Articular cavity
Tibia
Anterior ligament of head of fibula
Posterior ligament of head of fibula
Synovial membrane
Fibula
B. Transverse Section
Head of fibula
B
Posterior ligament of fibular head
Opening for anterior tibial vessels
Interosseous membrane
Tibia
Fibula
Opening for perforating branch of fibular artery
Posterior tibiofibular ligament
C
Inferior transverse ligament
A. Posterior View
Tibia
Anterior tibiofibular ligament
Interosseous ligament
Posterior tibiofibular ligament
Fibula
C. Transverse Section
Articular facet for tibia
Anterior border
Extensor surface for
Extensor digitorum longus
Fibularis (peroneus) tertius
Extensor hallucis longus
Interosseous border
Surface for tibialis posterior
Medial crest
Surface for flexor hallucis longus
For interosseous tibiofibular ligament
Articular facets for
Tibia
Talus
Malleolar fossa for posterior talofibular ligament
D. Fibula, Medial View
Articular facet for fibula
Anterior border
Extensor surface for tibialis anterior
Interosseous border
Surface for tibialis posterior
Tibia
Key for D
Proximal muscular attachment
Distal muscular attachment
Ligamentous/aponeurotic attachment
Fibular notch for interosseous tibiofibular ligament
Articular facets for fibula
Talus
Calcaneus
Lateral View

## 5.65 Superior tibiofibular joint and tibiofibular syndesmosis

**A.** Tibiofibular joints. **B.** Superior tibiofibular joint. **C.** Tibiofibular syndesmosis. **D.** Tibia and fibula, disarticulated.

- The superior tibiofibular joint (proximal tibiofibular joint) is a plane type of synovial joint between the flat facet on the fibular head and a similar facet located posterolaterally on the lateral tibial condyle. The tense joint capsule surrounds the joint and attaches to the margins of the articular surfaces of the fibula and tibia.
- The tibiofibular syndesmosis is a compound fibrous joint. This articulation is essential for stability of the ankle joint because it keeps the lateral malleolus firmly against the lateral surface of the talus. The strong interosseous tibiofibular ligament is continuous superiorly with the interosseous membrane and forms the principal connection between the distal ends of the tibia and fibula.

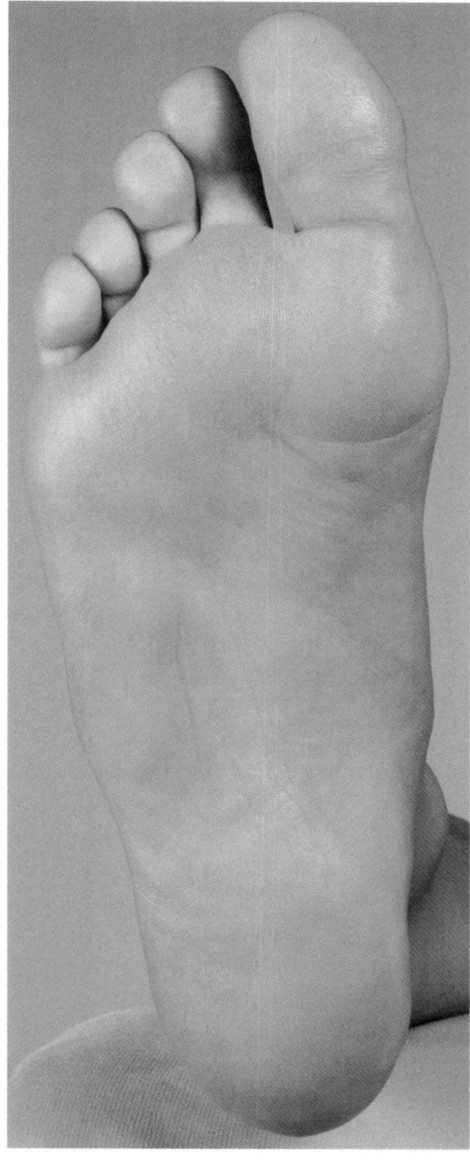

A. Plantar View

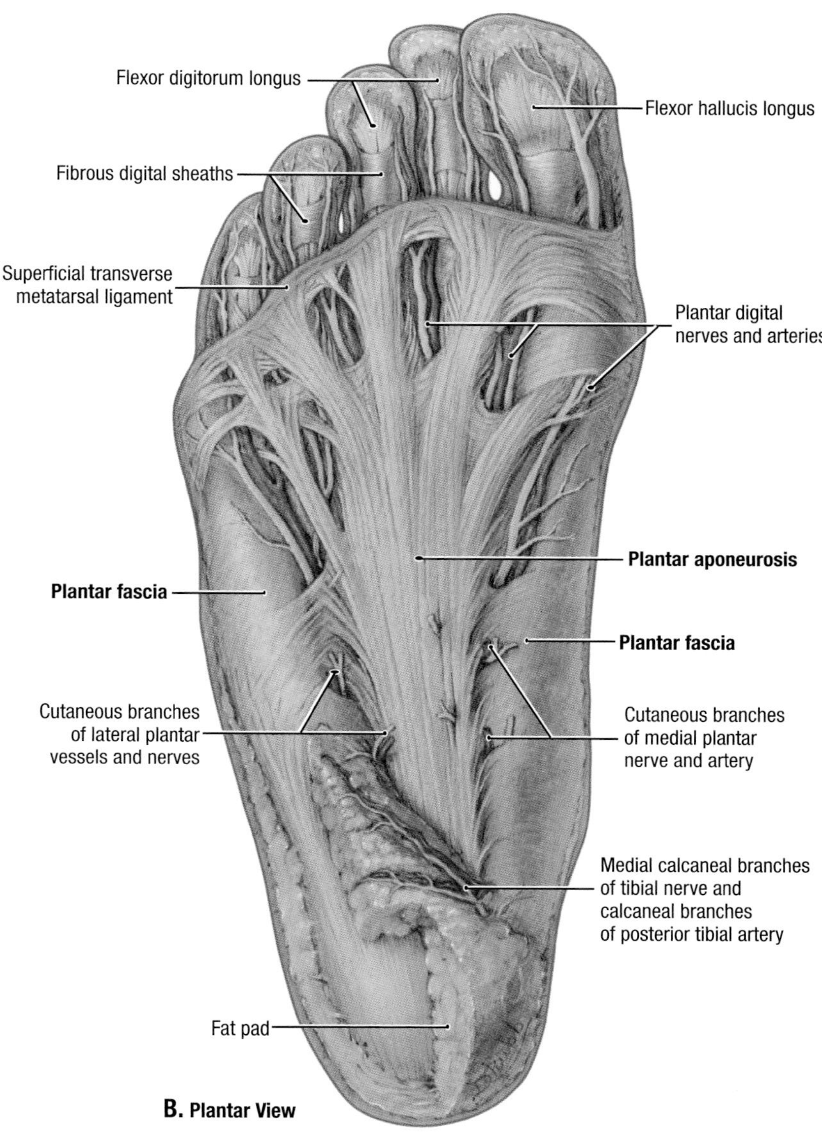
Flexor digitorum longus
Flexor hallucis longus
Fibrous digital sheaths
Superficial transverse metatarsal ligament
Plantar digital nerves and arteries
Plantar aponeurosis
Plantar fascia
Plantar fascia
Cutaneous branches of lateral plantar vessels and nerves
Cutaneous branches of medial plantar nerve and artery
Medial calcaneal branches of tibial nerve and calcaneal branches of posterior tibial artery
Fat pad

B. Plantar View

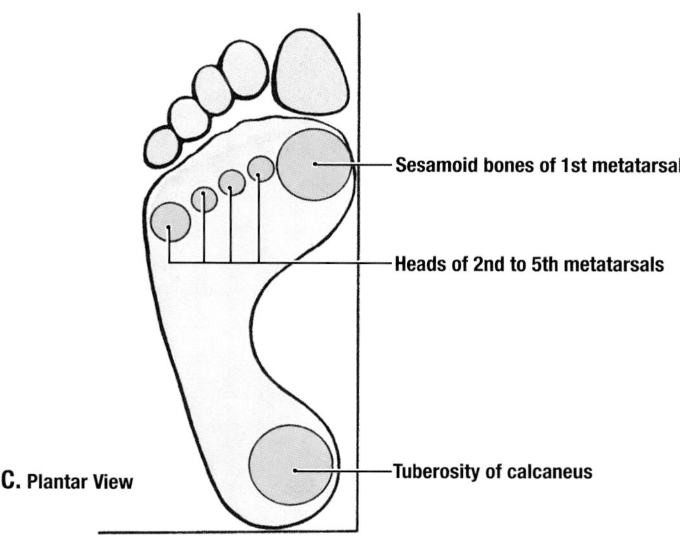
Sesamoid bones of 1st metatarsal
Heads of 2nd to 5th metatarsals
Tuberosity of calcaneus

C. Plantar View

## 5.66 Sole of foot, superficial

**A.** Surface anatomy. **B.** Dissection. Plantar aponeurosis and fascia, with neurovascular structures. **C.** Weight-bearing areas.

- The weight of the body is transmitted to the talus from the tibia and fibula. It is then transmitted to the tuberosity of the calcaneus, the heads of the second to fifth metatarsals, and the sesamoid bones of the first digit.

- Straining and inflammation of the plantar aponeurosis, a condition called plantar fasciitis, may result from running and high-impact aerobics, especially when inappropriate footwear is worn. It causes pain on the plantar surface of the heel and on the medial aspect of the foot. Point tenderness is located at the proximal attachment of the plantar aponeurosis to the medial tubercle of the calcaneus and on the medial surface of this bone. The pain increases with passive extension of the great toe and may be further exacerbated by dorsiflexion of the ankle and/or weight bearing.

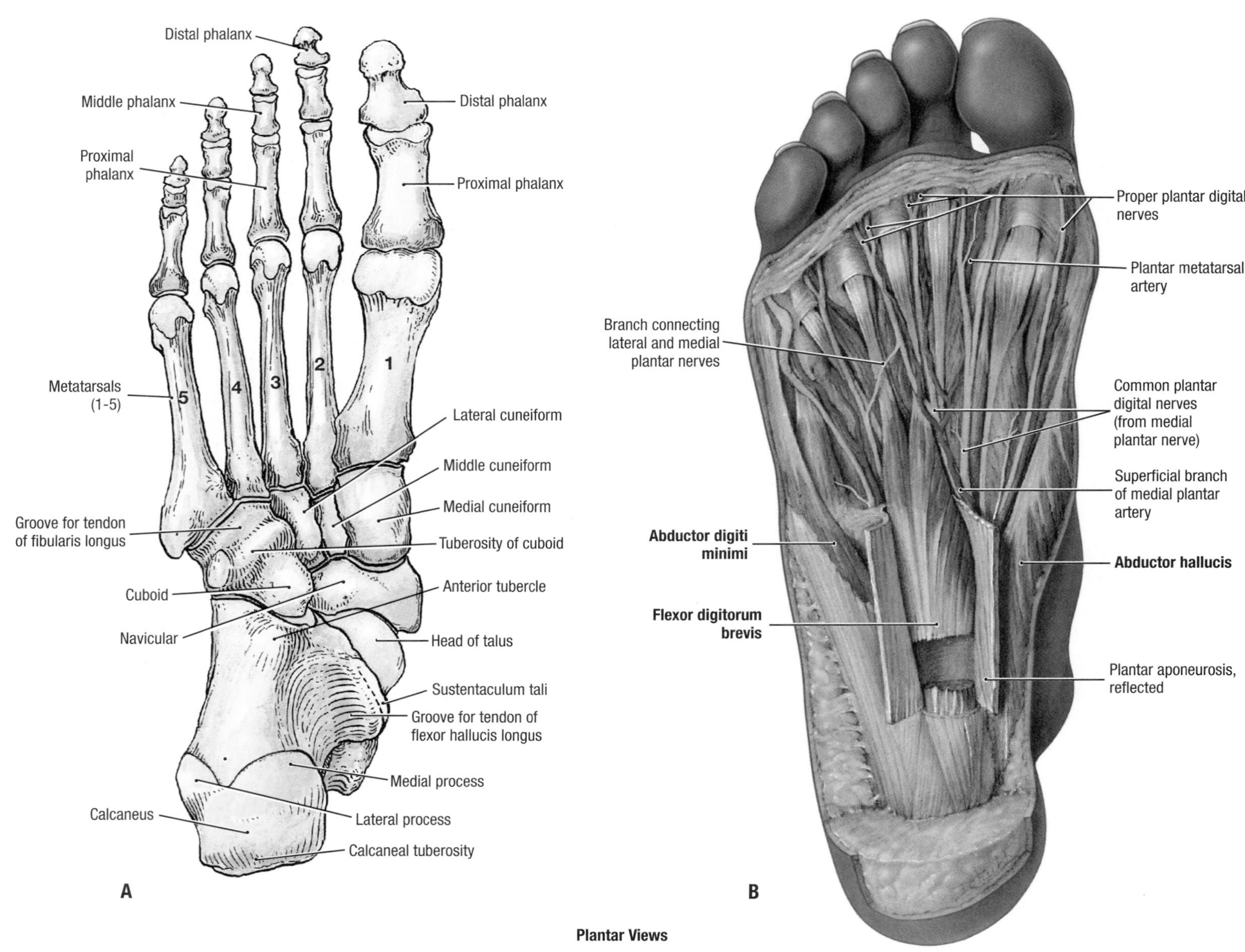
Distal phalanx
Middle phalanx
Proximal phalanx
Distal phalanx
Proximal phalanx
Metatarsals (1-5)
5
4
3
2
1
Lateral cuneiform
Middle cuneiform
Medial cuneiform
Groove for tendon of fibularis longus
Tuberosity of cuboid
Cuboid
Anterior tubercle
Navicular
Head of talus
Sustentaculum tali
Groove for tendon of flexor hallucis longus
Medial process
Calcaneus
Lateral process
Calcaneal tuberosity
A
Proper plantar digital nerves
Plantar metatarsal artery
Branch connecting lateral and medial plantar nerves
Common plantar digital nerves (from medial plantar nerve)
Superficial branch of medial plantar artery
Abductor digiti minimi
Abductor hallucis
Flexor digitorum brevis
Plantar aponeurosis, reflected
B
Plantar Views

## 5.67 First layer of muscles of sole of foot

**A.** Bones. **B.** Dissection. Muscles and neurovascular structures.

### TABLE 5.15 MUSCLES IN SOLE OF FOOT—FIRST LAYER

| Muscle | Proximal Attachment | Distal Attachment | Innervation | Actions[a] |
|---|---|---|---|---|
| **Abductor hallucis** | Medial process of tuberosity of calcaneus, flexor retinaculum, and plantar aponeurosis | Medial side of base of proximal phalanx of first digit | Medial plantar nerve (S2–S3) | Abducts and flexes |
| **Flexor digitorum brevis** | Medial process of tuberosity of calcaneus, plantar aponeurosis, and intermuscular septa | Both sides of middle phalanges of lateral four digits | | Flexes lateral four digits |
| **Abductor digiti minim** | Medial and lateral processes of tuberosity of calcaneus, plantar aponeurosis, and intermuscular septa | Lateral side of base of proximal phalanx of fifth digit | Lateral plantar nerve (S2–S3) | Abducts and flexes fifth digit |

[a]Although individual actions are described, the primary function of the intrinsic muscles of the foot is to act collectively to resist forces that stress (attempt to flatten) the arches of the foot.

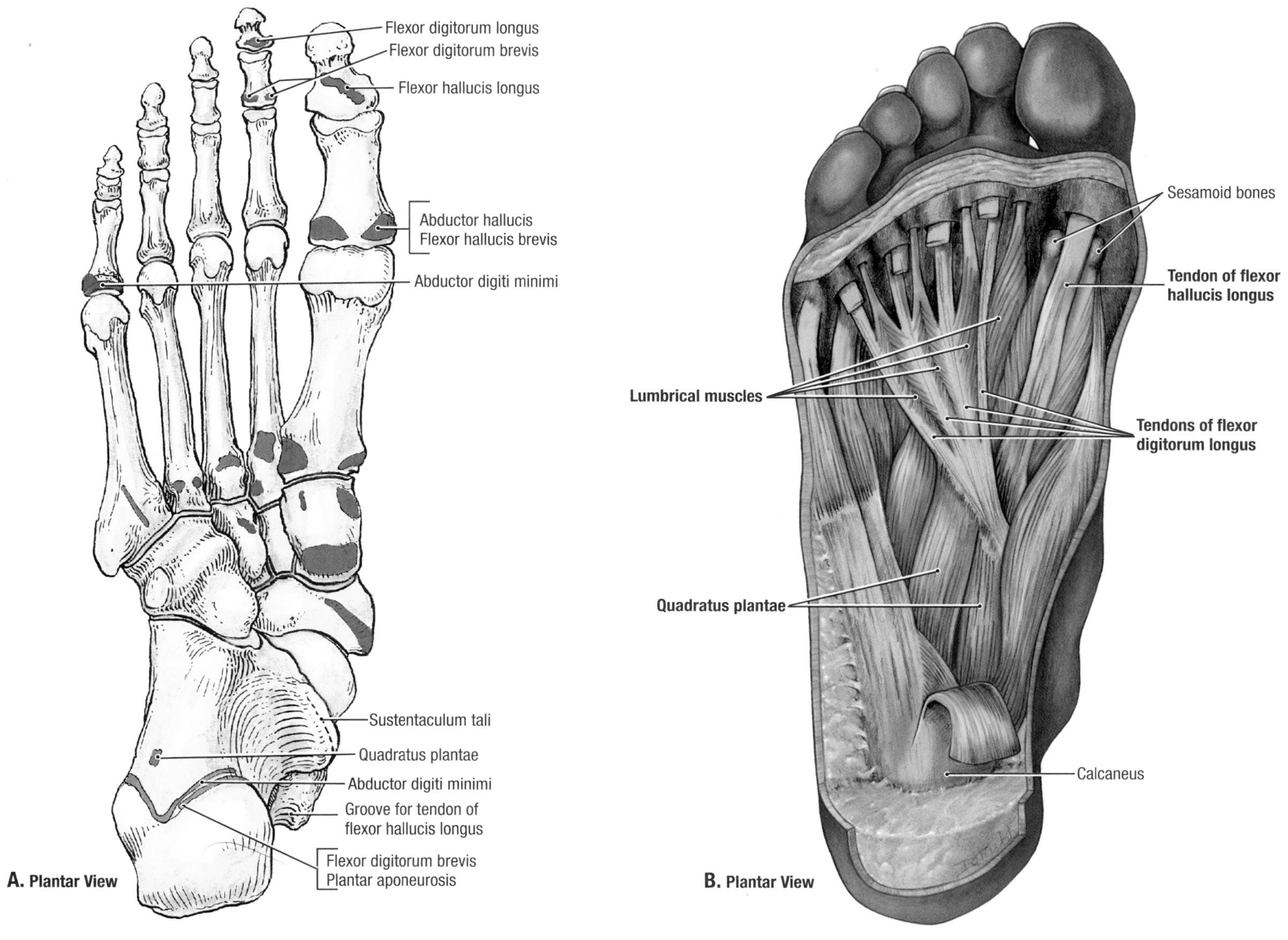

Flexor digitorum longus
Flexor digitorum brevis
Flexor hallucis longus
Abductor hallucis
Flexor hallucis brevis
Abductor digiti minimi
Sustentaculum tali
Quadratus plantae
Abductor digiti minimi
Groove for tendon of flexor hallucis longus
Flexor digitorum brevis
Plantar aponeurosis
A. Plantar View
Sesamoid bones
Tendon of flexor hallucis longus
Lumbrical muscles
Tendons of flexor digitorum longus
Quadratus plantae
Calcaneus
B. Plantar View


**5.68 Second layer of muscles of sole of foot**

**A.** Bony attachments. **B.** Dissection. Muscles.

**TABLE 5.16 MUSCLES IN SOLE OF FOOT—SECOND LAYER**

| Muscle | Proximal Attachment | Distal Attachment | Innervation | Actions[a] |
|---|---|---|---|---|
| **Quadratus plantae** | Medial surface and lateral margin of plantar surface of calcaneus | Posterolateral margin of tendon of flexor digitorum longus | Lateral plantar nerve (S2–**S3**) | Assists flexor digitorum longus in flexing lateral four digits |
| **Lumbricals** | Tendons of flexor digitorum longus | Medial aspect of extensor expansion over lateral four digits | *Medial one:* medial plantar nerve (S2–**S3**); *Lateral three:* lateral plantar nerve (S2–**S3**) | Flex proximal phalanges and extend middle and distal phalanges of lateral four digits |

[a]Although individual actions are described, the primary function of the intrinsic muscles of the foot is to act collectively to resist forces that stress (attempt to flatten) the arches of the foot.

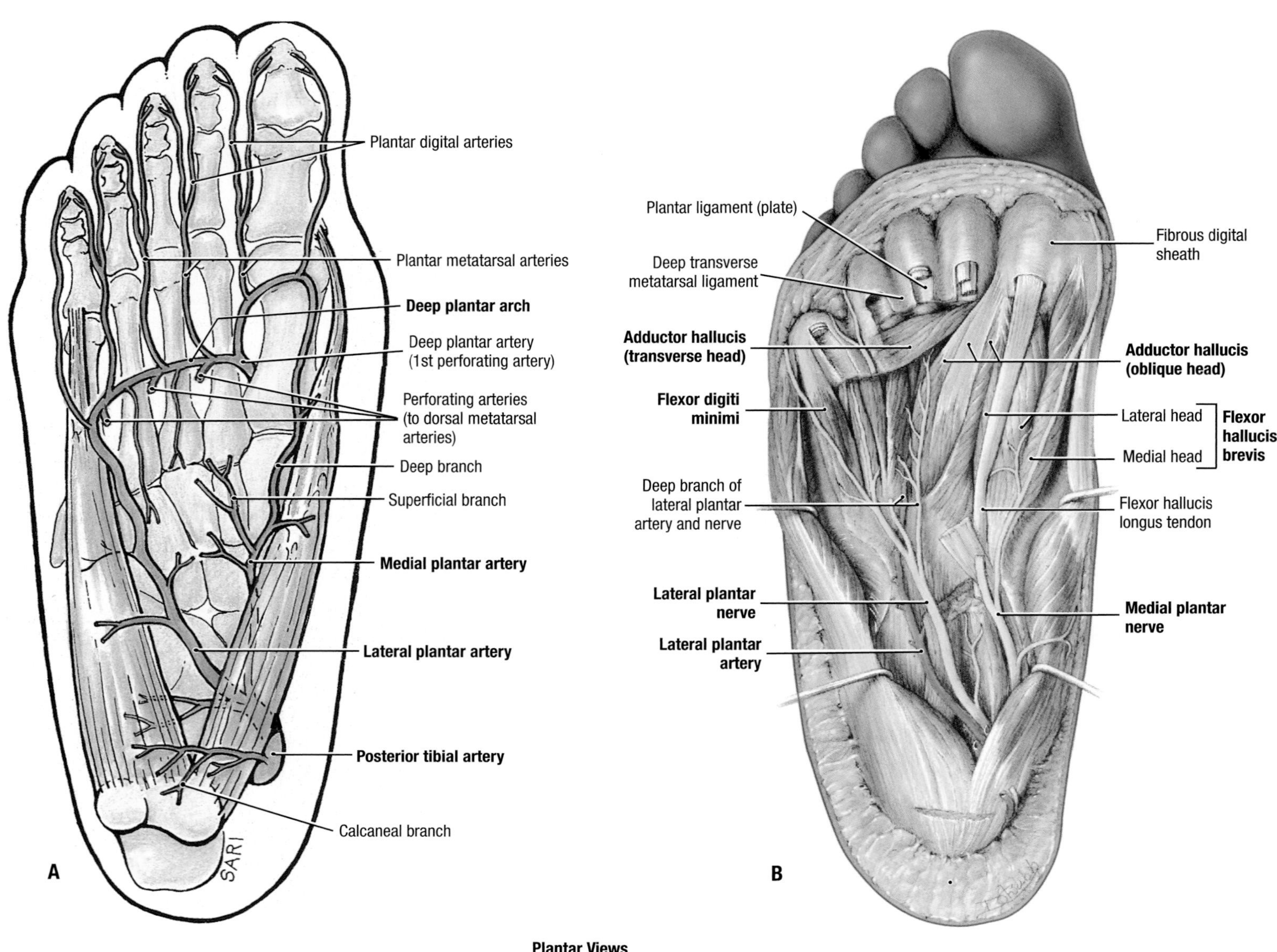
Plantar digital arteries
Plantar metatarsal arteries
Deep plantar arch
Deep plantar artery (1st perforating artery)
Perforating arteries (to dorsal metatarsal arteries)
Deep branch
Superficial branch
Medial plantar artery
Lateral plantar artery
Posterior tibial artery
Calcaneal branch
A
Plantar ligament (plate)
Deep transverse metatarsal ligament
Adductor hallucis (transverse head)
Flexor digiti minimi
Deep branch of lateral plantar artery and nerve
Lateral plantar nerve
Lateral plantar artery
Fibrous digital sheath
Adductor hallucis (oblique head)
Lateral head
Medial head
Flexor hallucis brevis
Flexor hallucis longus tendon
Medial plantar nerve
B
Plantar Views

**5.69 Third layer of muscles and arterial supply of sole of foot**

**A.** Arterial supply. **B.** Dissection. Muscles and neurovascular structures.

**TABLE 5.17 MUSCLES IN SOLE OF FOOT—THIRD LAYER**

| Muscle | Proximal Attachment | Distal Attachment | Innervation | Actions[a] |
|---|---|---|---|---|
| **Flexor hallucis brevis** | Plantar surfaces of cuboid and lateral cuneiforms | Both sides of base of proximal phalanx of first digit | Medial plantar nerve (S2 –**S3**) | Flexes proximal phalanx of first digit |
| **Adductor hallucis** | *Oblique head:* bases of metatarsals 2–4; *Transverse head:* plantar ligaments of metatarsophalangeal joints | Tendons of both heads attach to lateral side of base of proximal phalanx of first digit | Deep branch of lateral plantar nerve (S2–**S3**) | Adducts first digit; assists in maintaining transverse arch of foot |
| **Flexor digiti minimi** | Base of fifth metatarsal | Base of proximal phalanx of fifth digit | Superficial branch of lateral plantar nerve (S2–**S3**) | Flexes proximal phalanx of fifth digit, thereby assisting with its flexion |

[a]Although individual actions are described, the primary function of the intrinsic muscles of the foot is to act collectively to resist forces that stress (attempt to flatten) the arches of the foot.

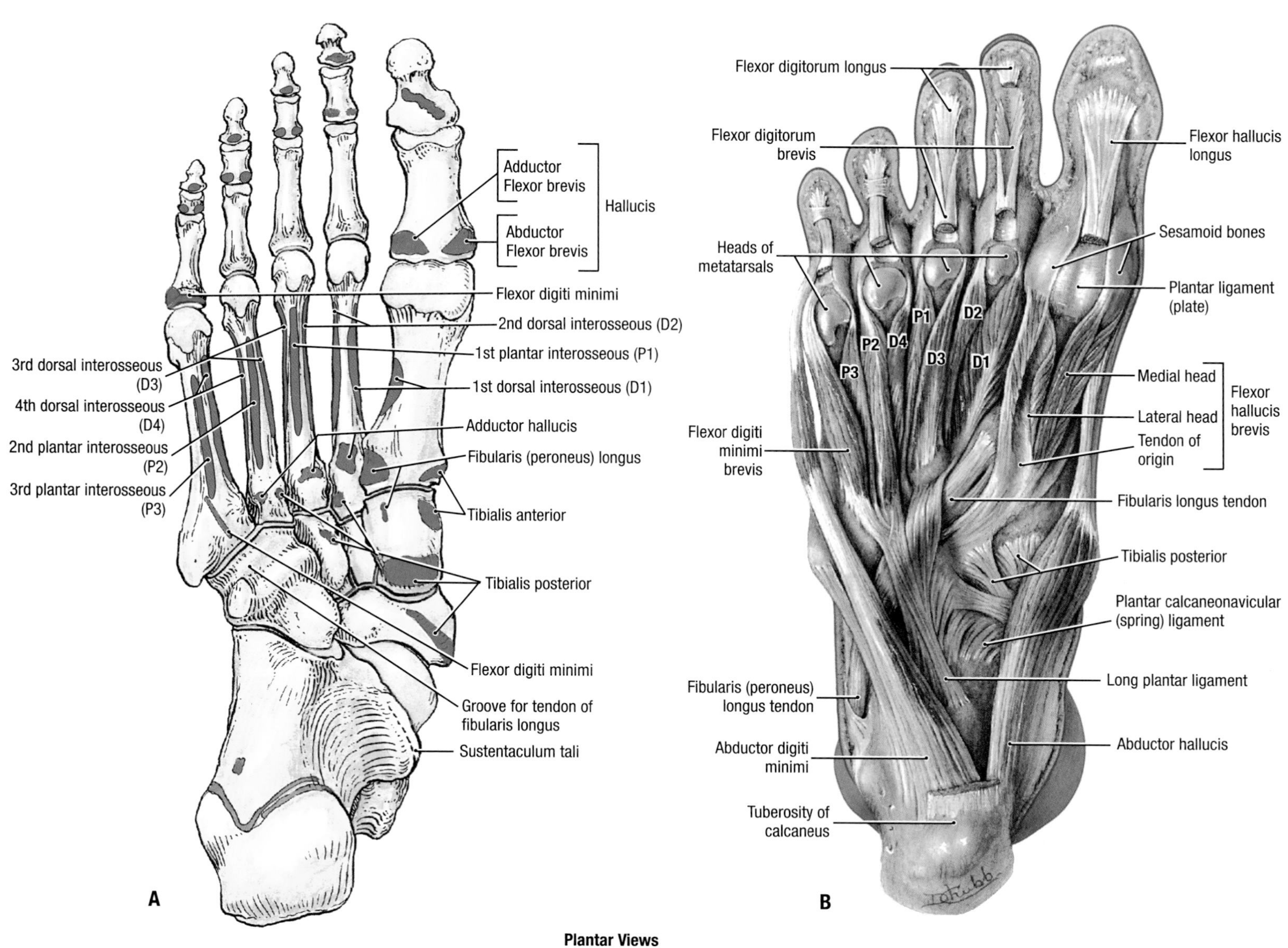
Adductor
Flexor brevis
Abductor
Flexor brevis
Hallucis
Flexor digiti minimi
2nd dorsal interosseous (D2)
1st plantar interosseous (P1)
1st dorsal interosseous (D1)
Adductor hallucis
Fibularis (peroneus) longus
Tibialis anterior
Tibialis posterior
Flexor digiti minimi
Groove for tendon of fibularis longus
Sustentaculum tali
3rd dorsal interosseous (D3)
4th dorsal interosseous (D4)
2nd plantar interosseous (P2)
3rd plantar interosseous (P3)
A
Flexor digitorum longus
Flexor digitorum brevis
Heads of metatarsals
Flexor digiti minimi brevis
Fibularis (peroneus) longus tendon
Abductor digiti minimi
Tuberosity of calcaneus
P1 D2 P2 D4 D3 D1 P3
Flexor hallucis longus
Sesamoid bones
Plantar ligament (plate)
Medial head
Lateral head
Tendon of origin
Flexor hallucis brevis
Fibularis longus tendon
Tibialis posterior
Plantar calcaneonavicular (spring) ligament
Long plantar ligament
Abductor hallucis
B
Plantar Views

**5.70 Fourth layer of muscles of sole of foot**

**A.** Bony attachments. **B.** Dissection. Muscles and ligaments.

**TABLE 5.18 MUSCLES IN SOLE OF FOOT—FOURTH LAYER**

| Muscle | Proximal Attachment | Distal Attachment | Innervation | Actions[a] |
|---|---|---|---|---|
| **Plantar interossei (three muscles; P1–P3)** | Bases and medial sides of metatarsals 3–5 | Medial sides of bases of proximal phalanges of third to fifth digits | Lateral plantar nerve (S2–S3) | Adduct digits (3–5) and flex metatarsophalangeal joints |
| **Dorsal interossei (four muscles; D1–D4)** | Adjacent sides of metatarsals 1–5 | First: medial side of proximal phalanx of second digit Second to fourth: lateral sides of second to fourth digits | | Abduct digits (2–4) and flex metatarsophalangeal joints |

[a]Although individual actions are described, the primary function of the intrinsic muscles of the foot is to act collectively to resist forces that stress (attempt to flatten) the arches of the foot.

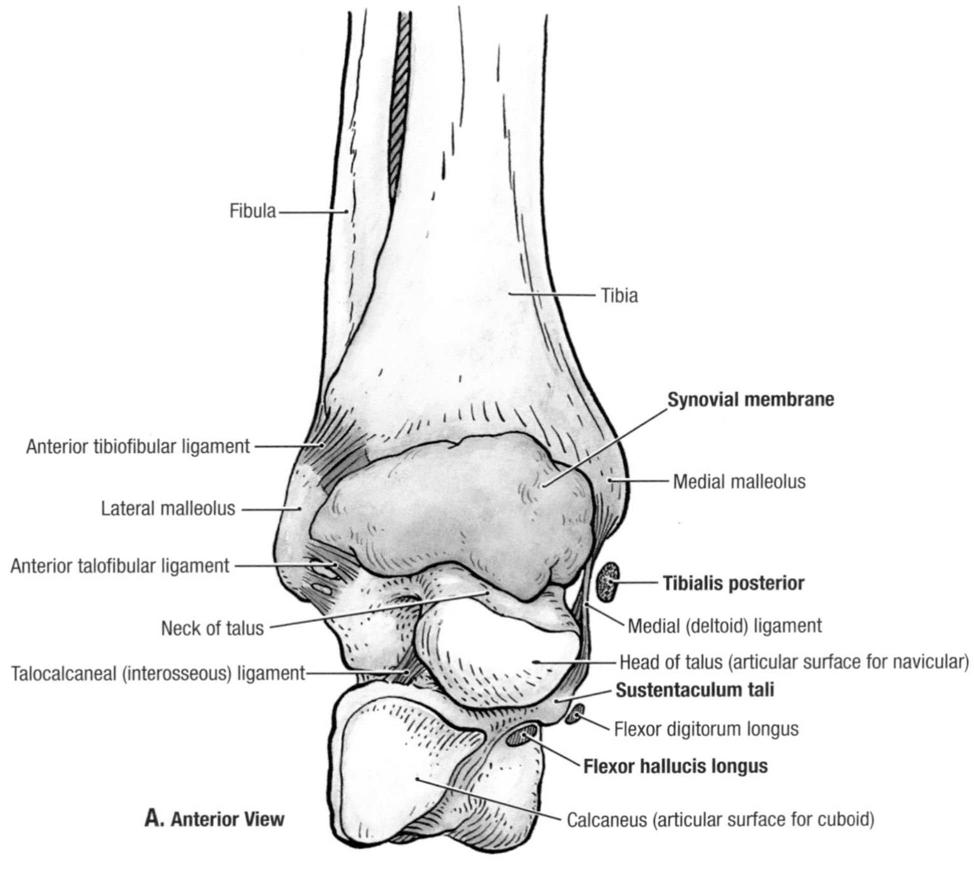
Fibula
Tibia
Synovial membrane
Anterior tibiofibular ligament
Medial malleolus
Lateral malleolus
Anterior talofibular ligament
Tibialis posterior
Neck of talus
Medial (deltoid) ligament
Head of talus (articular surface for navicular)
Talocalcaneal (interosseous) ligament
Sustentaculum tali
Flexor digitorum longus
Flexor hallucis longus
A. Anterior View
Calcaneus (articular surface for cuboid)

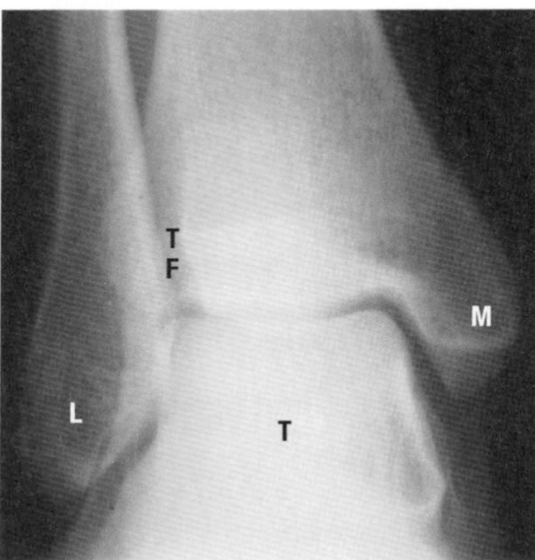
T
F
M
L
T

**B.** Anteroposterior View

## 5.71 Joint cavity of ankle joint

**A.** Ankle joint with joint cavity distended with injected latex. **B.** Radiograph of joints of ankle region. *L*, lateral malleolus; *M*, medial malleolus; *T*, talus; *TF*, tibiofibular syndesmosis.

- The anterior articular surfaces of the calcaneus and head of the talus are each convex from side to side; thus the foot can be inverted and everted at the transverse tarsal joint.
- Note the relations of the tendons to the sustentaculum tali: the flexor hallucis longus inferior to it, flexor digitorum longus along its medial aspect, and tibialis posterior superior to it and in contact with the medial (deltoid) ligament.

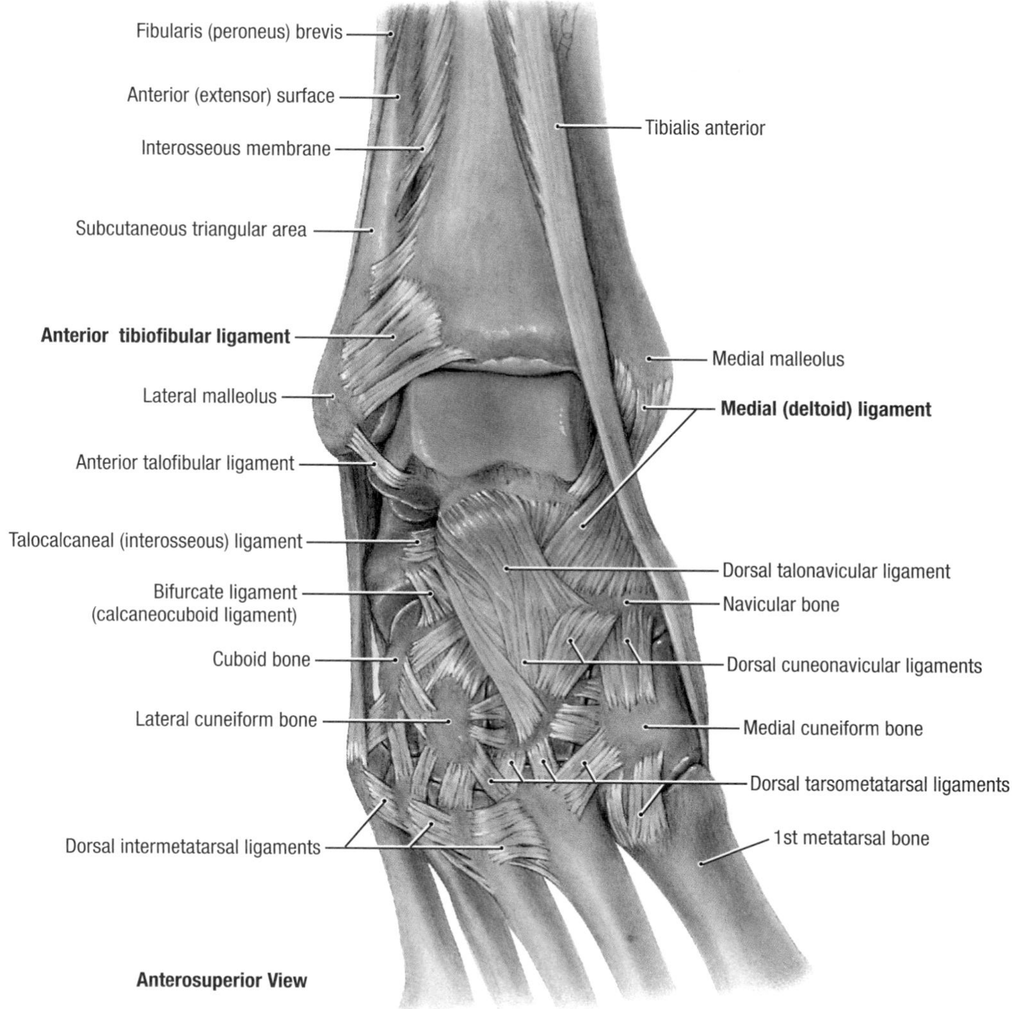
Fibularis (peroneus) brevis
Anterior (extensor) surface
Interosseous membrane
Subcutaneous triangular area
Anterior tibiofibular ligament
Lateral malleolus
Anterior talofibular ligament
Talocalcaneal (interosseous) ligament
Bifurcate ligament
(calcaneocuboid ligament)
Cuboid bone
Lateral cuneiform bone
Dorsal intermetatarsal ligaments
Tibialis anterior
Medial malleolus
Medial (deltoid) ligament
Dorsal talonavicular ligament
Navicular bone
Dorsal cuneonavicular ligaments
Medial cuneiform bone
Dorsal tarsometatarsal ligaments
1st metatarsal bone
Anterosuperior View

## 5.72 Ankle joint and ligaments of dorsum of foot

Dissection. The ankle joint is plantarflexed, and its anterior capsular fibers are removed.

- All muscles attached to the fibula except the biceps femoris pull inferiorly on the bone during contraction. The oblique fibers of the interosseous membrane and ligaments uniting the fibula to the tibia resist this inferior pull but allow the fibula to be forced superiorly during full dorsiflexion of the ankle.
- The anterior talofibular ligament (part of the lateral ligament of the ankle) is a weak band that is easily torn (see the legend for Fig. 5.77).
- The bifurcate ligament, a Y-shaped ligament consisting of calcaneocuboid and calcaneonavicular ligaments, and the talonavicular ligament are the primary dorsal ligaments of the transverse tarsal joint (Fig. 5.83).
- A Pott fracture-dislocation of the ankle occurs when the foot is forcibly everted. This action pulls on the extremely strong medial (deltoid) ligament, often avulsing the medial malleolus and compressing the lateral malleolus against the talus, shearing off the malleolus or, more often, fracturing the fibula superior to the tibiofibular syndesmosis.

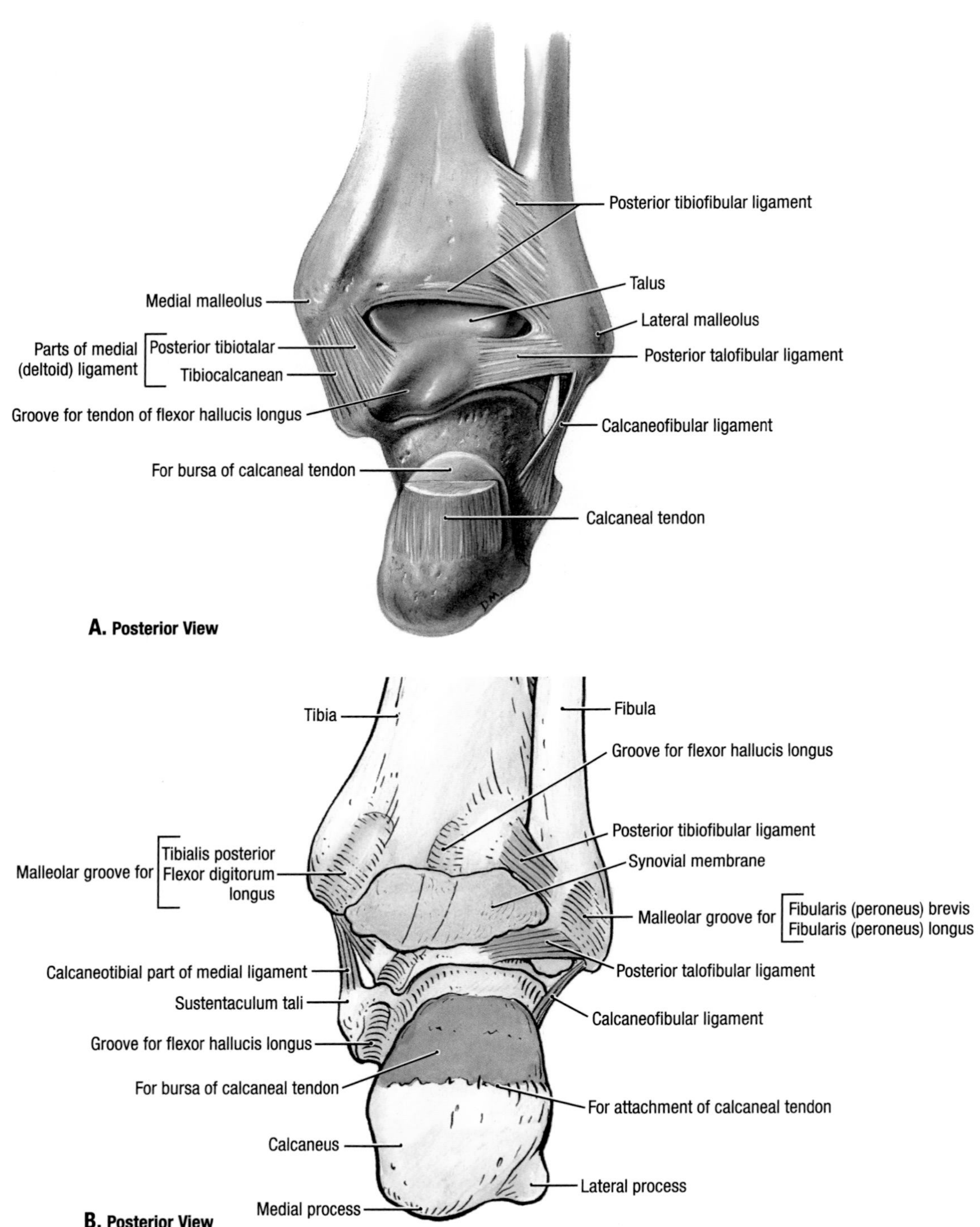
Posterior tibiofibular ligament
Talus
Medial malleolus
Lateral malleolus
Parts of medial (deltoid) ligament
Posterior tibiotalar
Tibiocalcanean
Posterior talofibular ligament
Groove for tendon of flexor hallucis longus
Calcaneofibular ligament
For bursa of calcaneal tendon
Calcaneal tendon
A. Posterior View
Tibia
Fibula
Groove for flexor hallucis longus
Posterior tibiofibular ligament
Synovial membrane
Malleolar groove for
Tibialis posterior
Flexor digitorum longus
Malleolar groove for
Fibularis (peroneus) brevis
Fibularis (peroneus) longus
Calcaneotibial part of medial ligament
Posterior talofibular ligament
Sustentaculum tali
Calcaneofibular ligament
Groove for flexor hallucis longus
For bursa of calcaneal tendon
For attachment of calcaneal tendon
Calcaneus
Lateral process
Medial process
B. Posterior View

## 5.73 Posterior aspect of ankle joint

**A.** Dissection. **B.** Ankle joint with joint cavity distended with latex. Observe the grooves for the flexor hallucis longus muscle, which crosses the middle of the ankle joint posteriorly, the two tendons posterior to the medial malleolus, and the two tendons posterior to the lateral malleolus.

- The posterior aspect of the ankle joint is strengthened by the transversely oriented posterior tibiofibular and posterior talofibular ligaments.
- The calcaneofibular ligament stabilizes the joint laterally, and the posterior tibiotalar and tibiocalcanean parts of the medial (deltoid) ligament stabilize it medially.
- The groove for the flexor hallucis tendon is between the medial and lateral tubercles of the talus and continues inferior to the sustentaculum tali.

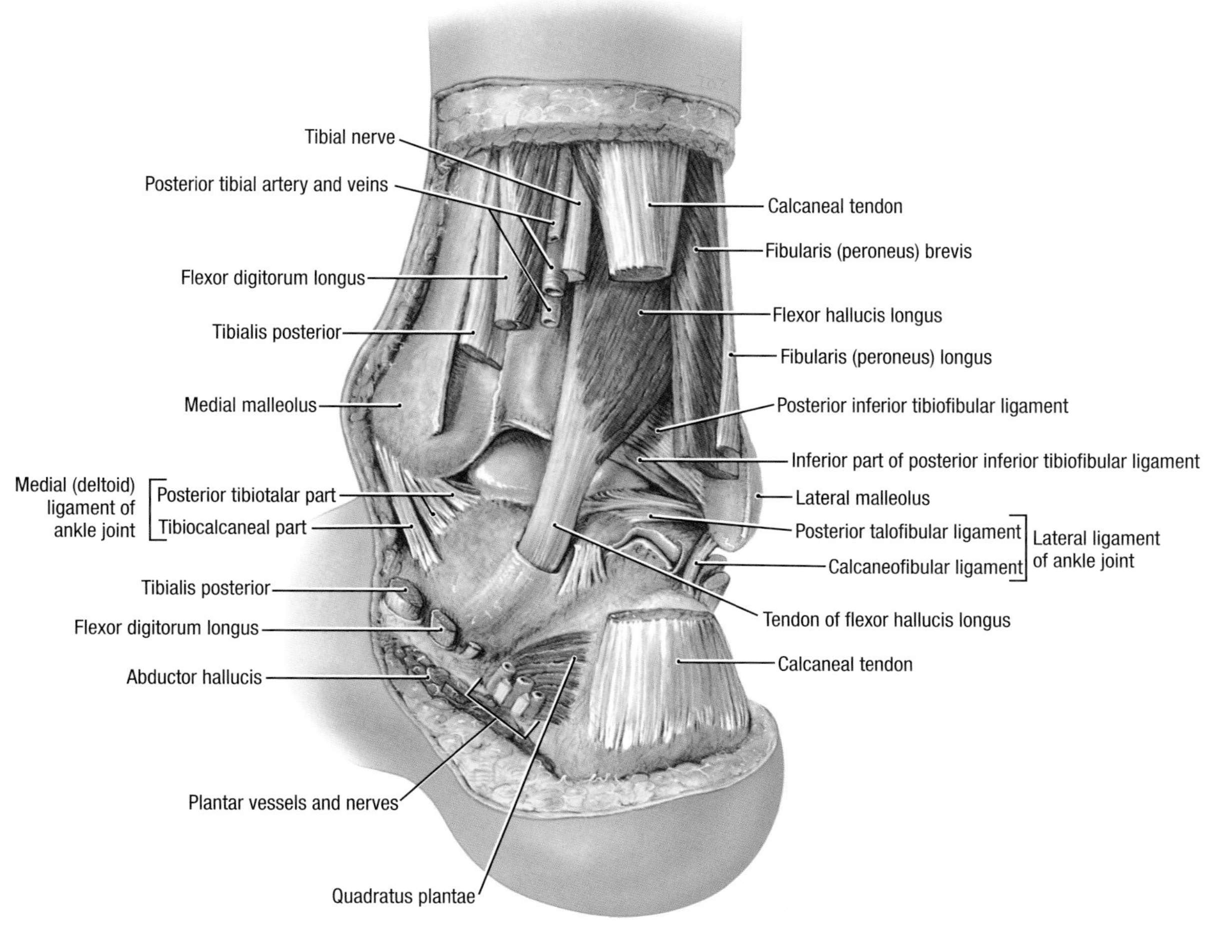
Tibial nerve
Posterior tibial artery and veins
Flexor digitorum longus
Tibialis posterior
Medial malleolus
Medial (deltoid) ligament of ankle joint
Posterior tibiotalar part
Tibiocalcaneal part
Tibialis posterior
Flexor digitorum longus
Abductor hallucis
Plantar vessels and nerves
Quadratus plantae
Calcaneal tendon
Fibularis (peroneus) brevis
Flexor hallucis longus
Fibularis (peroneus) longus
Posterior inferior tibiofibular ligament
Inferior part of posterior inferior tibiofibular ligament
Lateral malleolus
Posterior talofibular ligament
Calcaneofibular ligament
Lateral ligament of ankle joint
Tendon of flexor hallucis longus
Calcaneal tendon
Posteromedial View

## 5.74 Posteromedial ankle

- The flexor hallucis longus muscle is midway between the medial and lateral malleoli; the tendons of the flexor digitorum and tibialis posterior are medial to it, and the tendons of the fibularis longus and brevis are lateral to it.
- The posterior tibial artery and the tibial nerve lie medial to the flexor hallucis longus muscle proximally and distally, after bifurcating posterolateral to it.
- The strongest parts of the ligaments of the ankle are those that prevent anterior displacement of the leg bones, namely, the posterior part of the medial ligament (posterior tibiotalar), the posterior talofibular, the tibiocalcanean, and the calcaneofibular.

- Entrapment and compression of the tibial nerve (tarsal tunnel syndrome) occurs when there is edema and tightness in the ankle involving the synovial sheaths of the tendons of muscles in the posterior compartment of the leg. The area involved is from the medial malleolus to the calcaneus. The heel pain results from compression of the tibial nerve by the flexor retinaculum.

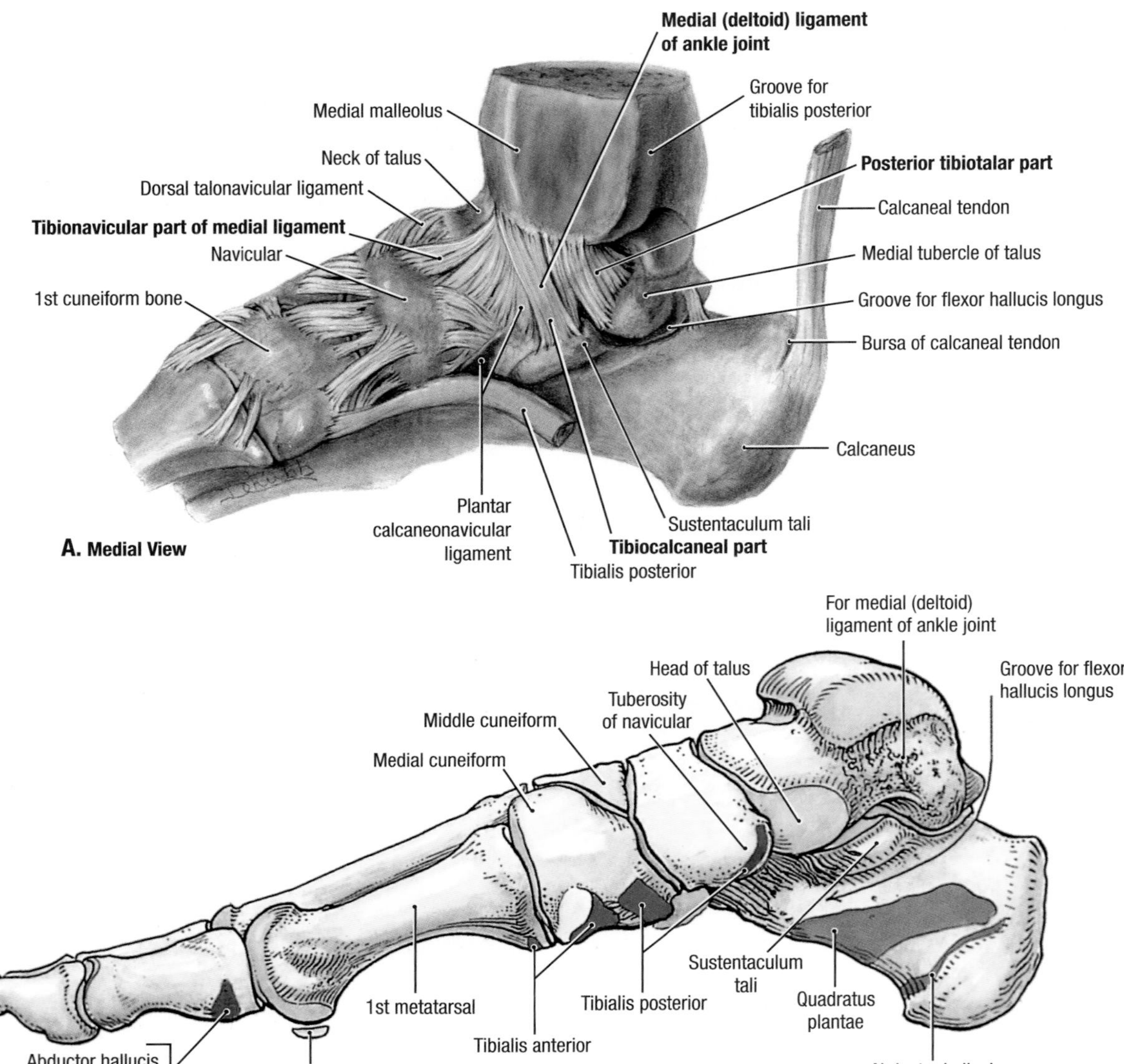

Medial (deltoid) ligament of ankle joint
Medial malleolus
Groove for tibialis posterior
Neck of talus
Posterior tibiotalar part
Dorsal talonavicular ligament
Calcaneal tendon
Tibionavicular part of medial ligament
Navicular
Medial tubercle of talus
1st cuneiform bone
Groove for flexor hallucis longus
Bursa of calcaneal tendon
Calcaneus
Plantar calcaneonavicular ligament
Sustentaculum tali
Tibiocalcaneal part
Tibialis posterior
A. Medial View
For medial (deltoid) ligament of ankle joint
Head of talus
Groove for flexor hallucis longus
Tuberosity of navicular
Middle cuneiform
Medial cuneiform
Sustentaculum tali
1st metatarsal
Tibialis posterior
Quadratus plantae
Tibialis anterior
B
Abductor hallucis
Flexor hallucis brevis
Medial sesamoid
Abductor hallucis


## 5.75 Medial ligaments of ankle region

**A.** Dissection. **B.** Bones. The joint capsule of the ankle joint is reinforced medially by the large, strong medial ligament of the ankle (deltoid ligament) that attaches proximally to the medial malleolus and fans out from it to attach distally to the talus, calcaneus, and navicular via four adjacent and continuous parts: the tibionavicular part, the tibiocalcaneal part, and the anterior and posterior tibiotalar parts. The medial ligament stabilizes the ankle joint during eversion of the foot and prevents subluxation (partial dislocation) of the ankle joint.

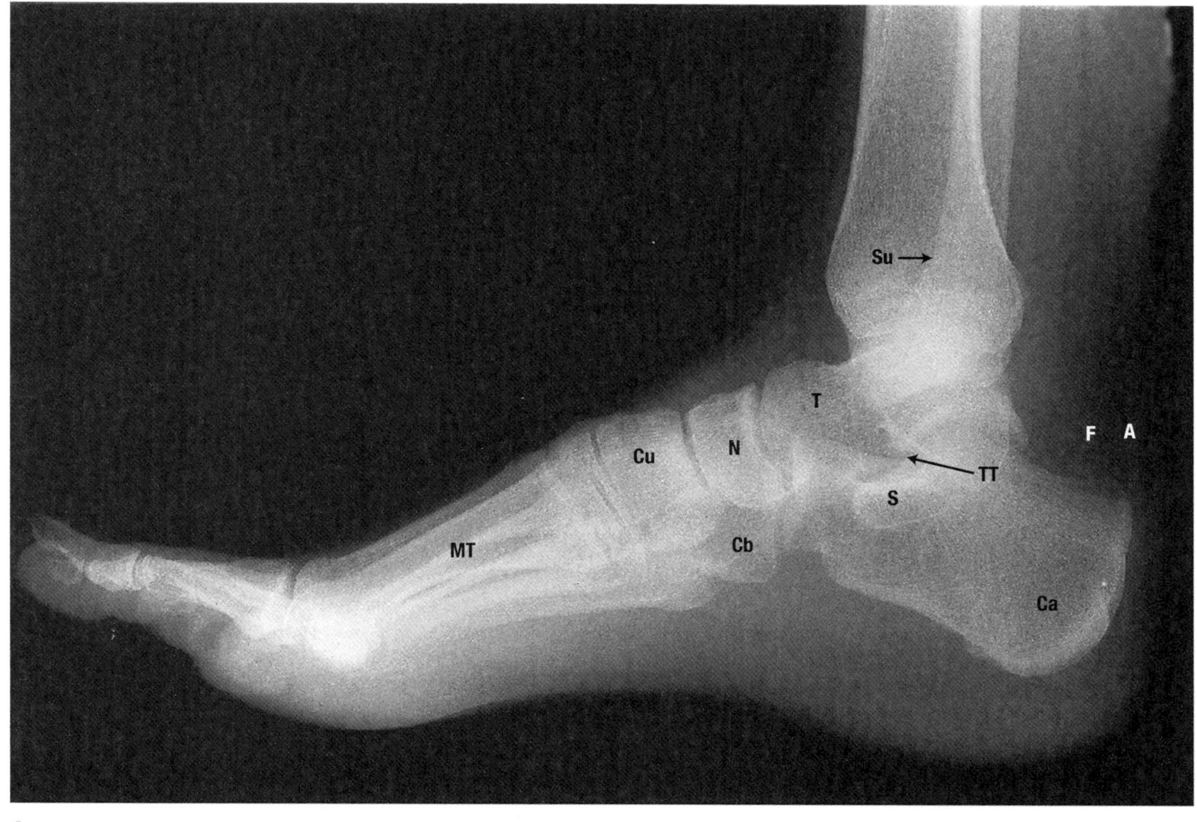
Su
T
F
A
Cu
N
TT
S
MT
Cb
Ca

A.

Medial Views

| | |
|---|---|
| A | Calcaneal (Achilles) tendon |
| Ca | Calcaneus |
| Cb | Cuboid |
| Cu | Cuneiforms |
| F | Fat |
| L | Lateral malleolus |
| MT | Metatarsal |
| N | Navicular |
| S | Sustentaculum tali |
| Su | Superimposed tibia and fibula |
| T | Talus |
| TT | Tarsal sinus |

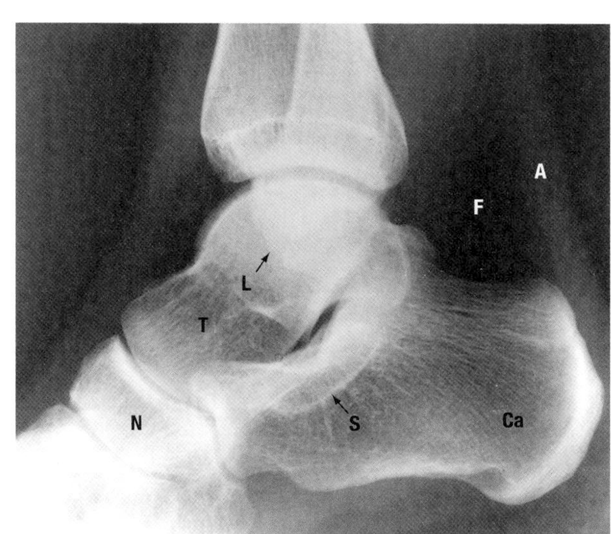
A
F
L
T
N
S
Ca

B.

**5.76 Radiographs of ankle and foot**

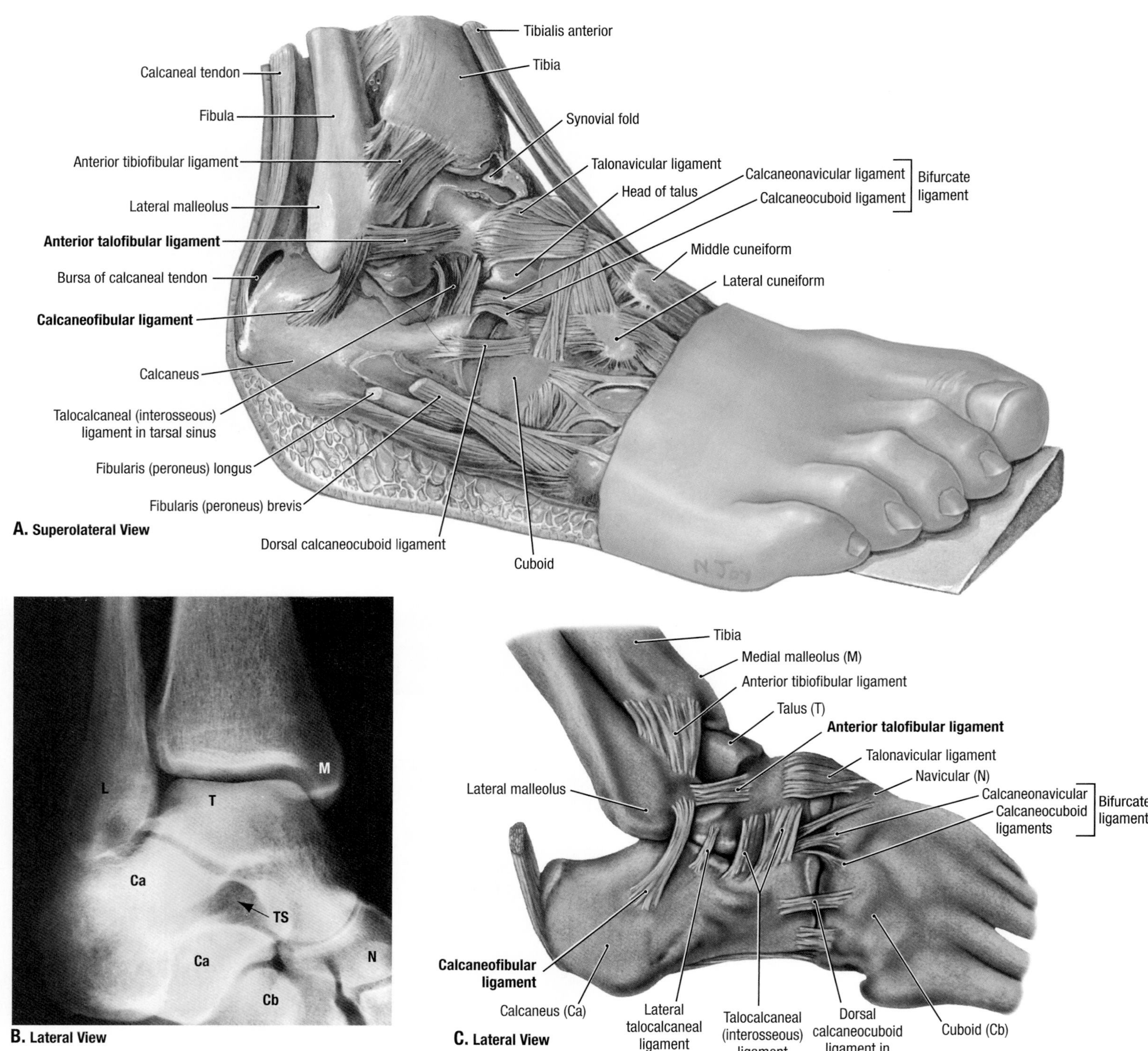
Tibialis anterior
Tibia
Calcaneal tendon
Fibula
Synovial fold
Anterior tibiofibular ligament
Talonavicular ligament
Head of talus
Calcaneonavicular ligament
Calcaneocuboid ligament
Bifurcate ligament
Lateral malleolus
Anterior talofibular ligament
Middle cuneiform
Bursa of calcaneal tendon
Lateral cuneiform
Calcaneofibular ligament
Calcaneus
Talocalcaneal (interosseous) ligament in tarsal sinus
Fibularis (peroneus) longus
Fibularis (peroneus) brevis
A. Superolateral View
Dorsal calcaneocuboid ligament
Cuboid
M
L
T
Ca
TS
Ca
N
Cb
B. Lateral View
Tibia
Medial malleolus (M)
Anterior tibiofibular ligament
Talus (T)
Anterior talofibular ligament
Talonavicular ligament
Navicular (N)
Lateral malleolus
Calcaneonavicular
Calcaneocuboid
ligaments
Bifurcate ligament
Calcaneofibular ligament
Calcaneus (Ca)
Lateral talocalcaneal ligament
Talocalcaneal (interosseous) ligament
Dorsal calcaneocuboid ligament in tarsal sinus (TS)
Cuboid (Cb)
C. Lateral View

## 5.77 Lateral ligaments of ankle region

**A.** Dissection with foot inverted by underlying wedge. **B.** Lateral radiograph. **C.** Dissection. (Abbreviations following some labels refer to structures identified in **B.**)

The ankle joint is reinforced laterally by the lateral ligament of the ankle, which consists of three separate ligaments: (1) anterior talofibular ligament, a flat, weak band; (2) calcaneofibular ligament, a round cord directed posteroinferiorly; and (3) posterior talofibular ligament, a strong, medially-directed horizontal ligament (see Fig. 5.74).

Ankle sprains (partial or fully torn ligaments) are common injuries. Ankle sprains nearly always result from forceful inversion of the weight-bearing plantarflexed foot. The anterior talofibular ligament is most commonly injured, resulting in instability of the ankle. The calcaneofibular is also often torn.

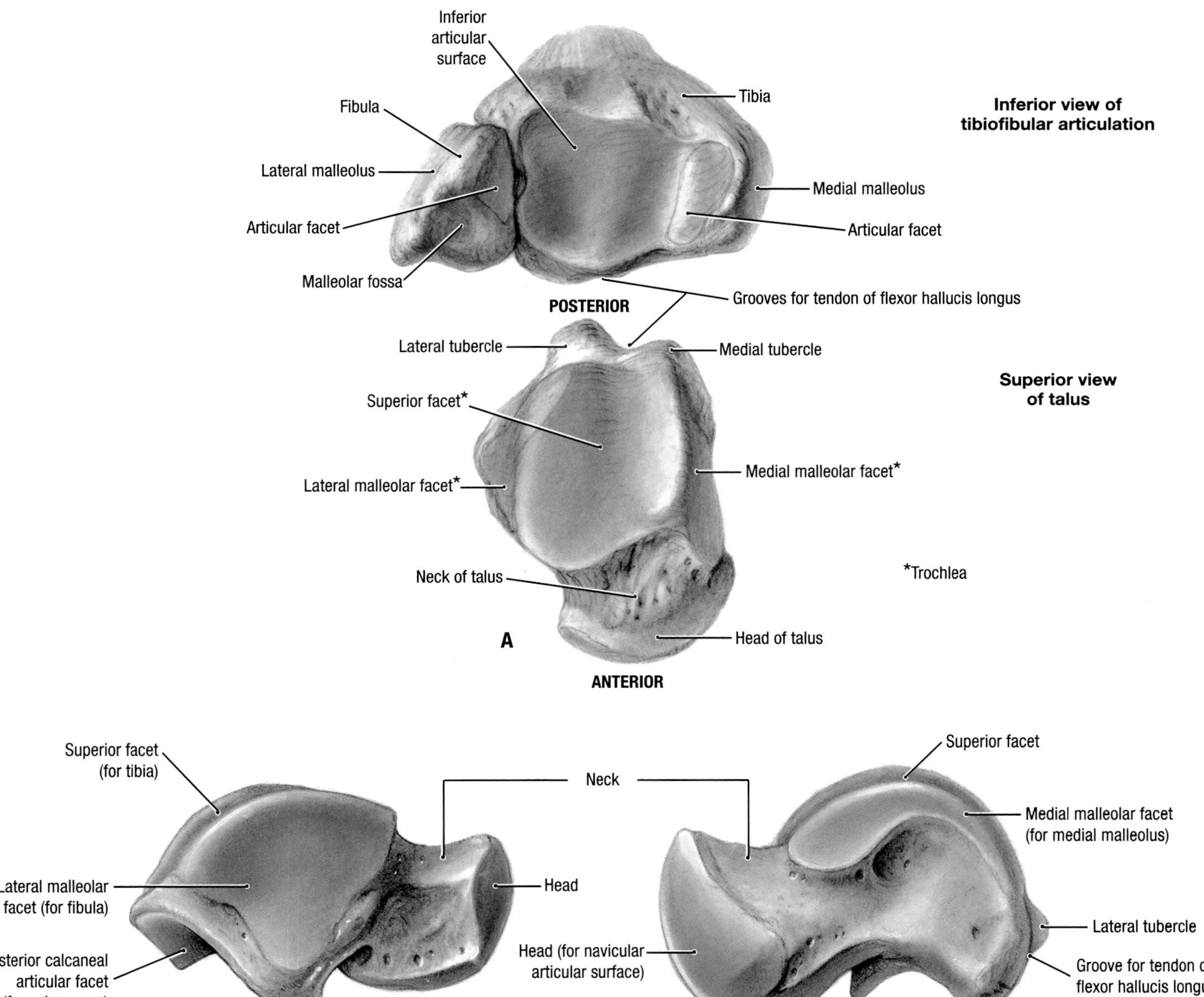
Inferior view of tibiofibular articulation
Inferior articular surface
Fibula
Tibia
Lateral malleolus
Medial malleolus
Articular facet
Articular facet
Malleolar fossa
POSTERIOR
Grooves for tendon of flexor hallucis longus
Superior view of talus
Lateral tubercle
Medial tubercle
Superior facet*
Lateral malleolar facet*
Medial malleolar facet*
Neck of talus
*Trochlea
A
Head of talus
ANTERIOR
Superior facet (for tibia)
Neck
Superior facet
Medial malleolar facet (for medial malleolus)
Lateral malleolar facet (for fibula)
Head
Head (for navicular articular surface)
Lateral tubercle
Posterior calcaneal articular facet (for calcaneous)
Groove for tendon of flexor hallucis longus
Medial tubercle
B. Lateral View
C. Medial View

## 5.78 Articular surfaces of ankle joint

**A.** Superior aspect of talus separated from distal ends of tibia and fibula. The superior articular surface of the talus is broader anteriorly than posteriorly; hence the medial and lateral malleoli, which grasp the sides of the talus, tend to be forced apart in dorsiflexion. The fully dorsiflexed position is stable compared with the fully plantar flexed position. In plantar flexion, when the tibia and fibula articulate with the narrower posterior part of the superior articular surface of the talus, some side-to-side movement of the joint is allowed, accounting for the instability of the joint in this position. **B.** Lateral aspect of talus. The lateral, triangular articular area is for articulation with the lateral malleolus. **C.** Medial aspect of talus. The comma-shaped articular area is for articulation with the medial malleolus.

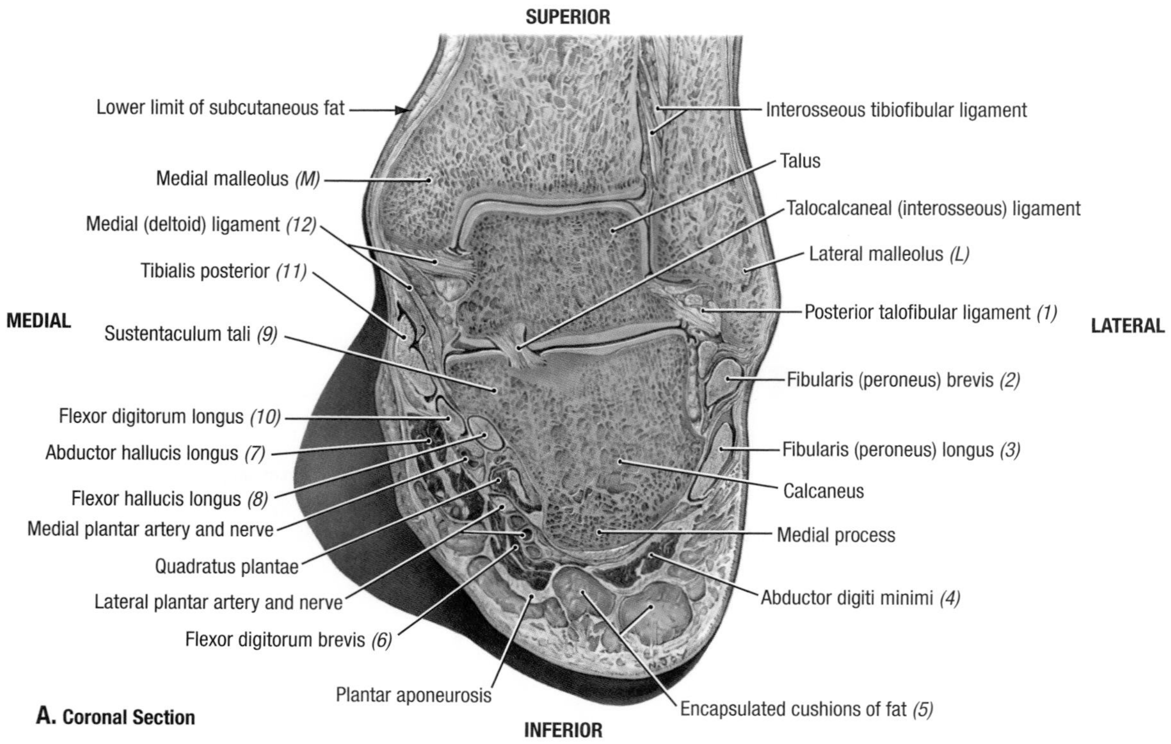
SUPERIOR
MEDIAL
LATERAL
INFERIOR
Lower limit of subcutaneous fat
Medial malleolus (M)
Medial (deltoid) ligament (12)
Tibialis posterior (11)
Sustentaculum tali (9)
Flexor digitorum longus (10)
Abductor hallucis longus (7)
Flexor hallucis longus (8)
Medial plantar artery and nerve
Quadratus plantae
Lateral plantar artery and nerve
Flexor digitorum brevis (6)
Plantar aponeurosis
Interosseous tibiofibular ligament
Talus
Talocalcaneal (interosseous) ligament
Lateral malleolus (L)
Posterior talofibular ligament (1)
Fibularis (peroneus) brevis (2)
Fibularis (peroneus) longus (3)
Calcaneus
Medial process
Abductor digiti minimi (4)
Encapsulated cushions of fat (5)

**A.** Coronal Section

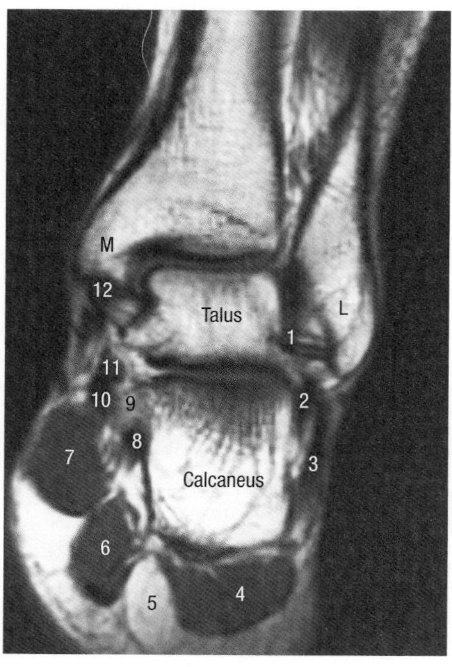
M
12
Talus
L
1
11
10
9
2
8
7
3
Calcaneus
6
5
4

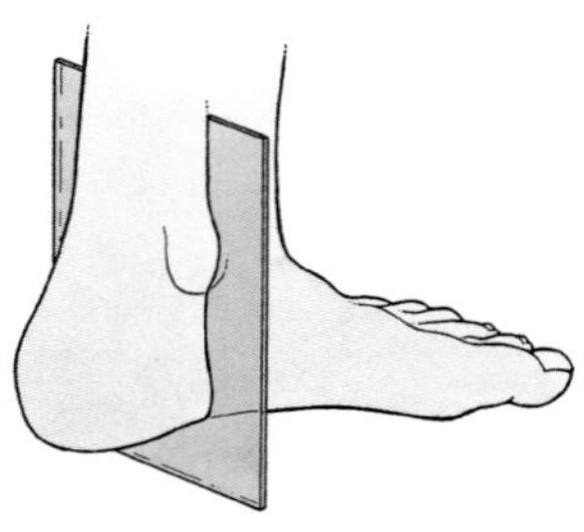

**B.** Coronal MRI

## 5.79 Coronal section and MRI through ankle

**A.** Coronal section. **B.** Coronal MRI (*numbers* in **B** refer to structures labeled in **A**).

- The tibia rests on the talus, and the talus rests on the calcaneus; between the calcaneus and the skin are several encapsulated cushions of fat.
- The lateral malleolus descends farther inferiorly than the medial malleolus.
- The talocalcaneal (interosseous) ligament between the talus and calcaneus separates the subtalar, or posterior, talocalcanean joint from the talocalcaneonavicular joint.
- The sustentaculum tali acts as a pulley for the flexor hallucis longus muscle and gives attachment to the calcaneotibial part of the medial (deltoid) ligament.

ANTERIOR

Anterior tibial artery and deep fibular (peroneal) nerve *(4)*

Extensor hallucis longus *(3)*

Extensor digitorum longus *(5)*

Tibialis anterior *(2)*

Fibularis (peroneus) tertius *(5)*

Saphenous nerve

Great (long) saphenous vein *(1)*

Medial malleolus *(M)*

Lateral malleolus *(L)*

Talus

Posterior talofibular ligament

Medial (deltoid) ligament

Tibialis posterior *(13)*

MEDIAL

LATERAL

Flexor digitorum longus *(12)*

Fibularis (peroneus) brevis *(6)*

Fibularis (peroneus) longus *(7)*

Medial tubercle

Posterior tibial artery and tibial nerve *(11)*

Sural nerve

Small (short) saphenous vein *(8)*

Medial calcaneal artery and nerve

Intermuscular fascial septum

Flexor hallucis longus *(10)*

Tubercle of calcaneus

Calcaneal tendon *(9)*

Lateral tubercle

Bursa of calcaneal tendon

Subcutaneous calcaneal bursa

POSTERIOR

**A. Transverse Section Superior View**

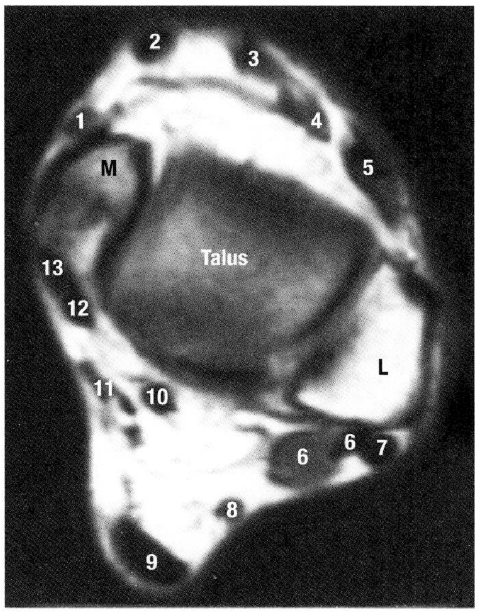
2
3
1
4
5
M
Talus
13
12
L
11
10
6
6
7
8
9

**B. Transverse MRI**

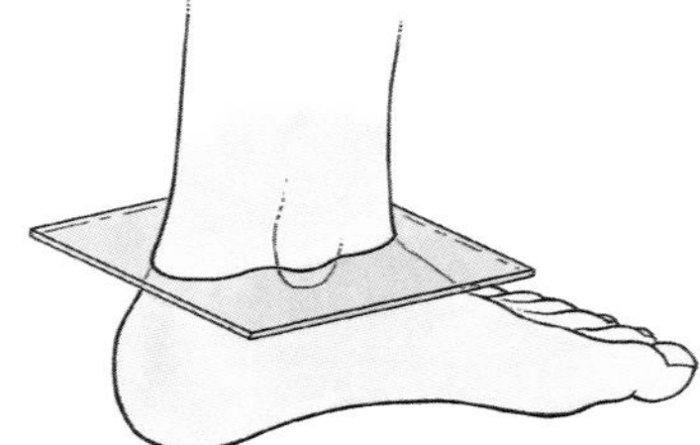

## 5.80 Transverse section and MRI through ankle

**A.** Transverse section. **B.** Transverse MRI (*numbers* in **B** refer to structures labeled in **A**).

- The body of the talus is wedge shaped and positioned between the malleoli, which are bound to it by the medial (deltoid) and posterior talofibular ligaments.
- The flexor hallucis longus muscle lies within its osseofibrous sheath between the medial and lateral tubercles of the talus.
- There is a small, inconstant subcutaneous bursa superficial to the calcaneal tendon and a large, constant bursa of calcaneal tendon deep to it.

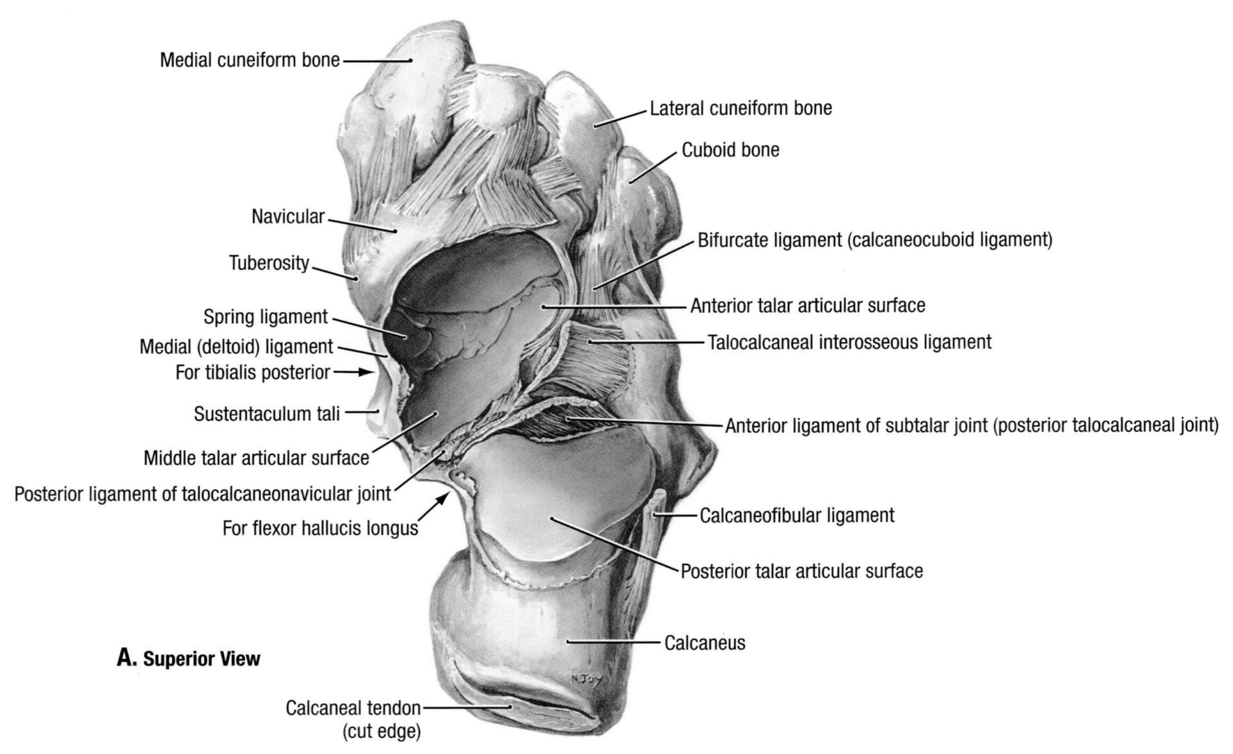
Medial cuneiform bone
Lateral cuneiform bone
Cuboid bone
Navicular
Tuberosity
Bifurcate ligament (calcaneocuboid ligament)
Anterior talar articular surface
Spring ligament
Talocalcaneal interosseous ligament
Medial (deltoid) ligament
For tibialis posterior
Sustentaculum tali
Anterior ligament of subtalar joint (posterior talocalcaneal joint)
Middle talar articular surface
Posterior ligament of talocalcaneonavicular joint
Calcaneofibular ligament
For flexor hallucis longus
Posterior talar articular surface
Calcaneus
Calcaneal tendon
(cut edge)

**A. Superior View**

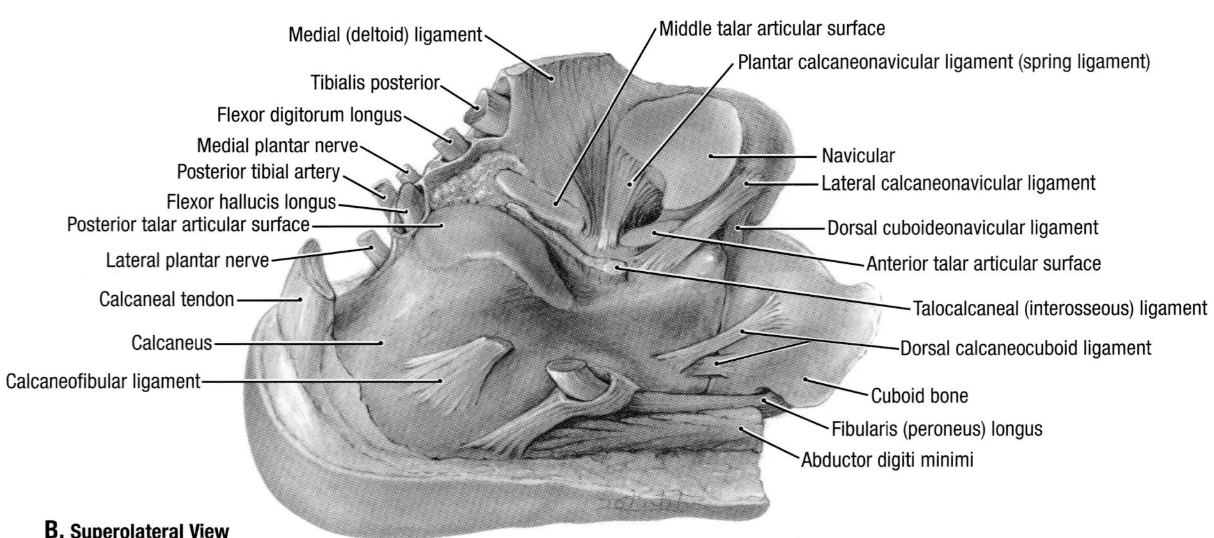
Medial (deltoid) ligament
Middle talar articular surface
Plantar calcaneonavicular ligament (spring ligament)
Tibialis posterior
Flexor digitorum longus
Medial plantar nerve
Navicular
Posterior tibial artery
Lateral calcaneonavicular ligament
Flexor hallucis longus
Posterior talar articular surface
Dorsal cuboideonavicular ligament
Lateral plantar nerve
Anterior talar articular surface
Calcaneal tendon
Talocalcaneal (interosseous) ligament
Calcaneus
Dorsal calcaneocuboid ligament
Calcaneofibular ligament
Cuboid bone
Fibularis (peroneus) longus
Abductor digiti minimi

**B. Superolateral View**

## 5.81 Joints of inversion and eversion

The joints of inversion and eversion are the subtalar (posterior talocalcanean) joint, talocalcaneonavicular joint, and transverse tarsal (combined calcaneocuboid and talonavicular) joint. **A.** Posterior and middle parts of foot with talus removed. **B.** Posterior part of foot with talus removed. The convex posterior talar facet is separated from the concave middle, and anterior facets by the talocalcaneal (interosseous) ligament within the tarsal sinus.

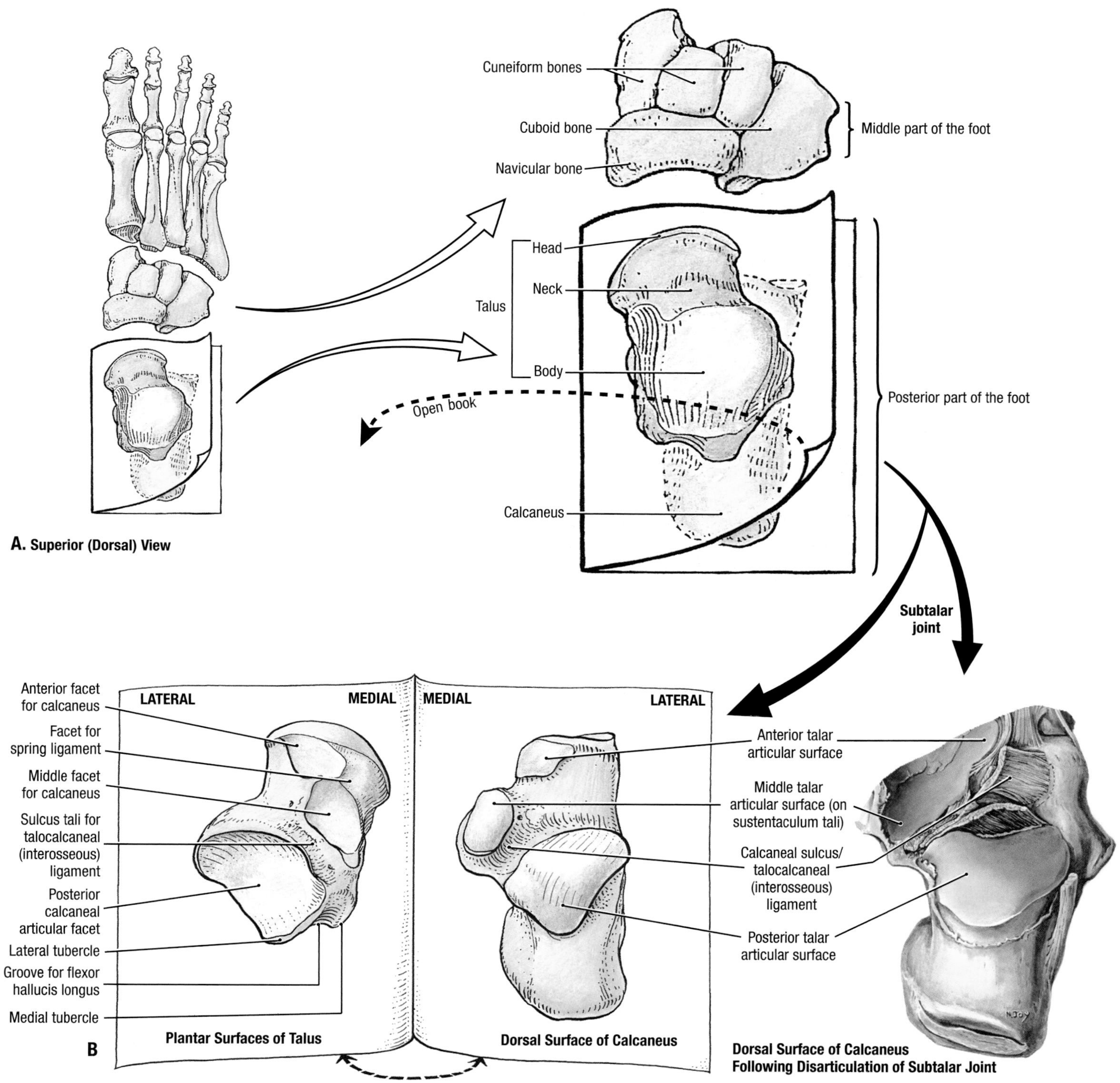
Cuneiform bones
Cuboid bone
Navicular bone
Middle part of the foot
Head
Neck
Talus
Body
Open book
Posterior part of the foot
Calcaneus
A. Superior (Dorsal) View
Subtalar joint
LATERAL
MEDIAL
MEDIAL
LATERAL
Anterior facet for calcaneus
Facet for spring ligament
Middle facet for calcaneus
Sulcus tali for talocalcaneal (interosseous) ligament
Posterior calcaneal articular facet
Lateral tubercle
Groove for flexor hallucis longus
Medial tubercle
B
Plantar Surfaces of Talus
Dorsal Surface of Calcaneus
Anterior talar articular surface
Middle talar articular surface (on sustentaculum tali)
Calcaneal sulcus/ talocalcaneal (interosseous) ligament
Posterior talar articular surface
Dorsal Surface of Calcaneus Following Disarticulation of Subtalar Joint

## 5.82 Talocalcanean joint

**A.** Bones of foot, dorsal view. **B.** Bony surfaces of talocalcanean joints. The plantar surface of the talus and dorsal surface of the calcaneus are displayed as pages in a book.

- The joints of inversion and eversion are the subtalar (posterior talocalcanean) joint, talocalcaneonavicular joint, and transverse tarsal (combined calcaneocuboid and talonavicular) joint.
- The talus is part of the ankle joint, of the posterior and anterior talocalcanean joints, and of the talonavicular joint.
- The posterior and anterior talocalcanean joints are separated from each other by the sulcus tarsi and calcaneal sulcus, which, when the talus and calcaneus are in articulation, become the tarsal sinus.

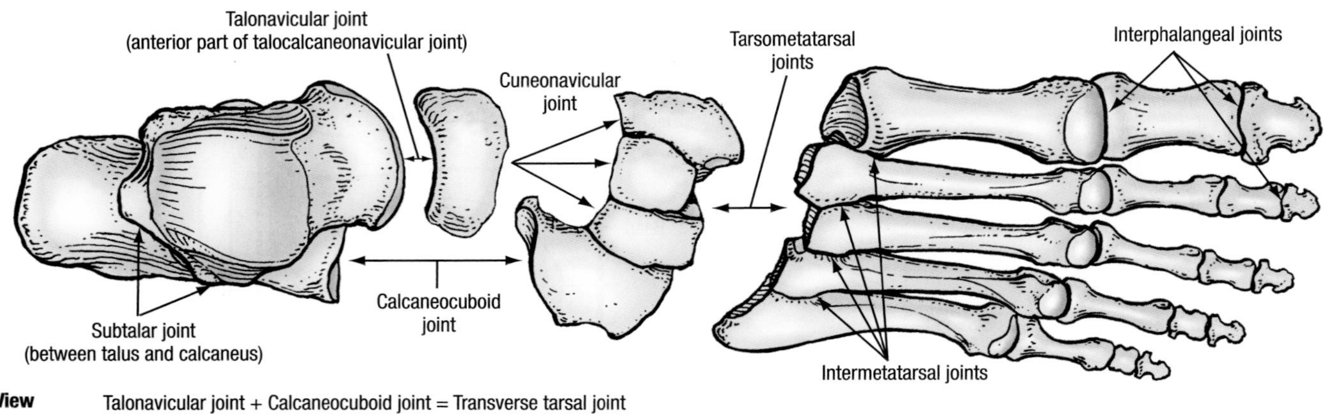
Talonavicular joint
(anterior part of talocalcaneonavicular joint)
Cuneonavicular joint
Tarsometatarsal joints
Interphalangeal joints
Subtalar joint
(between talus and calcaneus)
Calcaneocuboid joint
Intermetatarsal joints

**Superior View** Talonavicular joint + Calcaneocuboid joint = Transverse tarsal joint

**TABLE 5.19 JOINTS OF FOOT**

| Joint | Type | Articular Surface | Joint Capsule | Ligaments | Movements |
|---|---|---|---|---|---|
| **Subtalar** | Synovial (plane) joint | Inferior surface of body of talus articulates with superior surface of calcaneus | Attached to margins of articular surfaces | Medial, lateral, and posterior talocalcaneal ligaments support capsule; talocalcaneal (interosseous) ligament binds bones together | Inversion and eversion of foot |
| **Talocalcaneo-navicular** | Synovial joint; talonavicular part is ball-and-socket type | Head of talus articulates with calcaneus and navicular bones | Incompletely encloses joint | Plantar calcaneonavicular ("spring") ligament supports head of talus | Gliding and rotary movements |
| **Calcaneocuboid** | Synovial (plane) joint | Anterior end of calcaneus articulates with posterior surface of cuboid | Encloses joint | Dorsal calcaneocuboid ligament, plantar calcaneocuboid ligament, and long plantar ligament support fibrous capsule | Inversion and eversion of foot |
| **Cuneonavicular** | Synovial (plane) joint | Anterior navicular articulates with posterior surface of cuneiforms | Common joint capsule | Dorsal and plantar ligaments | Little movement |
| **Tarsometatarsal** | Synovial (plane) joint | Anterior tarsal bones articulate with bases of metatarsal bones | Encloses joint | Dorsal, plantar, and interosseous ligaments | Gliding or sliding |
| **Intermetatarsal** | Synovial (plane) joint | Bases of metatarsal bones articulate with each other | Encloses each joint | Dorsal, plantar, and interosseous ligaments bind bones together | Little individual movement |
| **Metatarsophalangeal** | Synovial (condyloid) joint | Heads of metatarsal bones articulate with bases of proximal phalanges | Encloses each joint ligament supports | Collateral ligaments support capsule on each side; plantar and circumduction plantar part of capsule | Flexion, extension, and some abduction, adduction, |
| **Interphalangeal** | Synovial (hinge) joint | Head of proximal or middle phalanx articulates with base of phalanx distal to it | Encloses each joint | Collateral and plantar ligaments support joints | Flexion and extension |

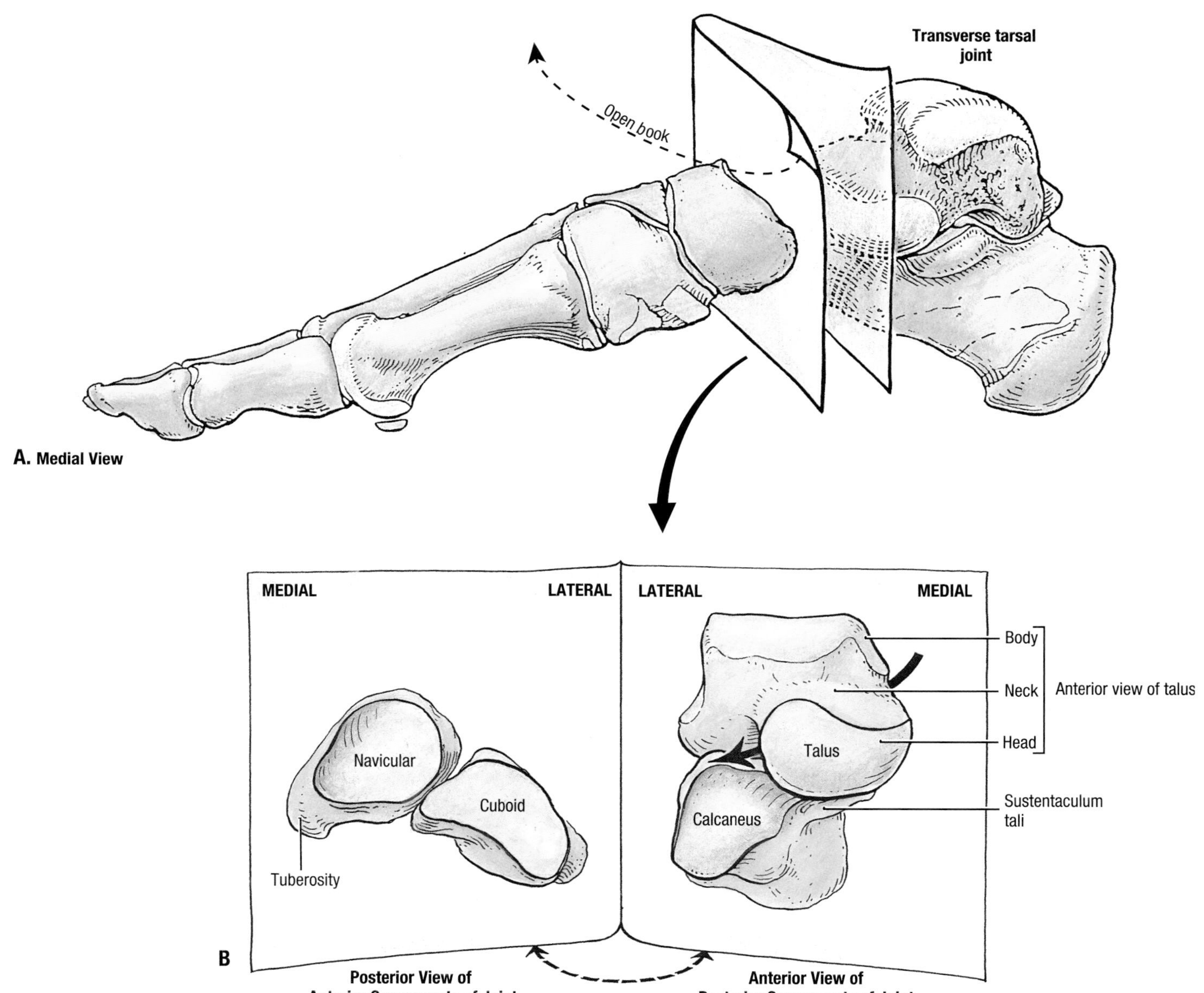
Transverse tarsal joint
Open book
A. Medial View
MEDIAL
LATERAL
LATERAL
MEDIAL
Navicular
Cuboid
Tuberosity
Body
Neck
Head
Anterior view of talus
Talus
Calcaneus
Sustentaculum tali
B
Posterior View of Anterior Components of Joint
Anterior View of Posterior Components of Joint

## 5.83 Transverse tarsal joint

**A.** Bones of foot, medial view. **B.** Articular surfaces of transverse tarsal joint. This compound joint includes the talonavicular and calcaneocuboid articulations. The posterior surfaces of the navicular and cuboid bones and the anterior surfaces of the talus and calcaneus are displayed as pages in a book. The *black arrow* traverses the tarsal sinus, in which the talocalcaneal (interosseous) ligament is located.

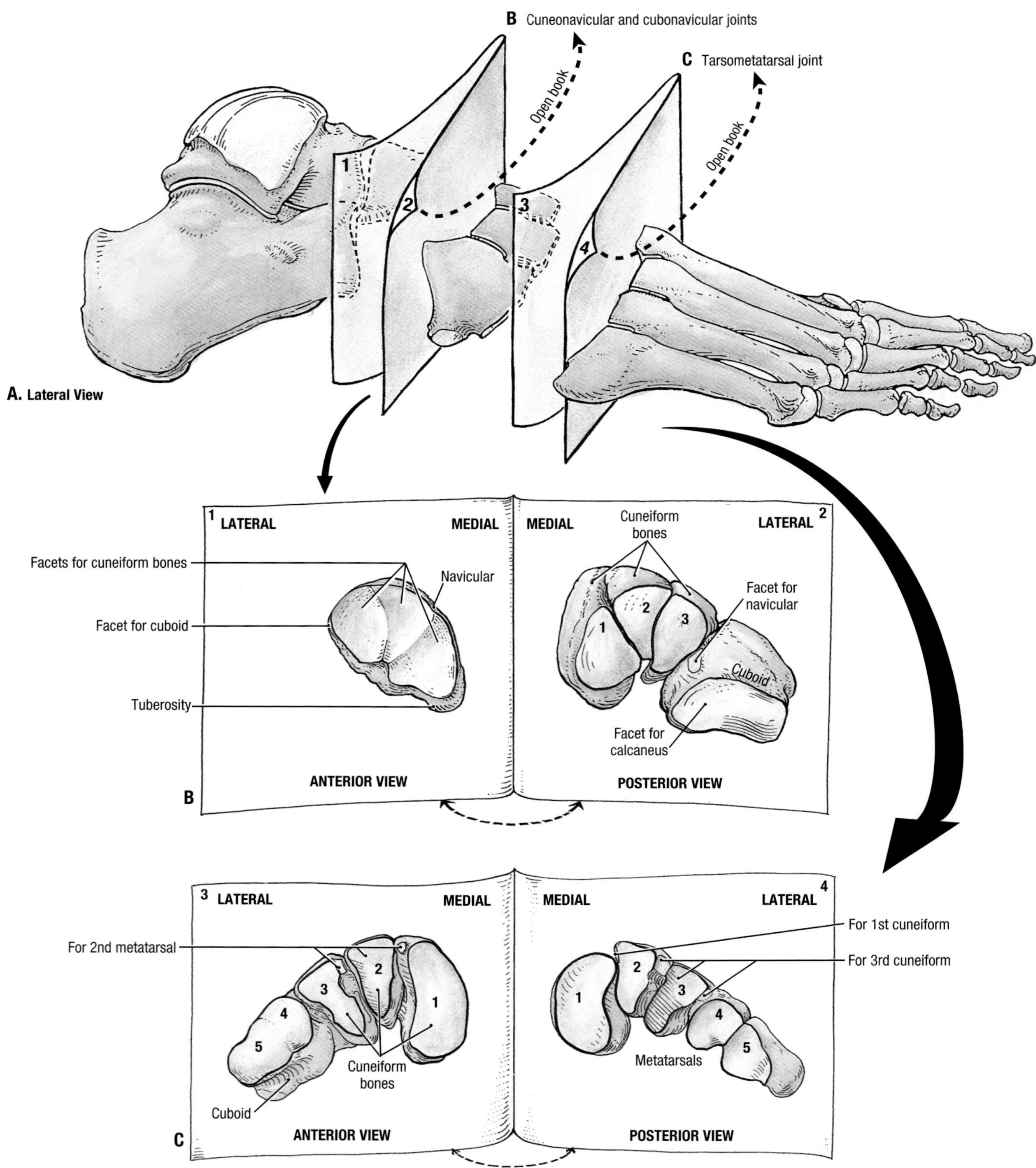
B Cuneonavicular and cubonavicular joints
C Tarsometatarsal joint
Open book
Open book
1
2
3
4
A. Lateral View
1 LATERAL
MEDIAL
MEDIAL
Cuneiform bones
LATERAL 2
Facets for cuneiform bones
Navicular
Facet for cuboid
Tuberosity
Facet for navicular
Cuboid
Facet for calcaneus
ANTERIOR VIEW
POSTERIOR VIEW
B
3 LATERAL
MEDIAL
MEDIAL
LATERAL 4
For 2nd metatarsal
For 1st cuneiform
For 3rd cuneiform
Cuneiform bones
Metatarsals
Cuboid
ANTERIOR VIEW
POSTERIOR VIEW
C

**5.84 Cuneonavicular, cubonavicular, and tarsometatarsal joints**

**A.** Bones of foot, lateral view. **B.** Bony surfaces of the cuneonavicular and cubonavicular joints. **C.** Bony surfaces of the tarsometatarsal joints.

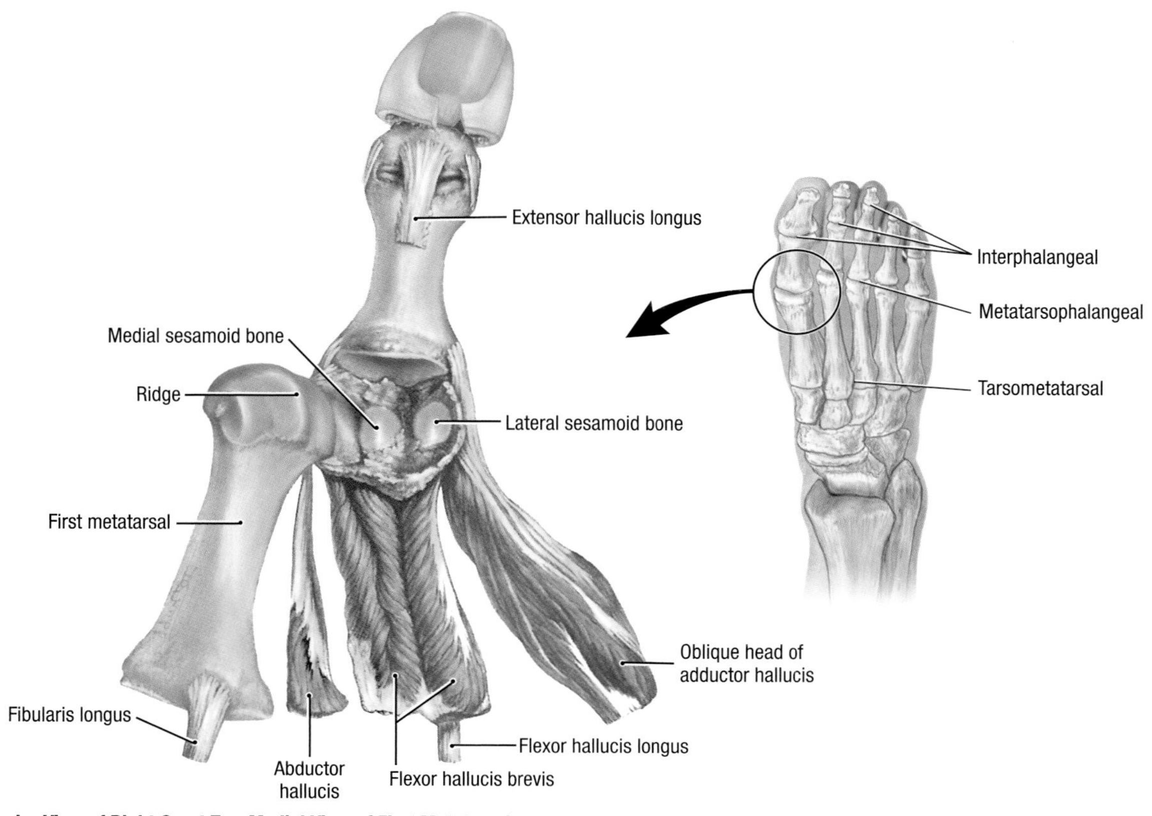
Extensor hallucis longus
Interphalangeal
Metatarsophalangeal
Tarsometatarsal
Medial sesamoid bone
Ridge
Lateral sesamoid bone
First metatarsal
Oblique head of adductor hallucis
Fibularis longus
Flexor hallucis longus
Abductor hallucis
Flexor hallucis brevis

**A. Superior View of Right Great Toe, Medial View of First Metetarsal**

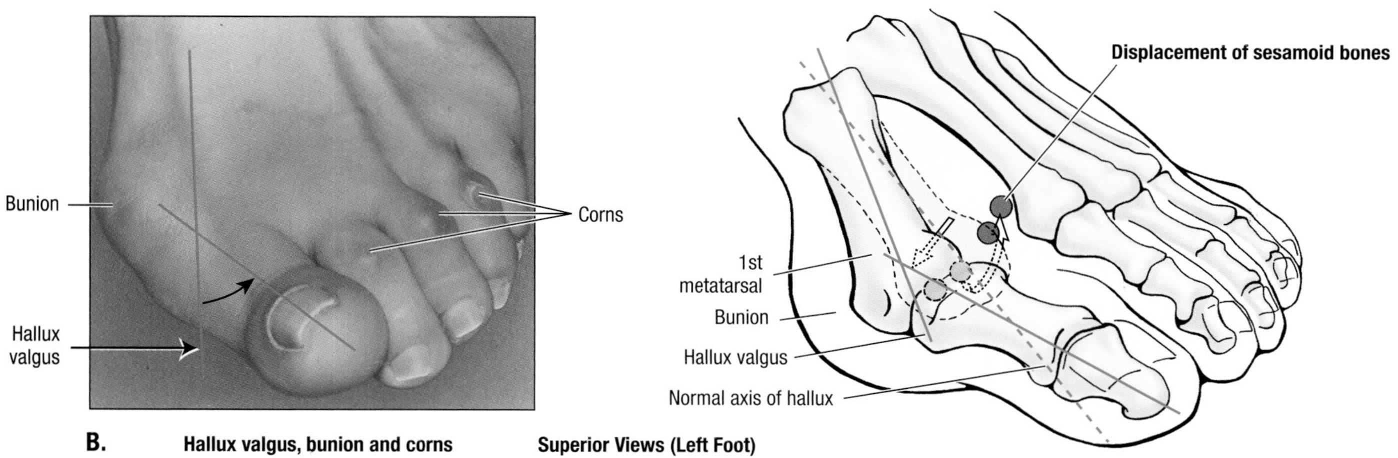
Bunion
Corns
Hallux valgus
Displacement of sesamoid bones
1st metatarsal
Bunion
Hallux valgus
Normal axis of hallux

**B.** **Hallux valgus, bunion and corns** **Superior Views (Left Foot)**

## 5.85 Metatarsophalangeal joint of great toe

**A.** First metatarsal and sesamoid bones of the right great toe. The sesamoid bones of the great toe (hallux) are bound together and located on each side of a bony ridge on the first metatarsal. **B.** Hallux valgus. Hallux valgus is a foot deformity caused by pressure from footwear and degenerative joint disease; it is characterized by lateral deviation of the great toe (L. *hallux*). In some people, the deviation is so great that the 1st toe overlaps the 2nd toe. These individuals are unable to move their 1st digit away from their 2nd digit because the sesamoid bones under the head of the 1st metatarsal are displaced and lie in the space between the heads of the 1st and 2nd metatarsals. In addition, a subcutaneous bursa may form owing to pressure and friction against the shoe. When tender and inflamed, the bursa is called a bunion.

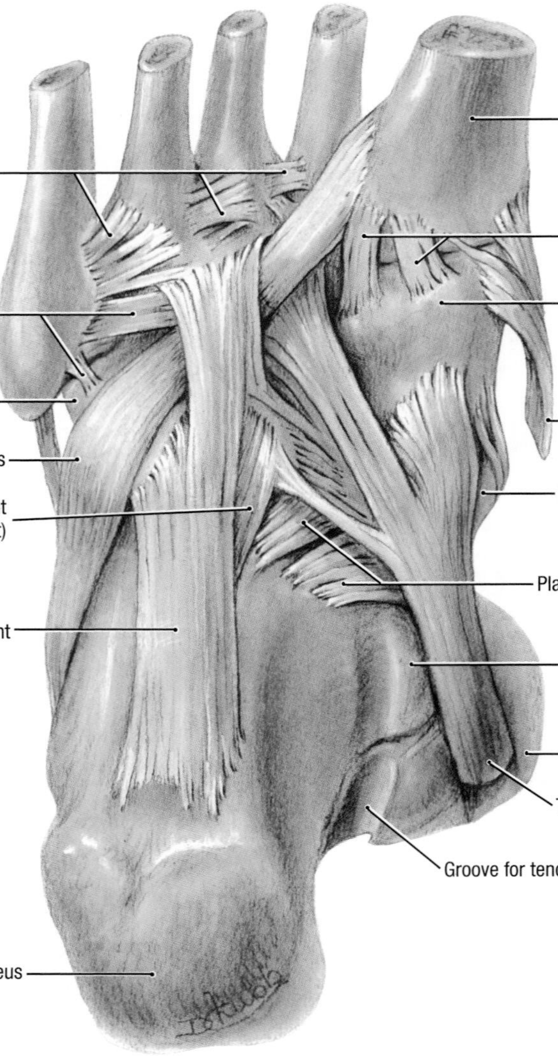

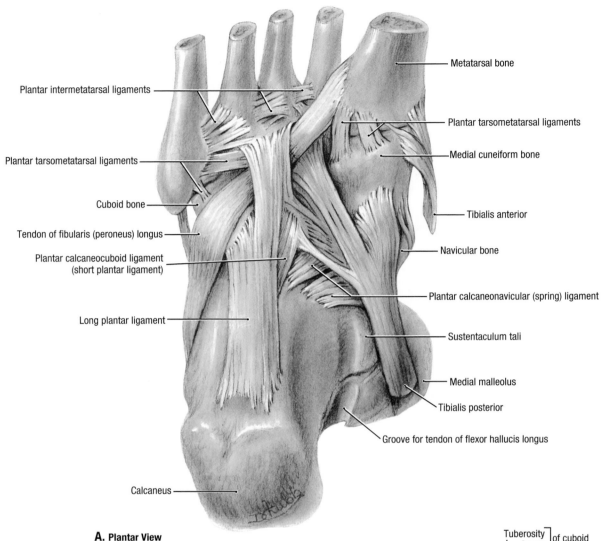

Metatarsal bone
Plantar intermetatarsal ligaments
Plantar tarsometatarsal ligaments
Medial cuneiform bone
Plantar tarsometatarsal ligaments
Cuboid bone
Tibialis anterior
Tendon of fibularis (peroneus) longus
Navicular bone
Plantar calcaneocuboid ligament (short plantar ligament)
Plantar calcaneonavicular (spring) ligament
Long plantar ligament
Sustentaculum tali
Medial malleolus
Tibialis posterior
Groove for tendon of flexor hallucis longus
Calcaneus

**A. Plantar View**

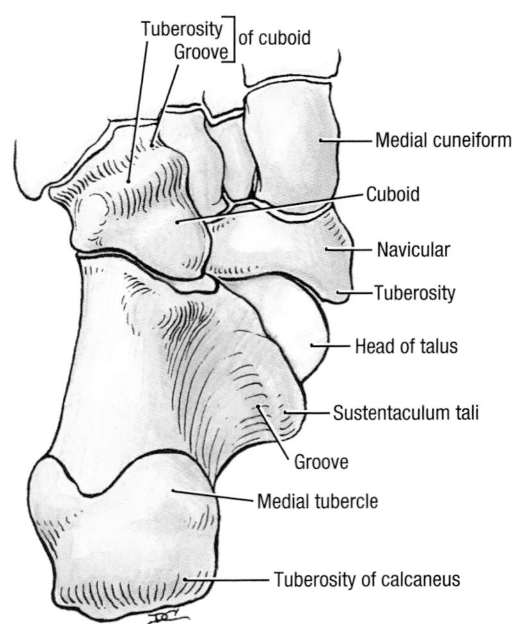
Tuberosity
Groove
of cuboid
Medial cuneiform
Cuboid
Navicular
Tuberosity
Head of talus
Sustentaculum tali
Groove
Medial tubercle
Tuberosity of calcaneus

**B. Plantar View**

## 5.86 Ligaments of sole of foot

**A.** Dissection of superficial ligaments. **B.** Bones lying deep to ligaments of **A.** In **A**:

- The head of the talus is exposed between the sustentaculum tali of the calcaneus and the navicular.
- Note the insertions of three long tendons: fibularis (peroneus) longus, tibialis anterior, and tibialis posterior.
- The tendon of the fibularis (peroneus) longus muscle crosses the sole of the foot in the groove anterior to the ridge of the cuboid, is bridged by some fibers of the long plantar ligament, and inserts into the base of the first metatarsal.
- Observe the slips of the tibialis posterior tendon extending to the bones anterior to the transverse tarsal joint.

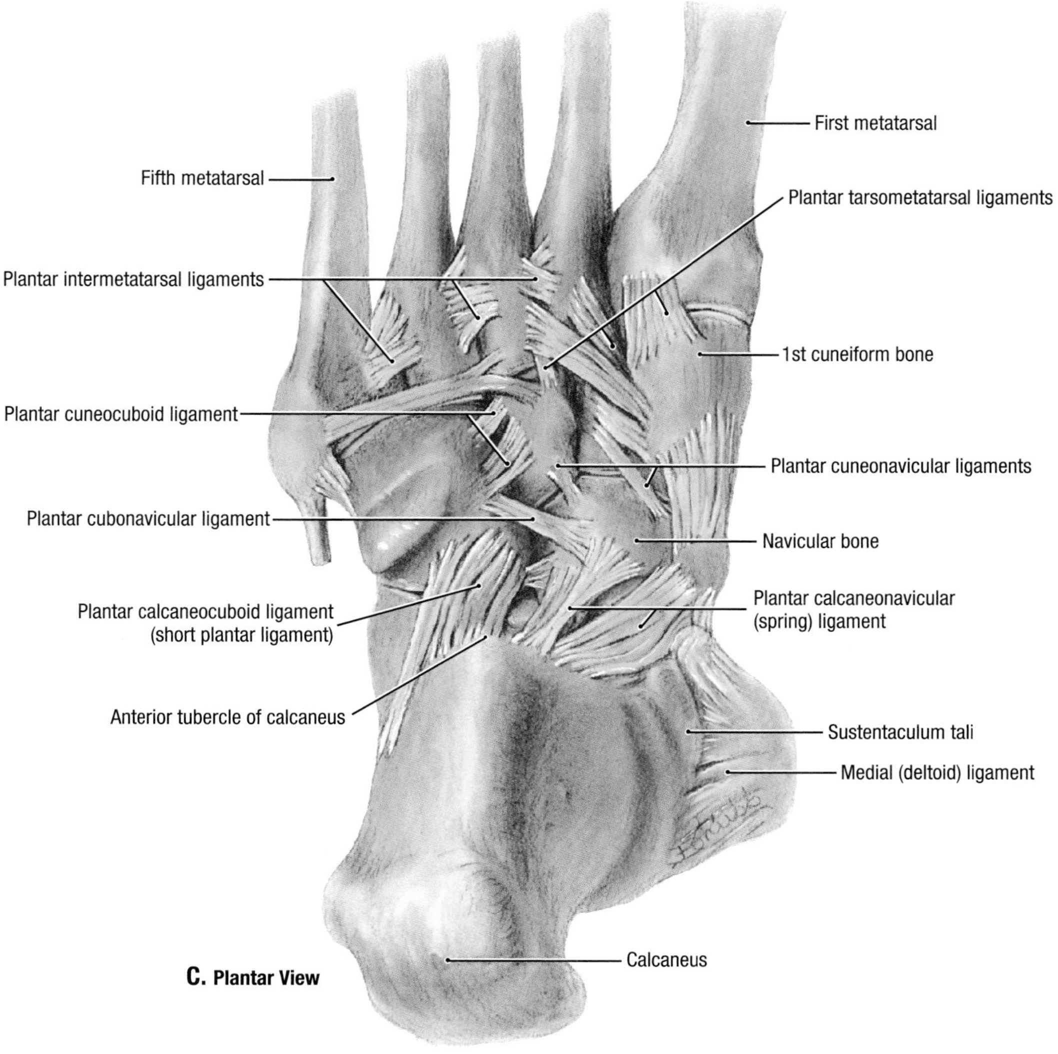
First metatarsal
Fifth metatarsal
Plantar tarsometatarsal ligaments
Plantar intermetatarsal ligaments
1st cuneiform bone
Plantar cuneocuboid ligament
Plantar cuneonavicular ligaments
Plantar cubonavicular ligament
Navicular bone
Plantar calcaneocuboid ligament
(short plantar ligament)
Plantar calcaneonavicular
(spring) ligament
Anterior tubercle of calcaneus
Sustentaculum tali
Medial (deltoid) ligament
Calcaneus

**C. Plantar View**

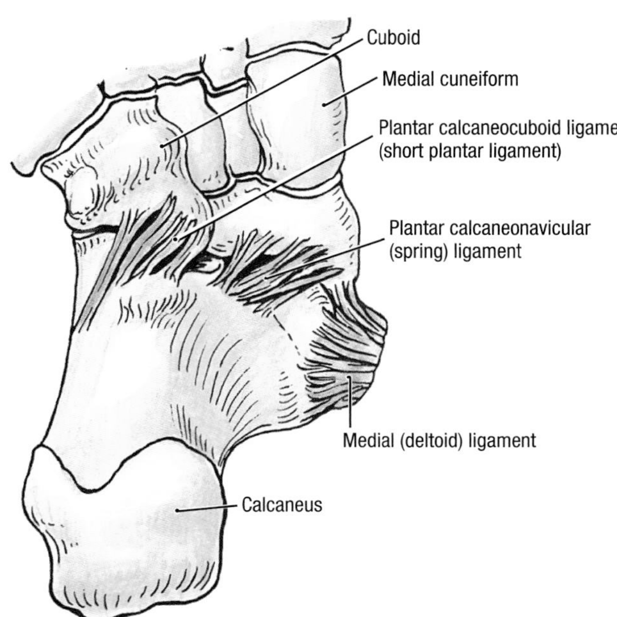
Cuboid
Medial cuneiform
Plantar calcaneocuboid ligament
(short plantar ligament)
Plantar calcaneonavicular
(spring) ligament
Medial (deltoid) ligament
Calcaneus

**D. Plantar View**

## 5.86 Ligaments of sole of foot *(continued)*

**C.** Dissection of the deep ligaments. **D.** Support for head of talus. The head of the talus is supported by the plantar calcaneonavicular ligament (spring ligament) and the tendon of the tibialis posterior.

- The plantar calcaneocuboid (short plantar) and plantar calcaneonavicular (spring) ligaments are the primary plantar ligaments of the transverse tarsal joint .
- The ligaments of the anterior foot diverge laterally and posteriorly from each side of the long axis of the third metatarsal and third cuneiform; hence a posterior thrust received by the first metatarsal, as when rising on the big toe while in walking, is transmitted directly to the navicular and talus by the first cuneiform and indirectly by the second metatarsal, second cuneiform, third metatarsal, and third cuneiform.
- A posterior thrust received by the fourth and fifth metatarsals is transmitted directly to the cuboid and calcaneus.

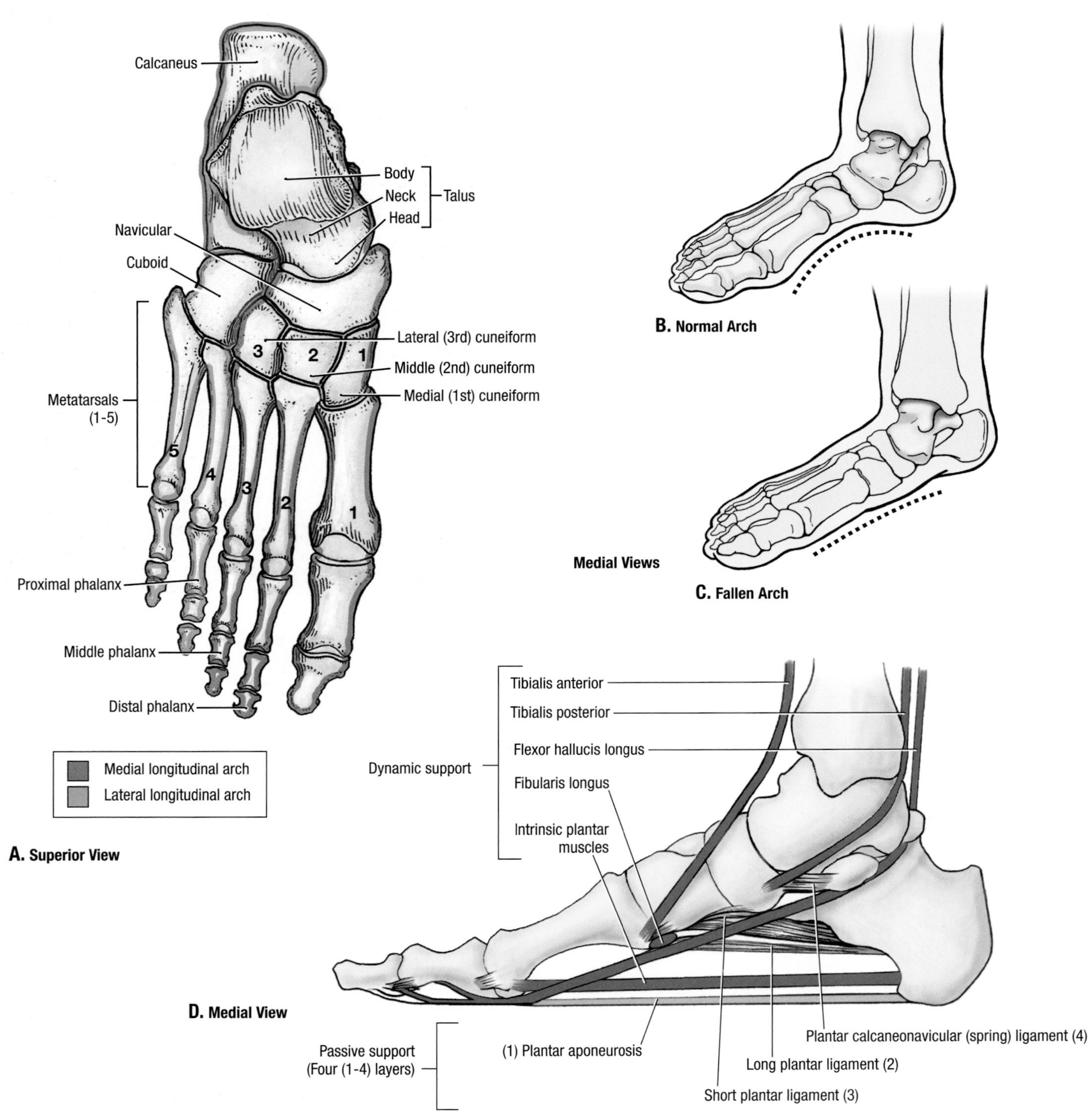
Calcaneus
Body
Neck
Head
Talus
Navicular
Cuboid
Lateral (3rd) cuneiform
Middle (2nd) cuneiform
Medial (1st) cuneiform
Metatarsals (1-5)
Proximal phalanx
Middle phalanx
Distal phalanx
Medial longitudinal arch
Lateral longitudinal arch
A. Superior View
B. Normal Arch
Medial Views
C. Fallen Arch
Dynamic support
Tibialis anterior
Tibialis posterior
Flexor hallucis longus
Fibularis longus
Intrinsic plantar muscles
D. Medial View
Passive support (Four (1-4) layers)
(1) Plantar aponeurosis
Plantar calcaneonavicular (spring) ligament (4)
Long plantar ligament (2)
Short plantar ligament (3)

## 5.87 Arches of foot

**A.** Medial and lateral longitudinal arches. **B.** Normal arch. **C.** Fallen arch. **D.** Supports of the longitudinal arches.

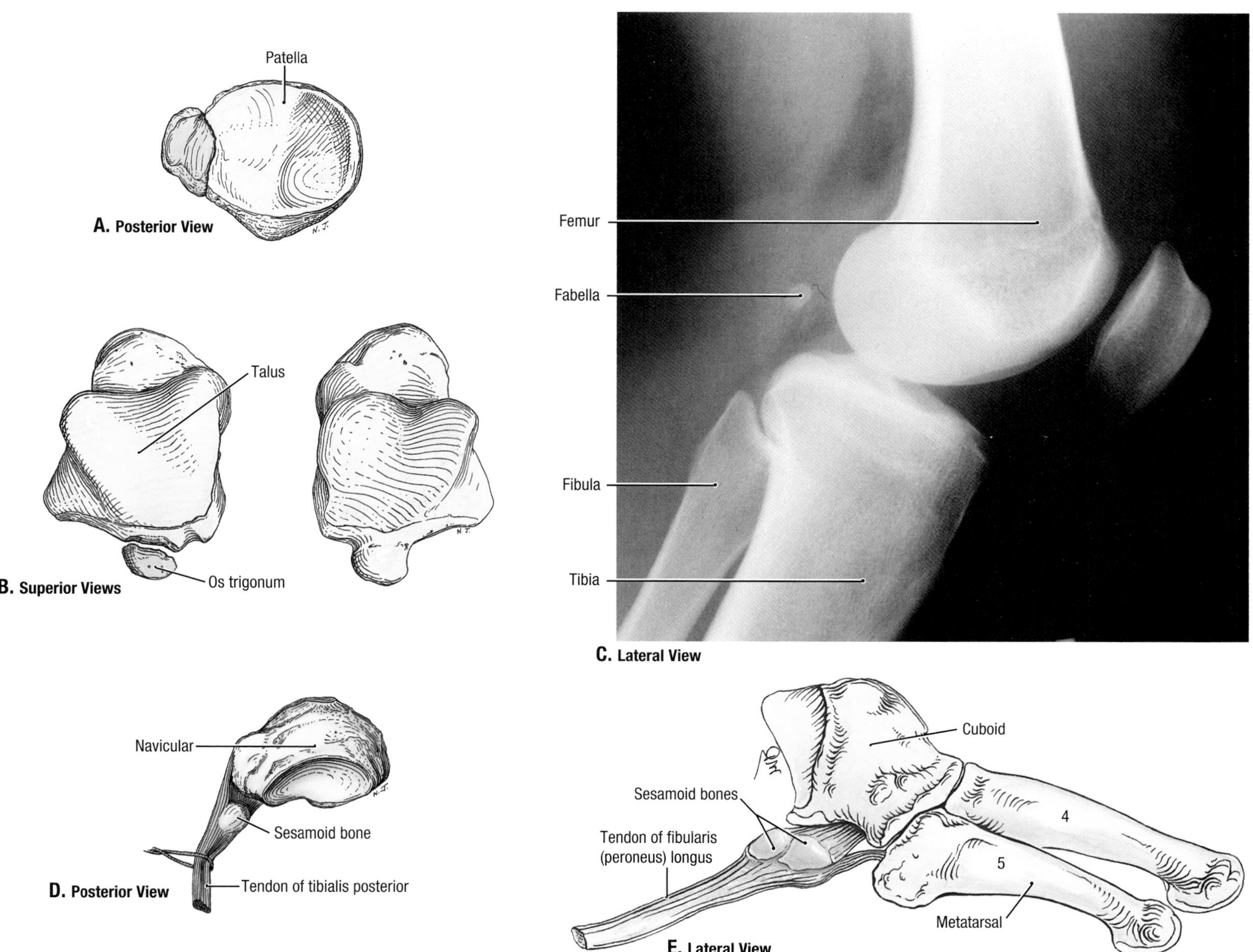
Patella
A. Posterior View
Talus
Os trigonum
B. Superior Views
Femur
Fabella
Fibula
Tibia
C. Lateral View
Navicular
Sesamoid bone
Tendon of tibialis posterior
D. Posterior View
Cuboid
Sesamoid bones
Tendon of fibularis
(peroneus) longus
4
5
Metatarsal
E. Lateral View

## 5.88 Bony anomalies

**A.** Bipartite patella. Occasionally, the superolateral angle of the patella ossifies independently and remains discrete. **B.** Os trigonum. The lateral (posterior) tubercle of the talus has a separate center of ossification that appears from the ages of 7 to 13 years; when this fails to fuse with the body of the talus, as in the left bone of this pair, it is called an *os trigonum*. It was found in 7.7% of 558 adult feet; 22 were paired, and 21 were unpaired. **C.** Fabella. A sesamoid bone in the lateral head of the gastrocnemius muscle was present in 21.6% of 116 limbs. **D.** Sesamoid bone in the tendon of tibialis posterior. A sesamoid bone was found in 23% of 348 adults. **E.** Sesamoid bone in the tendon of fibularis (peroneus) longus. A sesamoid bone was found in 26% of 92 feet. In this specimen, it is bipartite, and the fibularis (peroneus) longus muscle has an additional attachment to the 5th metatarsal bone.

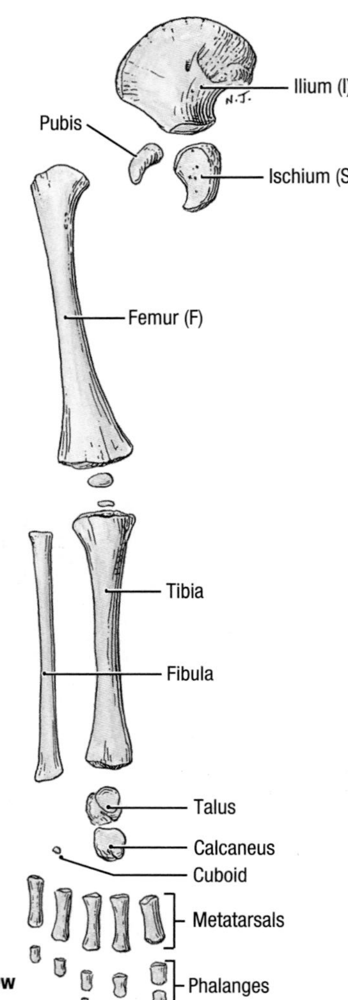
Ilium (I)
Pubis
Ischium (S)
Femur (F)
Tibia
Fibula
Talus
Calcaneus
Cuboid
Metatarsals
Phalanges

**A. Anterior View**

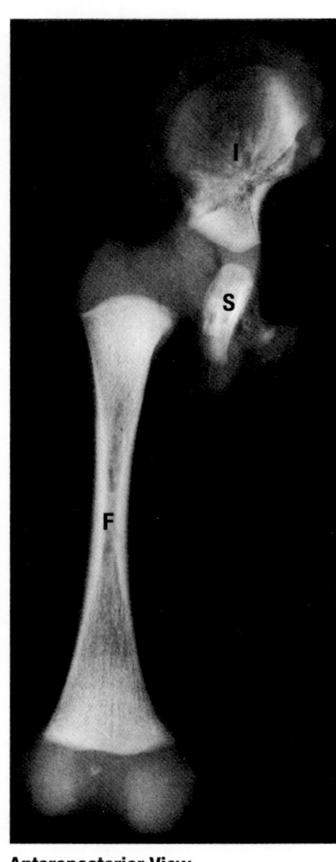
I
S
F

**B. Anteroposterior View**

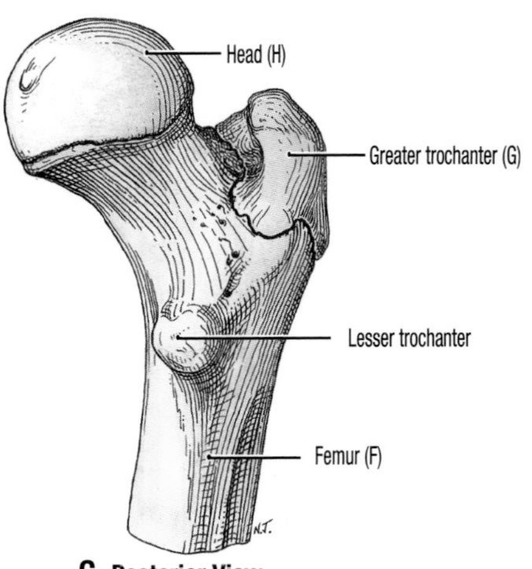
Head (H)
Greater trochanter (G)
Lesser trochanter
Femur (F)

**C. Posterior View**

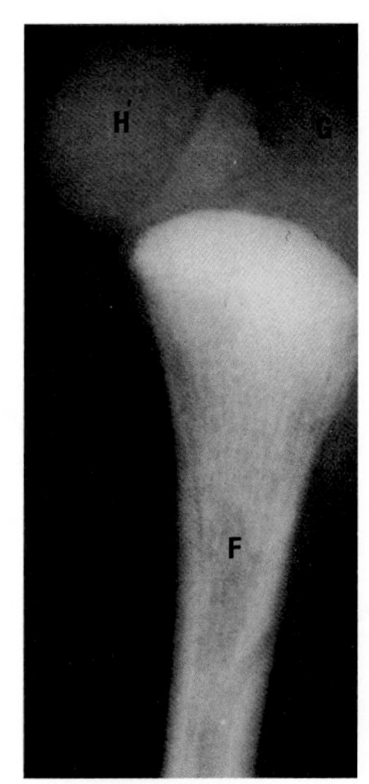
H
G
F

**D. Anteroposterior View**

## 5.89 Postnatal lower limb development

**A.** Bones of lower limb at birth. The hip bone can be divided into three primary parts: ilium, ischium, and pubis. The diaphyses (bodies) of the long bones are well ossified. Some epiphyses (growth plates) and tarsal bones have begun to ossify, including the distal epiphysis of the femur, proximal epiphysis of the tibia, calcaneus, talus, and cuboid. **B** and **D.** Anteroposterior radiographs of postmortem specimens of newborns show the bony *(white)* and cartilaginous *(gray)* components of the femur and hip bone. **C.** Epiphyses at proximal end of femur. The epiphysis of the head of the femur begins to ossify during the 1st year, that of the greater trochanter before the 5th year, and that of the lesser trochanter before the 14th year. These usually fuse completely with the body (shaft) before the end of the 18th year.

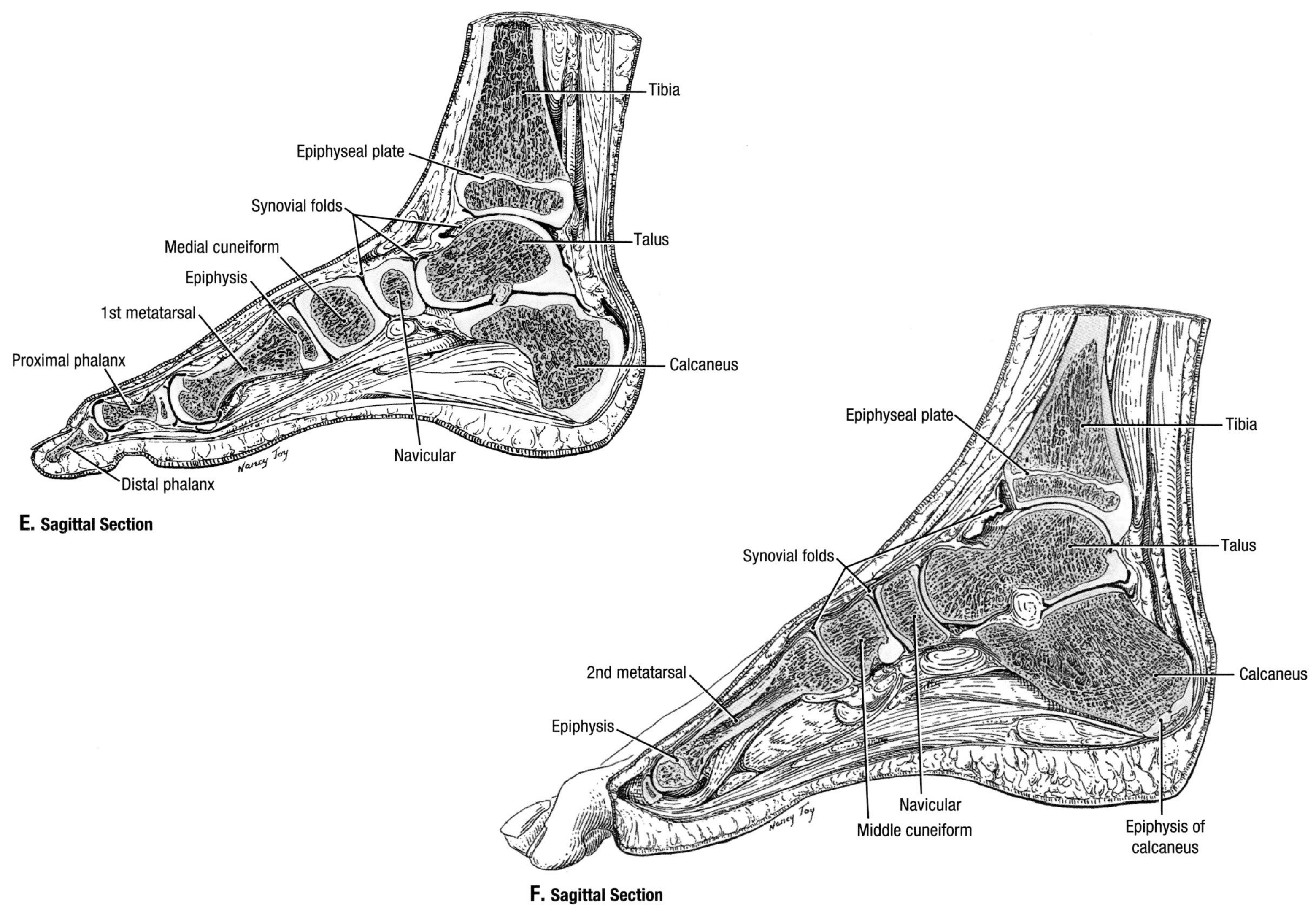
Tibia
Epiphyseal plate
Synovial folds
Talus
Medial cuneiform
Epiphysis
1st metatarsal
Proximal phalanx
Calcaneus
Navicular
Distal phalanx
Nancy Joy
Epiphyseal plate
Tibia
Synovial folds
Talus
2nd metatarsal
Calcaneus
Epiphysis
Navicular
Middle cuneiform
Epiphysis of calcaneus
Nancy Joy

**E. Sagittal Section**

**F. Sagittal Section**

## 5.89 Postnatal lower limb development *(continued)*

**E.** Foot of child age 4. **F.** Foot of child age 10.

- In the foot of the younger child **(E),** epiphyses of long bones (tibia, metatarsals, and phalanges) ossify like short bones, with the ossification centers being enveloped in cartilage. Ossification has already extended to the surface of the larger tarsal bones.
- In the foot of the older child **(F),** ossification has spread to the dorsal and plantar surfaces of all tarsal bones in view, and cartilage persists on the articular surfaces only.
- The traction epiphysis of the calcaneus for the calcaneal tendon and plantar aponeurosis begins to ossify from the ages of 6 to 10 years.
- The first metatarsal bone is similar to a phalanx in that its epiphysis is at the base instead of the head, as in the second and other metatarsal bones.
- The tuberosity of the calcaneus and the sesamoid bones of the first and the heads of the second to fifth metatarsals (here the second) support the longitudinal arch of the foot; the medial part of the longitudinal arch is higher and more mobile than the lateral.

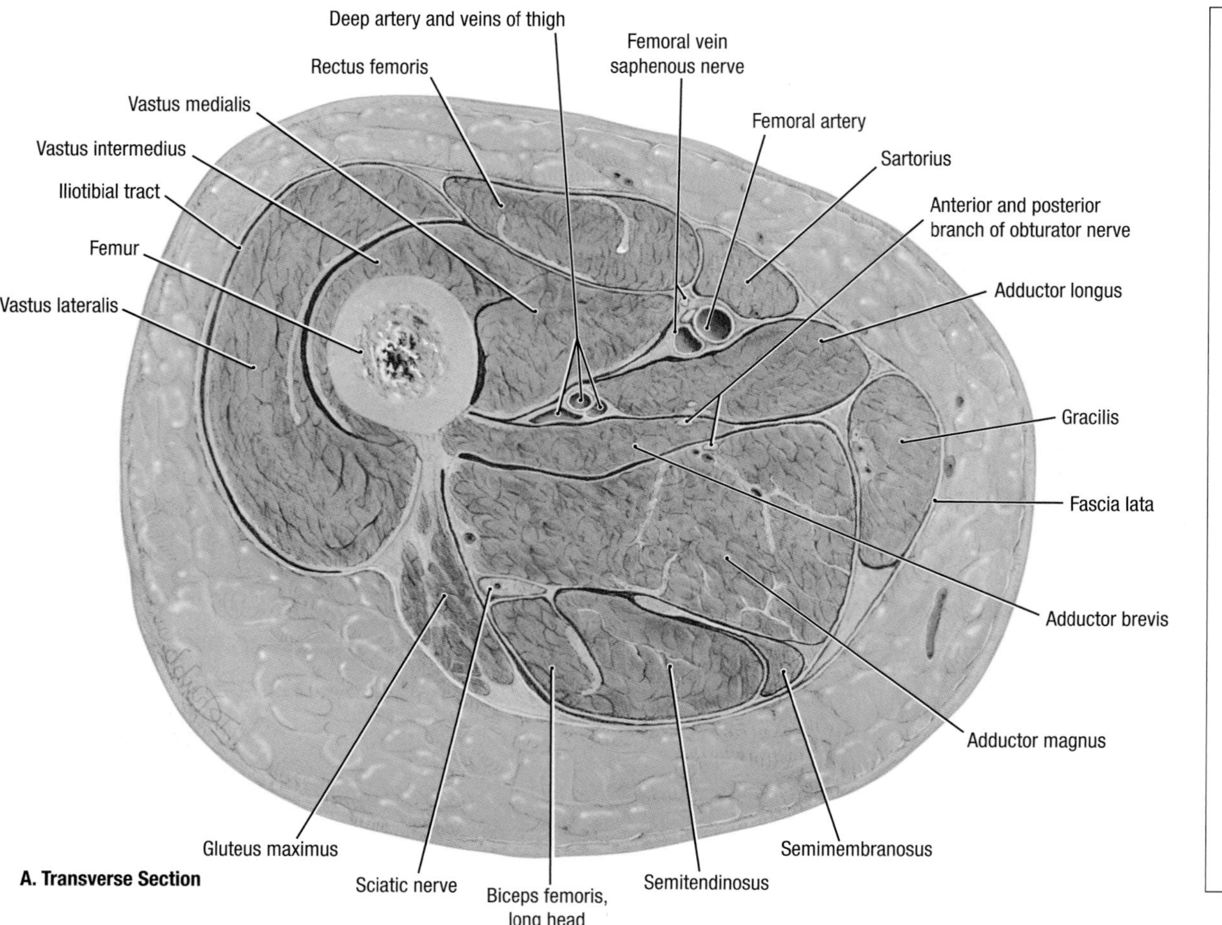

Deep artery and veins of thigh
Rectus femoris
Femoral vein
saphenous nerve
Vastus medialis
Femoral artery
Vastus intermedius
Sartorius
Iliotibial tract
Anterior and posterior
branch of obturator nerve
Femur
Adductor longus
Vastus lateralis
Gracilis
Fascia lata
Adductor brevis
Adductor magnus
Gluteus maximus
Semimembranosus
Sciatic nerve
Biceps femoris,
long head
Semitendinosus


A. Transverse Section

| Key | |
|---|---|
| AB | Adductor brevis |
| AL | Adductor longus |
| AM | Adductor magnus |
| AS | Anteriomedial intermuscular septum |
| BF | Biceps femoris |
| BFL | Long head of biceps femoris |
| BFS | Short head of biceps femoris |
| F | Femur |
| FA | Femoral artery |
| FL | Fascia lata |
| FV | Femoral vein |
| G | Gracilis |
| GM | Gluteus maximus |
| GSV | Great saphenous vein |
| H | Head of femur |
| IT | Iliotibial tract |
| LS | Lateral intermuscular septum |
| OE | Obturator externus |
| PS | Posterior intermuscular septum |
| RF | Rectus femoris |
| S | Sartorius |
| SM | Semimembranosus |
| SN | Sciatic nerve |
| ST | Semitendinosus |
| TFL | Tensor fasciae latae |
| UB | Urinary bladder |
| VI | Vastus intermedius |
| VL | Vastus lateralis |
| VM | Vastus medialis |

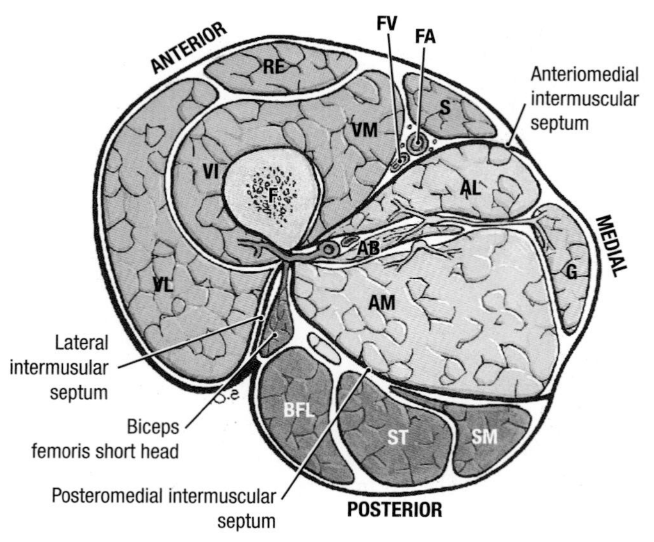

ANTERIOR
FV
FA
RF
S
VM
Anteriomedial
intermuscular
septum
VI
F
AL
MEDIAL
AB
VL
G
AM
Lateral
intermusular
septum
Biceps
femoris short head
BFL
ST
SM
Posteromedial intermuscular
septum
POSTERIOR


B. Transverse Section

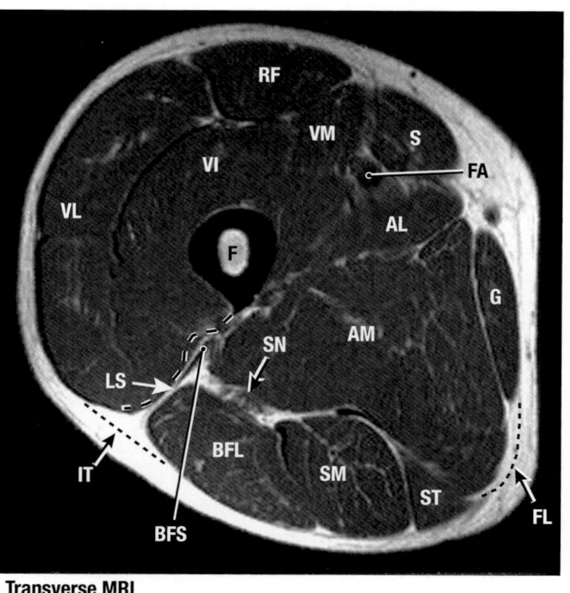

RF
VM
S
VI
FA
VL
AL
F
G
SN
AM
LS
BFL
SM
IT
ST
FL
BFS


C. Transverse MRI

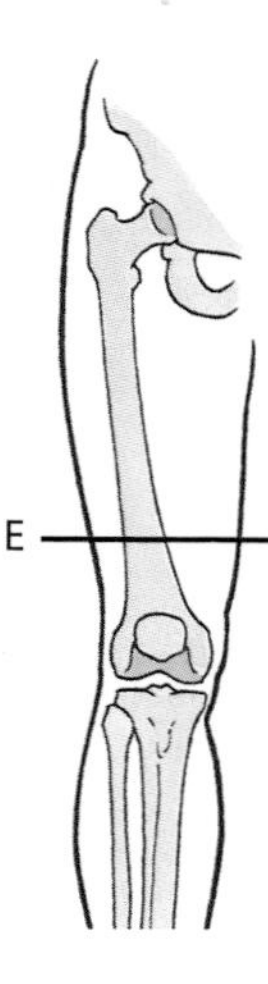

E


## 5.90 Transverse sections and MRIs of thigh

**A.** Anatomical section. **B.** Compartments of thigh. **C.** T1 transverse (axial) MRIs. The thigh has three compartments, each with its own nerve supply and primary function: anterior group extends the knee and is supplied by the femoral nerve; medial group adducts the hip and is supplied by the obturator nerve; posterior group flexes the knee and is supplied by the sciatic nerve.

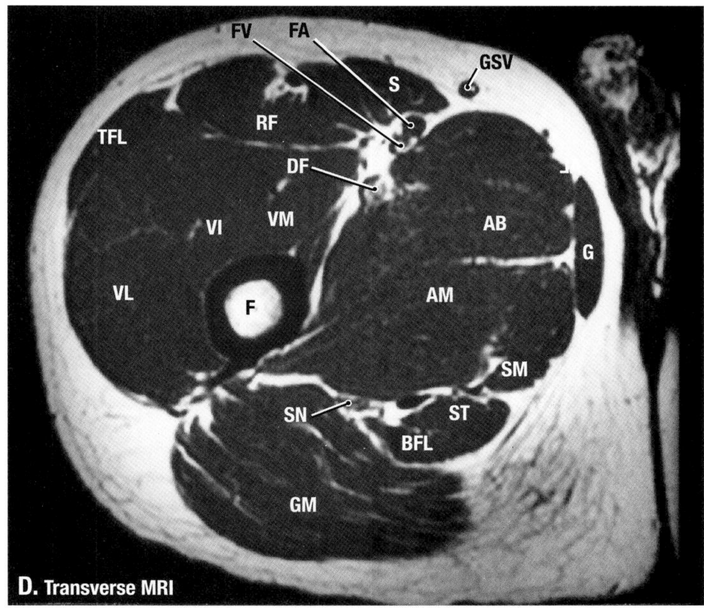
FV
FA
GSV
S
RF
TFL
DF
VI
VM
AB
G
VL
F
AM
SM
SN
ST
BFL
GM
D. Transverse MRI

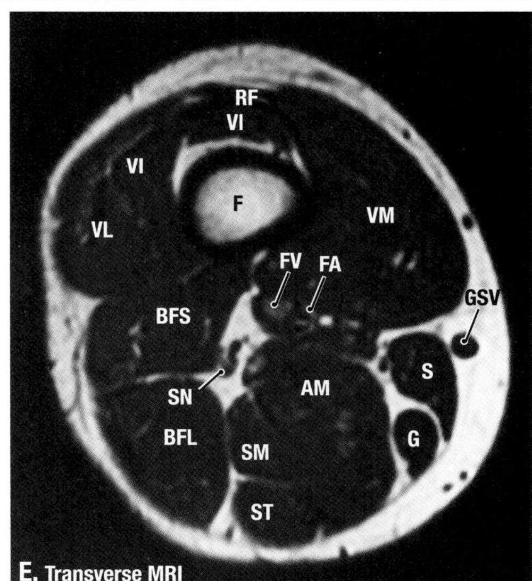
RF
VI
VI
F
VM
VL
FV
FA
GSV
BFS
S
SN
AM
BFL
SM
G
ST
E. Transverse MRI

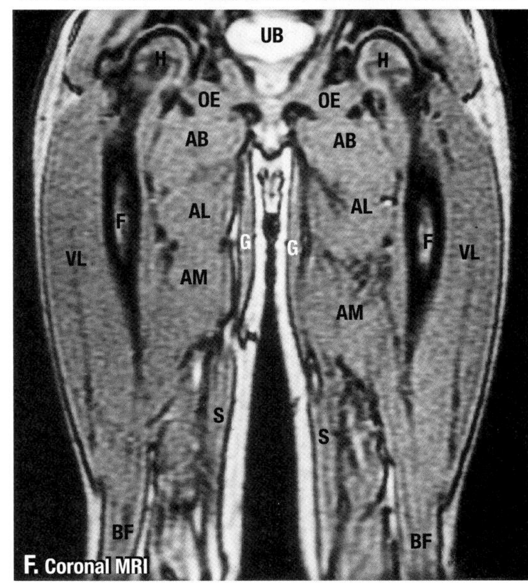
UB
H
H
OE
OE
AB
AB
AL
AL
F
G
G
F
VL
VL
AM
AM
S
S
BF
BF
F. Coronal MRI

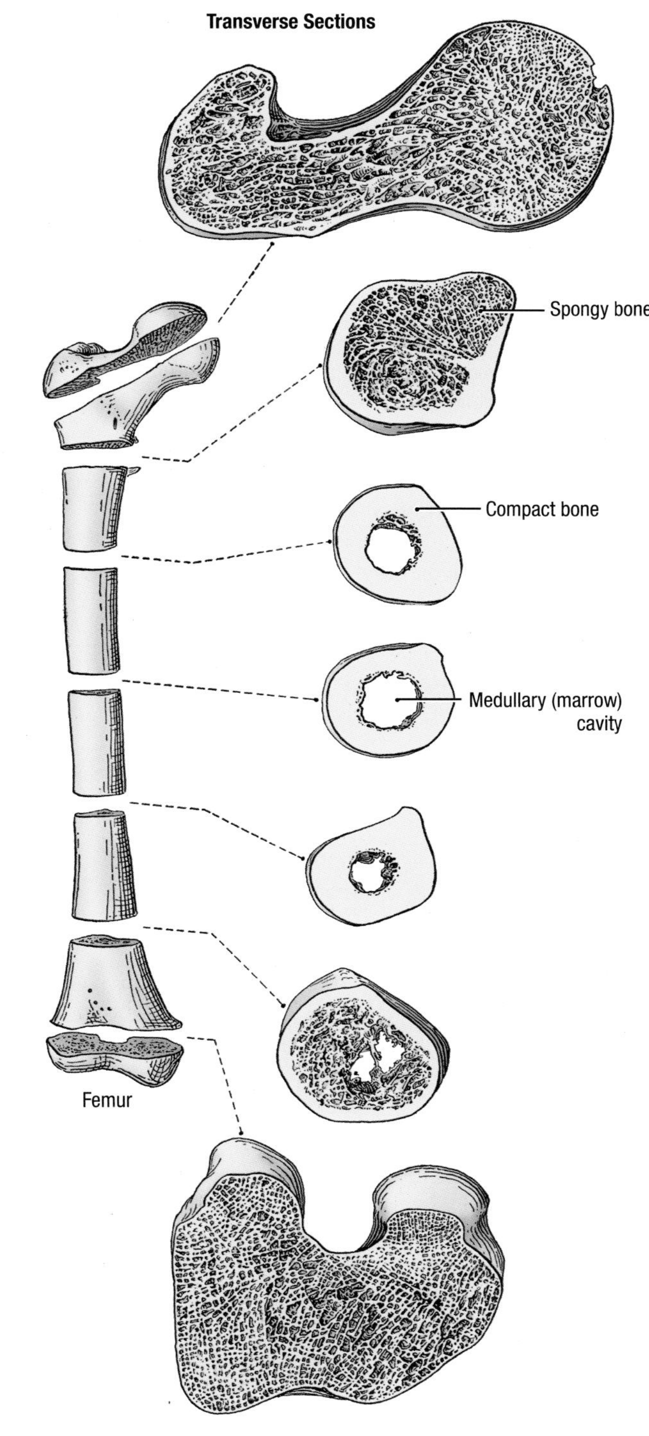
Transverse Sections
Spongy bone
Compact bone
Medullary (marrow) cavity
Femur
G. Anterior View

**5.90 Transverse sections and MRIs of thigh *(continued)***

**D** and **E.** T1 transverse MRIs. **F.** T1 coronal MRI. **G.** Transverse sections of femur. Note the differences in thickness of the compact and spongy bone and in the width of the medullary (marrow) cavity.

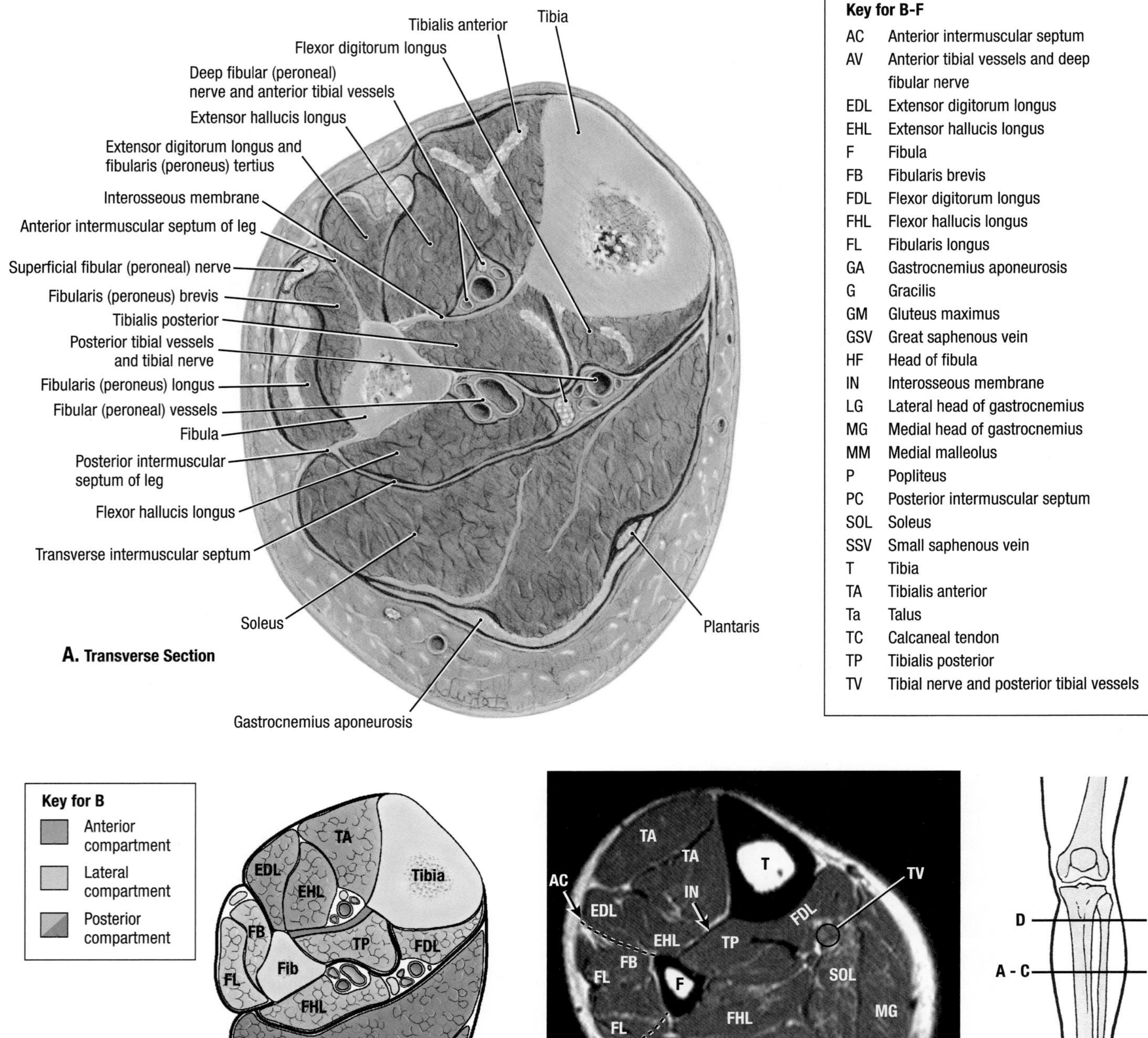
Tibialis anterior
Tibia
Flexor digitorum longus
Deep fibular (peroneal) nerve and anterior tibial vessels
Extensor hallucis longus
Extensor digitorum longus and fibularis (peroneus) tertius
Interosseous membrane
Anterior intermuscular septum of leg
Superficial fibular (peroneal) nerve
Fibularis (peroneus) brevis
Tibialis posterior
Posterior tibial vessels and tibial nerve
Fibularis (peroneus) longus
Fibular (peroneal) vessels
Fibula
Posterior intermuscular septum of leg
Flexor hallucis longus
Transverse intermuscular septum
Soleus
Plantaris
Gastrocnemius aponeurosis
A. Transverse Section
Key for B-F
AC Anterior intermuscular septum
AV Anterior tibial vessels and deep fibular nerve
EDL Extensor digitorum longus
EHL Extensor hallucis longus
F Fibula
FB Fibularis brevis
FDL Flexor digitorum longus
FHL Flexor hallucis longus
FL Fibularis longus
GA Gastrocnemius aponeurosis
G Gracilis
GM Gluteus maximus
GSV Great saphenous vein
HF Head of fibula
IN Interosseous membrane
LG Lateral head of gastrocnemius
MG Medial head of gastrocnemius
MM Medial malleolus
P Popliteus
PC Posterior intermuscular septum
SOL Soleus
SSV Small saphenous vein
T Tibia
TA Tibialis anterior
Ta Talus
TC Calcaneal tendon
TP Tibialis posterior
TV Tibial nerve and posterior tibial vessels
Key for B
Anterior compartment
Lateral compartment
Posterior compartment
TA
EDL
EHL
Tibia
FB
TP
FDL
Fib
FL
FHL
SOL
P
B. Transverse Section
TA
TA
T
AC
IN
TV
EDL
FDL
EHL
TP
FB
FL
F
SOL
FL
FHL
MG
PC
SOL
SOL
GA
C. Transverse Section
D
A - C
E

## 5.91 Transverse sections and MRI of leg

**A.** Anatomical section. **B.** Compartments of leg. **C.** T1 transverse (axial) MRI. The anterior compartment is bounded by the tibia, interosseous membrane, fibula, anterior intermuscular septum, and crural fascia. The lateral compartment is bounded by the fibula, anterior and posterior intermuscular septa, and the crural fascia. The posterior compartment is bounded by the tibia, interosseous membrane, fibula, posterior intermuscular septum, and crural fascia. This compartment is subdivided by the transverse intermuscular septum into superficial and deep subcompartments.

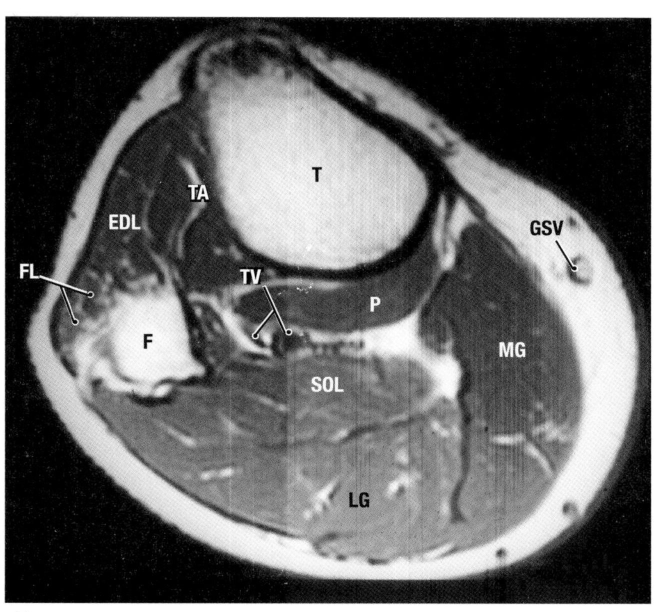
T
TA
EDL
GSV
FL
TV
P
F
MG
SOL
LG

**D.** Transverse MRI

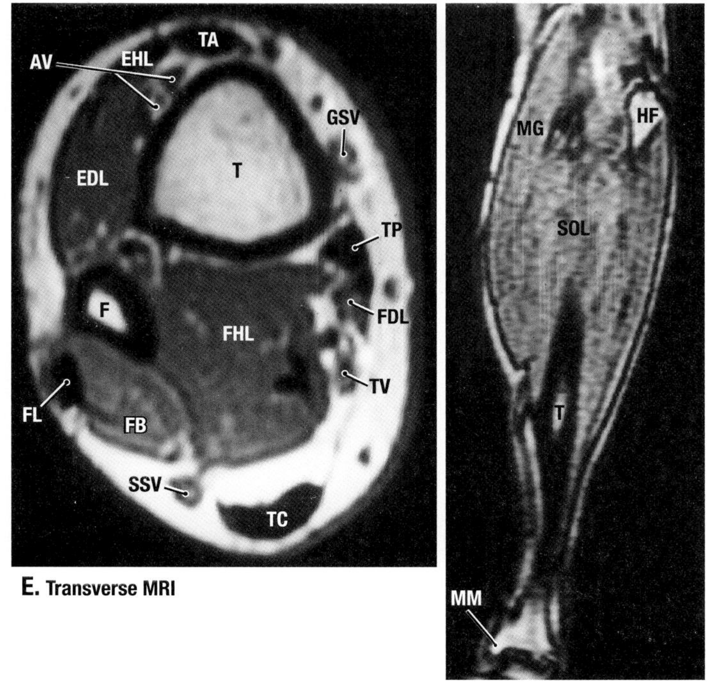
TA
AV
EHL
GSV
EDL
T
TP
F
FHL
FDL
TV
FL
FB
SSV
TC

**E.** Transverse MRI

**F.** Coronal MRI

Transverse Sections

Fibula (F)

Tibia (T)

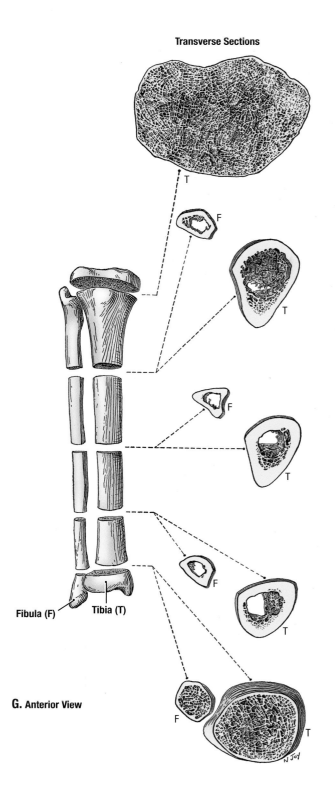

**G.** Anterior View

## 5.91 Transverse sections and MRI of leg *(continued)*

**D** and **E.** T1 transverse (axial) MRIs. **F.** T1 coronal MRI. **G.** Transverse sections of tibia and fibula.

CHAPTER 6

# UPPER LIMB

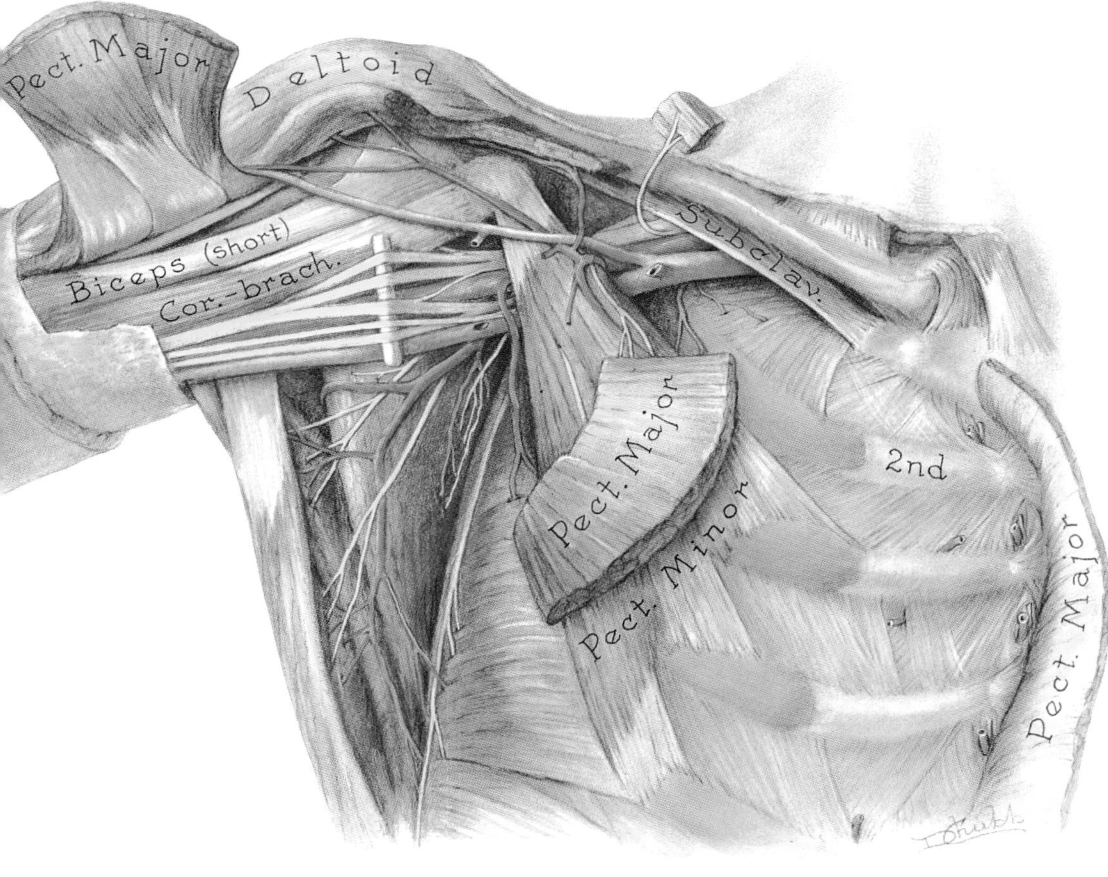

Pect. Major
Deltoid
Biceps (short)
Cor.-brach.
Subclav.
Pect. Major
2nd
Pect. Minor
Pect. Major



- Systemic Overview of Upper Limb **476**
  - Bones **476**
  - Nerves **480**
  - Blood Vessels **486**
  - Musculofascial Compartments **492**
- Pectoral Region **494**
- Axilla, Axillary Vessels, and Brachial Plexus **501**
- Scapular Region and Superficial Back **512**
- Arm and Rotator Cuff **516**
- Joints of Shoulder Region **530**
- Elbow Region **538**
- Elbow Joint **544**
- Anterior Aspect of Forearm **550**
- Anterior Aspect of Wrist and Palm of Hand **558**
- Posterior Aspect of Forearm **574**
- Posterior Aspect of Wrist and Dorsum of Hand **578**
- Lateral Aspect of Wrist and Hand **584**
- Medial Aspect of Wrist and Hand **587**
- Bones and Joints of Wrist and Hand **588**
- Function of Hand: Grips, Pinches, and Thumb Movements **596**
- Imaging and Sectional Anatomy **598**

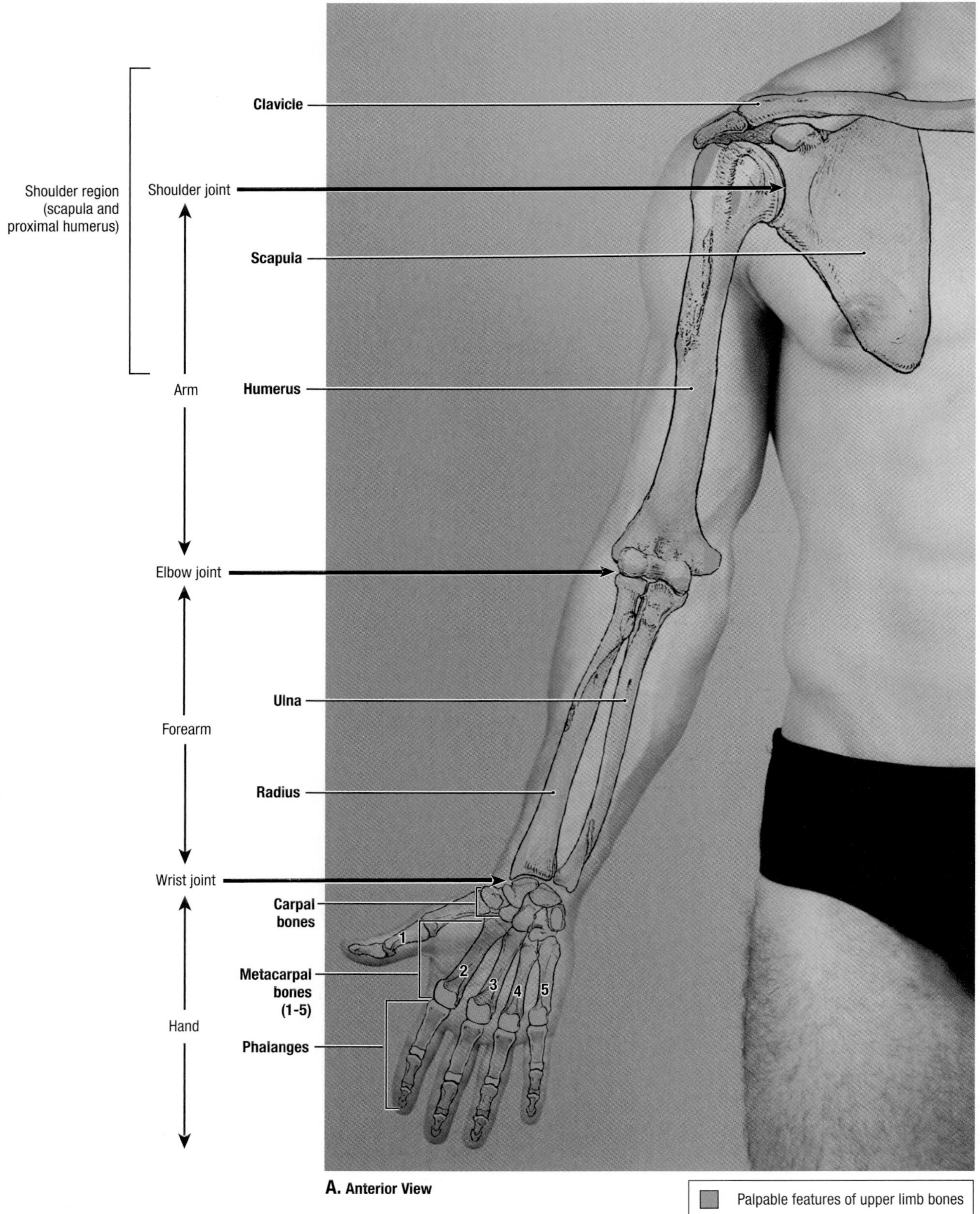
Shoulder region
(scapula and
proximal humerus)
Shoulder joint
Arm
Elbow joint
Forearm
Wrist joint
Hand
Clavicle
Scapula
Humerus
Ulna
Radius
Carpal
bones
Metacarpal
bones
(1-5)
Phalanges
1
2
3
4
5
Palpable features of upper limb bones

A. Anterior View

## 6.1 Regions, bones, and major joints of upper limb

The joints divide the upper limb into four main regions: the shoulder, arm, forearm, and hand.

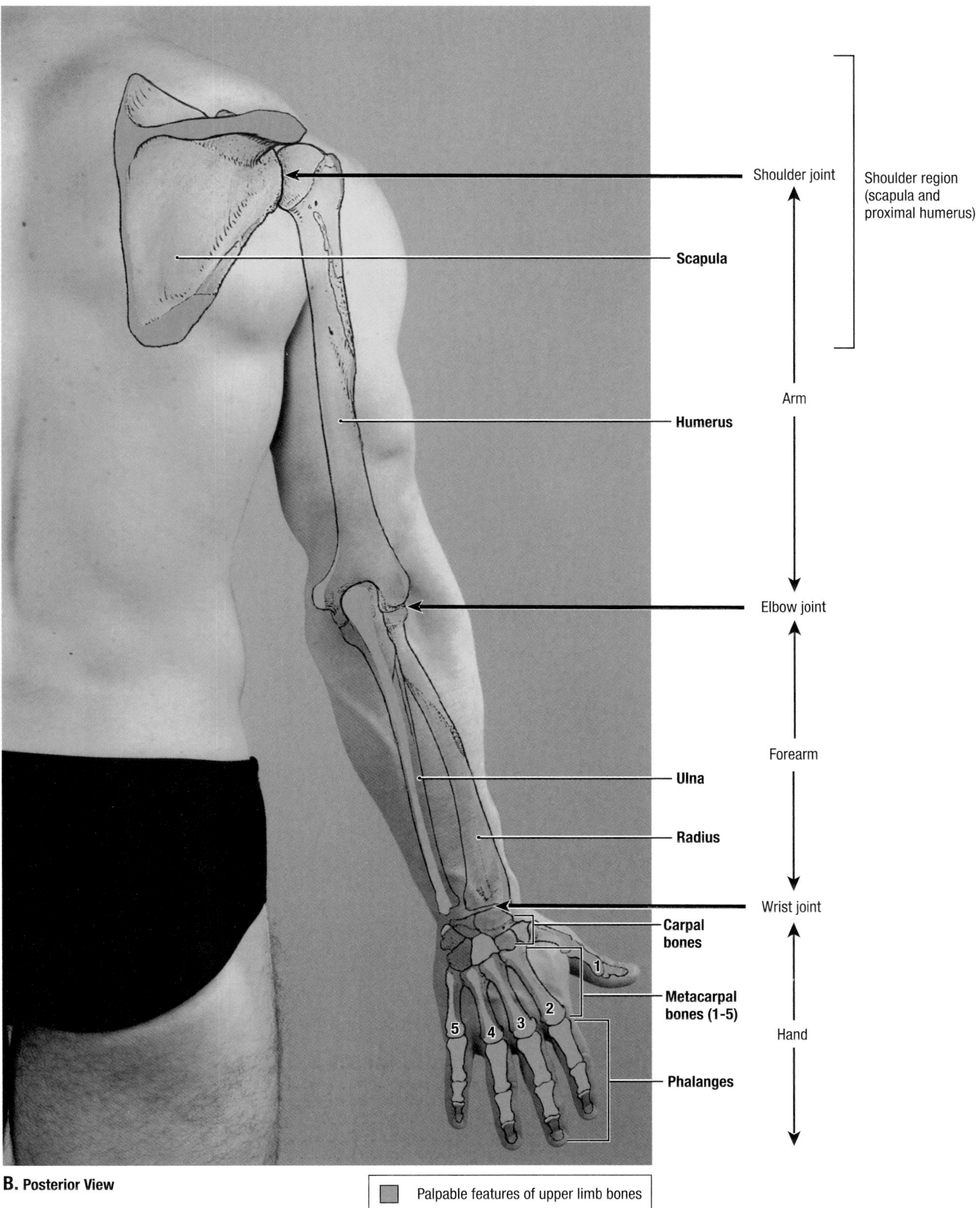
Shoulder joint
Shoulder region (scapula and proximal humerus)
Scapula
Humerus
Arm
Elbow joint
Forearm
Ulna
Radius
Wrist joint
Carpal bones
Metacarpal bones (1-5)
1
2
3
4
5
Phalanges
Hand
Palpable features of upper limb bones

B. Posterior View

## 6.1 Regions, bones, and major joints of upper limb *(continued)*

The pectoral (shoulder) girdle is an incomplete ring of bones formed by the right and left scapulae and clavicles and is joined medially to the manubrium of the sternum.

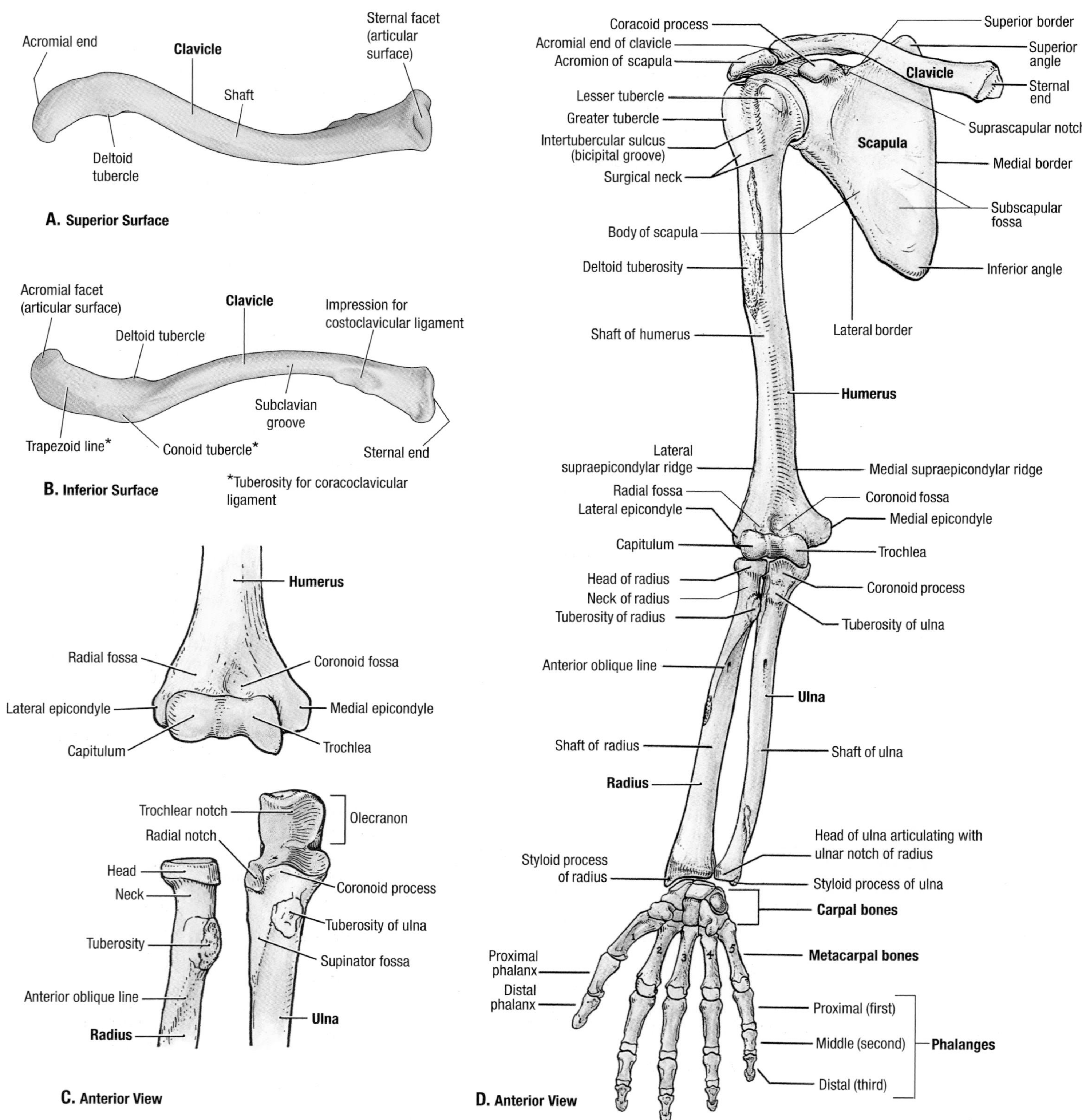
Acromial end
Clavicle
Sternal facet (articular surface)
Shaft
Deltoid tubercle
A. Superior Surface
Acromial facet (articular surface)
Clavicle
Impression for costoclavicular ligament
Deltoid tubercle
Subclavian groove
Trapezoid line*
Conoid tubercle*
Sternal end
B. Inferior Surface
*Tuberosity for coracoclavicular ligament
Humerus
Radial fossa
Coronoid fossa
Lateral epicondyle
Medial epicondyle
Capitulum
Trochlea
Trochlear notch
Olecranon
Radial notch
Head
Coronoid process
Neck
Tuberosity of ulna
Tuberosity
Supinator fossa
Anterior oblique line
Ulna
Radius
C. Anterior View
Coracoid process
Acromial end of clavicle
Acromion of scapula
Superior border
Superior angle
Clavicle
Sternal end
Lesser tubercle
Greater tubercle
Suprascapular notch
Intertubercular sulcus (bicipital groove)
Scapula
Medial border
Surgical neck
Subscapular fossa
Body of scapula
Deltoid tuberosity
Inferior angle
Shaft of humerus
Lateral border
Humerus
Lateral supraepicondylar ridge
Medial supraepicondylar ridge
Radial fossa
Coronoid fossa
Lateral epicondyle
Medial epicondyle
Capitulum
Trochlea
Head of radius
Coronoid process
Neck of radius
Tuberosity of radius
Tuberosity of ulna
Anterior oblique line
Ulna
Shaft of radius
Shaft of ulna
Radius
Head of ulna articulating with ulnar notch of radius
Styloid process of radius
Styloid process of ulna
Carpal bones
Metacarpal bones
Proximal phalanx
Distal phalanx
Proximal (first)
Middle (second)
Phalanges
Distal (third)
D. Anterior View

**6.2 Features of bones of upper limb**

**A** and **B.** Clavicle. **C.** Anterior aspect of disarticulated distal end of humerus and proximal end of radius and ulna. **D.** Anterior aspect of articulated upper limb.

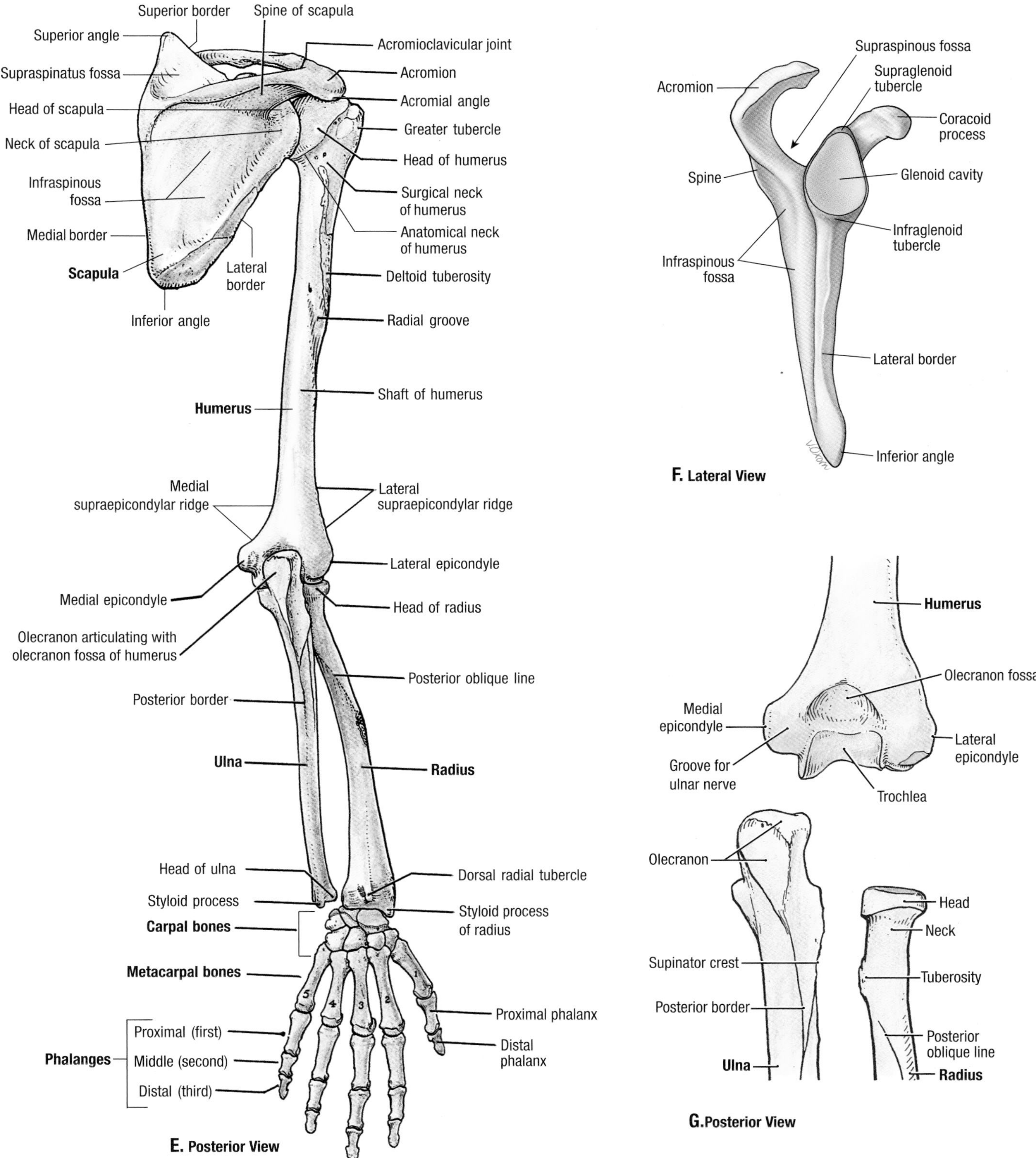
Superior border
Spine of scapula
Superior angle
Acromioclavicular joint
Supraspinatus fossa
Acromion
Head of scapula
Acromial angle
Greater tubercle
Neck of scapula
Head of humerus
Infraspinous fossa
Surgical neck of humerus
Anatomical neck of humerus
Medial border
Scapula
Lateral border
Deltoid tuberosity
Inferior angle
Radial groove
Shaft of humerus
Humerus
Medial supraepicondylar ridge
Lateral supraepicondylar ridge
Lateral epicondyle
Medial epicondyle
Head of radius
Olecranon articulating with olecranon fossa of humerus
Posterior oblique line
Posterior border
Ulna
Radius
Head of ulna
Dorsal radial tubercle
Styloid process
Styloid process of radius
Carpal bones
Metacarpal bones
Proximal phalanx
Proximal (first)
Distal phalanx
Phalanges
Middle (second)
Distal (third)
E. Posterior View
Supraspinous fossa
Supraglenoid tubercle
Acromion
Coracoid process
Glenoid cavity
Spine
Infraglenoid tubercle
Infraspinous fossa
Lateral border
Inferior angle
F. Lateral View
Humerus
Olecranon fossa
Medial epicondyle
Lateral epicondyle
Groove for ulnar nerve
Trochlea
Olecranon
Head
Neck
Supinator crest
Tuberosity
Posterior border
Posterior oblique line
Ulna
Radius
G. Posterior View

## 6.2 Features of bones of upper limb *(continued)*

**E.** Posterior aspect of articulated upper limb bones. **F.** Lateral aspect of scapula. **G.** Posterior aspect of disarticulated distal end of humerus and proximal ends of radius and ulna.

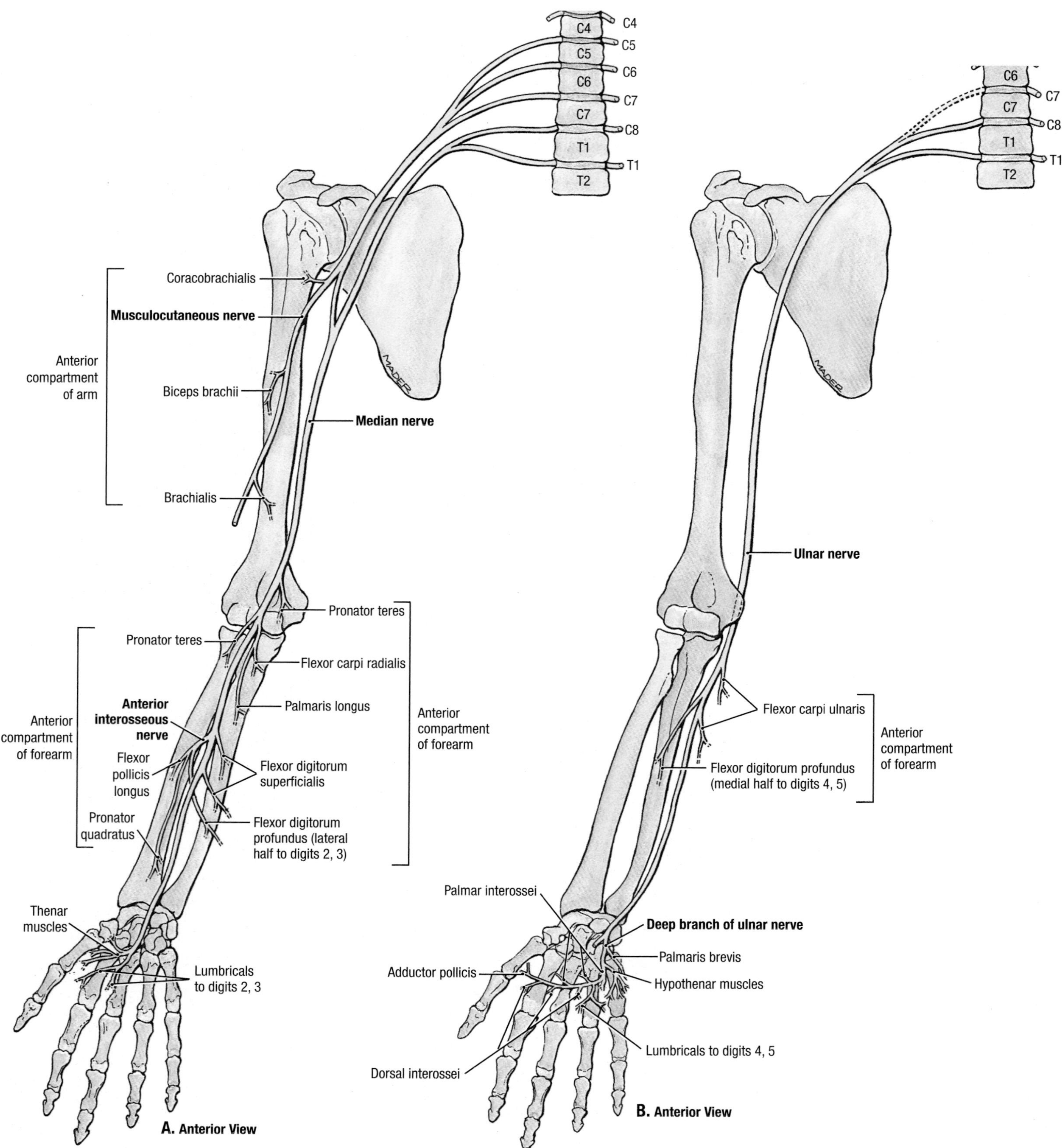
C4
C5
C6
C7
C8
T1
T2
Coracobrachialis
Musculocutaneous nerve
Anterior compartment of arm
Biceps brachii
Median nerve
Brachialis
Pronator teres
Pronator teres
Flexor carpi radialis
Anterior compartment of forearm
Anterior interosseous nerve
Palmaris longus
Anterior compartment of forearm
Flexor pollicis longus
Flexor digitorum superficialis
Pronator quadratus
Flexor digitorum profundus (lateral half to digits 2, 3)
Thenar muscles
Lumbricals to digits 2, 3
A. Anterior View
C6
C7
C8
T1
T2
Ulnar nerve
Flexor carpi ulnaris
Anterior compartment of forearm
Flexor digitorum profundus (medial half to digits 4, 5)
Palmar interossei
Deep branch of ulnar nerve
Palmaris brevis
Adductor pollicis
Hypothenar muscles
Lumbricals to digits 4, 5
Dorsal interossei
B. Anterior View

**6.3 Overview of motor innervation of upper limb**

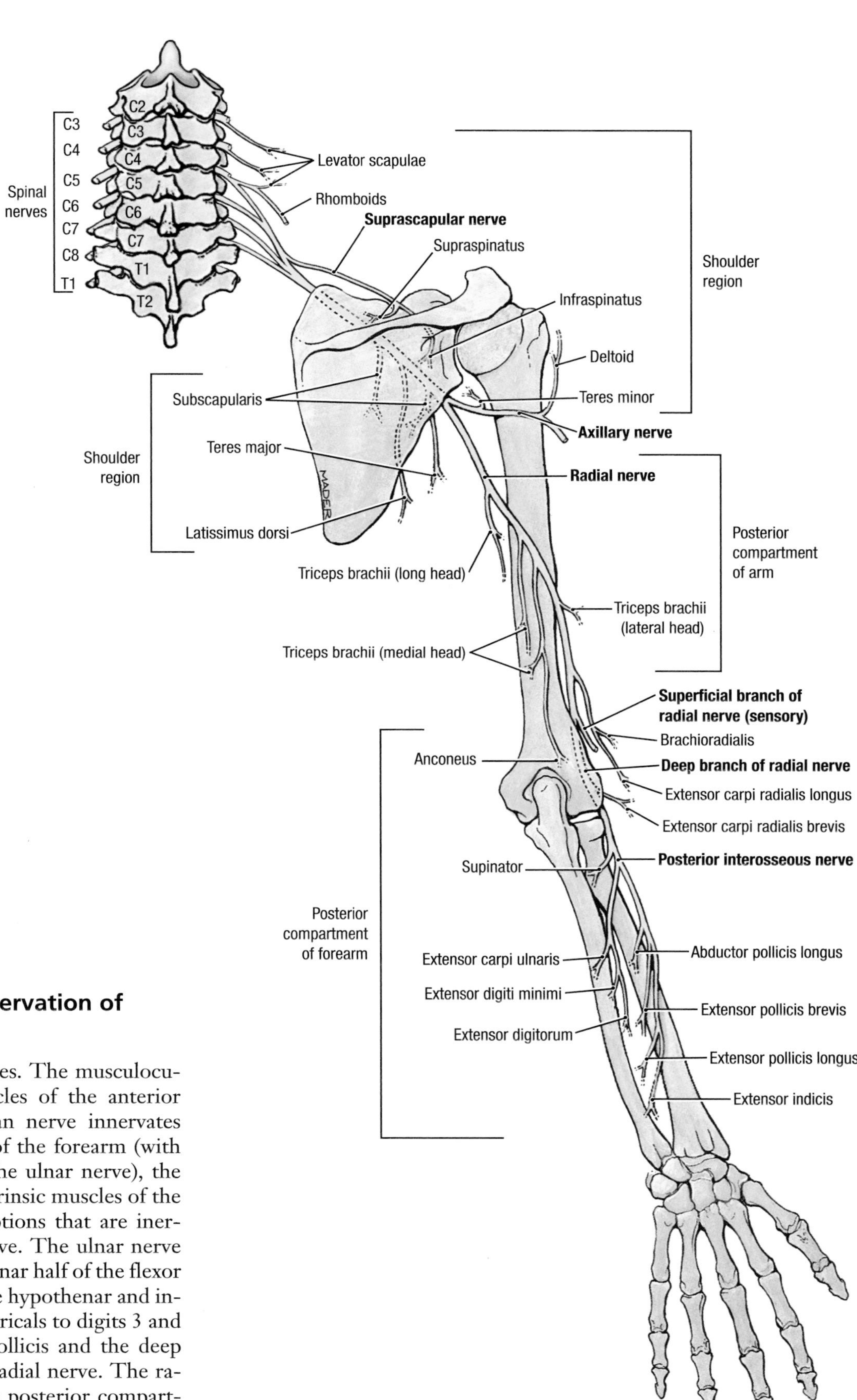
Spinal nerves
C3
C4
C5
C6
C7
C8
T1
C2
C3
C4
C5
C6
C7
T1
T2
Levator scapulae
Rhomboids
Suprascapular nerve
Supraspinatus
Shoulder region
Infraspinatus
Deltoid
Subscapularis
Teres minor
Axillary nerve
Shoulder region
Teres major
Radial nerve
Latissimus dorsi
Posterior compartment of arm
Triceps brachii (long head)
Triceps brachii (lateral head)
Triceps brachii (medial head)
Superficial branch of radial nerve (sensory)
Brachioradialis
Anconeus
Deep branch of radial nerve
Extensor carpi radialis longus
Extensor carpi radialis brevis
Supinator
Posterior interosseous nerve
Posterior compartment of forearm
Extensor carpi ulnaris
Abductor pollicis longus
Extensor digiti minimi
Extensor pollicis brevis
Extensor digitorum
Extensor pollicis longus
Extensor indicis
MADER
**C.** Posterior View

## 6.3 Overview of motor innervation of upper limb

**A.** Musculocutaneous and median nerves. The musculocutaneous nerve innervates all the muscles of the anterior compartment of the arm. The median nerve innervates muscles of the anterior compartment of the forearm (with 1½ exceptions that are innervated by the ulnar nerve), the lumbricals to digits 2 and 3, and the intrinsic muscles of the thumb (thenar muscles) with 1½ exceptions that are innervated by the ulnar nerve. **B.** Ulnar nerve. The ulnar nerve innervates the flexor carpi ulnaris and ulnar half of the flexor digitorum profundus in the forearm, the hypothenar and interosseus muscles of the hand, the lumbricals to digits 3 and 4, and 1½ thenar muscles (adductor pollicis and the deep head of the flexor pollicis brevis). **C.** Radial nerve. The radial nerve innervates all muscles of the posterior compartments of the arm and forearm.

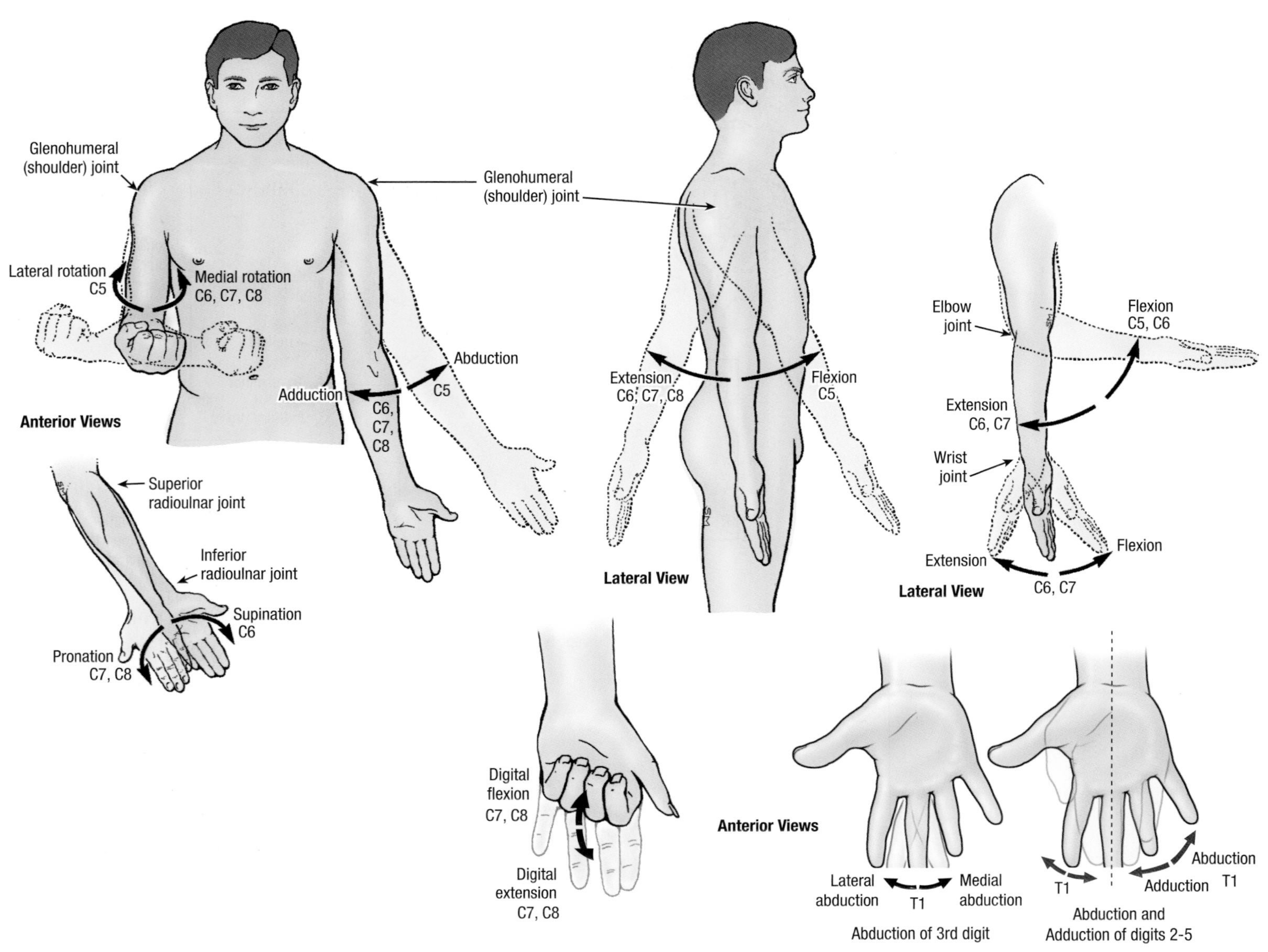
Glenohumeral (shoulder) joint
Glenohumeral (shoulder) joint
Lateral rotation C5
Medial rotation C6, C7, C8
Abduction
C5
Adduction
C6, C7, C8
Anterior Views
Superior radioulnar joint
Inferior radioulnar joint
Supination C6
Pronation C7, C8
Extension C6, C7, C8
Flexion C5
Lateral View
Elbow joint
Flexion C5, C6
Extension C6, C7
Wrist joint
Extension
Flexion
C6, C7
Lateral View
Digital flexion C7, C8
Digital extension C7, C8
Anterior Views
Lateral abduction
T1
Medial abduction
Abduction of 3rd digit
T1
Abduction
Adduction T1
Abduction and Adduction of digits 2-5

| Myotatic (deep tendon) reflex | Spinal cord segments |
|---|---|
| Biceps | C5/C6 |
| Brachioradialis | C5/C6 |
| Triceps | C6/C7 |

## 6.4 Myotomes and myotatic (deep tendon stretch) reflexes

**A.** Myotomes. Somatic motor (general somatic efferent) fibers transmit impulses to skeletal (voluntary) muscles. The unilateral muscle mass receiving information from the somatic motor fibers conveyed by a single spinal nerve is a myotome. The intrinsic muscles of the hand constitute a single myotome—myotome T1.
**B.** Myotatic reflexes. A myotatic reflex (deep tendon or stretch reflex) is an involuntary contraction of a muscle in response to sudden stretching. Myotatic reflexes are monosynaptic stretch reflexes that are elicited by briskly tapping the tendon with a reflex hammer. Each tendon reflex is mediated by specific spinal nerves. Stretch reflexes control muscle tone.

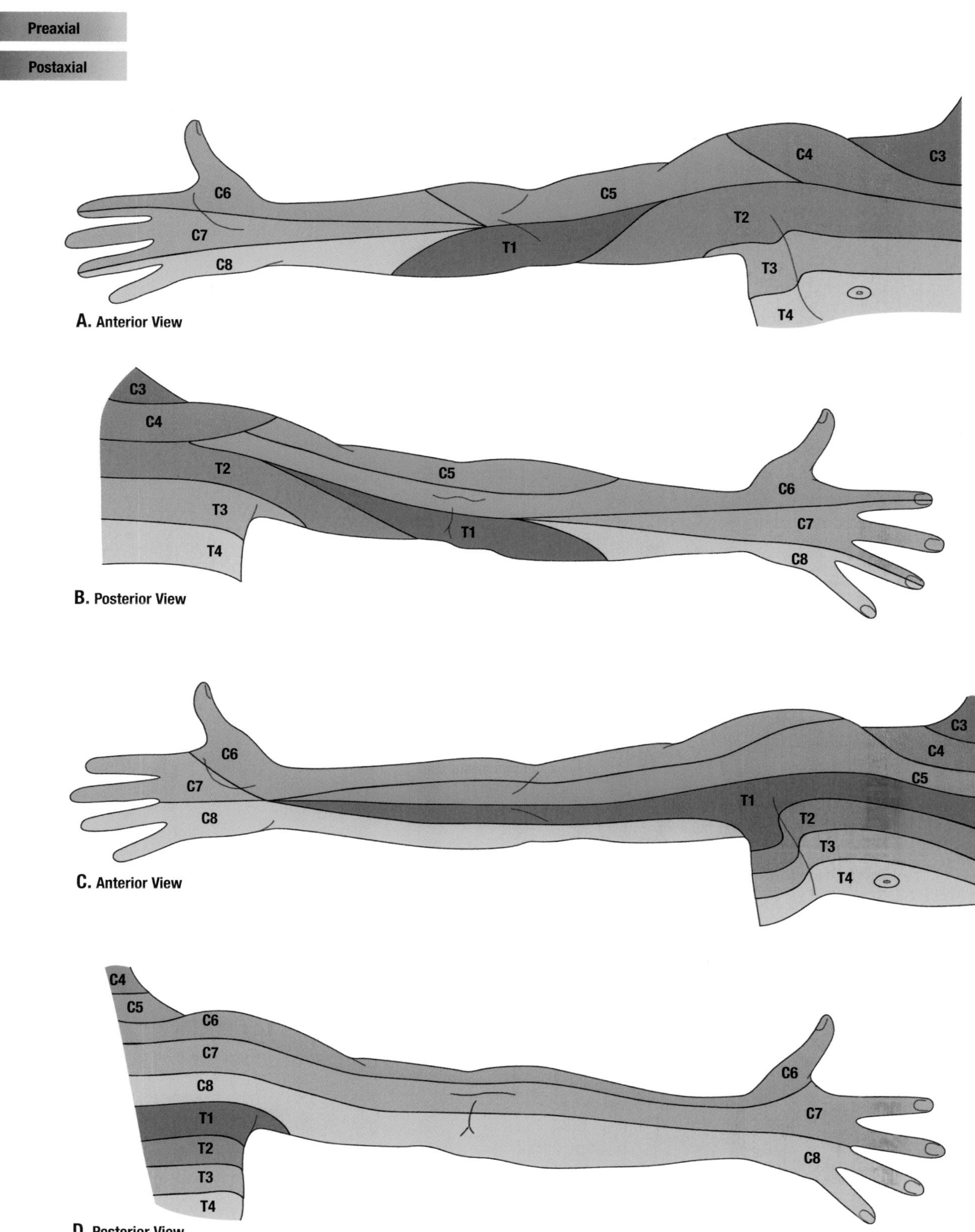
Preaxial
Postaxial
C6
C7
C8
T1
C5
C4
C3
T2
T3
T4
A. Anterior View
C3
C4
T2
T3
T4
C5
T1
C6
C7
C8
B. Posterior View
C6
C7
C8
T1
C3
C4
C5
T2
T3
T4
C. Anterior View
C4
C5
C6
C7
C8
T1
T2
T3
T4
C6
C7
C8
D. Posterior View

## 6.5 Dermatomes of upper limb

The dermatomal or segmental pattern of distribution of sensory nerve fibers persists despite the merging of spinal nerves in plexus formation during development. Two different dermatome maps are commonly used. **A** and **B**. The dermatome pattern of the upper limb according to Foerster (1933) is preferred by many because of its correlation with clinical findings. In the Foerster schema, dermatomes C6–T1 are displaced from the trunk to limbs. **C** and **D.** The dermatome pattern of the upper limb according to Keegan and Garrett (1948) is preferred by others for its correlation with development. Although depicted as distinct zones, adjacent dermatomes overlap considerably except along the axial line.

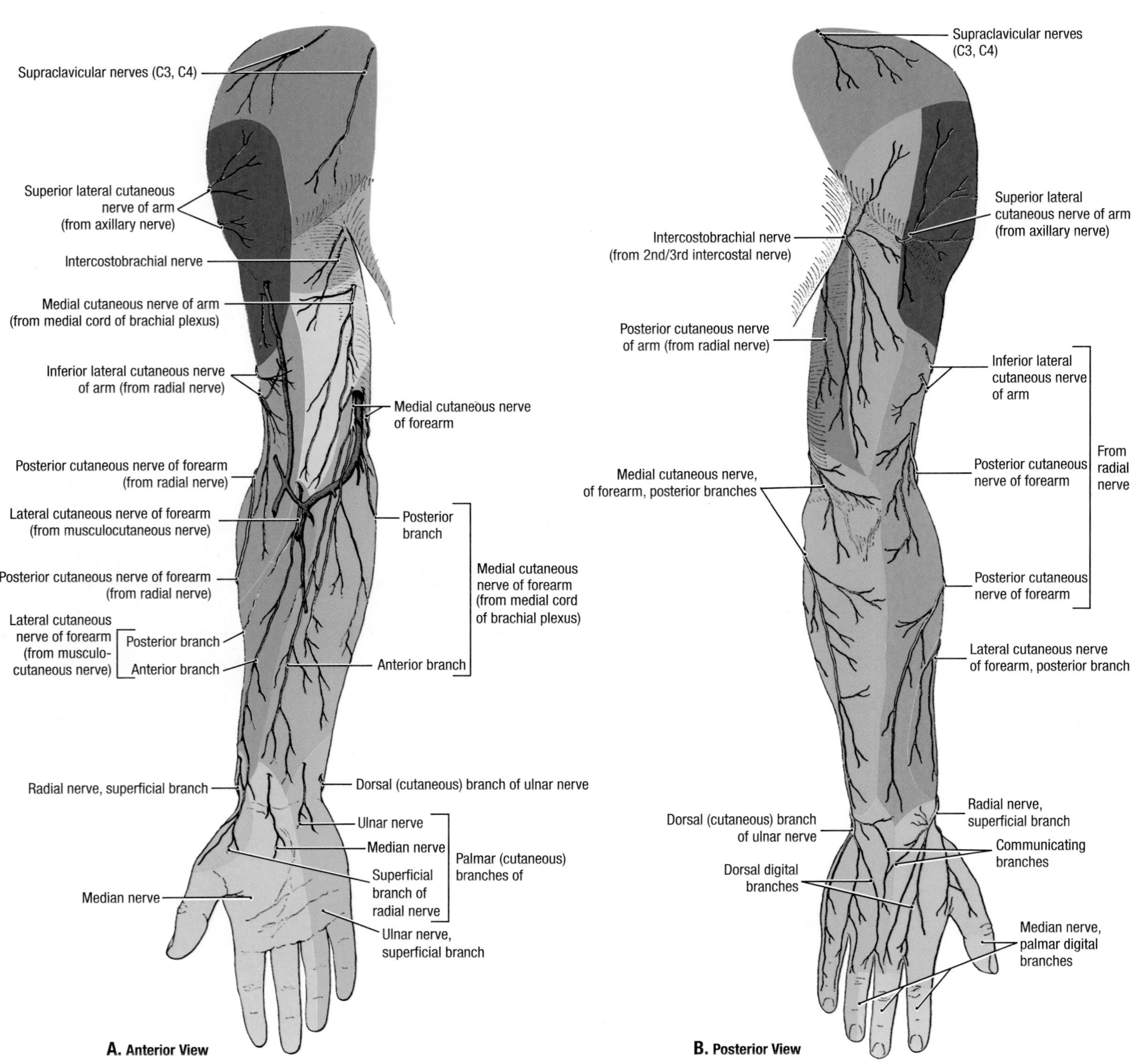
Supraclavicular nerves (C3, C4)
Superior lateral cutaneous nerve of arm (from axillary nerve)
Intercostobrachial nerve
Medial cutaneous nerve of arm (from medial cord of brachial plexus)
Inferior lateral cutaneous nerve of arm (from radial nerve)
Medial cutaneous nerve of forearm
Posterior cutaneous nerve of forearm (from radial nerve)
Lateral cutaneous nerve of forearm (from musculocutaneous nerve)
Posterior cutaneous nerve of forearm (from radial nerve)
Lateral cutaneous nerve of forearm (from musculo-cutaneous nerve)
Posterior branch
Anterior branch
Posterior branch
Anterior branch
Medial cutaneous nerve of forearm (from medial cord of brachial plexus)
Radial nerve, superficial branch
Dorsal (cutaneous) branch of ulnar nerve
Ulnar nerve
Median nerve
Superficial branch of radial nerve
Palmar (cutaneous) branches of
Median nerve
Ulnar nerve, superficial branch
A. Anterior View
Supraclavicular nerves (C3, C4)
Superior lateral cutaneous nerve of arm (from axillary nerve)
Intercostobrachial nerve (from 2nd/3rd intercostal nerve)
Posterior cutaneous nerve of arm (from radial nerve)
Inferior lateral cutaneous nerve of arm
Posterior cutaneous nerve of forearm
From radial nerve
Medial cutaneous nerve, of forearm, posterior branches
Posterior cutaneous nerve of forearm
Lateral cutaneous nerve of forearm, posterior branch
Radial nerve, superficial branch
Dorsal (cutaneous) branch of ulnar nerve
Communicating branches
Dorsal digital branches
Median nerve, palmar digital branches
B. Posterior View

**6.6 Cutaneous nerves of upper limb**

**TABLE 6.1 CUTANEOUS NERVES OF UPPER LIMB**

| Nerve | Spinal Nerve components | Source | Course/Distribution |
|---|---|---|---|
| **Supraclavicular nerves** | C3–C4 | Cervical plexus | Pass anterior to clavicle, immediately deep to platysma, and supply the skin over the clavicle and superolateral aspect of the pectoralis major muscle |
| **Superior lateral cutaneous nerve of arm** | C5–C6 | Axillary nerve (posterior cord of brachial plexus) | Emerges from posterior margin of deltoid to supply skin over lower part of this muscle and the lateral side of the midarm |
| **Inferior lateral cutaneous nerve of arm** | | Radial nerve (posterior cord of brachial plexus) | Arises with the posterior cutaneous nerve of forearm; pierces lateral head of triceps brachii to supply skin over the inferolateral aspect of the arm |
| **Posterior cutaneous nerve of arm** | | | Arises in axilla and supplies skin on posterior surface of the arm to olecranon |
| **Posterior cutaneous nerve of forearm** | C5–C8 | | Arises with the inferior lateral cutaneous nerve of the arm; pieces lateral head of triceps brachii to supply skin over the posterior aspect of the arm |
| **Superficial branch of radial nerve** | C6–C7 | | Arises in cubital fossa; supplies lateral (radial) half of the dorsal aspect of hand and thumb, and proximal portion of the dorsal aspects of digits 2 and 3, and the lateral (radial) half of dorsal aspect of digit 4 |
| **Lateral cutaneous nerve of forearm** | | Musculocutaneous nerve (lateral cord of brachial plexus) | Arises between biceps brachii and brachialis muscle as continuation of musculocutaneous nerve distal to branch to brachialis; emerges in cubital fossa lateral to biceps tendon and median cubital vein; supplies skin along radial (lateral) border of forearm to base of thenar eminence |
| **Median nerve** | C6–C7 (via lateral root); C8–T1 (via medial root) | Lateral and medial cords of brachial plexus | Courses with brachial artery in arm and deep to flexor digitorum superficialis in forearm; distal to origin of palmar cutaneous branch, traverses carpal tunnel to supply skin of palmar aspect of radial 3½ digits and adjacent palm, plus distal dorsal aspects of same, including nail beds |
| **Ulnar nerve** | (C7), C8–T1 | Medial cord of brachial plexus | Courses with brachial, superior ulnar collateral, and ulnar arteries; supplies skin of palmar and dorsal aspects of medial (ulnar) 1½ digits and palm and dorsum of hand proximal to those digits |
| **Medial cutaneous nerve of forearm** | C8–T1 | | Pierces deep fascia with basilic vein in midarm; divides into anterior and posterior branches supplying skin over anterior and medial surfaces of forearm to wrist |
| **Medial cutaneous nerve of arm** | C8–T2 | | Smallest and most medial branch of brachial plexus; communicates with intercostobrachial nerve, then descends medial to brachial artery and basilic vein to innervate skin of distal medial arm |
| **Intercostobrachial nerve** | T2 | Lateral cutaneous branch of 2nd intercostal nerve | Arises distal to angle of 2nd rib; supplies skin of axilla and proximal medial arm |

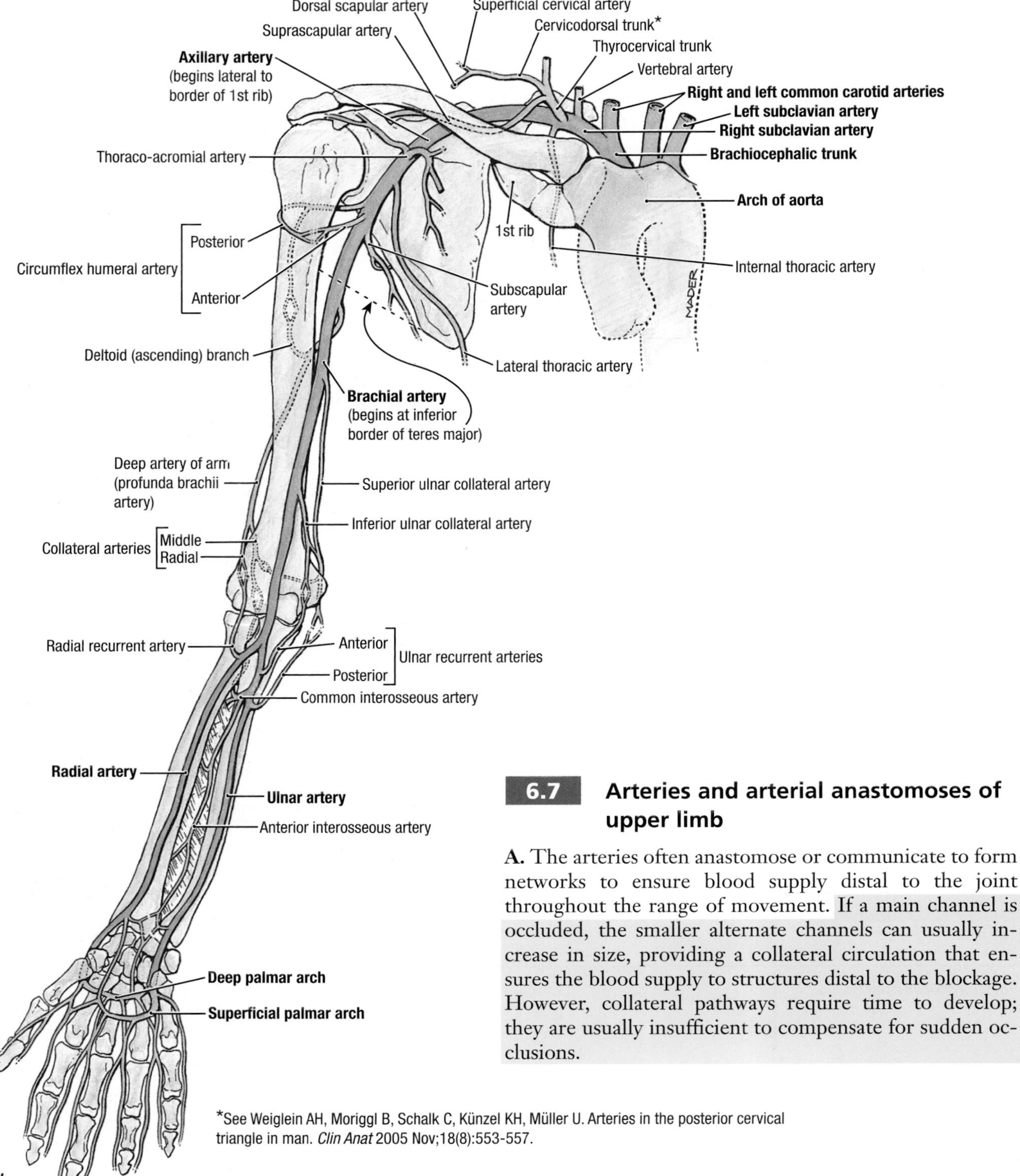
Dorsal scapular artery
Superficial cervical artery
Cervicodorsal trunk*
Suprascapular artery
Thyrocervical trunk
Axillary artery
(begins lateral to border of 1st rib)
Vertebral artery
Right and left common carotid arteries
Left subclavian artery
Right subclavian artery
Brachiocephalic trunk
Thoraco-acromial artery
Arch of aorta
1st rib
Posterior
Circumflex humeral artery
Anterior
Internal thoracic artery
Subscapular artery
MADER
Deltoid (ascending) branch
Lateral thoracic artery
Brachial artery
(begins at inferior border of teres major)
Deep artery of arm (profunda brachii artery)
Superior ulnar collateral artery
Inferior ulnar collateral artery
Collateral arteries
Middle
Radial
Radial recurrent artery
Anterior
Ulnar recurrent arteries
Posterior
Common interosseous artery
Radial artery
Ulnar artery
Anterior interosseous artery
Deep palmar arch
Superficial palmar arch

*See Weiglein AH, Moriggl B, Schalk C, Künzel KH, Müller U. Arteries in the posterior cervical triangle in man. *Clin Anat* 2005 Nov;18(8):553-557.

**A.** Anterior View

## 6.7 Arteries and arterial anastomoses of upper limb

**A.** The arteries often anastomose or communicate to form networks to ensure blood supply distal to the joint throughout the range of movement. If a main channel is occluded, the smaller alternate channels can usually increase in size, providing a collateral circulation that ensures the blood supply to structures distal to the blockage. However, collateral pathways require time to develop; they are usually insufficient to compensate for sudden occlusions.

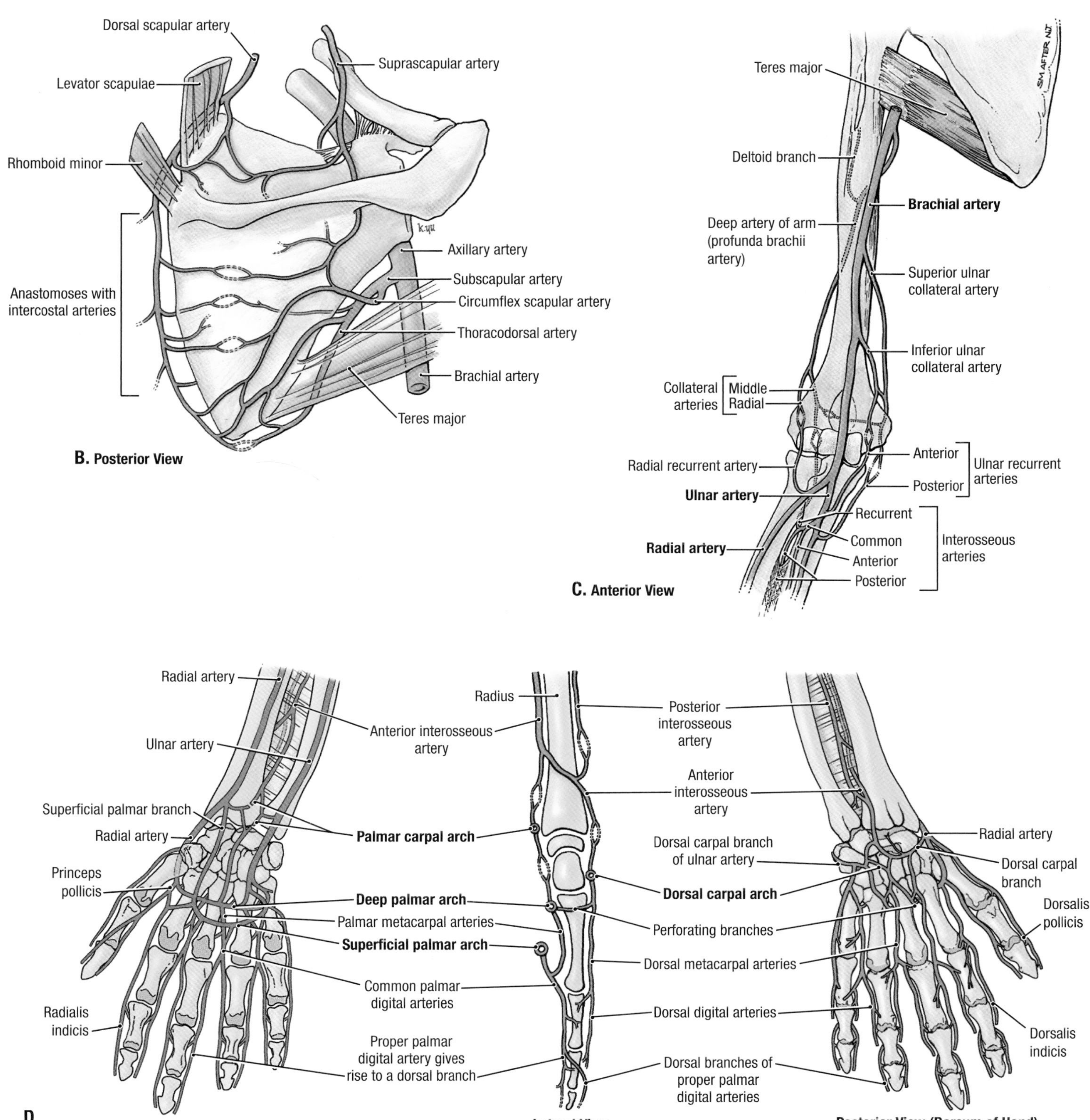

Dorsal scapular artery
Levator scapulae
Suprascapular artery
Rhomboid minor
Anastomoses with intercostal arteries
Axillary artery
Subscapular artery
Circumflex scapular artery
Thoracodorsal artery
Brachial artery
Teres major
B. Posterior View
Teres major
Deltoid branch
Brachial artery
Deep artery of arm (profunda brachii artery)
Superior ulnar collateral artery
Inferior ulnar collateral artery
Collateral arteries
Middle
Radial
Anterior
Posterior
Ulnar recurrent arteries
Radial recurrent artery
Ulnar artery
Recurrent
Common
Anterior
Posterior
Interosseous arteries
Radial artery
C. Anterior View
Radial artery
Ulnar artery
Anterior interosseous artery
Superficial palmar branch
Radial artery
Palmar carpal arch
Princeps pollicis
Deep palmar arch
Palmar metacarpal arteries
Superficial palmar arch
Common palmar digital arteries
Radialis indicis
Proper palmar digital artery gives rise to a dorsal branch
Radius
Posterior interosseous artery
Anterior interosseous artery
Dorsal carpal branch of ulnar artery
Dorsal carpal arch
Perforating branches
Dorsal metacarpal arteries
Dorsal digital arteries
Dorsal branches of proper palmar digital arteries
Radial artery
Dorsal carpal branch
Dorsalis pollicis
Dorsalis indicis
D
Anterior View (Palmar Aspect)
Lateral View (isolated third digit)
Posterior View (Dorsum of Hand)


**6.7 Arteries and periarterial anastomoses of upper limb *(continued)***

**B.** Scapular anastomoses. **C.** Anastomoses of the elbow. **D.** Anastomoses of the hand. Joints receive blood from articular arteries that arise from vessels around joints.

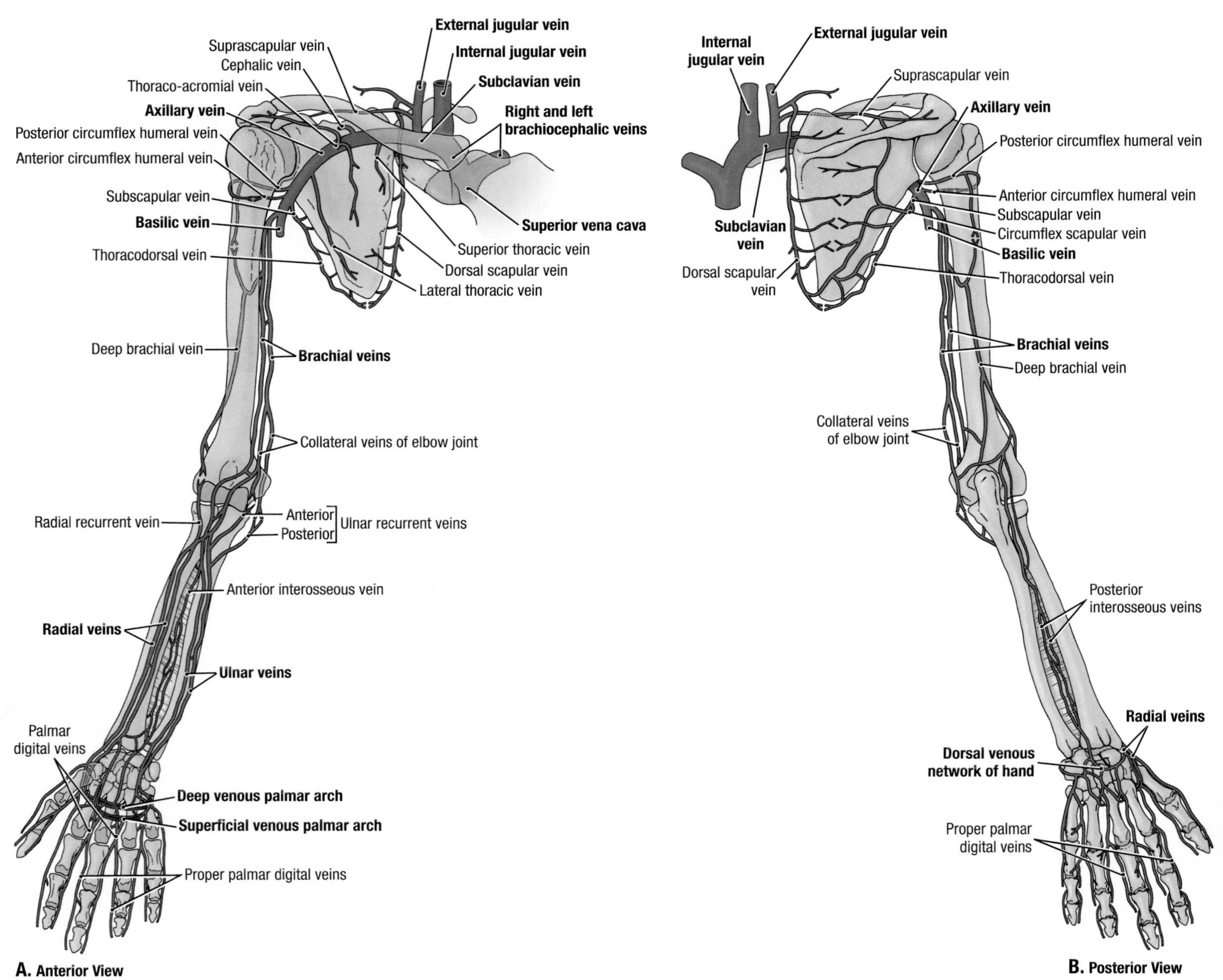
External jugular vein
Internal jugular vein
Subclavian vein
Right and left brachiocephalic veins
Suprascapular vein
Cephalic vein
Thoraco-acromial vein
Axillary vein
Posterior circumflex humeral vein
Anterior circumflex humeral vein
Subscapular vein
Basilic vein
Thoracodorsal vein
Superior vena cava
Superior thoracic vein
Dorsal scapular vein
Lateral thoracic vein
Deep brachial vein
Brachial veins
Collateral veins of elbow joint
Radial recurrent vein
Anterior
Posterior
Ulnar recurrent veins
Anterior interosseous vein
Radial veins
Ulnar veins
Palmar digital veins
Deep venous palmar arch
Superficial venous palmar arch
Proper palmar digital veins
A. Anterior View
Internal jugular vein
External jugular vein
Suprascapular vein
Axillary vein
Posterior circumflex humeral vein
Anterior circumflex humeral vein
Subscapular vein
Circumflex scapular vein
Basilic vein
Thoracodorsal vein
Subclavian vein
Dorsal scapular vein
Brachial veins
Deep brachial vein
Collateral veins of elbow joint
Posterior interosseous veins
Radial veins
Dorsal venous network of hand
Proper palmar digital veins
B. Posterior View

## 6.8 Overview of the deep veins of the upper limb

Deep veins lie internal to the deep fascia and occur as paired, continually interanastomosing "accompanying veins" (L., *venae comitantes*) surrounding and sharing the name of the artery they accompany.

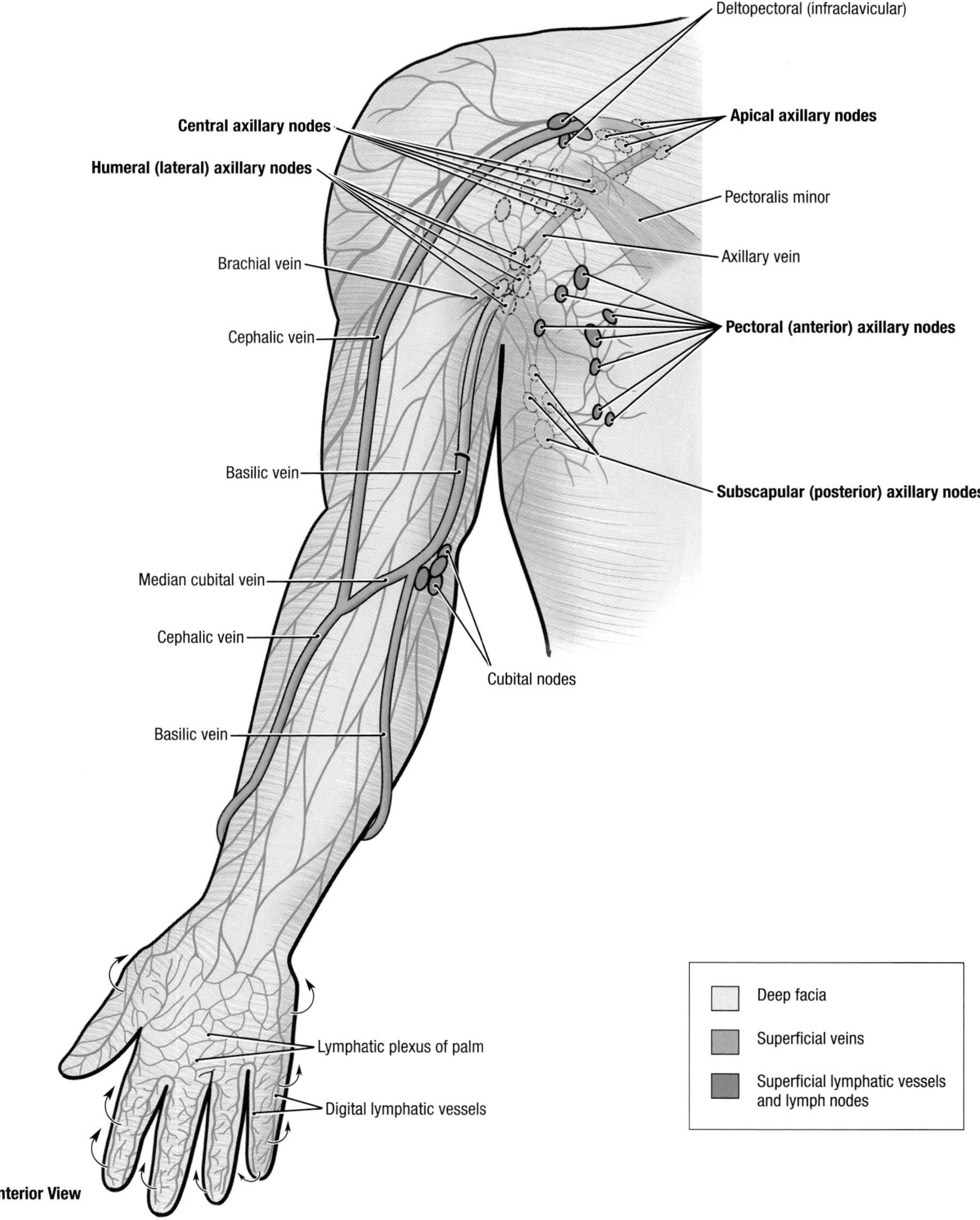
Deltopectoral (infraclavicular)
Central axillary nodes
Apical axillary nodes
Humeral (lateral) axillary nodes
Pectoralis minor
Axillary vein
Brachial vein
Pectoral (anterior) axillary nodes
Cephalic vein
Basilic vein
Subscapular (posterior) axillary nodes
Median cubital vein
Cephalic vein
Cubital nodes
Basilic vein
Deep facia
Superficial veins
Superficial lymphatic vessels and lymph nodes
Lymphatic plexus of palm
Digital lymphatic vessels
Anterior View

## 6.9 Superficial venous and lymphatic drainage of upper limb

Superficial lymphatic vessels arise from lymphatic plexuses in the digits, palm, and dorsum of the hand and ascend with the superficial veins of the upper limb. The superficial lymphatic vessels ascend through the forearm and arm, converging toward the cephalic and especially to the basilic vein to reach the axillary lymph nodes. Some lymph passes through the cubital nodes at the elbow and the deltopectoral (infraclavicular) nodes at the shoulder. Deep lymphatic vessels accompany the neurovascular bundles of the upper limb and end primarily in the humeral (lateral) and central axillary lymph nodes.

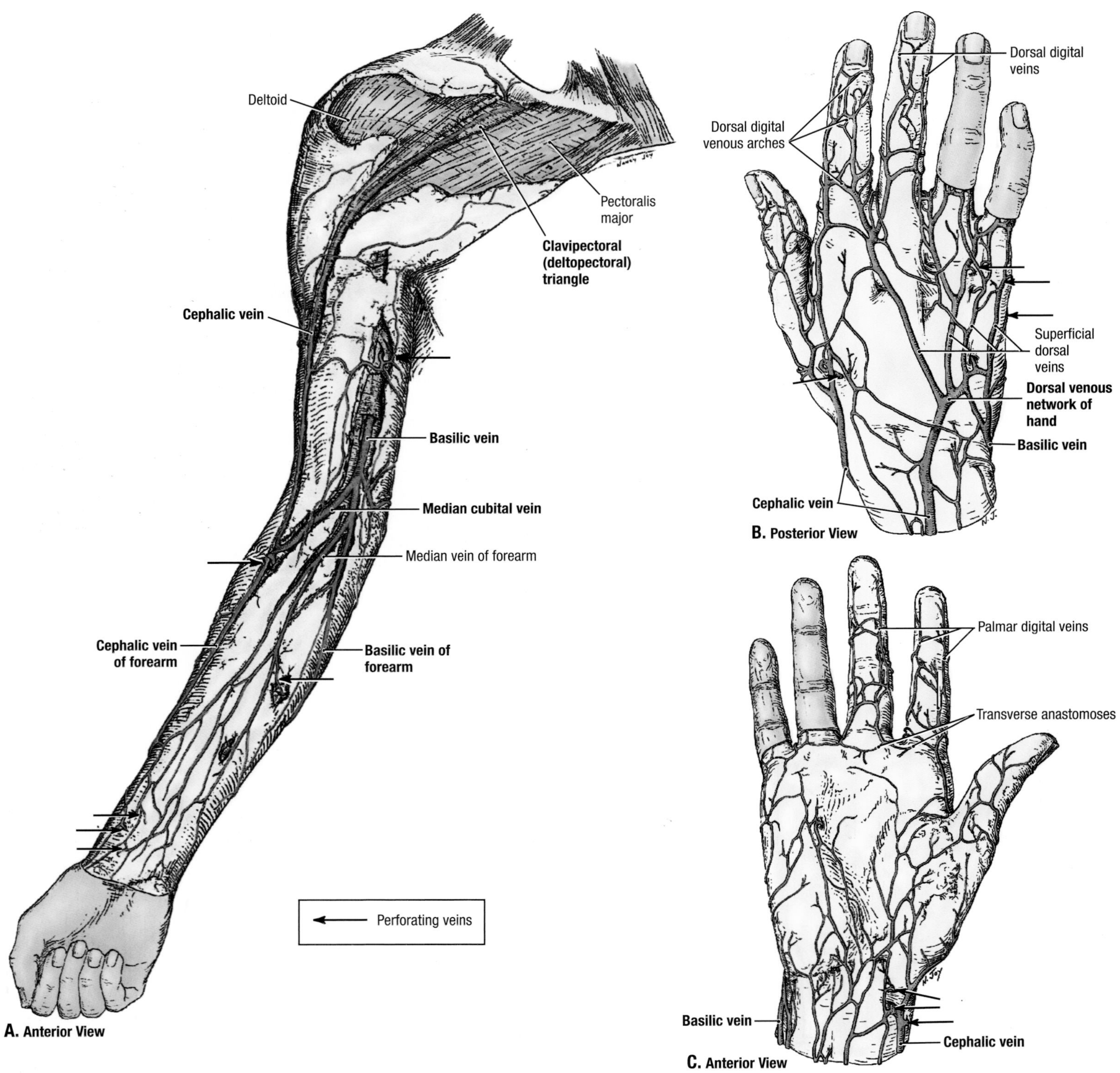
Deltoid
Pectoralis major
Clavipectoral (deltopectoral) triangle
Cephalic vein
Basilic vein
Median cubital vein
Median vein of forearm
Cephalic vein of forearm
Basilic vein of forearm
Perforating veins
A. Anterior View
Dorsal digital veins
Dorsal digital venous arches
Superficial dorsal veins
Dorsal venous network of hand
Basilic vein
Cephalic vein
B. Posterior View
Palmar digital veins
Transverse anastomoses
Basilic vein
Cephalic vein
C. Anterior View

## 6.10 Superficial venous drainage of upper limb

**A.** Forearm, arm, and pectoral region. **B.** Dorsal surface of hand. **C.** Palmar surface of hand. The *arrows* indicate where perforating veins penetrate the deep fascia. Blood is continuously shunted from these superficial veins in the subcutaneous tissue to deep veins via the perforating veins.

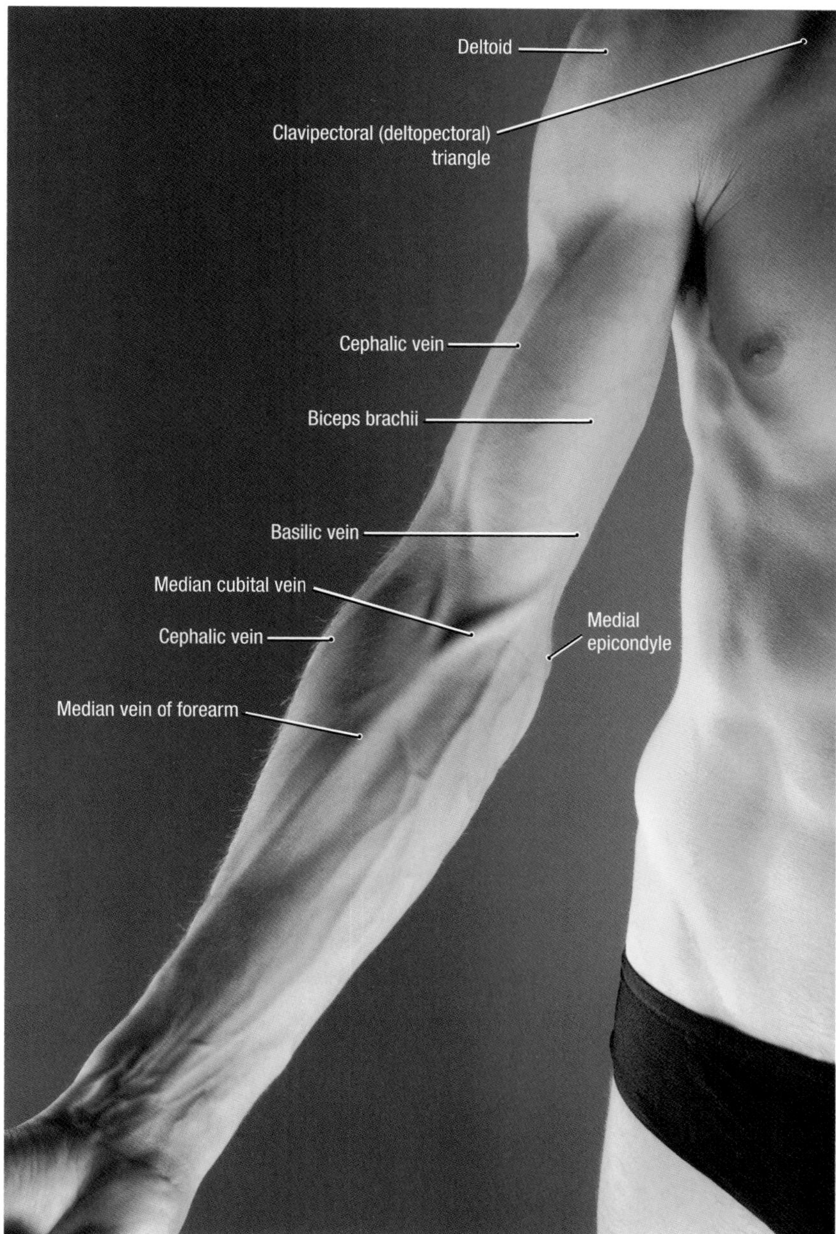
Deltoid
Clavipectoral (deltopectoral) triangle
Cephalic vein
Biceps brachii
Basilic vein
Median cubital vein
Cephalic vein
Medial epicondyle
Median vein of forearm

**D.** Anterior View

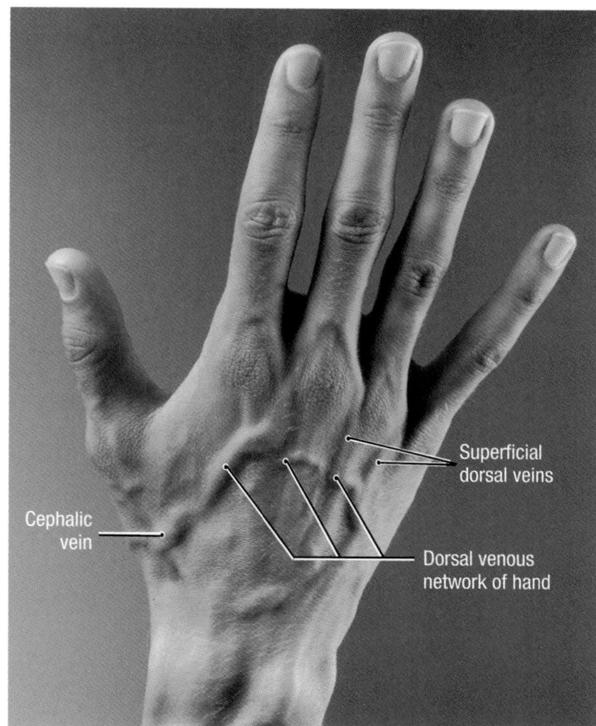
Superficial dorsal veins
Cephalic vein
Dorsal venous network of hand

**E.** Posterior View

## 6.10 Superficial venous drainage of upper limb *(continued)*

**D.** Surface anatomy of veins of forearm and arm. **E.** Surface anatomy of veins of the dorsal surface of hand.

Because of the prominence and accessibility of the superficial veins, they are commonly used for venipuncture (puncture of a vein to draw blood or inject a solution). By applying a tourniquet to the arm, the venous return is occluded, and the veins distend and usually are visible and/or palpable. Once a vein is punctured, the tourniquet is removed so that when the needle is removed the vein will not bleed extensively. The median cubital vein is commonly used for venipuncture. The veins forming the dorsal venous network of the hand and the cephalic and basilic veins arising from it are commonly used for long-term introduction of fluids (intravenous feeding). The cubital veins are also a site for the introduction of cardiac catheters to secure blood samples from the great vessels and chambers of the heart.

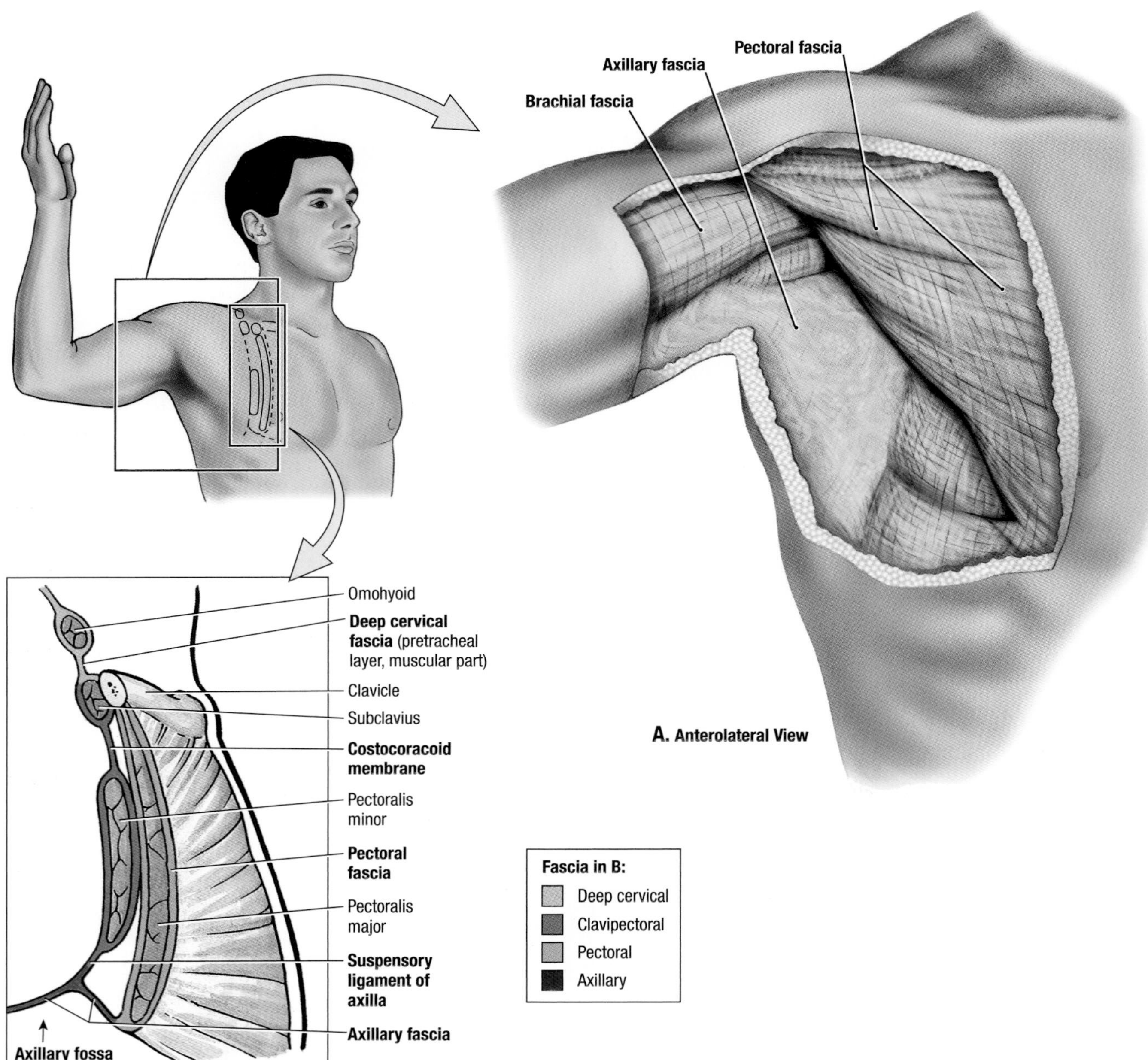
Pectoral fascia
Axillary fascia
Brachial fascia
A. Anterolateral View
Omohyoid
Deep cervical fascia (pretracheal layer, muscular part)
Clavicle
Subclavius
Costocoracoid membrane
Pectoralis minor
Pectoral fascia
Pectoralis major
Suspensory ligament of axilla
Axillary fascia
Axillary fossa
B. Sagittal Section
Fascia in B:
Deep cervical
Clavipectoral
Pectoral
Axillary

## 6.11 Deep fascia of upper limb—axillary and clavipectoral fascia

**A.** Axillary fascia. The axillary fascia forms the floor of the axillary fossa and is continuous with the pectoral fascia covering the pectoralis major muscle and the brachial fascia of the arm. **B.** Clavipectoral fascia. The clavipectoral fascia extends from the axillary fascia to enclose the pectoralis minor and subclavius muscles and then attaches to the clavicle. The part of the clavipectoral fascia superior to the pectoralis minor is the costocoracoid membrane and the part of the clavipectoral fascia inferior to the pectoralis minor is the suspensory ligament of the axilla. The suspensory ligament of the axilla, an extension of the axillary fascia, supports the axillary fascia and pulls the axillary fascia and the skin inferior to it superiorly when the arm is abducted, forming the axillary fossa or "armpit."

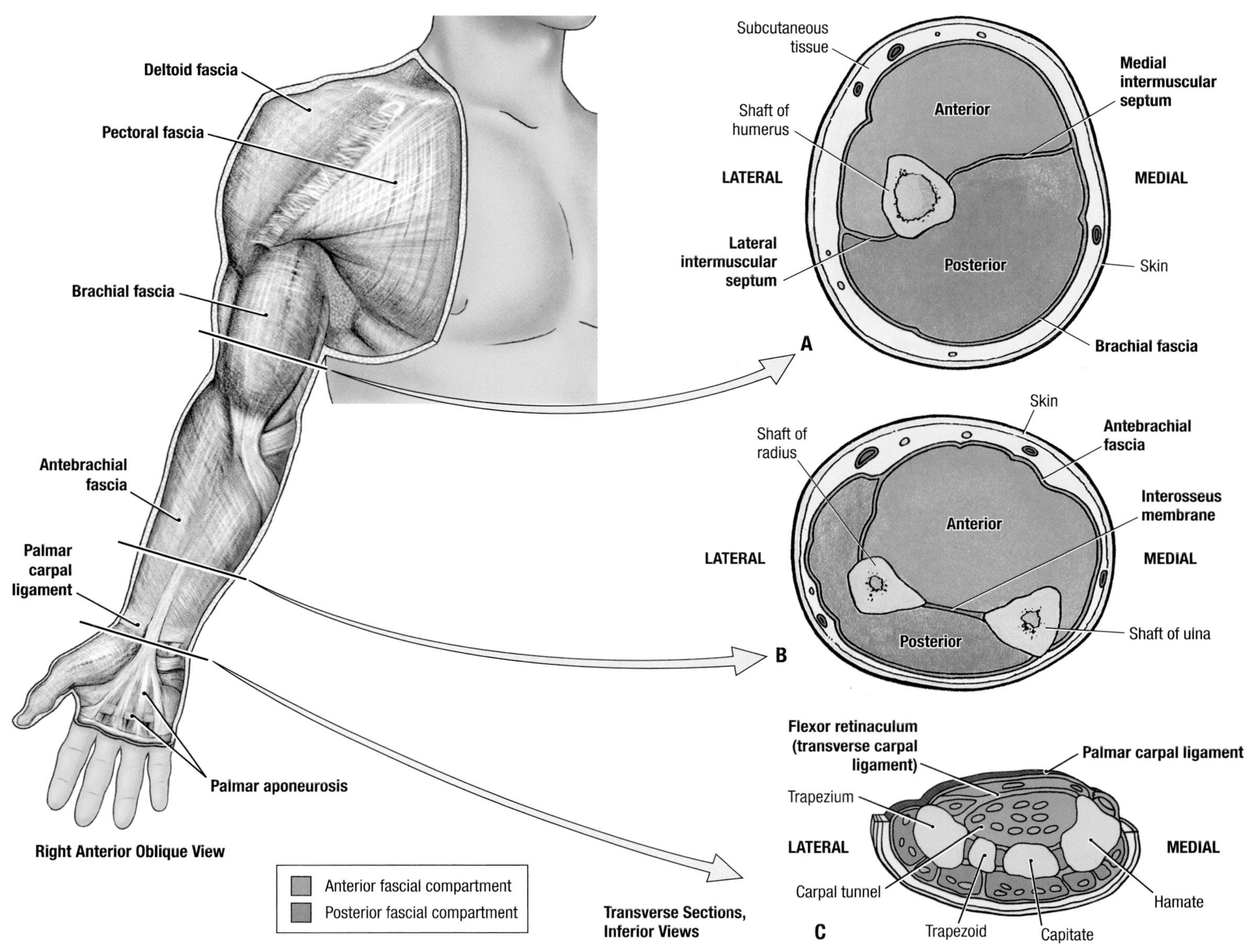
Deltoid fascia
Pectoral fascia
Brachial fascia
Antebrachial fascia
Palmar carpal ligament
Palmar aponeurosis
Right Anterior Oblique View
Anterior fascial compartment
Posterior fascial compartment
Subcutaneous tissue
Shaft of humerus
LATERAL
Lateral intermuscular septum
Anterior
Posterior
Medial intermuscular septum
MEDIAL
Skin
Brachial fascia
A
Shaft of radius
Skin
Antebrachial fascia
Interosseus membrane
LATERAL
Anterior
MEDIAL
Posterior
Shaft of ulna
B
Flexor retinaculum (transverse carpal ligament)
Palmar carpal ligament
Trapezium
LATERAL
MEDIAL
Carpal tunnel
Hamate
Trapezoid
Capitate
Transverse Sections, Inferior Views
C

## 6.12 Deep fascia of upper limb—brachial and antebrachial fascia

**A.** Brachial fascia. The brachial fascia is the deep fascia of the arm and is continuous superiorly with the pectoral and axillary layers of fascia. Medial and lateral intermuscular septa extend from the deep aspect of the brachial fascia to the humerus, dividing the arm into anterior and posterior musculofascial compartments. **B.** Antebrachial fascia. The antebrachial fascia surrounds the forearm and is continuous with the brachial fascia and deep fascia of the hand. The interosseous membrane separates the forearm into anterior and posterior musculofascial compartments. Distally the fascia thickens to form the palmar carpal ligament, which is continuous with the flexor retinaculum and dorsally with the extensor expansion. The deep fascia of the hand is continuous with the antebrachial fascia, and on the palmar surface of the hand it thickens to form the palmar aponeurosis. **C.** Flexor retinaculum (transverse carpal ligament). The flexor retinaculum extends between the medial and lateral carpal bones to form the carpal tunnel.

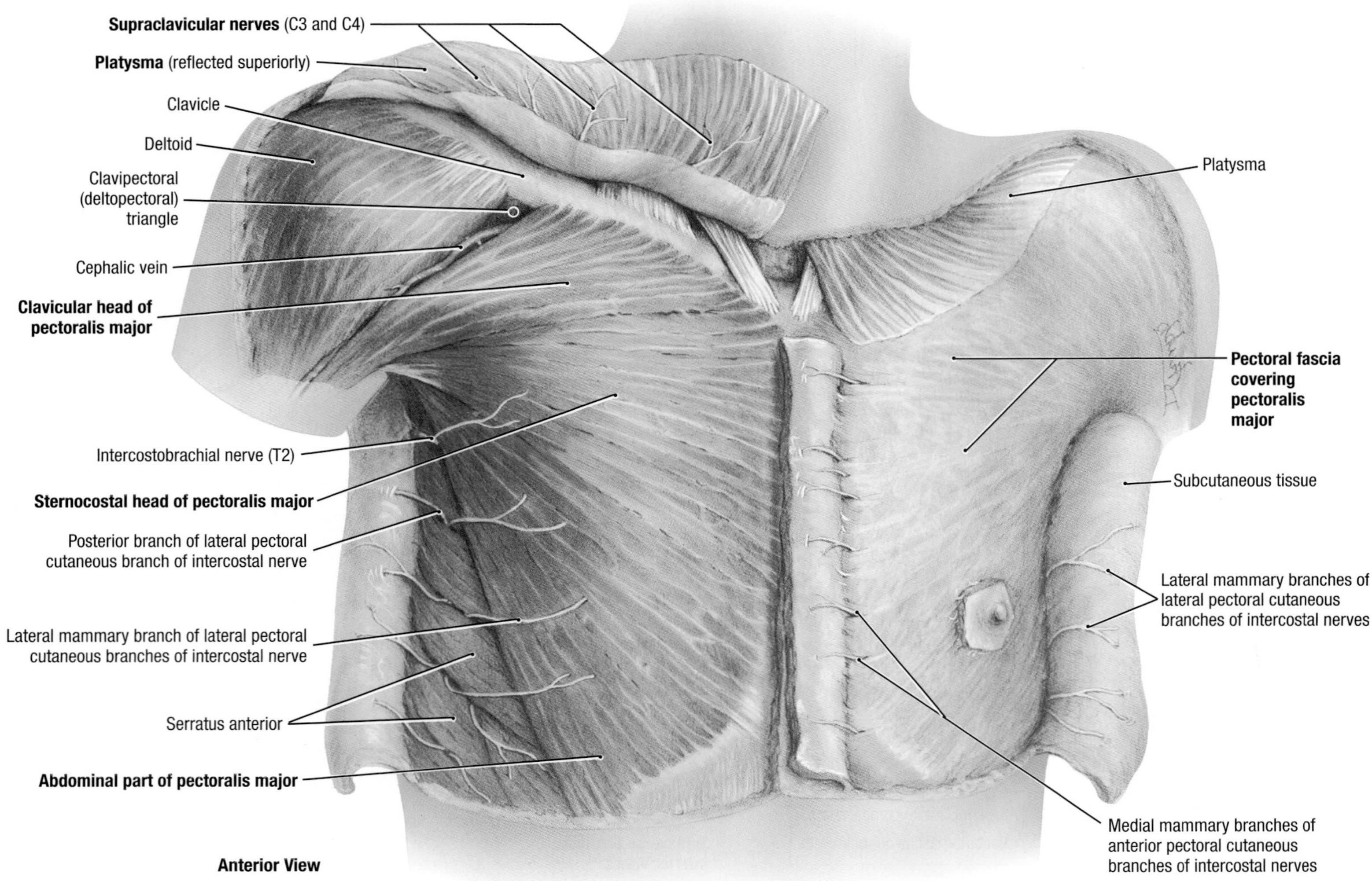
Supraclavicular nerves (C3 and C4)
Platysma (reflected superiorly)
Clavicle
Deltoid
Clavipectoral (deltopectoral) triangle
Cephalic vein
Clavicular head of pectoralis major
Intercostobrachial nerve (T2)
Sternocostal head of pectoralis major
Posterior branch of lateral pectoral cutaneous branch of intercostal nerve
Lateral mammary branch of lateral pectoral cutaneous branches of intercostal nerve
Serratus anterior
Abdominal part of pectoralis major
Anterior View
Platysma
Pectoral fascia covering pectoralis major
Subcutaneous tissue
Lateral mammary branches of lateral pectoral cutaneous branches of intercostal nerves
Medial mammary branches of anterior pectoral cutaneous branches of intercostal nerves

## 6.13 Superficial dissection, male pectoral region

- The platysma muscle, which usually descends to the 2nd or 3rd rib, is cut short on the right side and, together with the supraclavicular nerves, is reflected on the left side.
- The exposed intermuscular bony strip of the clavicle is subcutaneous and subplatysmal.
- The cephalic vein passes deeply to join the axillary vein in the clavipectoral (deltopectoral) triangle.
- The cutaneous innervation of the pectoral region by the supraclavicular nerves (C3 and C4) and upper thoracic nerves (T2 to T6); the brachial plexus (C5–T1) does not supply cutaneous branches to the pectoral region.

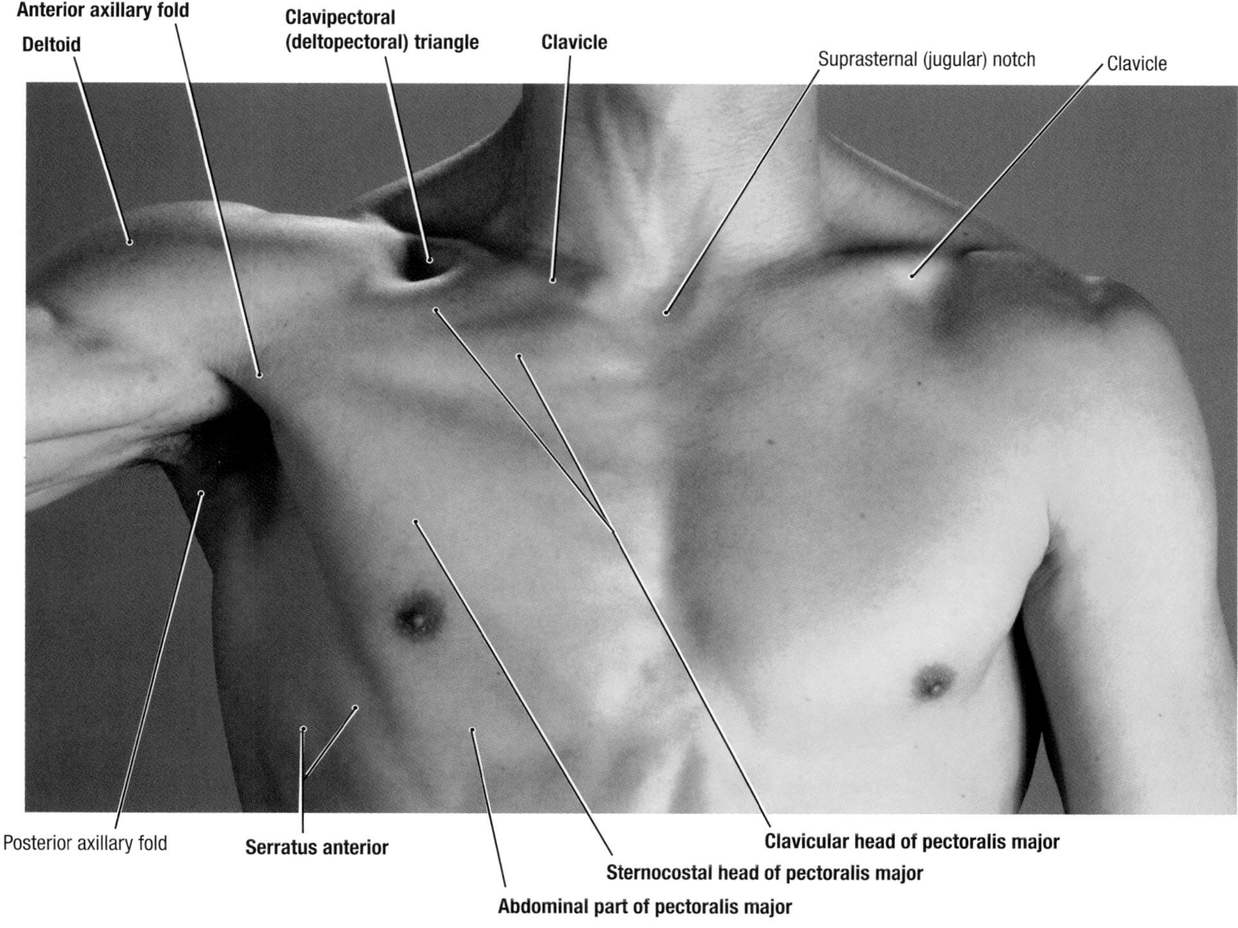
Anterior axillary fold
Deltoid
Clavipectoral (deltopectoral) triangle
Clavicle
Suprasternal (jugular) notch
Clavicle
Posterior axillary fold
Serratus anterior
Clavicular head of pectoralis major
Sternocostal head of pectoralis major
Abdominal part of pectoralis major

## 6.14 Surface anatomy, male pectoral region

The **clavipectoral** (deltopectoral) **triangle** is the depressed area just inferior to the lateral part of the clavicle. The clavipectoral triangle is bounded by the clavicle superiorly, the deltoid laterally, and the clavicular head of pectoralis major medially. When the arm is abducted and then adducted against resistance, the two heads of the pectoralis major are visible and palpable. As this muscle extends from the thoracic wall to the arm, it forms the anterior axillary fold. Digitations of the serratus anterior appear inferolateral to the pectoralis major. The coracoid process of the scapula is covered by the anterior part of deltoid; however, the tip of the process can be felt on deep palpation in the clavipectoral triangle. The deltoid forms the contour of the shoulder.

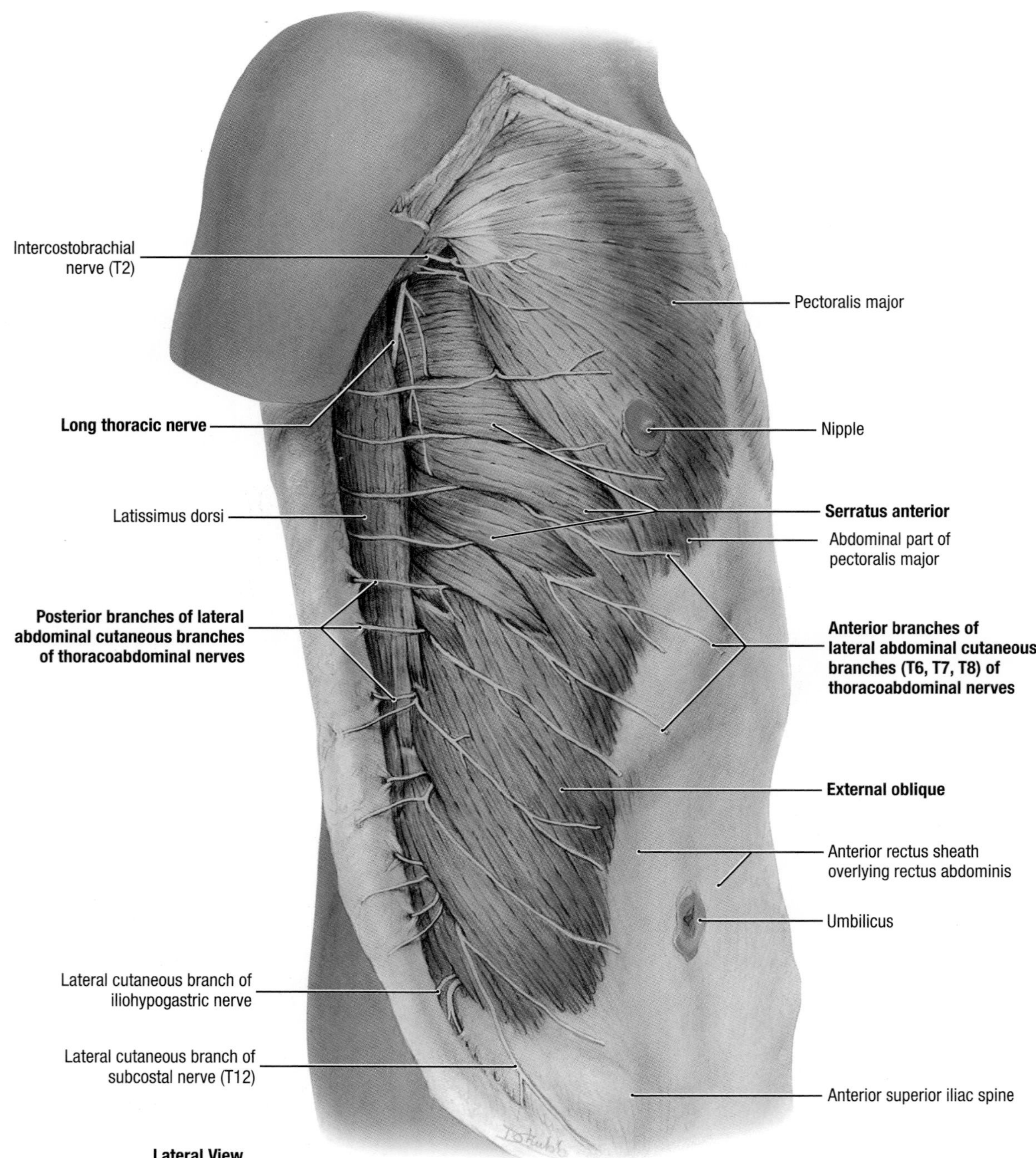
Intercostobrachial nerve (T2)
Pectoralis major
Long thoracic nerve
Nipple
Latissimus dorsi
Serratus anterior
Abdominal part of pectoralis major
Posterior branches of lateral abdominal cutaneous branches of thoracoabdominal nerves
Anterior branches of lateral abdominal cutaneous branches (T6, T7, T8) of thoracoabdominal nerves
External oblique
Anterior rectus sheath overlying rectus abdominis
Umbilicus
Lateral cutaneous branch of iliohypogastric nerve
Lateral cutaneous branch of subcostal nerve (T12)
Anterior superior iliac spine
Lateral View

## 6.15 Superficial dissection of trunk

- The slips of the serratus anterior interdigitate with the external oblique.
- The long thoracic nerve (nerve to serratus anterior) lies on the lateral (superficial) aspect of the serratus anterior; this nerve is vulnerable to damage from stab wounds and during surgery (e.g., radical mastectomy).
- The anterior and posterior branches of the lateral thoracic and abdominal cutaneous branches of intercostal and thoracoabdominal nerves are dissected.

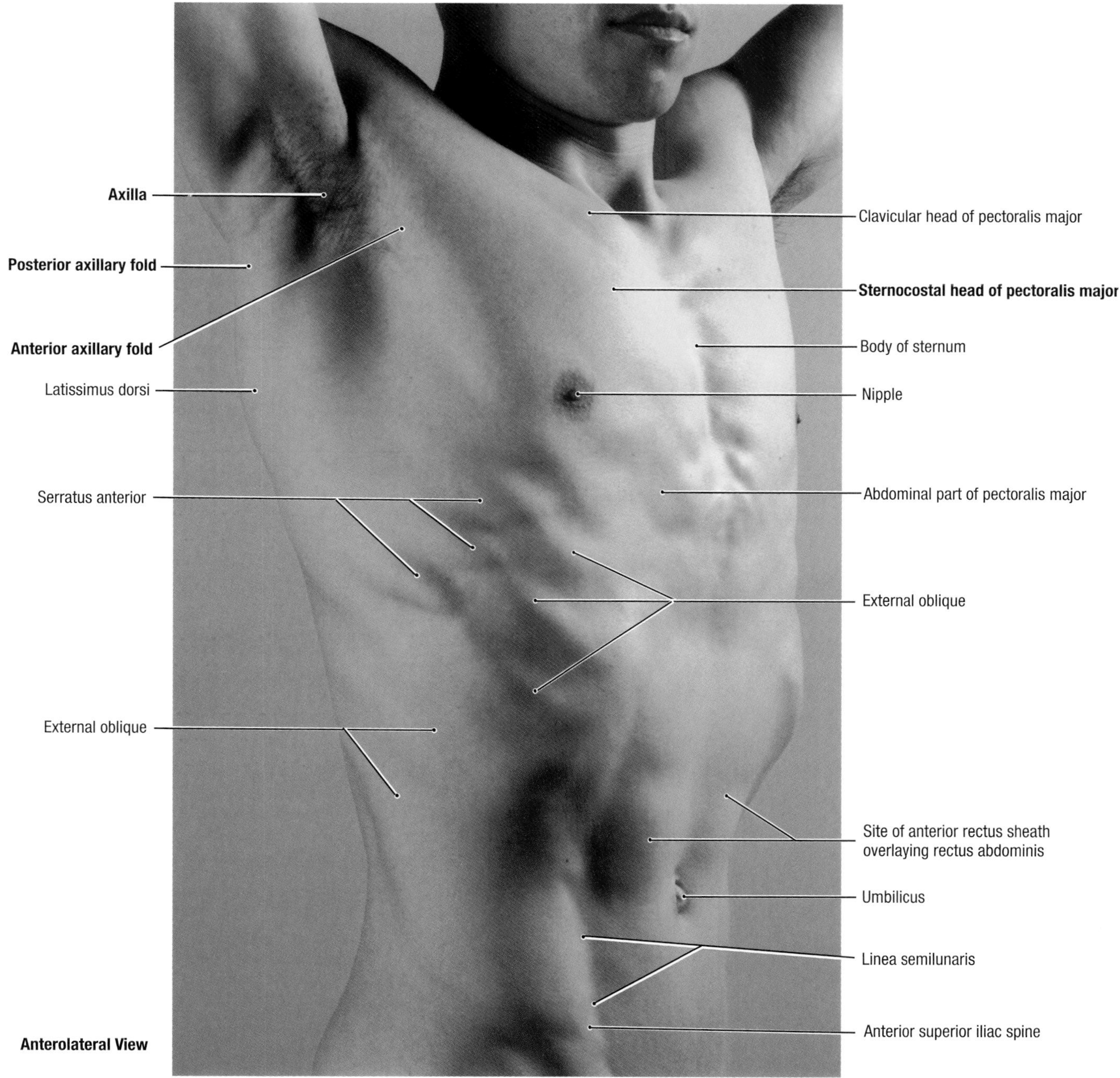
Axilla
Posterior axillary fold
Anterior axillary fold
Latissimus dorsi
Serratus anterior
External oblique
Anterolateral View
Clavicular head of pectoralis major
Sternocostal head of pectoralis major
Body of sternum
Nipple
Abdominal part of pectoralis major
External oblique
Site of anterior rectus sheath overlaying rectus abdominis
Umbilicus
Linea semilunaris
Anterior superior iliac spine

## 6.16 Surface anatomy of anterolateral aspect of the trunk

When the arm is abducted and then adducted against resistance, the sternocostal part of the pectoralis major can be seen and palpated. If the anterior axillary fold bounding the axilla is grasped between the fingers and thumb, the inferior border of the sternocostal head of the pectoralis major can be felt. Several digitations of the serratus anterior are visible inferior to the anterior axillary fold. The posterior axillary fold is composed of skin and muscular tissue (latissimus dorsi and teres major) bounding the axilla posteriorly.

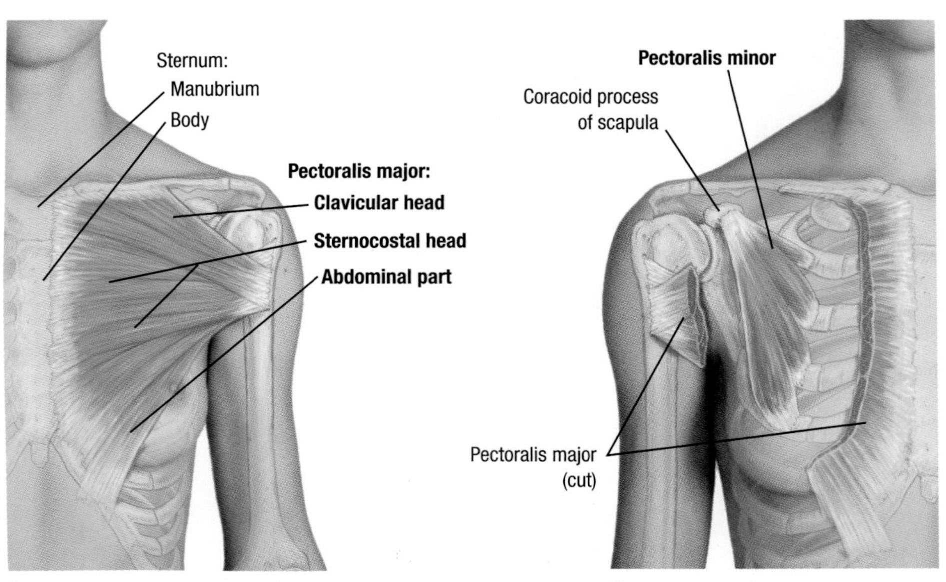
Sternum:
Manubrium
Body
Pectoralis major:
Clavicular head
Sternocostal head
Abdominal part
Pectoralis minor
Coracoid process of scapula
Pectoralis major (cut)
B. Anterior View

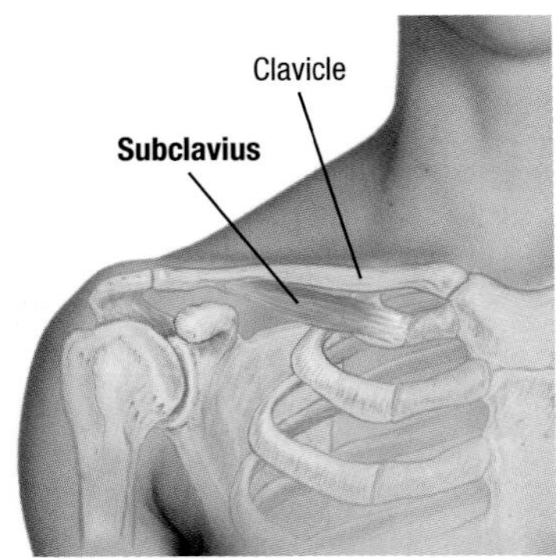
Clavicle
Subclavius
C. Anterior View

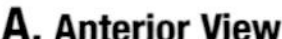
A. Anterior View

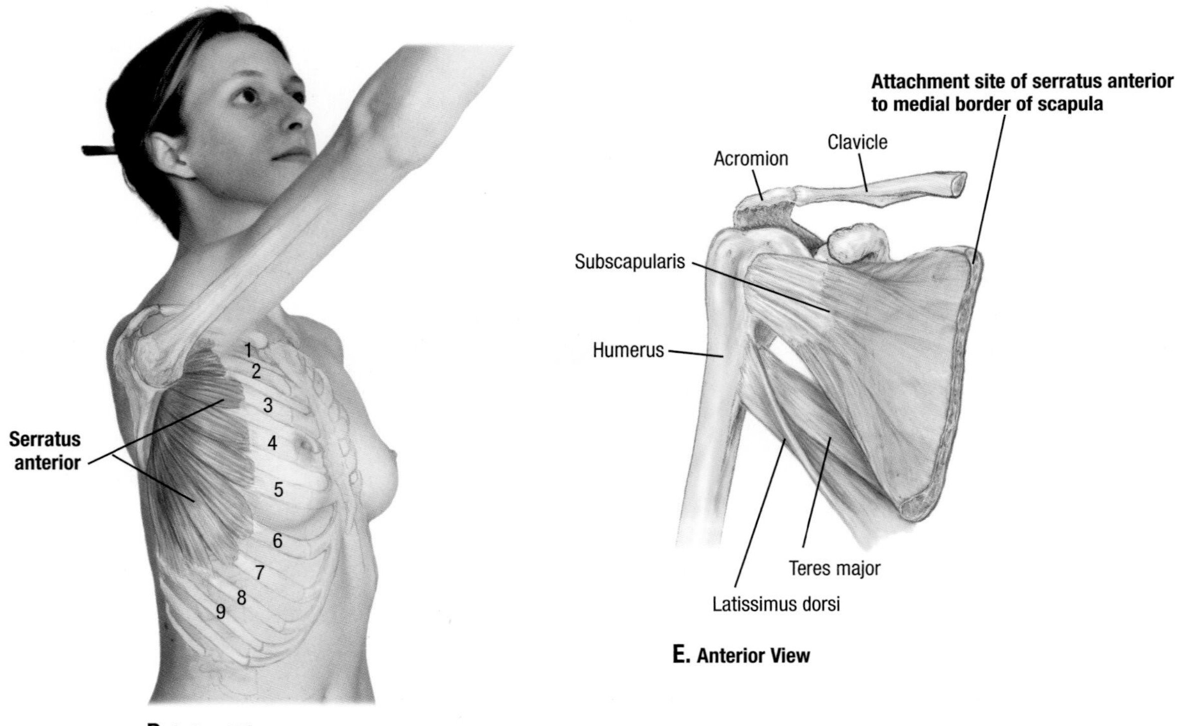
1
2
3
4
5
6
7
8
9
Serratus anterior
D. Lateral View
Attachment site of serratus anterior to medial border of scapula
Acromion
Clavicle
Subscapularis
Humerus
Teres major
Latissimus dorsi
E. Anterior View

## 6.17 Pectoralis major and minor and serratus anterior

**A.** Pectoralis major. **B.** Pectoralis minor. **C.** Subclavius. **D** and **E.** Serratus anterior and its scapular attachment.

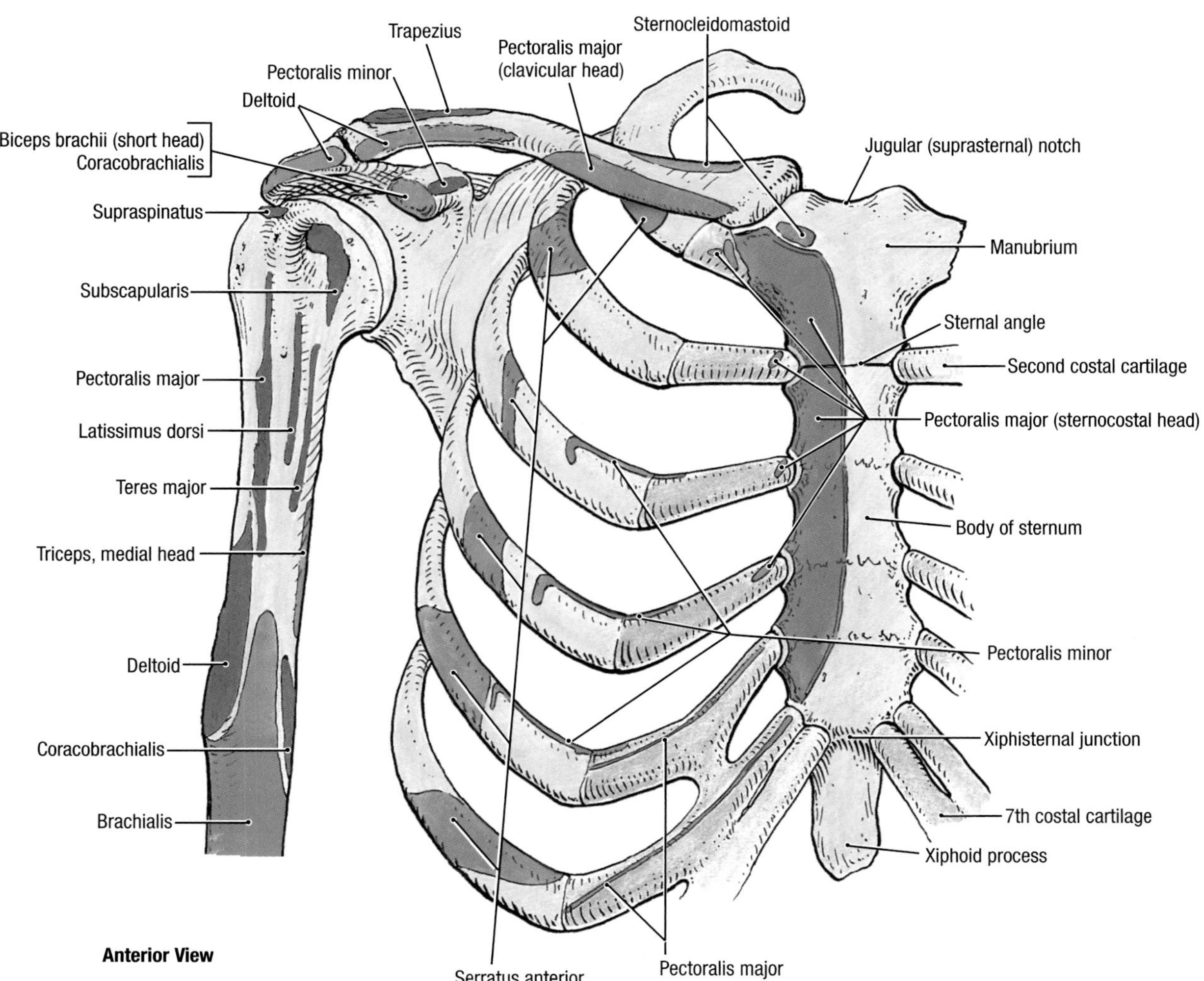
Trapezius
Sternocleidomastoid
Pectoralis major (clavicular head)
Pectoralis minor
Deltoid
Biceps brachii (short head)
Coracobrachialis
Jugular (suprasternal) notch
Supraspinatus
Manubrium
Subscapularis
Sternal angle
Second costal cartilage
Pectoralis major
Pectoralis major (sternocostal head)
Latissimus dorsi
Teres major
Body of sternum
Triceps, medial head
Pectoralis minor
Deltoid
Xiphisternal junction
Coracobrachialis
7th costal cartilage
Brachialis
Xiphoid process
Anterior View
Serratus anterior
Pectoralis major

## TABLE 6.2 ANTERIOR AXIOAPPENDICULAR MUSCLES

| Muscle | Proximal Attachment (red) | Distal Attachment (blue) | Innervation[a] | Main Actions |
|---|---|---|---|---|
| **Pectoralis major** | *Clavicular head:* anterior surface of medial half of clavicle<br>*Sternocostal head:* anterior surface of sternum, superior six costal cartilages<br>*Abdominal part:* aponeurosis of external oblique muscle | Crest of greater tubercle of intertubercular sulcus (lateral lip of bicipital groove) | Lateral and medial pectoral nerves; clavicular head (C5 and **C6**), sternocostal head (**C7**, **C8**, and T1) | Adducts and medially rotates humerus; draws scapula anteriorly and inferiorly<br>Acting alone: clavicular head flexes humerus and sternocostal head extends it from the flexed position |
| **Pectoralis minor** | 3rd to 5th ribs near their costal cartilages | Medial border and superior surface of coracoid process of scapula | Medial pectoral nerve (C8 and T1) | Stabilizes scapula by drawing it inferiorly and anteriorly against thoracic wall |
| **Subclavius** | Junction of 1st rib and its costal cartilage | Inferior surface of middle third of clavicle | Nerve to subclavius (**C5** and C6) | Anchors and depresses clavicle |
| **Serratus anterior** | External surfaces of lateral parts of 1st to 8th–9th ribs | Anterior surface of medial border of scapula | Long thoracic nerve (C5, **C6**, and **C7**) | Protracts scapula and holds it against thoracic wall; rotates scapula |

[a]Numbers indicate spinal cord segmental innervation (e.g., C5 and C6 indicate that nerves supplying the clavicular head of pectoralis major are derived from 5th and 6th cervical segments of spinal cord). Boldface numbers indicate the main segmental innervation. Damage to these segments or to motor nerve roots arising from them results in paralysis of the muscles concerned.

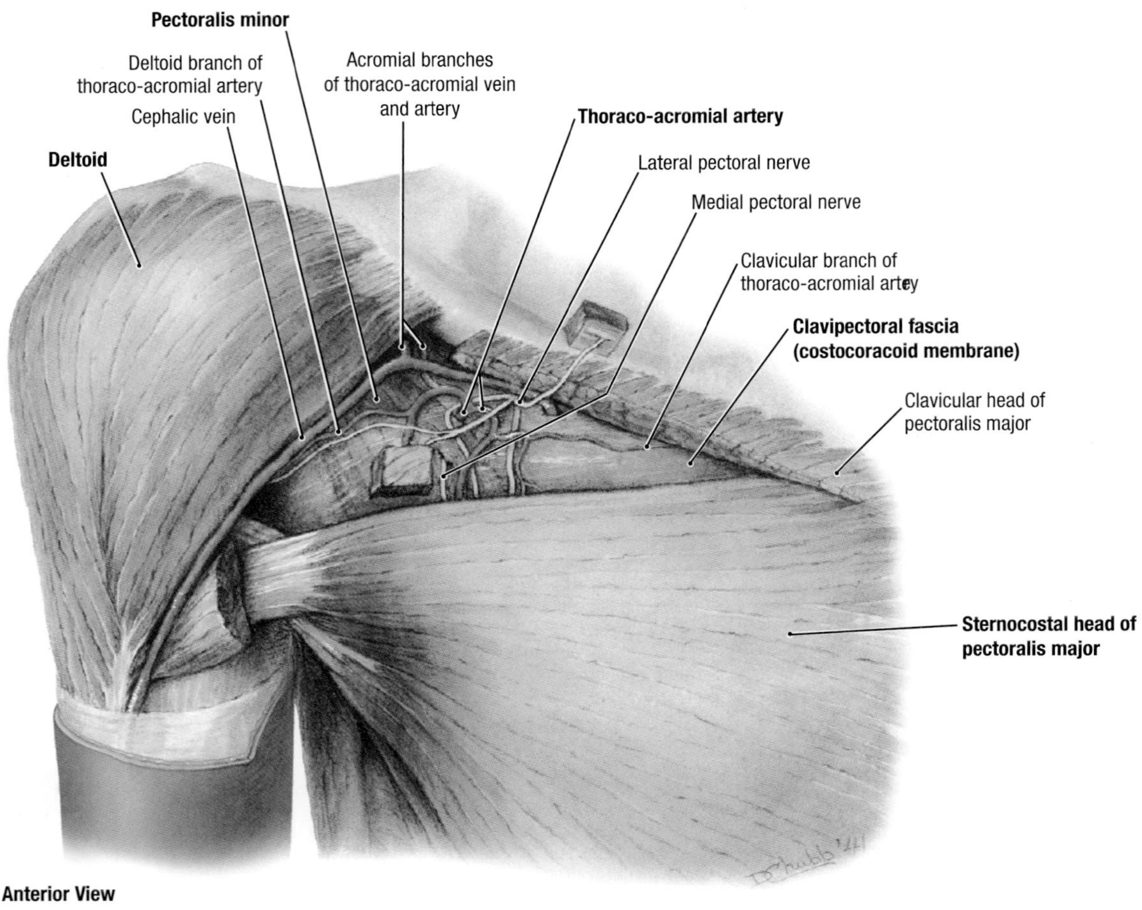

Pectoralis minor
Deltoid branch of thoraco-acromial artery
Acromial branches of thoraco-acromial vein and artery
Cephalic vein
Thoraco-acromial artery
Deltoid
Lateral pectoral nerve
Medial pectoral nerve
Clavicular branch of thoraco-acromial artey
Clavipectoral fascia (costocoracoid membrane)
Clavicular head of pectoralis major
Sternocostal head of pectoralis major
Anterior View


## 6.18 Anterior wall of axilla and clavipectoral fascia

**A.** Anterior wall of axilla. The clavicular head of the pectoralis major is excised, except for two cubes of muscle that remain to identify the branches of the lateral pectoral nerve.

- The clavipectoral fascia superior to the pectoralis minor (costocoracoid membrane) is pierced by the cephalic vein, the lateral pectoral nerve, and the thoraco-acromial vessels.
- The pectoralis minor and clavipectoral fascia are pierced by the medial pectoral nerve.
- Observe the trilaminar insertion of the pectoralis major from deep to superficial: inferior part of the sternocostal head, superior part of the sternocostal head, and clavicular head.

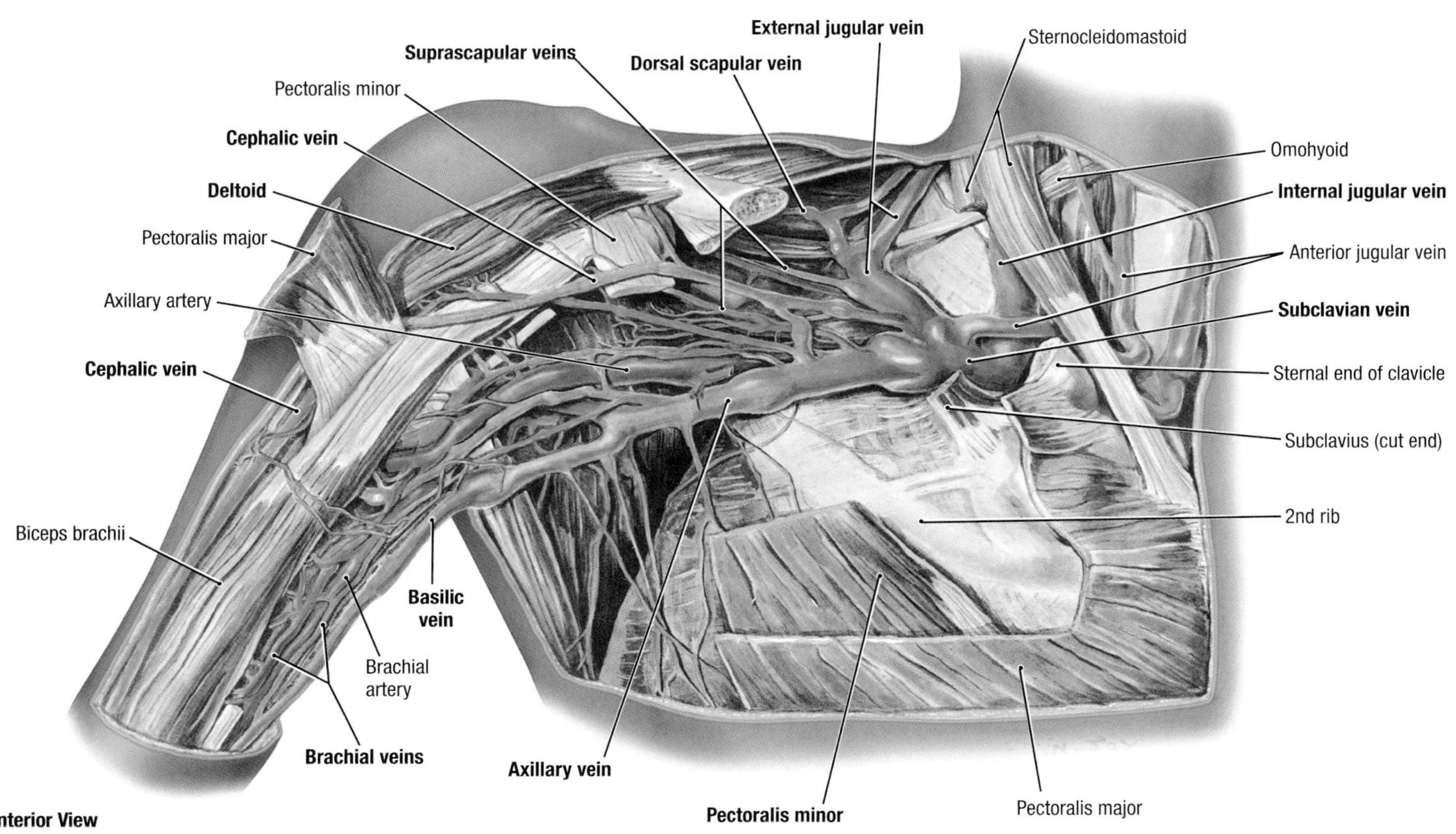
External jugular vein
Suprascapular veins
Dorsal scapular vein
Sternocleidomastoid
Pectoralis minor
Cephalic vein
Deltoid
Pectoralis major
Axillary artery
Cephalic vein
Biceps brachii
Basilic vein
Brachial artery
Brachial veins
Axillary vein
Pectoralis minor
Pectoralis major
Omohyoid
Internal jugular vein
Anterior jugular vein
Subclavian vein
Sternal end of clavicle
Subclavius (cut end)
2nd rib
Anterior View

## 6.19 Veins of axilla

- The basilic vein joins the brachial veins to become the axillary vein near the inferior border of teres major, the axillary vein becomes the subclavian vein at the lateral border of the 1st rib, and the subclavian joins the internal jugular to become the brachiocephalic vein posterior to the sternal end of the clavicle.
- Numerous valves, enlargements in the vein, are shown.
- The cephalic vein in this specimen bifurcates to end in the axillary and external jugular veins.

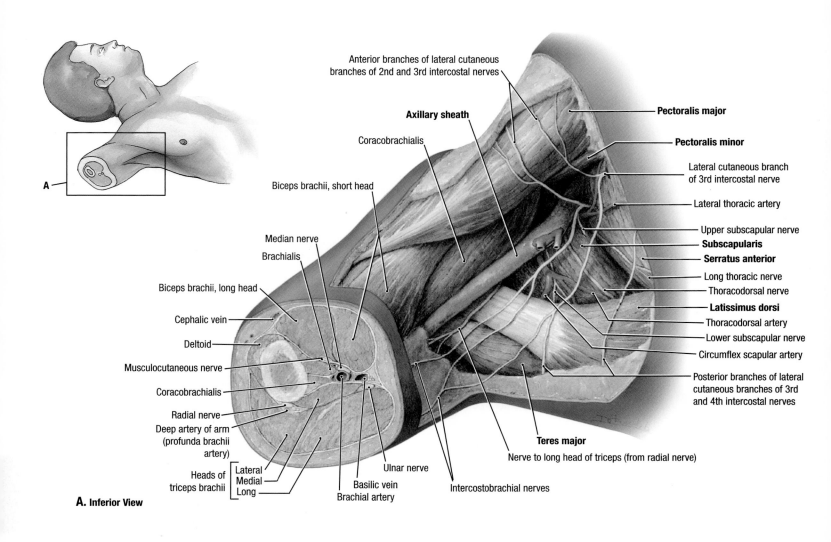

A
Anterior branches of lateral cutaneous branches of 2nd and 3rd intercostal nerves
Axillary sheath
Pectoralis major
Pectoralis minor
Coracobrachialis
Lateral cutaneous branch of 3rd intercostal nerve
Biceps brachii, short head
Lateral thoracic artery
Upper subscapular nerve
Subscapularis
Median nerve
Serratus anterior
Brachialis
Long thoracic nerve
Biceps brachii, long head
Thoracodorsal nerve
Latissimus dorsi
Cephalic vein
Thoracodorsal artery
Deltoid
Lower subscapular nerve
Circumflex scapular artery
Musculocutaneous nerve
Posterior branches of lateral cutaneous branches of 3rd and 4th intercostal nerves
Coracobrachialis
Radial nerve
Deep artery of arm (profunda brachii artery)
Teres major
Nerve to long head of triceps (from radial nerve)
Heads of triceps brachii: Lateral, Medial, Long
Ulnar nerve
Basilic vein
Brachial artery
Intercostobrachial nerves

**A. Inferior View**

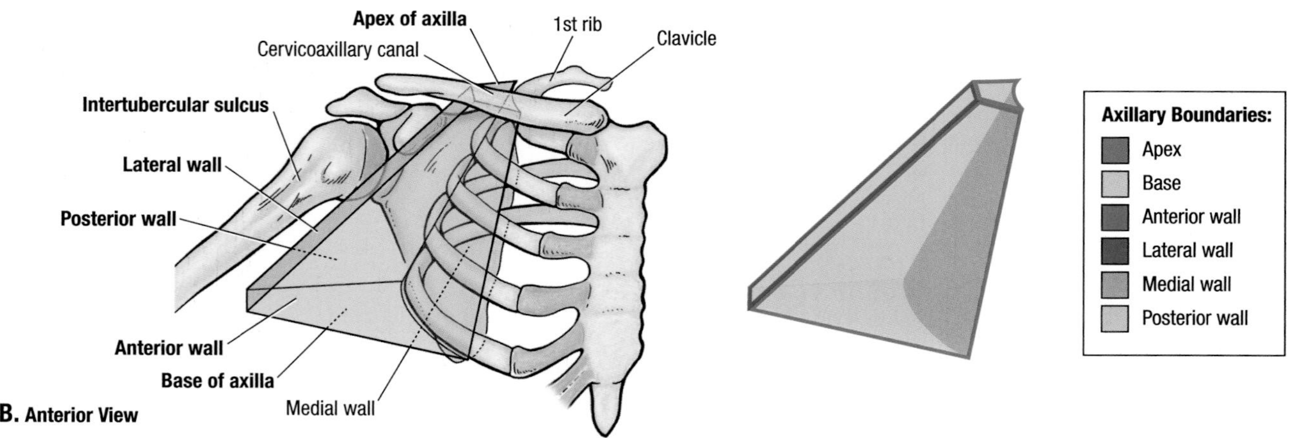
Apex of axilla
1st rib
Clavicle
Cervicoaxillary canal
Intertubercular sulcus
Lateral wall
Posterior wall
Anterior wall
Base of axilla
Medial wall
B. Anterior View
Axillary Boundaries:
Apex
Base
Anterior wall
Lateral wall
Medial wall
Posterior wall

## 6.20 Walls and contents of the axilla

**A.** Dissection. **B.** Location and walls of axilla, schematic diagram.

- The walls of the axilla are: anterior (formed by the pectoralis major, pectoralis minor, and subclavius muscles), posterior (formed by subscapularis, latissimus dorsi, and teres major muscles), medial (formed by the serratus anterior muscle), and lateral (formed by the intertubercular sulcus [bicipital groove] of the humerus [concealed by the biceps and coracobrachialis muscles]).
- The axillary sheath surrounds the nerves and vessels (neurovascular bundle) of the upper limb.

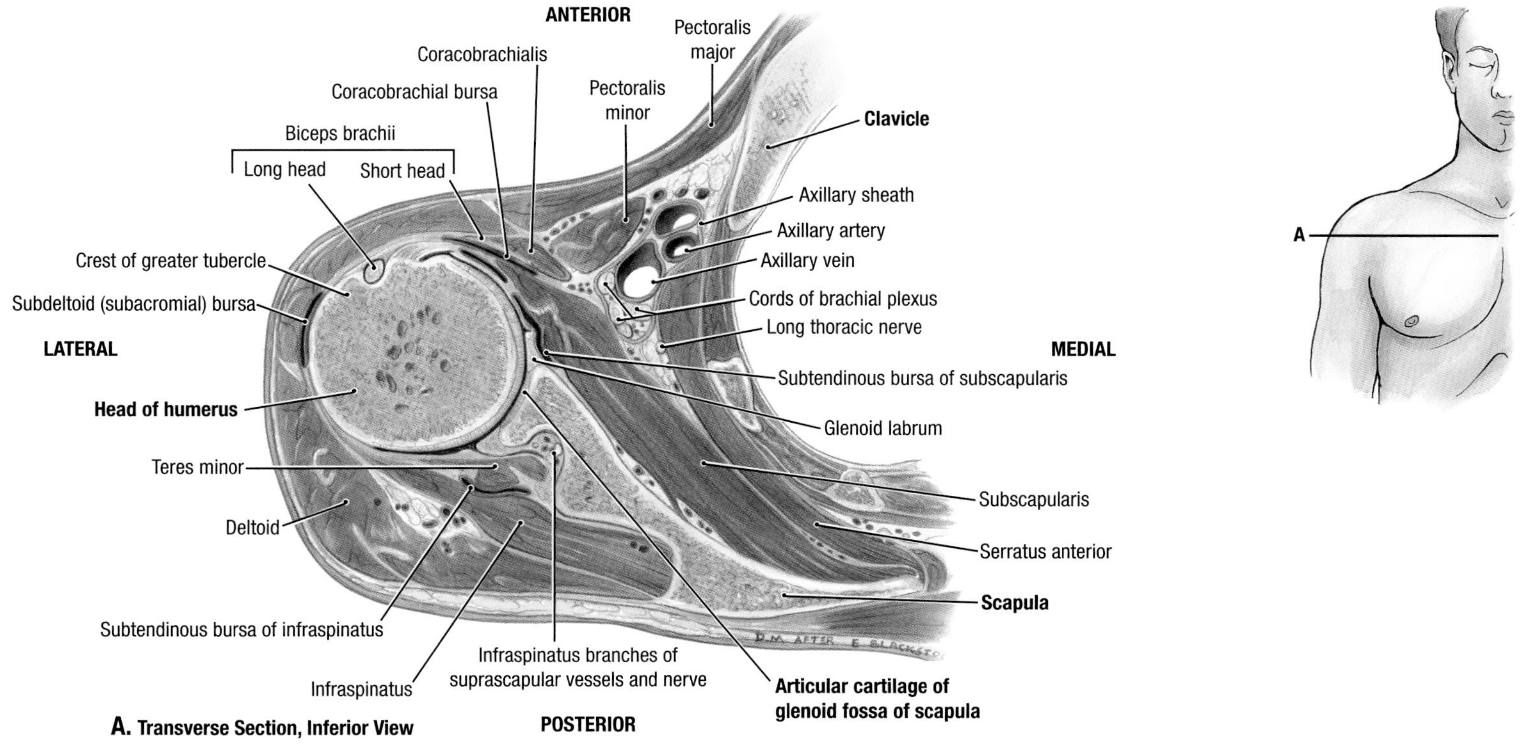
ANTERIOR
Pectoralis major
Coracobrachialis
Coracobrachial bursa
Pectoralis minor
Biceps brachii
Long head
Short head
Clavicle
Axillary sheath
Axillary artery
Axillary vein
Crest of greater tubercle
Subdeltoid (subacromial) bursa
Cords of brachial plexus
Long thoracic nerve
LATERAL
MEDIAL
Subtendinous bursa of subscapularis
Head of humerus
Glenoid labrum
Teres minor
Subscapularis
Deltoid
Serratus anterior
Scapula
Subtendinous bursa of infraspinatus
Infraspinatus branches of suprascapular vessels and nerve
Infraspinatus
Articular cartilage of glenoid fossa of scapula
POSTERIOR
A

A. Transverse Section, Inferior View

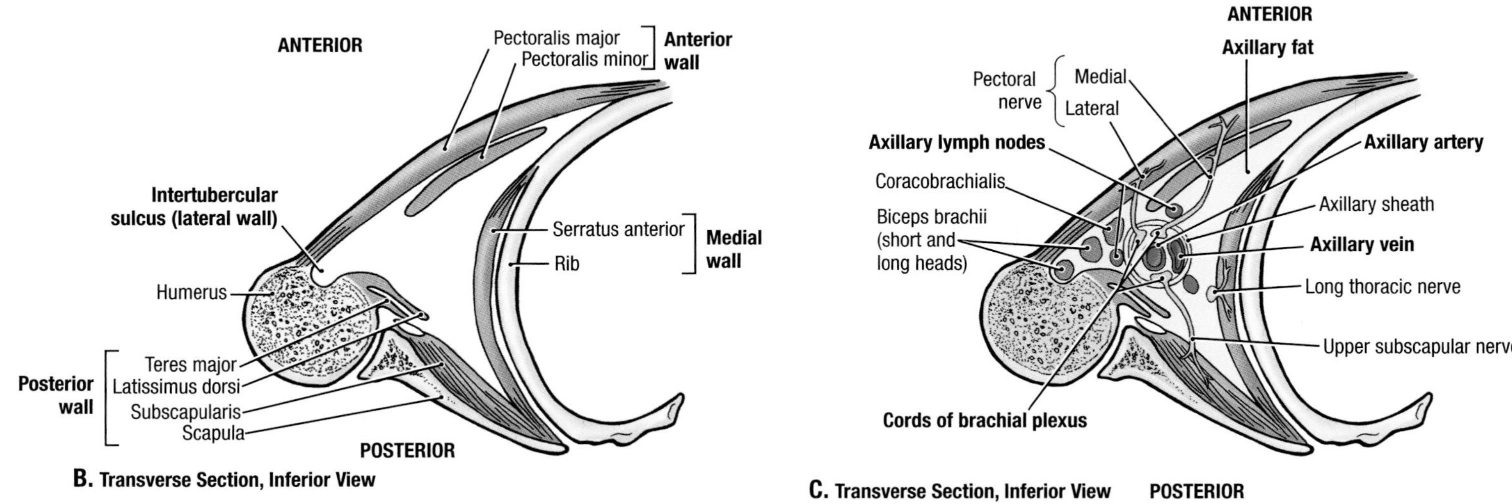
ANTERIOR
Pectoralis major
Pectoralis minor
Anterior wall
Intertubercular sulcus (lateral wall)
Serratus anterior
Rib
Medial wall
Humerus
Posterior wall
Teres major
Latissimus dorsi
Subscapularis
Scapula
POSTERIOR
ANTERIOR
Axillary fat
Pectoral nerve
Medial
Lateral
Axillary lymph nodes
Axillary artery
Coracobrachialis
Axillary sheath
Biceps brachii (short and long heads)
Axillary vein
Long thoracic nerve
Upper subscapular nerve
Cords of brachial plexus
POSTERIOR

B. Transverse Section, Inferior View

C. Transverse Section, Inferior View

## 6.21 Transverse sections through the shoulder joint and axilla

**A.** Anatomical section. **B.** Walls of axilla, schematic illustration. **C.** Walls and contents of axilla, schematic illustration.

- The intertubercular sulcus (bicipital groove) containing the tendon of the long head of the biceps brachii muscle is directed anteriorly; the short head of the biceps muscle and the coracobrachialis and pectoralis minor muscles are sectioned just inferior to their attachments to the coracoid process.
- The small glenoid cavity is deepened by the glenoid labrum.
- Bursae include the subdeltoid (subacromial) bursa, between the deltoid and greater tubercle; the subtendinous bursa of subscapularis, between the subscapularis tendon and scapula; and coracobrachial bursa, between the coracobrachialis and subscapularis.
- The axillary sheath encloses the axillary artery and vein and the three cords of the brachial plexus to form a neurovascular bundle, surrounded by axillary fat.

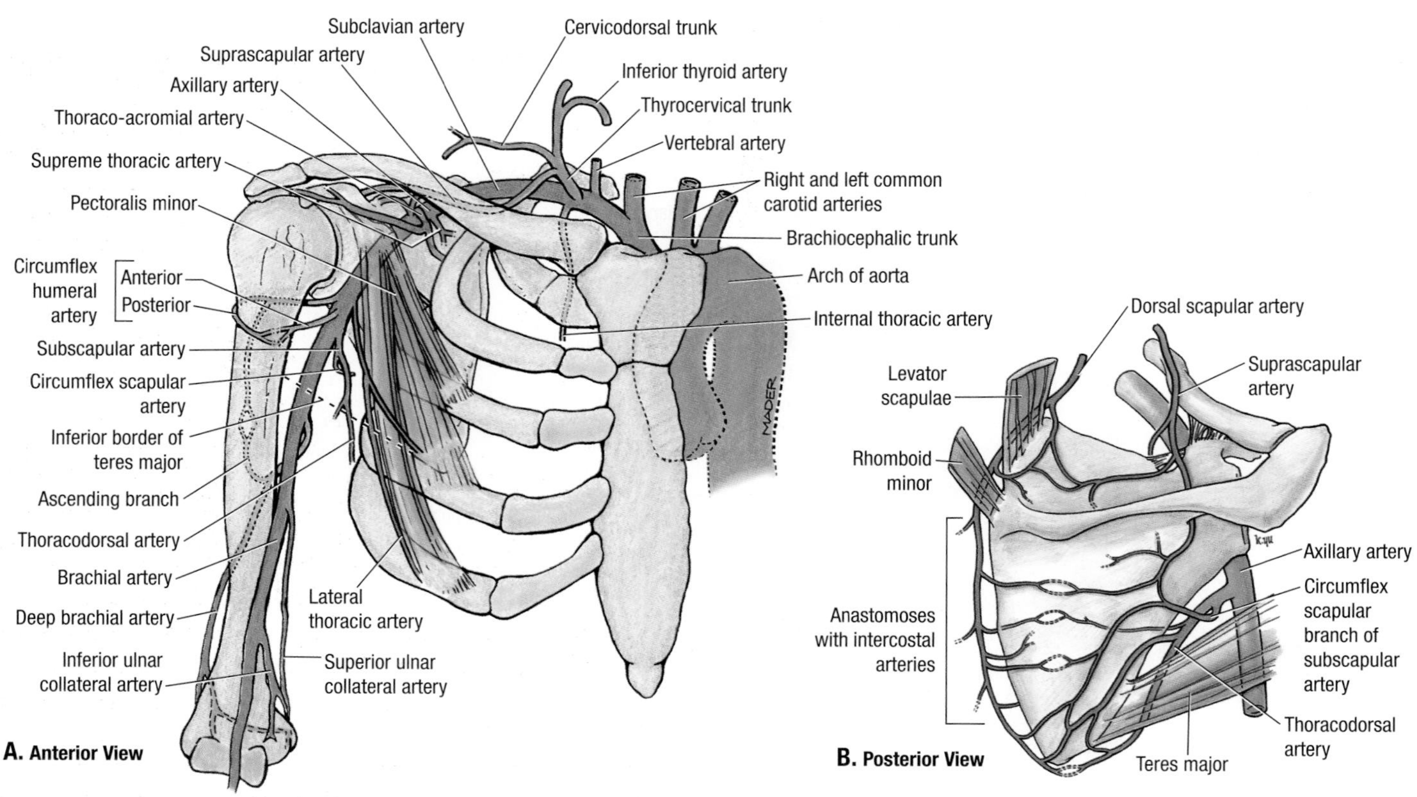
Subclavian artery
Cervicodorsal trunk
Suprascapular artery
Inferior thyroid artery
Axillary artery
Thyrocervical trunk
Thoraco-acromial artery
Vertebral artery
Supreme thoracic artery
Right and left common carotid arteries
Pectoralis minor
Brachiocephalic trunk
Circumflex humeral artery
Anterior
Posterior
Arch of aorta
Internal thoracic artery
Subscapular artery
Circumflex scapular artery
Inferior border of teres major
Ascending branch
Thoracodorsal artery
Brachial artery
Lateral thoracic artery
Deep brachial artery
Inferior ulnar collateral artery
Superior ulnar collateral artery
A. Anterior View
Dorsal scapular artery
Levator scapulae
Suprascapular artery
Rhomboid minor
Axillary artery
Circumflex scapular branch of subscapular artery
Anastomoses with intercostal arteries
Thoracodorsal artery
Teres major
B. Posterior View

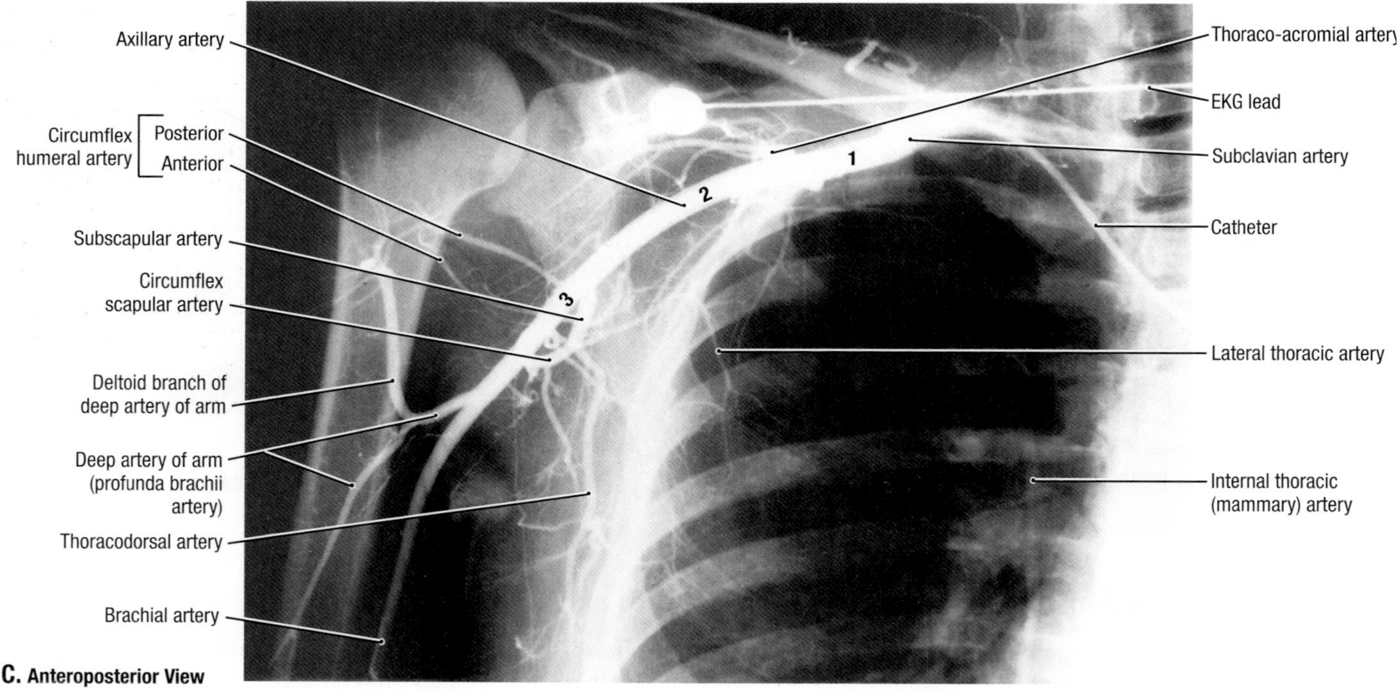
Axillary artery
Thoraco-acromial artery
EKG lead
Circumflex humeral artery
Posterior
Anterior
Subclavian artery
1
2
3
Catheter
Subscapular artery
Circumflex scapular artery
Lateral thoracic artery
Deltoid branch of deep artery of arm
Deep artery of arm (profunda brachii artery)
Internal thoracic (mammary) artery
Thoracodorsal artery
Brachial artery
C. Anteroposterior View

**1**: First part of the axillary artery is located between the lateral border of the 1st rib and the medial border of pectoralis minor.
**2**: Second part of the axillary artery lies posterior to pectoralis minor.
**3**: Third part of the axillary artery extends from the lateral border of pectoralis minor to the inferior border of teres major, where it becomes the brachial artery.

## 6.22 Arteries of the proximal upper limb

**A** and **B.** Schematic illustrations. **C.** Axillary arteriogram.

**TABLE 6.3 ARTERIES OF PROXIMAL UPPER LIMB (SHOULDER REGION AND ARM)**

| Artery | Origin | | Course |
|---|---|---|---|
| **Internal thoracic** | Subclavian artery | | Descends, inclining anteromedially, posterior to sternal end of clavicle and first costal cartilage; enters thorax to descend in parasternal plane; gives rise to perforating branches, anterior intercostal, musculophrenic, and superior epigastric arteries |
| **Thyrocervical trunk** | | | Ascends as a short, wide trunk, often giving rise to the suprascapular artery and/or cervicodorsal trunk and terminating by bifurcating into the ascending cervical and inferior thyroid arteries |
| **Suprascapular** | Cervicodorsal trunk from thyrocervical trunk (or as direct branch of subclavian artery[a]) | | Passes inferolaterally over anterior scalene muscle and phrenic nerve, subclavian artery and brachial plexus running laterally posterior and parallel to clavicle; next passes over transverse scapular ligament to supraspinous fossa, then lateral to scapular spine (deep to acromion) to infraspinous fossa |
| **Supreme thoracic** | 1st part (as only branch) | Axillary artery | Runs anteromedially along superior border of pectoralis minor; then passes between it and pectoralis major to thoracic wall; helps supply 1st and 2nd intercostal spaces and superior part of serratus anterior |
| **Thoraco-acromial** | 2nd part (medial branch) | | Curls around superomedial border of pectoralis minor, pierces costocaracoid membrane (clavipectoral fascia), and divides into four branches: pectoral, deltoid, acromial, and clavicular |
| **Lateral thoracic** | 2nd part (lateral branch) | | Descends along axillary border of pectoralis minor; follows it onto thoracic wall, supplying lateral aspect of breast |
| **Circumflex humeral (anterior and posterior)** | 3rd part (sometimes via a common trunk) | | Encircle surgical neck of humerus, anastomosing with each other laterally; larger posterior branch traverses quadrangular space |
| **Subscapular** | 3rd part (largest branch) | | Descends from level of inferior border of subscapularis along lateral border of scapula, dividing within 2-3 cm into terminal branches, the circumflex scapular and thoracodorsal arteries |
| **Circumflex scapular** | Subscapular artery | Brachial artery | Curves around lateral border of scapula to enter infraspinous fossa, anastomosing with subscapular artery |
| **Thoracodorsal** | Near its origin | | Continuation course of subscapular artery; accompanies thoracodorsal nerve to enter latissimus dorsi |
| **Deep brachial** | Near middle of arm | | Accompanies radial nerve through radial groove of humerus, supplying posterior compartment of arm and participating in periarticular arterial anastomosis around elbow joint |
| **Superior ulnar collateral** | Superior to medial epicondyle of humerus | | Accompanies ulnar nerve to posterior aspect of elbow; anastomoses with posterior ulnar recurrent artery |
| **Inferior ulnar collateral** | | | Passes anterior to medial epicondyle of humerus to anastomose with anterior ulnar collateral artery around elbow joint |

[a] See Weiglein AH, Moriggl B, Schalk C, et al. Arteries in the posterior cervical triangle. Clinical Anatomy 2005;18:533–537.

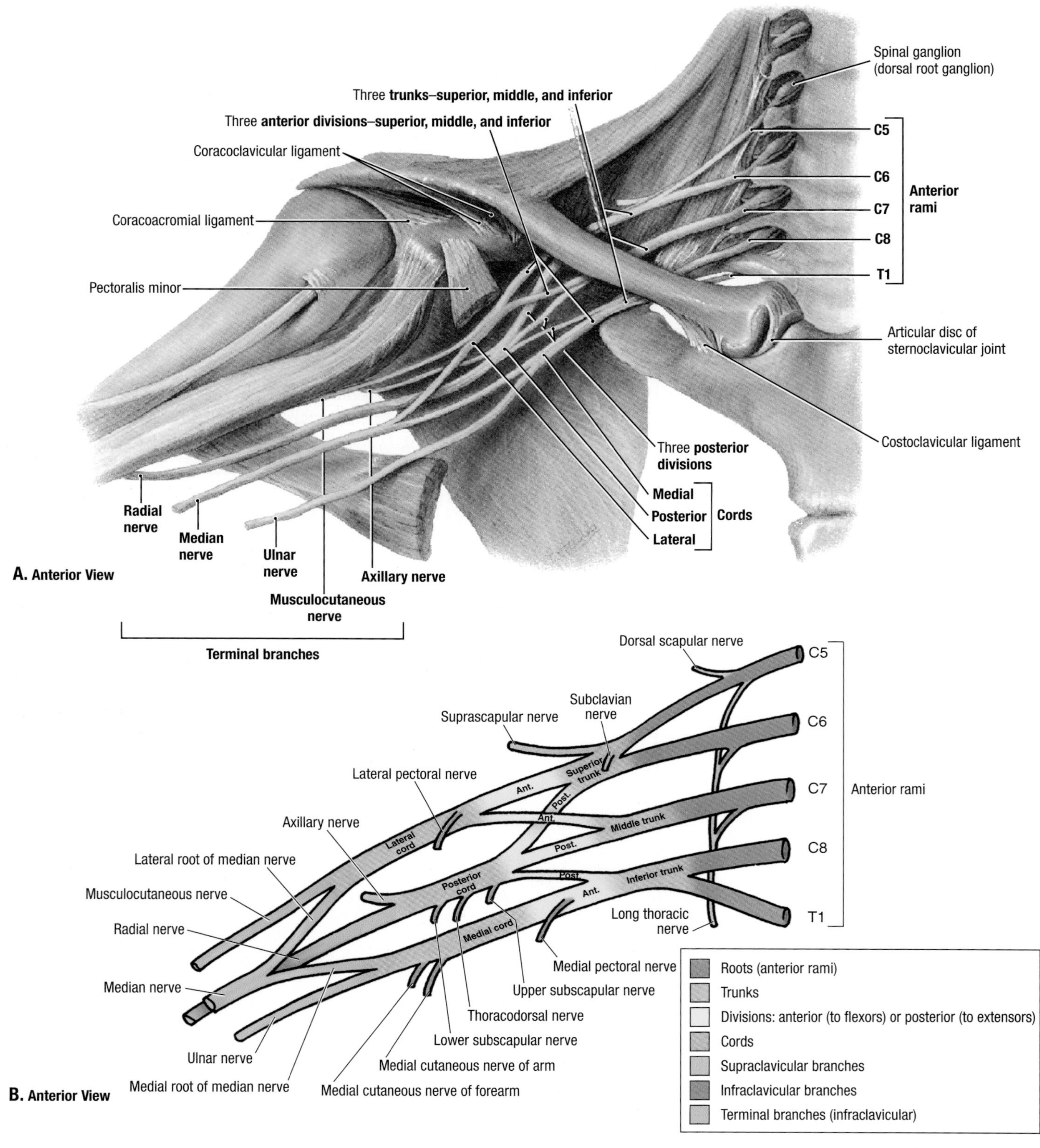

Spinal ganglion (dorsal root ganglion)
Three trunks–superior, middle, and inferior
Three anterior divisions–superior, middle, and inferior
Coracoclavicular ligament
Coracoacromial ligament
Pectoralis minor
C5
C6
C7
C8
T1
Anterior rami
Articular disc of sternoclavicular joint
Costoclavicular ligament
Three posterior divisions
Medial
Posterior
Lateral
Cords
Radial nerve
Median nerve
Ulnar nerve
Axillary nerve
Musculocutaneous nerve
Terminal branches
A. Anterior View
Dorsal scapular nerve
Subclavian nerve
Suprascapular nerve
Lateral pectoral nerve
Superior trunk
Ant.
Post.
Middle trunk
Inferior trunk
Axillary nerve
Lateral cord
Posterior cord
Medial cord
Lateral root of median nerve
Musculocutaneous nerve
Radial nerve
Median nerve
Ulnar nerve
Medial root of median nerve
Medial cutaneous nerve of forearm
Medial cutaneous nerve of arm
Lower subscapular nerve
Thoracodorsal nerve
Upper subscapular nerve
Medial pectoral nerve
Long thoracic nerve
Anterior rami
B. Anterior View
Roots (anterior rami)
Trunks
Divisions: anterior (to flexors) or posterior (to extensors)
Cords
Supraclavicular branches
Infraclavicular branches
Terminal branches (infraclavicular)


**6.23 Brachial plexus**

**A.** Dissection. **B.** Schematic illustration.

**TABLE 6.4 AXILLA, AXILLARY VESSELS, AND BRACHIAL PLEXUS**

| Nerve | Origin | Course | Distribution/Structure(s) Supplied |
|---|---|---|---|
| **Supraclavicular branches** | | | |
| Dorsal scapular | Anterior ramus of C5 with a frequent contribution from C4 | Pierces scalenus medius, descends deep to levator scapulae, and enters deep surface of rhomboids | Rhomboids and occasionally supplies levator scapulae |
| Long thoracic | Anterior rami of C5–C7 | Descends posterior to C8 and T1 rami and passes distally on external surface of serratus anterior | Serratus anterior |
| Subclavian | Superior trunk receiving fibers from C5 and C6 and often C4 | Descends posterior to clavicle and anterior to brachial plexus and subclavian artery | Subclavius and sternoclavicular joint |
| Suprascapular | Superior trunk receiving fibers from C5 and C6 and often C4 | Passes laterally across posterior triangle of neck, through suprascapular notch deep to superior transverse scapular ligament | Supraspinatus, infraspinatus, and glenohumeral (shoulder) joint |
| **Infraclavicular branches** | | | |
| Lateral pectoral | Lateral cord receiving fibers from C5–C7 | Pierces clavipectoral fascia to reach deep surface of pectoral muscles | Primarily pectoralis major but sends a loop to medial pectoral nerve that innervates pectoralis minor |
| Musculocutaneous | Lateral cord receiving fibers from C5–C7 | Enters deep surface of coracobrachialis and descends between biceps brachii and brachialis | Coracobrachialis, biceps brachii, and brachialis; continues as lateral cutaneous nerve of forearm |
| Median | Lateral root of median nerve is a terminal branch of lateral cord (C6, C7); medial root of median nerve is a terminal branch of medial cord (C8, T1) | Lateral and medial roots merge to form median nerve lateral to axillary artery; crosses anterior to brachial artery to lie medial to artery in cubital fossa | Flexor muscles in forearm (except flexor carpi ulnaris, ulnar half of flexor digitorum profundus, and five hand muscles) and skin of palm and 3½ digits lateral to a line bisecting 4th digit and the dorsum of the distal halves of these digits |
| Medial pectoral | Medial cord receiving fibers from C8, T1 | Passes between axillary artery and vein and enters deep surface of pectoralis minor | Pectoralis minor and part of pectoralis major |
| Medial cutaneous nerve of arm | Medial cord receiving fibers from C8, T1 | Runs along the medial side of axillary vein and communicates with intercosto-brachial nerve | Skin on medial side of arm |
| Medial cutaneous nerve of forearm | Medial cord receiving fibers from C8, T1 | Runs between axillary artery and vein | Skin over medial side of forearm |
| Ulnar | A terminal branch of medial cord receiving fibers from C8, T1 and often C7 | Passes down medial aspect of arm and runs posterior to medial epicondyle to enter forearm | Innervates 1½ flexor muscles in forearm, most small muscles in hand, and skin of hand medial to a line bisecting 4th digit (ring finger) anteriorly and posteriorly |
| Upper subscapular | Branch of posterior cord receiving fibers from C5 | Passes posteriorly and enters subscapularis | Superior portion of subscapularis |
| Thoracodorsal | Branch of posterior cord receiving fibers from C6–C8 | Arises between upper and lower subscapular nerves and runs inferolaterally to latissimus dorsi | Latissimus dorsi |
| Lower subscapular | Branch of posterior cord receiving fibers from C6 | Passes inferolaterally, deep to subscapular artery and vein, to subscapularis and teres major | Inferior portion of subscapularis and teres major |
| Axillary | Terminal branch of posterior cord receiving fibers from C5 and C6 | Passes to posterior aspect of arm through quadrangular space in company with posterior circumflex humeral artery and then winds around surgical neck of humerus; gives rise to lateral cutaneous nerve of arm | Teres minor and deltoid, glenohumeral (shoulder) joint, and skin of superolateral part of arm |
| Radial | Terminal branch of posterior cord receiving fibers from C5–T1 | Descends posterior to axillary artery; enters radial groove to pass between long and medial heads of triceps | Triceps brachii, anconeus, brachioradialis, and extensor muscles of forearm; supplies skin on posterior aspect of arm and forearm and dorsum of hand lateral to axial line of digit 4 |

[a] Quadrangular space is bounded superiorly by subscapularis and teres minor, inferiorly by teres major, medially by long head of triceps, and laterally by humerus.

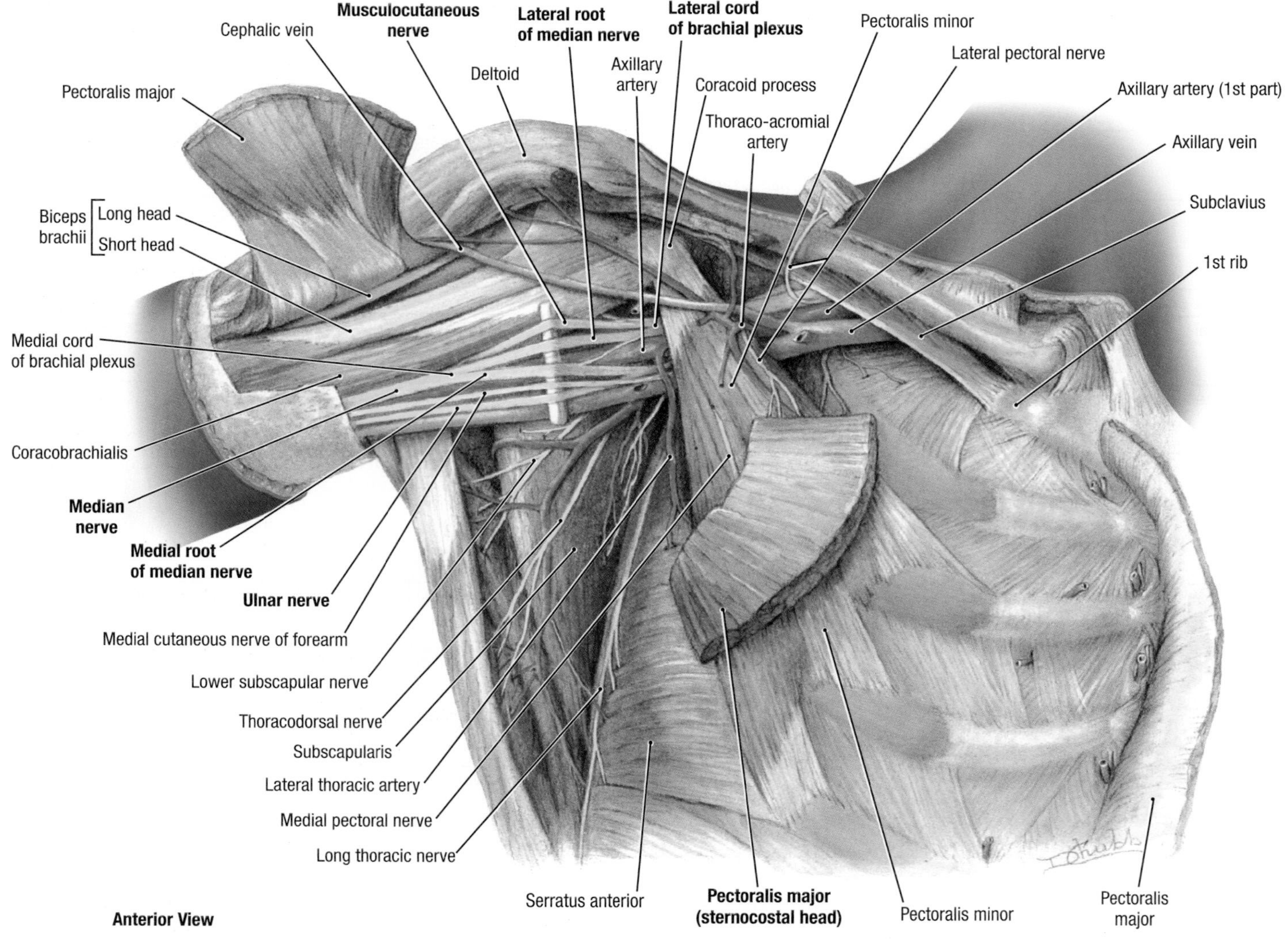
Cephalic vein
Musculocutaneous nerve
Lateral root of median nerve
Lateral cord of brachial plexus
Pectoralis minor
Lateral pectoral nerve
Deltoid
Axillary artery
Coracoid process
Thoraco-acromial artery
Axillary artery (1st part)
Axillary vein
Pectoralis major
Biceps brachii
Long head
Short head
Subclavius
1st rib
Medial cord of brachial plexus
Coracobrachialis
Median nerve
Medial root of median nerve
Ulnar nerve
Medial cutaneous nerve of forearm
Lower subscapular nerve
Thoracodorsal nerve
Subscapularis
Lateral thoracic artery
Medial pectoral nerve
Long thoracic nerve
Serratus anterior
Pectoralis major (sternocostal head)
Pectoralis minor
Pectoralis major
Anterior View

## 6.24 Structures of axilla: Deep dissection I

- The pectoralis major muscle is reflected, and the clavipectoral fascia is removed; the cube of muscle superior to the clavicle is cut from the clavicular head of the pectoralis major muscle.
- The subclavius and pectoralis minor are the two deep muscles of the anterior wall.
- The 2nd part axillary artery passes posterior to the pectoralis minor muscle, a fingerbreadth from the tip of the coracoid process; the axillary vein lies anterior and then medial to the axillary artery.
- The median nerve, followed proximally, leads by its lateral root to the lateral cord and musculocutaneous nerve and by its medial root to the medial cord and ulnar nerve. These four nerves and the medial cutaneous nerve of the forearm are derived from the anterior division of the brachial plexus and are raised on a stick. The lateral root of the median nerve may occur as several strands.
- The musculocutaneous nerve enters the flexor compartment of the arm by piercing the coracobrachialis muscle.

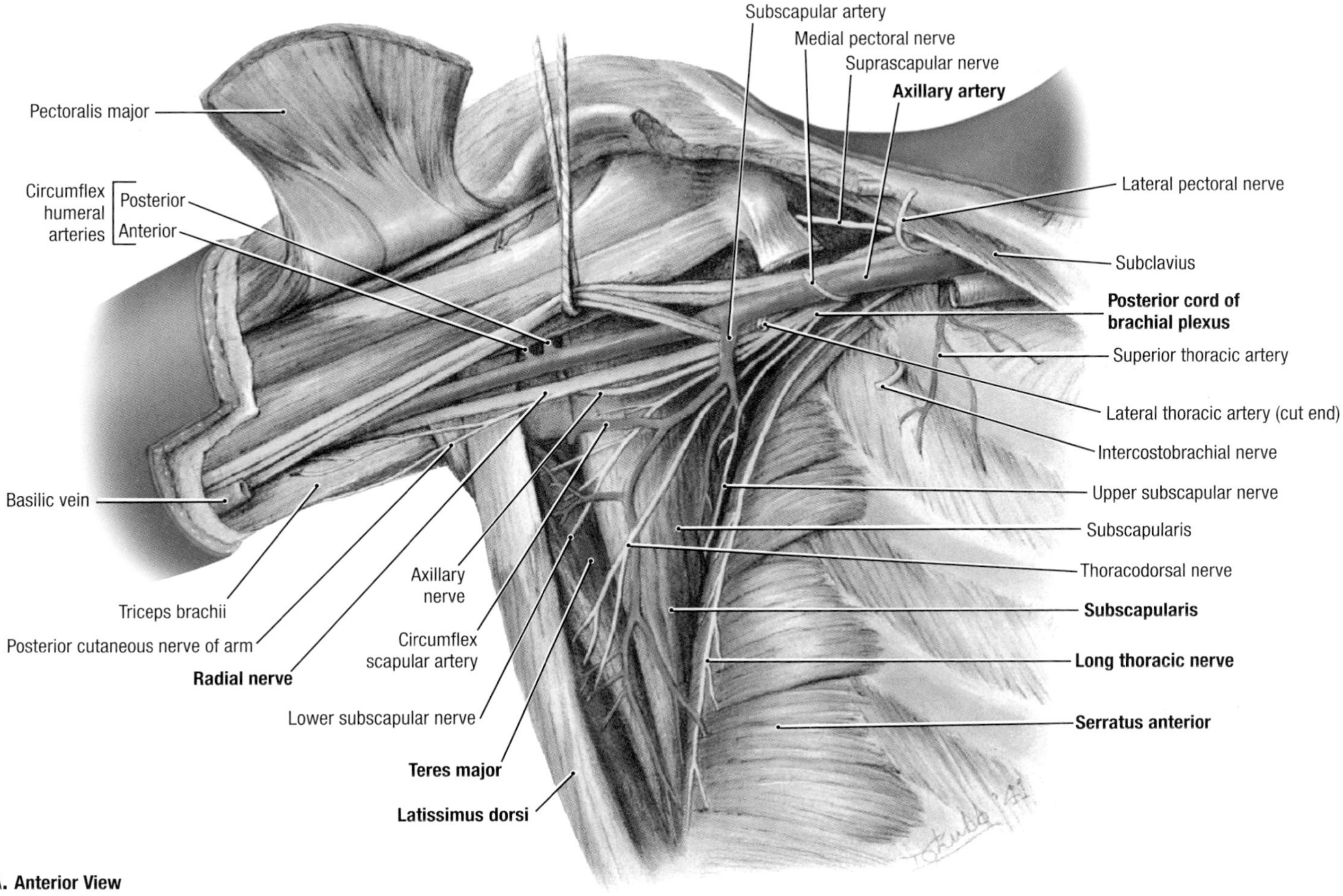

Subscapular artery
Medial pectoral nerve
Suprascapular nerve
**Axillary artery**
Pectoralis major
Circumflex humeral arteries: Posterior, Anterior
Lateral pectoral nerve
Subclavius
**Posterior cord of brachial plexus**
Superior thoracic artery
Lateral thoracic artery (cut end)
Intercostobrachial nerve
Basilic vein
Upper subscapular nerve
Subscapularis
Thoracodorsal nerve
Axillary nerve
**Subscapularis**
Triceps brachii
Posterior cutaneous nerve of arm
Circumflex scapular artery
**Long thoracic nerve**
**Radial nerve**
Lower subscapular nerve
**Serratus anterior**
**Teres major**
**Latissimus dorsi**

**A.** **Anterior View**

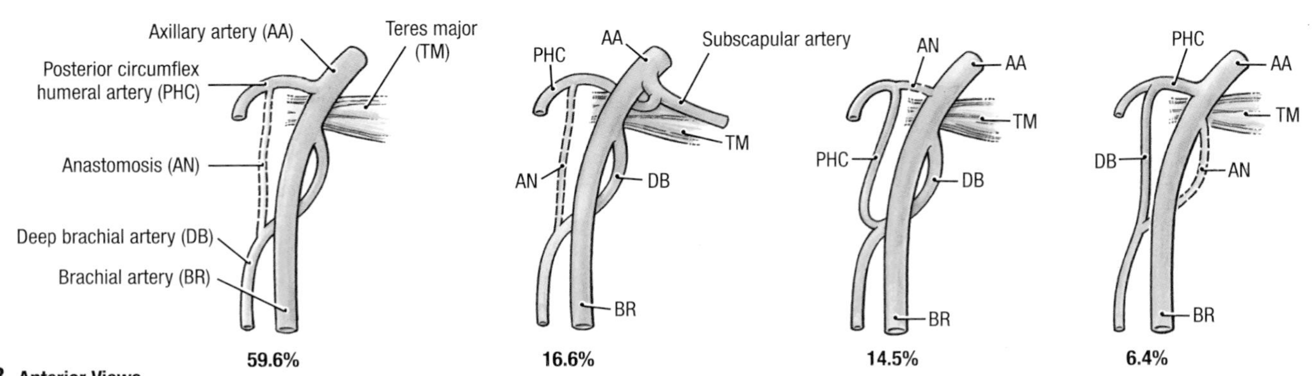
Axillary artery (AA)
Teres major (TM)
Posterior circumflex humeral artery (PHC)
Anastomosis (AN)
Deep brachial artery (DB)
Brachial artery (BR)
59.6%
PHC
AA
Subscapular artery
TM
AN
DB
BR
16.6%
AN
AA
TM
PHC
DB
BR
14.5%
PHC
AA
TM
DB
AN
BR
6.4%

**B.** **Anterior Views**

## 6.25 Posterior and medial walls of axilla: Deep dissection II

**A.** Dissection. The pectoralis minor muscle is excised, the lateral and medial cords of the brachial plexus are retracted, and the axillary vein is removed. **B.** Variations of the posterior circumflex humeral artery and deep artery of arm. Percentages are based on 235 specimens.

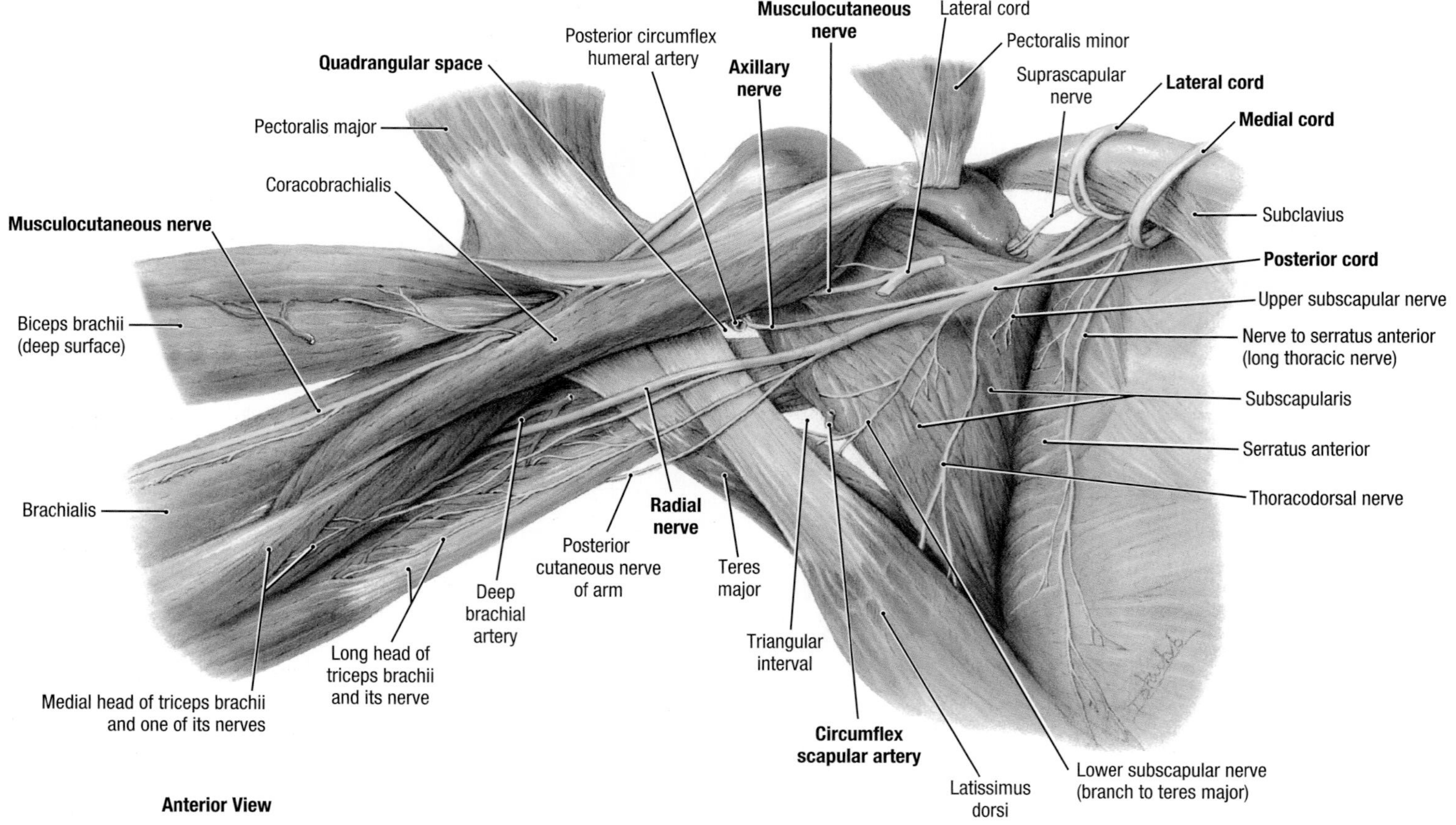
Musculocutaneous nerve
Lateral cord
Posterior circumflex humeral artery
Pectoralis minor
Quadrangular space
Axillary nerve
Suprascapular nerve
Lateral cord
Medial cord
Pectoralis major
Coracobrachialis
Subclavius
Musculocutaneous nerve
Posterior cord
Upper subscapular nerve
Biceps brachii (deep surface)
Nerve to serratus anterior (long thoracic nerve)
Subscapularis
Serratus anterior
Thoracodorsal nerve
Brachialis
Radial nerve
Posterior cutaneous nerve of arm
Teres major
Deep brachial artery
Long head of triceps brachii and its nerve
Triangular interval
Medial head of triceps brachii and one of its nerves
Circumflex scapular artery
Latissimus dorsi
Lower subscapular nerve (branch to teres major)
Anterior View

## 6.26 Posterior wall of axilla, musculocutaneous nerve, and posterior cord: Deep dissection III

- The pectoralis major and minor muscles are reflected laterally, the lateral and medial cords of the brachial plexus are reflected superiorly, and the arteries, veins, and median and ulnar nerves are removed.
- Coracobrachialis arises with the short head of the biceps brachii muscle from the tip of the coracoid process and attaches halfway down the medial aspect of the humerus.
- The musculocutaneous nerve pierces the coracobrachialis muscle and supplies it, the biceps, and the brachialis before becoming the lateral cutaneous nerve of the forearm.
- The posterior cord of the plexus is formed by the union of the three posterior divisions; it supplies the three muscles of the posterior wall of the axilla and then bifurcates into the radial and axillary nerves.
- In the axilla, the radial nerve gives off the nerve to the long head of the triceps brachii muscle and a cutaneous branch; in this specimen, it also gives off a branch to the medial head of the triceps. It then enters the radial groove of the humerus with the deep brachial (profunda brachii) artery.
- The axillary nerve passes through the quadrangular space along with the posterior circumflex humeral artery. The borders of the quadrangular space are superiorly, the lateral border of the scapula; inferiorly, the teres major; laterally, the humerus (surgical neck); and medially, the long head of triceps brachii. The circumflex scapular artery traverses the triangular interval.

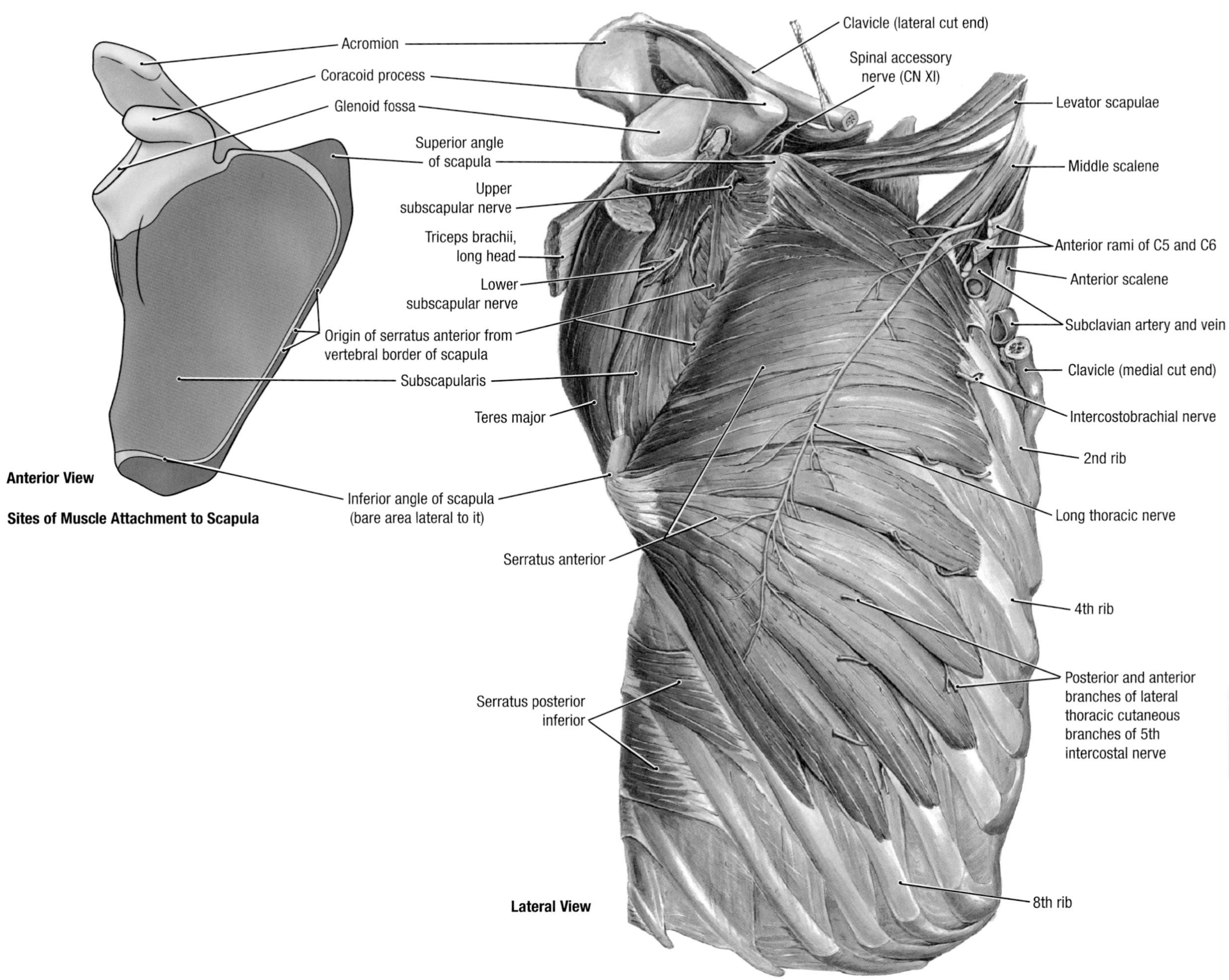
Acromion
Coracoid process
Glenoid fossa
Superior angle of scapula
Upper subscapular nerve
Triceps brachii, long head
Lower subscapular nerve
Origin of serratus anterior from vertebral border of scapula
Subscapularis
Teres major
Anterior View
Sites of Muscle Attachment to Scapula
Inferior angle of scapula (bare area lateral to it)
Serratus anterior
Serratus posterior inferior
Lateral View
Clavicle (lateral cut end)
Spinal accessory nerve (CN XI)
Levator scapulae
Middle scalene
Anterior rami of C5 and C6
Anterior scalene
Subclavian artery and vein
Clavicle (medial cut end)
Intercostobrachial nerve
2nd rib
Long thoracic nerve
4th rib
Posterior and anterior branches of lateral thoracic cutaneous branches of 5th intercostal nerve
8th rib

## 6.27 Serratus anterior and subscapularis

The serratus anterior muscle, which forms the medial wall of the axilla, has a fleshy belly extending from the superior 8 or 9 ribs in the midclavicular line *(right)* to the medial border of the scapula *(left)*.

- The fibers of the serratus anterior muscle from the 1st rib and the tendinous arch between the 1st and 2nd ribs (see Table 6.2) converge on the superior angle of the scapula; those from the 2nd and 3rd ribs diverge to spread thinly along the medial border; and the remainder (from the 4th to 9th ribs), which form the bulk of the muscle, converge on the inferior angle via a tendinous insertion.
- The long thoracic nerve to serratus anterior arises from spinal nerves C5, C6, and C7 and courses externally along most of the muscle's length.
- When the serratus anterior is paralyzed because of injury to the long thoracic nerve, the medial border of the scapula moves laterally and posteriorly, away from the thoracic wall. When the arm is abducted, the medial border and the inferior angle of the scapula pull away from the posterior thoracic wall, a deformation known as a winged scapula. In addition, the arm cannot be abducted above the horizontal position because the serratus anterior is unable to rotate the glenoid cavity superiorly.
- The trunks of the brachial plexus and the subclavian artery emerge between the anterior and middle scalene muscles (scalene triangle); the subclavian vein is separated from the artery by the anterior scalene muscle.

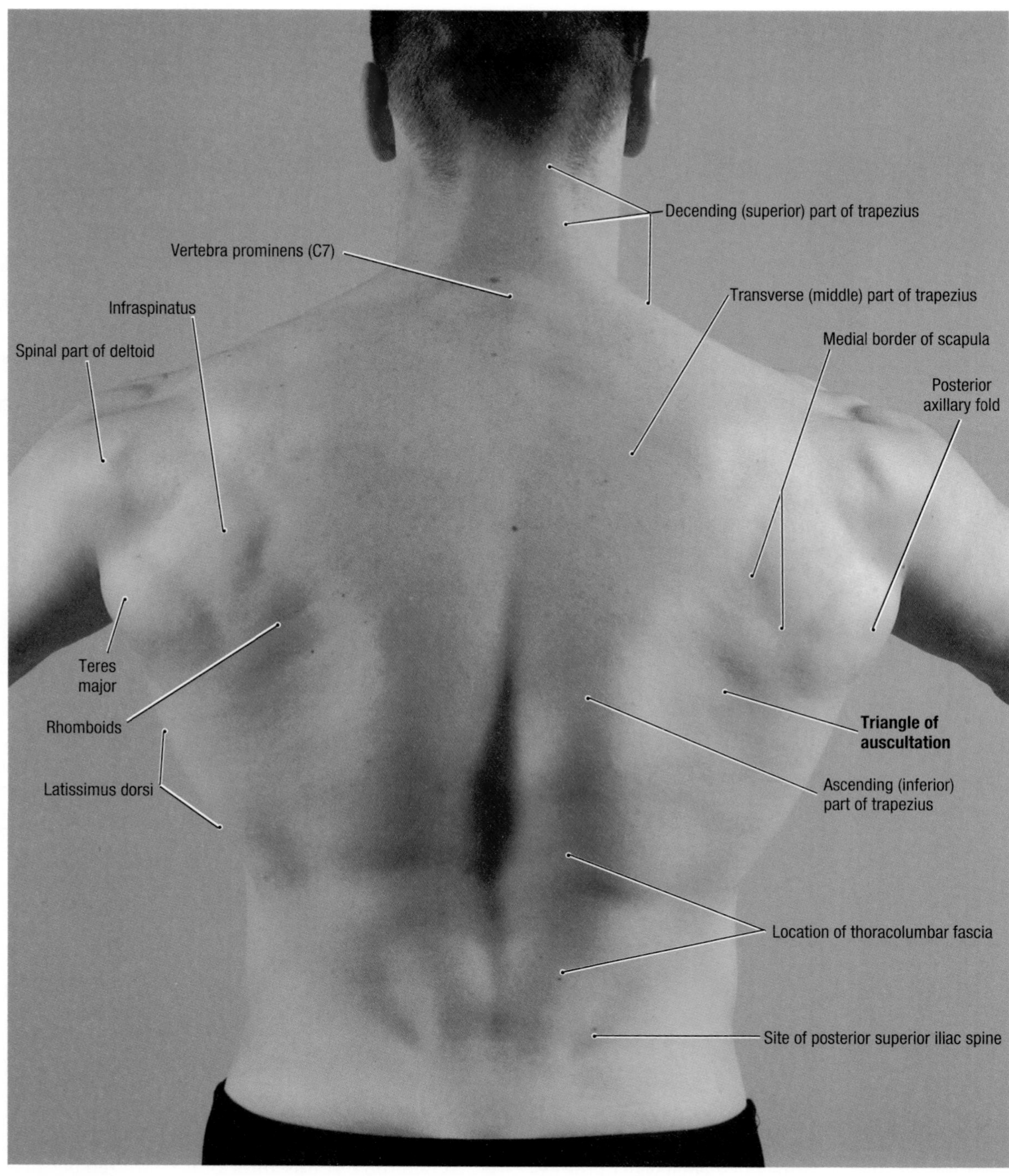
Decending (superior) part of trapezius
Vertebra prominens (C7)
Infraspinatus
Transverse (middle) part of trapezius
Spinal part of deltoid
Medial border of scapula
Posterior axillary fold
Teres major
Rhomboids
Triangle of auscultation
Latissimus dorsi
Ascending (inferior) part of trapezius
Location of thoracolumbar fascia
Site of posterior superior iliac spine

**Posterior View**

## 6.28 Surface anatomy of superficial back

The superior border of the latissimus dorsi and a part of the rhomboid major are overlapped by the trapezius. The area formed by the superior border of latissimus dorsi, the medial border of the scapula, and the inferolateral border of the trapezius is called the triangle of auscultation. This gap in the thick back musculature is a good place to examine posterior segments of the lungs with a stethoscope. When the scapulae are drawn anteriorly by folding the arms across the thorax and the trunk is flexed, the auscultatory triangle enlarges. The teres major forms a raised oval area on the inferolateral third of the posterior aspect of the scapula when the arm is adducted against resistance. The posterior axillary fold is formed by the teres major and the tendon of the latissimus dorsi.

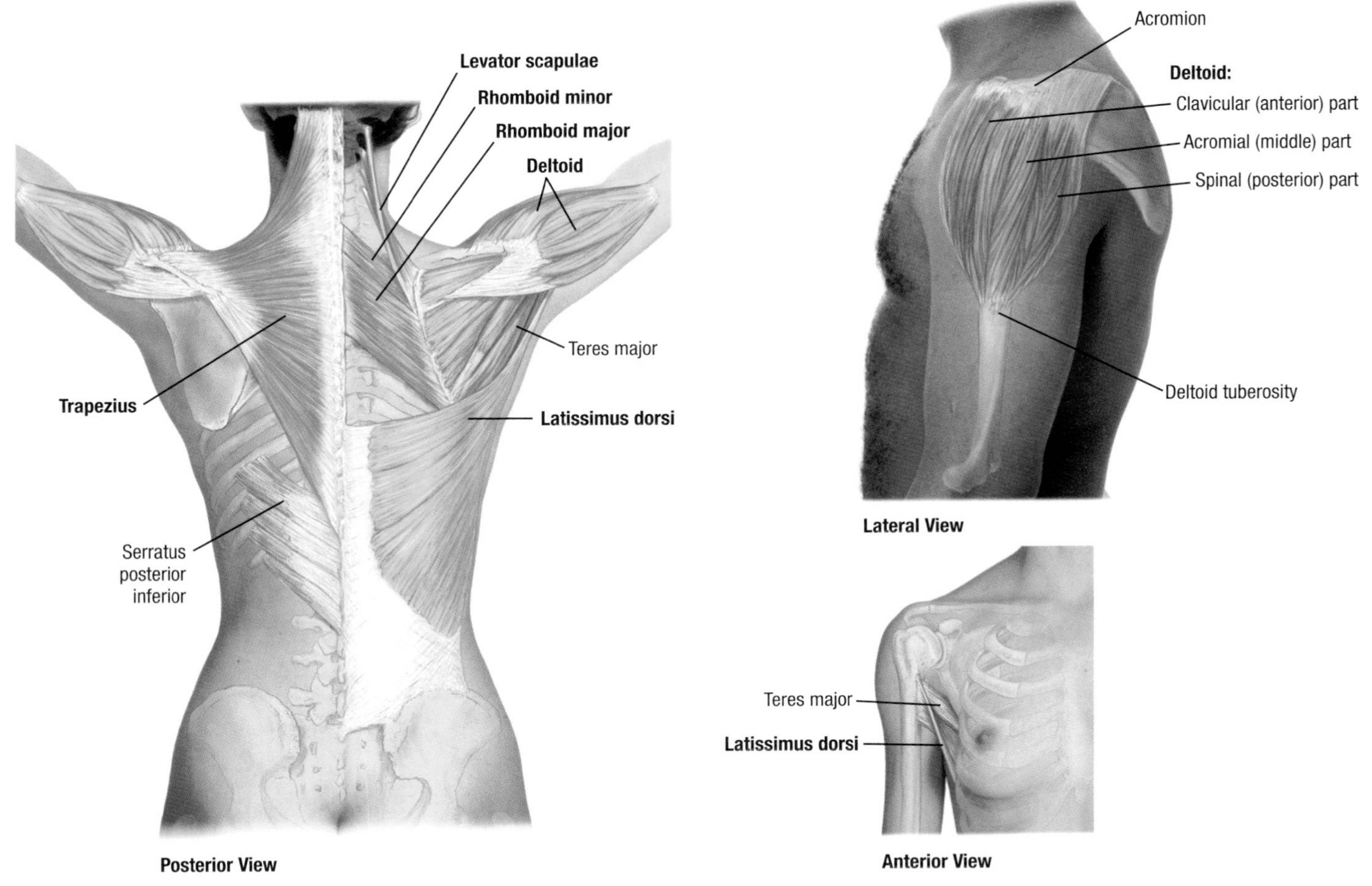
Levator scapulae
Rhomboid minor
Rhomboid major
Deltoid
Teres major
Trapezius
Latissimus dorsi
Serratus posterior inferior
Posterior View
Acromion
Deltoid:
Clavicular (anterior) part
Acromial (middle) part
Spinal (posterior) part
Deltoid tuberosity
Lateral View
Teres major
Latissimus dorsi
Anterior View

## TABLE 6.5 SUPERFICIAL BACK (POSTERIOR AXIOAPPENDICULAR) AND DELTOID MUSCLES

| Muscle | Proximal Attachment | Distal Attachment | Innervation | Main Actions |
|---|---|---|---|---|
| **Trapezius** | Medial third of superior nuchal line; external occipital protuberance, nuchal ligament, and spinous processes of T7–T12 | Lateral third of clavicle, acromion, and spine of scapula | Spinal accessory nerve (CN XI) and cervical nerves (C3–C4) | Elevates, retracts, and rotates scapula; *descending part* elevates, *transverse part* retracts, and *ascending part* depresses scapula; descending and ascending part act together in superior rotation of scapula |
| **Latissimus dorsi** | Spinous processes of inferior six thoracic vertebrae, thoracolumbar fascia, iliac crest, and inferior three or four ribs | Intertubercular sulcus (bicipital groove) of humerus | Thoracodorsal nerve (C6–C8) | Extends, adducts, and medially rotates humerus; raises body toward arms during climbing |
| **Levator scapulae** | Posterior tubercles of transverse processes of C1–C4 vertebrae | Superior part of medial border of scapula | Dorsal scapular (C5) and cervical (C3–C4) nerves | Elevates scapula and tilts its glenoid cavity inferiorly by rotating scapula |
| **Rhomboid minor and major** | *Minor:* nuchal ligament and spinous processes of C7 and T1 vertebrae<br>*Major:* spinous processes of T2–T5 vertebrae | Medial border of scapula from level of spine to inferior angle | Dorsal scapular nerve (C4–C5) | Retracts scapula and rotates it to depress glenoid cavity; fixes scapula to thoracic wall |
| **Deltoid** | Lateral third of clavicle *(clavicular part)*, acromion *(acromial part)*, and spine *(spinal part)* of scapula | Deltoid tuberosity of humerus | Axillary nerve (C5–C6) | *Clavicular (anterior) part:* flexes and medially rotates arm; *acromial (middle) part:* abducts arm; *spinal (posterior) part:* extends and laterally rotates arm |

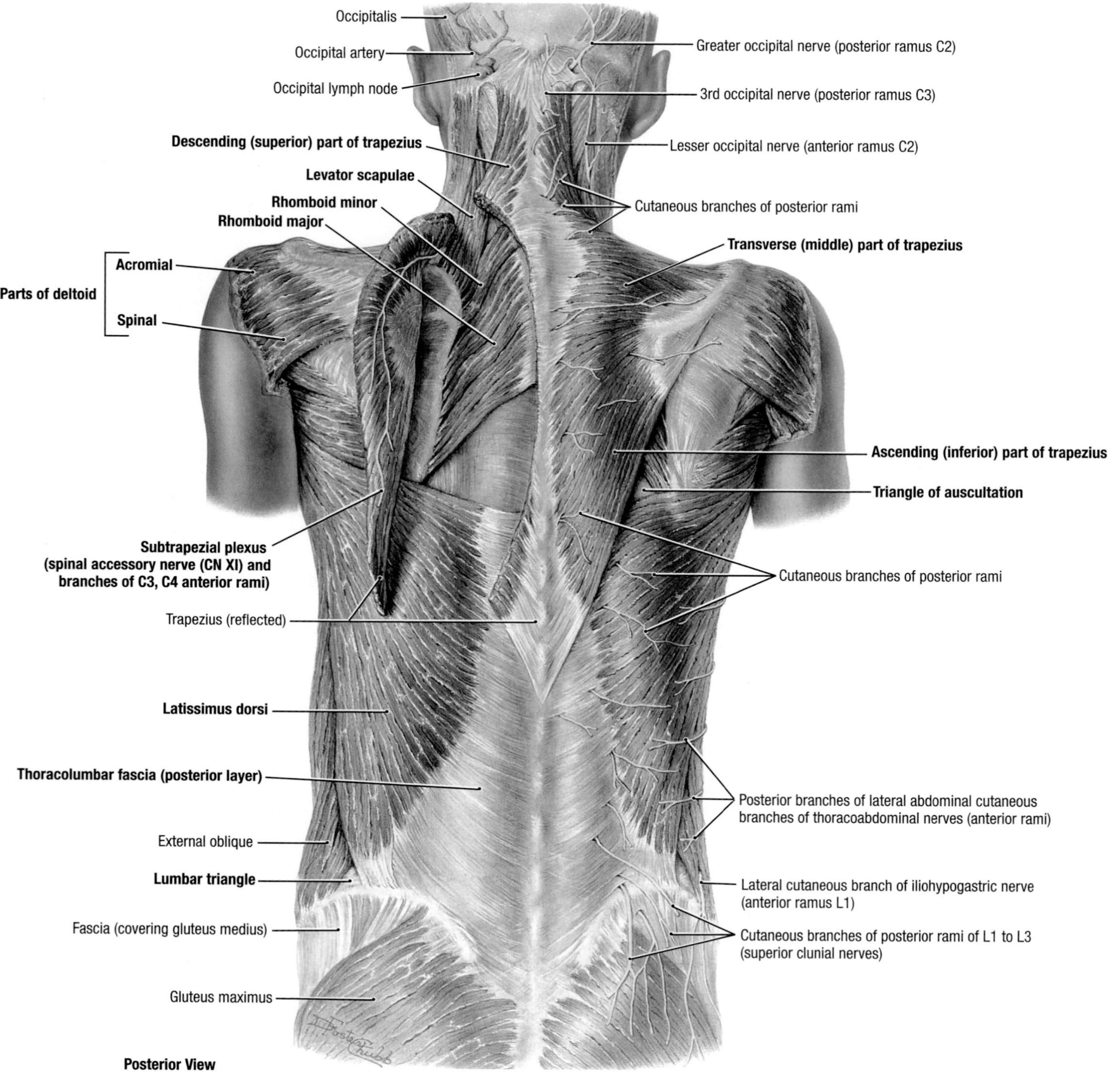
Occipitalis
Occipital artery
Occipital lymph node
Descending (superior) part of trapezius
Levator scapulae
Rhomboid minor
Rhomboid major
Parts of deltoid
Acromial
Spinal
Subtrapezial plexus (spinal accessory nerve (CN XI) and branches of C3, C4 anterior rami)
Trapezius (reflected)
Latissimus dorsi
Thoracolumbar fascia (posterior layer)
External oblique
Lumbar triangle
Fascia (covering gluteus medius)
Gluteus maximus
Posterior View
Greater occipital nerve (posterior ramus C2)
3rd occipital nerve (posterior ramus C3)
Lesser occipital nerve (anterior ramus C2)
Cutaneous branches of posterior rami
Transverse (middle) part of trapezius
Ascending (inferior) part of trapezius
Triangle of auscultation
Cutaneous branches of posterior rami
Posterior branches of lateral abdominal cutaneous branches of thoracoabdominal nerves (anterior rami)
Lateral cutaneous branch of iliohypogastric nerve (anterior ramus L1)
Cutaneous branches of posterior rami of L1 to L3 (superior clunial nerves)

## 6.29 Cutaneous nerves of superficial back and posterior axioapendicular muscles

The trapezius muscle is cut and reflected on the left side. A superficial or first muscle layer consists of the trapezius and latissimus dorsi muscles, and a second layer of the levator scapulae and rhomboids. Cutaneous branches of posterior rami penetrate but do not supply the superficial muscles.

## TABLE 6.6 MOVEMENTS OF SCAPULA

Boldface indicates prime movers. In the *middle* and *right columns* the *dotted outlines* represent the starting position for each movement.

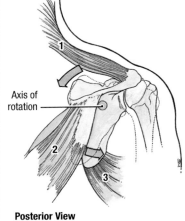

| | | |
|---|---|---|
| 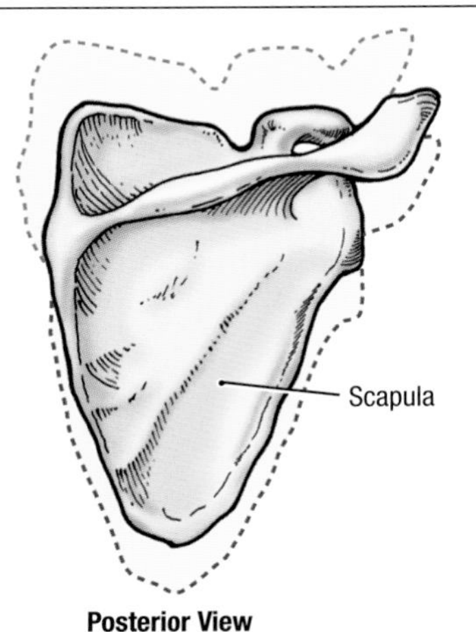 Scapula<br>**Posterior View**<br>Elevation (red)<br>Depression (green) | 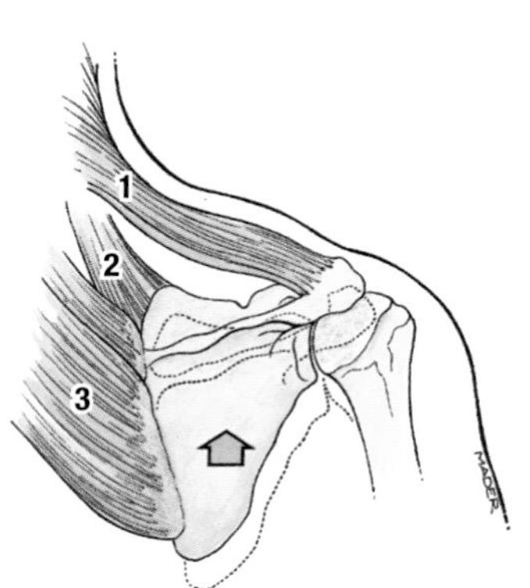<br>**Posterior View**<br>Elevation:<br>**Trapezius, superior part** (1)<br>Levator scapulae (2)<br>Rhomboids (3) | 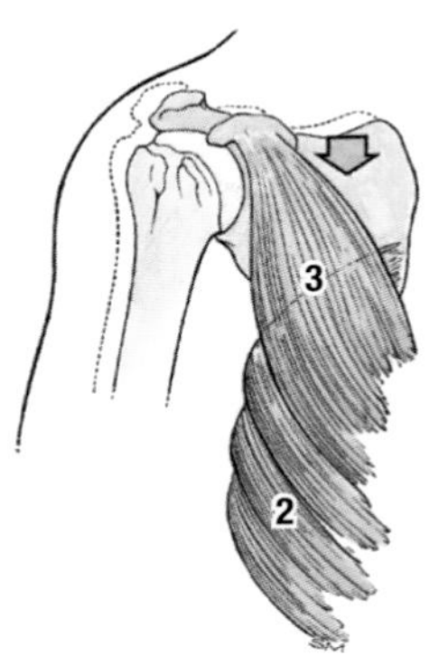<br>**Anterior View**<br>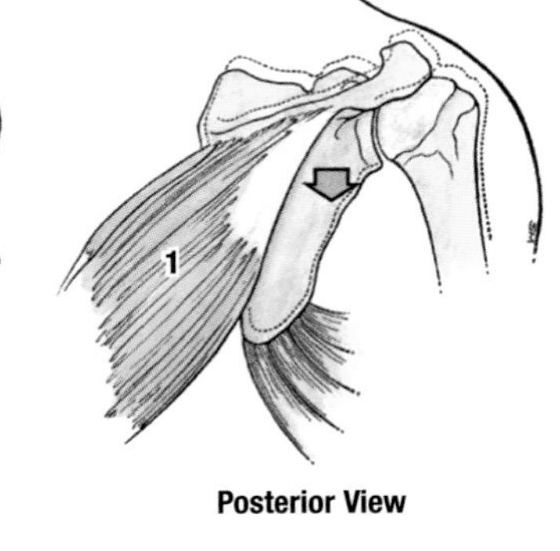<br>**Posterior View**<br>Depression:<br>Trapezius, inferior part (1)<br>Serratus anterior, inferior part<br>Pectoralis minor<br>Also: Gravity, Latissimus dorsi, Inferior sternocostal head of pectoralis major |
| 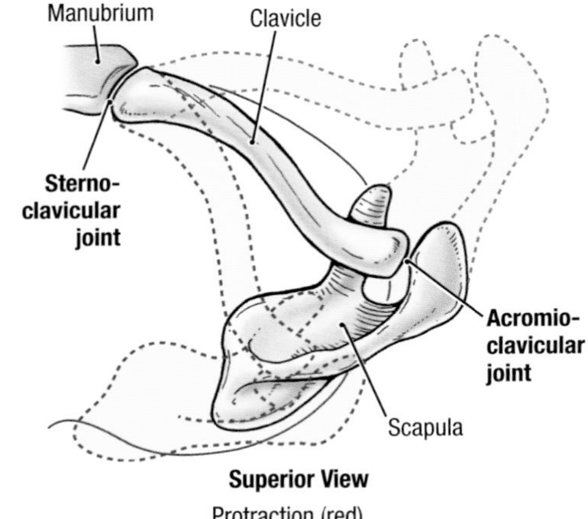 Manubrium<br>Clavicle<br>Sterno-clavicular joint<br>Acromio-clavicular joint<br>Scapula<br>**Superior View**<br>Protraction (red)<br>Retraction (green) | 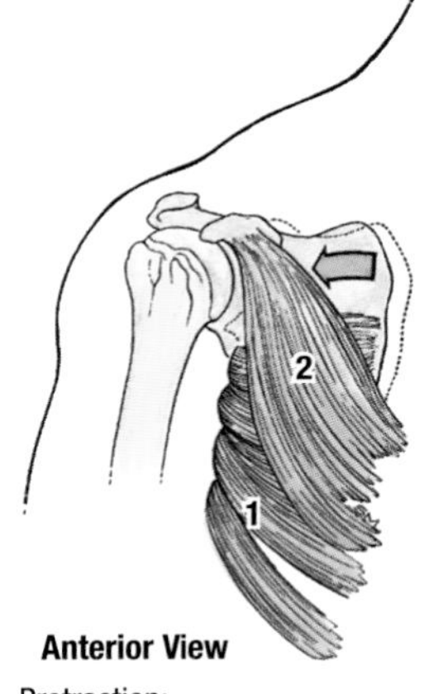<br>**Anterior View**<br>Protraction:<br>**Serratus anterior** (1)<br>Pectoralis minor (2)<br>Also: Pectoralis major | 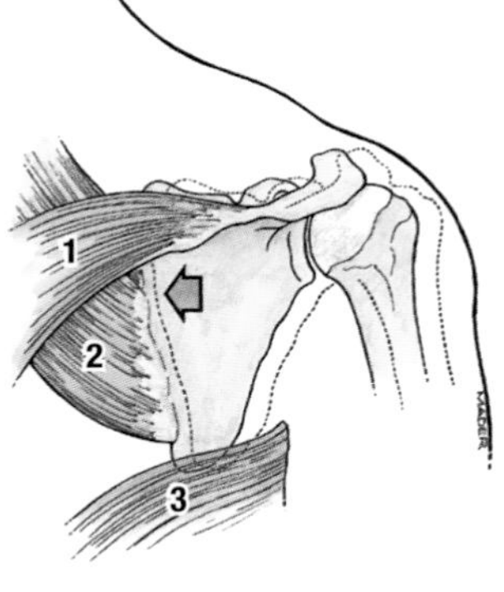<br>**Posterior View**<br>Retraction:<br>**Trapezius, middle part** (1)<br>Rhomboids(2)<br>Latissimus dorsi (3) |
| 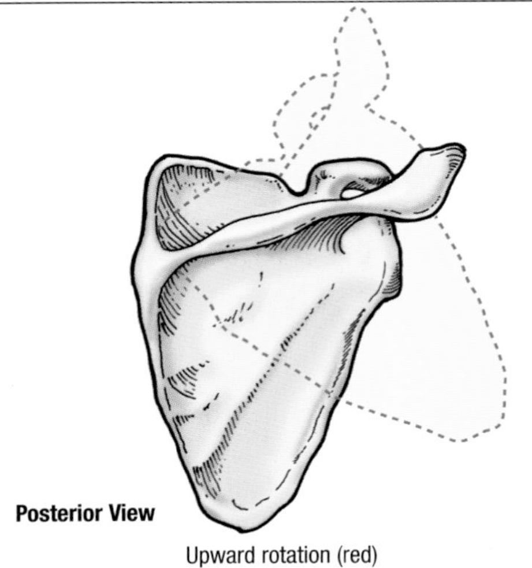<br>**Posterior View**<br>Upward rotation (red) | Axis of rotation<br>**Posterior View**<br>Upward rotation<br>**Trapezius, superior part** (1)<br>Trapezius, inferior part (2)<br>**Serratus anterior, inferior part(3)** | 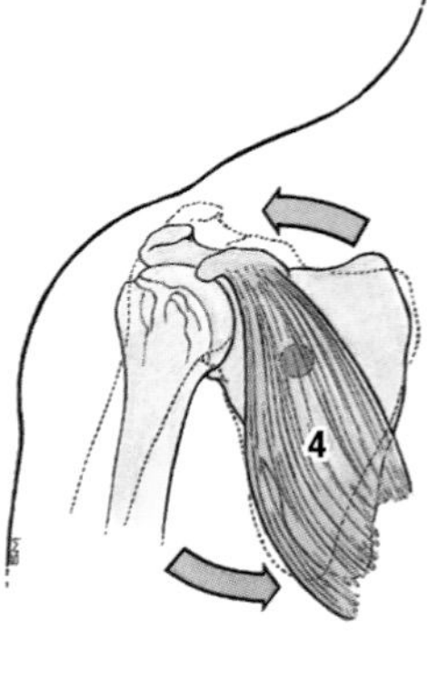<br>**Anterior View**<br>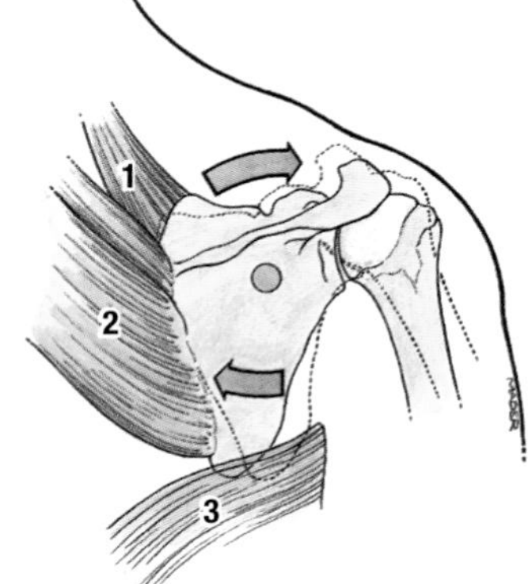<br>**Posterior View**<br>Downward rotation<br>Levator scapulae (1)<br>Rhomboids (2)<br>**Latissimus dorsi (3)**<br>Pectoralis minor (4)<br>Also: Gravity, Inferior sternocostal head of pectoralis major |

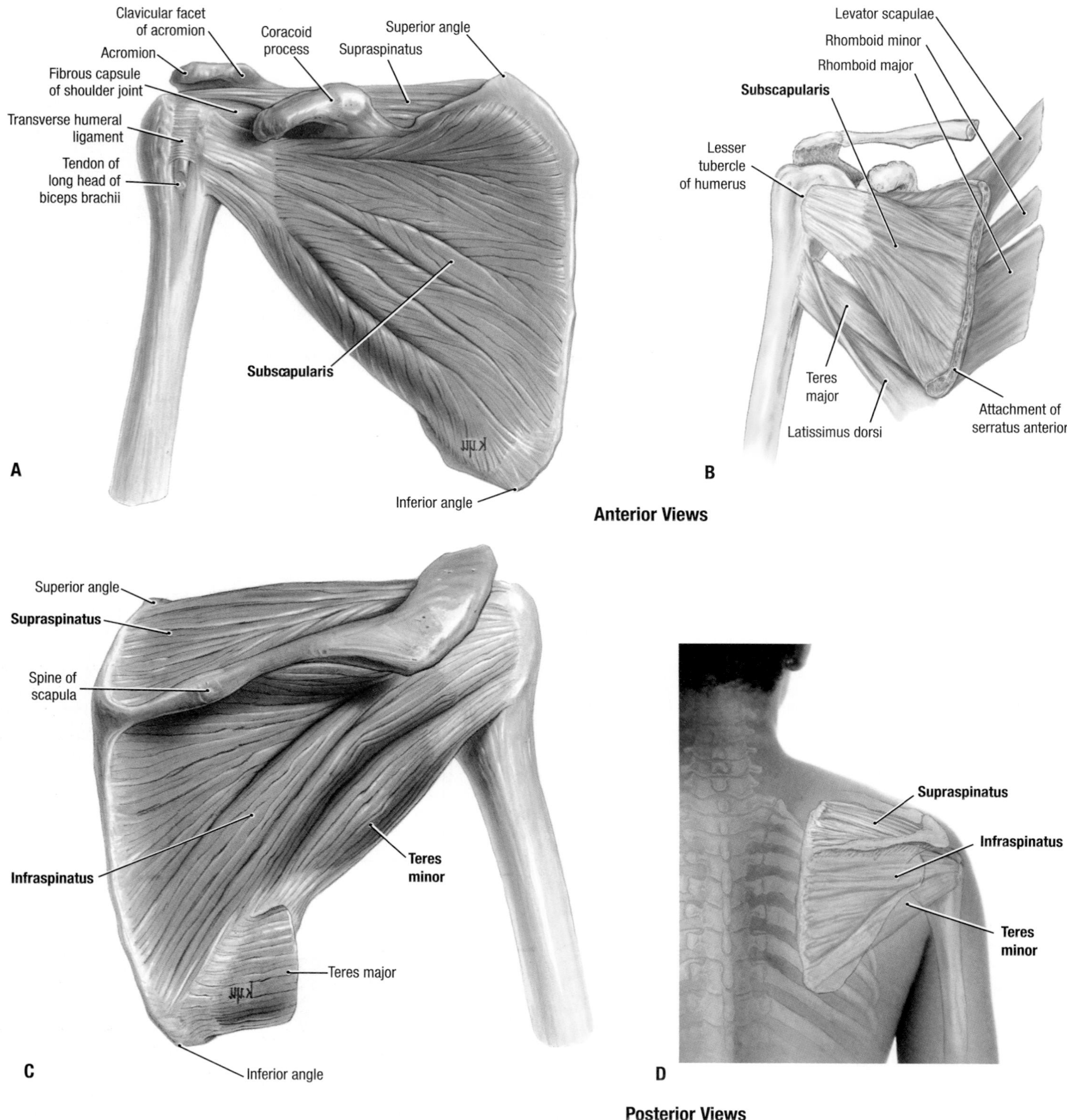
Clavicular facet of acromion
Acromion
Fibrous capsule of shoulder joint
Transverse humeral ligament
Tendon of long head of biceps brachii
Coracoid process
Supraspinatus
Superior angle
Subscapularis
Inferior angle
A
Levator scapulae
Rhomboid minor
Rhomboid major
Subscapularis
Lesser tubercle of humerus
Teres major
Latissimus dorsi
Attachment of serratus anterior
B
Anterior Views
Superior angle
Supraspinatus
Spine of scapula
Infraspinatus
Teres minor
Teres major
Inferior angle
C
Supraspinatus
Infraspinatus
Teres minor
D
Posterior Views

## 6.30 Rotator cuff

**A** and **B.** Subscapularis. **C** and **D.** Supraspinatus, infraspinatus, and teres minor.

Four of the scapulohumeral muscles—supraspinatus, infraspinatus, teres minor, and subscapularis—are called rotator cuff muscles because they form a musculotendinous rotator cuff around the glenohumeral joint. All except the supraspinatus are rotators of the humerus.

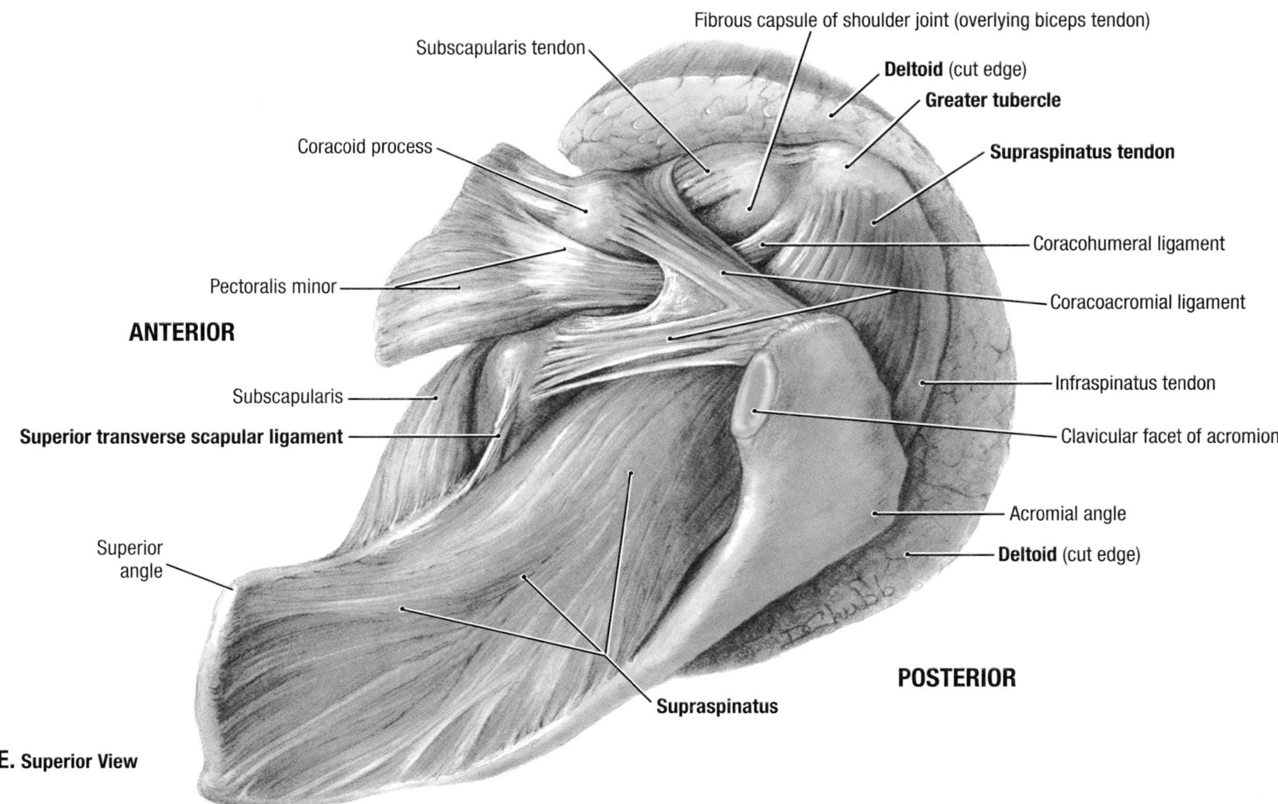
Fibrous capsule of shoulder joint (overlying biceps tendon)
Subscapularis tendon
Deltoid (cut edge)
Greater tubercle
Coracoid process
Supraspinatus tendon
Coracohumeral ligament
Pectoralis minor
Coracoacromial ligament
ANTERIOR
Infraspinatus tendon
Subscapularis
Superior transverse scapular ligament
Clavicular facet of acromion
Acromial angle
Superior angle
Deltoid (cut edge)
POSTERIOR
Supraspinatus
E. Superior View

## 6.30 Rotator cuff *(continued)*

**E.** Supraspinatus and supraspinatus tendon.

The supraspinatus, besides being part of the rotator cuff, initiates and assists the deltoid in the first 15° of abduction of the arm. The tendons of the rotator cuff muscles blend with the joint capsule of the glenohumeral joint, reinforcing it as the musculotendinous rotator cuff, which protects the joint and gives it stability.

Injury or disease may damage the rotator cuff, producing instability of the glenohumeral joint. Rupture or tear of the supraspinatus tendon is the most common injury of the rotator cuff. Degenerative tendinitis of the rotator cuff is common, especially in older people.

**TABLE 6.7 DEEP SCAPULOHUMERAL/SHOULDER MUSCLES**

| Muscle | Proximal Attachment | Distal Attachment | Innervation | Main Actions |
|---|---|---|---|---|
| **Supraspinatus (S)** | Supraspinous fossa of scapula | Superior facet on greater tubercle of humerus | Suprascapular nerve (C4, C5, and C6) | Helps deltoid to abduct arm and acts with rotator cuff muscles[a] |
| **Infraspinatus (I)** | Infraspinous fossa of scapula | Middle facet on greater tubercle of humerus | Suprascapular nerve (C5 and C6) | Laterally rotates arm; helps to hold humeral head in glenoid cavity of scapula |
| **Teres minor (T)** | Superior part of lateral border of scapula | Inferior facet on greater tubercle of humerus | Axillary nerve (C5 and C6) | |
| **Subscapularis(S)** | Subscapular fossa | Lesser tubercle of humerus | Upper and lower subscapular nerves (C5, C6, and C7) | Medially rotates arm and adducts it; helps to hold humeral head in glenoid cavity |
| **Teres major**[b] | Posterior surface of inferior angle of scapula | Crest of lesser tubercle (medial lip) of humerus | Lower subscapular nerve (C6 and C7) | Adducts and medially rotates arm |

[a]Collectively, the supraspinatus, infraspinatus, teres minor, and subscapularis muscles are referred to as the rotator cuff muscles or "SITS" muscles. They function together during all movements of the shoulder joint to hold the head of the humerus in the glenoid cavity of scapula.
[b]Not a rotator cuff muscle.

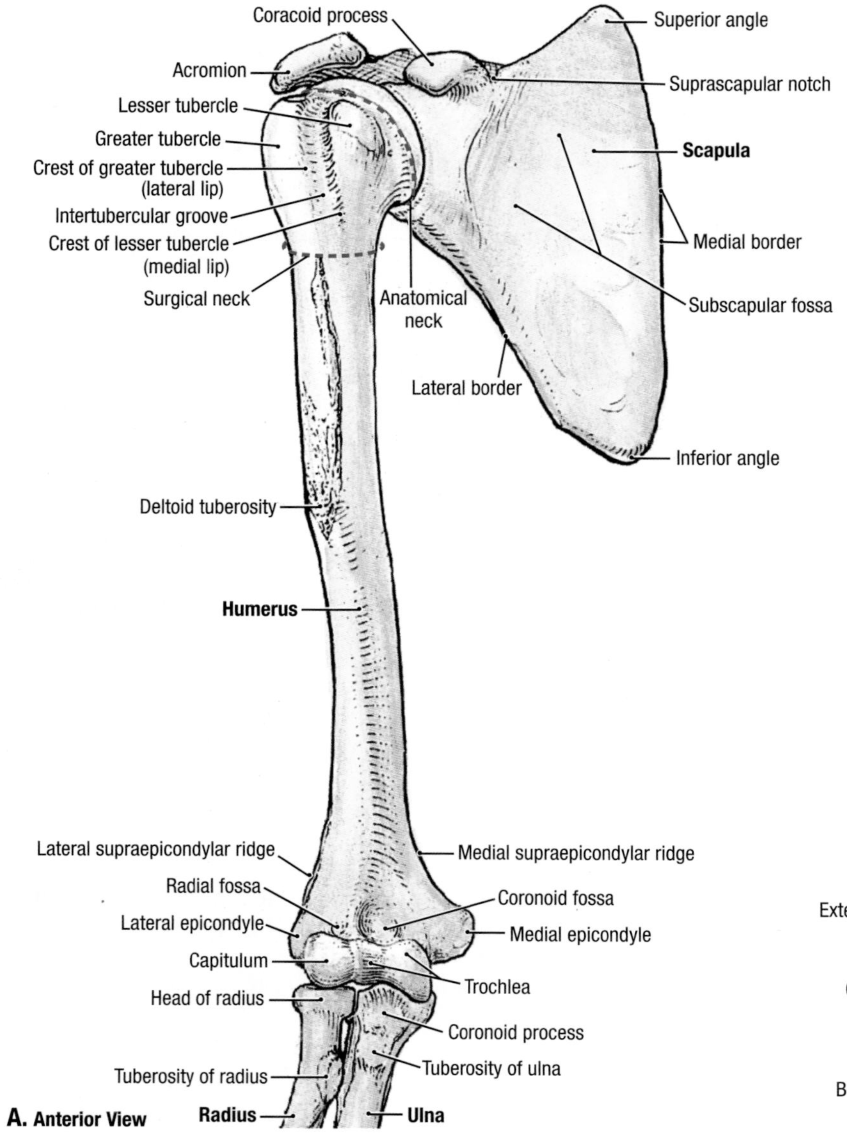

Coracoid process
Superior angle
Acromion
Suprascapular notch
Lesser tubercle
Greater tubercle
Scapula
Crest of greater tubercle (lateral lip)
Intertubercular groove
Medial border
Crest of lesser tubercle (medial lip)
Surgical neck
Anatomical neck
Subscapular fossa
Lateral border
Inferior angle
Deltoid tuberosity
Humerus
Lateral supraepicondylar ridge
Medial supraepicondylar ridge
Radial fossa
Coronoid fossa
Lateral epicondyle
Medial epicondyle
Capitulum
Trochlea
Head of radius
Coronoid process
Tuberosity of radius
Tuberosity of ulna
Radius
Ulna

**A. Anterior View**

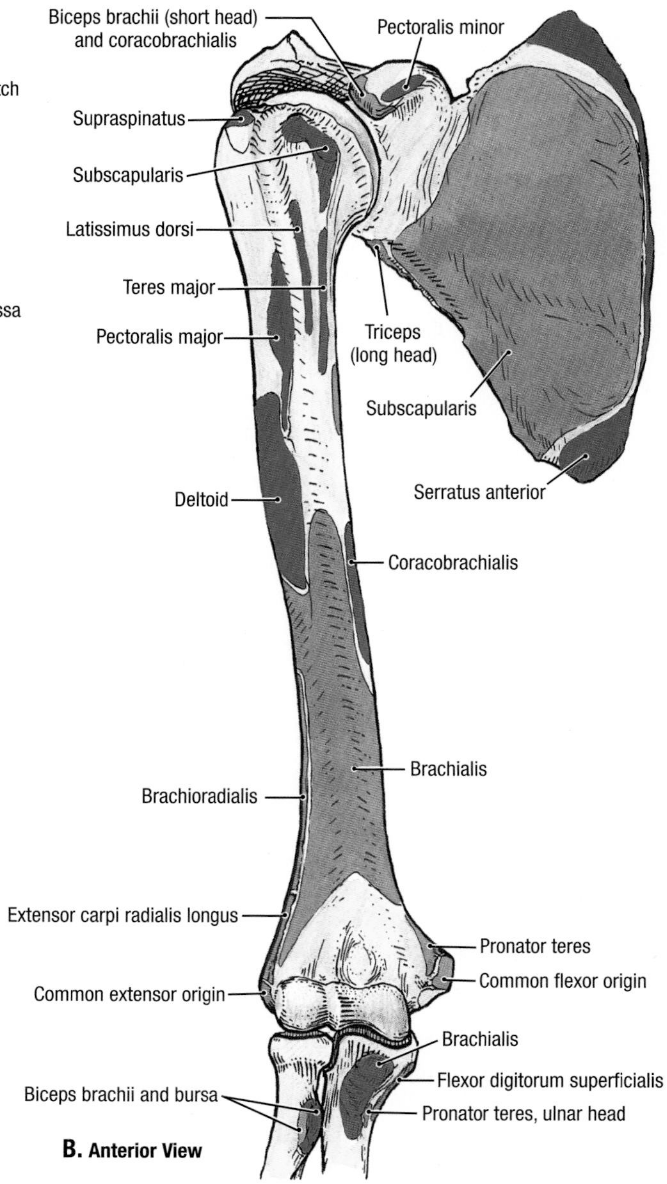

Biceps brachii (short head) and coracobrachialis
Pectoralis minor
Supraspinatus
Subscapularis
Latissimus dorsi
Teres major
Pectoralis major
Triceps (long head)
Subscapularis
Deltoid
Serratus anterior
Coracobrachialis
Brachialis
Brachioradialis
Extensor carpi radialis longus
Pronator teres
Common flexor origin
Common extensor origin
Brachialis
Flexor digitorum superficialis
Biceps brachii and bursa
Pronator teres, ulnar head

**B. Anterior View**

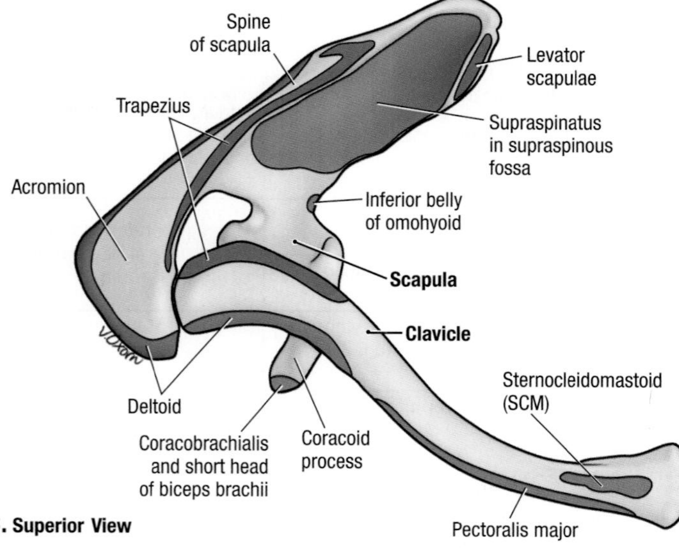
Spine of scapula
Levator scapulae
Trapezius
Supraspinatus in supraspinous fossa
Acromion
Inferior belly of omohyoid
Scapula
Clavicle
Sternocleidomastoid (SCM)
Deltoid
Coracobrachialis and short head of biceps brachii
Coracoid process
Pectoralis major

**C. Superior View**

## 6.31 Bones of proximal upper limb

**A.** Bony features, anterior aspect. **B.** Muscle attachment sites, anterior aspect. **C.** Muscle attachment sites, clavicle and scapula.

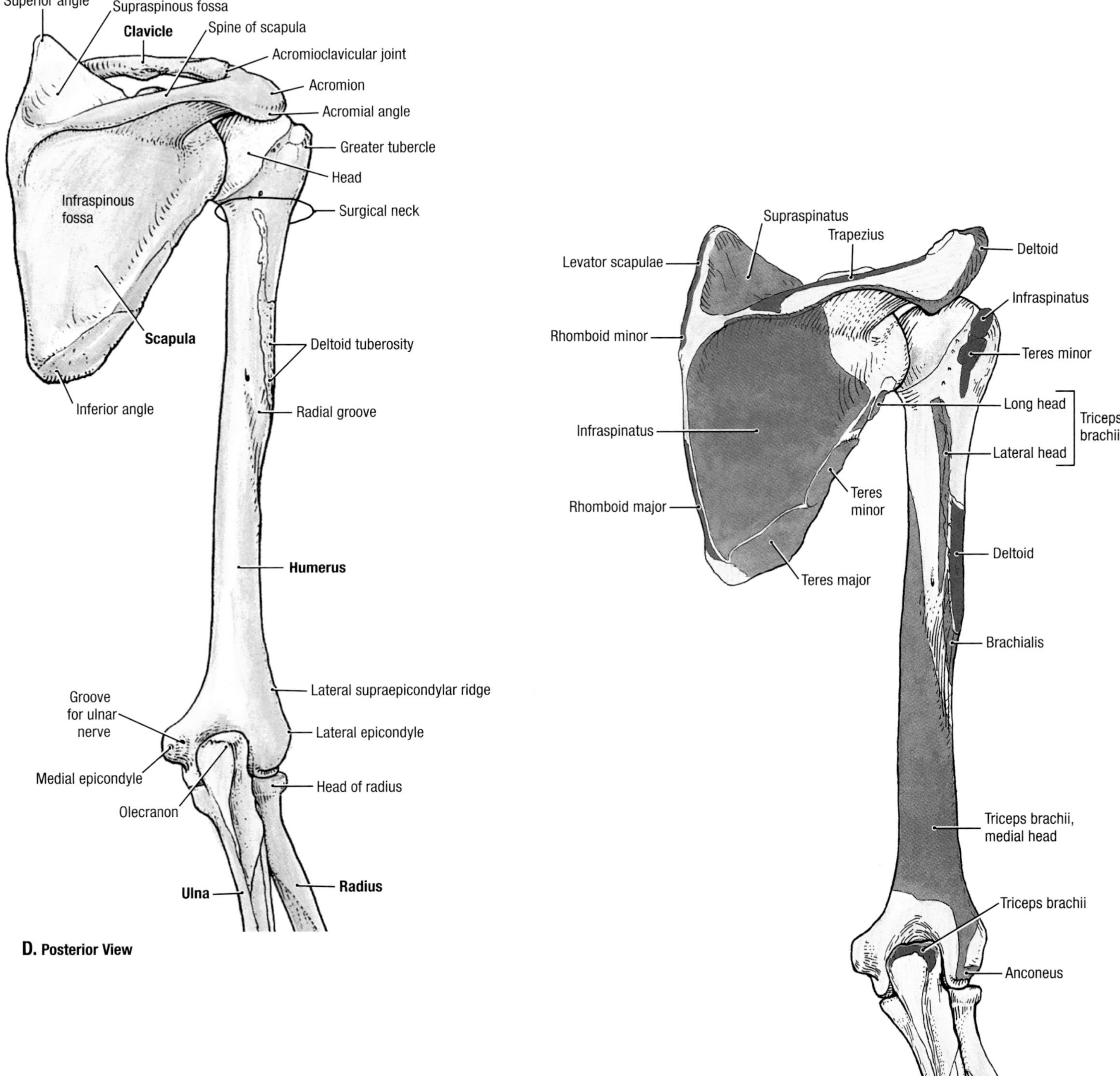
Superior angle
Supraspinous fossa
Clavicle
Spine of scapula
Acromioclavicular joint
Acromion
Acromial angle
Greater tubercle
Head
Surgical neck
Infraspinous fossa
Scapula
Deltoid tuberosity
Inferior angle
Radial groove
Humerus
Lateral supraepicondylar ridge
Groove for ulnar nerve
Lateral epicondyle
Medial epicondyle
Head of radius
Olecranon
Ulna
Radius
D. Posterior View
Supraspinatus
Trapezius
Levator scapulae
Deltoid
Infraspinatus
Rhomboid minor
Teres minor
Long head
Triceps brachii
Lateral head
Infraspinatus
Teres minor
Rhomboid major
Deltoid
Teres major
Brachialis
Triceps brachii, medial head
Triceps brachii
Anconeus
E. Posterior View

## 6.31 Bones of proximal upper limb *(continued)*

**D.** Bony features, posterior aspect. **E.** Muscle attachment sites, posterior aspect.

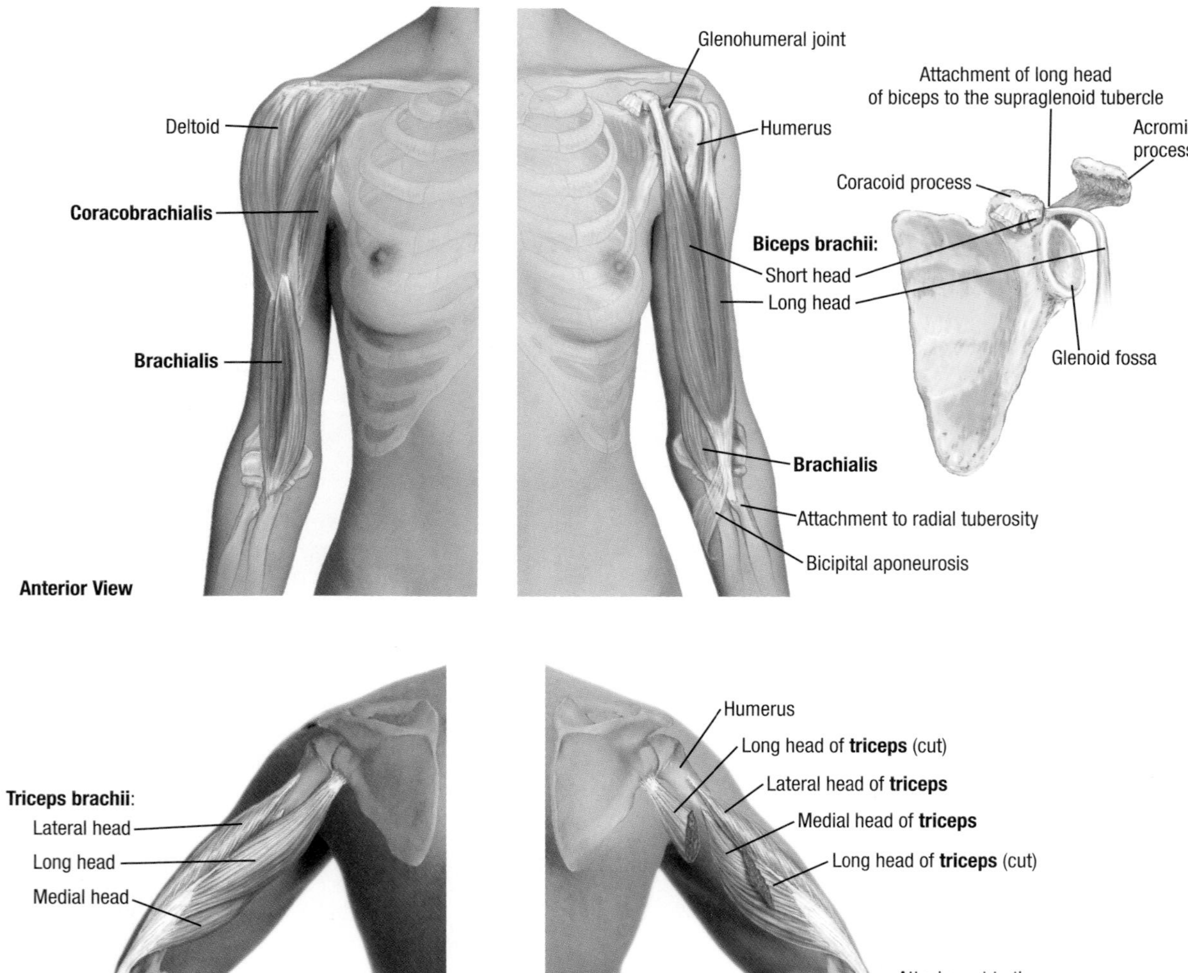

Deltoid
Coracobrachialis
Brachialis
Anterior View
Glenohumeral joint
Humerus
Attachment of long head of biceps to the supraglenoid tubercle
Acromion process
Coracoid process
Biceps brachii:
Short head
Long head
Glenoid fossa
Brachialis
Attachment to radial tuberosity
Bicipital aponeurosis
Triceps brachii:
Lateral head
Long head
Medial head
Posterior View
Humerus
Long head of triceps (cut)
Lateral head of triceps
Medial head of triceps
Long head of triceps (cut)
Attachment to the olecranon process of ulna


## TABLE 6.8 ARM MUSCLES

| Muscle | Proximal Attachment | Distal Attachment | Innervation | Main Actions |
|---|---|---|---|---|
| Biceps brachii | *Short head:* tip of coracoid process of scapula<br>*Long head:* supraglenoid tubercle of scapula | Tuberosity of radius and fascia of forearm through bicipital aponeurosis | Musculocutaneous nerve (C5–C6) | Supinates forearm and, when forearm is supine, flexes fore-arm |
| Brachialis | Distal half of anterior surface of humerus | Coronoid process and tuberosity of ulna | | Flexes forearm in all positions |
| Coracobrachialis | Tip of coracoid process of scapula | Middle third of medial surface of humerus | Musculocutaneous nerve (C5–C7) | Assists with flexion and adduction of arm |
| Triceps brachii | *Long head:* infraglenoid tubercle of scapula<br>*Lateral head:* posterior surface of humerus, superior to radial groove<br>*Medial head:* posterior surface of humerus, inferior to radial groove | Proximal end of olecranon of ulna and fascia of forearm | Radial nerve (C6–C8) | Extends the forearm; long head steadies head of abducted humerus |
| Anconeus | Lateral epicondyle of humerus | Lateral surface of olecranon and superior part of posterior surface of ulna | Radial nerve (C7–T1) | Assists triceps in extending forearm; stabilizes elbow joint; abducts ulna during pronation |

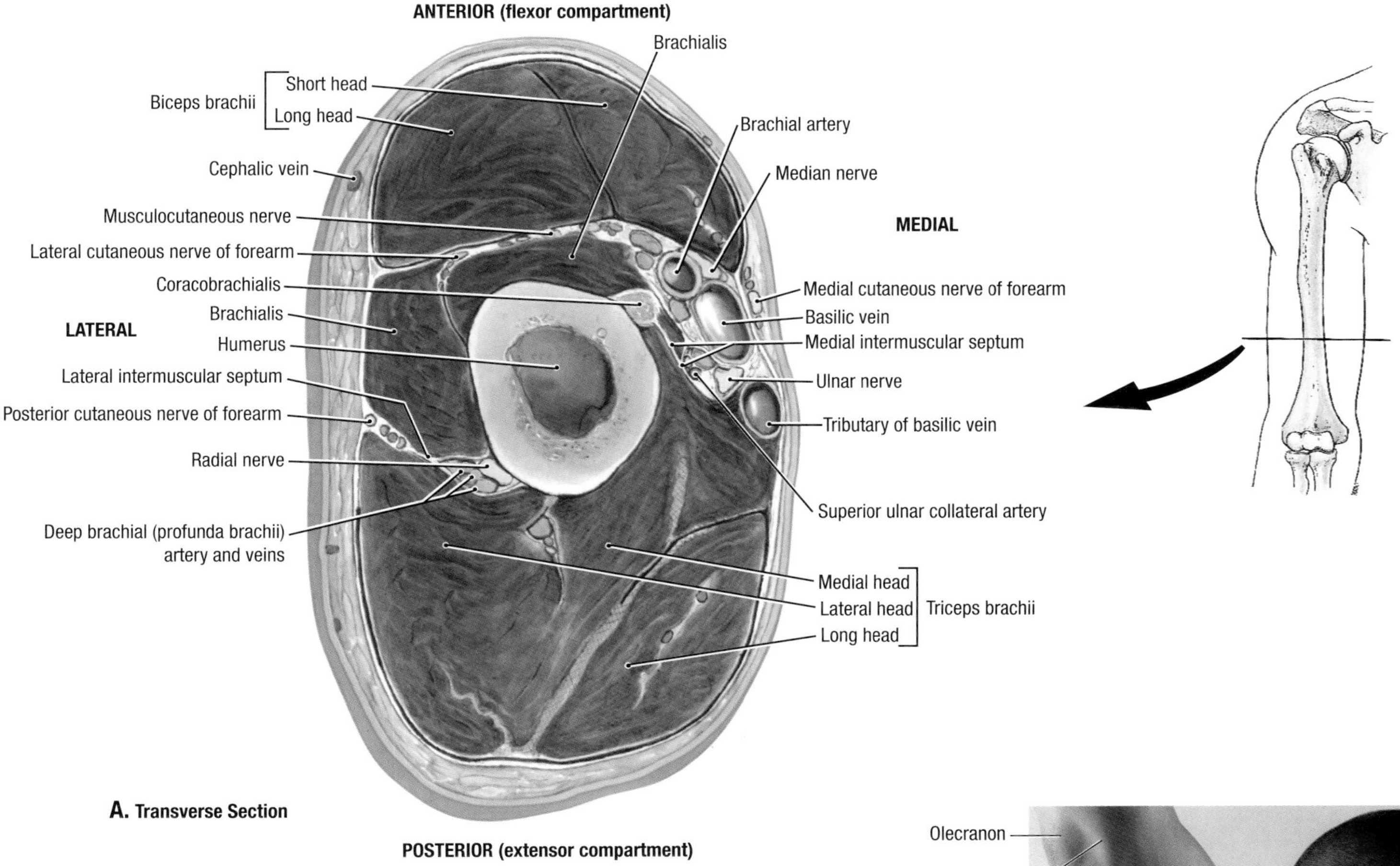

ANTERIOR (flexor compartment)
Brachialis
Biceps brachii
Short head
Long head
Brachial artery
Median nerve
Cephalic vein
MEDIAL
Musculocutaneous nerve
Lateral cutaneous nerve of forearm
Coracobrachialis
Medial cutaneous nerve of forearm
Brachialis
Basilic vein
LATERAL
Humerus
Medial intermuscular septum
Lateral intermuscular septum
Ulnar nerve
Posterior cutaneous nerve of forearm
Tributary of basilic vein
Radial nerve
Superior ulnar collateral artery
Deep brachial (profunda brachii) artery and veins
Medial head
Lateral head
Long head
Triceps brachii
POSTERIOR (extensor compartment)

**A.** Transverse Section

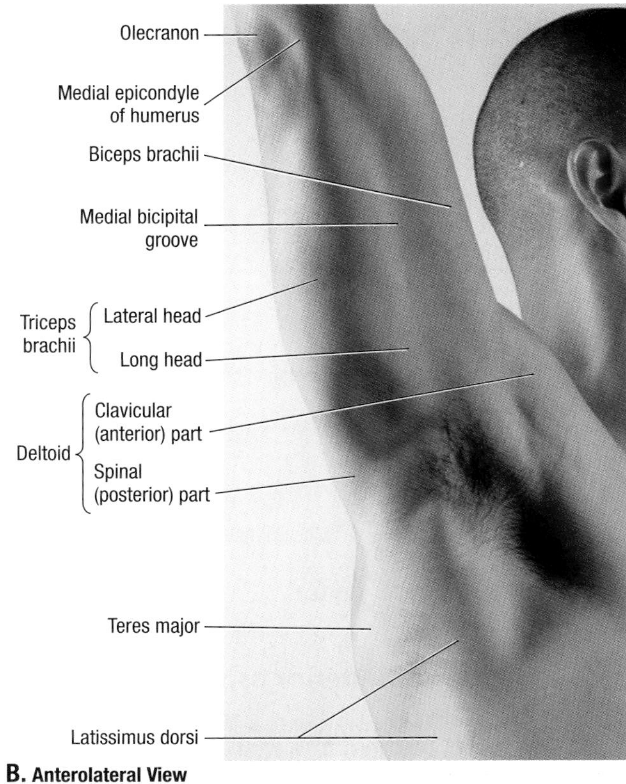
Olecranon
Medial epicondyle of humerus
Biceps brachii
Medial bicipital groove
Triceps brachii
Lateral head
Long head
Deltoid
Clavicular (anterior) part
Spinal (posterior) part
Teres major
Latissimus dorsi

**B.** Anterolateral View

## 6.32 Anterior and posterior compartments of arm

**A.** Anatomical section. **B.** Surface anatomy.

- Three muscles, the biceps, brachialis, and coracobrachialis, lie in the anterior compartment of the arm; the triceps brachii lies in the posterior compartment.
- The medial and lateral intermuscular septum separates these two muscle groups.
- The radial nerve and deep brachial artery and veins serving the posterior compartment lie in contact with the radial groove of the humerus.
- The musculocutaneous nerve serving the anterior compartment lies in the plane between the biceps and the brachialis muscles.
- The median nerve crosses to the medial side of the brachial artery.
- The ulnar nerve passes posteriorly onto the medial side of the triceps muscle.
- The basilic vein (appearing here as two vessels) has pierced the deep fascia.

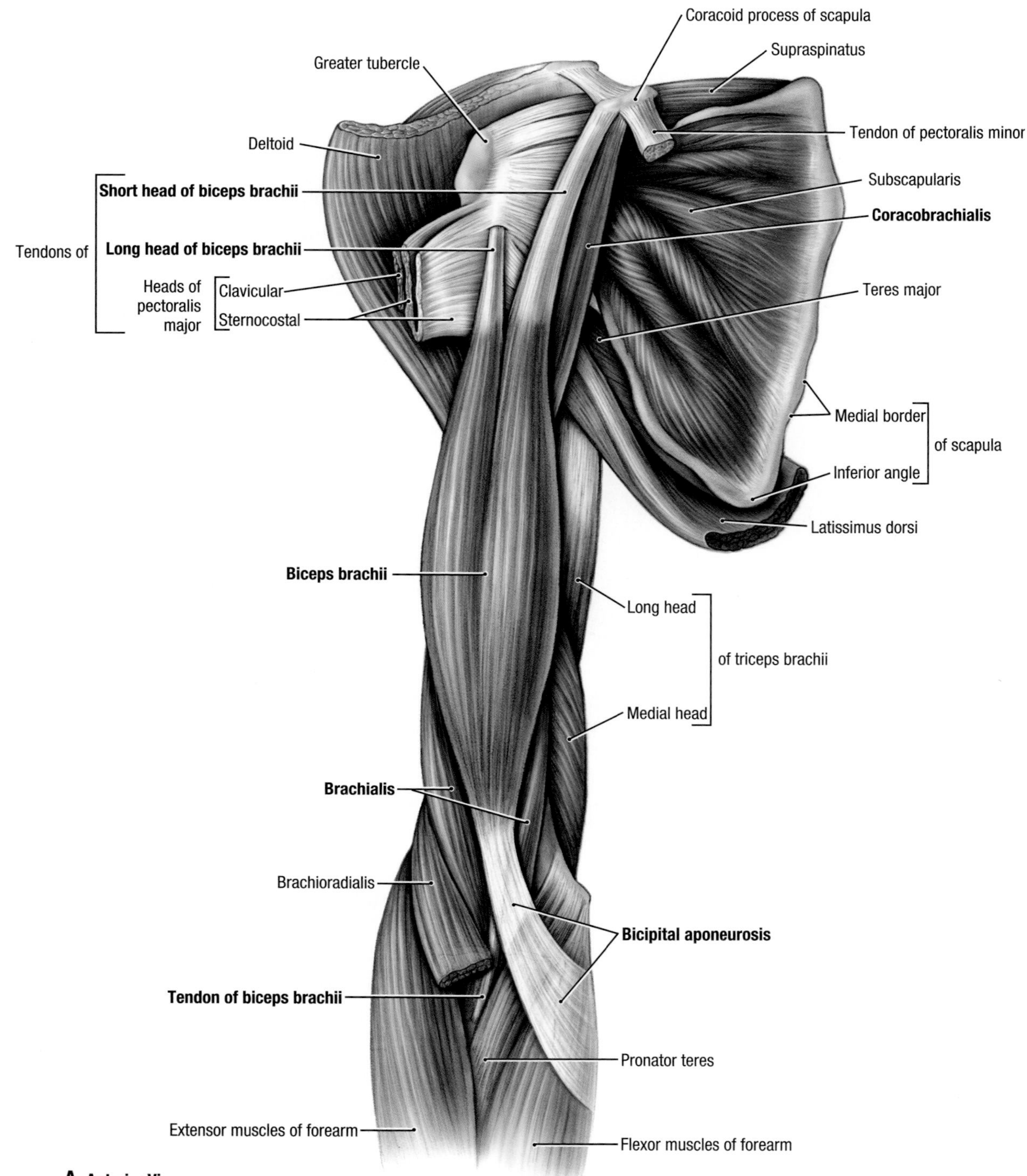
Coracoid process of scapula
Supraspinatus
Greater tubercle
Tendon of pectoralis minor
Deltoid
Subscapularis
Short head of biceps brachii
Coracobrachialis
Tendons of
Long head of biceps brachii
Heads of pectoralis major
Clavicular
Sternocostal
Teres major
Medial border
of scapula
Inferior angle
Latissimus dorsi
Biceps brachii
Long head
of triceps brachii
Medial head
Brachialis
Brachioradialis
Bicipital aponeurosis
Tendon of biceps brachii
Pronator teres
Extensor muscles of forearm
Flexor muscles of forearm

**A. Anterior View**

## 6.33 Muscles of anterior aspect of arm—I

- The biceps brachii has two heads: a long head and a short head.
- However, when the elbow is flexed approximately 90° the biceps is a flexor from the supinated position of the forearm but a very powerful supinator from the pronated position.
- A triangular membranous band, the bicipital aponeurosis runs from the biceps tendon across the cubital fossa and merges with the antebrachial (deep) fascia covering the flexor muscles on the medial side of the forearm.

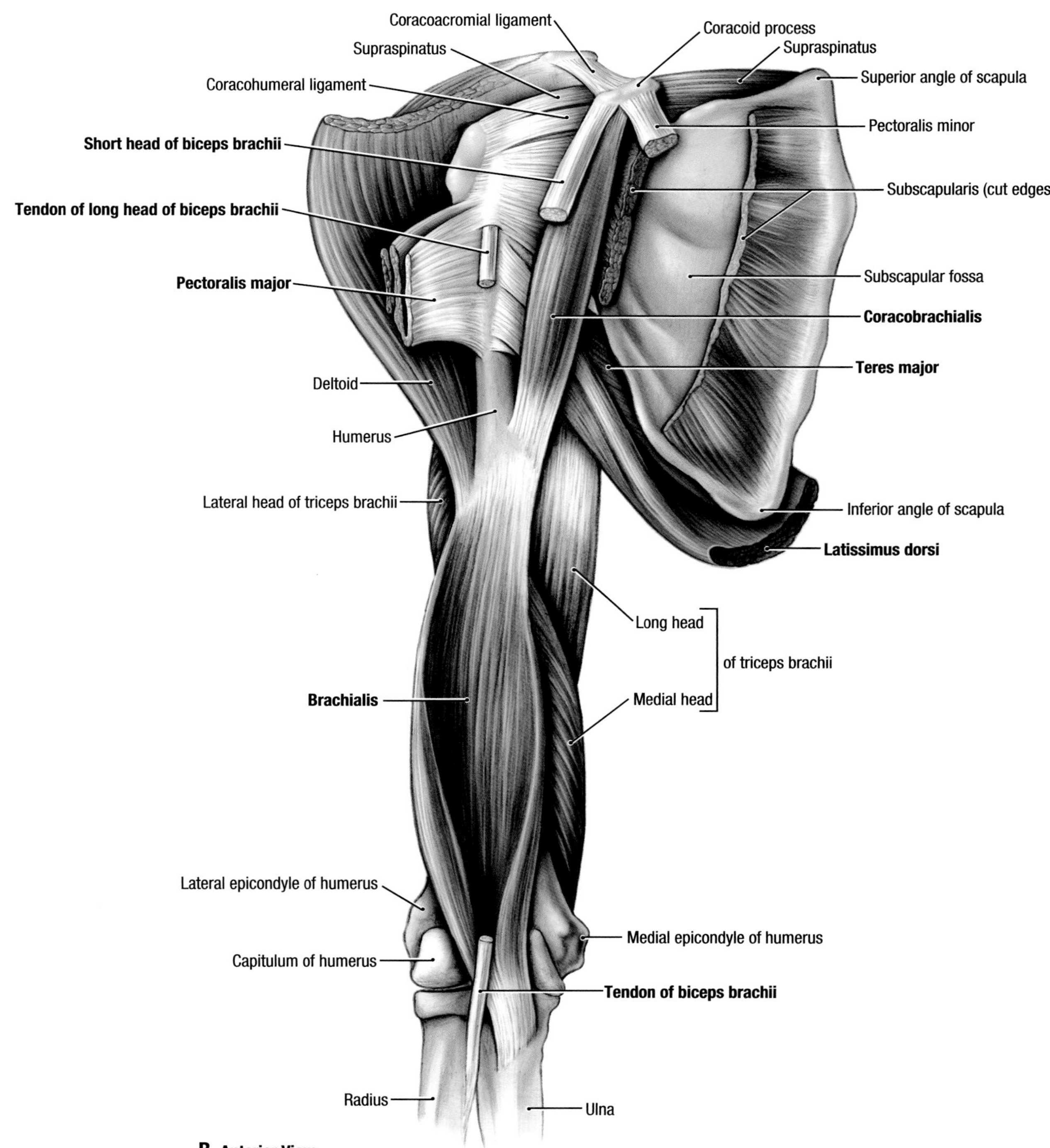
Coracoacromial ligament
Coracoid process
Supraspinatus
Supraspinatus
Superior angle of scapula
Coracohumeral ligament
Pectoralis minor
Short head of biceps brachii
Subscapularis (cut edges)
Tendon of long head of biceps brachii
Subscapular fossa
Pectoralis major
Coracobrachialis
Teres major
Deltoid
Humerus
Lateral head of triceps brachii
Inferior angle of scapula
Latissimus dorsi
Long head
of triceps brachii
Medial head
Brachialis
Lateral epicondyle of humerus
Medial epicondyle of humerus
Capitulum of humerus
Tendon of biceps brachii
Radius
Ulna

**B. Anterior View**

## 6.33 Muscles of anterior aspect of arm—II

- The **brachialis**, a flattened fusiform muscle, lies posterior (deep) to the biceps that produce the greatest amount of flexion force.
- The **coracobrachialis**, an elongated muscle in the superomedial part of the arm, is pierced by the musculocutaneous nerve. It helps flex and adduct the arm.

Rupture of the tendon of the long head of the biceps usually results from wear and tear of an inflamed tendon (*biceps tendinitis*). Normally, the tendon is torn from its attachment to the supraglenoid tubercle of the scapula. The detached muscle belly forms a ball near the center of the distal part of the anterior aspect of the arm.

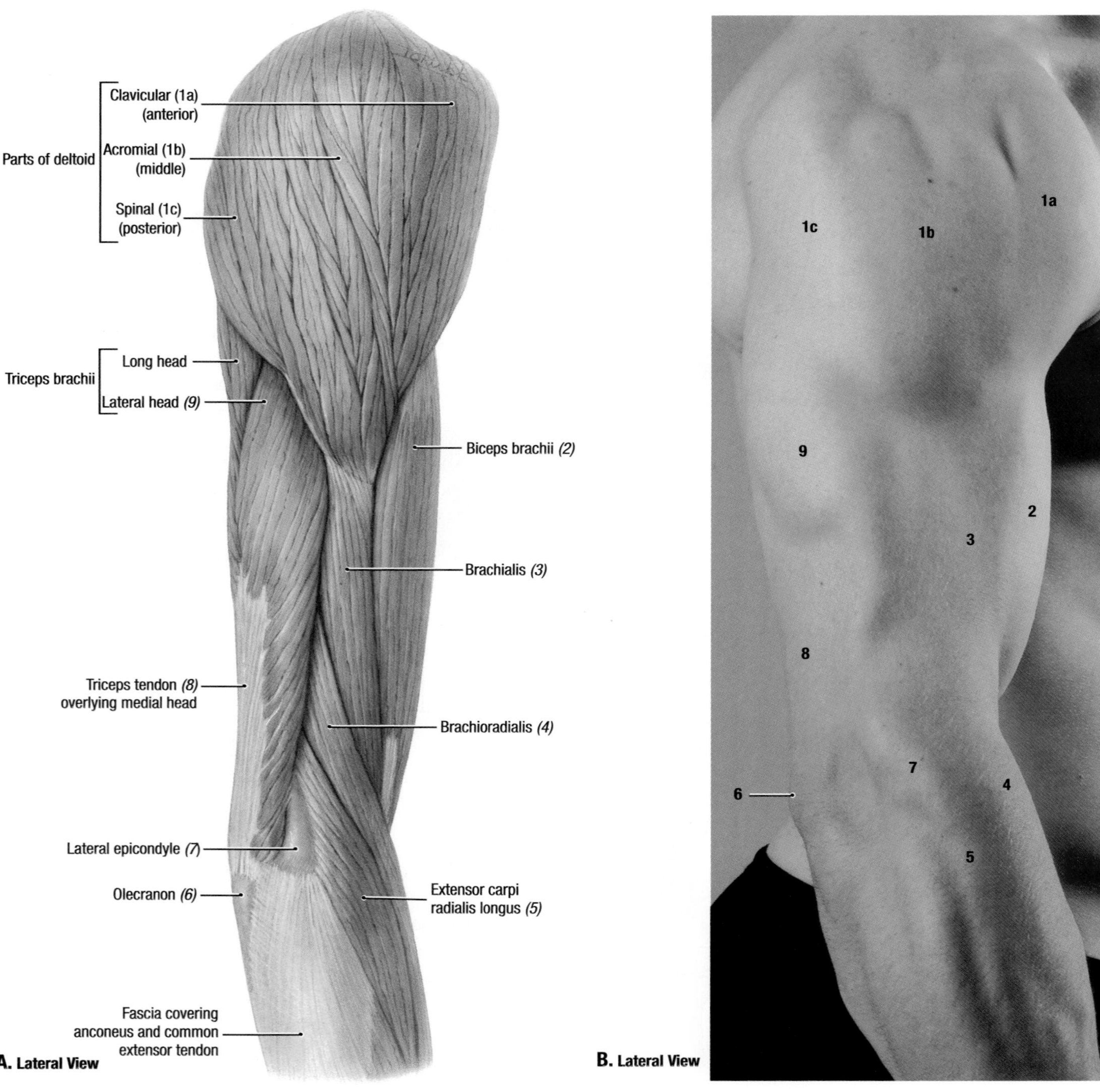
Parts of deltoid
Clavicular (1a) (anterior)
Acromial (1b) (middle)
Spinal (1c) (posterior)
Triceps brachii
Long head
Lateral head (9)
Biceps brachii (2)
Brachialis (3)
Triceps tendon (8) overlying medial head
Brachioradialis (4)
Lateral epicondyle (7)
Olecranon (6)
Extensor carpi radialis longus (5)
Fascia covering anconeus and common extensor tendon
A. Lateral View
1a
1c
1b
9
2
3
8
7
6
4
5
B. Lateral View

## 6.34 Lateral aspect of arm

**A.** Dissection (*numbers* in parentheses refer to structures in **B**). **B.** Surface anatomy.

Atrophy of the deltoid occurs when the axillary nerve (C5 and C6) is severely damaged (e.g., as might occur when the surgical neck of the humerus is fractured). As the deltoid atrophies, the rounded contour of the shoulder disappears. This gives the shoulder a flattened appearance and produces a slight hollow inferior to the acromion. A loss of sensation may occur over the lateral side of the proximal part of the arm, the area supplied by the superior lateral cutaneous nerve of the arm. To test the deltoid (or the function of the axillary nerve) the arm is abducted, against resistance, starting from approximately 15°. Supraspinatus initiates abduction.

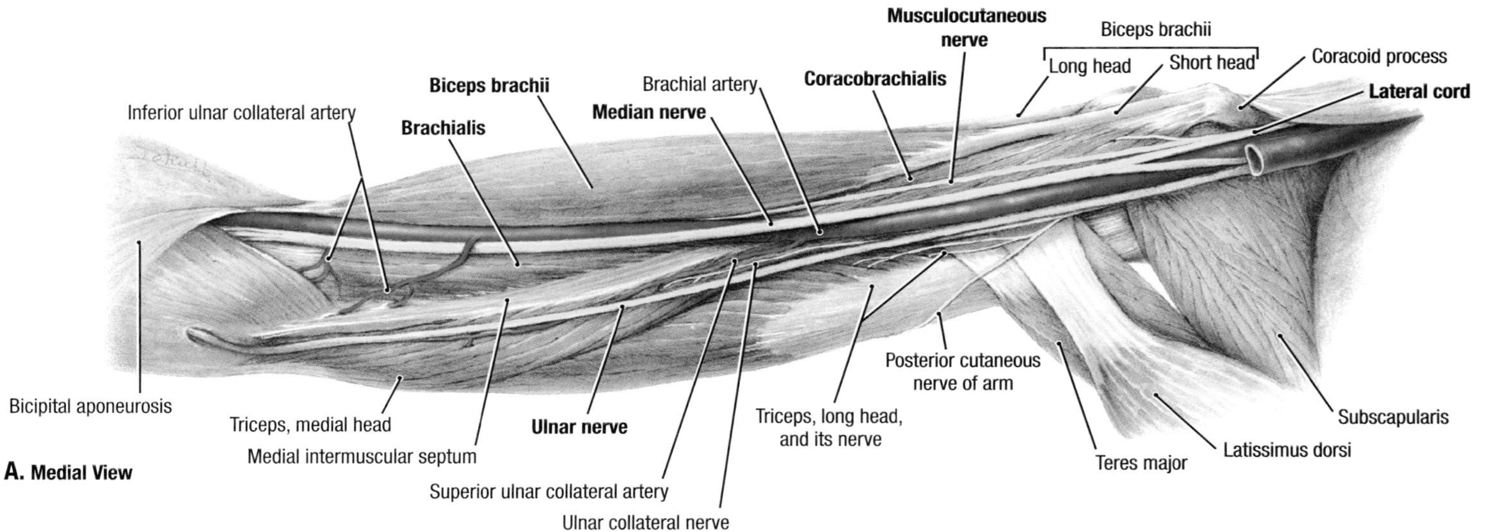
Musculocutaneous nerve
Biceps brachii
Long head
Short head
Coracoid process
Lateral cord
Coracobrachialis
Brachial artery
Biceps brachii
Median nerve
Brachialis
Inferior ulnar collateral artery
Bicipital aponeurosis
Triceps, medial head
Medial intermuscular septum
Ulnar nerve
Superior ulnar collateral artery
Ulnar collateral nerve
Triceps, long head, and its nerve
Posterior cutaneous nerve of arm
Teres major
Latissimus dorsi
Subscapularis
A. Medial View

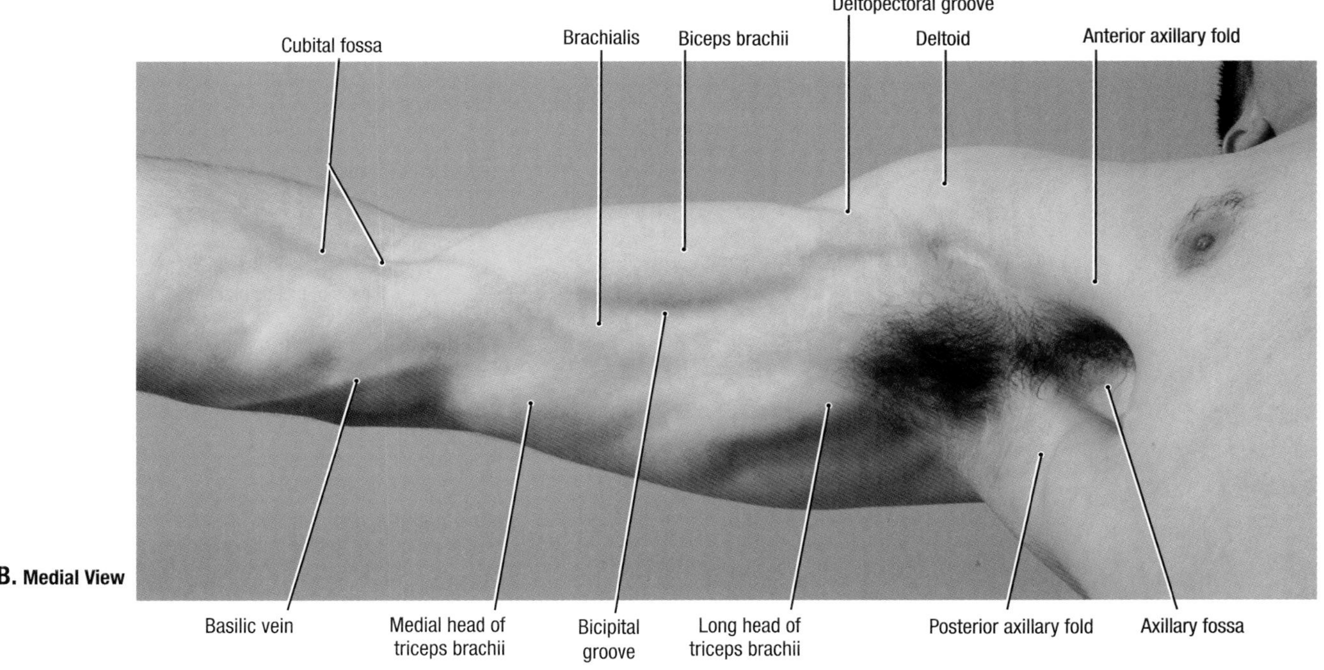
Deltopectoral groove
Cubital fossa
Brachialis
Biceps brachii
Deltoid
Anterior axillary fold
B. Medial View
Basilic vein
Medial head of triceps brachii
Bicipital groove
Long head of triceps brachii
Posterior axillary fold
Axillary fossa

## 6.35 Medial aspect of arm

**A.** Dissection. **B.** Surface anatomy.

- The axillary artery passes just inferior to the tip of the coracoid process and courses posterior to the coracobrachialis. At the inferior border of the teres major, the axillary artery changes names to become the brachial artery and continues distally on the anterior aspect of the brachialis.

- Although collateral pathways confer some protection against gradual temporary and partial occlusion, sudden complete occlusion or laceration of the brachial artery creates a surgical emergency because paralysis of muscles results from ischemia within a few hours.

- The median nerve lies adjacent to the axillary and brachial arteries and then crosses the artery from lateral to medial.
- Proximally, the ulnar nerve is adjacent to the medial side of the artery, passes posterior to the medial intermuscular septum, and descends on the medial head of triceps to pass posterior to the medial epicondyle; here, the ulnar nerve is palpable.
- The superior ulnar collateral artery and ulnar collateral branch of the radial nerve (to medial head of the triceps) accompany the ulnar nerve in the arm.

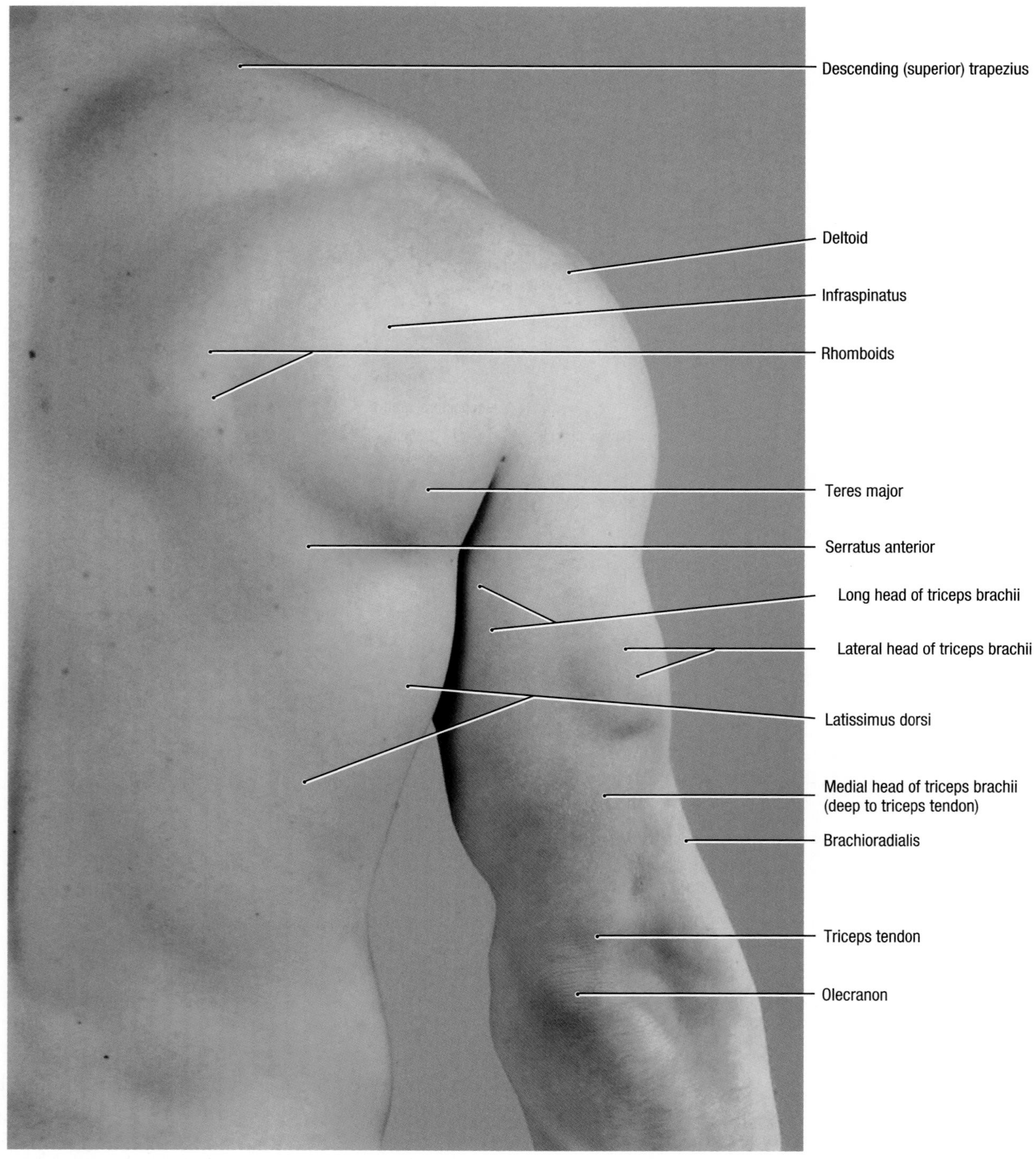
Descending (superior) trapezius
Deltoid
Infraspinatus
Rhomboids
Teres major
Serratus anterior
Long head of triceps brachii
Lateral head of triceps brachii
Latissimus dorsi
Medial head of triceps brachii (deep to triceps tendon)
Brachioradialis
Triceps tendon
Olecranon
Posterior View

## 6.36 Surface anatomy of the scapular region and posterior aspect of arm

The three heads of the triceps form a bulge on the posterior aspect of the arm and are identifiable when the forearm is extended from the flexed position against resistance.

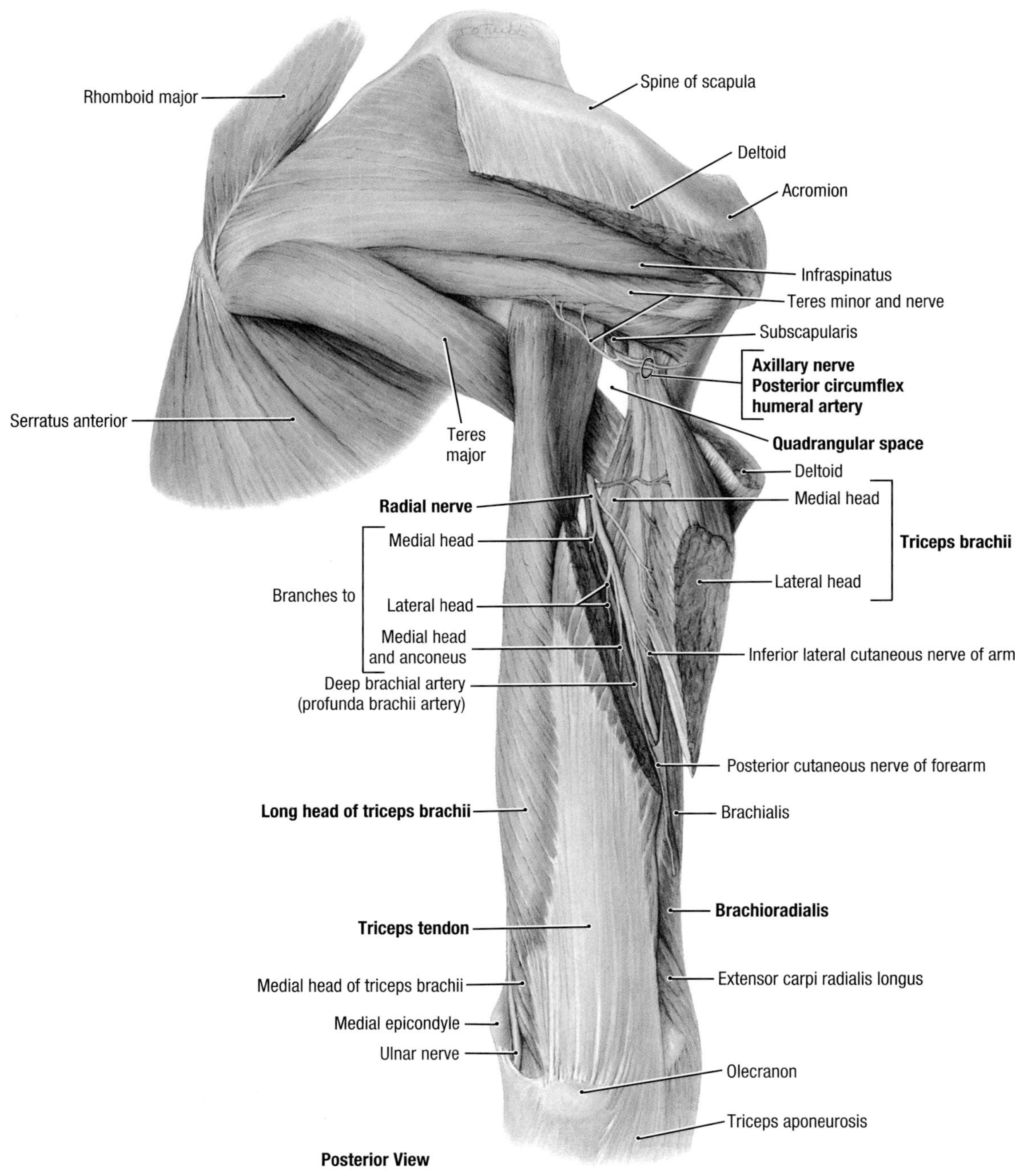
Rhomboid major
Spine of scapula
Deltoid
Acromion
Infraspinatus
Teres minor and nerve
Subscapularis
Axillary nerve
Posterior circumflex humeral artery
Serratus anterior
Teres major
Quadrangular space
Deltoid
Medial head
Radial nerve
Medial head
Triceps brachii
Branches to
Lateral head
Lateral head
Medial head and anconeus
Inferior lateral cutaneous nerve of arm
Deep brachial artery (profunda brachii artery)
Posterior cutaneous nerve of forearm
Long head of triceps brachii
Brachialis
Brachioradialis
Triceps tendon
Medial head of triceps brachii
Extensor carpi radialis longus
Medial epicondyle
Ulnar nerve
Olecranon
Triceps aponeurosis
Posterior View

## 6.37 Triceps brachii and related nerves

- The lateral head is reflected laterally, and the medial head is attached to the deep surface of the triceps tendon, which attaches to the olecranon.
- The radial nerve and deep brachial artery pass between the proximal attachments of the long and medial heads of the triceps brachii in the middle third of the arm, directly contacting the radial groove of the humerus.
- The middle third of the arm is a common site for fractures of the humerus, often with associated radial nerve trauma. When the radial nerve is injured in the radial groove, the triceps brachii muscle typically is only weakened because only the medial head is affected. However, the muscles in the posterior compartment of the forearm, supplied by more distal branches of the radial nerve, are paralyzed. The characteristic clinical sign of radial nerve injury is wrist drop (inability to extend the wrist and fingers at the metacarpophalangeal joints).
- The axillary nerve passes through the quadrangular space along with the posterior humeral circumflex artery.
- The ulnar nerve follows the medial border of the triceps then passes posterior to the medial epicondyle.

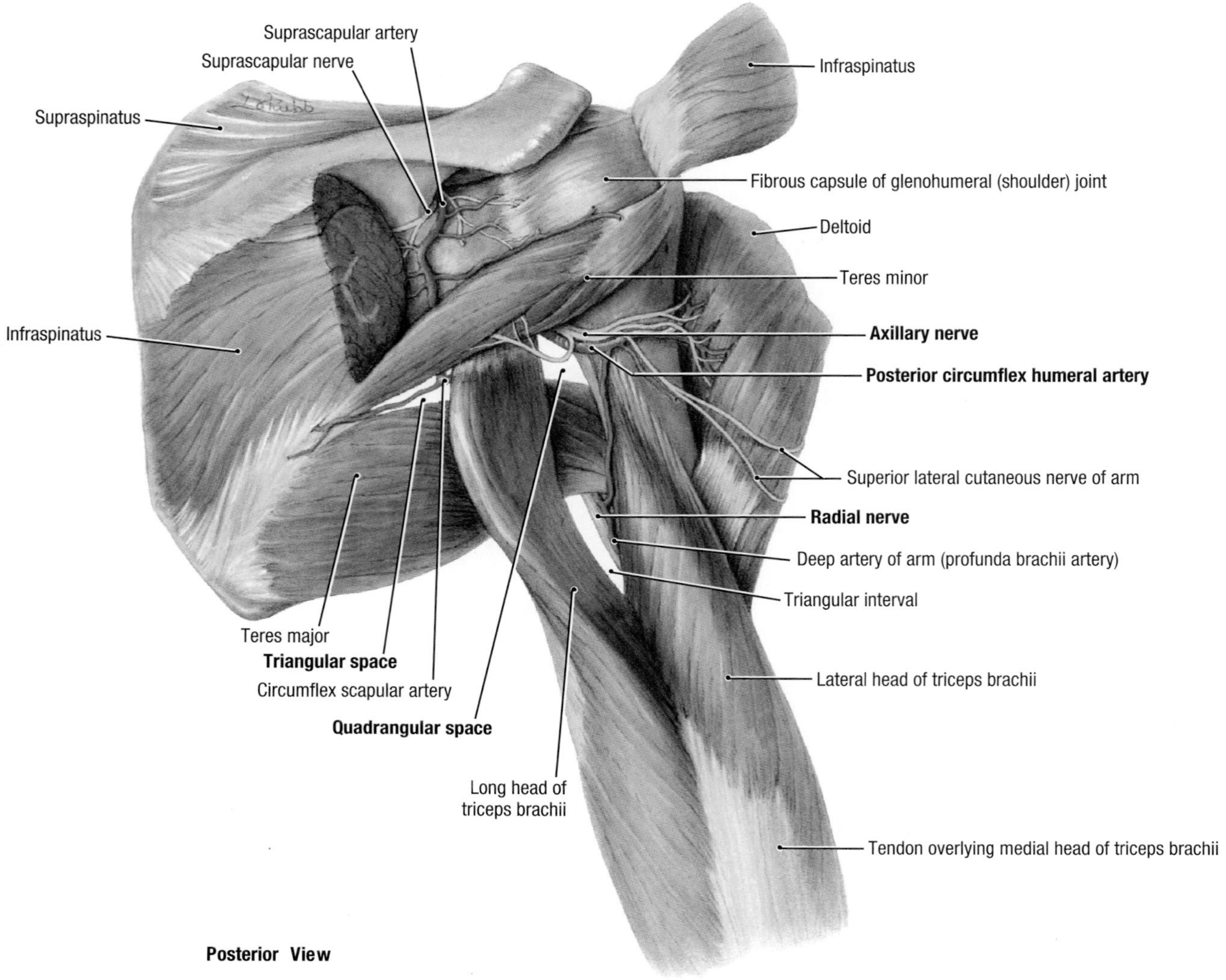
Suprascapular artery
Suprascapular nerve
Supraspinatus
Infraspinatus
Fibrous capsule of glenohumeral (shoulder) joint
Deltoid
Teres minor
Infraspinatus
Axillary nerve
Posterior circumflex humeral artery
Superior lateral cutaneous nerve of arm
Radial nerve
Deep artery of arm (profunda brachii artery)
Triangular interval
Teres major
Triangular space
Circumflex scapular artery
Quadrangular space
Lateral head of triceps brachii
Long head of
triceps brachii
Tendon overlying medial head of triceps brachii
Posterior View

## 6.38 Dorsal scapular and subdeltoid regions

- The infraspinatus muscle, aided by the teres minor and spinal (posterior) fibers of the deltoid muscle, rotates the humerus laterally.
- The long head of the triceps muscle passes between the teres minor (a lateral rotator) and teres major (a medial rotator) muscles.
- The long head of the triceps muscle separates the quadrangular space from the triangular space.
- Regarding the distribution of the suprascapular and axillary nerves, each comes from C5 and C6; each supplies two muscles—the suprascapular nerve innervates the supraspinatus and infraspinatus, and the axillary nerve innervates the teres minor and deltoid muscles. Both nerves supply the shoulder joint, but only the axillary nerve has a cutaneous branch.

- The axillary nerve may be injured when the glenohumeral joint dislocates because of its close relation to the inferior part of the joint capsule of this joint. The subglenoid displacement of the head of the humerus into the quadrangular space damages the axillary nerve. Axillary nerve injury is indicated by paralysis of the deltoid.

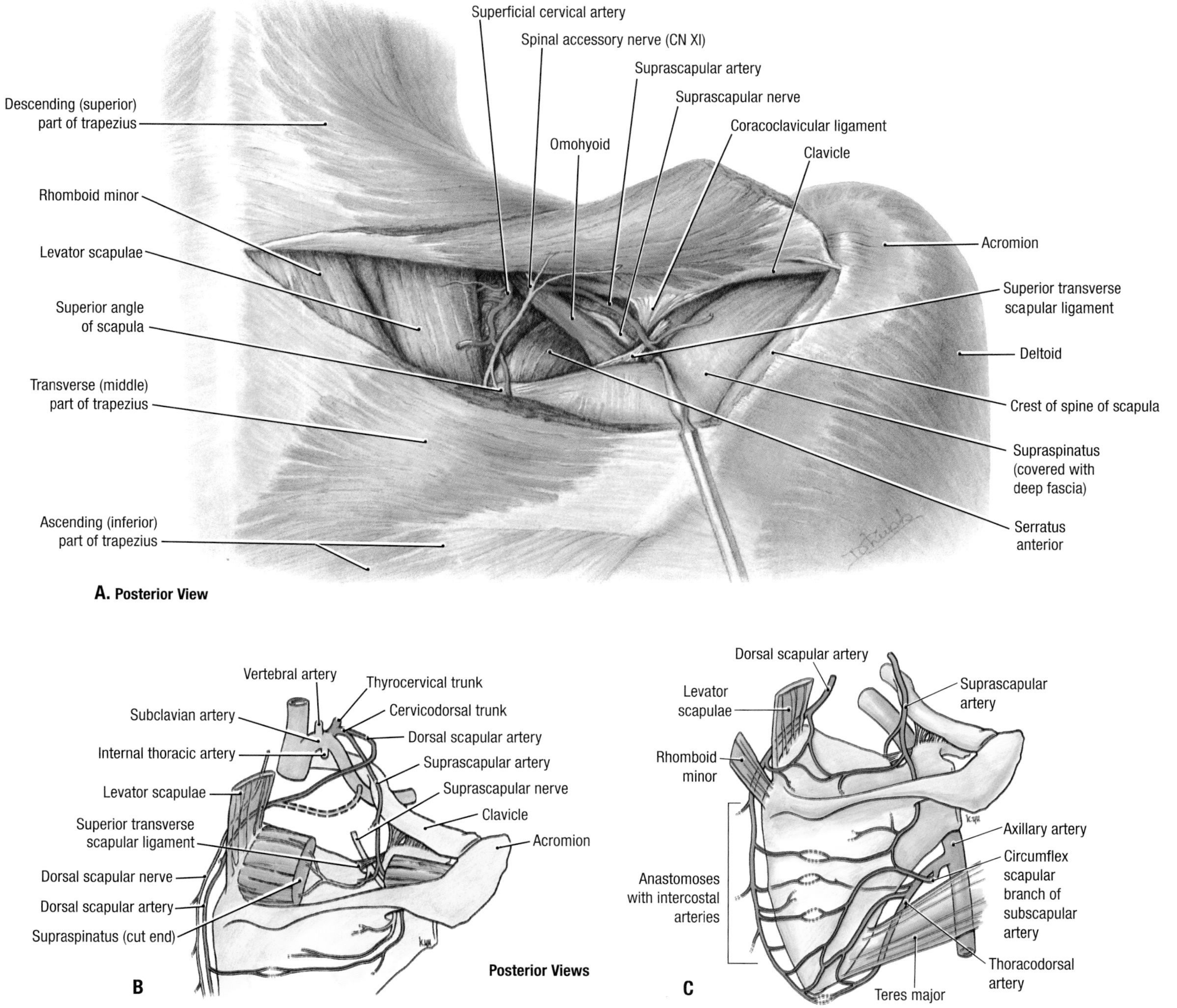

Superficial cervical artery
Spinal accessory nerve (CN XI)
Suprascapular artery
Suprascapular nerve
Coracoclavicular ligament
Clavicle
Omohyoid
Descending (superior) part of trapezius
Rhomboid minor
Levator scapulae
Superior angle of scapula
Transverse (middle) part of trapezius
Ascending (inferior) part of trapezius
Acromion
Superior transverse scapular ligament
Deltoid
Crest of spine of scapula
Supraspinatus (covered with deep fascia)
Serratus anterior

**A. Posterior View**

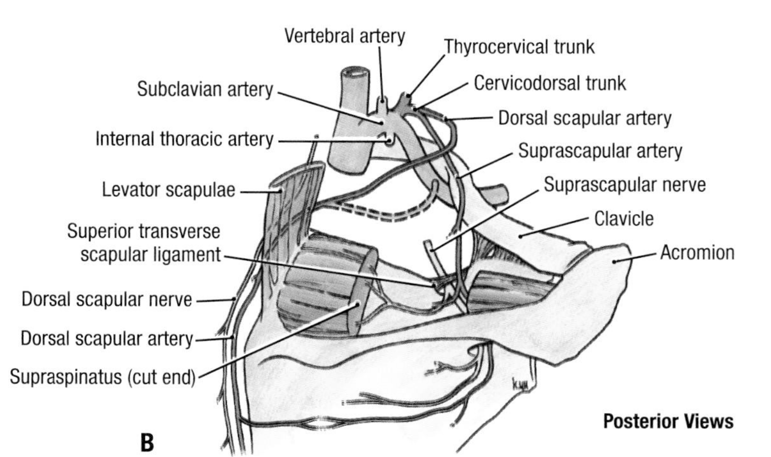
Vertebral artery
Thyrocervical trunk
Subclavian artery
Cervicodorsal trunk
Dorsal scapular artery
Internal thoracic artery
Suprascapular artery
Suprascapular nerve
Levator scapulae
Clavicle
Superior transverse scapular ligament
Acromion
Dorsal scapular nerve
Dorsal scapular artery
Supraspinatus (cut end)
B
Posterior Views

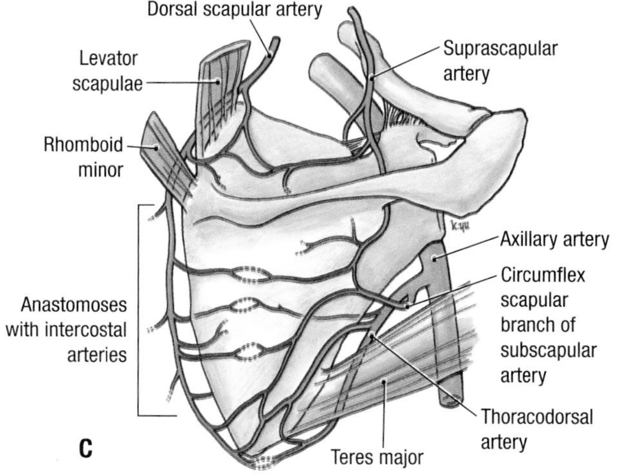
Dorsal scapular artery
Levator scapulae
Suprascapular artery
Rhomboid minor
Axillary artery
Circumflex scapular branch of subscapular artery
Anastomoses with intercostal arteries
Thoracodorsal artery
Teres major
C

## 6.39 Suprascapular region

**A.** Dissection. At the level of the superior angle of the scapula, the transverse part of the trapezius muscle is reflected. **B.** Suprascapular and dorsal scapular arteries. **C.** Scapular anastomosis.

Several arteries join to form anastomoses on the anterior and posterior surfaces of the scapula. The importance of the collateral circulation made possible by these anastomoses becomes apparent when ligation of a lacerated subclavian or axillary artery is necessary or there is occlusion of these vessels. The direction of blood flow in the subscapular artery is then reversed, enabling blood to reach the third part of the axillary artery. In contrast to a sudden occlusion, slow occlusion of an artery often enables sufficient lateral circulation to develop, preventing ischemia (deficiency of blood).

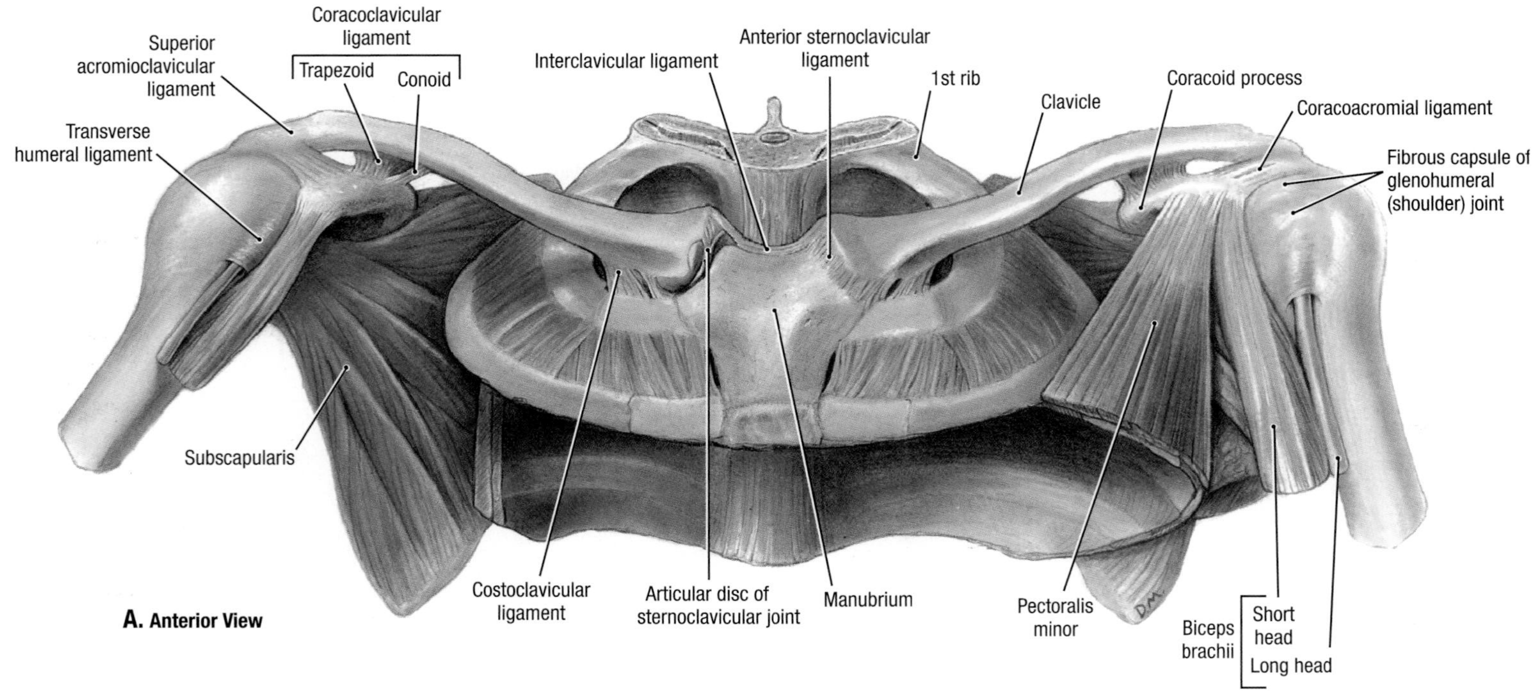
Coracoclavicular ligament
Trapezoid
Conoid
Superior acromioclavicular ligament
Transverse humeral ligament
Interclavicular ligament
Anterior sternoclavicular ligament
1st rib
Clavicle
Coracoid process
Coracoacromial ligament
Fibrous capsule of glenohumeral (shoulder) joint
Subscapularis
Costoclavicular ligament
Articular disc of sternoclavicular joint
Manubrium
Pectoralis minor
Biceps brachii
Short head
Long head
A. Anterior View

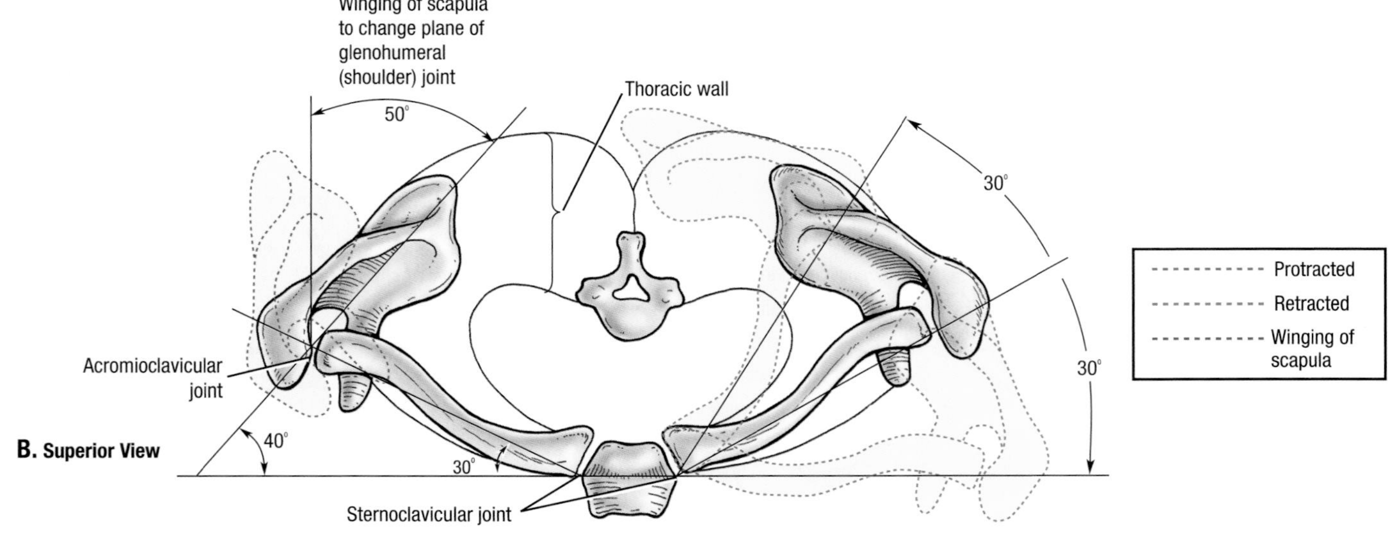
Winging of scapula to change plane of glenohumeral (shoulder) joint
50°
Thoracic wall
30°
30°
Protracted
Retracted
Winging of scapula
Acromioclavicular joint
40°
30°
B. Superior View
Sternoclavicular joint

## 6.40 Pectoral girdle

**A.** Dissection. **B.** Clavicular movements at the sternoclavicular and acromioclavicular joints during rotation, protraction, and retraction of the scapula on the thoracic wall *(left side)* and winging of the scapula *(right side)*.

- The shoulder region includes the sternoclavicular, acromioclavicular, and shoulder (glenohumeral) joints; the mobility of the clavicle is essential to the movement of the upper limb.
- The sternoclavicular joint is the only joint connecting the upper limb (appendicular skeleton) to the trunk (axial skeleton). The articular disc of the sternoclavicular joint divides the joint cavity into two parts and attaches superiorly to the clavicle and inferiorly to the first costal cartilage; the disc resists superior and medial displacement of the clavicle.

In **B,** note that when the serratus anterior is paralyzed because of injury to the long thoracic nerve, the medial border of the scapula moves laterally and posteriorly away from the thoracic wall, giving the scapula the appearance of a wing. The arm cannot be abducted beyond the horizontal position because the serratus anterior cannot rotate the glenoid cavity superiorly to allow complete abduction of the arm.

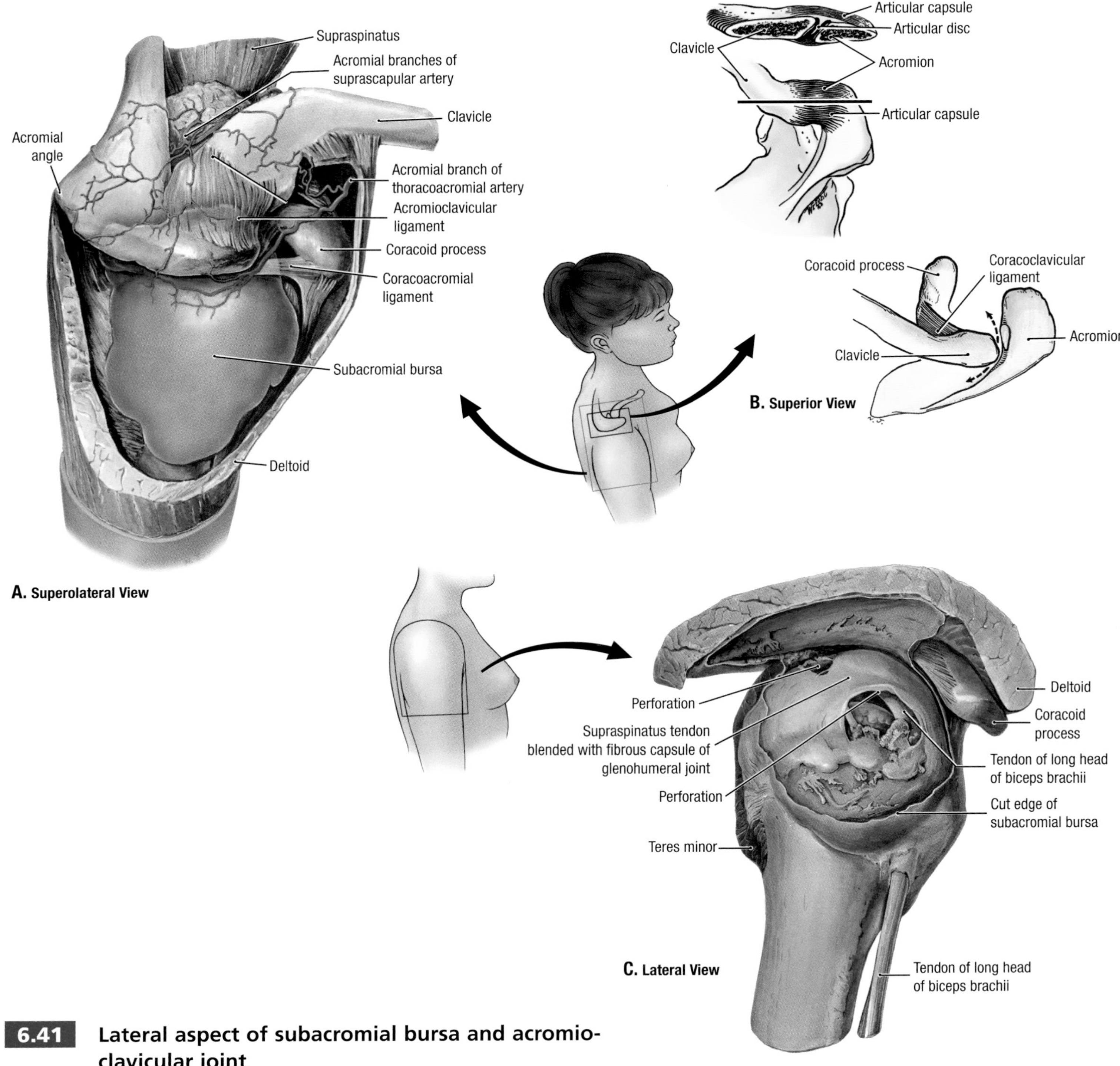
Supraspinatus
Acromial branches of suprascapular artery
Clavicle
Acromial angle
Acromial branch of thoracoacromial artery
Acromioclavicular ligament
Coracoid process
Coracoacromial ligament
Subacromial bursa
Deltoid
A. Superolateral View
Articular capsule
Articular disc
Clavicle
Acromion
Articular capsule
Coracoid process
Coracoclavicular ligament
Acromion
Clavicle
B. Superior View
Deltoid
Coracoid process
Perforation
Supraspinatus tendon blended with fibrous capsule of glenohumeral joint
Perforation
Tendon of long head of biceps brachii
Cut edge of subacromial bursa
Teres minor
C. Lateral View
Tendon of long head of biceps brachii

## 6.41 Lateral aspect of subacromial bursa and acromioclavicular joint

**A.** Subacromial bursa. The bursa has been injected with purple latex. **B.** Acromioclavicular joint. **C.** Attrition of supraspinatus tendon. As a result of wearing away of the supraspinatus tendon and underlying capsule, the subacromial bursa and shoulder joint come into communication. The intracapsular part of the tendon of the long head of biceps muscle becomes frayed, leaving it adherent to the intertubercular groove. Of 95 dissecting room subjects, none of the 18 younger than 50 years of age had a perforation, but 4 of the 19 who were 50 to 60 years and 23 of the 57 older than 60 years had perforations. The perforation was bilateral in 11 subjects and unilateral in 14.

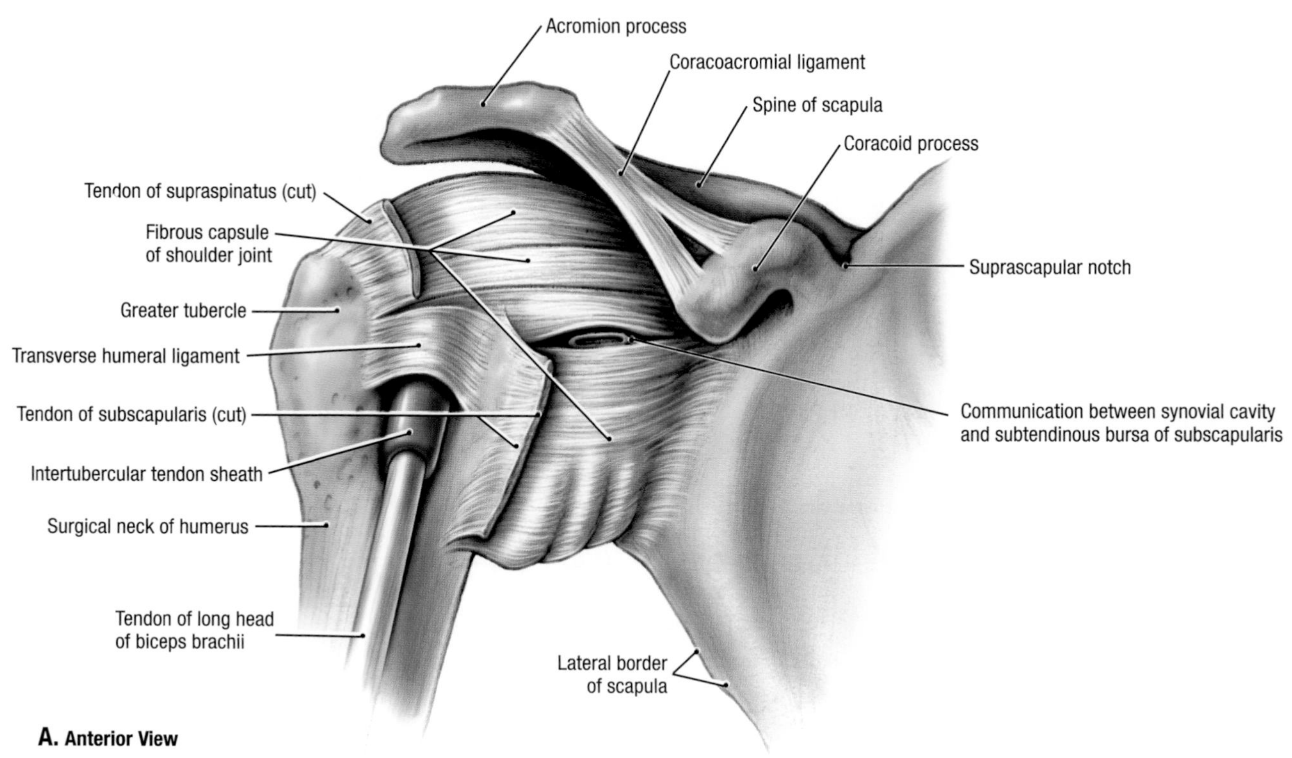
Acromion process
Coracoacromial ligament
Spine of scapula
Coracoid process
Tendon of supraspinatus (cut)
Fibrous capsule of shoulder joint
Suprascapular notch
Greater tubercle
Transverse humeral ligament
Tendon of subscapularis (cut)
Communication between synovial cavity and subtendinous bursa of subscapularis
Intertubercular tendon sheath
Surgical neck of humerus
Tendon of long head of biceps brachii
Lateral border of scapula

**A. Anterior View**

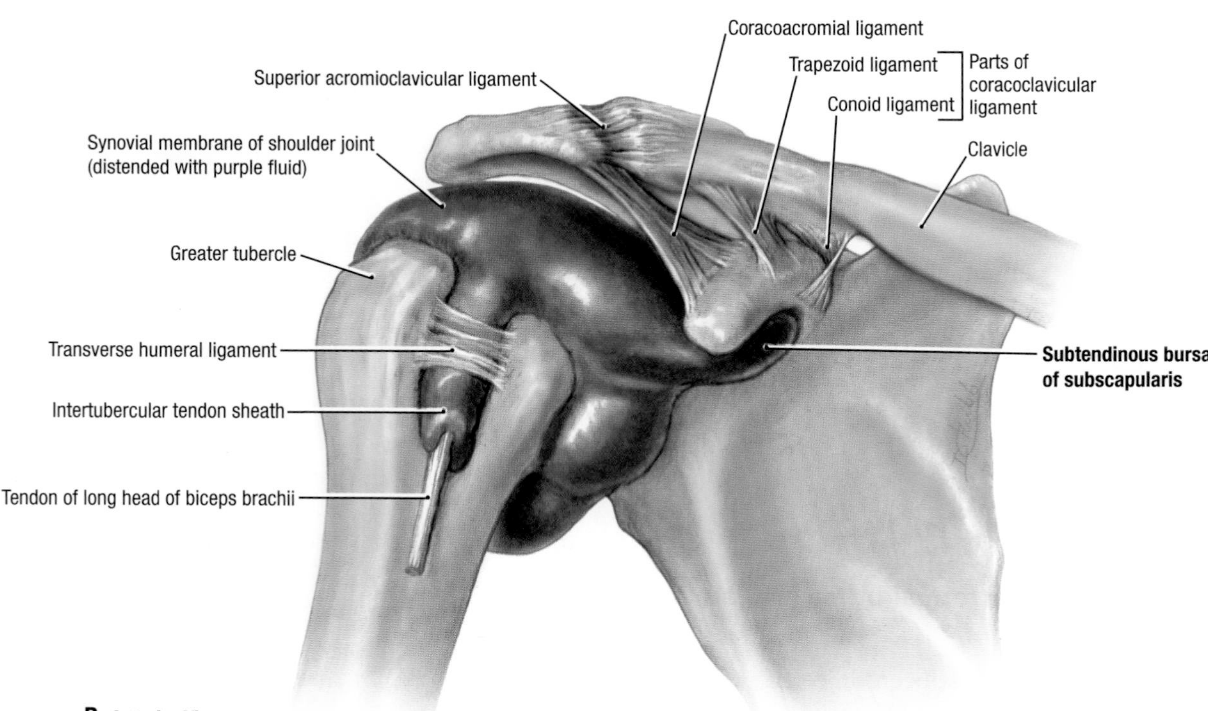
Coracoacromial ligament
Superior acromioclavicular ligament
Trapezoid ligament
Conoid ligament
Parts of coracoclavicular ligament
Synovial membrane of shoulder joint (distended with purple fluid)
Clavicle
Greater tubercle
Transverse humeral ligament
Subtendinous bursa of subscapularis
Intertubercular tendon sheath
Tendon of long head of biceps brachii

**B. Anterior View**

## 6.42 Ligaments and articular capsule of glenohumeral (shoulder) joint

**A.** Fibrous capsule.

- The loose fibrous capsule is attached to the margin of the glenoid cavity and to the anatomical neck of the humerus.
- The strong coracoclavicular ligament provides stability to the acromioclavicular joint and prevents the scapula from being driven medially and the acromion from being driven inferior to the clavicle.
- The coracoacromial ligament prevents superior displacement of the head of the humerus.

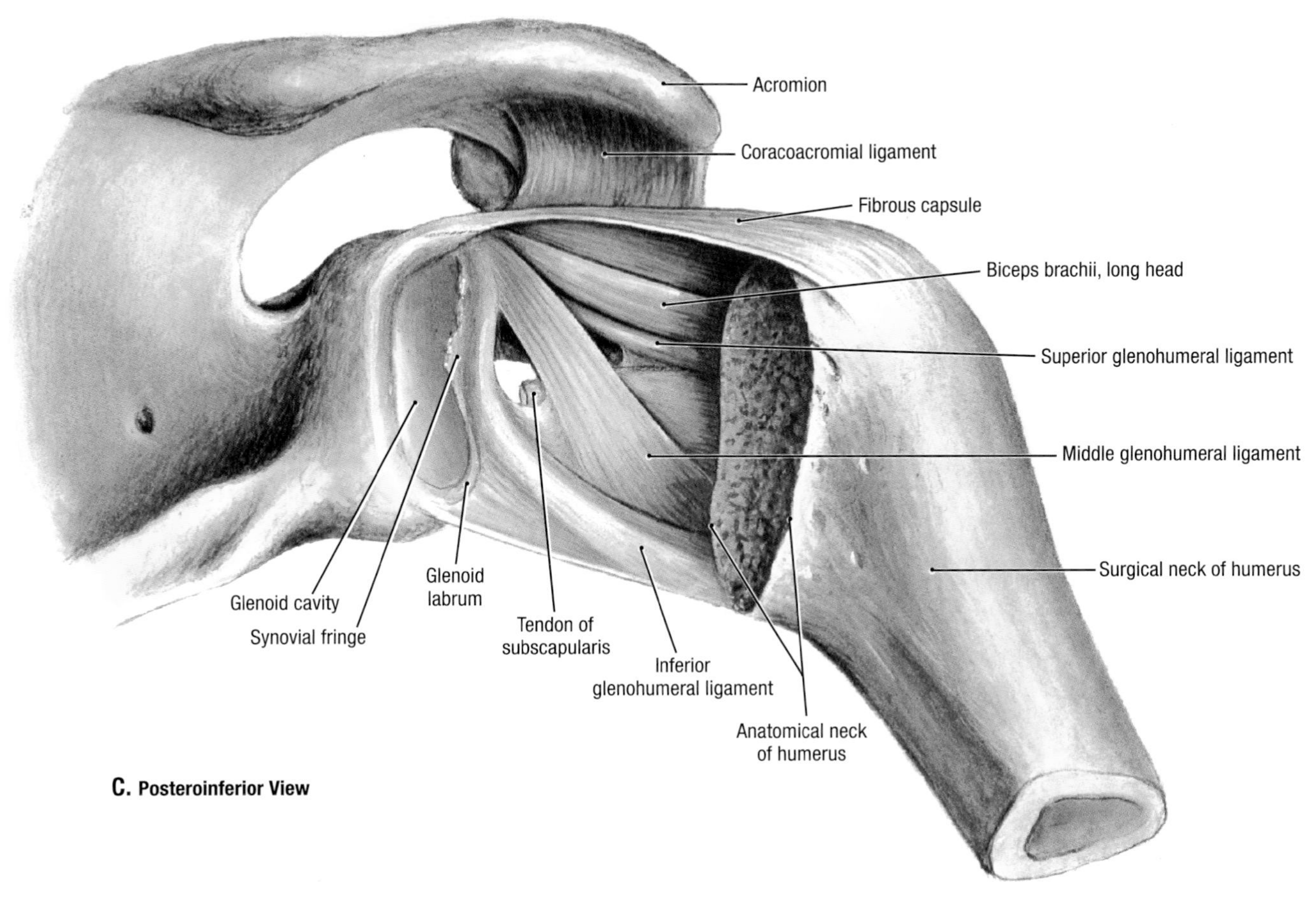
Acromion
Coracoacromial ligament
Fibrous capsule
Biceps brachii, long head
Superior glenohumeral ligament
Middle glenohumeral ligament
Surgical neck of humerus
Glenoid cavity
Synovial fringe
Glenoid labrum
Tendon of subscapularis
Inferior glenohumeral ligament
Anatomical neck of humerus
C. Posteroinferior View

## 6.42 Ligaments and articular capsule of glenohumeral (shoulder) joint *(continued)*

**B.** Synovial membrane of joint capsule. The synovial membrane lines the fibrous capsule and has two prolongations: (1) where it forms a synovial sheath for the tendon of the long head of the biceps muscle in its osseofibrous tunnel and (2) inferior to the coracoid process, where it forms a bursa between the subscapularis tendon and margin of the glenoid cavity—the subtendinous bursa of the subscapularis. **C.** Glenohumeral ligaments viewed from the interior of the shoulder joint.

- The joint is exposed from the posterior aspect by cutting away the thinner posteroinferior part of the capsule and sawing off the head of the humerus.
- The glenohumeral ligaments are visible from within the joint but are not easily seen externally.
- The glenohumeral ligaments and tendon of the long head of biceps brachii muscle converge on the supraglenoid tubercle.
- The slender superior glenohumeral ligament lies parallel to the tendon of the long head of biceps brachii. The middle ligament is free medially because the subtendinous bursa of subscapularis communicates with the joint cavity, usually there is only a single site of communication. In this individual there are openings on both sides of the ligament.

Because of its freedom of movement and instability, the glenohumeral joint is commonly dislocated by direct or indirect injury. Most dislocations of the humeral head occur in the downward (inferior) direction but are described clinically as anterior or (more rarely) posterior dislocations, indicating whether the humeral head has descended anterior or posterior to the infraglenoid tubercle and the long head of triceps. Anterior dislocation of the glenohumeral joint occurs most often in young adults, particularly athletes. It is usually caused by excessive extension and lateral rotation of the humerus.

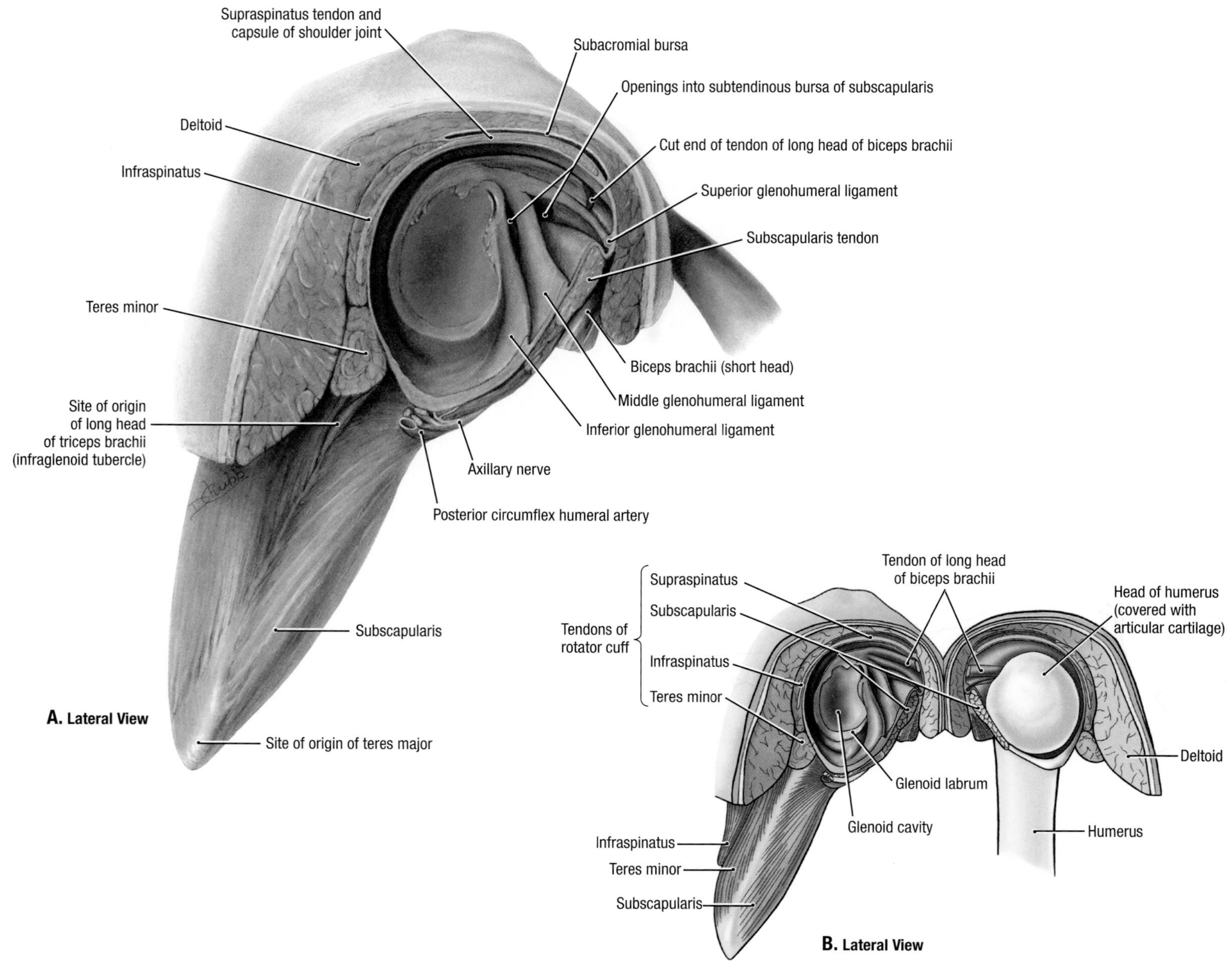
Supraspinatus tendon and capsule of shoulder joint
Subacromial bursa
Openings into subtendinous bursa of subscapularis
Deltoid
Cut end of tendon of long head of biceps brachii
Infraspinatus
Superior glenohumeral ligament
Subscapularis tendon
Teres minor
Biceps brachii (short head)
Middle glenohumeral ligament
Site of origin of long head of triceps brachii (infraglenoid tubercle)
Inferior glenohumeral ligament
Axillary nerve
Posterior circumflex humeral artery
Subscapularis
A. Lateral View
Site of origin of teres major
Tendons of rotator cuff
Supraspinatus
Subscapularis
Infraspinatus
Teres minor
Tendon of long head of biceps brachii
Head of humerus (covered with articular cartilage)
Deltoid
Glenoid labrum
Glenoid cavity
Humerus
Infraspinatus
Teres minor
Subscapularis
B. Lateral View

## 6.43 Interior of the glenohumeral (shoulder) joint and relationship of rotator cuff

**A.** Dissection. **B.** Schematic illustration.

- The fibrous capsule of the joint is thickened anteriorly by the three glenohumeral ligaments.
- The subacromial bursa is between the acromion and deltoid superiorly and the tendon of supraspinatus inferiorly.
- The four short rotator cuff muscles (supraspinatus, infraspinatus, teres minor, and subscapularis) cross the joint and blend with the capsule.
- The axillary nerve and posterior circumflex humeral artery are in contact with the capsule inferiorly and may be injured when the glenohumeral joint dislocates.

- Inflammation and calcification of the subacromial bursa result in pain, tenderness, and limitation of movement of the glenohumeral joint. This condition is also known as calcific scapulohumeral bursitis. Deposition of calcium in the supraspinatus tendon may irritate the overlying subacromial bursa, producing an inflammatory reaction, subacromial bursitis.

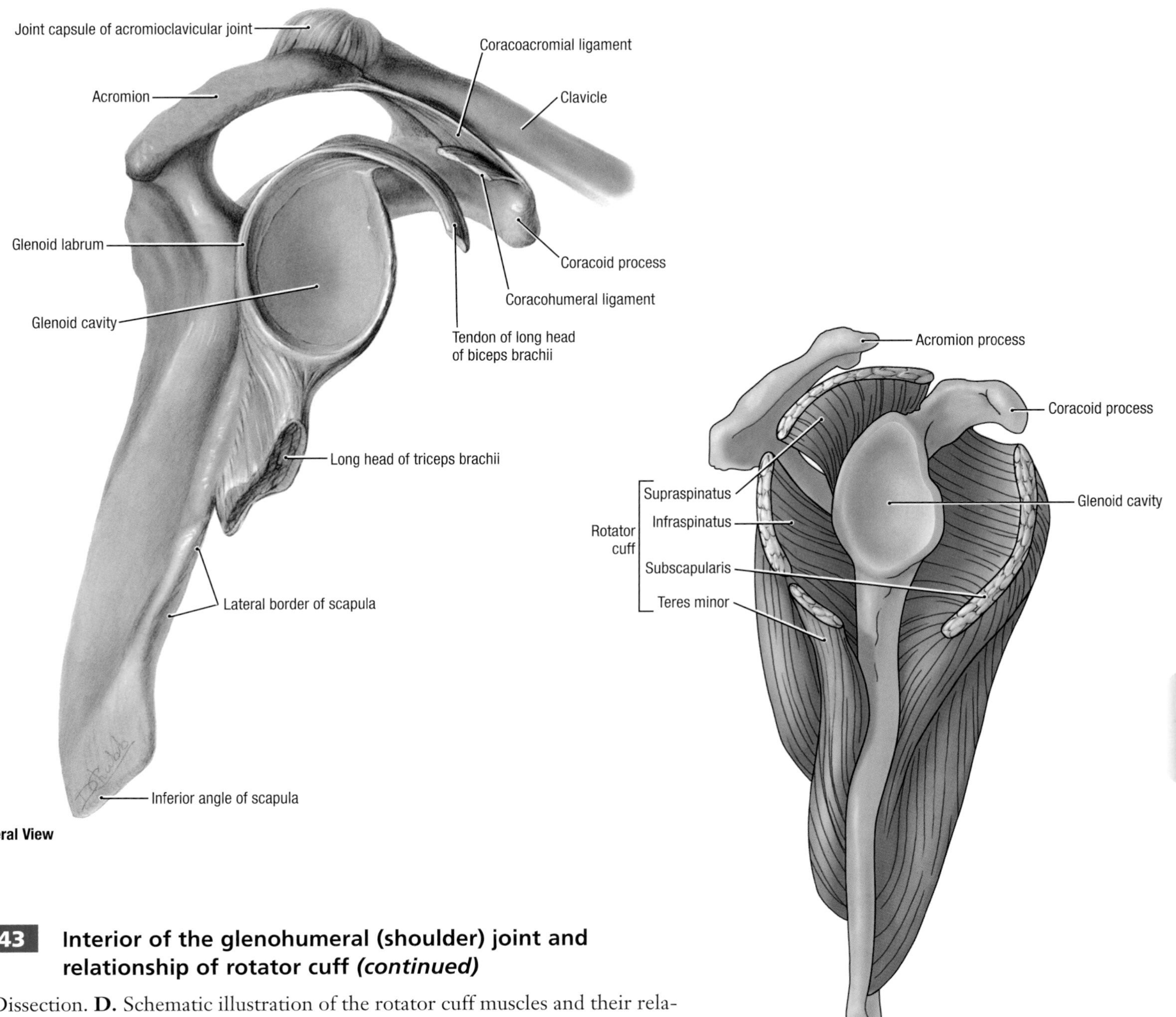
Joint capsule of acromioclavicular joint
Coracoacromial ligament
Acromion
Clavicle
Glenoid labrum
Coracoid process
Glenoid cavity
Coracohumeral ligament
Tendon of long head
of biceps brachii
Long head of triceps brachii
Lateral border of scapula
Inferior angle of scapula
C. Lateral View
Acromion process
Coracoid process
Supraspinatus
Infraspinatus
Rotator
cuff
Glenoid cavity
Subscapularis
Teres minor
D. Lateral View

## 6.43 Interior of the glenohumeral (shoulder) joint and relationship of rotator cuff *(continued)*

**C.** Dissection. **D.** Schematic illustration of the rotator cuff muscles and their relationship to the glenoid cavity.

- The coracoacromial arch (coracoid process, coracoacromial ligament, and acromion) prevents superior displacement of the head of the humerus.
- The long head of the triceps brachii muscle arises just inferior to the glenoid cavity; the long head of biceps just superior to it.
- The main function of the musculotendinous rotator cuff is to hold the large head of the humerus in the smaller and shallow glenoid cavity of the scapula, both during the relaxed state (by tonic contraction) and during active abduction.

Tearing of the fibrocartilaginous glenoid labrum commonly occurs in the athletes who throw (e.g., a baseball) and in those who have shoulder instability and subluxation (partial dislocation) of the glenohumeral joint. The tear often results from sudden contraction of the biceps or forceful subluxation of the humeral head over the glenoid labrum. Usually a tear occurs in the anterosuperior part of the labrum.

Acromion
Site of acromioclavicular joint
Spine of scapula
Clavicle
Superior border of scapula
Superior angle of scapula
Tubercle of 1st rib
Coracoid process
Greater tubercle
Shoulder joint
Deltoid muscle
Head of humerus
Surgical neck of humerus
Infraglenoid tubercle
Axillary fat
Lateral border of scapula
Vertebral border of scapula
Rim of glenoid fossa

**A. Anteroposterior View**

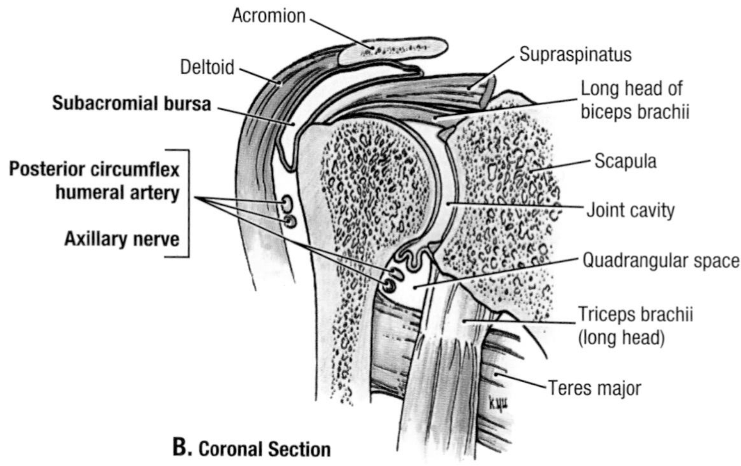

Acromion
Deltoid
Subacromial bursa
Posterior circumflex humeral artery
Axillary nerve
Supraspinatus
Long head of biceps brachii
Scapula
Joint cavity
Quadrangular space
Triceps brachii (long head)
Teres major


**B. Coronal Section**

## 6.44 Imaging of glenohumeral (shoulder) joint

**A.** Radiograph. **B.** Sectioned joint to show location of subacromial bursa and joint cavity.

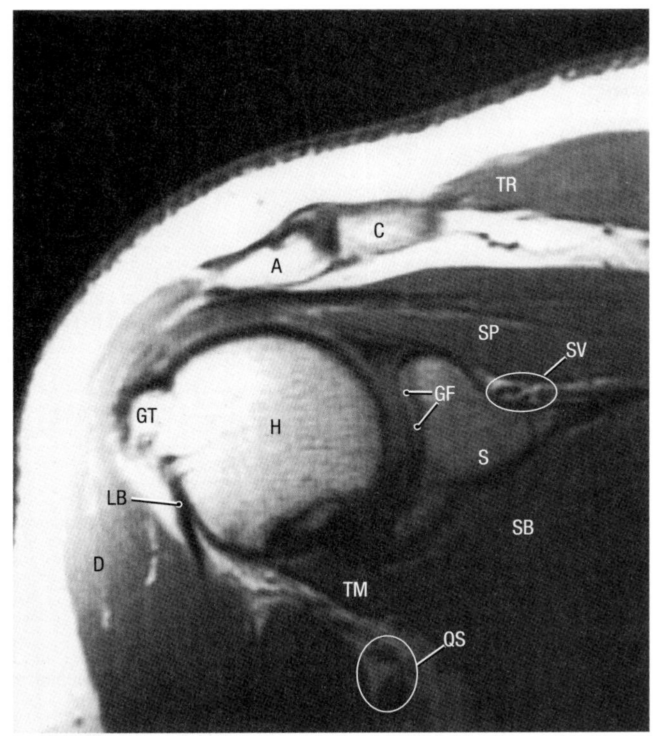
TR
C
A
SP
SV
GF
GT
H
S
LB
SB
D
TM
QS

**C.** Coronal MRI

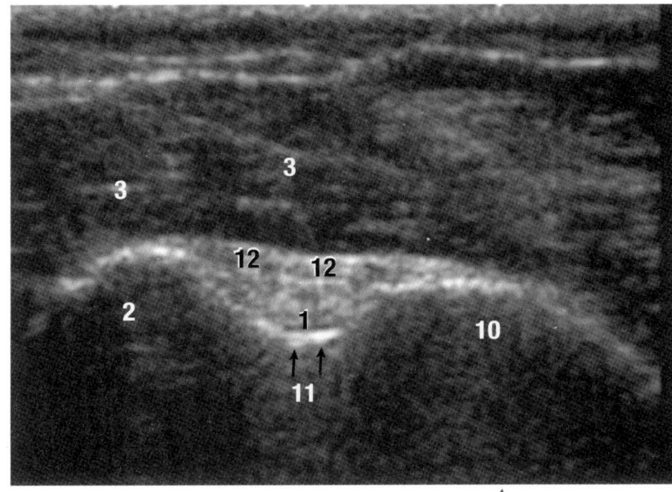
3
3
12
12
2
1
10
11

**D.** Transverse Scan

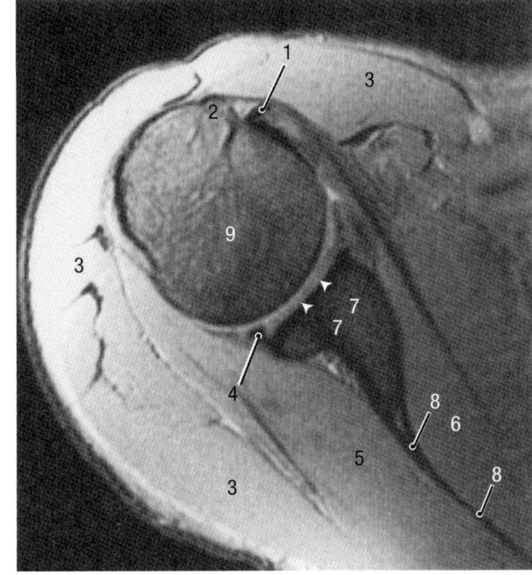
1
3
2
9
3
7
7
4
8
6
5
3
8

**E.** Transverse MRI

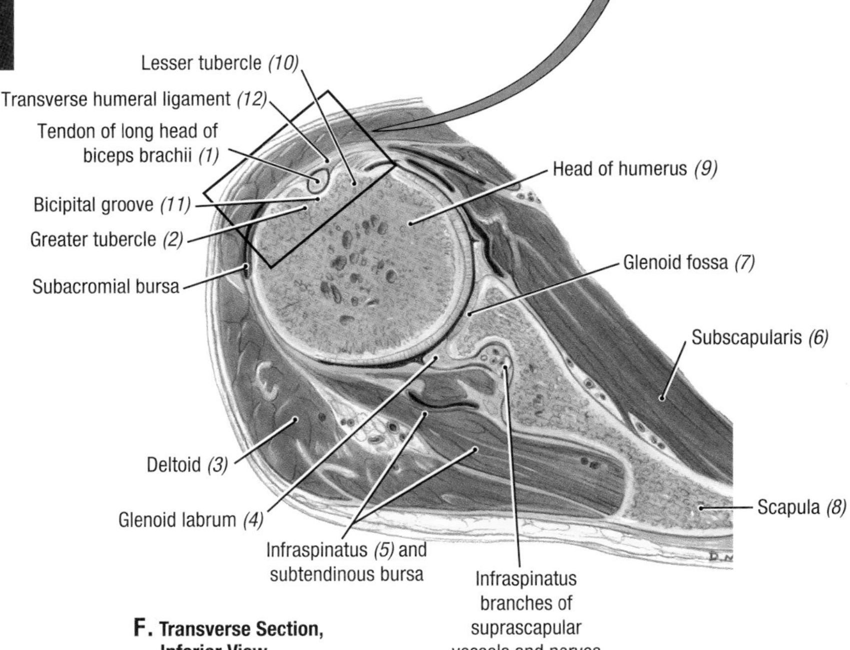
Lesser tubercle (10)
Transverse humeral ligament (12)
Tendon of long head of biceps brachii (1)
Bicipital groove (11)
Greater tubercle (2)
Subacromial bursa
Head of humerus (9)
Glenoid fossa (7)
Subscapularis (6)
Deltoid (3)
Glenoid labrum (4)
Infraspinatus (5) and subtendinous bursa
Infraspinatus branches of suprascapular vessels and nerves
Scapula (8)

**F.** Transverse Section, Inferior View

D
E, F

## 6.44 Imaging of glenohumeral (shoulder) joint *(continued)*

**C.** Coronal MRI. *A*, acromion; *C*, clavicle; *D*, deltoid; *GF*, glenoid cavity; *GT*, crest of greater tubercle; *H*, head of humerus; *LB*, long head of biceps brachii; *QS*, quadrangular space; *S*, scapula; *SB*, subscapularis; *SP*, supraspinatus; *SV*, suprascapular vessels and nerve; *TM*, teres minor; *TR*, trapezius. **D.** Transverse ultrasound scan of area indicated in **F. E.** Transverse MRI. **F.** Transverse section (*numbers* in **F** refer to structures labeled in **D** and **E**).

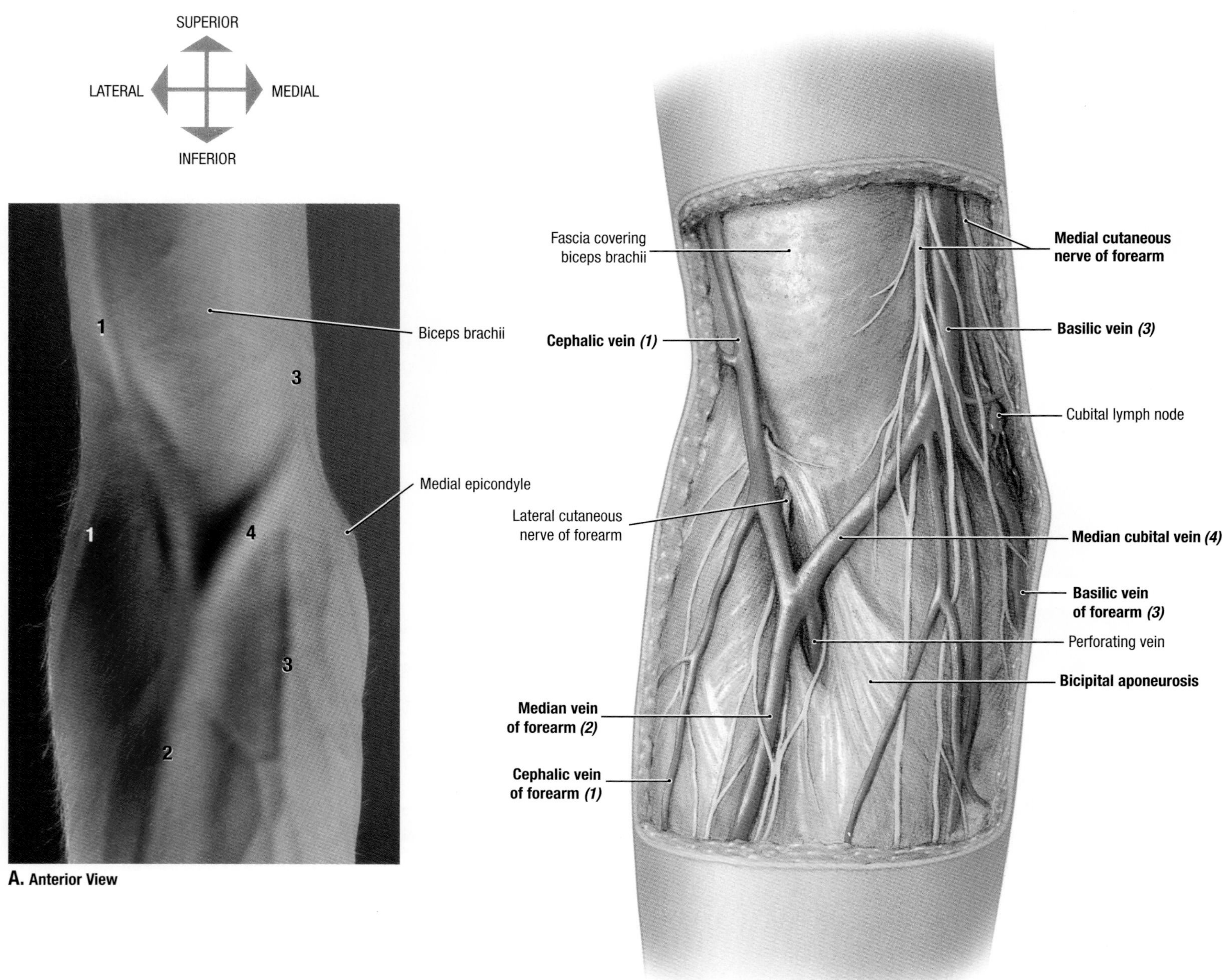
SUPERIOR
LATERAL
MEDIAL
INFERIOR
1
3
1
4
3
2
Biceps brachii
Medial epicondyle
A. Anterior View
Fascia covering biceps brachii
Cephalic vein (1)
Lateral cutaneous nerve of forearm
Median vein of forearm (2)
Cephalic vein of forearm (1)
Medial cutaneous nerve of forearm
Basilic vein (3)
Cubital lymph node
Median cubital vein (4)
Basilic vein of forearm (3)
Perforating vein
Bicipital aponeurosis
B. Anterior View

## 6.45 Cubital fossa: Surface anatomy and superficial dissection

**A.** Surface anatomy. **B.** Cutaneous nerves and superficial veins (*numbers* in parentheses refer to structures in **A**).

- The cubital fossa is a triangular space (compartment) inferior to the elbow crease, roofed by deep fascia.
- In the forearm, the superficial veins (cephalic, median, basilic, and their connecting veins) make a variable, M-shaped pattern.
- The cephalic and basilic veins occupy the bicipital grooves, one on each side of the biceps brachii. In the lateral bicipital groove, the lateral cutaneous nerve of the forearm appears just superior to the elbow crease; in the medial bicipital groove, the medial cutaneous nerve of the forearm becomes cutaneous at approximately the midpoint of the arm.
- The cubital fossa is the common site for sampling and transfusion of blood and intravenous injections because of the prominence and accessibility of veins. Usually, the median cubital vein or basilic vein is selected.

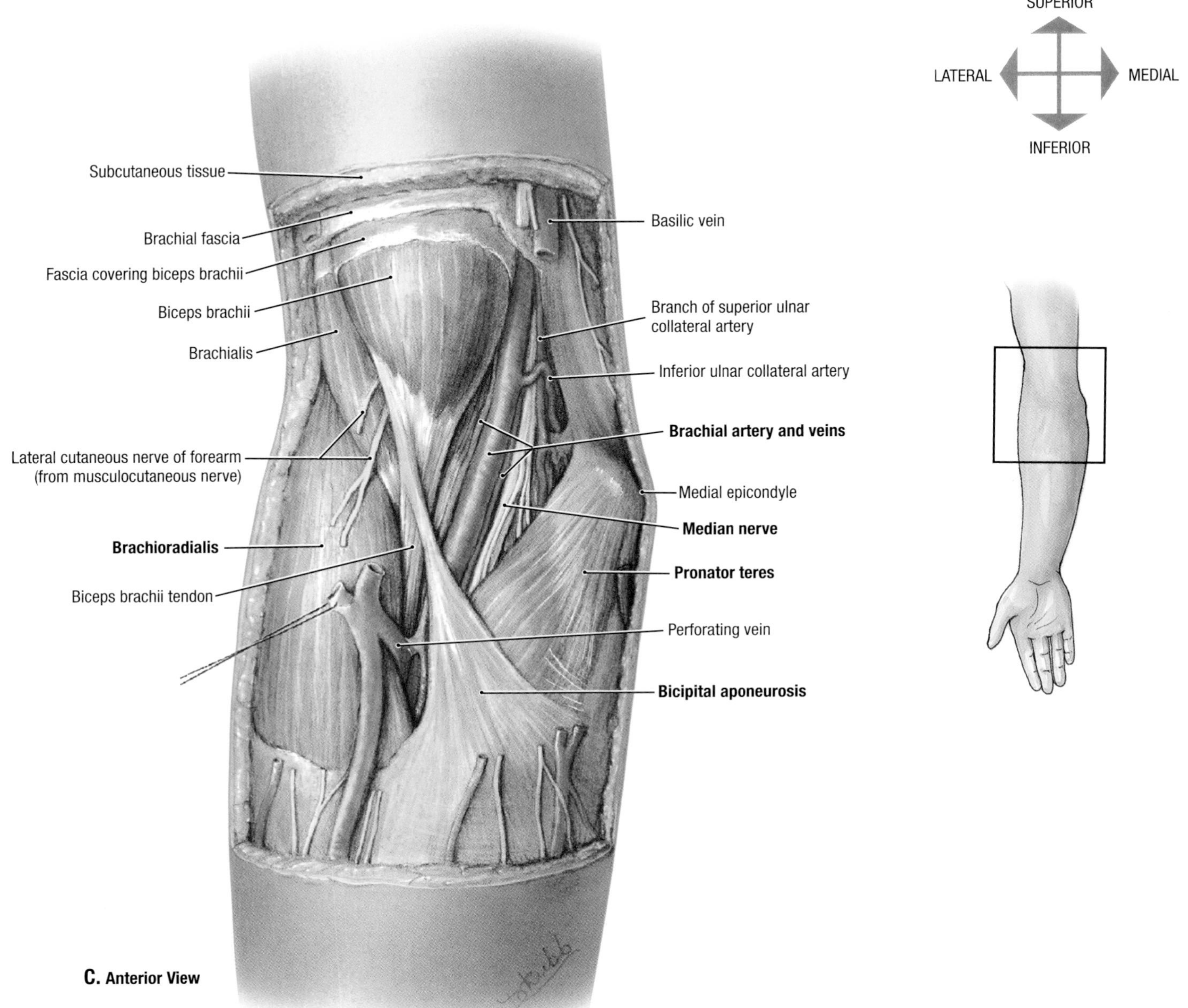
SUPERIOR
LATERAL
MEDIAL
INFERIOR
Subcutaneous tissue
Brachial fascia
Fascia covering biceps brachii
Biceps brachii
Brachialis
Lateral cutaneous nerve of forearm (from musculocutaneous nerve)
Brachioradialis
Biceps brachii tendon
Basilic vein
Branch of superior ulnar collateral artery
Inferior ulnar collateral artery
Brachial artery and veins
Medial epicondyle
Median nerve
Pronator teres
Perforating vein
Bicipital aponeurosis

C. Anterior View

## 6.45 Cubital fossa: Deep dissection I

C. Boundaries and contents of the cubital fossa.

- The cubital fossa is bound laterally by the brachioradialis and medially by the pronator teres and superiorly by a line joining the medial and lateral epicondyles.
- The three chief contents of the cubital fossa are the biceps brachii tendon, brachial artery, and median nerve.
- The biceps brachii tendon, on approaching its insertion, rotates through 90°, and the bicipital aponeurosis extends medially from the proximal part of the tendon.

- A fracture of the distal part of the humerus, near the supraepicondylar ridges, is called a *supraepicondylar fracture*. The distal bone fragment may be displaced anteriorly or posteriorly. Any of the nerves or branches of the brachial vessels related to the humerus may be injured by a displaced bone fragment.

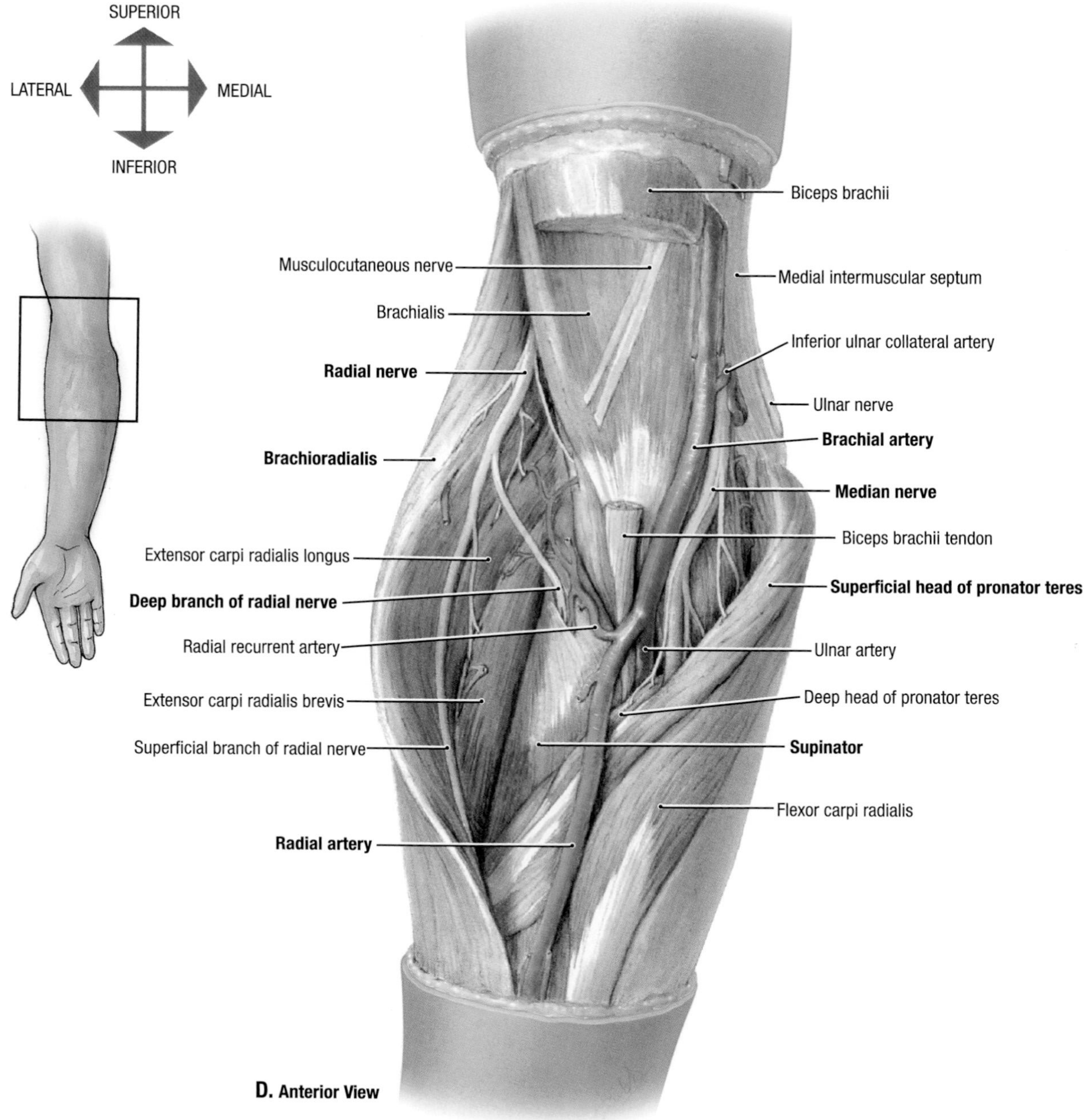
SUPERIOR
LATERAL
MEDIAL
INFERIOR
Biceps brachii
Musculocutaneous nerve
Medial intermuscular septum
Brachialis
Inferior ulnar collateral artery
Radial nerve
Ulnar nerve
Brachial artery
Brachioradialis
Median nerve
Biceps brachii tendon
Extensor carpi radialis longus
Superficial head of pronator teres
Deep branch of radial nerve
Radial recurrent artery
Ulnar artery
Extensor carpi radialis brevis
Deep head of pronator teres
Superficial branch of radial nerve
Supinator
Flexor carpi radialis
Radial artery
D. Anterior View

## 6.45 Cubital fossa: Deep dissection II

**D.** Floor of the cubital fossa.

- Part of the biceps brachii muscle is excised, and the cubital fossa is opened widely, exposing the brachialis and supinator muscles in the floor of the fossa.
- The deep branch of the radial nerve pierces the supinator.
- The brachial artery lies between the biceps tendon and median nerve and divides into two branches, the ulnar and radial arteries.
- The median nerve supplies the flexor muscles. With the exception of the twig to the deep head of pronator teres, its motor branches arise from its medial side.
- The radial nerve supplies the extensor muscles. With the exception of the twig to brachioradialis, its motor branches arise from its lateral side. In this specimen, the radial nerve has been displaced laterally, so here its lateral branches appear to run medially.

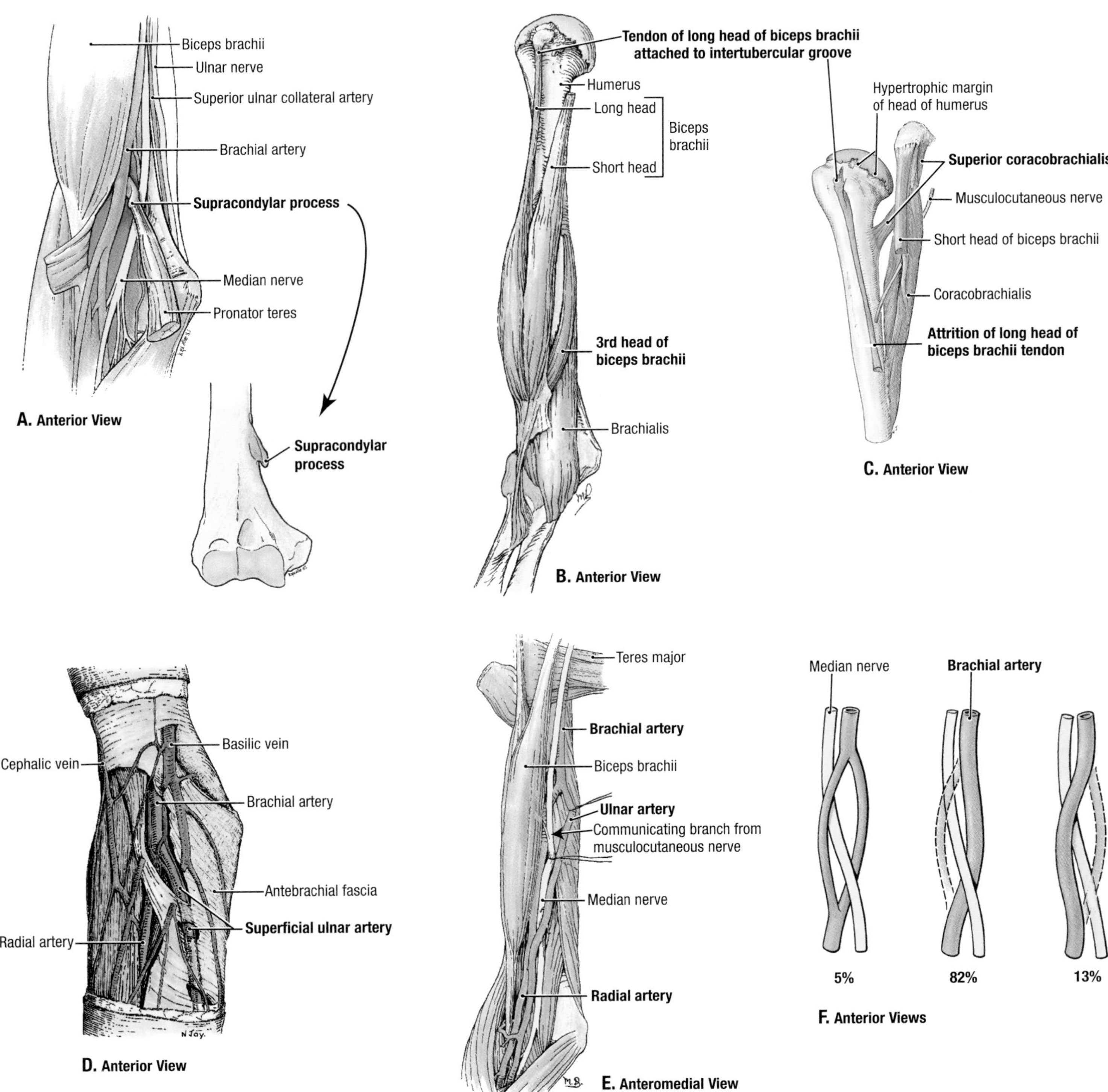
Biceps brachii
Ulnar nerve
Superior ulnar collateral artery
Brachial artery
Supracondylar process
Median nerve
Pronator teres
A. Anterior View
Supracondylar process
Tendon of long head of biceps brachii attached to intertubercular groove
Humerus
Long head
Short head
Biceps brachii
3rd head of biceps brachii
Brachialis
B. Anterior View
Hypertrophic margin of head of humerus
Superior coracobrachialis
Musculocutaneous nerve
Short head of biceps brachii
Coracobrachialis
Attrition of long head of biceps brachii tendon
C. Anterior View
Cephalic vein
Basilic vein
Brachial artery
Antebrachial fascia
Radial artery
Superficial ulnar artery
D. Anterior View
Teres major
Brachial artery
Biceps brachii
Ulnar artery
Communicating branch from musculocutaneous nerve
Median nerve
Radial artery
E. Anteromedial View
Median nerve
Brachial artery
5%
82%
13%
F. Anterior Views

## 6.46 Anomalies

**A.** Supracondylar process of humerus. A fibrous band, from which the pronator teres muscle arises, joins this supraepicondylar process to the medial epicondyle. The median nerve, often accompanied by the brachial artery, passes through the foramen formed by this band. This may be a cause of nerve entrapment. **B.** Third head of biceps brachii. In this case, there is also attrition of the biceps tendon. **C.** Attrition of the tendon of the long head of biceps brachii and presence of a coracobrachialis.

**D.** Superficial ulnar artery. **E.** Anomalous division of brachial artery. In this case, the median nerve passes between the radial and ulnar arteries, which arise high in the arm. **F.** Relationship of median nerve and brachial artery. The variable relationship of these two structures can be explained developmentally. In a study of 307 limbs, portions of both primitive brachial arteries persisted in 5%, the posterior in 82%, and the anterior in 13%.

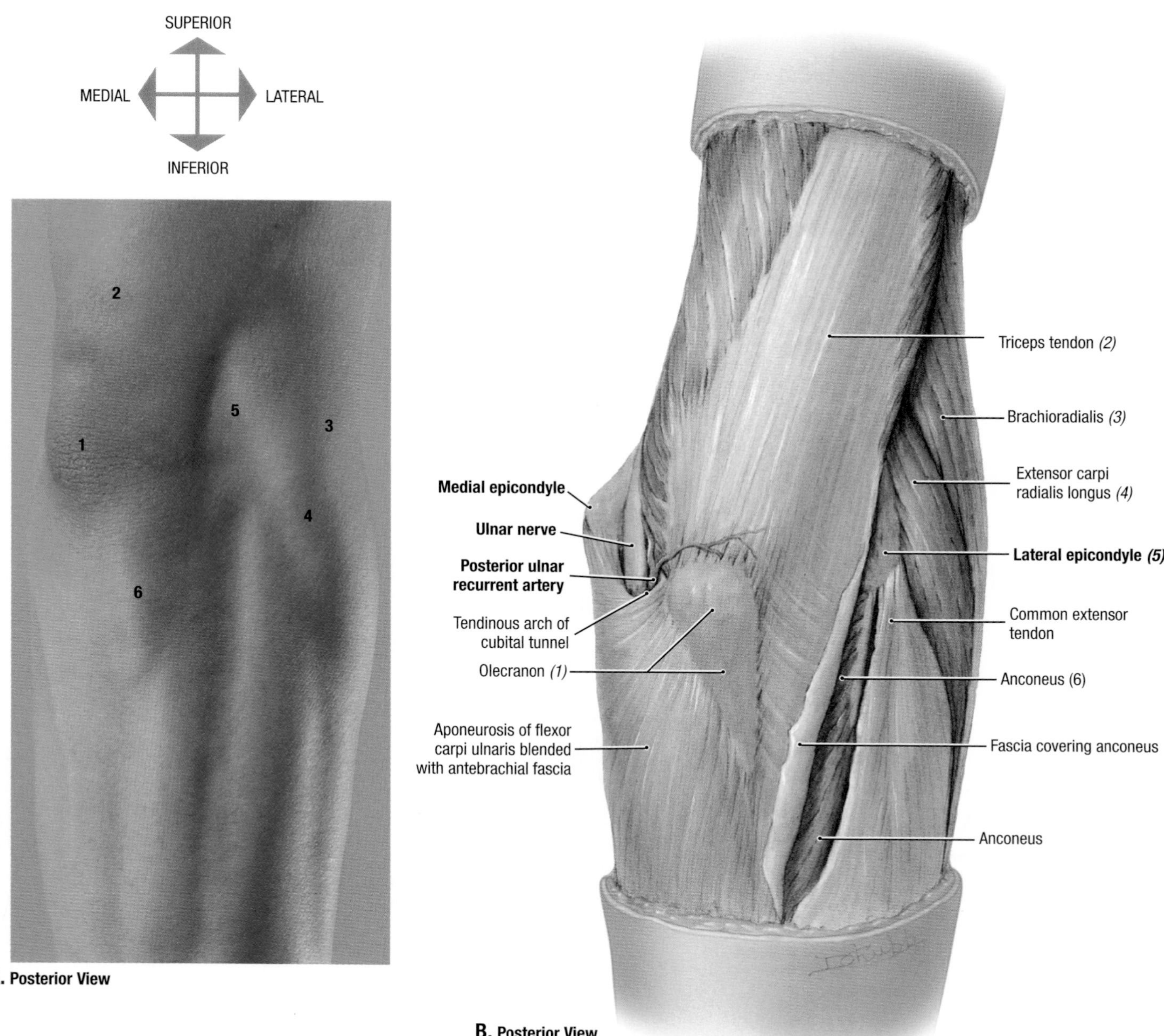
SUPERIOR
MEDIAL
LATERAL
INFERIOR
2
5
3
1
4
6
A. Posterior View
Triceps tendon (2)
Brachioradialis (3)
Extensor carpi radialis longus (4)
Medial epicondyle
Ulnar nerve
Lateral epicondyle (5)
Posterior ulnar recurrent artery
Tendinous arch of cubital tunnel
Common extensor tendon
Olecranon (1)
Anconeus (6)
Aponeurosis of flexor carpi ulnaris blended with antebrachial fascia
Fascia covering anconeus
Anconeus
B. Posterior View

## 6.47 Posterior aspect of elbow–I

**A.** Surface anatomy. **B.** Superficial dissection (*numbers* in parentheses refer to structures in **A**).

- The triceps brachii is attached distally to the superior surface of the olecranon and, through the deep fascia covering the anconeus, into the lateral border of olecranon.
- The posterior surfaces of the medial epicondyle, lateral epicondyle, and olecranon are subcutaneous and palpable.
- The ulnar nerve, also palpable, runs subfascially posterior to the medial epicondyle; distal to this point, it disappears deep to the two heads of the flexor carpi ulnaris.

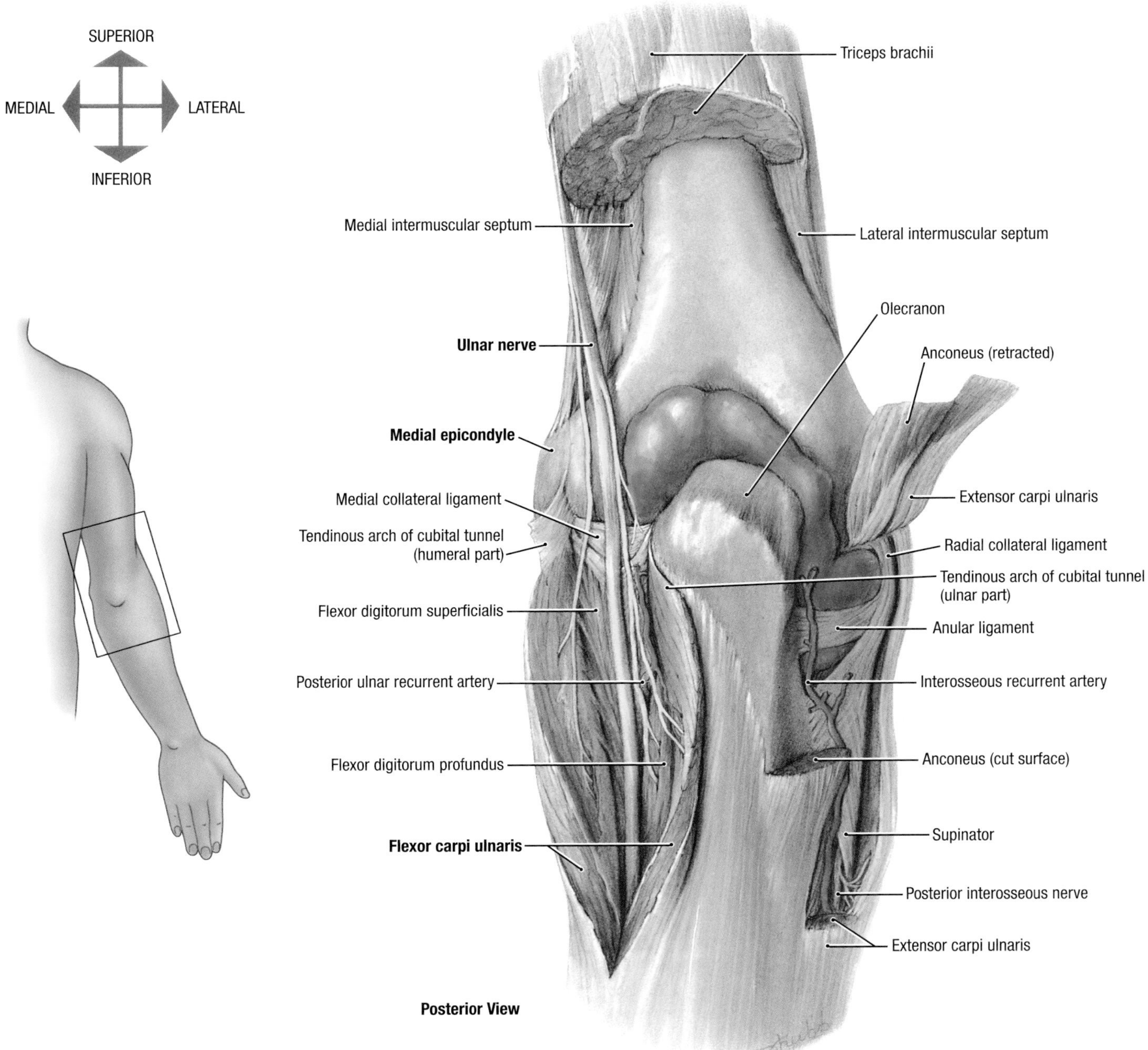
SUPERIOR
MEDIAL
LATERAL
INFERIOR
Triceps brachii
Medial intermuscular septum
Lateral intermuscular septum
Olecranon
Ulnar nerve
Anconeus (retracted)
Medial epicondyle
Medial collateral ligament
Extensor carpi ulnaris
Tendinous arch of cubital tunnel (humeral part)
Radial collateral ligament
Tendinous arch of cubital tunnel (ulnar part)
Flexor digitorum superficialis
Anular ligament
Posterior ulnar recurrent artery
Interosseous recurrent artery
Flexor digitorum profundus
Anconeus (cut surface)
Supinator
Flexor carpi ulnaris
Posterior interosseous nerve
Extensor carpi ulnaris
Posterior View

## 6.48 Posterior aspect of elbow–II

**C.** Deep dissection. The distal portion of the triceps brachii muscle was removed.

- The ulnar nerve descends subfascially within the posterior compartment of the arm, passing posterior to the medial epicondyle in the groove for the ulnar nerve. Next it passes posterior to the ulnar collateral ligament of the elbow joint and then between the flexor carpi ulnaris and flexor digitorum profundus muscles.

Ulnar nerve injury occurs most commonly where the nerve passes posterior to the medial epicondyle of the humerus. The injury results when the medial part of the elbow hits a hard surface, fracturing the medial epicondyle. The ulnar nerve may be compressed in the cubital tunnel (cubital tunnel syndrome) formed by the tendinous arch joining the humeral and ulnar heads of attachment of the flexor carpi ulnaris muscle. Ulnar nerve injury can result in extensive motor and sensory loss to the hand.

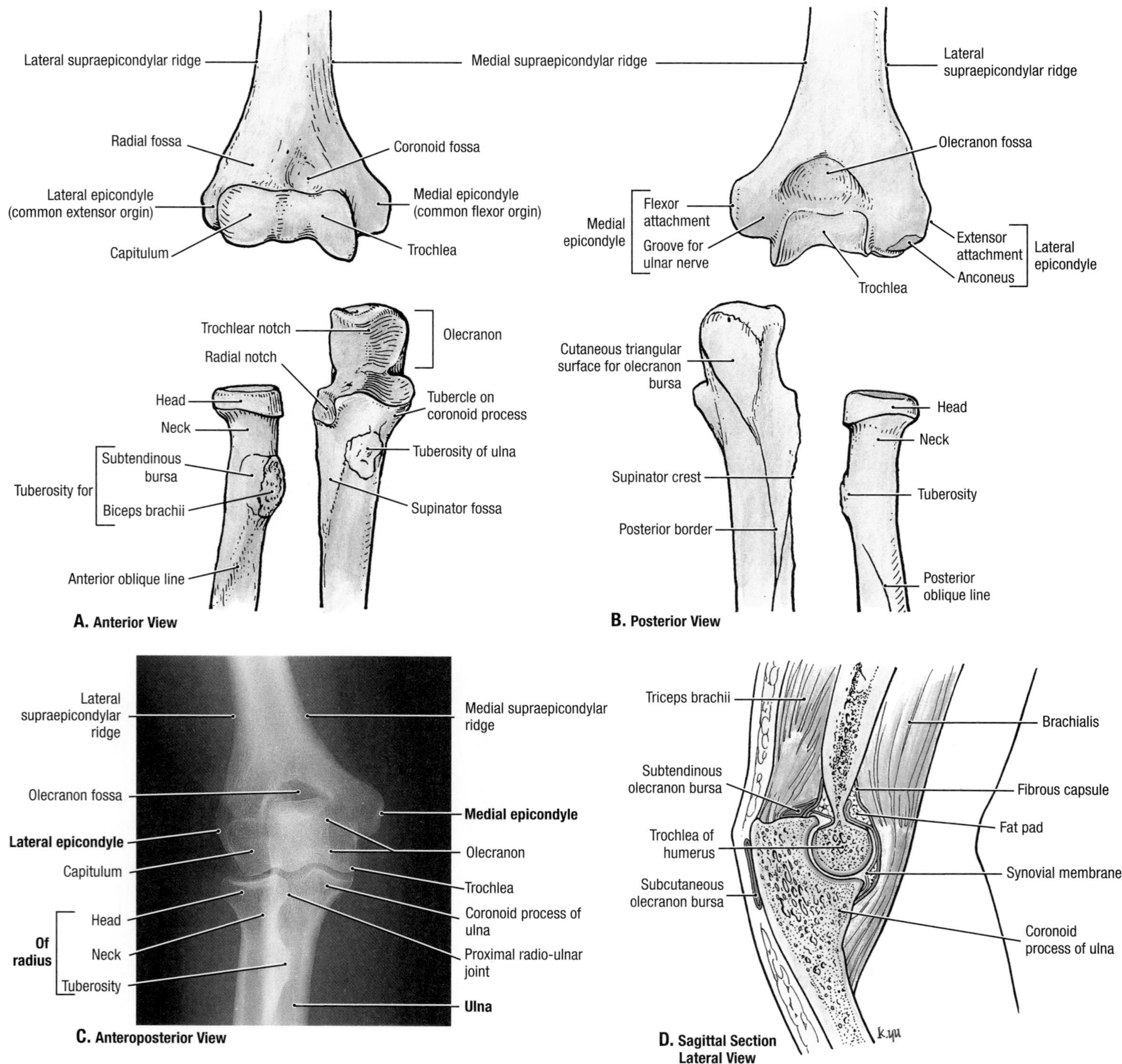
Lateral supraepicondylar ridge
Medial supraepicondylar ridge
Lateral supraepicondylar ridge
Radial fossa
Coronoid fossa
Olecranon fossa
Lateral epicondyle (common extensor orgin)
Medial epicondyle (common flexor orgin)
Capitulum
Trochlea
Medial epicondyle
Flexor attachment
Groove for ulnar nerve
Extensor attachment
Anconeus
Lateral epicondyle
Trochlea
Trochlear notch
Radial notch
Olecranon
Head
Neck
Tubercle on coronoid process
Tuberosity of ulna
Tuberosity for
Subtendinous bursa
Biceps brachii
Supinator fossa
Anterior oblique line
A. Anterior View
Cutaneous triangular surface for olecranon bursa
Head
Neck
Supinator crest
Tuberosity
Posterior border
Posterior oblique line
B. Posterior View
Lateral supraepicondylar ridge
Medial supraepicondylar ridge
Olecranon fossa
Medial epicondyle
Lateral epicondyle
Olecranon
Capitulum
Trochlea
Of radius
Head
Coronoid process of ulna
Neck
Proximal radio-ulnar joint
Tuberosity
Ulna
C. Anteroposterior View
Triceps brachii
Brachialis
Subtendinous olecranon bursa
Fibrous capsule
Fat pad
Trochlea of humerus
Synovial membrane
Subcutaneous olecranon bursa
Coronoid process of ulna
D. Sagittal Section Lateral View

## 6.49 Bones and imaging of elbow region

**A.** Anterior bony features. **B.** Posterior bony features. **C.** Radiograph of elbow joint. **D.** Section of humero-ulnar joint.

The subcutaneous olecranon bursa is exposed to injury during falls on the elbow and to infection from abrasions of the skin covering the olecranon. Repeated excessive pressure and friction produces a friction subcutaneous olecranon bursitis (e.g., "student's elbow"). Subtendinous olecranon bursitis results from excessive friction between the triceps tendon and the olecranon, for example, resulting from repeated flexion-extension of the forearm as occurs during certain assembly-line jobs. The pain is severe during flexion of the forearm because of pressure exerted on the inflamed subtendinous olecranon bursa by the triceps tendon.

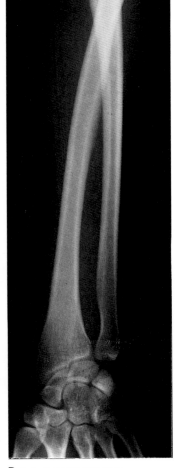

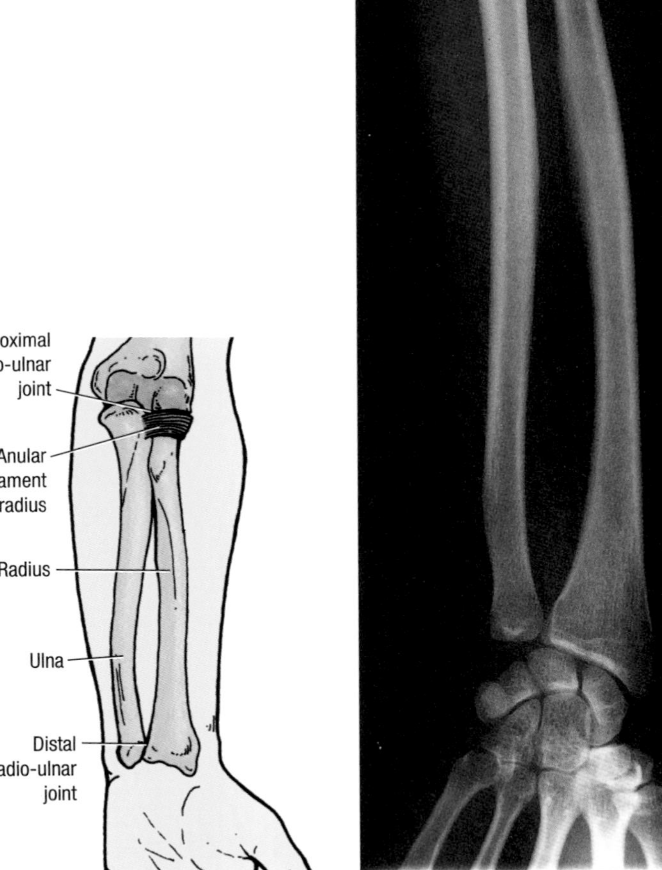
Proximal radio-ulnar joint
Anular ligament of radius
Radius
Ulna
Distal radio-ulnar joint

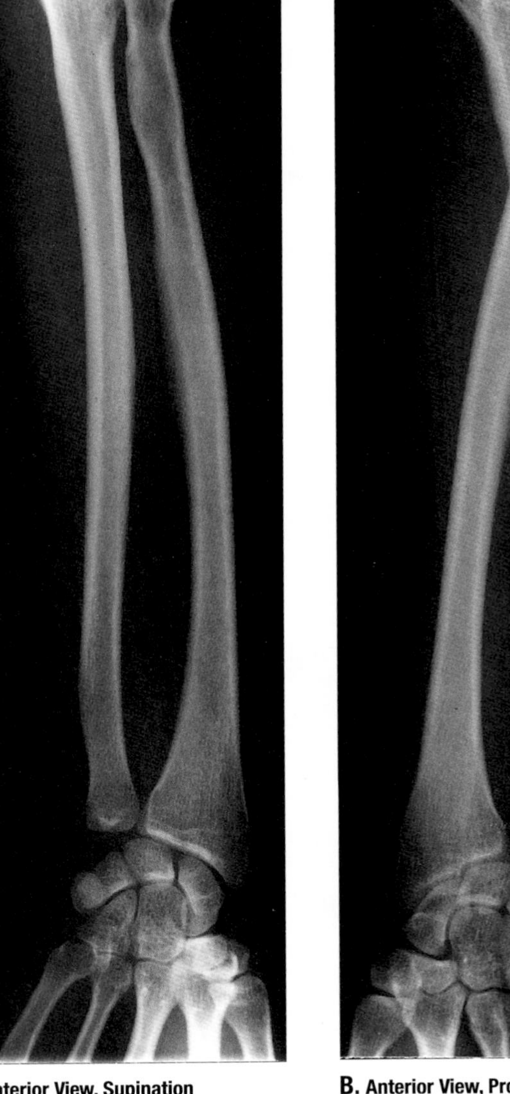

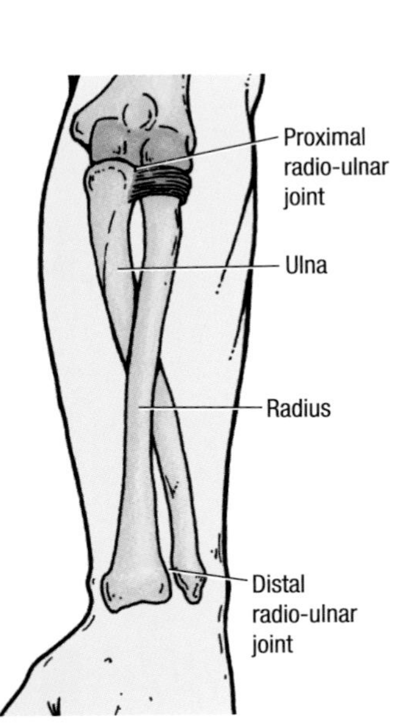
Proximal radio-ulnar joint
Ulna
Radius
Distal radio-ulnar joint

**A.** Anterior View, Supination

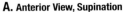

**B.** Anterior View, Pronation

## 6.50 Supination and pronation at superior, middle, and inferior radio-ulnar joints

**A.** Radiograph of forearm in supination. **B.** Radiograph of forearm in pronation. The radius crosses the ulna when the forearm is pronated. The superior and inferior radio-ulnar joints are synovial joints; the middle radio-ulnar joint is a syndesmosis (fibrous joint) in which the interosseous ligament connects the forearm bones.

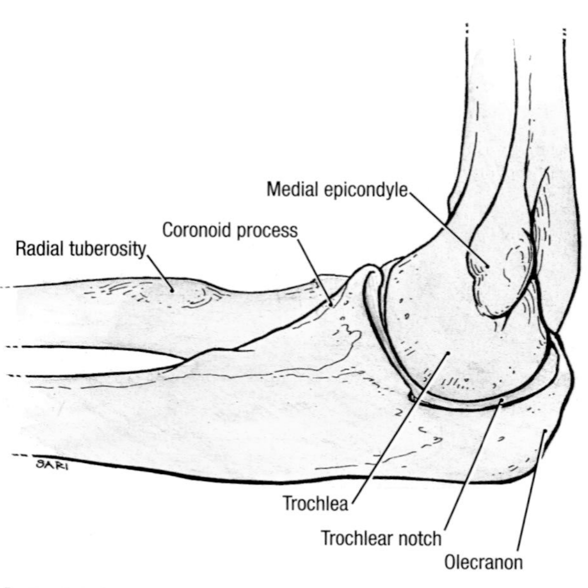

Medial epicondyle
Coronoid process
Radial tuberosity
Trochlea
Trochlear notch
Olecranon


**A. Medial View**

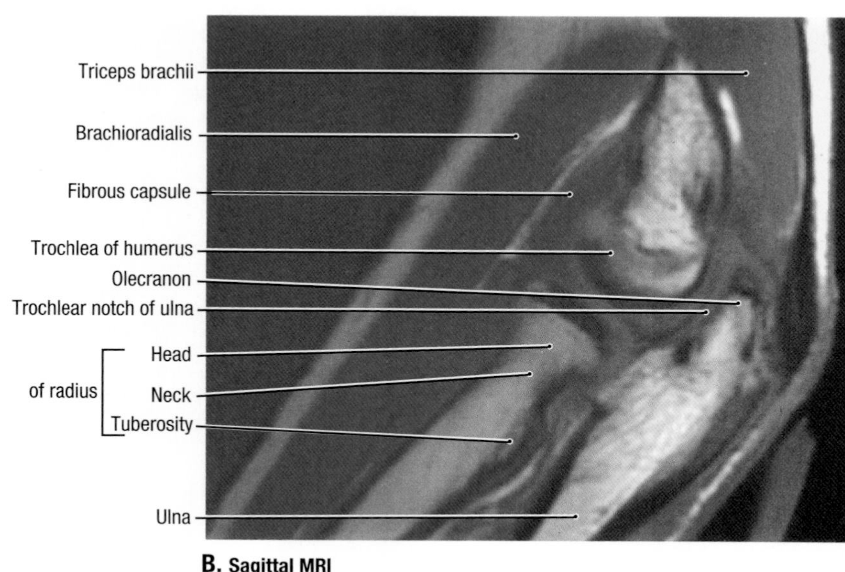

Triceps brachii
Brachioradialis
Fibrous capsule
Trochlea of humerus
Olecranon
Trochlear notch of ulna
Head
of radius
Neck
Tuberosity
Ulna


**B. Sagittal MRI**

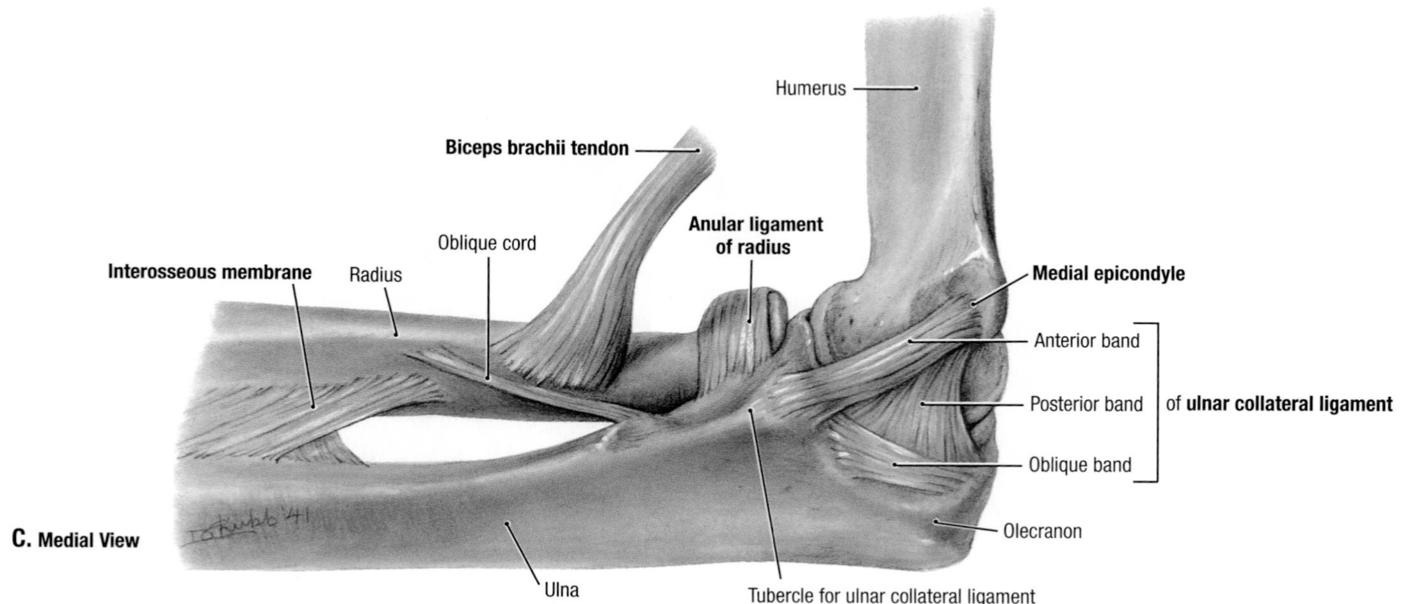

Humerus
Biceps brachii tendon
Oblique cord
Anular ligament of radius
Interosseous membrane
Radius
Medial epicondyle
Anterior band
Posterior band
of ulnar collateral ligament
Oblique band
Olecranon
Ulna
Tubercle for ulnar collateral ligament


**C. Medial View**

## 6.51 Medial aspect of bones and ligaments of elbow region

**A.** Bony features. **B.** MRI of elbow joint. **C.** Ligaments. The anterior band of the ulnar (medial) collateral ligament is a strong, round cord that is taut when the elbow joint is extended. The posterior band is a weak fan that is taut in flexion of the joint. The oblique fibers deepen the socket for the trochlea of the humerus.

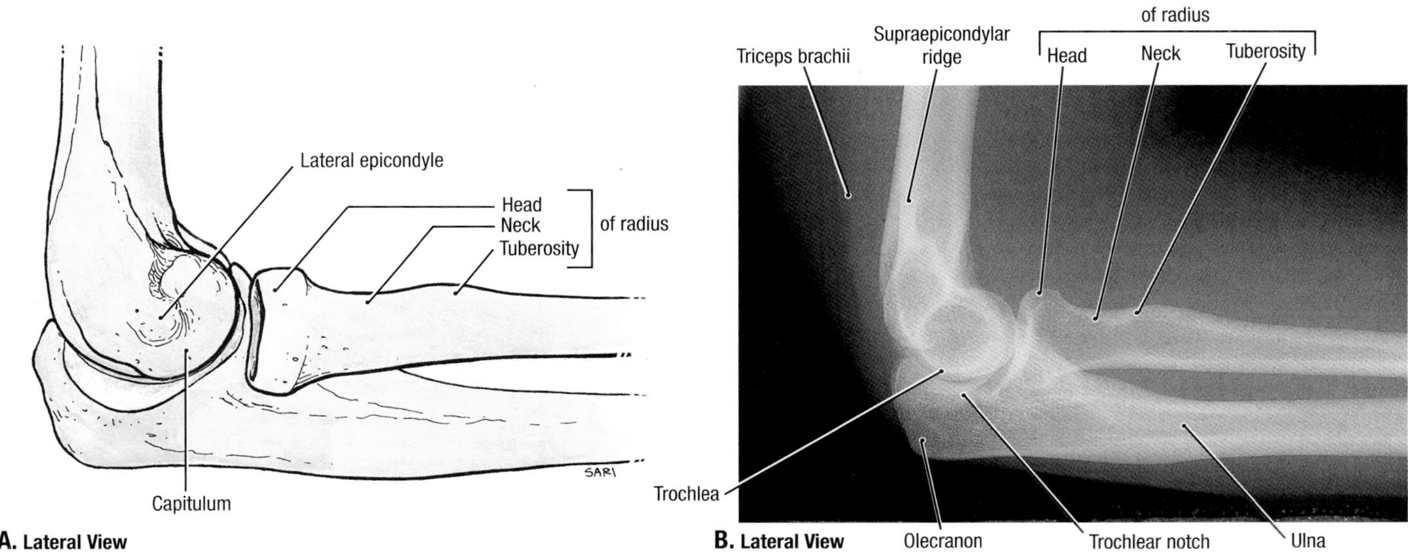
Lateral epicondyle
Head
Neck
Tuberosity
of radius
Capitulum
SARI
A. Lateral View
Triceps brachii
Supraepicondylar ridge
of radius
Head
Neck
Tuberosity
Trochlea
B. Lateral View
Olecranon
Trochlear notch
Ulna

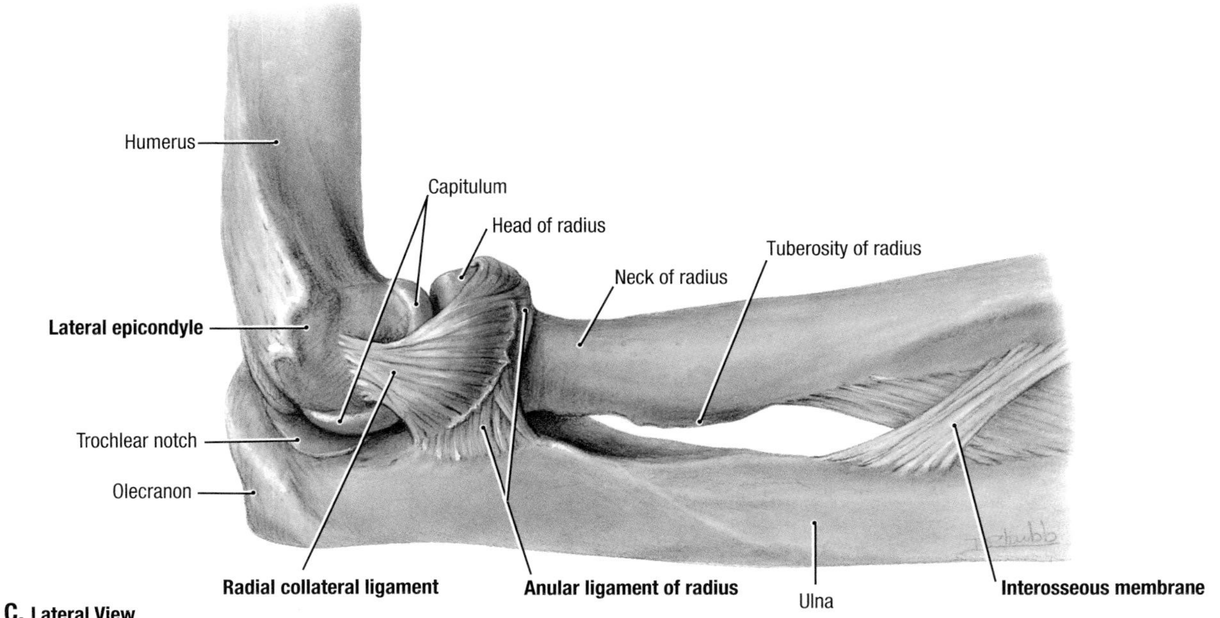
Humerus
Capitulum
Head of radius
Neck of radius
Tuberosity of radius
Lateral epicondyle
Trochlear notch
Olecranon
Radial collateral ligament
Anular ligament of radius
Ulna
Interosseous membrane
C. Lateral View

## 6.52 Lateral aspect of bones and ligaments of elbow region

**A.** Bony features. **B.** Lateral radiograph. **C.** Ligaments. The fan-shaped radial (lateral) collateral ligament is primarily attached to the anular ligament of the radius; superficial fibers of the lateral ligament blend with the fibrous capsule and continue onto the radius.

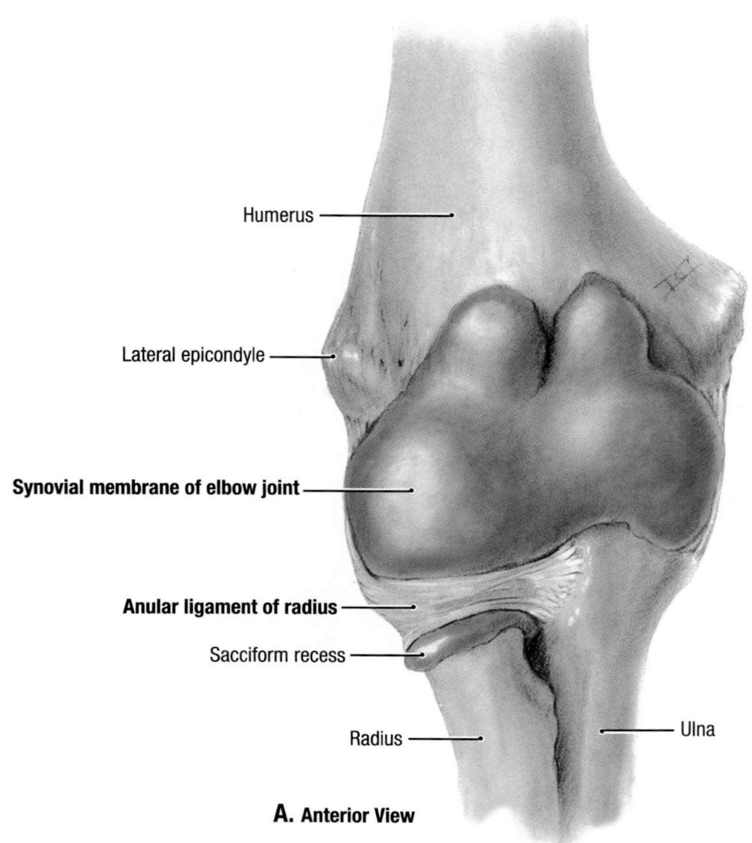
Humerus
Lateral epicondyle
Synovial membrane of elbow joint
Anular ligament of radius
Sacciform recess
Radius
Ulna
A. Anterior View

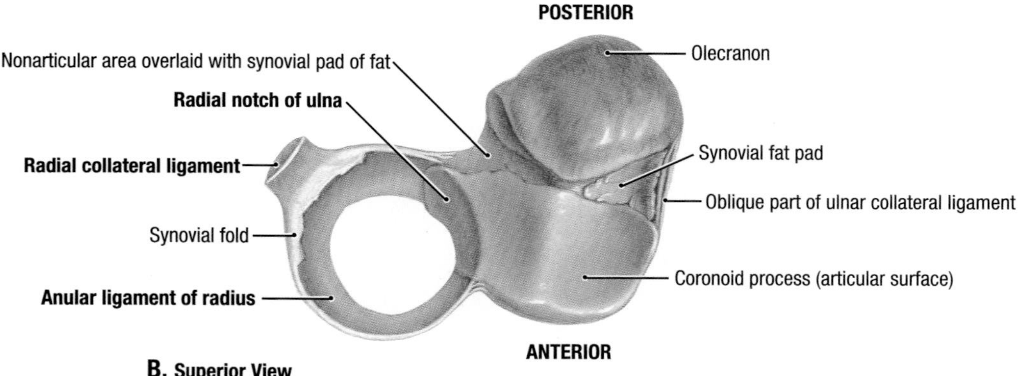
POSTERIOR
Nonarticular area overlaid with synovial pad of fat
Radial notch of ulna
Radial collateral ligament
Synovial fold
Anular ligament of radius
Olecranon
Synovial fat pad
Oblique part of ulnar collateral ligament
Coronoid process (articular surface)
ANTERIOR
B. Superior View

## 6.53 Synovial capsule of elbow joint and anular ligament

**A.** Synovial capsule of elbow and proximal radio-ulnar joints. The cavity of the elbow was injected with purple fluid (wax). The fibrous capsule was removed, and the synovial membrane remains. **B.** Anular ligament.

- The anular ligament secures the head of the radius to the radial notch of the ulna and with it forms a tapering columnar socket (i.e., wide superiorly, narrow inferiorly).
- The anular ligament is bound to the humerus by the radial collateral ligament of the elbow.

A common childhood injury is subluxation and dislocation of the head of the radius after traction on a pronated forearm (e.g., when lifting a child onto a bus). The sudden pulling of the upper limb tears or stretches the distal attachment of the less tapering anular ligament of a child. The radial head then moves distally, partially out of the anular ligament. The proximal part of the torn ligament may become trapped between the head of the radius and the capitulum of the humerus. The source of pain is the pinched anular ligament.

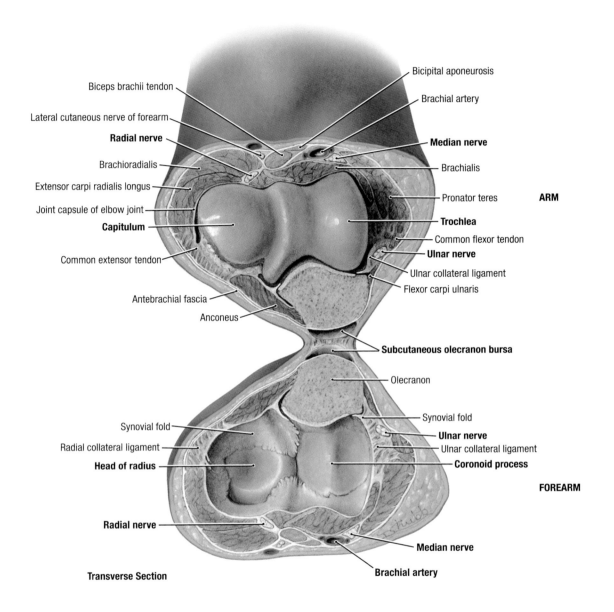

Biceps brachii tendon
Bicipital aponeurosis
Brachial artery
Lateral cutaneous nerve of forearm
Radial nerve
Median nerve
Brachioradialis
Brachialis
Extensor carpi radialis longus
Pronator teres
ARM
Joint capsule of elbow joint
Capitulum
Trochlea
Common flexor tendon
Ulnar nerve
Common extensor tendon
Ulnar collateral ligament
Flexor carpi ulnaris
Antebrachial fascia
Anconeus
Subcutaneous olecranon bursa
Olecranon
Synovial fold
Synovial fold
Ulnar nerve
Radial collateral ligament
Ulnar collateral ligament
Head of radius
Coronoid process
FOREARM
Radial nerve
Median nerve
Brachial artery
Transverse Section

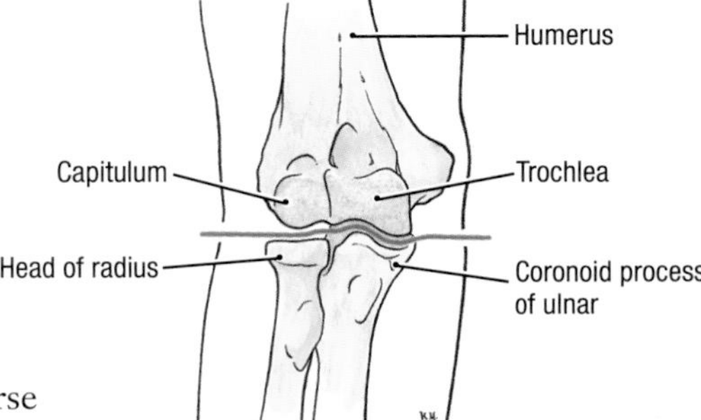
Humerus
Capitulum
Trochlea
Head of radius
Coronoid process of ulnar

## 6.54 Articular surfaces of elbow joint

The tissue surrounding the condyles of the humerus has been sectioned in a transverse plane, followed by disarticulation of the elbow joint, revealing the articular surfaces. Compare the forearm (inferior) component with Fig. 6.53B.

- Synovial folds containing fat overlie the periphery of the head of the radius and the nonarticular indentations on the trochlear notch of the ulna.
- The radial nerve is in contact with the joint capsule, the ulnar nerve is in contact with the ulnar collateral ligament, and the median nerve is separated from the joint capsule by the brachialis muscle.

**TABLE 6.9 ARTERIES OF FOREARM**

| Artery | Origin | Course/Distribution |
|---|---|---|
| Radial artery | In cubital fossa, as smaller terminal division of brachial artery | Runs distally under brachioradialis, lateral to flexor carpi radialis, defining boundary between the flexor and extensor compartments and supplying the radial aspect of both. Gives rise to a superficial palmar branch near the radio-carpal joint; it then transverses the anatomical snuff box to pass between the heads of the 1st dorsal interosseous muscle joining the deep branch of the ulnar artery to form the deep palmar arch |
| Ulanr artery | In cubital fossa, as larger terminal division of brachial artery | Passes distally between 2nd and 3rd layers of forearm flexor muscles, supplying ulnar aspect of flexor compartment; passes superficial to flexor retinaculum at wrist, continuing as the superficial palmar arch (with superficial branch of radial) after its deep palmar branch joins the deep palmar arch |
| Radial recurrent artery | In cubital fossa, as 1st (lateral) branch of radial artery | Courses proximally, superficial to supinator, passing between brachioradialis and brachialis to anastomose with radial collateral artery |
| Anterior and posterior ulnar recurrent arteries | In and immediately distal to cubital fossa, as 1st and 2nd medial branches of ulnar artery | Course proximally to anastomose with the inferior and superior ulnar collateral arteries, respectively, forming collateral pathways anterior and posterior to the medial epicondyle of the humerus |
| Common interosseous artery | Immediately distal to the cubital fossa, as 1st lateral branch of ulnar artery | Terminates almost immediately, dividing into anterior and posterior interosseous arteries |
| Anterior and posterior interosseous arteries | Distal to radial tubercle, as terminal branches of common interosseous | Pass to opposite sides of interosseous membrane; anterior artery runs on interosseous membrane; posterior artery runs between superficial and deep layers of extensor muscles as primary artery of compartment |
| Interosseous recurrent artery | Initial part of posterior interosseous artery | Courses proximally between lateral epicondyle and olecranon, deep to anconeus, to anastomose with middle collateral artery |

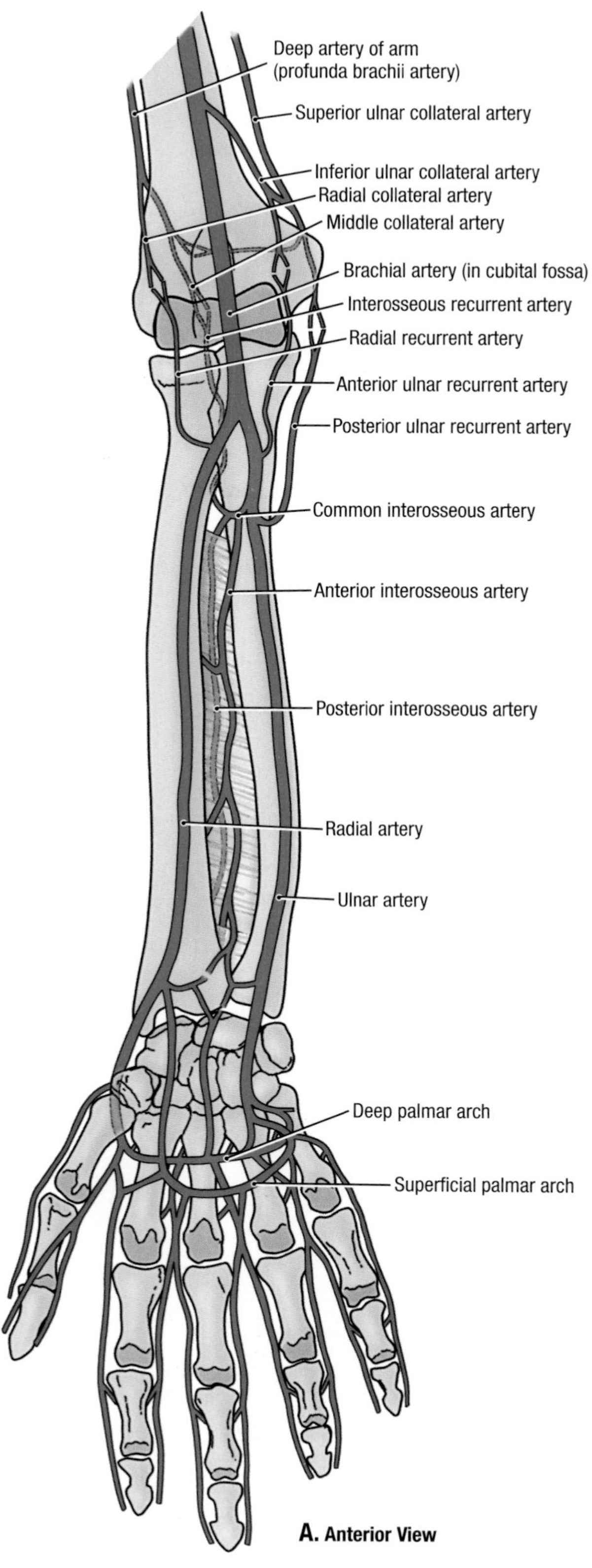
Deep artery of arm
(profunda brachii artery)
Superior ulnar collateral artery
Inferior ulnar collateral artery
Radial collateral artery
Middle collateral artery
Brachial artery (in cubital fossa)
Interosseous recurrent artery
Radial recurrent artery
Anterior ulnar recurrent artery
Posterior ulnar recurrent artery
Common interosseous artery
Anterior interosseous artery
Posterior interosseous artery
Radial artery
Ulnar artery
Deep palmar arch
Superficial palmar arch

**A. Anterior View**

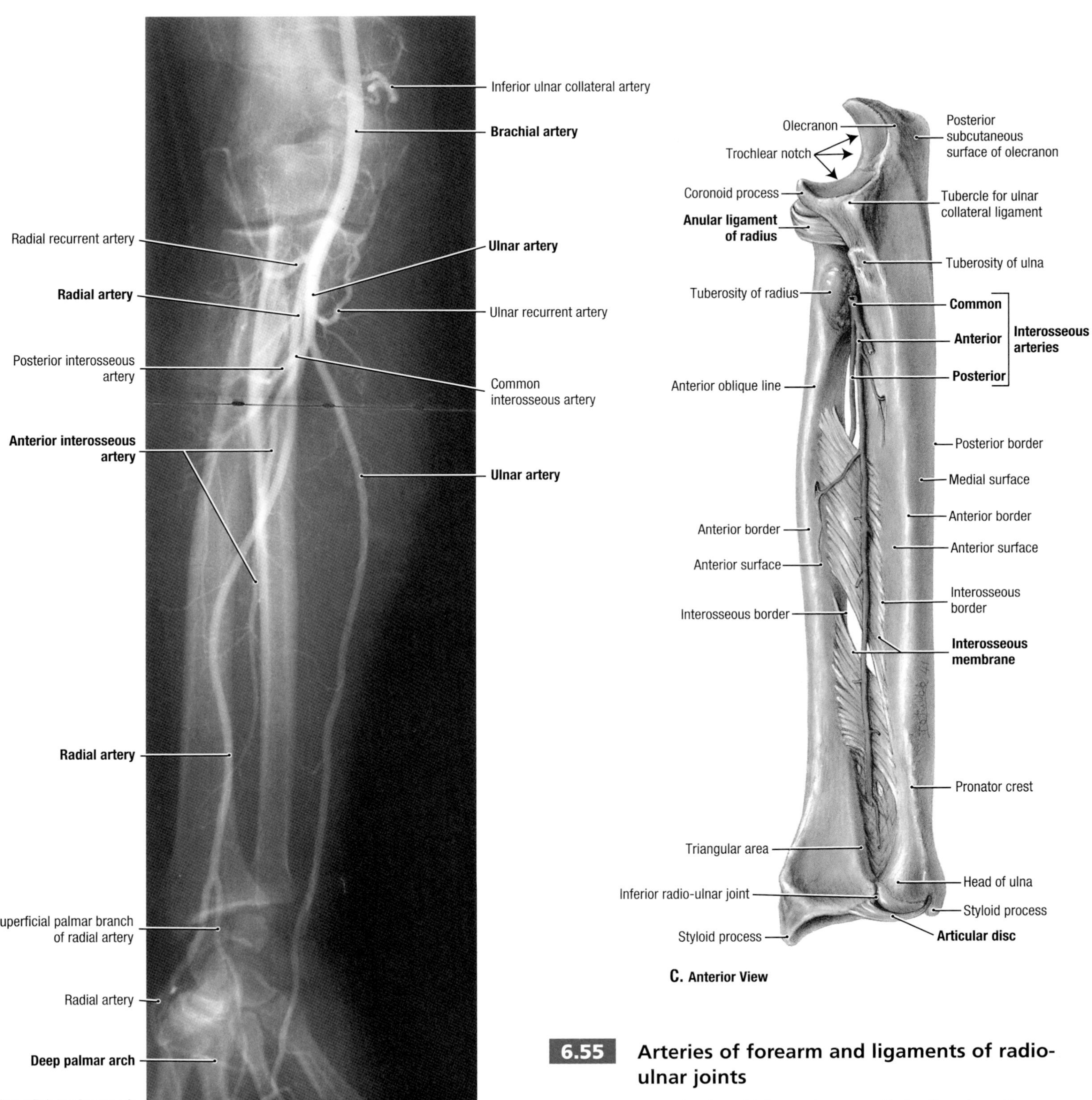
Inferior ulnar collateral artery
Brachial artery
Radial recurrent artery
Ulnar artery
Radial artery
Ulnar recurrent artery
Posterior interosseous artery
Common interosseous artery
Anterior interosseous artery
Ulnar artery
Radial artery
Superficial palmar branch of radial artery
Radial artery
Deep palmar arch
Superficial palmar arch
B. Anteroposterior View
Olecranon
Trochlear notch
Posterior subcutaneous surface of olecranon
Coronoid process
Tubercle for ulnar collateral ligament
Anular ligament of radius
Tuberosity of ulna
Tuberosity of radius
Common
Anterior
Posterior
Interosseous arteries
Anterior oblique line
Posterior border
Medial surface
Anterior border
Anterior border
Anterior surface
Anterior surface
Interosseous border
Interosseous border
Interosseous membrane
Pronator crest
Triangular area
Head of ulna
Inferior radio-ulnar joint
Styloid process
Styloid process
Articular disc
C. Anterior View

## 6.55 Arteries of forearm and ligaments of radio-ulnar joints

**A.** Anterior view **B.** Brachial arteriogram. **C.** Radio-ulnar ligaments and interosseous arteries. The ligament maintaining the proximal radio-ulnar joint is the anular ligament, that for the distal joint is the articular disc, and that for the middle joint is the interosseous membrane. The interosseous membrane is attached to the interosseous borders of the radius and ulna, but it also spreads onto their surfaces.

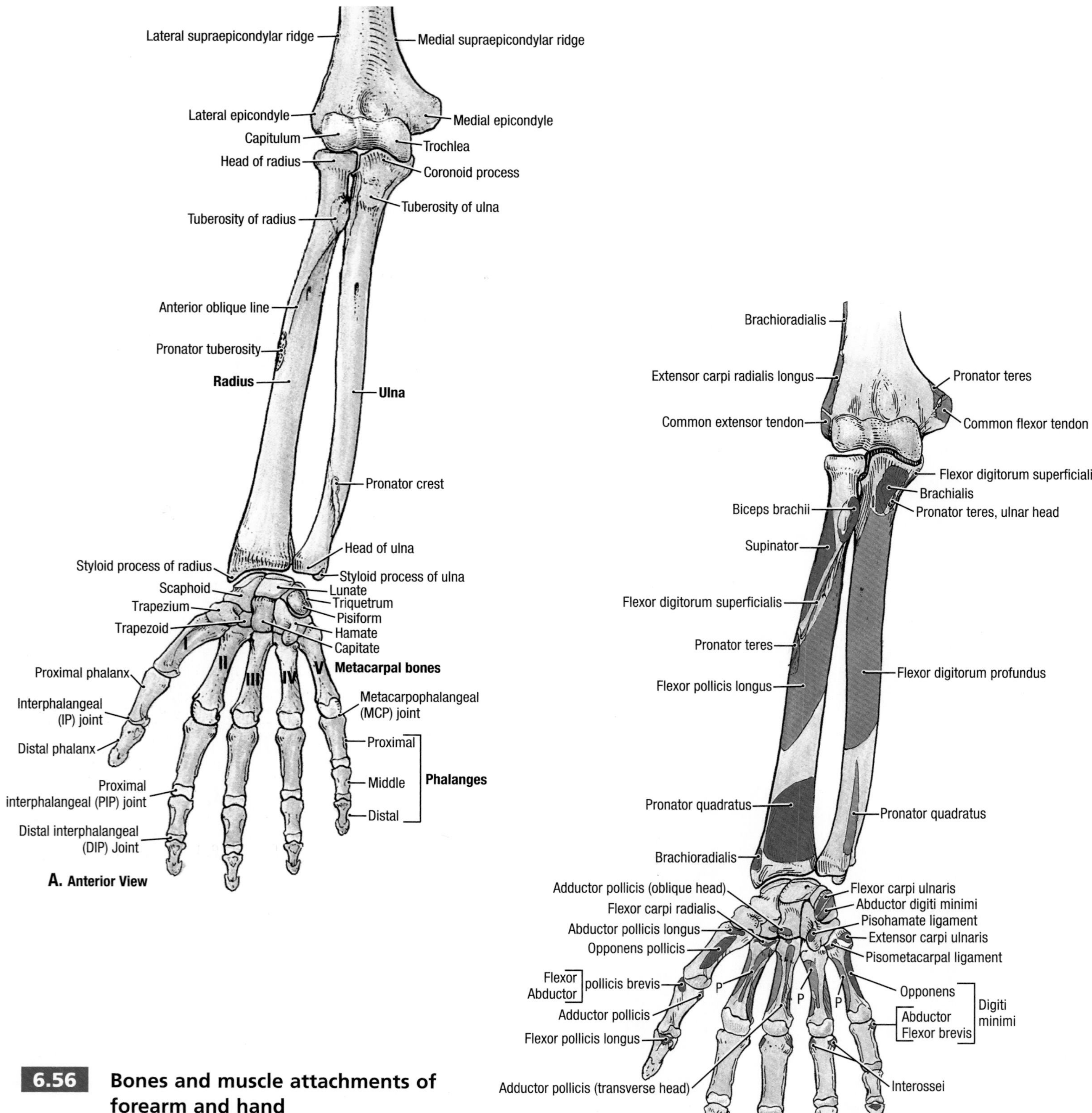

Lateral supraepicondylar ridge
Medial supraepicondylar ridge
Lateral epicondyle
Medial epicondyle
Capitulum
Trochlea
Head of radius
Coronoid process
Tuberosity of ulna
Tuberosity of radius
Anterior oblique line
Pronator tuberosity
Radius
Ulna
Pronator crest
Head of ulna
Styloid process of radius
Styloid process of ulna
Scaphoid
Lunate
Trapezium
Triquetrum
Pisiform
Trapezoid
Hamate
Capitate
I
II
III
IV
V
Metacarpal bones
Proximal phalanx
Interphalangeal (IP) joint
Metacarpophalangeal (MCP) joint
Distal phalanx
Proximal
Middle
Distal
Phalanges
Proximal interphalangeal (PIP) joint
Distal interphalangeal (DIP) Joint
A. Anterior View
Brachioradialis
Extensor carpi radialis longus
Pronator teres
Common extensor tendon
Common flexor tendon
Flexor digitorum superficialis
Brachialis
Biceps brachii
Pronator teres, ulnar head
Supinator
Flexor digitorum superficialis
Pronator teres
Flexor pollicis longus
Flexor digitorum profundus
Pronator quadratus
Pronator quadratus
Brachioradialis
Adductor pollicis (oblique head)
Flexor carpi ulnaris
Flexor carpi radialis
Abductor digiti minimi
Abductor pollicis longus
Pisohamate ligament
Opponens pollicis
Extensor carpi ulnaris
Pisometacarpal ligament
Flexor
Abductor
pollicis brevis
P
P
P
Opponens
Digiti minimi
Adductor pollicis
Abductor
Flexor brevis
Flexor pollicis longus
Interossei
Adductor pollicis (transverse head)
Flexor digitorum superficialis
Flexor digitorum profundus
B. Anterior View


## 6.56 Bones and muscle attachments of forearm and hand

**A.** Bony features. **B.** Sites of muscle attachments. The proximal attachments of the three palmar interossei are indicated by the letter *P;* those of the four dorsal interossei are indicated by color only.

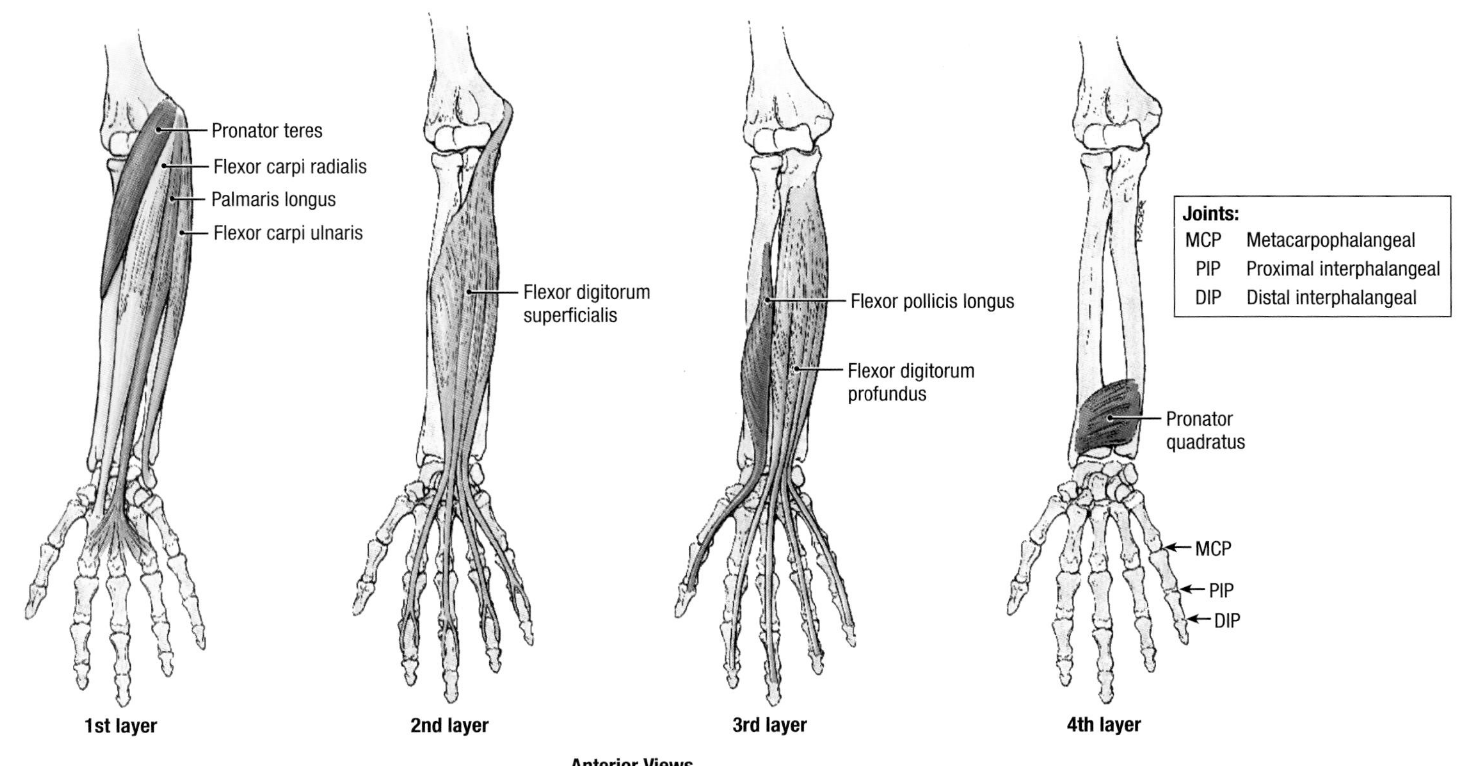
Pronator teres
Flexor carpi radialis
Palmaris longus
Flexor carpi ulnaris
Flexor digitorum superficialis
Flexor pollicis longus
Flexor digitorum profundus
Joints:
MCP Metacarpophalangeal
PIP Proximal interphalangeal
DIP Distal interphalangeal
Pronator quadratus
MCP
PIP
DIP
1st layer
2nd layer
3rd layer
4th layer

Anterior Views

## TABLE 6.10 MUSCLES OF ANTERIOR SURFACE OF FOREARM

| Muscle | Proximal Attachment | Distal Attachment | Innervation | Main Actions |
|---|---|---|---|---|
| **Pronator teres** | Medial epicondyle of humerus and coronoid process of ulna | Middle of lateral surface of radius (pronator tuberosity) | Median nerve (C6–**C7**) | Pronates forearm and flexes elbow |
| **Flexor carpi radialis** | Medial epicondyle of humerus | Base of 2nd metacarpal | | Flexes wrist and abducts hand |
| **Palmaris longus** | | Distal half of flexor retinaculum and palmar aponeurosis | Median nerve (C7–**C8**) | Flexes wrist and tightens palmar aponeurosis |
| **Flexor carpi ulnaris** | *Humeral head:* medial epicondyle of humerus; *Ulnar head:* olecranon and posterior border of ulna | Pisiform, hook of hamate, and 5th metacarpal | Ulnar nerve (C7–**C8**) | Flexes wrist and adducts hand |
| **Flexor digitorum superficialis** | *Humeroulnar head:* medial epicondyle of humerus, ulnar collateral ligament, and coronoid process of ulna *Radial head:* superior half of anterior border of radius | Bodies of middle phalanges of medial four digits | Median nerve (C7, **C8**, and T1) | Flexes PIPs of medial four digits; acting more strongly, it flexes MCPs and hand |
| **Flexor digitorum profundus** | Proximal three quarters of medial and anterior surfaces of ulna and interosseous membrane | Bases of distal phalanges of medial four digits | *Medial part:* ulnar nerve (**C8**–T1) *Lateral part:* median nerve (**C8**–T1) | Flexes DIPs of medial four digits; assists with flexion of wrist |
| **Flexor pollicis longus** | Anterior surface of radius and adjacent interosseous membrane | Base of distal phalanx of thumb | Anterior interosseous nerve from median (**C8**–T1) | Flexes phalanges of 1st digit (thumb) |
| **Pronator quadratus** | Distal fourth of anterior surface of ulna | Distal fourth of anterior surface of radius | | Pronates forearm; deep fibers bind radius and ulna together |

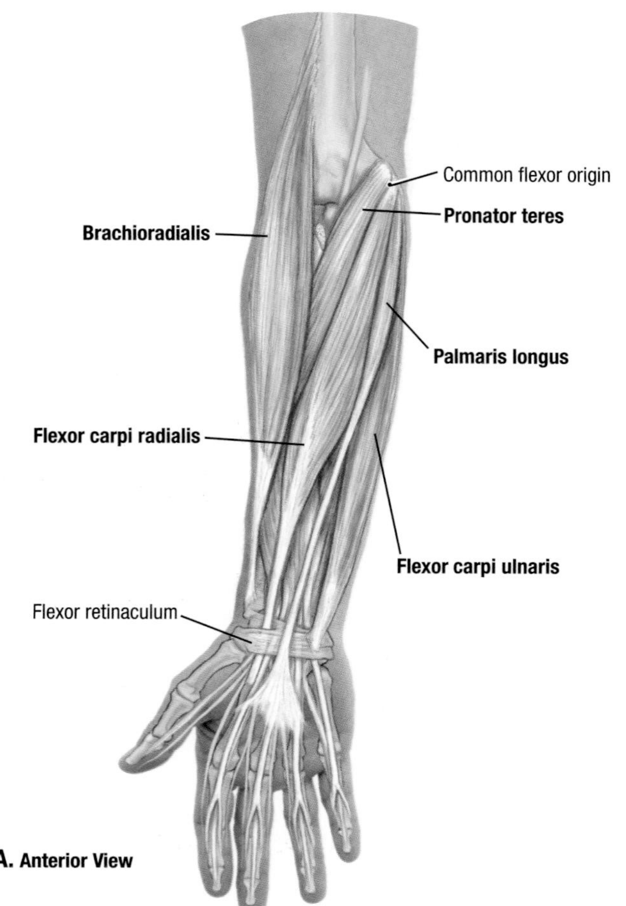
Common flexor origin
Pronator teres
Brachioradialis
Palmaris longus
Flexor carpi radialis
Flexor carpi ulnaris
Flexor retinaculum

**A.** Anterior View

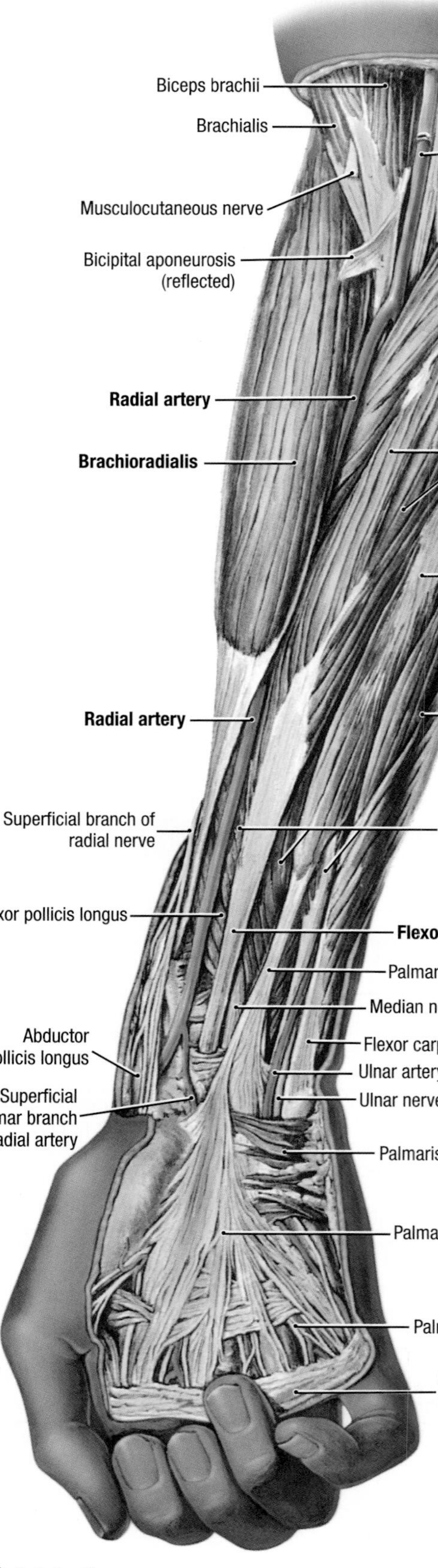

Biceps brachii
Brachialis
Musculocutaneous nerve
Bicipital aponeurosis (reflected)
Median nerve
Brachialis
Brachial artery
Medial epicondyle of humerus
Common flexor origin
Pronator teres
Radial artery
Brachioradialis
Flexor carpi radialis
Palmaris longus
Radial artery
Flexor carpi ulnaris
Superficial branch of radial nerve
Flexor digitorum superficialis
Flexor pollicis longus
Flexor carpi radiatis
Palmaris longus
Median nerve
Abductor pollicis longus
Flexor carpi ulnaris
Ulnar artery
Superficial palmar branch of radial artery
Ulnar nerve
Palmaris brevis
Palmar aponeurosis
Palmar digital arteries and nerves
Superficial transverse metacarpal ligament

**B.** Anterior View

## 6.57 Superficial muscles of the forearm and palmar aponeurosis

- At the elbow, the brachial artery lies between the biceps tendon and median nerve. It then bifurcates into the radial and ulnar arteries.
- At the wrist, the radial artery is lateral to the flexor carpi radialis tendon, and the ulnar artery is lateral to flexor carpi ulnaris tendon.
- In the forearm, the radial artery lies between the flexor and extensor compartments. The muscles lateral to the artery are supplied by the radial nerve, and those medial to it by the median and ulnar nerves; thus, no motor nerve crosses the radial artery.
- The brachioradialis muscle slightly overlaps the radial artery, which is otherwise superficial.
- The four superficial muscles (pronator teres, flexor carpi radialis, palmaris longus, and flexor carpi ulnaris) all attach proximally to the medial epicondyle of the humerus (common flexor origin).
- The palmaris longus muscle, in this specimen, has an anomalous distal belly; this muscle usually has a small belly at the common flexor origin and a long tendon that is continued into the palm as the palmar aponeurosis. The palmaris longus is absent in approximately 14% of limbs.

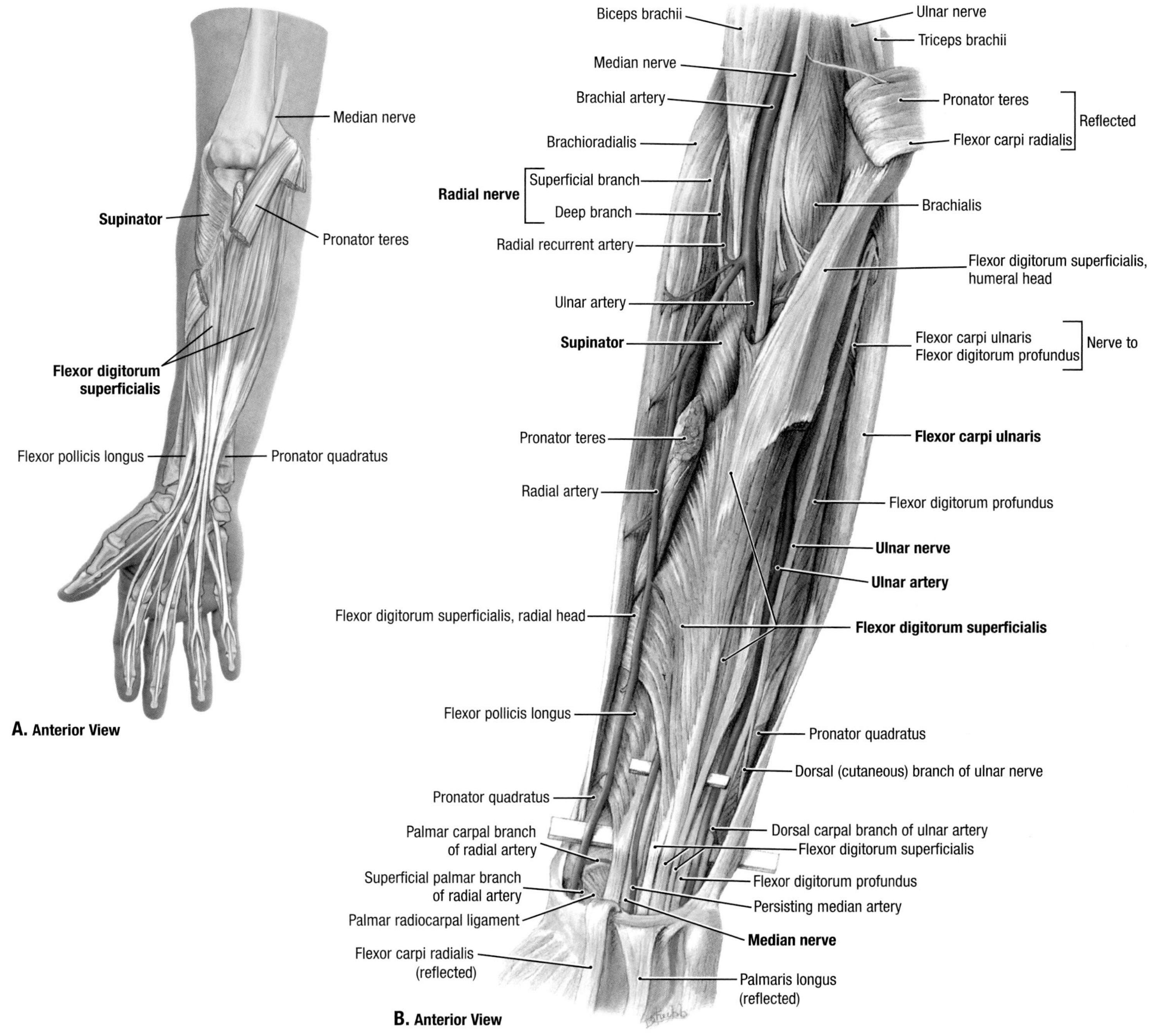
Median nerve
Supinator
Pronator teres
Flexor digitorum superficialis
Flexor pollicis longus
Pronator quadratus
A. Anterior View
Biceps brachii
Median nerve
Brachial artery
Brachioradialis
Radial nerve
Superficial branch
Deep branch
Radial recurrent artery
Ulnar artery
Supinator
Pronator teres
Radial artery
Flexor digitorum superficialis, radial head
Flexor pollicis longus
Pronator quadratus
Palmar carpal branch of radial artery
Superficial palmar branch of radial artery
Palmar radiocarpal ligament
Flexor carpi radialis (reflected)
Ulnar nerve
Triceps brachii
Pronator teres
Flexor carpi radialis
Reflected
Brachialis
Flexor digitorum superficialis, humeral head
Flexor carpi ulnaris
Flexor digitorum profundus
Nerve to
Flexor carpi ulnaris
Flexor digitorum profundus
Ulnar nerve
Ulnar artery
Flexor digitorum superficialis
Pronator quadratus
Dorsal (cutaneous) branch of ulnar nerve
Dorsal carpal branch of ulnar artery
Flexor digitorum superficialis
Flexor digitorum profundus
Persisting median artery
Median nerve
Palmaris longus (reflected)
B. Anterior View

## 6.58 Flexor digitorum superficialis and related structures

- The flexor digitorum superficialis muscle is attached proximally to the humerus, ulna, and radius.
- The ulnar artery passes obliquely posterior to the flexor digitorum superficialis; at the medial border of the muscle, the ulnar artery joins the ulnar nerve.
- The ulnar nerve lies between the flexor digitorum profundus and flexor carpi ulnaris.
- The median nerve descends vertically posterior to the flexor digitorum superficialis and appears distally at its lateral border.
- The median artery of this specimen is a variation resulting from persistence of an embryologic vessel that usually disappears.

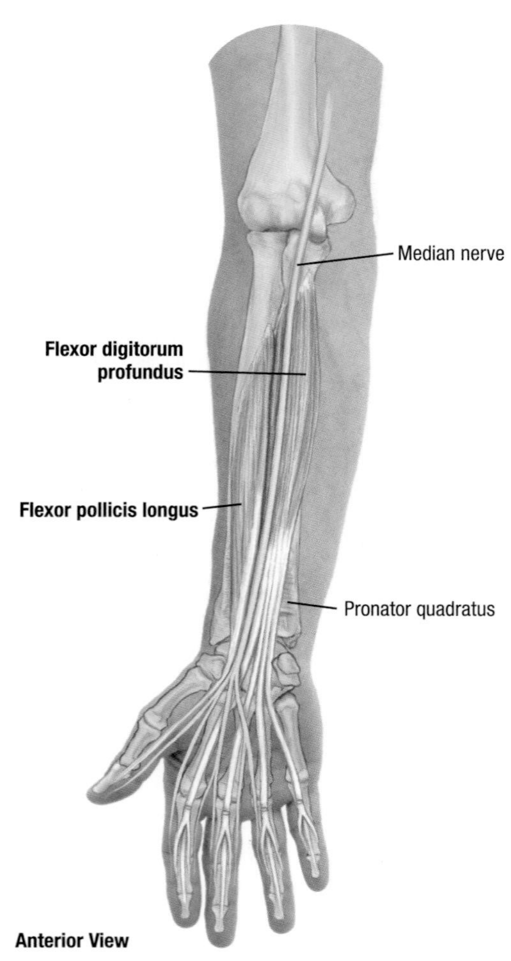
Median nerve
Flexor digitorum profundus
Flexor pollicis longus
Pronator quadratus
Anterior View

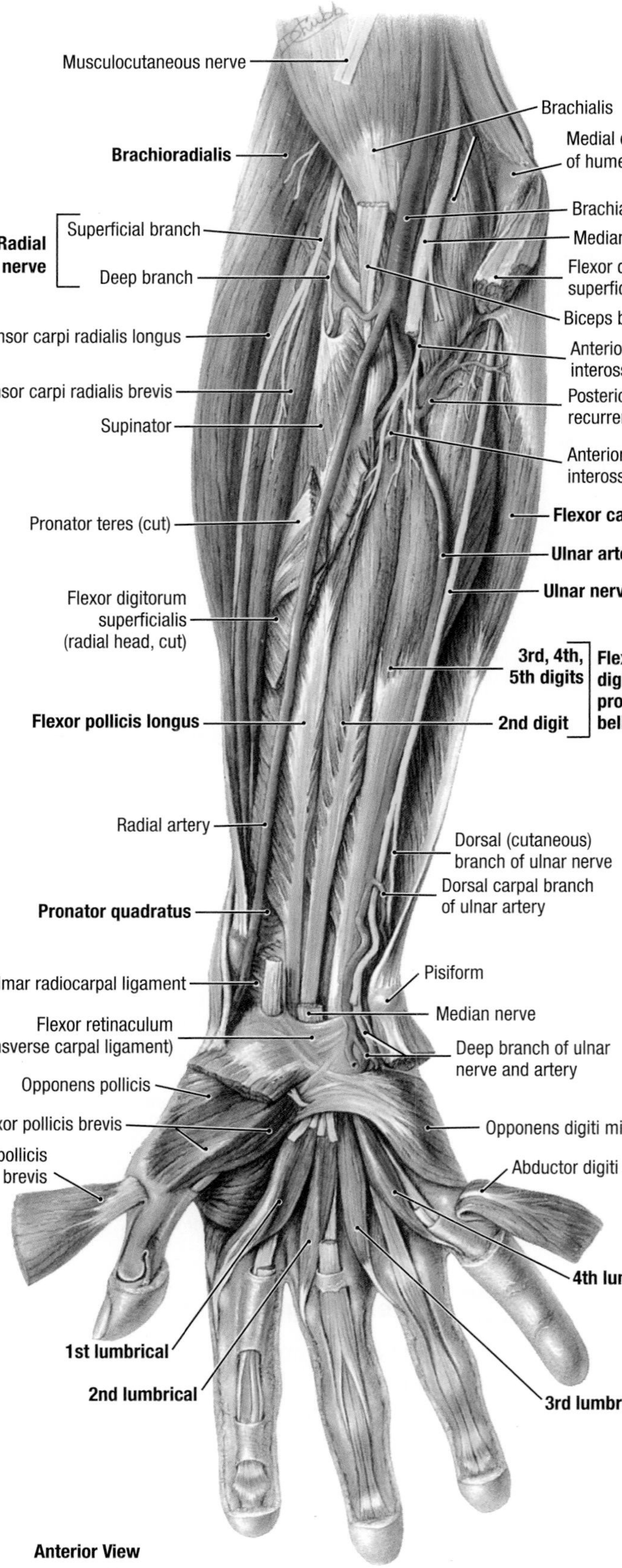

## 6.59 Deep flexors of the digits and related structures

- The two deep digital flexor muscles, flexor pollicis longus and flexor digitorum profundus, arise from the flexor aspects of the radius, interosseous membrane, and ulna between the origin of flexor digitorum superficialis proximally and pronator quadratus distally.
- The ulnar nerve enters the forearm posterior to the medial epicondyle, then descends between the flexor digitorum profundus and flexor carpi ulnaris and is joined by the ulnar artery. At the wrist the ulnar nerve and artery pass anterior to the flexor retinaculum and lateral to the pisiform to enter the palm.
- At the elbow, the ulnar nerve supplies the flexor carpi ulnaris and the medial half of the flexor digitorum profundus muscles; superior to the wrist, it gives off the dorsal (cutaneous) branch.
- The four lumbricals arise from the flexor digitorum profundus tendons.

Musculocutaneous nerve
Brachialis
Medial epicondyle of humerus
Brachioradialis
Brachial artery
Radial nerve
Superficial branch
Deep branch
Median nerve
Flexor digitorum superficialis
Biceps brachii tendon
Extensor carpi radialis longus
Anterior interosseous nerve
Extensor carpi radialis brevis
Posterior ulnar recurrent artery
Supinator
Anterior interosseous artery
Flexor carpi ulnaris
Pronator teres (cut)
Ulnar artery
Ulnar nerve
Flexor digitorum superficialis (radial head, cut)
3rd, 4th, 5th digits
2nd digit
Flexor digitorum profundus muscle belly for
Flexor pollicis longus
Radial artery
Dorsal (cutaneous) branch of ulnar nerve
Dorsal carpal branch of ulnar artery
Pronator quadratus
Pisiform
Palmar radiocarpal ligament
Median nerve
Flexor retinaculum (transverse carpal ligament)
Deep branch of ulnar nerve and artery
Opponens pollicis
Flexor pollicis brevis
Opponens digiti minimi
Abductor pollicis brevis
Abductor digiti minimi
4th lumbrical
1st lumbrical
2nd lumbrical
3rd lumbrical
Anterior View

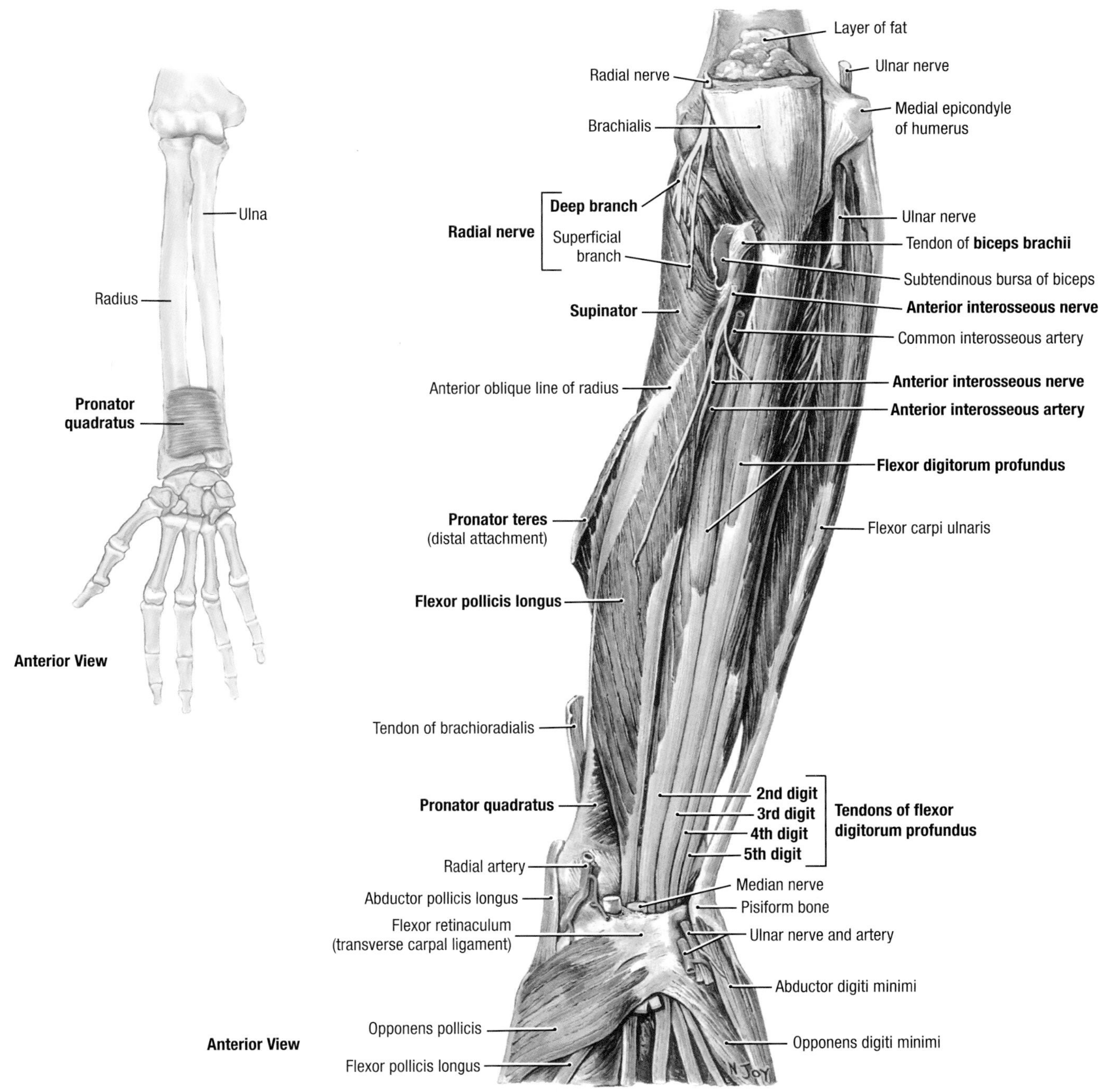
Ulna
Radius
Pronator quadratus
Anterior View
Layer of fat
Ulnar nerve
Radial nerve
Medial epicondyle of humerus
Brachialis
Deep branch
Radial nerve
Superficial branch
Ulnar nerve
Tendon of biceps brachii
Subtendinous bursa of biceps
Supinator
Anterior interosseous nerve
Common interosseous artery
Anterior oblique line of radius
Anterior interosseous nerve
Anterior interosseous artery
Flexor digitorum profundus
Pronator teres (distal attachment)
Flexor carpi ulnaris
Flexor pollicis longus
Tendon of brachioradialis
2nd digit
3rd digit
4th digit
5th digit
Tendons of flexor digitorum profundus
Pronator quadratus
Radial artery
Median nerve
Abductor pollicis longus
Pisiform bone
Flexor retinaculum (transverse carpal ligament)
Ulnar nerve and artery
Abductor digiti minimi
Opponens pollicis
Opponens digiti minimi
Anterior View
Flexor pollicis longus

## 6.60 Deep flexors of the digits and supinator

- The five tendons of the deep digital flexors (flexor pollicis longus and flexor digitorum profundus) lie side by side as they enter the carpal tunnel.
- The biceps brachii muscle attaches to the medial aspect of the radius; hence, it can supinate the forearm, whereas the pronator teres muscle, by attaching to the lateral surface, can pronate the forearm.
- The deep branch of the radial nerve pierces and innervates the supinator muscle.
- The anterior interosseous nerve and artery disappear between the flexor pollicis longus and flexor digitorum profundus muscles to lie on the interosseous membrane.

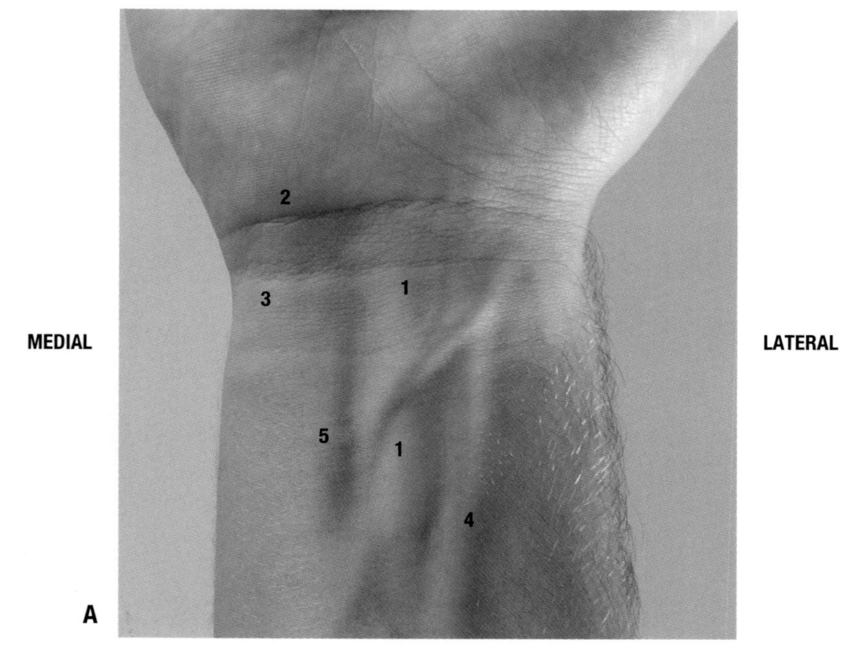
MEDIAL
LATERAL
1
2
3
4
5
1
A

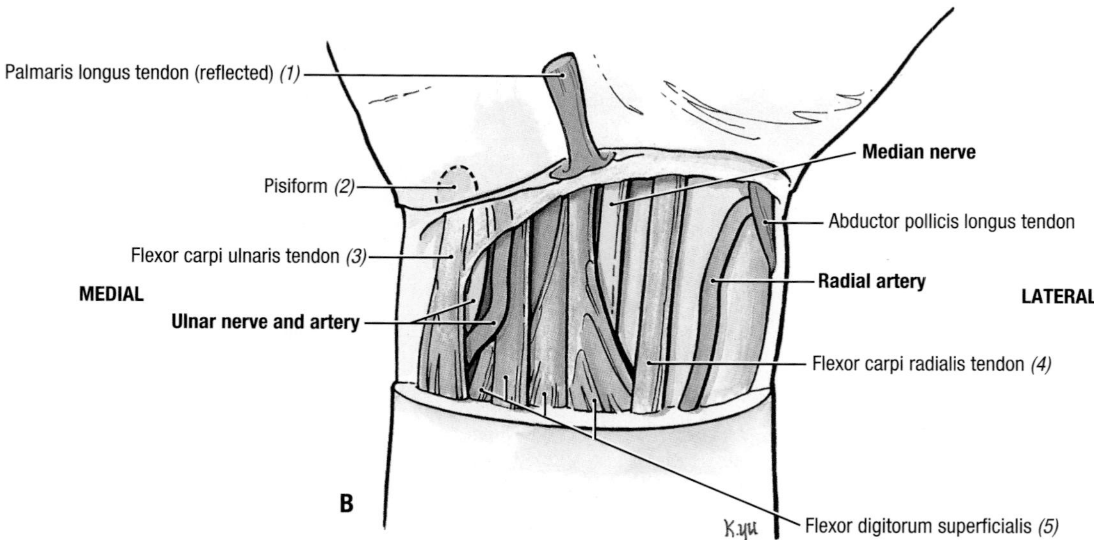
Palmaris longus tendon (reflected) (1)
Median nerve
Pisiform (2)
Abductor pollicis longus tendon
Flexor carpi ulnaris tendon (3)
Radial artery
MEDIAL
LATERAL
Ulnar nerve and artery
Flexor carpi radialis tendon (4)
B
Flexor digitorum superficialis (5)

Anterior Views of Right Hand and Wrist

## 6.61 Structures of anterior aspect of wrist

**A.** Surface anatomy. **B.** Schematic illustration. **C.** Dissection.

- The distal skin incision follows the transverse skin crease at the wrist. The incision crosses the pisiform, to which the flexor carpi ulnaris muscle attaches, and the tubercle of the scaphoid, to which the tendon of flexor carpi radialis muscle is a guide.
- The palmaris longus tendon bisects the transverse skin crease; deep to its lateral margin is the median nerve.
- The radial artery passes deep to the tendon of the abductor pollicis longus muscle.
- The flexor digitorum superficialis tendons to the 3rd and 4th digits become anterior to those of the 2nd and 5th digits.
- The recurrent branch of the median nerve to the thenar muscles lies within a circle whose center is 2.5 to 4 cm distal to the tubercle of the scaphoid.

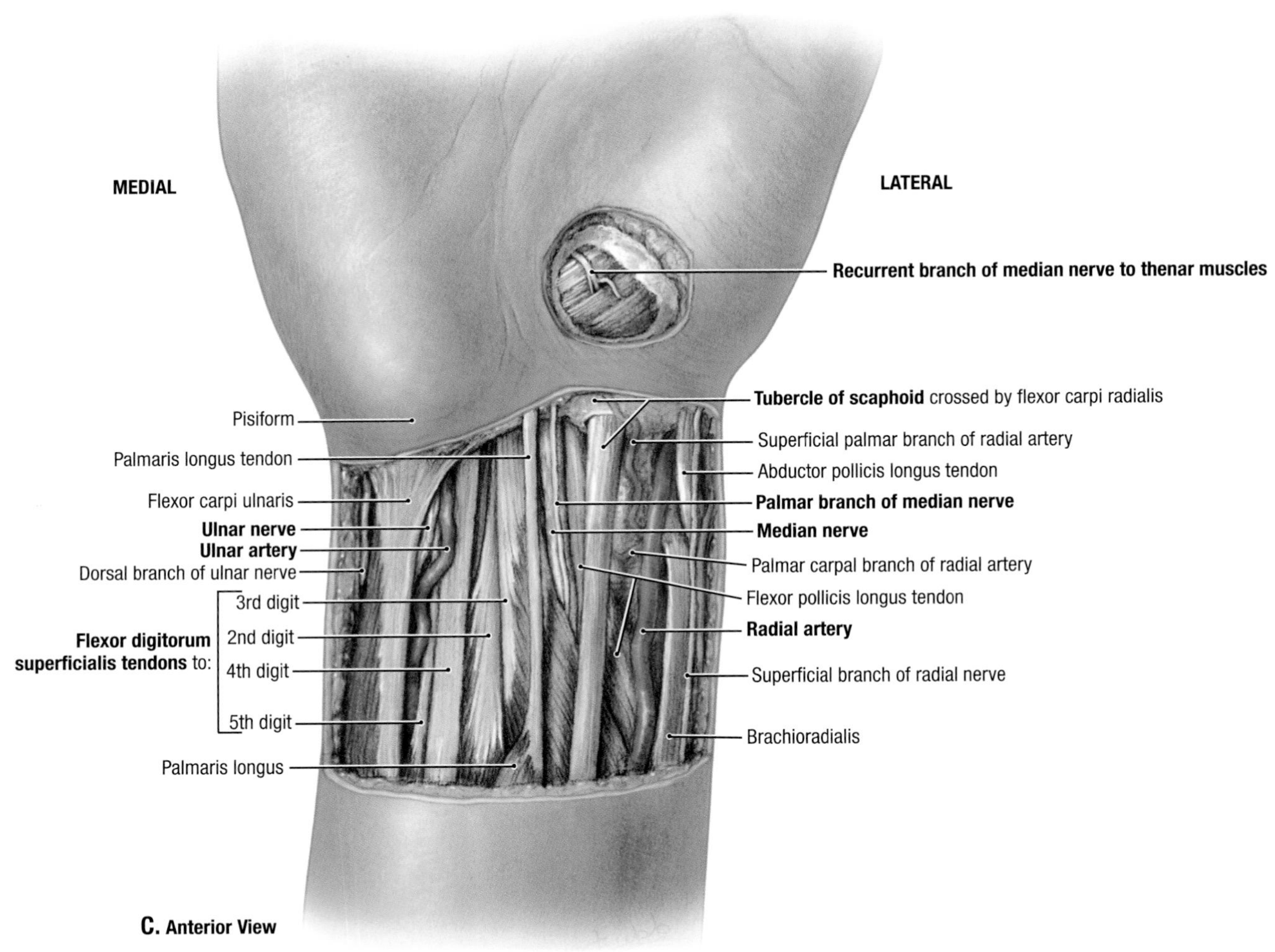
MEDIAL
LATERAL
Recurrent branch of median nerve to thenar muscles
Pisiform
Palmaris longus tendon
Flexor carpi ulnaris
Ulnar nerve
Ulnar artery
Dorsal branch of ulnar nerve
Flexor digitorum superficialis tendons to:
3rd digit
2nd digit
4th digit
5th digit
Palmaris longus
Tubercle of scaphoid crossed by flexor carpi radialis
Superficial palmar branch of radial artery
Abductor pollicis longus tendon
Palmar branch of median nerve
Median nerve
Palmar carpal branch of radial artery
Flexor pollicis longus tendon
Radial artery
Superficial branch of radial nerve
Brachioradialis
C. Anterior View

## 6.61 Structures of anterior aspect of wrist *(continued)*

Lesions of the median nerve usually occur in two places: the forearm and wrist. The most common site is where the nerve passes though the carpal tunnel. Lacerations of the wrist often cause median nerve injury because this nerve is relatively close to the surface. This results in paralysis of the thenar muscles and the first two lumbricals. Hence opposition of the thumb is not possible and fine control movements of the 2nd and 3rd digits are impaired. Sensation is also lost over the thumb and adjacent two and a half fingers.

Median nerve injury resulting from a perforating wound in the elbow region results in loss of flexion of the proximal and distal interphalangeal joints of the 2nd and 3rd digits. The ability to flex the metacarpophalangeal joints of these digits is also affected because digital branches of the median nerve supply the 1st and 2nd lumbricals. The palmar cutaneous branch of the median nerve does not traverse the carpal tunnel. It supplies the skin of the central palm, which remains sensitive in carpal tunnel syndrome.

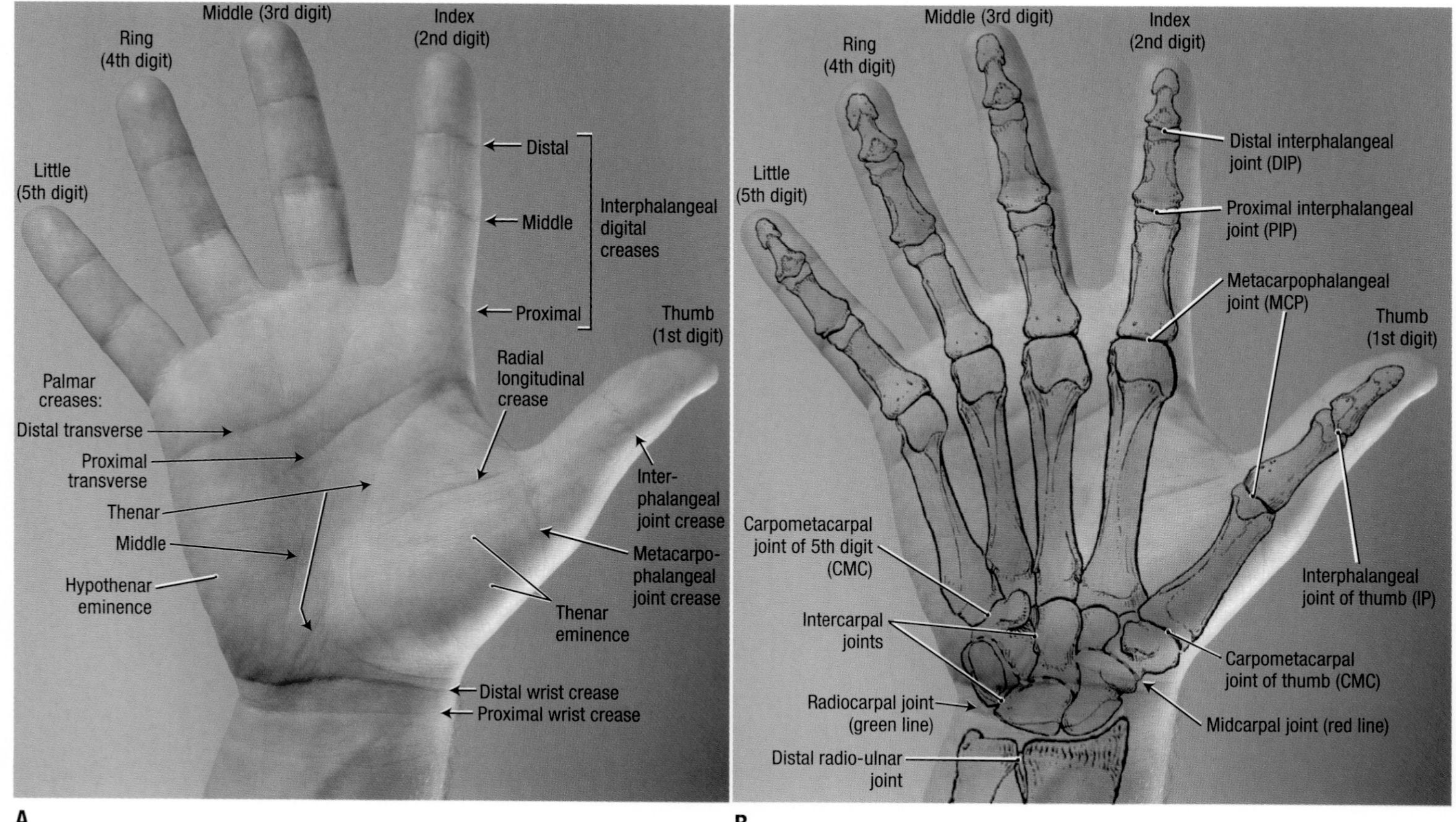
Middle (3rd digit)
Ring (4th digit)
Index (2nd digit)
Little (5th digit)
Distal
Middle
Proximal
Interphalangeal digital creases
Thumb (1st digit)
Palmar creases:
Distal transverse
Proximal transverse
Thenar
Middle
Hypothenar eminence
Radial longitudinal crease
Inter-phalangeal joint crease
Metacarpo-phalangeal joint crease
Thenar eminence
Distal wrist crease
Proximal wrist crease
A
Anterior Views
Middle (3rd digit)
Ring (4th digit)
Index (2nd digit)
Little (5th digit)
Distal interphalangeal joint (DIP)
Proximal interphalangeal joint (PIP)
Metacarpophalangeal joint (MCP)
Thumb (1st digit)
Carpometacarpal joint of 5th digit (CMC)
Intercarpal joints
Radiocarpal joint (green line)
Distal radio-ulnar joint
Interphalangeal joint of thumb (IP)
Carpometacarpal joint of thumb (CMC)
Midcarpal joint (red line)
B

## 6.62 Surface anatomy of skeleton of hand and wrist

**A.** Skin creases of wrist and hand. **B.** Surface projection of joints of wrist and hand. Note relationship of bones and joints to features of the hand.

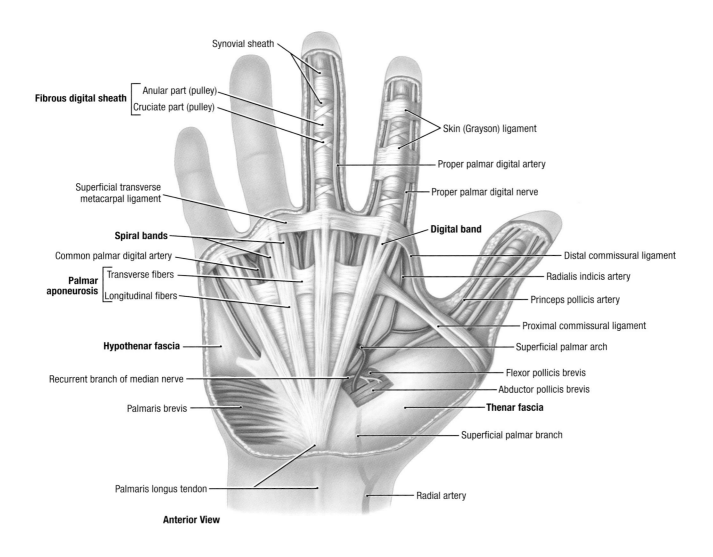

Synovial sheath
**Fibrous digital sheath**
Anular part (pulley)
Cruciate part (pulley)
Skin (Grayson) ligament
Proper palmar digital artery
Proper palmar digital nerve
Superficial transverse metacarpal ligament
**Spiral bands**
**Digital band**
Common palmar digital artery
Distal commissural ligament
**Palmar aponeurosis**
Transverse fibers
Longitudinal fibers
Radialis indicis artery
Princeps pollicis artery
Proximal commissural ligament
**Hypothenar fascia**
Superficial palmar arch
Recurrent branch of median nerve
Flexor pollicis brevis
Abductor pollicis brevis
Palmaris brevis
**Thenar fascia**
Superficial palmar branch
Palmaris longus tendon
Radial artery

**Anterior View**

## 6.63 Palmar (deep) fascia: palmar aponeurosis, thenar and hypothenar fascia

- The palmar fascia is thin over the thenar and hypothenar eminences, but thick centrally, where it forms the palmar aponeurosis, and in the digits, where it forms the fibrous digital sheaths.
- At the distal end (base) of the palmar aponeurosis, four bundles of digital and spiral bands continue to the bases and fibrous digital sheaths of digits 2–5.

- Dupuytren contracture is a disease of the palmar fascia resulting in progressive shortening, thickening, and fibrosis of the palmar fascia and palmar aponeurosis. The fibrous degeneration of the longitudinal digital bands of the aponeurosis on the medial side of the hand pulls the 4th and 5th fingers into partial flexion at the metacarpophalangeal and proximal interphalangeal joints. The contracture is frequently bilateral. Treatment of Dupuytren contracture usually involves surgical excision of all fibrotic parts of the palmar fascia to free the fingers.

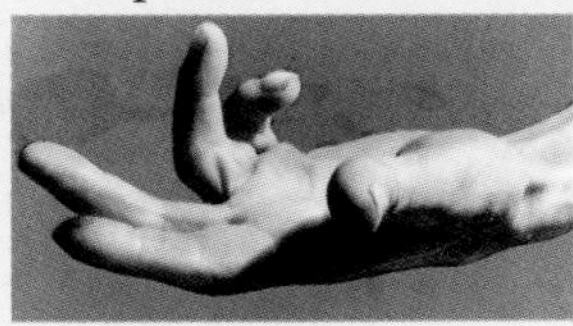

Dupuytren contracture

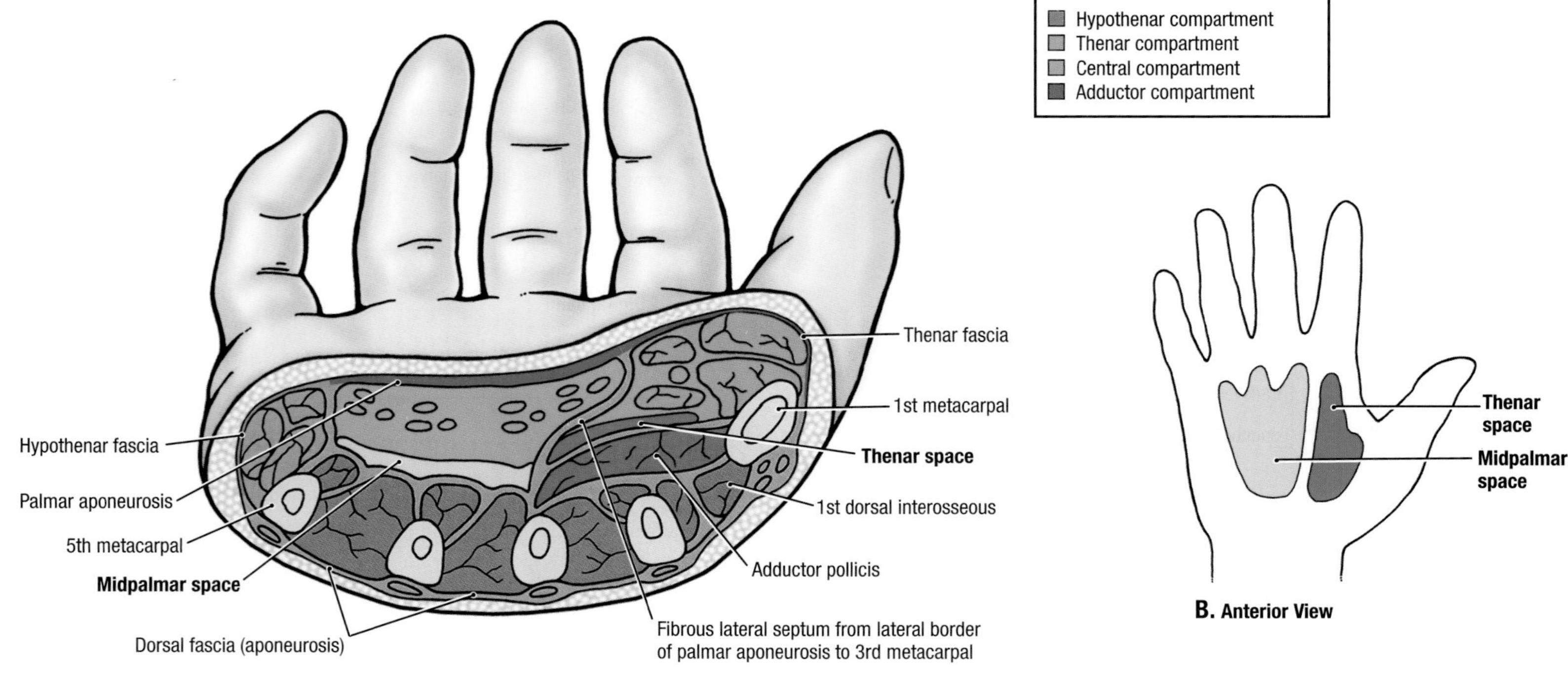
Hypothenar compartment
Thenar compartment
Central compartment
Adductor compartment
Thenar fascia
1st metacarpal
Thenar space
1st dorsal interosseous
Adductor pollicis
Fibrous lateral septum from lateral border of palmar aponeurosis to 3rd metacarpal
Hypothenar fascia
Palmar aponeurosis
5th metacarpal
Midpalmar space
Dorsal fascia (aponeurosis)
A. Transverse Section, Interior View
Thenar space
Midpalmar space
B. Anterior View

## 6.64 Compartments, spaces, and fascia of the palm

**A.** Transverse section through the middle of the palm showing the fascial compartments for the musculotendinous structures of the hand. **B.** Potential fascial spaces of palm.

- The potential midpalmar space lies posterior to the central compartment, is bounded medially by the hypothenar compartment, and is related distally to the synovial sheath of the 3rd, 4th, and 5th digits.
- The potential thenar space lies posterior to the thenar compartment and is related distally to the synovial sheath of the index finger.
- The potential midpalmar and thenar spaces are separated by a septum that passes from the palmar aponeurosis to the third metacarpal.

Because the palmar fascia is thick and strong, swellings resulting from hand infections usually appear on the dorsum of the hand where the fascia is thinner. The potential fascial spaces of the palm are important because they may become infected. The fascial spaces determine the extent and direction of the spread of pus formed in the infected areas. Depending on the site of infection, pus will accumulate in the thenar, hypothenar, or adductor compartments. Antibiotic therapy has made infections that spread beyond one of these fascial compartments rare, but an untreated infection can spread proximally through the carpal tunnel into the forearm anterior to the pronator quadratus and its fascia.

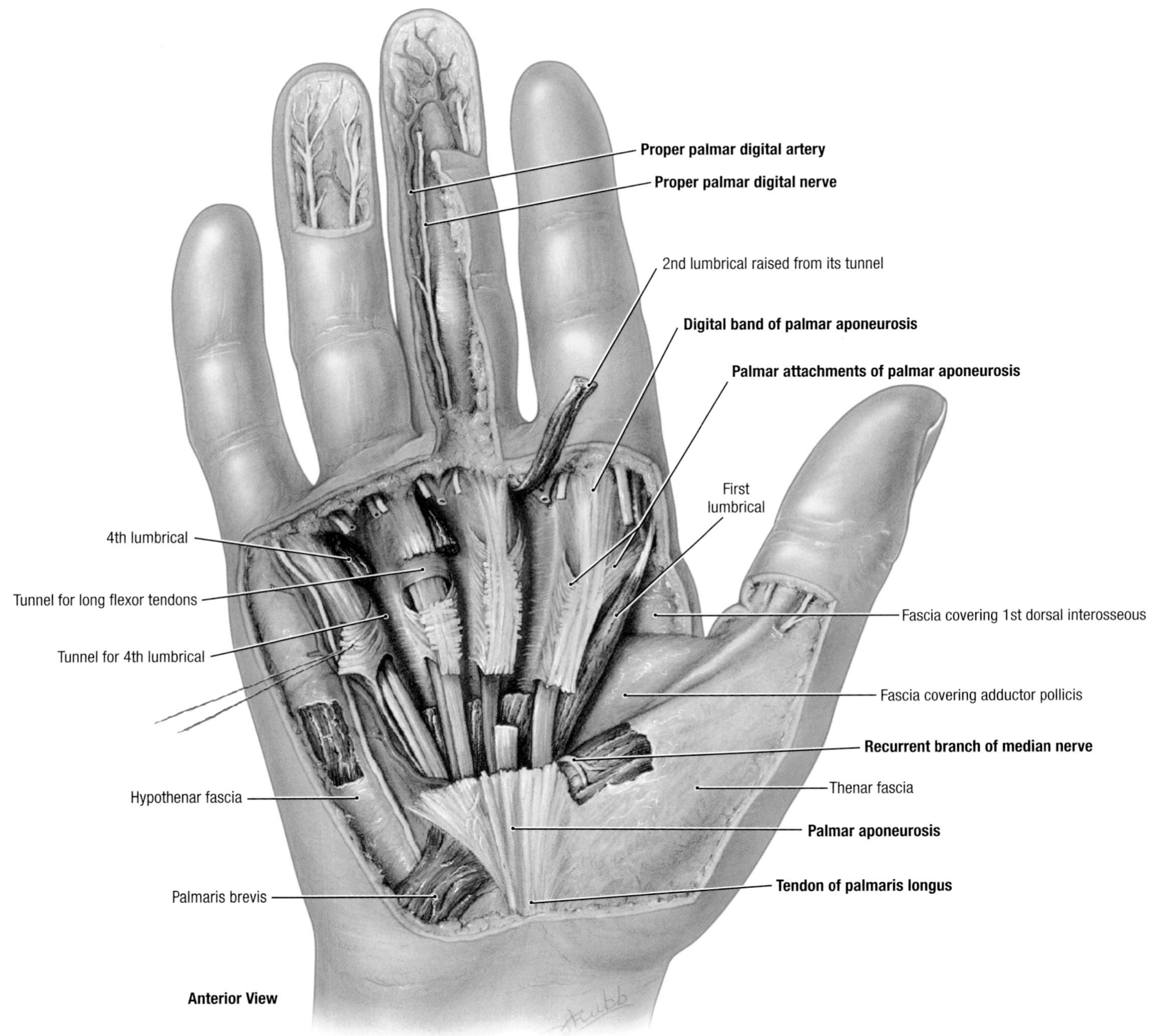
Proper palmar digital artery
Proper palmar digital nerve
2nd lumbrical raised from its tunnel
Digital band of palmar aponeurosis
Palmar attachments of palmar aponeurosis
First lumbrical
4th lumbrical
Tunnel for long flexor tendons
Fascia covering 1st dorsal interosseous
Tunnel for 4th lumbrical
Fascia covering adductor pollicis
Recurrent branch of median nerve
Hypothenar fascia
Thenar fascia
Palmar aponeurosis
Tendon of palmaris longus
Palmaris brevis
Anterior View

## 6.65 Attachments of palmar aponeurosis, digital vessels, and nerves

- From the palmar aponeurosis, four longitudinal digital bands enter the fingers; the other fibers form extensive fibroareolar septa that pass posteriorly to the palmar ligaments (see Fig. 6.71) and, more proximally, to the fascia covering the interossei. Thus, two sets of tunnels exist in the distal half of the palm: (1) tunnels for long flexor tendons and (2) tunnels for lumbricals, digital vessels, and digital nerves.
- In the dissected middle finger, note the absence of fat deep to the skin creases of the fingers.

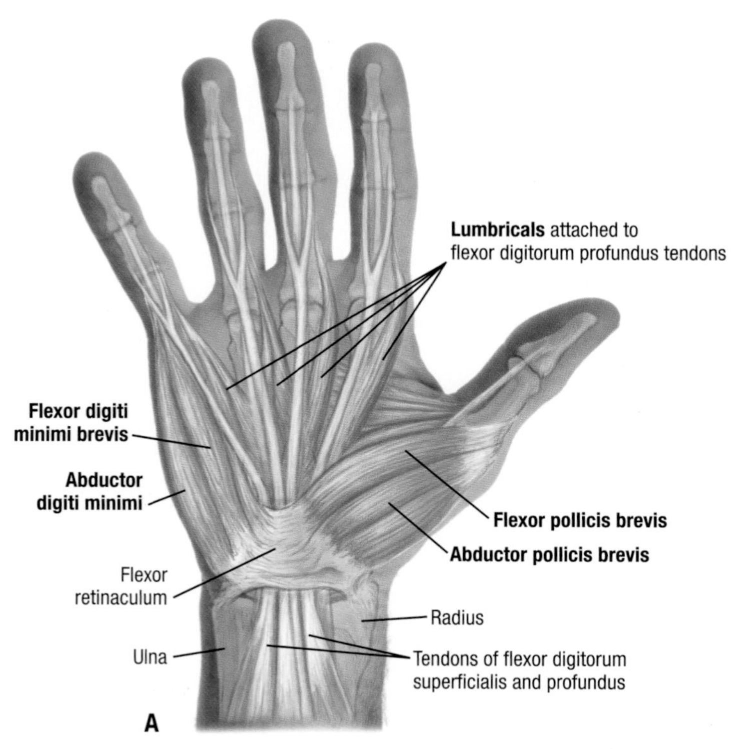
Lumbricals attached to flexor digitorum profundus tendons
Flexor digiti minimi brevis
Abductor digiti minimi
Flexor pollicis brevis
Abductor pollicis brevis
Flexor retinaculum
Radius
Ulna
Tendons of flexor digitorum superficialis and profundus
A

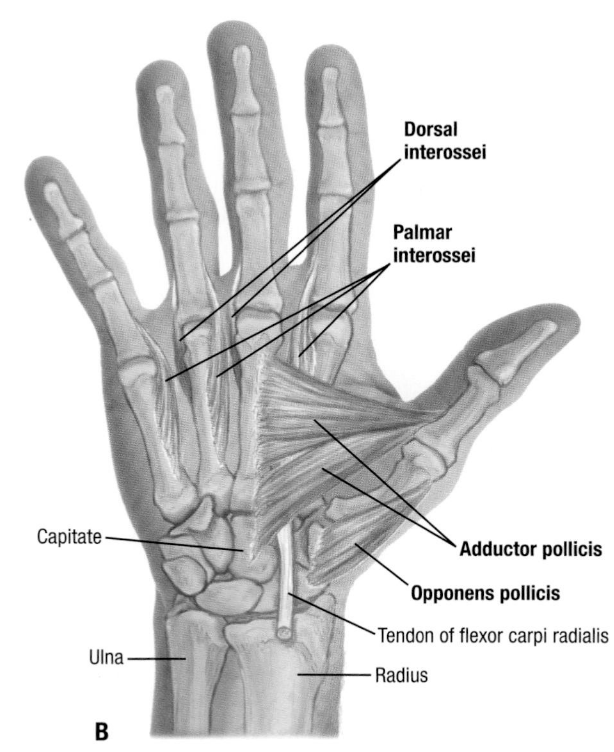
Dorsal interossei
Palmar interossei
Capitate
Adductor pollicis
Opponens pollicis
Tendon of flexor carpi radialis
Ulna
Radius
B

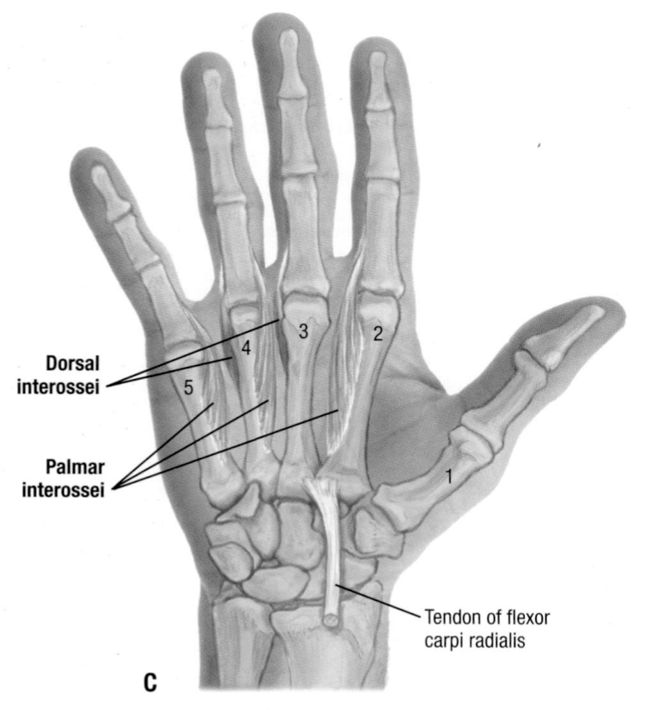
Dorsal interossei
Palmar interossei
1
2
3
4
5
Tendon of flexor carpi radialis
C

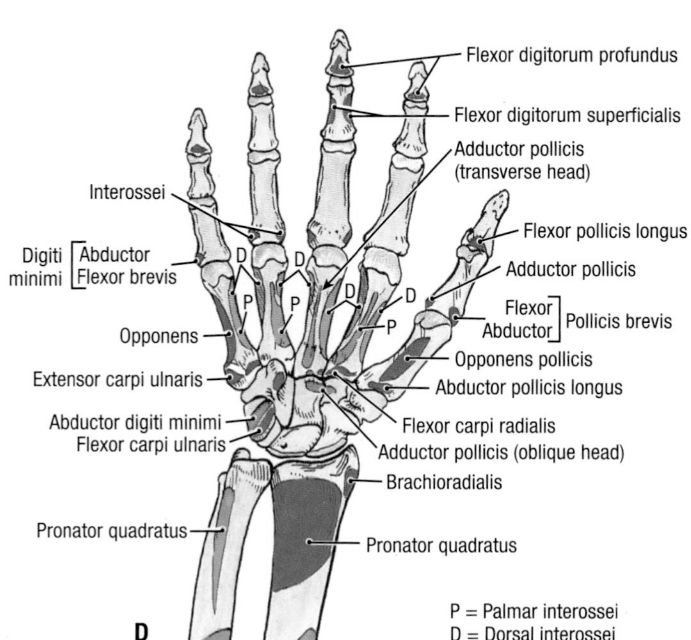
Flexor digitorum profundus
Flexor digitorum superficialis
Adductor pollicis (transverse head)
Interossei
Digiti minimi Abductor
Flexor brevis
Flexor pollicis longus
Adductor pollicis
Flexor
Abductor Pollicis brevis
Opponens
Opponens pollicis
Extensor carpi ulnaris
Abductor pollicis longus
Abductor digiti minimi
Flexor carpi ulnaris
Flexor carpi radialis
Adductor pollicis (oblique head)
Brachioradialis
Pronator quadratus
Pronator quadratus
D
P
D
P = Palmar interossei
D = Dorsal interossei

Anterior Views

**6.66 Muscular layers of palm**

**A.** Lumbricals. **B.** Adductor pollicis. **C.** Dorsal and palmar interossei. **D.** Bony attachments.

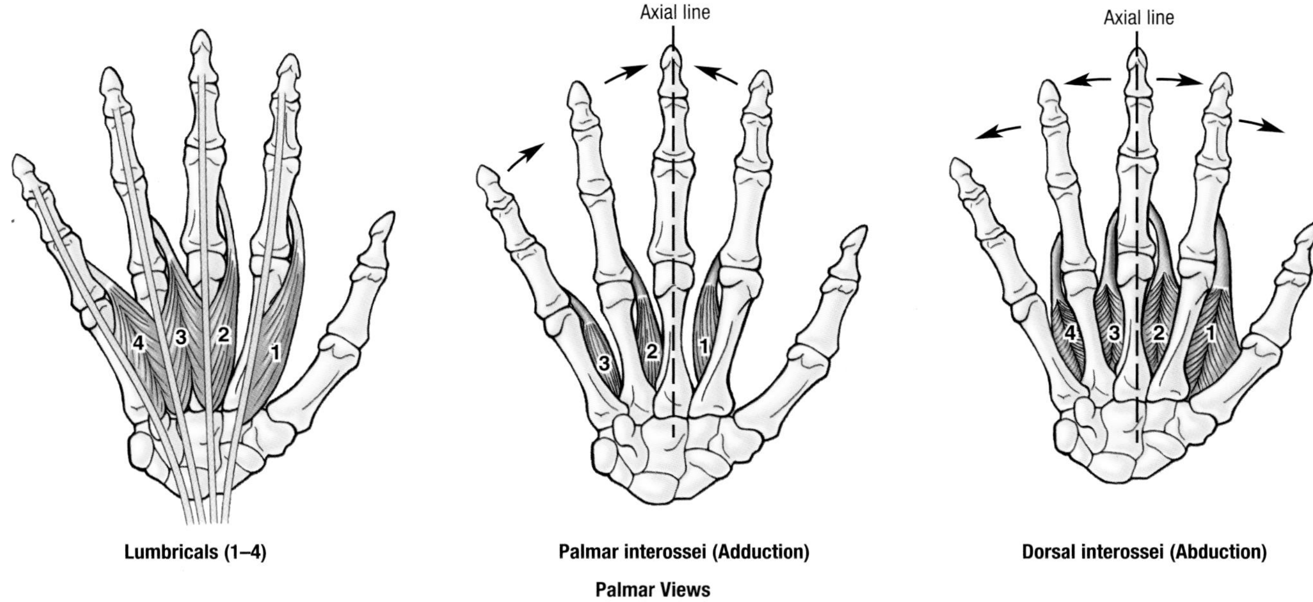
Axial line
Axial line
4
3
2
1
3
2
1
4
3
2
1

Lumbricals (1–4)

Palmar interossei (Adduction)

Dorsal interossei (Abduction)

Palmar Views

**TABLE 6.11 MUSCLES OF HAND**

| Muscle | Proximal Attachment | Distal Attachment | Innervation | Main Actions |
|---|---|---|---|---|
| **Abductor pollicis brevis** | Flexor retinaculum and tubercles of scaphoid and trapezium | Lateral side of base of proximal phalanx of thumb | Recurrent branch of median nerve (**C8** and T1) | Abducts thumb and helps oppose it |
| **Flexor pollicis brevis** | Flexor retinaculum (transverse carpal ligament) and tubercle of trapezium | | | Flexes thumb |
| **Opponens pollicis** | | Lateral side of first metacarpal | | Opposes thumb toward center of palm and rotates it medially |
| **Adductor pollicis** | *Oblique head:* bases of second and third metacarpals, capitate, and adjacent carpal bones<br>*Transverse head:* anterior surface of body of third metacarpal | Medial side of base of proximal phalanx of thumb | Deep branch of ulnar nerve (C8 and **T1**) | Adducts thumb toward middle digit |
| **Abductor digiti minimi** | Pisiform | Medial side of base of proximal phalanx of digit 5 | Deep branch of ulnar nerve (C8 and T1) | Abducts digit 5 |
| **Flexor digiti minimi brevis** | Hook of hamate and flexor retinaculum (transverse carpal ligament) | Medial border of fifth metacarpal | | Flexes proximal phalanx of digit 5 |
| **Opponens digiti minimi** | | | | Draws fifth metacarpal anteriorly and rotates it, bringing digit 5 into opposition with thumb |
| **Lumbricals 1 and 2** | Lateral two tendons of flexor digitorum profundus | Lateral sides of extensor expansions of digits 2–5 | Median nerve (C8 and **T1**) | Flex digits at metacarpophalangeal joints and extend interphalangeal joints |
| **Lumbricals 3 and 4** | Medial three tendons of flexor digitorum profundus | | Deep branch of ulnar nerve (C8 and **T1**) | |
| **Dorsal interossei 1–4** | Adjacent sides of two metacarpals | Extensor expansions and bases of proximal phalanges of digits 2–4 | | Abduct digits 2–5 and assist lumbricals |
| **Palmar interossei 1–3** | Palmar surfaces of second, fourth, and fifth metacarpals | Extensor expansions of digits and bases of proximal phalanges of digits 2, 4, and 5 | | Adduct digits 2, 4, and 5 and assist lumbricals |

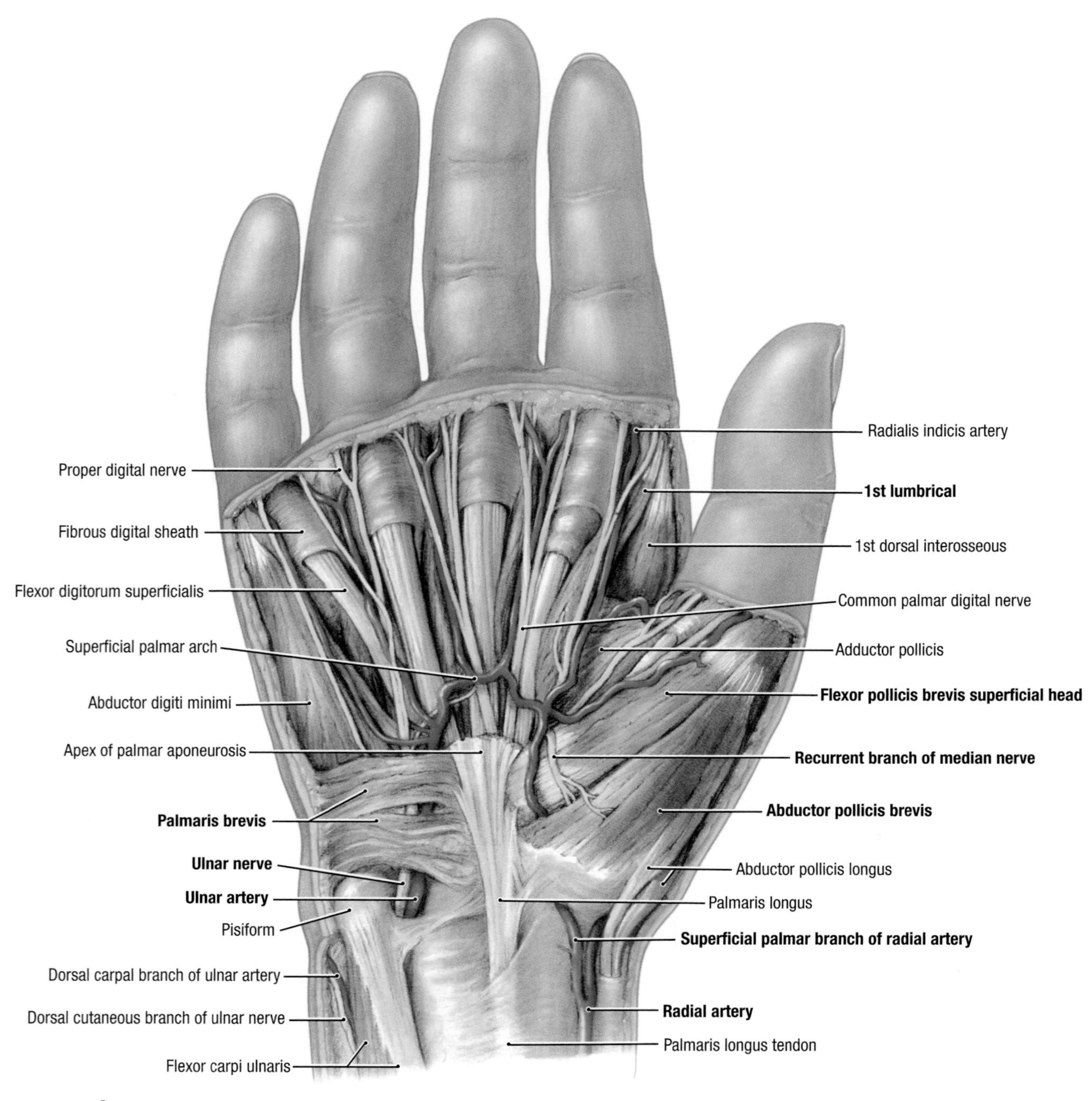
Radialis indicis artery
Proper digital nerve
1st lumbrical
Fibrous digital sheath
1st dorsal interosseous
Flexor digitorum superficialis
Common palmar digital nerve
Superficial palmar arch
Adductor pollicis
Abductor digiti minimi
Flexor pollicis brevis superficial head
Apex of palmar aponeurosis
Recurrent branch of median nerve
Palmaris brevis
Abductor pollicis brevis
Ulnar nerve
Abductor pollicis longus
Ulnar artery
Palmaris longus
Pisiform
Superficial palmar branch of radial artery
Dorsal carpal branch of ulnar artery
Radial artery
Dorsal cutaneous branch of ulnar nerve
Palmaris longus tendon
Flexor carpi ulnaris
A. Anterior View

## 6.67 Superficial dissection of palm, ulnar, and median nerves

**A.** Superficial palmar arch and digital nerves and vessels.

- The skin, superficial fascia, palmar aponeurosis, and thenar and hypothenar fasciae have been removed.
- The superficial palmar arch is formed by the ulnar artery and completed by the superficial palmar branch of the radial artery.

Bleeding is usually profuse when the palmar (arterial) arches are lacerated. It may not be sufficient to ligate (tie off) only one forearm artery when the arches are lacerated, because these vessels usually have numerous communications in the forearm and hand and thus bleed from both ends.

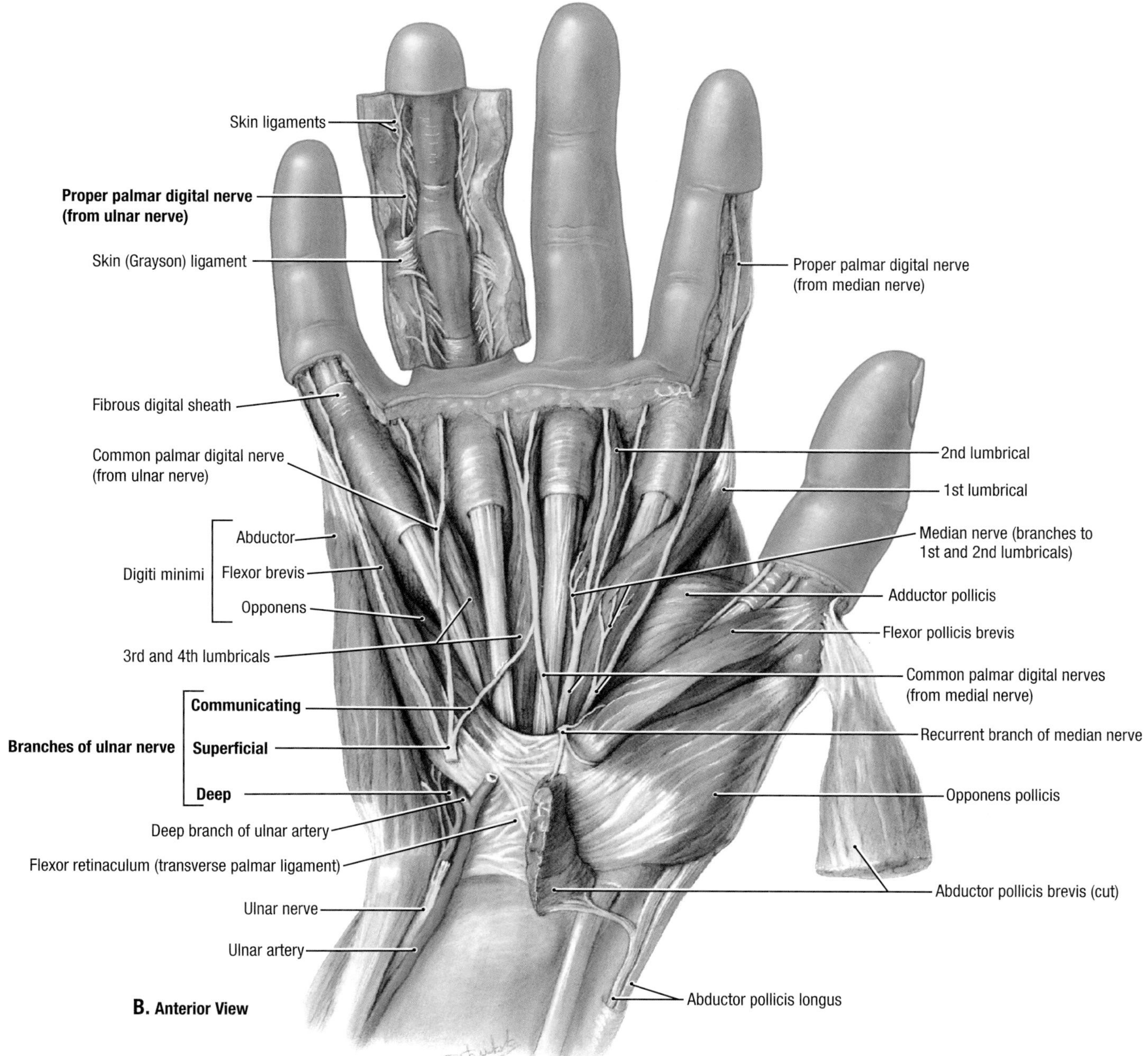

Skin ligaments
Proper palmar digital nerve (from ulnar nerve)
Skin (Grayson) ligament
Proper palmar digital nerve (from median nerve)
Fibrous digital sheath
Common palmar digital nerve (from ulnar nerve)
2nd lumbrical
1st lumbrical
Digiti minimi
Abductor
Flexor brevis
Opponens
Median nerve (branches to 1st and 2nd lumbricals)
Adductor pollicis
Flexor pollicis brevis
3rd and 4th lumbricals
Common palmar digital nerves (from medial nerve)
Branches of ulnar nerve
Communicating
Superficial
Deep
Recurrent branch of median nerve
Opponens pollicis
Deep branch of ulnar artery
Flexor retinaculum (transverse palmar ligament)
Abductor pollicis brevis (cut)
Ulnar nerve
Ulnar artery
Abductor pollicis longus
B. Anterior View


## 6.67 Superficial dissection of palm, ulnar, and median nerves *(continued)*

**B.** Ulnar and median nerves.

Carpal tunnel syndrome results from any lesion that significantly reduces the size of the carpal tunnel or, more commonly, increases the size of some of the structures (or their coverings) that pass though it (e.g., inflammation of the synovial sheaths). The median nerve is the most sensitive structure in the carpal tunnel. The median nerve has two terminal sensory branches that supply the skin of the hand; hence paresthesia (tingling), hypothesia (diminished sensation), or anesthesia (absence of tactile sensation) may occur in the lateral three and a half digits. Recall, however, that the palmar cutaneous branch of the median nerve arises proximal to and does not pass through the carpal tunnel; thus sensation in the central palm remains unaffected. This nerve also has one terminal motor branch, the recurrent branch, which innervates the three thenar muscles. Wasting of the thenar eminence and progressive loss of coordination and strength in the thumb may occur. To relieve the compression and resulting symptoms, partial or complete surgical division of the flexor retinaculum, a procedure called **carpal tunnel release**, may be necessary. The incision for carpal tunnel release is made toward the medial side of the wrist and flexor retinaculum to avoid possible injury to the recurrent branch of the median nerve.

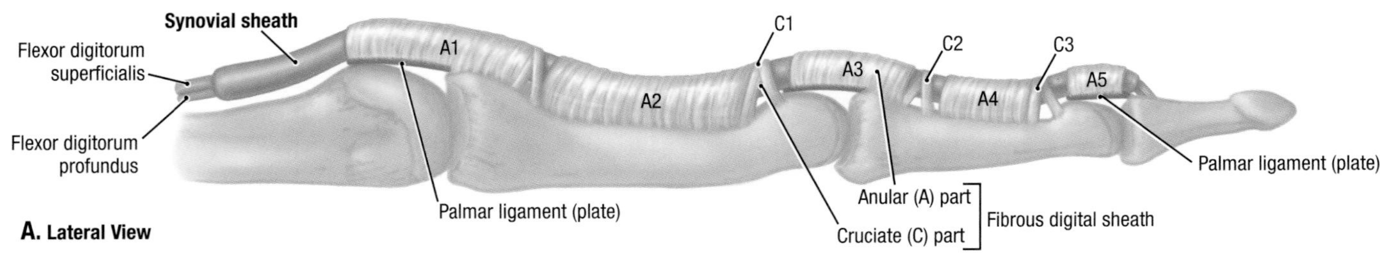
Synovial sheath
Flexor digitorum superficialis
Flexor digitorum profundus
A1
A2
C1
A3
C2
A4
C3
A5
Palmar ligament (plate)
Palmar ligament (plate)
Anular (A) part
Cruciate (C) part
Fibrous digital sheath
A. Lateral View

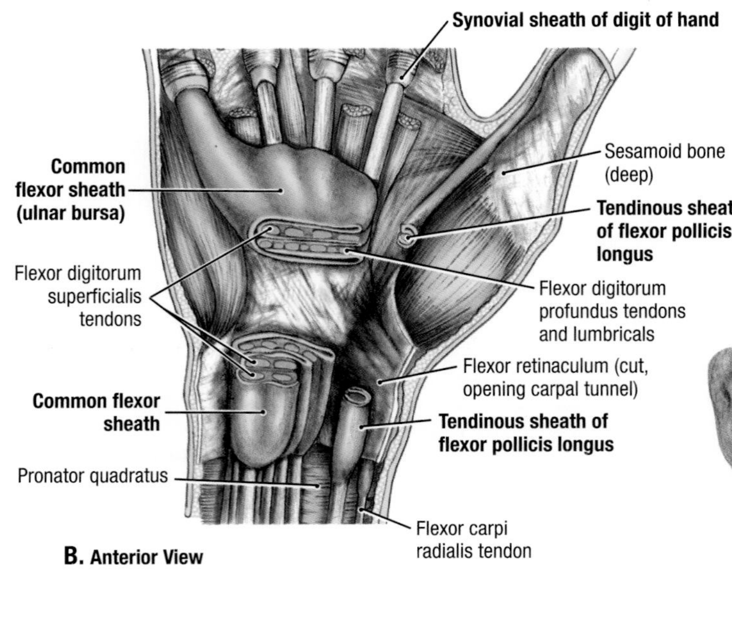
Synovial sheath of digit of hand
Common flexor sheath (ulnar bursa)
Sesamoid bone (deep)
Tendinous sheath of flexor pollicis longus
Flexor digitorum superficialis tendons
Flexor digitorum profundus tendons and lumbricals
Flexor retinaculum (cut, opening carpal tunnel)
Common flexor sheath
Tendinous sheath of flexor pollicis longus
Pronator quadratus
Flexor carpi radialis tendon
B. Anterior View

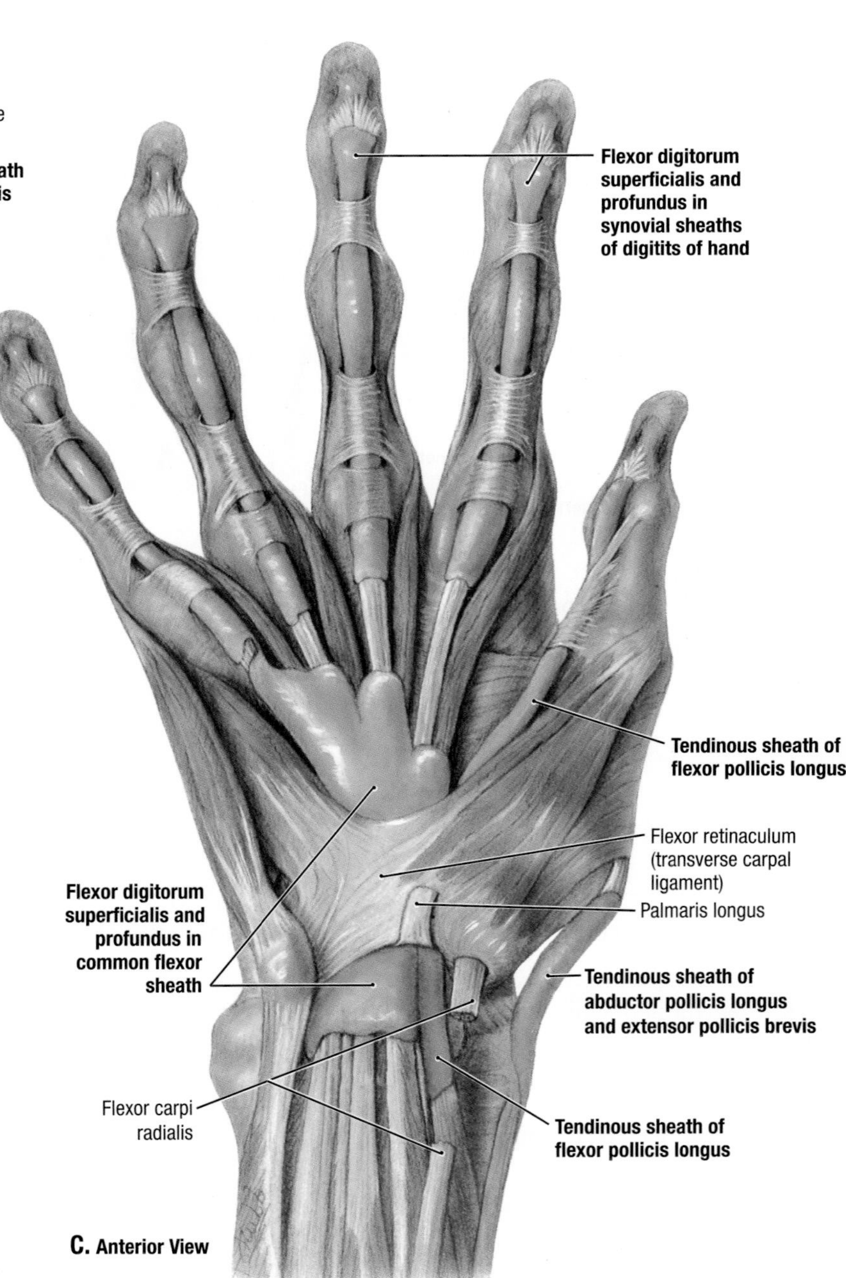
Flexor digitorum superficialis and profundus in synovial sheaths of digitits of hand
Tendinous sheath of flexor pollicis longus
Flexor retinaculum (transverse carpal ligament)
Palmaris longus
Flexor digitorum superficialis and profundus in common flexor sheath
Tendinous sheath of abductor pollicis longus and extensor pollicis brevis
Flexor carpi radialis
Tendinous sheath of flexor pollicis longus
C. Anterior View

## 6.68 Synovial sheaths of palm of hand

**A.** Anular and cruciate parts (pulleys) of the fibrous digital sheath. **B.** Common flexor sheath. **C.** Tendinous (synovial) sheaths of long flexor tendons of the digits.

Injuries such as puncture of a finger by a rusty nail can cause infection of the digital synovial sheaths. When inflammation of the tendon and synovial sheath (tenosynovitis) occurs, the digit swells and movement becomes painful. Because the tendons of the 2nd–4th digits nearly always have separate synovial sheaths, the infection usually is confined to the infected digits. If the infection is untreated, however, the proximal ends of these sheaths may rupture, allowing the infection to spread to the midpalmar space. Because the synovial sheath of the little finger is usually continuous with the common flexor sheath, tenosynovitis in this finger may spread to the common flexor sheath and thus through the palm and carpal tunnel to the anterior forearm. Likewise, tenosynovitis in the thumb may spread through the continuous tendinous sheath of flexor pollicis longus.

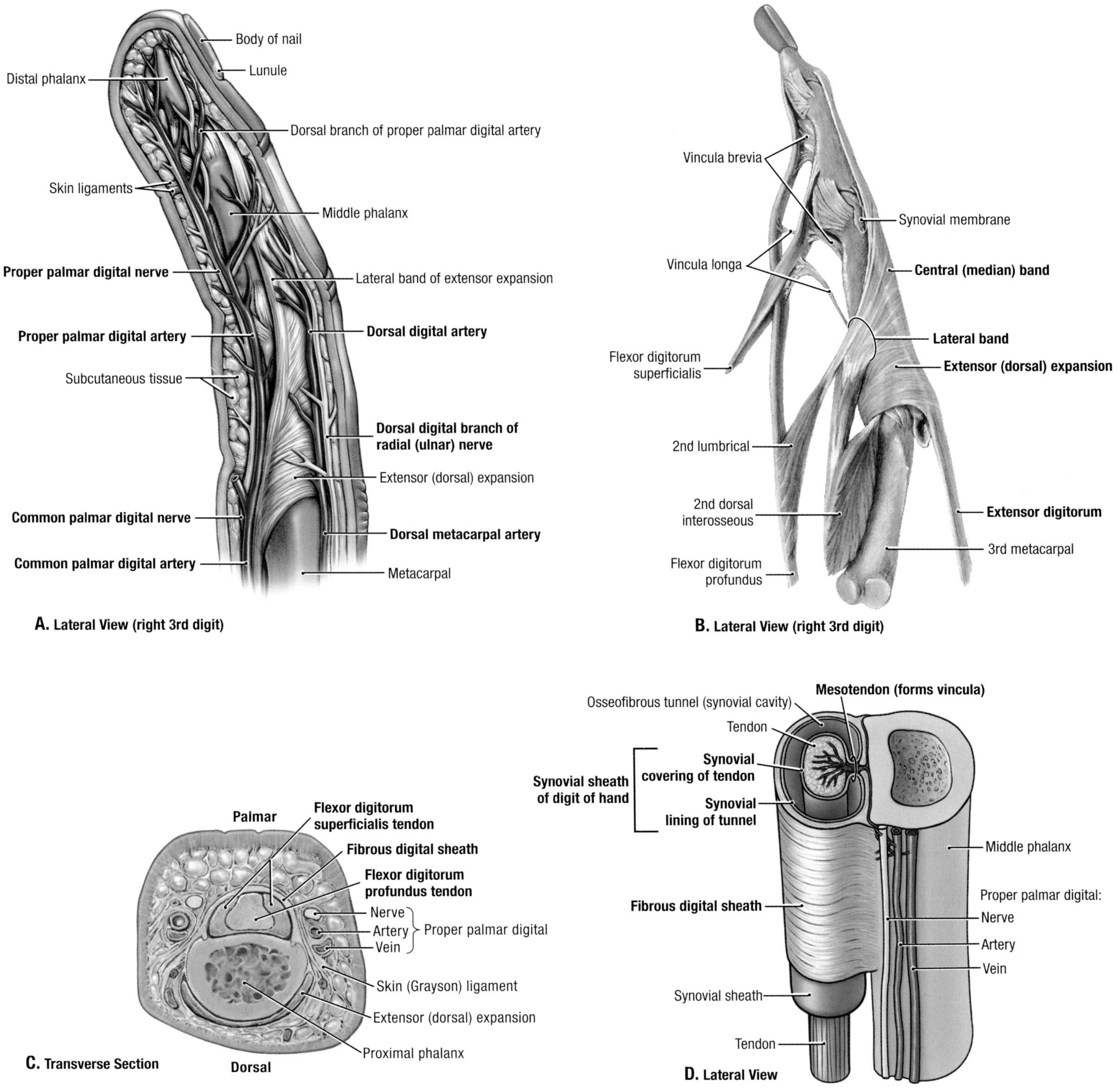

Body of nail
Lunule
Distal phalanx
Dorsal branch of proper palmar digital artery
Skin ligaments
Middle phalanx
**Proper palmar digital nerve**
Lateral band of extensor expansion
**Proper palmar digital artery**
**Dorsal digital artery**
Subcutaneous tissue
**Dorsal digital branch of radial (ulnar) nerve**
Extensor (dorsal) expansion
**Common palmar digital nerve**
**Dorsal metacarpal artery**
**Common palmar digital artery**
Metacarpal

**A.** Lateral View (right 3rd digit)

Vincula brevia
Synovial membrane
Vincula longa
**Central (median) band**
**Lateral band**
Flexor digitorum superficialis
**Extensor (dorsal) expansion**
2nd lumbrical
2nd dorsal interosseous
**Extensor digitorum**
3rd metacarpal
Flexor digitorum profundus

**B.** Lateral View (right 3rd digit)

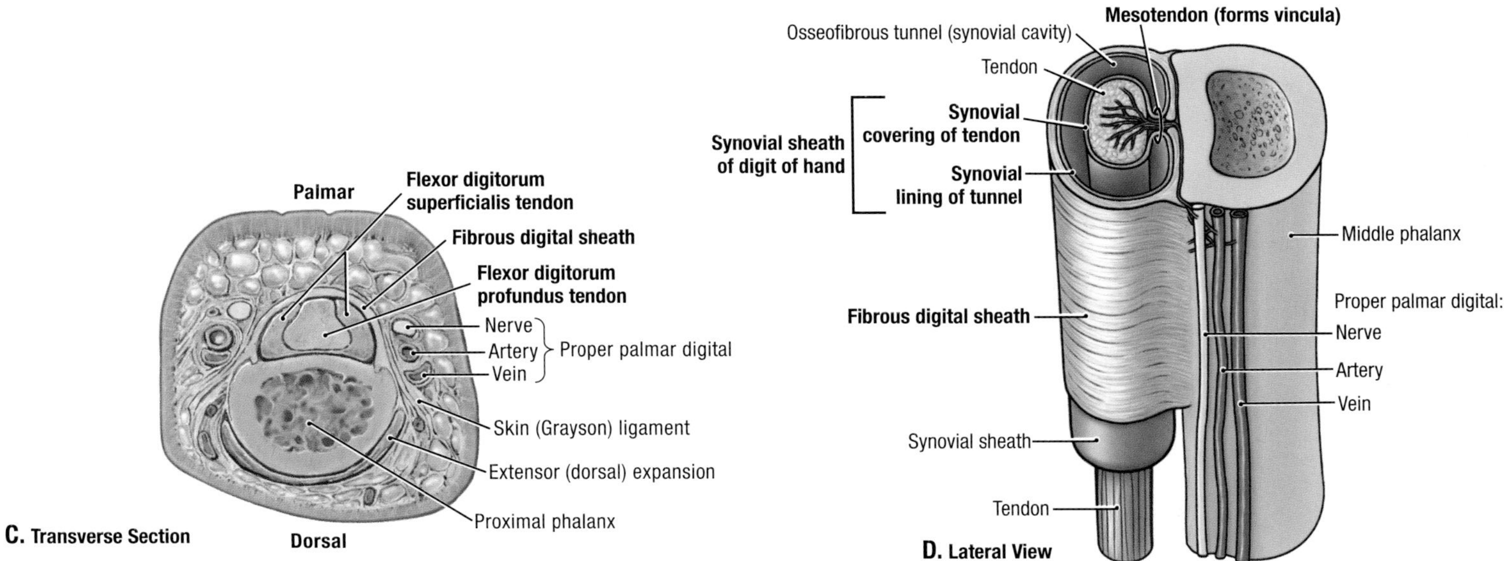
Palmar
Flexor digitorum superficialis tendon
Fibrous digital sheath
Flexor digitorum profundus tendon
Nerve
Artery
Vein
Proper palmar digital
Skin (Grayson) ligament
Extensor (dorsal) expansion
Proximal phalanx
Dorsal
Mesotendon (forms vincula)
Osseofibrous tunnel (synovial cavity)
Tendon
Synovial sheath of digit of hand
Synovial covering of tendon
Synovial lining of tunnel
Middle phalanx
Fibrous digital sheath
Proper palmar digital:
Nerve
Artery
Vein
Synovial sheath
Tendon

**C.** Transverse Section

**D.** Lateral View

## 6.69 Digital tendons, vessels, and nerves

**A.** Digital vessels and nerves. **B.** Extensor expansion of the 3rd (middle) digit. **C.** Transverse section through the proximal phalanx. **D.** Osseofibrous tunnel and tendinous (synovial) sheath.

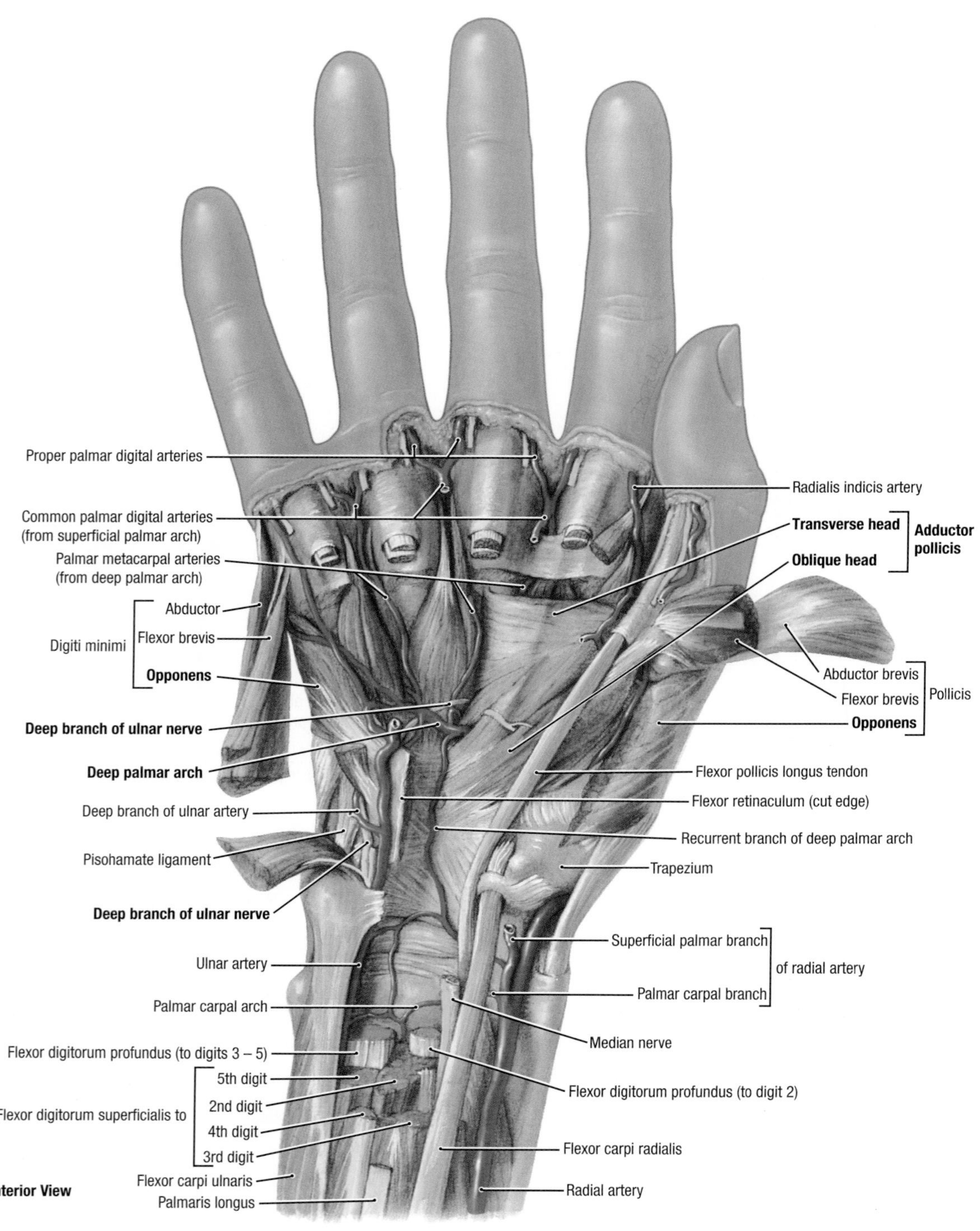
Proper palmar digital arteries
Common palmar digital arteries (from superficial palmar arch)
Palmar metacarpal arteries (from deep palmar arch)
Digiti minimi
Abductor
Flexor brevis
Opponens
Deep branch of ulnar nerve
Deep palmar arch
Deep branch of ulnar artery
Pisohamate ligament
Deep branch of ulnar nerve
Ulnar artery
Palmar carpal arch
Flexor digitorum profundus (to digits 3 – 5)
Flexor digitorum superficialis to
5th digit
2nd digit
4th digit
3rd digit
Flexor carpi ulnaris
Palmaris longus
Anterior View
Radialis indicis artery
Transverse head
Oblique head
Adductor pollicis
Abductor brevis
Flexor brevis
Opponens
Pollicis
Flexor pollicis longus tendon
Flexor retinaculum (cut edge)
Recurrent branch of deep palmar arch
Trapezium
Superficial palmar branch
Palmar carpal branch
of radial artery
Median nerve
Flexor digitorum profundus (to digit 2)
Flexor carpi radialis
Radial artery

## 6.70 Deep dissection of palm

- The deep branch of the ulnar artery joins the radial artery to form the deep palmar arch.

Compression of the ulnar nerve may occur at the wrist where it passes between the pisiform and the hook of hamate. The depression between these bones is converted by the pisohamate ligament into an osseofibrous ulnar canal (Guyon canal). Ulnar canal syndrome is manifest by hypoesthesia in the medial one and one half fingers and weakness of the intrinsic hand muscles. Clawing of the 4th and 5th fingers may occur, but in contrast to proximal nerve injury, their ability to flex is unaffected and there is no radical deviation of the hand.

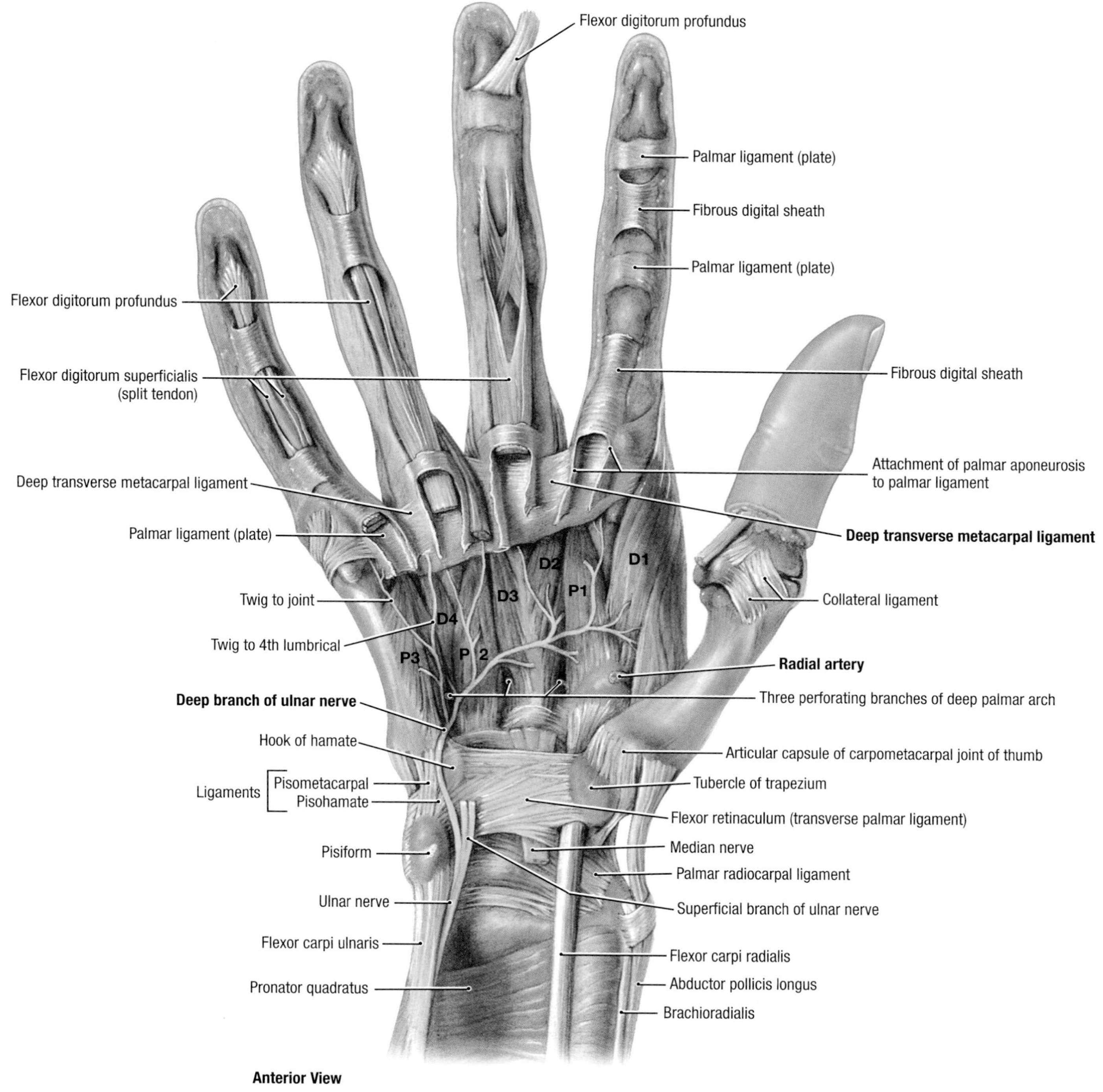
Flexor digitorum profundus
Palmar ligament (plate)
Fibrous digital sheath
Palmar ligament (plate)
Flexor digitorum profundus
Flexor digitorum superficialis (split tendon)
Fibrous digital sheath
Attachment of palmar aponeurosis to palmar ligament
Deep transverse metacarpal ligament
Deep transverse metacarpal ligament
Palmar ligament (plate)
D2
D1
D3
P1
Collateral ligament
Twig to joint
D4
Twig to 4th lumbrical
P3
P 2
Radial artery
Deep branch of ulnar nerve
Three perforating branches of deep palmar arch
Hook of hamate
Articular capsule of carpometacarpal joint of thumb
Ligaments
Pisometacarpal
Pisohamate
Tubercle of trapezium
Flexor retinaculum (transverse palmar ligament)
Pisiform
Median nerve
Palmar radiocarpal ligament
Ulnar nerve
Superficial branch of ulnar nerve
Flexor carpi ulnaris
Flexor carpi radialis
Pronator quadratus
Abductor pollicis longus
Brachioradialis
Anterior View

## 6.71 Deep dissection of palm and digits with deep branch of ulnar nerve

- Three unipennate palmar *(P1–3)* and four bipennate dorsal *(D1–4)* interosseous muscles are illustrated; the palmar interossei adduct the fingers, and the dorsal interossei abduct the fingers in relation to the axial line, an imaginary line drawn through the long axis of the 3rd digit (see Table 6.11).
- The deep transverse metacarpal ligaments unite the palmar ligaments; the lumbricals pass anterior to the deep transverse metacarpal ligament, and the interossei pass posterior to the ligament.
- Note the ulnar (Guyon) canal through which the ulnar vessels and nerve pass medial to the pisiform.

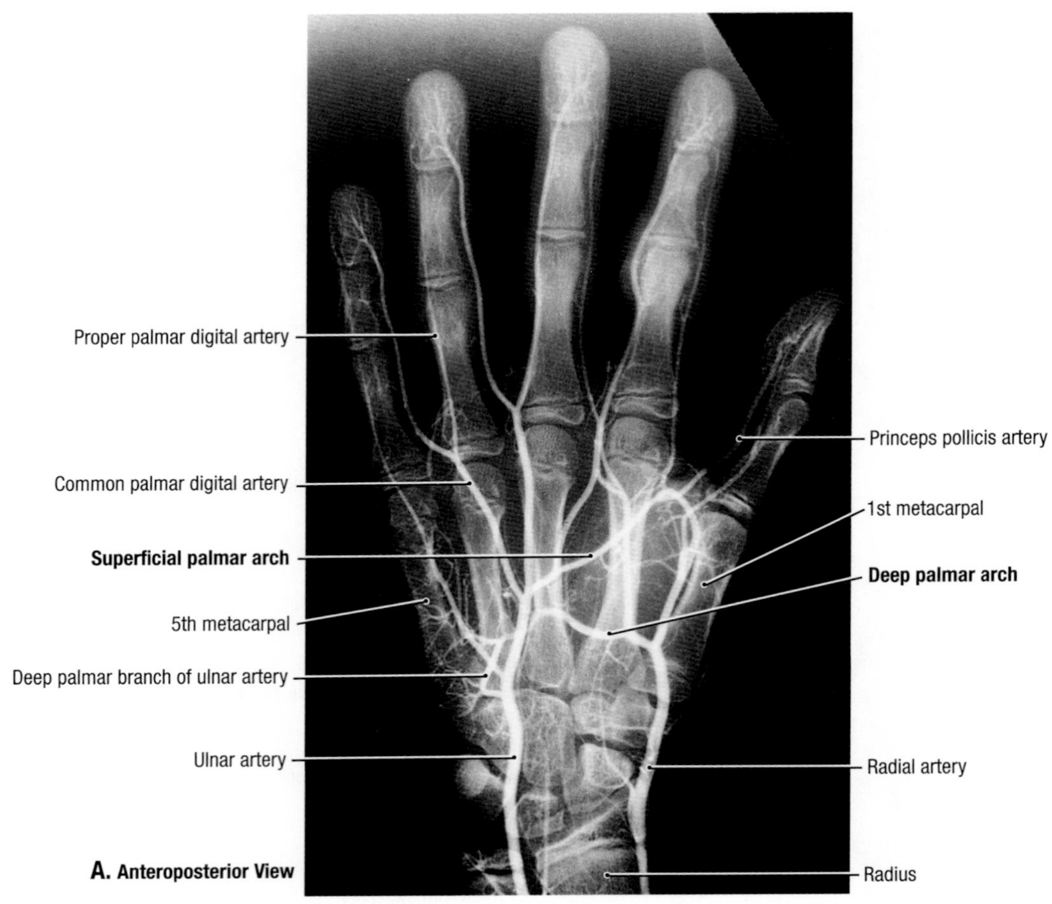
Proper palmar digital artery
Common palmar digital artery
Superficial palmar arch
5th metacarpal
Deep palmar branch of ulnar artery
Ulnar artery
Princeps pollicis artery
1st metacarpal
Deep palmar arch
Radial artery
Radius

**A.** Anteroposterior View

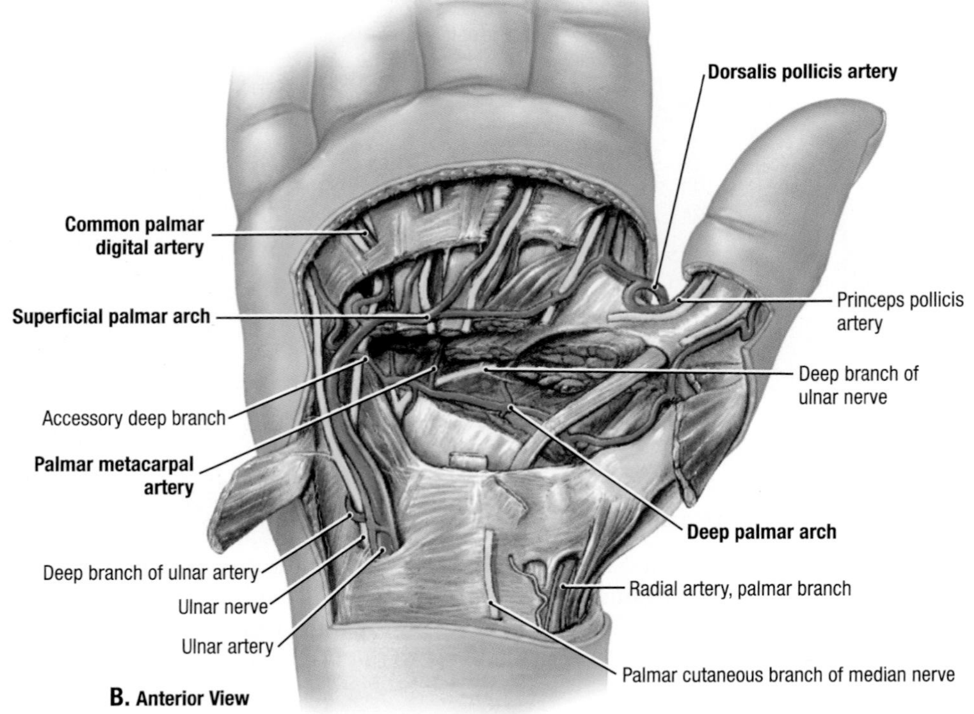
Common palmar digital artery
Superficial palmar arch
Accessory deep branch
Palmar metacarpal artery
Deep branch of ulnar artery
Ulnar nerve
Ulnar artery
Dorsalis pollicis artery
Princeps pollicis artery
Deep branch of ulnar nerve
Deep palmar arch
Radial artery, palmar branch
Palmar cutaneous branch of median nerve

**B.** Anterior View

## 6.72 Arterial supply of hand

**A.** Arteriogram of the hand. **B.** Dissection of palmar arterial arches.

- The superficial palmar arch is usually completed by the superficial palmar branch of the radial artery, but in this specimen the dorsalis pollicis artery completes the arch.

The superficial and deep palmar (arterial) arches are not palpable, but their surface markings are visible. The superficial palmar arch occurs at the level of the distal border of the fully extended thumb. The deep palmar arch lies approximately 1 cm proximal to the superficial palmar arch. The location of these arches should be borne in mind in wounds of the palm and when palmar incisions are made.

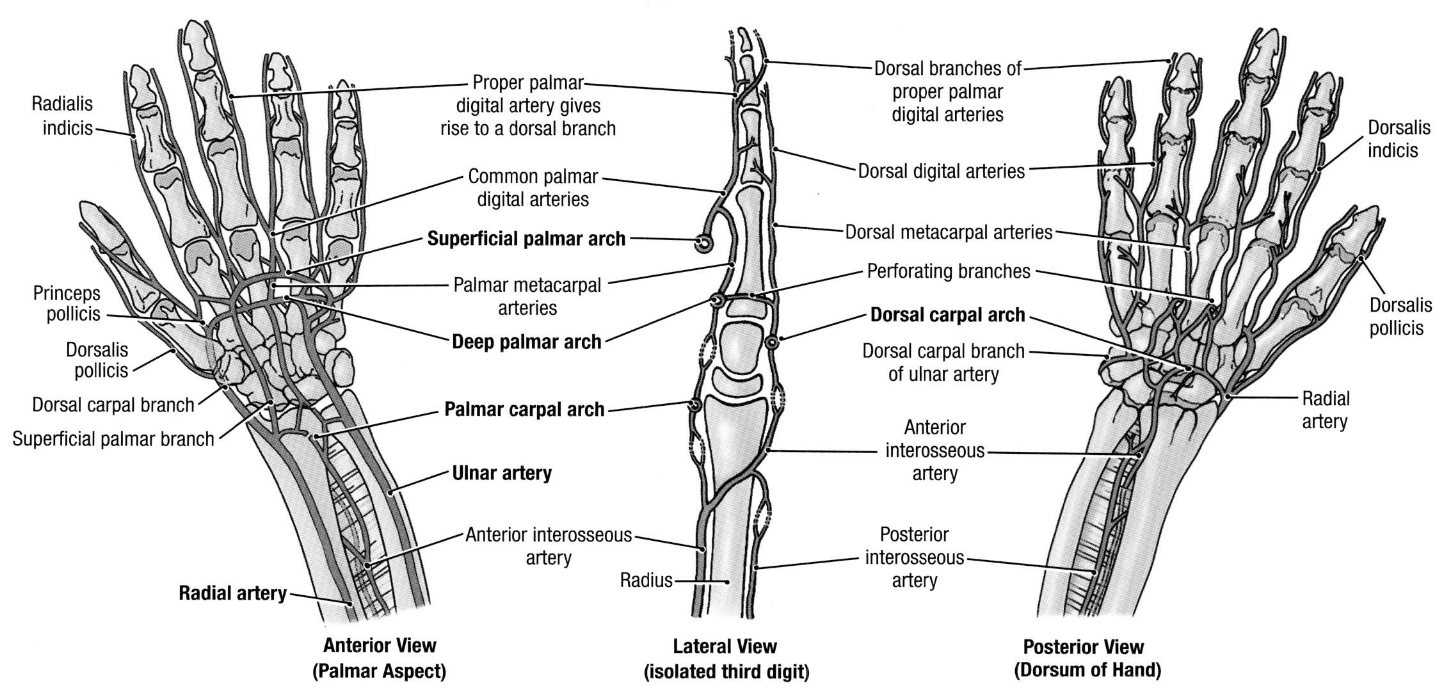
Radialis indicis
Proper palmar digital artery gives rise to a dorsal branch
Common palmar digital arteries
Superficial palmar arch
Princeps pollicis
Palmar metacarpal arteries
Dorsalis pollicis
Deep palmar arch
Dorsal carpal branch
Superficial palmar branch
Palmar carpal arch
Ulnar artery
Anterior interosseous artery
Radial artery
Radius
Dorsal branches of proper palmar digital arteries
Dorsal digital arteries
Dorsal metacarpal arteries
Perforating branches
Dorsal carpal arch
Dorsal carpal branch of ulnar artery
Anterior interosseous artery
Posterior interosseous artery
Dorsalis indicis
Dorsalis pollicis
Radial artery
Anterior View (Palmar Aspect)
Lateral View (isolated third digit)
Posterior View (Dorsum of Hand)

## TABLE 6.12 ARTERIES OF HAND

| Artery | Origin | Course |
|---|---|---|
| **Superficial palmar arch** | Direct continuation of ulnar artery; arch is completed on lateral side by superficial branch of radial artery or another of its branches | Curves laterally deep to palmar aponeurosis and superficial to long flexor tendons; curve of arch lies across palm at level of distal border of extended thumb |
| **Deep palmar arch** | Direct continuation of radial artery; arch is completed on medial side by deep branch of ulnar artery | Curves medially, deep to long flexor tendons and is in contact with bases of metacarpals |
| **Common palmar digitals** | Superficial palmar arch | Pass directly on lumbricals to webbings of digits |
| **Proper palmar digitals** | Common palmar digital arteries | Run along sides of digits 2–5 |
| **Princeps pollicis** | Radial artery as it turns into palm | Descends on palmar aspect of first metacarpal and divides at the base of proximal phalanx into two branches that run along sides of thumb |
| **Radialis indicis** | Radial artery, but may arise from princeps pollicis artery | Passes along lateral side of index finger to its distal end |
| **Dorsal carpal arch** | Radial and ulnar arteries | Arches within fascia on dorsum of hand |

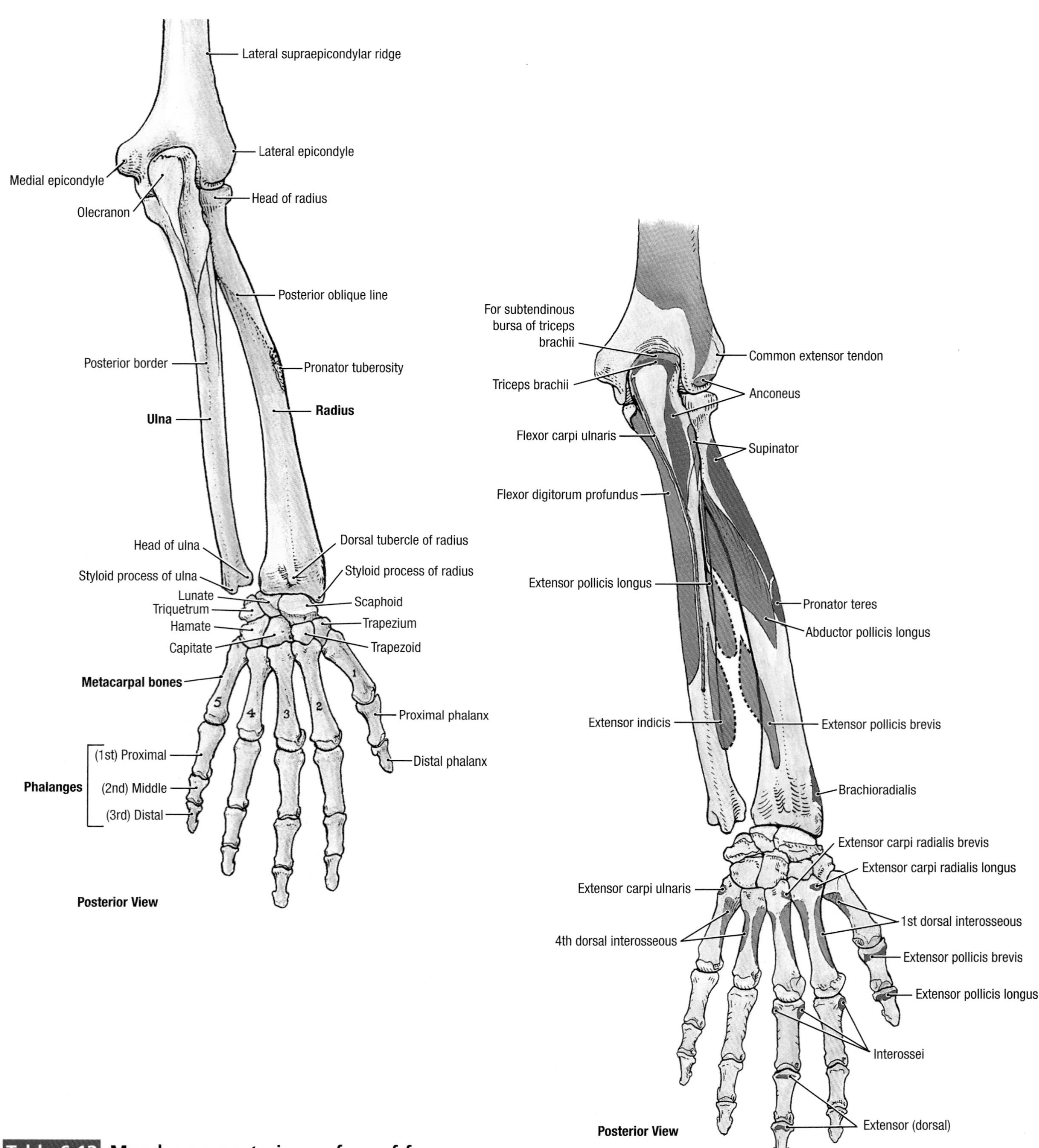
Lateral supraepicondylar ridge
Lateral epicondyle
Medial epicondyle
Olecranon
Head of radius
Posterior oblique line
Posterior border
Pronator tuberosity
Ulna
Radius
Head of ulna
Dorsal tubercle of radius
Styloid process of ulna
Styloid process of radius
Lunate
Triquetrum
Scaphoid
Hamate
Trapezium
Capitate
Trapezoid
Metacarpal bones
Proximal phalanx
(1st) Proximal
Phalanges
(2nd) Middle
(3rd) Distal
Distal phalanx
Posterior View
For subtendinous bursa of triceps brachii
Common extensor tendon
Triceps brachii
Anconeus
Flexor carpi ulnaris
Supinator
Flexor digitorum profundus
Extensor pollicis longus
Pronator teres
Abductor pollicis longus
Extensor indicis
Extensor pollicis brevis
Brachioradialis
Extensor carpi radialis brevis
Extensor carpi radialis longus
Extensor carpi ulnaris
1st dorsal interosseous
4th dorsal interosseous
Extensor pollicis brevis
Extensor pollicis longus
Interossei
Extensor (dorsal)
Posterior View

## Table 6.13 Muscles on posterior surface of forearm

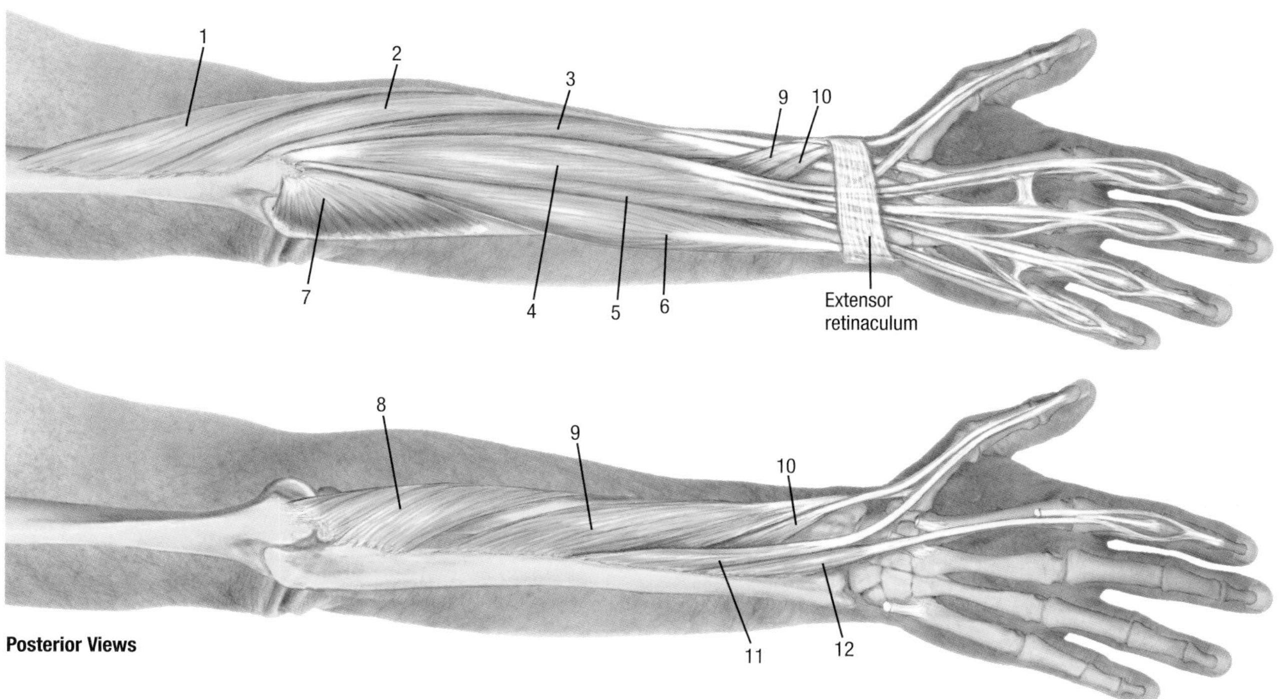
1
2
3
9
10
7
4
5
6
Extensor retinaculum
8
9
10
11
12

Posterior Views

### TABLE 6.13 MUSCLES OF POSTERIOR SURFACE OF FOREARM

| Muscle | Proximal Attachment | Distal Attachment | Innervation | Main Actions |
|---|---|---|---|---|
| **Brachioradialis *(1)*** | Proximal two thirds of lateral supraepicondylar ridge of humerus | Lateral surface of distal end of radius | Radial nerve (C5, **C6**, and C7) | Flexes forearm |
| **Extensor carpi radialis longus *(2)*** | Lateral supraepicondylar ridge of humerus | Base of second metacarpal bone | Radial nerve (C6 and C7) | Extend and abduct hand at wrist joint |
| **Extensor carpi radialis brevis *(3)*** | Lateral epicondyle of humerus | Base of third metacarpal bone | Deep branch of radial nerve (**C7** and C8) | |
| **Extensor digitorum *(4)*** | | Extensor expansions of medial four digits | Posterior interosseous nerve (C7 and C8), a branch of the radial nerve | Extends medial four digits at metacarpophalangeal joints; extends hand at wrist joint |
| **Extensor digiti minimi *(5)*** | | Extensor expansion of fifth digit | | Extends fifth digit at metacarpophalangeal and interphalangeal joints |
| **Extensor carpi ulnaris *(6)*** | Lateral epicondyle of humerus and posterior border of ulna | Base of fifth metacarpal bone | | Extends and adducts hand at wrist joint |
| **Anconeus *(7)*** | Lateral epicondyle of humerus | Lateral surface of olecranon and superior part of posterior surface of ulna | Radial nerve (C7, C8, and T1) | Assists triceps in extending elbow joint; stabilizes elbow joint; abducts ulna during pronation |
| **Supinator *(8)*** | Lateral epicondyle of humerus, radial collateral and anular ligaments, supinator fossa, and crest of ulna | Lateral, posterior, and anterior surfaces of proximal third of radius | Deep branch of radial nerve (C5 and **C6**) | Supinates forearm |
| **Abductor pollicis longus *(9)*** | Posterior surface of ulna, radius, and interosseous membrane | Base of first metacarpal bone | Posterior interosseous nerve (C7 and **C8**) | Abducts thumb and extends it at carpometacarpal joint |
| **Extensor pollicis brevis *(10)*** | Posterior surface of radius and interosseous membrane | Base of proximal phalanx of thumb | | Extends proximal phalanx of thumb at metacarpophalangeal **joint** |
| **Extensor pollicis longus *(11)*** | Posterior surface of middle third of ulna and interosseous membrane | Base of distal phalanx of thumb | | Extends distal phalanx of thumb at metacarpophalangeal and interphalangeal joints |
| **Extensor indicis *(12)*** | Posterior surface of ulna and interosseous membrane | Extensor expansion of second digit | | Extends second digit and helps to extend hand |

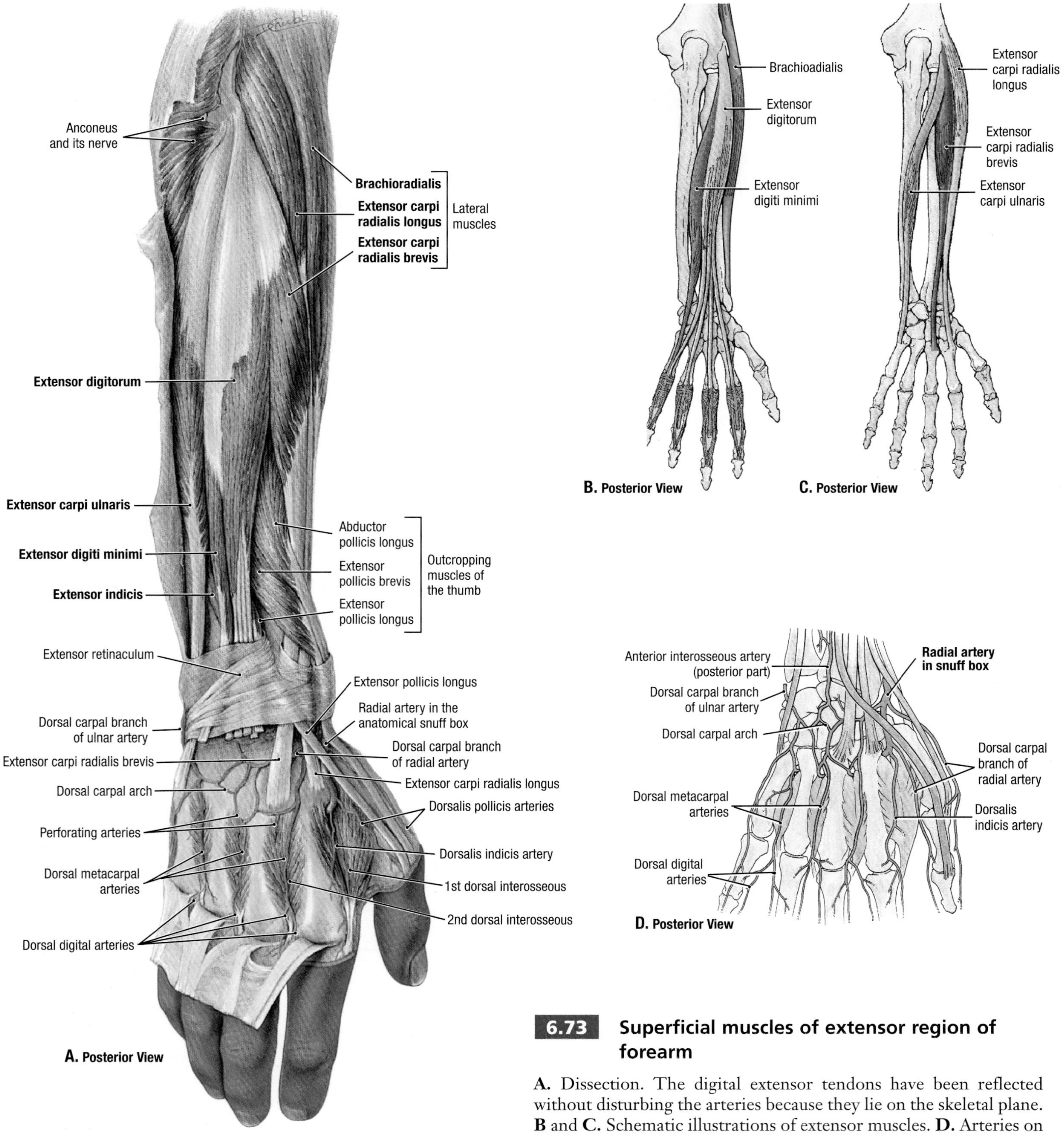

Anconeus and its nerve

**Brachioradialis**

**Extensor carpi radialis longus**

**Extensor carpi radialis brevis**

Lateral muscles

**Extensor digitorum**

**Extensor carpi ulnaris**

**Extensor digiti minimi**

**Extensor indicis**

Abductor pollicis longus

Extensor pollicis brevis

Extensor pollicis longus

Outcropping muscles of the thumb

Extensor retinaculum

Extensor pollicis longus

Radial artery in the anatomical snuff box

Dorsal carpal branch of ulnar artery

Dorsal carpal branch of radial artery

Extensor carpi radialis brevis

Extensor carpi radialis longus

Dorsal carpal arch

Dorsalis pollicis arteries

Perforating arteries

Dorsalis indicis artery

Dorsal metacarpal arteries

1st dorsal interosseous

2nd dorsal interosseous

Dorsal digital arteries

**A.** Posterior View

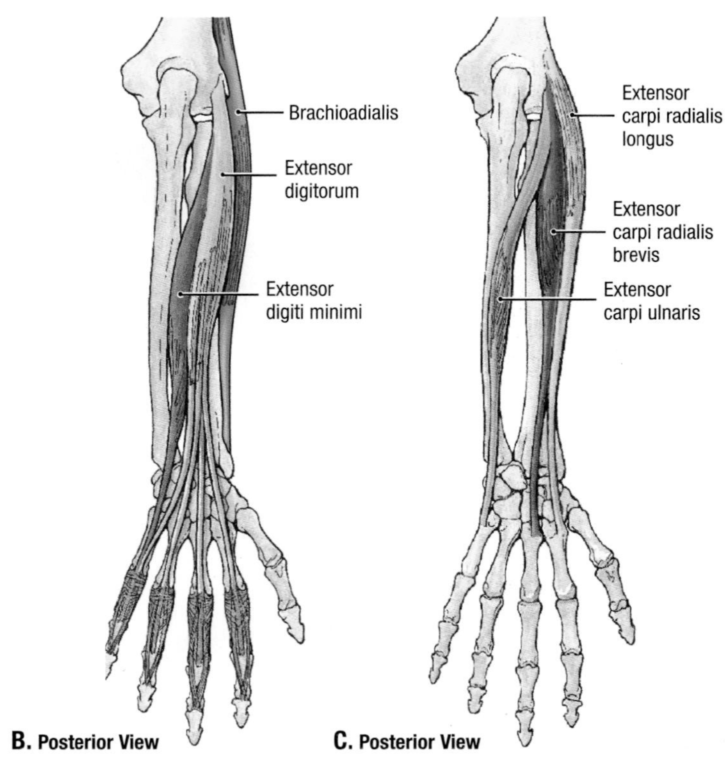
Brachioadialis
Extensor digitorum
Extensor digiti minimi
Extensor carpi radialis longus
Extensor carpi radialis brevis
Extensor carpi ulnaris
B. Posterior View
C. Posterior View

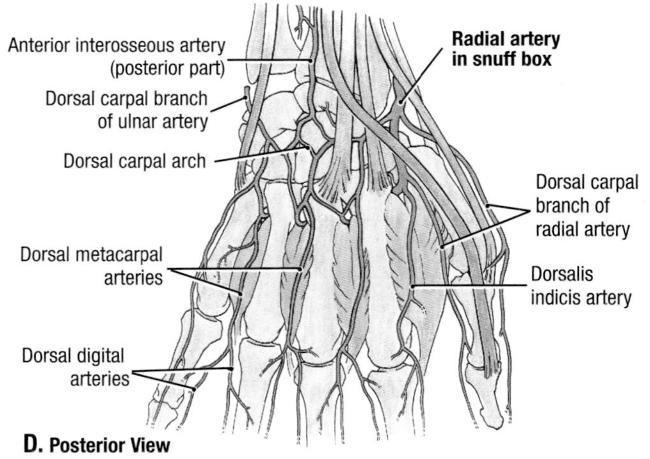
Anterior interosseous artery (posterior part)
Radial artery in snuff box
Dorsal carpal branch of ulnar artery
Dorsal carpal arch
Dorsal carpal branch of radial artery
Dorsal metacarpal arteries
Dorsalis indicis artery
Dorsal digital arteries
D. Posterior View

## 6.73 Superficial muscles of extensor region of forearm

**A.** Dissection. The digital extensor tendons have been reflected without disturbing the arteries because they lie on the skeletal plane. **B** and **C.** Schematic illustrations of extensor muscles. **D.** Arteries on dorsum of hand.

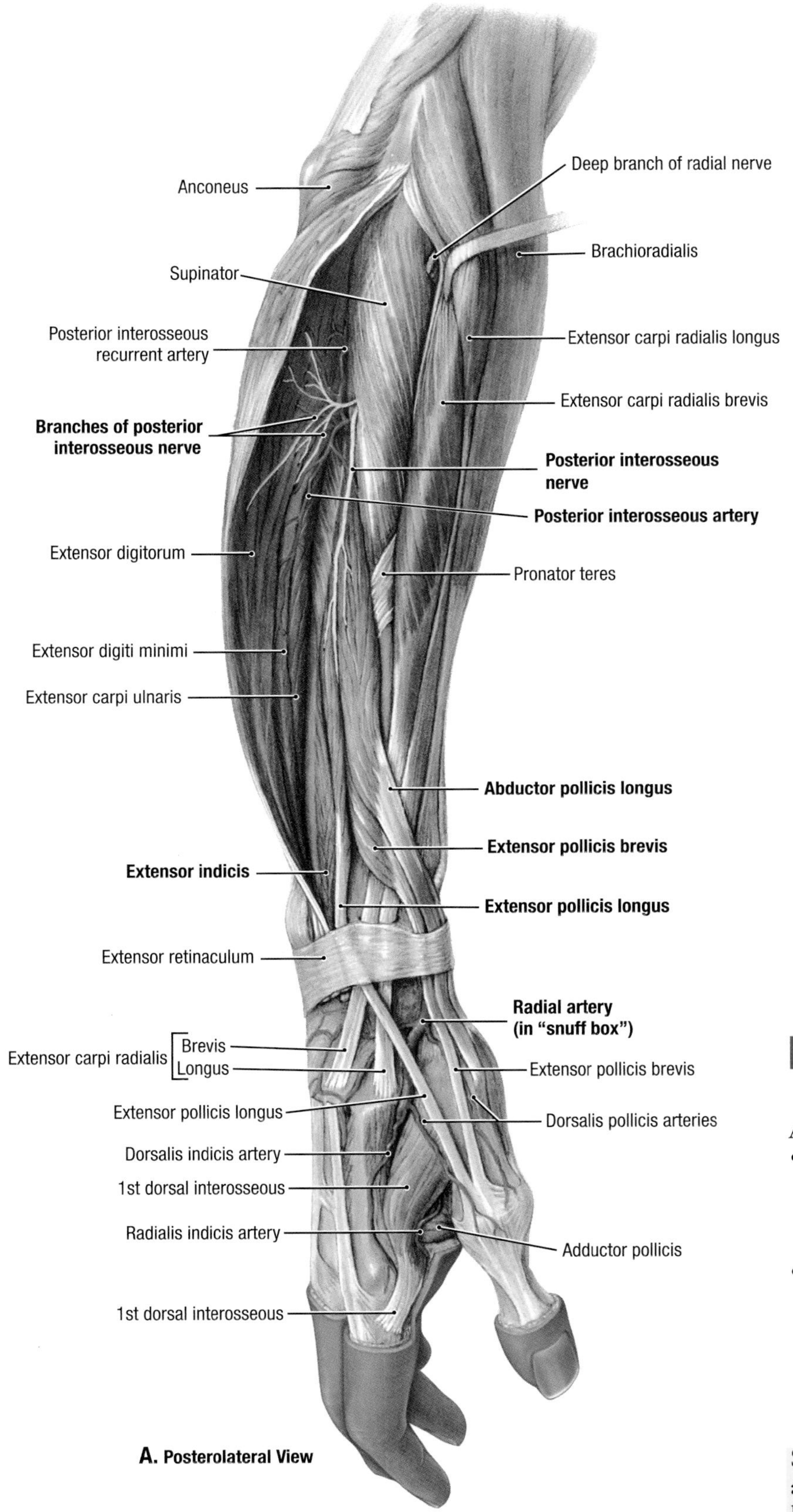

Anconeus
Deep branch of radial nerve
Brachioradialis
Supinator
Posterior interosseous recurrent artery
Extensor carpi radialis longus
Extensor carpi radialis brevis
Branches of posterior interosseous nerve
Posterior interosseous nerve
Posterior interosseous artery
Extensor digitorum
Pronator teres
Extensor digiti minimi
Extensor carpi ulnaris
Abductor pollicis longus
Extensor pollicis brevis
Extensor indicis
Extensor pollicis longus
Extensor retinaculum
Radial artery (in "snuff box")
Extensor carpi radialis Brevis
Longus
Extensor pollicis brevis
Extensor pollicis longus
Dorsalis pollicis arteries
Dorsalis indicis artery
1st dorsal interosseous
Radialis indicis artery
Adductor pollicis
1st dorsal interosseous

**A.** Posterolateral View

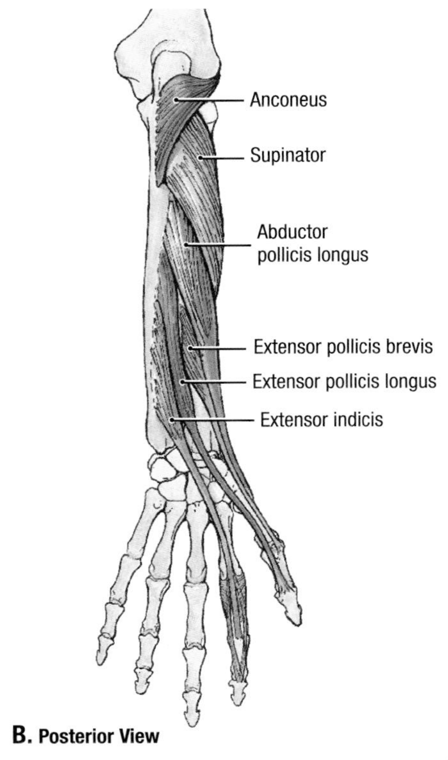
Anconeus
Supinator
Abductor pollicis longus
Extensor pollicis brevis
Extensor pollicis longus
Extensor indicis

**B.** Posterior View

## 6.74 Deep structures on extensor aspect of forearm

**A.** Dissection. **B.** Schematic illustration.

- Three "outcropping" muscles of the thumb (abductor pollicis longus, extensor pollicis brevis, and extensor pollicis longus) emerge between the extensor carpi radialis brevis and the extensor digitorum.
- The laterally retracted brachioradialis and extensor carpi radialis longus and brevis muscles and supinator muscles are innervated by the deep branch of the radial nerve; the other extensor muscles are supplied by the posterior interosseous nerve, which is a continuation of the deep branch of the radial nerve that pierced the supinator.

Severance of the deep branch of the radial nerve results in an inability to extend the thumb and the metacarpophalangeal joints of the other digits. Loss of sensation does not occur because the deep branch is entirely muscular and articular in distribution.

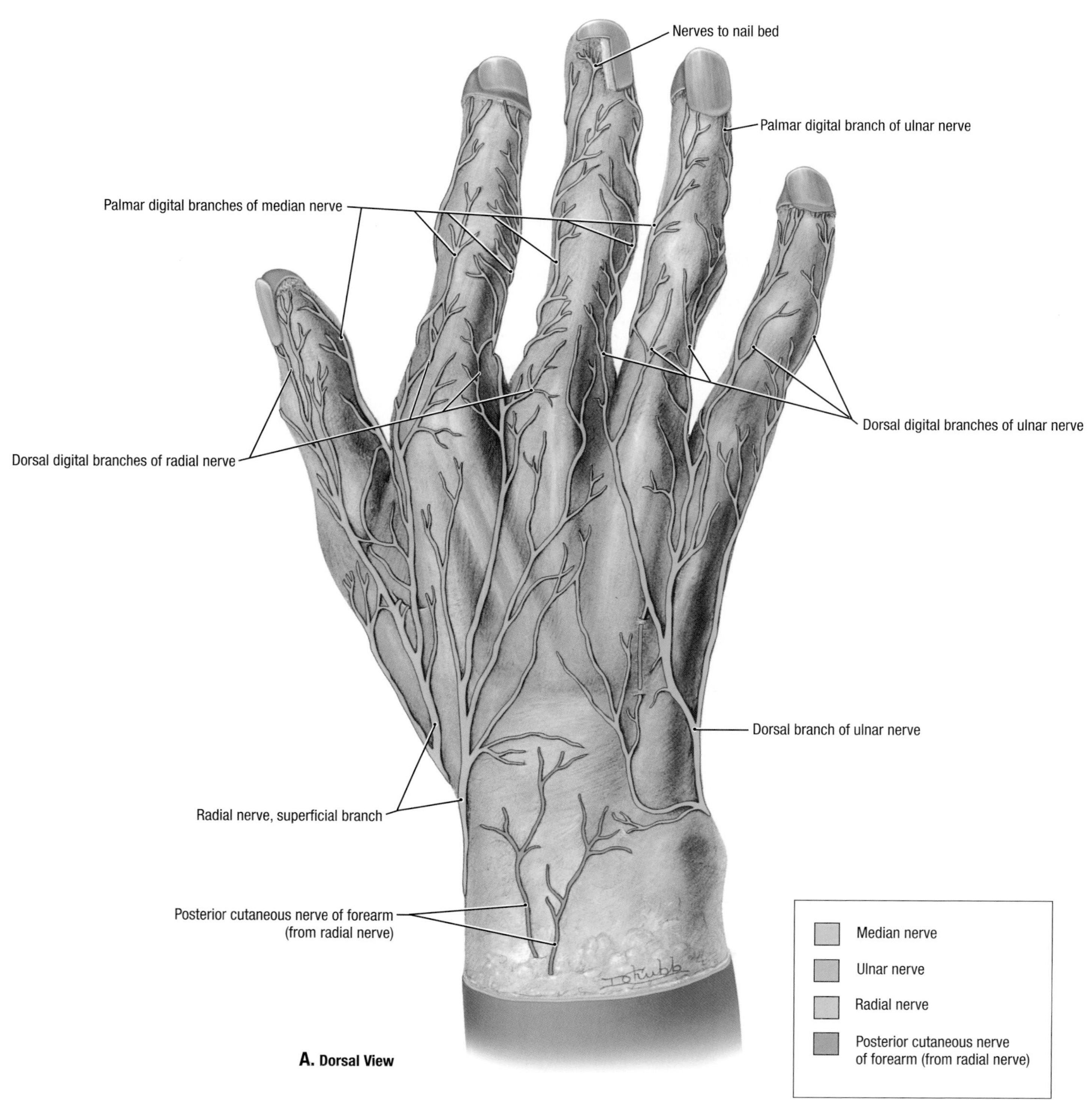
Nerves to nail bed
Palmar digital branch of ulnar nerve
Palmar digital branches of median nerve
Dorsal digital branches of ulnar nerve
Dorsal digital branches of radial nerve
Dorsal branch of ulnar nerve
Radial nerve, superficial branch
Posterior cutaneous nerve of forearm
(from radial nerve)
Median nerve
Ulnar nerve
Radial nerve
Posterior cutaneous nerve
of forearm (from radial nerve)
A. Dorsal View

## 6.75 Cutaneous innervation of hand

**A.** Dissection of nerves of dorsum of hand.

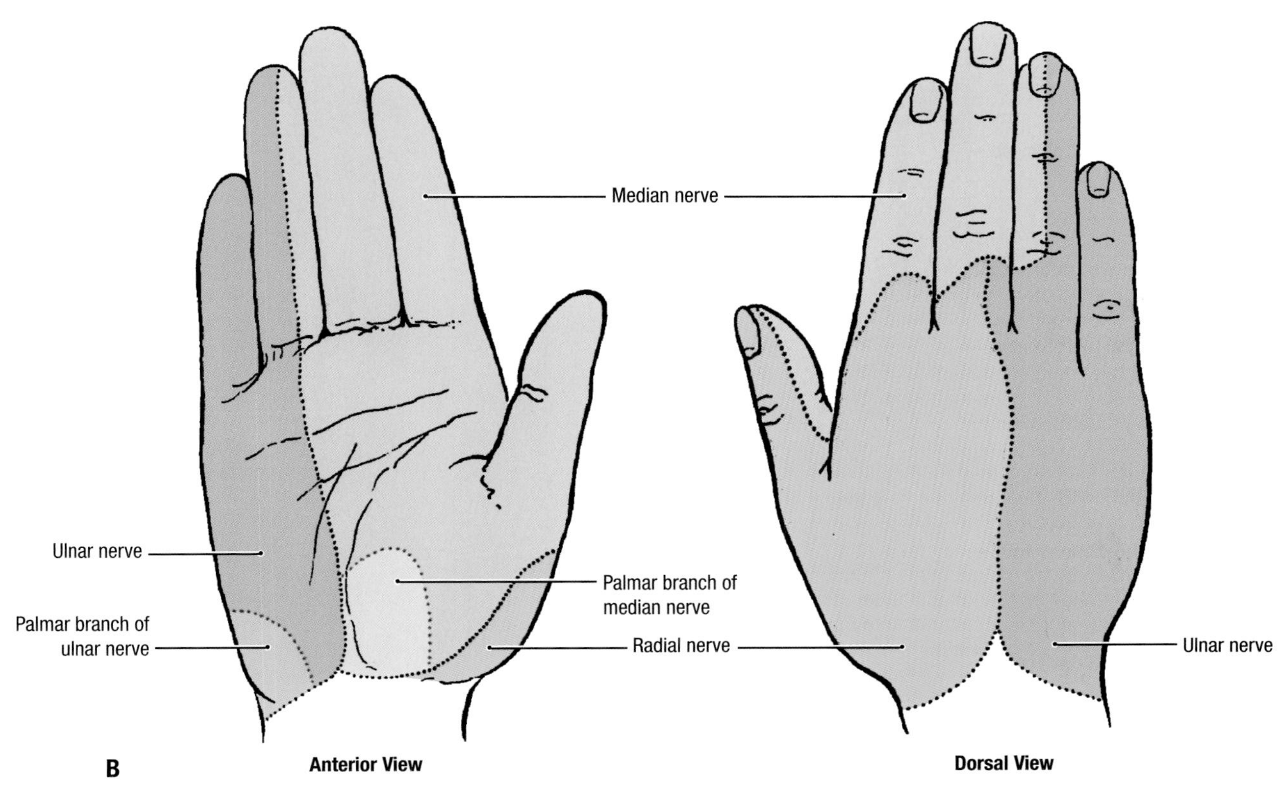
Median nerve
Ulnar nerve
Palmar branch of median nerve
Palmar branch of ulnar nerve
Radial nerve
Ulnar nerve
B
Anterior View
Dorsal View

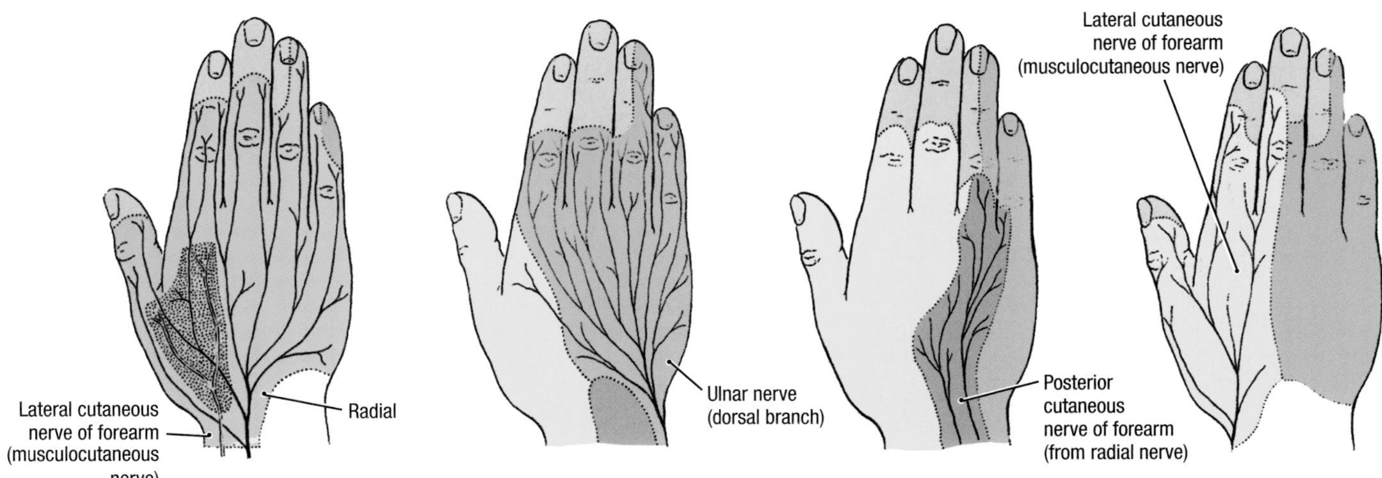
Lateral cutaneous nerve of forearm (musculocutaneous nerve)
Radial
Ulnar nerve (dorsal branch)
Posterior cutaneous nerve of forearm (from radial nerve)
Lateral cutaneous nerve of forearm (musculocutaneous nerve)
C. Dorsal Views

## 6.75 Cutaneous innervation of hand *(continued)*

**B.** Distribution of the cutaneous nerves to the palm and dorsum of the hand, schematic illustration. **C.** Variations in pattern of cutaneous nerves in dorsum of hand.

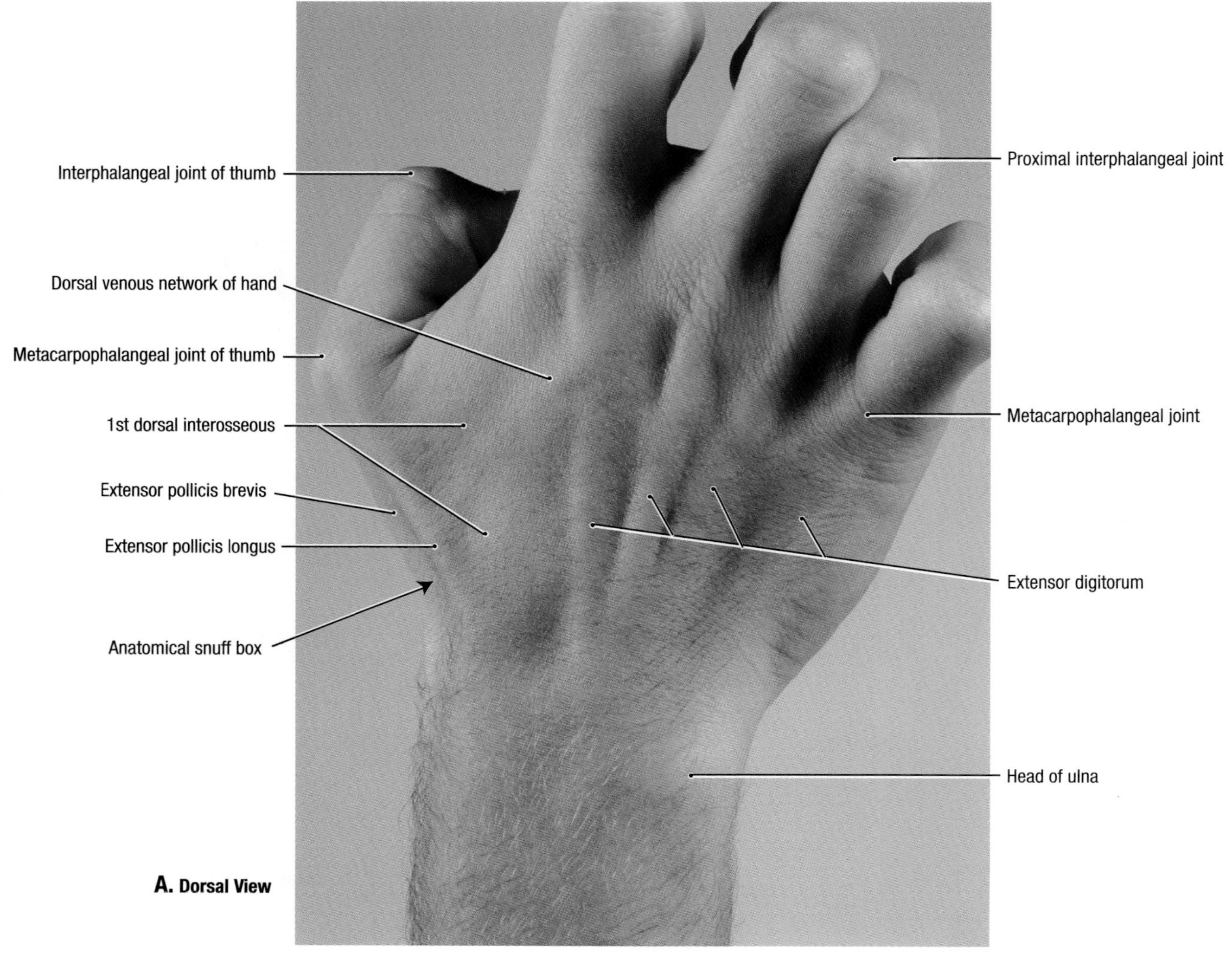
Interphalangeal joint of thumb
Dorsal venous network of hand
Metacarpophalangeal joint of thumb
1st dorsal interosseous
Extensor pollicis brevis
Extensor pollicis longus
Anatomical snuff box
Proximal interphalangeal joint
Metacarpophalangeal joint
Extensor digitorum
Head of ulna
A. Dorsal View

## 6.76 Dorsum of hand

**A.** Surface anatomy. The interphalangeal joints are flexed, and the metacarpophalangeal joints are hyperextended to demonstrate the extensor digitorum tendons. **B.** Tendinous (synovial) sheaths distended with blue fluid. **C.** Transverse section of distal forearm (*numbers* refer to structures labeled in B). **D.** Sites of bony attachments.

- Six tendinous sheaths occupy the six osseofibrous tunnels deep to the extensor retinaculum. They contain nine tendons: tendons for the thumb in sheaths 1 and 3, tendons for the extensors of the wrist in sheaths 2 and 6, and tendons for the extensors of the wrist and fingers in sheaths 4 and 5.
- The tendon of the extensor pollicis longus hooks around the dorsal tubercle of radius to pass obliquely across the tendons of the extensor carpi radialis longus and brevis to the thumb.

The tendons of the abductor pollicis longus and extensor pollicis brevis are in the same tendinous sheath on the dorsum of the wrist. Excessive friction of these tendons results in fibrous thickening of the sheath and stenosis of the osseofibrous tunnel, Quervain tenovaginitis stenosans. This condition causes pain in the wrist that radiates proximally to the forearm and distally to the thumb.

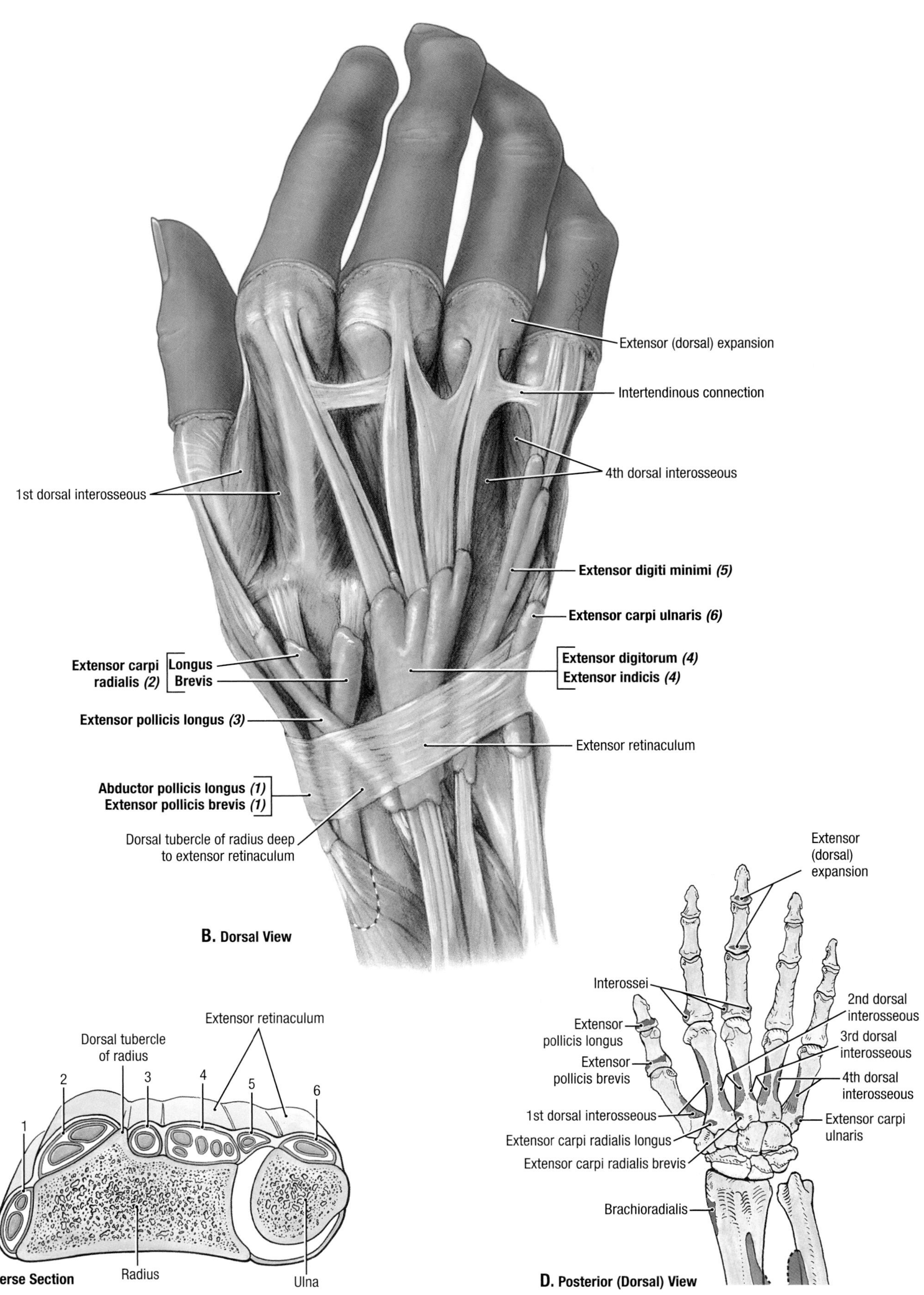
Extensor (dorsal) expansion
Intertendinous connection
4th dorsal interosseous
1st dorsal interosseous
Extensor digiti minimi (5)
Extensor carpi ulnaris (6)
Extensor carpi radialis (2) Longus
Brevis
Extensor digitorum (4)
Extensor indicis (4)
Extensor pollicis longus (3)
Extensor retinaculum
Abductor pollicis longus (1)
Extensor pollicis brevis (1)
Dorsal tubercle of radius deep to extensor retinaculum
Extensor (dorsal) expansion
Interossei
2nd dorsal interosseous
3rd dorsal interosseous
4th dorsal interosseous
Extensor pollicis longus
Extensor pollicis brevis
1st dorsal interosseous
Extensor carpi radialis longus
Extensor carpi radialis brevis
Extensor carpi ulnaris
Brachioradialis
Extensor retinaculum
Dorsal tubercle of radius
1
2
3
4
5
6
Radius
Ulna

**B.** Dorsal View

**C.** Transverse Section

**D.** Posterior (Dorsal) View

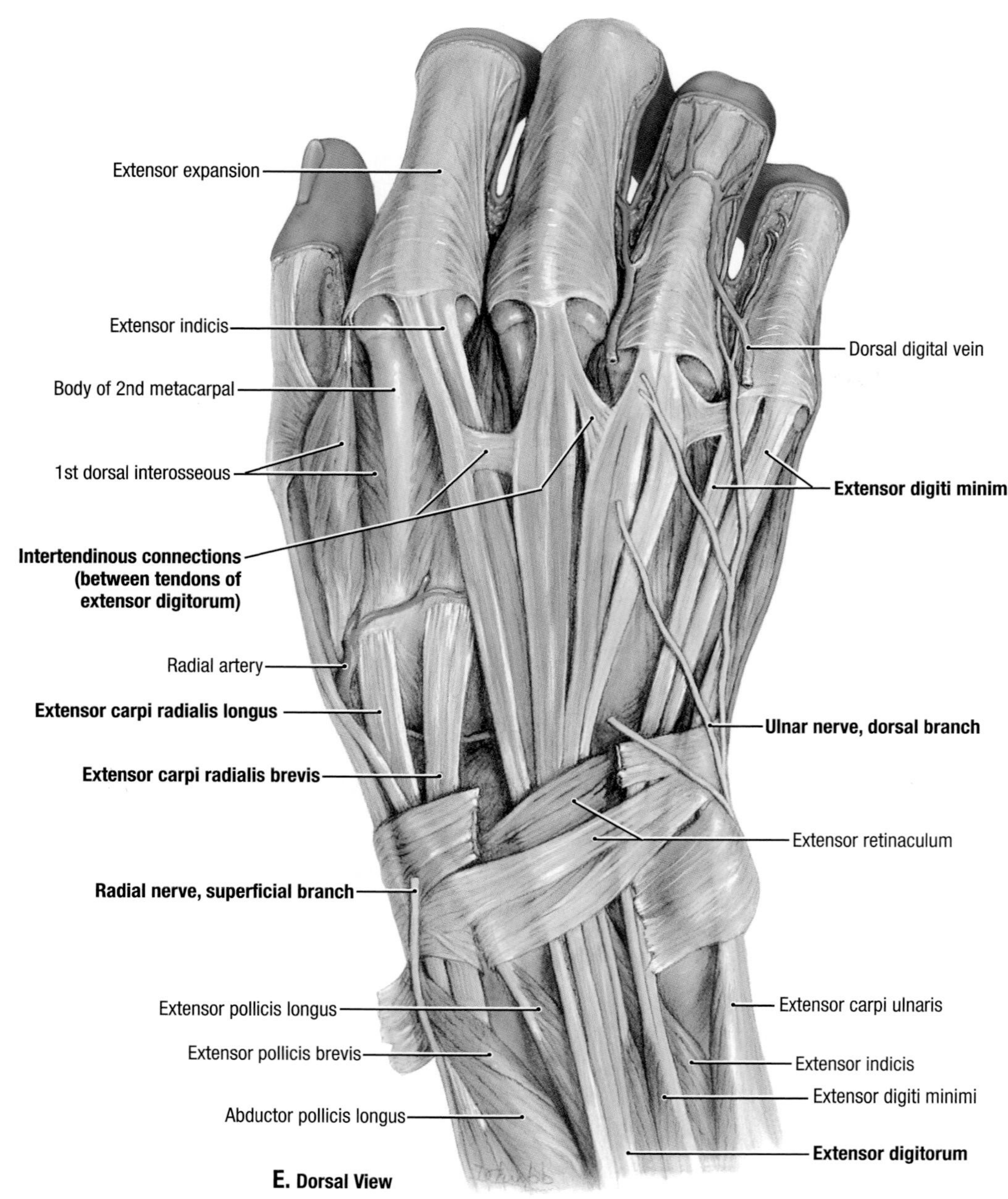
Extensor expansion
Extensor indicis
Body of 2nd metacarpal
1st dorsal interosseous
Intertendinous connections (between tendons of extensor digitorum)
Radial artery
Extensor carpi radialis longus
Extensor carpi radialis brevis
Radial nerve, superficial branch
Extensor pollicis longus
Extensor pollicis brevis
Abductor pollicis longus
Dorsal digital vein
Extensor digiti minimi
Ulnar nerve, dorsal branch
Extensor retinaculum
Extensor carpi ulnaris
Extensor indicis
Extensor digiti minimi
Extensor digitorum

**E.** Dorsal View

## 6.76 Dorsum of hand *(continued)*

**E.** Tendons on dorsum of hand and extensor retinaculum.

- The deep fascia is thickened to form the extensor retinaculum.
- Proximal to the knuckles, intertendinous connections extend between the tendons of the digital extensors and, thereby, restrict the independent action of the fingers.

Sometimes a nontender cystic swelling appears on the hand, most commonly on the dorsum of the wrist. The thin-walled cyst contains clear mucinous fluid. Clinically, this type of swelling is called a “ganglion” (G. swelling or knot). These synovial cysts are close to and often communicate with the synovial sheaths. The distal attachment of the extensor carpi radialis brevis tendon is a common site for such a cyst.

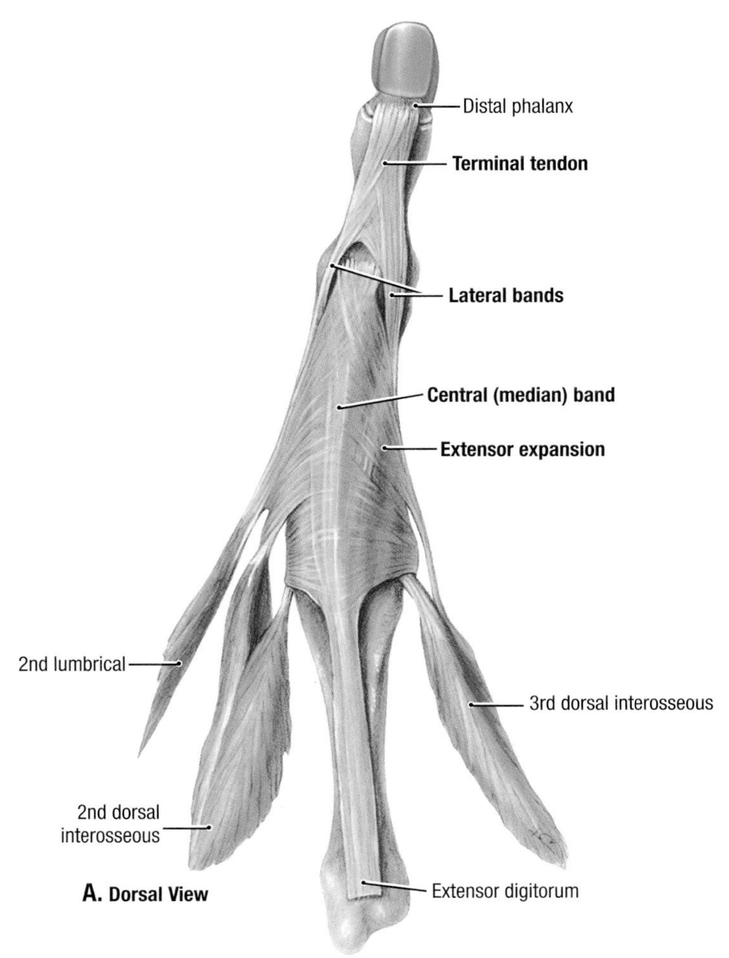
Distal phalanx
Terminal tendon
Lateral bands
Central (median) band
Extensor expansion
2nd lumbrical
3rd dorsal interosseous
2nd dorsal interosseous
Extensor digitorum
A. Dorsal View

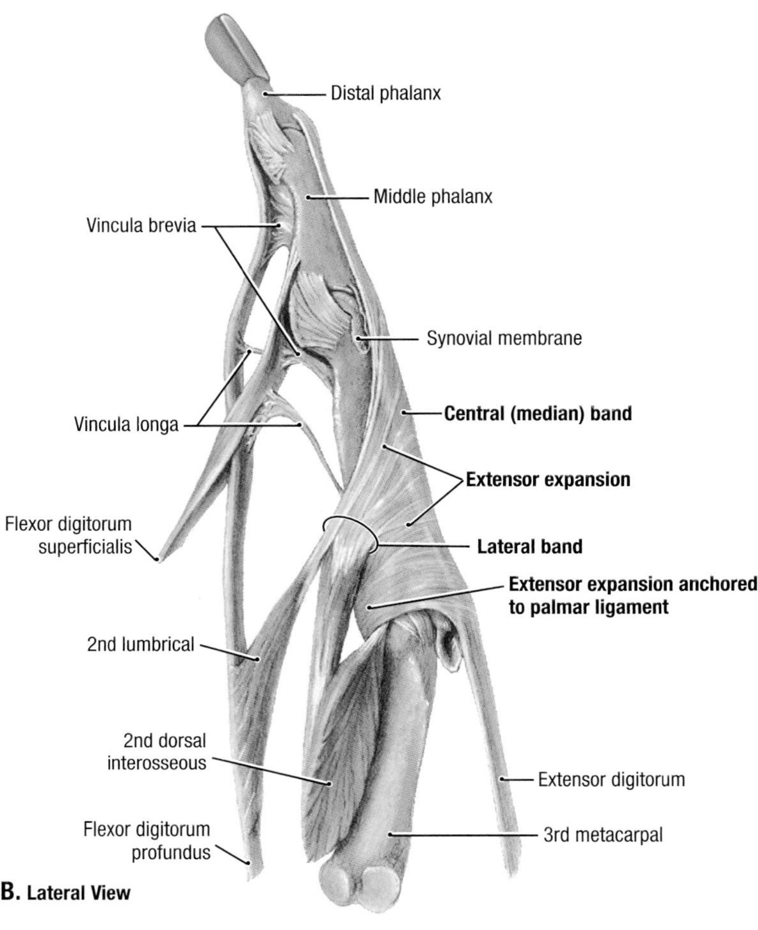
Distal phalanx
Middle phalanx
Vincula brevia
Synovial membrane
Central (median) band
Vincula longa
Extensor expansion
Flexor digitorum superficialis
Lateral band
Extensor expansion anchored to palmar ligament
2nd lumbrical
2nd dorsal interosseous
Extensor digitorum
Flexor digitorum profundus
3rd metacarpal
B. Lateral View

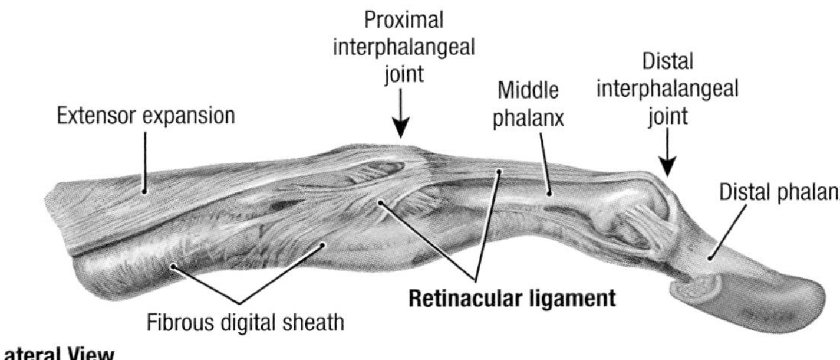
Proximal interphalangeal joint
Distal interphalangeal joint
Middle phalanx
Extensor expansion
Distal phalanx
Retinacular ligament
Fibrous digital sheath
C. Lateral View

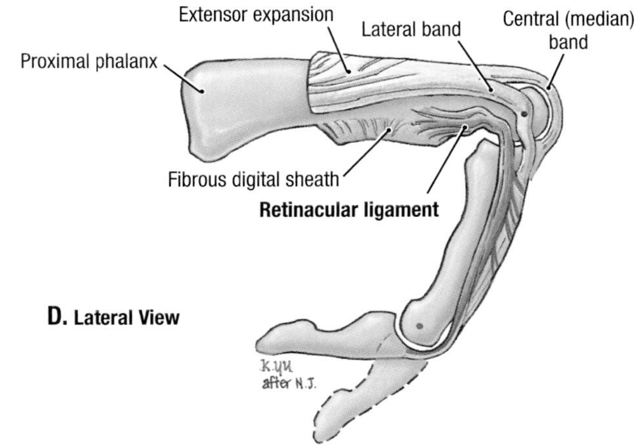
Extensor expansion
Lateral band
Central (median) band
Proximal phalanx
Fibrous digital sheath
Retinacular ligament
D. Lateral View

## 6.77 Extensor (dorsal) expansion of 3rd digit

**A.** Dorsal aspect. **B.** Lateral aspect. **C.** Retinacular ligaments of extended digit. **D.** Retinacular ligaments of flexed digit.

- The hood covering the head of the metacarpal is attached to the palmar ligament.
- Contraction of the muscles attaching to the lateral band will produce flexion of the metacarpophalangeal joint and extension of the interphalangeal joints.
- The retinacular ligament is a fibrous band that runs from the proximal phalanx and fibrous digital sheath obliquely across the middle phalanx and two interphalangeal joints to join the extensor (dorsal) expansion, and then to the distal phalanx.
- On flexion of the distal interphalangeal joint, the retinacular ligament becomes taut and pulls the proximal joint into flexion; on extension of the proximal joint, the distal joint is pulled by the ligament into nearly complete extension.

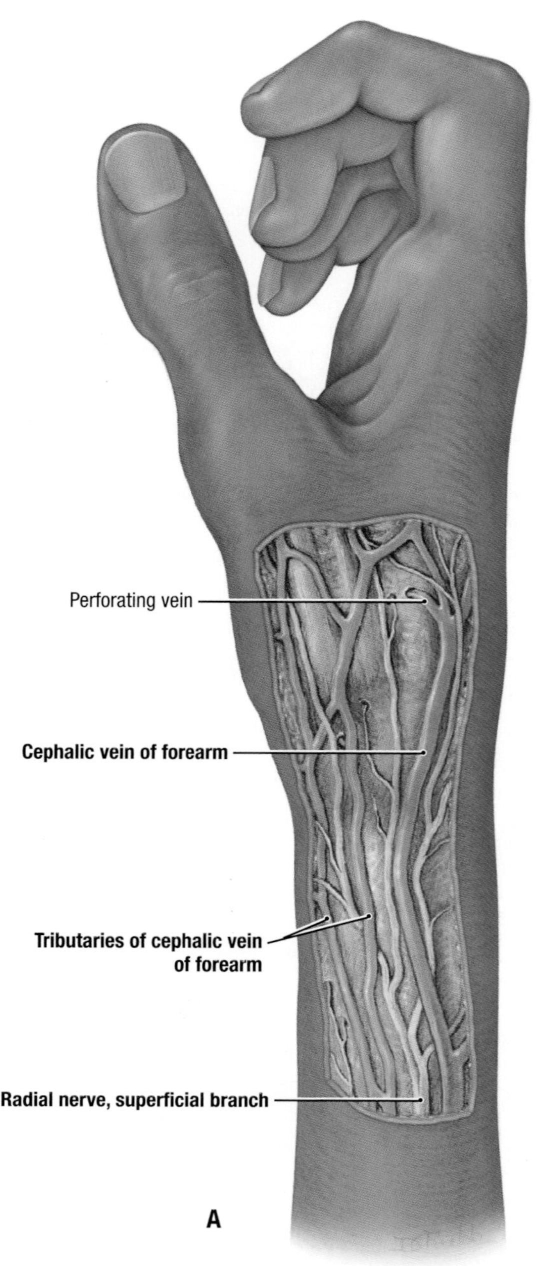
Perforating vein
Cephalic vein of forearm
Tributaries of cephalic vein of forearm
Radial nerve, superficial branch
A

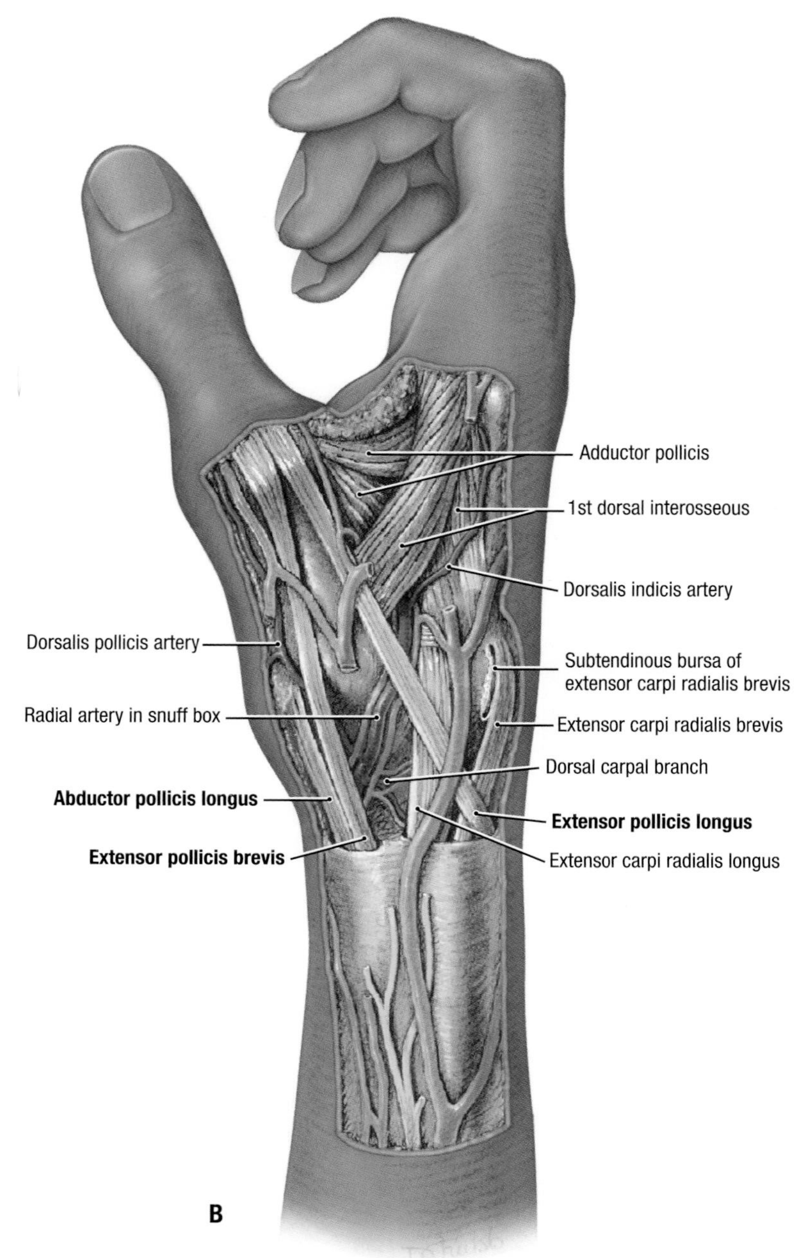
Adductor pollicis
1st dorsal interosseous
Dorsalis indicis artery
Dorsalis pollicis artery
Subtendinous bursa of extensor carpi radialis brevis
Radial artery in snuff box
Extensor carpi radialis brevis
Dorsal carpal branch
Abductor pollicis longus
Extensor pollicis longus
Extensor pollicis brevis
Extensor carpi radialis longus
B

Lateral Views

## 6.78 Lateral aspect of wrist and hand

**A.** Anatomical snuff box—I. **B.** Anatomical snuff box—II.

In **A**:

- The depression at the base of the thumb, the "anatomical snuff box," retains its name from an archaic habit.
- Note the superficial veins, including the cephalic vein of forearm and/or its tributaries, and cutaneous nerves crossing the snuff box.

In **B**:

- Three long tendons of the thumb form the boundaries of the snuff box; the extensor pollicis longus forms the medial boundary and the abductor pollicis longus and extensor pollicis brevis the lateral boundary.
- The radial artery crosses the floor of the snuff box and travels between the two heads of the 1st dorsal interosseous.
- The adductor pollicis and 1st dorsal interosseous are supplied by the ulnar nerve.

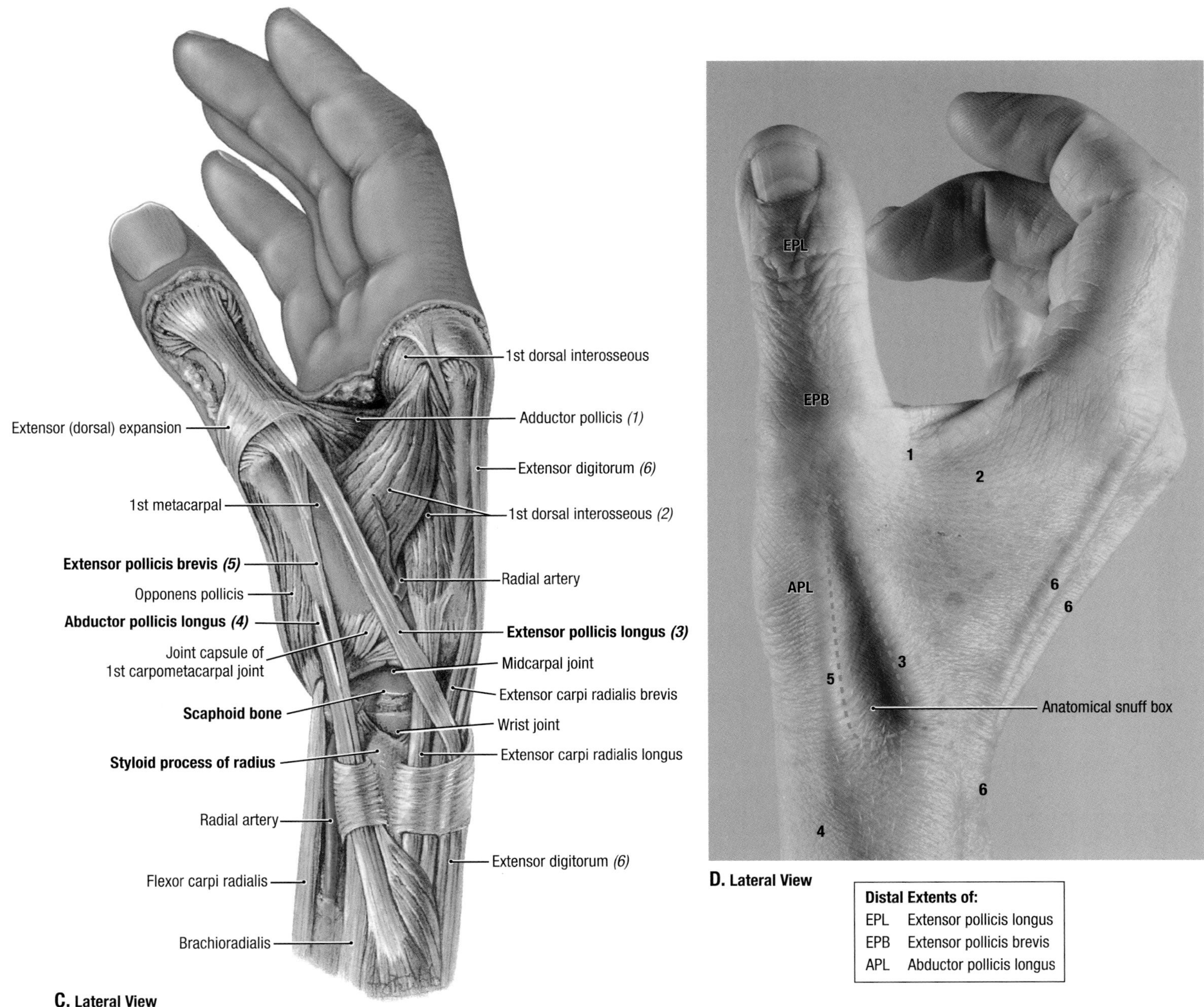
1st dorsal interosseous
Adductor pollicis (1)
Extensor (dorsal) expansion
Extensor digitorum (6)
1st metacarpal
1st dorsal interosseous (2)
Extensor pollicis brevis (5)
Radial artery
Opponens pollicis
Abductor pollicis longus (4)
Extensor pollicis longus (3)
Joint capsule of 1st carpometacarpal joint
Midcarpal joint
Extensor carpi radialis brevis
Scaphoid bone
Wrist joint
Styloid process of radius
Extensor carpi radialis longus
Radial artery
Extensor digitorum (6)
Flexor carpi radialis
Brachioradialis
C. Lateral View
EPL
EPB
APL
1
2
3
4
5
6
6
6
Anatomical snuff box
D. Lateral View
Distal Extents of:
EPL Extensor pollicis longus
EPB Extensor pollicis brevis
APL Abductor pollicis longus

## 6.78 Lateral aspect of wrist and hand *(continued)*

**C.** Anatomical snuff box—III. **D.** Surface anatomy.

In **C**: Note the scaphoid bone, the wrist joint proximal to the scaphoid, and the midcarpal joint distal to it.

Fracture of the scaphoid often results from a fall on the palm with the hand abducted. The fracture occurs across the narrow part ("waist") of the scaphoid. Pain occurs primarily on the lateral side of the wrist, especially during dorsiflexion and abduction of the hand. Initial radiographs of the wrist may not reveal a fracture, but radiographs taken 10–14 days later reveal a fracture because bone resorption has occurred. Owing to the poor blood supply to the proximal part of the scaphoid, union of the fractured parts may take several months. Avascular necrosis of the proximal fragment of the scaphoid (pathological death of bone resulting from poor blood supply) may occur and produce degenerative joint disease of the wrist.

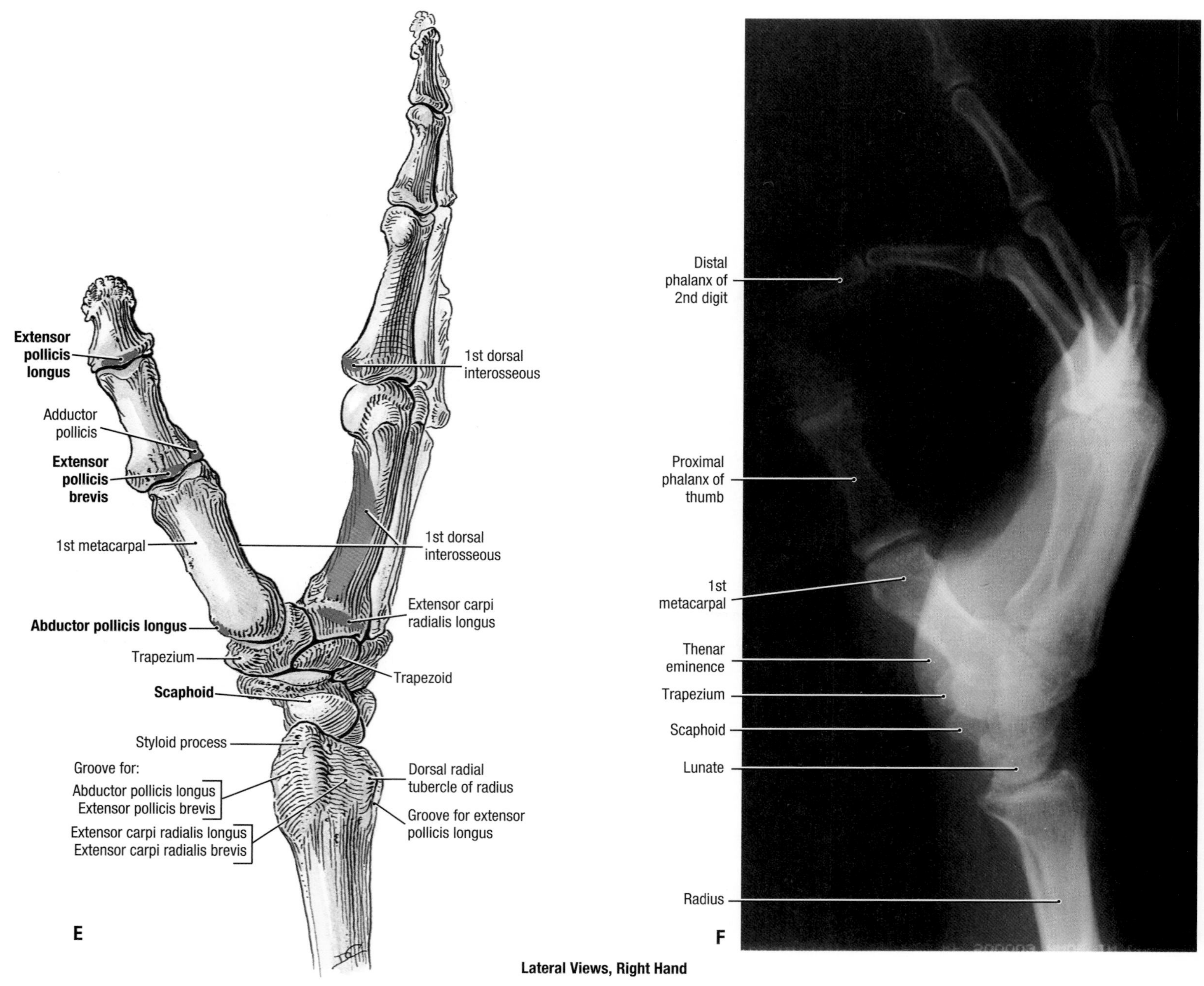
Extensor pollicis longus
Adductor pollicis
Extensor pollicis brevis
1st metacarpal
Abductor pollicis longus
Trapezium
Scaphoid
Styloid process
Groove for:
Abductor pollicis longus
Extensor pollicis brevis
Extensor carpi radialis longus
Extensor carpi radialis brevis
1st dorsal interosseous
1st dorsal interosseous
Extensor carpi radialis longus
Trapezoid
Dorsal radial tubercle of radius
Groove for extensor pollicis longus
E
Distal phalanx of 2nd digit
Proximal phalanx of thumb
1st metacarpal
Thenar eminence
Trapezium
Scaphoid
Lunate
Radius
F
Lateral Views, Right Hand

## 6.78 Lateral aspect of wrist and hand *(continued)*

**E.** Bony hand showing muscle attachments. **F.** Radiograph.

- The anatomical snuff box is limited proximally by the styloid process of the radius and distally by the base of the 1st metacarpal; aspects of the two lateral bones of the carpus (scaphoid and trapezium) form the floor of the snuff box.

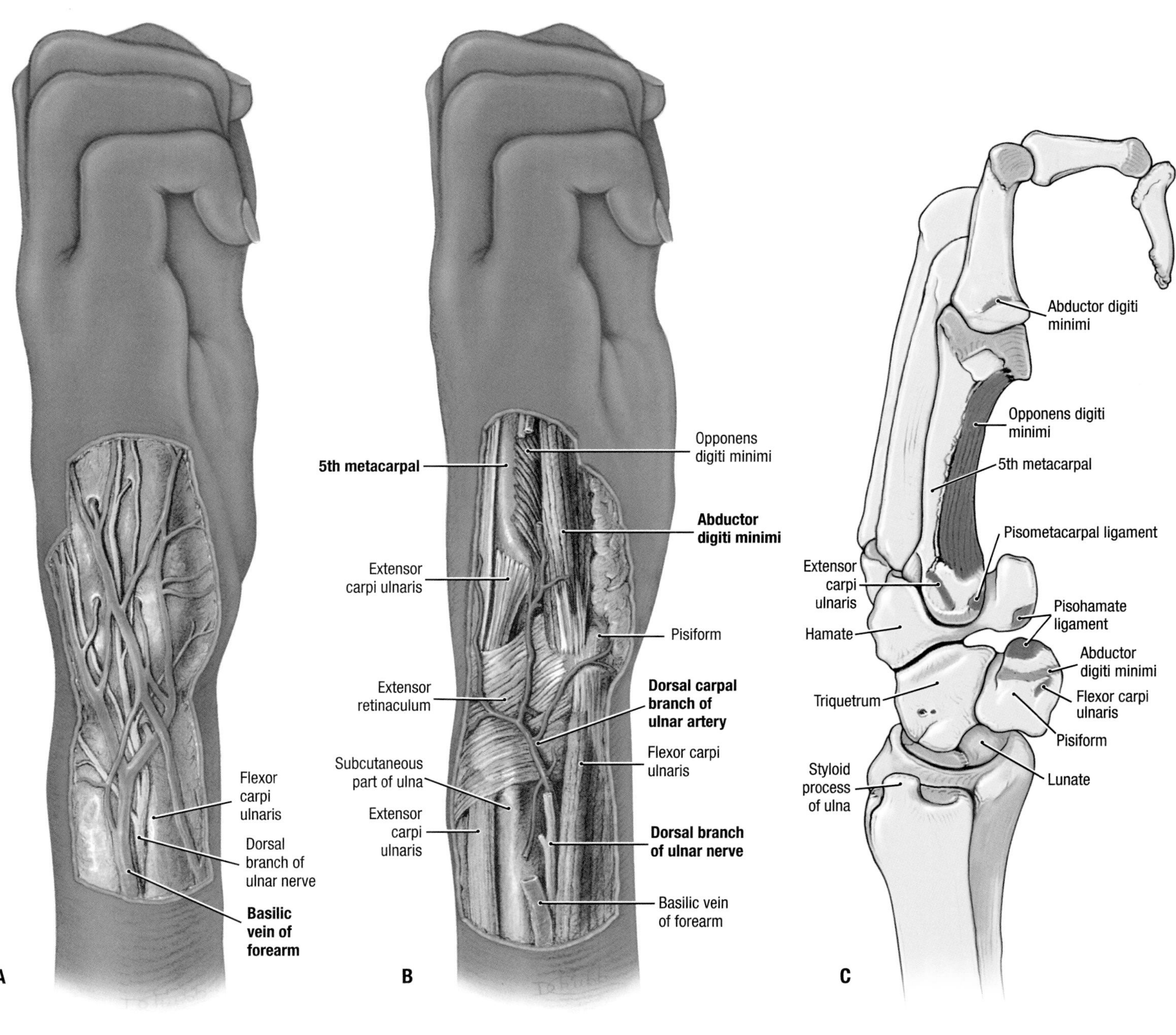
Flexor carpi ulnaris
Dorsal branch of ulnar nerve
Basilic vein of forearm
A
5th metacarpal
Extensor carpi ulnaris
Extensor retinaculum
Subcutaneous part of ulna
Extensor carpi ulnaris
Opponens digiti minimi
Abductor digiti minimi
Pisiform
Dorsal carpal branch of ulnar artery
Flexor carpi ulnaris
Dorsal branch of ulnar nerve
Basilic vein of forearm
B
Abductor digiti minimi
Opponens digiti minimi
5th metacarpal
Pisometacarpal ligament
Extensor carpi ulnaris
Hamate
Pisohamate ligament
Abductor digiti minimi
Flexor carpi ulnaris
Triquetrum
Pisiform
Styloid process of ulna
Lunate
C
Medial Views

## 6.79 Medial aspect of wrist and hand

**A.** Superficial dissection. **B.** Deep dissection. **C.** Bony hand showing sites of muscular and ligamentous attachments. The extensor carpi ulnaris is inserted directly into the base of the fifth metacarpal, but the flexor carpi ulnaris inserts indirectly to the base of the fifth metacarpal and the hook of the hamate through the pisiform and pisohamate and pisometacarpal ligaments.

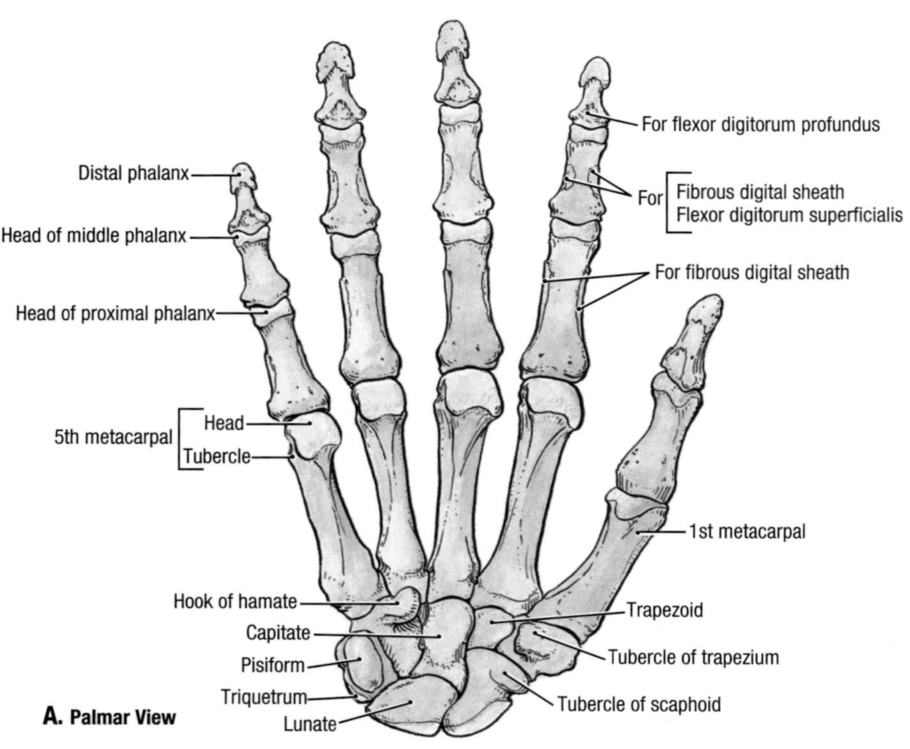
Distal phalanx
Head of middle phalanx
Head of proximal phalanx
5th metacarpal
Head
Tubercle
Hook of hamate
Capitate
Pisiform
Triquetrum
Lunate
For flexor digitorum profundus
For
Fibrous digital sheath
Flexor digitorum superficialis
For fibrous digital sheath
1st metacarpal
Trapezoid
Tubercle of trapezium
Tubercle of scaphoid

**A. Palmar View**

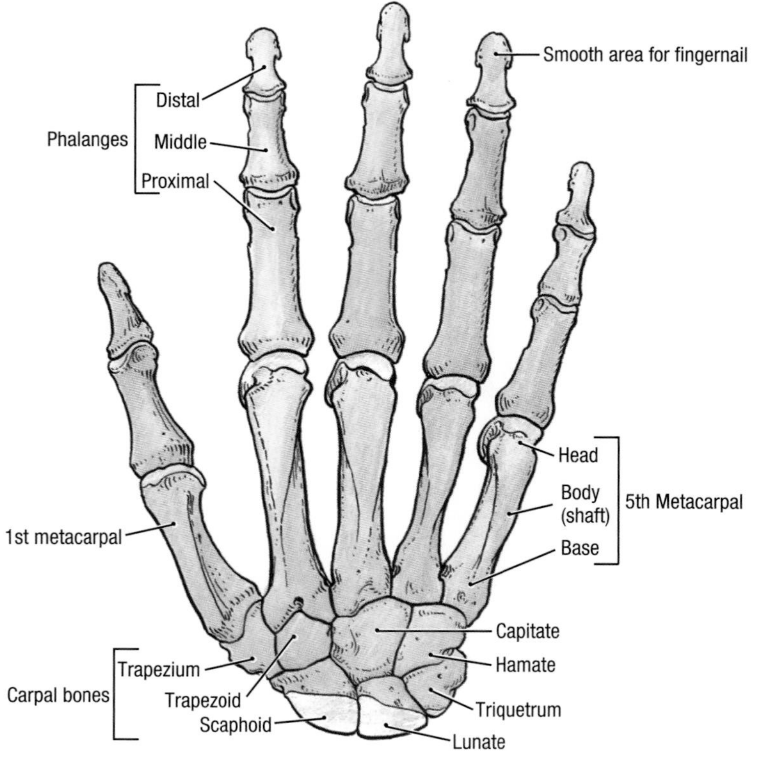
Smooth area for fingernail
Phalanges
Distal
Middle
Proximal
Head
Body (shaft)
Base
5th Metacarpal
1st metacarpal
Capitate
Hamate
Triquetrum
Lunate
Carpal bones
Trapezium
Trapezoid
Scaphoid

**B. Dorsal View**

## 6.80 Bones of hand

**A.** Palmar view. **B.** Dorsal view.
The eight carpal bones form two rows: in the distal row, the hamate, capitate, trapezoid, and trapezium; the trapezium forming a saddle-shaped joint with the 1st metacarpal; in the proximal row, the scaphoid, lunate, and pisiform; the pisiform is superimposed on the triquetrum.

Severe crushing injuries of the hand may produce multiple metacarpal fractures, resulting in instability of the hand. Similar injuries of the distal phalanges are common (e.g., when a finger is caught in a car door).

A fracture of a distal phalanx is usually comminuted, and a painful hematoma (collection of blood) develops. Fractures of the proximal and middle phalanges are usually the result of crushing or hypertension injuries.

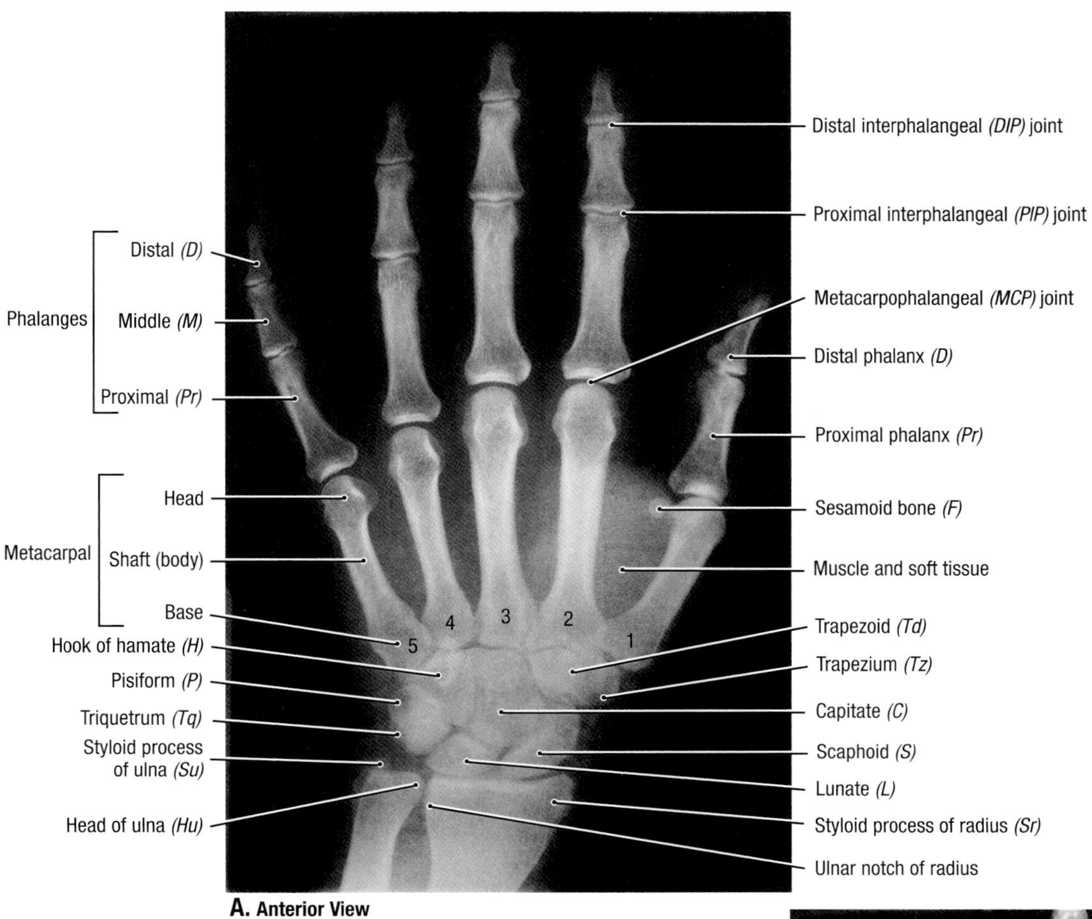
Distal interphalangeal (DIP) joint
Proximal interphalangeal (PIP) joint
Metacarpophalangeal (MCP) joint
Distal phalanx (D)
Proximal phalanx (Pr)
Sesamoid bone (F)
Muscle and soft tissue
Trapezoid (Td)
Trapezium (Tz)
Capitate (C)
Scaphoid (S)
Lunate (L)
Styloid process of radius (Sr)
Ulnar notch of radius
Phalanges
Distal (D)
Middle (M)
Proximal (Pr)
Metacarpal
Head
Shaft (body)
Base
Hook of hamate (H)
Pisiform (P)
Triquetrum (Tq)
Styloid process of ulna (Su)
Head of ulna (Hu)
1
2
3
4
5

**A.** Anterior View

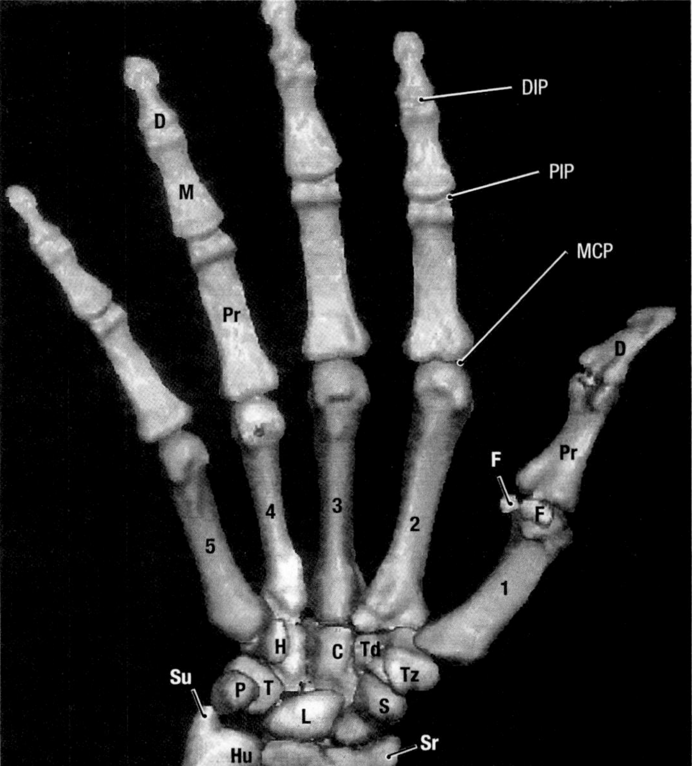
DIP
PIP
MCP
D
M
Pr
D
Pr
F
F
1
2
3
4
5
H
C
Td
Tz
Su
P
T
L
S
Hu
Sr

**B.** Anterior View

## 6.81 Imaging of bones of wrist and hand

**A.** Radiograph. **B.** Three-dimensional computer-generated image of wrist and hand (letters correspond to structures labeled in **A**).

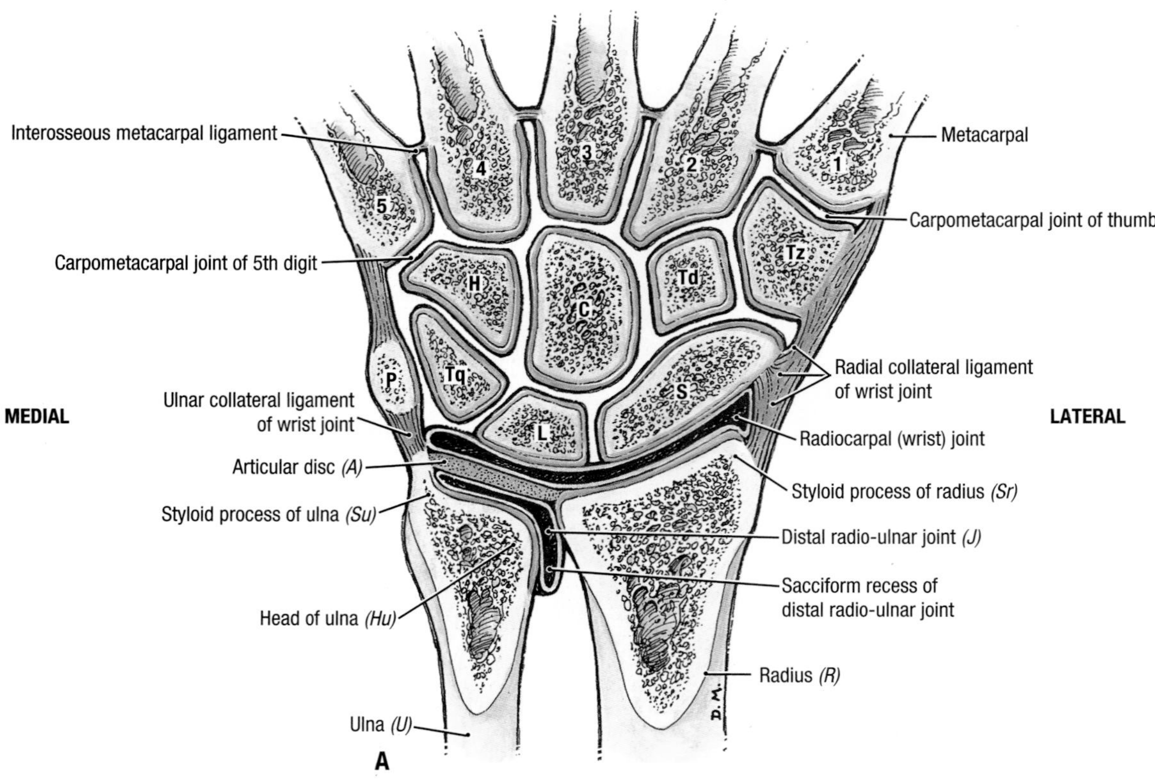
Interosseous metacarpal ligament
Metacarpal
5
4
3
2
1
Carpometacarpal joint of thumb
Carpometacarpal joint of 5th digit
H
C
Td
Tz
P
Tq
S
L
Radial collateral ligament of wrist joint
MEDIAL
Ulnar collateral ligament of wrist joint
LATERAL
Radiocarpal (wrist) joint
Articular disc (A)
Styloid process of radius (Sr)
Styloid process of ulna (Su)
Distal radio-ulnar joint (J)
Sacciform recess of distal radio-ulnar joint
Head of ulna (Hu)
Radius (R)
Ulna (U)
D.M.
A

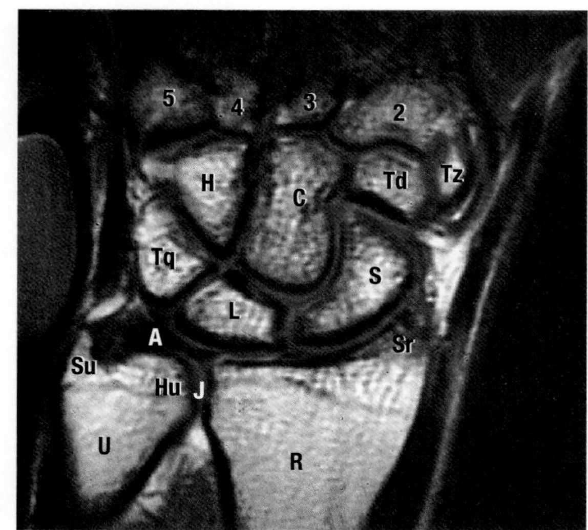
5
4
3
2
H
C
Td
Tz
Tq
S
L
A
Sr
Su
Hu
J
U
R
B

**6.82 Coronal section of wrist**

**A.** Schematic illustration. **B.** Coronal MRI. *A*, articular disc; *J*, distal radio-ulnar joint (letters correspond to structures labeled in **A** and Figure 6.81A).

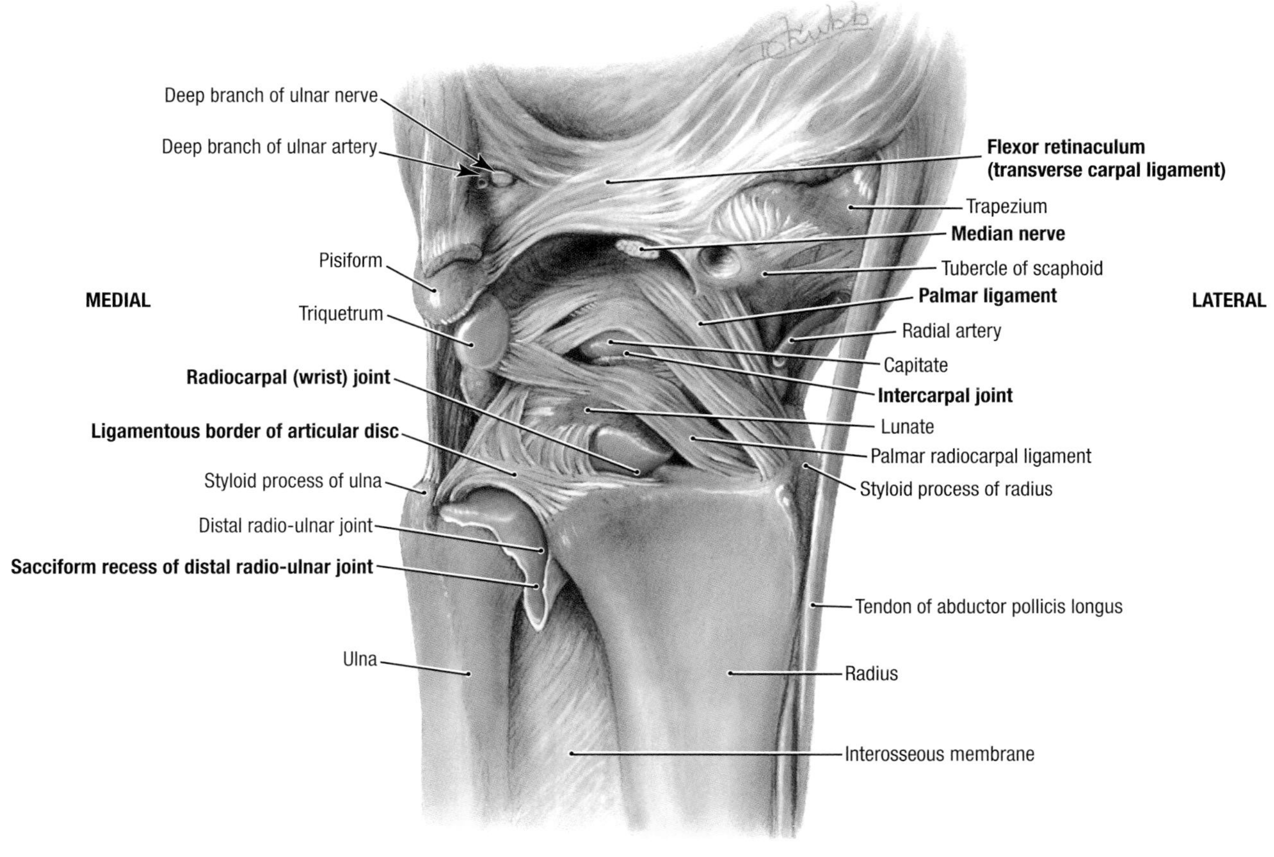
Deep branch of ulnar nerve
Deep branch of ulnar artery
Flexor retinaculum (transverse carpal ligament)
Trapezium
Median nerve
Pisiform
Tubercle of scaphoid
MEDIAL
Palmar ligament
LATERAL
Triquetrum
Radial artery
Capitate
Radiocarpal (wrist) joint
Intercarpal joint
Lunate
Ligamentous border of articular disc
Palmar radiocarpal ligament
Styloid process of ulna
Styloid process of radius
Distal radio-ulnar joint
Sacciform recess of distal radio-ulnar joint
Tendon of abductor pollicis longus
Ulna
Radius
Interosseous membrane
Anterior View

## 6.83 Ligaments of distal radio-ulnar, radiocarpal, and intercarpal joints

The hand is forcibly extended. Observe the palmar radiocarpal ligament passing from the radius to the two rows of carpal bones; they are strong and directed, so that the hand moves with the radius during supination.

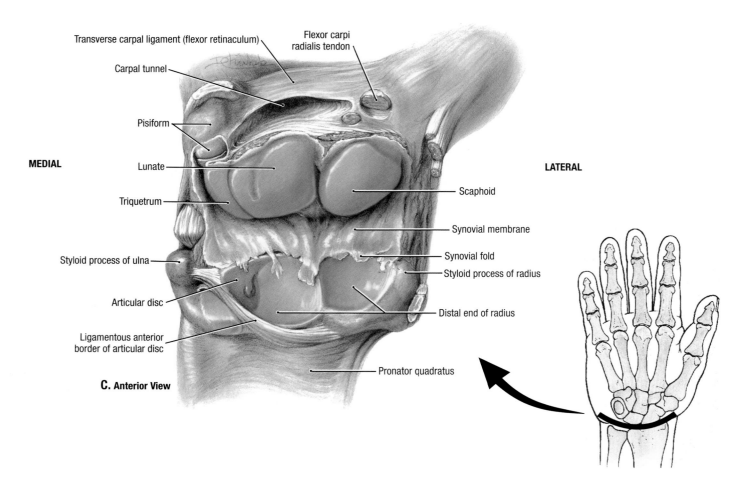

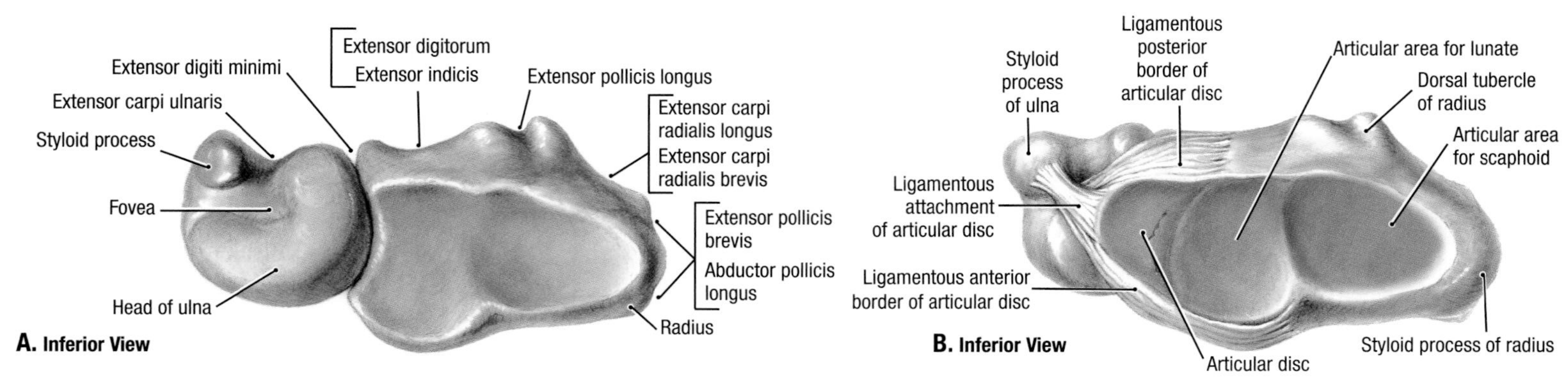
Extensor digitorum
Extensor indicis
Extensor digiti minimi
Extensor carpi ulnaris
Extensor pollicis longus
Styloid process
Extensor carpi radialis longus
Extensor carpi radialis brevis
Fovea
Extensor pollicis brevis
Abductor pollicis longus
Head of ulna
Radius
A. Inferior View
Ligamentous posterior border of articular disc
Styloid process of ulna
Articular area for lunate
Dorsal tubercle of radius
Articular area for scaphoid
Ligamentous attachment of articular disc
Ligamentous anterior border of articular disc
B. Inferior View
Articular disc
Styloid process of radius
Transverse carpal ligament (flexor retinaculum)
Flexor carpi radialis tendon
Carpal tunnel
Pisiform
MEDIAL
Lunate
LATERAL
Scaphoid
Triquetrum
Synovial membrane
Synovial fold
Styloid process of ulna
Styloid process of radius
Articular disc
Distal end of radius
Ligamentous anterior border of articular disc
Pronator quadratus
C. Anterior View

## 6.84 Radiocarpal (wrist) joint

**A.** Distal ends of radius and ulna showing grooves for tendons on the posterior aspects. **B.** Articular disc. The articular disc unites the distal ends of the radius and ulna; it is fibrocartilaginous at the triangular area between the head of the ulna and the lunate bone, but ligamentous and pliable elsewhere. The cartilaginous part commonly has a fissure or perforation, as shown here. **C.** Articular surface of the radiocarpal joint, which is opened anteriorly. The lunate articulates with the radius and articular disc; only during adduction of the wrist does the triquetrum come into articulation with the disc. The perforation in the disc and the associated roughened surface of the lunate are a common occurrence.

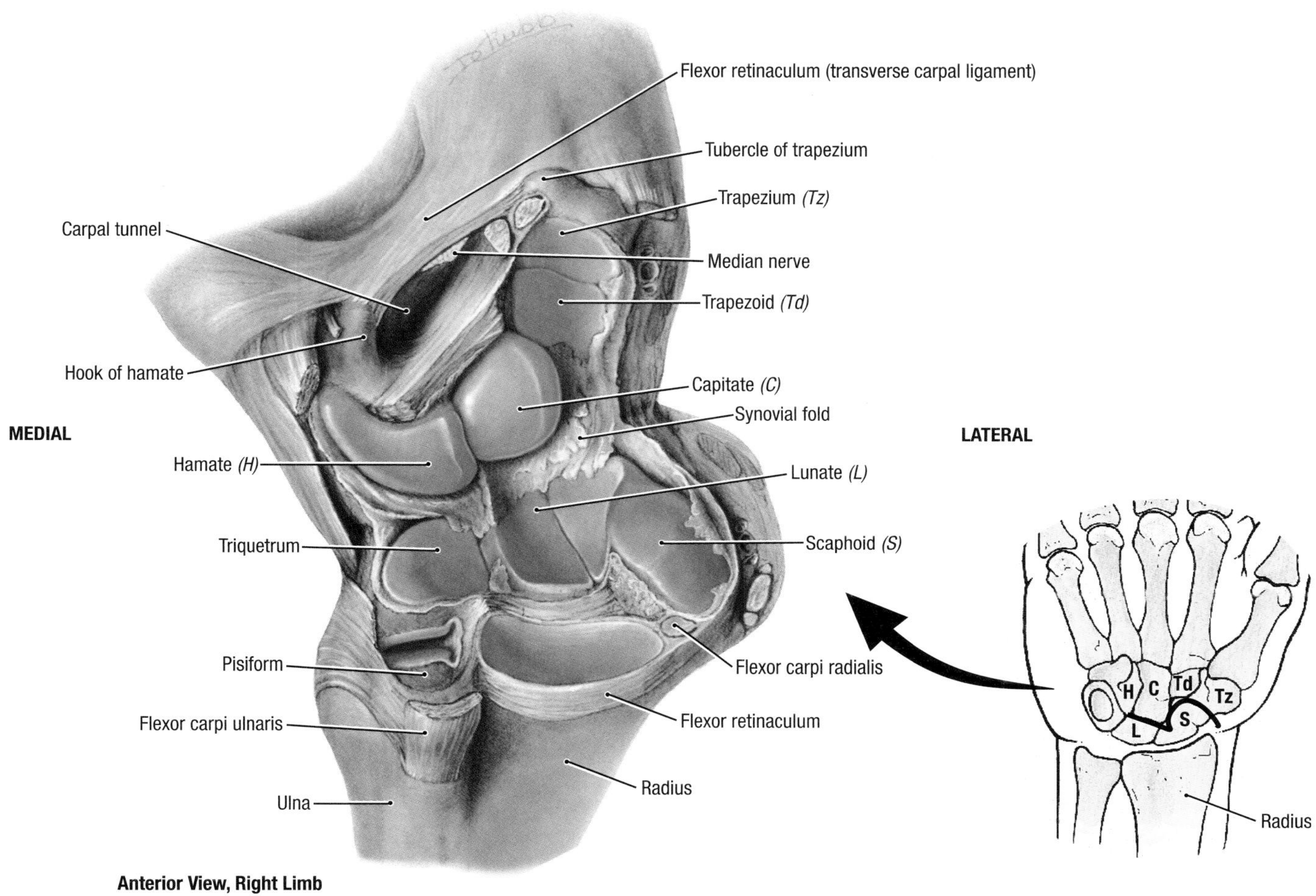
Flexor retinaculum (transverse carpal ligament)
Tubercle of trapezium
Trapezium (Tz)
Carpal tunnel
Median nerve
Trapezoid (Td)
Hook of hamate
Capitate (C)
Synovial fold
MEDIAL
LATERAL
Hamate (H)
Lunate (L)
Triquetrum
Scaphoid (S)
Pisiform
Flexor carpi radialis
Flexor carpi ulnaris
Flexor retinaculum
Radius
Ulna
H
C
Td
Tz
L
S
Radius
Anterior View, Right Limb

## 6.85 Articular surfaces of midcarpal (transverse carpal) joint, opened anteriorly

- The flexor retinaculum (transverse carpal ligament) is cut; the proximal part of the ligament, which spans from the pisiform to the scaphoid, is relatively weak; the distal part, which passes from the hook of the hamate to the tubercle of the trapezium, is strong.
- Observe the sinuous surfaces of the opposed bones: the trapezium and trapezoid together form a concave, oval surface for the scaphoid, and the capitate and hamate together form a convex surface for the scaphoid, lunate, and triquetrum.

Anterior dislocation of the lunate is a serious injury that usually results from a fall on the dorsiflexed wrist. The lunate is pushed to the palmar surface of the wrist and may compress the median nerve and lead to carpal tunnel syndrome. Because of poor blood supply, avascular necrosis of the lunate may occur.

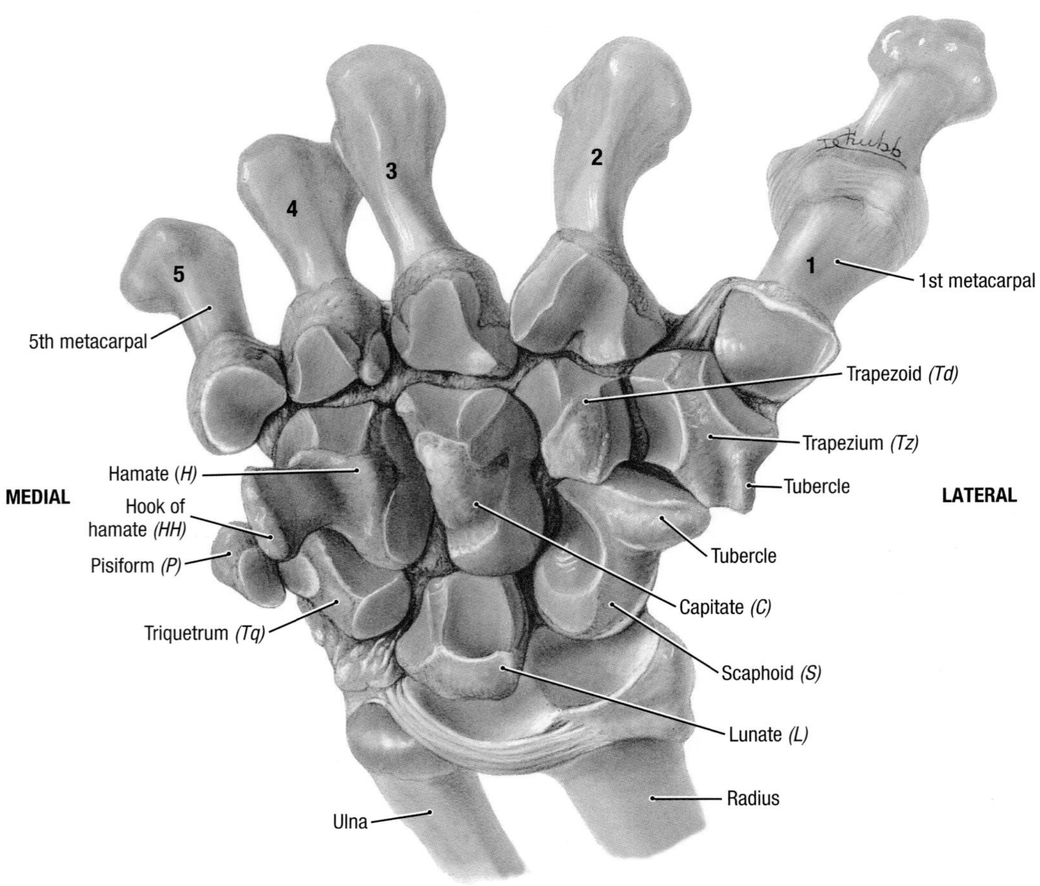
5
4
3
2
1
1st metacarpal
5th metacarpal
Trapezoid (Td)
Trapezium (Tz)
Hamate (H)
Tubercle
MEDIAL
LATERAL
Hook of hamate (HH)
Pisiform (P)
Tubercle
Capitate (C)
Triquetrum (Tq)
Scaphoid (S)
Lunate (L)
Radius
Ulna

**A. Anterior View, Right Limb**

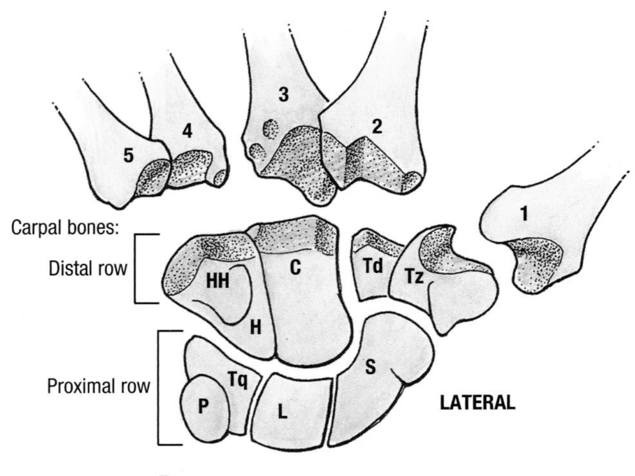
3
4
2
5
1
Carpal bones:
Distal row
HH
C
Td
Tz
H
Proximal row
Tq
S
P
L
LATERAL

**B. Anterior View**

## 6.86 Carpal bones and bases of metacarpals

**A.** Open intercarpal and carpometacarpal joints. The dorsal ligaments remain intact, and all the joints have been hyperextended, permitting study of articular facets. **B.** Diagram of the articular surfaces of the carpometacarpal joints (*letters* refer to structures labeled in **A**).

- The capitate articulates with three metacarpals (2nd, 3rd, and 4th).
- The 2nd metacarpal articulates with three carpals (trapezium, trapezoid, and capitate).
- The 2nd and 3rd carpometacarpal joints are practically immobile; the 1st is saddle-shaped, and the 4th and 5th are hinge-shaped synovial joints.

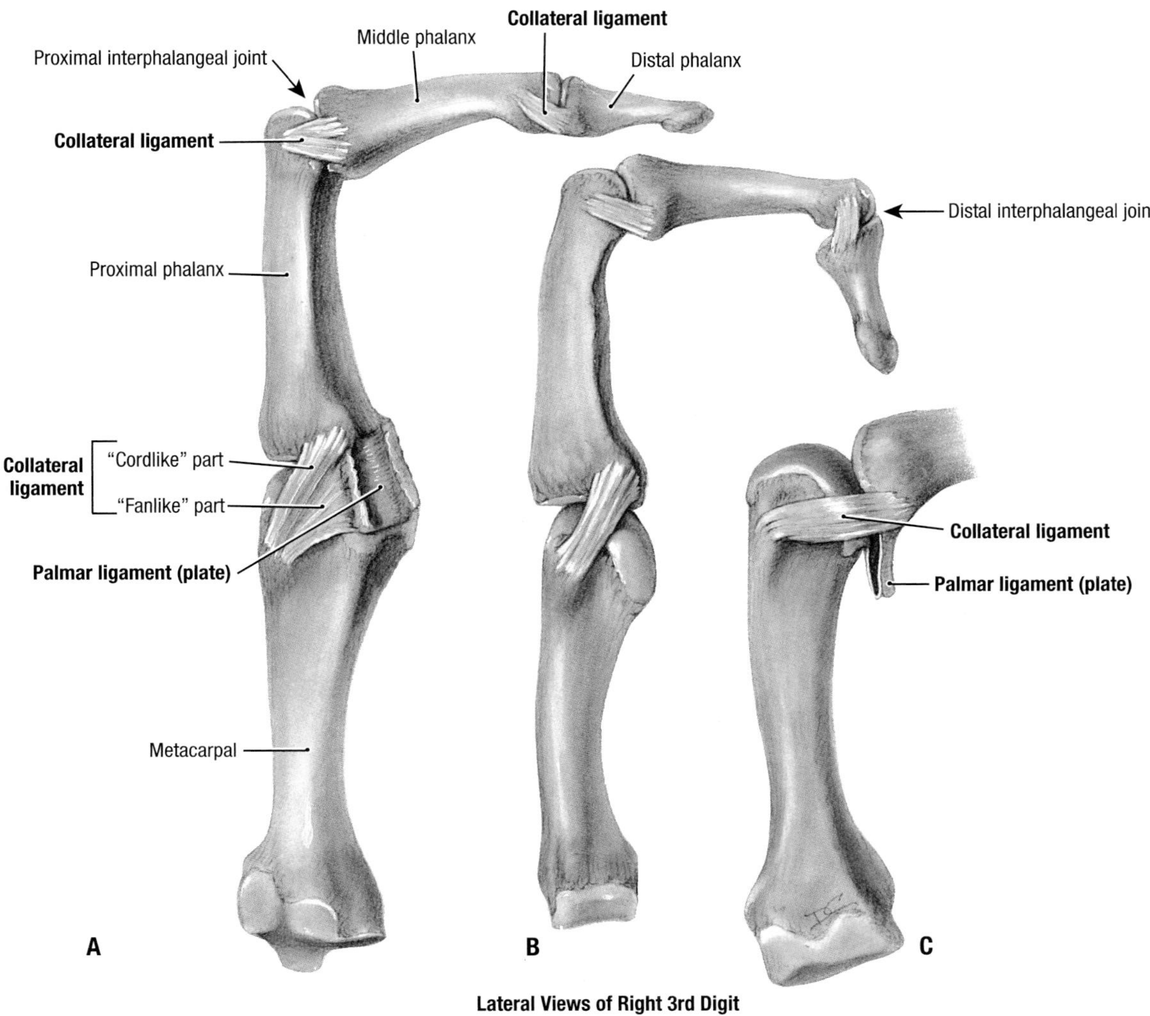
Collateral ligament
Middle phalanx
Proximal interphalangeal joint
Distal phalanx
Collateral ligament
Distal interphalangeal joint
Proximal phalanx
Collateral ligament
"Cordlike" part
"Fanlike" part
Palmar ligament (plate)
Collateral ligament
Palmar ligament (plate)
Metacarpal
A
B
C

Lateral Views of Right 3rd Digit

## 6.87 Collateral ligaments of metacarpophalangeal and interphalangeal joints of third digit

**A.** Extended metacarpophalangeal and distal interphalangeal joints. **B.** Flexed interphalangeal joints. **C.** Flexed metacarpophalangeal joint.

- A fibrocartilaginous plate, the palmar ligament, hangs from the base of the proximal phalanx; is fixed to the head of the metacarpal by the weaker, fanlike part of the collateral ligament (**A**); and moves like a visor across the metacarpal head (**C**).
- The extremely strong, cordlike parts of the collateral ligaments of this joint (**A** and **B**) are eccentrically attached to the metacarpal heads; they are slack during extension and taut during flexion (**C**), so the fingers cannot be spread (abducted) unless the hand is open; the interphalangeal joints have similar ligaments.

Skier's thumb refers to the rupture or chronic laxity of the collateral ligament of the 1st metacarpophalangeal joint. The injury results from hyperextension of the joint, which occurs when the thumb is held by the ski pole while the rest of the hand hits the ground or enters the snow.

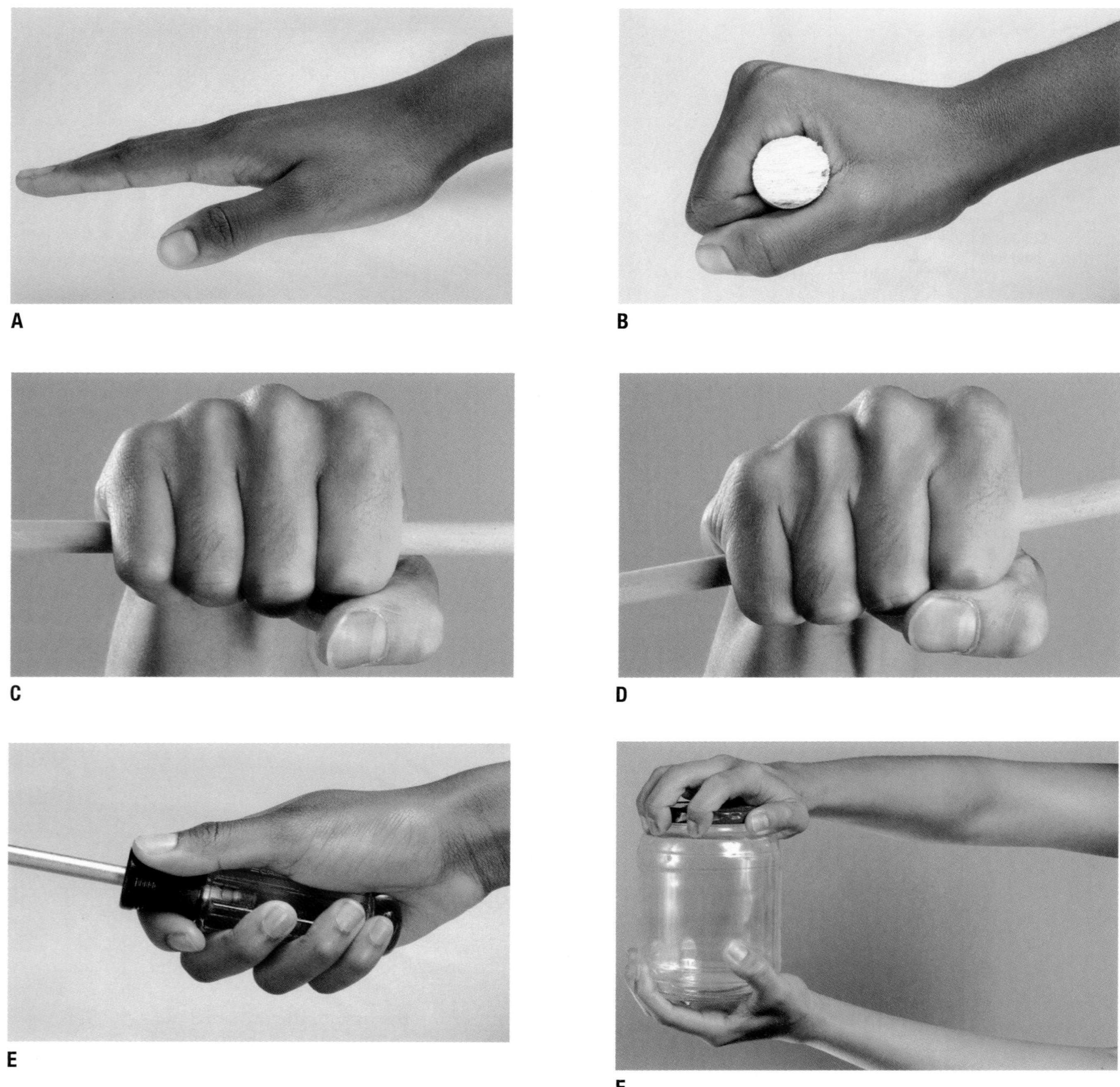
A
B
C
D
E
F

**6.88** **Grasp, pinch, and movements of the thumb**

**A.** The extended hand. **B.** Cylindrical (power) grasp. When grasping an object, the metacarpophalangeal and interphalangeal joints are flexed, but the radiocarpal joints are extended. Without wrist extension the grip is weak and insecure. **C.** Loose cylindrical grasp. **D.** Firm cylindrical (power) grasp. The heads of the 4th and 5th metacarpals have moved in a palmar direction. **E.** Centralized (power) grasp. **F.** Disc (power) grasp.

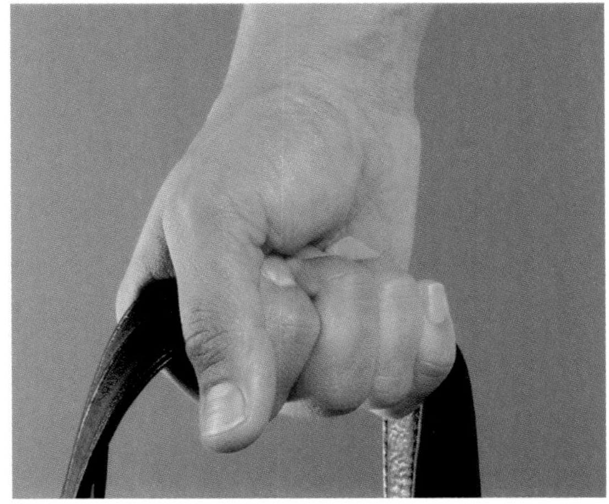

G

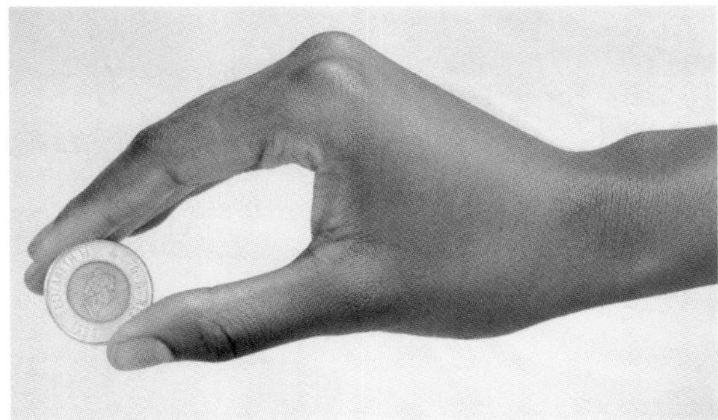

H

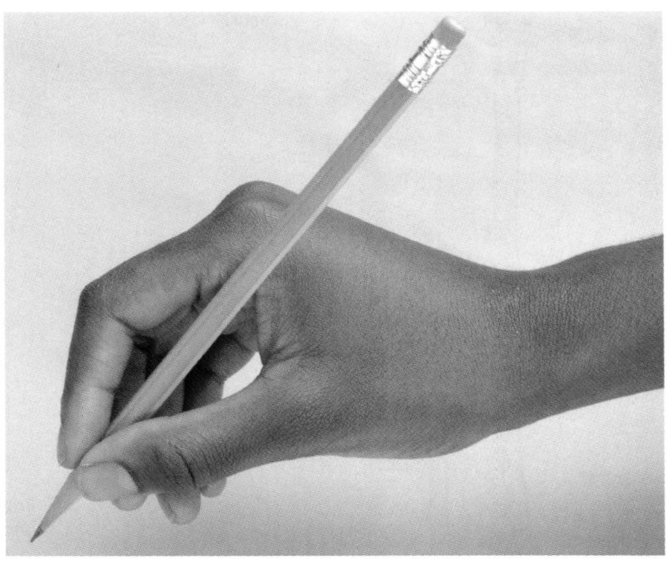

I

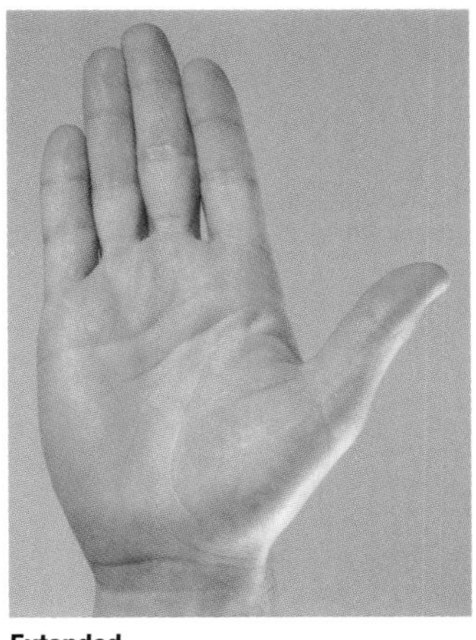

Extended

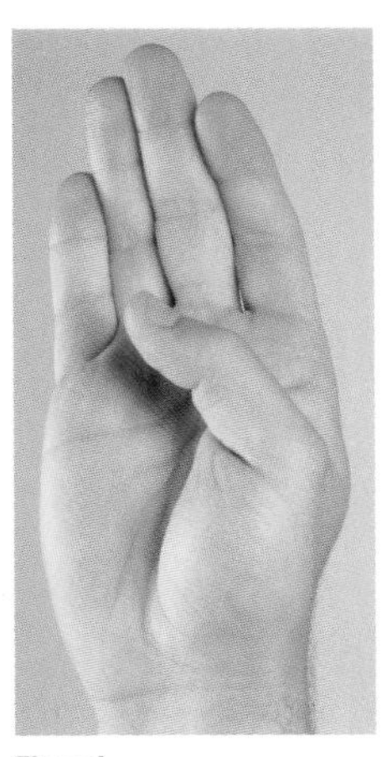

Flexed

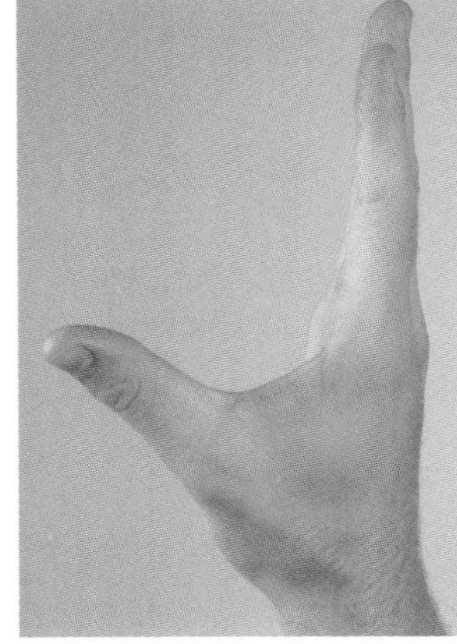

Abducted

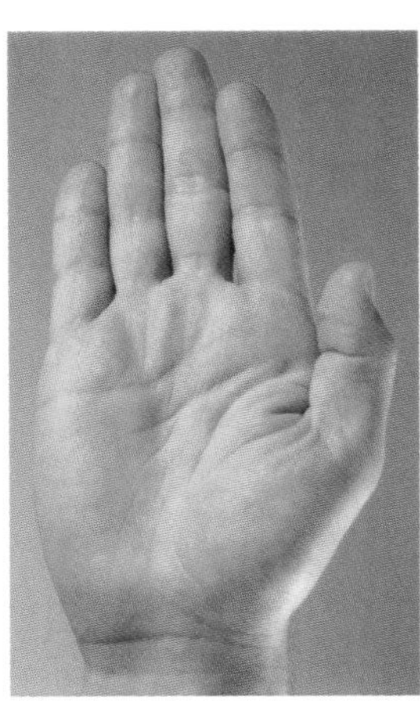

Adducted

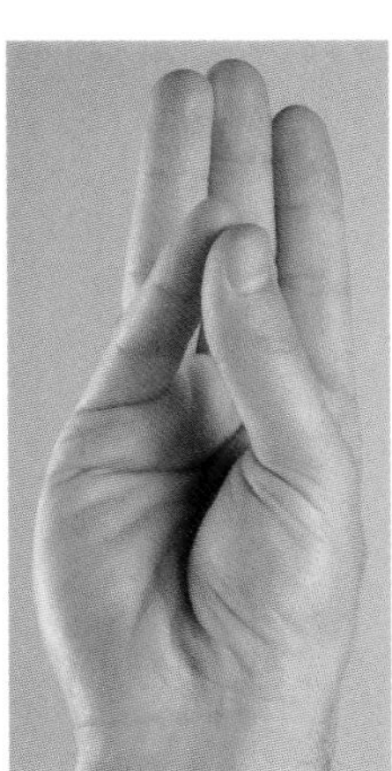

Opposed to little finger

J

## 6.88 Grasp, pinch, and movements of the thumb *(continued)*

**G.** Hook grasp. This grasp involves primarily the long flexors of the fingers, which are flexed to a varying degree depending on the size of the object. **H.** Fingertip pinch. **I.** Tripod (three-jaw chuck) pinch. **J.** Positions of the thumb.

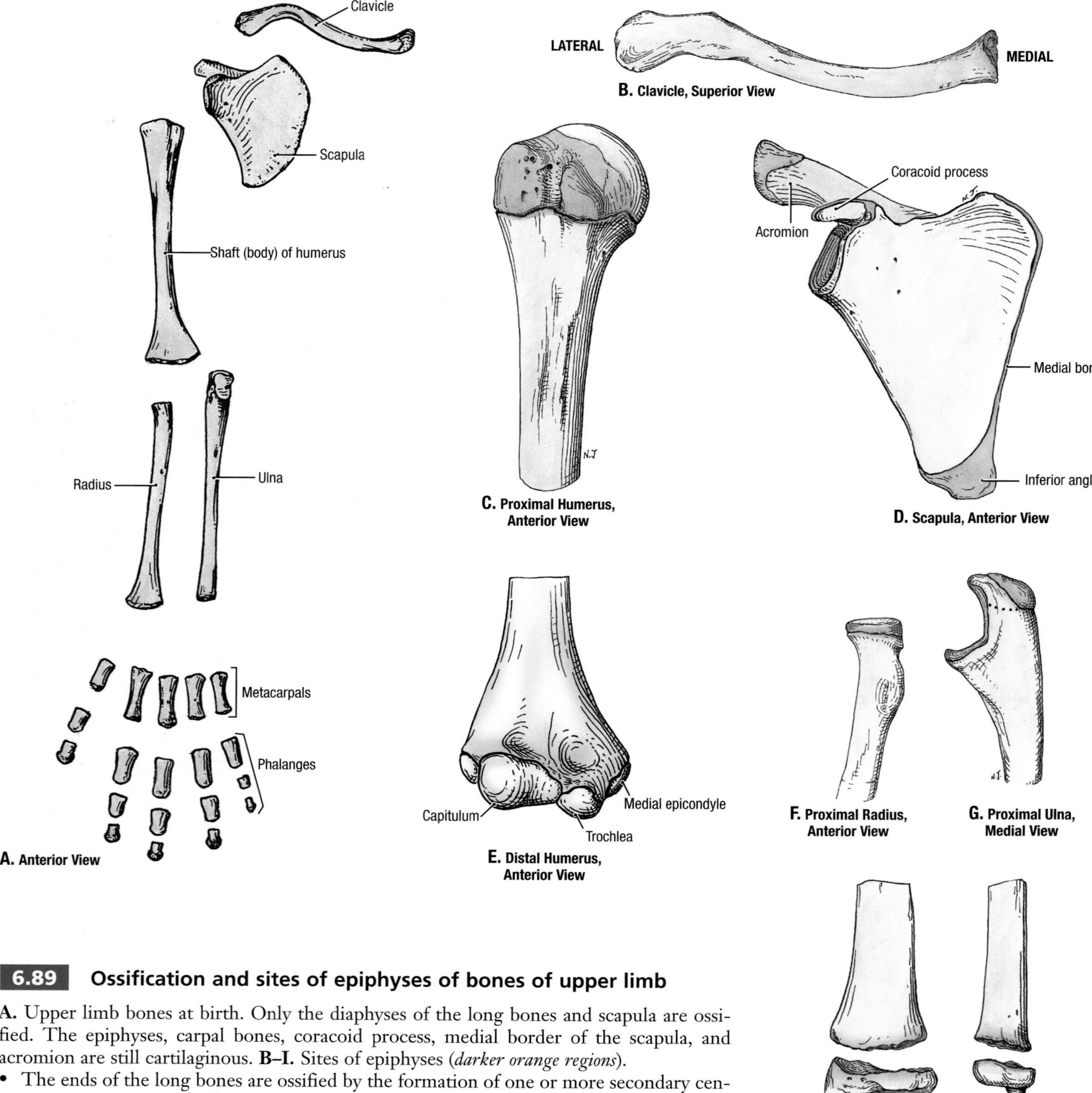
Clavicle
Scapula
Shaft (body) of humerus
Radius
Ulna
Metacarpals
Phalanges
A. Anterior View
LATERAL
MEDIAL
B. Clavicle, Superior View
C. Proximal Humerus, Anterior View
Coracoid process
Acromion
Medial border
Inferior angle
D. Scapula, Anterior View
Capitulum
Medial epicondyle
Trochlea
E. Distal Humerus, Anterior View
F. Proximal Radius, Anterior View
G. Proximal Ulna, Medial View
H. Distal Radius, Anterior View
I. Distal Ulna, Anterior View

## 6.89 Ossification and sites of epiphyses of bones of upper limb

**A.** Upper limb bones at birth. Only the diaphyses of the long bones and scapula are ossified. The epiphyses, carpal bones, coracoid process, medial border of the scapula, and acromion are still cartilaginous. **B–I.** Sites of epiphyses (*darker orange regions*).

- The ends of the long bones are ossified by the formation of one or more secondary centers of ossification; these epiphyses develop from birth to approximately 20 years of age in the clavicle, humerus, radius, ulna, metacarpals, and phalanges.

Without knowledge of bone growth and the appearance of bones in radiographic and other diagnostic images at various ages, a displaced epiphysial plate could be mistaken for a fracture, and separation of an epiphysis could be interpreted as a displaced piece of fractured bone. Knowledge of the patient's age and the location of epiphyses can prevent these errors.

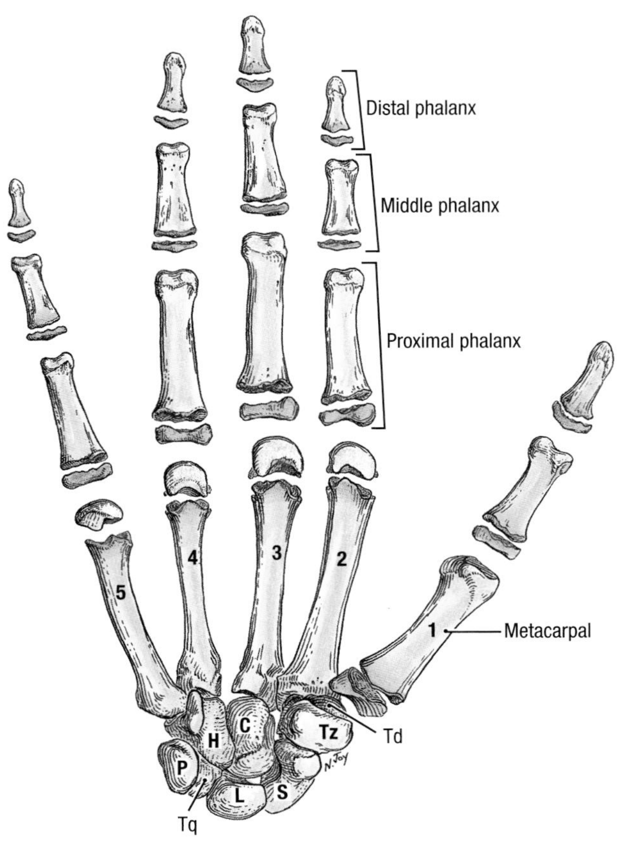
Distal phalanx
Middle phalanx
Proximal phalanx
Metacarpal
Td
Tz
C
H
P
L
S
Tq
1
2
3
4
5

**J. Anterior View (Right Hand)**

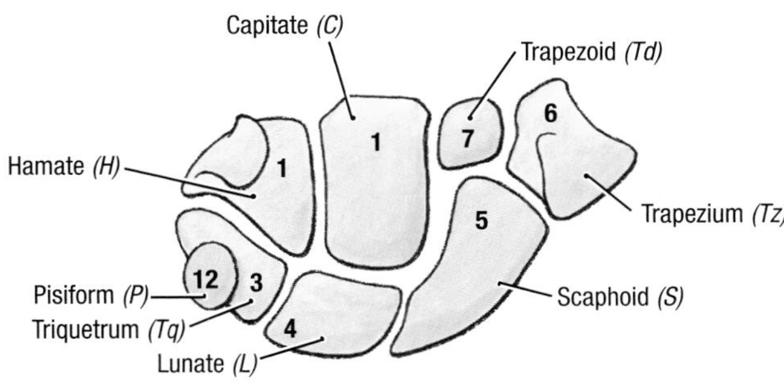
Capitate (C)
Trapezoid (Td)
Hamate (H)
Trapezium (Tz)
Pisiform (P)
Scaphoid (S)
Triquetrum (Tq)
Lunate (L)
1
1
7
6
5
12
3
4
Numbers: approximate age of ossification of carpal bones in years

**K. Anterior View**

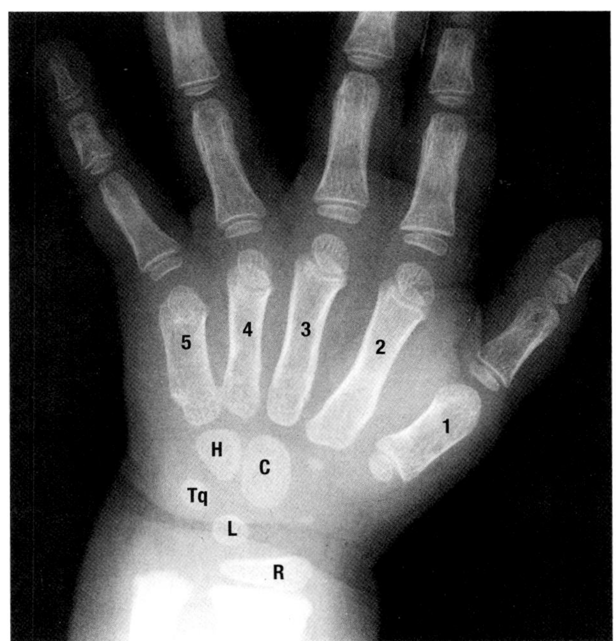
5
4
3
2
1
H
C
Tq
L
R

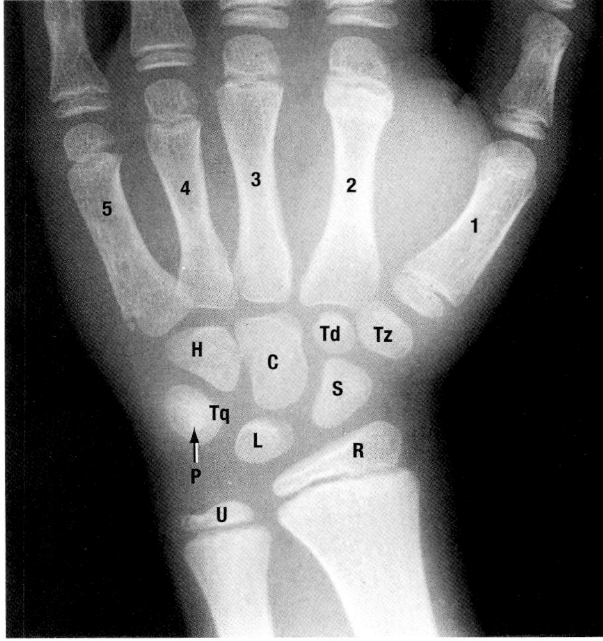
5
4
3
2
1
Td
Tz
H
C
S
Tq
L
R
P
U

**L. Anteroposterior View, Right Hand**

Epiphyses in radiographs appear as radiolucent lines

## 6.89 Ossification and sites of epiphyses of bones of upper limb *(continued)*

**J.** Sequence of ossification of carpal bones. **K.** Ossification of bones of hand. Note the phalanges have a single proximal epiphysis and metacarpals 2, 3, 4, and 5 have single distal epiphyses. The 1st metacarpal behaves as a phalanx by having proximal epiphysis. Short-lived epiphyses may appear at the other ends of metacarpals 1 and/or 2. There are individual and gender differences in sequence and timing of ossification. **L.** Radiographs of stages of ossification of wrist and hand. *Top*, a 2½-year-old child; the lunate is ossifying, and the distal radial epiphysis *(R)* is present (*C*, capitate; *H*, hamate; *Tq*, triquetrum; *L*, lunate). *Bottom*, an 11-year-old child. All carpal bones are ossified (*S*, scaphoid; *Td*, trapezoid; *Tz*, trapezium; *arrowhead*, pisiform), and the distal epiphysis of the ulna (*U*) has ossified.

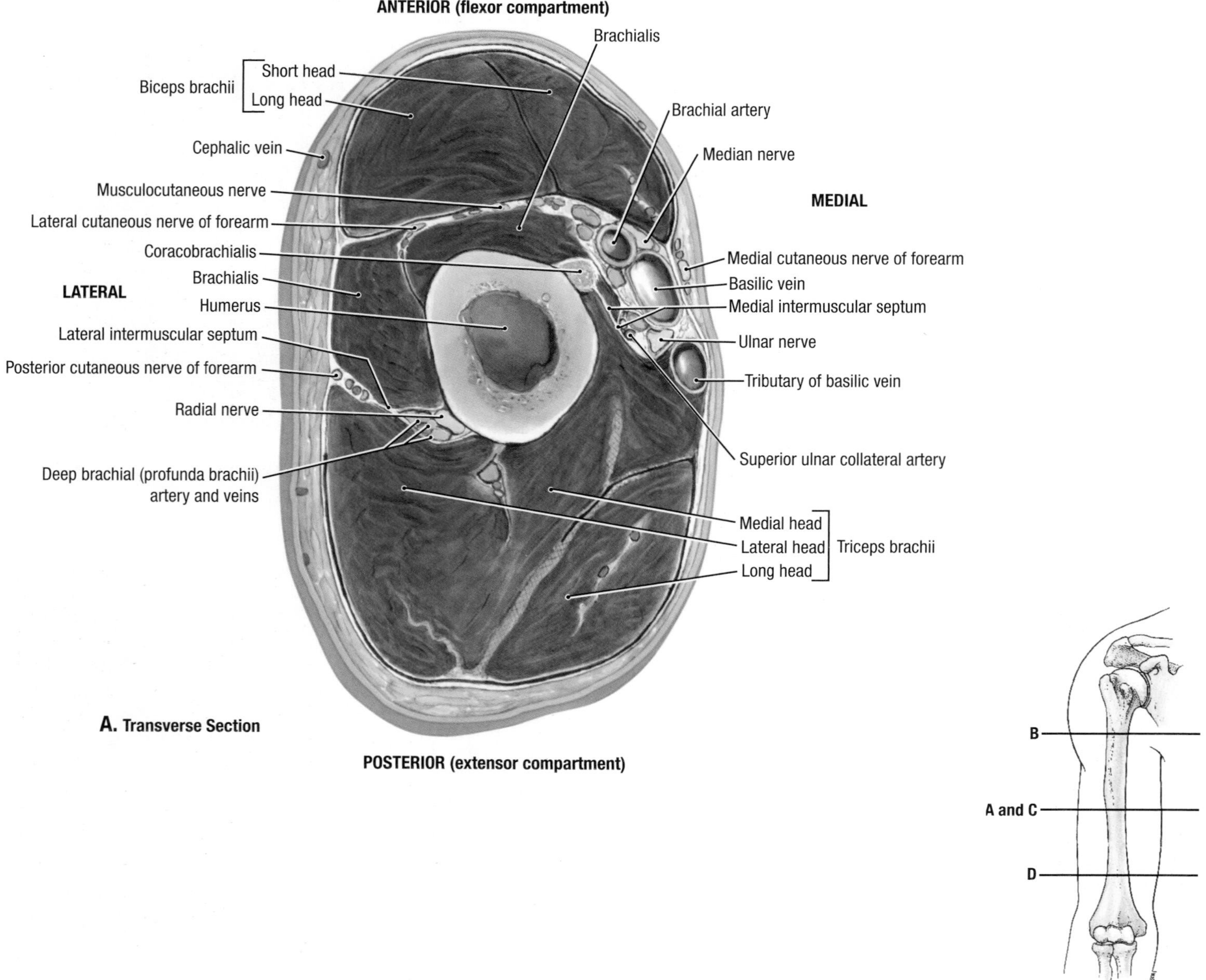
ANTERIOR (flexor compartment)
Brachialis
Biceps brachii
Short head
Long head
Brachial artery
Median nerve
Cephalic vein
Musculocutaneous nerve
MEDIAL
Lateral cutaneous nerve of forearm
Coracobrachialis
Medial cutaneous nerve of forearm
Brachialis
Basilic vein
LATERAL
Humerus
Medial intermuscular septum
Lateral intermuscular septum
Ulnar nerve
Posterior cutaneous nerve of forearm
Tributary of basilic vein
Radial nerve
Superior ulnar collateral artery
Deep brachial (profunda brachii) artery and veins
Medial head
Lateral head
Long head
Triceps brachii
POSTERIOR (extensor compartment)
B
A and C
D

A. Transverse Section

## 6.90 Transverse section and transverse (axial) MRIs of the arm

**A.** Transverse section through arm.

- The body (shaft) of the humerus is nearly circular, and its cortex is thickest at this level.
- Three heads (lateral, medial, and long) of the triceps muscle occupy the posterior compartment of the arm.
- The radial nerve and deep artery and veins of arm lie in contact with the radial groove of the humerus.
- The musculocutaneous nerve lies in the plane between the biceps and brachialis muscles.
- The median nerve crosses to the medial side of the brachial artery and veins, the ulnar nerve passes posteriorly onto the medial side of the triceps muscle, and the basilic vein (appearing here as two vessels) has pierced the deep fascia.

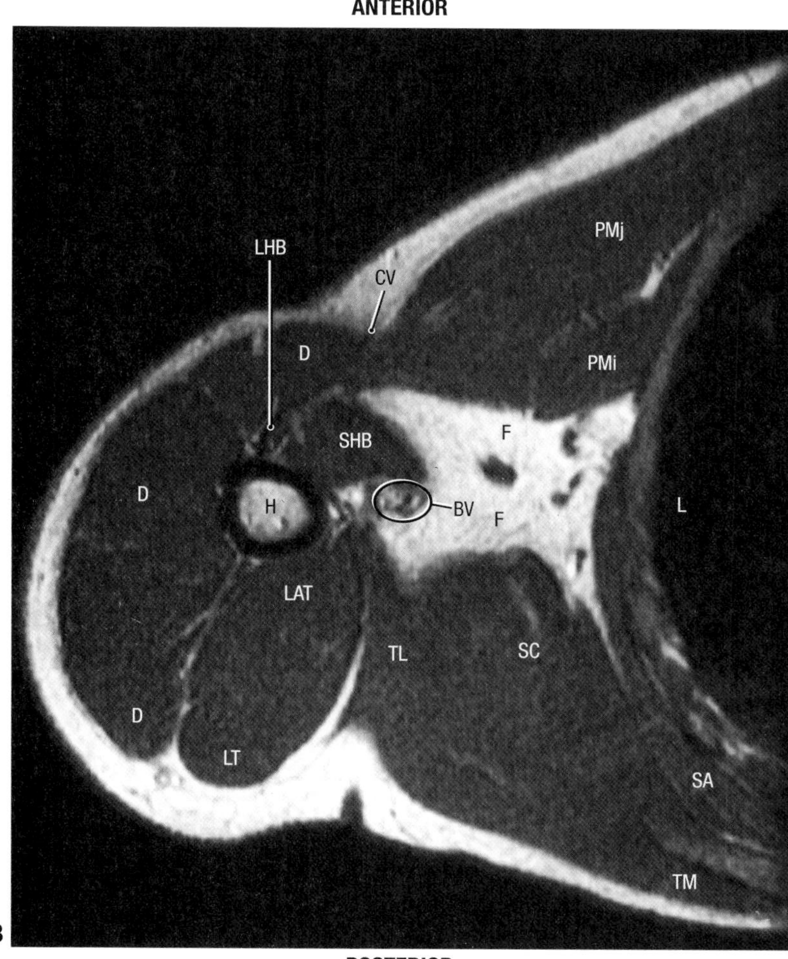
ANTERIOR
LHB
CV
PMj
D
PMi
SHB
F
D
H
BV
F
L
LAT
TL
SC
D
LT
SA
TM
B
POSTERIOR

ANTERIOR
CV
BB
BV
BC
LI
T
H
MT
D
LAT
LT
C
POSTERIOR

ANTERIOR
CV
BB
BV
BS
BR
BC
MI
TR
D
POSTERIOR

**Key for B, E, and D:**

| | | | |
|---|---|---|---|
| BB | Biceps brachii | LT | Long head of triceps brachii |
| BC | Brachialis | MI | Medial intermuscular septum |
| BR | Brachioradialis | MT | Medial head of triceps brachii |
| BS | Basilic vein | PMi | Pectoralis minor |
| BV | Brachial vessels and nerves | PMj | Pectoralis major |
| CV | Cephalic vein | SA | Serratus anterior |
| D | Deltoid | SC | Subscapularis |
| F | Fat in axilla | SHB | Short head of biceps brachii |
| H | Humerus | T | Deltoid tuberosity |
| L | Lung | TL | Teres major and latissimus dorsi |
| LAT | Lateral head of triceps brachii | TM | Teres minor |
| LHB | Long head of biceps brachii | TR | Triceps brachii |
| LI | Lateral intermuscular septum | | |

**6.90 Transverse section and transverse (axial) MRIs of the arm *(continued)***

**B.** Transverse MRI through the proximal arm. **C.** Transverse MRI though the middle of the arm. **D.** Transverse MRI through the distal arm.

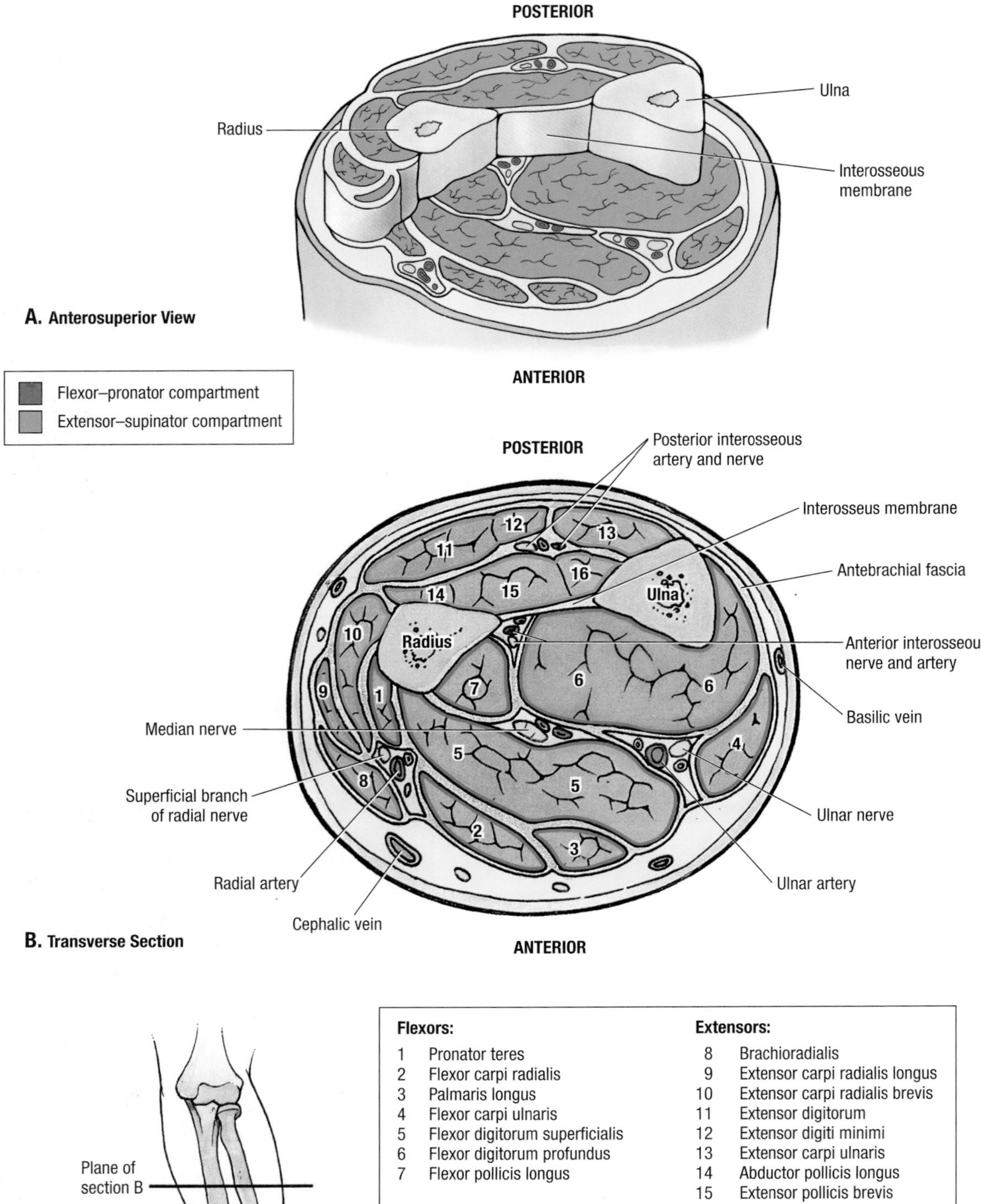
POSTERIOR
Radius
Ulna
Interosseous membrane
A. Anterosuperior View
ANTERIOR
Flexor–pronator compartment
Extensor–supinator compartment
POSTERIOR
Posterior interosseous artery and nerve
Interosseus membrane
Antebrachial fascia
Ulna
Radius
Anterior interosseous nerve and artery
Basilic vein
Median nerve
Superficial branch of radial nerve
Ulnar nerve
Radial artery
Cephalic vein
Ulnar artery
B. Transverse Section
ANTERIOR
Plane of section B

| Flexors: | | Extensors: | |
|---|---|---|---|
| 1 | Pronator teres | 8 | Brachioradialis |
| 2 | Flexor carpi radialis | 9 | Extensor carpi radialis longus |
| 3 | Palmaris longus | 10 | Extensor carpi radialis brevis |
| 4 | Flexor carpi ulnaris | 11 | Extensor digitorum |
| 5 | Flexor digitorum superficialis | 12 | Extensor digiti minimi |
| 6 | Flexor digitorum profundus | 13 | Extensor carpi ulnaris |
| 7 | Flexor pollicis longus | 14 | Abductor pollicis longus |
| | | 15 | Extensor pollicis brevis |
| | | 16 | Extensor pollicis longus and extensor indicis |

## 6.91 Transverse sections and transverse (axial) MRIs of forearm

**A.** Stepped transverse sections of the anterior and posterior compartments. **B.** Contents of the anterior and posterior compartments.

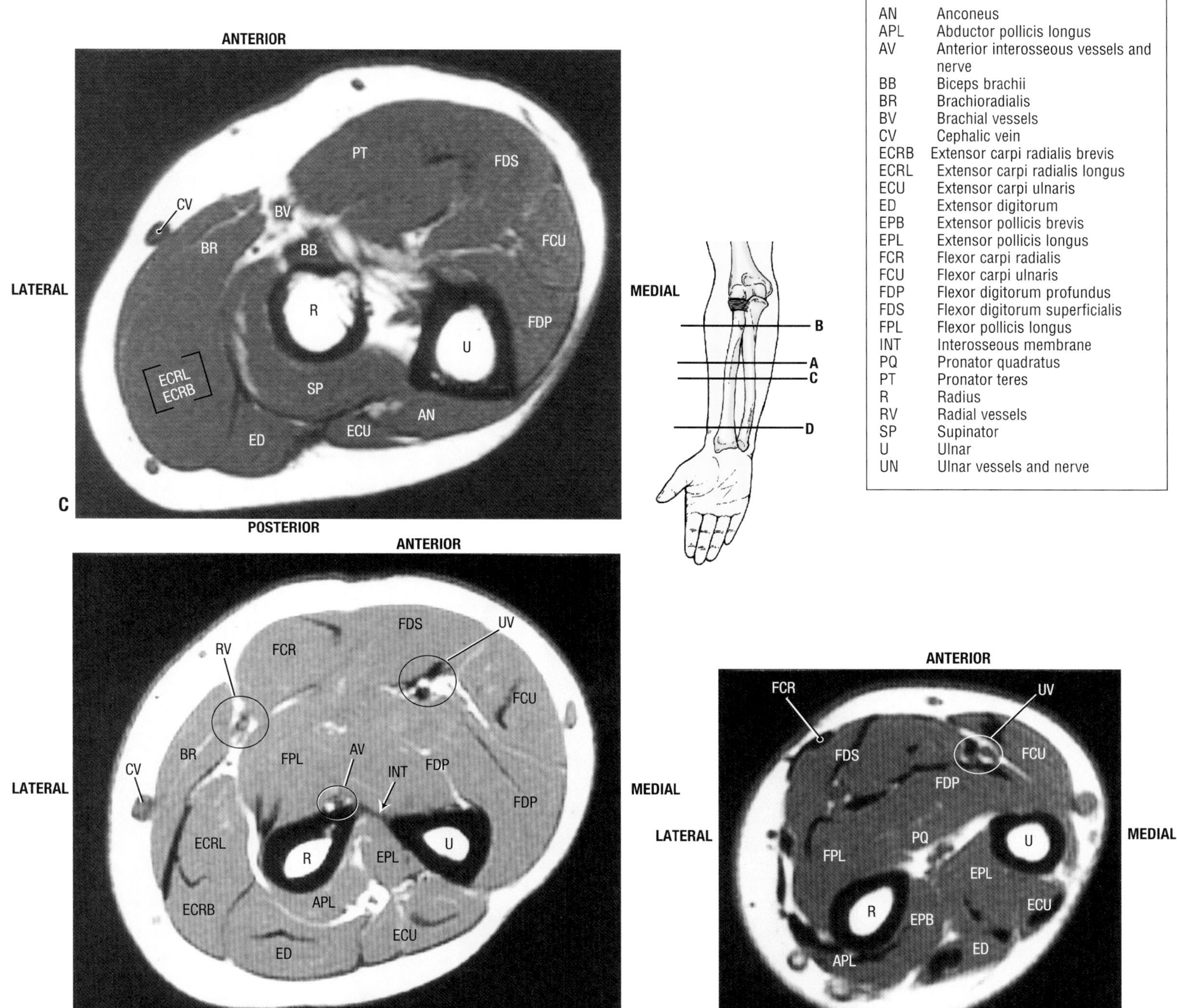
Key for C, D, and E:
AN Anconeus
APL Abductor pollicis longus
AV Anterior interosseous vessels and nerve
BB Biceps brachii
BR Brachioradialis
BV Brachial vessels
CV Cephalic vein
ECRB Extensor carpi radialis brevis
ECRL Extensor carpi radialis longus
ECU Extensor carpi ulnaris
ED Extensor digitorum
EPB Extensor pollicis brevis
EPL Extensor pollicis longus
FCR Flexor carpi radialis
FCU Flexor carpi ulnaris
FDP Flexor digitorum profundus
FDS Flexor digitorum superficialis
FPL Flexor pollicis longus
INT Interosseous membrane
PQ Pronator quadratus
PT Pronator teres
R Radius
RV Radial vessels
SP Supinator
U Ulnar
UN Ulnar vessels and nerve
ANTERIOR
POSTERIOR
LATERAL
MEDIAL
C
PT
FDS
CV
BV
BR
BB
FCU
R
FDP
U
ECRL
ECRB
SP
AN
ED
ECU
B
A
C
D
D
FDS
UV
RV
FCR
FCU
BR
FPL
AV
INT
FDP
CV
ECRL
R
EPL
U
ECRB
APL
ED
ECU
E
FCR
UV
FDS
FCU
FDP
PQ
FPL
U
EPL
R
EPB
ECU
ED
APL

## 6.91 Transverse section and transverse (axial) MRIs of forearm *(continued)*

**C.** Transverse MRI through the proximal forearm. **D.** Transverse MRI through the middle forearm. **E.** Transverse MRI through the distal forearm.

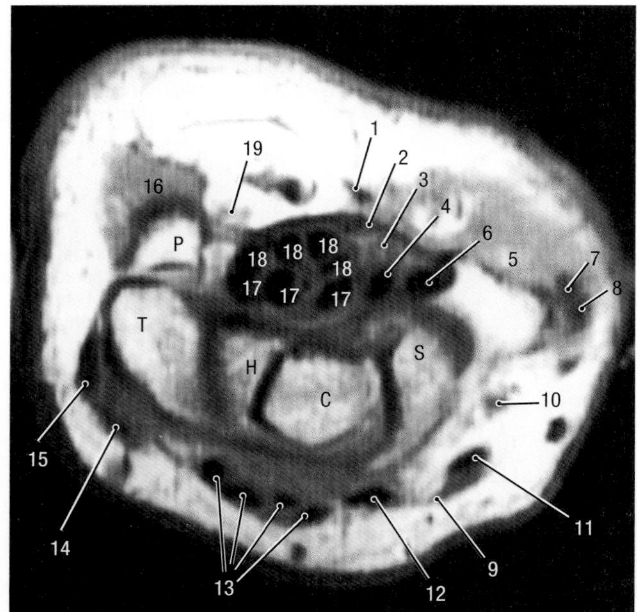
1
2
3
4
5
6
7
8
9
10
11
12
13
14
15
16
17
18
19
P
T
H
C
S

A. Transverse MRI

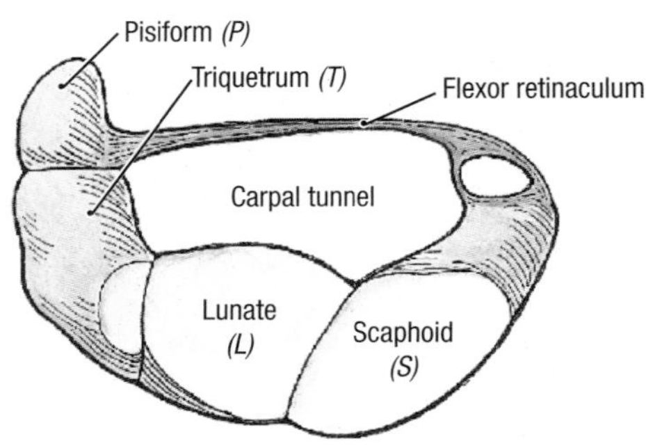
Pisiform (P)
Triquetrum (T)
Flexor retinaculum
Carpal tunnel
Lunate (L)
Scaphoid (S)

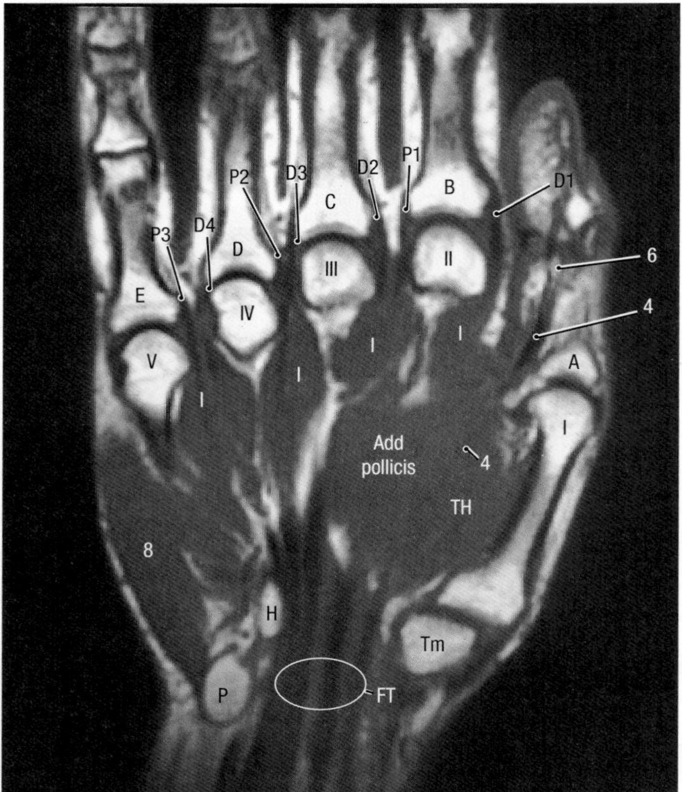
P1
P2
P3
D1
D2
D3
D4
B
C
D
E
A
II
III
IV
V
I
6
4
Add pollicis
TH
8
H
Tm
P
FT

B. Coronal MRI

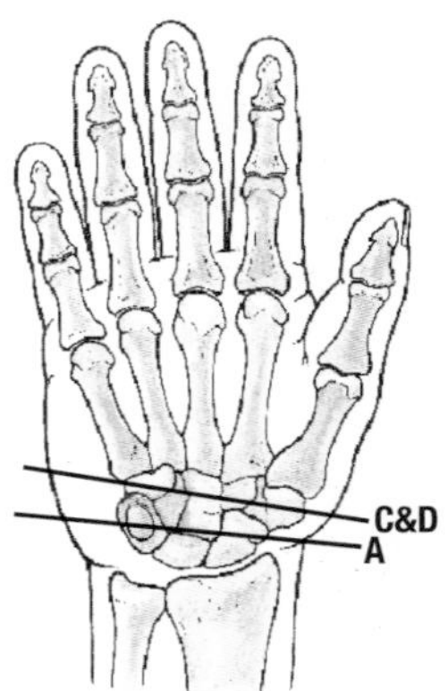
C&D
A

## 6.92 Transverse (axial) section and MRIs through carpal tunnel

**A.** Transverse MRI through the proximal carpal tunnel (*numbers* and *letters* in MRIs refer to structures in **D**). **B.** Coronal MRI of wrist and hand showing the course of the long flexor tendons in the carpal tunnel (*numbers* and *letters* in MRIs refer to structures in **D**). *FT*, long flexor tendons in carpal tunnel; *TH*, thenar muscles; *P*, pisiform; *H*, hook of hamate; *Tm*, trapezium; *I*, interossei, *A–E*, proximal phalanges.

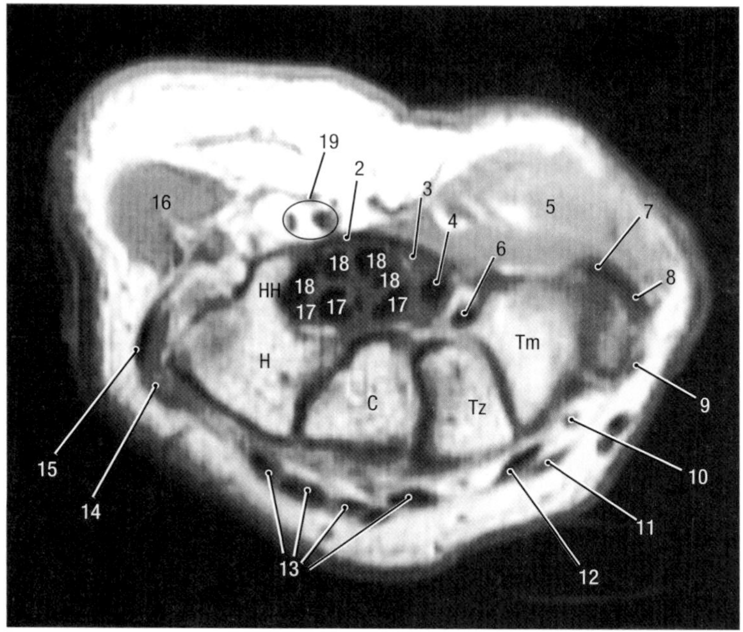
19
2
3
4
5
6
7
8
16
18 18
18
HH 18
17 17 17
H
Tm
C
Tz
9
10
11
12
13
14
15

C. Transverse MRI

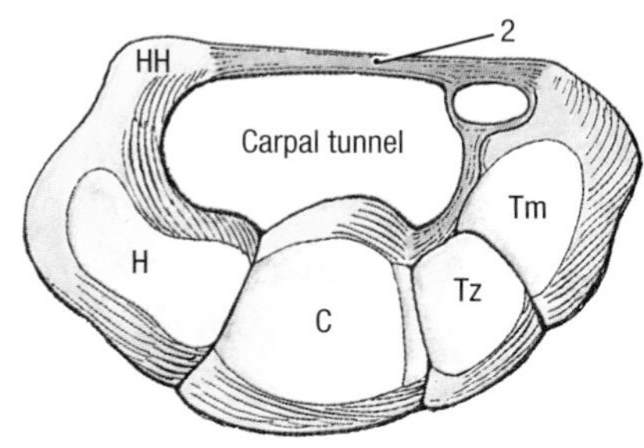
2
HH
Carpal tunnel
Tm
H
Tz
C

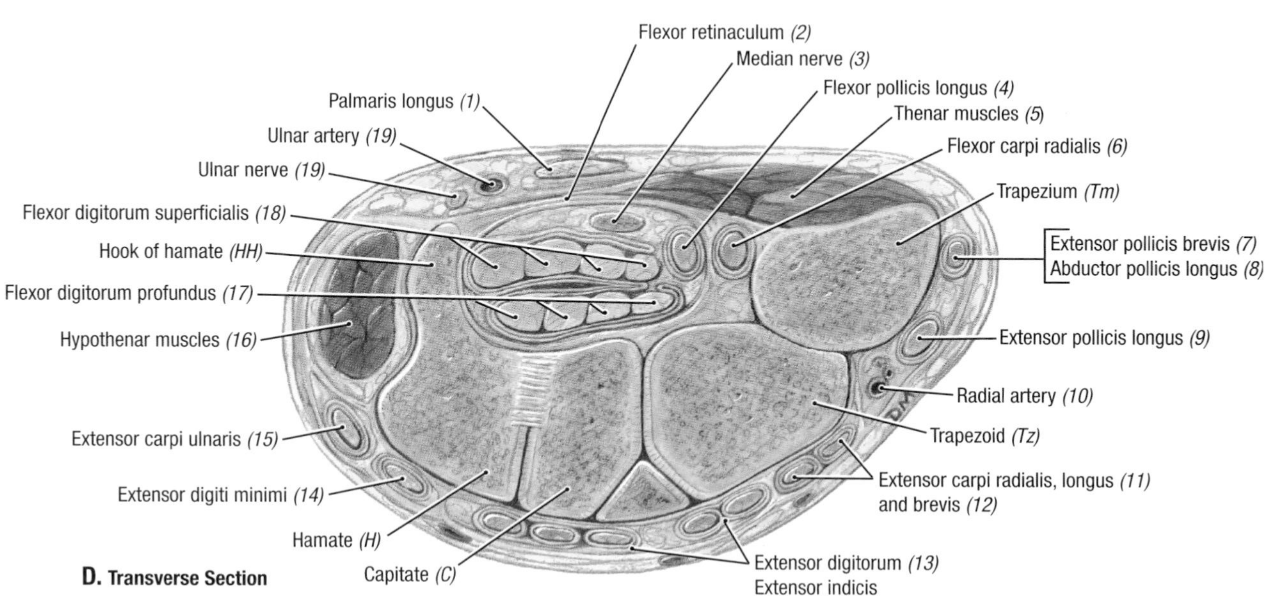
Flexor retinaculum (2)
Median nerve (3)
Flexor pollicis longus (4)
Palmaris longus (1)
Thenar muscles (5)
Ulnar artery (19)
Flexor carpi radialis (6)
Ulnar nerve (19)
Trapezium (Tm)
Flexor digitorum superficialis (18)
Hook of hamate (HH)
Extensor pollicis brevis (7)
Abductor pollicis longus (8)
Flexor digitorum profundus (17)
Hypothenar muscles (16)
Extensor pollicis longus (9)
Radial artery (10)
Extensor carpi ulnaris (15)
Trapezoid (Tz)
Extensor carpi radialis, longus (11) and brevis (12)
Extensor digiti minimi (14)
Hamate (H)
Capitate (C)
Extensor digitorum (13)
Extensor indicis

D. Transverse Section

## 6.92 Transverse (axial) section and MRIs through carpal tunnel *(continued)*

**C.** Transverse MRI through the distal carpal tunnel (*numbers* and *letters* in MRIs refer to structures in **D**). **D.** Transverse section of carpal tunnel through the distal row of carpal bones.

Flexor digitorum superficialis *(10)*
Flexor digitorum profundus *(9)*
Lumbrical *(1)* and digital artery and nerve *(2)*
Midpalmar space
Palmar aponeurosis *(3)*
Palmar space
Adductor pollicis *(AD)*
Flexor pollicis longus *(4)*
Abductor pollicis brevis *(5)*
Flexor pollicis brevis
Princeps pollicis arteries
1st metacarpal *(I)*
Sesamoid bone *(6)*
Extensor pollicis longus
Dorsalis pollicis artery
1st dorsal interosseous *(D1)*
Dorsalis indicis artery
2nd metacarpal *(II)*
1st palmar interosseous *(P1)*
2nd dorsal interosseous *(D2)*
Subaponeurotic areolar space
3rd metacarpal *(III)*
Extensor tendons *(7)*
3rd dorsal interosseous *(D3)*
4th metacarpal *(IV)*
2nd palmar interosseous *(P2)*
4th dorsal interosseous *(D4)*
3rd palmar interosseous *(P3)*
5th metacarpal *(V)*
Opponens digiti minimi
Abductor digiti minimi *(8)*
E. Blackstock
A

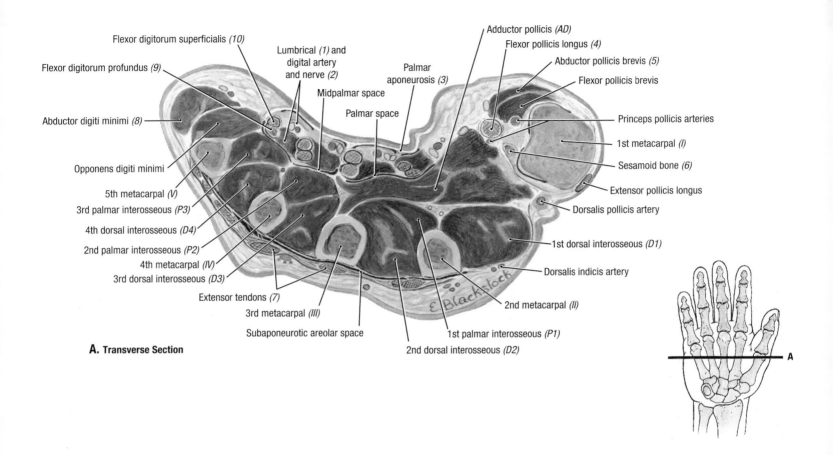

**A. Transverse Section**

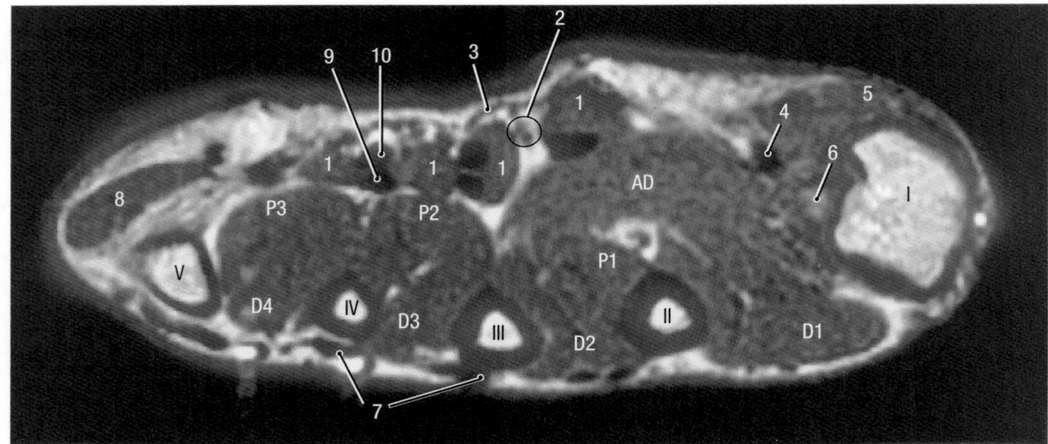
2
9
10
3
1
1
1
1
4
5
6
AD
I
8
P3
P2
P1
V
D4
IV
D3
III
D2
II
D1
7

**B. Transverse MRI**

**6.93 Transverse section and MRI through palm (metacarpals) at level of adductor pollicis**

CHAPTER 7

# HEAD

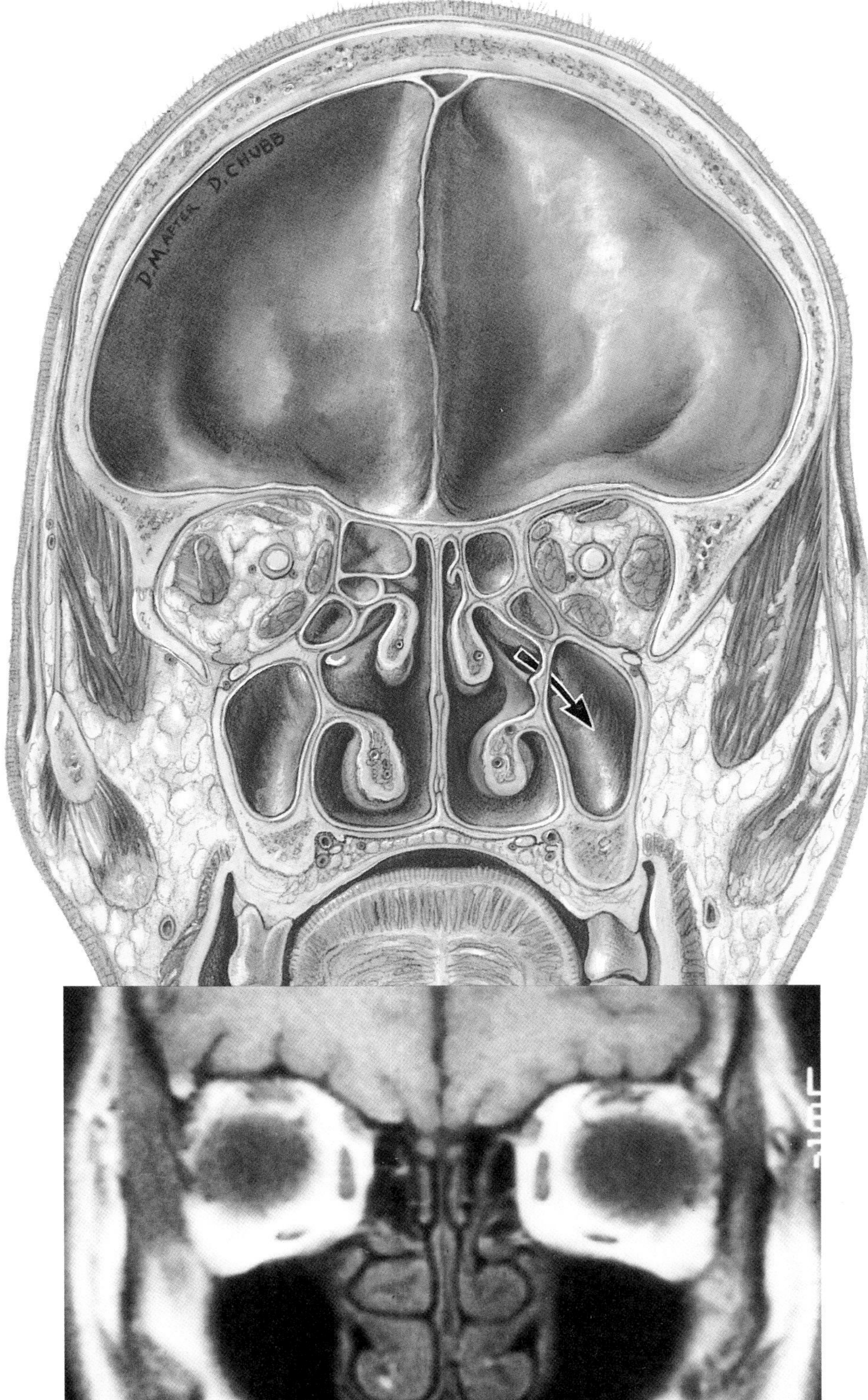
D.M.AFTER D.CHUBB


- Cranium **608**
- Face and Scalp **626**
- Circulation and Innervation of Cranial Cavity **632**
- Meninges and Meningeal Spaces **636**
- Cranial Base and Cranial Nerves **640**
- Blood Supply of Brain **646**
- Orbit and Eyeball **650**
- Parotid Region **662**
- Temporal Region and Infratemporal Fossa **664**
- Temporomandibular Joint **672**
- Tongue **676**
- Palate **682**
- Teeth **685**
- Nose, Paranasal Sinuses, and Pterygopalatine Fossa **690**
- Ear **703**
- Lymphatic Drainage of Head **716**
- Autonomic Innervation of Head **717**
- Imaging of Head **718**
- Neuroanatomy: Overview and Ventricular System **722**
- Telencephalon (Cerebrum) and Diencephalon **725**
- Brainstem and Cerebellum **734**
- Imaging of Brain **740**

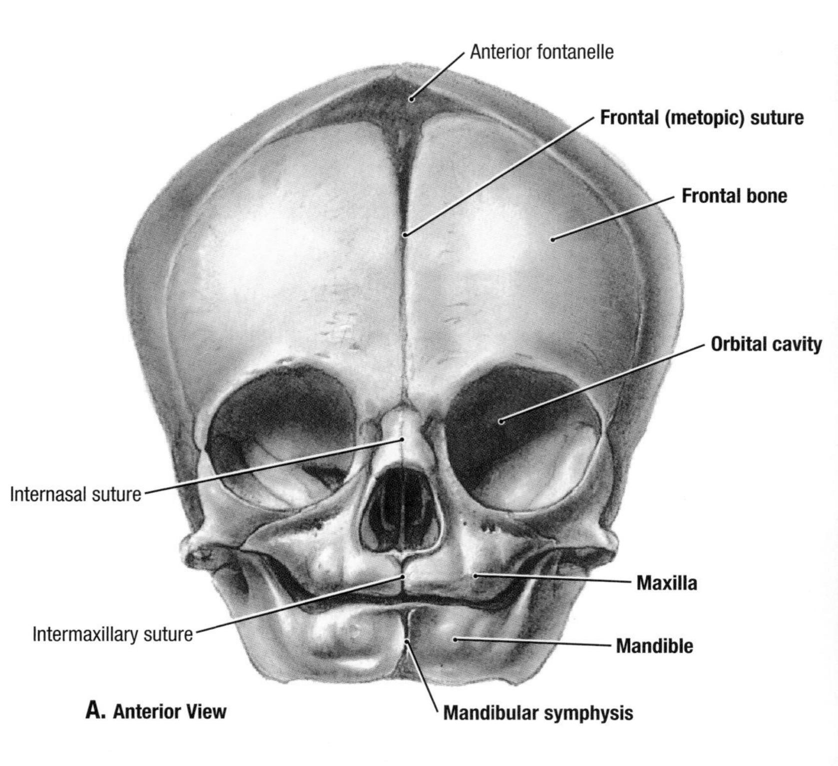
Anterior fontanelle
Frontal (metopic) suture
Frontal bone
Orbital cavity
Internasal suture
Maxilla
Intermaxillary suture
Mandible
Mandibular symphysis

A. Anterior View

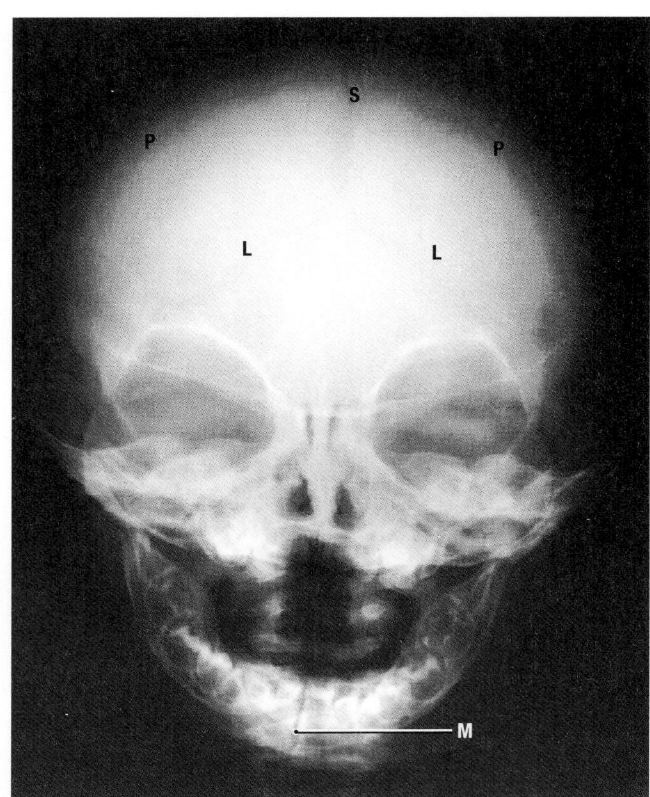
S
P
P
L
L
M

B. Anteroposterior View

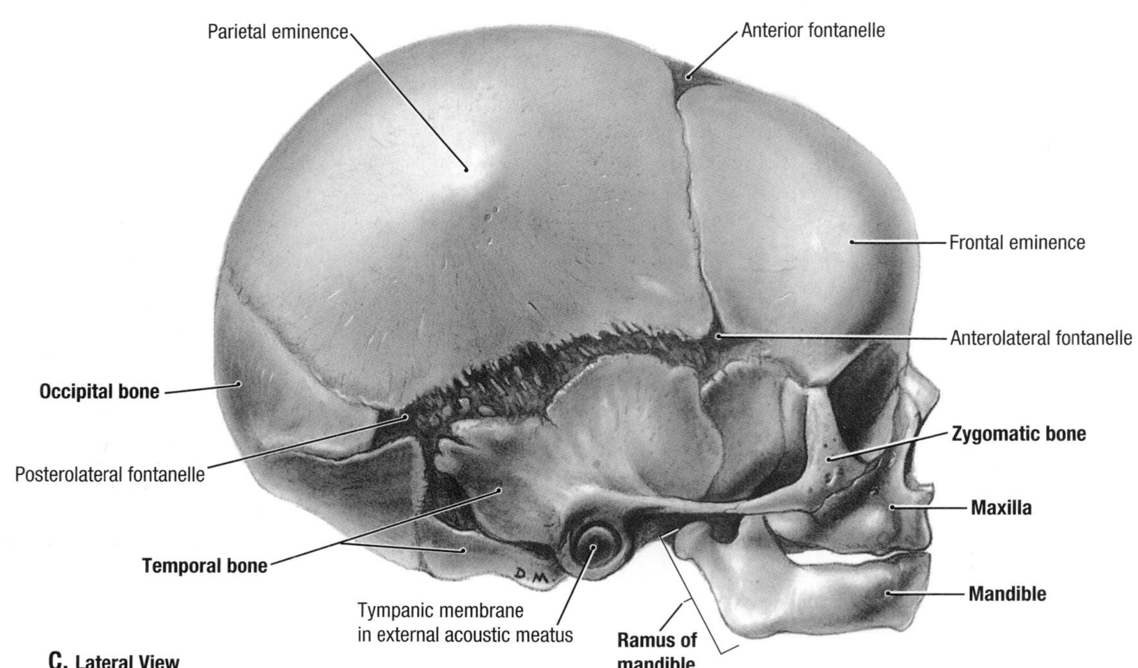
Parietal eminence
Anterior fontanelle
Frontal eminence
Anterolateral fontanelle
Occipital bone
Zygomatic bone
Posterolateral fontanelle
Maxilla
Temporal bone
D.M.
Mandible
Tympanic membrane
in external acoustic meatus
Ramus of
mandible

C. Lateral View

## 7.1 Cranium at birth and in early childhood

**A**. Cranium at birth, anterior aspect. **B.** Radiograph of $6\frac{1}{2}$-month-old child. **C.** Cranium at birth, lateral aspect.

Compared with the adult skull (Figs. 7.2–7.4):

- The maxilla and mandible are proportionately small.
- The mandibular symphysis, which closes during the second year, and the frontal suture, which closes during the sixth year, are still open (unfused).
- The orbital cavities are proportionately large, but the face is small; the facial skeleton forming only one eighth of the whole cranium, while in the adult, it forms one third.

Key for B, E and F

| | |
|---|---|
| A | Angle of mandible |
| B | Body of mandible |
| C | Coronal suture |
| F | Frontal bone |
| L | Lambdoid suture |
| M | Mandibular symphysis |
| O | Occipital bone |
| P | Parietal eminence |
| S | Sagittal suture |
| SP | Sphenoid |
| T | Temporal bone |
| X | Maxilla |
| Y | Mastoid process |
| Z | Zygomatic bone |

Arrowheads = Membranous outline of parietal bone

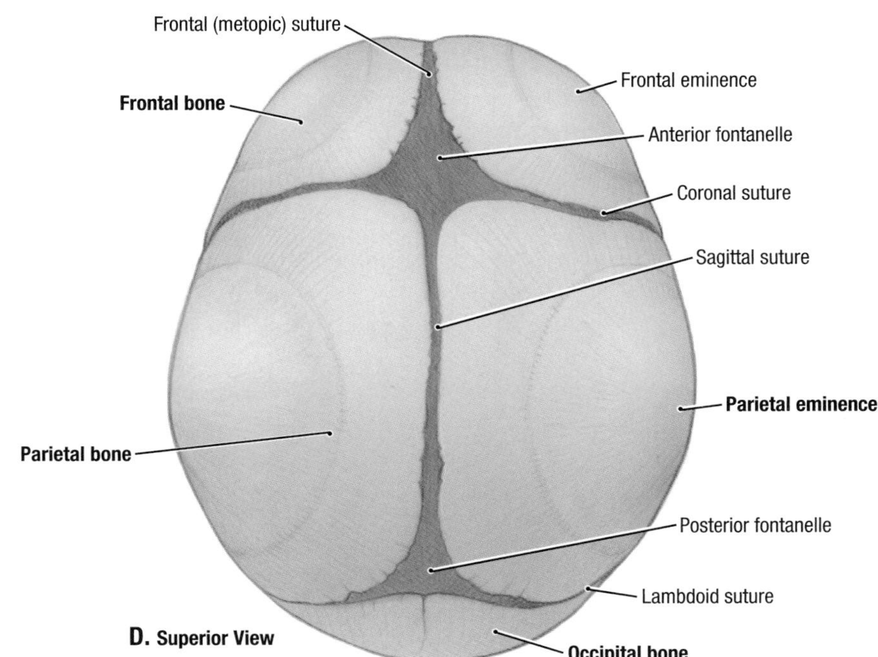
Frontal (metopic) suture
Frontal bone
Frontal eminence
Anterior fontanelle
Coronal suture
Sagittal suture
Parietal eminence
Parietal bone
Posterior fontanelle
Lambdoid suture
Occipital bone

D. Superior View

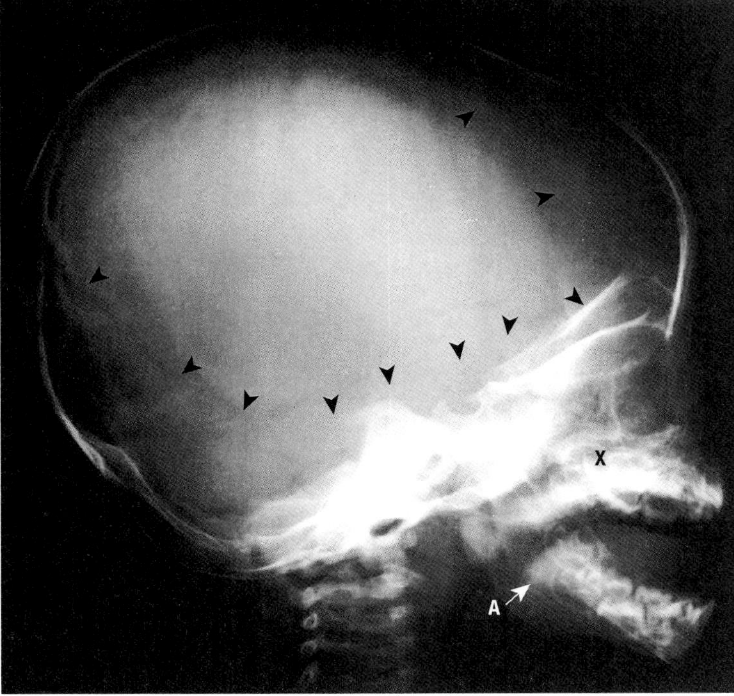
X
A

E. Lateral View

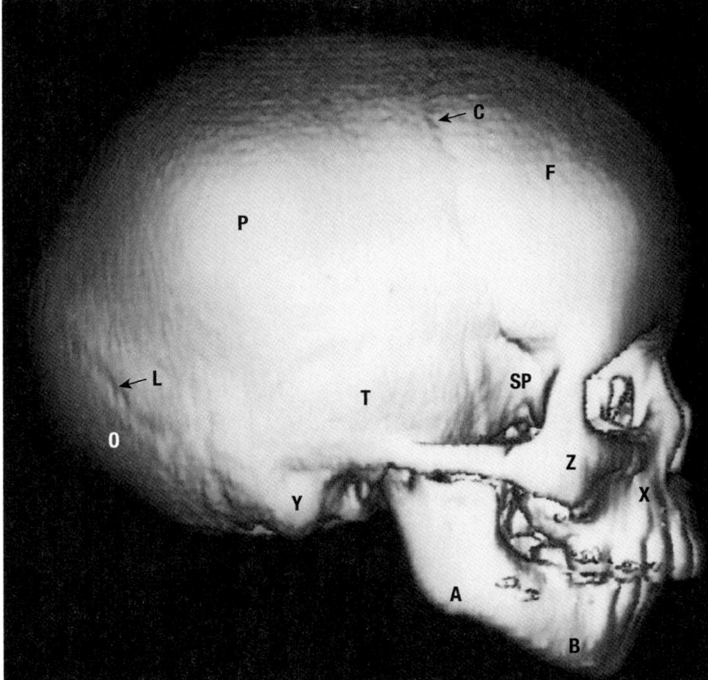
C
F
P
L
SP
T
O
Z
X
Y
A
B

F. Lateral View

## 7.1 Cranium at birth and in early childhood *(continued)*

**D.** Cranium at birth, superior aspect. **E.** Radiograph of 6½-month-old child. **F.** Three-dimensional computer-generated images of 3-year-old child's cranium.

- The parietal eminence is a rounded cone. Ossification, which starts at the eminences, has not yet reached the ultimate four angles of the parietal bone; accordingly, these regions are membranous, and the membrane is blended with the pericranium externally and the dura mater internally to form the fontanelles. The fontanelles are usually closed by the second year; there is no mastoid process until the second year.

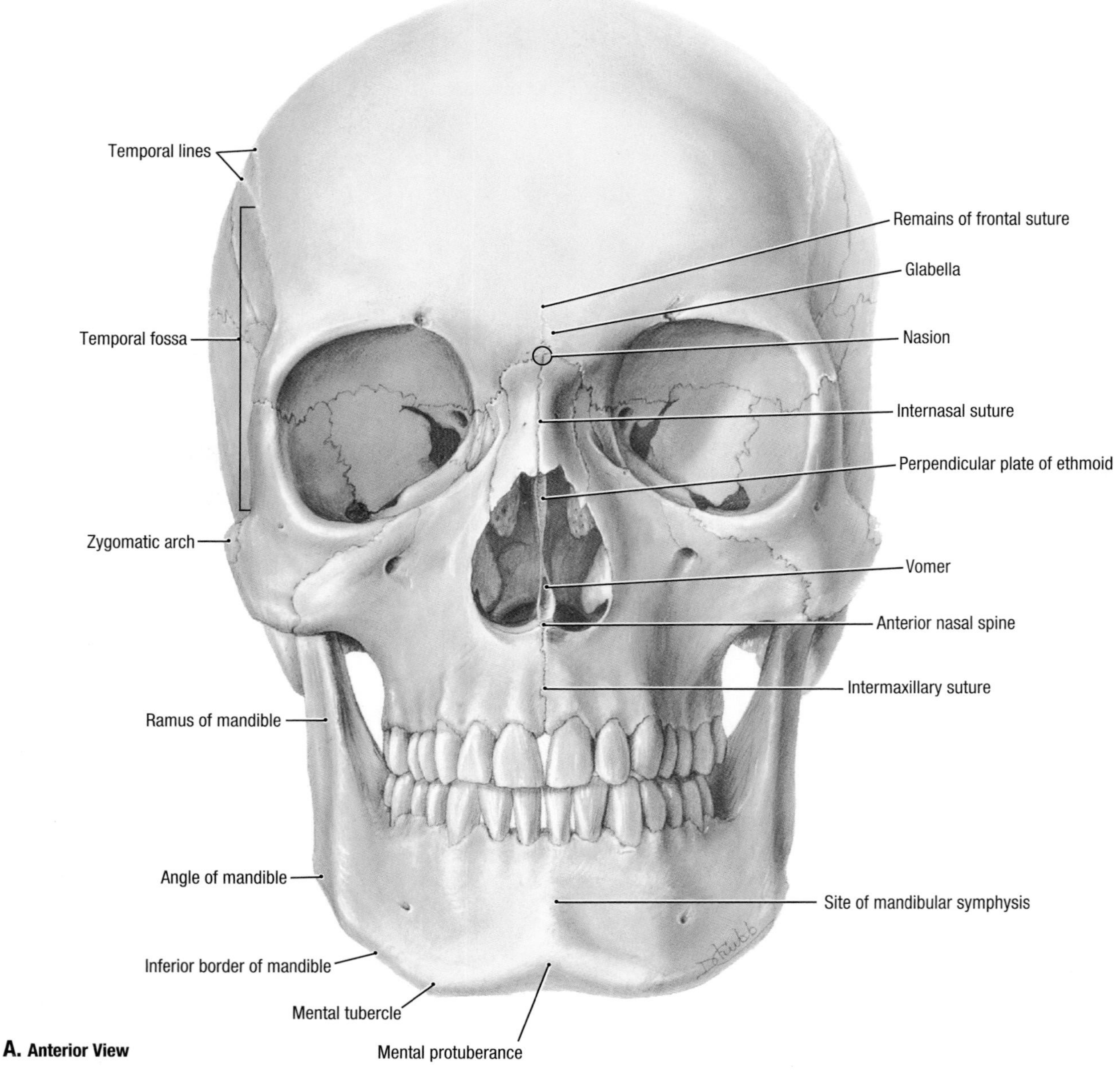
Temporal lines
Remains of frontal suture
Glabella
Temporal fossa
Nasion
Internasal suture
Perpendicular plate of ethmoid
Zygomatic arch
Vomer
Anterior nasal spine
Intermaxillary suture
Ramus of mandible
Angle of mandible
Site of mandibular symphysis
Inferior border of mandible
Mental tubercle
Mental protuberance
A. Anterior View

## 7.2 Cranium, facial (frontal) aspect

**A.** Formations of the bony cranium. **B.** Bones of cranium and their features. The individual bones forming the cranium are color coded. For the orbital cavity, see also Figure 7.31A.

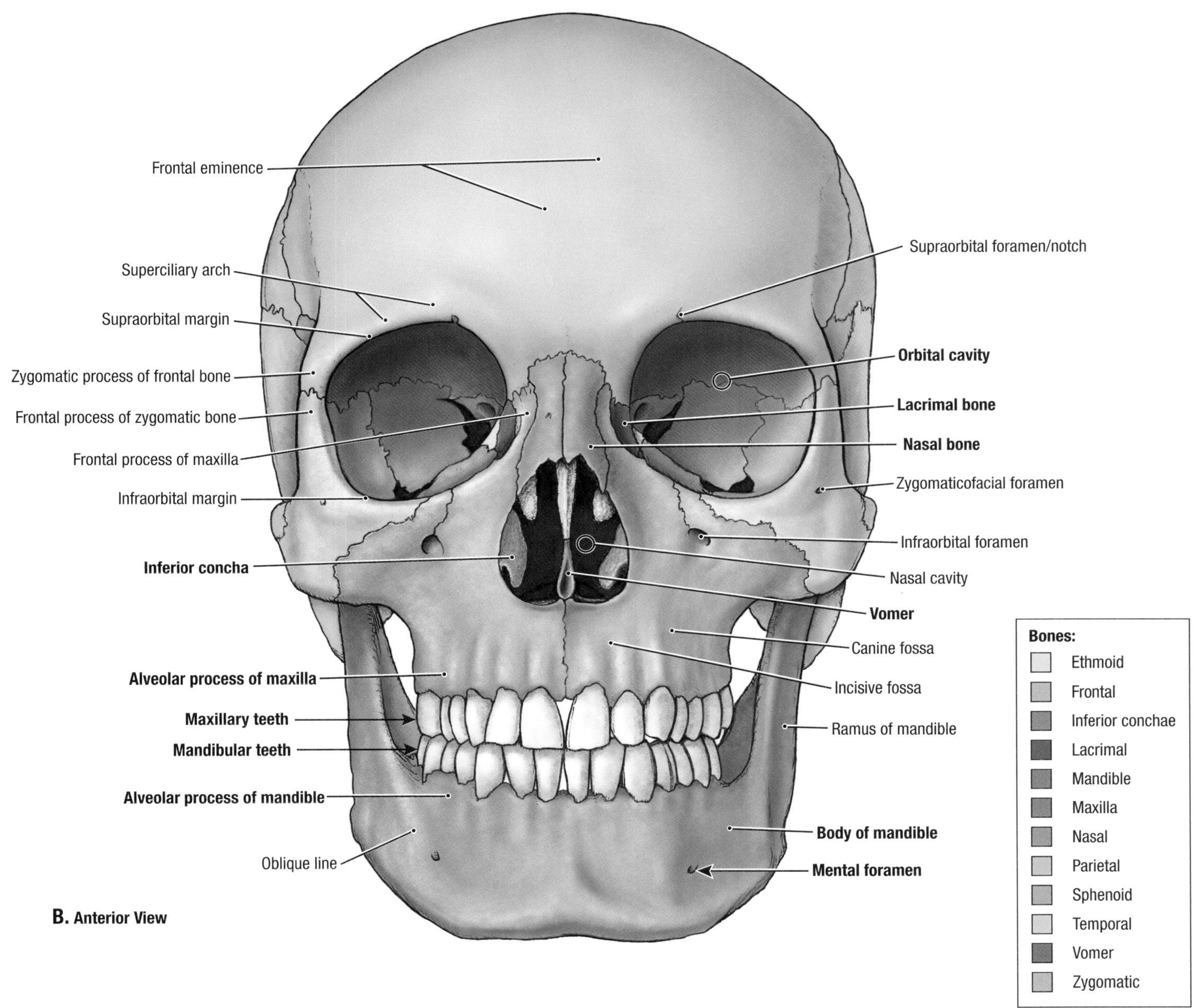
Frontal eminence
Superciliary arch
Supraorbital margin
Zygomatic process of frontal bone
Frontal process of zygomatic bone
Frontal process of maxilla
Infraorbital margin
Inferior concha
Alveolar process of maxilla
Maxillary teeth
Mandibular teeth
Alveolar process of mandible
Oblique line
Supraorbital foramen/notch
Orbital cavity
Lacrimal bone
Nasal bone
Zygomaticofacial foramen
Infraorbital foramen
Nasal cavity
Vomer
Canine fossa
Incisive fossa
Ramus of mandible
Body of mandible
Mental foramen
Bones:
Ethmoid
Frontal
Inferior conchae
Lacrimal
Mandible
Maxilla
Nasal
Parietal
Sphenoid
Temporal
Vomer
Zygomatic

**B.** **Anterior View**

## 7.2 Cranium, facial (frontal) aspect *(continued)*

Extraction of teeth causes the alveolar bone to resorb in the affected regions(s). Following complete loss or extraction of maxillary teeth, the sockets begin to fill in with bone, and the alveolar process begins to resorb. Similarly, extraction of mandibular teeth causes the bone to resorb. Gradually, the mental foramen lies near the superior border of the body of the mandible. In some cases, the mental foramina disappear, exposing the mental nerves to injury.

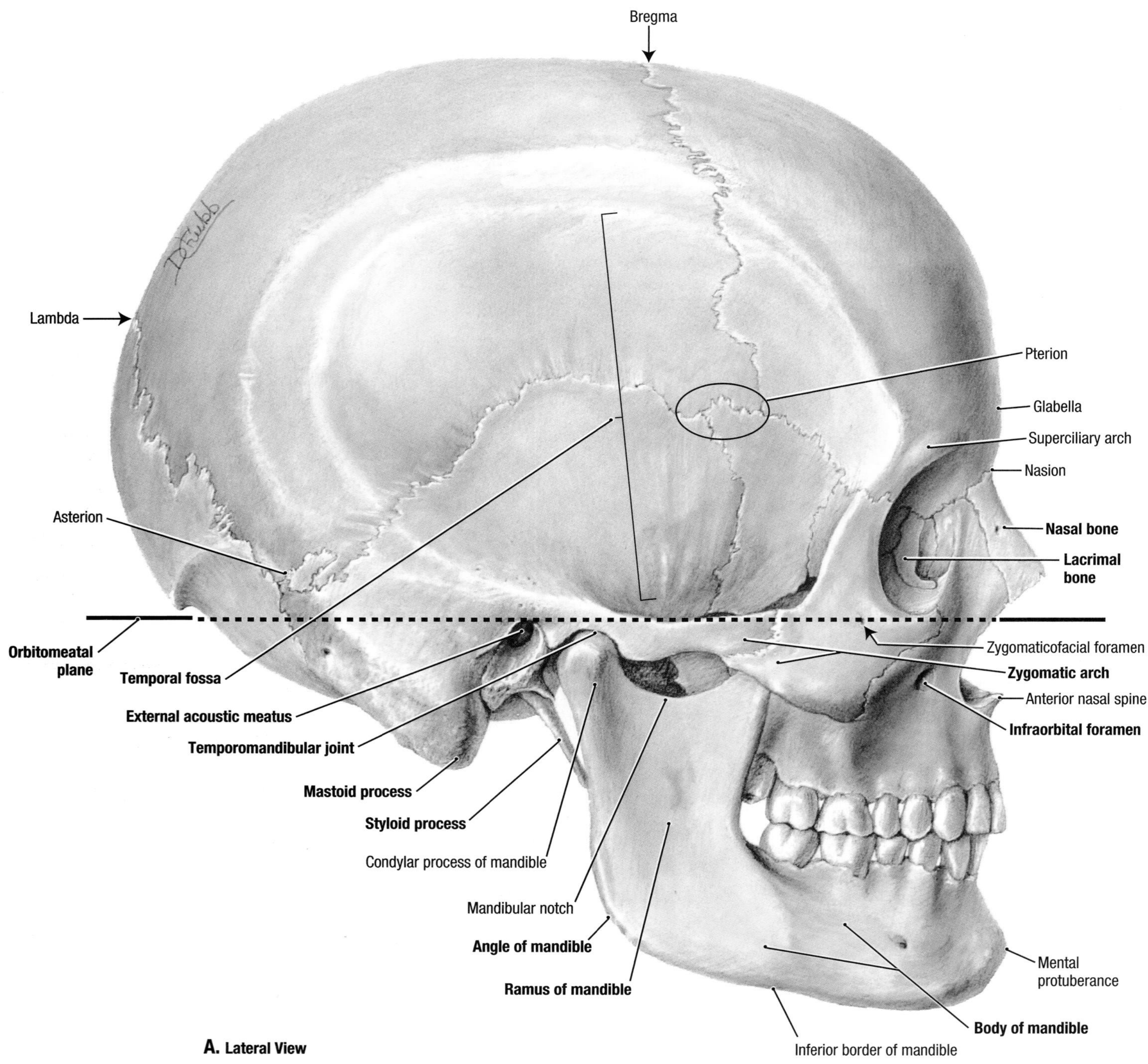
Bregma
Lambda
Pterion
Glabella
Superciliary arch
Nasion
Nasal bone
Lacrimal bone
Asterion
Orbitomeatal plane
Temporal fossa
Zygomaticofacial foramen
Zygomatic arch
Anterior nasal spine
External acoustic meatus
Infraorbital foramen
Temporomandibular joint
Mastoid process
Styloid process
Condylar process of mandible
Mandibular notch
Angle of mandible
Mental protuberance
Ramus of mandible
Body of mandible
Inferior border of mandible

**A.** Lateral View

## 7.3 Cranium, lateral aspect

**A**. Bony cranium. **B.** Cranium with bones color coded. The cranium is in the anatomical position when the orbitomeatal plane is horizontal.

The convexity of the neurocranium (braincase) distributes and thereby minimizes the effects of a blow to it. However, hard blows to the head in thin areas of the cranium (e.g., in the temporal fossa) are likely to produce depressed fractures, in which a fragment of bone is depressed inward, compressing and/or injuring the brain. In comminuted fractures, the bone is broken into several pieces. Linear fractures, the most frequent type, usually occur at the point of impact, but fracture lines often radiate away from it in two or more directions.

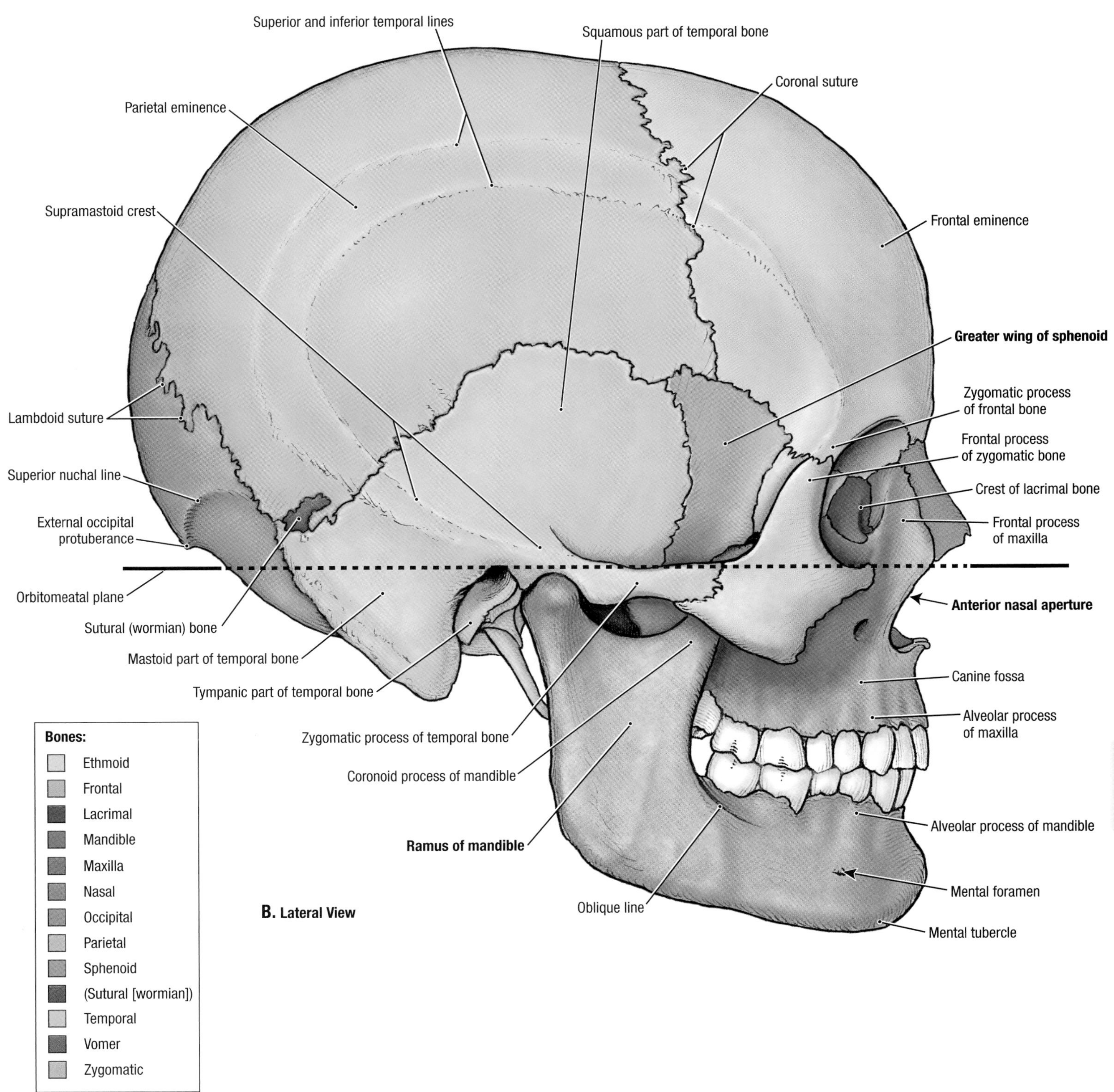
Superior and inferior temporal lines
Squamous part of temporal bone
Coronal suture
Parietal eminence
Supramastoid crest
Frontal eminence
Greater wing of sphenoid
Zygomatic process of frontal bone
Frontal process of zygomatic bone
Crest of lacrimal bone
Frontal process of maxilla
Lambdoid suture
Superior nuchal line
External occipital protuberance
Orbitomeatal plane
Anterior nasal aperture
Sutural (wormian) bone
Mastoid part of temporal bone
Tympanic part of temporal bone
Canine fossa
Alveolar process of maxilla
Zygomatic process of temporal bone
Coronoid process of mandible
Alveolar process of mandible
Ramus of mandible
Mental foramen
Oblique line
Mental tubercle
Bones:
Ethmoid
Frontal
Lacrimal
Mandible
Maxilla
Nasal
Occipital
Parietal
Sphenoid
(Sutural [wormian])
Temporal
Vomer
Zygomatic

**B.** Lateral View

## 7.3 Cranium, lateral aspect *(continued)*

If the area of the neurocranium is thick at the site of impact, the bone usually bends inward without fracturing; however, a fracture may occur some distance from the site of direct trauma where the calvaria is thinner. In a contrecoup (counterblow) fracture, the fracture occurs on the opposite side of the cranium rather than at the point of impact.

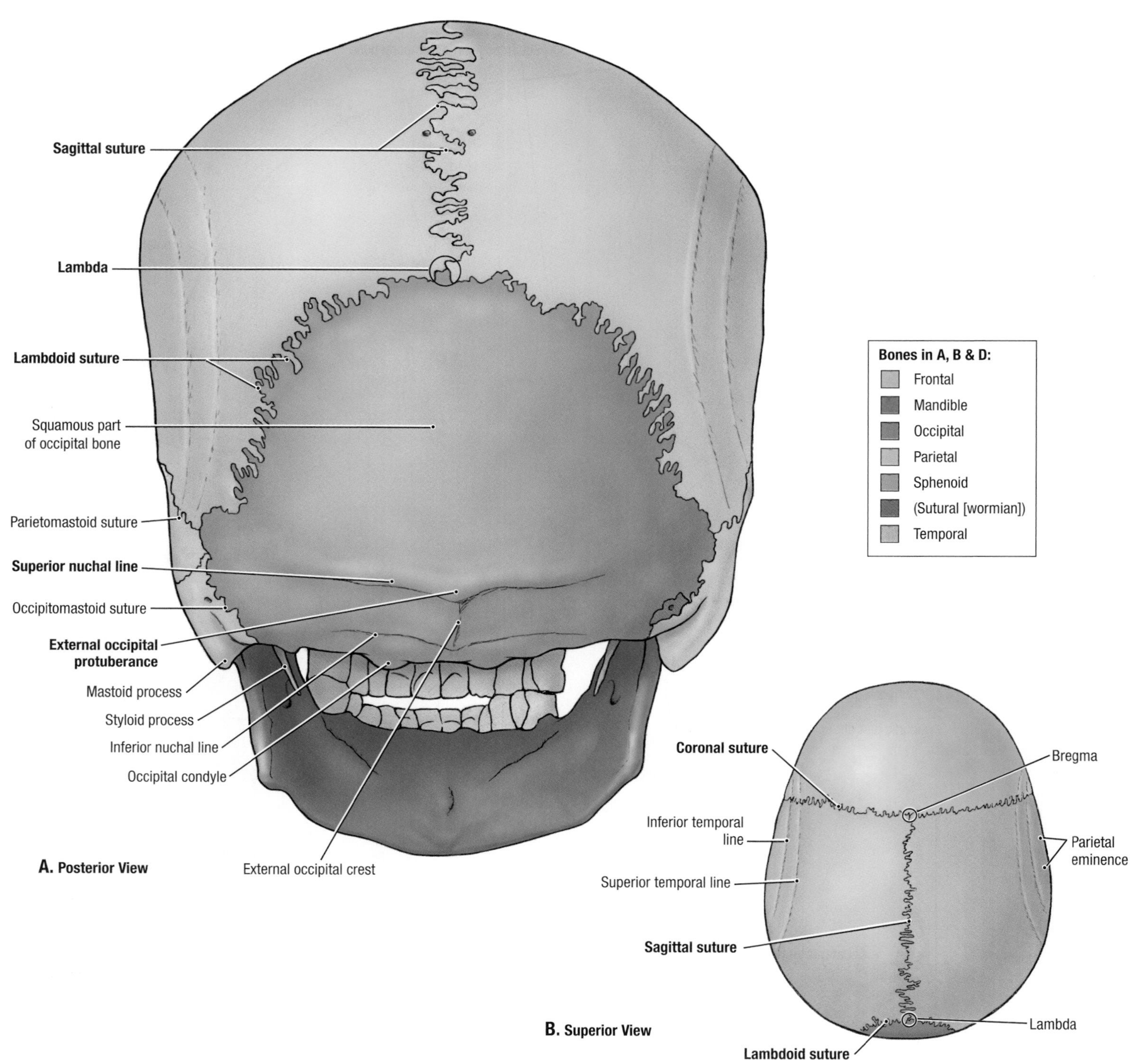
Sagittal suture
Lambda
Lambdoid suture
Squamous part of occipital bone
Parietomastoid suture
Superior nuchal line
Occipitomastoid suture
External occipital protuberance
Mastoid process
Styloid process
Inferior nuchal line
Occipital condyle
A. Posterior View
External occipital crest
Bones in A, B & D:
Frontal
Mandible
Occipital
Parietal
Sphenoid
(Sutural [wormian])
Temporal
Coronal suture
Bregma
Inferior temporal line
Parietal eminence
Superior temporal line
Sagittal suture
B. Superior View
Lambda
Lambdoid suture

## 7.4 Cranium, occipital aspect, calvaria, and anterior part of posterior cranial fossa

**A.** Posterior aspect. **B.** Superior aspect.

**A.** The lambda, near the center of this convex surface, is located at the junction of the superior and lambdoid sutures. **B.** The roof of the neurocranium, or calvaria (skullcap), is formed primarily by the paired parietal bones, the frontal bone, and the occipital bone.

Premature closure of the coronal suture results in a high, tower-like cranium, called oxycephaly or turricephaly. Premature closure of sutures usually does not affect brain development. When premature closure occurs on one side only, the cranium is asymmetrical, a condition known as plagiocephaly.

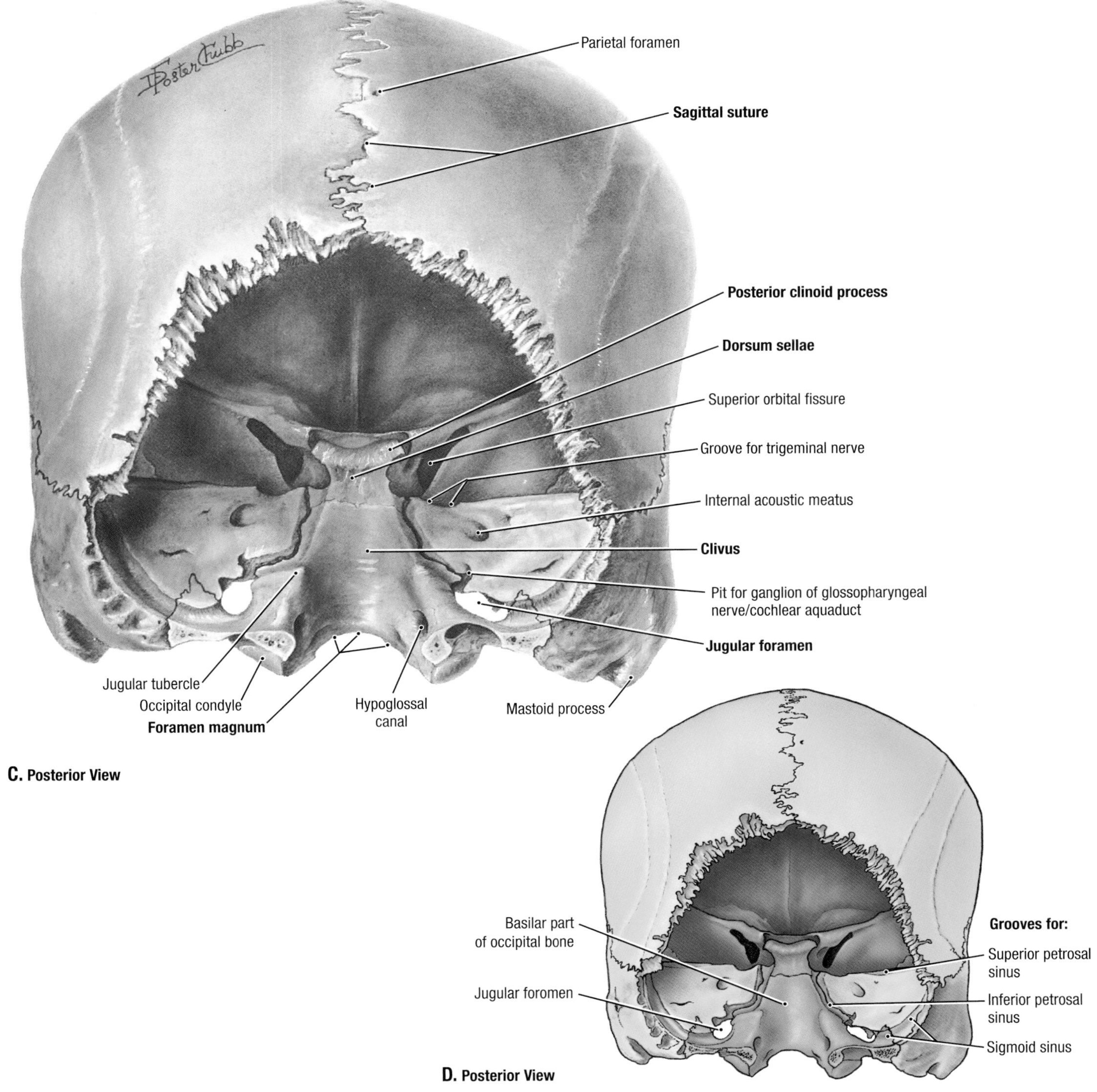
Parietal foramen
Sagittal suture
Posterior clinoid process
Dorsum sellae
Superior orbital fissure
Groove for trigeminal nerve
Internal acoustic meatus
Clivus
Pit for ganglion of glossopharyngeal nerve/cochlear aquaduct
Jugular foramen
Jugular tubercle
Occipital condyle
Foramen magnum
Hypoglossal canal
Mastoid process
Basilar part of occipital bone
Jugular foromen
Grooves for:
Superior petrosal sinus
Inferior petrosal sinus
Sigmoid sinus

**C.** Posterior View

**D.** Posterior View

## 7.4 Cranium, occipital aspect, calvaria, and anterior part of posterior cranial fossa *(continued)*

**C** and **D.** Cranium after removal of squamous part of occipital bone.

- The dorsum sellae projects from the body of the sphenoid; the posterior clinoid processes form its superolateral corners.
- The clivus is the slope descending from the dorsum sellae to the foramen magnum.
- The grooves for the sigmoid sinus and inferior petrosal sinus lead inferiorly to the jugular foramen.

Premature closure of the sagittal suture, in which the anterior fontanelle is small or absent, results in a long, narrow, wedge-shaped cranium, a condition called scaphocephaly.

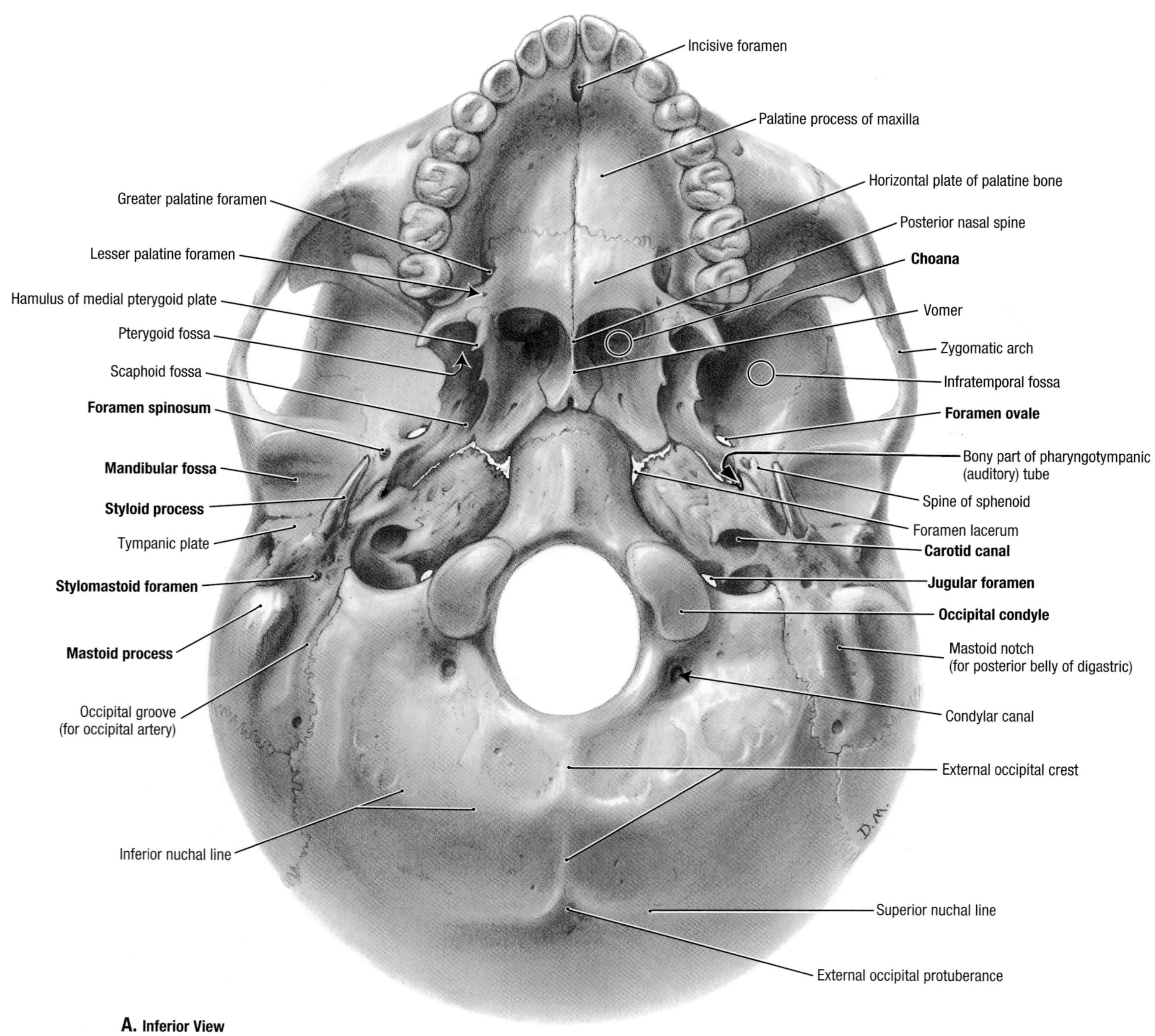
Incisive foramen
Palatine process of maxilla
Horizontal plate of palatine bone
Posterior nasal spine
Choana
Vomer
Zygomatic arch
Infratemporal fossa
Foramen ovale
Bony part of pharyngotympanic (auditory) tube
Spine of sphenoid
Foramen lacerum
Carotid canal
Jugular foramen
Occipital condyle
Mastoid notch (for posterior belly of digastric)
Condylar canal
External occipital crest
Superior nuchal line
External occipital protuberance
Greater palatine foramen
Lesser palatine foramen
Hamulus of medial pterygoid plate
Pterygoid fossa
Scaphoid fossa
Foramen spinosum
Mandibular fossa
Styloid process
Tympanic plate
Stylomastoid foramen
Mastoid process
Occipital groove (for occipital artery)
Inferior nuchal line
D.M.
A. Inferior View

## 7.5 Cranium, inferior aspect

**A.** Bony cranium. **B.** Diagram of cranium with bones color coded.

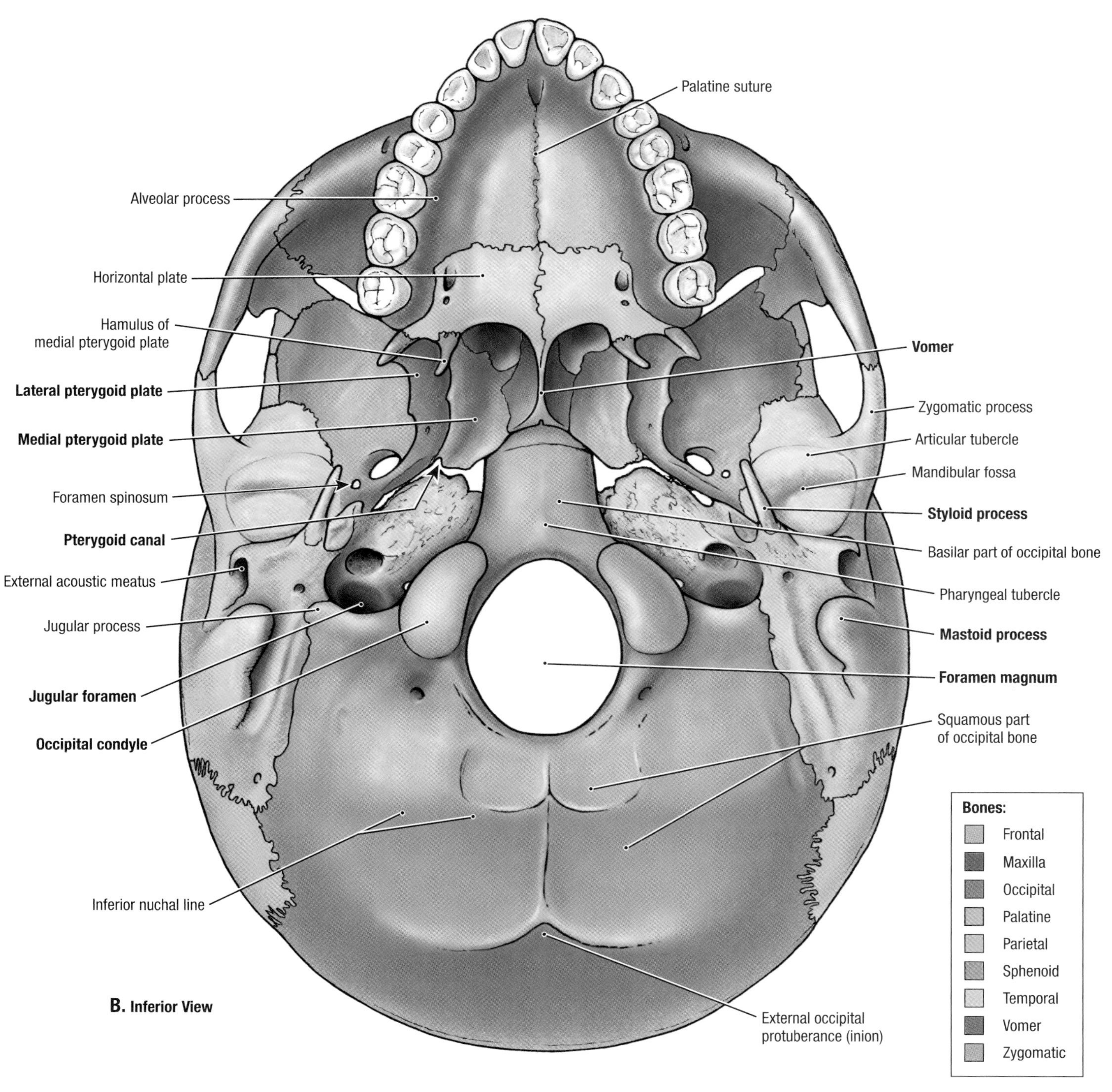
Palatine suture
Alveolar process
Horizontal plate
Hamulus of
medial pterygoid plate
Vomer
Lateral pterygoid plate
Zygomatic process
Medial pterygoid plate
Articular tubercle
Mandibular fossa
Foramen spinosum
Styloid process
Pterygoid canal
Basilar part of occipital bone
External acoustic meatus
Pharyngeal tubercle
Jugular process
Mastoid process
Foramen magnum
Jugular foramen
Squamous part
of occipital bone
Occipital condyle
Bones:
Frontal
Maxilla
Occipital
Palatine
Parietal
Sphenoid
Temporal
Vomer
Zygomatic
Inferior nuchal line
B. Inferior View
External occipital
protuberance (inion)

**7.5 Cranium, inferior aspect *(continued)***

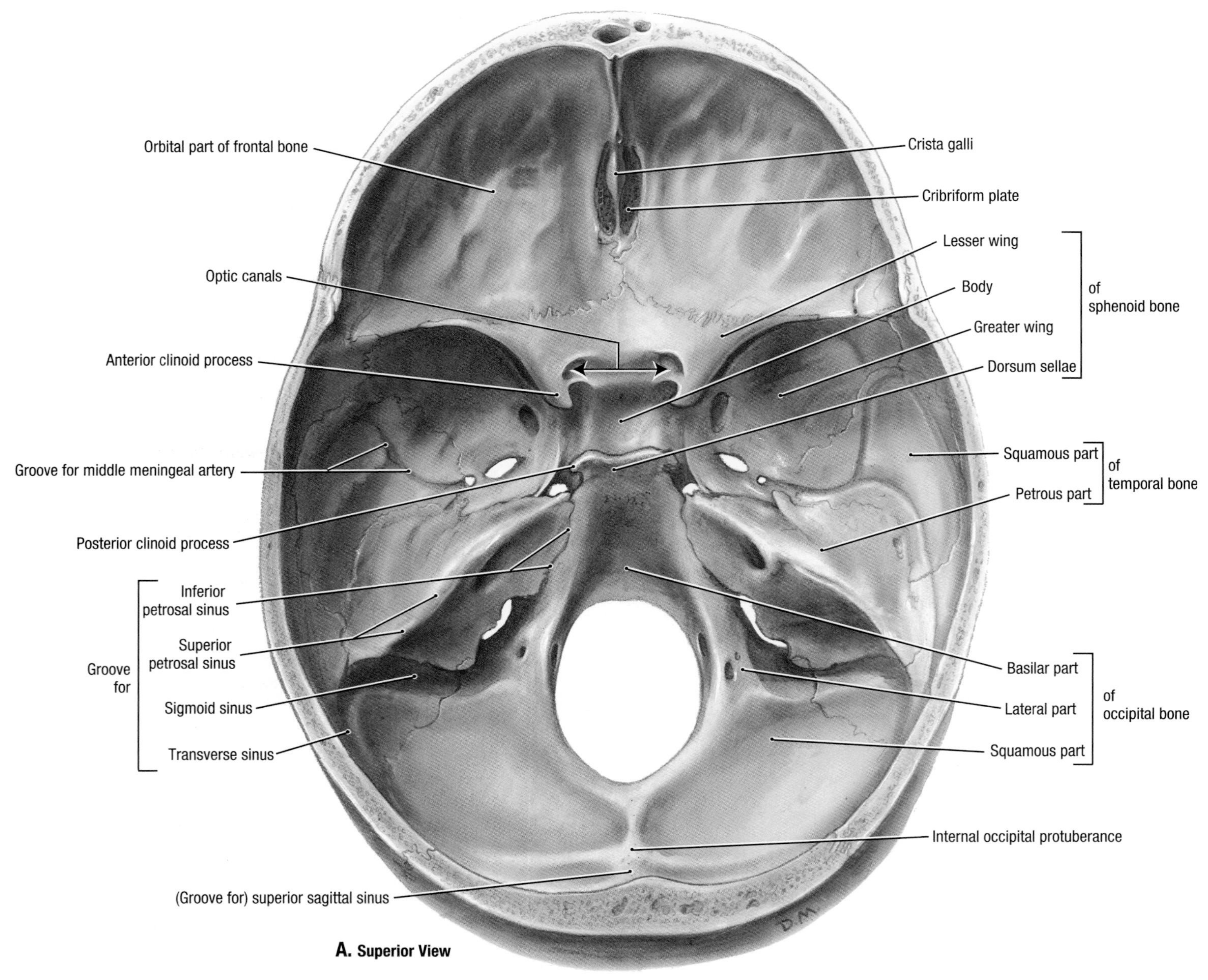
Orbital part of frontal bone
Crista galli
Cribriform plate
Lesser wing
Body
Greater wing
Dorsum sellae
of sphenoid bone
Optic canals
Anterior clinoid process
Groove for middle meningeal artery
Squamous part
Petrous part
of temporal bone
Posterior clinoid process
Inferior petrosal sinus
Superior petrosal sinus
Sigmoid sinus
Transverse sinus
Groove for
Basilar part
Lateral part
Squamous part
of occipital bone
Internal occipital protuberance
(Groove for) superior sagittal sinus
D.M.

**A.** Superior View

## 7.6 Interior of the cranial base

**A.** Bony cranial base. **B.** Diagrammatic cranial base with bones color coded.

In **A:**

- Three bones contribute to the anterior cranial fossa: the orbital part of the frontal bone, the cribriform plate of the ethmoid, and the lesser wing of the sphenoid.
- The four parts of the occipital bone are the basilar, right and left lateral, and squamous.
- Fractures in the floor of the anterior cranial fossa may involve the cribriform plate of the ethmoid, resulting in leakage of CSF through the nose (CSF rhinorrhea). CSF rhinorrhea may be a primary indication of a cranial base fracture which increases the risk of meningitis, because an infection could spread to the meninges from the ear or nose.

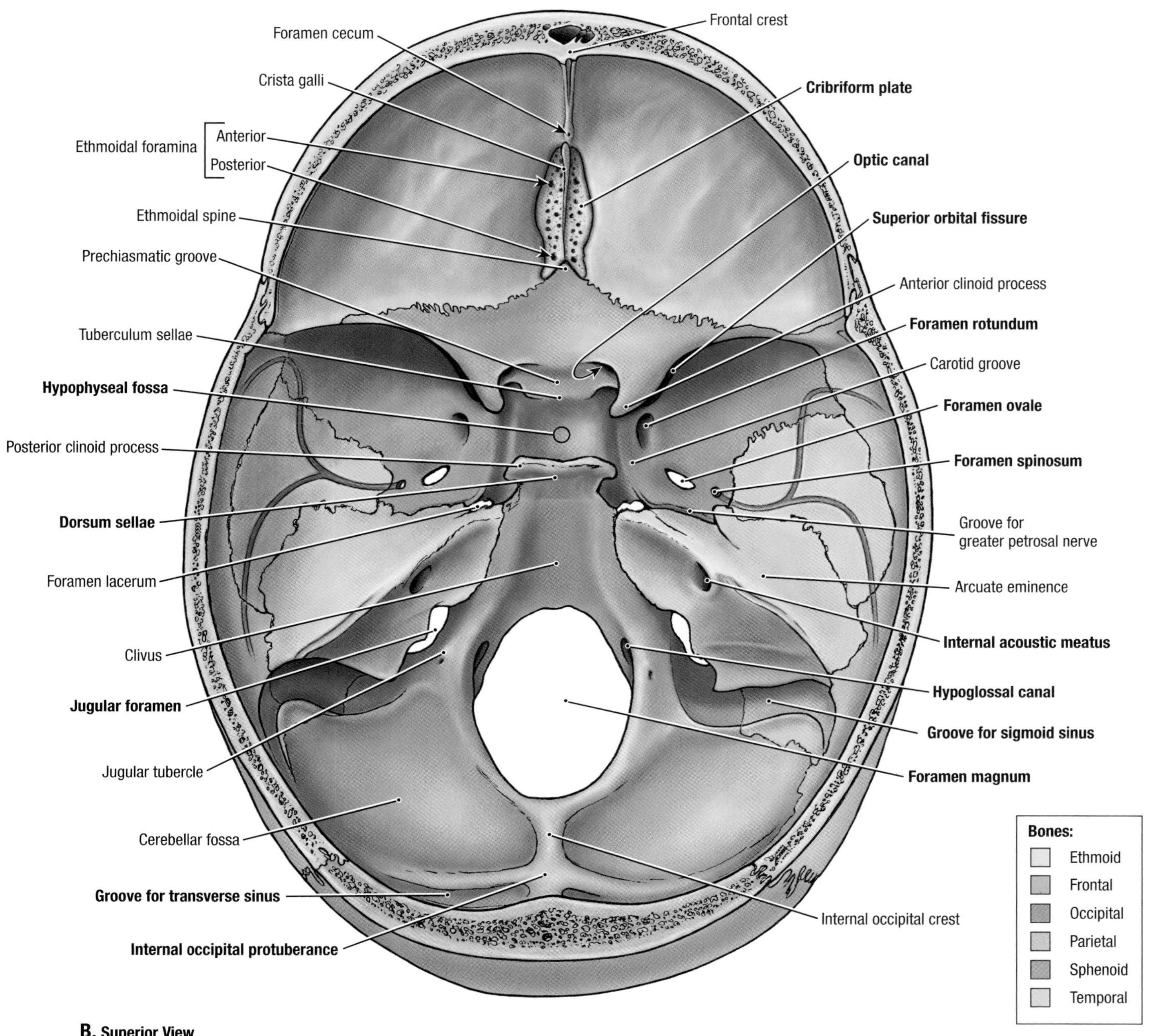
Foramen cecum
Frontal crest
Crista galli
Cribriform plate
Ethmoidal foramina
Anterior
Posterior
Optic canal
Ethmoidal spine
Superior orbital fissure
Prechiasmatic groove
Anterior clinoid process
Tuberculum sellae
Foramen rotundum
Carotid groove
Hypophyseal fossa
Foramen ovale
Posterior clinoid process
Foramen spinosum
Dorsum sellae
Groove for greater petrosal nerve
Foramen lacerum
Arcuate eminence
Internal acoustic meatus
Clivus
Hypoglossal canal
Jugular foramen
Groove for sigmoid sinus
Jugular tubercle
Foramen magnum
Bones:
Ethmoid
Frontal
Occipital
Parietal
Sphenoid
Temporal
Cerebellar fossa
Groove for transverse sinus
Internal occipital crest
Internal occipital protuberance

**B.** Superior View

## 7.6 Interior of the cranial base *(continued)*

In **B,** note the following midline features:

- In the anterior cranial fossa, the frontal crest and crista galli for anterior attachment of the falx cerebri have between them the foramen cecum, which, during development, transmits a vein connecting the superior sagittal sinus with the veins of the frontal sinus and root of the nose.
- In the middle cranial fossa, the tuberculum sellae, hypophyseal fossa, dorsum sellae, and posterior clinoid processes constitute the sella turcica (L. Turkish saddle).
- In the posterior cranial fossa, note the clivus, foramen magnum, internal occipital crest for attachment of the falx cerebelli, and the internal occipital protuberance, from which the grooves for the transverse sinuses course laterally.

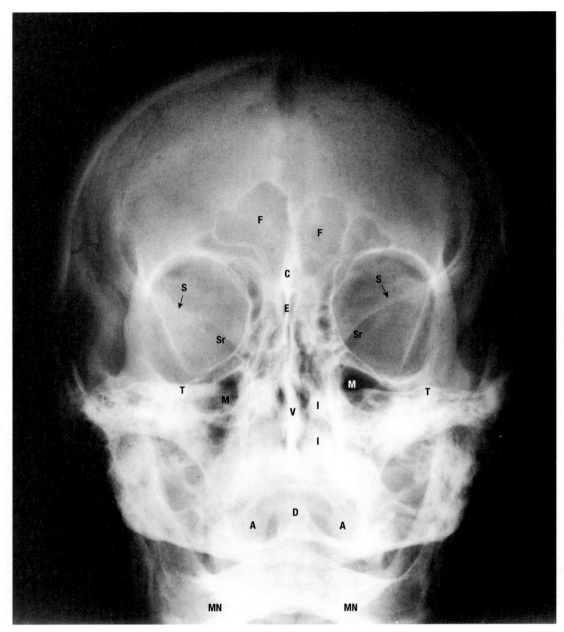

**A.** Anteroposterior View

## 7.7 Radiographs of the cranium

**A.** Posteroanterior (Caldwell) radiograph. This view places the orbits centrally in the head and is used to examine the orbits and paranasal sinuses. Observe in **A:**

- The labeled features include the superior orbital fissure *(Sr)*, lesser wing of the sphenoid *(S)*, superior surface of the petrous part of the temporal bone *(T)*, crista galli *(C)*, frontal sinus *(F)*, mandible *(MN)*, and maxillary sinus *(M)*.
- The nasal septum is formed by the perpendicular plate of the ethmoid *(E)* and the vomer *(V)*; note the inferior and middle conchae *(I)* of the lateral wall of the nose.
- Superimposed on the facial skeleton are the dens *(D)* and lateral masses of the atlas *(A)*.

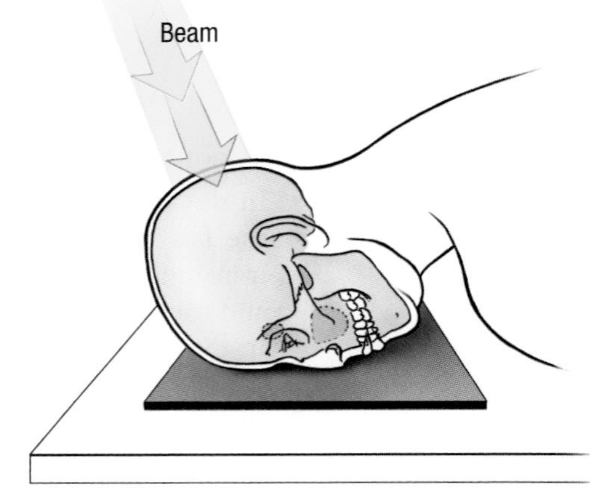
Beam

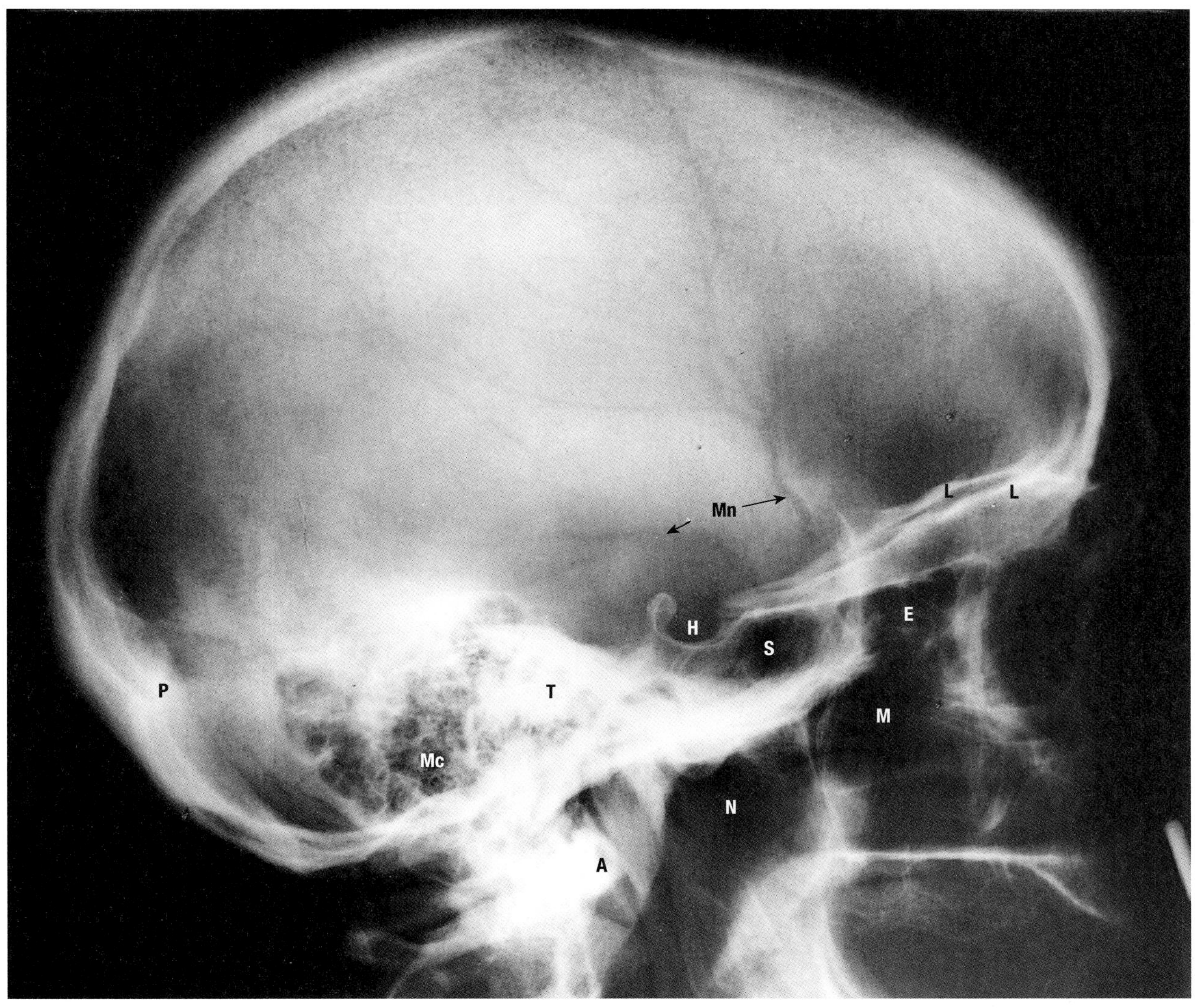
Mn
L
L
H
E
S
P
T
M
Mc
N
A

**B. Lateral View**

## 7.7 Radiographs of the cranium *(continued)*

**B.** Lateral radiograph of the cranium. Most of the relatively thin bone of the facial skeleton (viscerocranium) is radiolucent (appears black).

- The labeled features include the ethmoidal cells (*E* ), sphenoidal (*S* ) and maxillary (*M* ) sinuses, the hypophyseal fossa (*H* ) for the pituitary gland, the petrous part of the temporal bone (*T* ), mastoid cells (*Mc* ), grooves for the branches of the middle meningeal vessels (*Mn*), arch of the atlas (*A*), internal occipital protuberance (*P* ), and the nasopharynx (*N* ).
- The right and left orbital plates of the frontal bone are not superimposed; thus, the floor of the anterior cranial fossa appears as two lines (*L*).

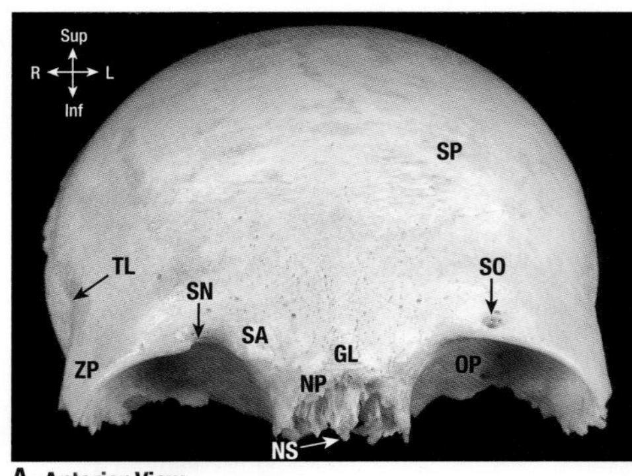
Sup
R
L
Inf
SP
TL
SN
SO
SA
GL
ZP
NP
OP
NS

**A. Anterior View**

Ant
R
L
Post
NP
SU
RE
FS
ZP
FL
OP
TS
EN
SM

**B. Inferior View**

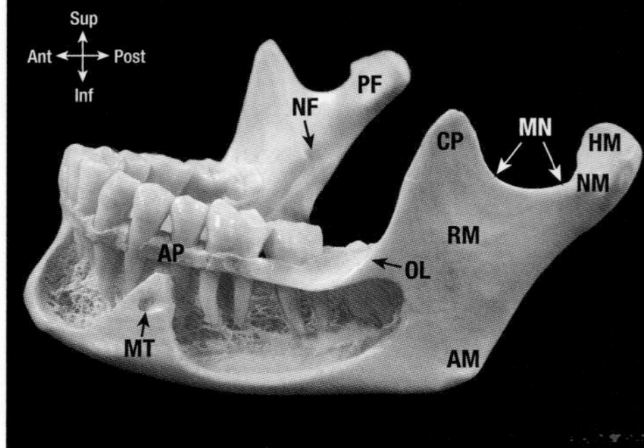
Sup
Ant
Post
Inf
PF
NF
MN
CP
HM
NM
RM
AP
OL
MT
AM

**C. Lateral View**

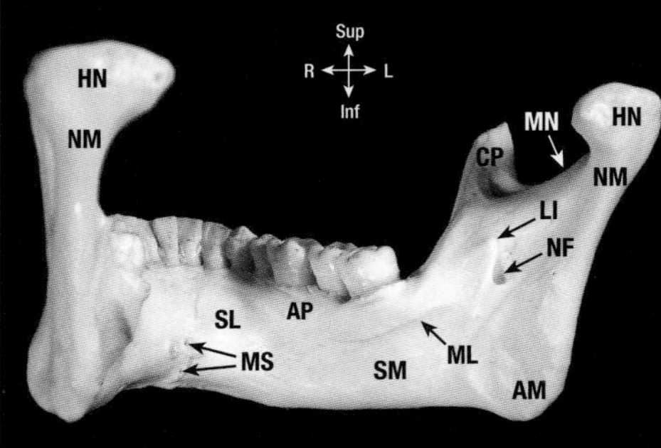
HN
Sup
R
L
Inf
NM
MN
HN
CP
NM
LI
NF
AP
SL
MS
ML
SM
AM

**D. Posteromedial View**

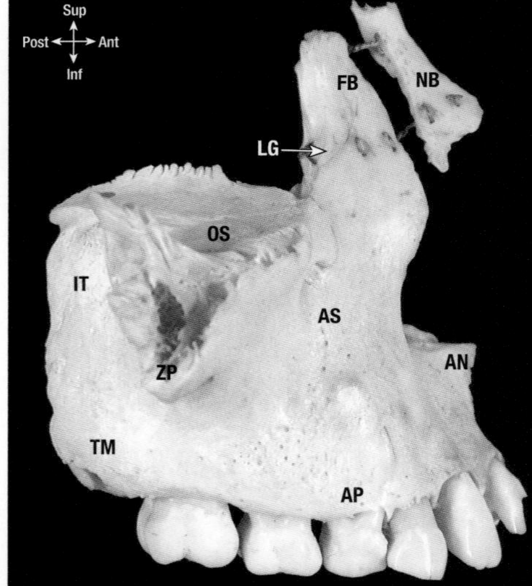
Sup
Post
Ant
Inf
NB
FB
LG
OS
IT
AS
AN
ZP
TM
AP

**E. Lateral View**

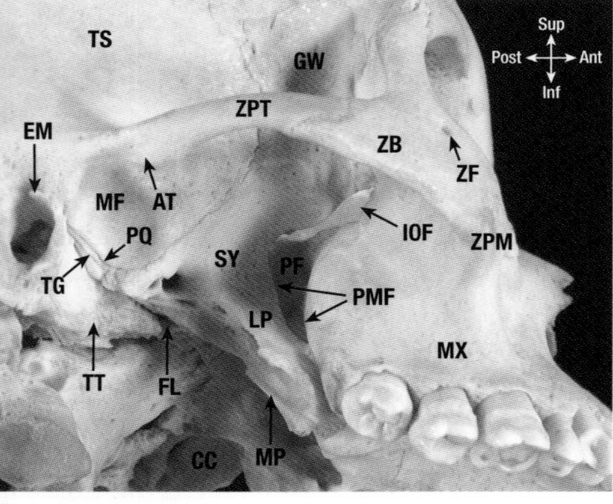
TS
GW
Sup
Post
Ant
Inf
ZPT
EM
ZB
ZF
MF
AT
IOF
PQ
SY
PF
ZPM
TG
PMF
LP
MX
TT
FL
CC
MP

**F. Inferolateral View**

**Maxilla and nasal bone**

| | |
|---|---|
| AN | Anterior nasal spine |
| AP | Alveolar part |
| AS | Anterior surface of maxilla |
| FP | Frontal process of maxilla |
| IT | Infratemporal surface of maxilla |
| LG | Lacrimal groove |
| NB | Nasal bone |
| OS | Orbital surface |
| TM | Tuberosity |
| ZP | Zygomatic process |

**Key**

**Frontal Bone**

| | |
|---|---|
| EN | Ethmoidal notch |
| FL | Fossa for lacrimal gland |
| FS | Opening of frontal sinus |
| GL | Glabella |
| NP | Nasal part |
| NS | Nasal spine |
| OP | Orbital part |
| RE | Root of ethmoid cells |
| SA | Superciliary arch |
| SM | Sphenoidal margin |
| SN | Supra-orbital notch |
| SO | Supra-orbital foramen |
| SP | Squamous part |
| SU | Supra-orbital margin |
| TL | Temporal line |
| TS | Temporal surface |
| ZP | Zygomatic process |

**Mandible**

| | |
|---|---|
| AM | Angle of mandible |
| AP | Alveolar part |
| CP | Coronoid process |
| HM | Head of mandible |
| LI | Lingula |
| ML | Mylohyoid groove |
| MN | Mandibular notch |
| MS | Superior and inferior mental spines |
| MT | Mental foramen |
| NF | Mandibular foramen |
| NM | Neck of mandible |
| PF | Pterygoid fovea |
| RM | Ramus of mandible |
| SL | Sublingual fossa |
| SM | Submandibular fossa |

**Pterygopalatine fossa**

| | |
|---|---|
| PF | Pterygopalatine fossa |
| MF | Mandibular fossa |
| AT | Articular tubercle |
| ZPT | Zygomatic process of temporal bone |
| CC | Carotid canal |
| FL | Foramen lacerum |
| ZF | Zygomaticofacial foramen |
| PQ | Petrosquamous fissure |
| TG | Tegmen tympani |
| TT | Temporal bone (tympanic part) |
| ZB | Zygomatic bone |
| MX | Maxilla |
| IOF | Inferior orbital fissure |
| PMF | Pterygomaxillary fissure |
| ZPM | Zygomatic process of maxilla |
| EM | External acoustic meatus |
| GW | Greater wing of sphenoid |
| LP | Lateral pterygoid plate |
| MP | Medial pterygoid plate |
| SY | Stylomastoid foramen |

## 7.8 Superficial bones of facial skeleton

**A** and **B.** Frontal bone. **C** and **D.** Mandible. **E.** Maxilla. **F.** Infratemporal fossa.

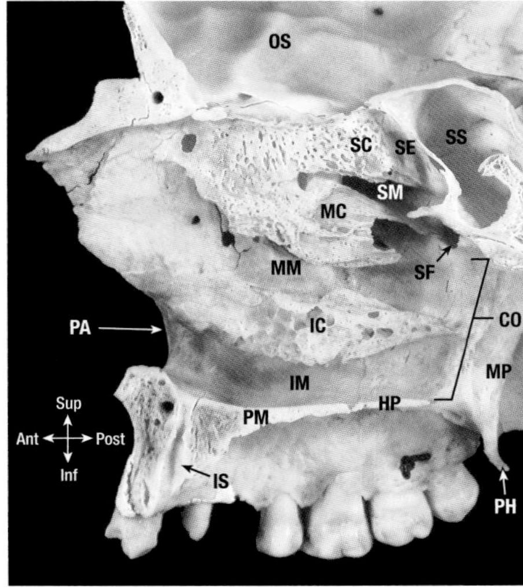
OS
SC
SE
SS
SM
MC
MM
SF
PA
IC
CO
MP
IM
HP
PM
Sup
Ant
Post
Inf
IS
PH

**A. Medial View**

**C. Anterior View**

**B. Anterior View**

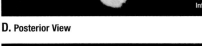

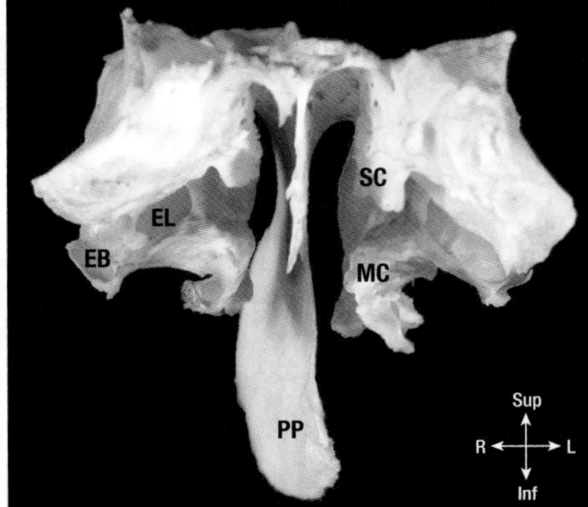
SC
EL
EB
MC
PP
Sup
R
L
Inf

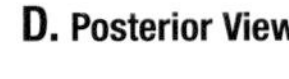

**D. Posterior View**

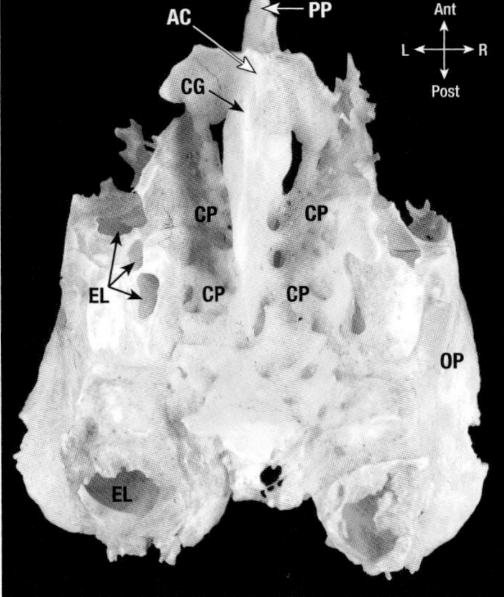
AC
PP
Ant
L
R
Post
CG
CP
CP
EL
CP
CP
OP
EL

**E. Superior View**

**Key**

**Lateral Wall of Nose**

| | |
|---|---|
| CO | Choana (posterior nasal aperture) |
| HP | Horizontal plate of palatine bone |
| IC | Inferior nasal concha |
| IS | Incisive canal |
| IM | Inferior nasal meatus |
| MC | Middle nasal concha |
| MM | Middle nasal meatus |
| PH | Pterygoid hamulus |
| PM | Palatine process of maxilla |
| OS | Orbital surface of frontal bone |
| PA | Piriform aperture |
| PM | Palatine process of maxilla |
| SC | Superior nasal concha |
| SE | Spheno-ethmoidal recess |
| SF | Sphenopalatine foramen |
| SM | Superior nasal meatus |
| SS | Sphenoidal sinus |

**Palatine Bone**

| | |
|---|---|
| HP | Horizontal plate |
| NC | Nasal crest |
| OP | Orbital process |
| PP | Perpendicular plate |
| PY | Pyramidal process |

**Ethmoid Bone**

| | |
|---|---|
| AC | Ala of crista galli |
| CG | Crista galli |
| CP | Cribriform plate |
| EB | Ethmoidal bulla |
| EL | Ethmoidal labyrinth (ethmoidal cells) |
| MC | Middle nasal concha |
| OP | Orbital plate |
| PP | Perpendicular plate |
| SC | Superior nasal concha |

**7.9 Deep bones of facial skeleton**

**A.** Lateral wall of nose. **B.** Palatine bone. **C–E.** Ethmoid bone.

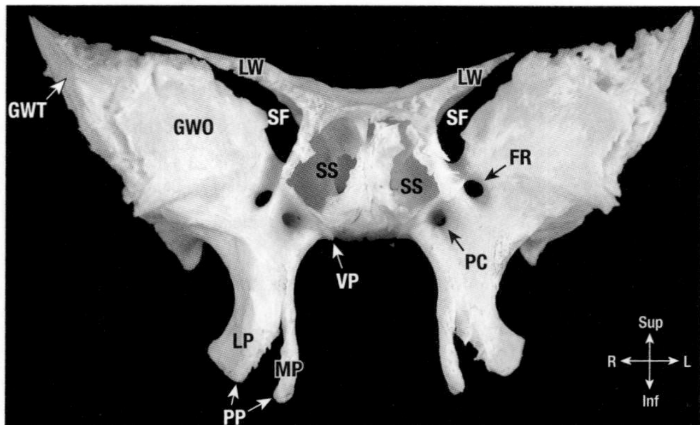

LW
LW
GWT
GWO
SF
SF
SS
SS
FR
VP
PC
LP
MP
PP
Sup
R
L
Inf


**A.** Anterior View

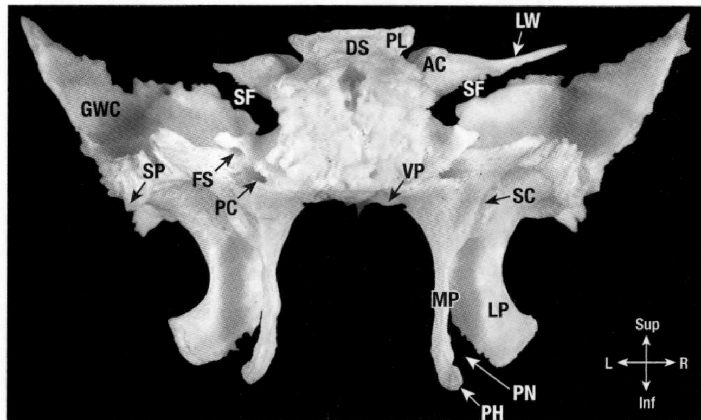

LW
DS
PL
AC
SF
SF
GWC
SP
FS
PC
VP
SC
MP
LP
PN
PH
Sup
L
R
Inf


**B.** Posterior View

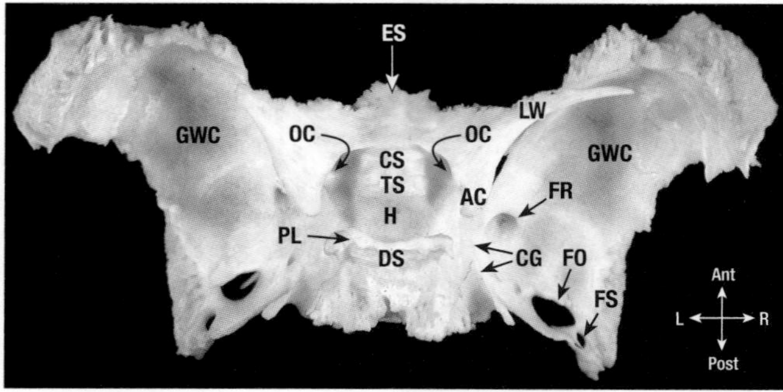

ES
LW
GWC
OC
OC
GWC
CS
TS
H
AC
FR
PL
DS
CG
FO
FS
Ant
L
R
Post


**C.** Superior View

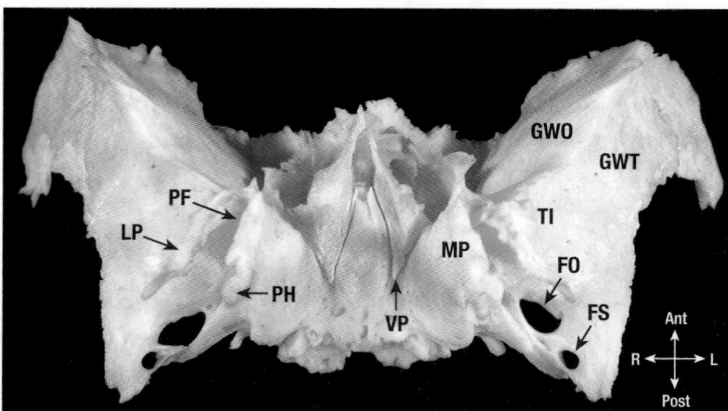

GWO
GWT
PF
TI
LP
MP
FO
PH
VP
FS
Ant
R
L
Post


**D.** Inferior View

**Key**

| | |
|---|---|
| AC | Anterior clinoid process |
| CG | Carotid sulcus |
| CS | Prechiasmatic sulcus |
| DS | Dorsum sellae |
| ES | Ethmoidal spine |
| FO | Foramen ovale |
| FR | Foramen rotundum |
| FS | Foramen spinosum |
| GWC | Greater wing (cerebral surface) |
| GWO | Greater wing (orbital surface) |
| GWT | Greater wing (temporal surface) |
| H | Hypophysial fossa |
| LP | Lateral pterygoid plate |
| LW | Lesser wing |
| MP | Medial pterygoid plate |
| OC | Optic canal |
| PC | Pterygoid canal |
| PF | Pterygoid fossa |
| PH | Pterygoid hamulus |
| PL | Posterior clinoid process |
| PN | Pterygoid notch |
| PP | Pterygoid process |
| SC | Scaphoid fossa |
| SF | Superior orbital fissure |
| SP | Spine of sphenoid bone |
| SS | Sphenoidal sinus (in body of sphenoid) |
| TI | Greater wing of sphenoid (Infratemporal surface) |
| TS | Tuberculum sellae |
| VP | Vaginal process |

**7.10 Sphenoid bone**

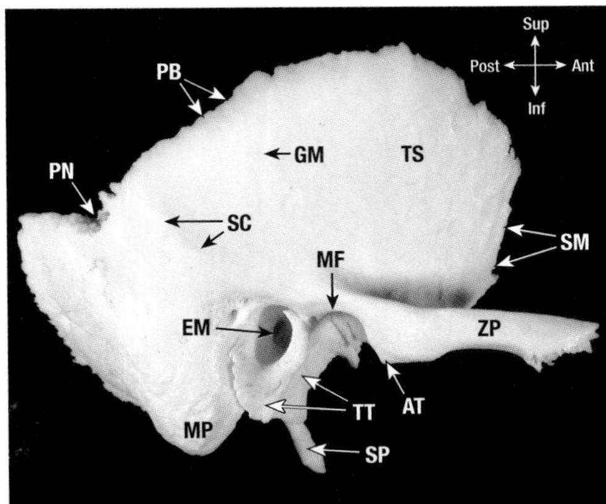
Sup
Post
Ant
Inf
PB
PN
GM
TS
SC
SM
MF
EM
ZP
TT
AT
MP
SP

A. Lateral View

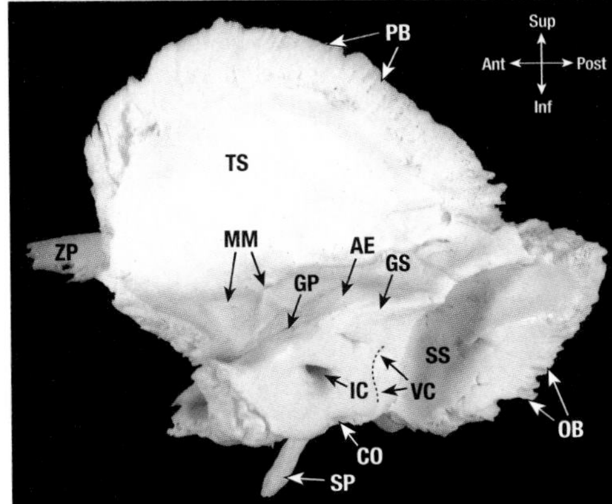
Sup
Ant
Post
Inf
PB
TS
ZP
MM
AE
GS
GP
SS
IC
VC
OB
CO
SP

B. Medial View

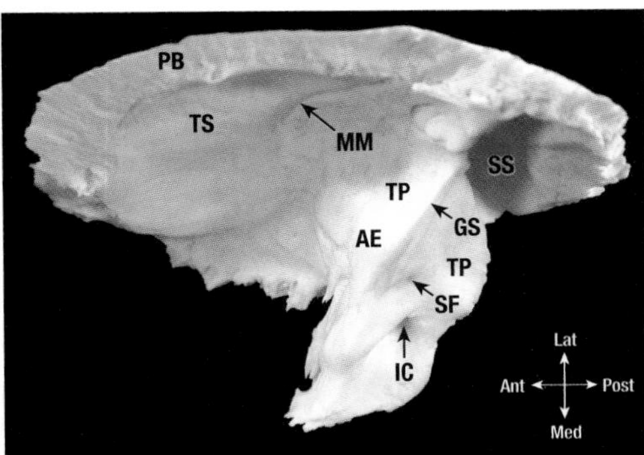
PB
TS
MM
SS
TP
GS
AE
TP
SF
IC
Lat
Ant
Post
Med

C. Superior View

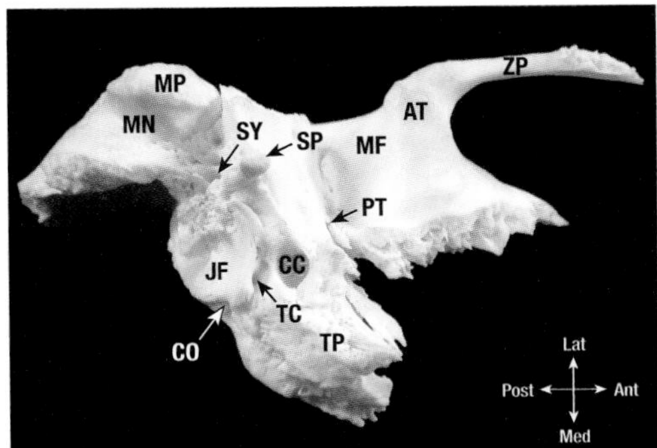
MP
MN
SY
SP
MF
AT
ZP
PT
JF
CC
TC
CO
TP
Lat
Post
Ant
Med

D. Inferior View

**Key**

| | |
|---|---|
| AE | Arcuate eminence |
| AT | Articular tubercle |
| CC | Carotid canal |
| CO | Cochlear canaliculus |
| EM | External acoustic meatus |
| GM | Groove for middle temporal artery |
| GP | Hiatus for greater petrosal nerve |
| GS | Groove for superior petrosal sinus |
| IC | Internal acoustic meatus |
| JF | Jugular fossa |
| MF | Mandibular fossa |
| MM | Groove for middle meningeal artery |
| MN | Mastoid notch |
| MP | Mastoid process |
| OB | Occipital border |
| PB | Parietal border |
| PN | Parietal notch |
| PT | Petrotympanic fissure |
| SC | Supramastoid crest |
| SF | Subarcuate fossa |
| SM | Sphenoid margin |
| SP | Styloid process |
| SS | Groove for sigmoid sinus |
| SY | Stylomastoid foramen |
| TC | Tympanic canaliculus |
| TP | Temporal bone (petrous part) |
| TS | Temporal bone (squamous part) |
| TT | Temporal bone (tympanic part) |
| VC | Vestibular canaliculus |
| ZP | Zygomatic process |

**7.11 Temporal bone**

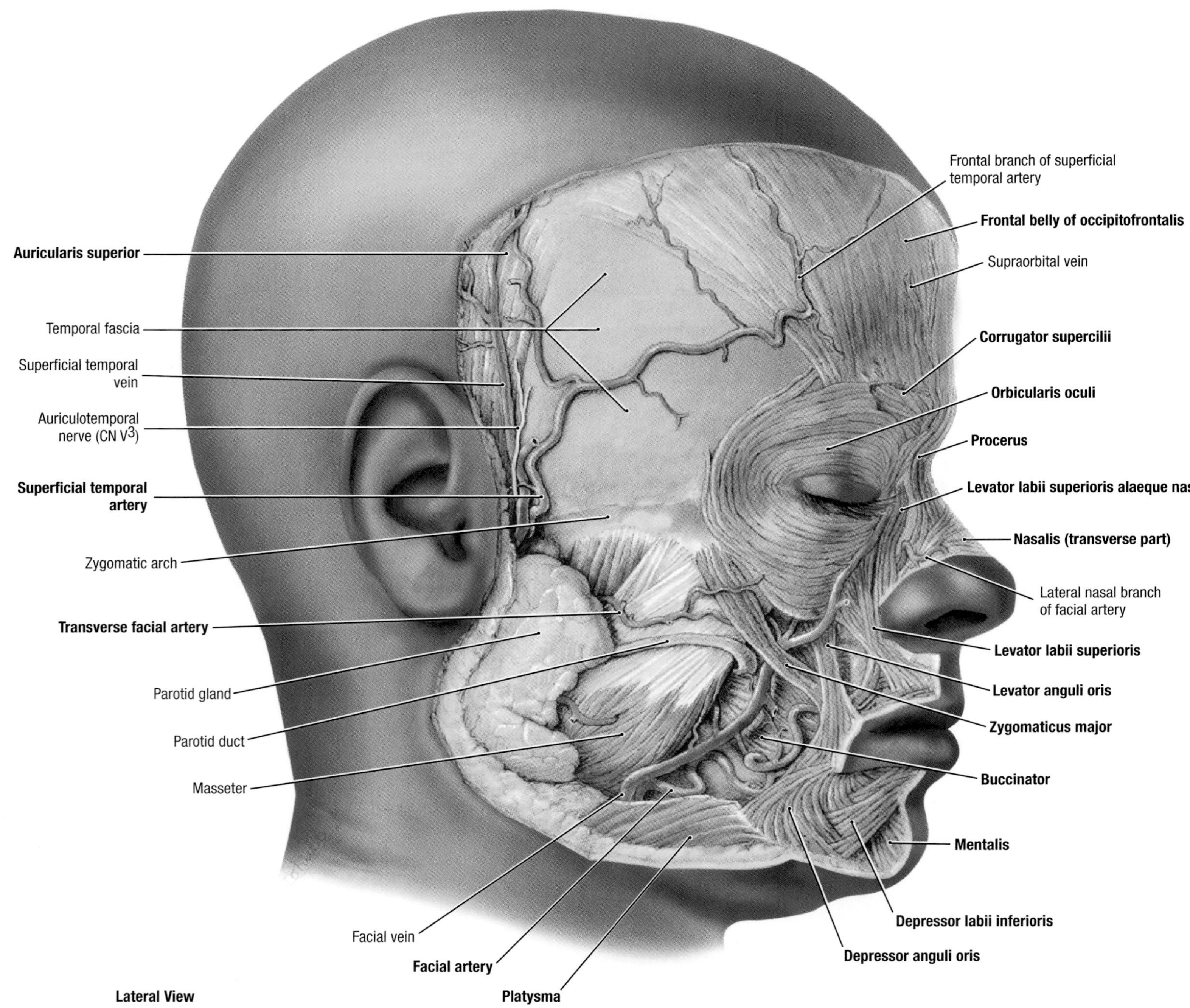
Frontal branch of superficial temporal artery
Frontal belly of occipitofrontalis
Auricularis superior
Supraorbital vein
Temporal fascia
Corrugator supercilii
Superficial temporal vein
Orbicularis oculi
Auriculotemporal nerve (CN V3)
Procerus
Superficial temporal artery
Levator labii superioris alaeque nasi
Nasalis (transverse part)
Zygomatic arch
Lateral nasal branch of facial artery
Transverse facial artery
Levator labii superioris
Levator anguli oris
Parotid gland
Zygomaticus major
Parotid duct
Buccinator
Masseter
Mentalis
Depressor labii inferioris
Facial vein
Depressor anguli oris
Facial artery
Lateral View
Platysma

## 7.12 Muscles of facial expression and arteries of the face

- The muscles of facial expression are the superficial sphincters and dilators of the openings of the head; all are supplied by the facial nerve (CN VII). The masseter and temporalis (the latter covered here by temporal fascia) are muscles of mastication that are innervated by the trigeminal nerve (CN V).
- The pulses of the superficial temporal and facial arteries can be used for taking the pulse. For example, anesthesiologists at the head of the operating table often take the temporal pulse anterior to the auricle as the artery crosses the zygomatic arch to supply the scalp. The facial pulse can be palpated where the facial artery crosses the inferior border of the mandible immediately anterior to the masseter.

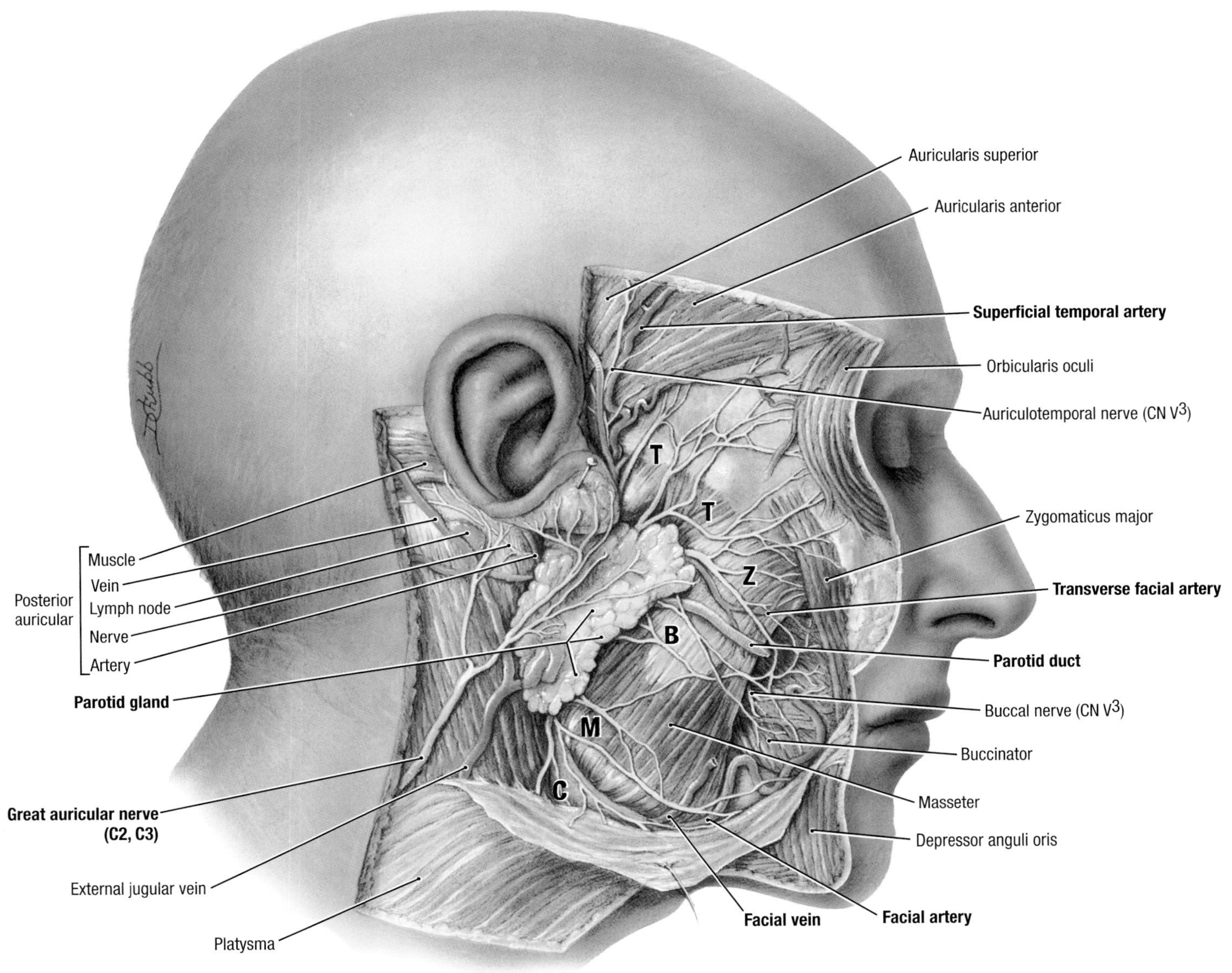
Auricularis superior
Auricularis anterior
Superficial temporal artery
Orbicularis oculi
Auriculotemporal nerve (CN V3)
T
T
Zygomaticus major
Z
Transverse facial artery
B
Parotid duct
Buccal nerve (CN V3)
M
Buccinator
C
Masseter
Depressor anguli oris
Facial vein
Facial artery
Posterior auricular
Muscle
Vein
Lymph node
Nerve
Artery
Parotid gland
Great auricular nerve (C2, C3)
External jugular vein
Platysma
Lateral View

## 7.13 Relationships of the branches of the facial nerve and vessels to the parotid gland and duct

- The parotid duct extends across the masseter muscle just inferior to the zygomatic arch; the duct turns medially to pierce the buccinator.
- The facial nerve (CN VII) innervates the muscles of facial expression; it forms a plexus within the parotid gland, the branches of which radiate over the face, anastomosing with each other and the branches of the trigeminal nerve. After emerging from the stylomastoid foramen, the main stem of the facial nerve has posterior auricular, digastric, and stylohyoid branches; the parotid plexus gives rise to temporal (T), zygomatic (Z), buccal (B), marginal mandibular (M), cervical (C), and posterior auricular branches.
- During parotidectomy (surgical excision of the parotid gland), identification, dissection, and preservation of the branches of the facial nerve are critical.
- The parotid gland may become infected by infectious agents that pass through the bloodstream, as occurs in mumps, an acute communicable viral disease. Infection of the gland causes inflammation (parotiditis) and swelling of the gland. Severe pain occurs because the parotid sheath, innervated by the great auricular nerve, limits swelling.

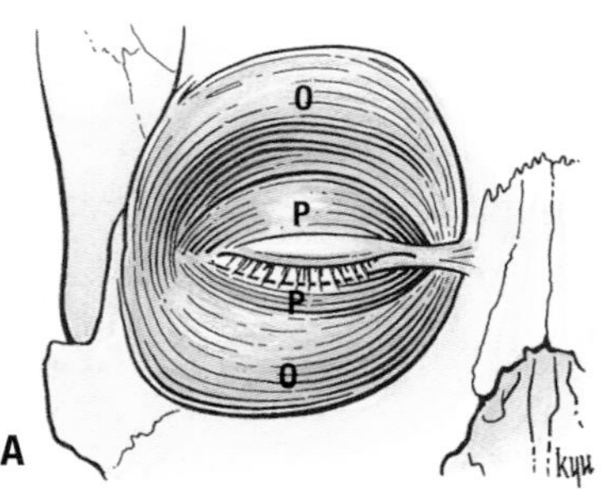
O
P
P
O

A

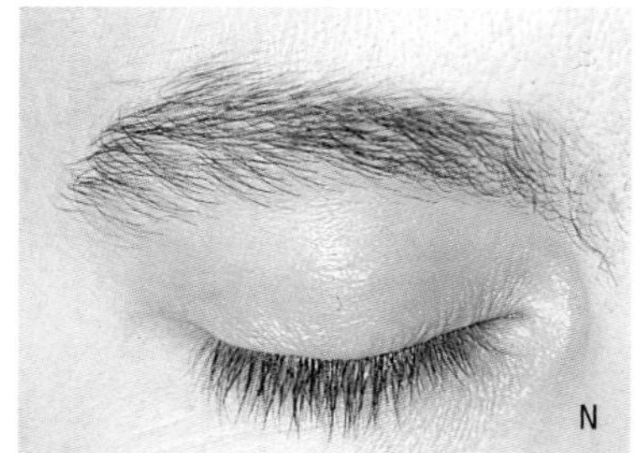
N

B

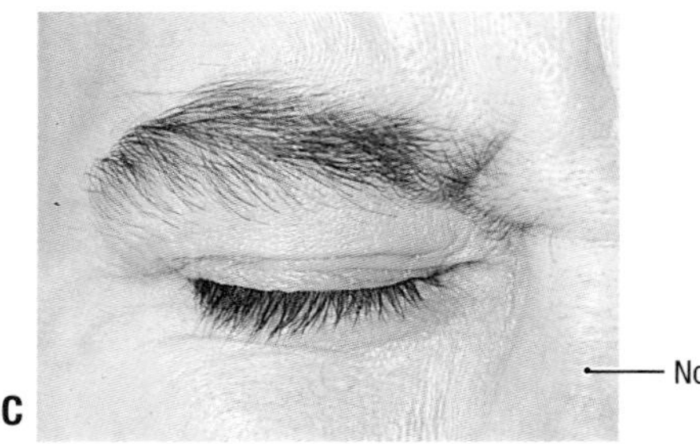
Nose (N)

C

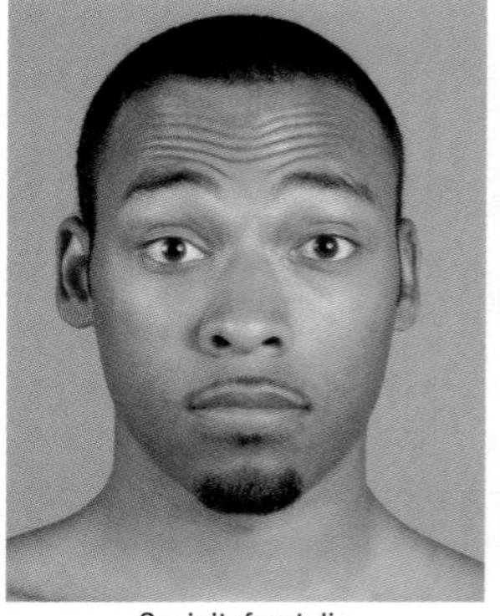

Occipitofrontalis

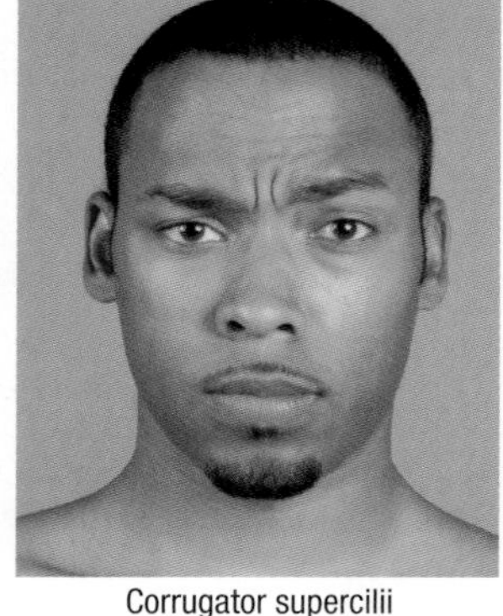

Corrugator supercilii

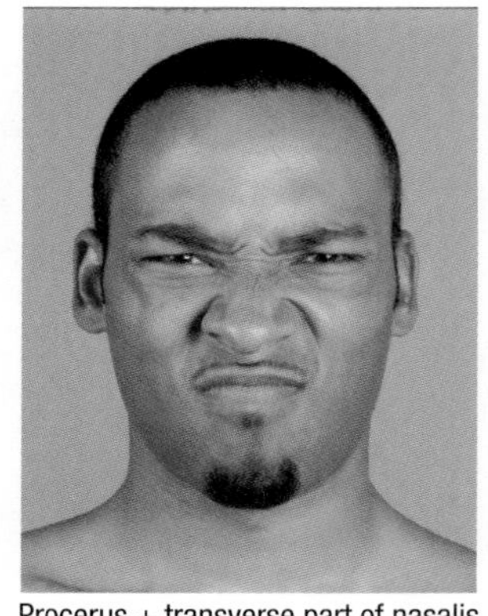

Procerus + transverse part of nasalis

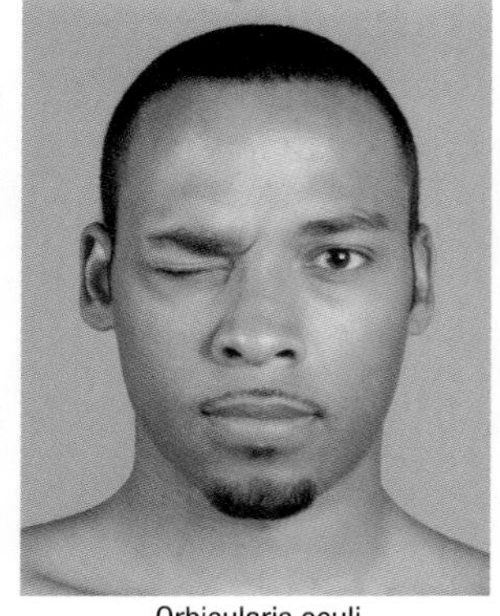

Orbicularis oculi

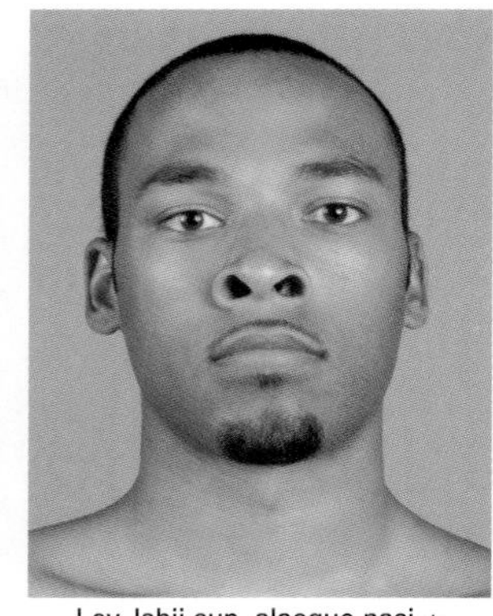

Lev. labii sup. alaeque nasi + alar part of nasalis

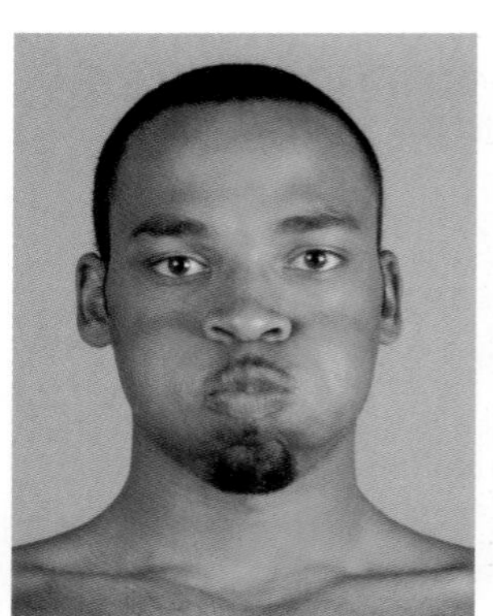

Buccinator + orbicularis oris

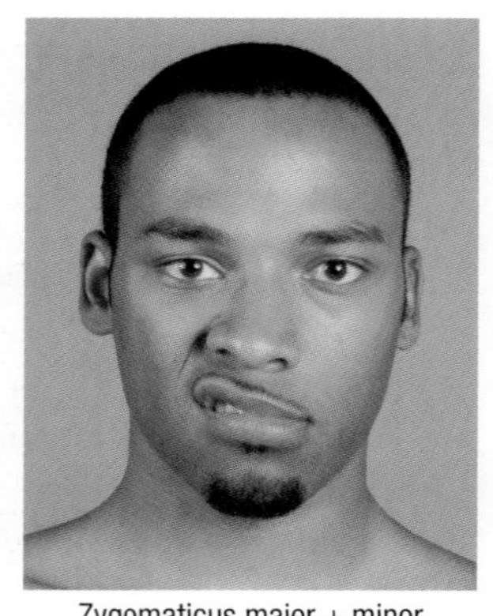

Zygomaticus major + minor

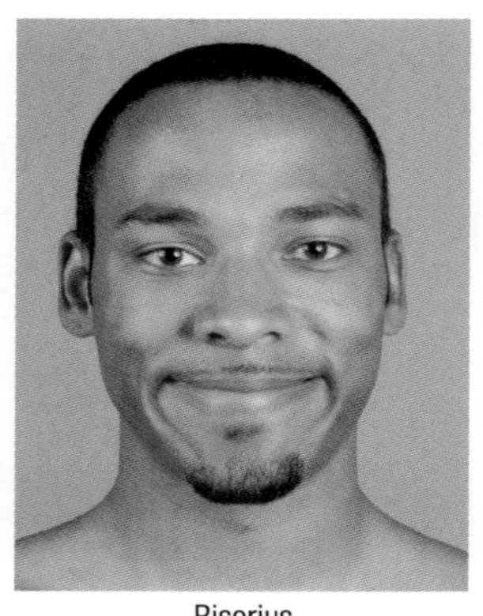

Risorius

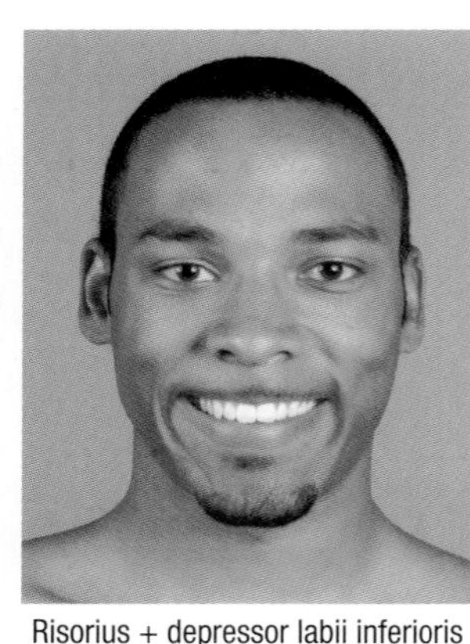

Risorius + depressor labii inferioris

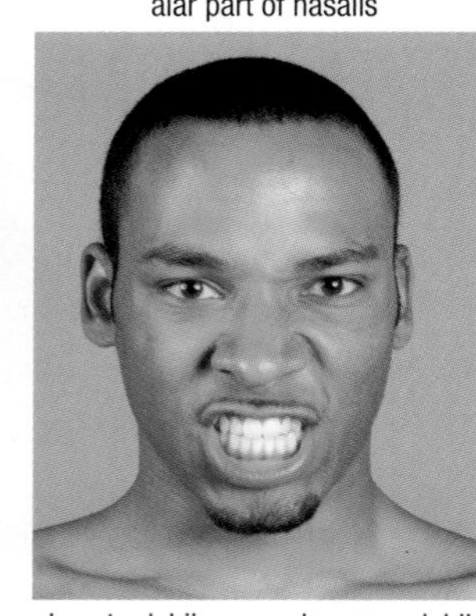

Levator labii sup. + depressor labii

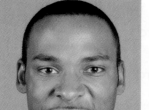

Dilators of mouth: Risorius plus levator labii superioris + depressor labii inferioris

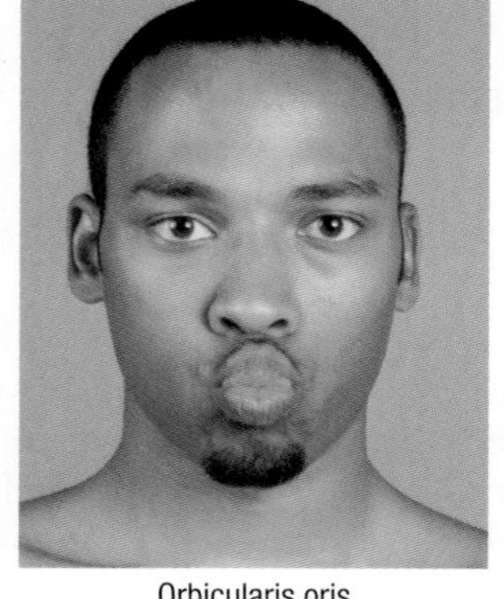

Orbicularis oris

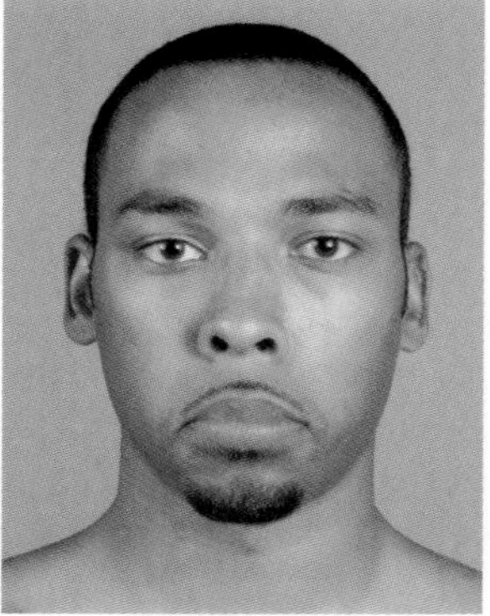

Depressor anguli oris

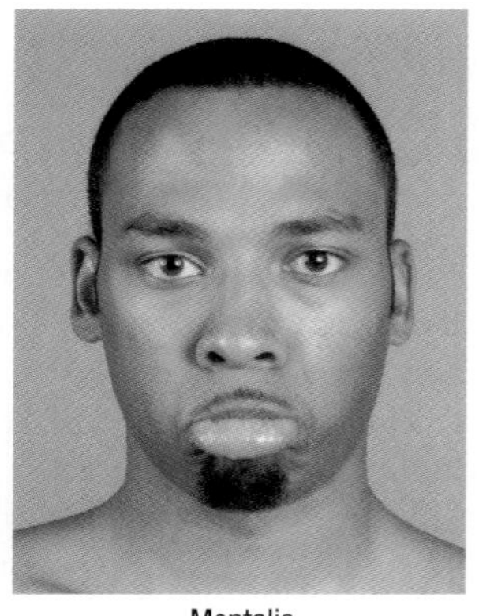

Mentalis

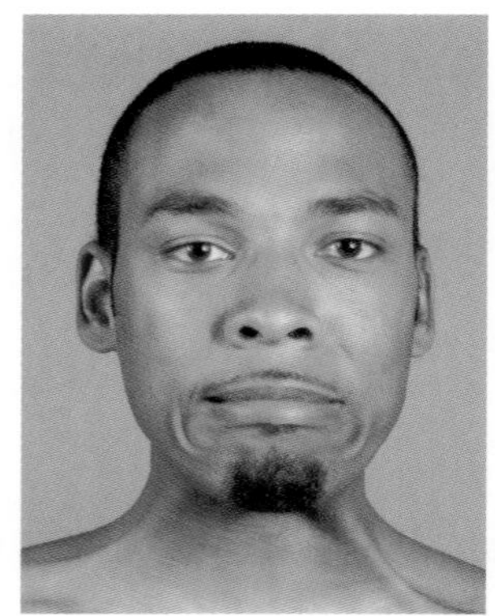

Platysma

D

**Anterior Views**

## 7.14 Muscles of facial expression

**A.** Orbicularis oculi: palpebral (P) and orbital (O) parts. The lacrimal portion (not shown) passes posterior to the lacrimal sac and helps spread of lacrimal secretions. **B.** Gentle closure of eyelid—palpebral part. **C.** Tight closure of eyelid—orbital part. **D.** Actions of selected muscles of facial expression.

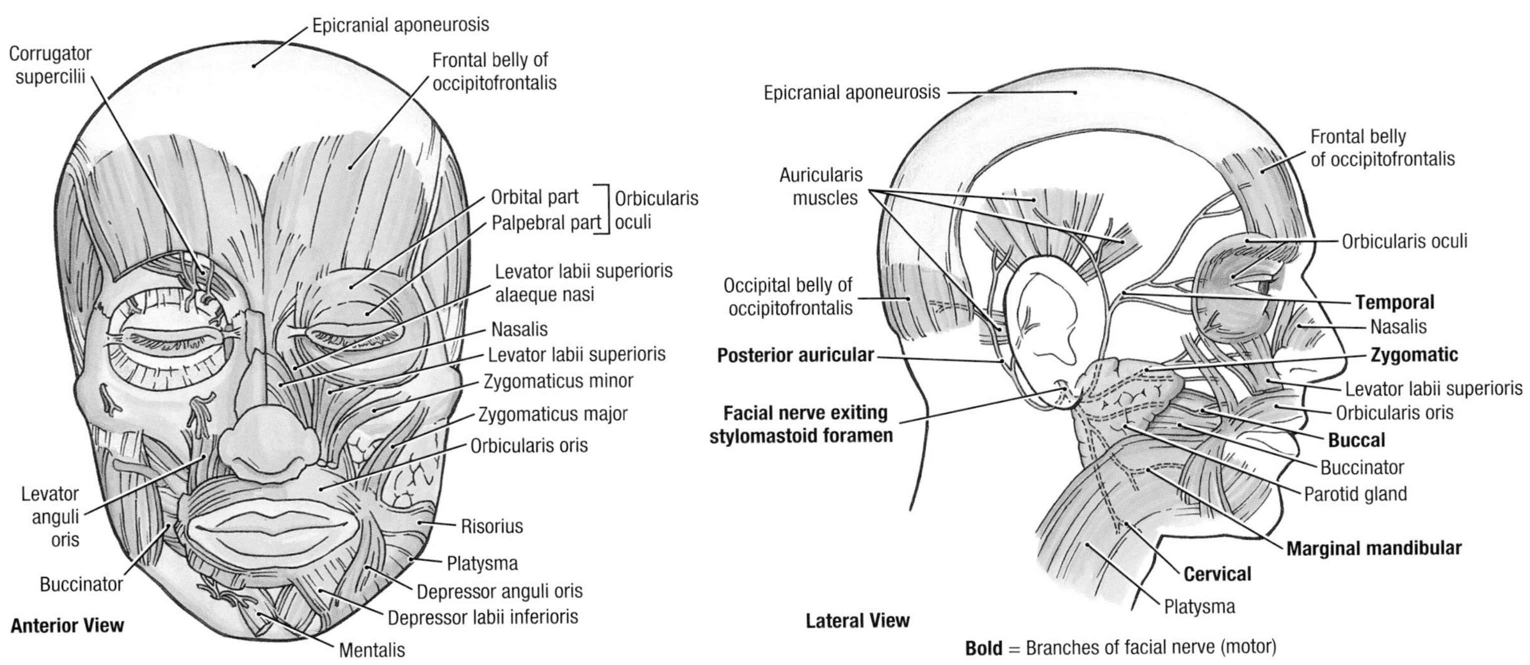
Epicranial aponeurosis
Corrugator supercilii
Frontal belly of occipitofrontalis
Orbital part
Palpebral part
Orbicularis oculi
Levator labii superioris alaeque nasi
Nasalis
Levator labii superioris
Zygomaticus minor
Zygomaticus major
Orbicularis oris
Levator anguli oris
Risorius
Platysma
Buccinator
Depressor anguli oris
Depressor labii inferioris
Mentalis
Anterior View
Epicranial aponeurosis
Frontal belly of occipitofrontalis
Auricularis muscles
Orbicularis oculi
Occipital belly of occipitofrontalis
Temporal
Nasalis
Zygomatic
Posterior auricular
Levator labii superioris
Orbicularis oris
Facial nerve exiting stylomastoid foramen
Buccal
Buccinator
Parotid gland
Marginal mandibular
Cervical
Platysma
Lateral View
Bold = Branches of facial nerve (motor)

**TABLE 7.1 MAIN MUSCLES OF FACIAL EXPRESSION[a]**

| Muscle | Origin | Insertion | Action |
|---|---|---|---|
| **Frontal belly of occipitofrontalis** | Epicranial aponeurosis | Skin of forehead | Elevates eyebrows and forehead |
| **Orbicularis oculi** | Medial orbital margin, medial palpebral ligament, and lacrimal bone | Skin around margin of orbit; tarsal plate | Closes eyelids |
| **Nasalis** | Superior part of canine ridge of maxilla | Nasal cartilages | Flares nostrils |
| **Orbicularis oris** | Some fibers arise near median plane of maxilla superiorly and mandible inferiorly; other fibers arise from deep surface of skin | Mucous membrane of lips | Compresses and protrudes lips (e.g., purses them during whistling, sucking, and kissing) |
| **Levator labii superioris** | Frontal process of maxilla and infraorbital region | Skin of upper lip and alar cartilage of nose | Elevates lip, dilates nostril, and raises angle of mouth |
| **Platysma** | Superficial fascia of deltoid and pectoral regions | Mandible, skin of cheek, angle of mouth, and orbicularis oris | Depresses mandible and tenses skin of lower face and neck |
| **Mentalis** | Incisive fossa of mandible | Skin of chin | Protrudes lower lip |
| **Buccinator** | Mandible, pterygomandibular raphe, and alveolar processes of maxilla and mandible | Angle of mouth | Presses cheek against molar teeth to keep food between teeth; expels air from oral cavity as occurs when playing a wind instrument |

**[a]All of these muscles are supplied by the facial nerve (CN VII).**

Injury to the facial nerve (CN VII) or its branches produces paralysis of some or all of the facial muscles on the affected side (Bell palsy). The affected area sags, and facial expression is distorted. The loss of tonus of the orbicularis oculi causes the inferior lid to evert (fall away from the surface of the eyeball). As a result, the lacrimal fluid is not spread over the cornea, preventing adequate lubrication, hydration, and flushing of the cornea. This makes the cornea vulnerable to ulceration. If the injury weakens or paralyzes the buccinator and orbicularis oris, food will accumulate in the oral vestibule during chewing, usually requiring continual removal with a finger. When the sphincters or dilators of the mouth are affected, displacement of the mouth (drooping of the corner) is produced by gravity and contraction of unopposed contralateral facial muscles, resulting in food and saliva dribbling out of the side of the mouth. Weakened lip muscles affect speech. Affected people cannot whistle or blow a wind instrument effectively. They frequently dab their eyes and mouth with a handkerchief to wipe the fluid (tears and saliva) that runs from the drooping lid and mouth.

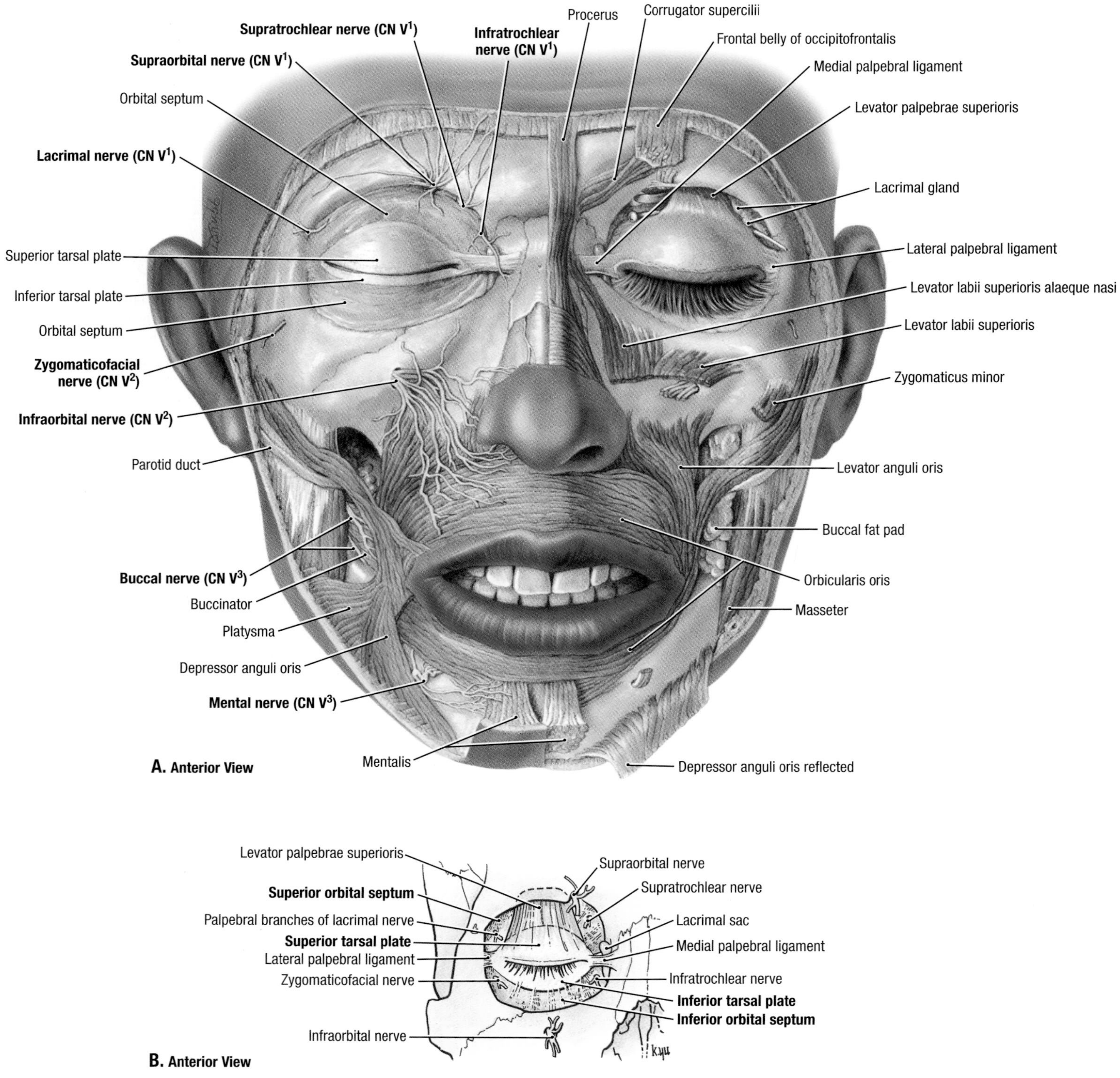

Procerus
Corrugator supercilii
Supratrochlear nerve (CN V1)
Infratrochlear nerve (CN V1)
Frontal belly of occipitofrontalis
Supraorbital nerve (CN V1)
Medial palpebral ligament
Orbital septum
Levator palpebrae superioris
Lacrimal nerve (CN V1)
Lacrimal gland
Superior tarsal plate
Lateral palpebral ligament
Inferior tarsal plate
Levator labii superioris alaeque nasi
Orbital septum
Levator labii superioris
Zygomaticofacial nerve (CN V2)
Zygomaticus minor
Infraorbital nerve (CN V2)
Parotid duct
Levator anguli oris
Buccal fat pad
Buccal nerve (CN V3)
Orbicularis oris
Buccinator
Masseter
Platysma
Depressor anguli oris
Mental nerve (CN V3)
Mentalis
Depressor anguli oris reflected

**A.** Anterior View

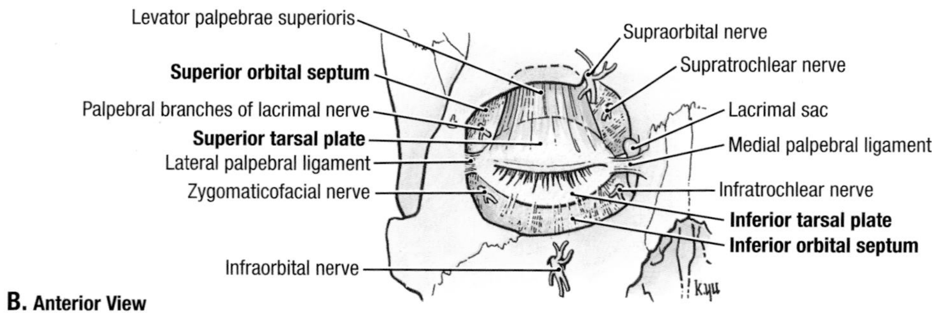
Levator palpebrae superioris
Supraorbital nerve
Superior orbital septum
Supratrochlear nerve
Palpebral branches of lacrimal nerve
Lacrimal sac
Superior tarsal plate
Medial palpebral ligament
Lateral palpebral ligament
Zygomaticofacial nerve
Infratrochlear nerve
Inferior tarsal plate
Inferior orbital septum
Infraorbital nerve

**B.** Anterior View

## 7.15 Cutaneous branches of trigeminal nerve, muscles of facial expression, and eyelid

**A.** Dissection of face. **B.** Orbital septum and eyelid.

Because the face does not have a distinct layer of deep fascia and the subcutaneous tissue is loose between the attachments of facial muscles, facial lacerations tend to gap (part widely). Consequently, the skin must be sutured carefully to prevent scarring. The looseness of the subcutaneous tissue also enables fluid and blood to accumulate in the loose connective tissue after bruising of the face.

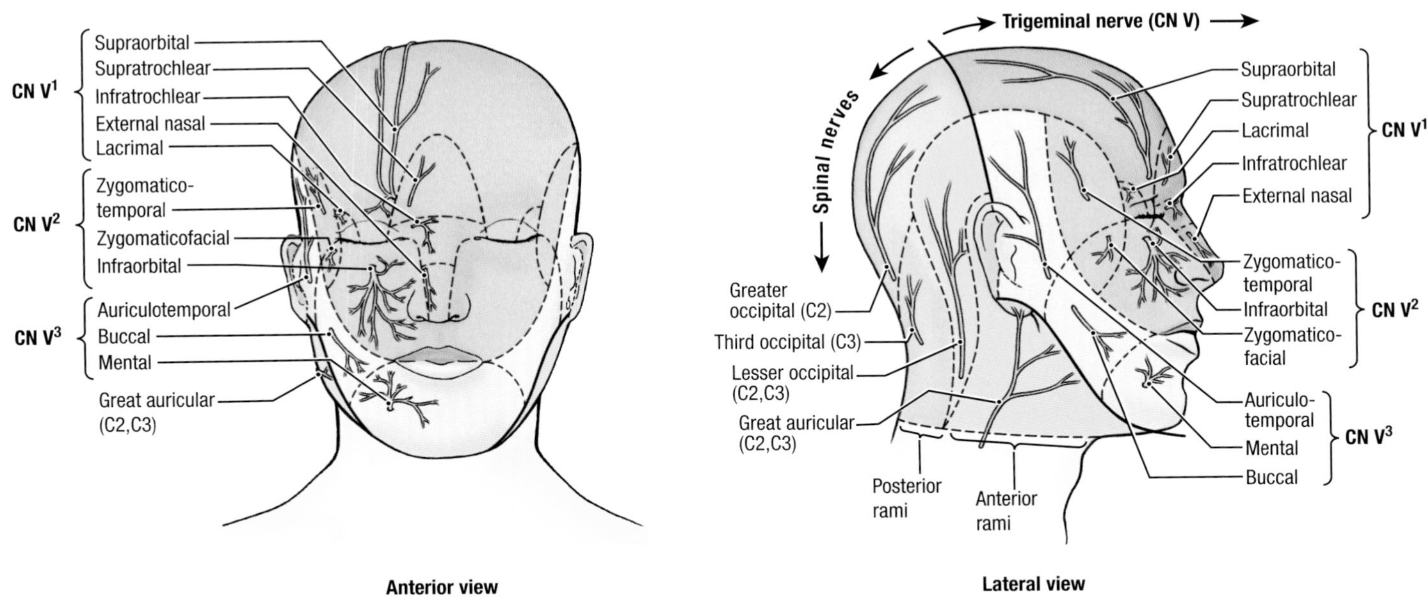
CN V1
Supraorbital
Supratrochlear
Infratrochlear
External nasal
Lacrimal
CN V2
Zygomatico-temporal
Zygomaticofacial
Infraorbital
CN V3
Auriculotemporal
Buccal
Mental
Great auricular (C2,C3)
Anterior view
Trigeminal nerve (CN V)
Spinal nerves
Greater occipital (C2)
Third occipital (C3)
Lesser occipital (C2,C3)
Great auricular (C2,C3)
Posterior rami
Anterior rami
Supraorbital
Supratrochlear
Lacrimal
Infratrochlear
External nasal
CN V1
Zygomatico-temporal
Infraorbital
Zygomatico-facial
CN V2
Auriculo-temporal
Mental
Buccal
CN V3
Lateral view

## TABLE 7.2 NERVES OF FACE AND SCALP

| Nerve | Origin | Course | Distribution |
|---|---|---|---|
| **Frontal** | Ophthalmic nerve (CN $V^1$) | Crosses orbit on superior aspect of levator palpebrae superioris; divides into supraorbital and supratrochlear branches | Skin of forehead, scalp, superior eyelid, and nose; conjunctiva of superior lid and mucosa of frontal sinus |
| **Supraorbital** | Continuation of frontal nerve (CN $V^1$) | Emerges through supraorbital notch, or foramen, and and breaks up into small branches | Mucous membrane of frontal sinus and conjunctiva (lining) of superior eyelid; skin of forehead as far as vertex |
| **Supratrochlear** | Frontal nerve (CN $V^1$) | Continues anteromedially along roof of orbit, passing lateral to trochlea | Skin in middle of forehead to hairline |
| **Infratrochlear** | Nasociliary nerve (CN $V^1$) | Follows medial wall of orbit passing inferior to trochlea to superior eyelid | Skin and conjunctiva (lining) of superior eye lid |
| **Lacrimal** | Ophthalmic nerve (CN $V^1$) | Passes through palpebral fascia of superior eyelid near lateral angle (canthus) of eye | Lacrimal gland and small area of skin and conjunctiva of lateral part of superior eyelid |
| **External nasal** | Anterior ethmoidal nerve (CN $V^1$) | Runs in nasal cavity and emerges on face between nasal bone and lateral nasal cartilage | Skin on dorsum of nose, including tip of nose |
| **Zygomatic** | Maxillary nerve (CN $V^2$) | Arises in floor of orbit, divides into zygomaticofacial and zygomaticotemporal nerves, which traverse foramina of same name | Skin over zygomatic arch and anterior temporal region; carries postsynaptic parasympathetic fibers from pterygopalatine ganglion to lacrimal nerve |
| **Infraorbital** | Terminal branch of maxillary nerve (CN $V^2$) | Runs in floor of orbit and emerges at infraorbital foramen | Skin of cheek, inferior lid, lateral side of nose and inferior septum and superior lip, upper premolar incisors and canine teeth; mucosa of maxillary sinus and superior lip |
| **Auriculotemporal** | Mandibular nerve (CN $V^3$) | From posterior division of CN $V^3$, it passes between neck of mandible and external acoustic meatus to accompany superficial temporal artery | Skin anterior to ear and posterior temporal region, tragus and part of helix of auricle, and roof of external acoustic meatus and upper tympanic membrane |
| **Buccal** | Mandibular nerve (CN $V^3$) | From the anterior division of CN $V^3$ in infratemporal fossa, it passes anteriorly to reach cheek | Skin and mucosa of cheek, buccal gingiva adjacent to 2nd and 3rd molar teeth |
| **Mental** | Terminal branch of inferior alveolar nerve (CN $V^3$) | Emerges from mandibular canal at mental foramen | Skin of chin and inferior lip and mucosa of lower lip |

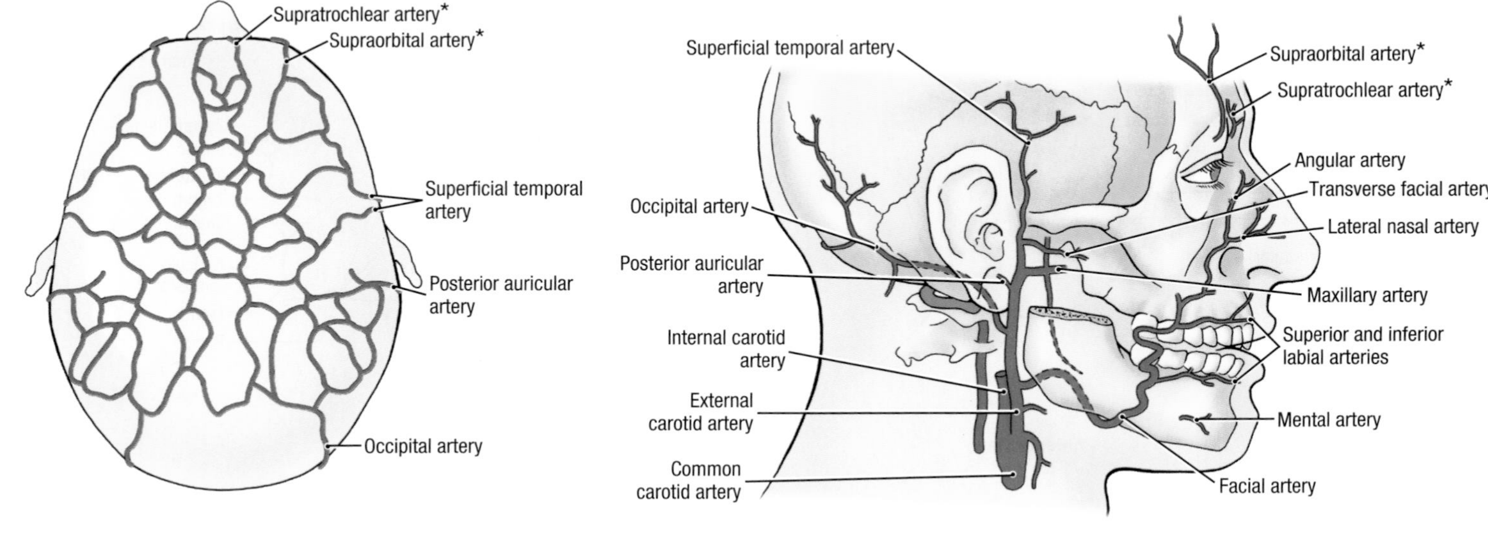
Supratrochlear artery*
Supraorbital artery*
Superficial temporal artery
Posterior auricular artery
Occipital artery
Superior View
Superficial temporal artery
Supraorbital artery*
Supratrochlear artery*
Angular artery
Transverse facial artery
Occipital artery
Lateral nasal artery
Posterior auricular artery
Maxillary artery
Internal carotid artery
Superior and inferior labial arteries
External carotid artery
Mental artery
Common carotid artery
Facial artery
Lateral View

*Source= internal carotid artery (ophthalmic artery); all other labeled arteries are from external carotid

**TABLE 7.3 ARTERIES OF FACE AND SCALP**

| Artery | Origin | Course | Distribution |
|---|---|---|---|
| **Facial** | External carotid artery | Ascends deep to submandibular gland, winds around inferior border of mandible and enters face | Muscles of facial expression and face |
| **Inferior labial** | Facial artery near angle of mouth | Runs medially in lower lip | Lower lip and chin |
| **Superior labial** | | Runs medially in upper lip | Upper lip and ala (side) and septum of nose |
| **Lateral nasal** | Facial artery as it ascends alongside nose | Passes to ala of nose | Skin on ala and dorsum of nose |
| **Angular** | Terminal branch of facial artery | Passes to medial angle (canthus) of eye | Superior part of cheek and lower eyelid |
| **Occipital** | External carotid artery | Passes medial to posterior belly of digastric and mastoid process; accompanies occipital nerve in occipital region | Scalp of back of head, as far as vertex |
| **Posterior auricular** | | Passes posteriorly, deep to parotid, along styloid process between mastoid and ear | Scalp posterior to auricle and auricle |
| **Superficial temporal** | Smaller terminal branch of external carotid artery | Ascends anterior to ear to temporal region and ends in scalp | Facial muscles and skin of frontal and temporal regions |
| **Transverse facial** | Superficial temporal artery within parotid gland | Crosses face superficial to masseter and inferior to zygomatic arch | Parotid gland and duct, muscles and skin of face |
| **Mental** | Terminal branch of inferior alveolar artery | Emerges from mental foramen and passes to chin | Facial muscles and skin of chin |
| ***Supraorbital** | Terminal branch of ophthalmic artery, a branch of internal carotid artery | Passes superiorly from supraorbital foramen | Muscles and skin of forehead and scalp |
| ***Supratrochlear** | | Passes superiorly from supratrochlear notch | Muscles and skin of scalp |

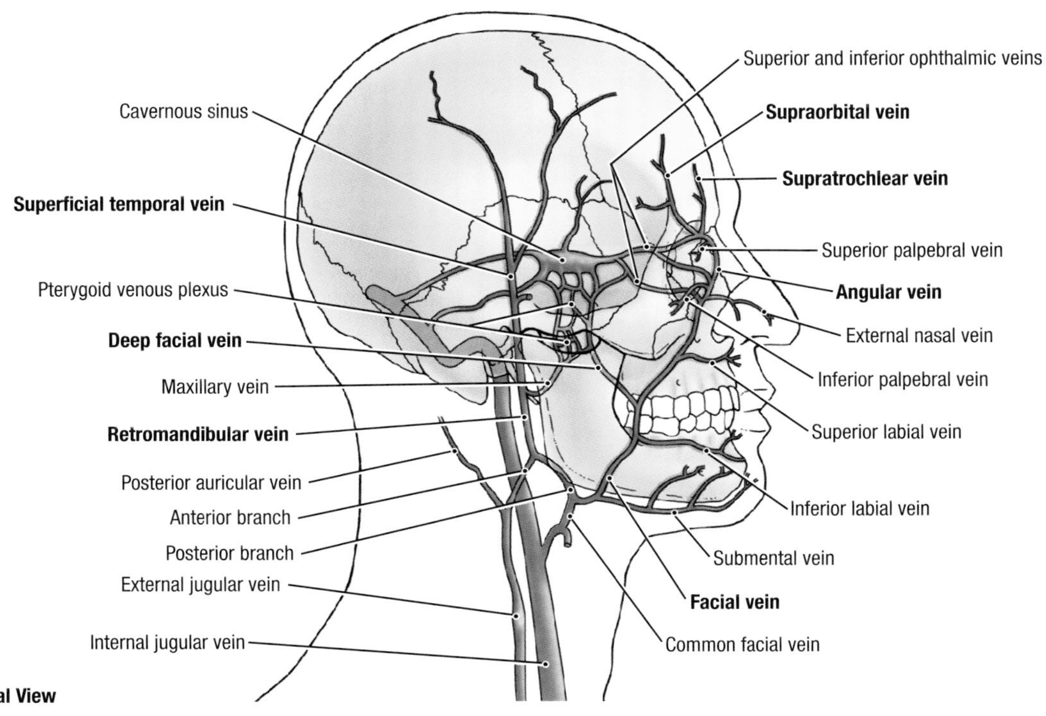
Cavernous sinus
Superficial temporal vein
Pterygoid venous plexus
Deep facial vein
Maxillary vein
Retromandibular vein
Posterior auricular vein
Anterior branch
Posterior branch
External jugular vein
Internal jugular vein
Superior and inferior ophthalmic veins
Supraorbital vein
Supratrochlear vein
Superior palpebral vein
Angular vein
External nasal vein
Inferior palpebral vein
Superior labial vein
Inferior labial vein
Submental vein
Facial vein
Common facial vein

Lateral View

## TABLE 7.4 VEINS OF FACE

| Vein | Origin | Course | Termination | Area Drained |
|---|---|---|---|---|
| **Supratrochlear** | Begins from a venous plexus on the forehead and scalp, through which it communicates with the frontal branch of the superficial temporal vein, its contralateral partner, and the supraorbital vein | Descends near the midline of the forehead to the root of the nose where it joins the supraorbital vein | Angular vein at the root of the nose | Anterior part of scalp and forehead |
| **Supraorbital** | Begins in the forehead by anastomosing with a frontal tributary of the superficial temporal vein | Passes medially superior to the orbit and joins the supratrochlear vein; a branch passes through the supraorbital notch and joins with the superior ophthalmic vein | | |
| **Angular** | Begins at root of nose by union of supratrochlear and supraorbital veins | Descends obliquely along the root and side of the nose to the inferior margin of the orbit | Becomes the facial vein at the inferior margin of the orbit | In addition to above, drains upper and lower lids and conjunctiva; may receive drainage from cavernous sinus |
| **Facial** | Continuation of angular vein past inferior margin of orbit | Descends along lateral border of the nose, receiving external nasal and inferior palpebral veins, then obliquely across face to mandible; receives anterior division of retromandibular vein, after which it is sometimes called the common facial vein | Internal jugular vein opposite or inferior to the level of the hyoid bone | Anterior scalp and forehead, eyelids, external nose, and anterior cheek, lips, chin, and submandibular gland |
| **Deep facial** | Pterygoid venous plexus | Runs anteriorly on maxilla above buccinator and deep to masseter, emerging medial to anterior border of masseter onto face | Enters posterior aspect of facial vein | Infratemporal fossa (most areas supplied by maxillary artery) |
| **Superficial temporal** | Begins from a widespread plexus of veins on the side of the scalp and along the zygomatic arch | Its frontal and parietal tributaries unite anterior to the auricle; it crosses the temporal root of the zygomatic arch to pass from the temporal region and enters the substance of the parotid gland | Joins the maxillary vein posterior to the neck of the mandible to form the retromandibular vein | Side of the scalp, superficial aspect of the temporal muscle, and external ear |
| **Retromandibular** | Formed anterior to the ear by the union of the superficial temporal and maxillary veins | Runs posterior and deep to the ramus of the mandible through the substance of the parotid gland; communicates at its inferior end with the facial vein | *Anterior branch* unites with facial vein to form common facial vein; *posterior branch* unites with the posterior auricular vein to form the external jugular vein | Parotid gland and masseter muscle |

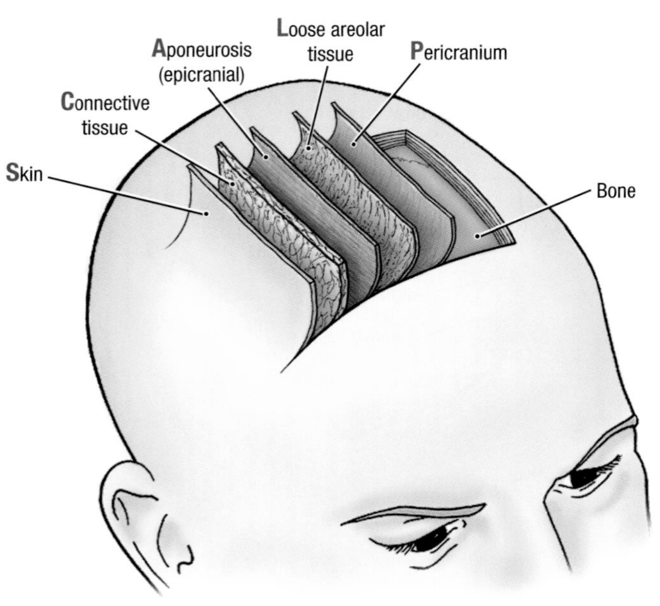
Skin
Connective tissue
Aponeurosis (epicranial)
Loose areolar tissue
Pericranium
Bone

A. Superolateral view

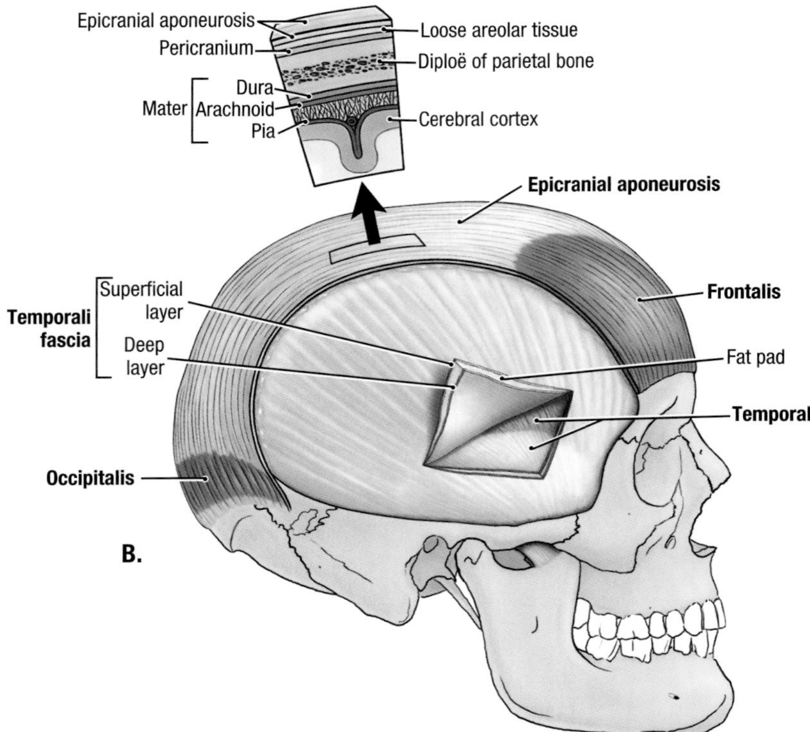
Epicranial aponeurosis
Pericranium
Mater
Dura
Arachnoid
Pia
Loose areolar tissue
Diploë of parietal bone
Cerebral cortex
Epicranial aponeurosis
Temporali fascia
Superficial layer
Deep layer
Frontalis
Fat pad
Temporalis
Occipitalis

B.

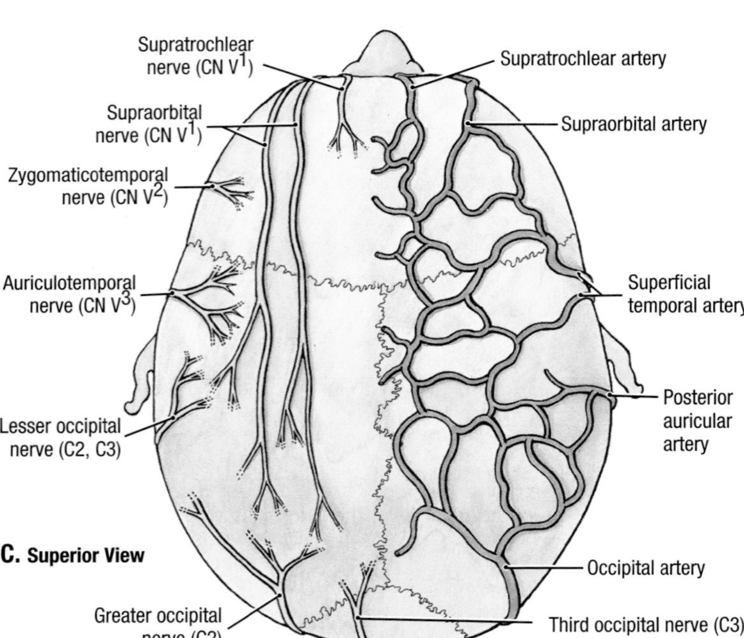
Supratrochlear nerve (CN V1)
Supraorbital nerve (CN V1)
Zygomaticotemporal nerve (CN V2)
Auriculotemporal nerve (CN V3)
Lesser occipital nerve (C2, C3)
Greater occipital nerve (C2)
Supratrochlear artery
Supraorbital artery
Superficial temporal artery
Posterior auricular artery
Occipital artery
Third occipital nerve (C3)

C. Superior View

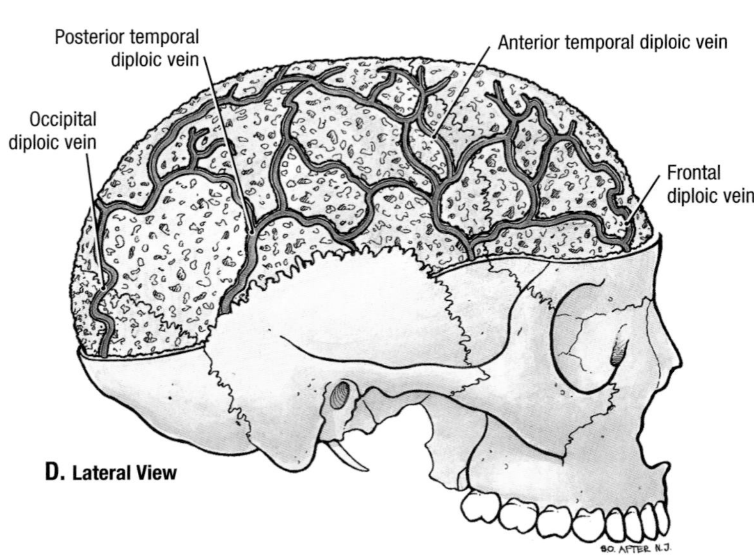
Posterior temporal diploic vein
Occipital diploic vein
Anterior temporal diploic vein
Frontal diploic vein

D. Lateral View

## 7.16 Branches of facial nerve, muscles of facial expression, and scalp

**A.** Layers of scalp. **B.** Occipitofrontalis and temporal muscles and fascia. **C.** Sensory nerves and arteries of the scalp. **D.** Diploic veins. The outer layer of the compact bone of the cranium has been filed away, exposing the channels for the diploic veins in the cancellous bone that composes the diploë.

The loose areolar tissue layer is the danger area of the scalp because pus or blood spreads easily in it. Infection in this layer can pass into the cranial cavity through emissary veins, which pass through parietal foramina in the calvaria and reach intracranial structures such as the meninges. An infection cannot pass into the neck because the occipital belly of the occipitofrontalis attaches to the occipital bone and mastoid parts of the temporal bones. Neither can a scalp infection spread laterally beyond the zygomatic arches because the epicranial aponeurosis is continuous with the temporalis fascia that attaches to these arches. An infection or fluid (e.g., pus or blood) can enter the eyelids and the root of the nose because the frontal belly of the occipitofrontalis inserts into the skin and dense subcutaneous tissue and does not attach to the bone. Ecchymoses, or purple patches, develop as a result of extravasation of blood into the subcutaneous tissue and skin of the eyelids and surrounding regions.

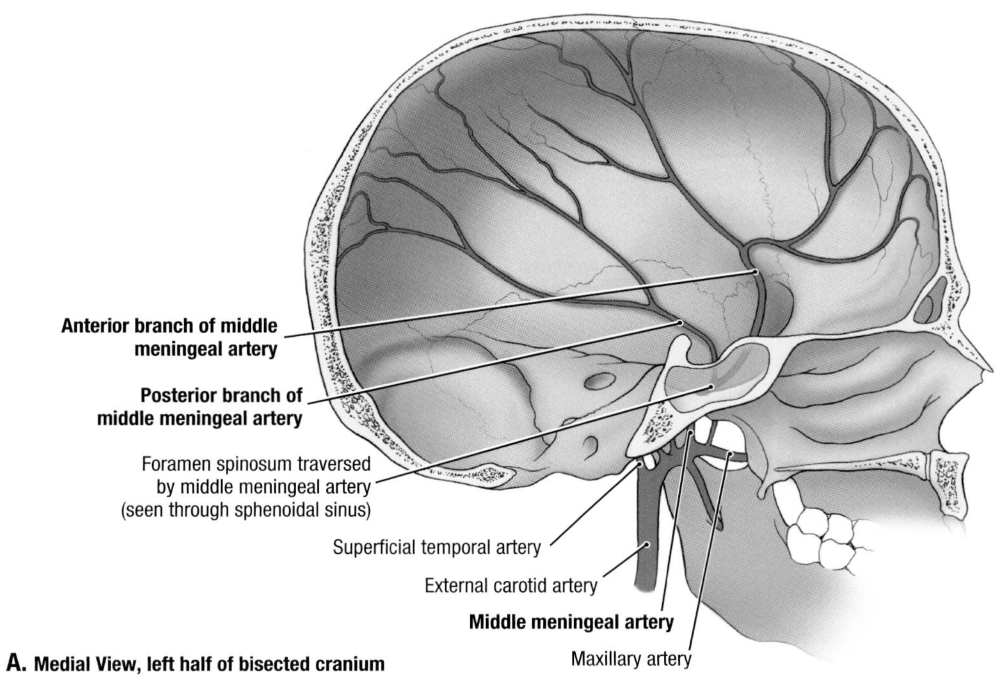
Anterior branch of middle meningeal artery
Posterior branch of middle meningeal artery
Foramen spinosum traversed by middle meningeal artery (seen through sphenoidal sinus)
Superficial temporal artery
External carotid artery
Middle meningeal artery
Maxillary artery
A. Medial View, left half of bisected cranium

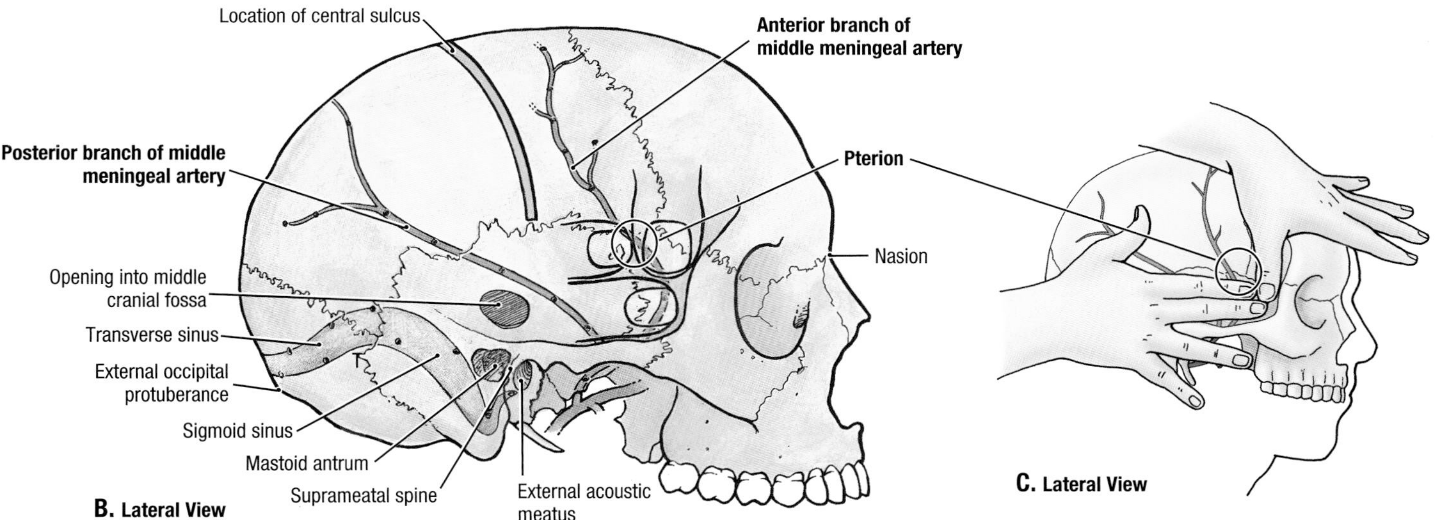
Location of central sulcus
Anterior branch of middle meningeal artery
Posterior branch of middle meningeal artery
Pterion
Nasion
Opening into middle cranial fossa
Transverse sinus
External occipital protuberance
Sigmoid sinus
Mastoid antrum
Suprameatal spine
External acoustic meatus
B. Lateral View
C. Lateral View

## 7.17 Middle meningeal artery and pterion

**A.** Course of the middle meningeal artery in the cranium. **B.** Surface projections of internal features of the neurocranium. **C.** Locating the pterion. The pterion is located two fingers breadth superior to the zygomatic arch and one thumb breadth posterior to the frontal process of the zygomatic bone (approximately 4 cm superior to the midpoint of the zygomatic arch); the anterior branch of the middle meningeal artery crosses the pterion.

A hard blow to the side of the head may fracture the thin bones forming the pterion, rupturing the anterior branch of the middle meningeal artery crossing the pterion. The resulting extradural (epidural) hematoma exerts pressure on the underlying cerebral cortex. Untreated middle meningeal artery hemorrhage may cause death in a few hours.

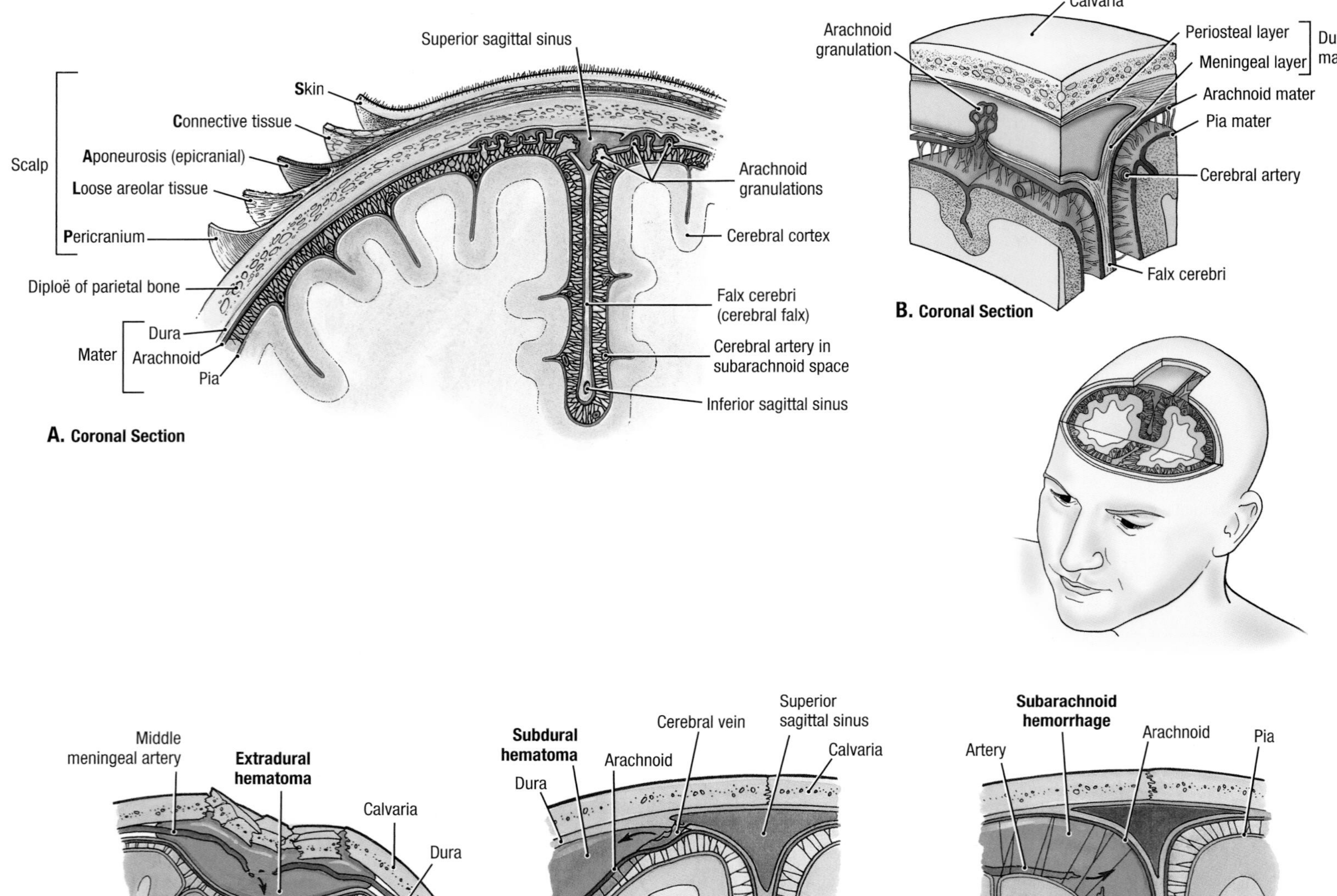
Superior sagittal sinus
Skin
Connective tissue
Aponeurosis (epicranial)
Loose areolar tissue
Pericranium
Scalp
Diploë of parietal bone
Mater
Dura
Arachnoid
Pia
Arachnoid granulations
Cerebral cortex
Falx cerebri (cerebral falx)
Cerebral artery in subarachnoid space
Inferior sagittal sinus
A. Coronal Section
Calvaria
Arachnoid granulation
Periosteal layer
Meningeal layer
Dura mater
Arachnoid mater
Pia mater
Cerebral artery
Falx cerebri
B. Coronal Section
Middle meningeal artery
Extradural hematoma
Calvaria
Dura
C. Coronal Section
Subdural hematoma
Dura
Arachnoid
Cerebral vein
Superior sagittal sinus
Calvaria
D. Coronal Section
Subarachnoid hemorrhage
Artery
Arachnoid
Pia
E. Coronal Section

## 7.18 Layers of the scalp and meninges

**A.** Scalp, cranium, and meninges. **B.** Meninges and their relationship to the calvaria. The three meningeal spaces include the extradural (epidural) space between the cranial bones and dura, which is a potential space normally (it becomes a real space pathologically if blood accumulates in it); the similarly potential subdural space between the dura and arachnoid; and the subarachnoid space, the normal realized space between the arachnoid and pia, which contains cerebrospinal fluid (CSF). **C.** Extradural (epidural) hematomas result from bleeding from a torn middle meningeal artery. **D.** Subdural hematomas commonly result from tearing of a cerebral vein as it enters the superior sagittal sinus. E. Subarachnoid hemorrhage results from bleeding within the subarachnoid space, e.g., from rupture of an aneurysm.

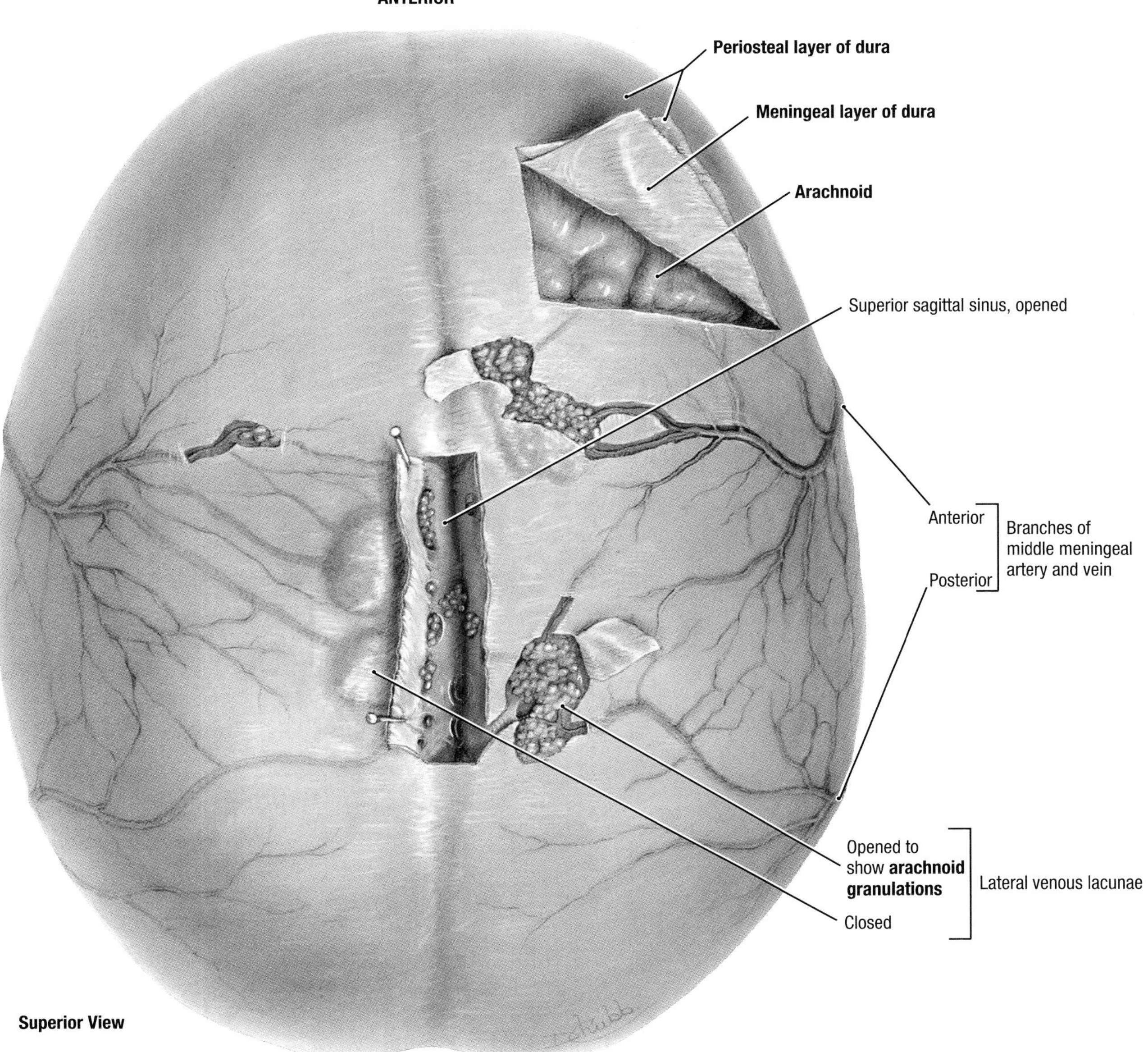
ANTERIOR
Periosteal layer of dura
Meningeal layer of dura
Arachnoid
Superior sagittal sinus, opened
Anterior
Posterior
Branches of middle meningeal artery and vein
Opened to show arachnoid granulations
Closed
Lateral venous lacunae
Superior View
POSTERIOR

## 7.19 Dura mater and arachnoid granulations

- The calvaria is removed. In the median plane, the thick roof of the superior sagittal sinus is partly pinned aside, and laterally, the thin roofs of two lateral lacunae are reflected.
- The middle meningeal artery lies in a venous channel (middle meningeal vein), which enlarges superiorly into a lateral lacunae. Other channels drain the lateral lacunae into the superior sagittal sinus.
- Arachnoid granulations in the lacunae are responsible for absorption of CSF from the subarachnoid space into the venous system.
- The dura is sensitive to pain, especially where it is related to the dural venous sinuses and meningeal arteries. Although the causes of headache are numerous, distention of the scalp or meningeal vessels (or both) is believed to be one cause of headache. Many headaches appear to be dural in origin, such as the headache occurring after a lumbar spinal puncture for removal of CSF. These headaches are thought to result from stimulation of sensory nerve endings in the dura.

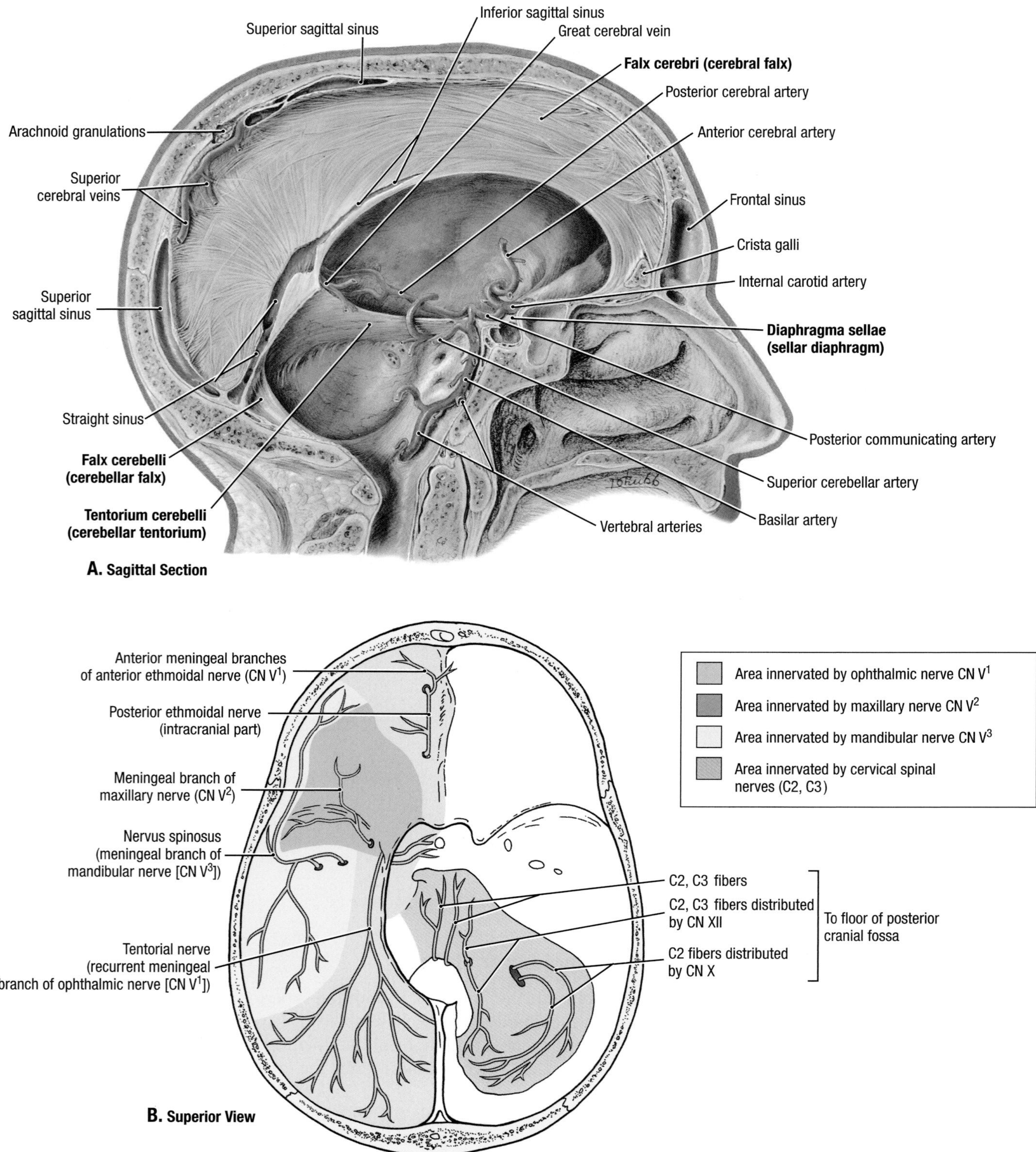

Superior sagittal sinus
Inferior sagittal sinus
Great cerebral vein
Falx cerebri (cerebral falx)
Posterior cerebral artery
Anterior cerebral artery
Arachnoid granulations
Superior cerebral veins
Frontal sinus
Crista galli
Internal carotid artery
Superior sagittal sinus
Diaphragma sellae (sellar diaphragm)
Straight sinus
Posterior communicating artery
Falx cerebelli (cerebellar falx)
Superior cerebellar artery
Tentorium cerebelli (cerebellar tentorium)
Vertebral arteries
Basilar artery
A. Sagittal Section
Anterior meningeal branches of anterior ethmoidal nerve (CN V[1])
Posterior ethmoidal nerve (intracranial part)
Meningeal branch of maxillary nerve (CN V[2])
Nervus spinosus (meningeal branch of mandibular nerve [CN V[3]])
Tentorial nerve (recurrent meningeal branch of ophthalmic nerve [CN V[1]])
Area innervated by ophthalmic nerve CN V[1]
Area innervated by maxillary nerve CN V[2]
Area innervated by mandibular nerve CN V[3]
Area innervated by cervical spinal nerves (C2, C3)
C2, C3 fibers
C2, C3 fibers distributed by CN XII
C2 fibers distributed by CN X
To floor of posterior cranial fossa
B. Superior View


## 7.20 Dura mater

**A.** Reflections of the dura mater. **B.** Innervation of the dura of the cranial base. The dura of the cranial base is innervated by branches of the trigeminal nerve and sensory fibers of cervical spinal nerves (C2, C3) passing directly from those nerves or via meningeal branches of the vagus (CN X) and hypoglossal (CN XII) nerves.

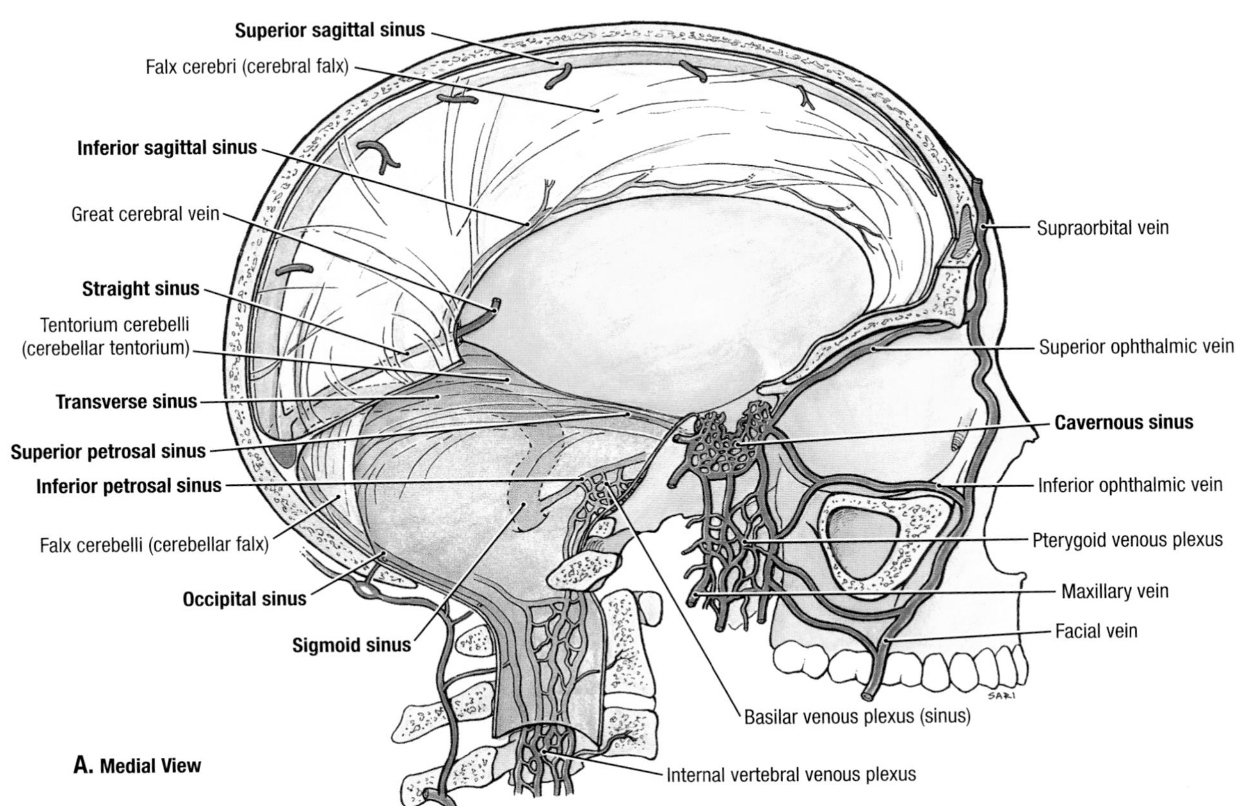
Superior sagittal sinus
Falx cerebri (cerebral falx)
Inferior sagittal sinus
Great cerebral vein
Straight sinus
Tentorium cerebelli (cerebellar tentorium)
Transverse sinus
Superior petrosal sinus
Inferior petrosal sinus
Falx cerebelli (cerebellar falx)
Occipital sinus
Sigmoid sinus
Supraorbital vein
Superior ophthalmic vein
Cavernous sinus
Inferior ophthalmic vein
Pterygoid venous plexus
Maxillary vein
Facial vein
Basilar venous plexus (sinus)
Internal vertebral venous plexus
A. Medial View

## 7.21 Venous sinuses of the dura mater

**A.** Schematic of left half of cranial cavity and right facial skeleton. **B.** Venous sinuses of the cranial base.

- The superior sagittal sinus is at the superior border of the falx cerebri, and the inferior sagittal sinus is in its free border. The great cerebral vein joins the inferior sagittal sinus to form the straight sinus.
- The superior sagittal sinus usually becomes the right transverse sinus, right sigmoid sinus, and right internal jugular vein; the straight sinus similarly drains through the left transverse sinus, left sigmoid sinus, and left internal jugular vein.
- The cavernous sinus communicates with the veins of the face through the ophthalmic veins and pterygoid plexus of veins and with the sigmoid sinus through the superior and inferior petrosal sinuses.
- The basilar and occipital sinuses communicate through the foramen magnum with the internal vertebral venous plexuses. Because these venous channels are valveless, compression of the thorax, abdomen, or pelvis, as occurs during heavy coughing and straining, may force venous blood from these regions into the internal vertebral venous system and from it into the dural venous sinuses. As a result, pus in abscesses and tumor cells in these regions may spread to the vertebrae and brain.

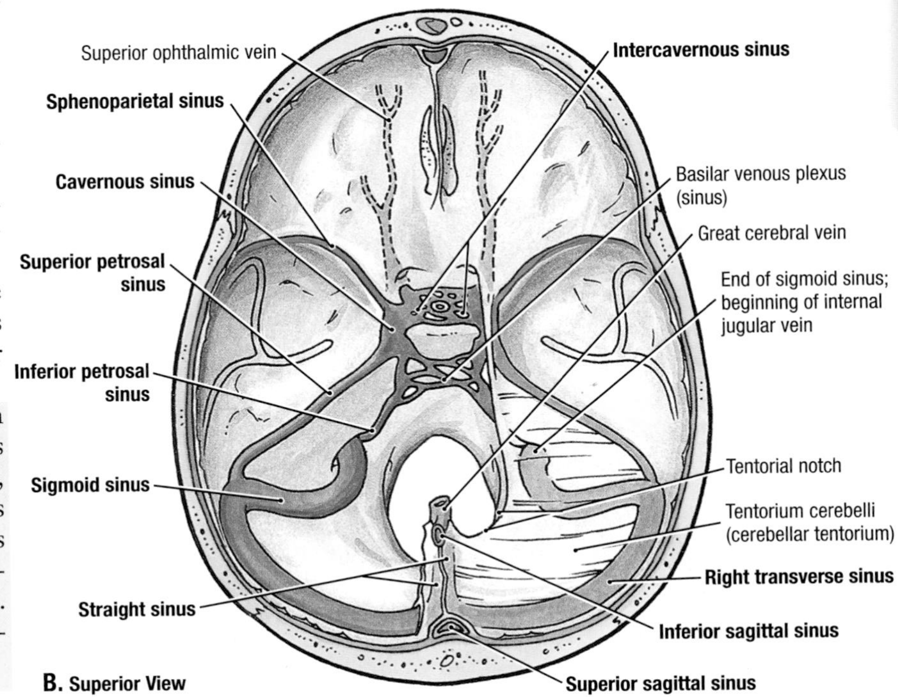
Superior ophthalmic vein
Sphenoparietal sinus
Cavernous sinus
Superior petrosal sinus
Inferior petrosal sinus
Sigmoid sinus
Straight sinus
Intercavernous sinus
Basilar venous plexus (sinus)
Great cerebral vein
End of sigmoid sinus; beginning of internal jugular vein
Tentorial notch
Tentorium cerebelli (cerebellar tentorium)
Right transverse sinus
Inferior sagittal sinus
Superior sagittal sinus
B. Superior View

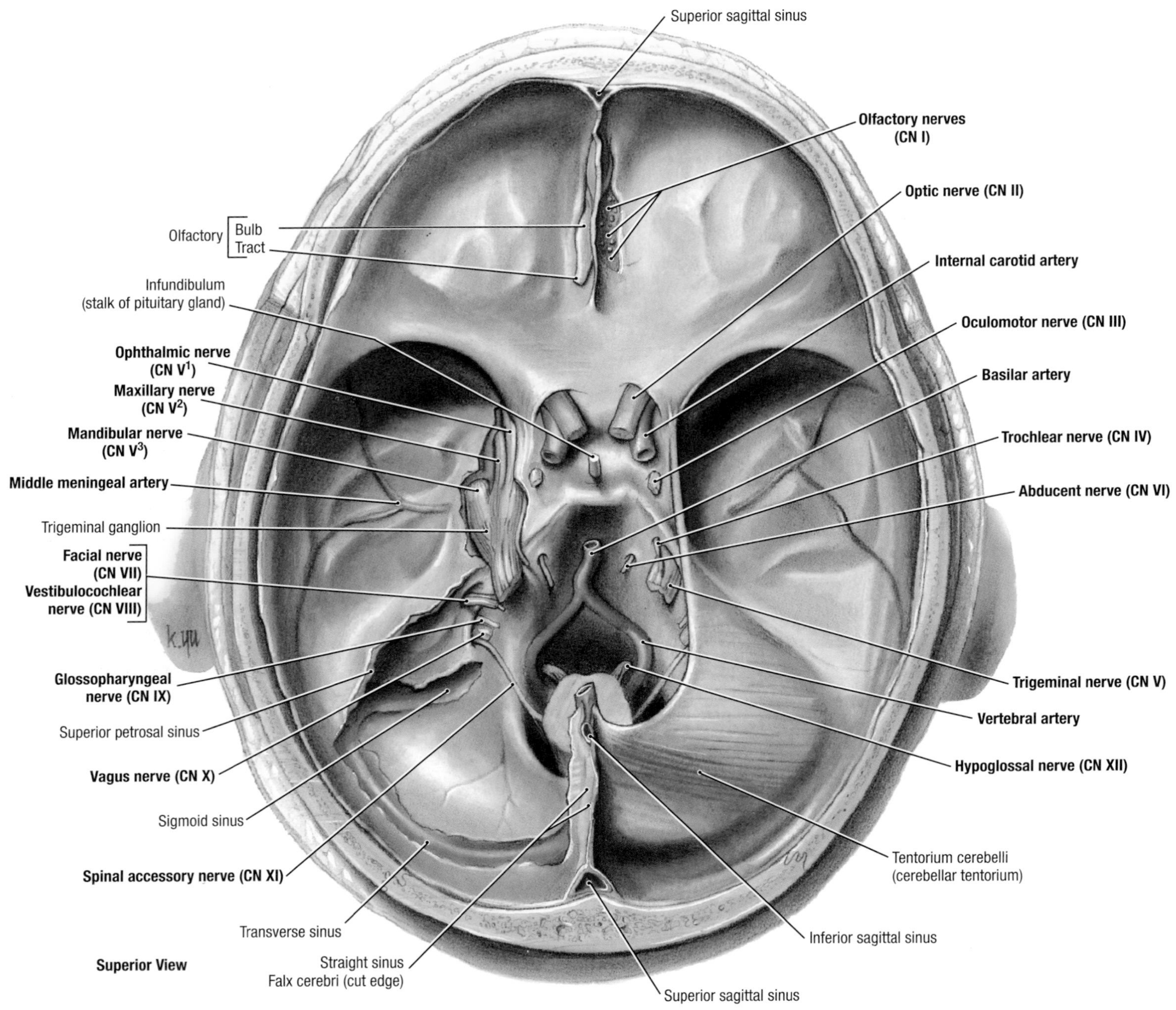
Superior sagittal sinus
Olfactory nerves (CN I)
Optic nerve (CN II)
Internal carotid artery
Oculomotor nerve (CN III)
Basilar artery
Trochlear nerve (CN IV)
Abducent nerve (CN VI)
Olfactory Bulb
Tract
Infundibulum (stalk of pituitary gland)
Ophthalmic nerve (CN V1)
Maxillary nerve (CN V2)
Mandibular nerve (CN V3)
Middle meningeal artery
Trigeminal ganglion
Facial nerve (CN VII)
Vestibulocochlear nerve (CN VIII)
Glossopharyngeal nerve (CN IX)
Superior petrosal sinus
Vagus nerve (CN X)
Sigmoid sinus
Spinal accessory nerve (CN XI)
Transverse sinus
Superior View
Straight sinus
Falx cerebri (cut edge)
Superior sagittal sinus
Inferior sagittal sinus
Tentorium cerebelli (cerebellar tentorium)
Hypoglossal nerve (CN XII)
Vertebral artery
Trigeminal nerve (CN V)

## 7.22 Nerves and vessels of the interior of the base of the cranium

- On the left of the specimen, the dura mater forming the roof of the trigeminal cave is cut away to expose the trigeminal nerve and its three branches and the sigmoid sinus. The tentorium cerebelli is removed to reveal the transverse and superior petrosal sinuses.
- The frontal lobes of the cerebrum are located in the anterior cranial fossa, the temporal lobes in the middle cranial fossa, and the brainstem and cerebellum in the posterior cranial fossa; the occipital lobes rest on the tentorium cerebelli.
- The sites wherre the 12 cranial nerves and the internal carotid, vertebral, basilar, and middle meningeal arteries penetrate the dura mater are shown.

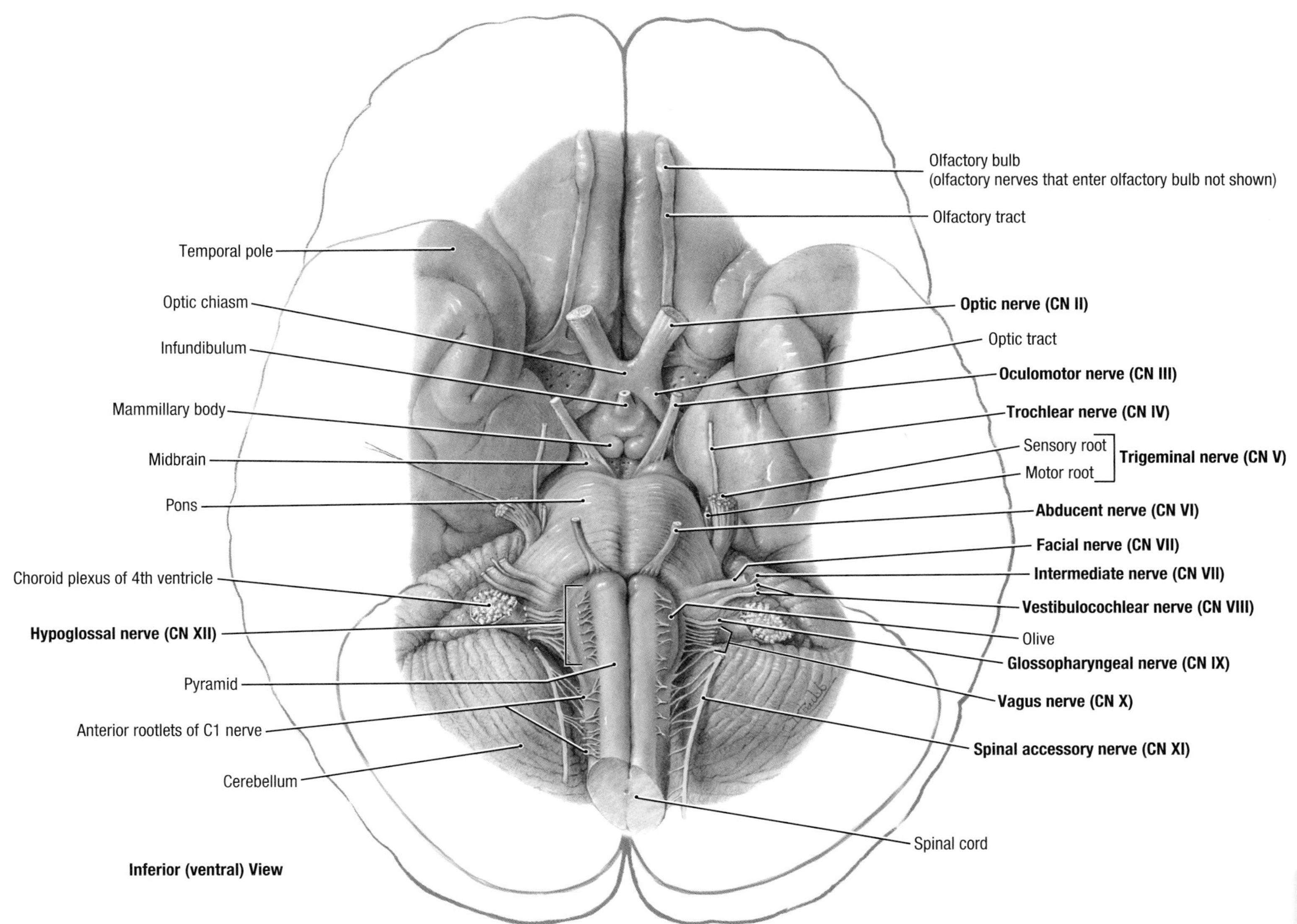
Olfactory bulb
(olfactory nerves that enter olfactory bulb not shown)
Olfactory tract
Temporal pole
Optic chiasm
Infundibulum
Mammillary body
Midbrain
Pons
Choroid plexus of 4th ventricle
Hypoglossal nerve (CN XII)
Pyramid
Anterior rootlets of C1 nerve
Cerebellum
Optic nerve (CN II)
Optic tract
Oculomotor nerve (CN III)
Trochlear nerve (CN IV)
Sensory root
Motor root
Trigeminal nerve (CN V)
Abducent nerve (CN VI)
Facial nerve (CN VII)
Intermediate nerve (CN VII)
Vestibulocochlear nerve (CN VIII)
Olive
Glossopharyngeal nerve (CN IX)
Vagus nerve (CN X)
Spinal accessory nerve (CN XI)
Spinal cord
Inferior (ventral) View

**7.23 Base of brain and superficial origins of cranial nerves**

Foramina of skull and their associated cranial nerve(s) are listed below.

### OPENINGS BY WHICH CRANIAL NERVES EXIT CRANIAL CAVITY

| Foramina/Apertures | Cranial nerve |
|---|---|
| **Anterior cranial fossa** | |
| Cribriform foramina in cribriform plate | Axons of olfactory cells in olfactory epithelium form olfactory nerves (CN I) |
| **Middle cranial fossa** | |
| Optic canal | Optic nerve (CN II) |
| Superior orbital fissure | Opthalmic nerve (CN $V^1$), oculomotor nerve (CN III), trochlear nerve (CN IV), abducent nerve (CN VI) and branches of opthalmic nerve (CN $V^1$) |
| Foramen rotundum | Maxillary nerve (CN $V^2$) |
| Foramen ovale | Mandibular nerve (CN $V^3$) |
| **Posterior cranial fossa** | |
| Foramen magnum | Spinal accessory nerve (CN XI) |
| Jugular foramen | Glossopharyngeal nerve (CN IX), vagus nerve (CN X), and spinal accessory nerve (CN XI) |
| Hypoglossal canal | Hypoglossal nerve (CN XII) |

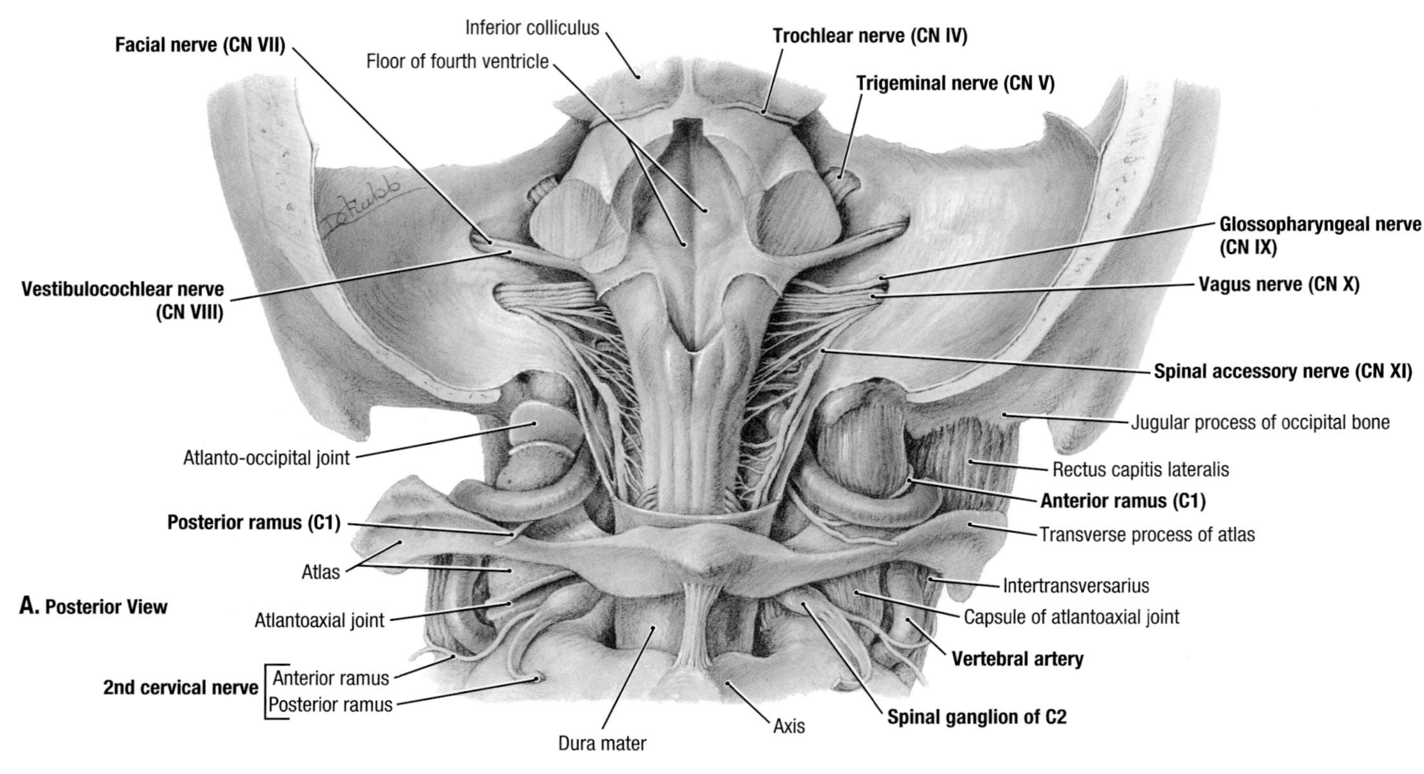
Inferior colliculus
Facial nerve (CN VII)
Floor of fourth ventricle
Trochlear nerve (CN IV)
Trigeminal nerve (CN V)
Glossopharyngeal nerve (CN IX)
Vestibulocochlear nerve (CN VIII)
Vagus nerve (CN X)
Spinal accessory nerve (CN XI)
Jugular process of occipital bone
Atlanto-occipital joint
Rectus capitis lateralis
Anterior ramus (C1)
Posterior ramus (C1)
Transverse process of atlas
Atlas
Intertransversarius
A. Posterior View
Atlantoaxial joint
Capsule of atlantoaxial joint
Vertebral artery
2nd cervical nerve
Anterior ramus
Posterior ramus
Axis
Spinal ganglion of C2
Dura mater

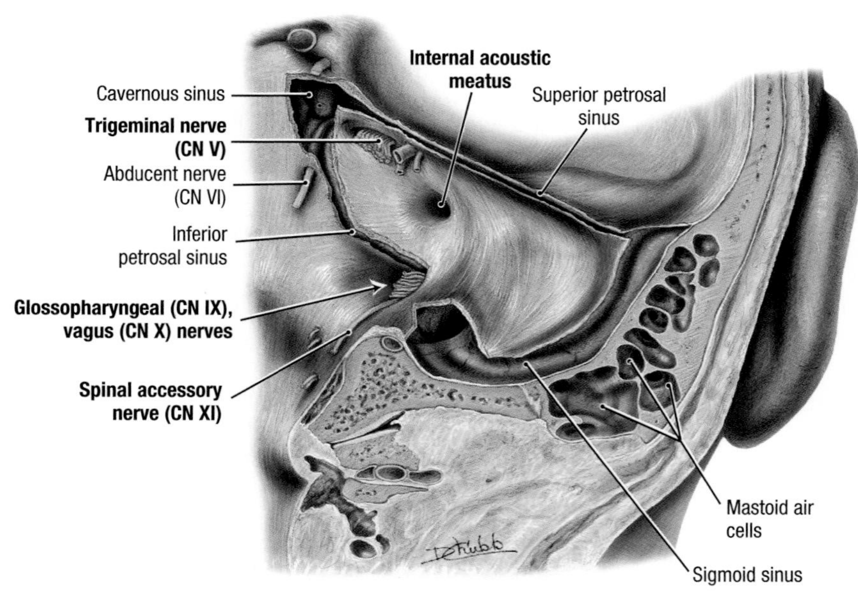
Internal acoustic meatus
Cavernous sinus
Superior petrosal sinus
Trigeminal nerve (CN V)
Abducent nerve (CN VI)
Inferior petrosal sinus
Glossopharyngeal (CN IX), vagus (CN X) nerves
Spinal accessory nerve (CN XI)
Mastoid air cells
Sigmoid sinus
B. Posterior View

## 7.24 Posterior exposures of cranial nerves

**A** and **B.** Squamous part of occipital bone has been removed posterior to foramen magnum to reveal posterior cranial fossa. **A.** Brainstem in situ. **B.** Right side, with brainstem removed. The trochlear nerves (CN IV) arise from the dorsal aspect of the midbrain, just inferior to the inferior colliculi.

- The sensory and motor roots of the trigeminal nerves (CN V) pass anterolaterally to enter the mouth of the trigeminal cave.
- The facial (CN VII) and vestibulocochlear (CN VIII) nerves course laterally to enter the internal acoustic meatus.
- The glossopharyngeal nerve (CN IX) pierces the dura mater separately but passes with the vagus (CN X) and spinal accessory (CN XI) nerves through the jugular foramen.

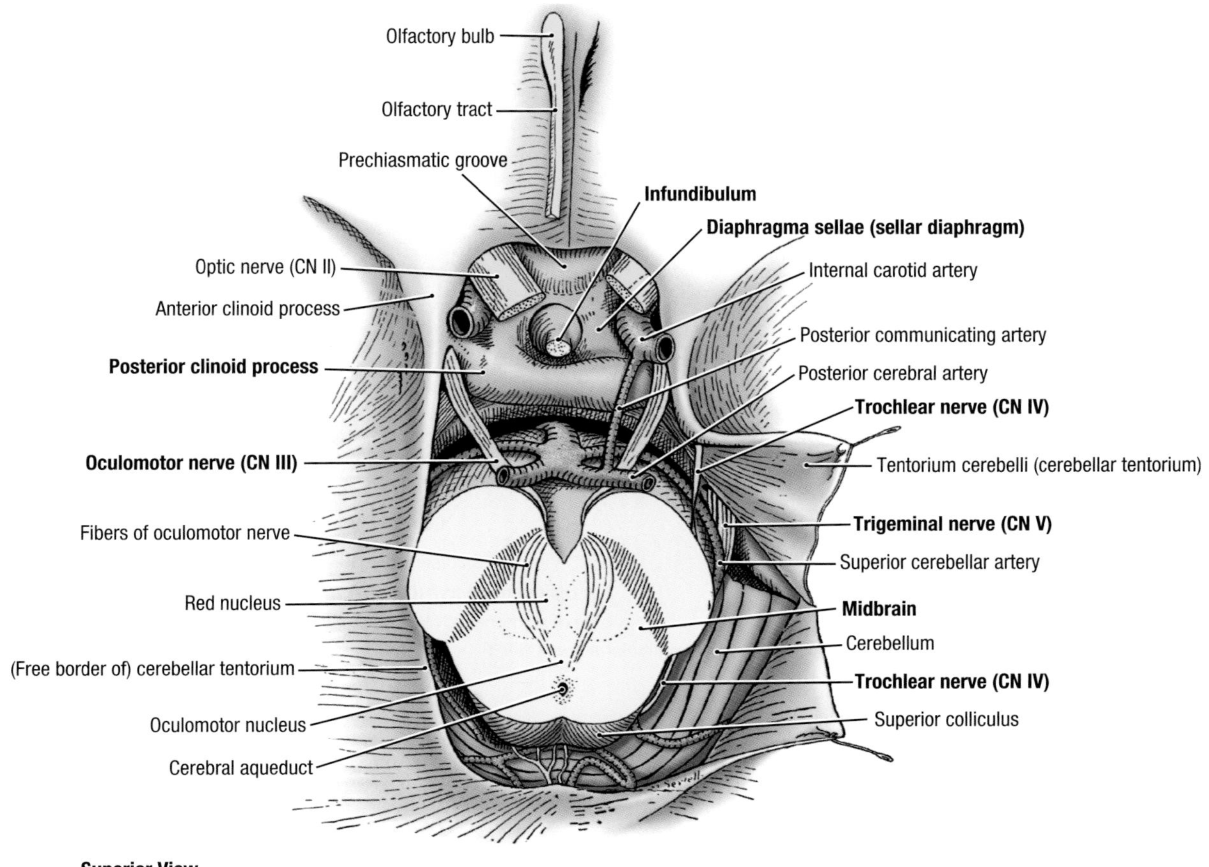
Olfactory bulb
Olfactory tract
Prechiasmatic groove
Infundibulum
Diaphragma sellae (sellar diaphragm)
Optic nerve (CN II)
Internal carotid artery
Anterior clinoid process
Posterior communicating artery
Posterior clinoid process
Posterior cerebral artery
Trochlear nerve (CN IV)
Oculomotor nerve (CN III)
Tentorium cerebelli (cerebellar tentorium)
Fibers of oculomotor nerve
Trigeminal nerve (CN V)
Superior cerebellar artery
Red nucleus
Midbrain
Cerebellum
(Free border of) cerebellar tentorium
Trochlear nerve (CN IV)
Oculomotor nucleus
Superior colliculus
Cerebral aqueduct
Superior View

## 7.25 Tentorial notch

- The brain has been removed by cutting through the midbrain, revealing the tentorial notch through which the brainstem extends from the posterior into the middle cranial fossa.
- On the right side of the specimen, the tentorium cerebelli is divided and reflected. The trochlear nerve (CN IV) passes around the midbrain under the free edge of the tentorium cerebelli; the roots of the trigeminal nerve (CN V) enter the mouth of the trigeminal cave.
- There is a circular opening in the diaphragma sellae for the infundibulum, the stalk of the pituitary gland.
- The oculomotor nerve (CN III) passes between the posterior cerebral and superior cerebellar arteries and then laterally around the posterior clinoid process.
- The tentorial notch is the opening in the tentorium cerebelli for the brainstem, which is slightly larger than is necessary to accommodate the midbrain. Hence, space-occupying lesions, such as tumors in the supratentorial compartment, produce increased intracranial pressure that may cause part of the adjacent temporal lobe of the brain to herniate through the tentorial notch. During tentorial herniation, the temporal lobe may be lacerated by the tough tentorium cerebelli, and the oculomotor nerve (CN III) may be stretched, compressed, or both. Oculomotor lesions may produce paralysis of the extrinsic eye muscles supplied by CN III.

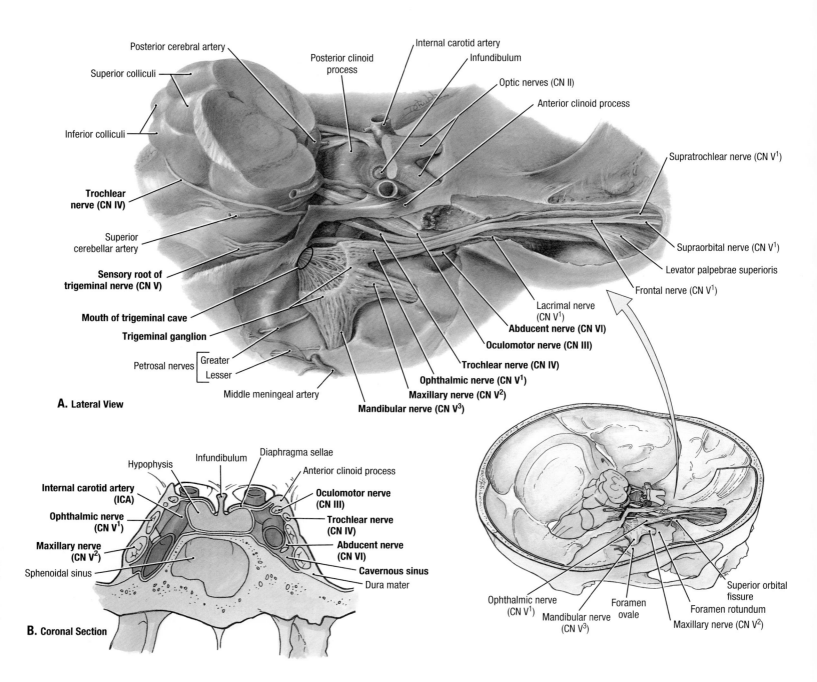

Posterior cerebral artery
Superior colliculi
Inferior colliculi
Trochlear nerve (CN IV)
Superior cerebellar artery
Sensory root of trigeminal nerve (CN V)
Mouth of trigeminal cave
Trigeminal ganglion
Petrosal nerves
Greater
Lesser
Middle meningeal artery
Posterior clinoid process
Internal carotid artery
Infundibulum
Optic nerves (CN II)
Anterior clinoid process
Supratrochlear nerve (CN V[1])
Supraorbital nerve (CN V[1])
Levator palpebrae superioris
Frontal nerve (CN V[1])
Lacrimal nerve (CN V[1])
Abducent nerve (CN VI)
Oculomotor nerve (CN III)
Trochlear nerve (CN IV)
Ophthalmic nerve (CN V[1])
Maxillary nerve (CN V[2])
Mandibular nerve (CN V[3])

**A.** Lateral View

Ophthalmic nerve (CN V[1])
Mandibular nerve (CN V[3])
Foramen ovale
Foramen rotundum
Maxillary nerve (CN V[2])
Superior orbital fissure

Hypophysis
Infundibulum
Diaphragma sellae
Anterior clinoid process
Internal carotid artery (ICA)
Ophthalmic nerve (CN V[1])
Maxillary nerve (CN V[2])
Sphenoidal sinus
Oculomotor nerve (CN III)
Trochlear nerve (CN IV)
Abducent nerve (CN VI)
Cavernous sinus
Dura mater

**B.** Coronal Section

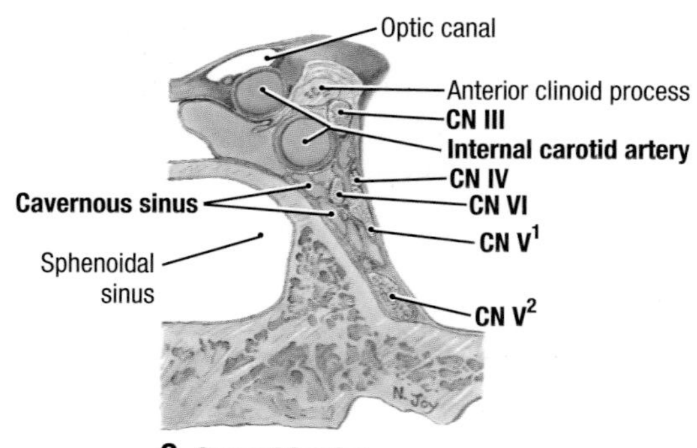
Optic canal
Anterior clinoid process
CN III
Internal carotid artery
CN IV
Cavernous sinus
CN VI
CN V1
Sphenoidal sinus
CN V2

**C.** Coronal Section

## 7.26 Nerves and vessels of middle cranial fossa—I

**A.** Superficial dissection. The tentorium cerebelli is cut away . The dura mater is largely removed from the middle cranial fossa. The roof of the orbit is partly removed. **B** and **C.** Coronal sections through the cavernous sinus.

In fractures of the cranial base, the internal carotid artery may be torn, producing an arteriovenous fistula within the cavernous sinus. Arterial blood rushes into the sinus, enlarging it and forcing retrograde blood flow into its venous tributaries, especially the ophthalmic veins. As a result, the eyeball protrudes (exophthalmos) and the conjunctiva becomes engorged (chemosis). Because CN III, CN IV, CN VI, CN V1, and CN V2 lie in or close to the lateral wall of the cavernous sinus, these nerves may also be affected.

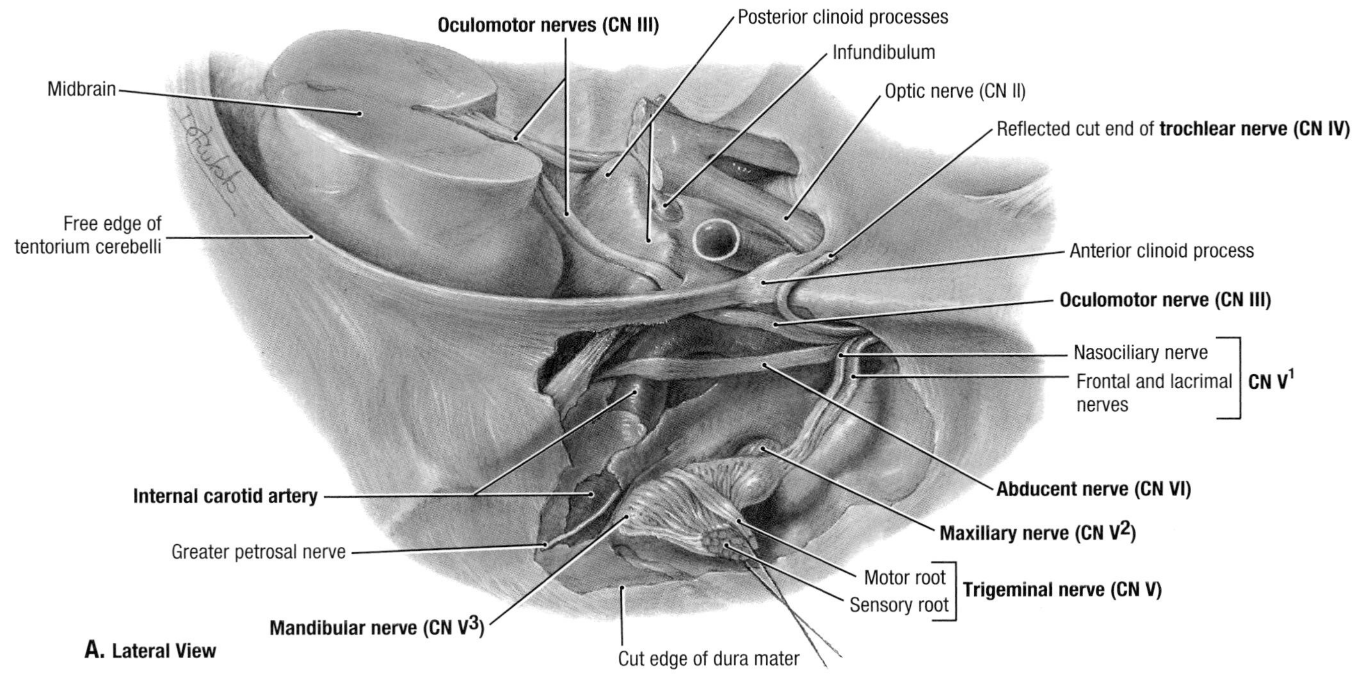
Oculomotor nerves (CN III)
Posterior clinoid processes
Infundibulum
Optic nerve (CN II)
Reflected cut end of trochlear nerve (CN IV)
Midbrain
Free edge of tentorium cerebelli
Anterior clinoid process
Oculomotor nerve (CN III)
Nasociliary nerve
Frontal and lacrimal nerves
CN V1
Abducent nerve (CN VI)
Maxillary nerve (CN V2)
Motor root
Sensory root
Trigeminal nerve (CN V)
Internal carotid artery
Greater petrosal nerve
Mandibular nerve (CN V3)
Cut edge of dura mater
A. Lateral View

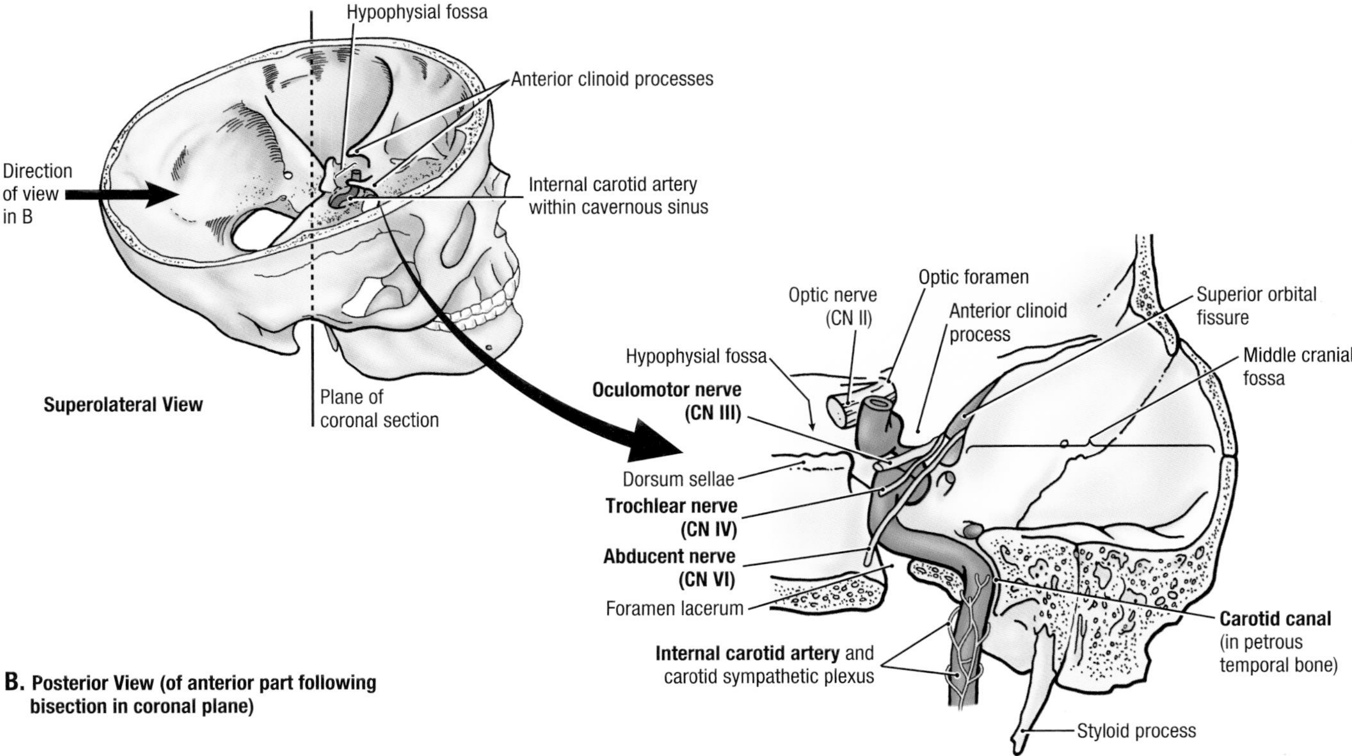
Hypophysial fossa
Anterior clinoid processes
Direction of view in B
Internal carotid artery within cavernous sinus
Superolateral View
Plane of coronal section
Optic nerve (CN II)
Optic foramen
Anterior clinoid process
Superior orbital fissure
Middle cranial fossa
Hypophysial fossa
Oculomotor nerve (CN III)
Dorsum sellae
Trochlear nerve (CN IV)
Abducent nerve (CN VI)
Foramen lacerum
Internal carotid artery and carotid sympathetic plexus
Carotid canal (in petrous temporal bone)
Styloid process
B. Posterior View (of anterior part following bisection in coronal plane)

## 7.27 Nerves and vessels of middle cranial fossa—II

**A.** Deep dissection. The roots of the trigeminal nerve are divided, withdrawn from the mouth of the trigeminal cave, and turned anteriorly. The trochlear nerve is reflected anteriorly. **B.** Course of the internal carotid artery.

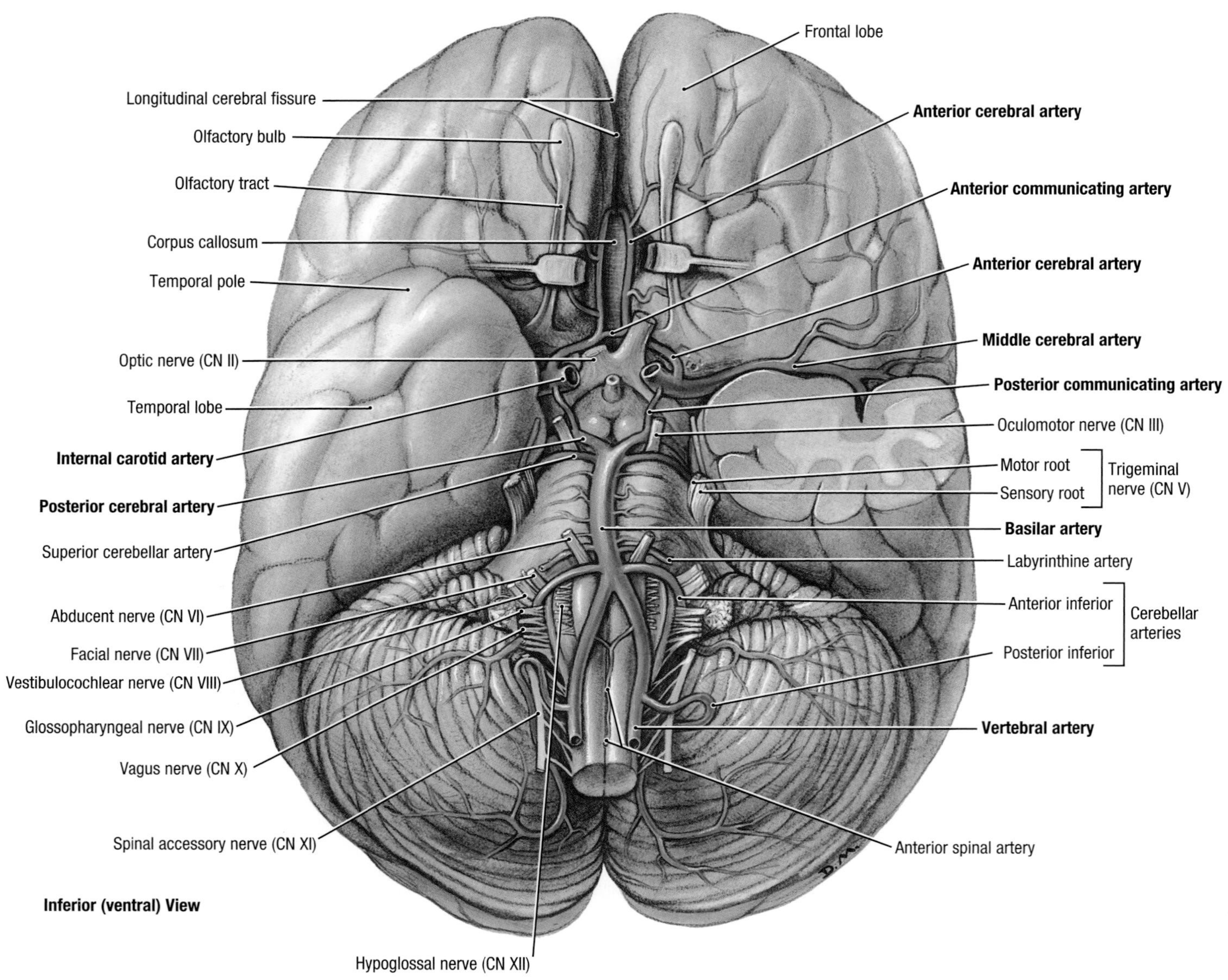
Frontal lobe
Longitudinal cerebral fissure
Anterior cerebral artery
Olfactory bulb
Olfactory tract
Anterior communicating artery
Corpus callosum
Anterior cerebral artery
Temporal pole
Middle cerebral artery
Optic nerve (CN II)
Posterior communicating artery
Temporal lobe
Oculomotor nerve (CN III)
Internal carotid artery
Motor root
Sensory root
Trigeminal nerve (CN V)
Posterior cerebral artery
Basilar artery
Superior cerebellar artery
Labyrinthine artery
Abducent nerve (CN VI)
Anterior inferior
Posterior inferior
Cerebellar arteries
Facial nerve (CN VII)
Vestibulocochlear nerve (CN VIII)
Glossopharyngeal nerve (CN IX)
Vertebral artery
Vagus nerve (CN X)
Spinal accessory nerve (CN XI)
Anterior spinal artery
Inferior (ventral) View
Hypoglossal nerve (CN XII)

## 7.28 Base of brain and cerebral arterial circle

The left temporal pole is removed to enable visualization of the middle cerebral artery in the lateral fissure. The frontal lobes are separated to expose the anterior cerebral arteries and corpus callosum.

An ischemic stroke denotes the sudden development of neurological deficits that are consequences of impaired cerebral blood flow. The most common causes of strokes are spontaneous cerebrovascular accidents such as cerebral embolism, cerebral thrombosis, cerebral hemorrhage, and subarachnoid hemorrhage (Rowland, 2000). The cerebral arterial circle is an important means of collateral circulation in the event of gradual obstruction of one of the major arteries forming the circle. Sudden occlusion, even if only partial, results in neurological deficits. In elderly persons, the anastomoses are often inadequate when a large artery (e.g., internal carotid) is occluded, even if the occlusion is gradual. In such cases function is impaired at least to some degree.

Hemorrhagic stroke follows the rupture of an artery or a saccular aneurysm, a saclike dilation on a weak part of the arterial wall. The most common type of saccular aneurysm is a berry aneurysm, occurring in the vessels of or near the cerebral arterial circle. In time, especially in people with hypertension (high blood pressure), the weak part of the arterial wall expands and may rupture, allowing blood to enter the subarachnoid space.

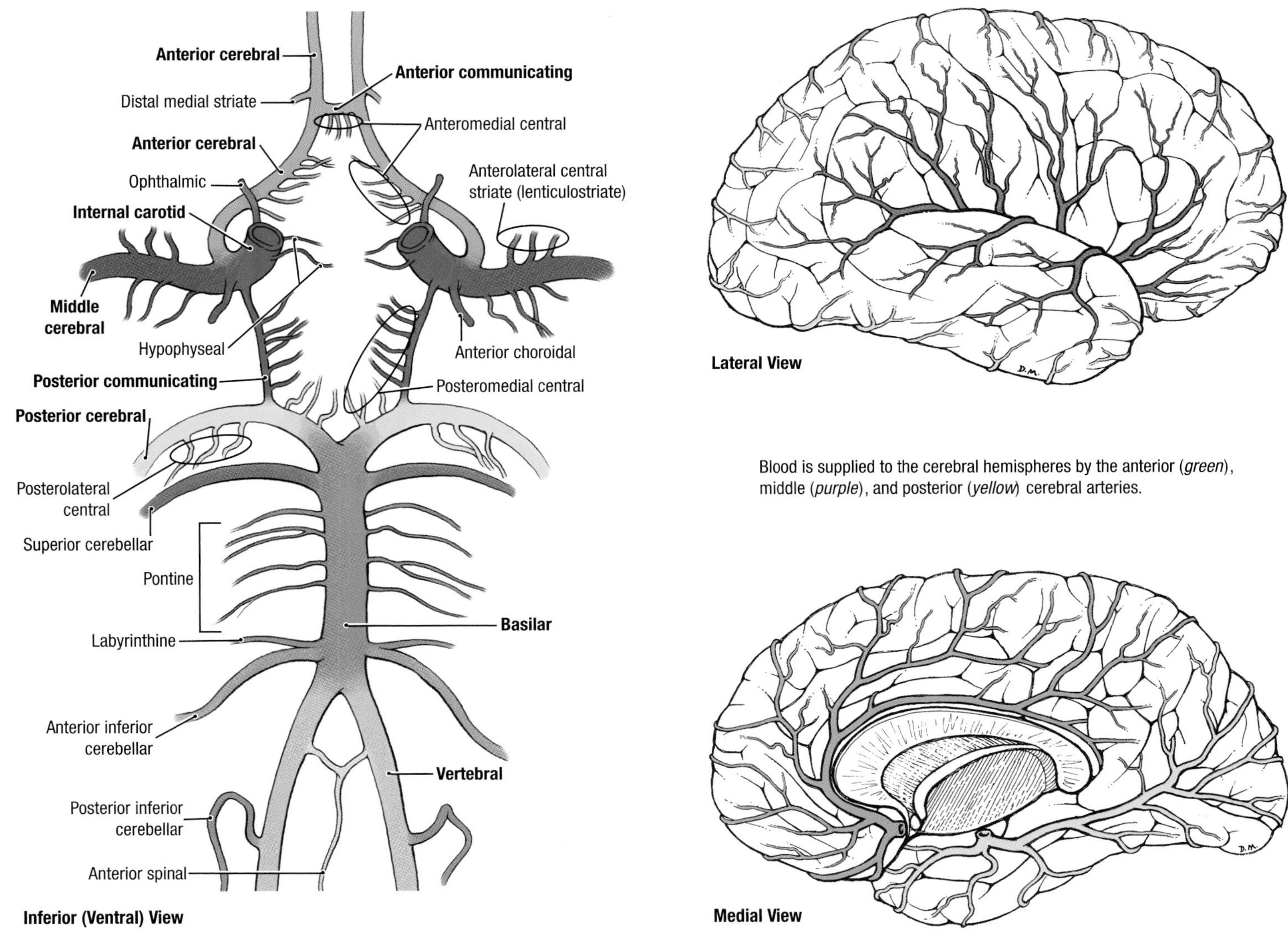
Anterior cerebral
Anterior communicating
Distal medial striate
Anteromedial central
Anterior cerebral
Anterolateral central striate (lenticulostriate)
Ophthalmic
Internal carotid
Middle cerebral
Hypophyseal
Anterior choroidal
Posterior communicating
Posteromedial central
Posterior cerebral
Posterolateral central
Superior cerebellar
Pontine
Basilar
Labyrinthine
Anterior inferior cerebellar
Vertebral
Posterior inferior cerebellar
Anterior spinal
Inferior (Ventral) View
Lateral View
Medial View

Blood is supplied to the cerebral hemispheres by the anterior (*green*), middle (*purple*), and posterior (*yellow*) cerebral arteries.

**TABLE 7.5 ARTERIAL SUPPLY TO BRAIN**

| Artery | Origin | Distribution |
|---|---|---|
| Vertebral | Subclavian artery | Cranial meninges and cerebellum |
| Posterior inferior cerebellar | Vertebral artery | Posteroinferior aspect of cerebellum |
| Basilar | Formed by junction of vertebral arteries | Brainstem, cerebellum, and cerebrum |
| Pontine | Basilar artery | Numerous branches to brainstem |
| Anterior inferior cerebellar | | Inferior aspect of cerebellum |
| Superior cerebellar | | Superior aspect of cerebellum |
| Internal carotid | Common carotid artery at superior border of thyroid cartilage | Gives branches in cavernous sinus and provides supply to brain |
| Anterior cerebral | Internal carotid artery | Cerebral hemispheres, except for occipital lobes |
| Middle cerebral | Continuation of the internal carotid artery distal to anterior cerebral artery | Most of lateral surface of cerebral hemispheres |
| Posterior cerebral | Terminal branch of basilar artery | Inferior aspect of cerebral hemisphere and occipital lobe |
| Anterior communicating | Anterior cerebral artery | Cerebral arterial circle |
| Posterior communicating | Internal carotid artery | |

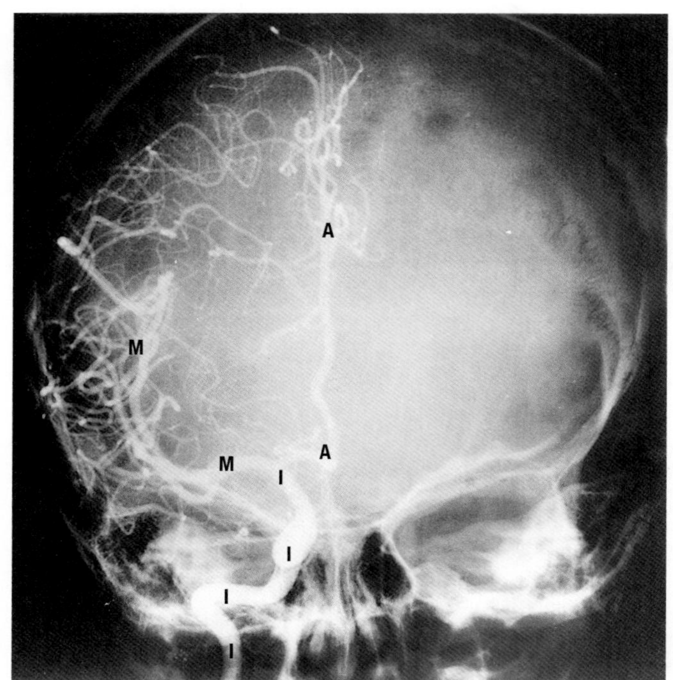
A
M
M
I
A
I
I
I

A. Posteroanterior View

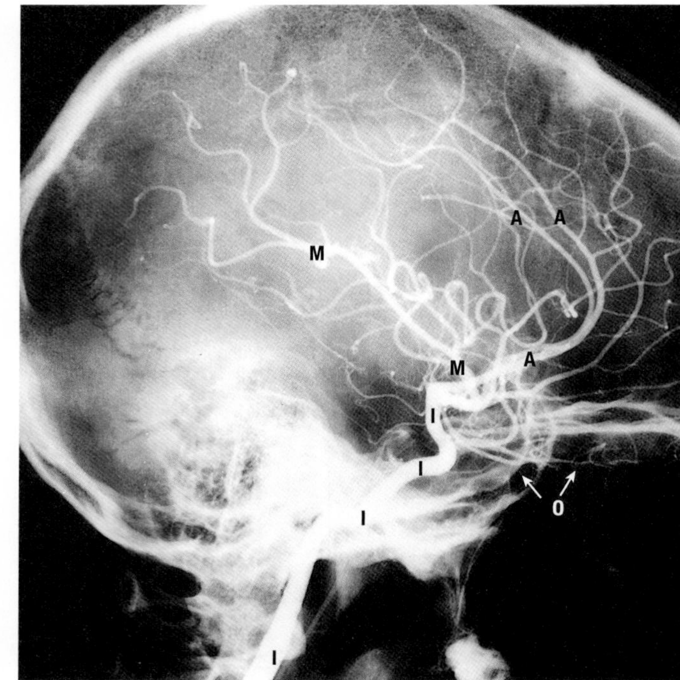
M
A
A
M
A
I
I
I
0
I

B. Lateral View

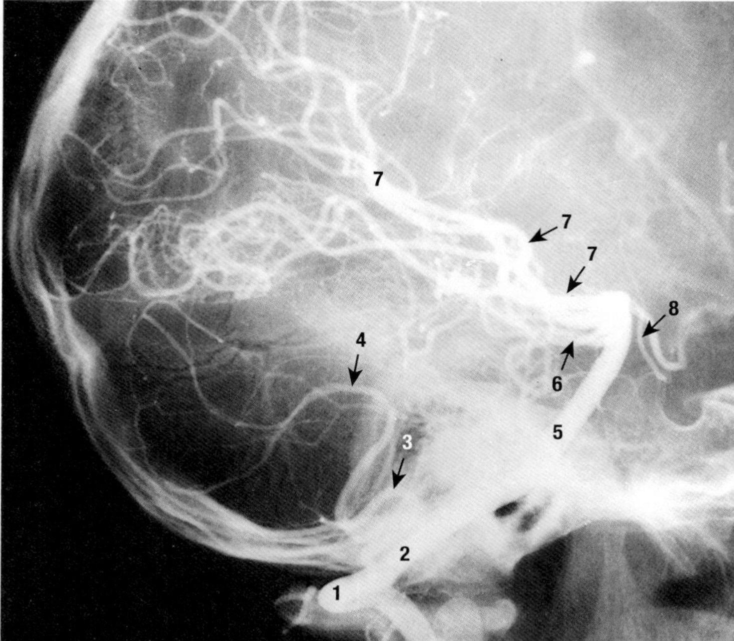
7
7
7
8
4
6
5
3
2
1

C. Lateral View

| | |
|---|---|
| A | Anterior cerebral artery |
| M | Middle cerebral artery |
| I | Internal carotid artery |
| 0 | Ophthalmic artery |
| 1 | Vertebral artery on posterior arch of atlas |
| 2 | Vertebral artery entering skull through foramen magnum |
| 3 | Posterior inferior cerebellar artery |
| 4 | Anterior inferior cerebellar artery |
| 5 | Basilar artery |
| 6 | Superior cerebellar artery |
| 7 | Posterior cerebellar artery |
| 8 | Posterior communicating artery |

## 7.29 Arteriograms

**A** and **B.** Carotid arteriogram. The four letter Is indicate the parts of the internal carotid artery: cervical, before entering the cranium; petrous, within the temporal bone; cavernous, within the sinus; and cerebral, within the cranial subarachnoid space. **C.** Vertebral arteriogram. Transient ischemic attacks (TIAs) refer to neurological symptoms resulting from ischemia (deficient blood supply) of the brain. The symptoms of a TIA may be ambiguous: staggering, dizziness, light-headedness, fainting, and paresthesias (e.g., tingling in a limb). Most TIAs last a few minutes, but some persist longer. Individuals with TIAs are at increased risk for myocardial infarction and ischemic stroke (Brust, 2000).

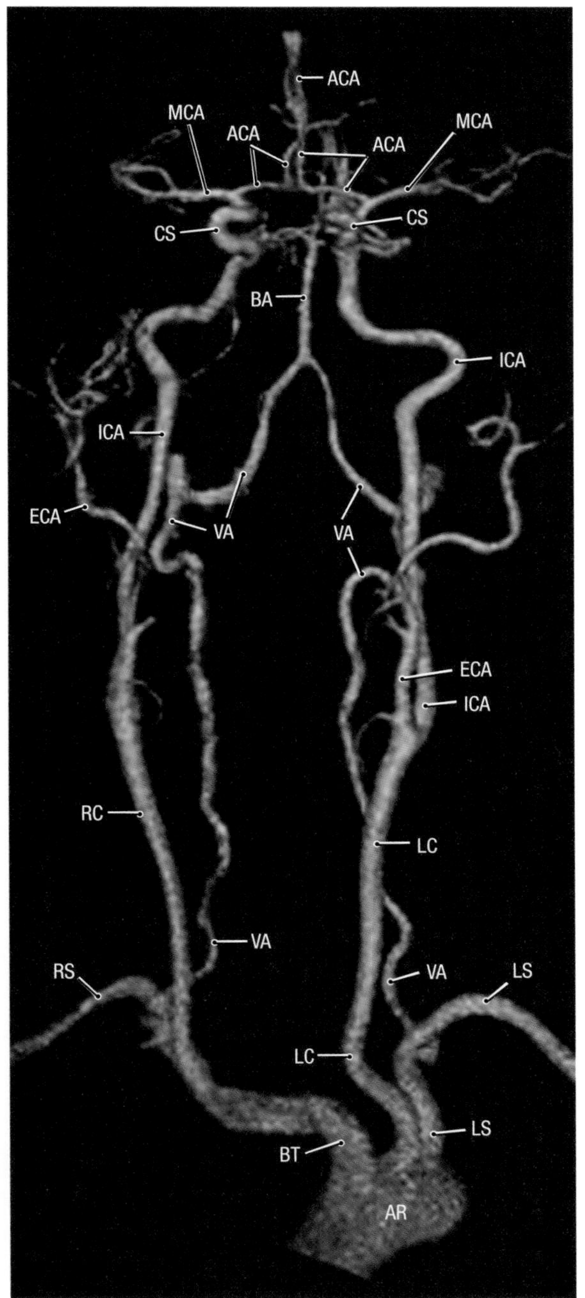
ACA
MCA
ACA
ACA
MCA
CS
CS
BA
ICA
ICA
ECA
VA
VA
ECA
ICA
RC
LC
VA
RS
VA
LS
LC
LS
BT
AR

A. Anterior View

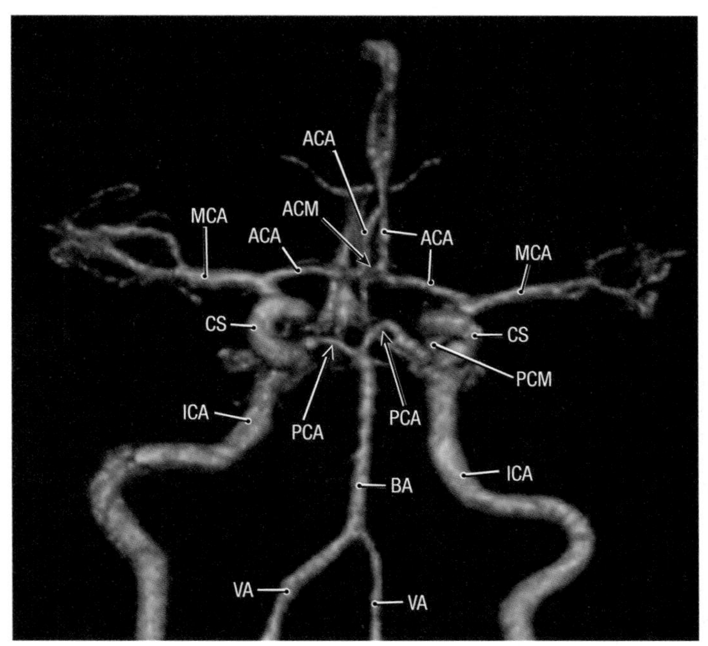
ACA
MCA
ACM
ACA
ACA
MCA
CS
CS
PCM
ICA
PCA
PCA
ICA
BA
VA
VA

B. Anterior View

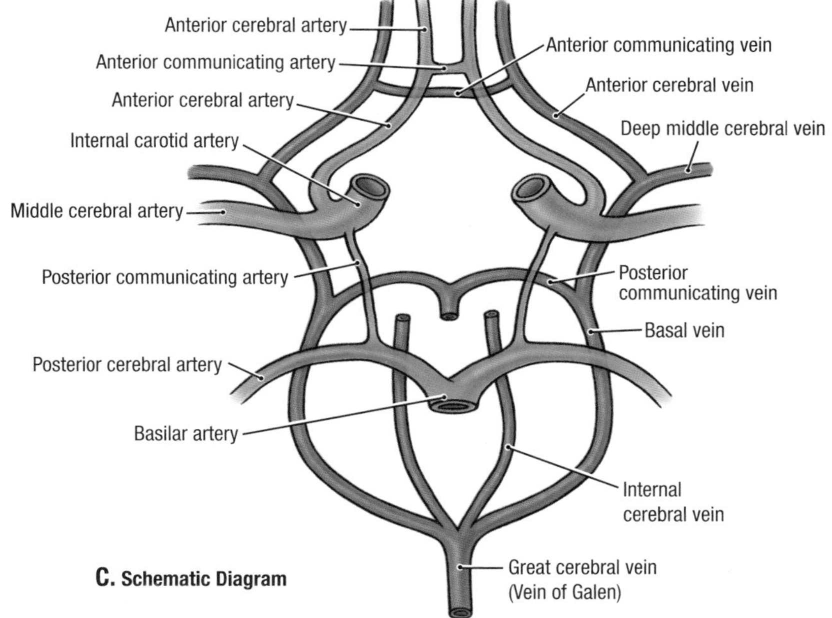
Anterior cerebral artery
Anterior communicating artery
Anterior cerebral artery
Internal carotid artery
Middle cerebral artery
Posterior communicating artery
Posterior cerebral artery
Basilar artery
Anterior communicating vein
Anterior cerebral vein
Deep middle cerebral vein
Posterior communicating vein
Basal vein
Internal cerebral vein
Great cerebral vein (Vein of Galen)

C. Schematic Diagram

| | | | | | | | |
|---|---|---|---|---|---|---|---|
| ACM | Anterior communicating artery | BT | Brachiocephalic trunk | LC | Left common carotid artery | PCM | Posterior communicating artery |
| ACA | Anterior cerebral artery | CS | Carotid siphon | LS | Left subclavian artery | RC | Right common carotid artery |
| AR | Arch of aorta | ECA | External carotid artery | MCA | Middle cerebral artery | RS | Right subclavian artery |
| BA | Basilar artery | ICA | Internal carotid artery | PCA | Posterior cerebral artery | VA | Vertebral artery |

**7.30 Blood supply of head and neck**

**A.** CT angiogram of arteries of head and neck. **B.** CT angiogram of cerebral arterial circle (circle of Willis). **C.** Schematic diagram of cerebral arterial circle and veins of cerebral base.

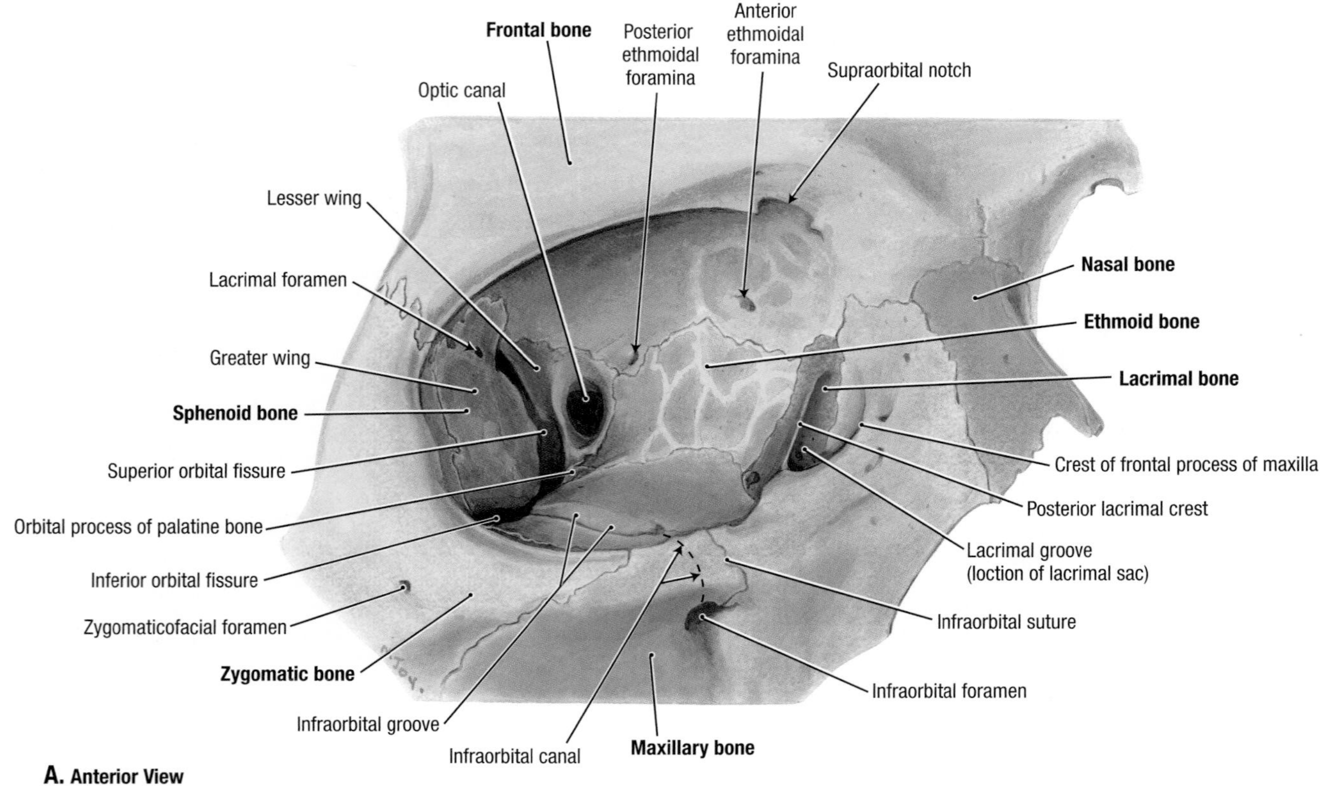

Frontal bone
Posterior ethmoidal foramina
Anterior ethmoidal foramina
Supraorbital notch
Optic canal
Lesser wing
Lacrimal foramen
Greater wing
Sphenoid bone
Superior orbital fissure
Orbital process of palatine bone
Inferior orbital fissure
Zygomaticofacial foramen
Zygomatic bone
Infraorbital groove
Infraorbital canal
Maxillary bone
Nasal bone
Ethmoid bone
Lacrimal bone
Crest of frontal process of maxilla
Posterior lacrimal crest
Lacrimal groove (loction of lacrimal sac)
Infraorbital suture
Infraorbital foramen
A. Anterior View


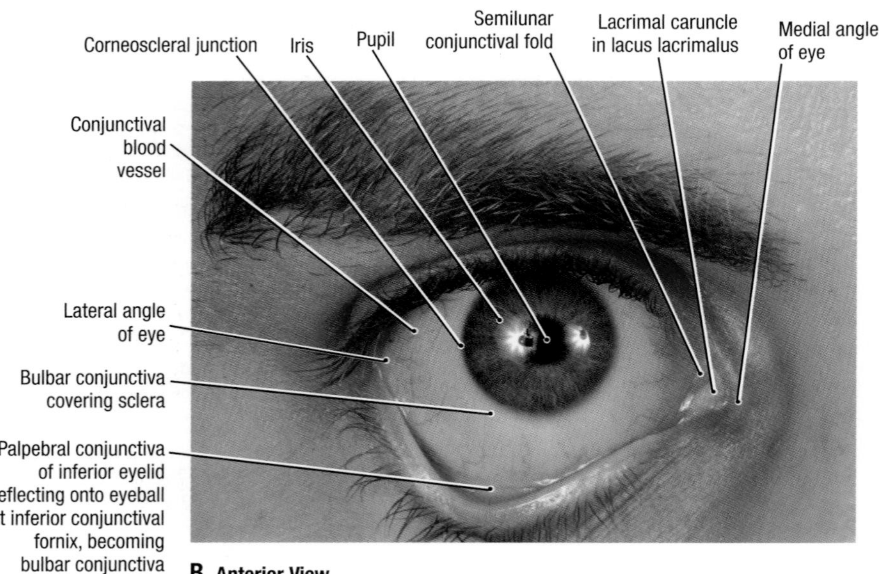

Corneoscleral junction
Iris
Pupil
Semilunar conjunctival fold
Lacrimal caruncle in lacus lacrimalus
Medial angle of eye
Conjunctival blood vessel
Lateral angle of eye
Bulbar conjunctiva covering sclera
Palpebral conjunctiva of inferior eyelid reflecting onto eyeball at inferior conjunctival fornix, becoming bulbar conjunctiva
B. Anterior View


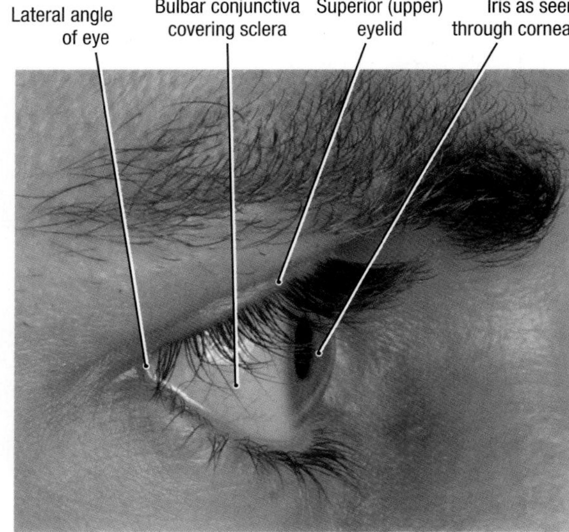

Lateral angle of eye
Bulbar conjunctiva covering sclera
Superior (upper) eyelid
Iris as seen through cornea
C. Lateral View


## 7.31 Orbital cavity and surface anatomy of the eye

**A.** Bones and features of the orbital cavity. **B** and **C.** Surface anatomy of the eye. In **B,** the inferior eyelid is everted to demonstrate the palpebral conjunctiva. When powerful blows impact directly on the bony rim of the orbit, the resulting fractures usually occur at the sutures between the bones forming the orbital margin. Fractures of the medial wall may involve the ethmoidal and sphenoidal sinuses, whereas fractures in the inferior wall may involve the maxillary sinus. Although the superior wall is stronger than the medial and inferior walls, it is thin enough to be translucent and may be readily penetrated. Thus, a sharp object may pass through it into the frontal lobe of the brain. Orbital fractures often result in intraorbital bleeding, which exerts pressure on the eyeball, causing exophthalmos (protrusion of the eyeball).

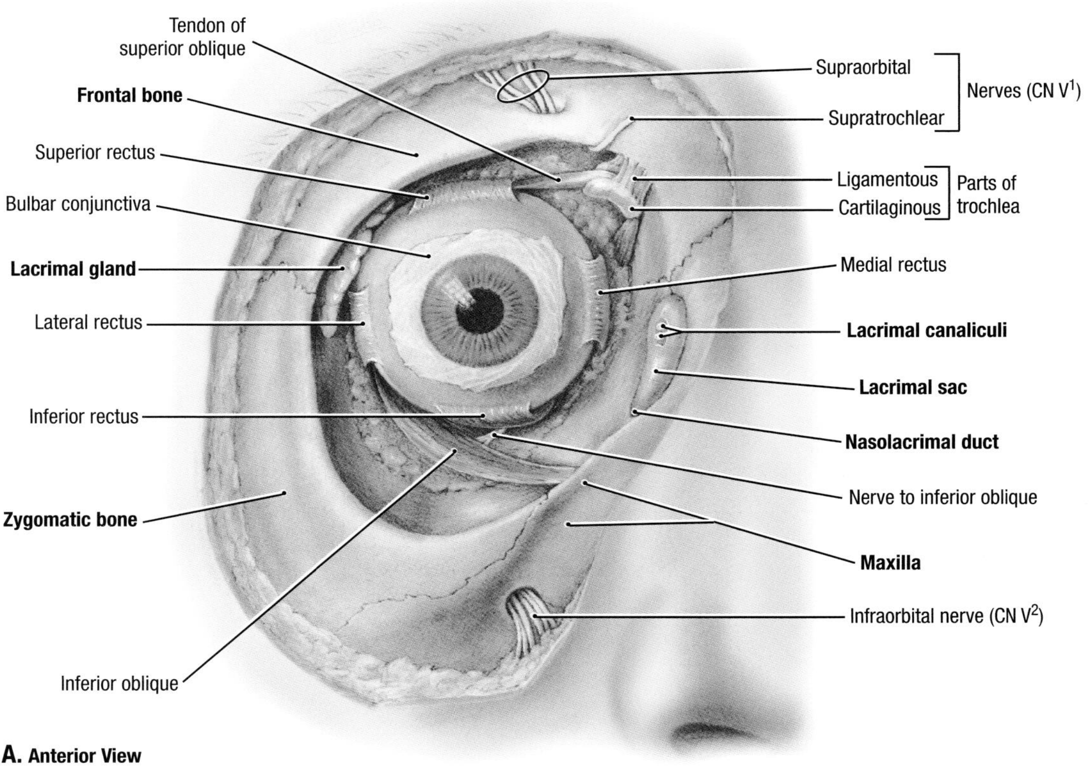
Tendon of superior oblique
Frontal bone
Superior rectus
Bulbar conjunctiva
Lacrimal gland
Lateral rectus
Inferior rectus
Zygomatic bone
Inferior oblique
Supraorbital
Supratrochlear
Nerves (CN V1)
Ligamentous
Cartilaginous
Parts of trochlea
Medial rectus
Lacrimal canaliculi
Lacrimal sac
Nasolacrimal duct
Nerve to inferior oblique
Maxilla
Infraorbital nerve (CN V2)

**A.** Anterior View

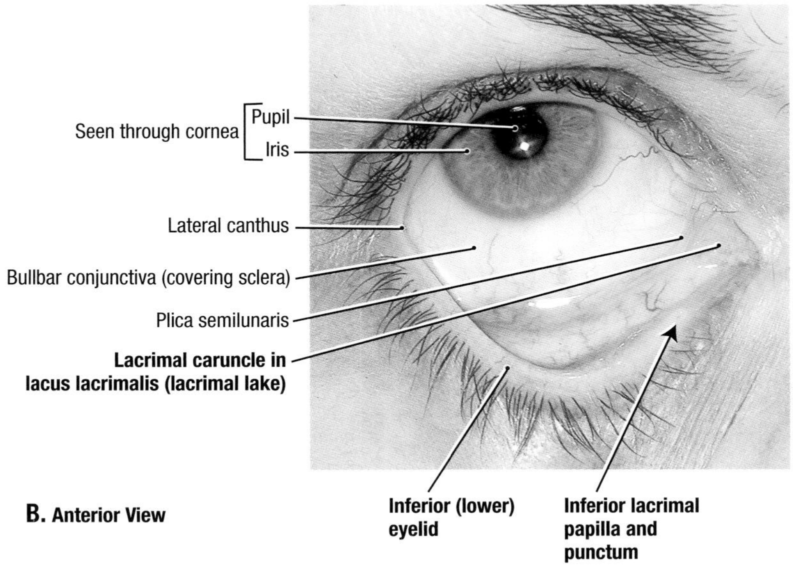
Seen through cornea
Pupil
Iris
Lateral canthus
Bullbar conjunctiva (covering sclera)
Plica semilunaris
Lacrimal caruncle in lacus lacrimalis (lacrimal lake)
Inferior (lower) eyelid
Inferior lacrimal papilla and punctum

**B.** Anterior View

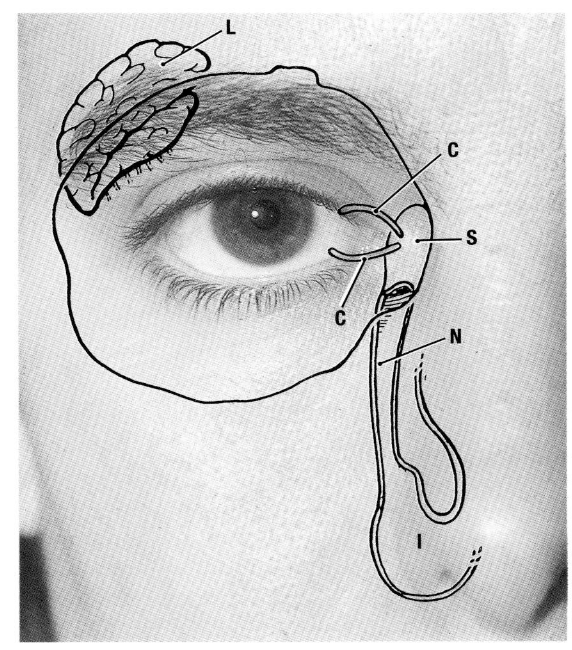
L
C
S
C
N
I

**C.** Anterior View

## 7.32 Eye and lacrimal apparatus

**A.** Anterior dissection of orbital cavity. The eyelids, orbital septum, levator palpebrae superioris, and some fat are removed. **B.** Surface features, with the inferior eyelid everted. **C.** Surface projection of lacrimal apparatus. Tears, secreted by the lacrimal gland *(L)* in the superolateral angle of the bony orbit, pass across the eyeball and enter the lacus lacrimalis (lacrimal lake) at the medial angle of the eye; from here they drain through the lacrimal puncta and lacrimal canaliculi *(C)* to the lacrimal sac *(S)*. The lacrimal sac drains into the nasolacrimal duct *(N)*, which empties into the inferior meatus *(I)* of the nose.

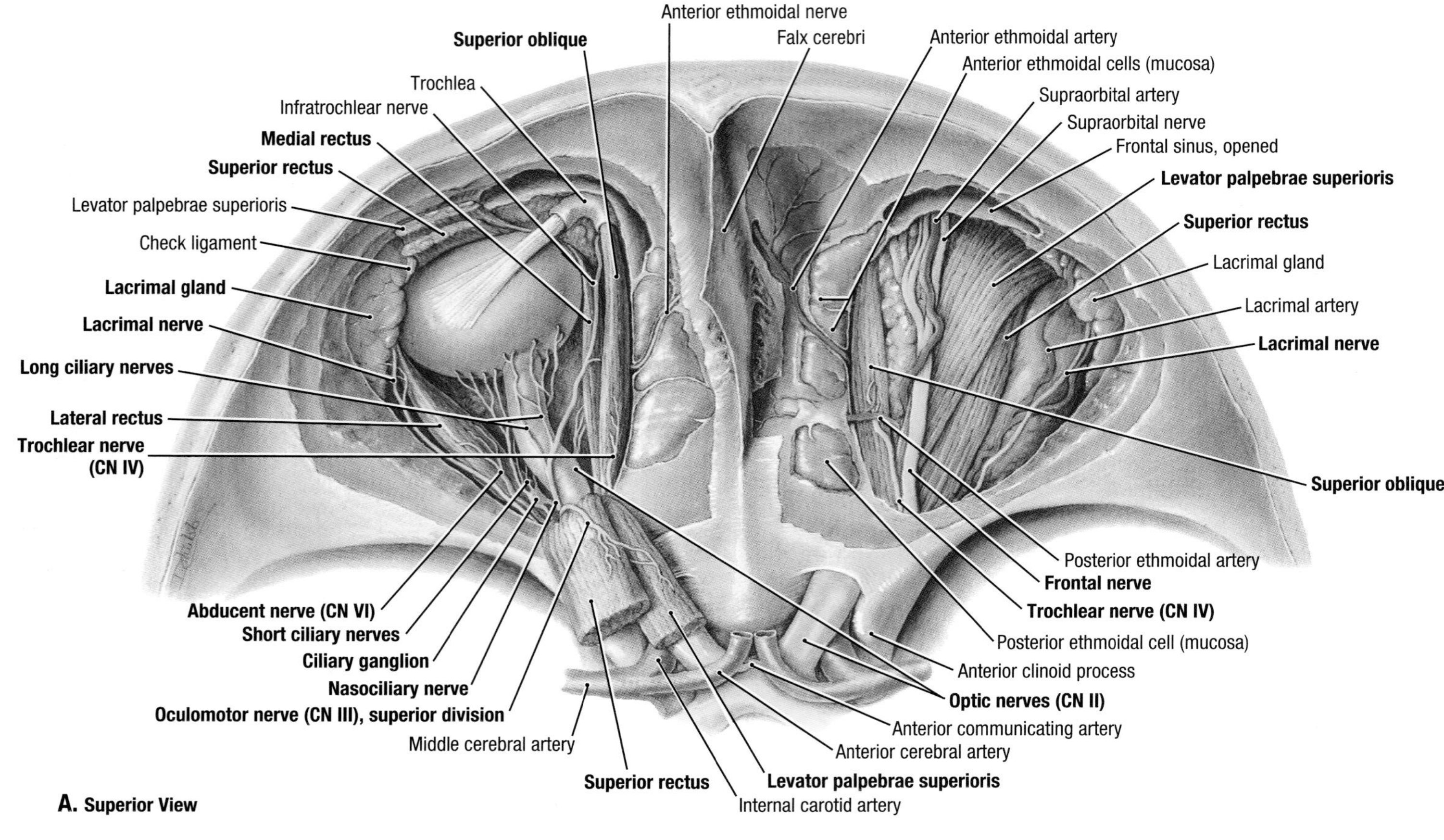
Anterior ethmoidal nerve
Superior oblique
Falx cerebri
Anterior ethmoidal artery
Anterior ethmoidal cells (mucosa)
Trochlea
Infratrochlear nerve
Supraorbital artery
Supraorbital nerve
Medial rectus
Frontal sinus, opened
Superior rectus
Levator palpebrae superioris
Levator palpebrae superioris
Superior rectus
Check ligament
Lacrimal gland
Lacrimal gland
Lacrimal artery
Lacrimal nerve
Lacrimal nerve
Long ciliary nerves
Lateral rectus
Trochlear nerve (CN IV)
Superior oblique
Posterior ethmoidal artery
Frontal nerve
Abducent nerve (CN VI)
Trochlear nerve (CN IV)
Short ciliary nerves
Posterior ethmoidal cell (mucosa)
Ciliary ganglion
Anterior clinoid process
Nasociliary nerve
Optic nerves (CN II)
Oculomotor nerve (CN III), superior division
Anterior communicating artery
Middle cerebral artery
Anterior cerebral artery
Superior rectus
Levator palpebrae superioris
Internal carotid artery

**A.** Superior View

## 7.33 Orbital cavity, superior approach

**A.** Superficial dissection.

On the right side of figure **A:**

- The orbital plate of the frontal bone is removed.
- The levator palpebrae superioris muscle lies superficial to the superior rectus muscle.
- The trochlear, frontal, and lacrimal nerves lie immediately inferior to the roof of the orbital cavity.

On the left side of figure **A:**

- The levator palpebrae and superior rectus muscles are reflected.
- The superior division of the oculomotor nerve (CN III) supplies the superior rectus and levator palpebrae muscles.
- The trochlear nerve (CN IV) lies on the medial side of the superior oblique muscle, and the abducent nerve (CN VI) on the medial side of the lateral rectus muscle.
- The lacrimal nerve runs superior to the lateral rectus muscle supplying sensory fibers to the conjunctiva and skin of the superior eyelid; it receives a communicating branch of the zygomaticotemporal nerve carrying secretory motor fibers from the pterygopalatine ganglion to the lacrimal gland.
- The parasympathetic ciliary ganglion, placed between the lateral rectus muscle and the optic nerve (CN II), gives rise to many short ciliary nerves; the nasociliary nerve gives rise to two long ciliary nerves that anastomose with each other and the short ciliary nerves.

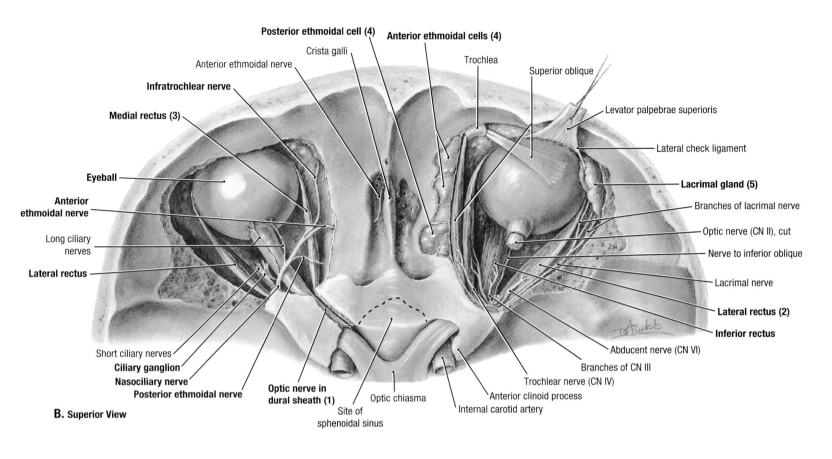

Posterior ethmoidal cell (4)
Anterior ethmoidal cells (4)
Crista galli
Anterior ethmoidal nerve
Trochlea
Superior oblique
Infratrochlear nerve
Levator palpebrae superioris
Medial rectus (3)
Lateral check ligament
Eyeball
Lacrimal gland (5)
Anterior ethmoidal nerve
Branches of lacrimal nerve
Optic nerve (CN II), cut
Long ciliary nerves
Nerve to inferior oblique
Lateral rectus
Lacrimal nerve
Lateral rectus (2)
Inferior rectus
Abducent nerve (CN VI)
Short ciliary nerves
Branches of CN III
Ciliary ganglion
Nasociliary nerve
Trochlear nerve (CN IV)
Posterior ethmoidal nerve
Optic nerve in dural sheath (1)
Optic chiasma
Anterior clinoid process
Site of sphenoidal sinus
Internal carotid artery

**B.** Superior View

## 7.33 Orbital cavity, superior approach *(continued)*

**B.** Deep dissection before *(left side)* and after *(right side)* section of the optic nerve (CN II). **C.** Transverse (axial) MRI of orbital cavity. (The *numbers* refer to structures labeled in **B**).

Observe on the right side of figure **B:**

- The eyeball occupies the anterior half of the orbital cavity.
- Nerves supplying the four recti (superior, medial, inferior, lateral) enter their ocular surfaces (the superior rectus is not shown).

Observe on the left of figure **B:**

- The parasympathetic ciliary ganglion lies posteriorly between the lateral rectus muscle and the sheath of the optic nerve.
- The nasociliary nerve (CN $V^1$) sends a branch to the ciliary ganglion and crosses the optic nerve (CN II), where it gives off two long ciliary nerves (sensory to the eyeball and cornea) and the posterior ethmoidal nerve (to the sphenoidal sinus and posterior ethmoidal cells). The nasociliary nerve then divides into the anterior ethmoidal and infratrochlear nerves.

Because of the closeness of the optic nerve to the sphenoidal sinus and posterior ethmoidal cell, a malignant tumor in these sinuses may erode the thin bony walls of the orbit and compress the optic nerve and orbital contents. Tumors in the orbit produce exophthalmos. A tumor in the middle cranial fossa may enter the orbital cavity through the superior orbital fissure.

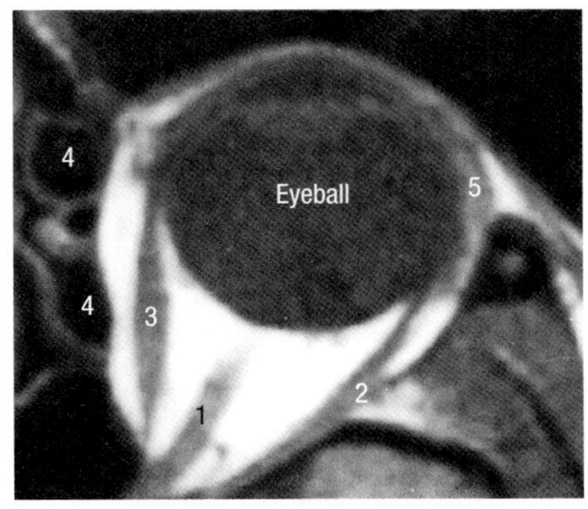
4
Eyeball
5
4
3
2
1

**C.** Axial MRI

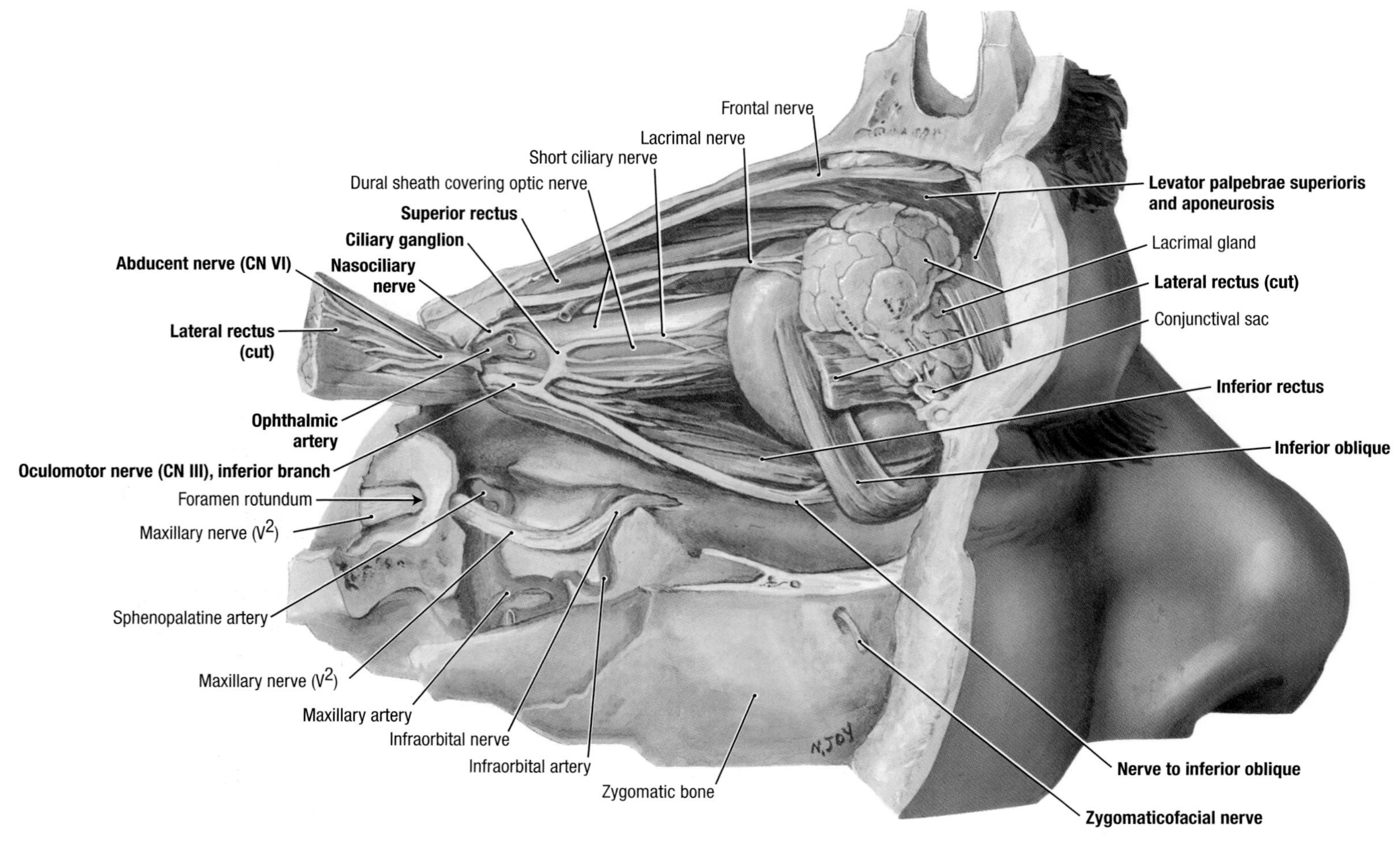
Frontal nerve
Lacrimal nerve
Short ciliary nerve
Dural sheath covering optic nerve
Superior rectus
Ciliary ganglion
Abducent nerve (CN VI)
Nasociliary nerve
Lateral rectus (cut)
Ophthalmic artery
Oculomotor nerve (CN III), inferior branch
Foramen rotundum
Maxillary nerve (V2)
Sphenopalatine artery
Maxillary nerve (V2)
Maxillary artery
Infraorbital nerve
Infraorbital artery
Zygomatic bone
Levator palpebrae superioris and aponeurosis
Lacrimal gland
Lateral rectus (cut)
Conjunctival sac
Inferior rectus
Inferior oblique
Nerve to inferior oblique
Zygomaticofacial nerve
N. JOY

## 7.34 Lateral aspect of the orbit and structure of the eyelid

- The ciliary ganglion receives sensory fibers from the nasociliary branches of VI, postsynaptic sympathetic fibers from the continuation of the internal carotid plexus extending along the ophthalmic artery, and presynaptic parasympathetic fibers from the inferior branch of the oculomotor nerve; only the latter synapse in the ganglion.
- Complete oculomotor nerve palsy affects most of the ocular muscles, the levator palpebrae superioris, and the sphincter pupillae. The superior eyelid droops (ptosis) and cannot be raised voluntarily because of the unopposed activity of the orbicularis oculi (supplied by the facial nerve). The pupil is also fully dilated and nonreactive because of the unopposed dilator pupillae. The pupil is fully abducted and depressed ("down and out") because of the unopposed activity of the lateral rectus and superior oblique, respectively.
- A lesion of the abducent nerve results in loss of lateral gaze to the ipsilateral side because of paralysis of the lateral rectus muscle. On forward gaze, the eye is diverted medially because of the lack of normal resting tone in the lateral rectus, resulting in diplopia (double vision). Horner syndrome results from interruption of a cervical sympathetic trunk and is manifest by the absence of sympathetically stimulated functions on the ipsilateral side of the head. The syndrome includes the following signs: constriction of the pupil (miosis), drooping of the superior eyelid (ptosis), redness and increased temperature of the skin (vasodilatation), and absence of sweating (anhydrosis).

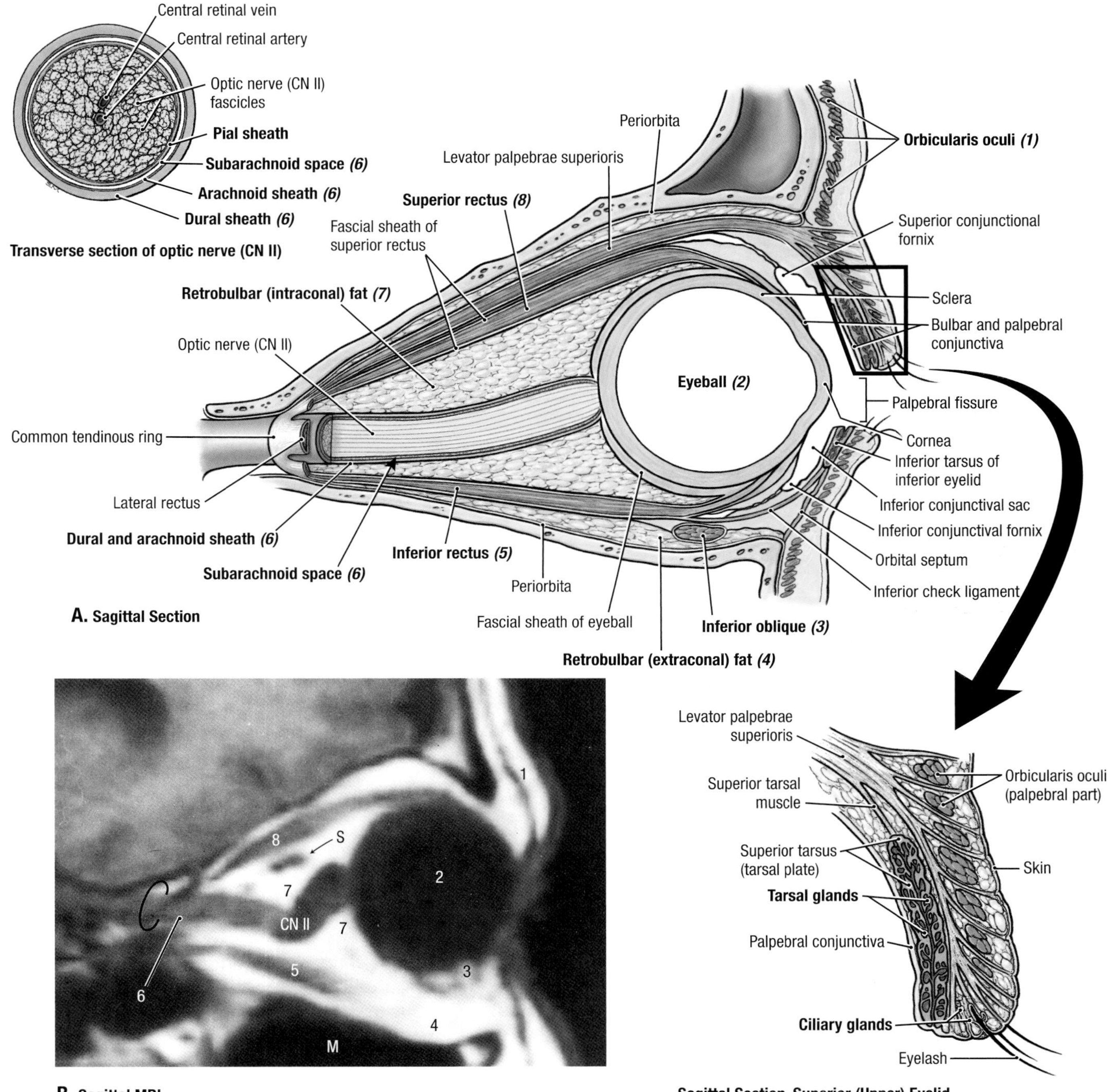
Central retinal vein
Central retinal artery
Optic nerve (CN II) fascicles
Pial sheath
Subarachnoid space (6)
Arachnoid sheath (6)
Dural sheath (6)
Transverse section of optic nerve (CN II)
Periorbita
Levator palpebrae superioris
Orbicularis oculi (1)
Superior rectus (8)
Fascial sheath of superior rectus
Superior conjunctional fornix
Retrobulbar (intraconal) fat (7)
Sclera
Bulbar and palpebral conjunctiva
Optic nerve (CN II)
Eyeball (2)
Palpebral fissure
Common tendinous ring
Cornea
Inferior tarsus of inferior eyelid
Lateral rectus
Inferior conjunctival sac
Inferior conjunctival fornix
Dural and arachnoid sheath (6)
Inferior rectus (5)
Orbital septum
Subarachnoid space (6)
Periorbita
Inferior check ligament
A. Sagittal Section
Fascial sheath of eyeball
Inferior oblique (3)
Retrobulbar (extraconal) fat (4)
1
8
S
2
7
CN II
7
5
3
6
4
M
B. Sagittal MRI
Levator palpebrae superioris
Superior tarsal muscle
Orbicularis oculi (palpebral part)
Superior tarsus (tarsal plate)
Skin
Tarsal glands
Palpebral conjunctiva
Ciliary glands
Eyelash
Sagittal Section, Superior (Upper) Eyelid

## 7.35 Lateral aspect of the orbit and structure of the eyelid

**A.** Schematic sagittal and cross-section through optic nerve. **B.** Sagittal MRI. The *numbers* refer to structures labeled in **A;** *S*, superior ophthalmic vein; *M*, maxillary sinus; *circled*, optic foramen.

- Foreign objects, such as sand or metal filings, produce corneal abrasions that cause sudden, stabbing eye pain and tears. Opening and closing the eyelids is also painful. Corneal lacerations are caused by sharp objects such as fingernails or the corner of a page of a book.
- Any of the glands in the eyelid may become inflamed and swollen from infection or obstruction of their ducts. If the ducts of the ciliary glands are obstructed, a painful red suppurative (pus-producing) swelling, a sty (hordeolum), develops on the eyelid. Obstruction of a tarsal gland produces inflammation, a tarsal chalazion, that protrudes toward the eyeball and rubs against it as the eyelids blink.

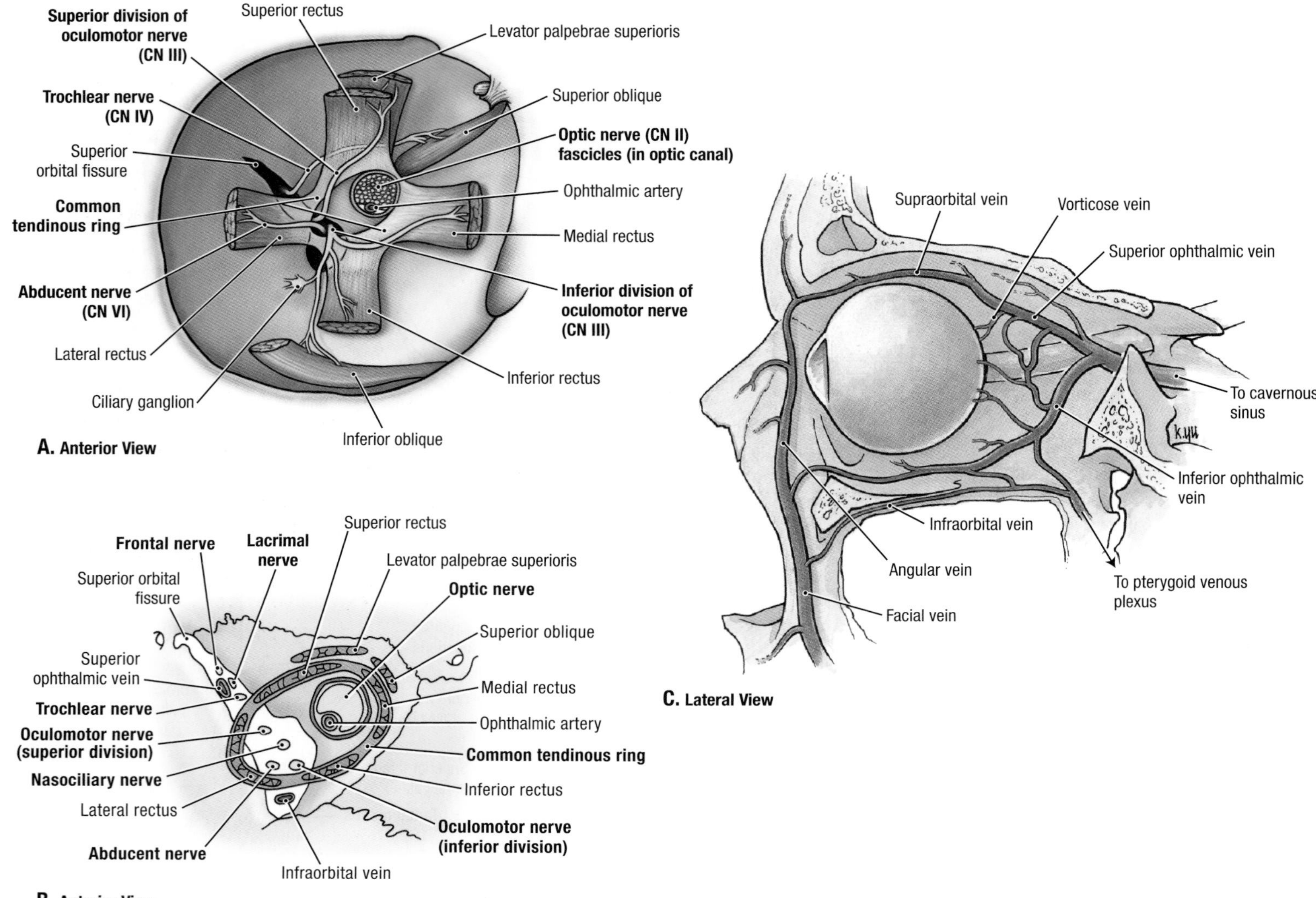
Superior division of oculomotor nerve (CN III)
Superior rectus
Levator palpebrae superioris
Trochlear nerve (CN IV)
Superior oblique
Superior orbital fissure
Optic nerve (CN II) fascicles (in optic canal)
Common tendinous ring
Ophthalmic artery
Medial rectus
Abducent nerve (CN VI)
Inferior division of oculomotor nerve (CN III)
Lateral rectus
Inferior rectus
Ciliary ganglion
Inferior oblique
A. Anterior View
Frontal nerve
Lacrimal nerve
Superior rectus
Levator palpebrae superioris
Superior orbital fissure
Optic nerve
Superior oblique
Superior ophthalmic vein
Trochlear nerve
Medial rectus
Oculomotor nerve (superior division)
Ophthalmic artery
Common tendinous ring
Nasociliary nerve
Inferior rectus
Lateral rectus
Oculomotor nerve (inferior division)
Abducent nerve
Infraorbital vein
B. Anterior View
Supraorbital vein
Vorticose vein
Superior ophthalmic vein
To cavernous sinus
Inferior ophthalmic vein
Infraorbital vein
Angular vein
To pterygoid venous plexus
Facial vein
C. Lateral View

## 7.36 Nerves and veins of the orbit

**A** and **B.** Nerves of orbit in relation to the orbital fissures and the common tendinous ring. The common tendinous ring is formed by the origin of the four recti and encircles the dural sheath of the optic nerve, CN VI, and the superior and inferior branches of CN III; the nasociliary nerve (CN $V^1$) also passes through this cuff. **C.** Ophthalmic veins. The superior and inferior ophthalmic veins receive the vorticose veins from the eyeball and drain into the cavernous sinus posteriorly and the pterygoid plexus inferiorly. They communicate with the facial and supraorbital veins anteriorly.

- The facial veins make clinically important connections with the cavernous sinus through the superior ophthalmic veins. Cavernous sinus thrombosis usually results from infections in the orbit, nasal sinuses, and superior part of the face (the danger triangle). In persons with thrombophlebitis of the facial vein, pieces of an infected thrombus may extend into the cavernous sinus, producing thrombophlebitis of the cavernous sinus. The infection usually involves only one sinus initially but may spread to the opposite side through the intercavernous sinuses.

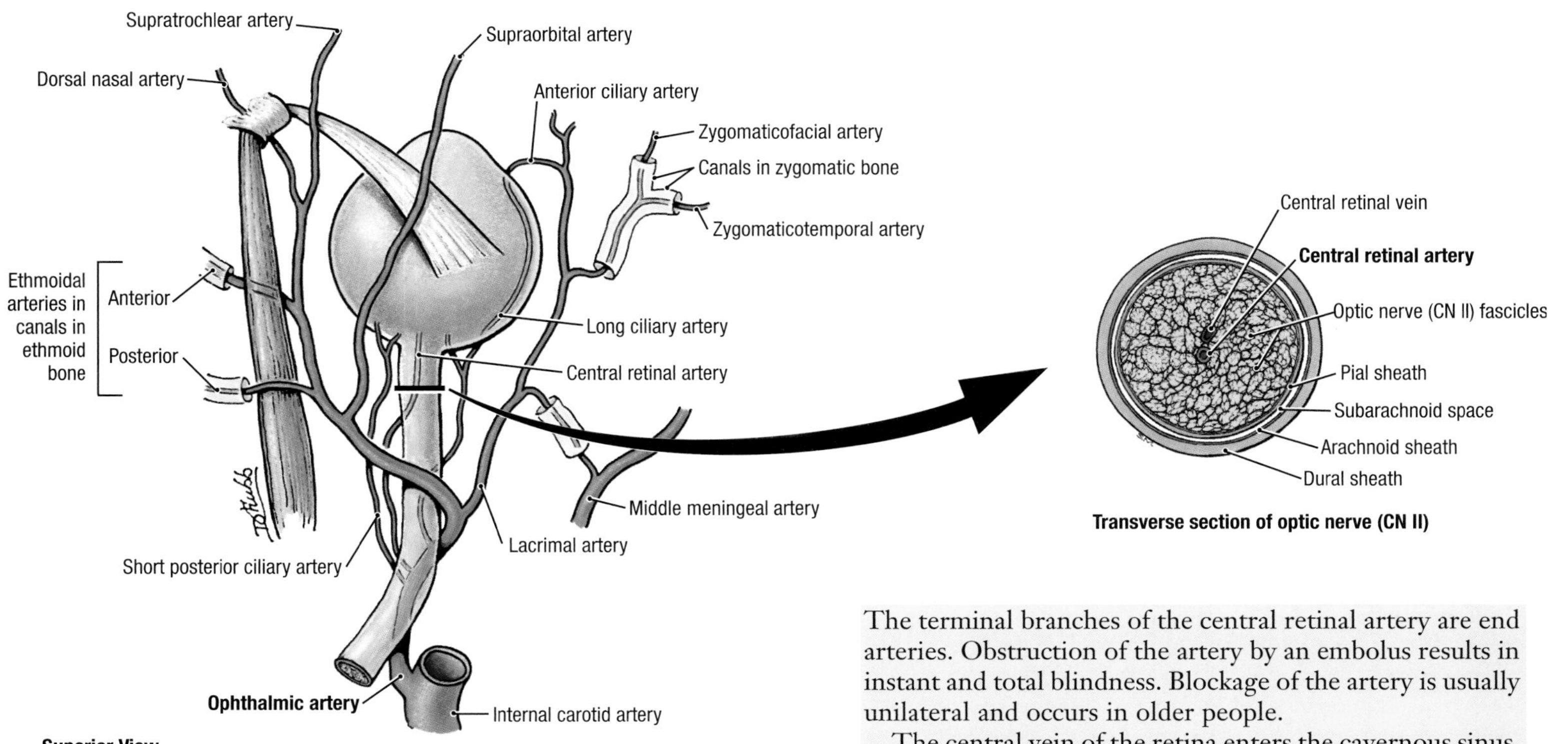
Supratrochlear artery
Dorsal nasal artery
Supraorbital artery
Anterior ciliary artery
Zygomaticofacial artery
Canals in zygomatic bone
Zygomaticotemporal artery
Ethmoidal arteries in canals in ethmoid bone
Anterior
Posterior
Long ciliary artery
Central retinal artery
Middle meningeal artery
Lacrimal artery
Short posterior ciliary artery
Ophthalmic artery
Internal carotid artery
Superior View
Central retinal vein
Central retinal artery
Optic nerve (CN II) fascicles
Pial sheath
Subarachnoid space
Arachnoid sheath
Dural sheath
Transverse section of optic nerve (CN II)

The terminal branches of the central retinal artery are end arteries. Obstruction of the artery by an embolus results in instant and total blindness. Blockage of the artery is usually unilateral and occurs in older people.

The central vein of the retina enters the cavernous sinus. Thrombophlebitis of this sinus may result in passage of a thrombus to the central retinal vein and produce a blockage in one of the small retinal veins. Occlusion of a branch of the central vein of the retina usually results in slow, painless loss of vision.

**TABLE 7.6 ARTERIES OF ORBIT**

| Artery | Origin | Courseand Distribution |
|---|---|---|
| **Ophthalmic** | Internal carotid artery | Traverses optic foramen to reach orbital cavity |
| **Central retinal** | Ophthalmic artery | Runs in dural sheath of optic nerve, entering nerve near eyeball; appears at center of optic disc; supplies optic retina (except cones and rods) |
| **Supraorbital** | | Passes superiorly and posteriorly from supraorbital foramen to supply forehead and scalp |
| **Supratrochlear** | | Passes from supraorbital margin to forehead and scalp |
| **Lacrimal** | | Passes along superior border of lateral rectus muscle to supply lacrimal gland, conjunctiva, and eyelids |
| **Dorsal nasal** | | Courses along dorsal aspect of nose and supplies its surface |
| **Short posterior ciliary** | | Pierces sclera at periphery of optic nerve to supply choroid, which, in turn, supplies cones and rods of optic retina |
| **Long posterior ciliary** | | Pierces sclera to supply ciliary body and iris |
| **Posterior ethmoidal** | | Passes through posterior ethmoidal foramen to posterior ethmoidal cells |
| **Anterior ethmoidal** | | Passes through anterior ethmoidal foramen to anterior cranial fossa; supplies anterior and middle ethmoidal cells, frontal sinus, nasal cavity, and skin on dorsum of nose |
| **Anterior ciliary** | Muscular branches of ophthalmic artery | Pierces sclera at attachments of rectus muscles and forms network in iris and ciliary body |
| **Infraorbital** | Third part of maxillary artery | Passes along infraorbital groove and exits through infraorbital foramen to face |

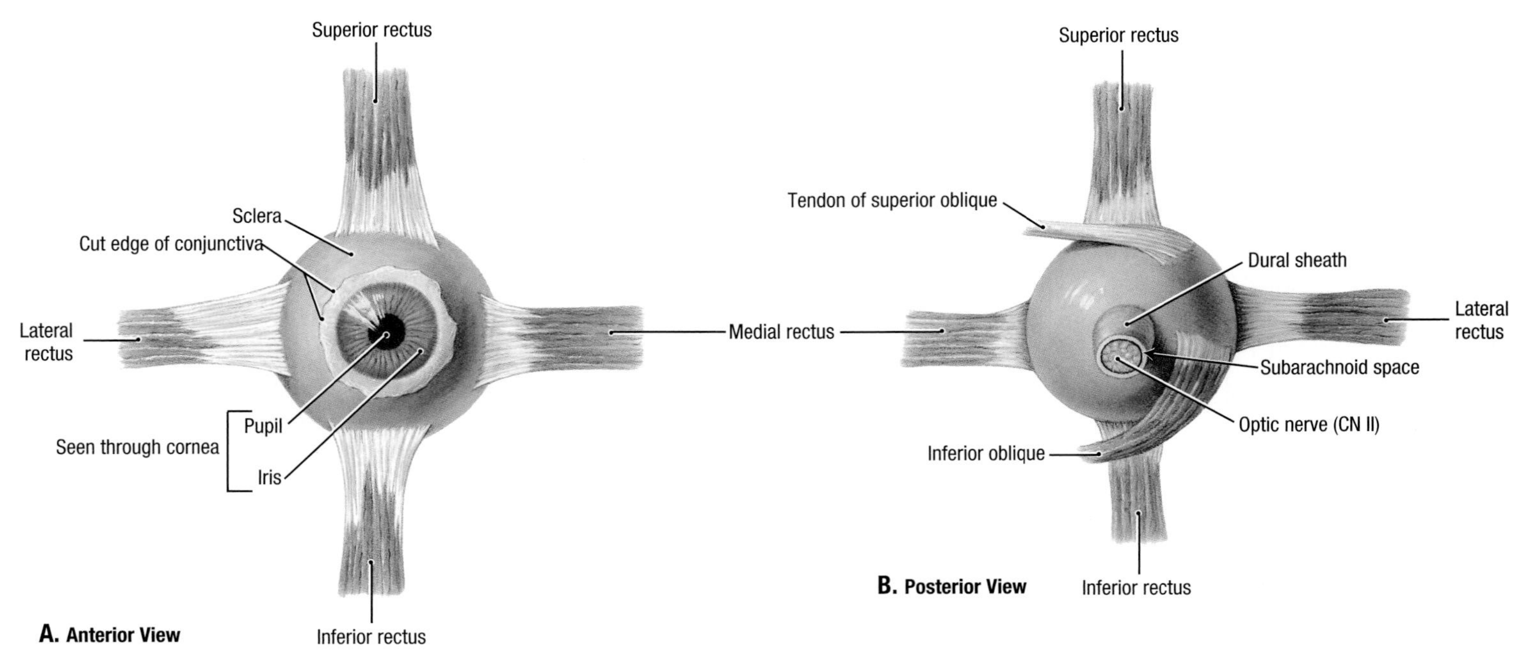
Superior rectus
Sclera
Cut edge of conjunctiva
Lateral rectus
Medial rectus
Seen through cornea
Pupil
Iris
Inferior rectus
A. Anterior View
Superior rectus
Tendon of superior oblique
Dural sheath
Lateral rectus
Subarachnoid space
Optic nerve (CN II)
Inferior oblique
Inferior rectus
B. Posterior View

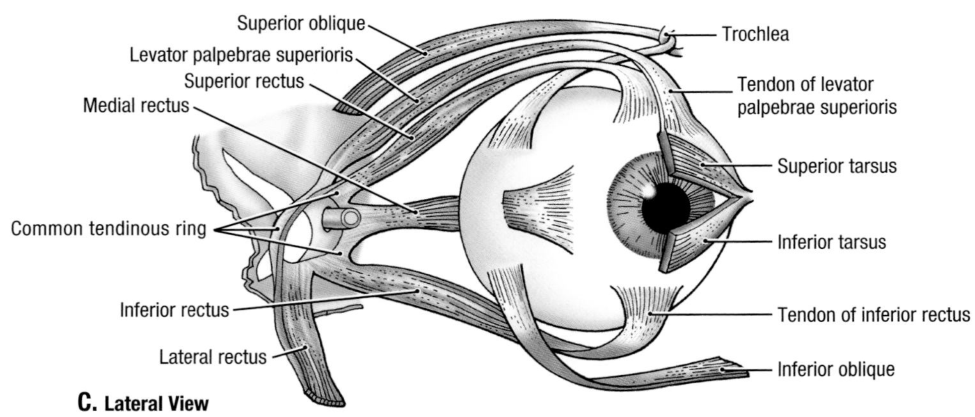
Superior oblique
Levator palpebrae superioris
Superior rectus
Medial rectus
Trochlea
Tendon of levator palpebrae superioris
Superior tarsus
Common tendinous ring
Inferior tarsus
Inferior rectus
Tendon of inferior rectus
Lateral rectus
Inferior oblique
C. Lateral View

## TABLE 7.7 MUSCLES OF ORBIT

| Muscle | Origin | Insertion | Innervation | Main Action |
|---|---|---|---|---|
| **Levator palpebrae superioris** | Lesser wing of sphenoid bone, superior and anterior to optic canal | Tarsal plate and skin of superior (upper) eyelid | Oculomotor nerve (CN III); deep layer (superior tarsal muscle) is supplied by sympathetic fibers | Elevates superior (upper) eyelid |
| **Superior rectus** | Common tendinous ring | Sclera just posterior to cornea | Oculomotor nerve (CN III) | Elevates, adducts, and rotates eyeball medially |
| **Inferior rectus** | | | | Depresses, adducts, and rotates eyeball laterally |
| **Lateral rectus** | | | Abducent nerve (CN VI) | Abducts eyeball |
| **Medial rectus** | | | Oculomotor nerve (CN III) | Adducts eyeball |
| **Superior oblique** | Body of sphenoid bone | Its tendon passes through the trochlea (fibrous ring), changes its direction, and inserts into sclera deep to superior rectus muscle | Trochlear nerve (CN IV) | Abducts, depresses, and medially rotates eyeball |
| **Inferior oblique** | Anterior part of floor of orbit | Sclera deep to lateral rectus muscle | Oculomotor nerve (CN III) | Abducts, elevates, and laterally rotates eyeball |

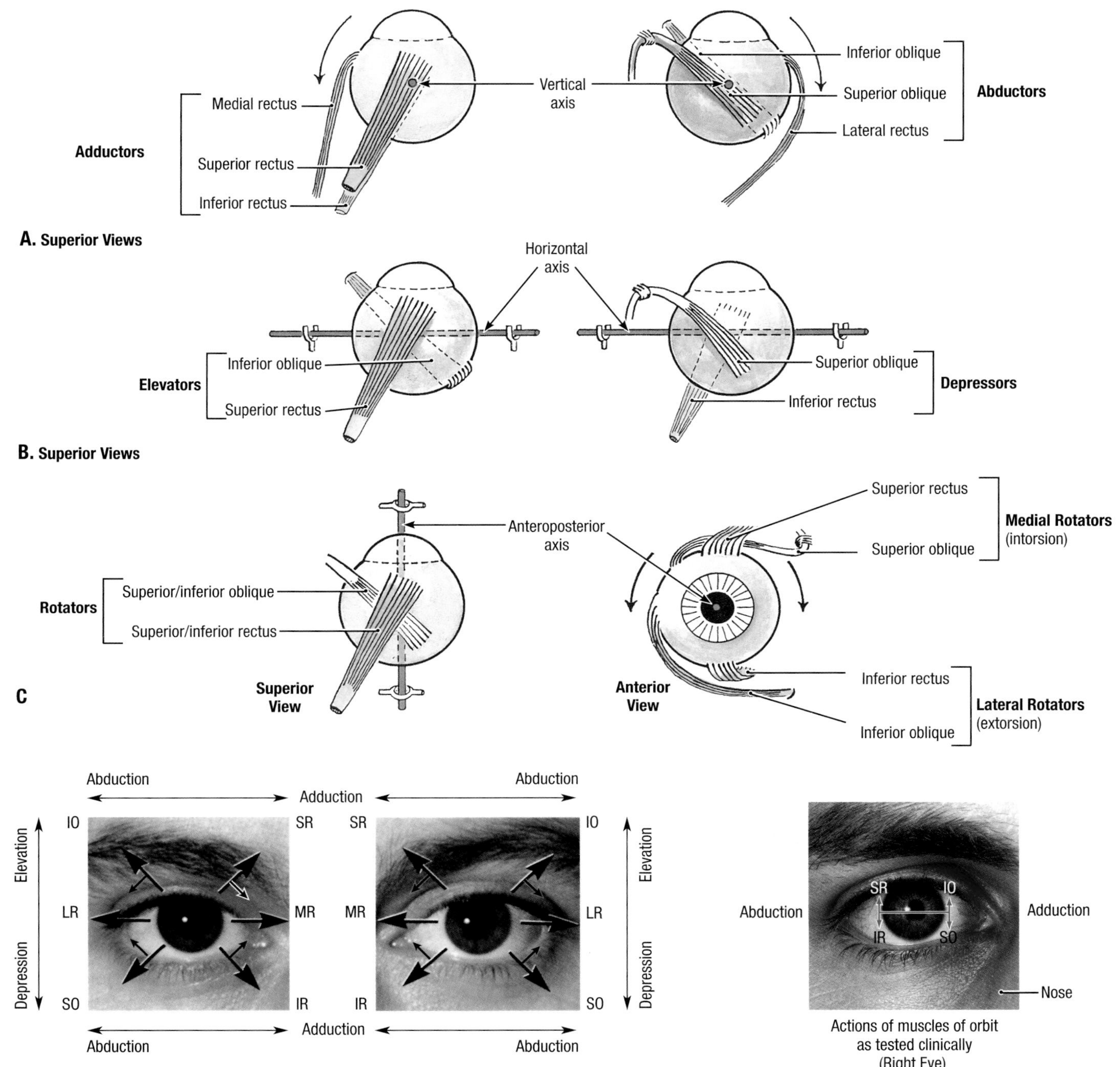

Medial rectus
Adductors
Superior rectus
Inferior rectus
Vertical axis
Inferior oblique
Superior oblique
Lateral rectus
Abductors
A. Superior Views
Horizontal axis
Elevators
Inferior oblique
Superior rectus
Superior oblique
Inferior rectus
Depressors
B. Superior Views
Anteroposterior axis
Superior rectus
Superior oblique
Medial Rotators (intorsion)
Rotators
Superior/inferior oblique
Superior/inferior rectus
C
Superior View
Anterior View
Inferior rectus
Inferior oblique
Lateral Rotators (extorsion)
Abduction
Adduction
Abduction
IO
SR
SR
IO
Elevation
LR
MR
MR
LR
Depression
SO
IR
IR
SO
Abduction
Adduction
Abduction
Anterior View
Abduction
SR
IO
IR
SO
Adduction
Nose


Actions of muscles of orbit as tested clinically (Right Eye)

Movement from the primary position always involves more than one muscle acting synergistically. When testing muscles, it is desirable to test actions produced by one muscle acting independently. Because the axes of the orbits diverge and do not correspond to the axis of gaze in the primary position, responsibility for elevation and depression changes with abduction and adduction. When the eye is adducted, the oblique muscles are solely responsible; when the eye is abducted, the rectus muscles are solely responsible.

## TABLE 7.8 ACTIONS OF MUSCLES OF THE ORBIT STARTING FROM PRIMARY POSITION[a]

| Muscle | Main Action | | |
|---|---|---|---|
| | Vertical Axis (A) | Horizontal Axis (B) | Anteroposterior Axis (C) |
| Superior rectus (SR) | Elevates | Adducts | Rotates medially (intorsion) |
| Inferior rectus (IR) | Depresses | Adducts | Rotates laterally (extorsion) |
| Superior oblique (SO) | Depresses | Abducts | Rotates medially (intorsion) |
| Inferior oblique (IO) | Elevates | Abducts | Rotates laterally (extorsion) |
| Medial rectus (MR) | N/A | Adducts | N/A |
| Lateral rectus (LR) | N/A | Abducts | N/A |

[a] Primary position, gaze directed anteriorly.

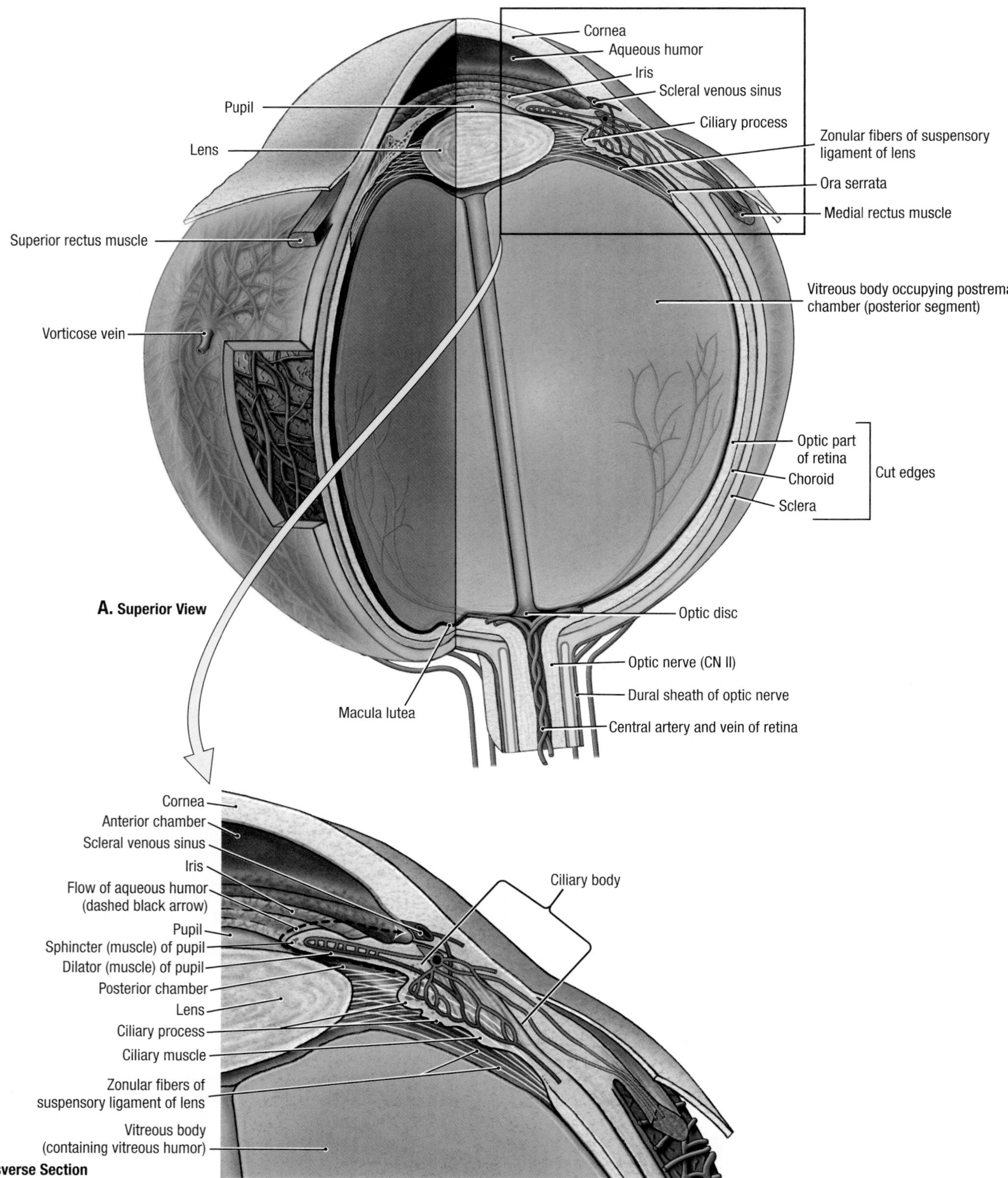
Cornea
Aqueous humor
Iris
Scleral venous sinus
Pupil
Ciliary process
Lens
Zonular fibers of suspensory ligament of lens
Ora serrata
Medial rectus muscle
Superior rectus muscle
Vitreous body occupying postremal chamber (posterior segment)
Vorticose vein
Optic part of retina
Choroid
Sclera
Cut edges
A. Superior View
Optic disc
Optic nerve (CN II)
Dural sheath of optic nerve
Macula lutea
Central artery and vein of retina
Cornea
Anterior chamber
Scleral venous sinus
Iris
Ciliary body
Flow of aqueous humor (dashed black arrow)
Pupil
Sphincter (muscle) of pupil
Dilator (muscle) of pupil
Posterior chamber
Lens
Ciliary process
Ciliary muscle
Zonular fibers of suspensory ligament of lens
Vitreous body (containing vitreous humor)
B. Transverse Section

## 7.37 Illustration of a dissected eyeball

**A.** Parts of the eyeball. **B.** Ciliary region. The aqueous humor is produced by the ciliary processes and provides nutrients for the avascular cornea and lens; the aqueous humor drains into the scleral venous sinus (also called the *sinus venosus sclerae* or *canal of Schlemm*). If drainage of the aqueous humor is reduced significantly, pressure builds up in the chambers of the eye (glaucoma). Blindness can result from compression of the inner layer of the retina and retinal arteries if aqueous humor production is not reduced to maintain normal intraocular pressure.

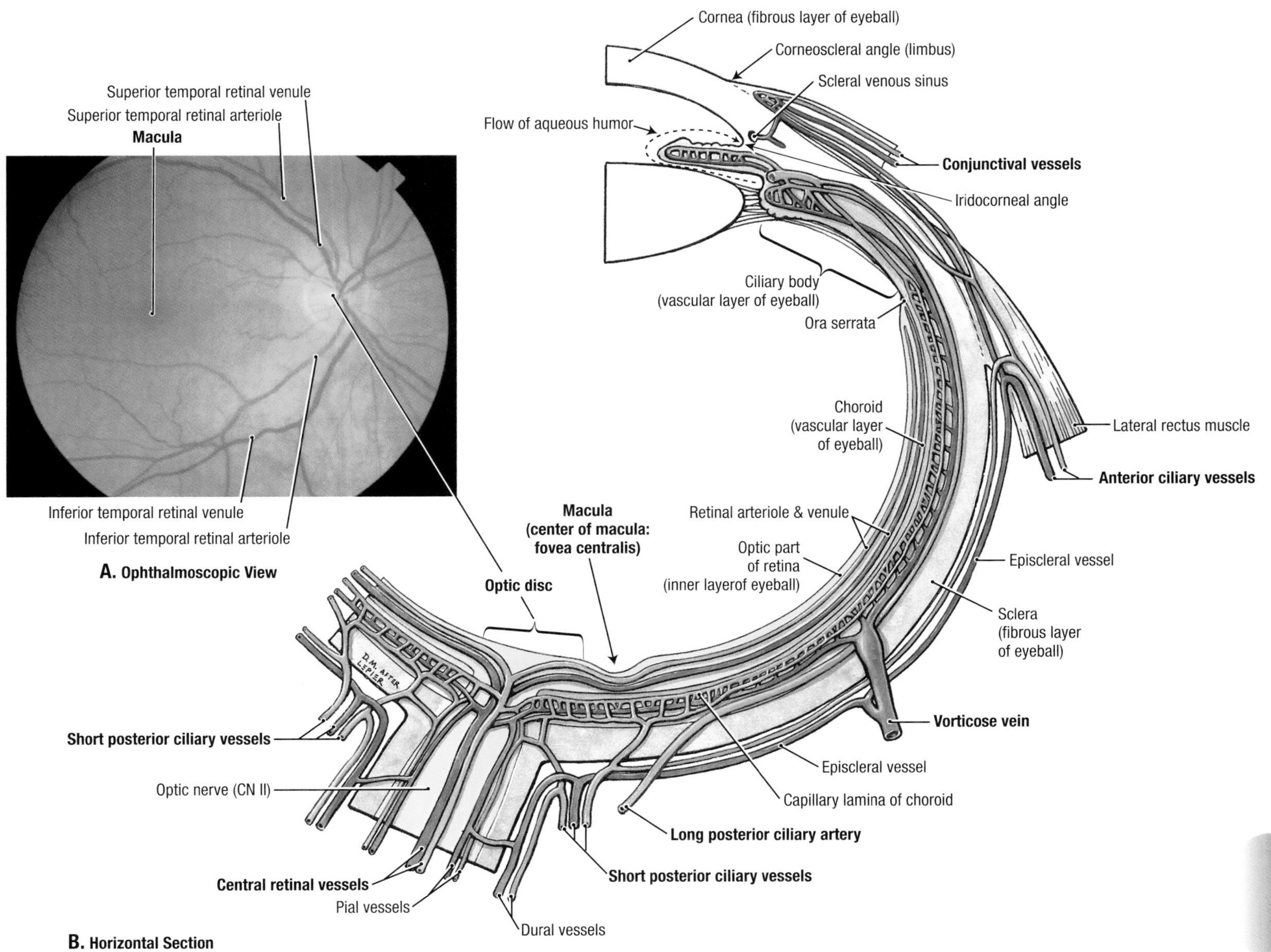
Superior temporal retinal venule
Superior temporal retinal arteriole
Macula
Inferior temporal retinal venule
Inferior temporal retinal arteriole
A. Ophthalmoscopic View
Cornea (fibrous layer of eyeball)
Corneoscleral angle (limbus)
Scleral venous sinus
Flow of aqueous humor
Conjunctival vessels
Iridocorneal angle
Ciliary body
(vascular layer of eyeball)
Ora serrata
Choroid
(vascular layer
of eyeball)
Lateral rectus muscle
Anterior ciliary vessels
Macula
(center of macula:
fovea centralis)
Retinal arteriole & venule
Optic part
of retina
(inner layerof eyeball)
Optic disc
Episcleral vessel
Sclera
(fibrous layer
of eyeball)
Vorticose vein
Short posterior ciliary vessels
Optic nerve (CN II)
Episcleral vessel
Capillary lamina of choroid
Long posterior ciliary artery
Short posterior ciliary vessels
Central retinal vessels
Pial vessels
Dural vessels
B. Horizontal Section

## 7.38 Ocular fundus and blood supply to the eyeball

**A.** Right ocular fundus, ophthalmoscopic view. Retinal venules (wider) and retinal arterioles (narrower) radiate from the center of the oval optic disc, formed in relation to the entry of the optic nerve into the eyeball. The round, dark area lateral to the disc is the macula; branches of vessels extend to this area, but do not reach its center, the fovea centralis, a depressed spot that is the area of most acute vision. It is avascular but, like the rest of the outermost (cones and rods) layer of the retina, is nourished by the adjacent choriocapillaris. An increase in CSF pressure slows venous return from the retina, causing edema of the retina (fluid accumulation). The edema is viewed during ophthalmoscopy as swelling of the optic disc, a condition called papilledema. **B.** Blood supply to eyeball. The eyeball has three layers: (a) the external, fibrous layer is the sclera and cornea; (b) the middle, vascular layer is the choroid, ciliary body, and iris; and (c) the internal, neural layer or retina consists of a pigment cell layer and a neural layer. The central artery of the retina, a branch of the ophthalmic artery, is an end artery. Of the eight posterior ciliary arteries, six are short posterior ciliary arteries and supply the choroid, which in turn nourishes the outer, nonvascular layer of the retina. Two long posterior ciliary arteries, one on each side of the eyeball, run between the sclera and choroid to anastomose with the anterior ciliary arteries, which are derived from muscular branches. The choroid is drained by posterior ciliary veins, and four to five vorticose veins drain into the ophthalmic veins.

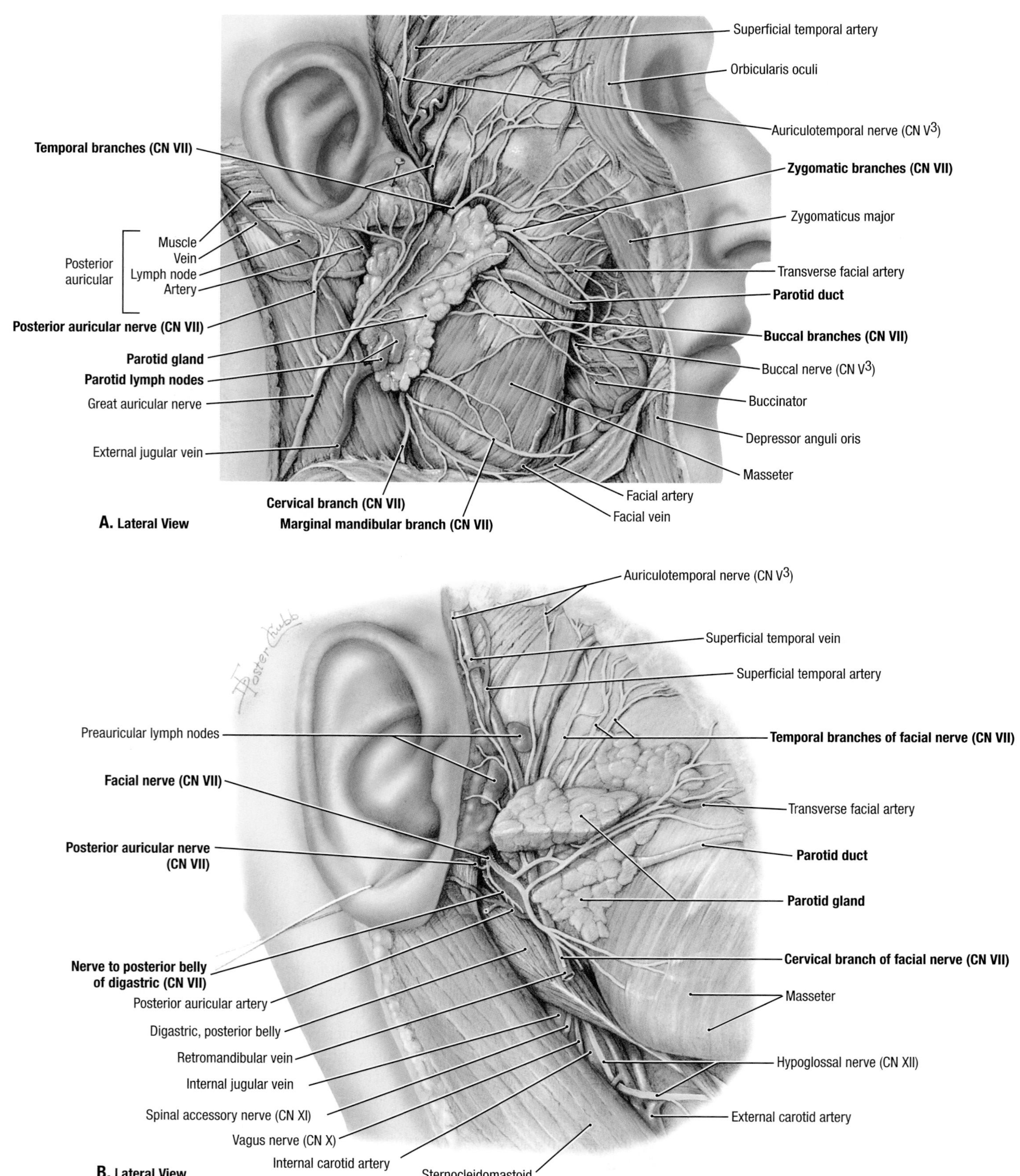
Superficial temporal artery
Orbicularis oculi
Auriculotemporal nerve (CN V3)
Temporal branches (CN VII)
Zygomatic branches (CN VII)
Zygomaticus major
Posterior auricular
Muscle
Vein
Lymph node
Artery
Transverse facial artery
Parotid duct
Posterior auricular nerve (CN VII)
Buccal branches (CN VII)
Parotid gland
Parotid lymph nodes
Buccal nerve (CN V3)
Great auricular nerve
Buccinator
Depressor anguli oris
External jugular vein
Masseter
Facial artery
Cervical branch (CN VII)
Facial vein
Marginal mandibular branch (CN VII)
Auriculotemporal nerve (CN V3)
Superficial temporal vein
Superficial temporal artery
Preauricular lymph nodes
Temporal branches of facial nerve (CN VII)
Facial nerve (CN VII)
Transverse facial artery
Posterior auricular nerve (CN VII)
Parotid duct
Parotid gland
Nerve to posterior belly of digastric (CN VII)
Cervical branch of facial nerve (CN VII)
Posterior auricular artery
Masseter
Digastric, posterior belly
Retromandibular vein
Hypoglossal nerve (CN XII)
Internal jugular vein
Spinal accessory nerve (CN XI)
External carotid artery
Vagus nerve (CN X)
Internal carotid artery
Sternocleidomastoid

**A.** Lateral View

**B.** Lateral View

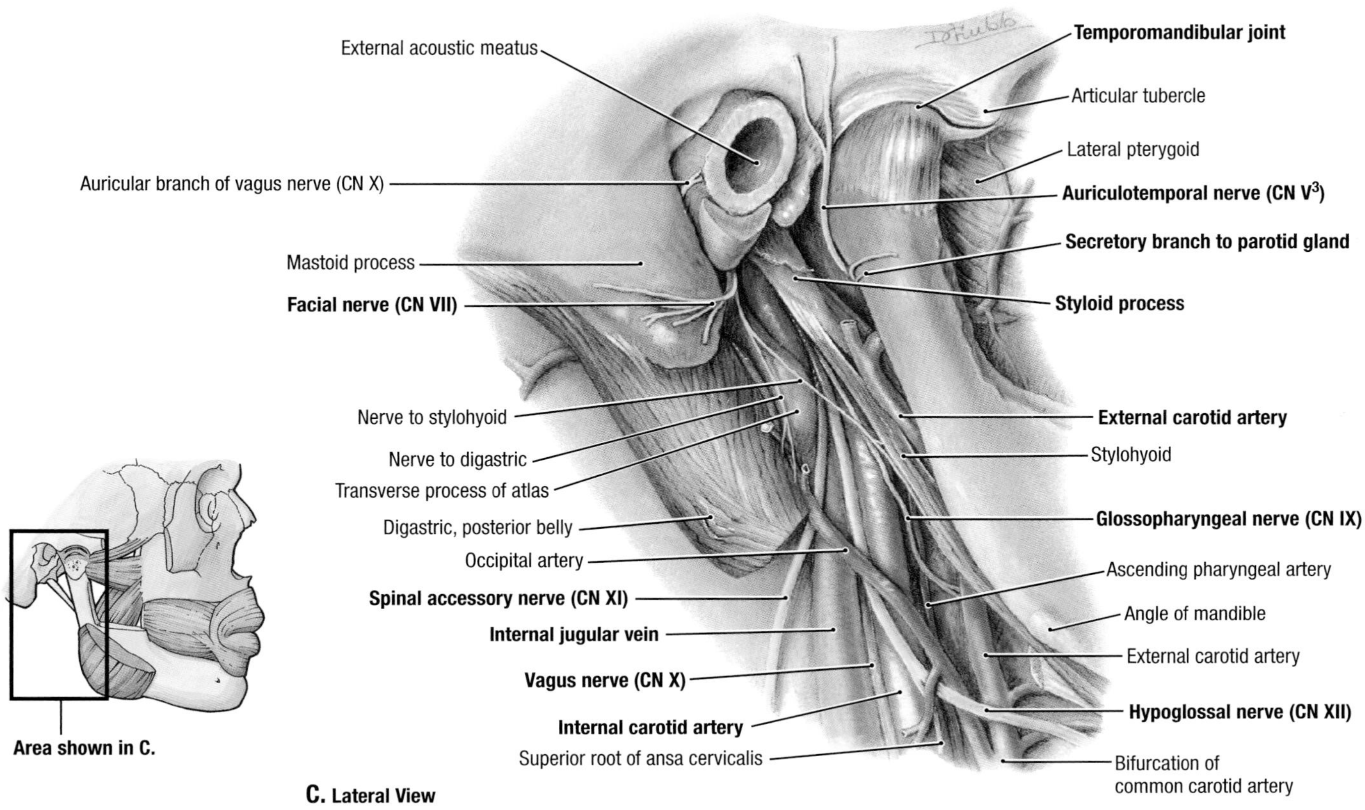
External acoustic meatus
Auricular branch of vagus nerve (CN X)
Mastoid process
Facial nerve (CN VII)
Nerve to stylohyoid
Nerve to digastric
Transverse process of atlas
Digastric, posterior belly
Occipital artery
Spinal accessory nerve (CN XI)
Internal jugular vein
Vagus nerve (CN X)
Internal carotid artery
Superior root of ansa cervicalis
Temporomandibular joint
Articular tubercle
Lateral pterygoid
Auriculotemporal nerve (CN V3)
Secretory branch to parotid gland
Styloid process
External carotid artery
Stylohyoid
Glossopharyngeal nerve (CN IX)
Ascending pharyngeal artery
Angle of mandible
External carotid artery
Hypoglossal nerve (CN XII)
Bifurcation of common carotid artery
Area shown in C.

**C. Lateral View**

## 7.39 Parotid region

**A.** Superficial dissection. **B.** Deep dissection with part of the gland removed. The facial nerve (CN VII) supplies motor innervation to the muscles of facial expression; it forms a plexus within the parotid gland and the branches of which radiate over the face, anastomosing with each other and the branches of the trigeminal nerve. During parotidectomy (surgical excision of the parotid gland), identification, dissection, and preservation of the facial nerve are critical. **C.** Deep dissection following removal of the parotid gland. The facial nerve, posterior belly of the digastric muscle, and its nerve are retracted; the external carotid artery, stylohyoid muscle, and the nerve to the stylohyoid remain in situ. The internal jugular vein, internal carotid artery, and glossopharyngeal (CN IX), vagus (CN X), accessory (CN XI), and hypoglossal (CN XII) nerves cross anterior to the transverse process of the atlas and deep to the styloid process.

Care must be taken during surgical procedures involving the temporomandibular joint to preserve the branches of the facial nerve that overlie the joint and the articular branches of the auriculotemporal nerve that enter the joint.

Trauma, such as a fractured mandible, may injure the hypoglossal nerve (CN XII), resulting in paralysis and eventual atrophy of one side of the tongue. The tongue deviates to the paralyzed side during protrusion.

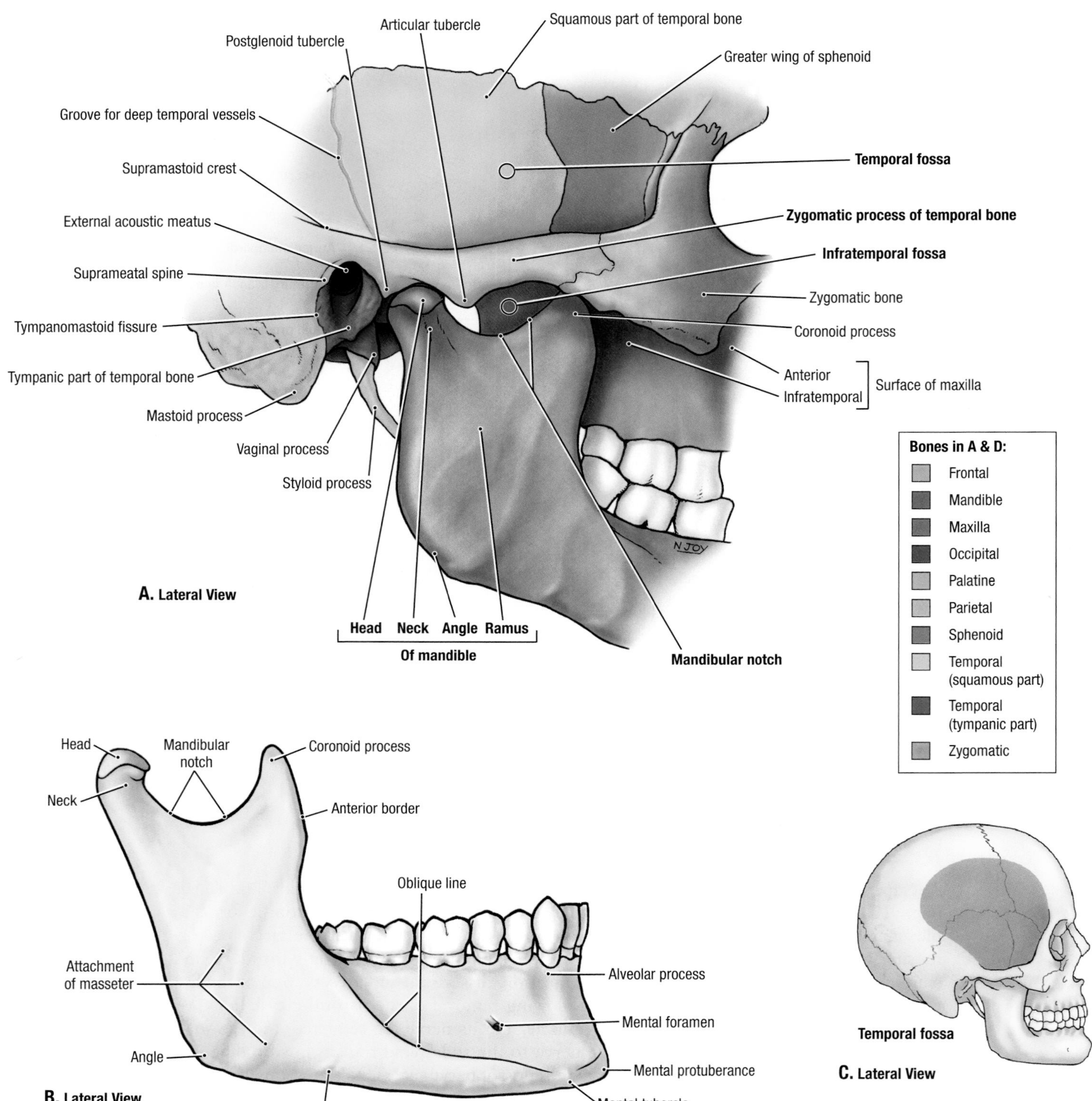
Postglenoid tubercle
Articular tubercle
Squamous part of temporal bone
Greater wing of sphenoid
Groove for deep temporal vessels
Supramastoid crest
External acoustic meatus
Suprameatal spine
Tympanomastoid fissure
Tympanic part of temporal bone
Mastoid process
Vaginal process
Styloid process
Temporal fossa
Zygomatic process of temporal bone
Infratemporal fossa
Zygomatic bone
Coronoid process
Anterior
Infratemporal
Surface of maxilla
A. Lateral View
Head Neck Angle Ramus
Of mandible
Mandibular notch
Bones in A & D:
Frontal
Mandible
Maxilla
Occipital
Palatine
Parietal
Sphenoid
Temporal (squamous part)
Temporal (tympanic part)
Zygomatic
Head
Mandibular notch
Coronoid process
Neck
Anterior border
Oblique line
Attachment of masseter
Alveolar process
Mental foramen
Angle
Mental protuberance
B. Lateral View
Groove for facial artery
Mental tubercle
Temporal fossa
C. Lateral View

**7.40 Temporal and infratemporal fossa and mandible**

**A.** Bones and bony features. Note that superficially the zygomatic process of the temporal bone is the boundary between the temporal fossa superiorly and the infratemporal fossa inferiorly. **B.** External surface of the mandible. **C.** Temporal fossa (gray area).

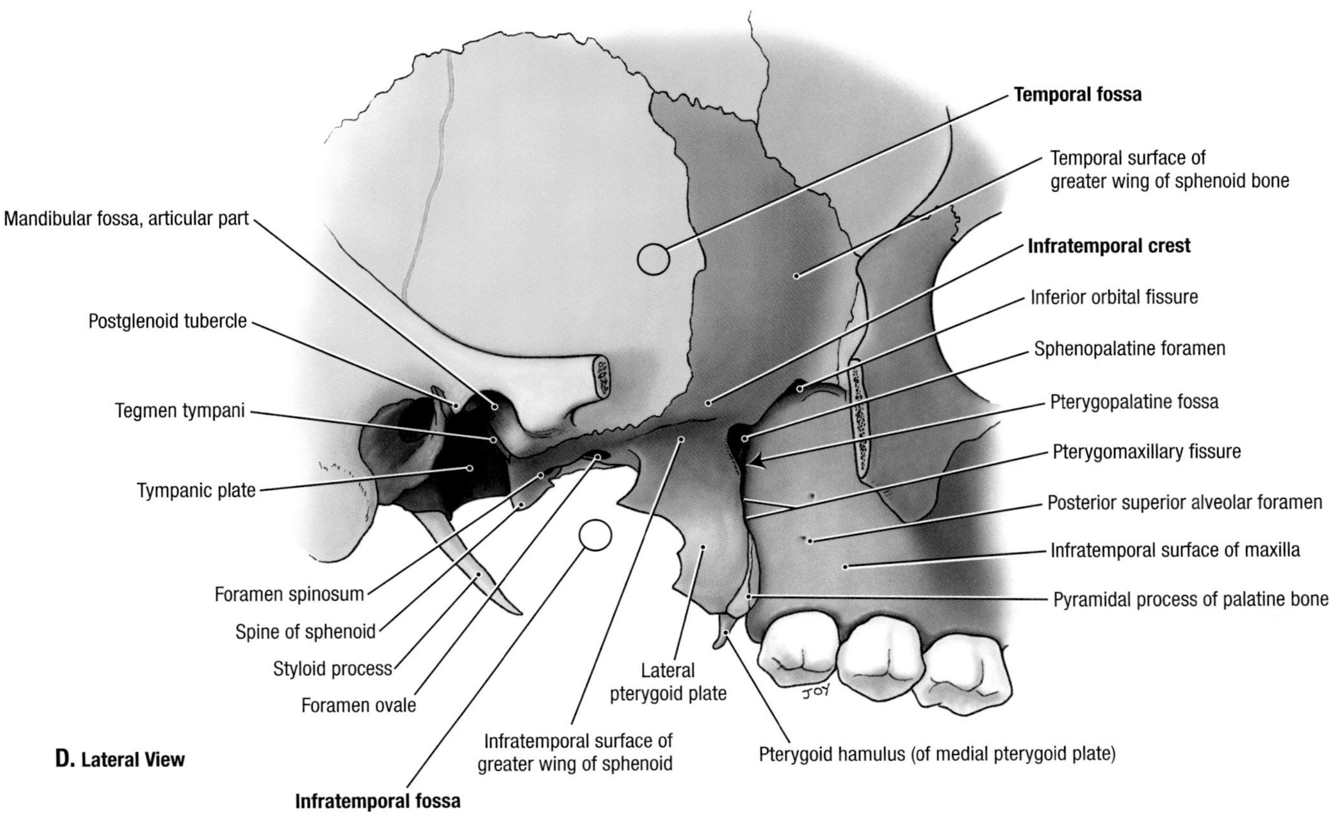
Temporal fossa
Temporal surface of greater wing of sphenoid bone
Infratemporal crest
Inferior orbital fissure
Sphenopalatine foramen
Pterygopalatine fossa
Pterygomaxillary fissure
Posterior superior alveolar foramen
Infratemporal surface of maxilla
Pyramidal process of palatine bone
Mandibular fossa, articular part
Postglenoid tubercle
Tegmen tympani
Tympanic plate
Foramen spinosum
Spine of sphenoid
Styloid process
Foramen ovale
Lateral pterygoid plate
Infratemporal surface of greater wing of sphenoid
Pterygoid hamulus (of medial pterygoid plate)
Infratemporal fossa

D. Lateral View

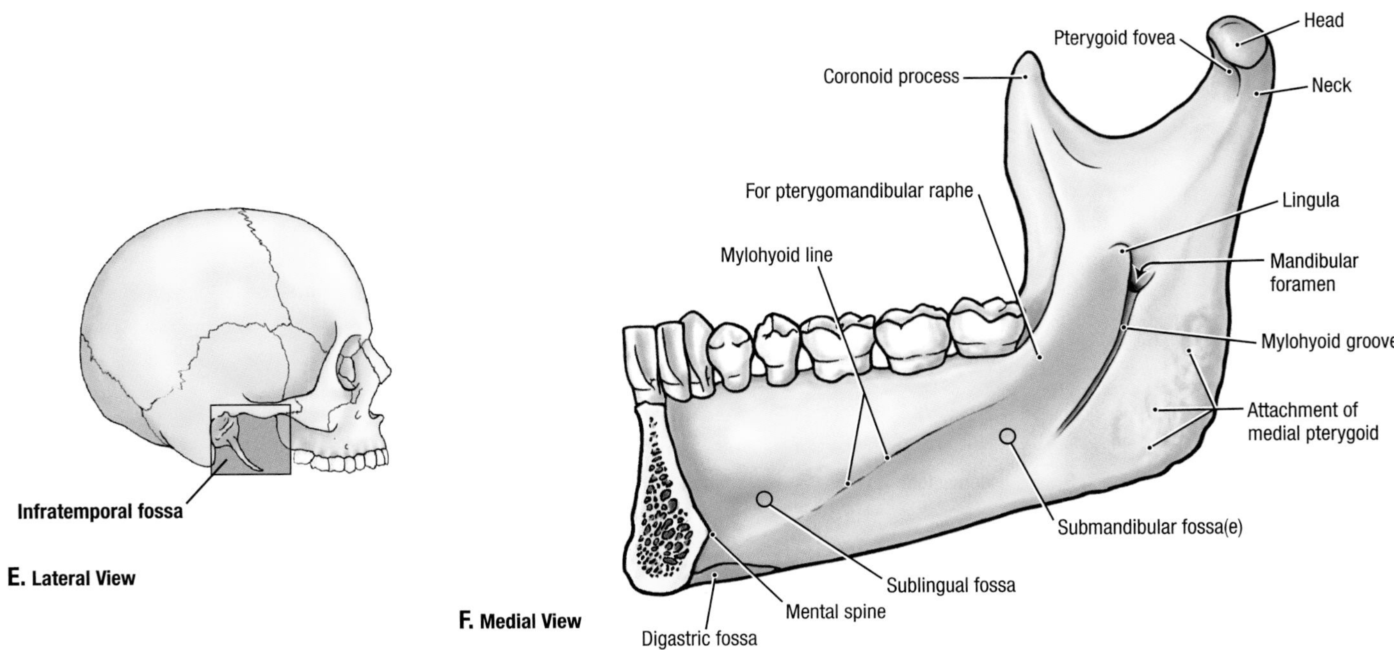
Head
Pterygoid fovea
Coronoid process
Neck
For pterygomandibular raphe
Lingula
Mylohyoid line
Mandibular foramen
Mylohyoid groove
Attachment of medial pterygoid
Submandibular fossa(e)
Sublingual fossa
Mental spine
Digastric fossa
Infratemporal fossa

E. Lateral View

F. Medial View

**7.40 Temporal and infratemporal fossa and mandible *(continued)***

**D.** Bones and bony features of the infratemporal fossa. The mandible and part of the zygomatic arch have been removed. Deeply, the infratemporal crest separates the temporal and infratemporal fossae. **E.** Infratemporal fossa (gray area). **F.** Internal surface of the mandible.

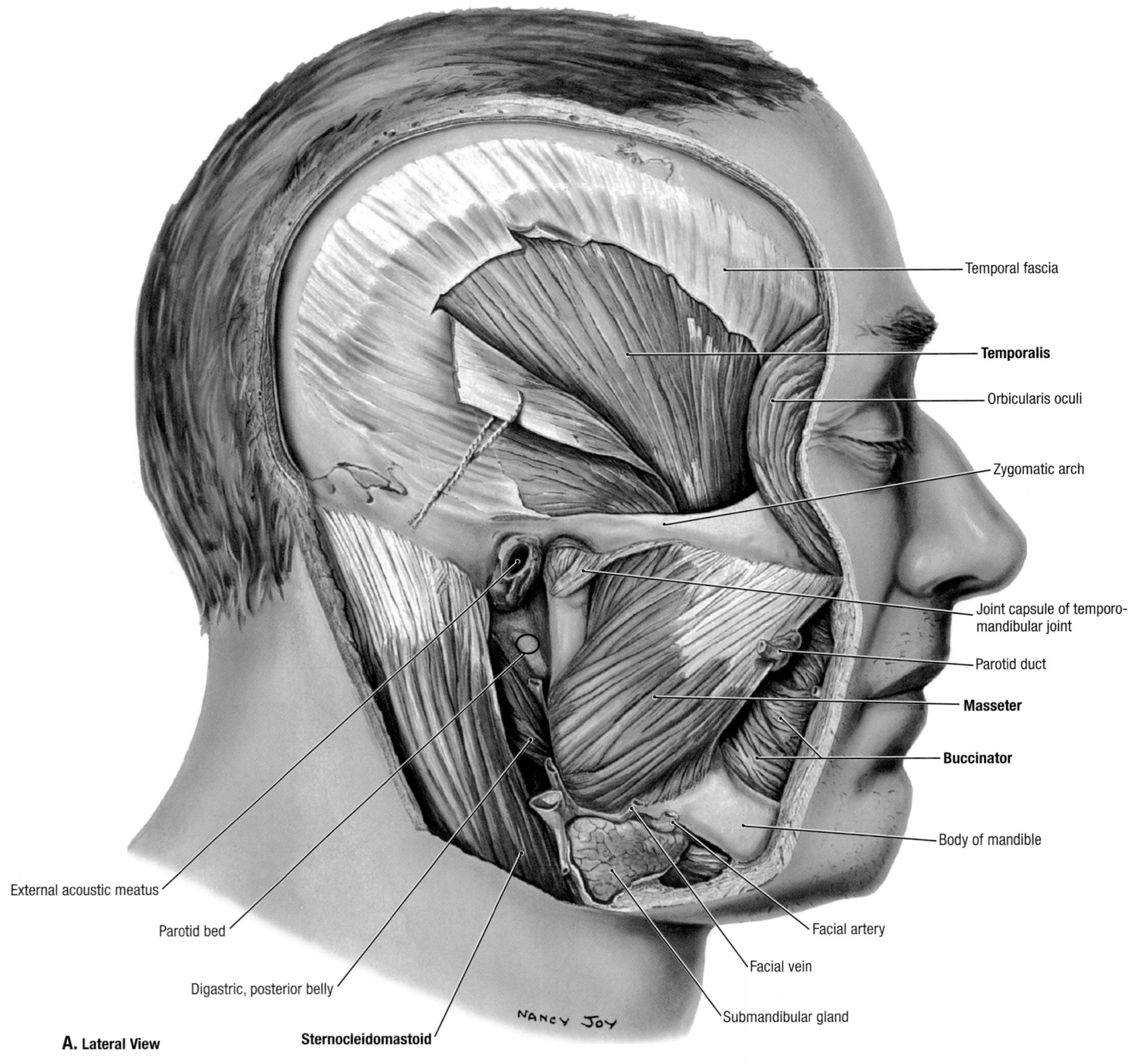
Temporal fascia
Temporalis
Orbicularis oculi
Zygomatic arch
Joint capsule of temporo-mandibular joint
Parotid duct
Masseter
Buccinator
Body of mandible
External acoustic meatus
Parotid bed
Digastric, posterior belly
Sternocleidomastoid
Facial artery
Facial vein
Submandibular gland
NANCY JOY
A. Lateral View

## 7.41 Temporalis and masseter

**A.** Superficial dissection.

- The temporalis and masseter muscles are supplied by the trigeminal nerve (CN V), and both elevate the mandible. The buccinator muscle, supplied by the facial nerve (CN VII), functions during chewing to keep food between the teeth but does not act on the mandible.
- The sternocleidomastoid muscle, supplied by the spinal accessory nerve (CN XI), is the chief flexor of the head and neck; it forms the lateral part of the posterior boundary of the parotid region/parotid bed.

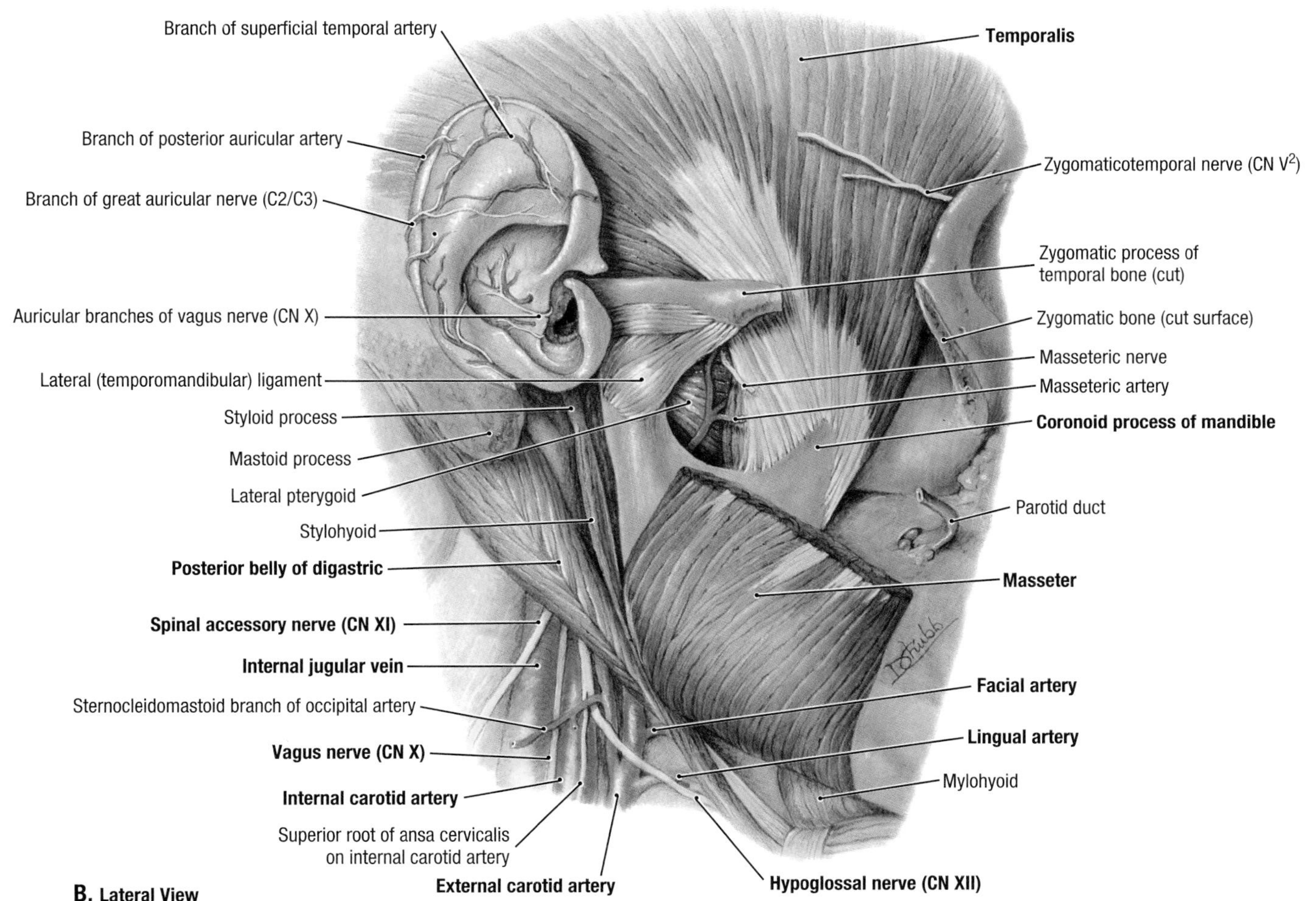
Branch of superficial temporal artery
Temporalis
Branch of posterior auricular artery
Zygomaticotemporal nerve (CN V2)
Branch of great auricular nerve (C2/C3)
Zygomatic process of temporal bone (cut)
Auricular branches of vagus nerve (CN X)
Zygomatic bone (cut surface)
Masseteric nerve
Lateral (temporomandibular) ligament
Masseteric artery
Styloid process
Coronoid process of mandible
Mastoid process
Lateral pterygoid
Parotid duct
Stylohyoid
Posterior belly of digastric
Masseter
Spinal accessory nerve (CN XI)
Internal jugular vein
Facial artery
Sternocleidomastoid branch of occipital artery
Lingual artery
Vagus nerve (CN X)
Mylohyoid
Internal carotid artery
Superior root of ansa cervicalis on internal carotid artery
External carotid artery
Hypoglossal nerve (CN XII)

**B.** **Lateral View**

## 7.41 Temporalis and masseter *(continued)*

**B.** Deep dissection.

- Parts of the zygomatic arch and the masseter muscle have been removed to expose the attachment of the temporalis muscle to the coronoid process of the mandible.
- The carotid sheath surrounding the internal jugular vein, internal carotid artery, and the vagus nerve (CN X) has been removed. The external carotid artery and its lingual, facial, and occipital branches, and the spinal accessory (CN XI) and hypoglossal (CN XII) nerves pass deep to the posterior belly of the digastric muscle.

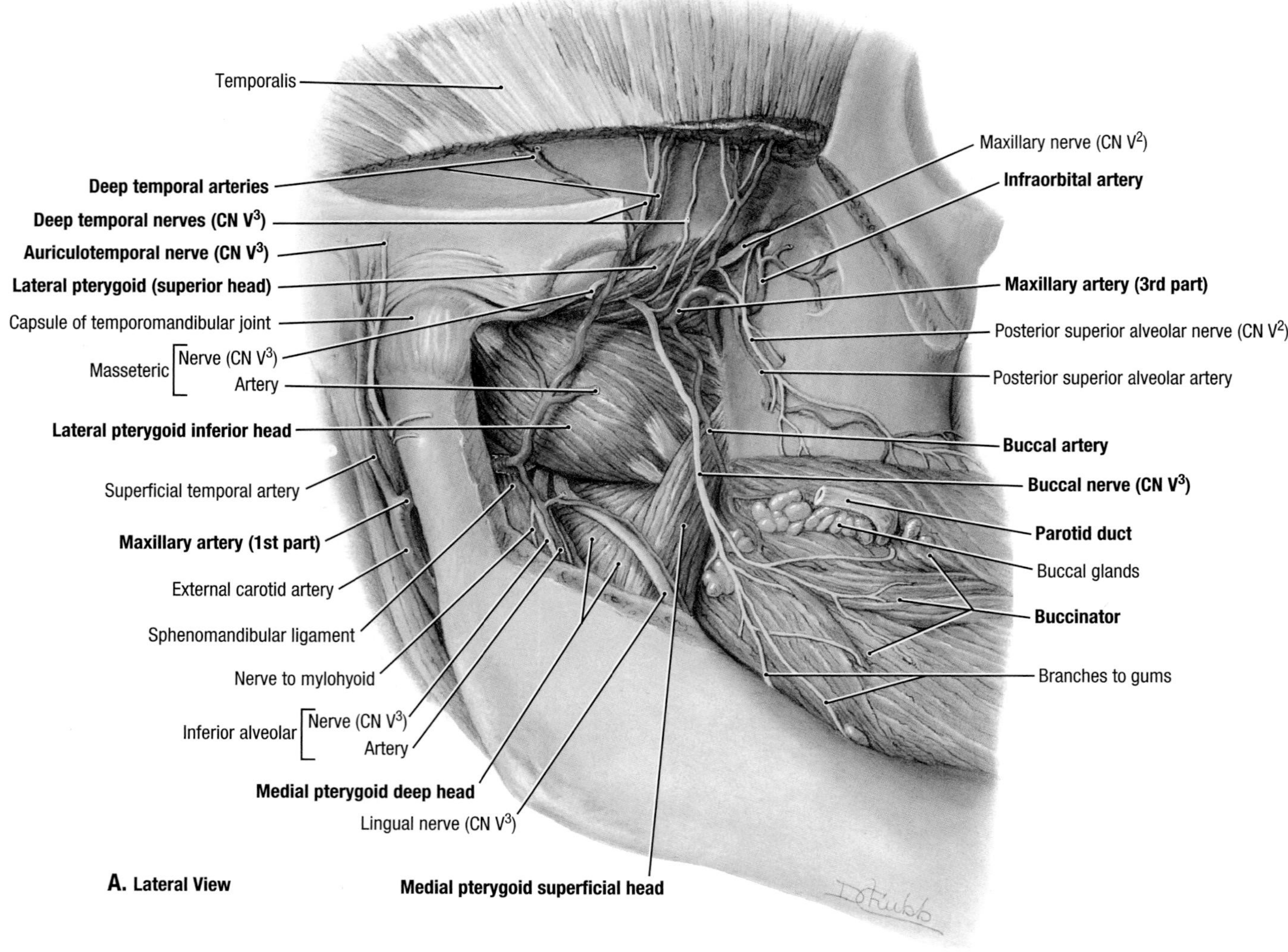
Temporalis
Deep temporal arteries
Deep temporal nerves (CN V3)
Auriculotemporal nerve (CN V3)
Lateral pterygoid (superior head)
Capsule of temporomandibular joint
Masseteric
Nerve (CN V3)
Artery
Lateral pterygoid inferior head
Superficial temporal artery
Maxillary artery (1st part)
External carotid artery
Sphenomandibular ligament
Nerve to mylohyoid
Inferior alveolar
Nerve (CN V3)
Artery
Medial pterygoid deep head
Lingual nerve (CN V3)
Medial pterygoid superficial head
Maxillary nerve (CN V2)
Infraorbital artery
Maxillary artery (3rd part)
Posterior superior alveolar nerve (CN V2)
Posterior superior alveolar artery
Buccal artery
Buccal nerve (CN V3)
Parotid duct
Buccal glands
Buccinator
Branches to gums

**A.** Lateral View

## 7.42 Infratemporal region

**A.** Superficial dissection.

- The maxillary artery, the larger of two terminal branches of the external carotid, is divided into three parts relative to the lateral pterygoid muscle.
- The buccinator is pierced by the parotid duct, the ducts of the buccal glands, and sensory branches of the buccal nerve.
- The lateral pterygoid muscle arises by two heads (parts), one head from the roof, and the other head from the medial wall of the infratemporal fossa; both heads insert in relation to the temporomandibular joint—the superior head attaching primarily to the articular disc of the joint and the inferior head primarily to the anterior aspect of the neck of the mandible (pterygoid fovea).
- Because of the close relationship of the facial and auriculotemporal nerves to the temporomandibular joint (TMJ), care must be taken during surgical procedures to preserve both the branches of the facial nerve overlying it and the articular branches of the auriculotemporal nerve that enter the posterior part of the joint. Injury to articular branches of the auriculotemporal nerve supplying the TMJ—associated with traumatic dislocation and rupture of the joint capsule and lateral ligament—leads to laxity and instability of the TMJ.

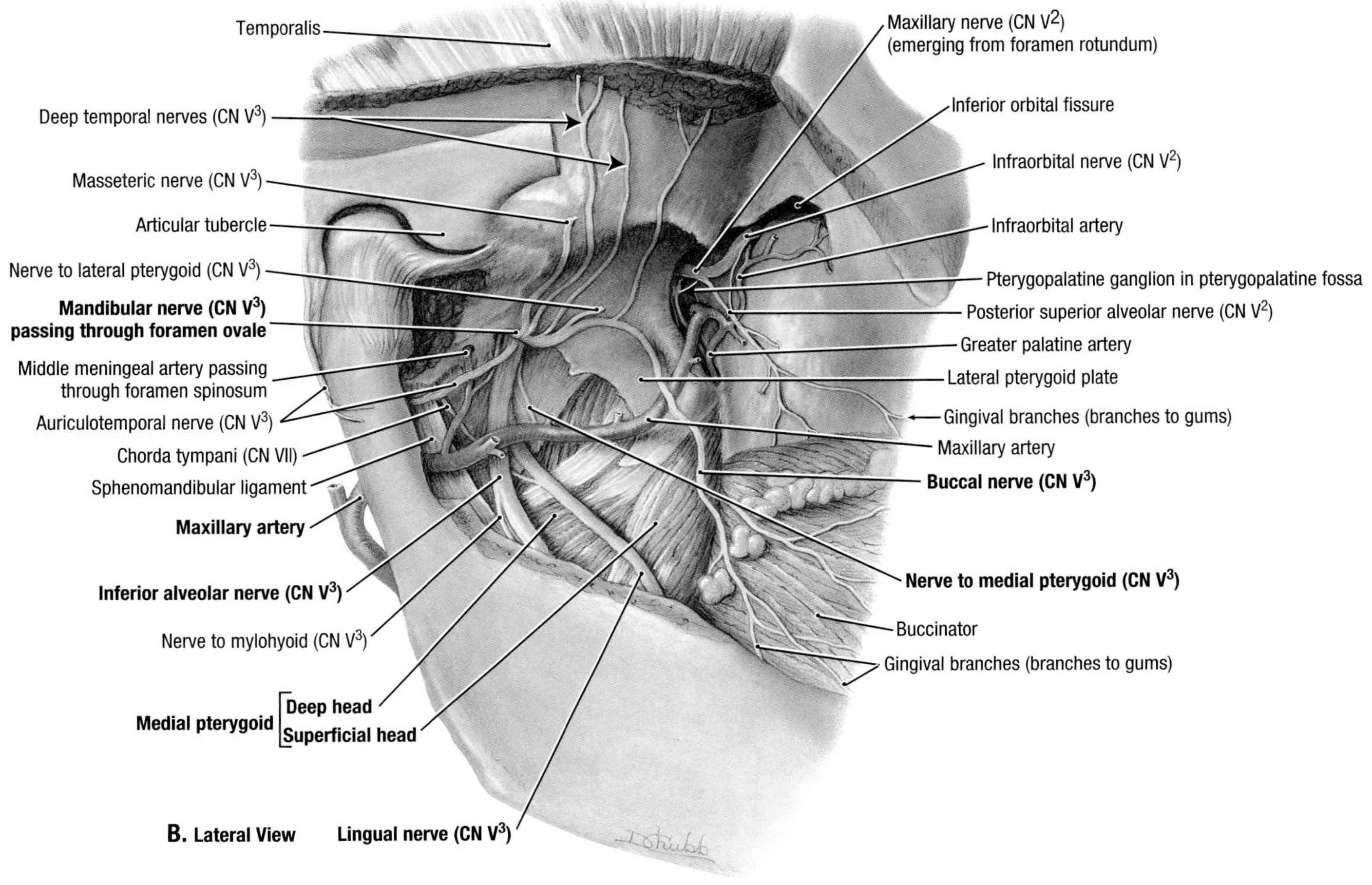
Temporalis
Deep temporal nerves (CN V3)
Masseteric nerve (CN V3)
Articular tubercle
Nerve to lateral pterygoid (CN V3)
Mandibular nerve (CN V3) passing through foramen ovale
Middle meningeal artery passing through foramen spinosum
Auriculotemporal nerve (CN V3)
Chorda tympani (CN VII)
Sphenomandibular ligament
Maxillary artery
Inferior alveolar nerve (CN V3)
Nerve to mylohyoid (CN V3)
Medial pterygoid
Deep head
Superficial head
B. Lateral View
Lingual nerve (CN V3)
Maxillary nerve (CN V2) (emerging from foramen rotundum)
Inferior orbital fissure
Infraorbital nerve (CN V2)
Infraorbital artery
Pterygopalatine ganglion in pterygopalatine fossa
Posterior superior alveolar nerve (CN V2)
Greater palatine artery
Lateral pterygoid plate
Gingival branches (branches to gums)
Maxillary artery
Buccal nerve (CN V3)
Nerve to medial pterygoid (CN V3)
Buccinator
Gingival branches (branches to gums)

## 7.42 Infratemporal region (continued)

**B.** Deeper dissection.

- The lateral pterygoid muscle and most of the branches of the maxillary artery have been removed to expose the mandibular nerve (CN $V^3$) entering the infratemporal fossa through the foramen ovale and the middle meningeal artery passing through the foramen spinosum.
- The deep head of the medial pterygoid muscle arises from the medial surface of the lateral pterygoid plate and the pyramidal process of the palatine bone. It has a small, superficial head that arises from the tuberosity of the maxilla.
- The inferior alveolar and lingual nerves descend on the medial pterygoid muscle. The inferior alveolar nerve gives off the nerve to mylohyoid and nerve to anterior belly of the digastric muscle, and the lingual nerve receives the chorda tympani, which carries secretory parasympathetic fibers and fibers of taste.
- Motor nerves arising from CN $V^3$ supply the four muscles of mastication: the masseter, temporalis, and lateral and medial pterygoids. The buccal nerve from the mandibular nerve is sensory; the buccal branch of the facial nerve is the motor supply to the buccinator muscle.
- To perform a mandibular nerve block, an anesthetic agent is injected near the mandibular nerve where it enters the infratemporal fossa. This block usually anesthetizes the auriculotemporal, inferior alveolar, lingual, and buccal branches of the mandibular nerve.

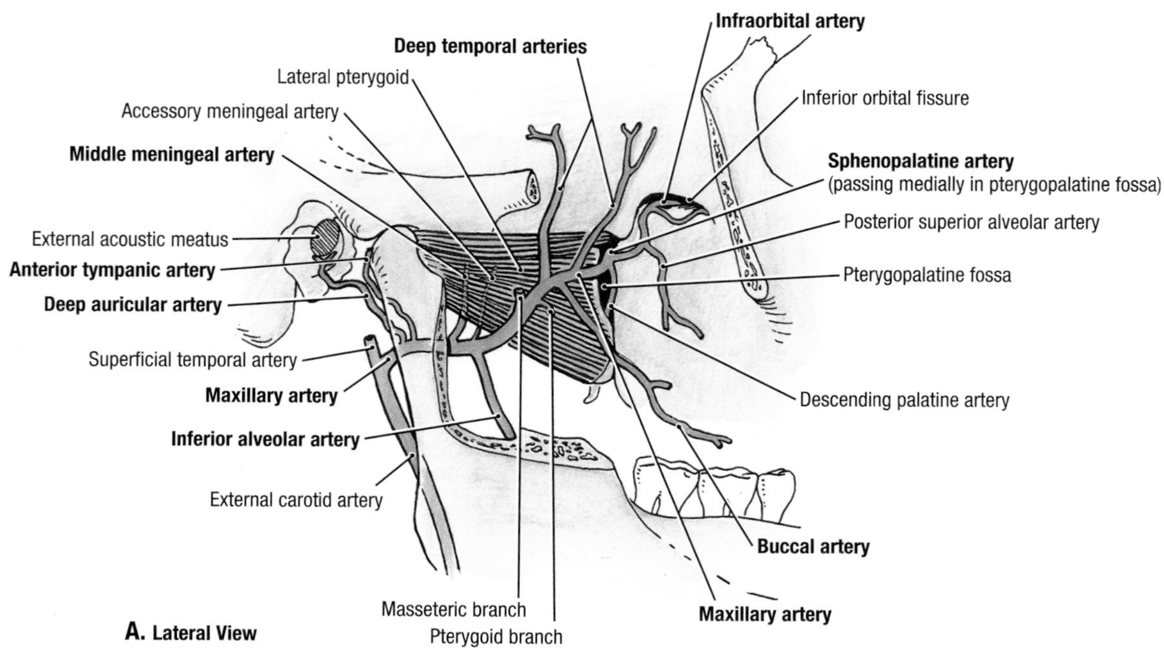
Infraorbital artery
Deep temporal arteries
Lateral pterygoid
Inferior orbital fissure
Accessory meningeal artery
Middle meningeal artery
Sphenopalatine artery
(passing medially in pterygopalatine fossa)
Posterior superior alveolar artery
External acoustic meatus
Anterior tympanic artery
Pterygopalatine fossa
Deep auricular artery
Superficial temporal artery
Maxillary artery
Descending palatine artery
Inferior alveolar artery
External carotid artery
Buccal artery
Masseteric branch
Maxillary artery
Pterygoid branch
A. Lateral View

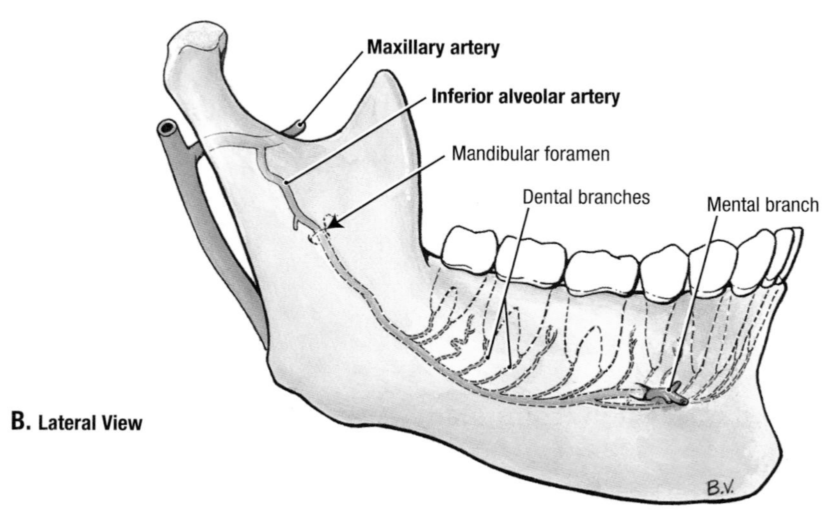
Maxillary artery
Inferior alveolar artery
Mandibular foramen
Dental branches
Mental branch
B. Lateral View
B.V.

## 7.43 Branches of maxillary artery

**A.** Infratemporal region. **B.** Mandible.

- The maxillary artery arises at the neck of the mandible and is divided into three parts by the lateral pterygoid; it can pass medial or lateral to the lateral pterygoid.
- The branches of the first or retromandibular part pass through foramina or canals: the deep auricular to the external acoustic meatus, the anterior tympanic to the tympanic cavity, the middle and accessory meningeal to the cranial cavity, and the inferior alveolar to the mandible and teeth.
- The branches of the second part (directly related to the lateral pterygoid) supply muscles via the masseteric, deep temporal, pterygoid, and buccal branches.
- The branches of the third (pterygopalatine) part (posterior superior alveolar, infraorbital, descending palatine, and sphenopalatine arteries) arise immediately proximal to and within the pterygopalatine fossa.

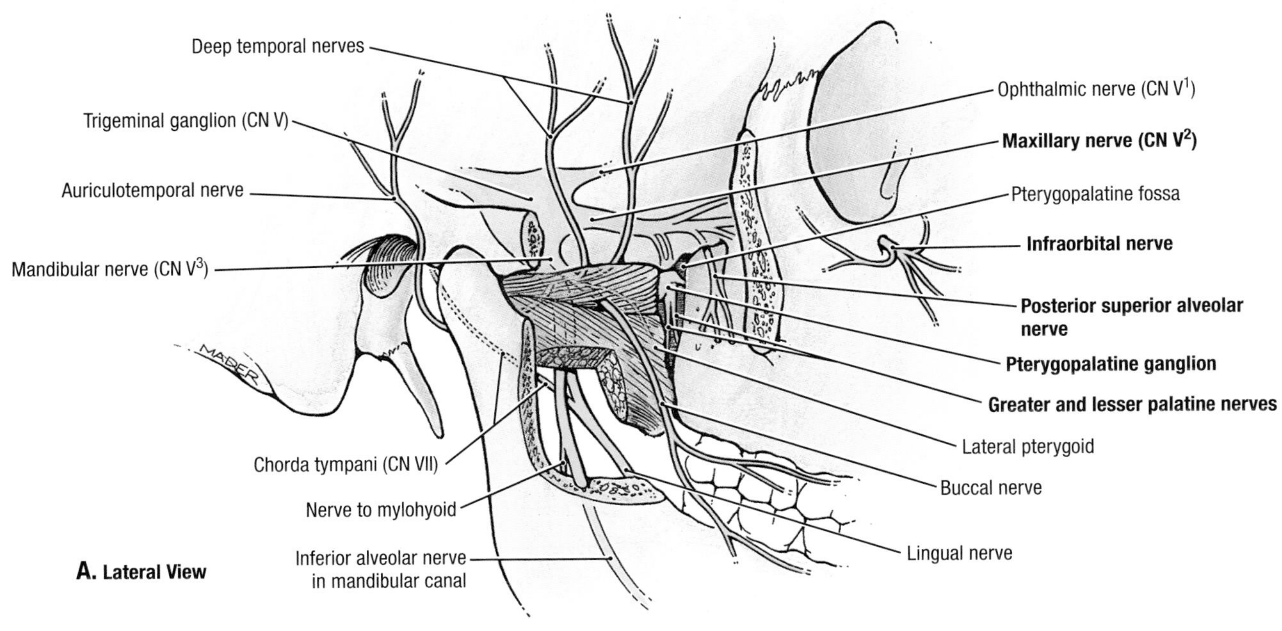
Deep temporal nerves
Trigeminal ganglion (CN V)
Auriculotemporal nerve
Mandibular nerve (CN V3)
MADER
Chorda tympani (CN VII)
Nerve to mylohyoid
Inferior alveolar nerve in mandibular canal
Ophthalmic nerve (CN V1)
Maxillary nerve (CN V2)
Pterygopalatine fossa
Infraorbital nerve
Posterior superior alveolar nerve
Pterygopalatine ganglion
Greater and lesser palatine nerves
Lateral pterygoid
Buccal nerve
Lingual nerve

**A. Lateral View**

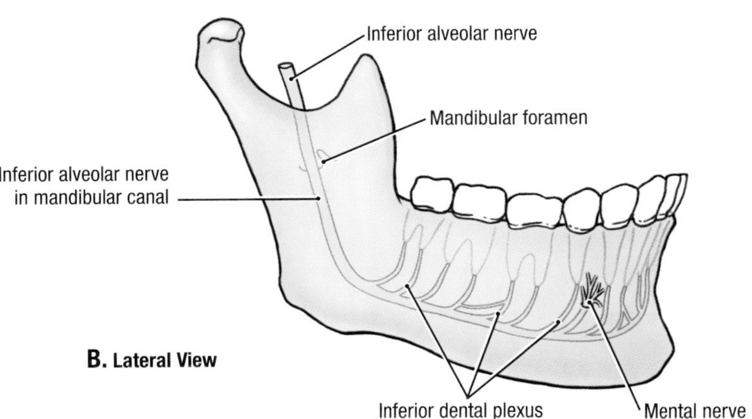
Inferior alveolar nerve
Mandibular foramen
Inferior alveolar nerve in mandibular canal
Inferior dental plexus
Mental nerve

**B. Lateral View**

## 7.44 Branches of maxillary and mandibular nerves

**A.** Infratemporal region and pterygopalatine fossa. Branches of the maxillary (CN $V^2$) and mandibular (CN $V^3$) nerves accompany branches from the three parts of the maxillary artery. **B.** Mandible and inferior alveolar nerve.

An alveolar nerve block—commonly used by dentists when repairing mandibular teeth—anesthetizes the inferior alveolar nerve, a branch of CN $V^3$. The anesthetic agent is injected around the mandibular foramen, the opening into the mandibular canal on the medial aspect of the ramus of the mandible. This canal gives passage to the inferior alveolar nerve, artery, and vein. When this nerve block is successful, all mandibular teeth are anesthetized to the median plane. The skin and mucous membrane of the lower lip, the labial alveolar mucosa and gingiva, and the skin of the chin are also anesthetized because they are supplied by the mental branch of this nerve.

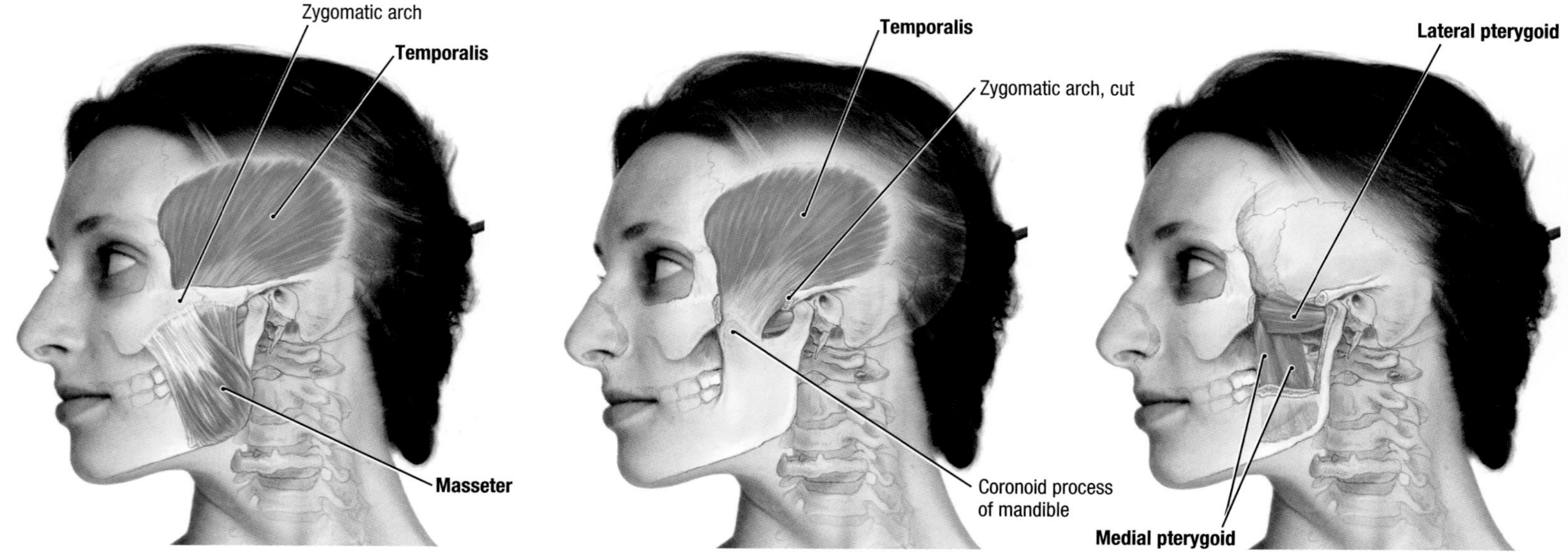
Zygomatic arch
Temporalis
Masseter
Temporalis
Zygomatic arch, cut
Coronoid process of mandible
Lateral pterygoid
Medial pterygoid

Lateral Views

**TABLE 7.9 MUSCLES OF MASTICATION (ACTING ON TEMPOROMANDIBULAR JOINT)**

| Muscle | Origin | Insertion | Innervation | Main Action |
|---|---|---|---|---|
| **Temporalis** | Floor of temporal fossa and deep surface of temporal fascia | Tip and medial surface of coronoid process and anterior border of ramus of mandible | Deep temporal branches of mandibular nerve (CN $V^3$) | Elevates mandible, closing jaws; posterior fibers retrude mandible after protrusion |
| **Masseter** | Inferior border and medial surface of zygomatic arch | Lateral surface of ramus of mandible and coronoid process | Mandibular nerve (CN $V^3$) through masseteric nerve that enters deep surface of the muscle | Elevates and protrudes mandible, thus closing jaws; deep fibers retrude it |
| **Lateral pterygoid** | *Superior head:* infratemporal surface and infratemporal crest of greater wing of sphenoid bone<br>*Inferior head:* lateral surface of lateral pterygoid plate | Neck of mandible, articular disc, and capsule of temporomandibular joint | Mandibular nerve (CN $V^3$) through lateral pterygoid nerve which enters its deep surface | *Acting bilaterally,* protrude mandible and depress chin; *Acting unilaterally* alternately, they produce side-to-side movements of mandible |
| **Medial pterygoid** | *Deep head:* medial surface of lateral pterygoid plate and pyramidal process of palatine bone<br>*Superficial head:* tuberosity of maxilla | Medial surface of ramus of mandible, inferior to mandibular foramen | Mandibular nerve (CN $V^3$) through medial pterygoid nerve | Helps elevate mandible, closing jaws; *acting bilaterally* protrude mandible; *acting unilaterally,* protrudes side of jaw; acting alternately, they produce a grinding motion |

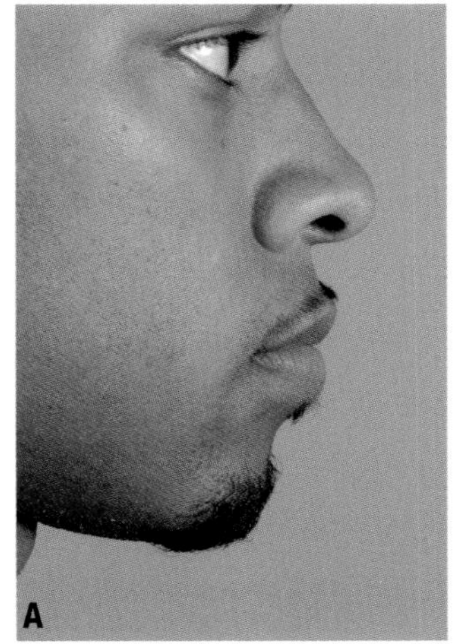
A
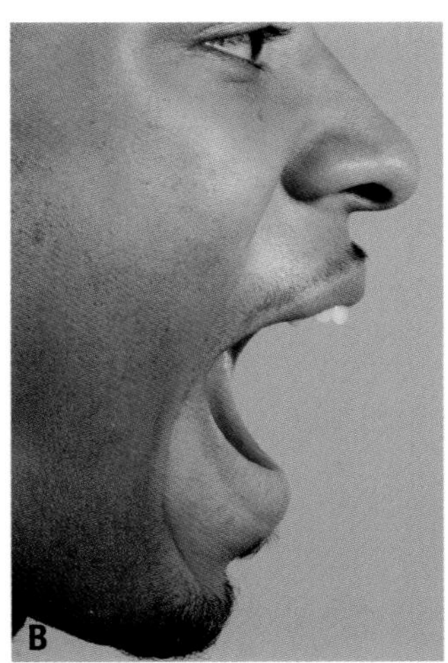
B
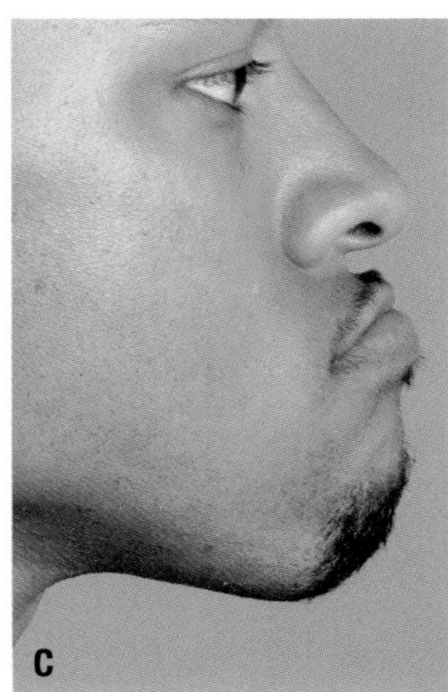
C
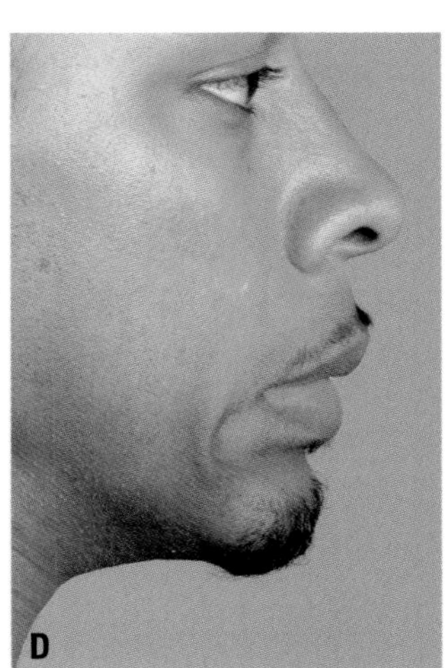
D

**Lateral Views**

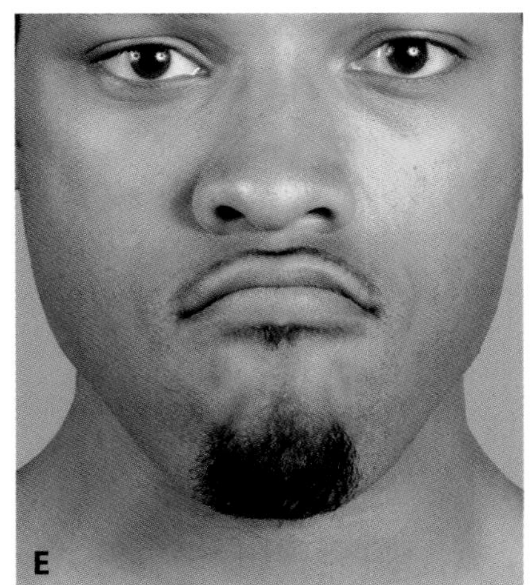
E
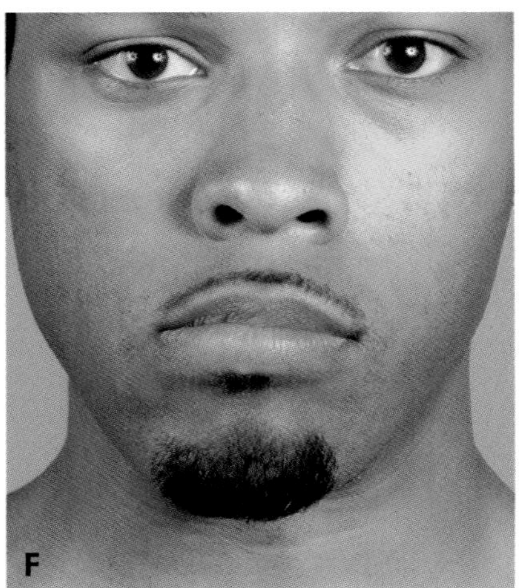
F
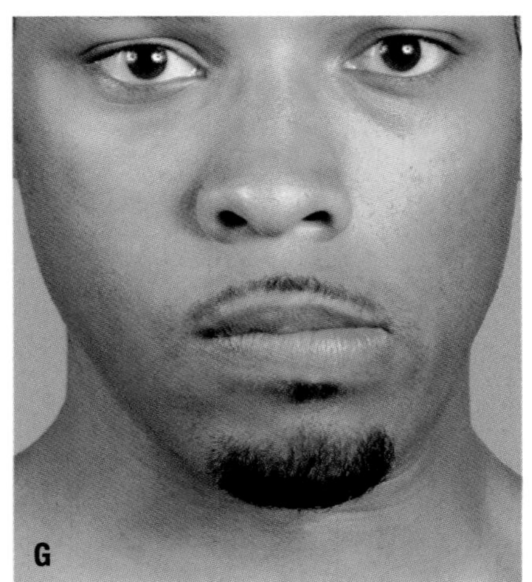
G

**Anterior Views**

**TABLE 7.10 MOVEMENTS OF THE TEMPOROMANDIBULAR JOINT**

| Movements | Muscles |
|---|---|
| Elevation (close mouth) (A) | Temporalis, masseter, and medial pterygoid |
| Depression (open mouth) (B) | Lateral pterygoid; suprahyoid and infrahyoid muscles; gravity |
| Protrusion (protrude chin) (C and E) | Lateral pterygoid, masseter, and medial pterygoid |
| Retrusion (retrude chin) (D) | Temporalis (posterior oblique and near horizontal fibers) and masseter |
| Lateral movements (grinding and chewing) (F and G) | Temporalis of same side, pterygoids of opposite side, and masseter |

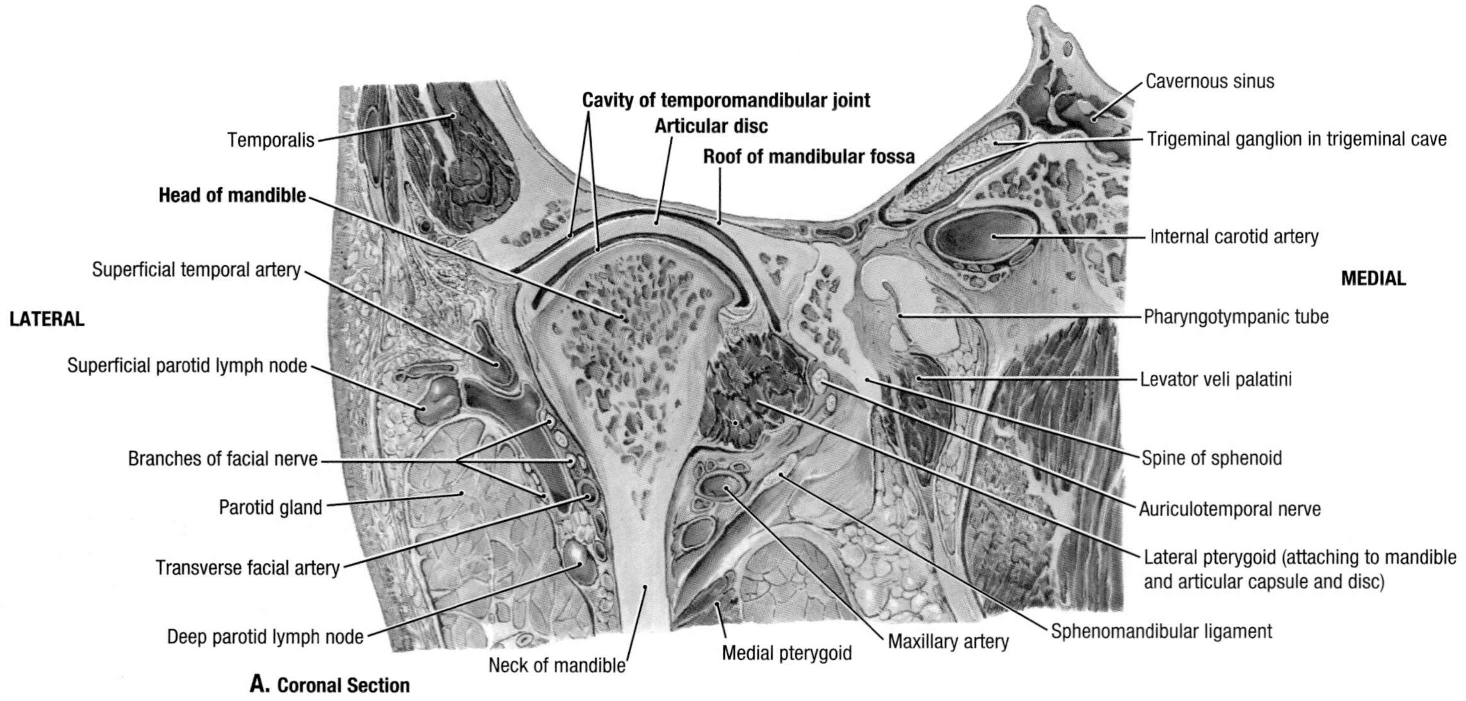
Cavity of temporomandibular joint
Articular disc
Roof of mandibular fossa
Temporalis
Head of mandible
Superficial temporal artery
LATERAL
Superficial parotid lymph node
Branches of facial nerve
Parotid gland
Transverse facial artery
Deep parotid lymph node
Neck of mandible
Medial pterygoid
Maxillary artery
Sphenomandibular ligament
Cavernous sinus
Trigeminal ganglion in trigeminal cave
Internal carotid artery
MEDIAL
Pharyngotympanic tube
Levator veli palatini
Spine of sphenoid
Auriculotemporal nerve
Lateral pterygoid (attaching to mandible and articular capsule and disc)
A. Coronal Section

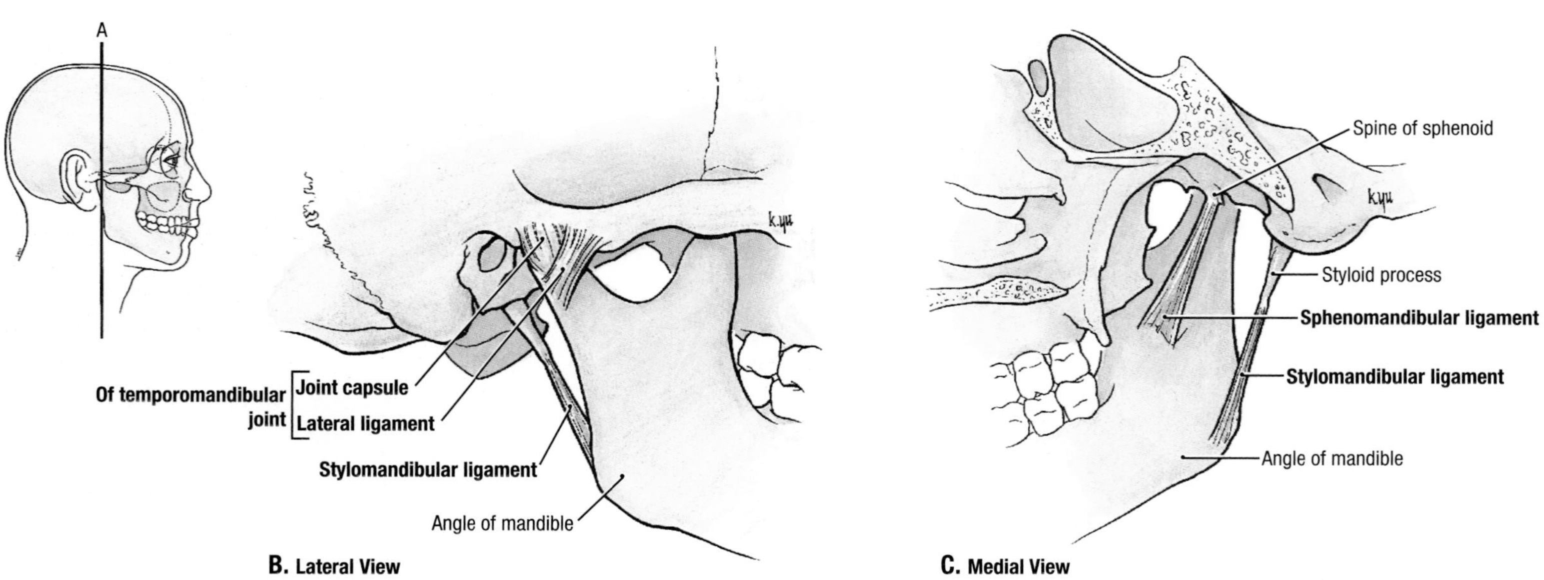
A
Of temporomandibular joint
Joint capsule
Lateral ligament
Stylomandibular ligament
Angle of mandible
B. Lateral View
Spine of sphenoid
Styloid process
Sphenomandibular ligament
Stylomandibular ligament
Angle of mandible
C. Medial View

## 7.45 Temporomandibular joint

**A.** Coronal section. **B.** Temporomandibular joint and stylomandibular ligament. The joint capsule of the temporomandibular joint attaches to the margins of the mandibular fossa and articular tubercle of the temporal bone and around the neck of the mandible; the lateral (temporomandibular) ligament strengthens the lateral aspect of the joint. **C.** Stylomandibular and sphenomandibular ligaments. The strong sphenomandibular ligament descends from near the spine of the sphenoid to the lingula of the mandible and is the "swinging hinge" by which the mandible is suspended; the weaker stylomandibular ligament is a thickened part of the parotid sheath that joins the styloid process to the angle of the mandible.

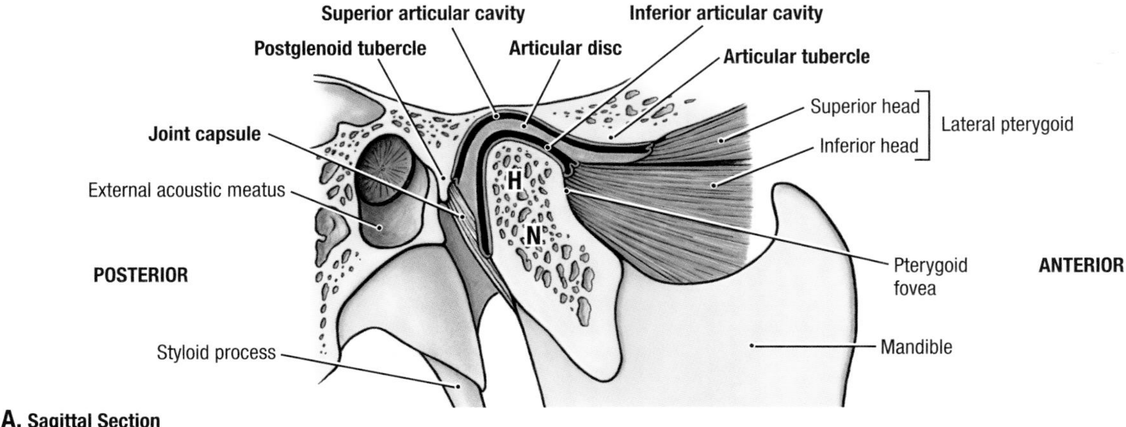
Superior articular cavity
Inferior articular cavity
Postglenoid tubercle
Articular disc
Articular tubercle
Joint capsule
Superior head
Inferior head
Lateral pterygoid
External acoustic meatus
H
N
POSTERIOR
Pterygoid fovea
ANTERIOR
Styloid process
Mandible

A. Sagittal Section

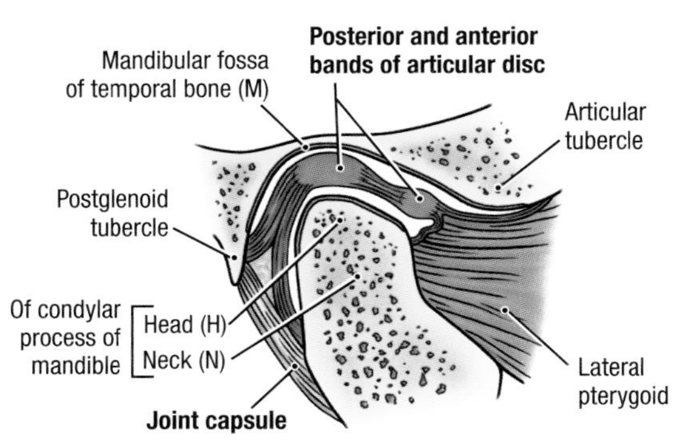
Mandibular fossa of temporal bone (M)
Posterior and anterior bands of articular disc
Articular tubercle
Postglenoid tubercle
Of condylar process of mandible
Head (H)
Neck (N)
Lateral pterygoid
Joint capsule

B. Closed Mouth, Sagittal Section

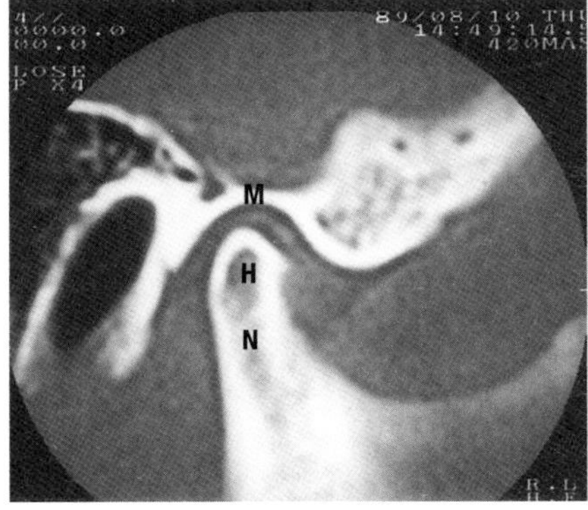
M
H
N

Sagittal CT

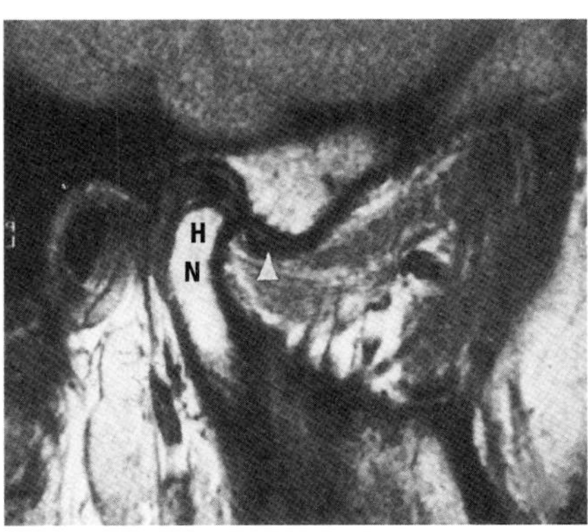
H
N

Sagittal MRI

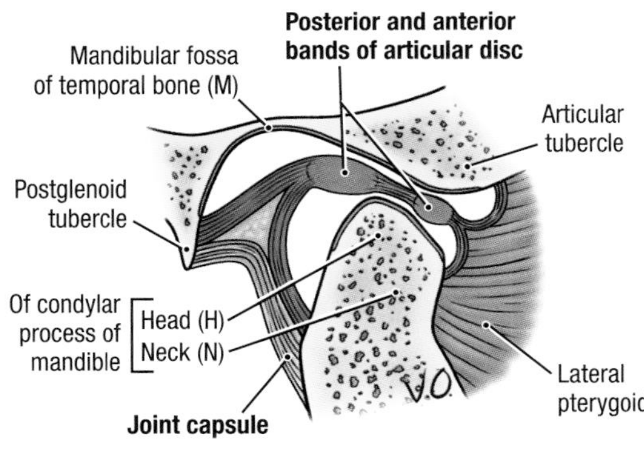
Mandibular fossa of temporal bone (M)
Posterior and anterior bands of articular disc
Articular tubercle
Postglenoid tubercle
Of condylar process of mandible
Head (H)
Neck (N)
Lateral pterygoid
Joint capsule

C. Open Mouth, Sagittal Section

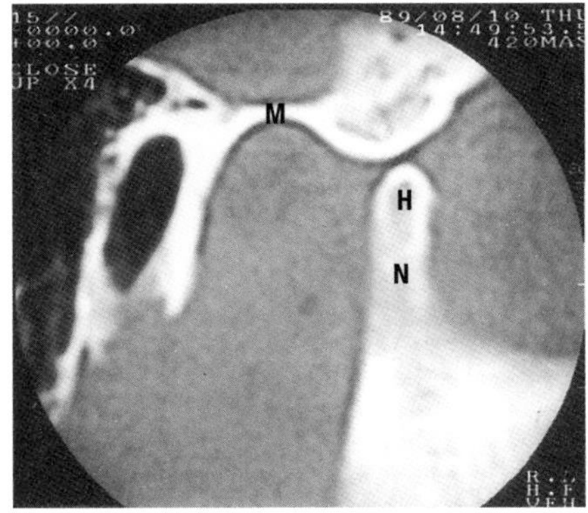
M
H
N

Sagittal CT

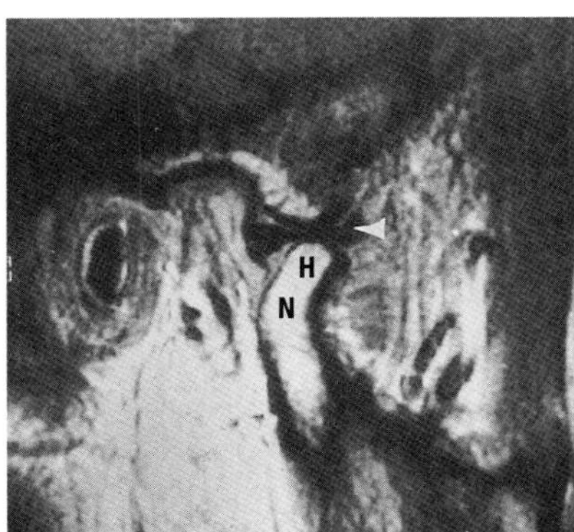
H
N

Sagittal MRI

## 7.46 Sectional anatomy of temporomandibular joint (TMJ)

**A.** TMJ and related structures, sagittal section. **B.** Sagittal orientation figure, CT, and MRI—mouth closed. **C.** Sagittal orientation figure, CT, and MRI—mouth opened widely. The articular disc divides the articular cavity into superior and inferior compartments, each lined by a separate synovial membrane.

During yawning or taking large bites, excessive contraction of the lateral pterygoids can cause the head of the mandible to dislocate (pass anterior to the articular tubercle). In this position, the mouth remains wide open, and the person cannot close it without manual distraction.

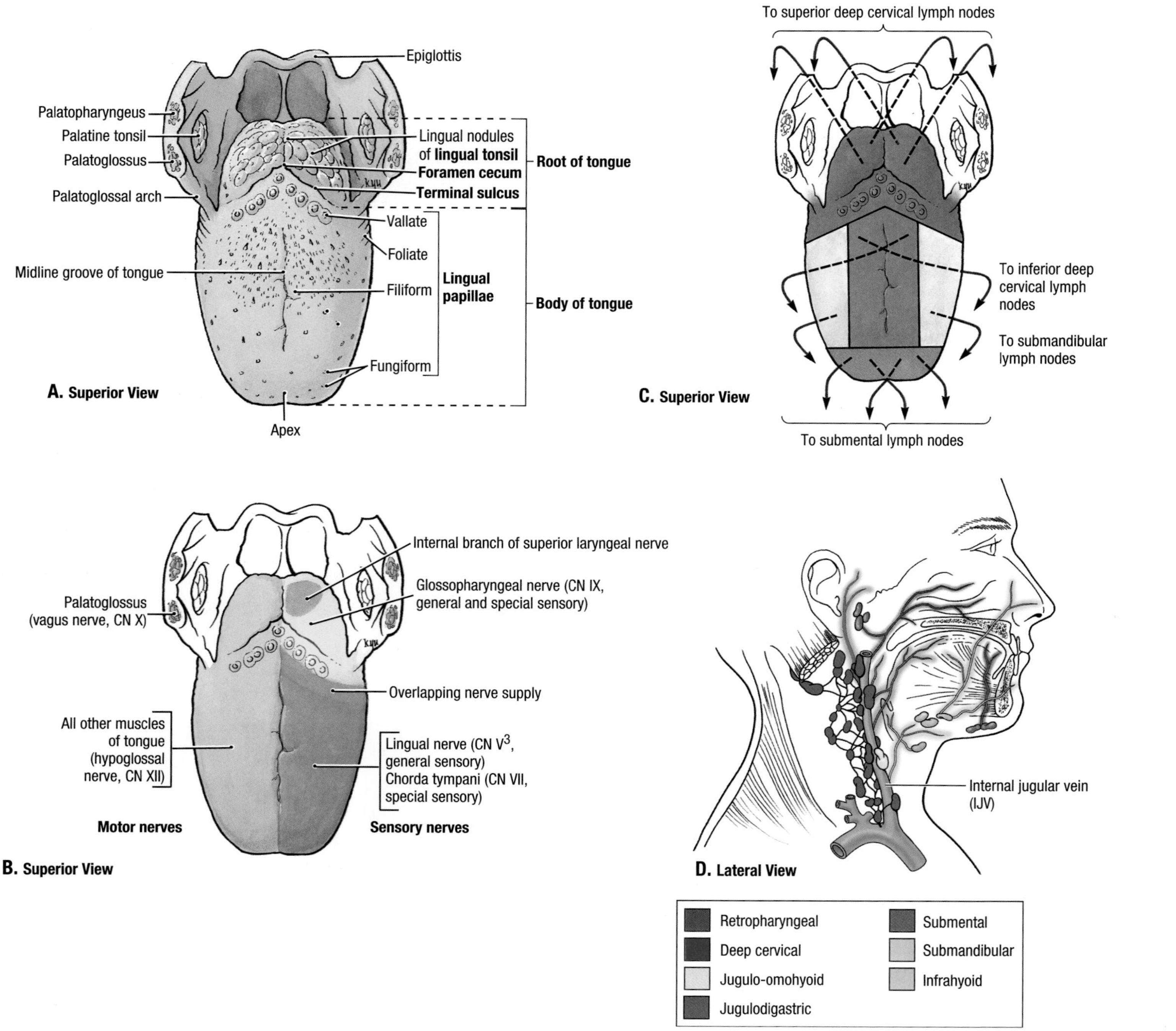

## 7.47 Tongue

**A.** Features of dorsum of the tongue. The foramen cecum is the upper end of the primitive thyroglossal duct; the arms of the V-shaped terminal sulcus diverge from the foramen, demarcating the posterior third of the tongue from the anterior two thirds. **B.** General sensory, special sensory (taste), and motor innervation of tongue. **C.** Lymphatic drainage of dorsum of tongue. **D.** Lymphatic drainage of tongue, mouth, nasal cavity, and nose.

Malignant tumors in the posterior part of the tongue metastasize to the superior deep cervical lymph nodes on both sides. In contrast, tumors in the apex and anterolateral parts usually do not metastasize to the inferior deep cervical nodes until late in the disease. Because the deep nodes are closely related to the internal jugular vein (IJV), metastases from the carcinoma may spread to the submental and submandibular regions and along the IJV into the neck.

One may touch the anterior part of the tongue without feeling discomfort; however, when the posterior part is touched, one usually gags. CN IX and CN X are responsible for the muscular contraction of each side of the pharynx. Glossopharyngeal branches (CN IX) provide the afferent limb of the gag reflex.

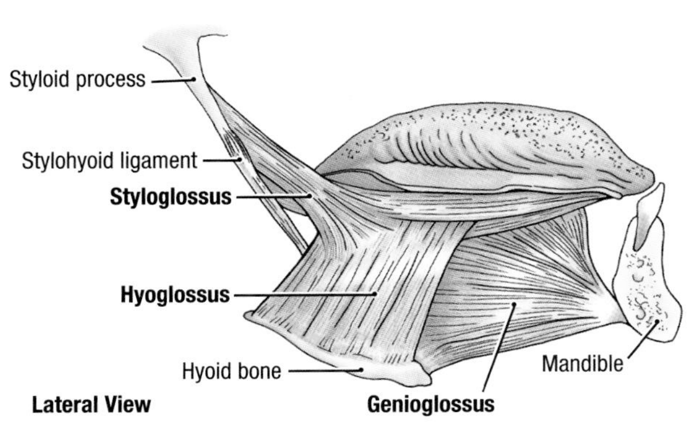
Styloid process
Stylohyoid ligament
Styloglossus
Hyoglossus
Hyoid bone
Mandible
Lateral View
Genioglossus

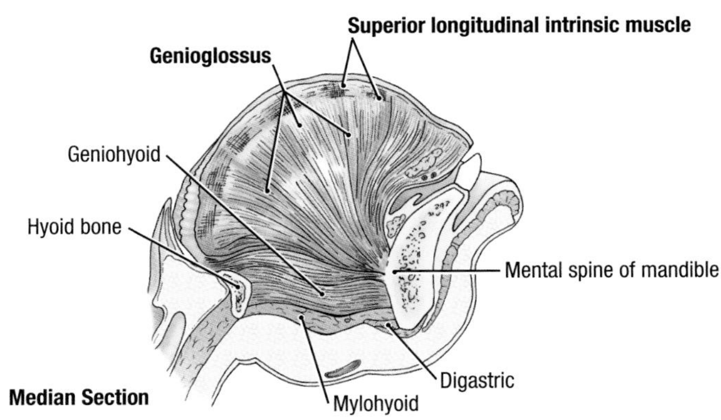
Superior longitudinal intrinsic muscle
Genioglossus
Geniohyoid
Hyoid bone
Mental spine of mandible
Digastric
Median Section
Mylohyoid

## TABLE 7.11 MUSCLES OF TONGUE

**Extrinsic Muscles**

| Muscle | Origin | Insertion | Innervation | Main Action |
|---|---|---|---|---|
| **Genioglossus** | Superior part of mental spine of mandible | Dorsum of tongue and body of hyoid bone | Hypoglossal nerve (CN XII) | Depresses tongue; its posterior part pulls tongue anteriorly for protrusion[a] |
| **Hyoglossus** | Body and greater horn of hyoid bone | Side and inferior aspect of tongue | | Depresses and retracts tongue |
| **Styloglossus** | Styloid process of temporal bone and stylohyoid ligament | Side and inferior aspect of tongue | | Retracts tongue and draws it up to create a trough for swallowing |
| **Palatoglossus** | Palatine aponeurosis of soft palate | Side of tongue | CN X and pharyngeal plexus | Elevates posterior part of tongue |

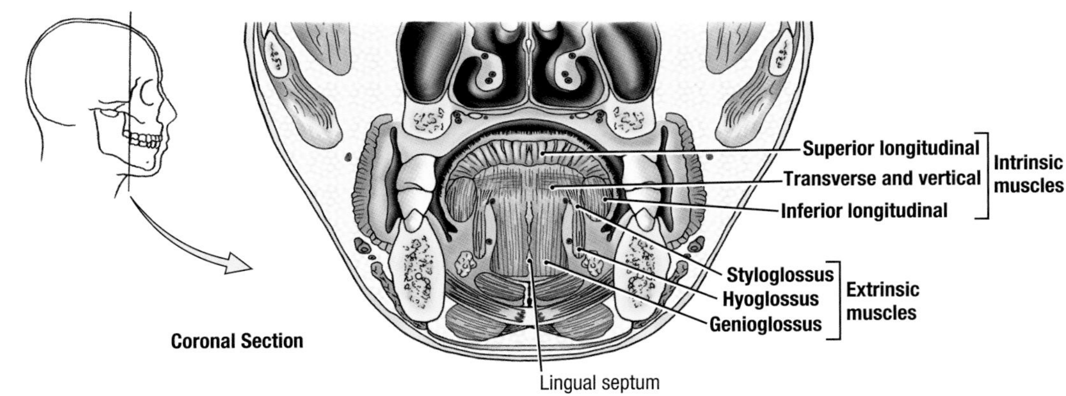
Superior longitudinal
Transverse and vertical
Inferior longitudinal
Intrinsic muscles
Styloglossus
Hyoglossus
Genioglossus
Extrinsic muscles
Coronal Section
Lingual septum

**Intrinsic Muscles**

| Muscle | Origin | Insertion | Innervation | Main Action |
|---|---|---|---|---|
| **Superior longitudinal** | Submucous fibrous layer and lingual septum | Margins and mucous membrane of tongue | Hypoglossal nerve (CN XII) | Curls tip and sides of tongue superiorly and shortens tongue |
| **Inferior longitudinal** | Root of tongue and body of hyoid bone | Apex of tongue | | Curls tip of tongue inferiorly and shortens tongue |
| **Transverse** | Lingual septum | Fibrous tissue at margins of tongue | | Narrows and elongates the tongue[a] |
| **Vertical** | Superior surface of borders of tongue | Inferior surface of borders of tongue | | Flattens and broadens the tongue[a] |

[a]Acts simultaneously to protrude tongue.

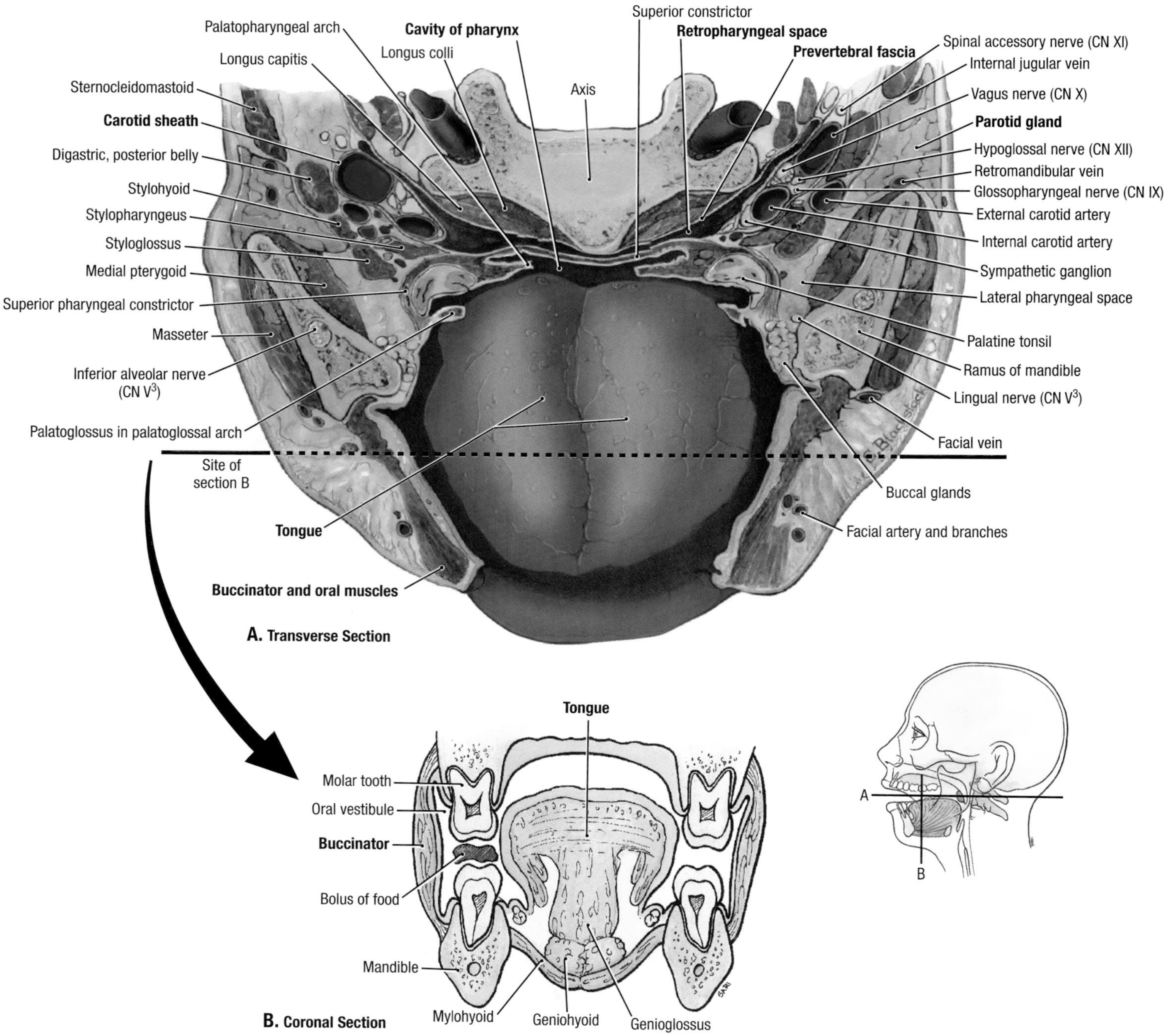
Palatopharyngeal arch
Longus capitis
Cavity of pharynx
Longus colli
Superior constrictor
Retropharyngeal space
Prevertebral fascia
Axis
Spinal accessory nerve (CN XI)
Internal jugular vein
Vagus nerve (CN X)
Parotid gland
Hypoglossal nerve (CN XII)
Retromandibular vein
Glossopharyngeal nerve (CN IX)
External carotid artery
Internal carotid artery
Sympathetic ganglion
Lateral pharyngeal space
Palatine tonsil
Ramus of mandible
Lingual nerve (CN V3)
Facial vein
Buccal glands
Facial artery and branches
Sternocleidomastoid
Carotid sheath
Digastric, posterior belly
Stylohyoid
Stylopharyngeus
Styloglossus
Medial pterygoid
Superior pharyngeal constrictor
Masseter
Inferior alveolar nerve (CN V3)
Palatoglossus in palatoglossal arch
Site of section B
Tongue
Buccinator and oral muscles
A. Transverse Section
Tongue
Molar tooth
Oral vestibule
Buccinator
Bolus of food
Mandible
Mylohyoid
Geniohyoid
Genioglossus
B. Coronal Section
A
B

## 7.48 Sections through mouth

**A.** The viscerocranium has been sectioned at the C1 vertebral level, the plane of section passing through the oral fissure anteriorly. The retropharyngeal space (opened up in this specimen) allows the pharynx to contract and relax during swallowing; the retropharyngeal space is closed laterally at the carotid sheath and limited posteriorly by the prevertebral fascia. The beds of the parotid glands are also demonstrated. **B.** Schematic coronal section demonstrating how the tongue and buccinator (or, anteriorly, the orbicularis oris) work together to retain food between the teeth when chewing. The buccinator and superior part of the orbicularis oris are innervated by the buccal branch of the facial nerve (CN VII).

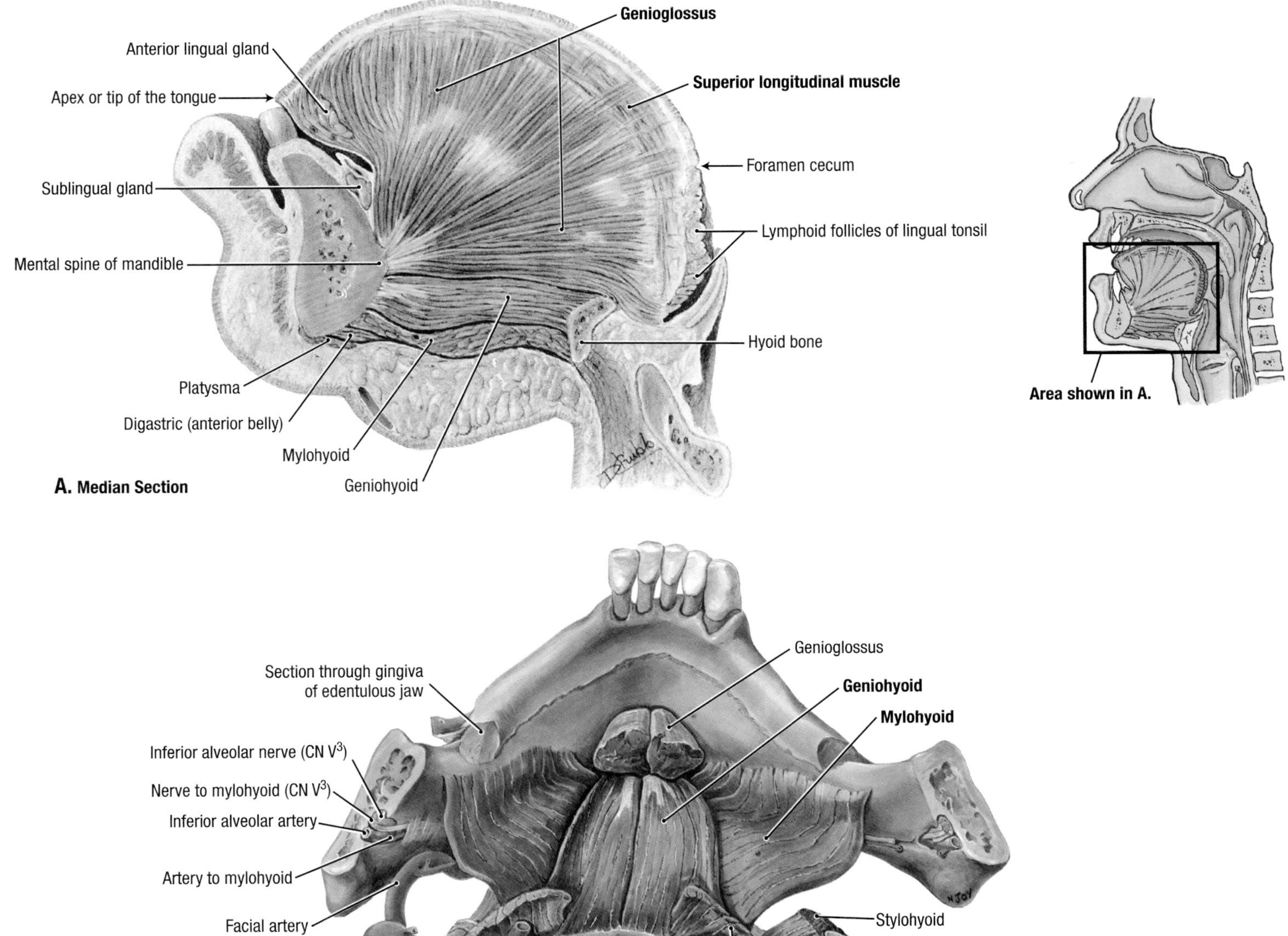
Genioglossus
Anterior lingual gland
Superior longitudinal muscle
Apex or tip of the tongue
Foramen cecum
Sublingual gland
Lymphoid follicles of lingual tonsil
Mental spine of mandible
Hyoid bone
Platysma
Digastric (anterior belly)
Mylohyoid
Geniohyoid
A. Median Section
Area shown in A.
Genioglossus
Section through gingiva of edentulous jaw
Geniohyoid
Mylohyoid
Inferior alveolar nerve (CN V3)
Nerve to mylohyoid (CN V3)
Inferior alveolar artery
Artery to mylohyoid
Facial artery
Stylohyoid
Lesser horn of hyoid
Digastric (intermediate tendon)
Lingual artery
Stylohyoid ligament
Middle constrictor
Body of hyoid
Greater horn of hyoid
Hyoglossus
Epiglottis
Vallecula
B. Posterosuperior View
External carotid artery

## 7.49 Tongue and floor of mouth

**A.** Median section though the tongue and lower jaw. The tongue is composed mainly of muscle; extrinsic muscles alter the position of the tongue, and intrinsic muscles alter its shape. The genioglossus is the extrinsic muscle apparent in this plane, and the superior longitudinal muscle is the intrinsic muscle. **B.** Muscles of the floor of the mouth viewed posterosuperiorly. The mylohyoid muscle extends between the two mylohyoid lines of the mandible. It has a thick, free posterior border and becomes thinner anteriorly.

When the genioglossus is paralyzed, the tongue mass has a tendency to shift posteriorly, obstructing the airway and presenting the risk of suffocation. Total relaxation of the genioglossus muscles occurs during general anesthesia; therefore, the tongue of an anesthetized patient must be prevented from relapsing by inserting an airway.

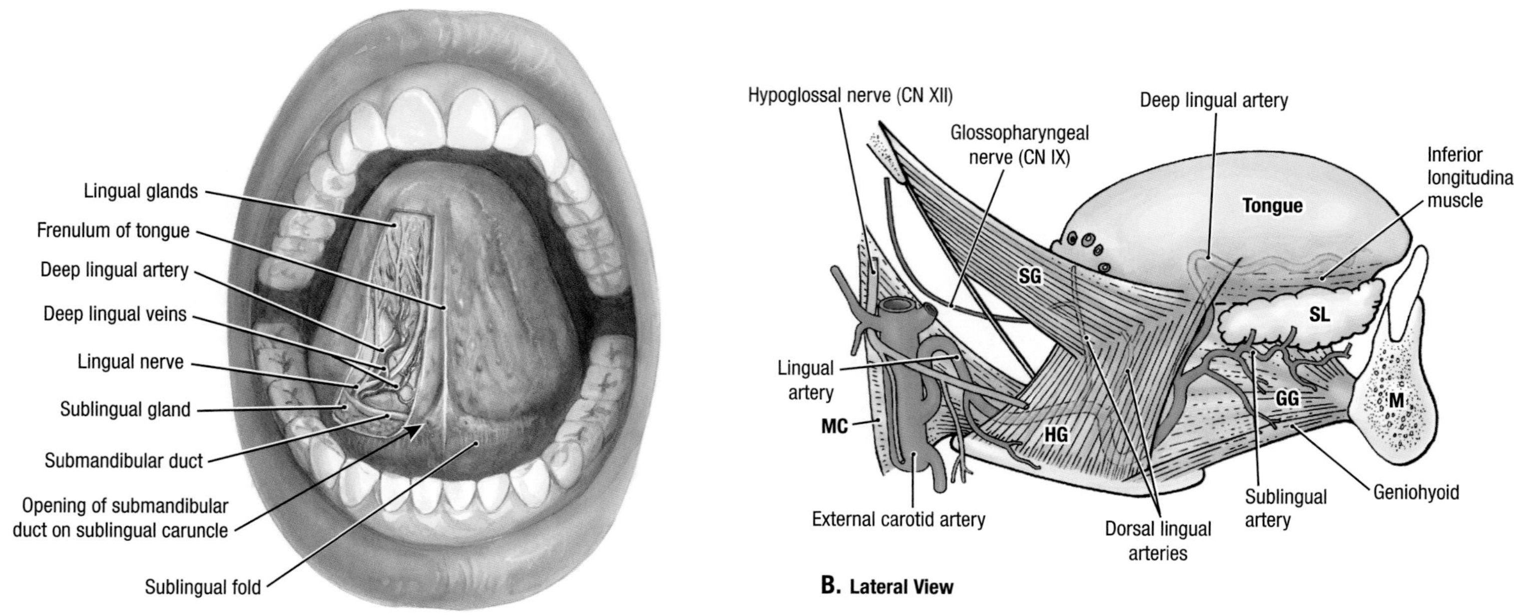
Lingual glands
Frenulum of tongue
Deep lingual artery
Deep lingual veins
Lingual nerve
Sublingual gland
Submandibular duct
Opening of submandibular duct on sublingual caruncle
Sublingual fold
A. Anterior View
Hypoglossal nerve (CN XII)
Glossopharyngeal nerve (CN IX)
Deep lingual artery
Inferior longitudinal muscle
Tongue
SG
SL
Lingual artery
MC
HG
GG
M
External carotid artery
Dorsal lingual arteries
Sublingual artery
Geniohyoid
B. Lateral View

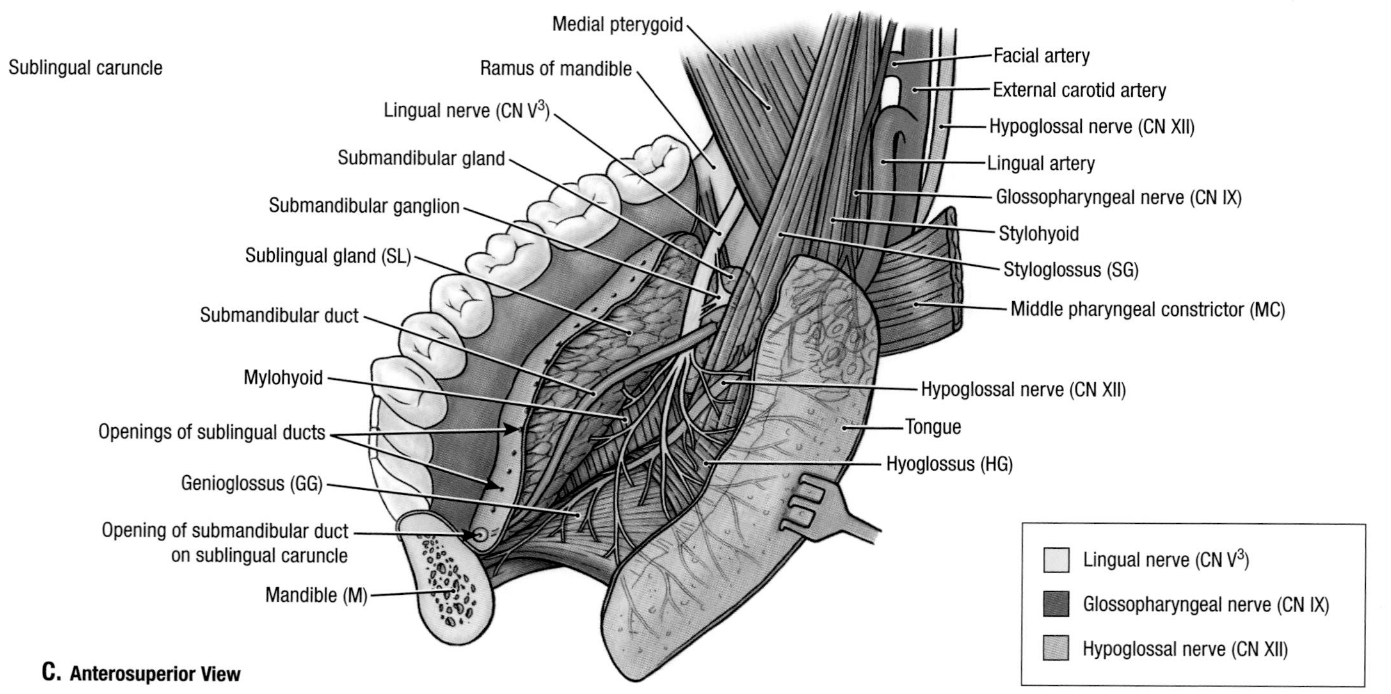
Sublingual caruncle
Medial pterygoid
Ramus of mandible
Lingual nerve (CN V3)
Submandibular gland
Submandibular ganglion
Sublingual gland (SL)
Submandibular duct
Mylohyoid
Openings of sublingual ducts
Genioglossus (GG)
Opening of submandibular duct on sublingual caruncle
Mandible (M)
Facial artery
External carotid artery
Hypoglossal nerve (CN XII)
Lingual artery
Glossopharyngeal nerve (CN IX)
Stylohyoid
Styloglossus (SG)
Middle pharyngeal constrictor (MC)
Hypoglossal nerve (CN XII)
Tongue
Hyoglossus (HG)
Lingual nerve (CN V3)
Glossopharyngeal nerve (CN IX)
Hypoglossal nerve (CN XII)
C. Anterosuperior View

## 7.50 Arteries and nerves of the tongue

**A.** Inferior surface of the tongue and floor of the mouth. The thin sublingual mucosa has been removed on the left side. **B.** Course and distribution of the lingual artery. **C.** Dissection of right side of floor of mouth. Letters in parentheses refer to **B.**

The parotid and submandibular salivary glands may be examined radiographically after the injection of a contrast medium into their ducts. This special type of radiograph (sialogram) demonstrates the salivary ducts and some secretory units. Because of the small size and number of sublingual ducts of the sublingual glands, one cannot usually inject contrast medium into them.

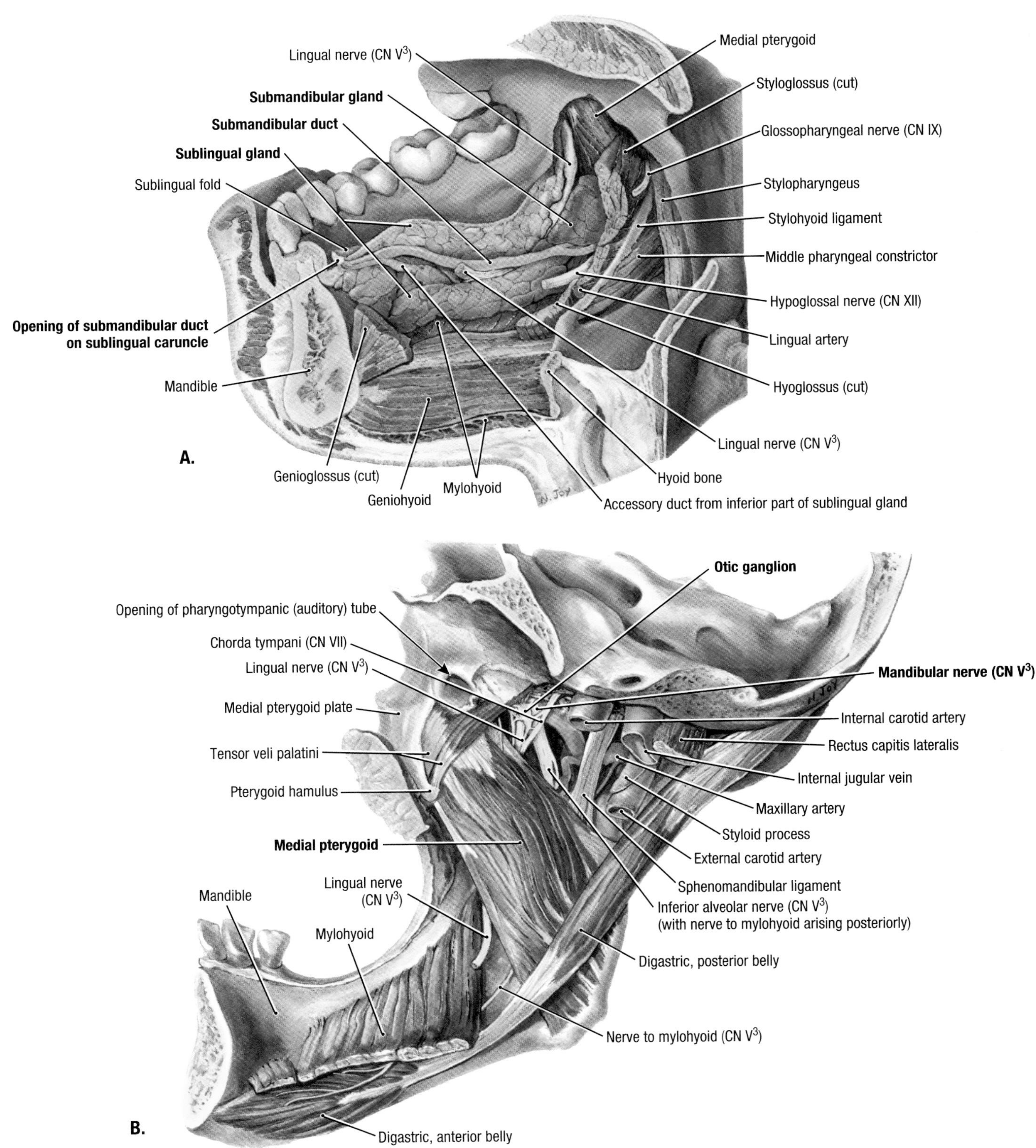
Lingual nerve (CN V3)
Submandibular gland
Submandibular duct
Sublingual gland
Sublingual fold
Opening of submandibular duct on sublingual caruncle
Mandible
A.
Genioglossus (cut)
Geniohyoid
Mylohyoid
Medial pterygoid
Styloglossus (cut)
Glossopharyngeal nerve (CN IX)
Stylopharyngeus
Stylohyoid ligament
Middle pharyngeal constrictor
Hypoglossal nerve (CN XII)
Lingual artery
Hyoglossus (cut)
Lingual nerve (CN V3)
Hyoid bone
Accessory duct from inferior part of sublingual gland
Opening of pharyngotympanic (auditory) tube
Chorda tympani (CN VII)
Lingual nerve (CN V3)
Medial pterygoid plate
Tensor veli palatini
Pterygoid hamulus
Medial pterygoid
Mandible
Lingual nerve (CN V3)
Mylohyoid
B.
Digastric, anterior belly
Otic ganglion
Mandibular nerve (CN V3)
Internal carotid artery
Rectus capitis lateralis
Internal jugular vein
Maxillary artery
Styloid process
External carotid artery
Sphenomandibular ligament
Inferior alveolar nerve (CN V3) (with nerve to mylohyoid arising posteriorly)
Digastric, posterior belly
Nerve to mylohyoid (CN V3)
Medial Views

## 7.51 Muscles, glands, and vessels of floor of mouth and medial aspect of mandible

**A.** Sublingual and submandibular glands. The tongue has been excised. **B.** Structures related to the medial surface of the mandible. The otic ganglion lies medial to the mandibular nerve (CN $V^3$) and between the foramen ovale superiorly and the medial pterygoid muscle inferiorly.

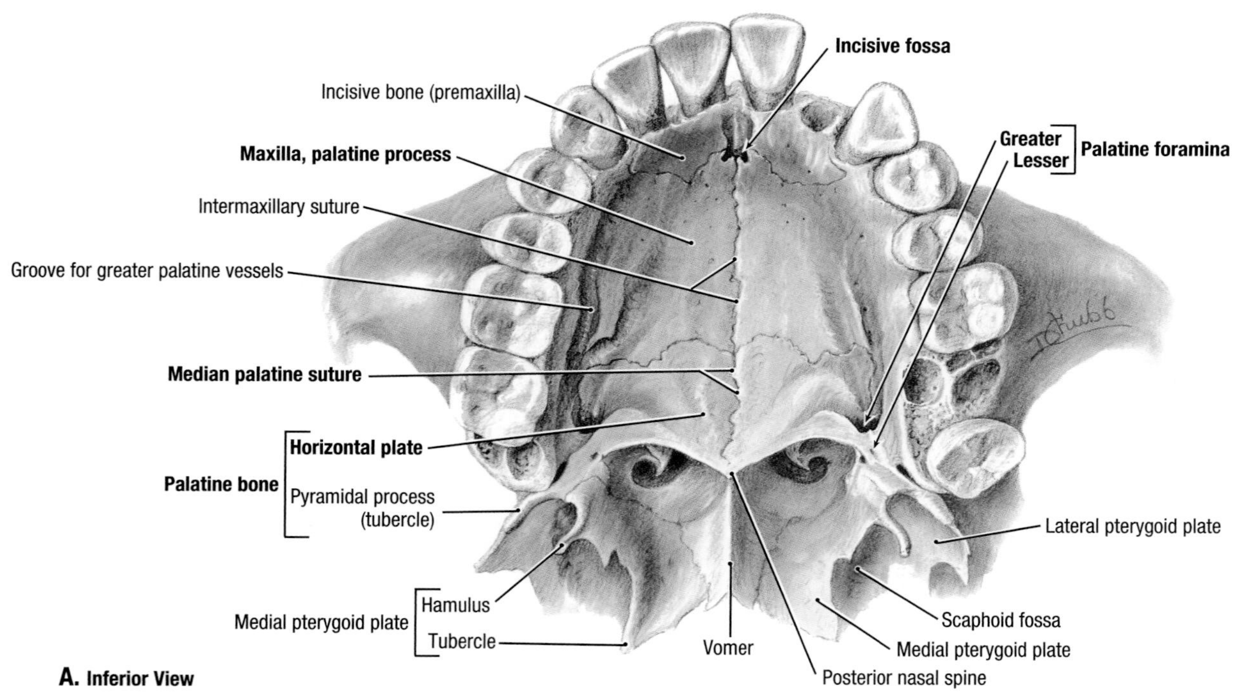
Incisive fossa
Incisive bone (premaxilla)
Maxilla, palatine process
Greater
Lesser
Palatine foramina
Intermaxillary suture
Groove for greater palatine vessels
Median palatine suture
Horizontal plate
Palatine bone
Pyramidal process (tubercle)
Lateral pterygoid plate
Hamulus
Medial pterygoid plate
Tubercle
Scaphoid fossa
Medial pterygoid plate
Vomer
Posterior nasal spine
A. Inferior View

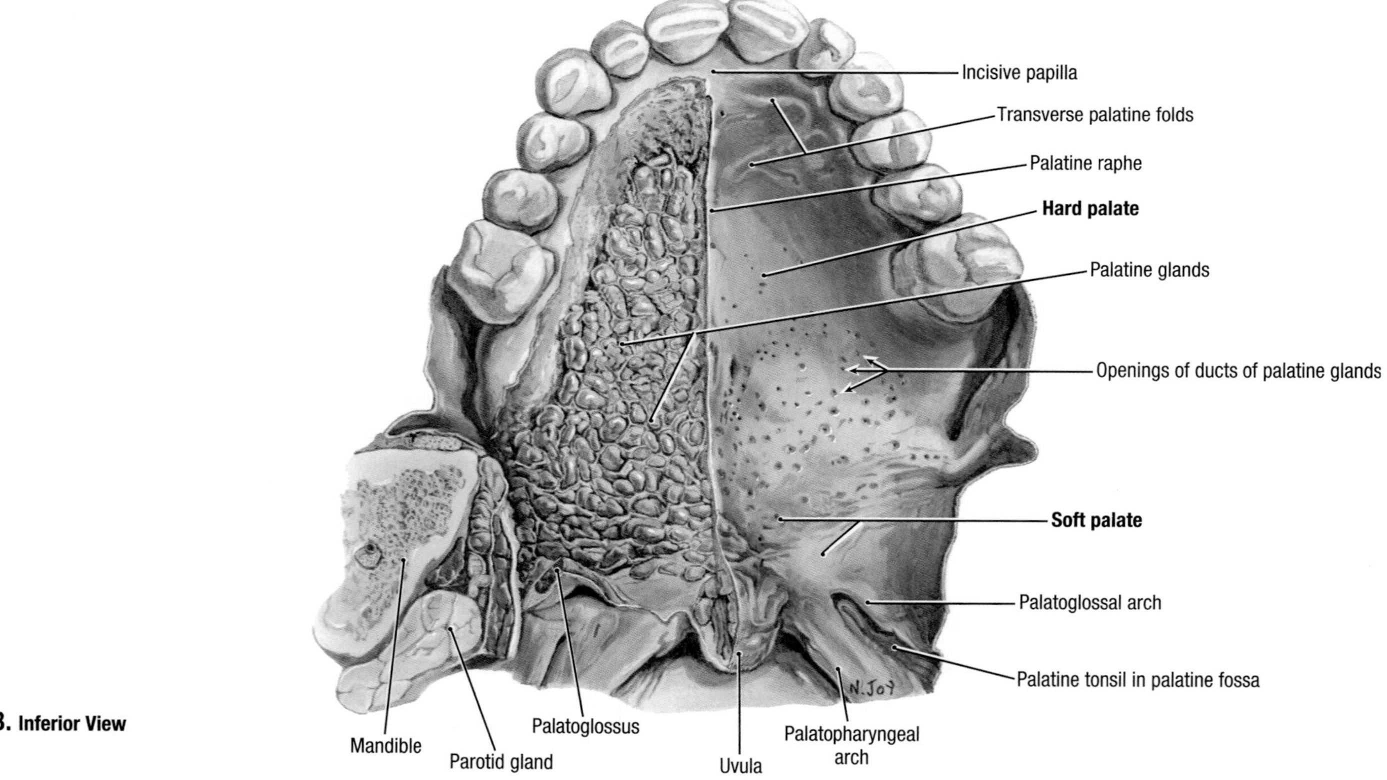
Incisive papilla
Transverse palatine folds
Palatine raphe
Hard palate
Palatine glands
Openings of ducts of palatine glands
Soft palate
Palatoglossal arch
Palatine tonsil in palatine fossa
B. Inferior View
Mandible
Parotid gland
Palatoglossus
Uvula
Palatopharyngeal arch

## 7.52 Palate

**A.** Bones of the hard palate. The palatine aponeurosis, which forms the fibrous "skeleton" of the soft palate, stretches between the hamuli of the medial pterygoid plates. **B.** Mucous membrane and glands of palate.

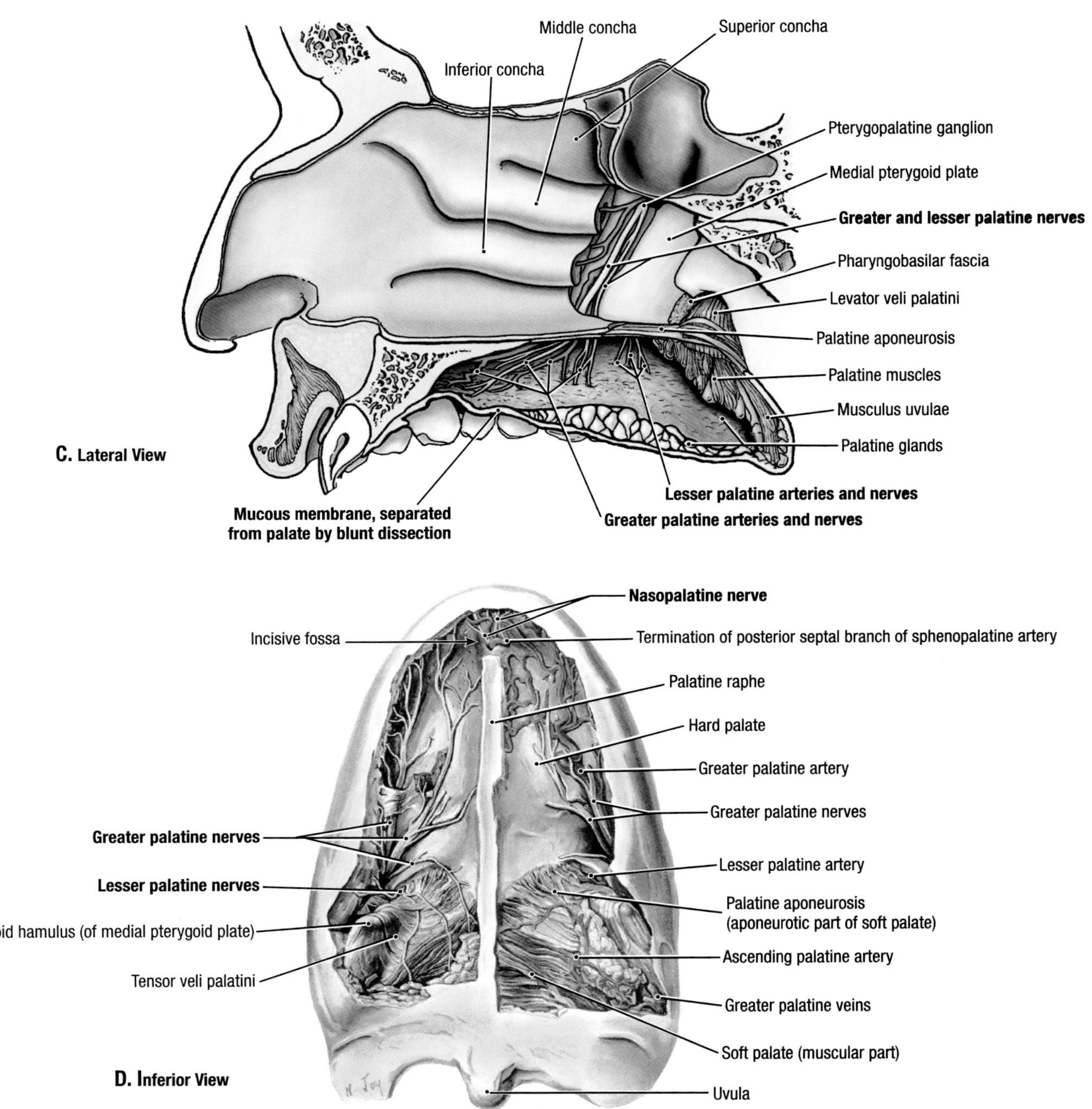
Middle concha
Superior concha
Inferior concha
Pterygopalatine ganglion
Medial pterygoid plate
Greater and lesser palatine nerves
Pharyngobasilar fascia
Levator veli palatini
Palatine aponeurosis
Palatine muscles
Musculus uvulae
Palatine glands
C. Lateral View
Lesser palatine arteries and nerves
Mucous membrane, separated from palate by blunt dissection
Greater palatine arteries and nerves
Nasopalatine nerve
Incisive fossa
Termination of posterior septal branch of sphenopalatine artery
Palatine raphe
Hard palate
Greater palatine artery
Greater palatine nerves
Greater palatine nerves
Lesser palatine artery
Lesser palatine nerves
Palatine aponeurosis (aponeurotic part of soft palate)
Pterygoid hamulus (of medial pterygoid plate)
Ascending palatine artery
Tensor veli palatini
Greater palatine veins
Soft palate (muscular part)
D. Inferior View
Uvula

## 7.52 Palate *(continued)*

**C.** Nerves and vessels of palatine canal. The lateral wall of the nasal cavity is shown. The posterior ends of the middle and inferior conchae are excised along with the mucoperiosteum; the thin, perpendicular plate of the palatine bone is removed to expose the palatine nerves and arteries. **D.** Dissection of an edentulous palate. The greater palatine nerve supplies the gingivae and hard palate, the nasopalatine nerve the incisive region, and the lesser palatine nerves the soft palate. The nasopalatine nerves can be anesthetized by injecting anesthetic into the mouth of the incisive fossa in the hard palate. The anesthetized tissues are the palatal mucosa, the lingual gingivae, the six anterior maxillary teeth, and associated alveolar bone. The greater palatine nerve can be anesthetized by injecting anesthetic into the greater palatine foramen. The nerve emerges between the second and third maxillary molar teeth. This nerve block anesthetizes the palatal mucosa and lingual gingivae posterior to the maxillary canine teeth, and the underlying bone of the palate.

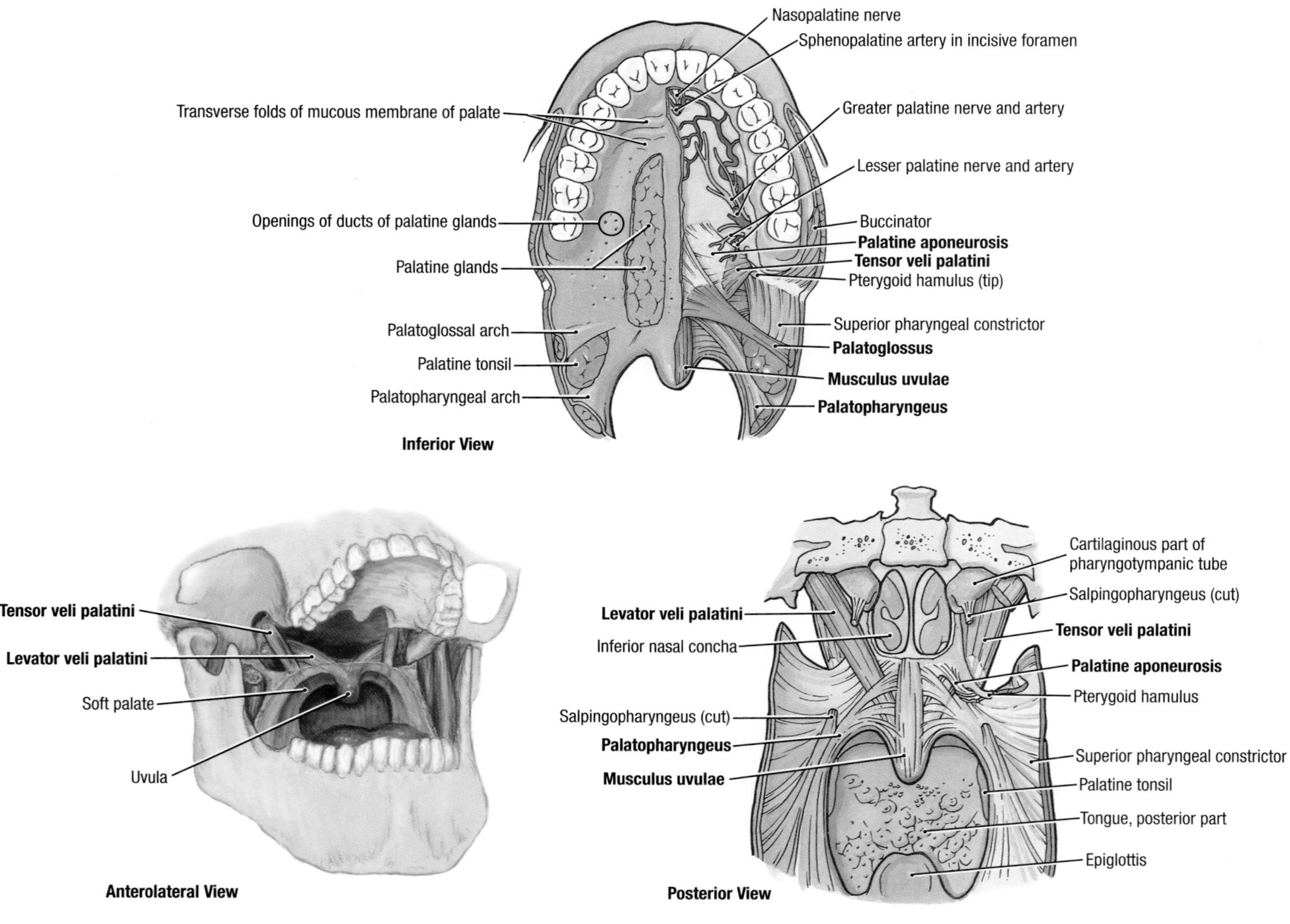
Nasopalatine nerve
Sphenopalatine artery in incisive foramen
Transverse folds of mucous membrane of palate
Greater palatine nerve and artery
Lesser palatine nerve and artery
Openings of ducts of palatine glands
Buccinator
Palatine aponeurosis
Tensor veli palatini
Pterygoid hamulus (tip)
Palatine glands
Superior pharyngeal constrictor
Palatoglossal arch
Palatoglossus
Palatine tonsil
Musculus uvulae
Palatopharyngeal arch
Palatopharyngeus
Inferior View
Tensor veli palatini
Levator veli palatini
Soft palate
Uvula
Anterolateral View
Cartilaginous part of pharyngotympanic tube
Salpingopharyngeus (cut)
Levator veli palatini
Tensor veli palatini
Inferior nasal concha
Palatine aponeurosis
Pterygoid hamulus
Salpingopharyngeus (cut)
Palatopharyngeus
Superior pharyngeal constrictor
Musculus uvulae
Palatine tonsil
Tongue, posterior part
Epiglottis
Posterior View

## TABLE 7.12 MUSCLES OF SOFT PALATE

| Muscle | Superior Attachment | Inferior Attachment | Innervation | Main Action(s) |
|---|---|---|---|---|
| **Levator veli palatini** | Cartilage of pharyngotympanic tube and petrous part of temporal bone | Palatine aponeurosis | Pharyngeal branch of vagus nerve through pharyngeal plexus | Elevates soft palate during swallowing and yawning |
| **Tensor veli palatini** | Scaphoid fossa of medial pterygoid plate, spine of sphenoid bone, and cartilage of pharyngotympanic tube | | Medial pterygoid nerve (CN $V^3$) through otic ganglion | Tenses soft palate and opens mouth of pharyngotympanic tube during swallowing and yawning |
| **Palatoglossus** | Palatine aponeurosis | Side of tongue | Pharyngeal branch of vagus nerve (CN X) via pharyngeal plexus | Elevates posterior part of tongue and draws soft palate onto tongue |
| **Palatopharyngeus** | Hard palate and palatine aponeurosis | Lateral wall of pharynx | | Tenses soft palate and pulls walls of pharynx superiorly, anteriorly, and medially during swallowing |
| **Musculus uvulae** | Posterior nasal spine and palatine aponeurosis | Mucosa of uvula | | Shortens uvula and pulls it superiorly |

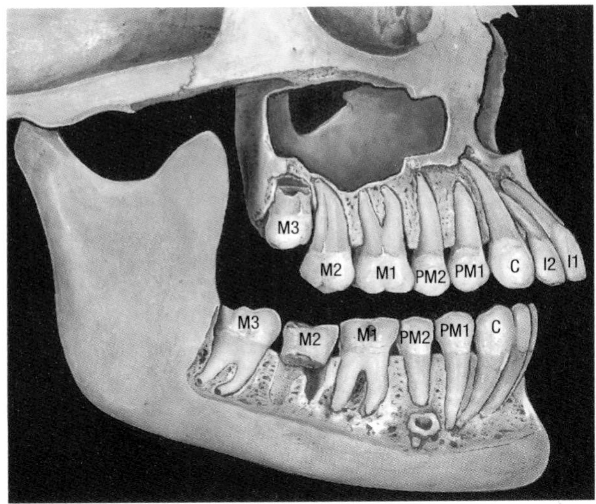
M3
M2
M1
PM2
PM1
C
I2
I1
M3
M2
M1
PM2
PM1
C

A. Lateral View

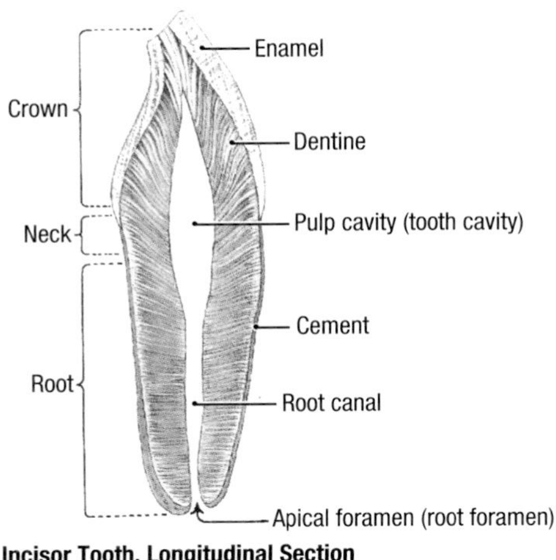
Crown
Neck
Root
Enamel
Dentine
Pulp cavity (tooth cavity)
Cement
Root canal
Apical foramen (root foramen)

Incisor Tooth, Longitudinal Section

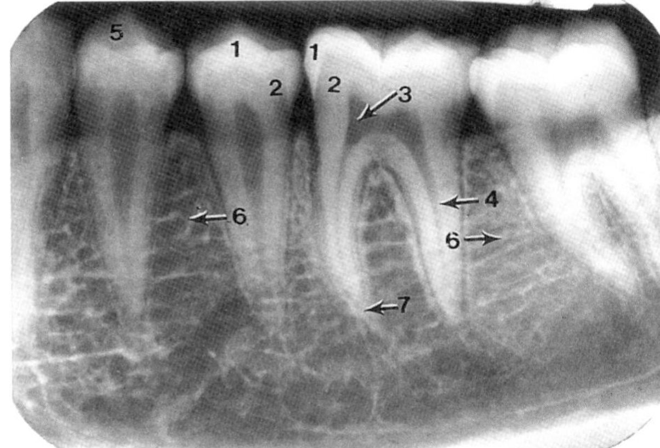
5
1
1
2
2
3
4
6
6
7

B. Lateral Radiograph

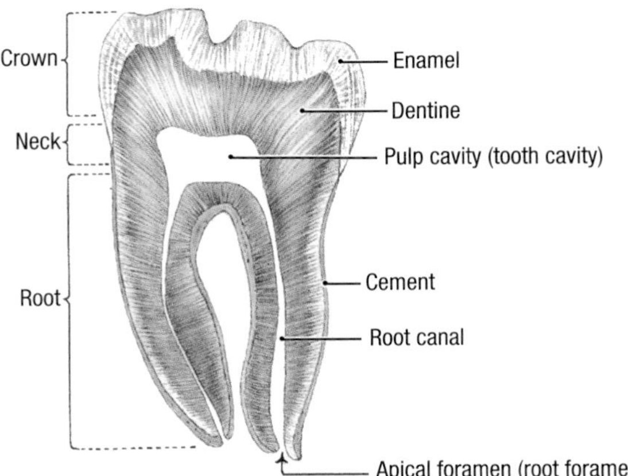
Crown
Neck
Root
Enamel
Dentine
Pulp cavity (tooth cavity)
Cement
Root canal
Apical foramen (root foramen)

C. Molar Tooth, Longitudinal Section

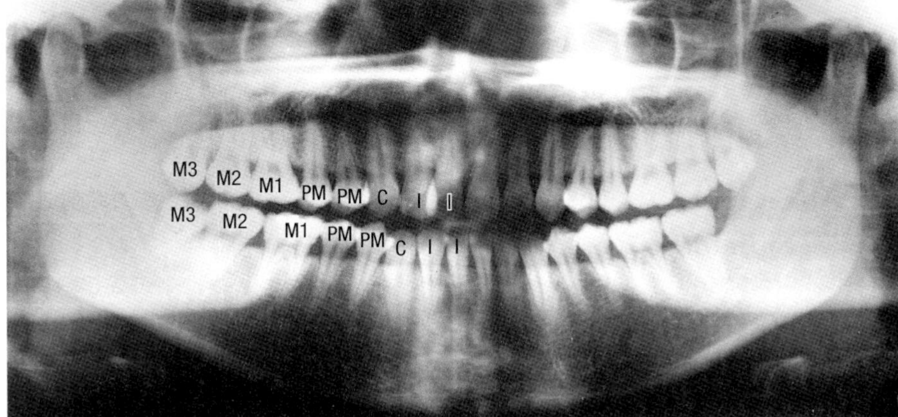
M3
M2
M1
PM
PM
C
I
I
M3
M2
M1
PM
PM
C
I
I

D. Pantomographic Radiograph

## 7.53 Permanent teeth—I

**A.** Teeth in situ with roots exposed. Incisors *(I1, I2)*, canine *(C1)*, premolars *(PM1, PM2)*, and molars *(M1, M2, M3)*. The roots of the 2nd lower molar have been removed. **B.** Lateral radiograph. *(1)* enamel, *(2)* dentin, *(3)* pulp chamber, *(4)* pulp canal, *(5)* buccal cusp, *(6)* alveolar bone, and *(7)* root apex. **C.** Longitudinal sections of an incisor and a molar tooth. **D.** Pantomographic radiograph of mandible and maxilla. The left lower third molar is not present.

Decay of the hard tissues of a tooth results in the formation of dental caries (cavities). Invasion of the pulp of the tooth by a carious lesion (cavity) results in infection and irritation of the tissues in the pulp cavity. This condition causes an inflammatory process (pulpitis). Because the pulp cavity is a rigid space, the swollen pulpal tissues cause pain (toothache).

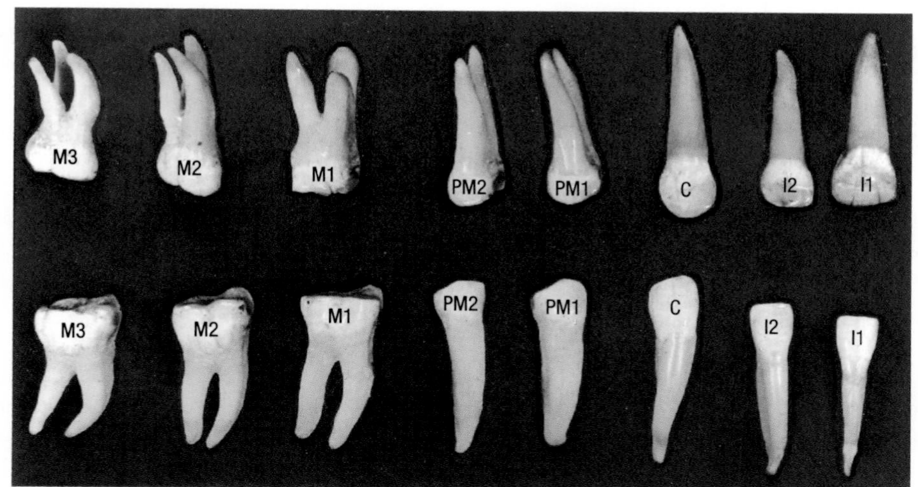
M3
M2
M1
PM2
PM1
C
I2
I1
Maxillary Teeth
M3
M2
M1
PM2
PM1
C
I2
I1
Mandibular Teeth

**A.** Vestibular View

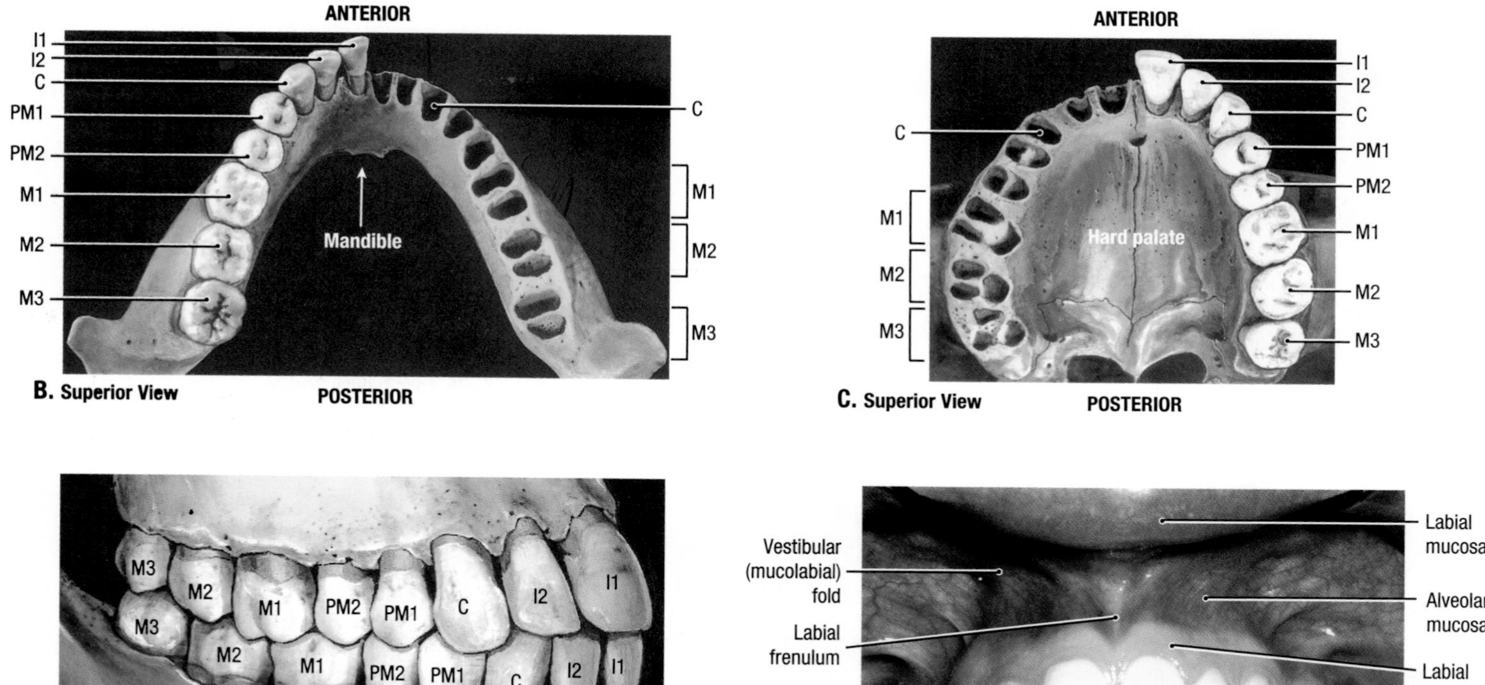
ANTERIOR
I1
I2
C
PM1
PM2
M1
M2
M3
Mandible
C
M1
M2
M3
POSTERIOR
ANTERIOR
I1
I2
C
PM1
PM2
M1
M2
M3
Hard palate
C
M1
M2
M3
POSTERIOR
M3
M2
M1
PM2
PM1
C
I2
I1
M3
M2
M1
PM2
PM1
C
I2
I1
Vestibular (mucolabial) fold
Labial frenulum
Labial mucosa
Alveolar mucosa
Labial maxillary gingiva
PM
I1
I2
C

**B.** Superior View

**C.** Superior View

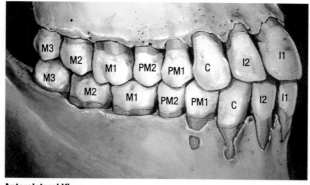

**D.** Anterolateral View

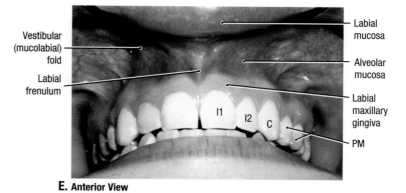

**E.** Anterior View

## 7.54 Permanent teeth—II

**A.** Removed teeth, displaying roots. There are 32 permanent teeth; 8 are on each side of each dental arch on the top (maxillary teeth) and bottom (mandibular teeth): 2 incisors *(I1–2)*, 1 canine *(C)*, 2 premolars *(PM1–2)*, and 3 molars *(M1–3)*. **B.** Permanent mandibular teeth and their sockets. **C.** Permanent maxillary teeth and their sockets. **D.** Teeth in occlusion. **E.** Vestibule and gingivae of the maxilla

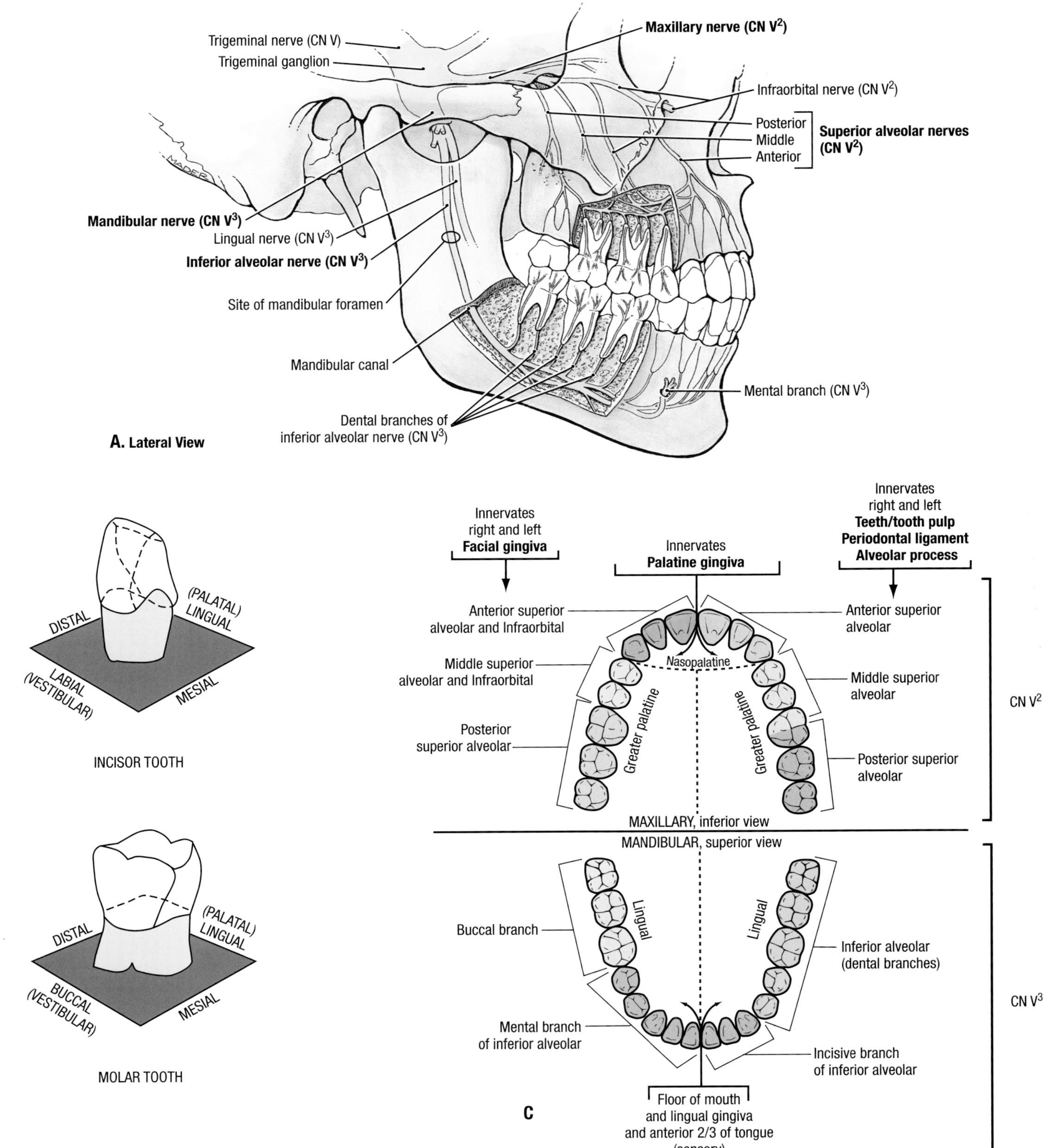
Trigeminal nerve (CN V)
Trigeminal ganglion
Maxillary nerve (CN V²)
Infraorbital nerve (CN V²)
Posterior
Middle
Anterior
Superior alveolar nerves (CN V²)
Mandibular nerve (CN V³)
Lingual nerve (CN V³)
Inferior alveolar nerve (CN V³)
Site of mandibular foramen
Mandibular canal
Mental branch (CN V³)
Dental branches of inferior alveolar nerve (CN V³)
A. Lateral View
DISTAL
(PALATAL) LINGUAL
LABIAL (VESTIBULAR)
MESIAL
INCISOR TOOTH
DISTAL
(PALATAL) LINGUAL
BUCCAL (VESTIBULAR)
MESIAL
B
MOLAR TOOTH
Innervates right and left Facial gingiva
Innervates Palatine gingiva
Innervates right and left Teeth/tooth pulp Periodontal ligament Alveolar process
Anterior superior alveolar and Infraorbital
Middle superior alveolar and Infraorbital
Posterior superior alveolar
Nasopalatine
Greater palatine
Greater palatine
Anterior superior alveolar
Middle superior alveolar
Posterior superior alveolar
CN V²
MAXILLARY, inferior view
MANDIBULAR, superior view
Buccal branch
Lingual
Lingual
Inferior alveolar (dental branches)
Mental branch of inferior alveolar
Incisive branch of inferior alveolar
CN V³
Floor of mouth and lingual gingiva and anterior 2/3 of tongue (sensory)
C

## 7.55 Innervation of teeth

**A.** Superior and inferior alveolar nerves. **B.** Surfaces of an incisor and molar tooth. **C.** Innervation of the mouth and teeth.

Improper oral hygiene results in food deposits in tooth and gingival crevices, which may cause inflammation of the gingivae (gingivitis). If untreated, the disease spreads to other supporting structures (including the alveolar bone), producing periodontitis. Periodontitis results in inflammation of the gingivae and may result in absorption of alveolar bone and gingival recession. Gingival recession exposes the sensitive cement of the teeth.

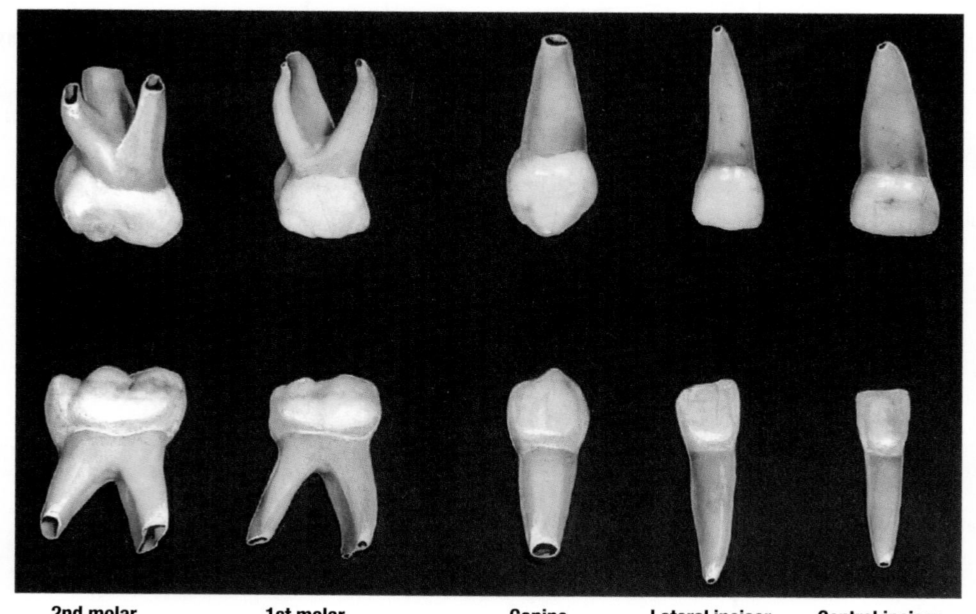
MAXILLARY TEETH
MANDIBULAR TEETH
A. Vestibular View
2nd molar
1st molar
Canine
Lateral incisor
Central incisor

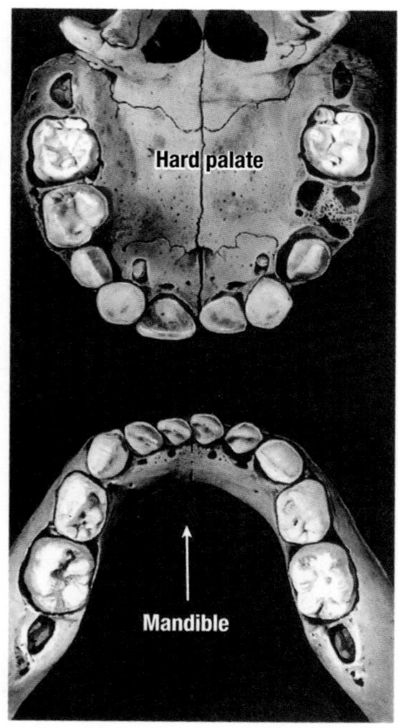
INFERIOR VIEW OF MAXILLARY TEETH
Hard palate
SUPERIOR VIEW OF MANDIBULAR TEETH
Mandible
B

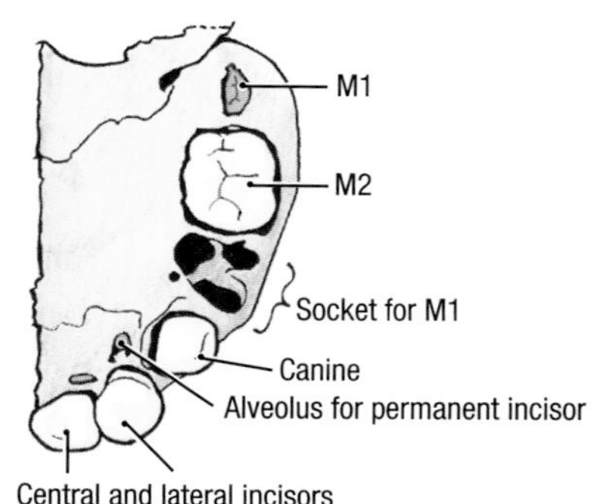
M1
M2
Socket for M1
Canine
Alveolus for permanent incisor
Central and lateral incisors

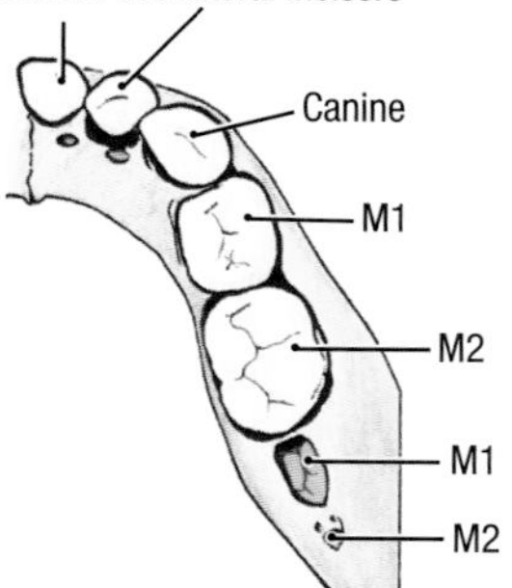
Canine
M1
M2
M1
M2

## 7.56 Primary teeth

**A.** Removed teeth. There are 20 primary (deciduous) teeth, 5 in each half of the mandible and 5 in each maxilla. They are named central incisor, lateral incisor, canine, 1st molar *(M1)*, and 2nd molar *(M2)*. Primary teeth differ from permanent teeth in that the primary teeth are smaller and whiter; the molars also have more bulbous crowns and more divergent roots. **B.** Teeth in situ, younger than 2 years of age. Permanent teeth are colored orange; the crowns of the unerupted 1st and 2nd permanent molars are partly visible.

**TABLE 7.13 PRIMARY AND SECONDARY DENTITION**

| Deciduous Teeth | Medial Incisor | Lateral Incisor | Canine | First Molar | Second Molar |
|---|---|---|---|---|---|
| Eruption (months)[a] | 6–8 | 8–10 | 16–20 | 12–16 | 20–24 |
| Shedding (years) | 6–7 | 7–8 | 10–12 | 9–11 | 10–12 |

[a]In some normal infants, the first teeth (medial incisors) may not erupt until 12 to 13 months of age

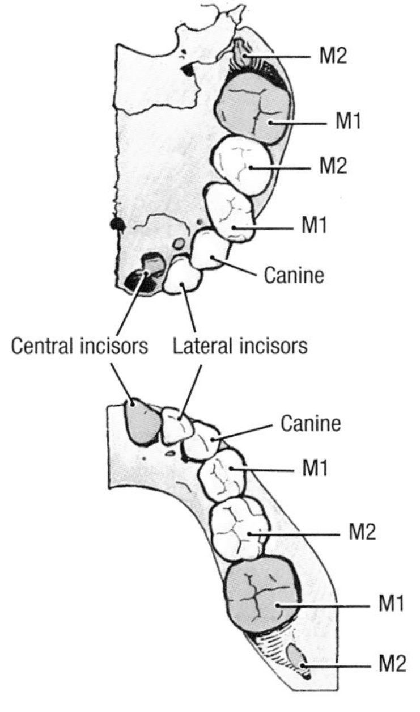
M2
M1
M2
M1
Canine
Central incisors
Lateral incisors
Canine
M1
M2
M1
M2

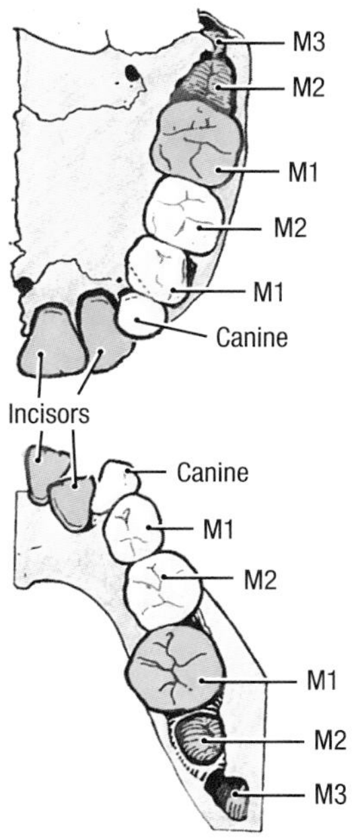
M3
M2
M1
M2
M1
Canine
Incisors
Canine
M1
M2
M1
M2
M3

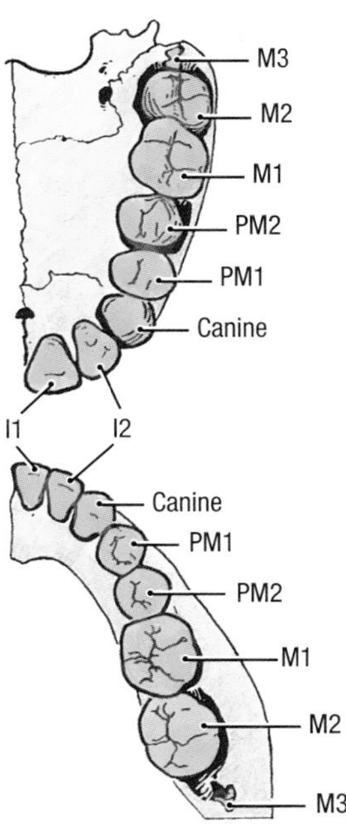
M3
M2
M1
PM2
PM1
Canine
I1
I2
Canine
PM1
PM2
M1
M2
M3

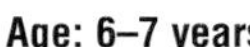

**Age: 6–7 years**

The 1st molars (6-year molars) have fully erupted, the primary central incisor has been shed, the lower central incisor is almost fully erupted, and the upper central incisor is descending into the vacated socket.

**Age: 8 years**

All of the permanent incisors have erupted; however, the lower lateral incisor is only partially erupted.

**Age: 12 years**

The primary teeth have been replaced by 20 permanent teeth, and the 1st and 2nd molars (12-year molars) have erupted; the canines, 2nd premolars, and 2nd molars (especially those in the upper jaw) have not erupted fully, nor have their bony sockets closed around them. By age 12, 28 permanent teeth are in evidence; the last 4 teeth, the 3rd molars, may erupt any time after this, or never.

| Permanent Teeth | Medial Incisor | Lateral Incisor | Canine | First Premolar | Second Premolar | First Molar | Second Molar | Third Molar |
|---|---|---|---|---|---|---|---|---|
| Eruption (years) | 7–8 | 8–9 | 10–12 | 10–11 | 11–12 | 6–7 | 12 | 13–25 |

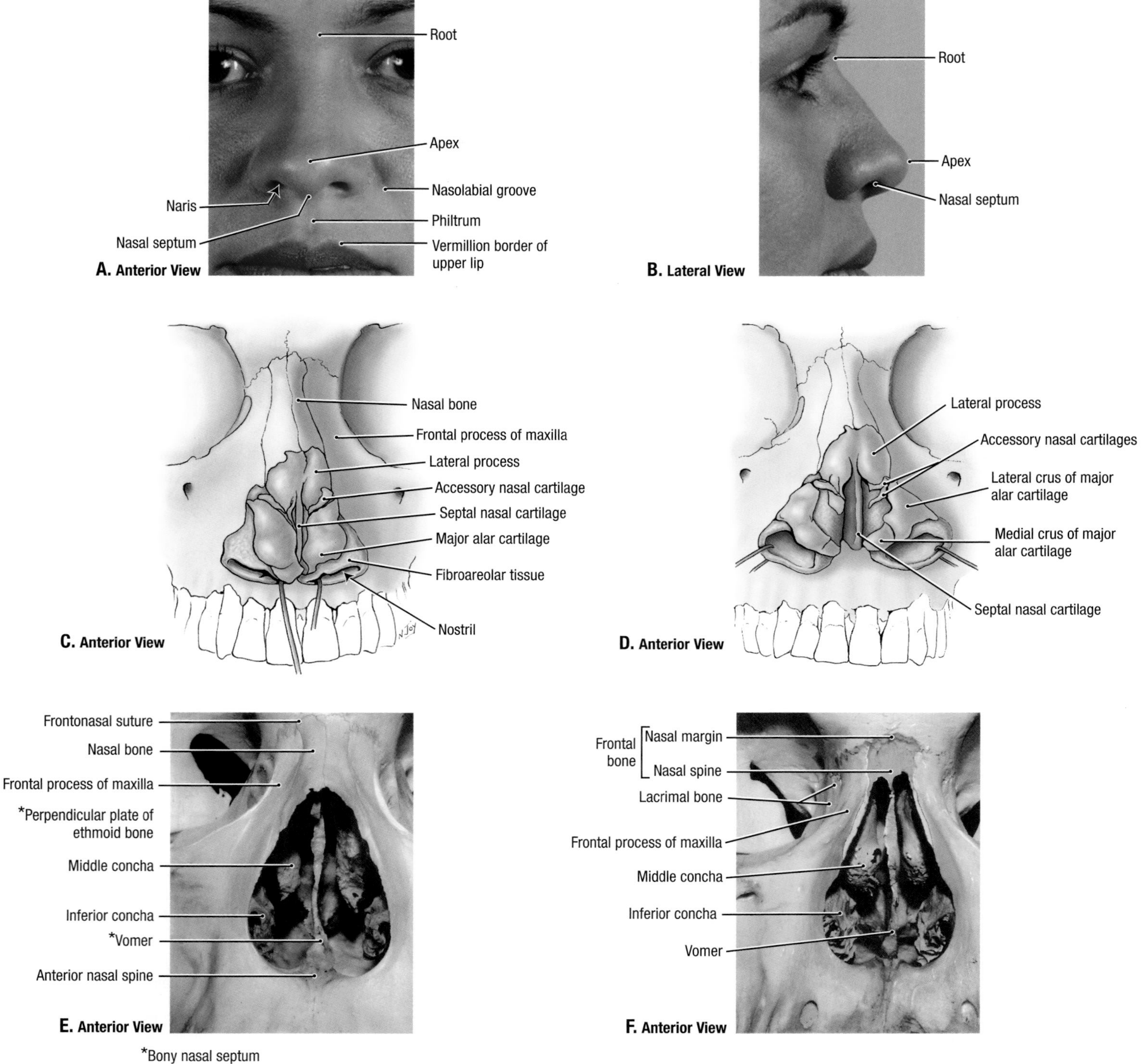
Root
Apex
Naris
Nasolabial groove
Nasal septum
Philtrum
Vermillion border of upper lip
A. Anterior View
Root
Apex
Nasal septum
B. Lateral View
Nasal bone
Frontal process of maxilla
Lateral process
Accessory nasal cartilage
Septal nasal cartilage
Major alar cartilage
Fibroareolar tissue
Nostril
C. Anterior View
Lateral process
Accessory nasal cartilages
Lateral crus of major alar cartilage
Medial crus of major alar cartilage
Septal nasal cartilage
D. Anterior View
Frontonasal suture
Nasal bone
Frontal process of maxilla
*Perpendicular plate of ethmoid bone
Middle concha
Inferior concha
*Vomer
Anterior nasal spine
E. Anterior View
*Bony nasal septum
Frontal bone
Nasal margin
Nasal spine
Lacrimal bone
Frontal process of maxilla
Middle concha
Inferior concha
Vomer
F. Anterior View

## 7.57 Surface anatomy, cartilages, and bones of nose

**A.** Surface features of anterior aspect of nose. **B.** Surface features of lateral aspect of nose. **C.** Nasal cartilages, with the septum pulled inferiorly. **D.** Nasal cartilages, separated and retracted laterally. **E.** Lower conchae and bony septum seen through the piriform aperture. The margin of the piriform aperture is sharp and formed by the maxillae and nasal bones. **F.** Nasal bones removed. The areas of the frontal processes of the maxillae *(yellow)* and of the frontal bone *(blue)* that articulate with the nasal bones can be seen.

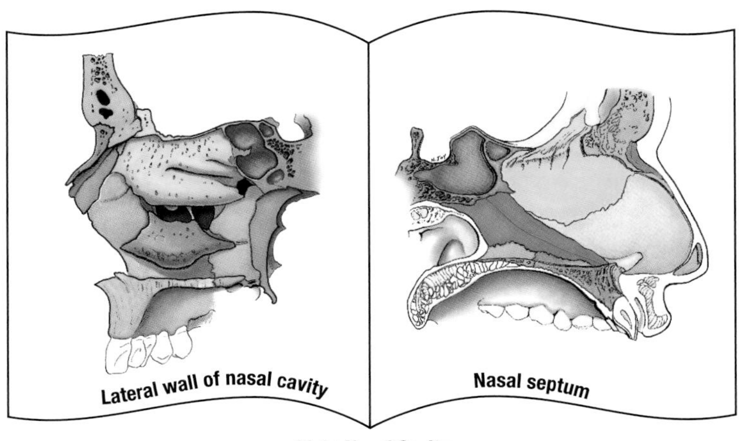
Lateral wall of nasal cavity
Nasal septum
Right Nasal Cavity

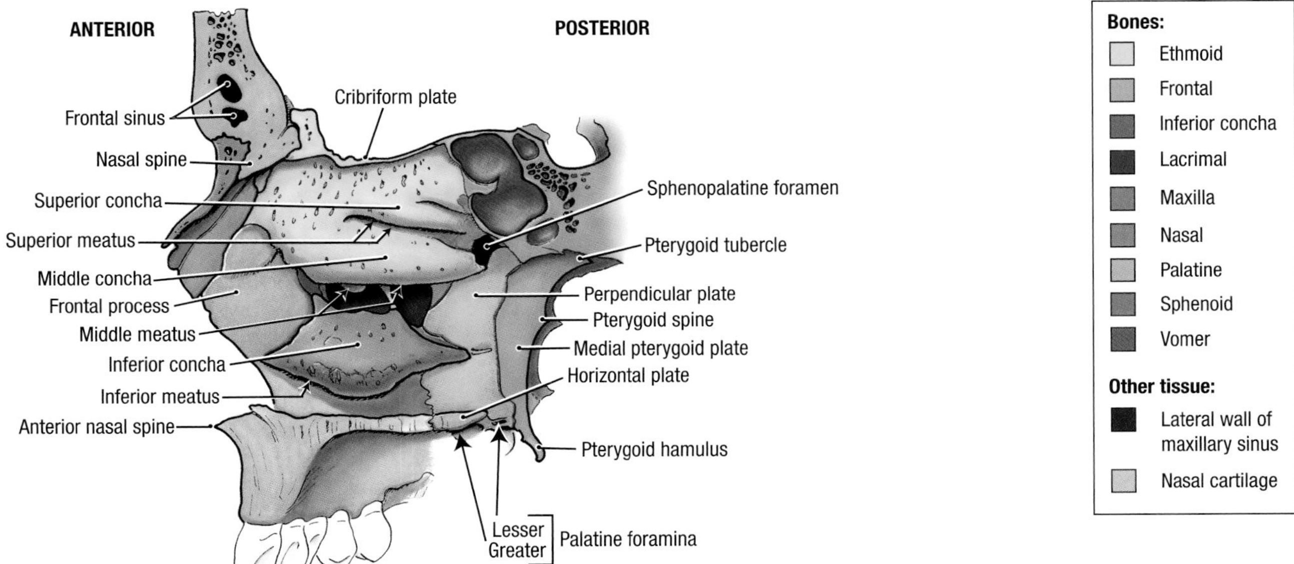
ANTERIOR
POSTERIOR
Frontal sinus
Cribriform plate
Nasal spine
Superior concha
Sphenopalatine foramen
Superior meatus
Pterygoid tubercle
Middle concha
Frontal process
Perpendicular plate
Pterygoid spine
Middle meatus
Medial pterygoid plate
Inferior concha
Horizontal plate
Inferior meatus
Anterior nasal spine
Pterygoid hamulus
Lesser
Greater
Palatine foramina
Bones:
Ethmoid
Frontal
Inferior concha
Lacrimal
Maxilla
Nasal
Palatine
Sphenoid
Vomer
Other tissue:
Lateral wall of maxillary sinus
Nasal cartilage

**A.** Medial View of Lateral Wall

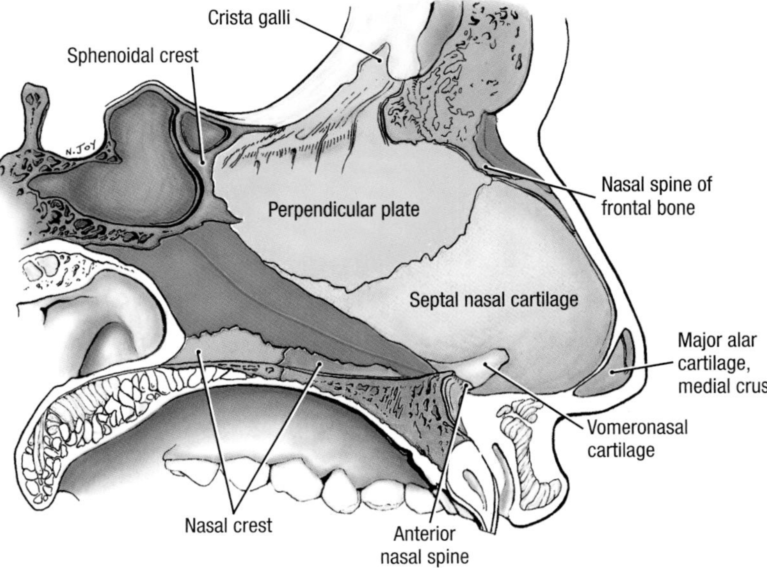
Crista galli
Sphenoidal crest
Perpendicular plate
Nasal spine of frontal bone
Septal nasal cartilage
Major alar cartilage, medial crus
Vomeronasal cartilage
Nasal crest
Anterior nasal spine

**B.** Lateral View of Nasal Septum

## 7.58 Bones of the lateral wall and septum of the nose

**A.** Lateral wall of nose. The superior and middle conchae are parts of the ethmoid bone, whereas the inferior concha is itself a bone. **B.** Nasal septum.

Deformity of the external nose usually is present with a fracture, particularly when a lateral force is applied by someone's elbow, for example. When the injury results from a direct blow (e.g., from a hockey stick), the cribriform plate of the ethmoid bone may fracture, resulting in CSF rhinorrhea.

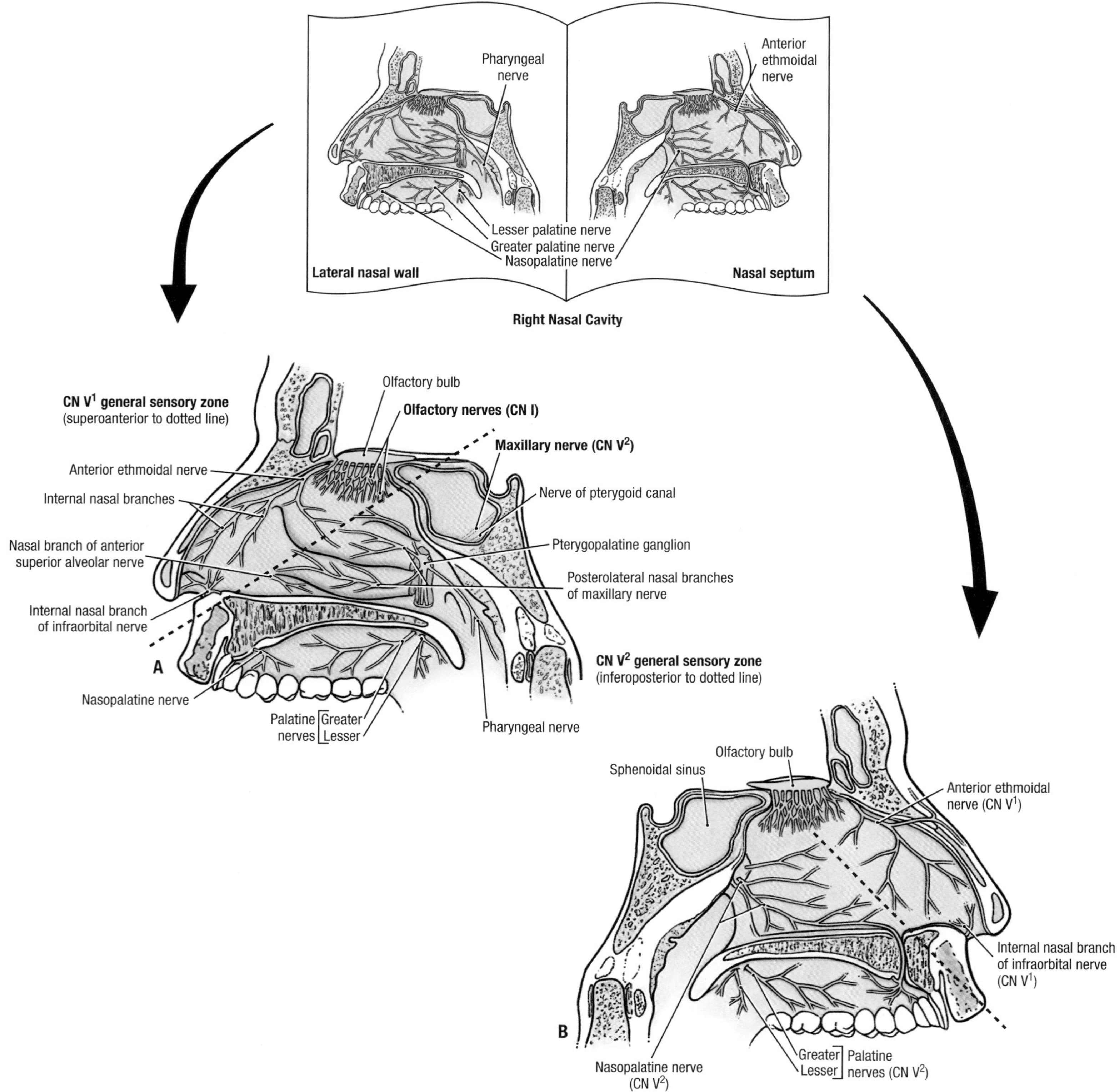
Pharyngeal nerve
Anterior ethmoidal nerve
Lesser palatine nerve
Greater palatine nerve
Nasopalatine nerve
Lateral nasal wall
Nasal septum
Right Nasal Cavity
CN V1 general sensory zone (superoanterior to dotted line)
Olfactory bulb
Olfactory nerves (CN I)
Maxillary nerve (CN V2)
Anterior ethmoidal nerve
Internal nasal branches
Nerve of pterygoid canal
Pterygopalatine ganglion
Nasal branch of anterior superior alveolar nerve
Posterolateral nasal branches of maxillary nerve
Internal nasal branch of infraorbital nerve
A
CN V2 general sensory zone (inferoposterior to dotted line)
Nasopalatine nerve
Palatine nerves Greater Lesser
Pharyngeal nerve
Olfactory bulb
Sphenoidal sinus
Anterior ethmoidal nerve (CN V1)
Internal nasal branch of infraorbital nerve (CN V1)
B
Nasopalatine nerve (CN V2)
Greater Lesser Palatine nerves (CN V2)

## 7.59 Innervation of lateral wall and septum of the nose

**A.** Lateral wall of nose. *Dotted diagonal lines* demarcate CN $V^1$ and CN $V^2$ general sensory zones. The olfactory neuroepithelium is in the superior part of the lateral and septal walls of the nasal cavity. The central processes of the olfactory neurosensory cells of each side form approximately 20 bundles that together form an olfactory nerve (CN I). **B.** Nasal septum. The nasopalatine nerve from the pterygopalatine ganglion supplies the posteroinferior septum, and the anterior ethmoidal nerve (branch of $V^1$) supplies the anterosuperior septum.

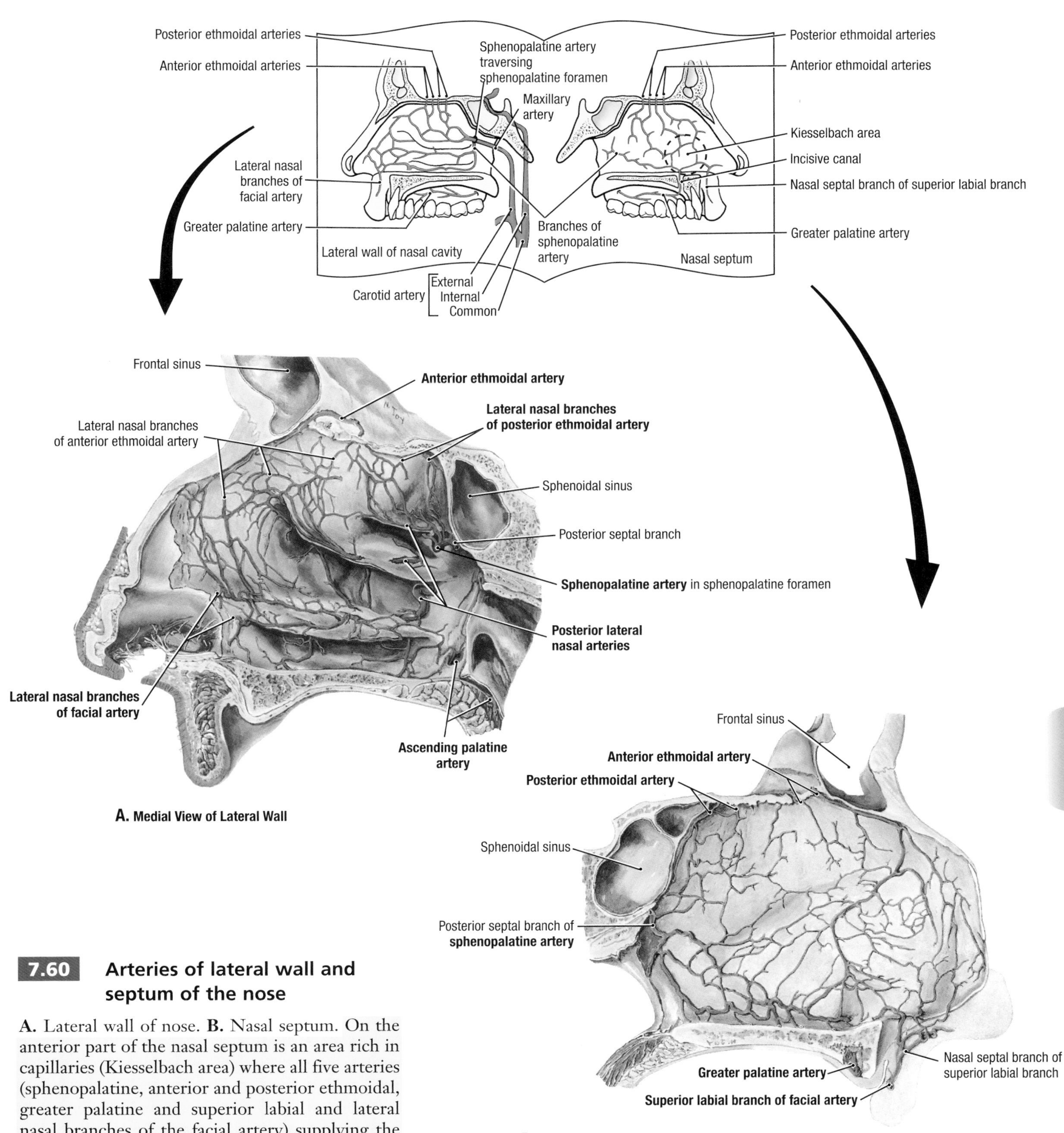
Posterior ethmoidal arteries
Anterior ethmoidal arteries
Sphenopalatine artery traversing sphenopalatine foramen
Maxillary artery
Lateral nasal branches of facial artery
Greater palatine artery
Lateral wall of nasal cavity
Branches of sphenopalatine artery
Carotid artery
External
Internal
Common
Posterior ethmoidal arteries
Anterior ethmoidal arteries
Kiesselbach area
Incisive canal
Nasal septal branch of superior labial branch
Greater palatine artery
Nasal septum
Frontal sinus
Anterior ethmoidal artery
Lateral nasal branches of posterior ethmoidal artery
Lateral nasal branches of anterior ethmoidal artery
Sphenoidal sinus
Posterior septal branch
Sphenopalatine artery in sphenopalatine foramen
Posterior lateral nasal arteries
Lateral nasal branches of facial artery
Ascending palatine artery
A. Medial View of Lateral Wall
Frontal sinus
Anterior ethmoidal artery
Posterior ethmoidal artery
Sphenoidal sinus
Posterior septal branch of sphenopalatine artery
Greater palatine artery
Nasal septal branch of superior labial branch
Superior labial branch of facial artery
B. Lateral View of Nasal Septum

## 7.60 Arteries of lateral wall and septum of the nose

**A.** Lateral wall of nose. **B.** Nasal septum. On the anterior part of the nasal septum is an area rich in capillaries (Kiesselbach area) where all five arteries (sphenopalatine, anterior and posterior ethmoidal, greater palatine and superior labial and lateral nasal branches of the facial artery) supplying the nasal septum anastomose. This area is often where profuse bleeding from the nose (epistaxis) occurs.

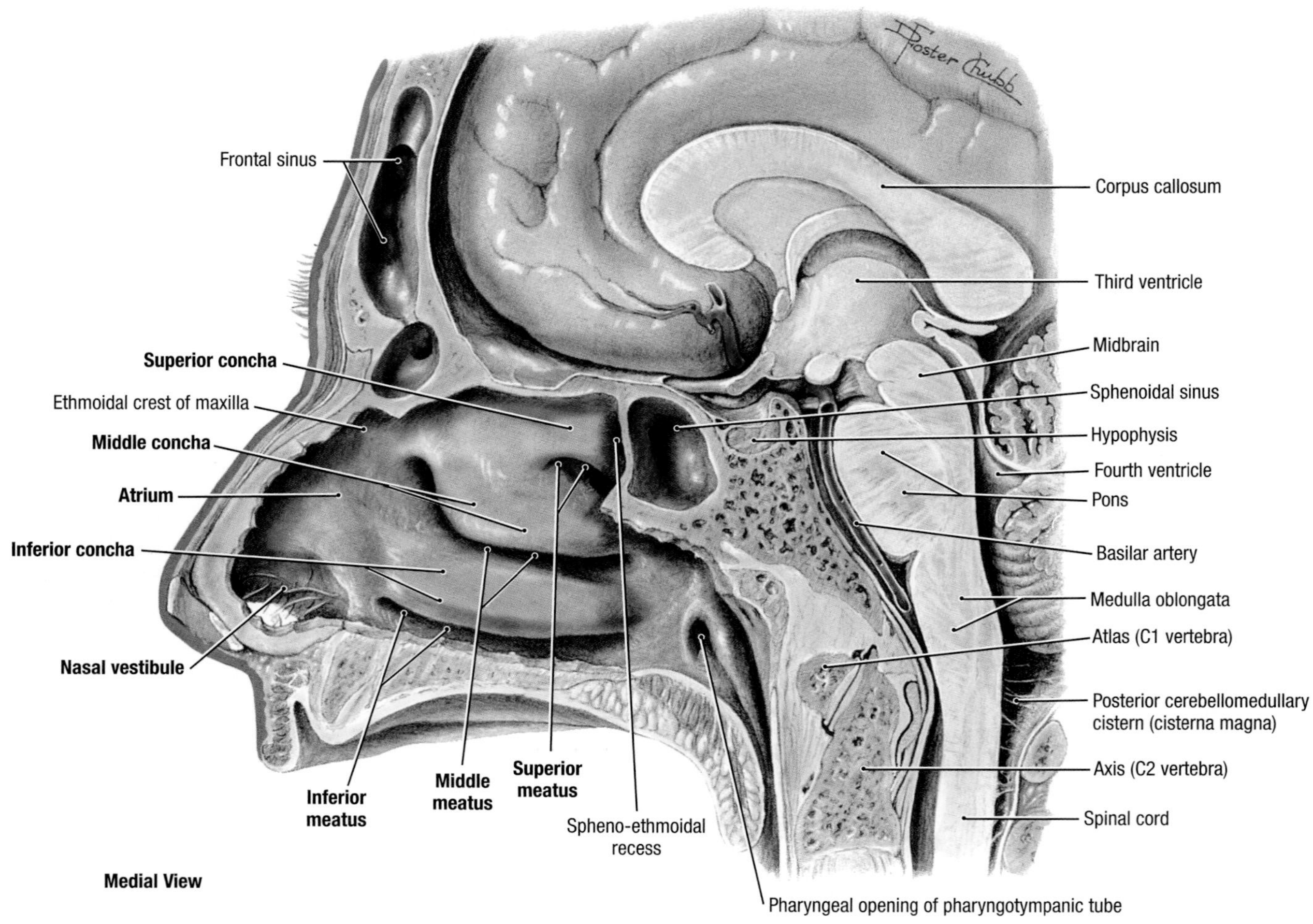
Frontal sinus
Superior concha
Ethmoidal crest of maxilla
Middle concha
Atrium
Inferior concha
Nasal vestibule
Inferior meatus
Middle meatus
Superior meatus
Spheno-ethmoidal recess
Medial View
Pharyngeal opening of pharyngotympanic tube
Corpus callosum
Third ventricle
Midbrain
Sphenoidal sinus
Hypophysis
Fourth ventricle
Pons
Basilar artery
Medulla oblongata
Atlas (C1 vertebra)
Posterior cerebellomedullary cistern (cisterna magna)
Axis (C2 vertebra)
Spinal cord

## 7.61 Right half of hemisected head demonstrating upper respiratory tract

- The vestibule is superior to the nostril and anterior to the inferior meatus; hairs grow from its skin-lined surface. The atrium is superior to the vestibule and anterior to the middle meatus.
- The inferior and middle conchae curve inferiorly and medially from the lateral wall, dividing it into three nearly equal parts and covering the inferior and middle meatuses, respectively. The middle concha ends inferior to the sphenoidal sinus, and the inferior concha ends inferior to the middle concha, just anterior to the orifice of the auditory tube. The superior concha is small and anterior to the sphenoidal sinus.
- The roof comprises an anterior sloping part corresponding to the bridge of the nose; an intermediate horizontal part; a perpendicular part anterior to the sphenoidal sinus; and a curved part, inferior to the sinus, that is continuous with the roof of the nasopharynx.

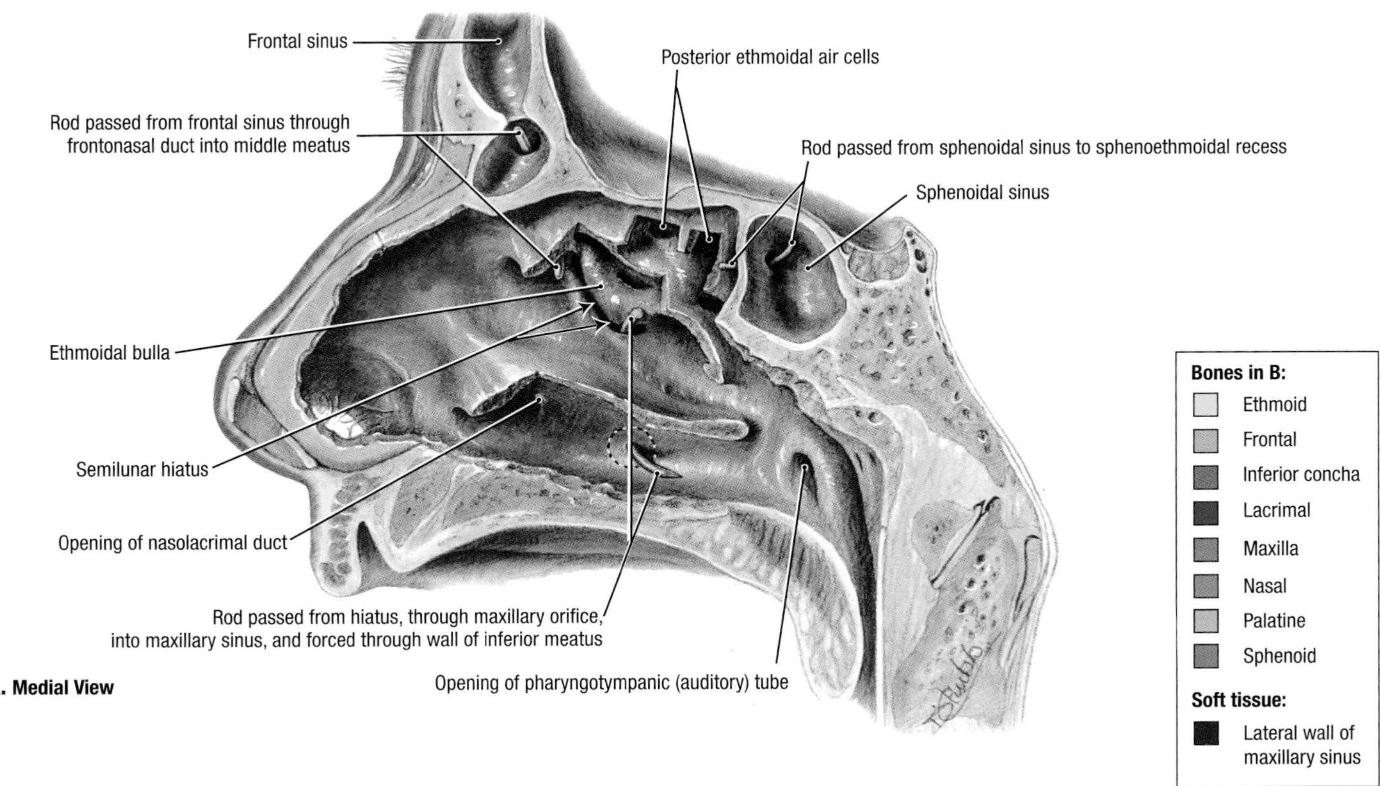

Frontal sinus
Rod passed from frontal sinus through frontonasal duct into middle meatus
Posterior ethmoidal air cells
Rod passed from sphenoidal sinus to sphenoethmoidal recess
Sphenoidal sinus
Ethmoidal bulla
Semilunar hiatus
Opening of nasolacrimal duct
Rod passed from hiatus, through maxillary orifice, into maxillary sinus, and forced through wall of inferior meatus
Opening of pharyngotympanic (auditory) tube
A. Medial View
Bones in B:
Ethmoid
Frontal
Inferior concha
Lacrimal
Maxilla
Nasal
Palatine
Sphenoid
Soft tissue:
Lateral wall of maxillary sinus


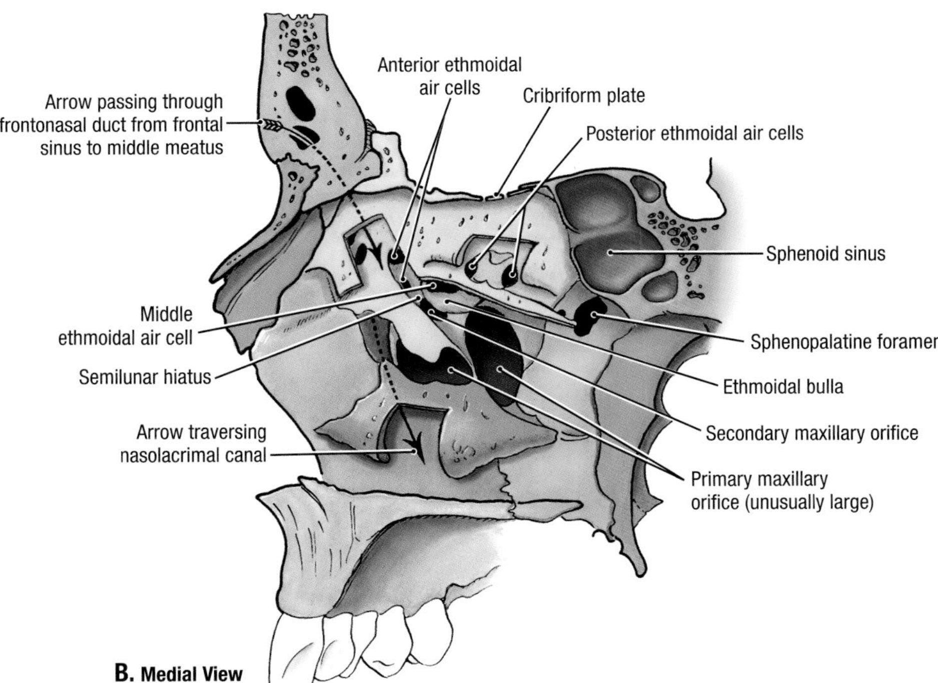

Arrow passing through frontonasal duct from frontal sinus to middle meatus
Anterior ethmoidal air cells
Cribriform plate
Posterior ethmoidal air cells
Sphenoid sinus
Middle ethmoidal air cell
Semilunar hiatus
Sphenopalatine foramen
Ethmoidal bulla
Arrow traversing nasolacrimal canal
Secondary maxillary orifice
Primary maxillary orifice (unusually large)
B. Medial View


## 7.62 Communications through the lateral wall of the nasal cavity

**A.** Dissection. Parts of the superior, middle, and inferior conchae are cut away to reveal the openings of the air sinuses. **B.** Diagrams of the bones and openings of the lateral wall of nasal cavity following dissection. Note one *arrow* passing from the frontal sinus through the frontonasal duct into the middle meatus and another *arrow* coming from the antero-medial orbit via the nasolacrimal canal.

The nasal mucosa becomes swollen and inflamed (rhinitis) during upper respiratory infections and allergic reactions (e.g., hay fever). Swelling of this mucous membrane occurs readily because of its vascularity and abundant mucosal glands. Infections of the nasal cavities may spread to the anterior cranial fossa through the cribriform plate, nasopharynx and retropharyngeal soft tissues, middle ear through the pharyngotympanic (auditory) tube, paranasal sinuses, lacrimal apparatus, and conjunctiva.

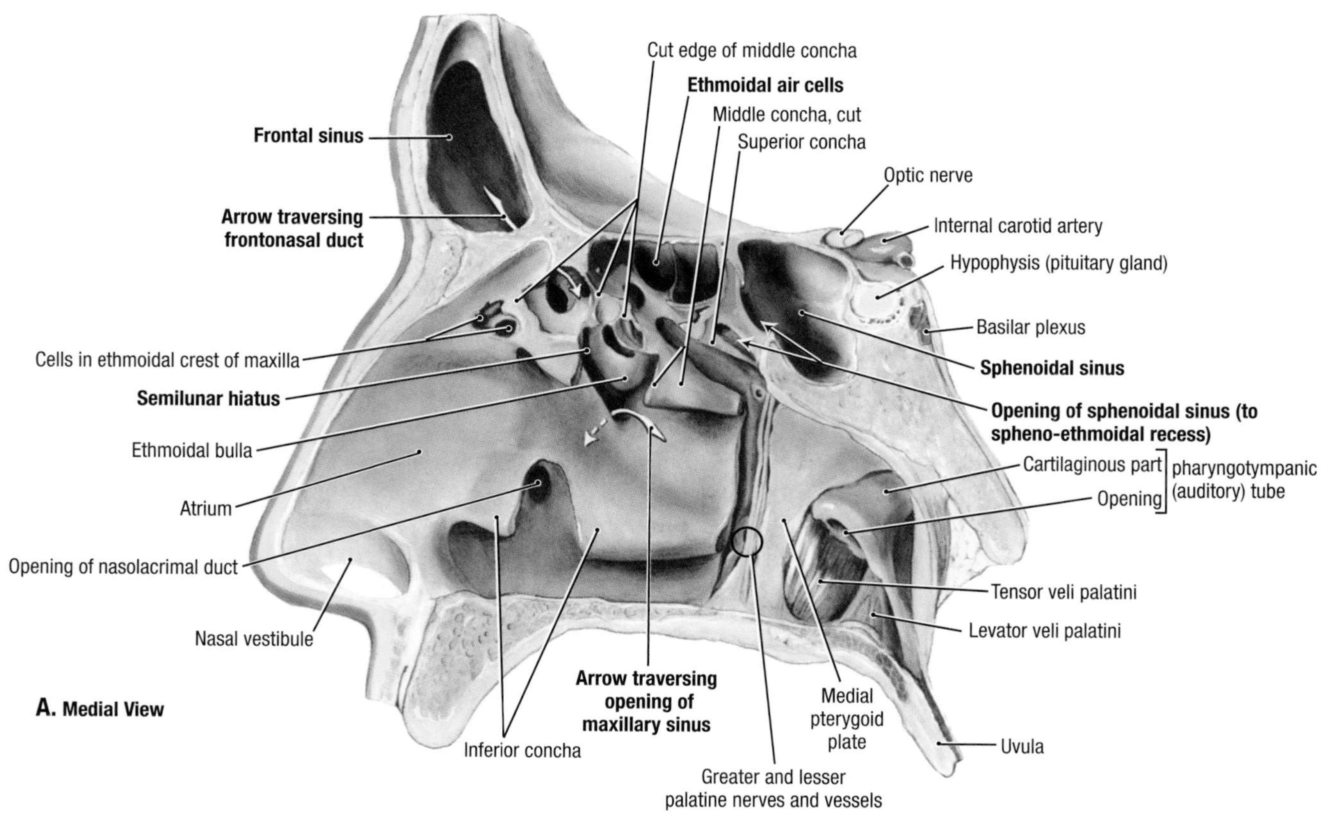
Cut edge of middle concha
Ethmoidal air cells
Middle concha, cut
Superior concha
Frontal sinus
Optic nerve
Arrow traversing frontonasal duct
Internal carotid artery
Hypophysis (pituitary gland)
Basilar plexus
Cells in ethmoidal crest of maxilla
Sphenoidal sinus
Semilunar hiatus
Opening of sphenoidal sinus (to spheno-ethmoidal recess)
Ethmoidal bulla
Cartilaginous part
Opening
pharyngotympanic (auditory) tube
Atrium
Opening of nasolacrimal duct
Tensor veli palatini
Levator veli palatini
Nasal vestibule
Arrow traversing opening of maxillary sinus
Medial pterygoid plate
A. Medial View
Uvula
Inferior concha
Greater and lesser palatine nerves and vessels

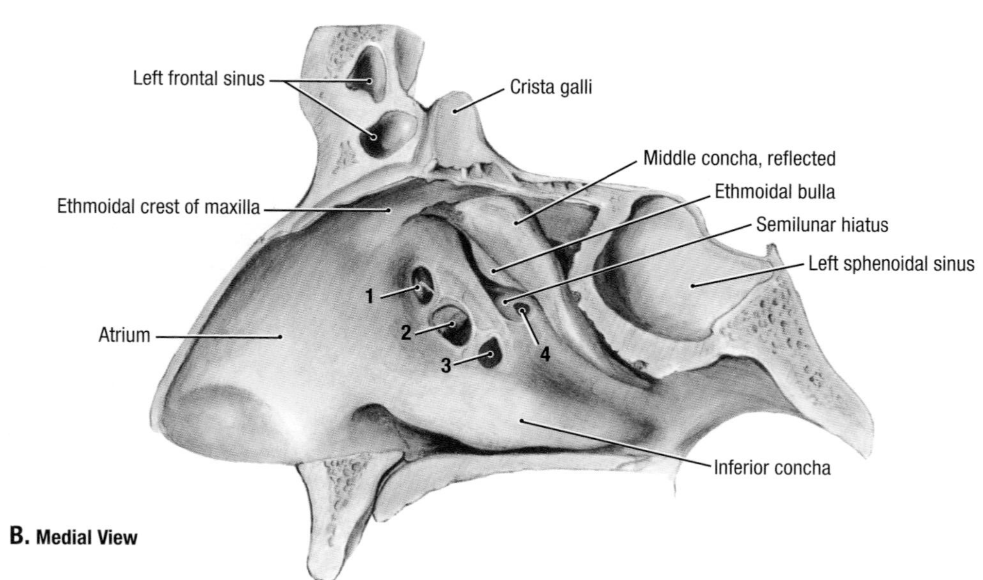
Left frontal sinus
Crista galli
Middle concha, reflected
Ethmoidal crest of maxilla
Ethmoidal bulla
Semilunar hiatus
Left sphenoidal sinus
1
2
3
4
Atrium
Inferior concha
B. Medial View

## 7.63 Paranasal sinuses, openings, and palatine muscles in the lateral wall of the nasal cavity

**A.** Dissection. Parts of the middle and inferior conchae and lateral wall of the nasal cavity are cut away to expose the nerves and vessels in the palatine canal and the extrinsic palatine muscles. **B.** Accessory maxillary orifices. In addition to the primary, or normal, ostium (not shown), there are four secondary, or acquired, ostia (numbered 1–4).

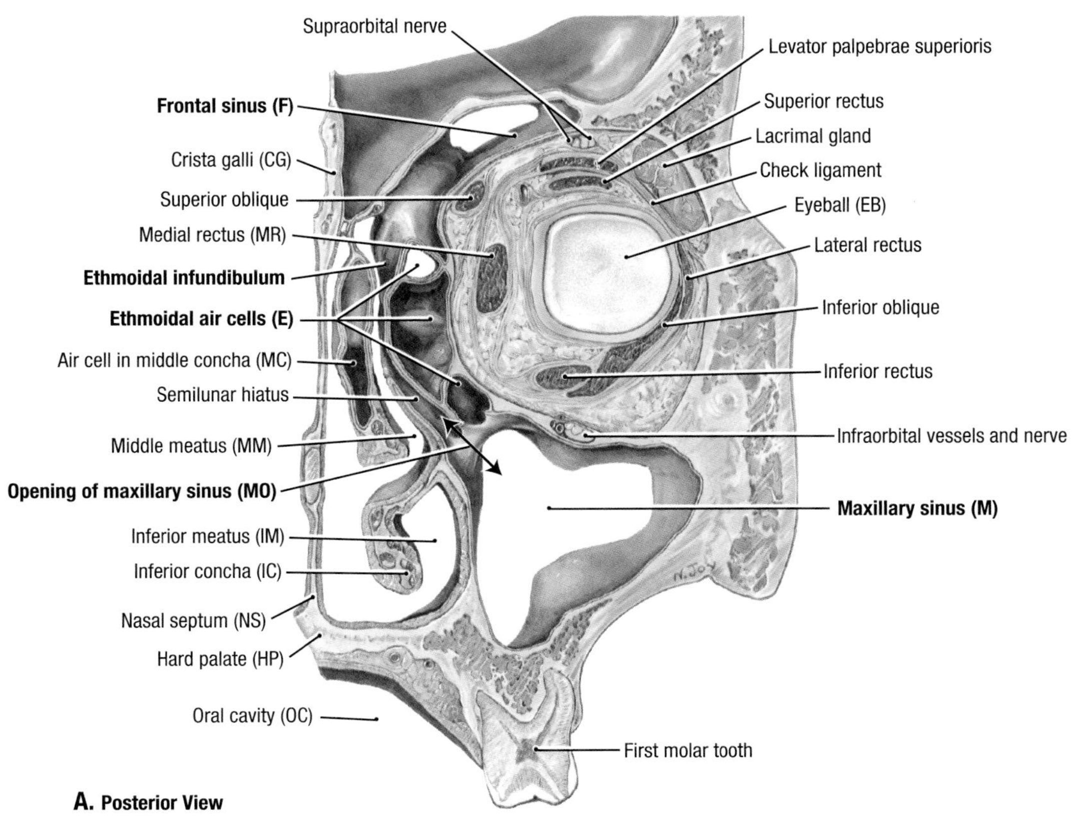
Supraorbital nerve
Levator palpebrae superioris
Frontal sinus (F)
Superior rectus
Lacrimal gland
Crista galli (CG)
Check ligament
Superior oblique
Eyeball (EB)
Medial rectus (MR)
Lateral rectus
Ethmoidal infundibulum
Ethmoidal air cells (E)
Inferior oblique
Air cell in middle concha (MC)
Inferior rectus
Semilunar hiatus
Infraorbital vessels and nerve
Middle meatus (MM)
Opening of maxillary sinus (MO)
Maxillary sinus (M)
Inferior meatus (IM)
Inferior concha (IC)
Nasal septum (NS)
Hard palate (HP)
Oral cavity (OC)
First molar tooth

A. Posterior View

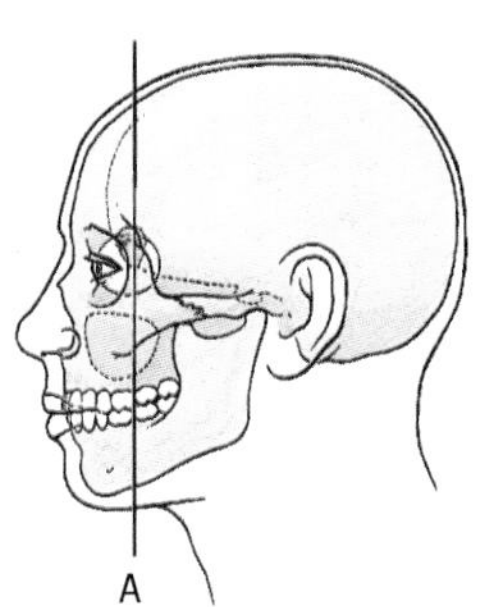
A

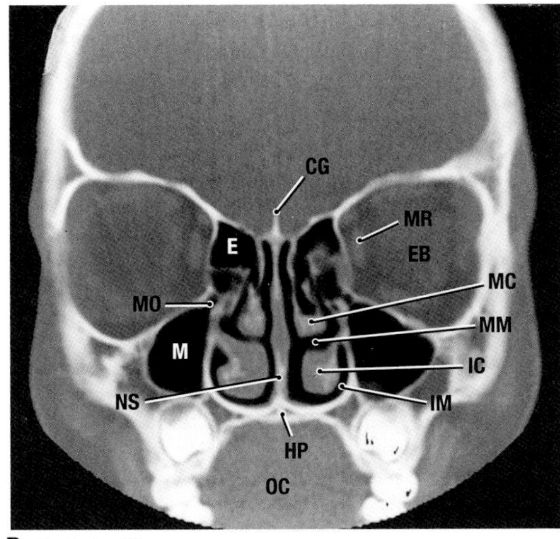
CG
MR
E
EB
MC
MO
MM
M
IC
NS
IM
HP
OC

B. Posterior View

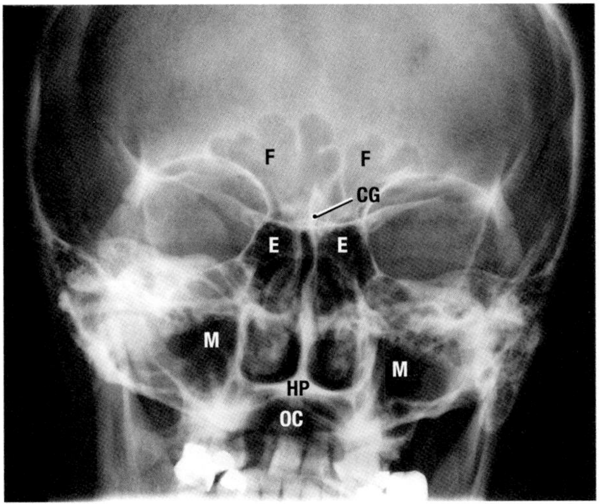
F
F
CG
E
E
M
M
HP
OC

C. Anteroposterior View

## 7.64 Paranasal sinuses and nasal cavity

**A.** Coronal section of right side of the head. **B.** CT scan. **C.** Radiograph of cranium. Letters in **B** and **C** refer to structures labeled in **A.**

If nasal drainage is blocked, infections of the ethmoidal cells of the ethmoidal sinuses may break through the fragile medial wall of the orbit. Severe infections from this source may cause blindness but could also affect the dural sheath of the optic nerve, causing optic neuritis.

During removal of a maxillary molar tooth, a fracture of a root may occur. If proper retrieval methods are not used, a piece of the root may be driven superiorly into the maxillary sinus.

Wall of optic canal
Optic nerve (CN II)
Internal carotid artery
Hypophysis
Dorsum sellae
Recess in anterior clinoid process
Fullness over internal carotid artery
Roof of pterygoid canal
Sphenopalatine foramen (to pterygopalatine fossa)
Greater and lesser palatine nerves in palatine canal
Palatine canal
Medial pterygoid plate
Lesser palatine nerve
Greater palatine nerves
Hard palate
Superciliary arch
Left frontal sinus
Lateral nasal cartilage
Accessory or sesamoid cartilage
Mobile part of nasal septum

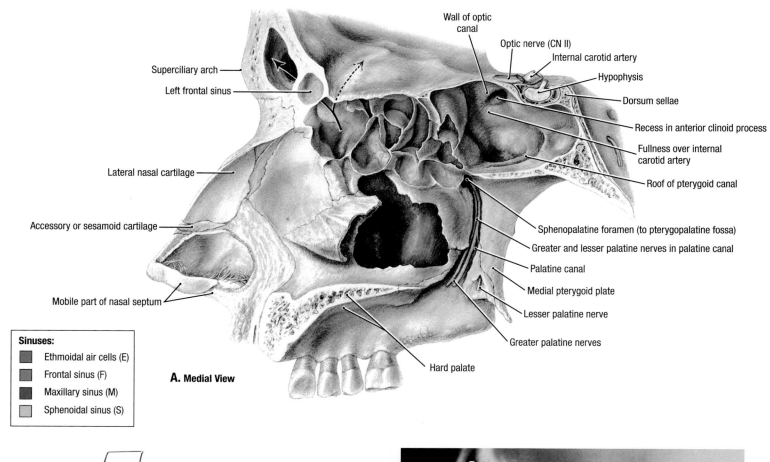

**Sinuses:**
- Ethmoidal air cells (E)
- Frontal sinus (F)
- Maxillary sinus (M)
- Sphenoidal sinus (S)

**A. Medial View**

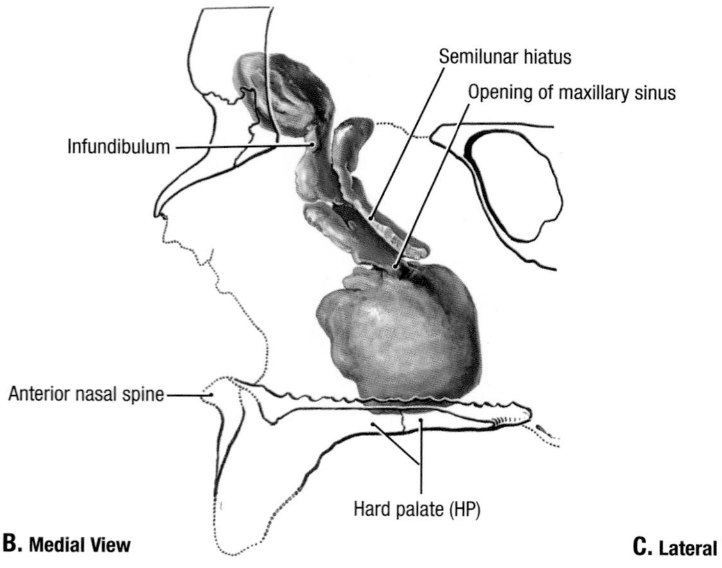
Semilunar hiatus
Opening of maxillary sinus
Infundibulum
Anterior nasal spine
Hard palate (HP)

**B. Medial View**

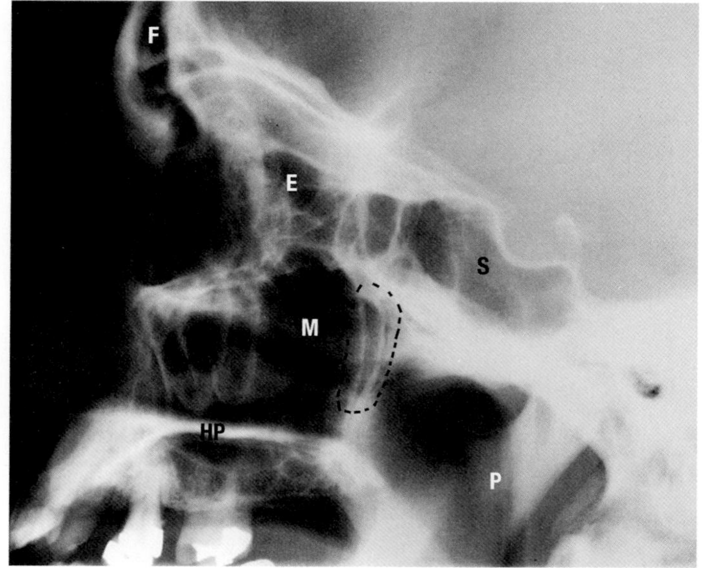
F
E
S
M
HP
P

**C. Lateral View**

## 7.65 Paranasal sinuses

**A.** Opened sinuses, color coded. **B.** Cast of frontal and maxillary sinuses. **C.** Radiograph of cranium. *P*, pharynx; *dotted lines*, pterygopalatine fossa. Letters refer to structures labeled in **B.** The maxillary sinuses are the most commonly infected, probably because their ostia are small and located high on their superomedial walls, a poor location for natural drainage of the sinus. When the mucous membrane of the sinus is congested, the maxillary ostia often are obstructed. The maxillary sinus can be cannulated and drained by passing a canula from the nares through the maxillary ostium into the sinus.

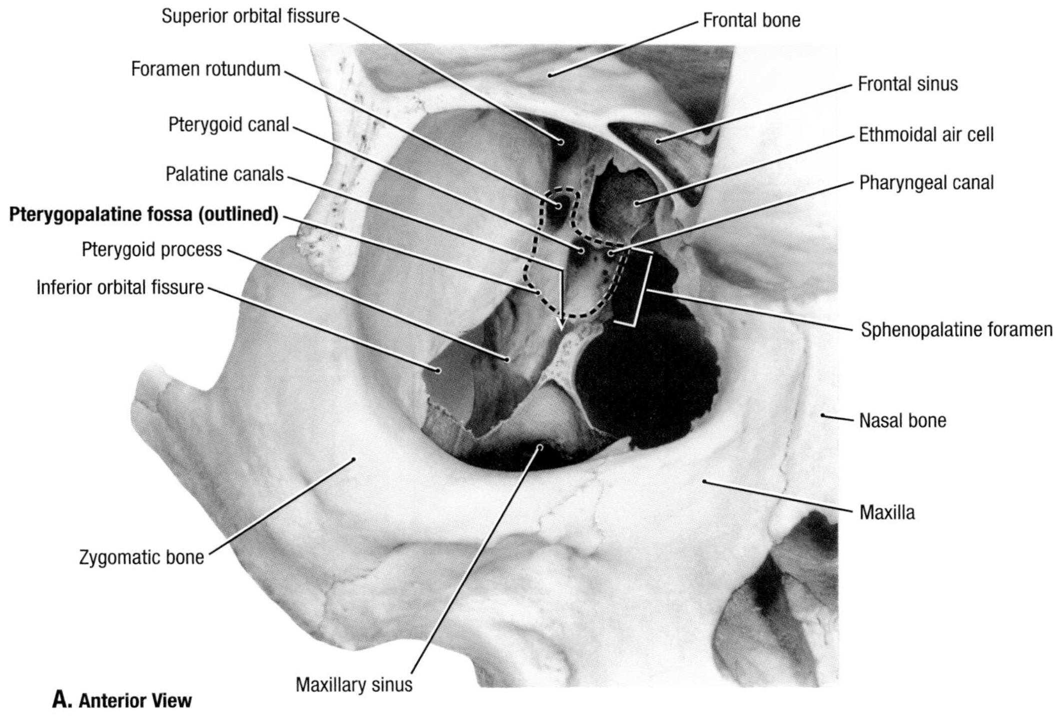
Superior orbital fissure
Foramen rotundum
Pterygoid canal
Palatine canals
Pterygopalatine fossa (outlined)
Pterygoid process
Inferior orbital fissure
Frontal bone
Frontal sinus
Ethmoidal air cell
Pharyngeal canal
Sphenopalatine foramen
Nasal bone
Maxilla
Zygomatic bone
Maxillary sinus
A. Anterior View

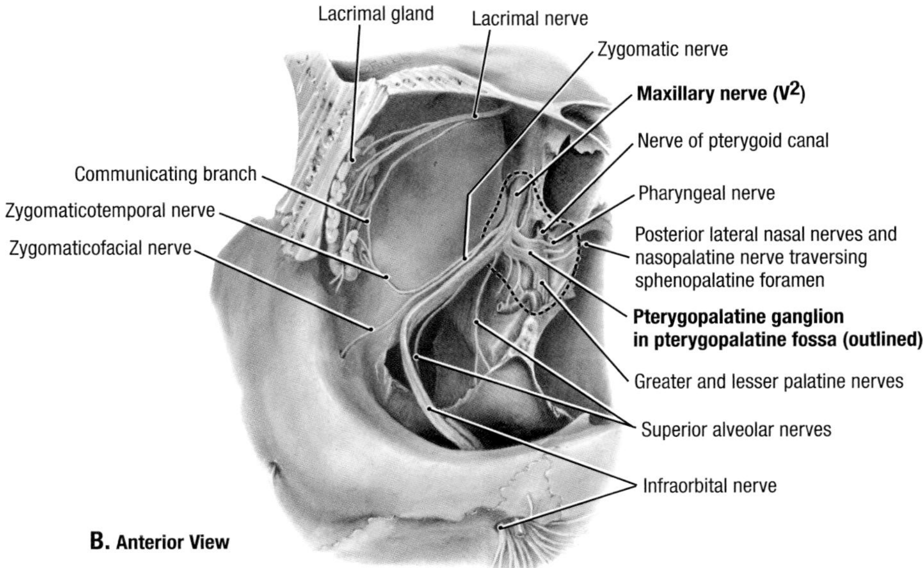
Lacrimal gland
Lacrimal nerve
Zygomatic nerve
Maxillary nerve (V2)
Nerve of pterygoid canal
Pharyngeal nerve
Posterior lateral nasal nerves and nasopalatine nerve traversing sphenopalatine foramen
Pterygopalatine ganglion in pterygopalatine fossa (outlined)
Greater and lesser palatine nerves
Superior alveolar nerves
Infraorbital nerve
Communicating branch
Zygomaticotemporal nerve
Zygomaticofacial nerve
B. Anterior View

## 7.66 Pterygopalatine fossa, orbital approach

**A.** Bones and foramina. **B.** Maxillary nerve. In **A** and **B,** the pterygopalatine fossa has been exposed through the floor of the orbit and maxillary sinus.

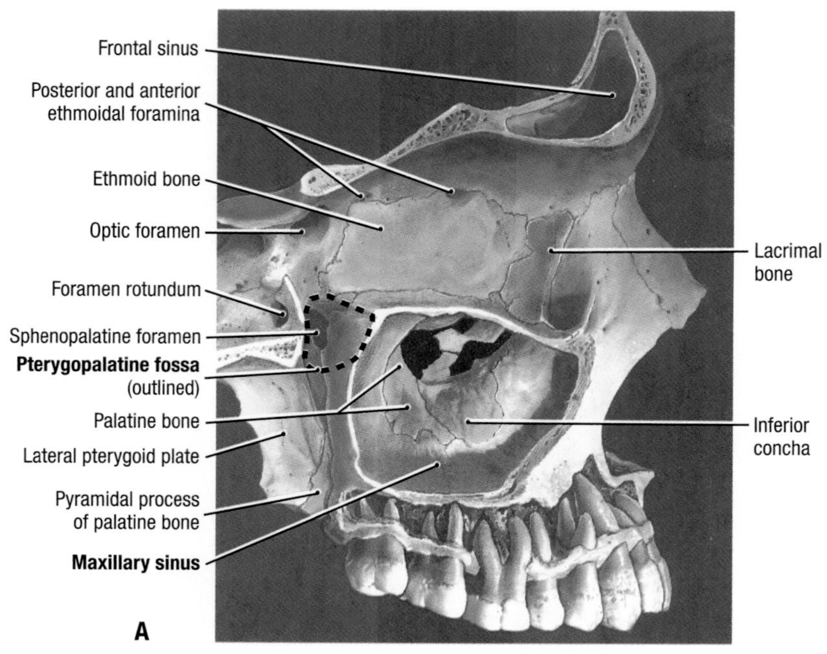
Frontal sinus
Posterior and anterior ethmoidal foramina
Ethmoid bone
Optic foramen
Foramen rotundum
Sphenopalatine foramen
Pterygopalatine fossa (outlined)
Palatine bone
Lateral pterygoid plate
Pyramidal process of palatine bone
Maxillary sinus
A
Lacrimal bone
Inferior concha

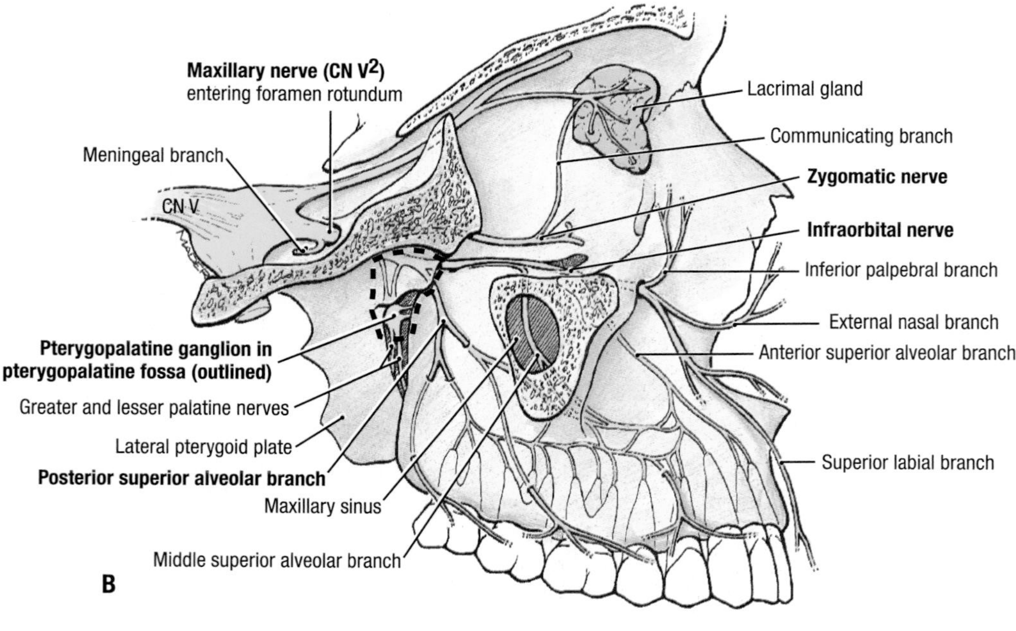
Maxillary nerve (CN V2) entering foramen rotundum
Meningeal branch
CN V
Pterygopalatine ganglion in pterygopalatine fossa (outlined)
Greater and lesser palatine nerves
Lateral pterygoid plate
Posterior superior alveolar branch
Maxillary sinus
Middle superior alveolar branch
B
Lacrimal gland
Communicating branch
Zygomatic nerve
Infraorbital nerve
Inferior palpebral branch
External nasal branch
Anterior superior alveolar branch
Superior labial branch

**Lateral Views**

## 7.67 Nerves of the pterygopalatine fossa

**A.** Medial half of the right viscerocranium following sagittal sectioning through the maxillary sinus. The inferior concha *(orange)* and palatine bone *(pink)* form part of the medial wall of the maxillary sinus. Note the ethmoid *(yellow)* and lacrimal *(blue)* bones of the medial wall of the orbital cavity and the sphenopalatine foramen opening into the nasal cavity from the pterygopalatine fossa. **B.** Maxillary nerve (CN $V^2$) and branches.

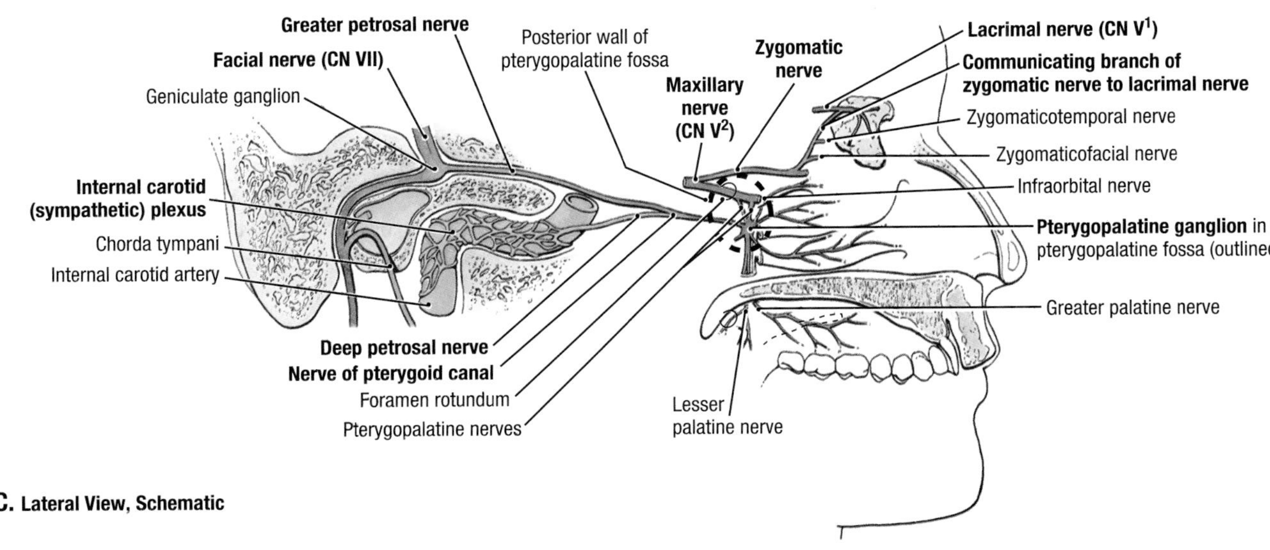
Greater petrosal nerve
Facial nerve (CN VII)
Geniculate ganglion
Internal carotid (sympathetic) plexus
Chorda tympani
Internal carotid artery
Posterior wall of pterygopalatine fossa
Maxillary nerve (CN V²)
Zygomatic nerve
Lacrimal nerve (CN V¹)
Communicating branch of zygomatic nerve to lacrimal nerve
Zygomaticotemporal nerve
Zygomaticofacial nerve
Infraorbital nerve
Pterygopalatine ganglion in pterygopalatine fossa (outlined)
Greater palatine nerve
Deep petrosal nerve
Nerve of pterygoid canal
Foramen rotundum
Pterygopalatine nerves
Lesser palatine nerve

C. Lateral View, Schematic

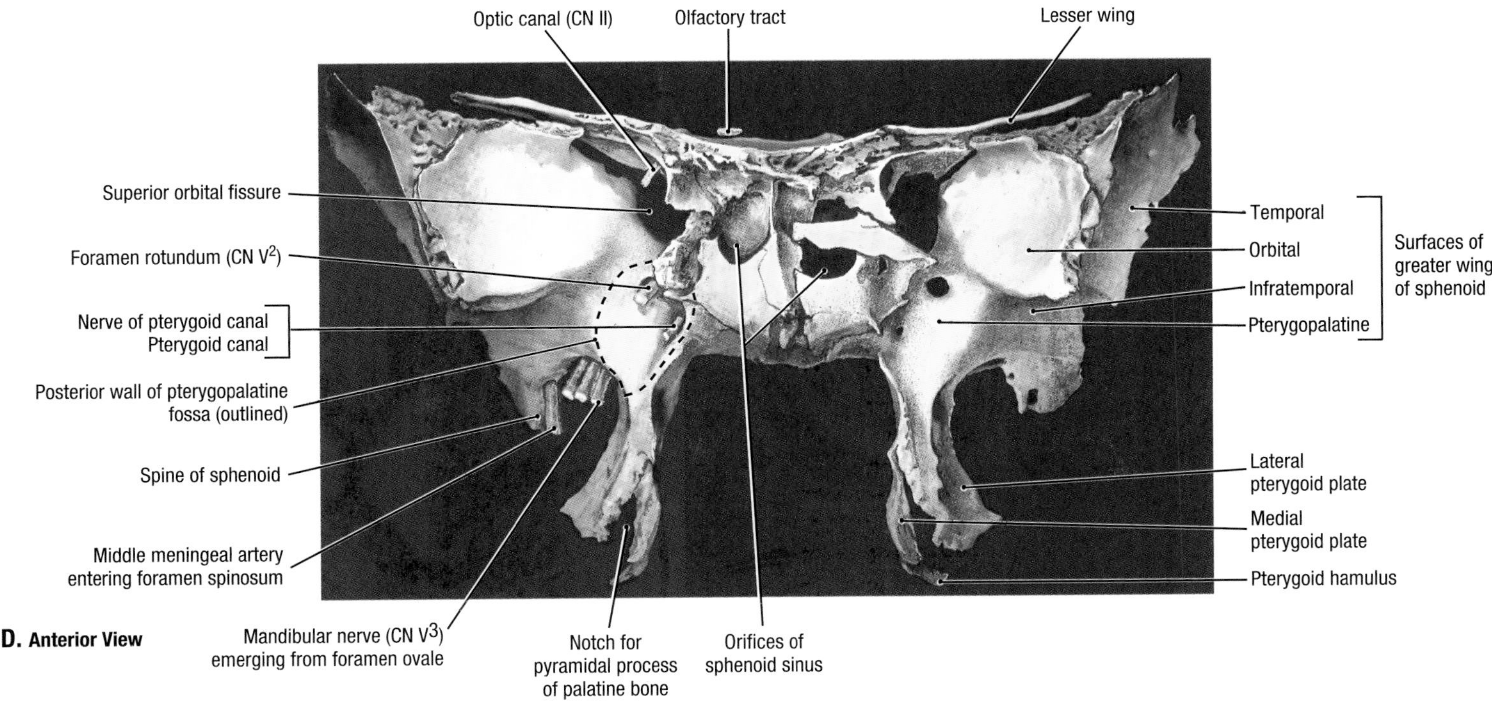
Optic canal (CN II)
Olfactory tract
Lesser wing
Superior orbital fissure
Foramen rotundum (CN V²)
Nerve of pterygoid canal
Pterygoid canal
Posterior wall of pterygopalatine fossa (outlined)
Spine of sphenoid
Middle meningeal artery entering foramen spinosum
Mandibular nerve (CN V³) emerging from foramen ovale
Notch for pyramidal process of palatine bone
Orifices of sphenoid sinus
Temporal
Orbital
Infratemporal
Pterygopalatine
Surfaces of greater wing of sphenoid
Lateral pterygoid plate
Medial pterygoid plate
Pterygoid hamulus

D. Anterior View

## 7.67 Nerves of the pterygopalatine fossa *(continued)*

**C.** Autonomic innervation of the lacrimal gland and glands of the palatine and nasal mucosa. **D.** Sphenoid bone, anterior surface of the body, pterygoid process, and central parts of the greater and lesser wings.

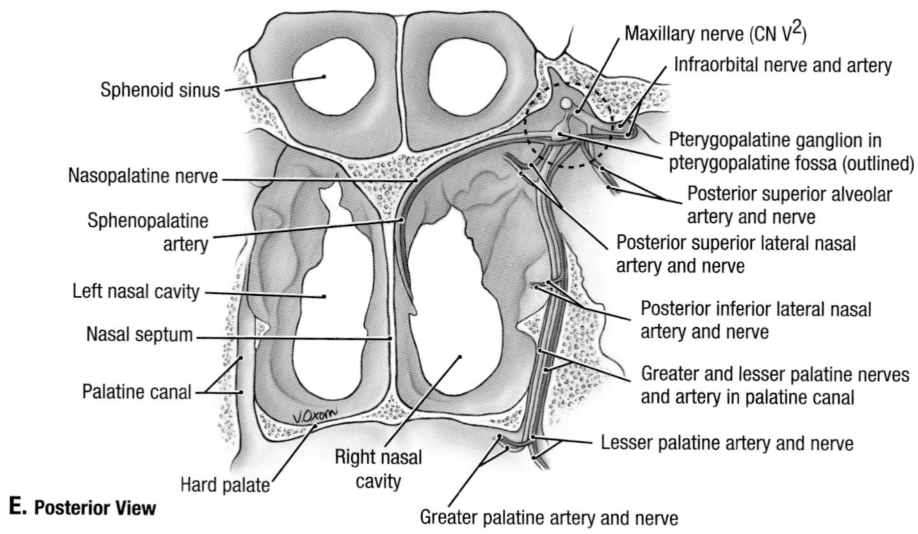
Sphenoid sinus
Maxillary nerve (CN V2)
Infraorbital nerve and artery
Pterygopalatine ganglion in pterygopalatine fossa (outlined)
Nasopalatine nerve
Posterior superior alveolar artery and nerve
Sphenopalatine artery
Posterior superior lateral nasal artery and nerve
Left nasal cavity
Posterior inferior lateral nasal artery and nerve
Nasal septum
Greater and lesser palatine nerves and artery in palatine canal
Palatine canal
Lesser palatine artery and nerve
Right nasal cavity
Hard palate
Greater palatine artery and nerve
E. Posterior View

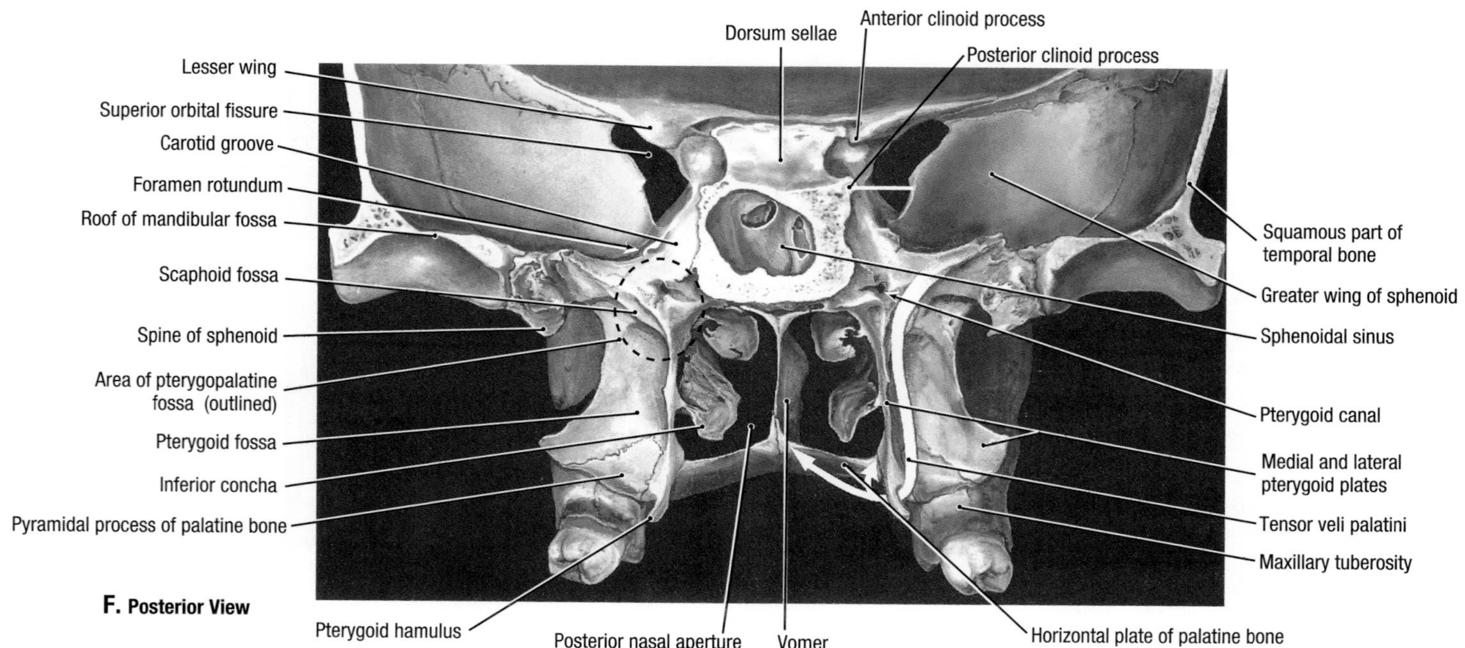
Dorsum sellae
Anterior clinoid process
Posterior clinoid process
Lesser wing
Superior orbital fissure
Carotid groove
Foramen rotundum
Roof of mandibular fossa
Squamous part of temporal bone
Scaphoid fossa
Greater wing of sphenoid
Spine of sphenoid
Sphenoidal sinus
Area of pterygopalatine fossa (outlined)
Pterygoid canal
Pterygoid fossa
Medial and lateral pterygoid plates
Inferior concha
Tensor veli palatini
Pyramidal process of palatine bone
Maxillary tuberosity
Pterygoid hamulus
Posterior nasal aperture
Vomer
Horizontal plate of palatine bone
F. Posterior View

## 7.67 Nerves of the pterygopalatine fossa *(continued)*

**E.** Coronal section through nasal cavities, sphenoidal sinuses, and right pterygopalatine fossa, in the plane of the palatine canal, demonstrating the course of the nasopalatine and greater and lesser palatine nerves. **F.** Anterior part of cranium following coronal sectioning in the plane of the foramen lacerum demonstrating the posterior wall of the pterygopalatine fossa.

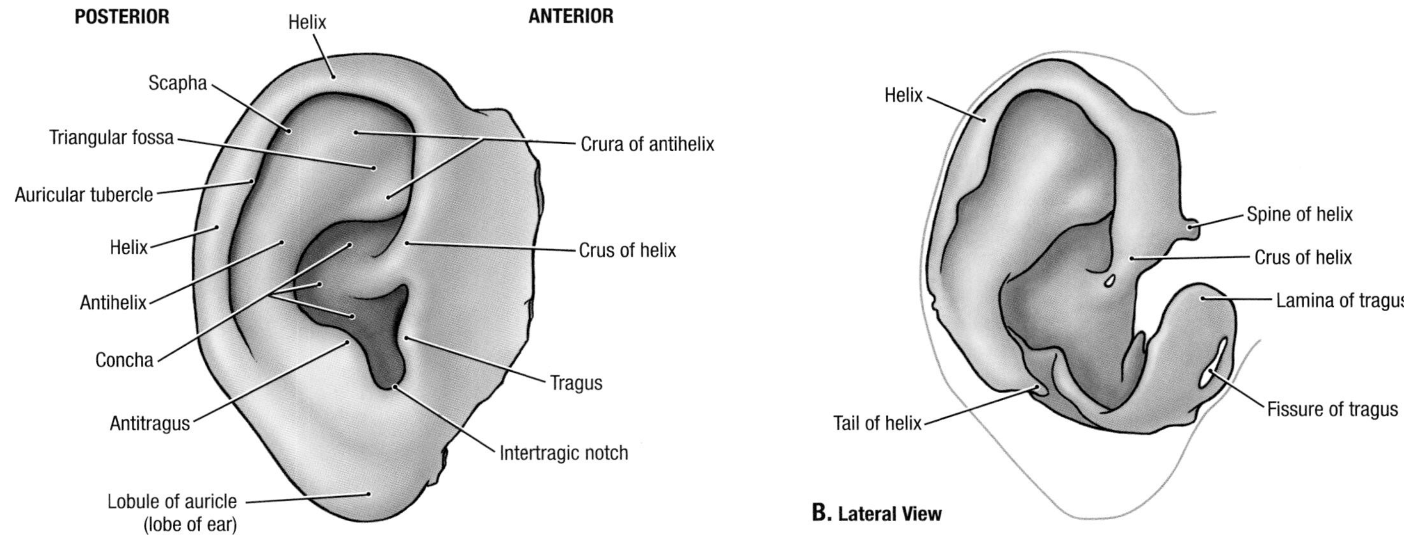
POSTERIOR
ANTERIOR
Helix
Scapha
Triangular fossa
Auricular tubercle
Helix
Antihelix
Concha
Antitragus
Lobule of auricle (lobe of ear)
Crura of antihelix
Crus of helix
Tragus
Intertragic notch
A. Lateral View
Helix
Spine of helix
Crus of helix
Lamina of tragus
Fissure of tragus
Tail of helix
B. Lateral View

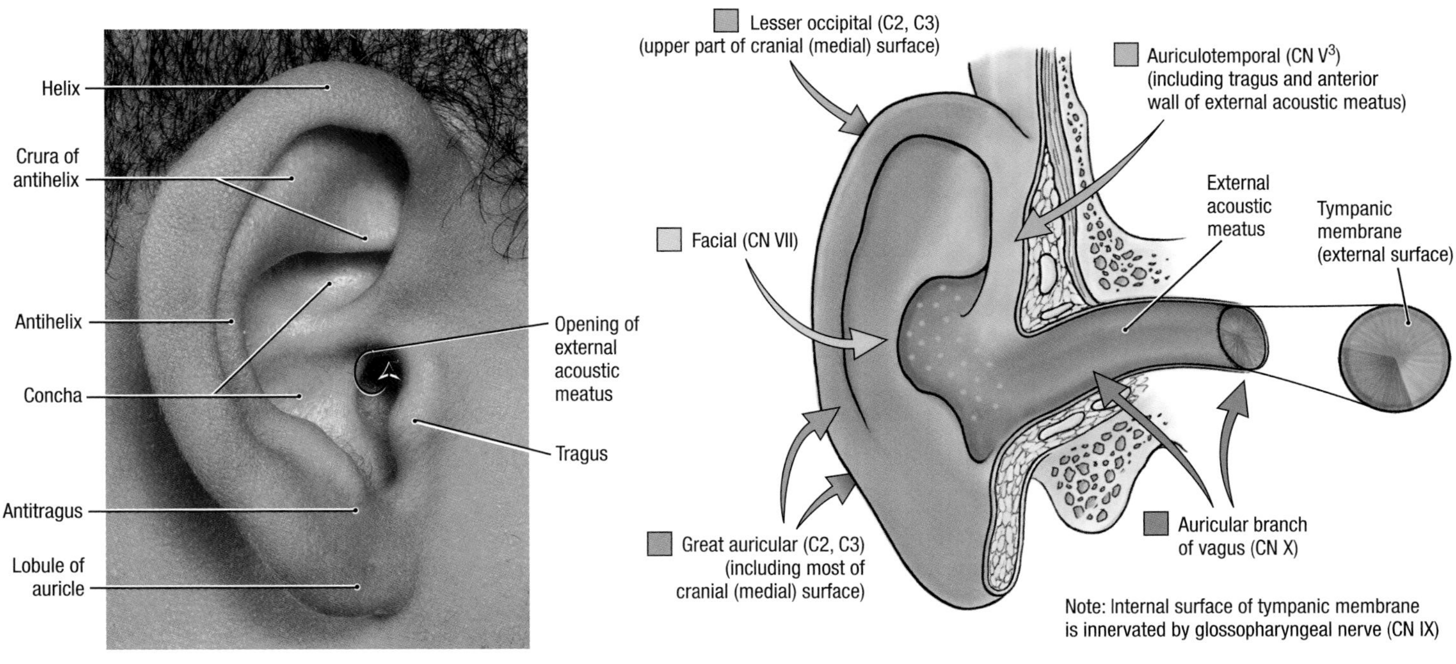
Helix
Crura of antihelix
Antihelix
Concha
Antitragus
Lobule of auricle
Opening of external acoustic meatus
Tragus
C. Lateral View
Lesser occipital (C2, C3) (upper part of cranial (medial) surface)
Auriculotemporal (CN V3) (including tragus and anterior wall of external acoustic meatus)
Facial (CN VII)
External acoustic meatus
Tympanic membrane (external surface)
Great auricular (C2, C3) (including most of cranial (medial) surface)
Auricular branch of vagus (CN X)
Note: Internal surface of tympanic membrane is innervated by glossopharyngeal nerve (CN IX)
D. Schematic Section

**7.68 Auricle**

**A.** Features of auricle. **B.** Cartilage of auricle. **C.** Surface anatomy of auricle.

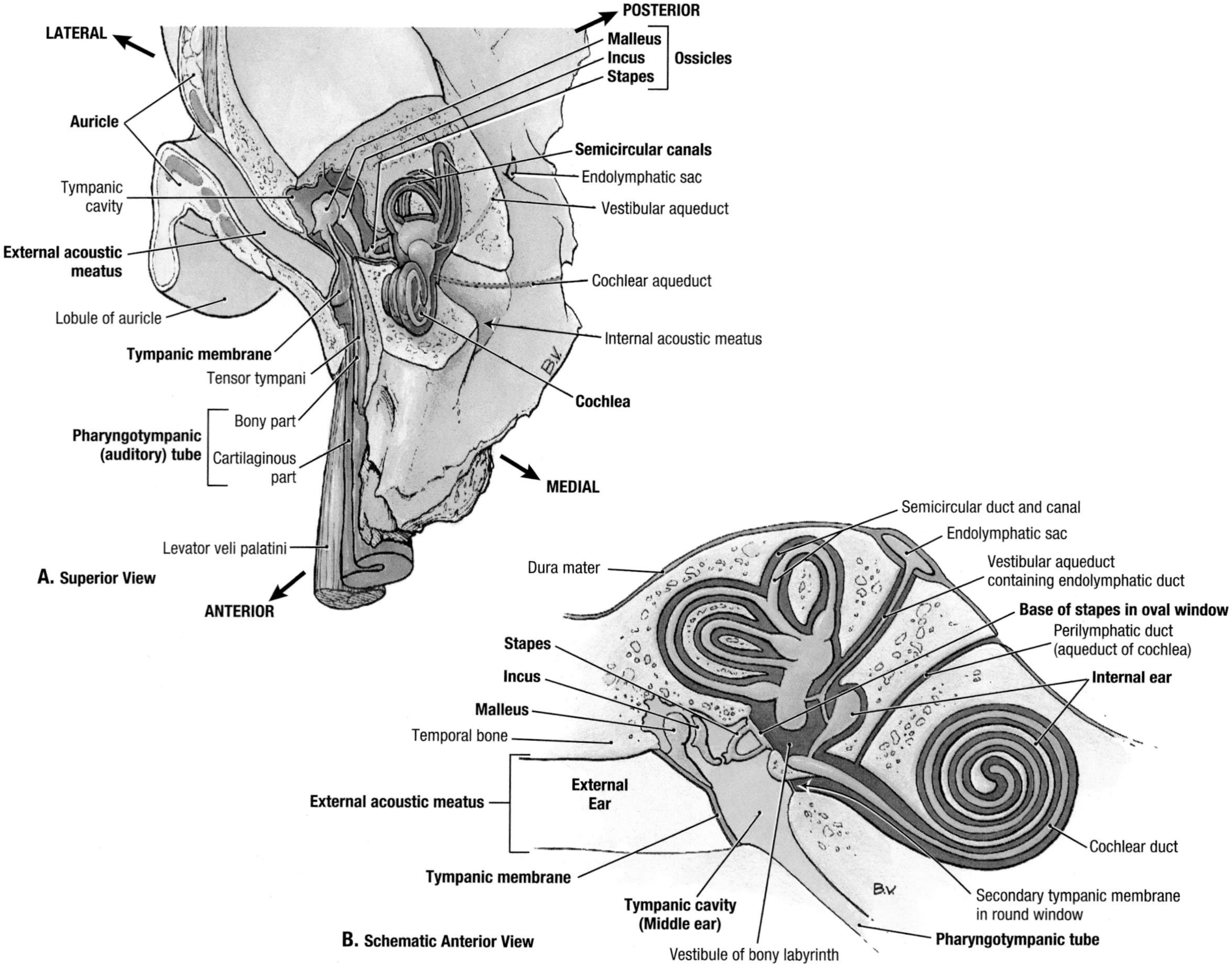

POSTERIOR
LATERAL
Malleus
Incus
Stapes
Ossicles
Auricle
Semicircular canals
Endolymphatic sac
Tympanic cavity
Vestibular aqueduct
External acoustic meatus
Cochlear aqueduct
Lobule of auricle
Internal acoustic meatus
Tympanic membrane
Tensor tympani
Cochlea
Bony part
Pharyngotympanic (auditory) tube
Cartilaginous part
MEDIAL
Levator veli palatini
ANTERIOR

A. Superior View

Semicircular duct and canal
Endolymphatic sac
Dura mater
Vestibular aqueduct containing endolymphatic duct
Base of stapes in oval window
Perilymphatic duct (aqueduct of cochlea)
Stapes
Incus
Internal ear
Malleus
Temporal bone
External acoustic meatus
External Ear
Cochlear duct
Tympanic membrane
Secondary tympanic membrane in round window
Tympanic cavity (Middle ear)
Pharyngotympanic tube
Vestibule of bony labyrinth

B. Schematic Anterior View

## 7.69 External, middle, and internal ear—I: overviews

**A.** Right temporal bone and auricle, sectioned in planes of (1) externa acoustic meatus and (2) pharyngotympanic tube. **B.** Schematic section of petrous temporal bone.

- The external ear comprises the auricle and external acoustic (auditory) meatus.
- The middle ear (tympanum) lies between the tympanic membrane and internal ear. Three ossicles extend from the lateral to the medial walls of the tympanum. Of these, the malleus is attached to the tympanic membrane. The stapes is attached by the anular ligament to the fenestra vestibuli (oval window), and the incus connects to the malleus and stapes. The pharyngotympanic tube, extending from the nasopharynx, opens into the anterior wall of the tympanic cavity.
- The membranous labyrinth comprises a closed system of membranous tubes and bulbs filled with fluid (endolymph) and bathed in surrounding fluid, called *perilymph* (*purple* in **B**); both membranous labyrinth and perilymph are contained within the bony labyrinth.

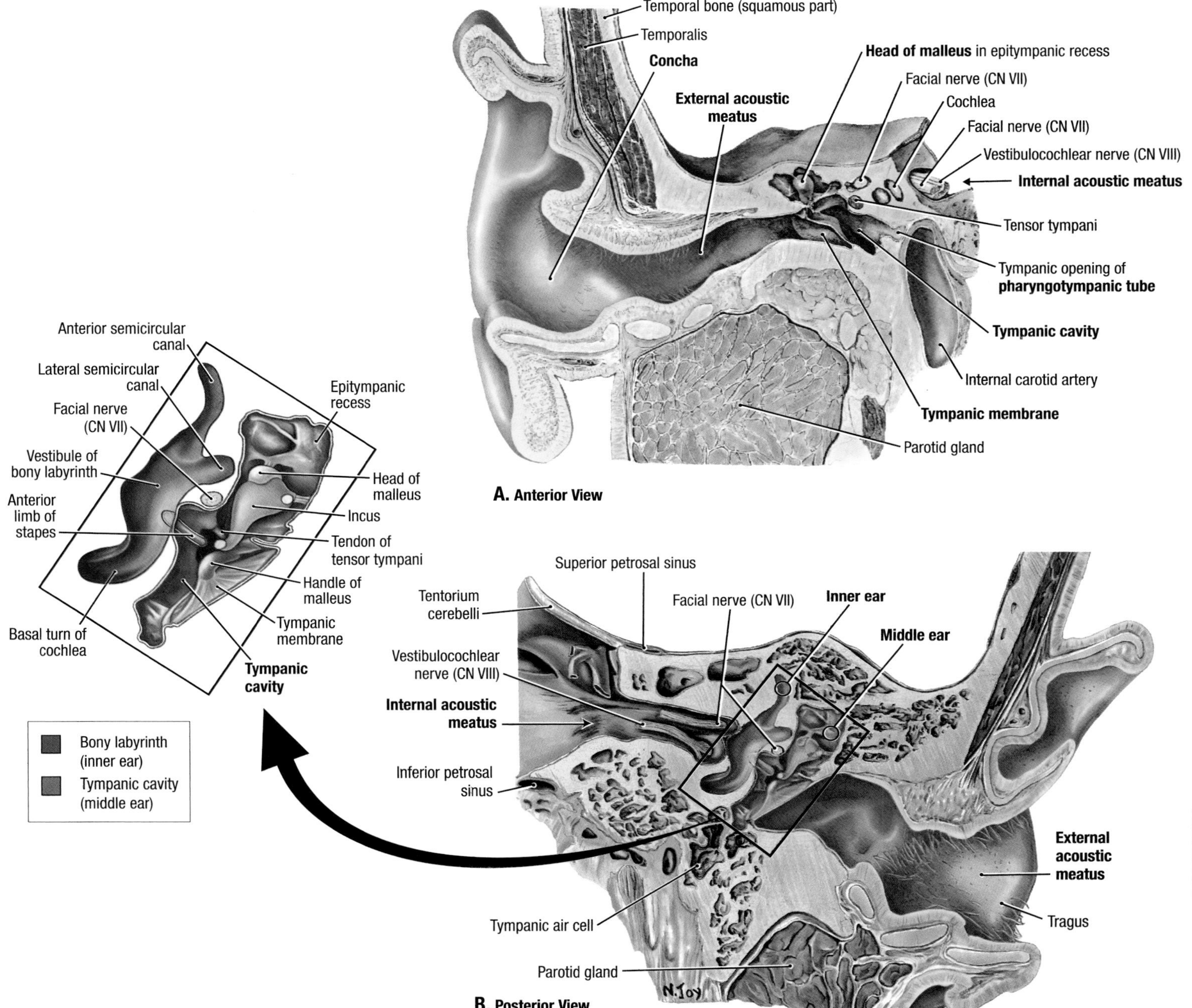
Temporal bone (squamous part)
Temporalis
Concha
External acoustic meatus
Head of malleus in epitympanic recess
Facial nerve (CN VII)
Cochlea
Facial nerve (CN VII)
Vestibulocochlear nerve (CN VIII)
Internal acoustic meatus
Tensor tympani
Tympanic opening of pharyngotympanic tube
Tympanic cavity
Internal carotid artery
Tympanic membrane
Parotid gland
A. Anterior View
Anterior semicircular canal
Lateral semicircular canal
Facial nerve (CN VII)
Vestibule of bony labyrinth
Anterior limb of stapes
Basal turn of cochlea
Epitympanic recess
Head of malleus
Incus
Tendon of tensor tympani
Handle of malleus
Tympanic membrane
Tympanic cavity
Bony labyrinth (inner ear)
Tympanic cavity (middle ear)
Superior petrosal sinus
Tentorium cerebelli
Facial nerve (CN VII)
Inner ear
Middle ear
Vestibulocochlear nerve (CN VIII)
Internal acoustic meatus
Inferior petrosal sinus
External acoustic meatus
Tragus
Tympanic air cell
Parotid gland
N.Joy
B. Posterior View

## 7.70 External, middle, and internal ear—II: coronally sectioned

**A.** Anterior portion. **B.** Posterior portion. The inset *(outlined by the box)* is an enlargement of the structures of the middle and internal ear as they appear in B.

- The external acoustic meatus is about 3 cm long; half is cartilaginous and half is bony. It is narrowest at the isthmus, near the junction of the cartilaginous and bony parts.
- The external acoustic meatus is innervated by the auriculotemporal branch of the mandibular nerve (CN $V^3$) and the auricular branches of the vagus nerve (CN X); the middle ear is innervated by the glossopharyngeal nerve (CN IX).
- The cartilaginous part of the external acoustic meatus is lined with thick skin; the bony part is lined with thin epithelium that adheres to the periosteum and forms the outermost layer of the tympanic membrane.

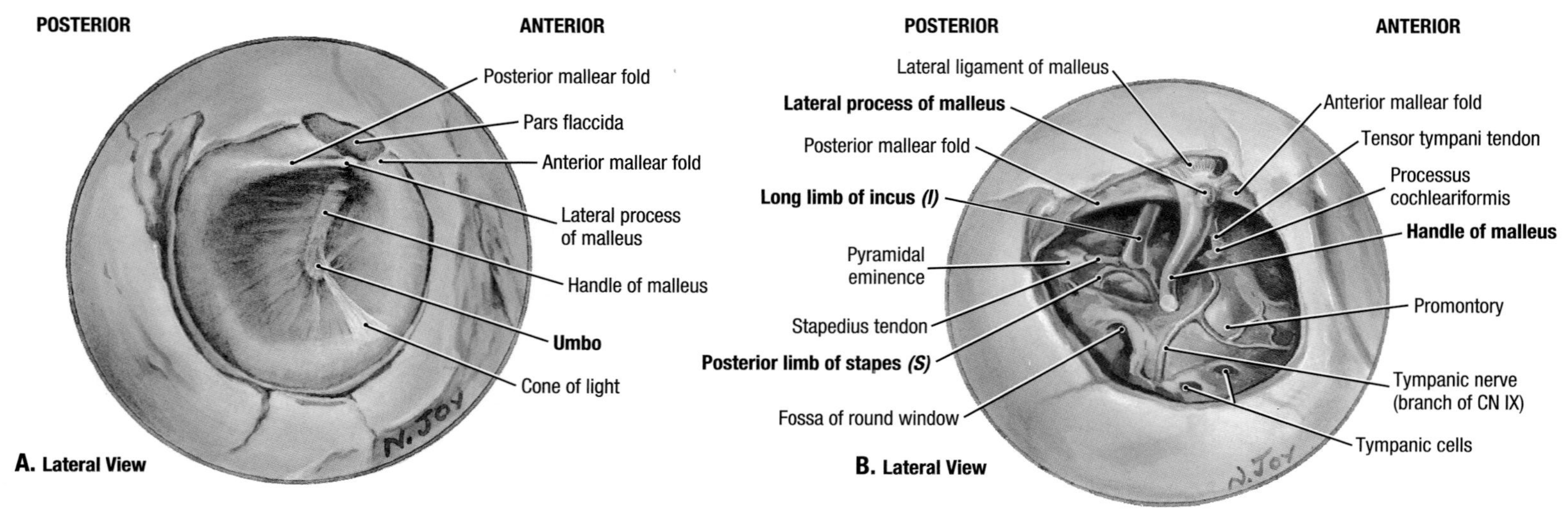
POSTERIOR
ANTERIOR
Posterior mallear fold
Pars flaccida
Anterior mallear fold
Lateral process of malleus
Handle of malleus
Umbo
Cone of light
A. Lateral View
POSTERIOR
ANTERIOR
Lateral ligament of malleus
Lateral process of malleus
Posterior mallear fold
Long limb of incus (I)
Pyramidal eminence
Stapedius tendon
Posterior limb of stapes (S)
Fossa of round window
Anterior mallear fold
Tensor tympani tendon
Processus cochleariformis
Handle of malleus
Promontory
Tympanic nerve (branch of CN IX)
Tympanic cells
B. Lateral View

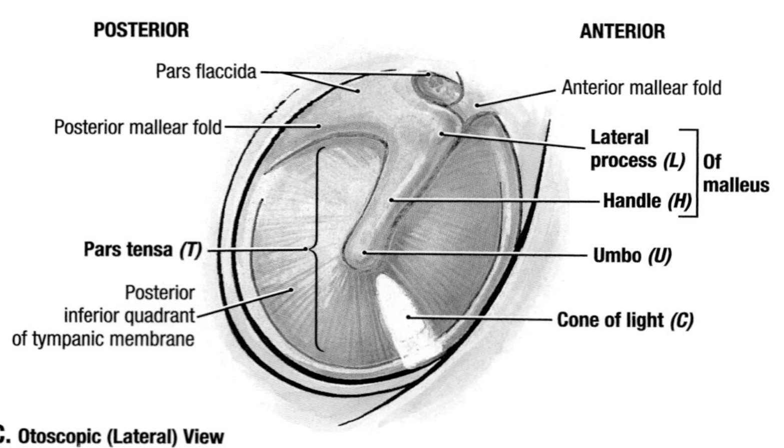
POSTERIOR
ANTERIOR
Pars flaccida
Posterior mallear fold
Anterior mallear fold
Lateral process (L)
Handle (H)
Of malleus
Pars tensa (T)
Umbo (U)
Posterior inferior quadrant of tympanic membrane
Cone of light (C)

C. Otoscopic (Lateral) View

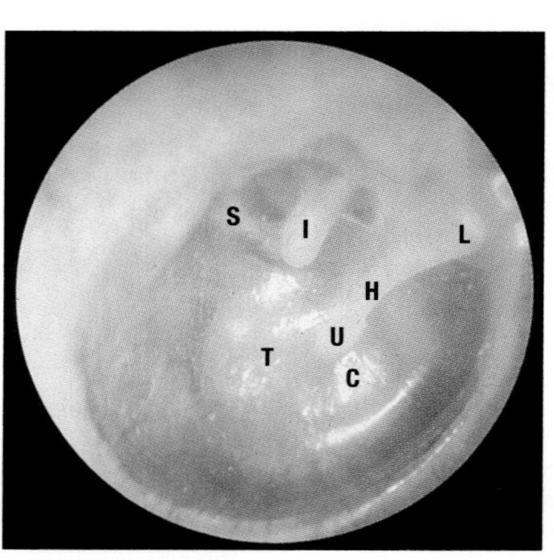
S
I
L
H
U
T
C

D. Otoscopic (Lateral) View

## 7.71 Tympanic membrane

**A.** External (lateral) surface of tympanic membrane. **B.** Tympanic membrane removed, demonstrating structures that lie medially. **C.** Diagram of otoscopic view of tympanic membrane. **D.** Otoscopic view of tympanic membrane. Letter labels are identified in **C.**

- The oval tympanic membrane is a shallow cone deepest at the central apex, the umbo, where the membrane is attached to the tip of the handle of the malleus. The handle of the malleus is attached to the membrane along its entire length as it extends anterosuperiorly toward the periphery of the membrane.
- Superior to the lateral process of the malleus, the membrane is thin (pars flaccida); the flaccid part lacks the radial and circular fibers present in the remainder of the membrane (pars tensa). The junction between the two parts is marked by anterior and posterior mallear folds.
- The lateral surface of the tympanic membrane is innervated by the auricular branch of the auriculotemporal nerve (CN $V^3$) and the auricular branch of the vagus nerve (CN X); the medial surface is innervated by tympanic branches of CN IX.

Examination of the external acoustic meatus and tympanic membrane begins by straightening the meatus. In adults, the helix is grasped and pulled posterosuperiorly (up, out, and back). These movements reduce the curvature of the external acoustic meatus, facilitating insertion of the otoscope. The external acoustic meatus is relatively short in infants; therefore, extra care must be taken to prevent damage to the tympanic membrane.

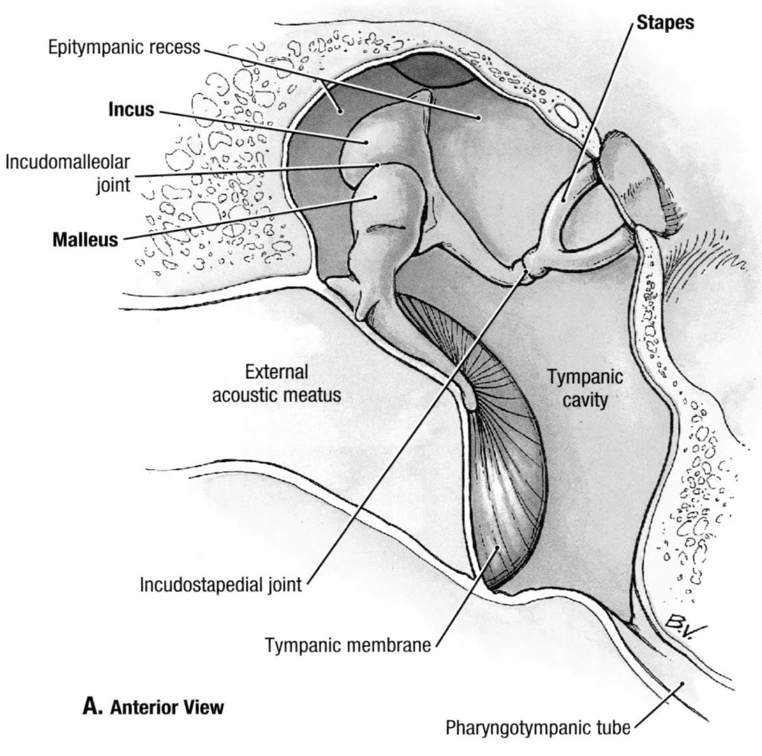
Stapes
Epitympanic recess
Incus
Incudomalleolar joint
Malleus
External acoustic meatus
Tympanic cavity
Incudostapedial joint
Tympanic membrane
Pharyngotympanic tube
B.V.

**A.** Anterior View

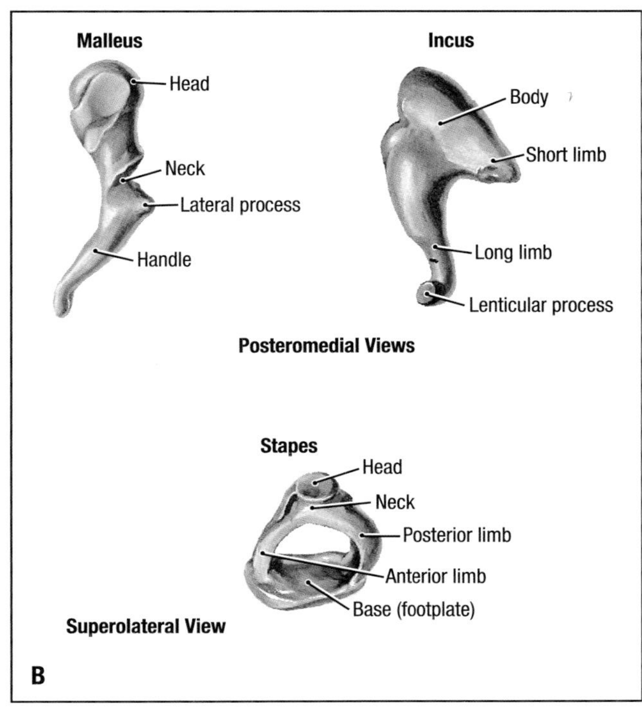
Malleus
Head
Neck
Lateral process
Handle
Incus
Body
Short limb
Long limb
Lenticular process
Posteromedial Views
Stapes
Head
Neck
Posterior limb
Anterior limb
Base (footplate)
Superolateral View
B

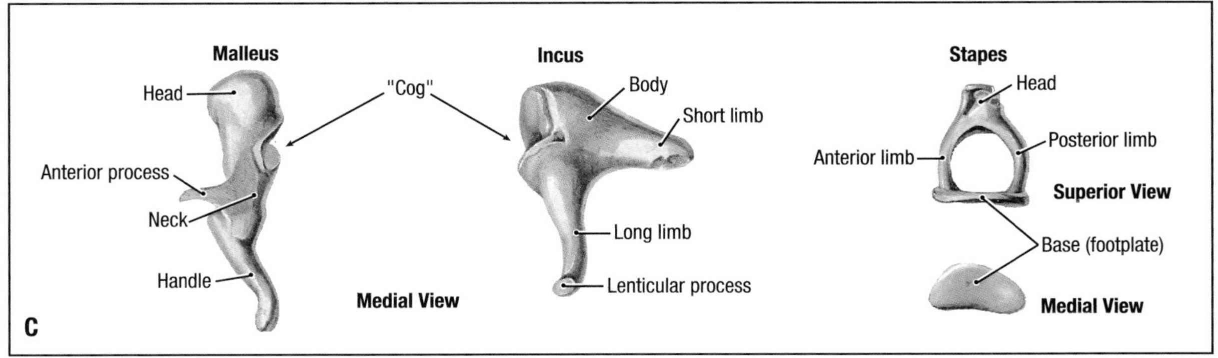
Malleus
Head
Anterior process
Neck
Handle
"Cog"
Incus
Body
Short limb
Long limb
Lenticular process
Medial View
Stapes
Head
Anterior limb
Posterior limb
Superior View
Base (footplate)
Medial View
C

## 7.72 Ossicles of the middle ear

**A.** Ossicles in situ, as revealed by a coronal section of the temporal bone. **B** and **C.** Isolated ossicles.

- The head of the malleus and body and short process of the incus lie in the epitympanic recess, and the handle of the malleus is embedded in the tympanic membrane.
- The saddle-shaped articular surface of the head of the malleus and the reciprocally shaped articular surface of the body of the incus form the incudomalleolar synovial joint.
- A convex articular facet at the end of the long process of the incus articulates with the head of the stapes to compose the incudostapedial synovial joint.

- An earache and bulging red tympanic membrane may indicate pus or fluid in the middle ear, a sign of otitis media. Infection of the middle ear often is secondary to upper respiratory infections. Inflammation and swelling of the mucous membrane lining the tympanic cavity may cause partial or complete blockage of the pharyngotympanic tube. The tympanic membrane becomes red and bulges, and the person may complain of "ear popping." If untreated, otitis media may produce impaired hearing as the result of scarring of the auditory ossicles, limiting the ability of these bones to move in response to sound.

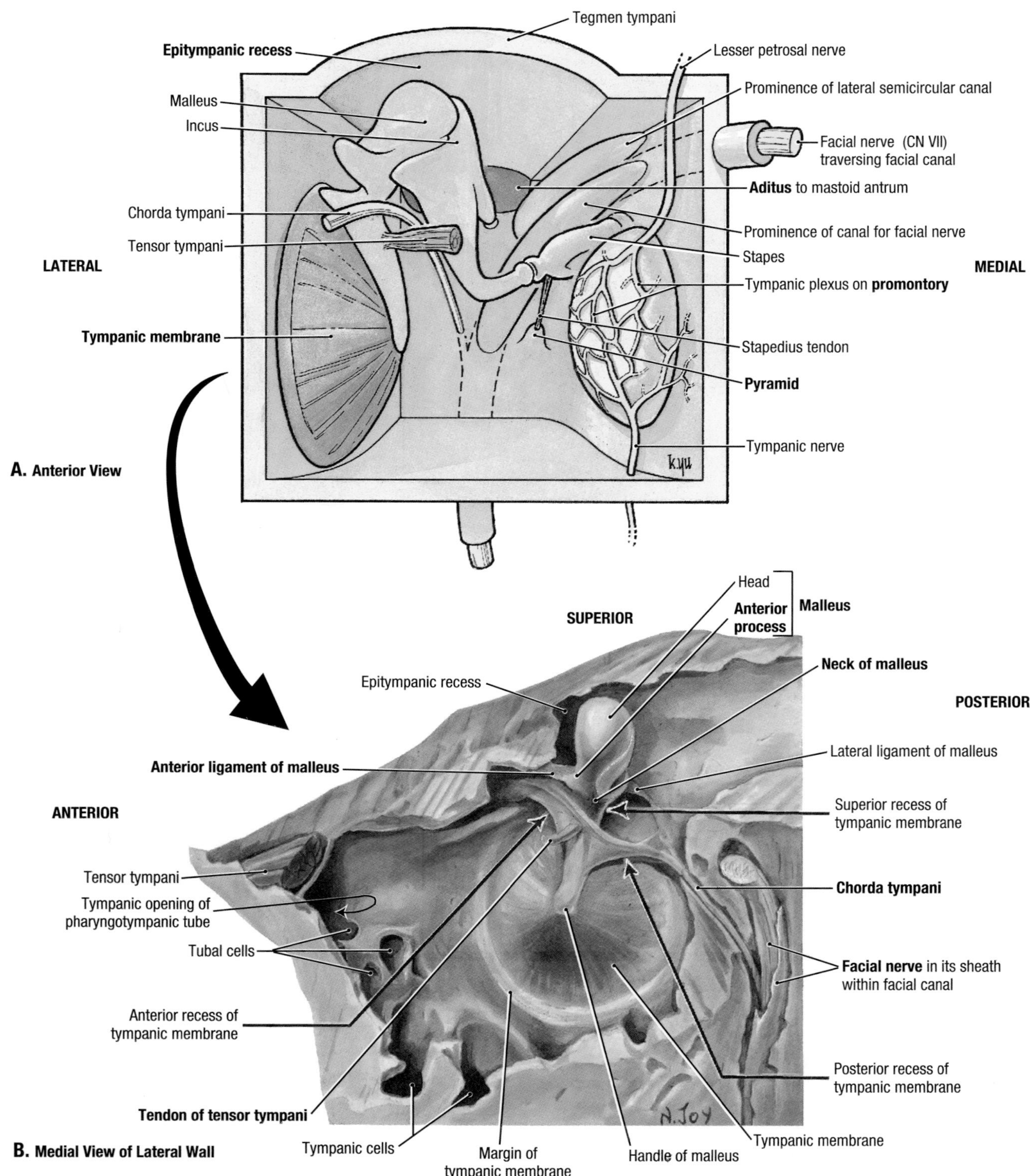
Tegmen tympani
Epitympanic recess
Lesser petrosal nerve
Prominence of lateral semicircular canal
Malleus
Incus
Facial nerve (CN VII) traversing facial canal
Aditus to mastoid antrum
Chorda tympani
Prominence of canal for facial nerve
Tensor tympani
Stapes
LATERAL
MEDIAL
Tympanic plexus on promontory
Tympanic membrane
Stapedius tendon
Pyramid
Tympanic nerve
A. Anterior View
Head
Anterior process
Malleus
SUPERIOR
Neck of malleus
Epitympanic recess
POSTERIOR
Lateral ligament of malleus
Anterior ligament of malleus
ANTERIOR
Superior recess of tympanic membrane
Tensor tympani
Chorda tympani
Tympanic opening of pharyngotympanic tube
Tubal cells
Facial nerve in its sheath within facial canal
Anterior recess of tympanic membrane
Posterior recess of tympanic membrane
Tendon of tensor tympani
B. Medial View of Lateral Wall
Tympanic cells
Margin of tympanic membrane
Handle of malleus
Tympanic membrane

## 7.73 Structures of the tympanic cavity

**A.** Schematic illustration of the tympanic cavity with the anterior wall removed. **B.** Lateral wall of the tympanic cavity. The facial nerve lies within the facial canal surrounded by a tough periosteal tube; the chorda tympani leaves the facial nerve and lies within two crescentic folds of mucous membrane, crossing the neck of the malleus superior to the tendon of tensor tympani.

Perforation of the tympanic membrane (ruptured eardrum) may result from otitis media. Perforation may also result from foreign bodies in the external acoustic meatus, trauma, or excessive pressure. Because the superior half of the tympanic membrane is much more vascular than the inferior half, incisions are made posteroinferiorly through the membrane. This incision also avoids injury to the chorda tympani nerve and auditory ossicles.

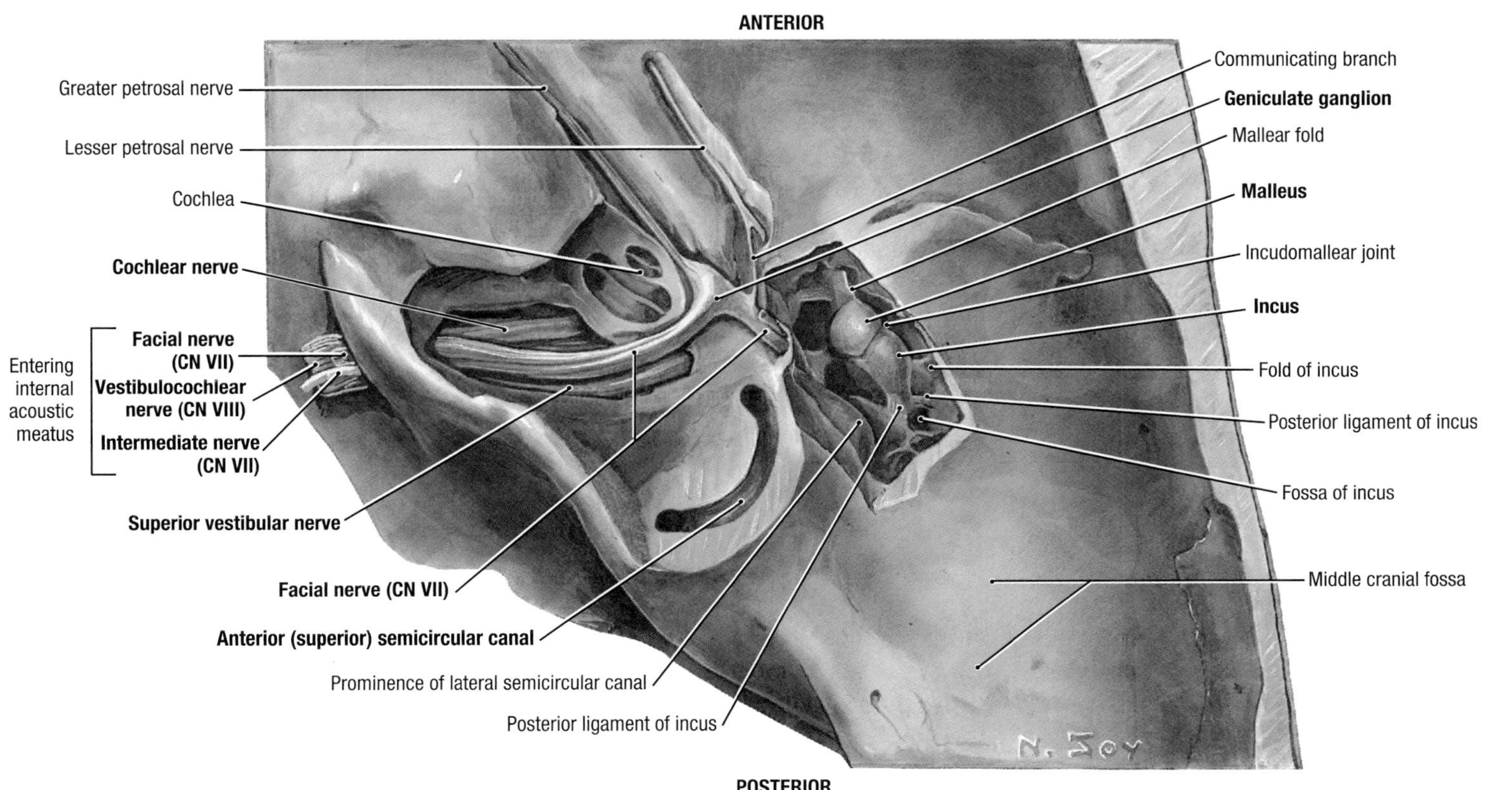
ANTERIOR
Greater petrosal nerve
Lesser petrosal nerve
Cochlea
Cochlear nerve
Entering internal acoustic meatus
Facial nerve (CN VII)
Vestibulocochlear nerve (CN VIII)
Intermediate nerve (CN VII)
Superior vestibular nerve
Facial nerve (CN VII)
Anterior (superior) semicircular canal
Prominence of lateral semicircular canal
Posterior ligament of incus
POSTERIOR
Communicating branch
Geniculate ganglion
Mallear fold
Malleus
Incudomallear joint
Incus
Fold of incus
Posterior ligament of incus
Fossa of incus
Middle cranial fossa

## 7.74 Middle and inner ear *in situ*

The tegmen tympani has been removed to expose the middle ear, the arcuate eminence has been removed to expose the anterior semicircular canal, and the course of the facial and vestibulocochlear nerves through the internal acoustic meatus and internal ear is demonstrated. At the geniculate ganglion, the facial nerve executes a sharp bend, called the genu, and then curves posteroinferiorly within the bony facial canal; the thin lateral wall of the facial canal separates the facial nerve from the tympanic cavity of the middle ear.

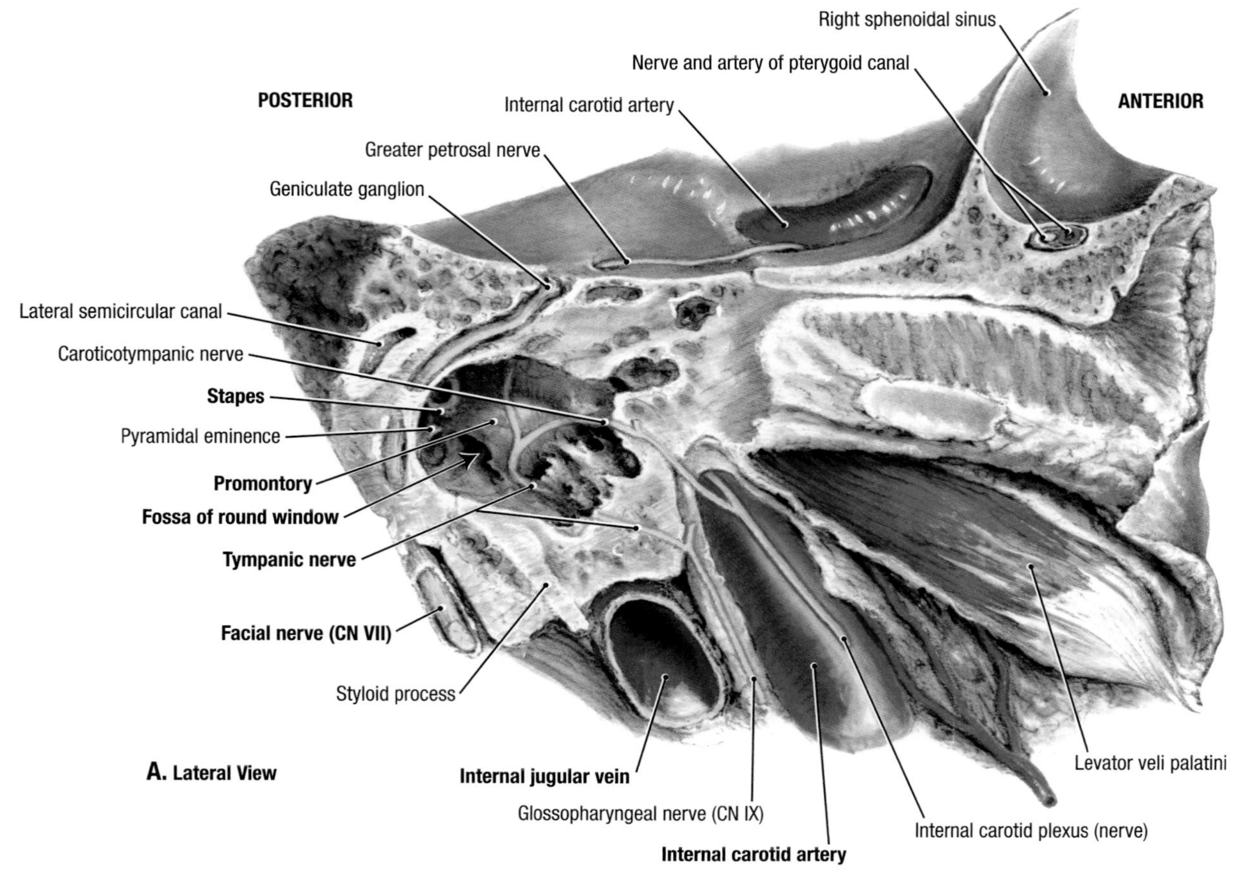

Right sphenoidal sinus
Nerve and artery of pterygoid canal
POSTERIOR
Internal carotid artery
ANTERIOR
Greater petrosal nerve
Geniculate ganglion
Lateral semicircular canal
Caroticotympanic nerve
Stapes
Pyramidal eminence
Promontory
Fossa of round window
Tympanic nerve
Facial nerve (CN VII)
Styloid process
A. Lateral View
Internal jugular vein
Glossopharyngeal nerve (CN IX)
Internal carotid artery
Internal carotid plexus (nerve)
Levator veli palatini


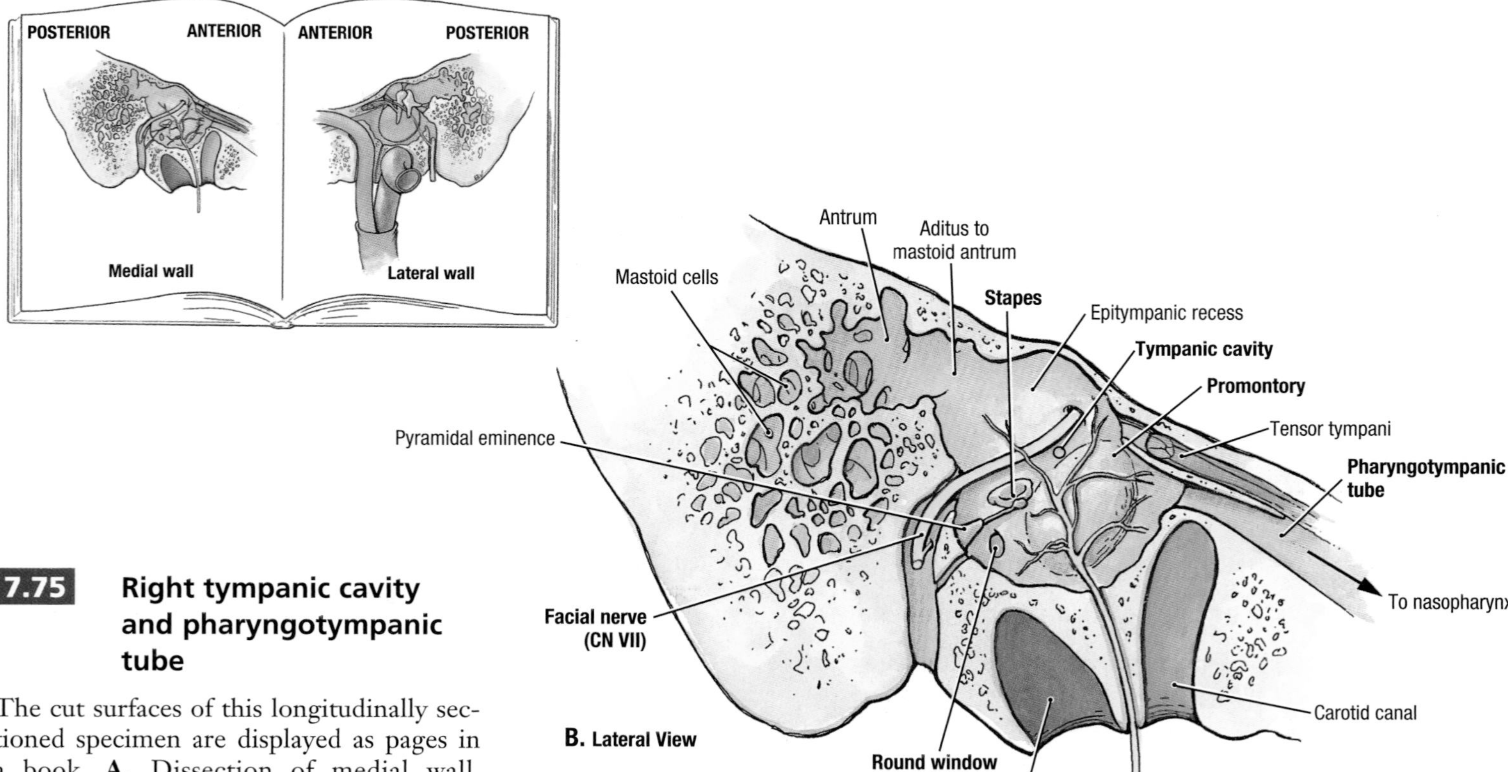

POSTERIOR
ANTERIOR
ANTERIOR
POSTERIOR
Medial wall
Lateral wall
Antrum
Aditus to mastoid antrum
Mastoid cells
Stapes
Epitympanic recess
Tympanic cavity
Promontory
Tensor tympani
Pharyngotympanic tube
Pyramidal eminence
To nasopharynx
Facial nerve (CN VII)
Carotid canal
B. Lateral View
Round window
Jugular foramen
Tympanic nerve (CN IX)


## 7.75 Right tympanic cavity and pharyngotympanic tube

The cut surfaces of this longitudinally sectioned specimen are displayed as pages in a book. **A.** Dissection of medial wall. **B.** Schematic illustration of medial wall.

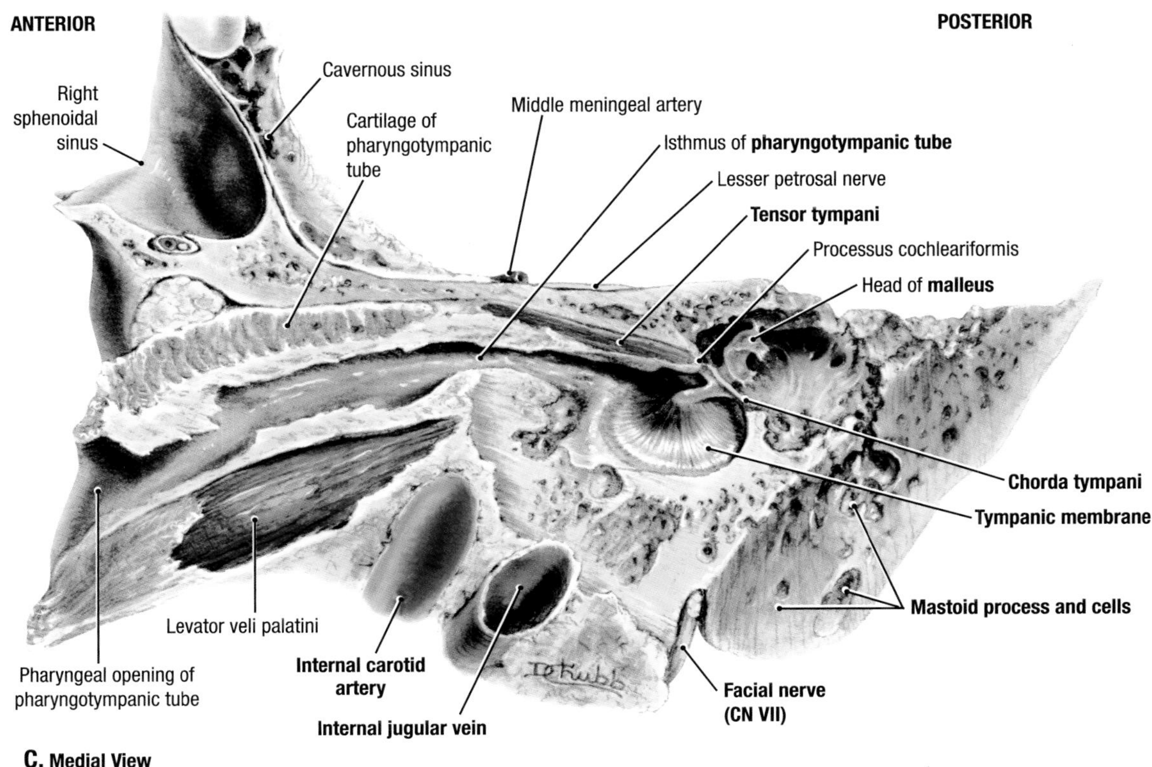
ANTERIOR
POSTERIOR
Right sphenoidal sinus
Cavernous sinus
Cartilage of pharyngotympanic tube
Middle meningeal artery
Isthmus of pharyngotympanic tube
Lesser petrosal nerve
Tensor tympani
Processus cochleariformis
Head of malleus
Chorda tympani
Tympanic membrane
Mastoid process and cells
Facial nerve (CN VII)
Internal jugular vein
Internal carotid artery
Levator veli palatini
Pharyngeal opening of pharyngotympanic tube

**C.** Medial View

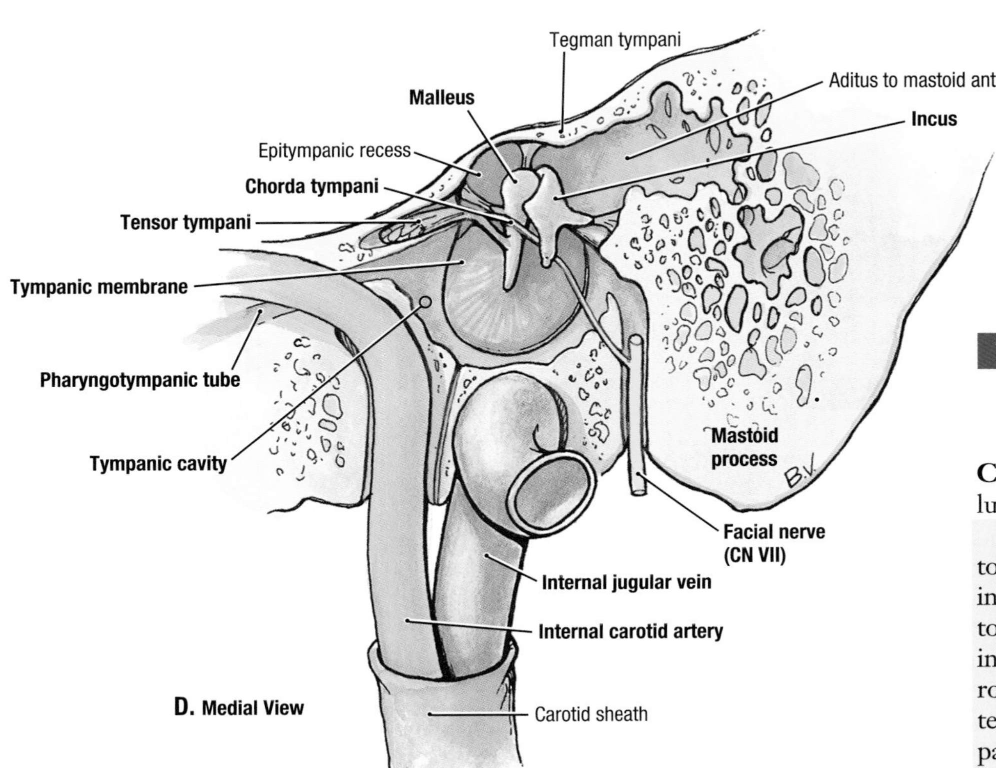
Tegman tympani
Aditus to mastoid antrum
Malleus
Incus
Epitympanic recess
Chorda tympani
Tensor tympani
Tympanic membrane
Pharyngotympanic tube
Tympanic cavity
Mastoid process
Facial nerve (CN VII)
Internal jugular vein
Internal carotid artery
Carotid sheath

**D.** Medial View

## 7.75 Right tympanic cavity and pharyngotympanic tube *(continued)*

**C.** Dissection of lateral wall. **D.** Schematic illustration of lateral wall.

Infections of the mastoid antrum and mastoid cells (mastoiditis) result from middle ear infections that cause inflammation of the mastoid process. Infections may spread superiorly into the middle cranial fossa through the petrosquamous fissure in children or may cause osteomyelitis (bone infection) of the tegmen tympani. Since the advent of antibiotics, mastoiditis is uncommon.

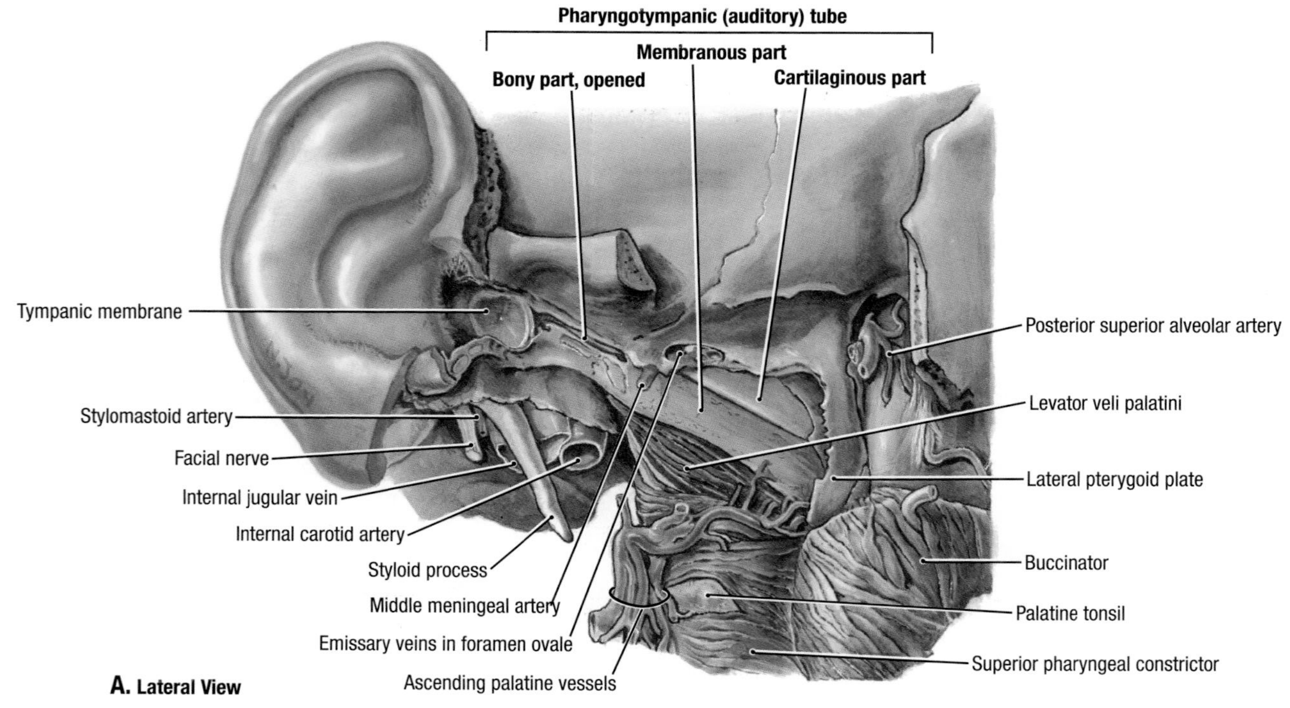
Pharyngotympanic (auditory) tube
Membranous part
Bony part, opened
Cartilaginous part
Tympanic membrane
Posterior superior alveolar artery
Stylomastoid artery
Levator veli palatini
Facial nerve
Internal jugular vein
Lateral pterygoid plate
Internal carotid artery
Buccinator
Styloid process
Middle meningeal artery
Palatine tonsil
Emissary veins in foramen ovale
Superior pharyngeal constrictor
Ascending palatine vessels
A. Lateral View

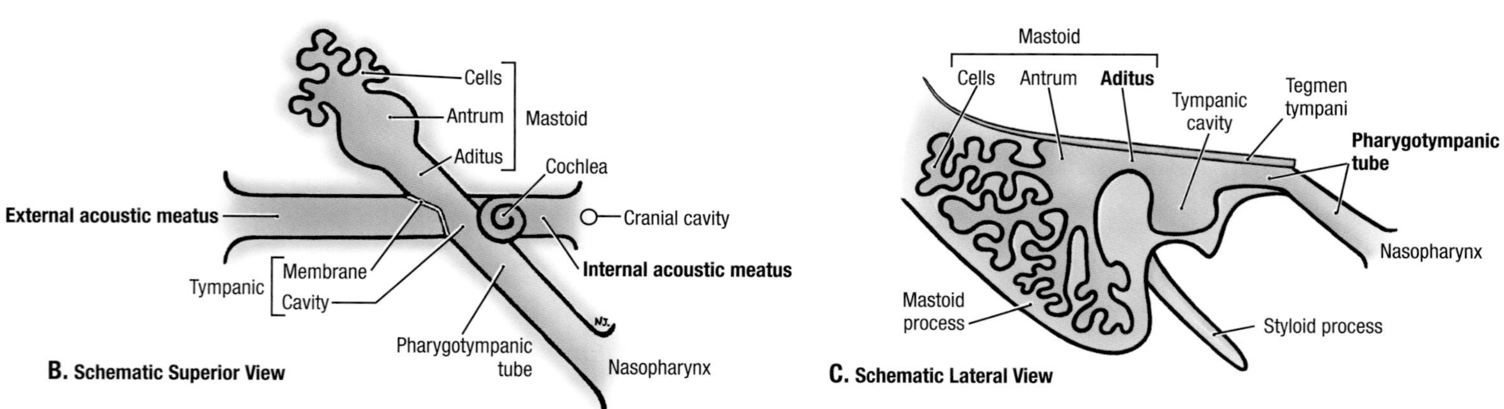
Cells
Antrum
Mastoid
Aditus
Cochlea
External acoustic meatus
Cranial cavity
Tympanic
Membrane
Cavity
Internal acoustic meatus
Pharygotympanic tube
Nasopharynx
B. Schematic Superior View
Mastoid
Cells
Antrum
Aditus
Tympanic cavity
Tegmen tympani
Pharygotympanic tube
Nasopharynx
Mastoid process
Styloid process
C. Schematic Lateral View

## 7.76 Right tympanic cavity and pharyngotympanic tube

**A.** Dissection demonstrating lateral aspect of pharyngotympanic tube and structures located medially. **B.** Schematic illustration demonstrating relationship between internal and external acoustic meatuses. **C.** Diagram of tegmen tympani. **D.** Spaces of tympanic bone. **E.** Relationship of tympanic cavity to internal carotid artery, sigmoid sinus, and middle cranial fossa.

- The general direction of the pharyngotympanic tube is superior, posterior, and lateral from the nasopharynx to the tympanic cavity.
- The cartilaginous part of the tube rests throughout its length on the levator veli palatini muscle.
- The line of the meatuses and the line of the airway, from nasopharynx to mastoid cells, intersect at the tympanic cavity.
- The tegmen tympani forms the roof of the tympanic cavity and mastoid antrum.
- The internal carotid artery is the primary relationship of the anterior wall, the internal jugular vein is the primary relationship of the floor, and the facial nerve is the primary relationship of the posterior wall.

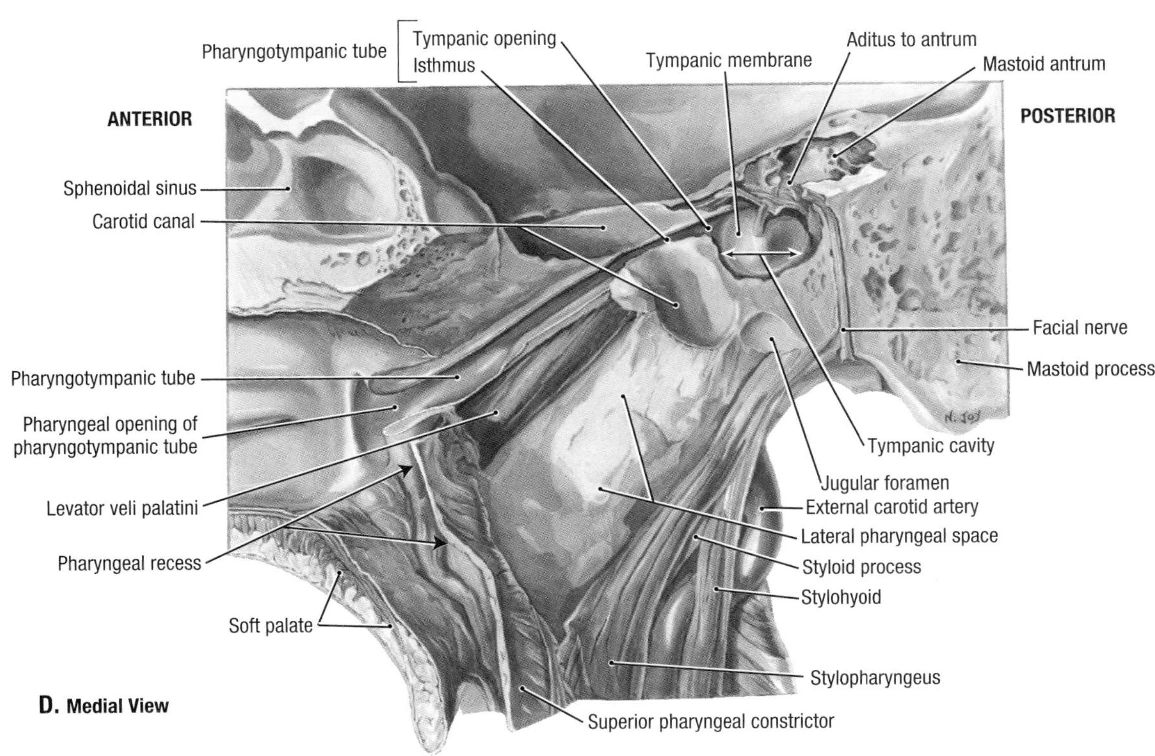
Pharyngotympanic tube
Tympanic opening
Isthmus
Tympanic membrane
Aditus to antrum
Mastoid antrum
ANTERIOR
POSTERIOR
Sphenoidal sinus
Carotid canal
Facial nerve
Mastoid process
Pharyngotympanic tube
Pharyngeal opening of pharyngotympanic tube
Tympanic cavity
Jugular foramen
Levator veli palatini
External carotid artery
Lateral pharyngeal space
Pharyngeal recess
Styloid process
Stylohyoid
Soft palate
Stylopharyngeus
Superior pharyngeal constrictor
N. Joy

**D. Medial View**

SUPERIOR
Facial nerve (CN VII)
Tegmen tympani
Mastoid antrum
Tendon of tensor tympani
ANTERIOR
POSTERIOR
Tympanic opening of pharyngotympanic (auditory) tube
Internal carotid artery in carotid canal
Superior bulb of internal jugular vein
Sigmoid sinus
N. Joy.

**E. Medial View**

**7.76 Right tympanic cavity and pharyngotympanic tube *(continued)***

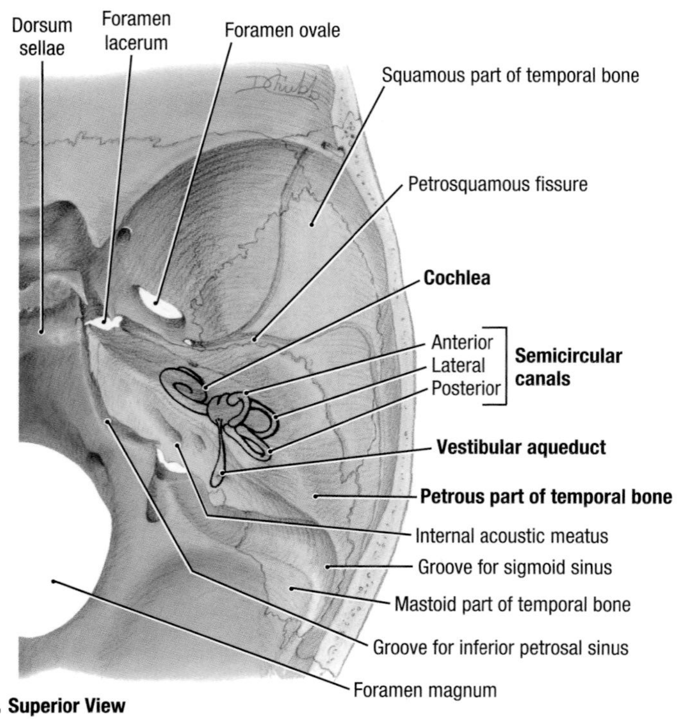
Dorsum sellae
Foramen lacerum
Foramen ovale
Squamous part of temporal bone
Petrosquamous fissure
Cochlea
Anterior
Lateral
Posterior
Semicircular canals
Vestibular aqueduct
Petrous part of temporal bone
Internal acoustic meatus
Groove for sigmoid sinus
Mastoid part of temporal bone
Groove for inferior petrosal sinus
Foramen magnum

**A.** Superior View

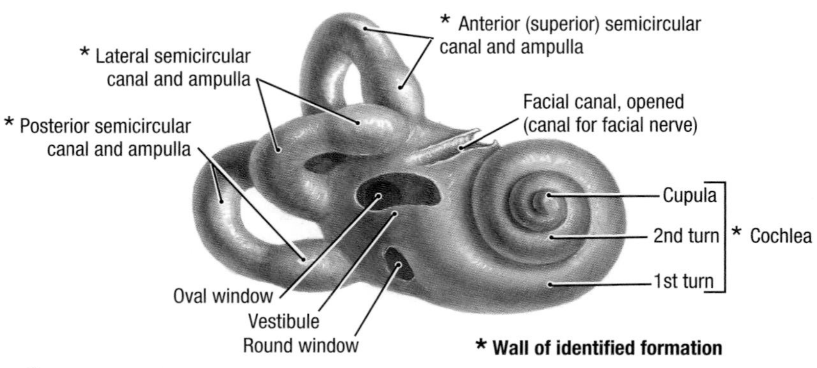
* Anterior (superior) semicircular canal and ampulla
* Lateral semicircular canal and ampulla
* Posterior semicircular canal and ampulla
Facial canal, opened (canal for facial nerve)
Cupula
2nd turn
1st turn
* Cochlea
Oval window
Vestibule
Round window
* Wall of identified formation

**C.** Anterolateral View

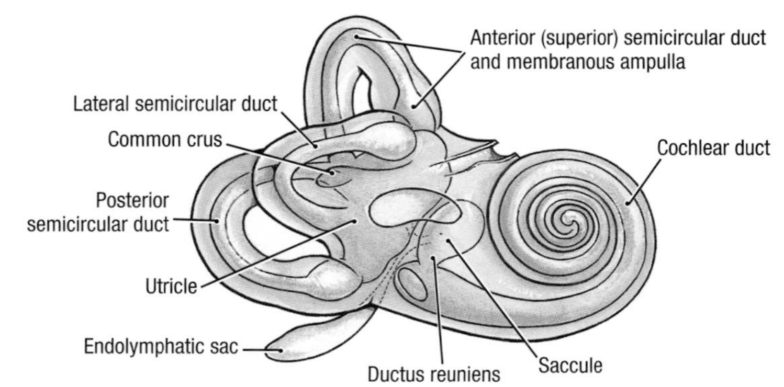
Anterior (superior) semicircular duct and membranous ampulla
Lateral semicircular duct
Common crus
Cochlear duct
Posterior semicircular duct
Utricle
Endolymphatic sac
Ductus reuniens
Saccule

**D.** Anterolateral View

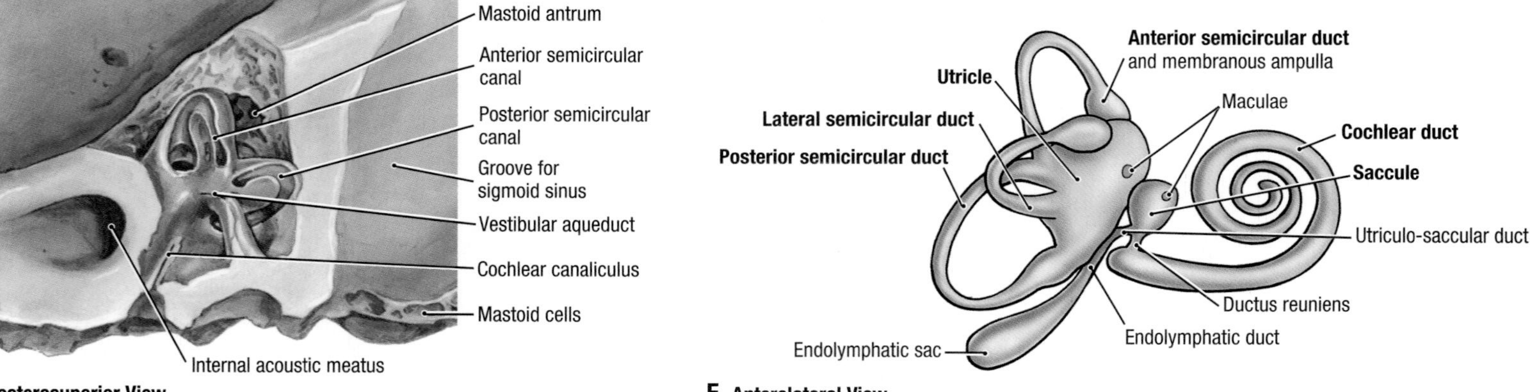
Mastoid antrum
Anterior semicircular canal
Posterior semicircular canal
Groove for sigmoid sinus
Vestibular aqueduct
Cochlear canaliculus
Mastoid cells
Internal acoustic meatus
Anterior semicircular duct and membranous ampulla
Utricle
Maculae
Lateral semicircular duct
Cochlear duct
Posterior semicircular duct
Saccule
Utriculo-saccular duct
Ductus reuniens
Endolymphatic duct
Endolymphatic sac

**B.** Posterosuperior View

**E.** Anterolateral View

## 7.77 Bony and membranous labyrinths

**A.** Location and orientation of bony labyrinth within petrous temporal bone. **B.** Semicircular canals and aqueducts *in situ*. The tegmen tympani has been excised, and the softer bone surrounding the harder bone of the otic capsule has been drilled away. **C.** Walls of left bony labyrinth (otic capsule). The bony labyrinth is the fluid-filled space contained within this formation. **D.** Membranous labyrinth as it lies within the surrounding bony labyrinth. **E.** Isolated left membranous labyrinth.

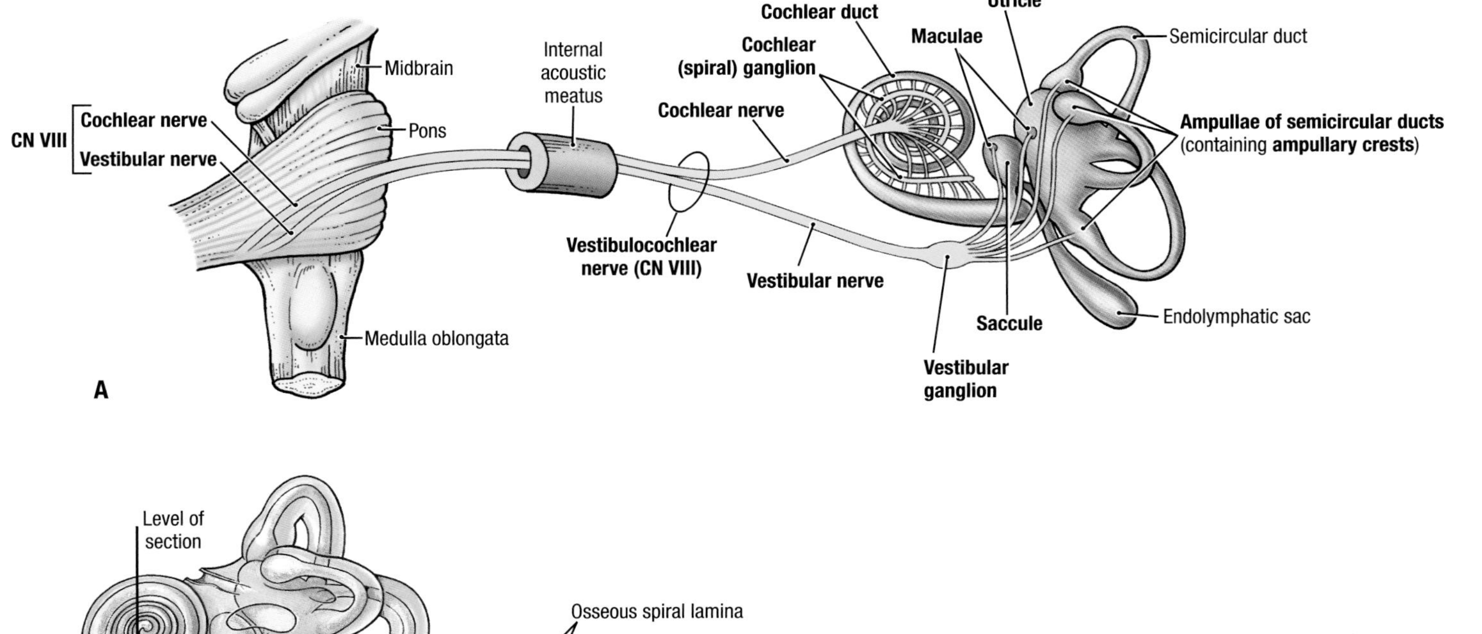
CN VIII
Cochlear nerve
Vestibular nerve
Midbrain
Pons
Medulla oblongata
A
Internal acoustic meatus
Vestibulocochlear nerve (CN VIII)
Vestibular nerve
Cochlear duct
Cochlear (spiral) ganglion
Cochlear nerve
Maculae
Utricle
Semicircular duct
Ampullae of semicircular ducts (containing ampullary crests)
Endolymphatic sac
Saccule
Vestibular ganglion

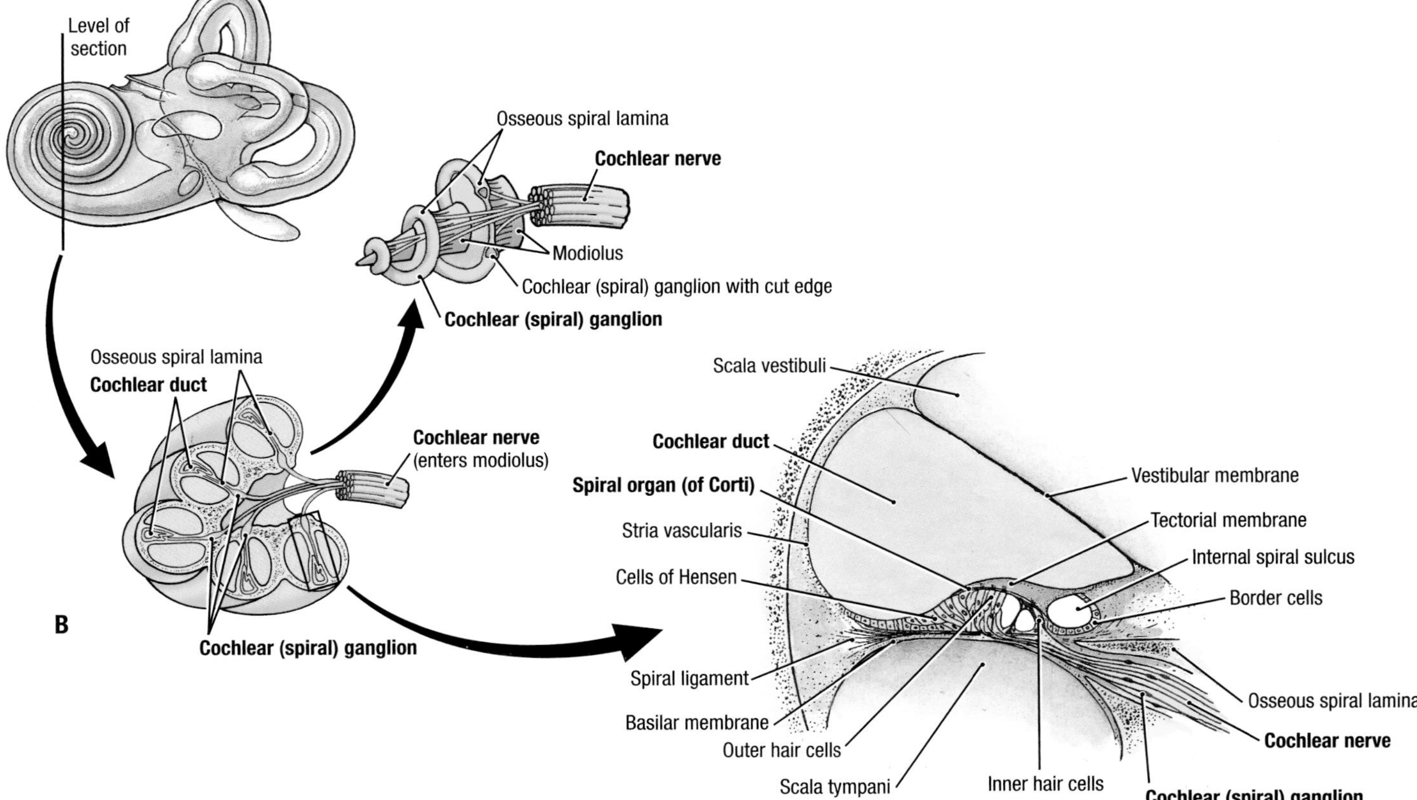
Level of section
Osseous spiral lamina
Cochlear nerve
Modiolus
Cochlear (spiral) ganglion with cut edge
Cochlear (spiral) ganglion
Osseous spiral lamina
Cochlear duct
Cochlear nerve (enters modiolus)
Cochlear (spiral) ganglion
B
Scala vestibuli
Cochlear duct
Spiral organ (of Corti)
Stria vascularis
Cells of Hensen
Spiral ligament
Basilar membrane
Outer hair cells
Scala tympani
Inner hair cells
Vestibular membrane
Tectorial membrane
Internal spiral sulcus
Border cells
Osseous spiral lamina
Cochlear nerve
Cochlear (spiral) ganglion

## 7.78 Vestibulocochlear nerve and structure of cochlea

**A.** Distribution of vestibulocochlear nerve (schematic). **B.** Structure of cochlea. The cochlea has been sectioned along the bony core of the cochlea (modiolus), the axis about which the cochlea winds. An isolated modiolus is shown after the turns of the cochlea are removed, leaving only the spiral lamina winding around it. The *large drawing* shows the details of the *area enclosed in the rectangle*, including a cross-section of the cochlear duct of the membranous labyrinth.

- The maculae of the membranous labyrinth are primarily static organs, which have small dense particles (otoliths) embedded among the hair cells. Under the influence of gravity, the otoliths cause bending of the hair cells, which stimulate the vestibular nerve and provide awareness of the position of the head in space; the hairs also respond to quick tilting movements and to linear acceleration and deceleration. Motion sickness results mainly from discordance between vestibular and visual stimuli.
- Persistent exposure to excessively loud sound causes degenerative changes in the spiral organ, resulting in high-tone deafness. This type of hearing loss commonly occurs in workers who are exposed to loud noises and do not wear protective earmuffs.

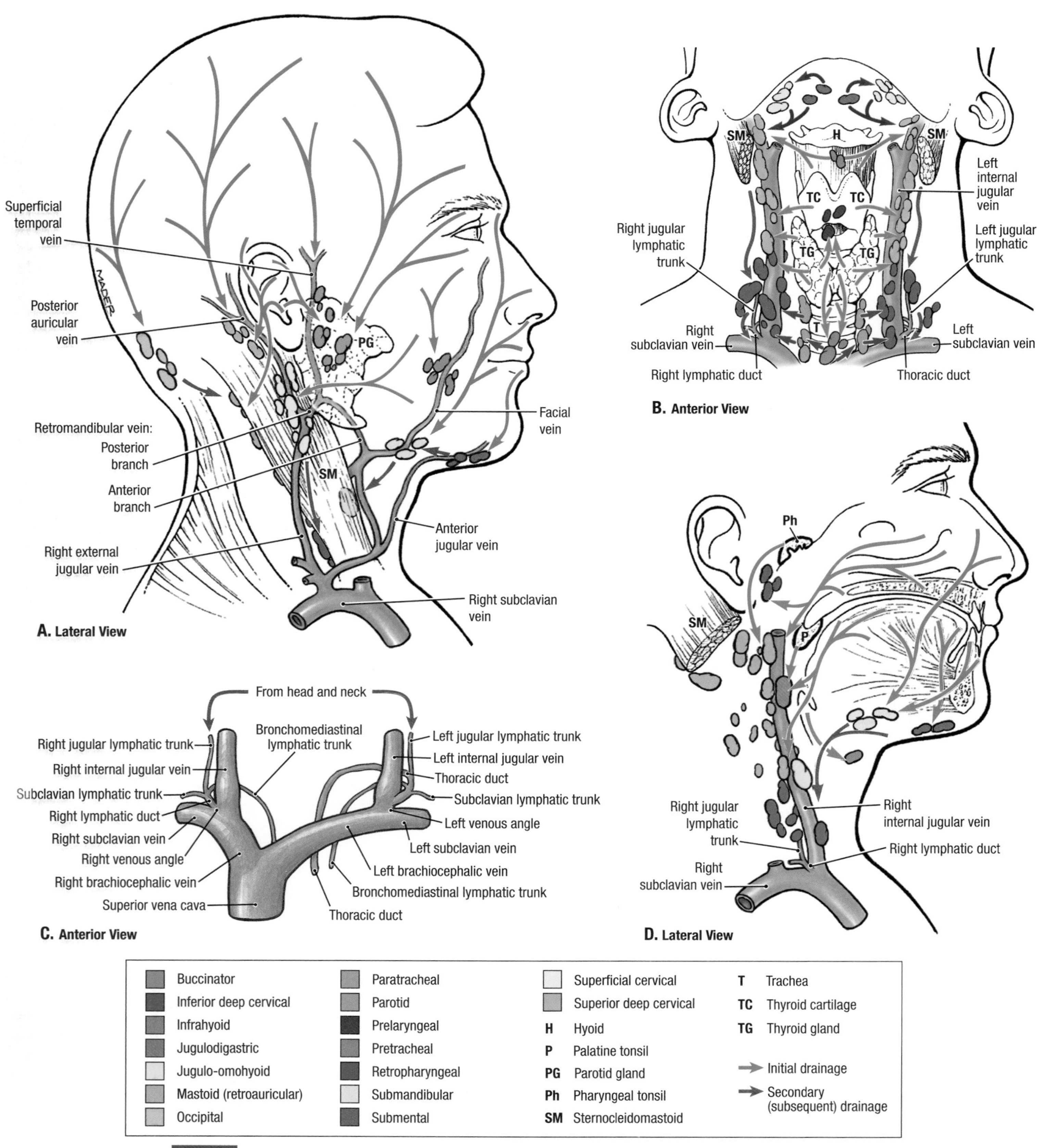
Superficial temporal vein
Posterior auricular vein
PG
SM
Retromandibular vein:
Posterior branch
Anterior branch
Right external jugular vein
Facial vein
Anterior jugular vein
Right subclavian vein
A. Lateral View
SM
H
SM
TC
TC
TG
TG
T
Left internal jugular vein
Right jugular lymphatic trunk
Left jugular lymphatic trunk
Right subclavian vein
Left subclavian vein
Right lymphatic duct
Thoracic duct
B. Anterior View
From head and neck
Bronchomediastinal lymphatic trunk
Right jugular lymphatic trunk
Right internal jugular vein
Subclavian lymphatic trunk
Right lymphatic duct
Right subclavian vein
Right venous angle
Right brachiocephalic vein
Superior vena cava
Left jugular lymphatic trunk
Left internal jugular vein
Thoracic duct
Subclavian lymphatic trunk
Left venous angle
Left subclavian vein
Left brachiocephalic vein
Bronchomediastinal lymphatic trunk
Thoracic duct
C. Anterior View
Ph
SM
P
Right jugular lymphatic trunk
Right subclavian vein
Right internal jugular vein
Right lymphatic duct
D. Lateral View
Buccinator
Inferior deep cervical
Infrahyoid
Jugulodigastric
Jugulo-omohyoid
Mastoid (retroauricular)
Occipital
Paratracheal
Parotid
Prelaryngeal
Pretracheal
Retropharyngeal
Submandibular
Submental
Superficial cervical
Superior deep cervical
H Hyoid
P Palatine tonsil
PG Parotid gland
Ph Pharyngeal tonsil
SM Sternocleidomastoid
T Trachea
TC Thyroid cartilage
TG Thyroid gland
Initial drainage
Secondary (subsequent) drainage

**7.79 Lymphatic and venous drainage of the head and neck**

**A.** Superficial drainage. **B.** Drainage of the trachea, thyroid gland, larynx, and floor of mouth. **C.** Termination of right and left jugular lymphatic trunks. **D.** Deep drainage.

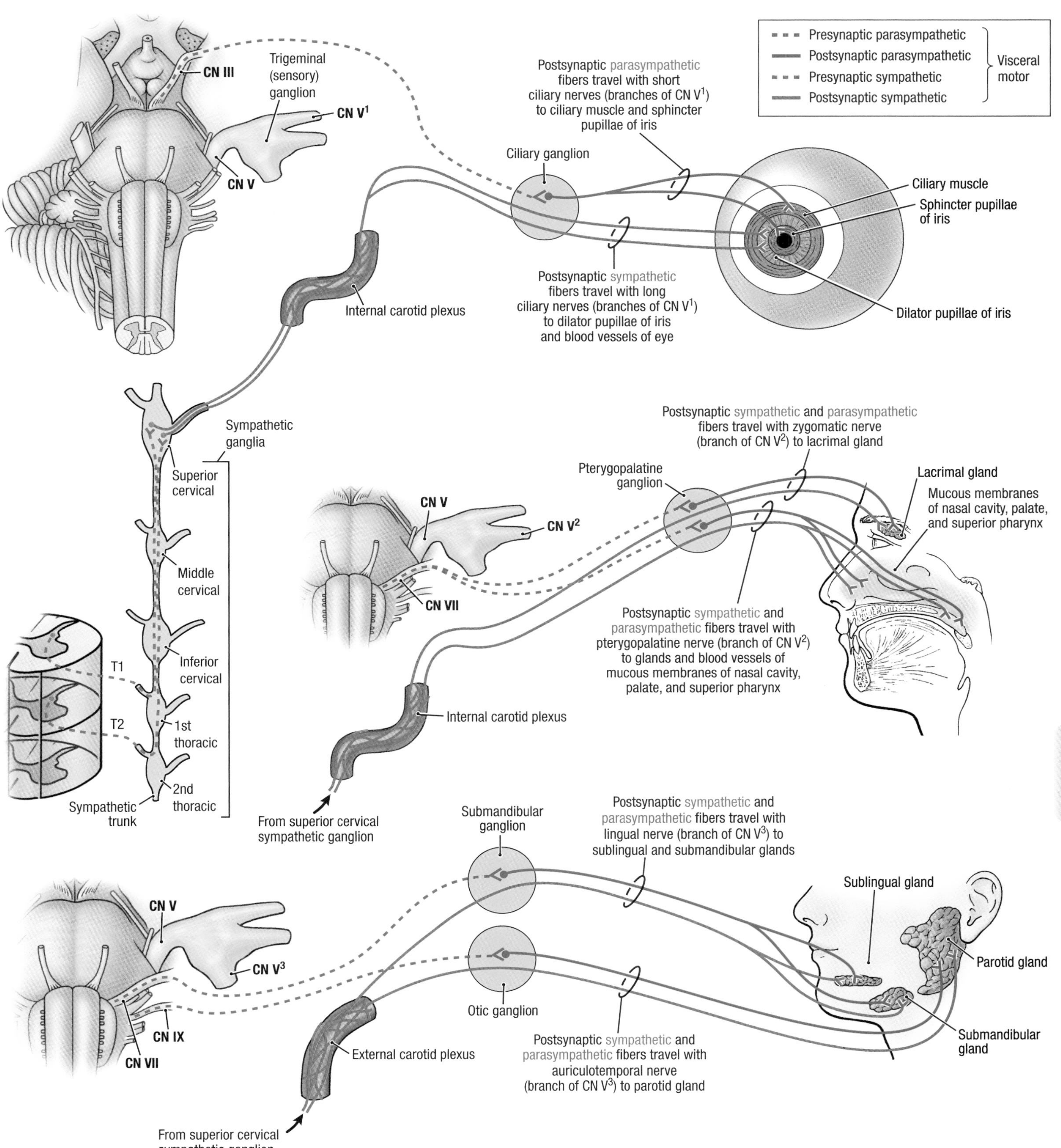
Presynaptic parasympathetic
Postsynaptic parasympathetic
Presynaptic sympathetic
Postsynaptic sympathetic
Visceral motor
CN III
Trigeminal (sensory) ganglion
CN V$^1$
CN V
Postsynaptic parasympathetic fibers travel with short ciliary nerves (branches of CN V$^1$) to ciliary muscle and sphincter pupillae of iris
Ciliary ganglion
Ciliary muscle
Sphincter pupillae of iris
Dilator pupillae of iris
Internal carotid plexus
Postsynaptic sympathetic fibers travel with long ciliary nerves (branches of CN V$^1$) to dilator pupillae of iris and blood vessels of eye
Sympathetic ganglia
Superior cervical
Middle cervical
Inferior cervical
1st thoracic
2nd thoracic
Sympathetic trunk
T1
T2
Postsynaptic sympathetic and parasympathetic fibers travel with zygomatic nerve (branch of CN V$^2$) to lacrimal gland
Pterygopalatine ganglion
Lacrimal gland
Mucous membranes of nasal cavity, palate, and superior pharynx
CN V
CN V$^2$
CN VII
Postsynaptic sympathetic and parasympathetic fibers travel with pterygopalatine nerve (branch of CN V$^2$) to glands and blood vessels of mucous membranes of nasal cavity, palate, and superior pharynx
Internal carotid plexus
From superior cervical sympathetic ganglion
Submandibular ganglion
Postsynaptic sympathetic and parasympathetic fibers travel with lingual nerve (branch of CN V$^3$) to sublingual and submandibular glands
Sublingual gland
Parotid gland
Submandibular gland
CN V
CN V$^3$
CN IX
CN VII
Otic ganglion
External carotid plexus
Postsynaptic sympathetic and parasympathetic fibers travel with auriculotemporal nerve (branch of CN V$^3$) to parotid gland
From superior cervical sympathetic ganglion

**7.80 Autonomic innervation of the head**

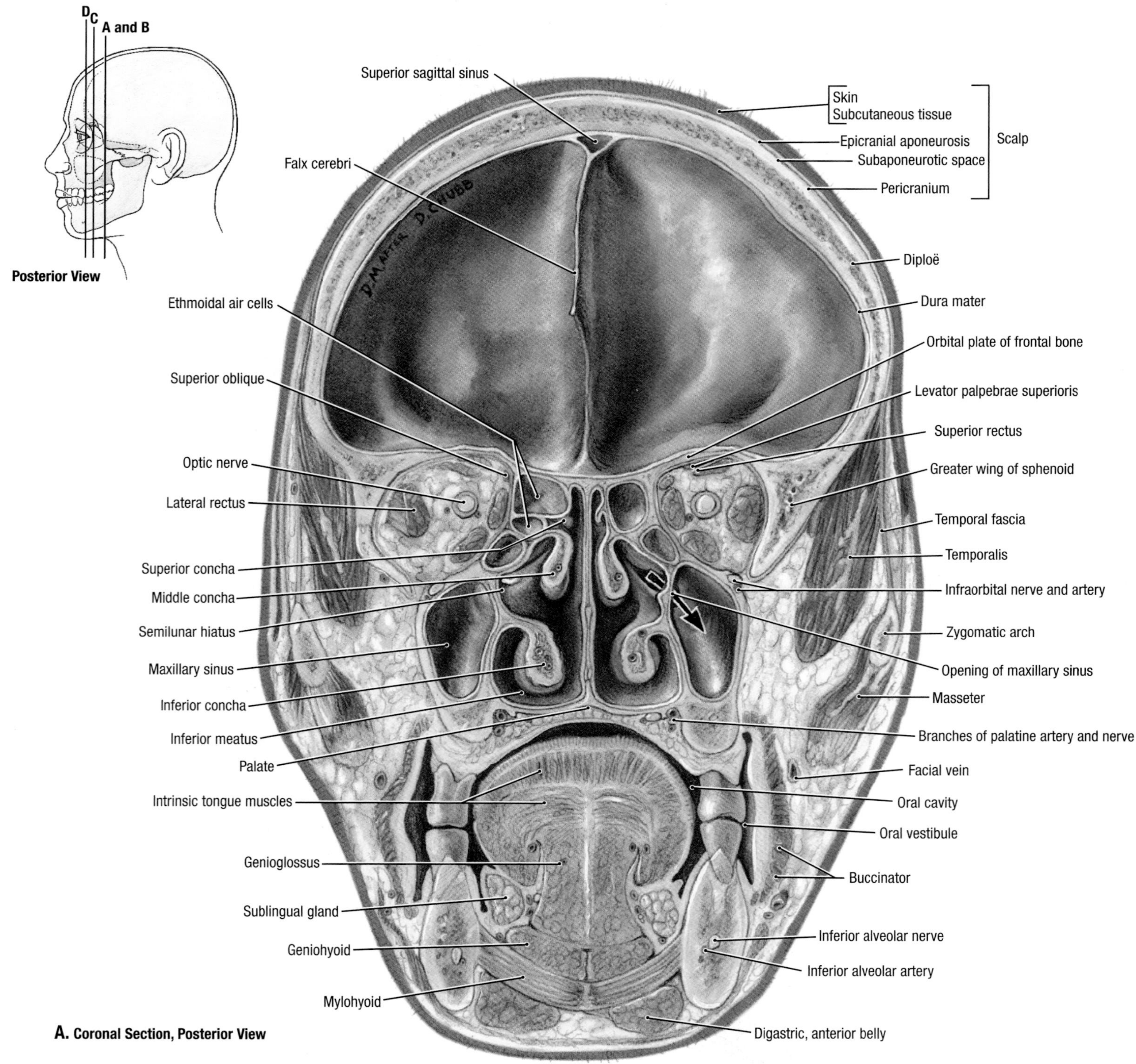
D
C
A and B
Posterior View
Superior sagittal sinus
Skin
Subcutaneous tissue
Epicranial aponeurosis
Subaponeurotic space
Pericranium
Scalp
Falx cerebri
Diploë
Dura mater
Ethmoidal air cells
Orbital plate of frontal bone
Superior oblique
Levator palpebrae superioris
Superior rectus
Optic nerve
Greater wing of sphenoid
Lateral rectus
Temporal fascia
Temporalis
Superior concha
Middle concha
Infraorbital nerve and artery
Semilunar hiatus
Zygomatic arch
Maxillary sinus
Opening of maxillary sinus
Inferior concha
Masseter
Inferior meatus
Branches of palatine artery and nerve
Palate
Facial vein
Intrinsic tongue muscles
Oral cavity
Oral vestibule
Genioglossus
Buccinator
Sublingual gland
Inferior alveolar nerve
Geniohyoid
Inferior alveolar artery
Mylohyoid
Digastric, anterior belly
A. Coronal Section, Posterior View

**7.81 Coronal section and MRI imaging of nasopharynx and oral cavity**

**A.** Coronal section. **B–D.** Coronal MRIs.

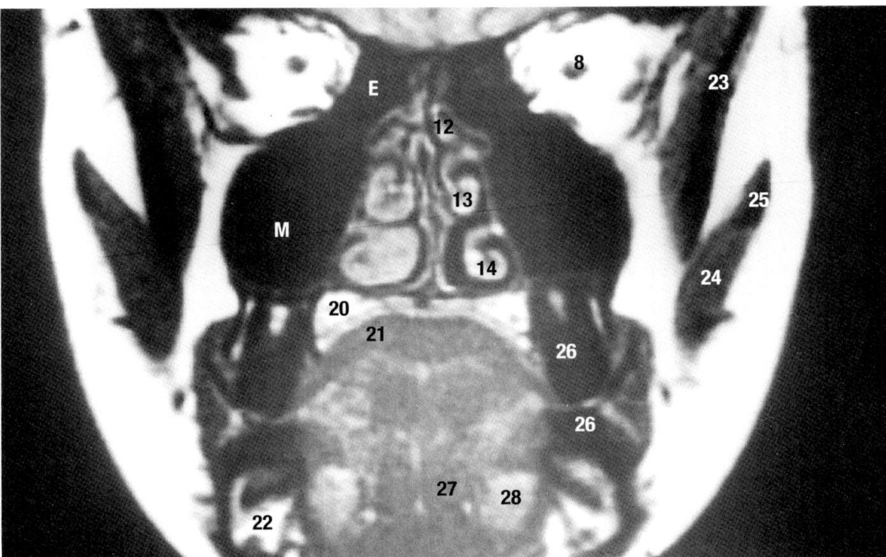
8
E
23
12
13
25
M
14
24
20
21
26
26
27
28
22
B

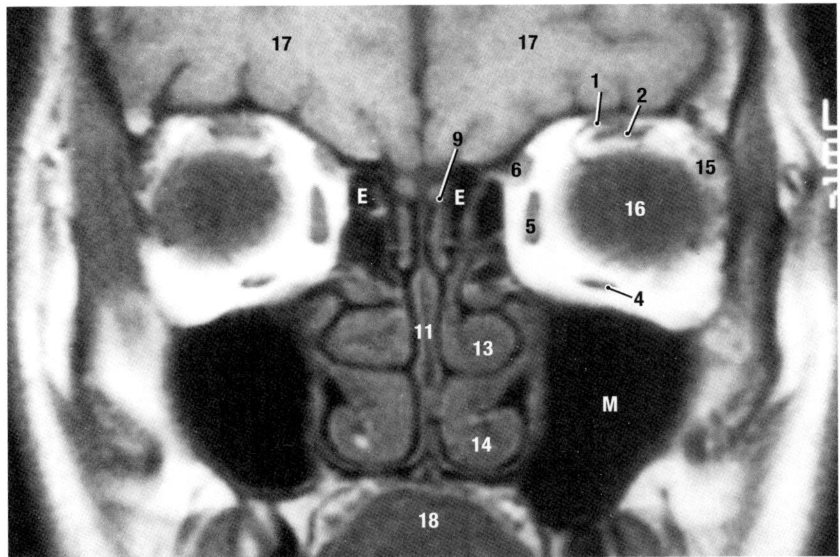
17
17
1
2
9
6
15
E
E
16
5
4
11
13
M
14
18
C

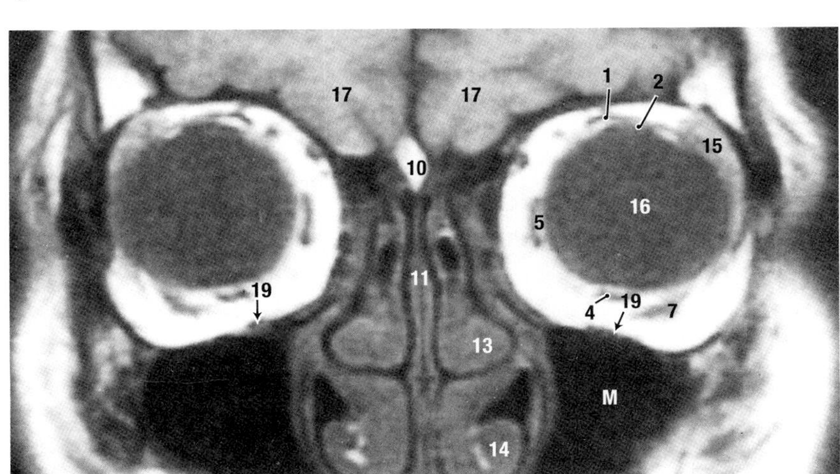
17
17
1
2
15
10
16
5
11
19
4
19
7
13
M
14
D

Posterior Views

| | |
|---|---|
| 1 | Levator palpebrae superioris |
| 2 | Superior rectus |
| 3 | Lateral rectus |
| 4 | Inferior rectus |
| 5 | Medial rectus |
| 6 | Superior oblique |
| 7 | Inferior oblique |
| 8 | Optic nerve |
| 9 | Olfactory bulb |
| 10 | Crista galli |
| 11 | Nasal septum |
| 12 | Superior concha |
| 13 | Middle concha |
| 14 | Inferior concha |
| 15 | Lacrimal gland |
| 16 | Eyeball |
| 17 | Frontal lobe |
| 18 | Tongue |
| 19 | Infraorbital vessels and nerve |
| 20 | Hard palate |
| 21 | Intrinsic muscles of tongue |
| 22 | Mandible |
| 23 | Temporalis |
| 24 | Masseter |
| 25 | Zygomatic arch |
| 26 | Molar teeth |
| 27 | Genioglossus |
| 28 | Sublingual gland |
| M | Maxillary sinus |
| E | Ethmoidal air cell |

**7.81 Coronal section and MRI imaging of nasopharynx and oral cavity *(continued)***

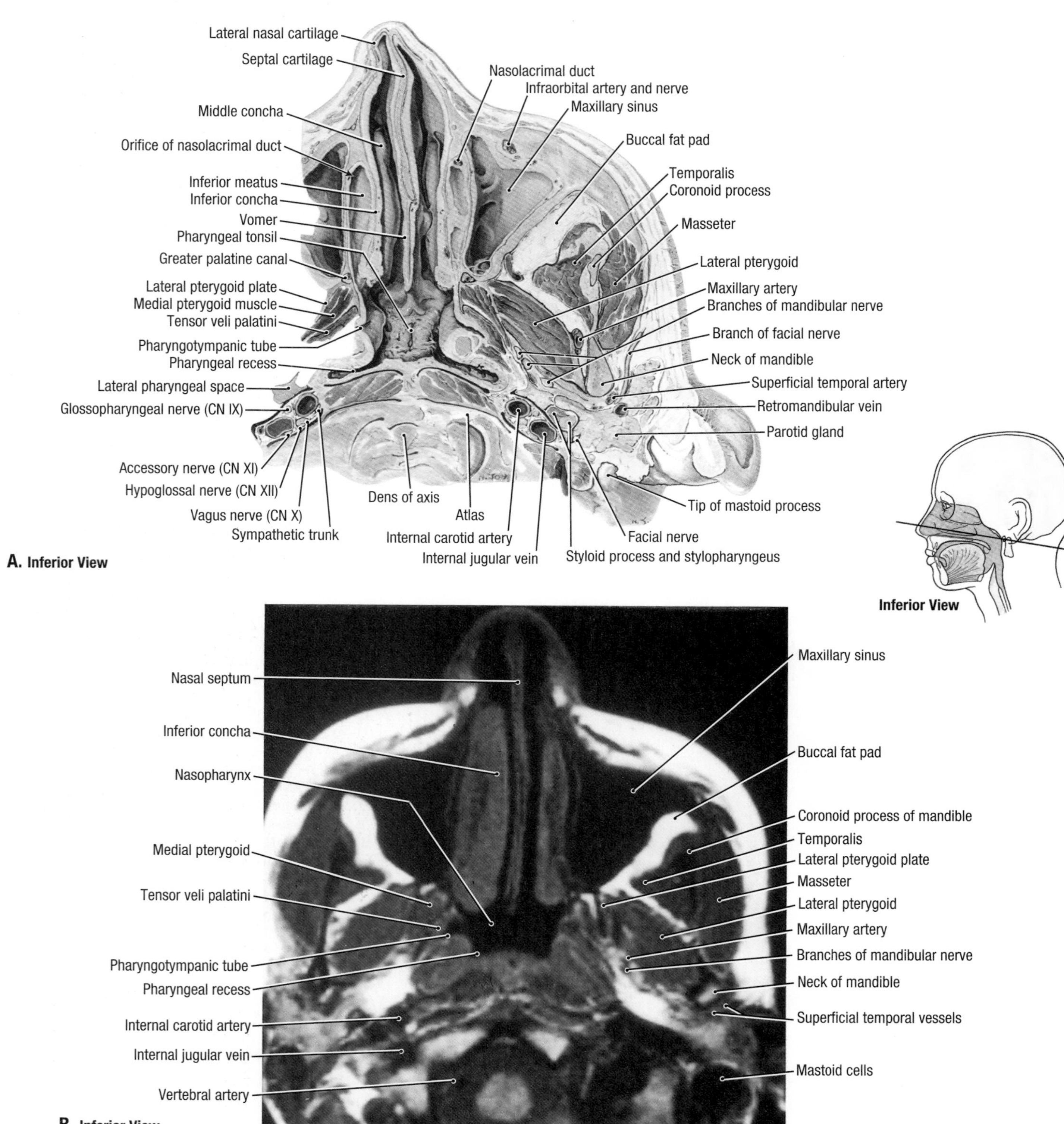
Lateral nasal cartilage
Septal cartilage
Middle concha
Orifice of nasolacrimal duct
Inferior meatus
Inferior concha
Vomer
Pharyngeal tonsil
Greater palatine canal
Lateral pterygoid plate
Medial pterygoid muscle
Tensor veli palatini
Pharyngotympanic tube
Pharyngeal recess
Lateral pharyngeal space
Glossopharyngeal nerve (CN IX)
Accessory nerve (CN XI)
Hypoglossal nerve (CN XII)
Vagus nerve (CN X)
Sympathetic trunk
Dens of axis
Atlas
Internal carotid artery
Internal jugular vein
Styloid process and stylopharyngeus
Facial nerve
Tip of mastoid process
Nasolacrimal duct
Infraorbital artery and nerve
Maxillary sinus
Buccal fat pad
Temporalis
Coronoid process
Masseter
Lateral pterygoid
Maxillary artery
Branches of mandibular nerve
Branch of facial nerve
Neck of mandible
Superficial temporal artery
Retromandibular vein
Parotid gland
A. Inferior View
Inferior View
Nasal septum
Inferior concha
Nasopharynx
Medial pterygoid
Tensor veli palatini
Pharyngotympanic tube
Pharyngeal recess
Internal carotid artery
Internal jugular vein
Vertebral artery
Maxillary sinus
Buccal fat pad
Coronoid process of mandible
Temporalis
Lateral pterygoid plate
Masseter
Lateral pterygoid
Maxillary artery
Branches of mandibular nerve
Neck of mandible
Superficial temporal vessels
Mastoid cells
B. Inferior View

**7.82 Transverse section and MRI imaging of nasal cavity and nasopharynx**

**A.** Transverse section of left side of head. **B.** Transverse (axial) MRI scan.

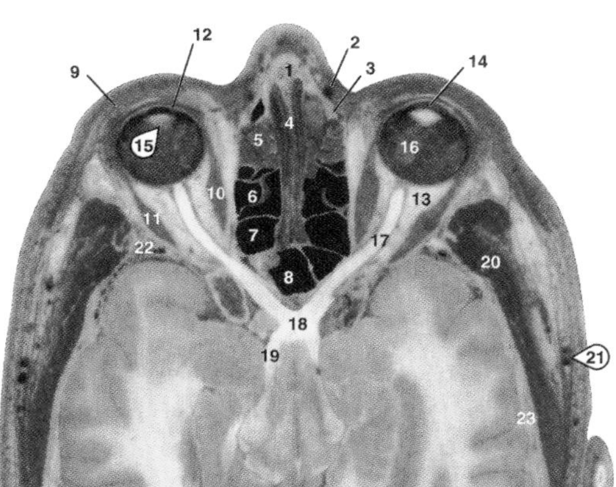
12
2
9
1
3
14
4
15
5
16
10
6
13
11
7
17
22
20
8
18
19
21
23

**A.** **Transverse Section**

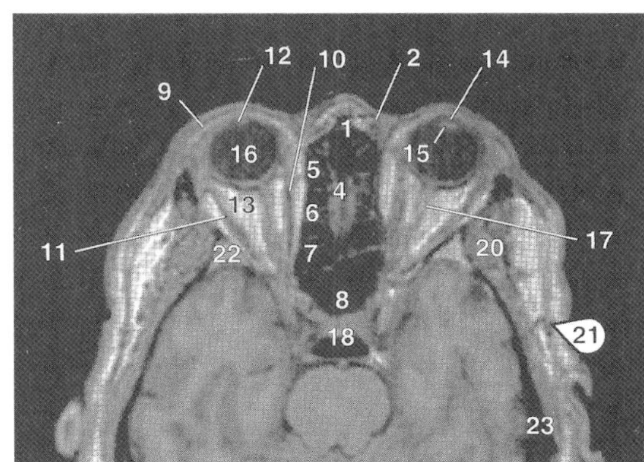
12
10
2
14
9
1
16
15
5
4
13
6
11
22
7
20
17
8
18
21
23

**B.** **Transverse (axial) MRI Scan**

**Key**

1 Nasal bones
2 Angular artery
3 Frontal process of maxilla
4 Nasal septum
5 Anterior ethmoidal cell
6 Middle ethmoidal cell
7 Posterior ethmoidal air cell
8 Sphenoid sinus
9 Orbicularis oculi muscle
10 Medial rectus muscle
11 Lateral rectus muscle
12 Cornea
13 Retrobulbar fat
14 Anterior chamber
15 Lens
16 Vitreous body
17 Optic nerve
18 Optic chiasm
19 Optic tract
20 Temporalis muscle
21 Superficial temporal vessels
22 Greater wing of sphenoid
23 Squamous portion of temporal bone

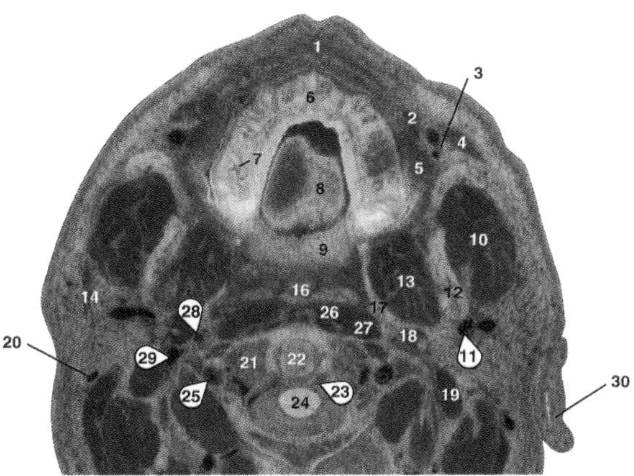
1
3
6
2
4
7
5
8
10
9
13
16
12
14
28
26
17
27
18
20
29
21
22
11
25
24
23
19
30

**C.** **Transverse Section**

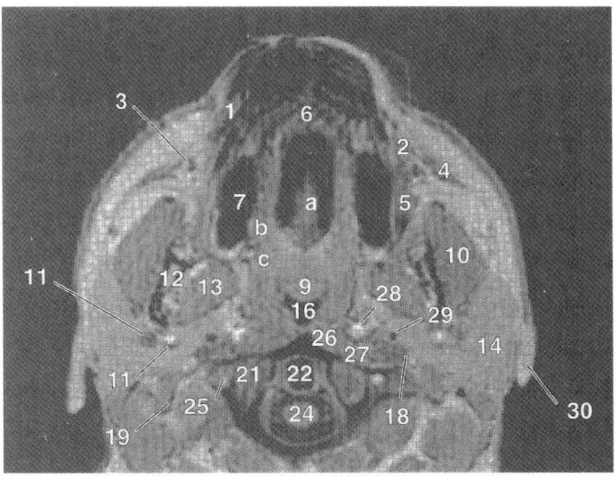
3
1
6
2
4
7
a
5
b
c
10
11
12
13
9
28
16
29
26
14
27
11
21
22
30
25
24
18
19

**D.** **Transverse (axial) MRI Scan**

**Key**

1 Orbicularis oris muscle
2 Levator anguli oris muscle
3 Facial artery and vein
4 Zygomaticus major muscle
5 Buccinator muscle
6 Maxilla
7 Alveolar process of maxilla
8 Dorsum of the tongue
9 Soft palate (uvula apparent in radiographs)
10 Masseter muscle
11 Retromandibular vein
12 Ramus of mandible
13 Lateral pterygoid muscle
14 Parotid gland
15 Superficial temporal vessels
16 Region of pharyngeal tubercle
17 Sphenoid bone
18 Stylohyoid ligament and muscle
19 Posterior belly of digastric muscle
20 Occipital artery
21 First cervical vertebrae (Atlas)
22 Dens (Axis)
23 Transverse ligament of Atlas
24 Spinal cord
25 Vertebral artery in foramina transversaria
26 Longus colli muscle
27 Longus capitis muscle
28 Internal carotid artery
29 Internal jugular vein
30 Interior portion of helix of auricle
a Hard palate
b Palatoglossus muscle
c Palatopharyngeus muscle

**7.83** **MRIs of oropharynx**

**A** and **B.** Transverse (axial) MRIs. **C** and **D.** Coronal MRIs. **E.** Sagittal MRI

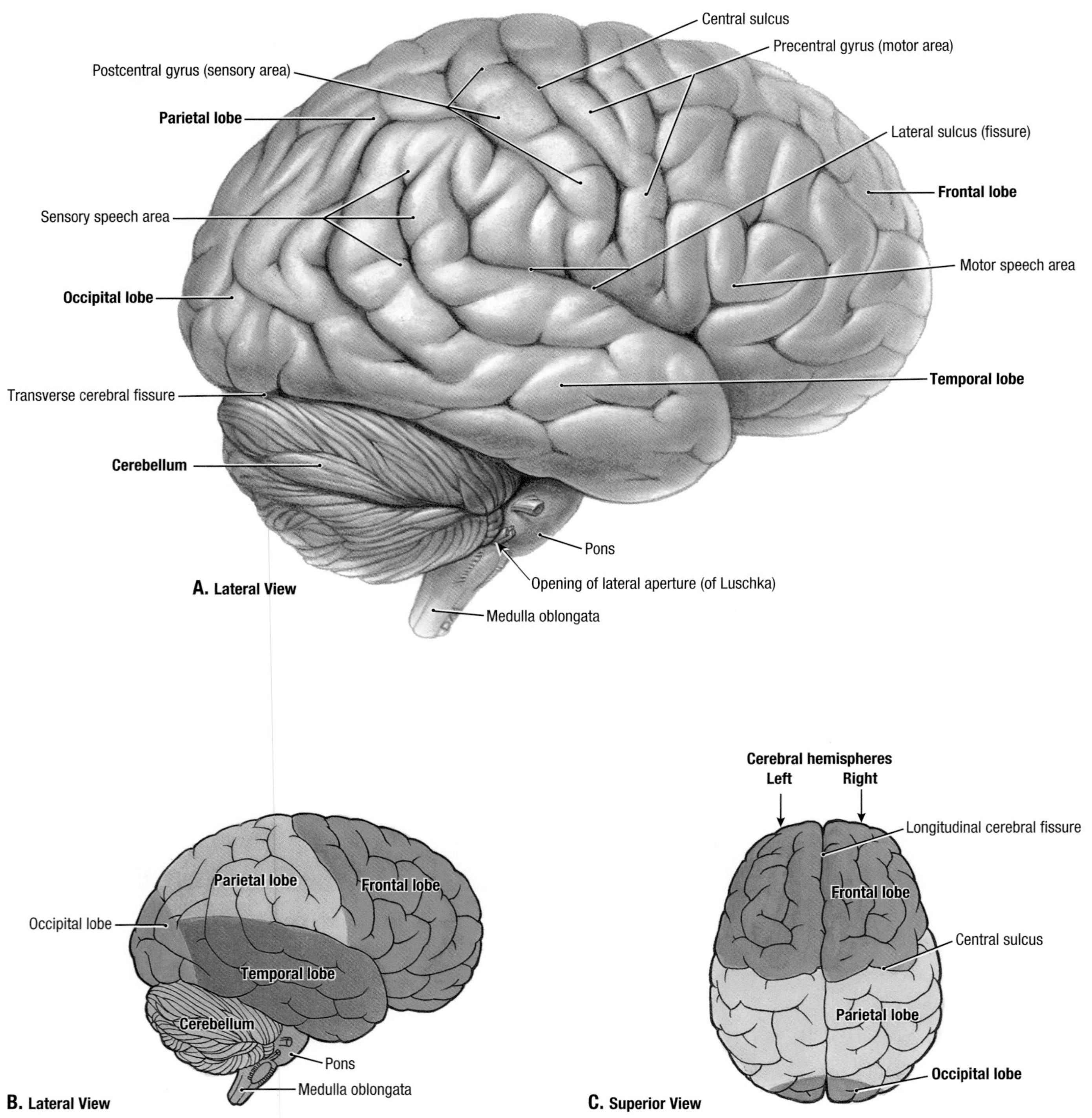
Central sulcus
Precentral gyrus (motor area)
Postcentral gyrus (sensory area)
Parietal lobe
Lateral sulcus (fissure)
Frontal lobe
Sensory speech area
Motor speech area
Occipital lobe
Temporal lobe
Transverse cerebral fissure
Cerebellum
Pons
Opening of lateral aperture (of Luschka)
Medulla oblongata
A. Lateral View
Parietal lobe
Frontal lobe
Occipital lobe
Temporal lobe
Cerebellum
Pons
Medulla oblongata
B. Lateral View
Cerebral hemispheres
Left
Right
Longitudinal cerebral fissure
Frontal lobe
Central sulcus
Parietal lobe
Occipital lobe
C. Superior View

## 7.84 Brain

**A.** Cerebrum, cerebellum, and brainstem, lateral aspect. **B.** Lobes of the cerebral hemispheres, lateral aspect. **C.** Lobes of the cerebral hemispheres, superior aspect.

Cerebral contusion (bruising) results from brain trauma in which the pia is stripped from the injured surface of the brain and may be torn, allowing blood to enter the subarachnoid space. The bruising results from the sudden impact of the moving brain against the stationary cranium or from the suddenly moving cranium against the stationary brain. Cerebral contusion may result in an extended loss of consciousness

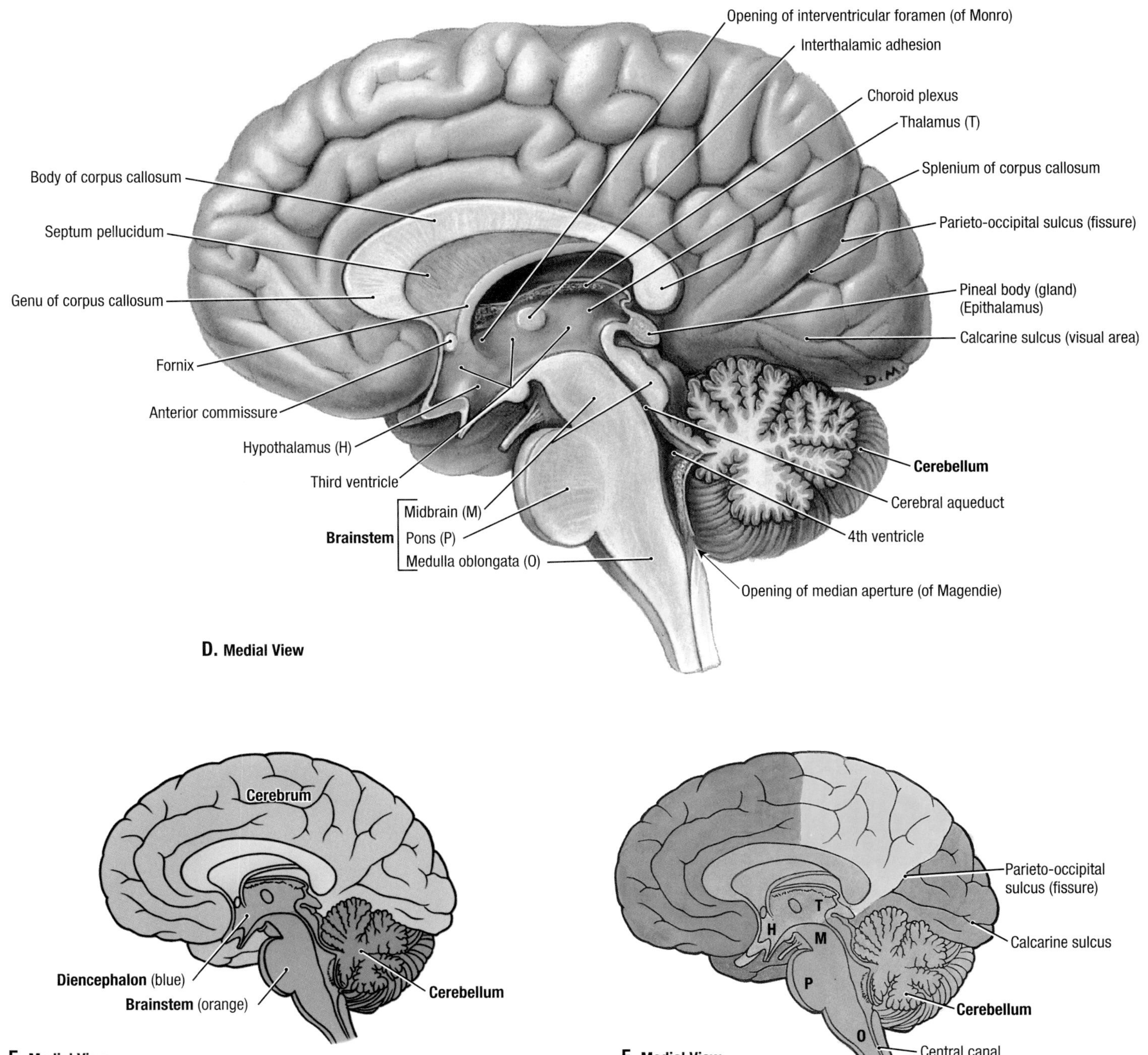
Opening of interventricular foramen (of Monro)
Interthalamic adhesion
Choroid plexus
Thalamus (T)
Splenium of corpus callosum
Parieto-occipital sulcus (fissure)
Pineal body (gland) (Epithalamus)
Calcarine sulcus (visual area)
Body of corpus callosum
Septum pellucidum
Genu of corpus callosum
Fornix
Anterior commissure
Hypothalamus (H)
Third ventricle
Brainstem
Midbrain (M)
Pons (P)
Medulla oblongata (O)
Cerebellum
Cerebral aqueduct
4th ventricle
Opening of median aperture (of Magendie)
D. Medial View
Cerebrum
Diencephalon (blue)
Brainstem (orange)
Cerebellum
E. Medial View
T
H
M
P
O
Parieto-occipital sulcus (fissure)
Calcarine sulcus
Cerebellum
Central canal
F. Medial View

## 7.84 Brain *(continued)*

**D.** Cerebrum, cerebellum, and brainstem, median section. **E.** Parts of the brain, median section. **F.** Lobes of the cerebral hemisphere, median section. See **D** for labeling key.

Cerebral compression may be produced by intracranial collections of blood, obstruction of CSF circulation or absorption, intracranial tumors or abscesses, and brain swelling caused by brain edema, an increase in brain volume resulting from an increase in water and sodium content.

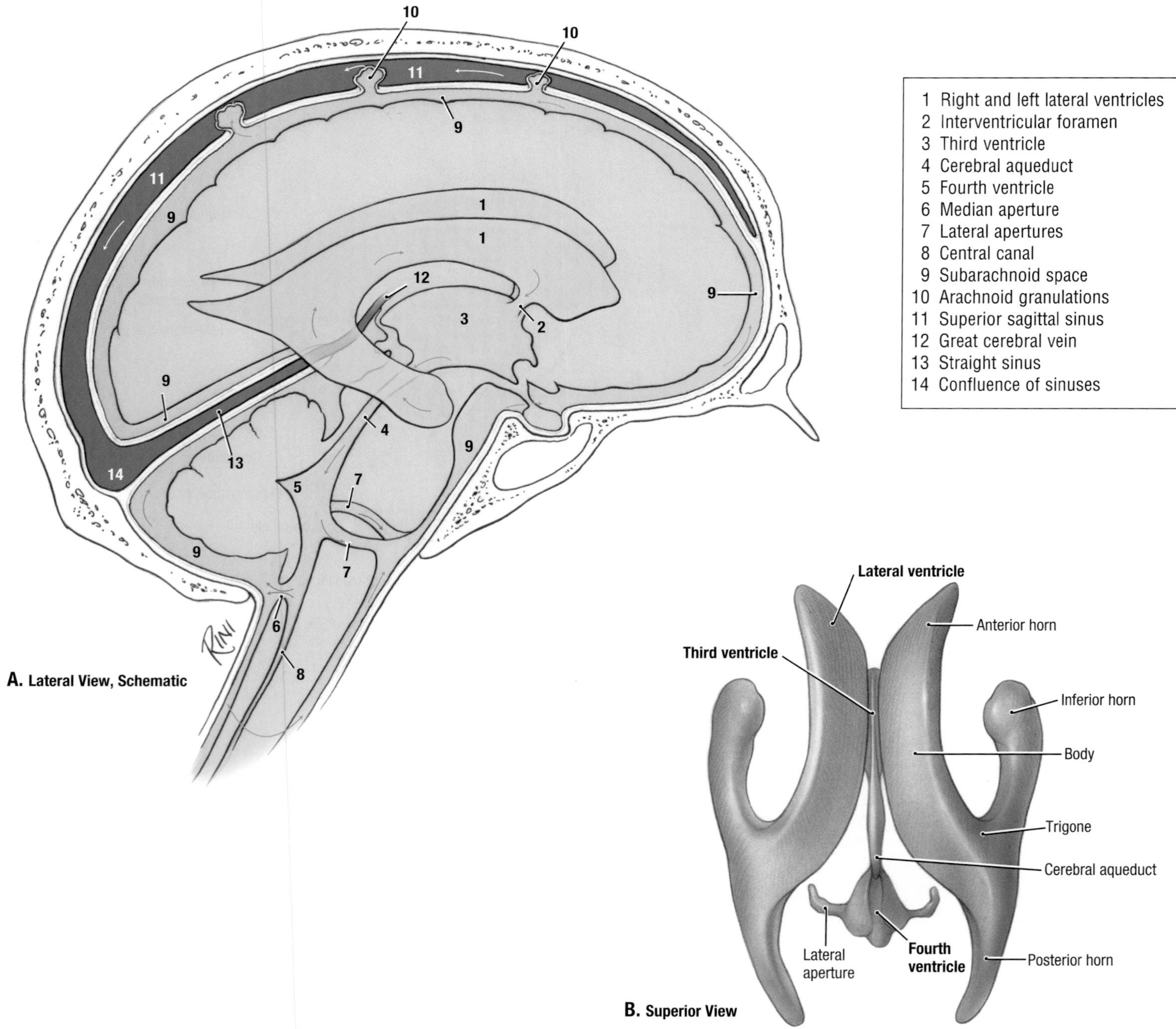
1 Right and left lateral ventricles
2 Interventricular foramen
3 Third ventricle
4 Cerebral aqueduct
5 Fourth ventricle
6 Median aperture
7 Lateral apertures
8 Central canal
9 Subarachnoid space
10 Arachnoid granulations
11 Superior sagittal sinus
12 Great cerebral vein
13 Straight sinus
14 Confluence of sinuses
A. Lateral View, Schematic
Lateral ventricle
Anterior horn
Third ventricle
Inferior horn
Body
Trigone
Cerebral aqueduct
Lateral aperture
Fourth ventricle
Posterior horn
B. Superior View

## 7.85 Ventricular system

**A.** Circulation of cerebrospinal fluid (CSF). **B.** Ventricles: lateral, third, and fourth.

- The ventricular system consists of two lateral ventricles located in the cerebral hemispheres, a third ventricle located between the right and left halves of the diencephalon, and a fourth ventricle located in the posterior parts of the pons and medulla.
- CSF secreted by choroid plexus in the ventricles drains via the interventricular foramen from the lateral to the third ventricle, via the cerebral aqueduct from the third to the fourth ventricle, and via median and lateral apertures into the subarachnoid space. CSF is absorbed by arachnoid granulations into the venous sinuses (especially the superior sagittal sinus).
- Overproduction of CSF, obstruction of its flow, or interference with its absorption results in an excess of CSF in the ventricles and enlargement of the head, a condition known as hydrocephalus. Excess CSF dilates the ventricles; thins the brain; and, in infants, separates the bones of the calvaria because the sutures and fontanelles are still open.

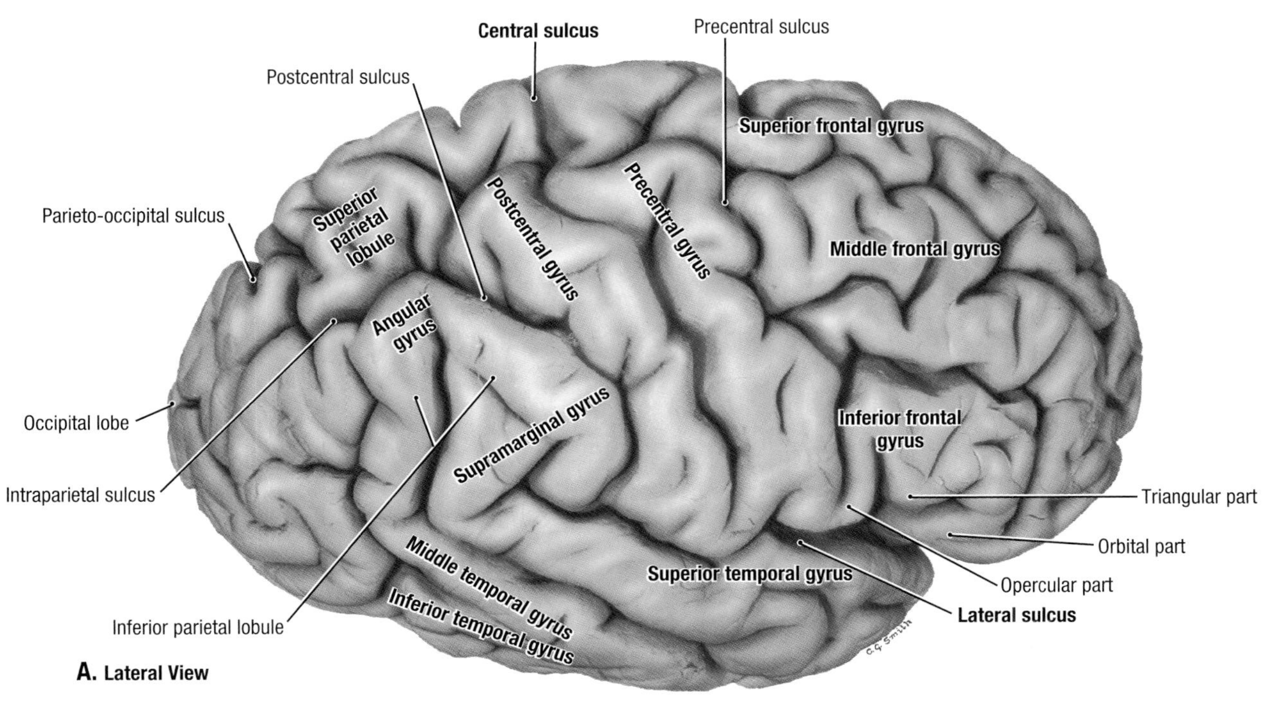
Central sulcus
Precentral sulcus
Postcentral sulcus
Superior frontal gyrus
Parieto-occipital sulcus
Superior parietal lobule
Postcentral gyrus
Precentral gyrus
Middle frontal gyrus
Angular gyrus
Occipital lobe
Supramarginal gyrus
Inferior frontal gyrus
Intraparietal sulcus
Triangular part
Orbital part
Middle temporal gyrus
Superior temporal gyrus
Opercular part
Inferior temporal gyrus
Lateral sulcus
Inferior parietal lobule
A. Lateral View

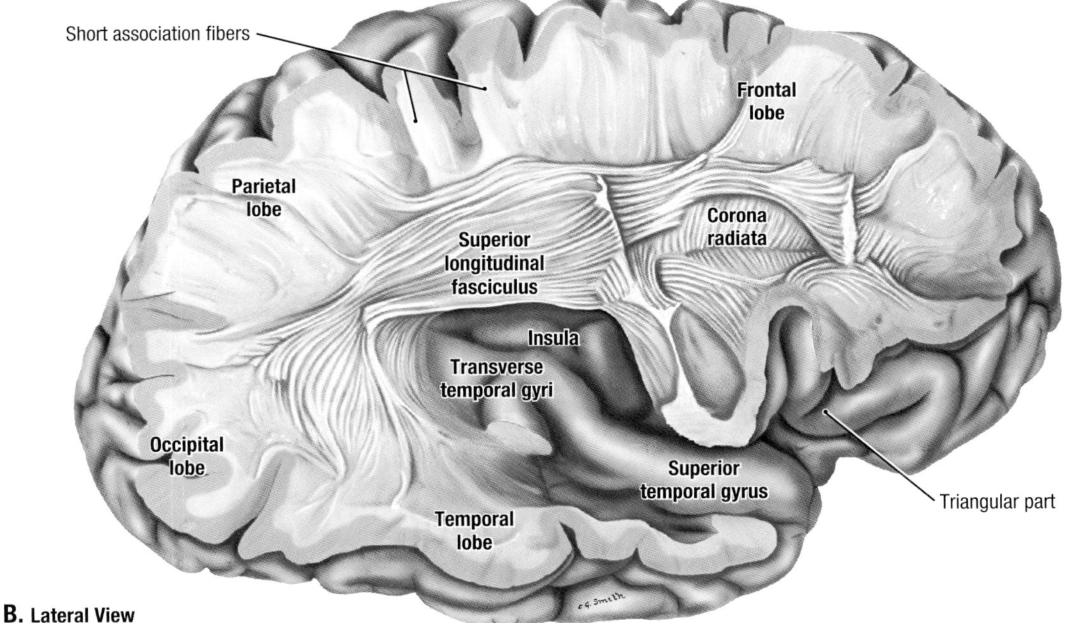
Short association fibers
Frontal lobe
Parietal lobe
Corona radiata
Superior longitudinal fasciculus
Insula
Transverse temporal gyri
Occipital lobe
Superior temporal gyrus
Triangular part
Temporal lobe
B. Lateral View

## 7.86 Serial dissections of the lateral aspect of the cerebral hemisphere

The dissections begin from the lateral surface of the cerebral hemisphere **(A)** and proceed sequentially medially **(B–F)**.

**A.** Sulci and gyri of the lateral surface of one cerebral hemisphere. Each gyrus is a fold of cerebral cortex with a core of white matter. The furrows are called *sulci*. The pattern of sulci and gyri formed shortly before birth is recognizable in some adult brains, as shown in this specimen. Usually the expanding cortex acquires secondary foldings, which make identification of this basic pattern more difficult. **B.** Superior longitudinal fasciculus, transverse temporal gyri, and insula. The cortex and short association fiber bundles around the lateral fissure have been removed.

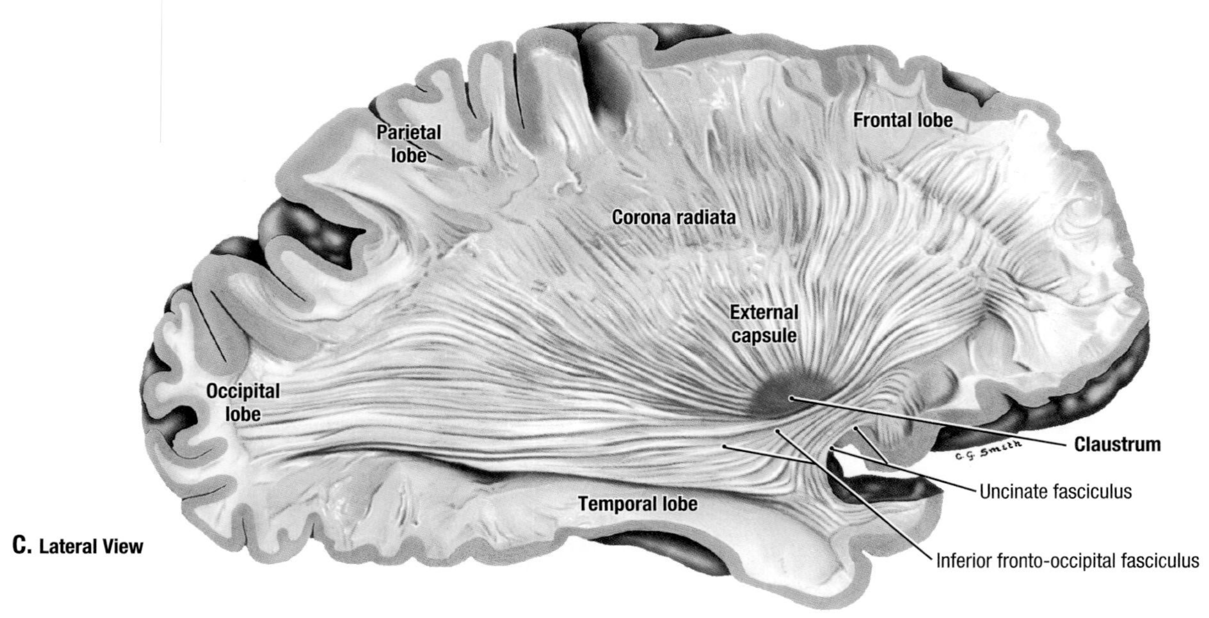
Parietal lobe
Frontal lobe
Corona radiata
External capsule
Occipital lobe
Claustrum
Uncinate fasciculus
Temporal lobe
Inferior fronto-occipital fasciculus
C. Lateral View

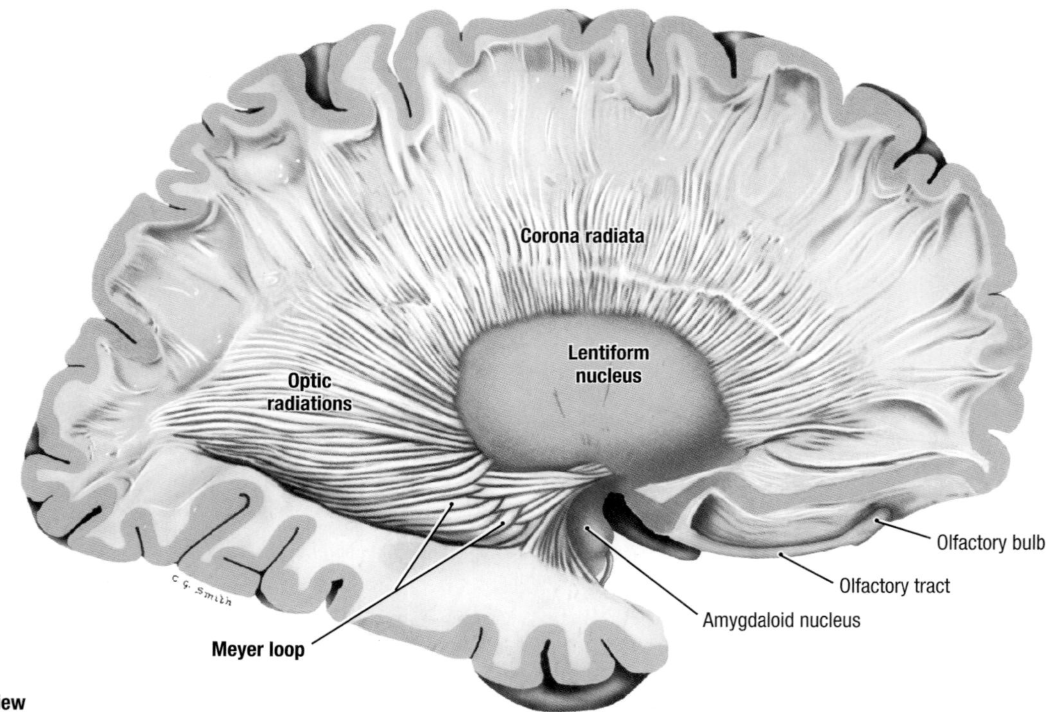
Corona radiata
Lentiform nucleus
Optic radiations
Olfactory bulb
Olfactory tract
Amygdaloid nucleus
Meyer loop
D. Lateral View

**7.86 Serial dissections of the lateral aspect of the cerebral hemisphere *(continued)***

**C.** Uncinate and inferior fronto-occipital fasciculi and external capsule. The external capsule consists of projection fibers that pass between the claustrum laterally and the lentiform nucleus medially. **D.** Lentiform nucleus and corona radiata. The inferior longitudinal and uncinate fasciculi, claustrum, and external capsule have been removed. The fibers of the optic radiations convey impulses from the right half of the retina of each eye; the fibers extending closest to the temporal pole (Meyer's loop) carry impulses from the lower portion of each retina.

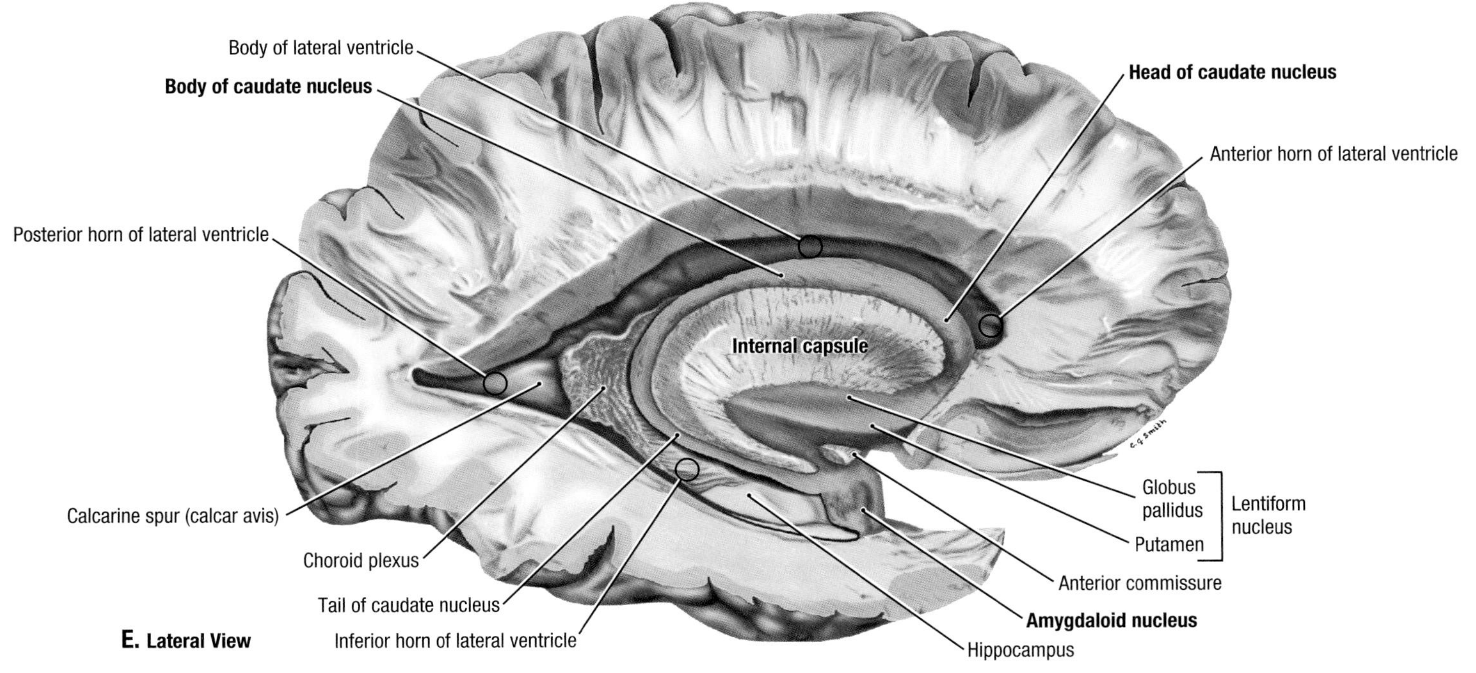
Body of lateral ventricle
Body of caudate nucleus
Head of caudate nucleus
Anterior horn of lateral ventricle
Posterior horn of lateral ventricle
Internal capsule
Calcarine spur (calcar avis)
Choroid plexus
Tail of caudate nucleus
Inferior horn of lateral ventricle
Globus pallidus
Putamen
Lentiform nucleus
Anterior commissure
Amygdaloid nucleus
Hippocampus
E. Lateral View

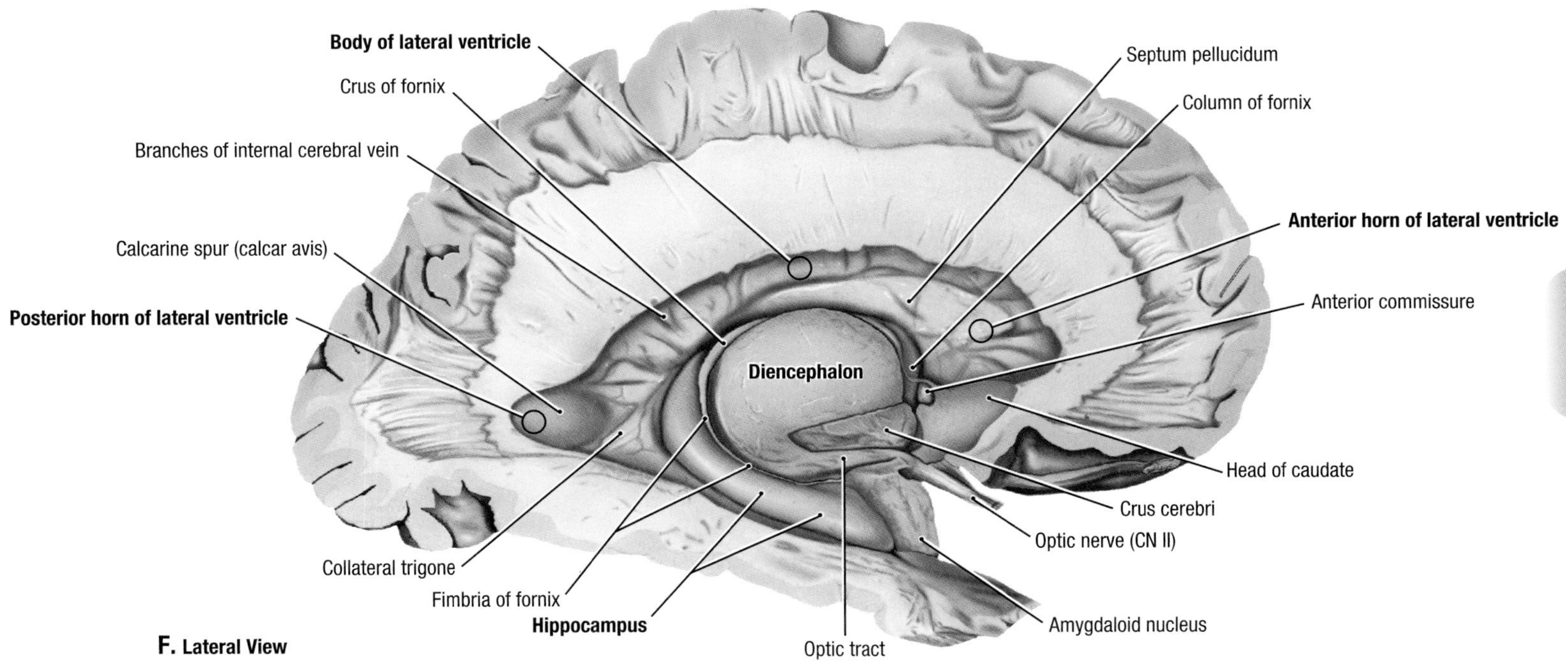
Body of lateral ventricle
Crus of fornix
Branches of internal cerebral vein
Calcarine spur (calcar avis)
Posterior horn of lateral ventricle
Septum pellucidum
Column of fornix
Anterior horn of lateral ventricle
Anterior commissure
Diencephalon
Head of caudate
Crus cerebri
Optic nerve (CN II)
Collateral trigone
Fimbria of fornix
Hippocampus
Optic tract
Amygdaloid nucleus
F. Lateral View

## 7.86 Serial dissections of the lateral aspect of the cerebral hemisphere *(continued)*

**E.** Caudate and amygdaloid nuclei and internal capsule. The lateral wall of the lateral ventricle, the marginal part of the internal capsule, the anterior commissure, and the superior part of the lentiform nucleus have been removed. **F.** Lateral ventricle, hippocampus, and diencephalon. The inferior parts of the lentiform nucleus, internal capsule, and caudate nucleus have been removed.

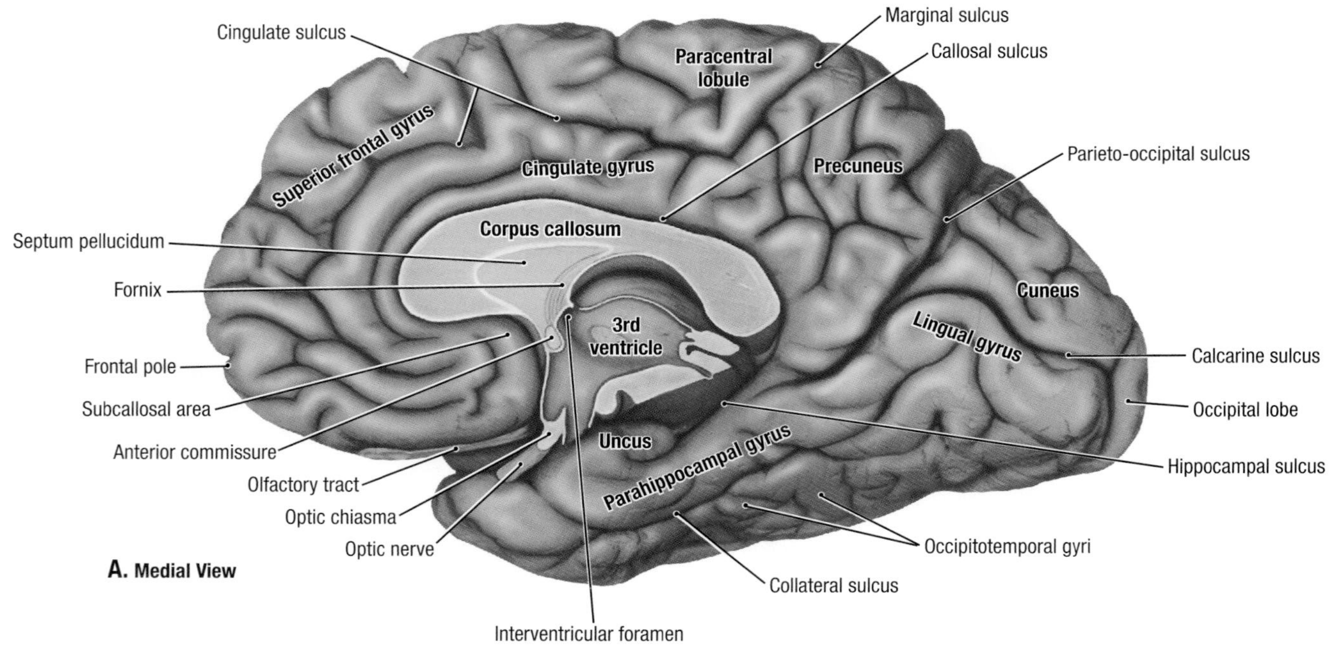
Cingulate sulcus
Marginal sulcus
Callosal sulcus
Paracentral lobule
Superior frontal gyrus
Cingulate gyrus
Precuneus
Parieto-occipital sulcus
Corpus callosum
Septum pellucidum
Fornix
Cuneus
3rd ventricle
Lingual gyrus
Calcarine sulcus
Frontal pole
Occipital lobe
Subcallosal area
Anterior commissure
Uncus
Hippocampal sulcus
Olfactory tract
Parahippocampal gyrus
Optic chiasma
Optic nerve
Occipitotemporal gyri
A. Medial View
Collateral sulcus
Interventricular foramen

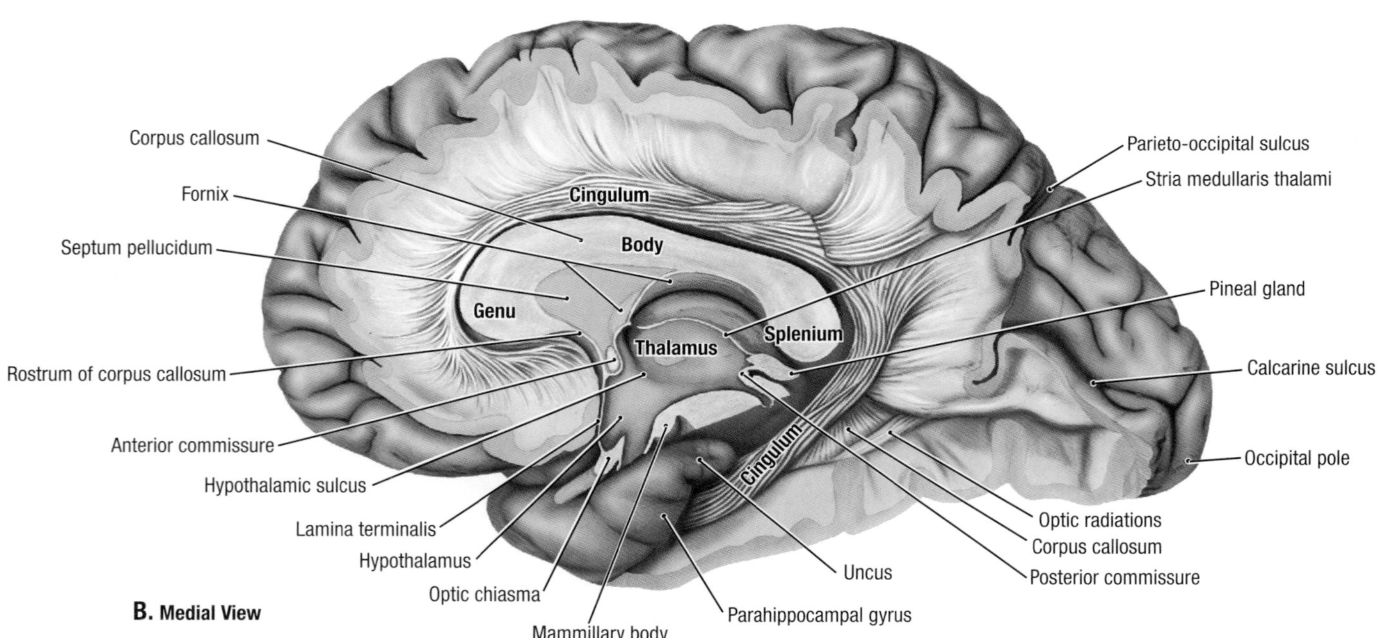
Corpus callosum
Parieto-occipital sulcus
Stria medullaris thalami
Fornix
Cingulum
Body
Septum pellucidum
Pineal gland
Genu
Thalamus
Splenium
Rostrum of corpus callosum
Calcarine sulcus
Anterior commissure
Occipital pole
Hypothalamic sulcus
Cingulum
Lamina terminalis
Optic radiations
Corpus callosum
Hypothalamus
Uncus
Posterior commissure
Optic chiasma
B. Medial View
Parahippocampal gyrus
Mammillary body

## 7.87 Serial dissections of the medial aspect of cerebral hemisphere

The dissections begin from the medial surface of the cerebral hemisphere **(A)** and proceed sequentially laterally **(B–D)**.

**A.** Sulci and gyri of medial surface of cerebral hemisphere. The corpus callosum consists of the rostrum, genu, body, and splenium; the cingulate and parahippocampal gyri from the limbic lobe. **B.** Cingulum. The cortex and short association fibers were removed from the medial aspect of the hemisphere. The cingulum is a long association fiber bundle that lies in the core of the cingulate and parahippocampal gyri.

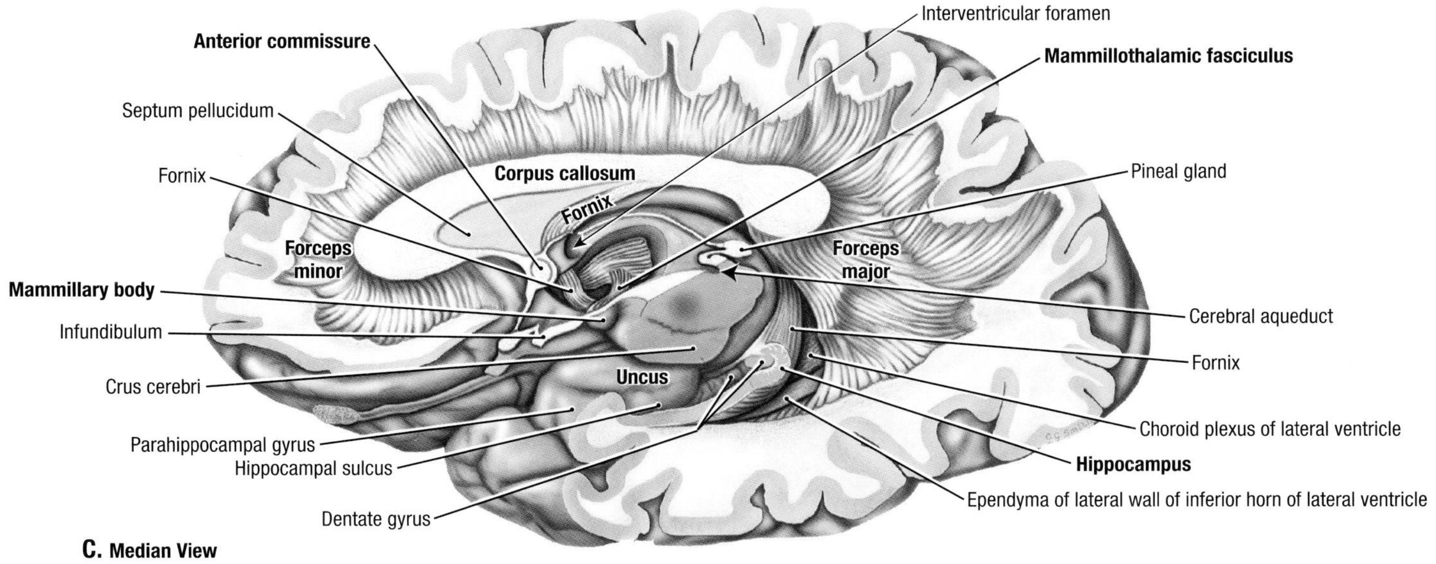

Interventricular foramen
Anterior commissure
Mammillothalamic fasciculus
Septum pellucidum
Fornix
Corpus callosum
Fornix
Pineal gland
Forceps minor
Forceps major
Mammillary body
Cerebral aqueduct
Infundibulum
Fornix
Crus cerebri
Uncus
Choroid plexus of lateral ventricle
Parahippocampal gyrus
Hippocampal sulcus
Hippocampus
Ependyma of lateral wall of inferior horn of lateral ventricle
Dentate gyrus


C. Median View

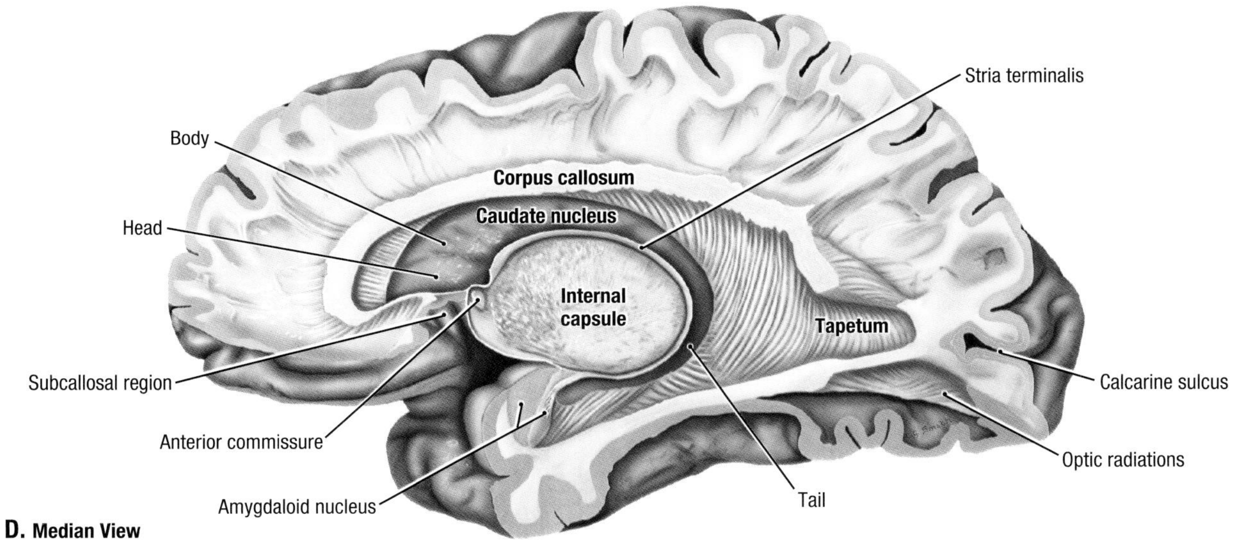

Stria terminalis
Body
Corpus callosum
Caudate nucleus
Head
Internal capsule
Tapetum
Subcallosal region
Calcarine sulcus
Anterior commissure
Optic radiations
Amygdaloid nucleus
Tail


D. Median View

## 7.87 Serial dissections of the medial aspect of cerebral hemisphere *(continued)*

**C.** Fornix, mamillothalamic fasciculus, and forceps major and minor. The cingulum and a portion of the wall of the third ventricle have been removed. The fornix begins at the hippocampus and terminates in the mammillary body by passing anterior to the interventricular foramen and posterior to the anterior commissure. The mamillothalamic fasciculus emerges from the mammillary body and terminates in the anterior nucleus of the thalamus. **D.** Caudate nucleus and internal capsule. The diencephalon was removed, along with the ependyma of the lateral ventricle, except where it covers the caudate and amygdaloid nuclei. **E.** Corpus callosum. The body of the corpus callosum connects the two cerebral hemispheres; the minor (frontal) forceps (at the genu of corpus callosum) connects the frontal lobes, and the major (occipital) forceps (at splenium) connects the occipital lobes.

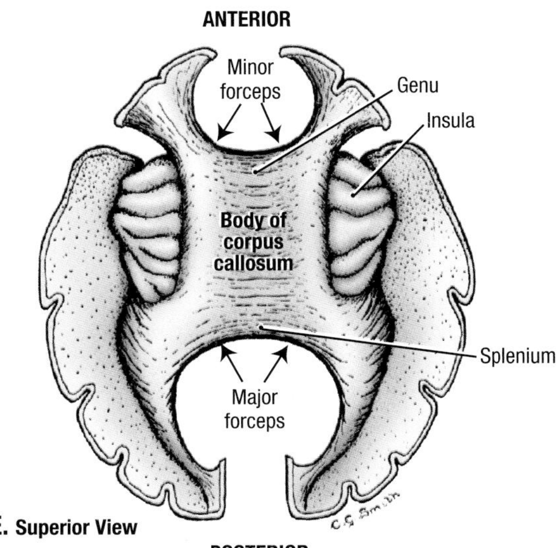

ANTERIOR
Minor forceps
Genu
Insula
Body of corpus callosum
Splenium
Major forceps
POSTERIOR


E. Superior View

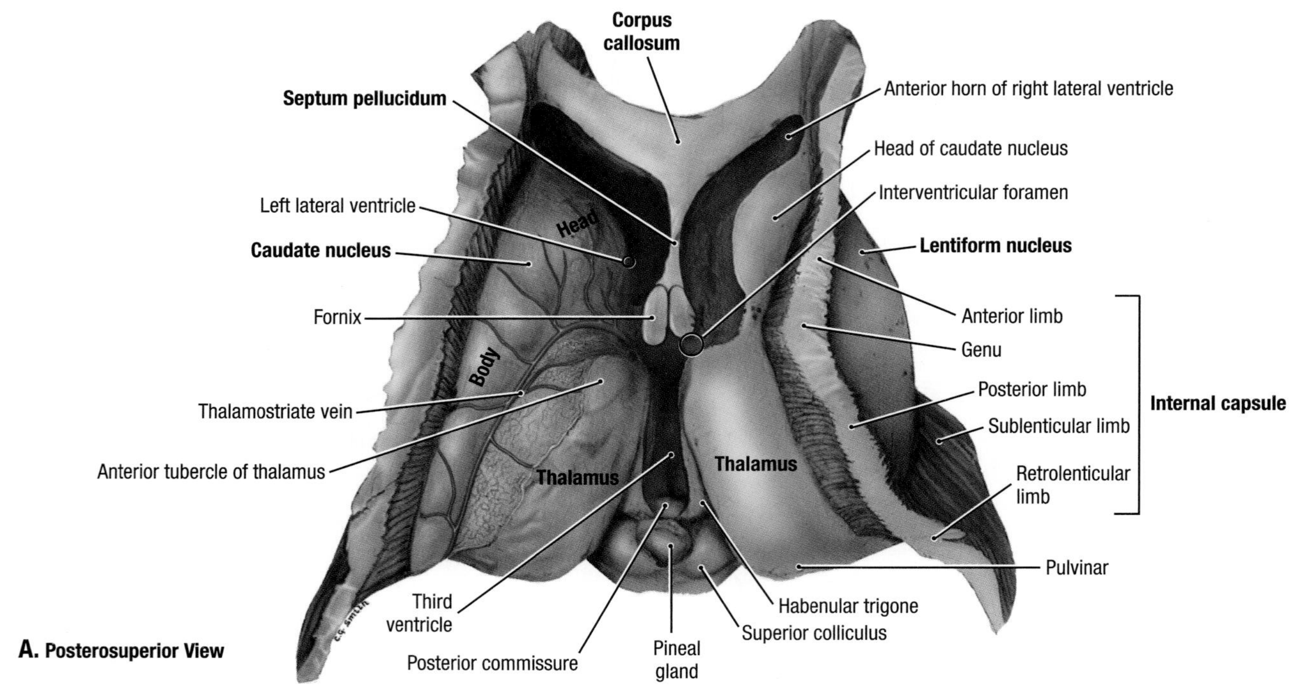
Corpus callosum
Septum pellucidum
Anterior horn of right lateral ventricle
Head of caudate nucleus
Interventricular foramen
Left lateral ventricle
Caudate nucleus
Head
Lentiform nucleus
Fornix
Anterior limb
Genu
Body
Posterior limb
Thalamostriate vein
Sublenticular limb
Internal capsule
Anterior tubercle of thalamus
Thalamus
Thalamus
Retrolenticular limb
Pulvinar
Third ventricle
Habenular trigone
Superior colliculus
A. Posterosuperior View
Posterior commissure
Pineal gland

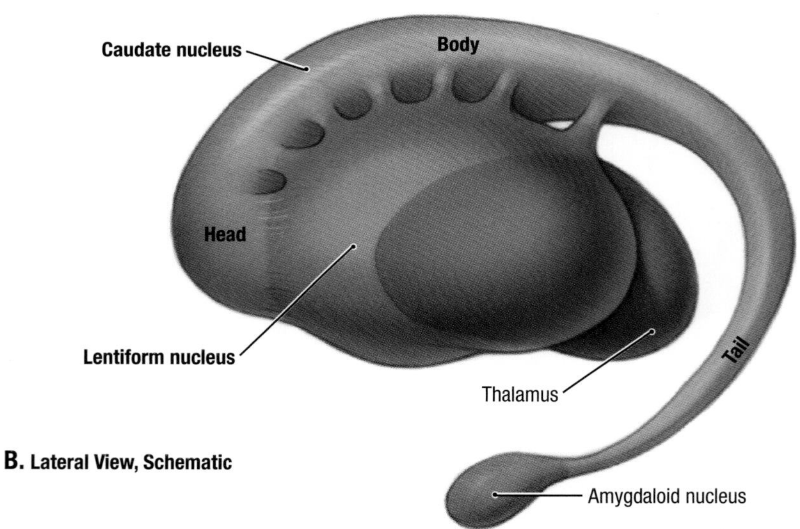
Caudate nucleus
Body
Head
Lentiform nucleus
Tail
Thalamus
B. Lateral View, Schematic
Amygdaloid nucleus

## 7.88 Caudate and lentiform nuclei

**A.** Relationship to the lateral ventricles and internal capsule. The dorsal surface of the diencephalon has been exposed by dissecting away the two cerebral hemispheres, except the anterior part of the corpus callosum, the inferior part of the septum pellucidum, the internal capsule, and the caudate and lentiform nuclei. On the right side of the specimen, the thalamus, caudate, and lentiform nuclei have been cut horizontally at the level of the interventricular foramen. The parts of the internal capsule include the anterior, posterior, retrolenticular sublenticular limbs, and genu. **B.** Schematic illustration of nuclei.

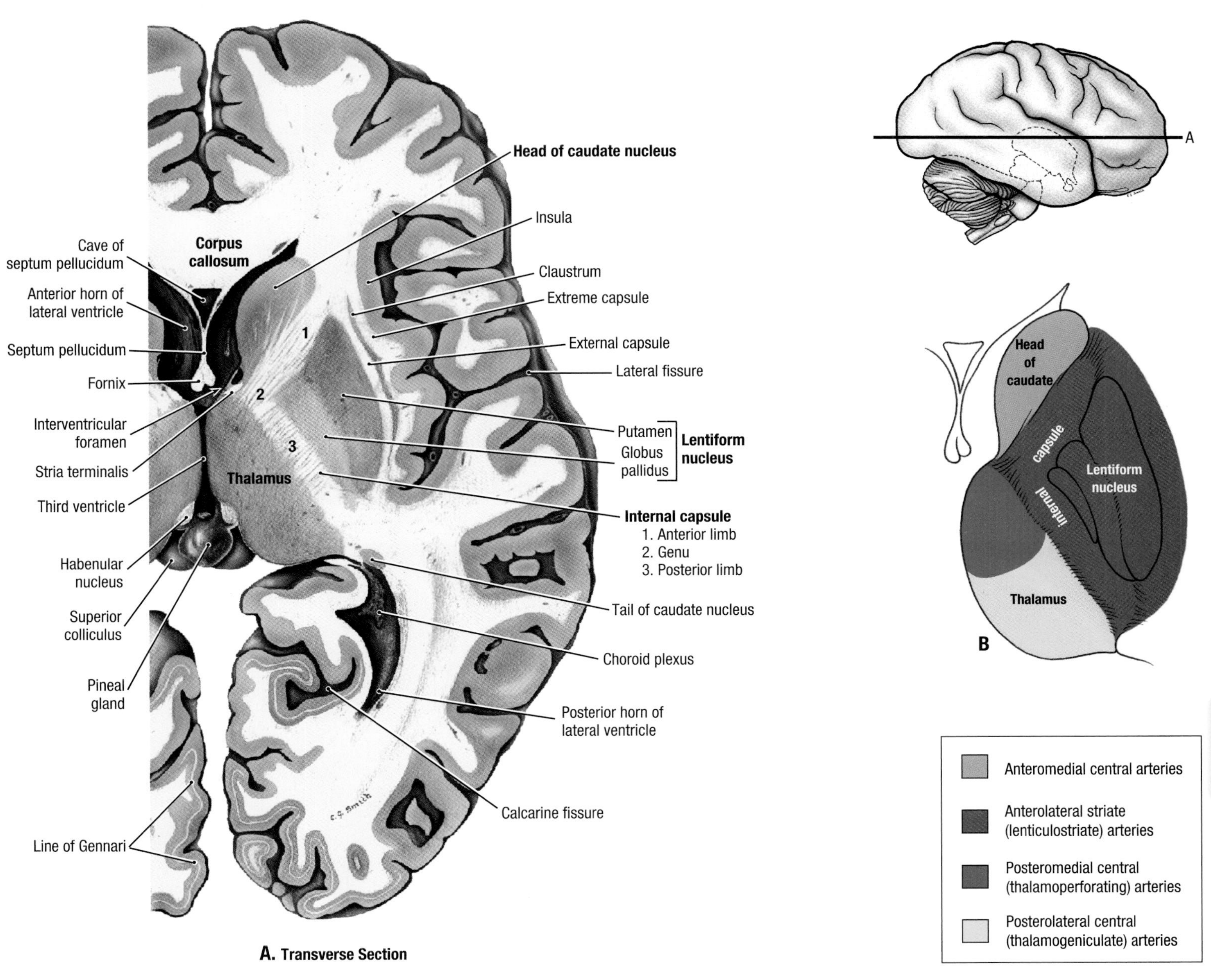
Head of caudate nucleus
Insula
Claustrum
Extreme capsule
External capsule
Lateral fissure
Putamen
Globus pallidus
Lentiform nucleus
Internal capsule
1. Anterior limb
2. Genu
3. Posterior limb
Tail of caudate nucleus
Choroid plexus
Posterior horn of lateral ventricle
Calcarine fissure
Cave of septum pellucidum
Corpus callosum
Anterior horn of lateral ventricle
Septum pellucidum
Fornix
Interventricular foramen
Stria terminalis
Third ventricle
Thalamus
Habenular nucleus
Superior colliculus
Pineal gland
Line of Gennari
1
2
3
A. Transverse Section
A
Head of caudate
Internal capsule
Lentiform nucleus
Thalamus
B
Anteromedial central arteries
Anterolateral striate (lenticulostriate) arteries
Posteromedial central (thalamoperforating) arteries
Posterolateral central (thalamogeniculate) arteries

## 7.89 Axial sections through the thalamus, caudate nucleus, and lentiform nucleus

**A.** Relationships of the internal capsule. **B.** Blood supply of region.

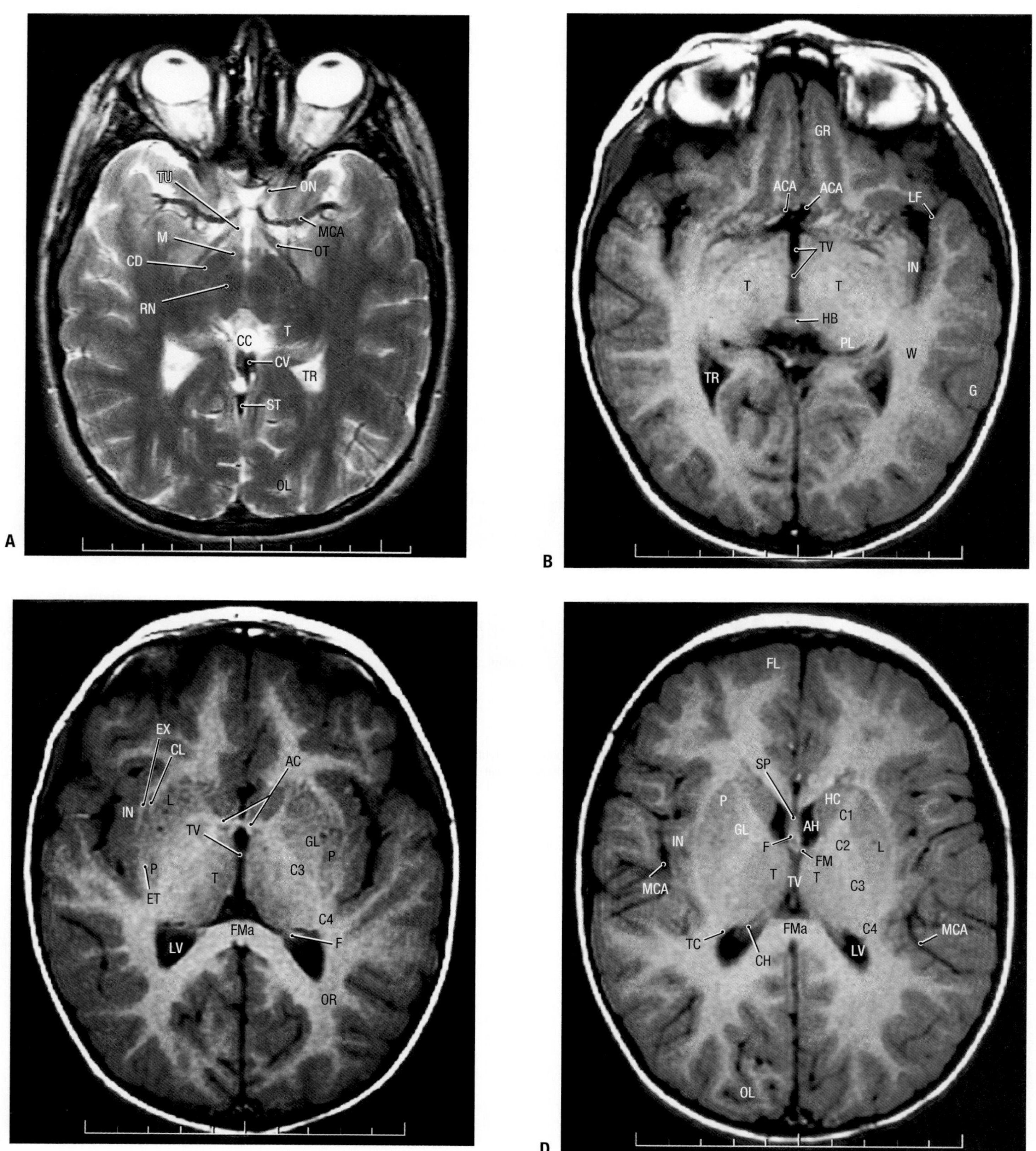
A
TU
ON
MCA
M
OT
CD
RN
T
CC
CV
TR
ST
OL
B
GR
ACA
ACA
LF
TV
IN
T
T
HB
PL
W
TR
G
C
EX
CL
AC
IN
L
TV
GL
P
P
T
C3
ET
C4
FMa
F
LV
OR
D
FL
SP
HC
P
C1
AH
GL
IN
F
C2
L
FM
MCA
T
TV
T
C3
FMa
C4
MCA
TC
LV
CH
OL

**7.90 Axial (transverse) MRIs through the cerebral hemispheres**

See orientation drawing for sites of scans **A–F. A** is T2 weighted, and **B–F** are T1 weighted.

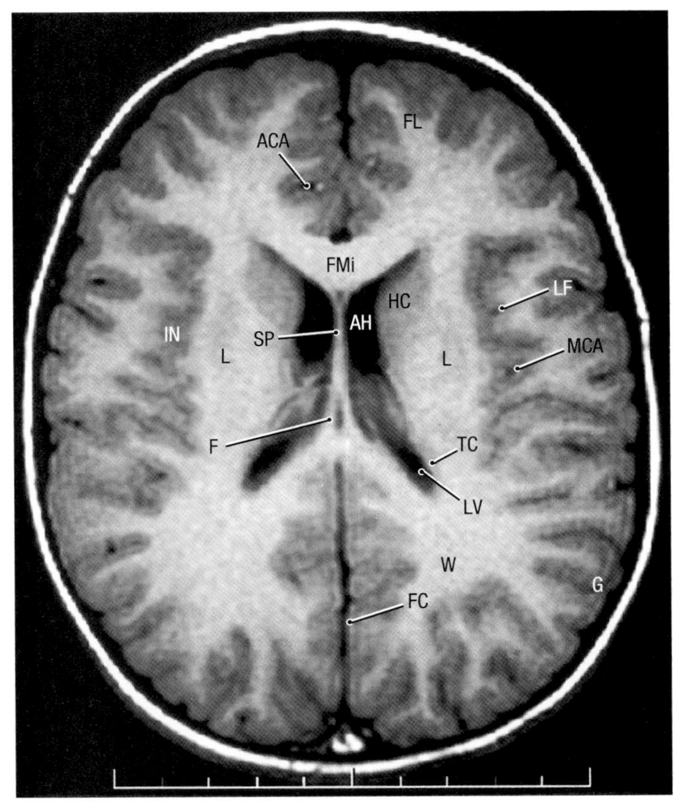
ACA
FL
FMi
HC
LF
IN
SP
AH
L
L
MCA
F
TC
LV
W
G
FC

E

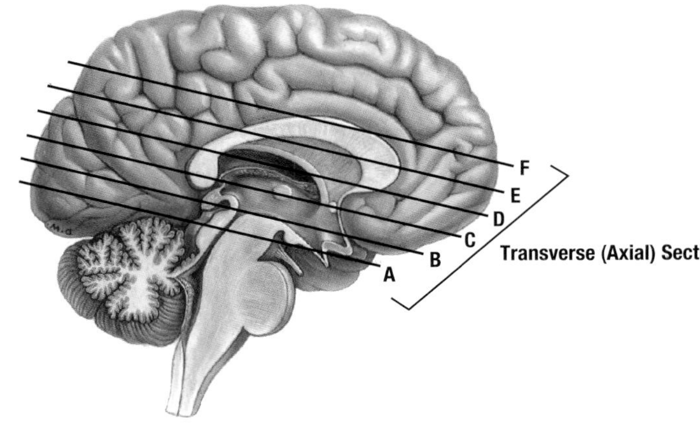
F
E
D
C
B
A
Transverse (Axial) Secti

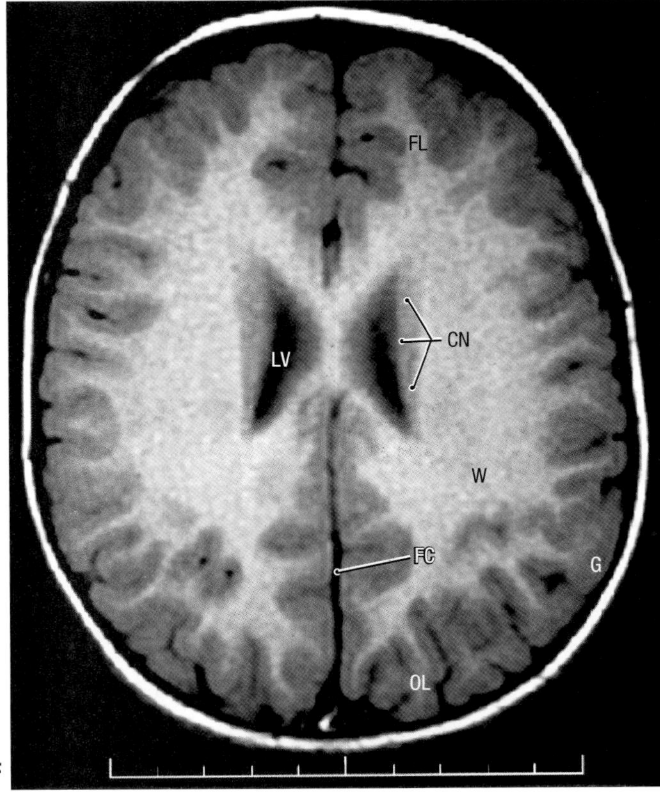
FL
CN
LV
W
FC
G
OL

F

| | | | |
|---|---|---|---|
| AC | Anterior commissure | GL | Globus pallidus |
| ACA | Anterior cerebral artery | GR | Gyrus rectus |
| AH | Anterior horn of lateral ventricle | HB | Habenular commissure |
| C1 | Anterior limb of internal capsule | HC | Head of caudate nucleus |
| | | IN | Insular cortex |
| C2 | Genu of internal capsule | L | Lentiform nucleus |
| C3 | Posterior limb of internal capsule | LF | Lateral fissure |
| | | LV | Lateral ventricle |
| C4 | Retrolenticular limb of internal capsule | M | Mammillary body |
| | | MCA | Middle cerebral artery |
| CC | Collicular cistern | OL | Occipital lobe |
| CD | Cerebral peduncle | ON | Optic nerve |
| CH | Choroid plexus | OR | Optic radiations |
| CL | Claustrum | OT | Optic tract |
| CN | Caudate nucleus | P | Putamen |
| CV | Great cerebral vein | PL | Pulvinar |
| ET | External capsule | RN | Red nucleus |
| EX | Extreme capsule | SP | Septum pellucidum |
| F | Fornix | ST | Straight sinus |
| FC | Falx cerebri | T | Thalamus |
| FL | Frontal lobe | TC | Tail of caudate nucleus |
| FM | Interventricular foramen | TR | Trigone of lateral ventricle |
| FMa | Forceps major | TU | Tuber cinereum |
| FMi | Forceps minor | TV | Third ventricle |
| G | Gray matter | W | White matter |

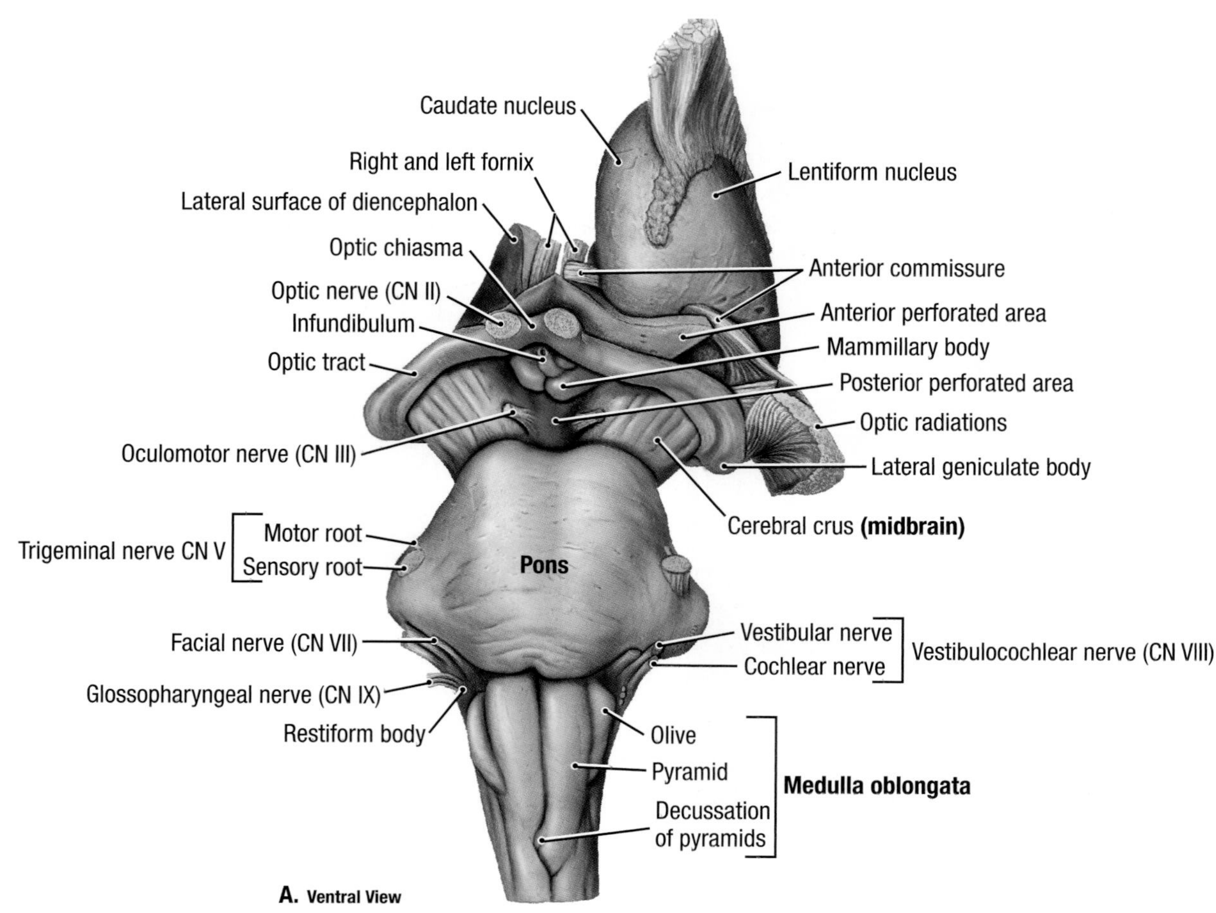
Caudate nucleus
Right and left fornix
Lateral surface of diencephalon
Optic chiasma
Optic nerve (CN II)
Infundibulum
Optic tract
Oculomotor nerve (CN III)
Lentiform nucleus
Anterior commissure
Anterior perforated area
Mammillary body
Posterior perforated area
Optic radiations
Lateral geniculate body
Cerebral crus (midbrain)
Trigeminal nerve CN V
Motor root
Sensory root
Pons
Facial nerve (CN VII)
Glossopharyngeal nerve (CN IX)
Restiform body
Vestibular nerve
Cochlear nerve
Vestibulocochlear nerve (CN VIII)
Olive
Pyramid
Decussation of pyramids
Medulla oblongata

**A.** Ventral View

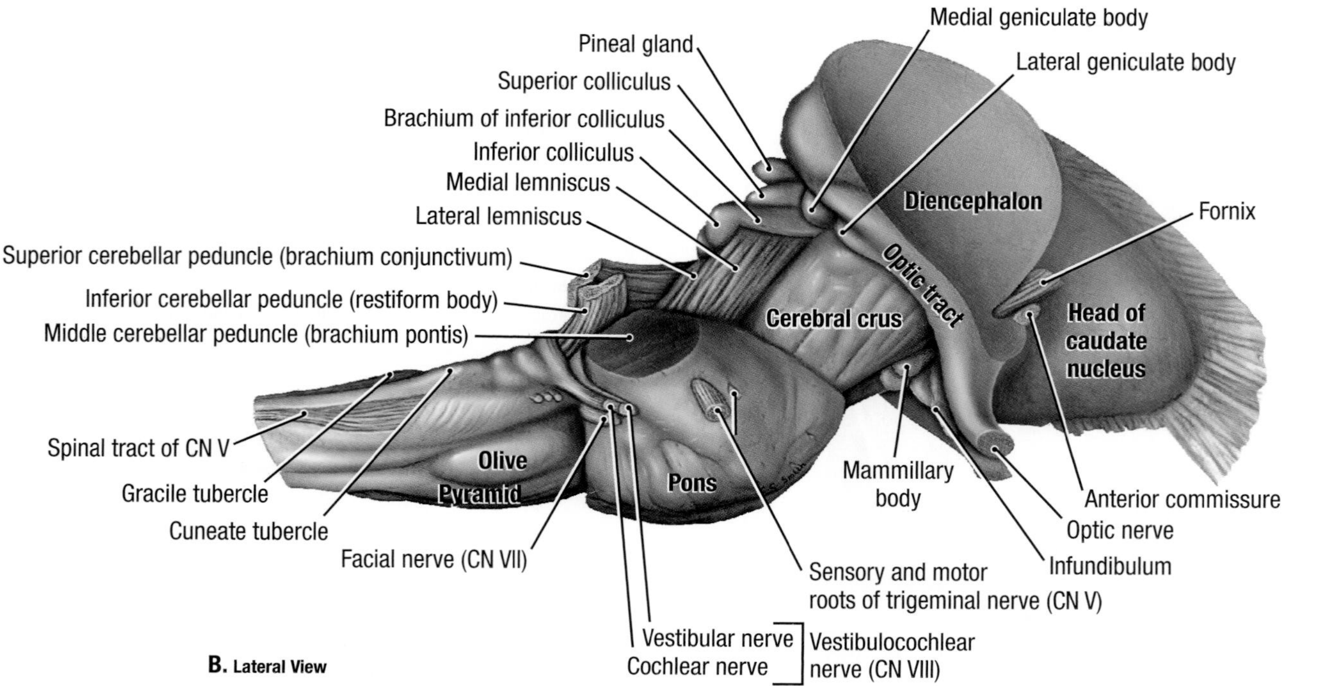
Pineal gland
Superior colliculus
Brachium of inferior colliculus
Inferior colliculus
Medial lemniscus
Lateral lemniscus
Superior cerebellar peduncle (brachium conjunctivum)
Inferior cerebellar peduncle (restiform body)
Middle cerebellar peduncle (brachium pontis)
Spinal tract of CN V
Gracile tubercle
Cuneate tubercle
Facial nerve (CN VII)
Medial geniculate body
Lateral geniculate body
Diencephalon
Optic tract
Cerebral crus
Fornix
Head of caudate nucleus
Olive
Pyramid
Pons
Mammillary body
Anterior commissure
Optic nerve
Infundibulum
Sensory and motor roots of trigeminal nerve (CN V)
Vestibular nerve
Cochlear nerve
Vestibulocochlear nerve (CN VIII)

**B.** Lateral View

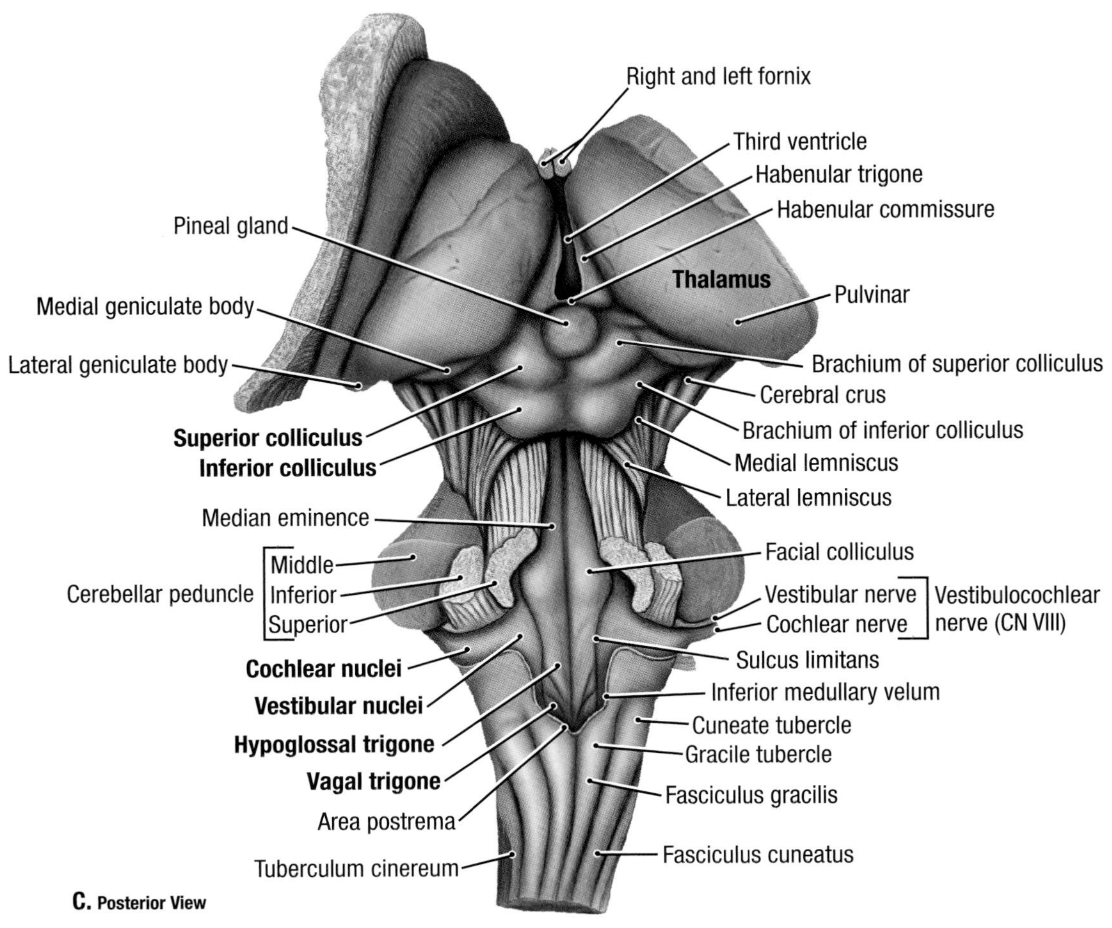
Right and left fornix
Third ventricle
Habenular trigone
Habenular commissure
Pineal gland
Thalamus
Pulvinar
Medial geniculate body
Lateral geniculate body
Brachium of superior colliculus
Cerebral crus
Superior colliculus
Inferior colliculus
Brachium of inferior colliculus
Medial lemniscus
Lateral lemniscus
Median eminence
Facial colliculus
Cerebellar peduncle
Middle
Inferior
Superior
Vestibular nerve
Cochlear nerve
Vestibulocochlear nerve (CN VIII)
Sulcus limitans
Cochlear nuclei
Vestibular nuclei
Inferior medullary velum
Hypoglossal trigone
Cuneate tubercle
Gracile tubercle
Vagal trigone
Fasciculus gracilis
Area postrema
Tuberculum cinereum
Fasciculus cuneatus

**C.** Posterior View

## 7.91 Brainstem

The brainstem has been exposed by removing the cerebellum, all of the right cerebral hemisphere, and the major portion of the left hemisphere. **A.** Ventral aspect.

- The brainstem consists of the medulla oblongata, pons, and midbrain.
- The pyramid is on the ventral surface of the medulla; the decussation of the pyramids is formed by the decussating (crossing) lateral corticospinal tract.
- The trigeminal nerve (CN V) emerges as sensory and motor roots.
- The crus cerebri are part of the midbrain;
- The oculomotor nerve emerges from the interpeduncular fossa.

**B.** Lateral aspect.

- The vestibulocochlear nerve (CN VIII) consists of two nerves, the vestibular and cochlear nerves.
- The spinal tract of the trigeminal nerve is exposed where it comes to the surface of the medulla to form the tuber cinereum.
- The three are cerebellar peduncles: superior, middle, and inferior.
- The medial and lateral lemnisci on the lateral aspect of the midbrain

**C.** Dorsal aspect.

- Ridges are formed by the fasciculus gracilis and cuneatus.
- The gracile and cuneate tubercles are the site of the nucleus cuneatus and nucleus gracilis.
- The diamond-shaped floor of the fourth ventricle; lateral to the sulcus limitans are the vestibular and cochlear nuclei and medially are the hypoglossal and vagal trigones and the facial colliculus.
- The superior and inferior colliculi form the dorsal surface of the midbrain.

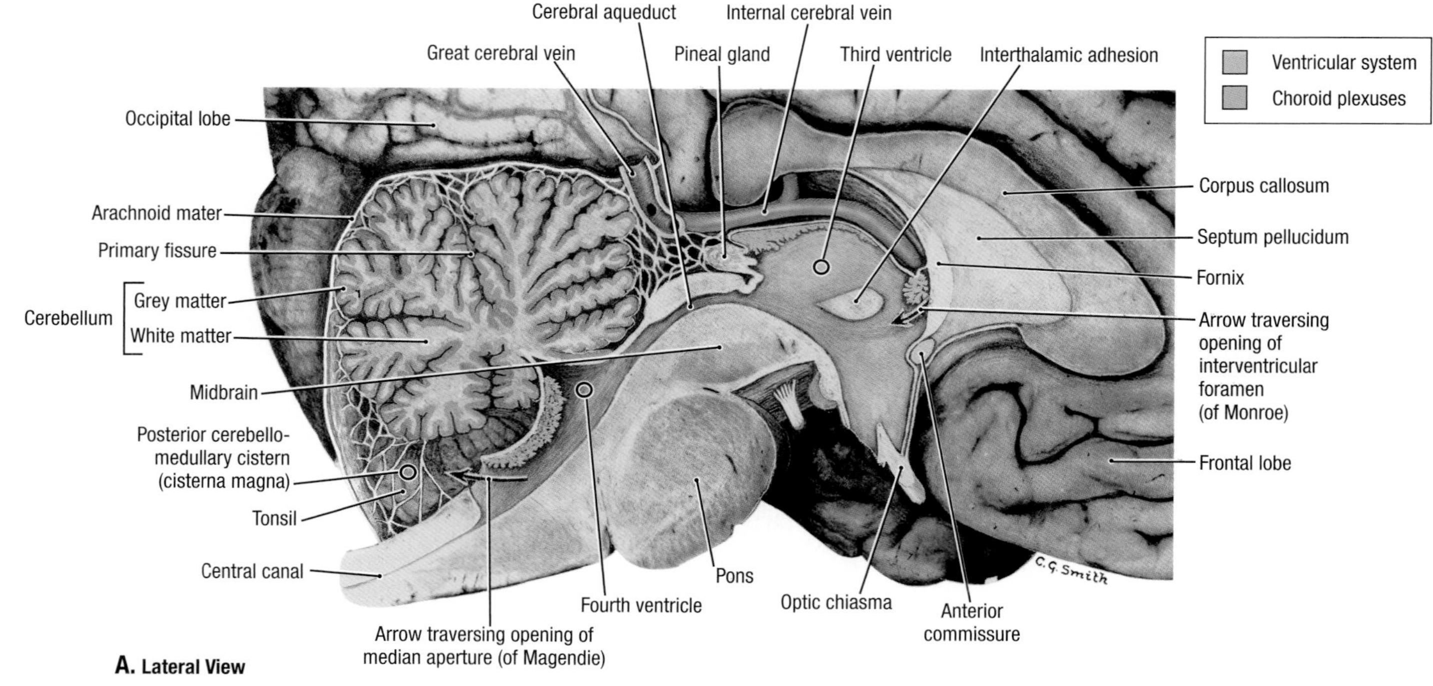
Cerebral aqueduct
Internal cerebral vein
Great cerebral vein
Pineal gland
Third ventricle
Interthalamic adhesion
Ventricular system
Choroid plexuses
Occipital lobe
Corpus callosum
Arachnoid mater
Septum pellucidum
Primary fissure
Fornix
Cerebellum
Grey matter
White matter
Arrow traversing opening of interventricular foramen (of Monroe)
Midbrain
Posterior cerebello-medullary cistern (cisterna magna)
Frontal lobe
Tonsil
C.G. Smith
Central canal
Pons
Fourth ventricle
Optic chiasma
Anterior commissure
Arrow traversing opening of median aperture (of Magendie)
A. Lateral View

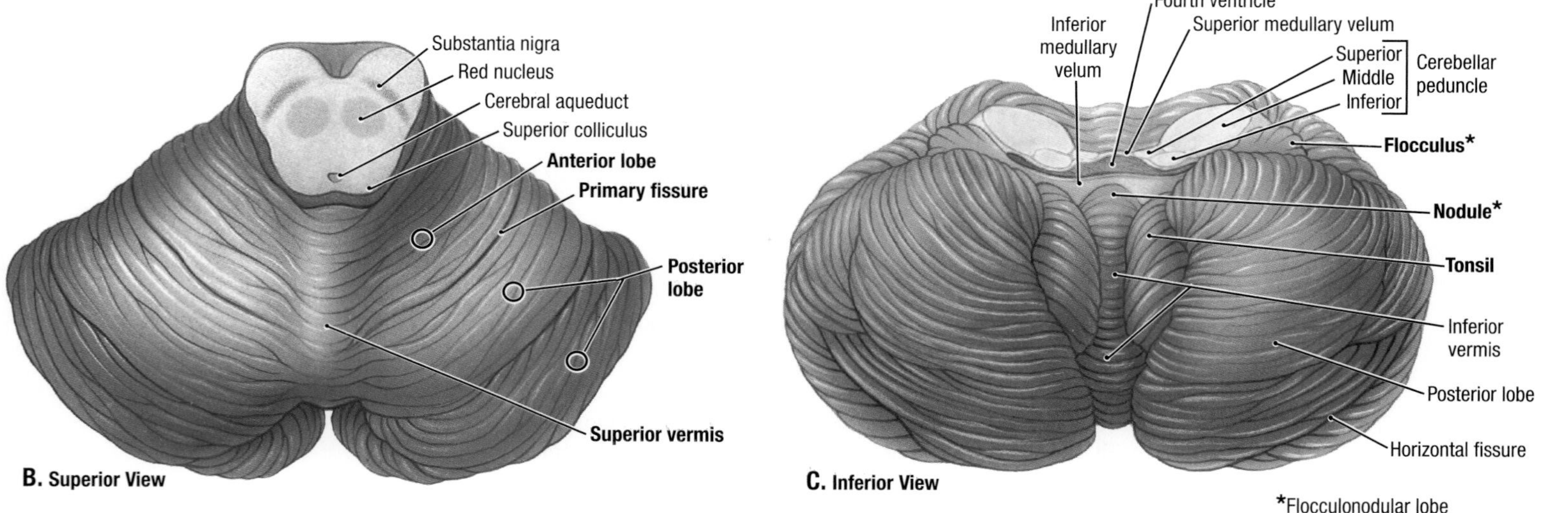
Substantia nigra
Red nucleus
Cerebral aqueduct
Superior colliculus
Anterior lobe
Primary fissure
Posterior lobe
Superior vermis
B. Superior View
Fourth ventricle
Inferior medullary velum
Superior medullary velum
Superior
Middle
Inferior
Cerebellar peduncle
Flocculus*
Nodule*
Tonsil
Inferior vermis
Posterior lobe
Horizontal fissure
C. Inferior View
*Flocculonodular lobe

## 7.92 Cerebellum

**A.** Median section. The arachnoid mater was removed except where it covered the cerebellum and the occipital lobe. CSF may be obtained, for diagnostic purposes, from the posterior cerebellomedullary cistern, using a procedure known as cisternal puncture. The subarachnoid space or the ventricular system may also be entered for measuring or monitoring CSF pressure, injecting antibiotics, or administering contrast media for radiography. **B.** Superior view of the cerebellum. The right and left cerebellar hemispheres are united by the superior vermis; the anterior and posterior lobes are separated by the primary fissure. **C.** Inferior view of cerebellum. The flocculonodular lobe, the oldest part of the cerebellum, consists of the flocculus and nodule; the cerebellar tonsils typically extend into the foramen magnum.

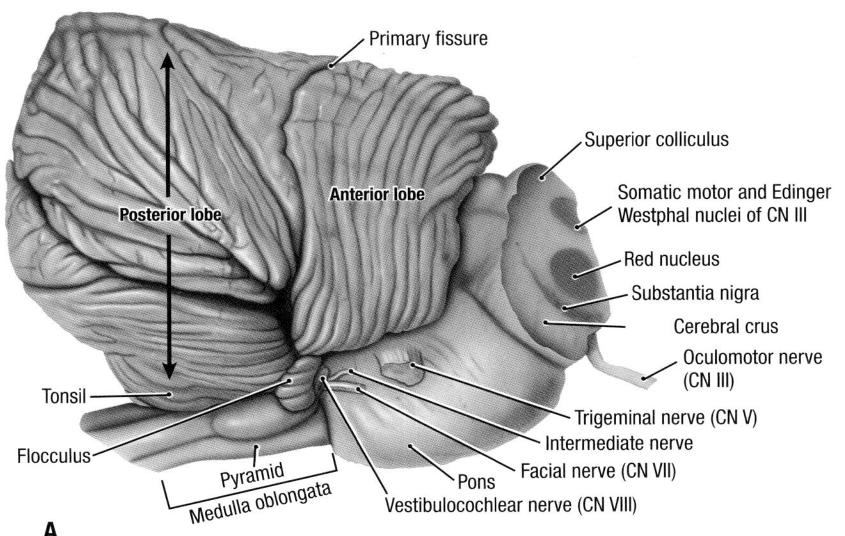
Primary fissure
Superior colliculus
Somatic motor and Edinger Westphal nuclei of CN III
Red nucleus
Substantia nigra
Cerebral crus
Oculomotor nerve (CN III)
Anterior lobe
Posterior lobe
Tonsil
Flocculus
Pyramid
Medulla oblongata
Pons
Trigeminal nerve (CN V)
Intermediate nerve
Facial nerve (CN VII)
Vestibulocochlear nerve (CN VIII)
A

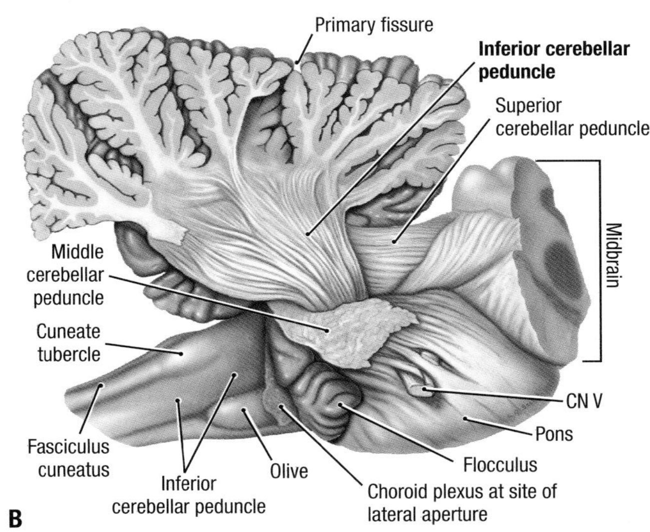
Primary fissure
Inferior cerebellar peduncle
Superior cerebellar peduncle
Midbrain
Middle cerebellar peduncle
Cuneate tubercle
Fasciculus cuneatus
Inferior cerebellar peduncle
Olive
Choroid plexus at site of lateral aperture
Flocculus
Pons
CN V
B

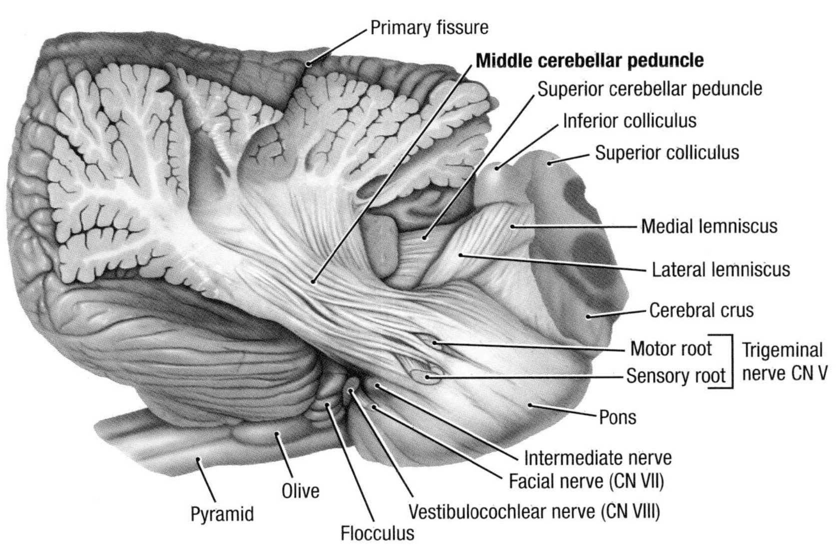
Primary fissure
Middle cerebellar peduncle
Superior cerebellar peduncle
Inferior colliculus
Superior colliculus
Medial lemniscus
Lateral lemniscus
Cerebral crus
Motor root
Sensory root
Trigeminal nerve CN V
Pons
Intermediate nerve
Facial nerve (CN VII)
Vestibulocochlear nerve (CN VIII)
Pyramid
Olive
Flocculus
C

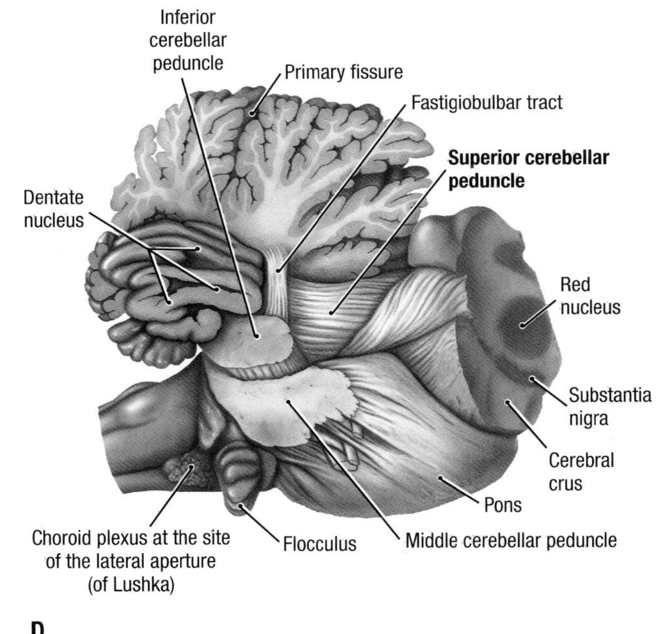
Inferior cerebellar peduncle
Primary fissure
Fastigiobulbar tract
Superior cerebellar peduncle
Dentate nucleus
Red nucleus
Substantia nigra
Cerebral crus
Pons
Middle cerebellar peduncle
Flocculus
Choroid plexus at the site of the lateral aperture (of Lushka)
D

**Lateral Views**

## 7.93 Serial dissections of the cerebellum

The series begins with the lateral surface of the cerebellar hemispheres **(A)** and proceeds medially in sequence **(B–D)**.

**A.** Cerebellum and brainstem. **B.** Inferior cerebellar peduncle. The fibers of the middle cerebellar peduncle were cut dorsal to the trigeminal nerve and peeled away to expose the fibers of the inferior cerebellar peduncle. **C.** Middle cerebellar peduncle. The fibers of the middle cerebellar peduncle were exposed by peeling away the lateral portion of the lobules of the cerebellar hemisphere. **D.** Superior cerebellar peduncle and dentate nucleus. The fibers of the inferior cerebellar peduncle were cut just dorsal to the previously sectioned middle cerebellar peduncle and peeled away until the gray matter of the dentate nucleus could be seen.

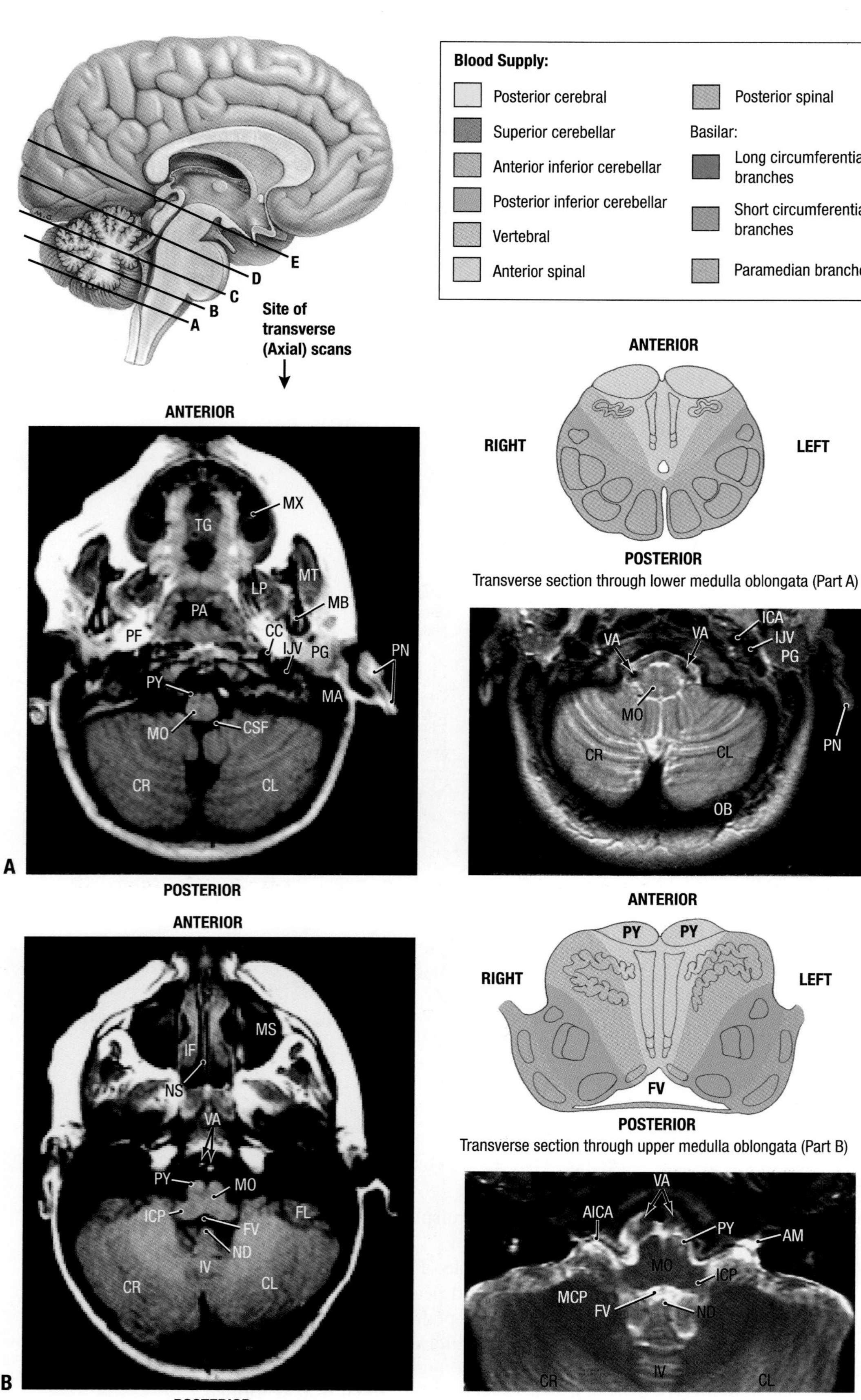
Blood Supply:
Posterior cerebral
Superior cerebellar
Anterior inferior cerebellar
Posterior inferior cerebellar
Vertebral
Anterior spinal
Posterior spinal
Basilar:
Long circumferential branches
Short circumferential branches
Paramedian branches
A
B
C
D
E
Site of transverse (Axial) scans
ANTERIOR
POSTERIOR
RIGHT
LEFT
Transverse section through lower medulla oblongata (Part A)
Transverse section through upper medulla oblongata (Part B)
MX
TG
MT
LP
MB
PA
PF
CC
IJV
PG
PN
PY
MA
MO
CSF
CR
CL
ICA
VA
OB
MS
IF
NS
FL
ICP
FV
ND
IV
AICA
AM
MCP
A
B

| | |
|---|---|
| AICA | Anterior inferior cerebellar artery |
| AM | Internal acoustic meatus |
| BA | Basilar artery |
| C | Cerebral crus |
| CA | Cerebral aqueduct |
| CB | Ciliary body |
| CC | Common carotid artery |
| CI | Colliculi |
| CL | Left cerebellar hemisphere |
| CP | Cochlear perilymph |
| CR | Right cerebellar hemisphere |
| CSF | CSF in subarachnoid space |
| DS | Dorsum sellae |
| EB | Eyeball |
| F | CN VII and CN VIII |
| FC | Facial colliculus |
| FI | Fat in infratemporal fossa |
| FL | Flocculus |
| FV | Fourth ventricle |
| G | Gray matter |
| HF | Hypophyseal fossa |
| HP | Hippocampus |
| IN | Infundibulum |
| IC | Interpeduncular cistern |
| ICA | Internal carotid artery |
| ICP | Inferior cerebellar peduncle |
| IF | Inferior concha |
| IH | Inferior horn (lateral ventricle) |
| IJV | Internal jugular vein |
| IP | Interpeduncular fossa |
| IV | Inferior vermis |
| L | Lens |
| LP | Lateral pterygoid |
| MA | Mastoid air cells |
| MB | Mandible |
| MC | Middle concha |
| MCP | Middle cerebellar peduncle |
| MD | Midbrain |
| MO | Medulla oblongata |
| MS | Maxillary sinus |
| MT | Masseter |
| MX | Maxilla |
| ND | Nodule of cerebellum |
| NS | Nasal septum |
| OB | Occipital bone |
| OC | Optic chiasm |

**7.94** Axial (transverse) MRIs through the brainstem, inferior views

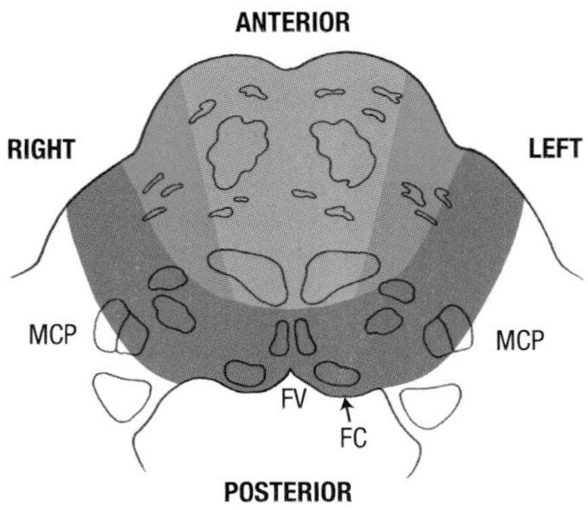

ANTERIOR

RIGHT LEFT

MCP MCP

FV FC

POSTERIOR

Transverse section through pons (Parts C & D)

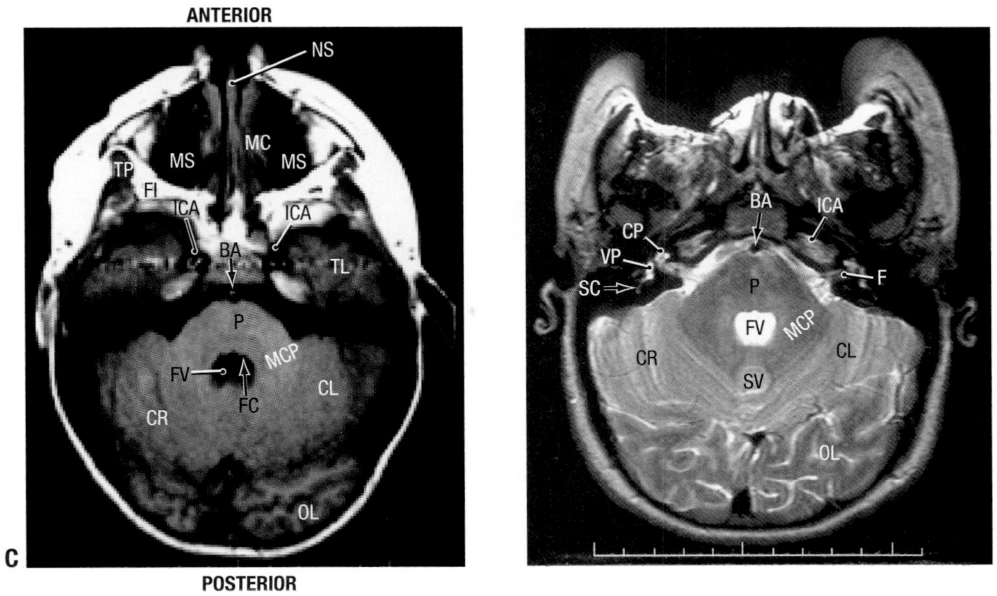

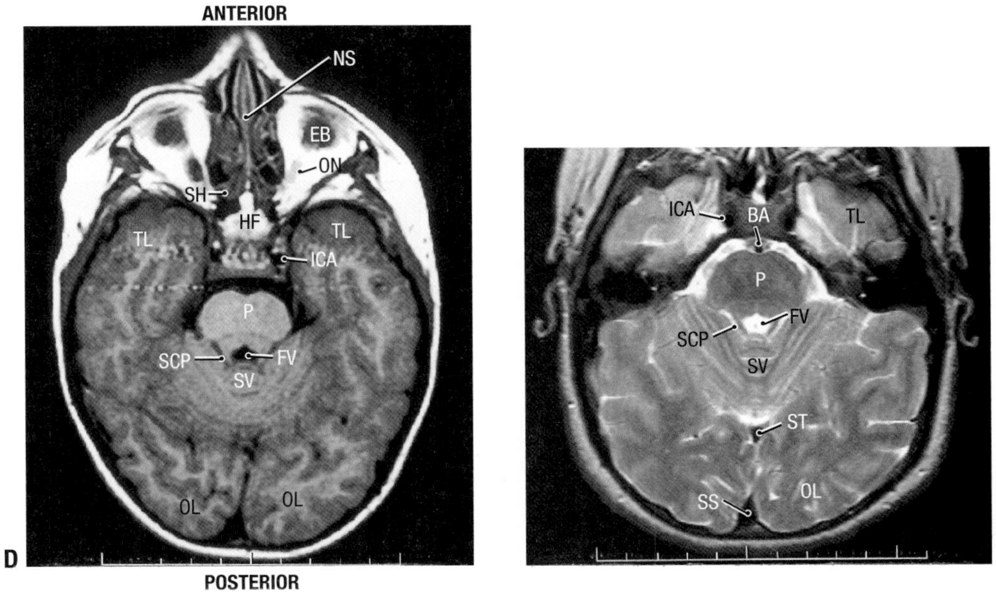

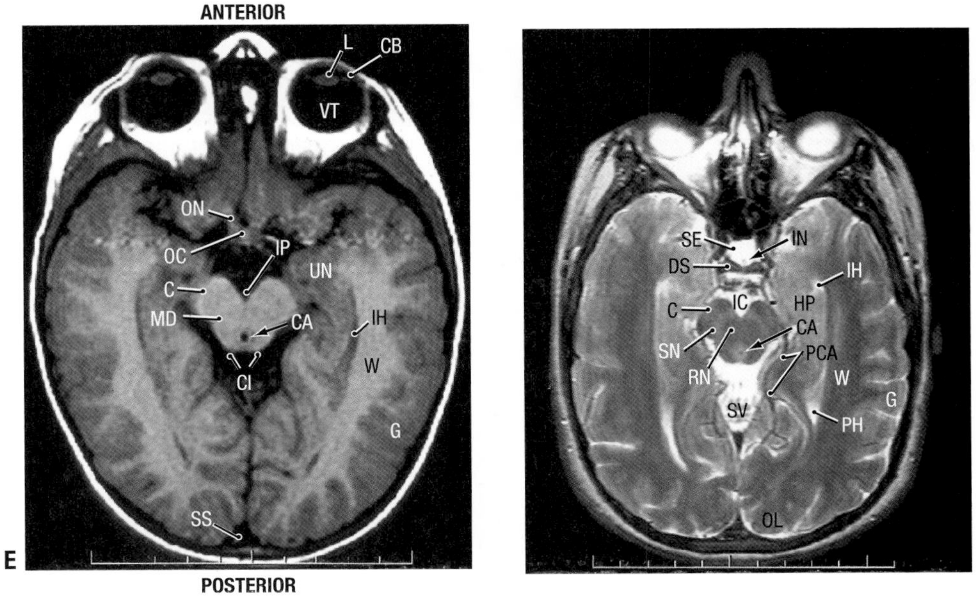

| | |
|---|---|
| OL | Occipital lobe |
| ON | Optic nerve (CN II) |
| P | Pons |
| PA | Pharynx |
| PCA | Posterior cerebral artery |
| PF | Parapharyngeal fat |
| PG | Parotid gland |
| PH | Posterior horn (lateral ventricle) |
| PN | Pinna |
| PY | Pyramid |
| RN | Red nucleus |
| SC | Semicircular canal |
| SCP | Superior cerebellar peduncle |
| SE | Suprasellar cistern |
| SH | Superior concha |
| SN | Substantia nigra |
| SS | Superior sagittal sinus |
| ST | Straight sinus |
| SV | Superior vermis |
| TG | Tongue |
| TL | Temporal lobe |
| TP | Temporalis |
| UN | Uncus |
| VA | Vertebral artery |
| VP | Vestibular perilymph |
| VT | Vitreous body |
| W | White matter |

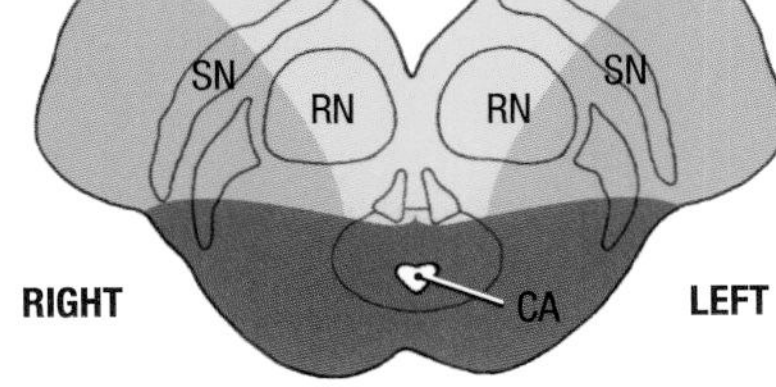
ANTERIOR
SN
RN
RN
SN
RIGHT
CA
LEFT
POSTERIOR

Transverse section through midbrain (Part E)

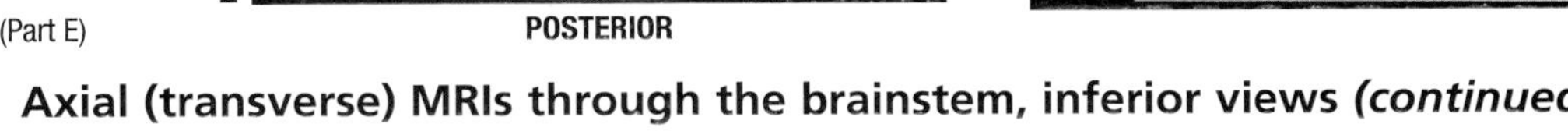

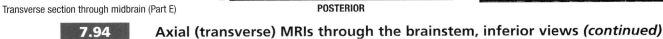

**7.94 Axial (transverse) MRIs through the brainstem, inferior views *(continued)***

Images on left side of page are T1 weighted, and images on the right side are T2 weighted.

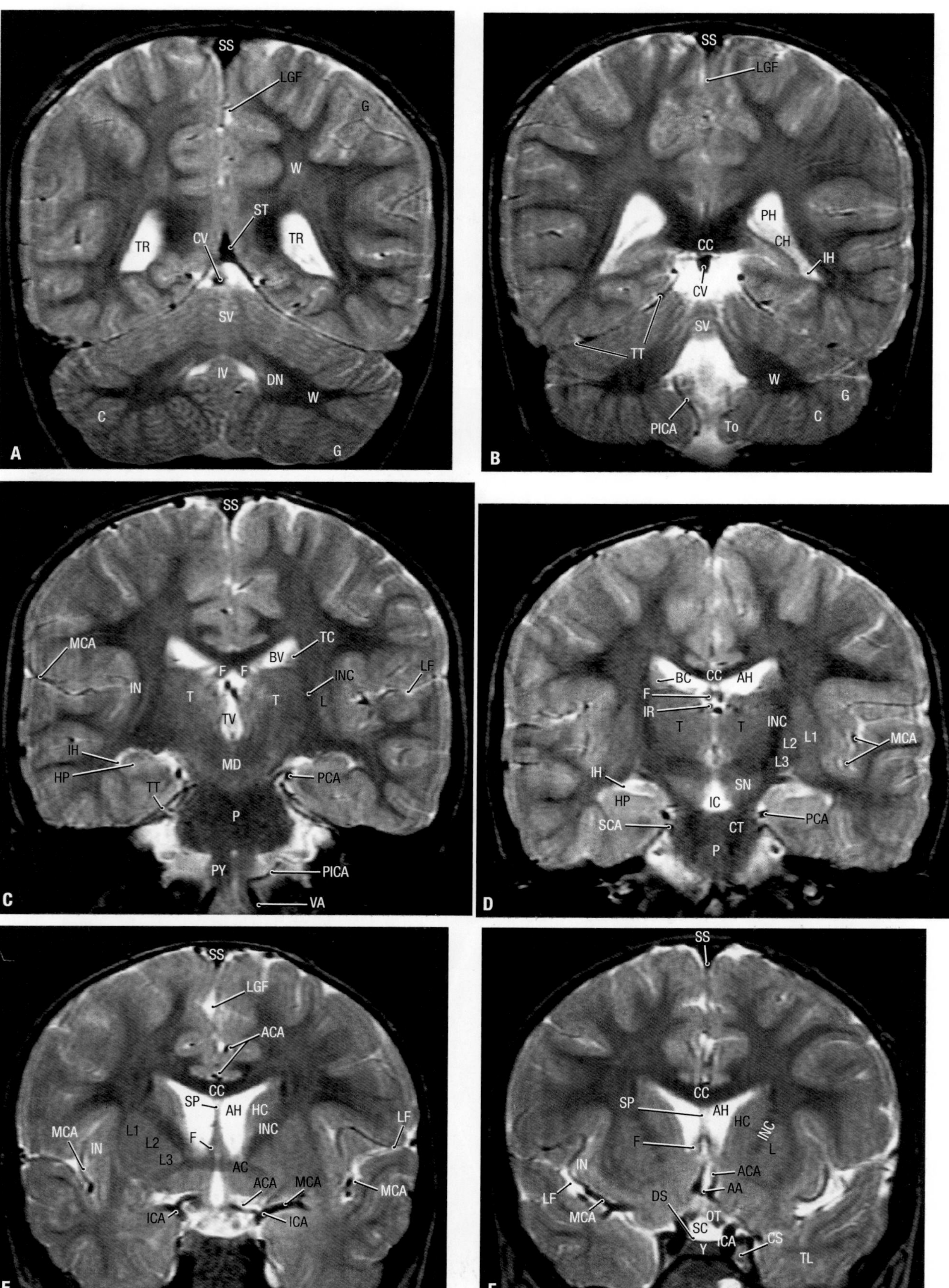
SS
LGF
G
W
ST
TR
CV
TR
SV
IV
DN
W
C
G
A
SS
LGF
PH
CC
CH
IH
CV
SV
TT
W
G
C
PICA
To
B
SS
MCA
TC
BV
F F
INC
LF
IN
T
T
L
TV
IH
HP
MD
PCA
TT
P
PY
PICA
VA
C
BC
CC
AH
F
IR
T
T
INC
L2
L1
L3
MCA
IH
SN
HP
IC
PCA
SCA
CT
P
D
SS
LGF
ACA
CC
SP
AH
HC
INC
MCA
IN
L1
L2
L3
F
LF
AC
ACA
MCA
MCA
ICA
ICA
E
SS
CC
SP
AH
HC
INC
L
F
IN
ACA
AA
LF
MCA
DS
OT
SC
ICA
CS
Y
TL
F

AA Anterior communicating artery
AC Anterior commissure
ACA Anterior cerebral artery
AH Anterior horn of lateral ventricle
BC Body of caudate nucleus
BV Body of lateral ventricle
C Cerebellum
CC Corpus callosum
CH Choroid plexus
CS Cavernous sinus
CT Corticospinal tract
CV Great cerebral vein
DN Dentate nucleus
DS Diaphragma sellae
F Fornix
FV Fourth ventricle
G Gray matter
HC Head of caudate nucleus
HP Hippocampus
IC Interpeduncular cistern
ICA Internal carotid artery
IH Interior horn of lateral ventricle
IN Insular cortex
INC Internal capsule
IR Intervertebral vein
IV Inferior vermis
L Lentiform nucleus
L1 Putamen
L2 External (lateral) segment of globus pallidus
L3 Internal (medial) segment of globus pallidus
LF Lateral fissure
LGF Longitudinal fissure
MCA Middle cerebral artery
MD Midbrain
OT Optic tract
P Pons
PCA Posterior cerebral artery
PH Posterior horn of lateral ventricle
PICA Posterior inferior cerebellar artery
PY Pyramid
S Carotid siphon
SC Supracellebellar cistern
SCA Superior cerebellar artery
SN Substantia nigra
SP Septum pellucidum
SS Superior sagittal sinus
ST Straight sinus
SV Superior vermis
T Thalamus
TC Tail of caudate nucleus
TL Temporal lobe
To Cerebellar tonsil
TR Trigone of lateral ventricle
TT Tentorium cerebelli
TV Third ventricle
VA Vertebral artery
W White matter
Y Hypophysis

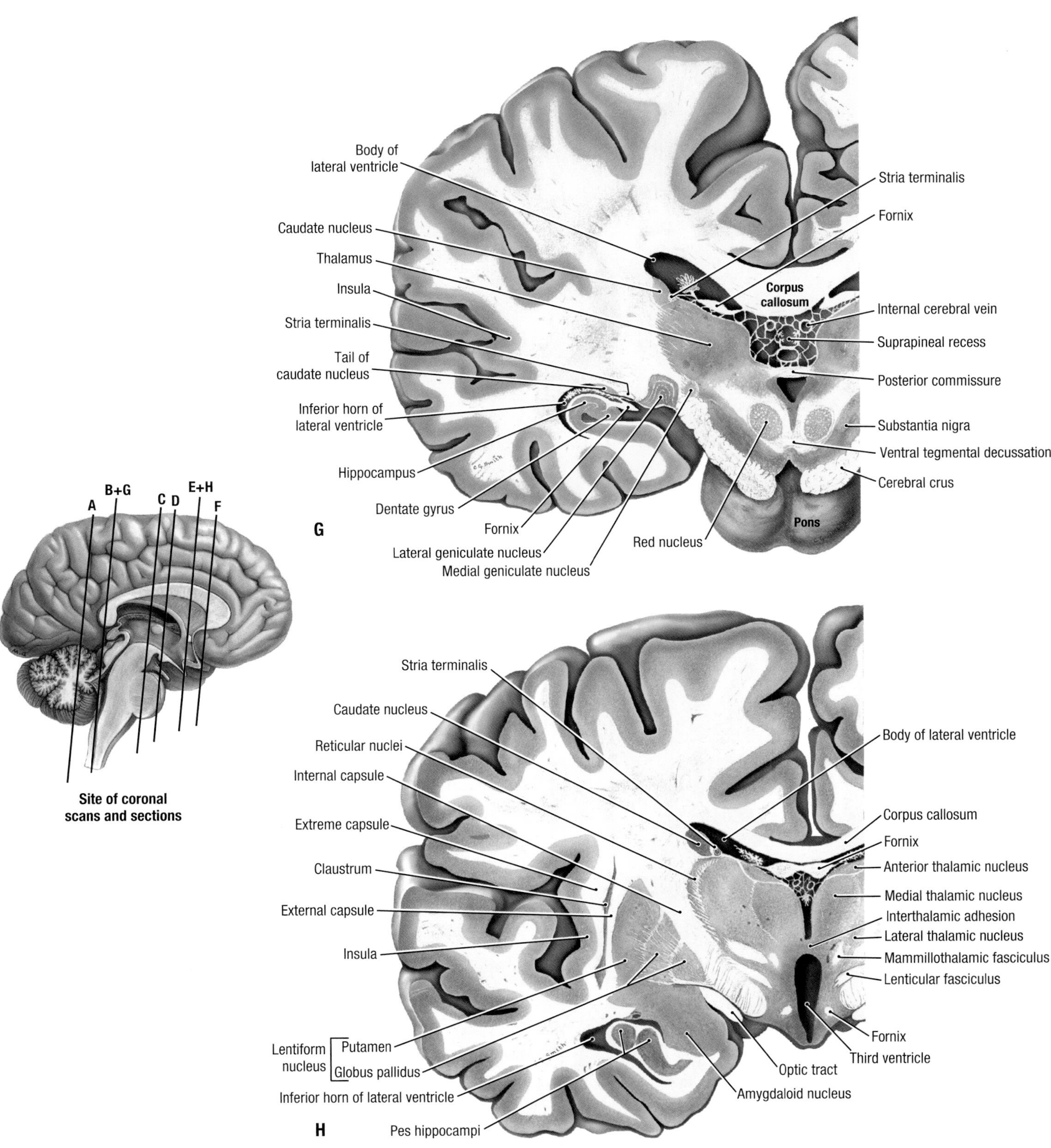
Body of lateral ventricle
Caudate nucleus
Thalamus
Insula
Stria terminalis
Tail of caudate nucleus
Inferior horn of lateral ventricle
Hippocampus
Dentate gyrus
Fornix
Lateral geniculate nucleus
Medial geniculate nucleus
Red nucleus
Pons
G
Stria terminalis
Fornix
Corpus callosum
Internal cerebral vein
Suprapineal recess
Posterior commissure
Substantia nigra
Ventral tegmental decussation
Cerebral crus
A
B+G
C
D
E+H
F
Site of coronal scans and sections
Stria terminalis
Caudate nucleus
Reticular nuclei
Internal capsule
Extreme capsule
Claustrum
External capsule
Insula
Lentiform nucleus
Putamen
Globus pallidus
Inferior horn of lateral ventricle
Pes hippocampi
H
Body of lateral ventricle
Corpus callosum
Fornix
Anterior thalamic nucleus
Medial thalamic nucleus
Interthalamic adhesion
Lateral thalamic nucleus
Mammillothalamic fasciculus
Lenticular fasciculus
Fornix
Third ventricle
Optic tract
Amygdaloid nucleus

**7.95 Coronal MRIs (T2 weighted) and sections of brain**

**A–F.** Coronal MRIs. **G–H.** Coronal sections, posterior views.

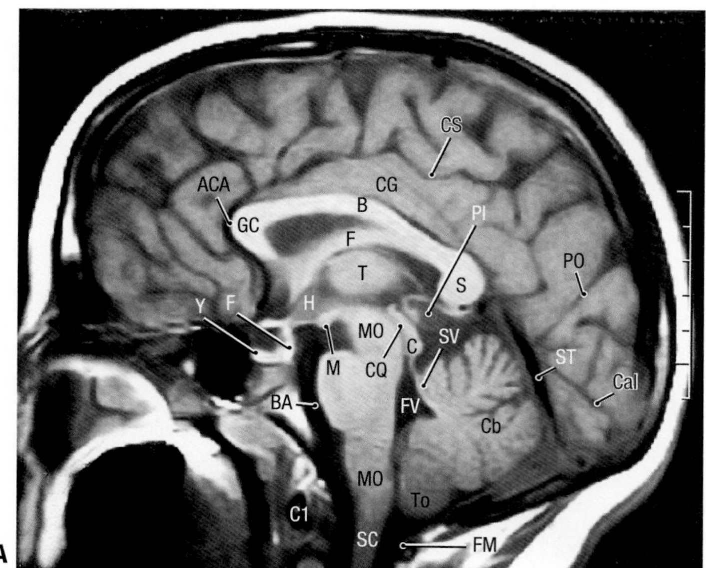
CS
ACA
CG
B
GC
PI
F
T
PO
S
Y
F
H
MO
C
SV
M
CQ
ST
Cal
BA
FV
Cb
MO
To
C1
SC
FM

A

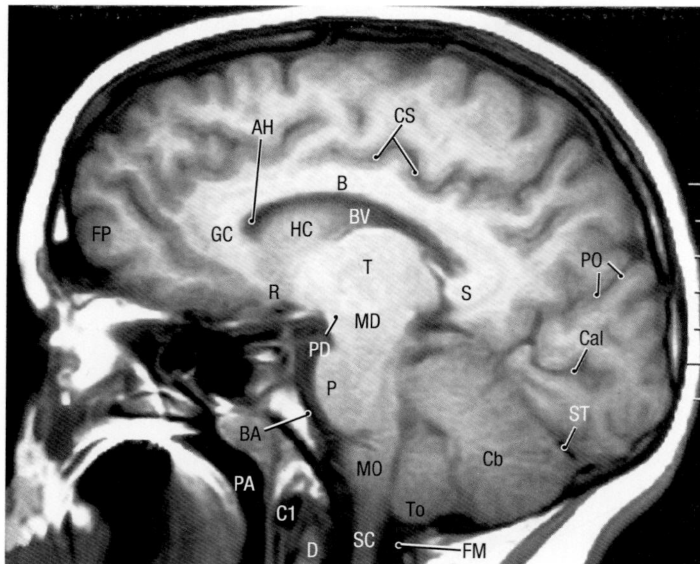
CS
AH
B
FP
GC
HC
BV
T
PO
R
S
MD
PD
Cal
P
ST
BA
Cb
MO
PA
C1
To
D
SC
FM

B

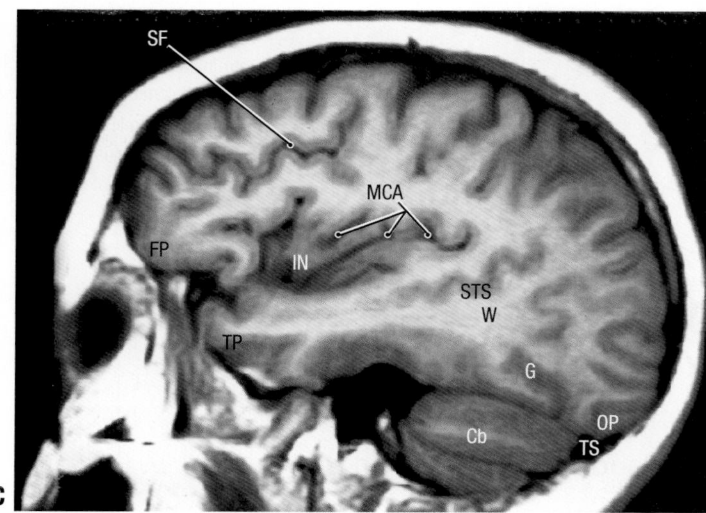
SF
MCA
FP
IN
STS
W
TP
G
OP
Cb
TS

C

| | |
|---|---|
| ACA | Anterior cerebral artery |
| AH | Anterior horn of lateral ventricle |
| B | Body of corpus callosum |
| BA | Basilar artery |
| BV | Body of lateral ventricle |
| C | Colliculi |
| C1 | Anterior tubercle of atlas |
| Cal | Calcarine sulcus |
| Cb | Cerebellum |
| CG | Cingulate nucleus |
| CQ | Cerebral aqueduct |
| CS | Cingulate sulcus |
| D | Dens (odontoid process) |
| F | Fornix |
| FM | Foramen magnum |
| FP | Frontal pole |
| FV | Fourth ventricle |
| G | Cerebral cortex (gray matter) |
| GC | Genus of corpus callosum |
| H | Hypothalamus |
| HC | Head of caudate nucleus |
| I | Infundibulum |
| IN | Insular cortex |
| M | Mammillary body |
| MCA | Middle cerebral artery |
| MD | Midbrain |
| OP | Occipital pole |
| P | Pons |
| PA | Pharynx |
| PD | Cerebral peduncle |
| PI | Pineal |
| PO | Parieto-occipital fissure |
| R | Rostrum of corpus callosum |
| S | Splenium of corpus callosum |
| SC | Spinal cord |
| SF | Superior frontal sulcus |
| ST | Straight sinus |
| STS | Superior temporal sulcus |
| SV | Superior medullary vellum |
| T | Thalamus |
| To | Cerebral tonsil |
| TP | Temporal pole |
| TS | Transverse sinus |
| W | White matter |
| Y | Hypophysis |

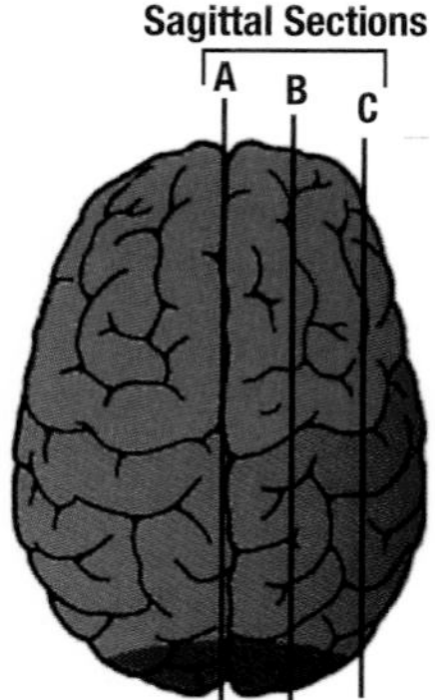
Sagittal Sections
A
B
C

**7.96 Sagittal MRIs (T1 weighted) and median section of brain**

See orientation drawing for sites of scans **A–C.**

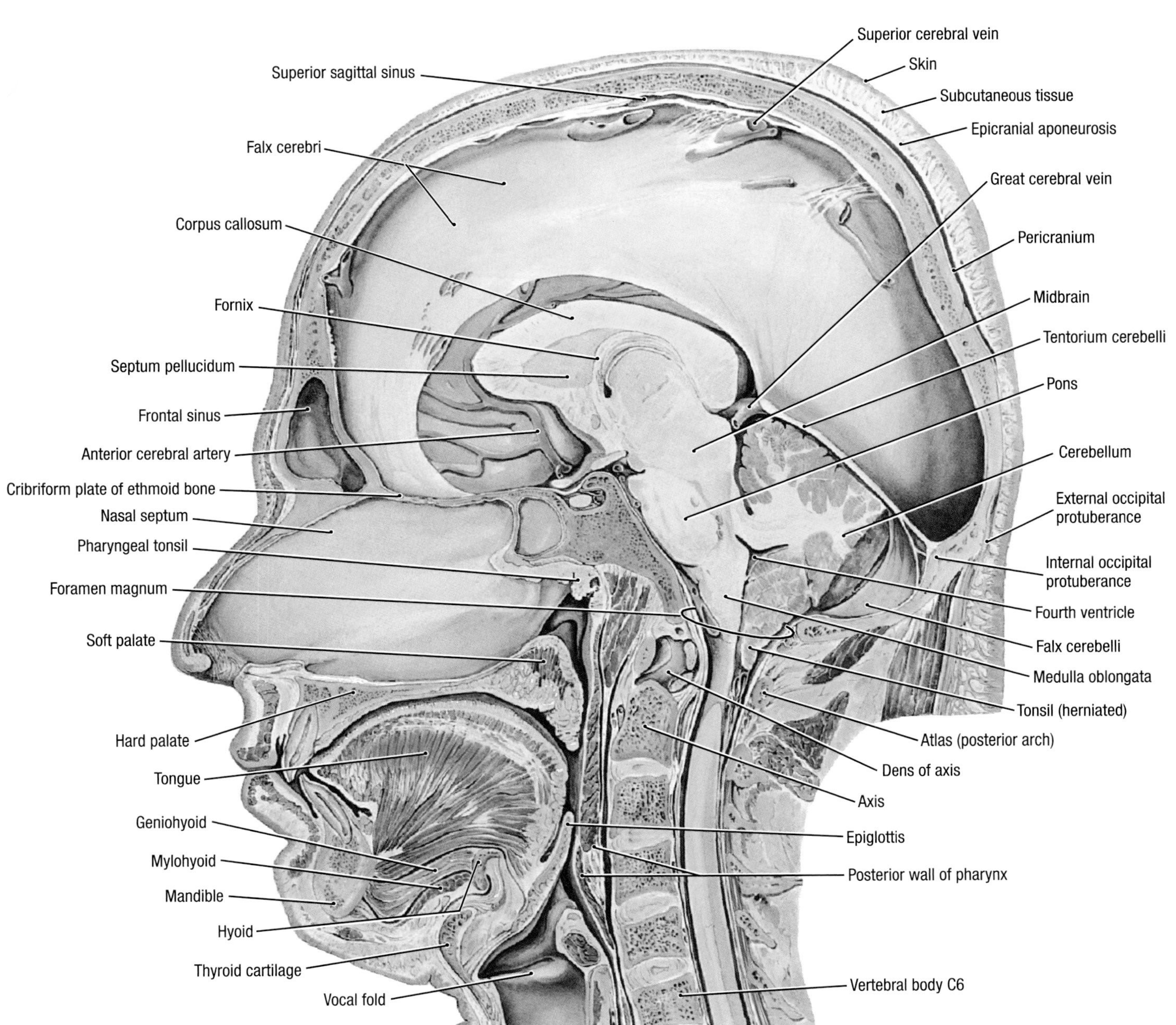
Superior cerebral vein
Skin
Subcutaneous tissue
Epicranial aponeurosis
Great cerebral vein
Pericranium
Midbrain
Tentorium cerebelli
Pons
Cerebellum
External occipital protuberance
Internal occipital protuberance
Fourth ventricle
Falx cerebelli
Medulla oblongata
Tonsil (herniated)
Atlas (posterior arch)
Dens of axis
Axis
Epiglottis
Posterior wall of pharynx
Vertebral body C6
Superior sagittal sinus
Falx cerebri
Corpus callosum
Fornix
Septum pellucidum
Frontal sinus
Anterior cerebral artery
Cribriform plate of ethmoid bone
Nasal septum
Pharyngeal tonsil
Foramen magnum
Soft palate
Hard palate
Tongue
Geniohyoid
Mylohyoid
Mandible
Hyoid
Thyroid cartilage
Vocal fold

**D.** **Median Section**

## 7.96 Sagittal MRIs (T1 weighted) and median section of brain *(continued)*

Increased intracranial pressure (e.g., due to a tumor) may cause displacement of the cerebellar tonsils through the foramen magnum, resulting in a formial (tonsillar) herniation. Compression of the brainstem, if severe, may result in respiratory and cardiac arrest.

CHAPTER 8

# NECK

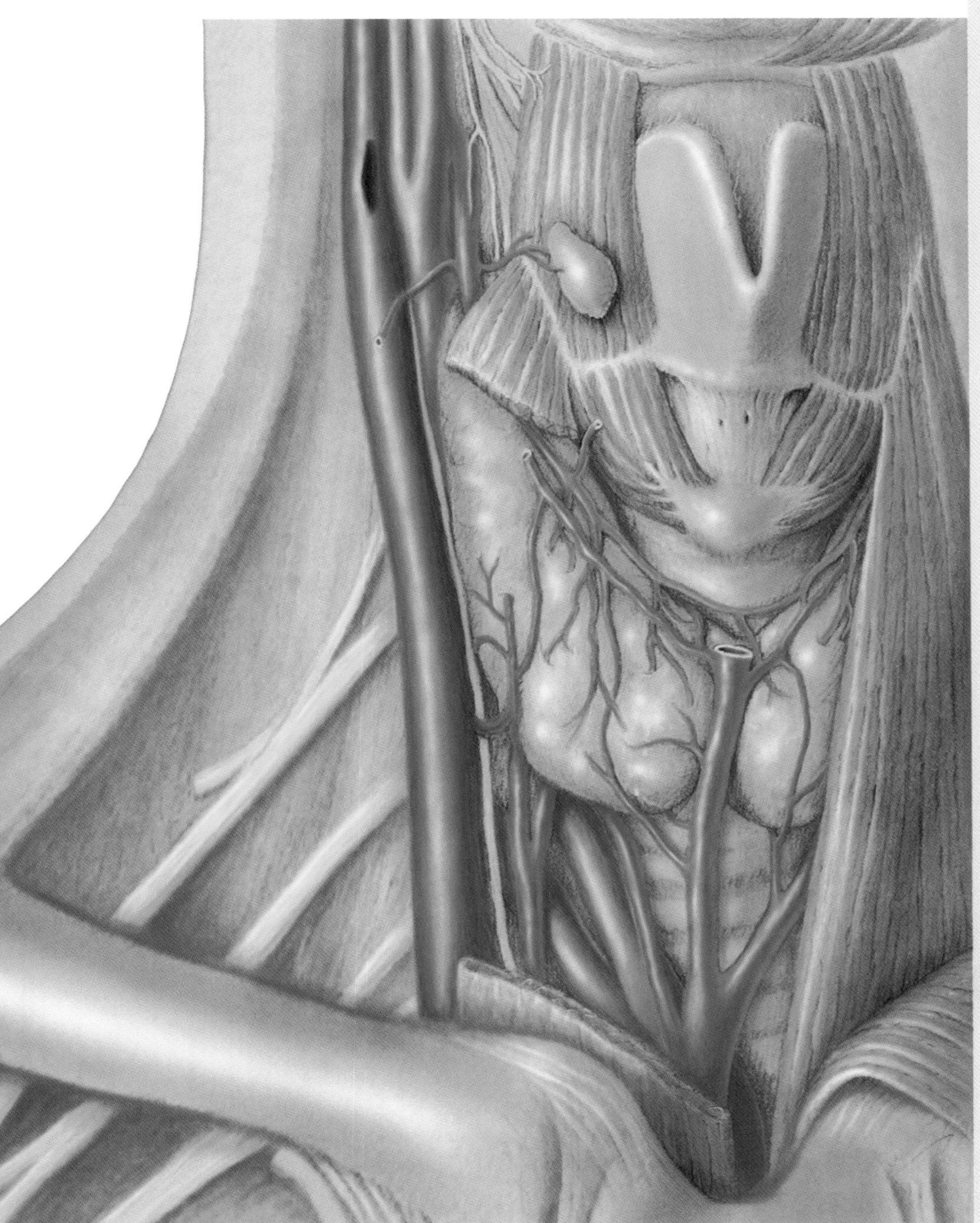


- Subcutaneous Structures and Cervical Fascia **746**
- Skeleton of Neck **750**
- Regions of Neck **752**
  - Lateral Region (Posterior Triangle) of Neck **754**
  - Anterior Region (Anterior Triangle) of Neck **758**
    - Neurovascular Structures of Neck **762**
    - Visceral Compartment of Neck **768**
    - Root and Prevertebral Region of Neck **772**
    - Submandibular Region and Floor of Mouth **778**
  - Posterior Cervical Region **783**
- Pharynx **786**
- Isthmus of Fauces **792**
- Larynx **798**
- Sectional Anatomy and Imaging of Neck **806**

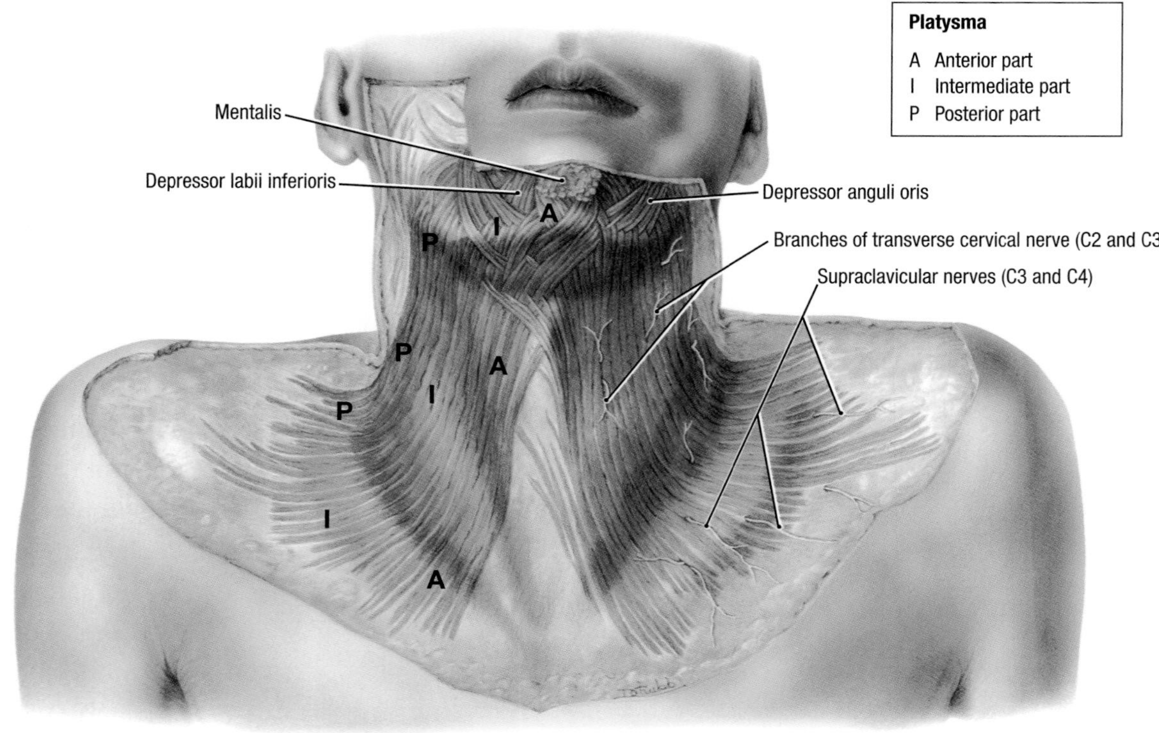
Platysma
A Anterior part
I Intermediate part
P Posterior part
Mentalis
Depressor labii inferioris
Depressor anguli oris
Branches of transverse cervical nerve (C2 and C3)
Supraclavicular nerves (C3 and C4)
A
I
P
P
A
I
P
I
A

A. Anterior View

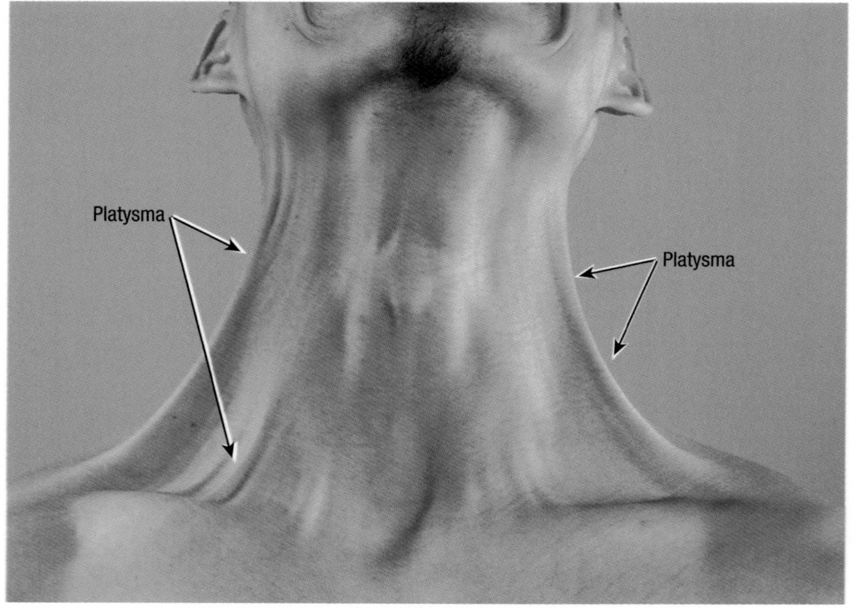
Platysma
Platysma

**TABLE 8.1 PLATYSMA**

| Muscle | Superior Attachment | Inferior Attachment | Innervation | Main Action |
|---|---|---|---|---|
| **Platysma** | *Anterior part:* Fibers interlace with contralateral muscle<br>*Intermediate part:* Fibers pass deep to depressors anguli oris and labii inferioris to attach to inferior border of mandible<br>*Posterior part:* Skin/subcutaneous tissue of lower face lateral to mouth | Subcutaneous tissue overlying superior parts of pectoralis major and sometimes deltoid muscles | Cervical branch of facial nerve (CN VII) | Draws corner of mouth inferiorly and widens it as in expressions of sadness and fright; draws the skin of the neck superiorly, forming tense vertical and oblique ridges over the anterior neck |

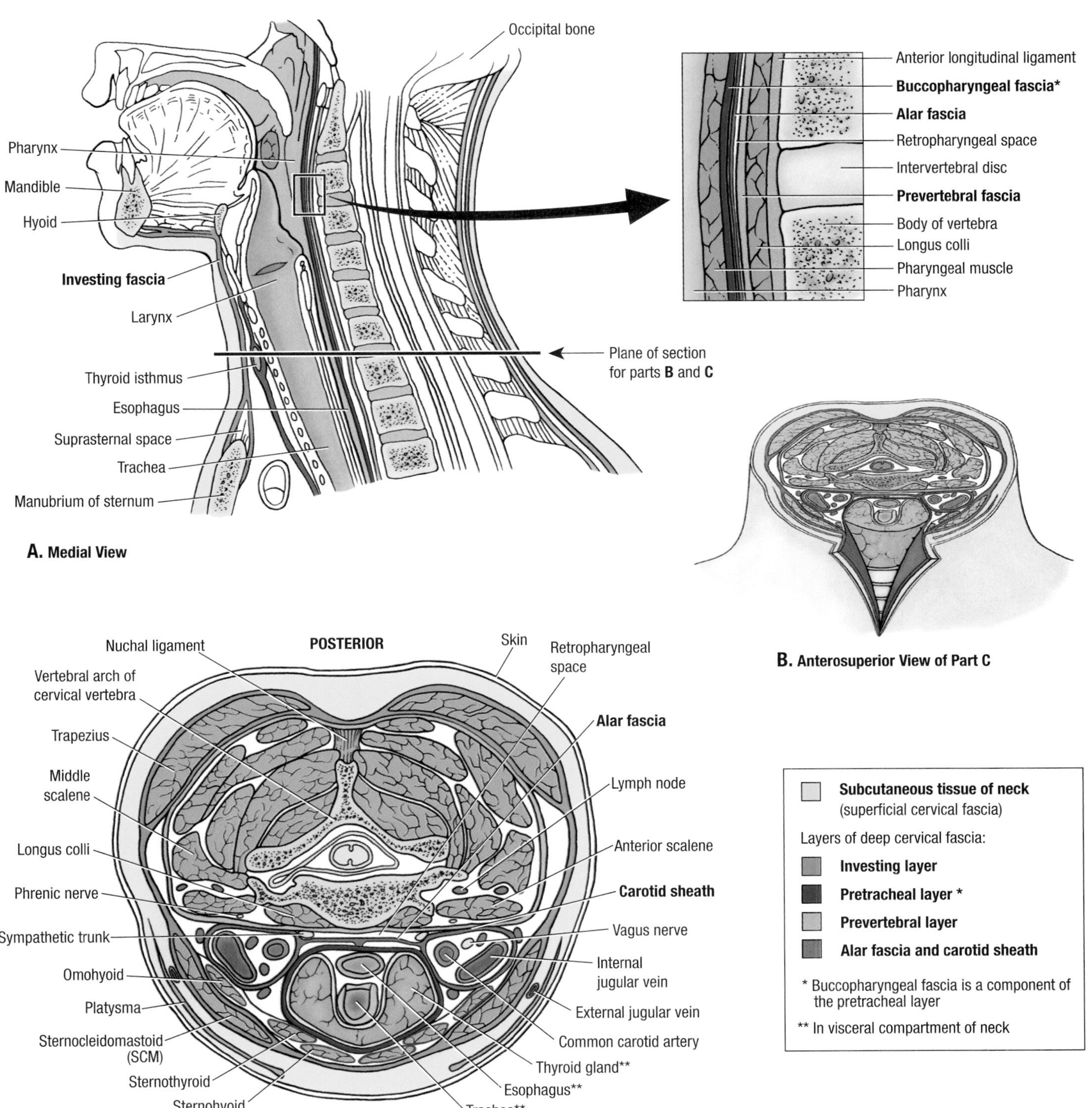
Occipital bone
Pharynx
Mandible
Hyoid
Investing fascia
Larynx
Thyroid isthmus
Esophagus
Suprasternal space
Trachea
Manubrium of sternum
Plane of section for parts B and C
Anterior longitudinal ligament
Buccopharyngeal fascia*
Alar fascia
Retropharyngeal space
Intervertebral disc
Prevertebral fascia
Body of vertebra
Longus colli
Pharyngeal muscle
Pharynx
A. Medial View
B. Anterosuperior View of Part C
POSTERIOR
Nuchal ligament
Skin
Retropharyngeal space
Vertebral arch of cervical vertebra
Alar fascia
Trapezius
Middle scalene
Lymph node
Longus colli
Anterior scalene
Phrenic nerve
Carotid sheath
Sympathetic trunk
Vagus nerve
Omohyoid
Internal jugular vein
Platysma
External jugular vein
Sternocleidomastoid (SCM)
Common carotid artery
Sternothyroid
Thyroid gland**
Sternohyoid
Esophagus**
Trachea**
ANTERIOR
Subcutaneous tissue of neck (superficial cervical fascia)
Layers of deep cervical fascia:
Investing layer
Pretracheal layer *
Prevertebral layer
Alar fascia and carotid sheath
* Buccopharyngeal fascia is a component of the pretracheal layer
** In visceral compartment of neck

C. Superior View of Transverse Section (at level of C7 vertebra)

## 8.1 Subcutaneous tissue and deep fascia of neck

Sectional demonstrations of the fasciae of the neck. **A.** Fasciae of the neck are continuous inferiorly and superiorly with thoracic and cranial fasciae. The *inset* illustrates the fascia of the retropharyngeal region. **B.** Relationship of the main layers of deep cervical fascia and the carotid sheath. Midline access to the cervical viscera is possible with minimal disruption of tissues. **C.** The concentric layers of fascia are apparent in this transverse section of neck at the level indicated in **A.**

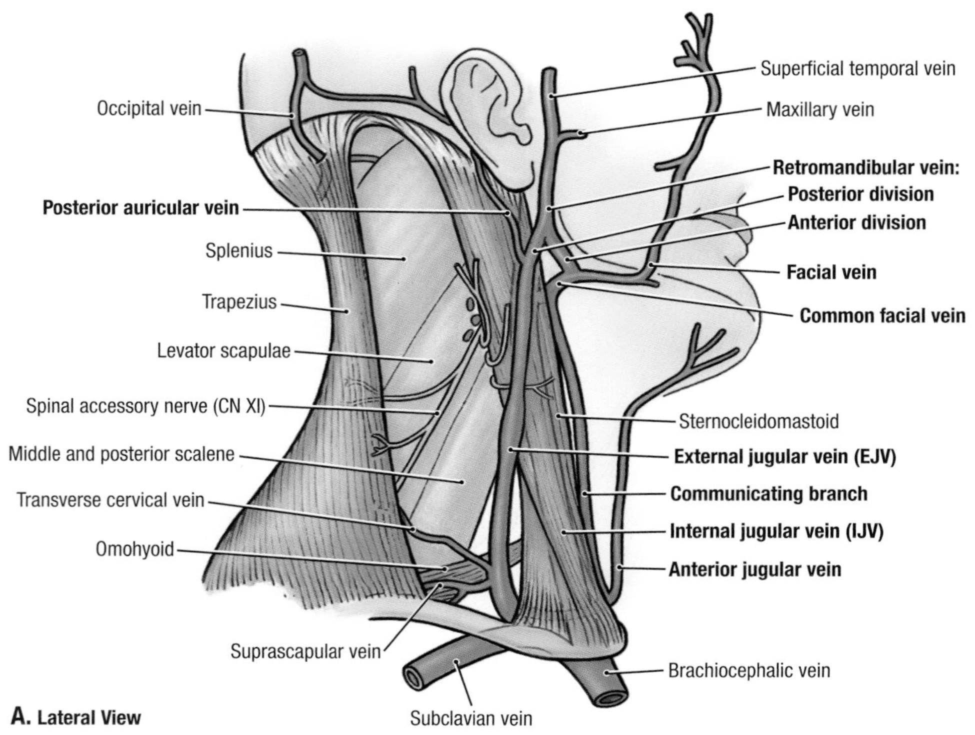
Superficial temporal vein
Maxillary vein
Retromandibular vein:
Posterior division
Anterior division
Facial vein
Common facial vein
Occipital vein
Posterior auricular vein
Splenius
Trapezius
Levator scapulae
Spinal accessory nerve (CN XI)
Middle and posterior scalene
Transverse cervical vein
Omohyoid
Suprascapular vein
Subclavian vein
Brachiocephalic vein
Sternocleidomastoid
External jugular vein (EJV)
Communicating branch
Internal jugular vein (IJV)
Anterior jugular vein
A. Lateral View

## 8.2 Superficial veins of the neck

**A.** Schematic illustration of superficial veins of the neck. The superficial temporal and maxillary veins merge to form the retromandibular vein. The posterior division of the retromandibular vein unites with the posterior auricular vein to form the external jugular vein (EJV). The facial vein receives the anterior division of the retromandibular vein, forming the common facial vein that empties into the internal jugular vein. **B.** Surface anatomy of the external jugular vein and the muscles bounding the lateral cervical region (posterior triangle) of the neck.

The EJV may serve as an "internal barometer." When venous pressure is in the normal range, the EJV is usually visible superior to the clavicle for only a short distance. However, when venous pressure rises (e.g., as in heart failure) the vein is prominent throughout its course along the side of the neck. Consequently, routine observation for distention of the EJVs during physical examinations may reveal diagnostic signs of heart failure, obstruction of the superior vena cava, enlarged supraclavicular lymph nodes, or increased intrathoracic pressure.

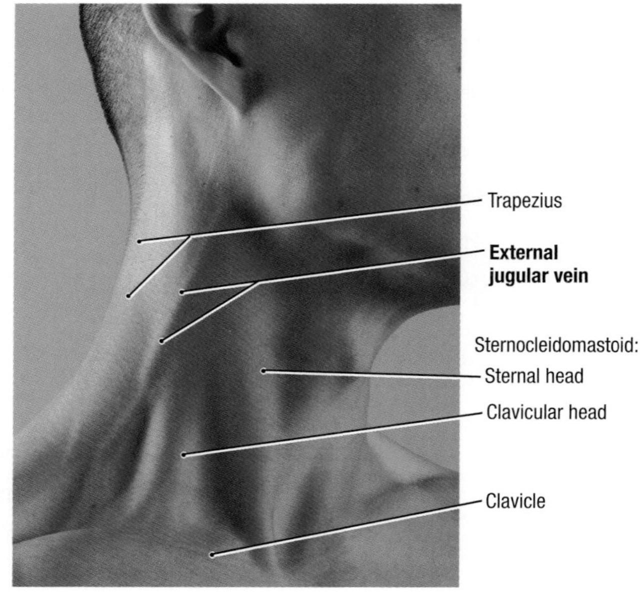
Trapezius
External jugular vein
Sternocleidomastoid:
Sternal head
Clavicular head
Clavicle
B. Lateral View

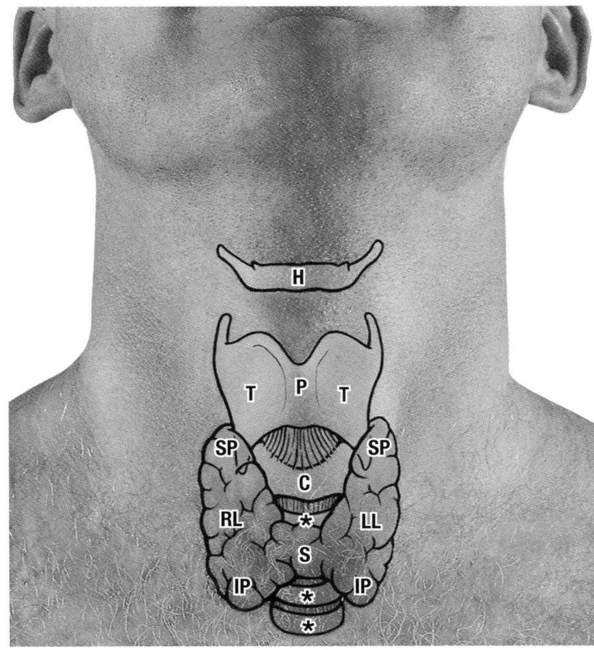
H
T
P
T
SP
SP
C
RL
LL
*
S
IP
IP
*
*

**Anterior View**

| | | | |
|---|---|---|---|
| C | Cricoid cartilage | RL | Right lobe of thyroid gland |
| H | Hyoid | S | Isthmus |
| IP | Inferior pole of thyroid gland | SP | Superior pole of thyroid gland |
| LL | Left lobe of thyroid gland | T | Thyroid cartilage |
| P | Laryngeal prominence | * | Tracheal rings |

## 8.3 Surface anatomy of hyoid and cartilages of anterior neck

The U-shaped hyoid lies superior to the thyroid cartilage at the level of the C4 and C5 vertebrae. The laryngeal prominence is produced by the fused laminae of the thyroid cartilage, which meet in the median plane. The cricoid cartilage can be felt inferior to the laryngeal prominence. It lies at the level of the C6 vertebra. The cartilaginous tracheal rings are palpable in the inferior part of the neck. The 2nd–4th rings cannot be felt because the isthmus of the thyroid, connecting its right and left lobes, covers them. The first tracheal ring is just superior to the isthmus.

### Tracheostomy

A transverse incision through the skin of the neck and anterior wall of the trachea (*tracheostomy*) establishes an airway in patients with upper airway obstruction or respiratory failure. The infrahyoid muscles are retracted laterally, and the isthmus of the thyroid gland is either divided or retracted superiorly. An opening is made in the trachea between the 1st and 2nd tracheal rings or through the 2nd through 4th rings. A *tracheostomy tube* is then inserted into the trachea and secured. To avoid complications during a tracheostomy, the following anatomical relationships are important:

- The *inferior thyroid veins* arise from a venous plexus on the thyroid gland and descend anterior to the trachea (see Fig. 8.13).
- A small *thyroid ima artery* is present in approximately 10% of people; it ascends from the brachiocephalic trunk or the arch of the aorta to the isthmus of the thyroid gland (see Fig. 8.15).
- The *left brachiocephalic vein*, jugular venous arch, and pleurae may be encountered, particularly in infants and children.
- The *thymus* covers the inferior part of the trachea in infants and children.
- The trachea is small, mobile, and soft in infants, making it easy to cut through its posterior wall and damage the esophagus.

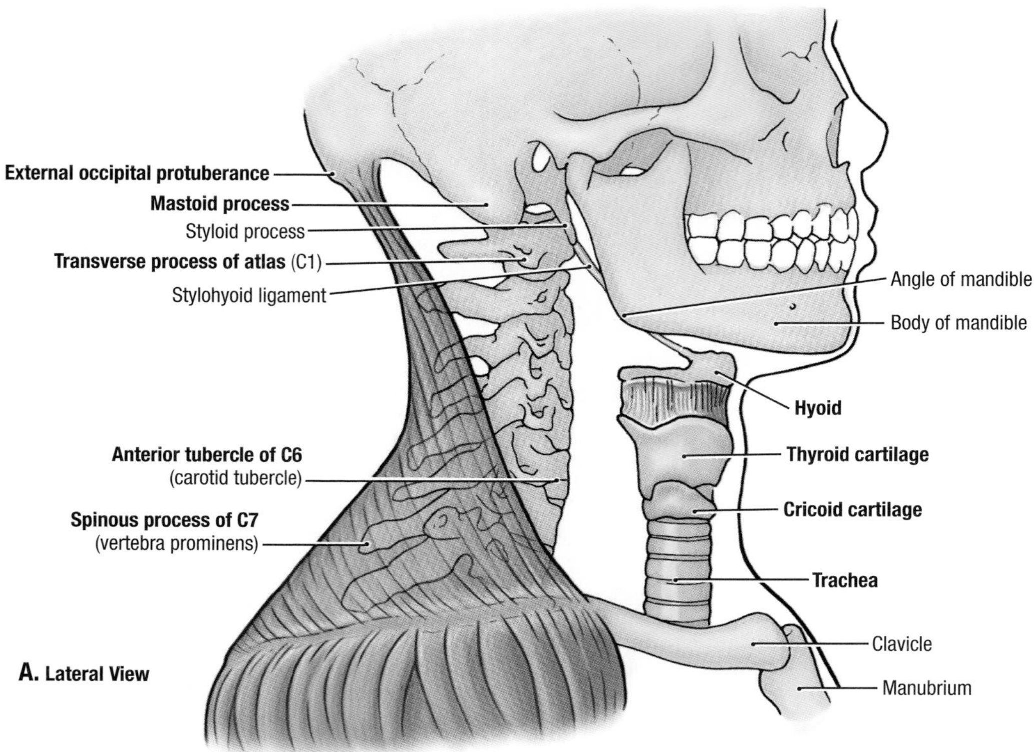
External occipital protuberance
Mastoid process
Styloid process
Transverse process of atlas (C1)
Stylohyoid ligament
Angle of mandible
Body of mandible
Hyoid
Thyroid cartilage
Cricoid cartilage
Trachea
Clavicle
Manubrium
Anterior tubercle of C6 (carotid tubercle)
Spinous process of C7 (vertebra prominens)
A. Lateral View

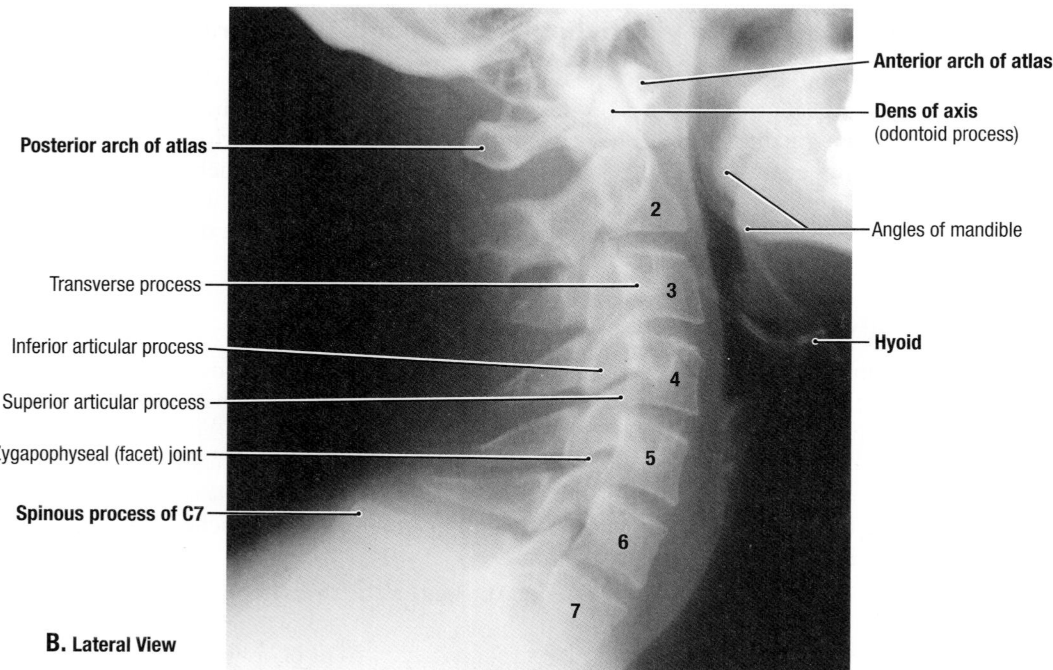
Anterior arch of atlas
Dens of axis (odontoid process)
Posterior arch of atlas
Angles of mandible
Transverse process
Hyoid
Inferior articular process
Superior articular process
Zygapophyseal (facet) joint
Spinous process of C7
2
3
4
5
6
7
B. Lateral View

## 8.4 Bones and cartilages of the neck

**A.** Bony and cartilaginous landmarks of the neck. **B.** Radiograph of hyoid bone and cervical vertebrae. Because the upper cervical vertebrae lie posterior to the upper and lower jaws and teeth, they are best seen radiographically in lateral views.

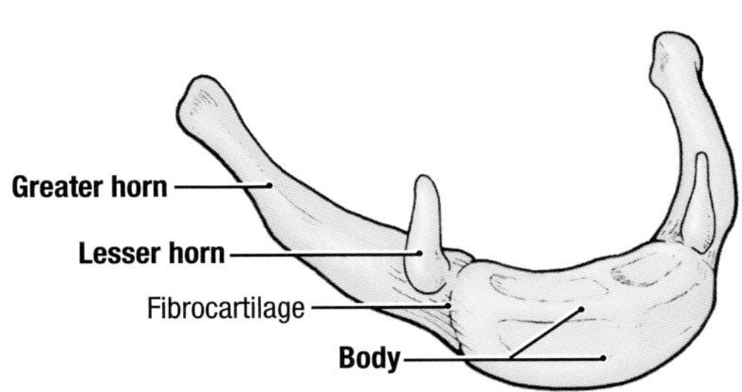
Greater horn
Lesser horn
Fibrocartilage
Body

C. Right Anterolateral View of Hyoid

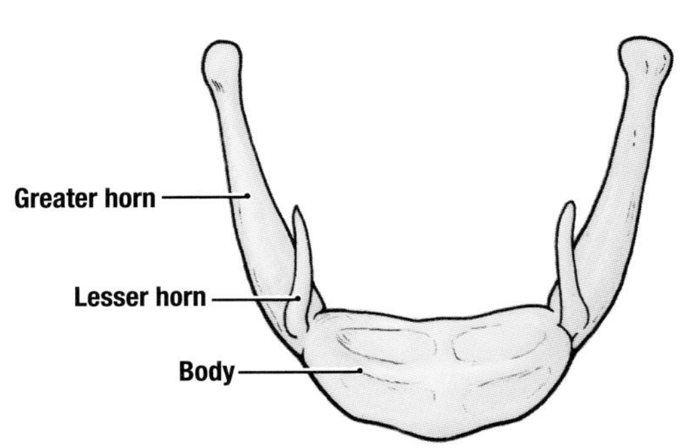
Greater horn
Lesser horn
Body

D. Anterosuperior View of Hyoid

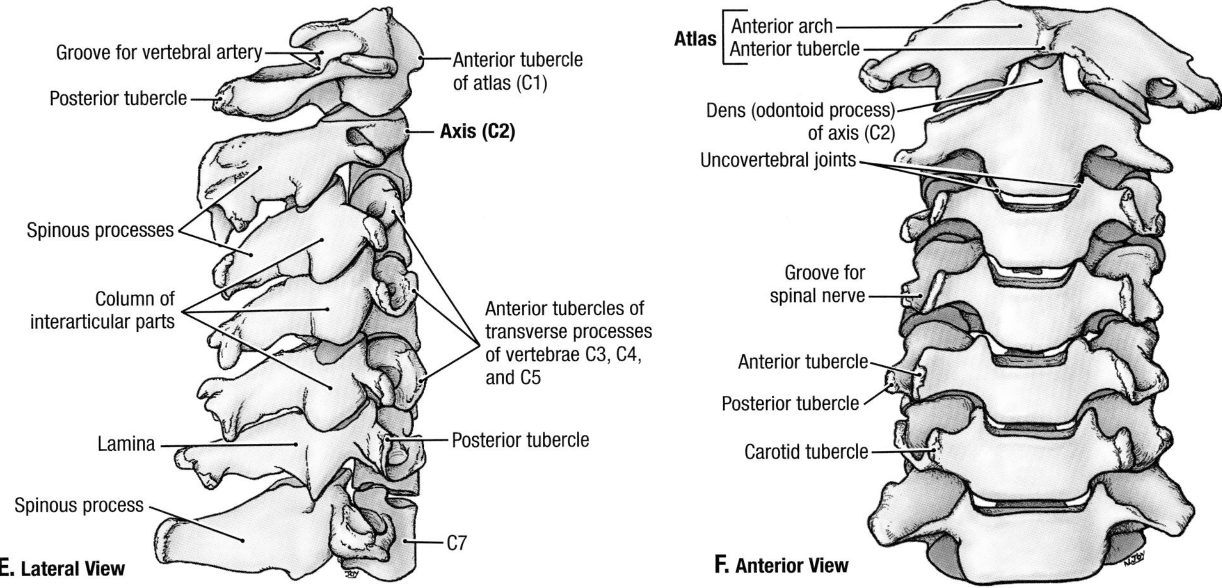
Groove for vertebral artery
Posterior tubercle
Anterior tubercle of atlas (C1)
Axis (C2)
Spinous processes
Column of interarticular parts
Anterior tubercles of transverse processes of vertebrae C3, C4, and C5
Lamina
Posterior tubercle
Spinous process
C7
Atlas
Anterior arch
Anterior tubercle
Dens (odontoid process) of axis (C2)
Uncovertebral joints
Groove for spinal nerve
Anterior tubercle
Posterior tubercle
Carotid tubercle

E. Lateral View

F. Anterior View

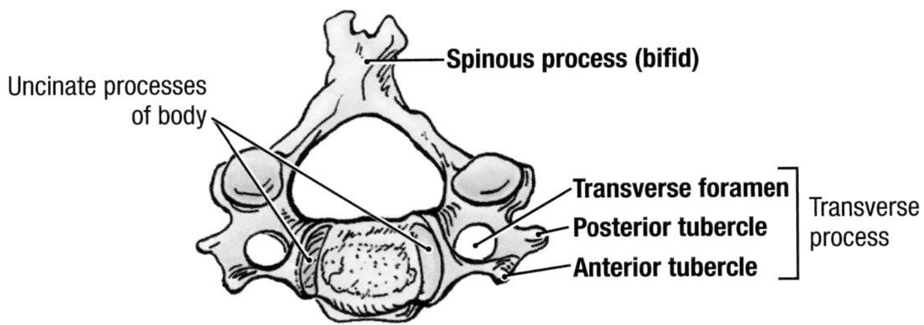
Uncinate processes of body
Spinous process (bifid)
Transverse foramen
Posterior tubercle
Anterior tubercle
Transverse process

G. Superior View of Typical Cervical Vertebra (e.g., C4)

## 8.4 Bones and cartilages of the neck *(continued)*

**C** and **D.** Features of hyoid bone. **E** and **F.** Articulated cervical vertebrae. **G.** Features of typical cervical vertebrae.

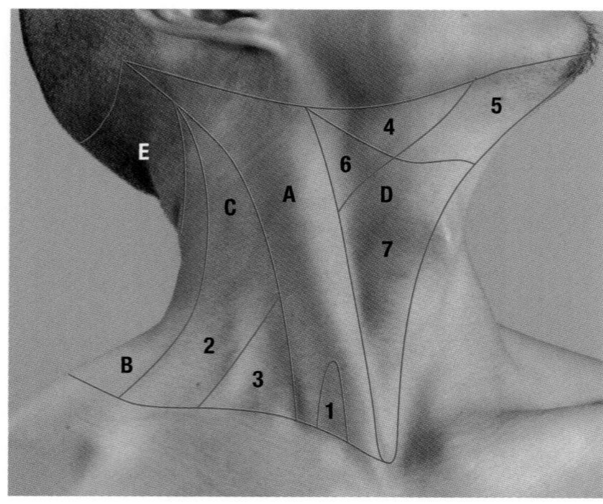

E
C
A
6
4
5
D
7
B
2
3
1


**A** Anterolateral view

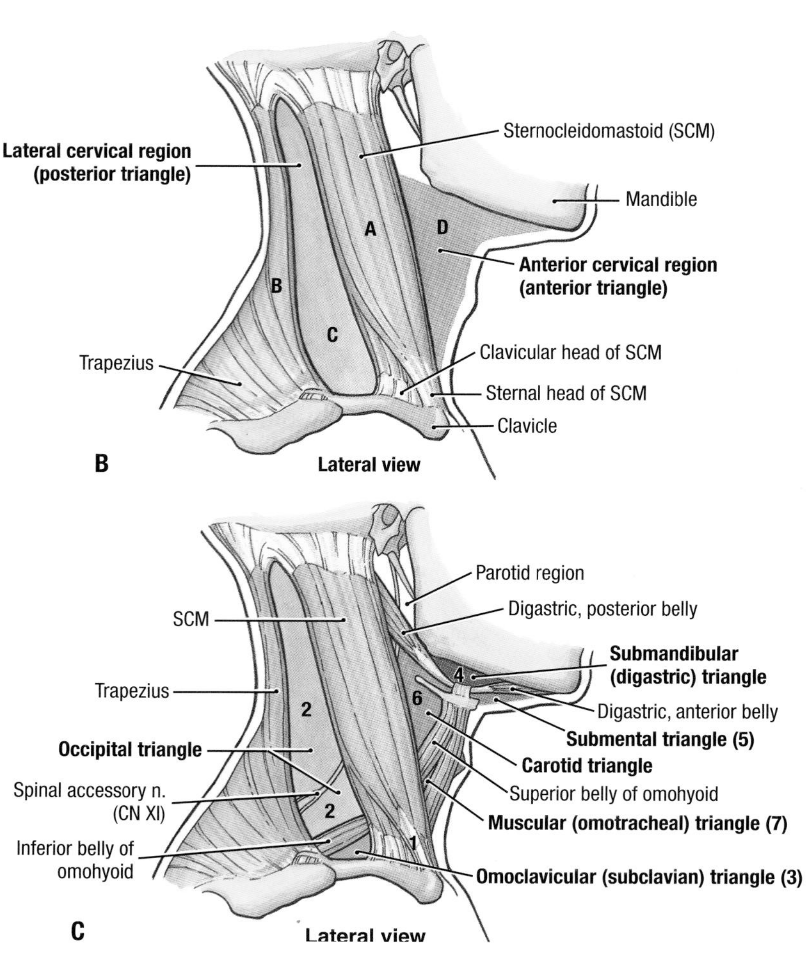

Lateral cervical region (posterior triangle)
Sternocleidomastoid (SCM)
Mandible
A
D
Anterior cervical region (anterior triangle)
B
C
Trapezius
Clavicular head of SCM
Sternal head of SCM
Clavicle
Lateral view
Parotid region
Digastric, posterior belly
SCM
Submandibular (digastric) triangle
Trapezius
Digastric, anterior belly
Submental triangle (5)
Occipital triangle
Carotid triangle
Spinal accessory n. (CN XI)
Superior belly of omohyoid
Muscular (omotracheal) triangle (7)
Inferior belly of omohyoid
Omoclavicular (subclavian) triangle (3)
Lateral view


**B**

**C**

**TABLE 8.2 CERVICAL REGIONS AND CONTENTS**[a]

| Region | Main Contents and Underlying Structures |
|---|---|
| **Sternocleidomastoid region** *(A)* | Sternocleidomastoid (SCM) muscle; superior part of the external jugular vein; greater auricular nerve; transverse cervical nerve |
| Lesser supraclavicular fossa *(1)* | Inferior part of internal jugular vein |
| **Posterior cervical region** *(B)* | Trapezius muscle; cutaneous branches of posterior rami of cervical spinal nerves; suboccipital region (E) lies deep to superior part of this region |
| **Lateral cervical region (posterior triangle)** *(C)* | |
| Occipital triangle *(2)* | Part of external jugular vein; posterior branches of cervical plexus of nerves; spinal accessory nerve; trunks of brachial plexus; transverse cervical artery; cervical lymph nodes |
| Omoclavicular triangle | Subclavian artery (3rd part); part of subclavian vein (variable); suprascapular artery; supraclavicular lymph nodes |
| **Anterior cervical region (anterior triangle)** *(D)* | |
| Submandibular (digastric) triangle *(4)* | Submandibular gland almost fills triangle; submandibular lymph nodes; hypoglossal nerve; mylohyoid nerve; parts of facial artery and vein |
| Submental triangle *(5)* | Submental lymph nodes and small veins that unite to form anterior jugular vein |
| Carotid triangle *(6)* | Common carotid artery and its branches; internal jugular vein and its tributaries; vagus nerve; external carotid artery and some of its branches; hypoglossal nerve and superior root of ansa cervicalis; spinal accessory nerve; thyroid gland, larynx, and pharynx; deep cervical lymph nodes; branches of cervical plexus |
| **Muscular (omotracheal) triangle** *(7)* | Sternothyroid and sternohyoid muscles; thyroid and parathyroid glands |

[a]Letters and numbers in parentheses refer to Figures A and B.

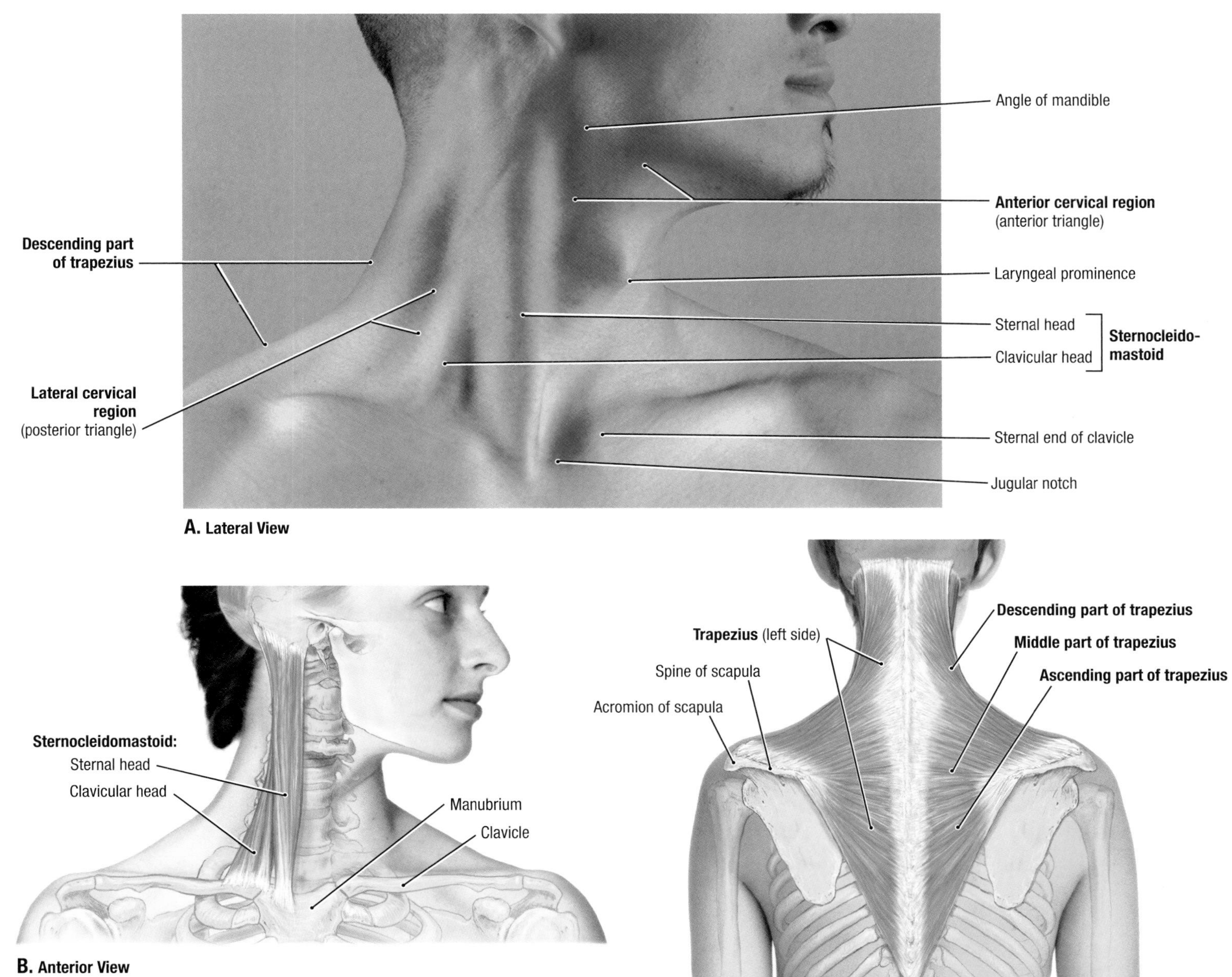

Angle of mandible
Anterior cervical region (anterior triangle)
Descending part of trapezius
Laryngeal prominence
Sternal head
Clavicular head
Sternocleido-mastoid
Lateral cervical region (posterior triangle)
Sternal end of clavicle
Jugular notch
Sternocleidomastoid:
Sternal head
Clavicular head
Manubrium
Clavicle
Trapezius (left side)
Spine of scapula
Acromion of scapula
Descending part of trapezius
Middle part of trapezius
Ascending part of trapezius


**A.** Lateral View

**B.** Anterior View

**C.** Posterior View

## TABLE 8.3 STERNOCLEIDOMASTOID AND TRAPEZIUS

| Muscle | Superior Attachment | Inferior Attachment | Innervation | Main Action |
|---|---|---|---|---|
| **Sternocleidomastoid** | Lateral surface of mastoid process of temporal bone; lateral half of superior nuchal line | *Sternal head:* anterior surface of manubrium of sternum *Clavicular head:* superior surface of medial third of clavicle | Spinal accessory nerve (CN XI) [motor] and C2 and C3 nerves (pain and proprioception) | *Unilateral contraction:* laterally flexes neck; rotates neck so face is turned superiorly toward opposite side; *Bilateral contraction:* (1) extends neck at atlanto-occipital joints, (2) flexes cervical vertebrae so that chin approaches manubrium, or (3) extends superior cervical vertebrae while flexing inferior vertebrae, so chin is thrust forward with head kept level; with cervical vertebrae fixed, may elevate manubrium and medial end of clavicles, assisting deep respiration. |
| **Trapezius** | Medial third of superior nuchal line, external occipital protuberance, nuchal ligament, spinous processes of C7–T12 vertebrae, lumbar and sacral spinous processes | Lateral third of clavicle, acromion, spine of scapula | Spinal accessory nerve (CN XI) [motor] and C2 and C3 nerves (pain and proprioception) | *Superior fibers* elevate pectoral girdle, maintain level of shoulders against gravity or resistance; *middle fibers* retract scapula; and *inferior fibers* depress shoulders; *superior* and *inferior fibers* work together to rotate scapula upward; *when shoulders are fixed*, bilateral contraction extends neck; unilateral contraction produces lateral flexion to same |

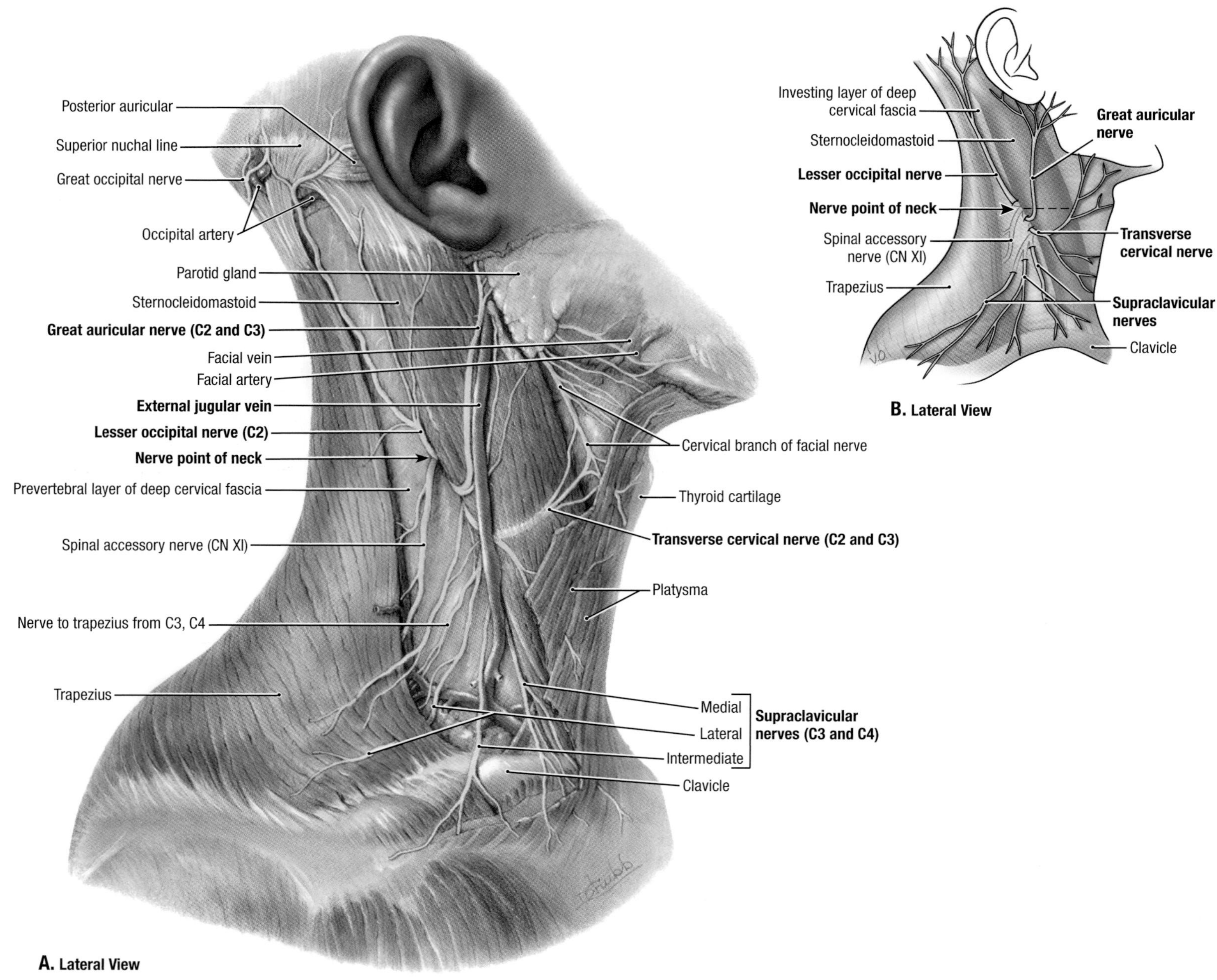
Posterior auricular
Superior nuchal line
Great occipital nerve
Occipital artery
Parotid gland
Sternocleidomastoid
Great auricular nerve (C2 and C3)
Facial vein
Facial artery
External jugular vein
Lesser occipital nerve (C2)
Nerve point of neck
Prevertebral layer of deep cervical fascia
Spinal accessory nerve (CN XI)
Nerve to trapezius from C3, C4
Trapezius
Cervical branch of facial nerve
Thyroid cartilage
Transverse cervical nerve (C2 and C3)
Platysma
Medial
Lateral
Intermediate
Supraclavicular nerves (C3 and C4)
Clavicle
A. Lateral View
Investing layer of deep cervical fascia
Sternocleidomastoid
Lesser occipital nerve
Nerve point of neck
Spinal accessory nerve (CN XI)
Trapezius
Great auricular nerve
Transverse cervical nerve
Supraclavicular nerves
Clavicle
B. Lateral View

## 8.5 Serial dissection of lateral cervical region (posterior triangle of neck)

**A.** External jugular vein and cutaneous branches of cervical plexus. Subcutaneous fat, the part of the plasma overlying the inferior part of the lateral cervical region, and the investing layer of deep cervical fascia have all been removed. The external jugular vein descends vertically across the sternocleidomastoid and pierces the prevertebral layer of deep cervical fascia superior to the clavicle.

**B** and **C.** Branches of the cervical plexus

- Branches arising from the nerve loop between the anterior rami of C2 and C3 are the lesser occipital, great auricular, and transverse cervical nerves.
- Branches arising from the loop formed between the anterior rami of C3 and C4 are the supraclavicular nerves, which emerge as a common trunk under cover of the SCM.

Regional anesthesia is often used for surgical procedures in the neck region or upper limb. In a cervical plexus block, an anesthetic agent is injected at several points along the posterior border of the SCM, mainly at its midpoint, the nerve point of the neck.

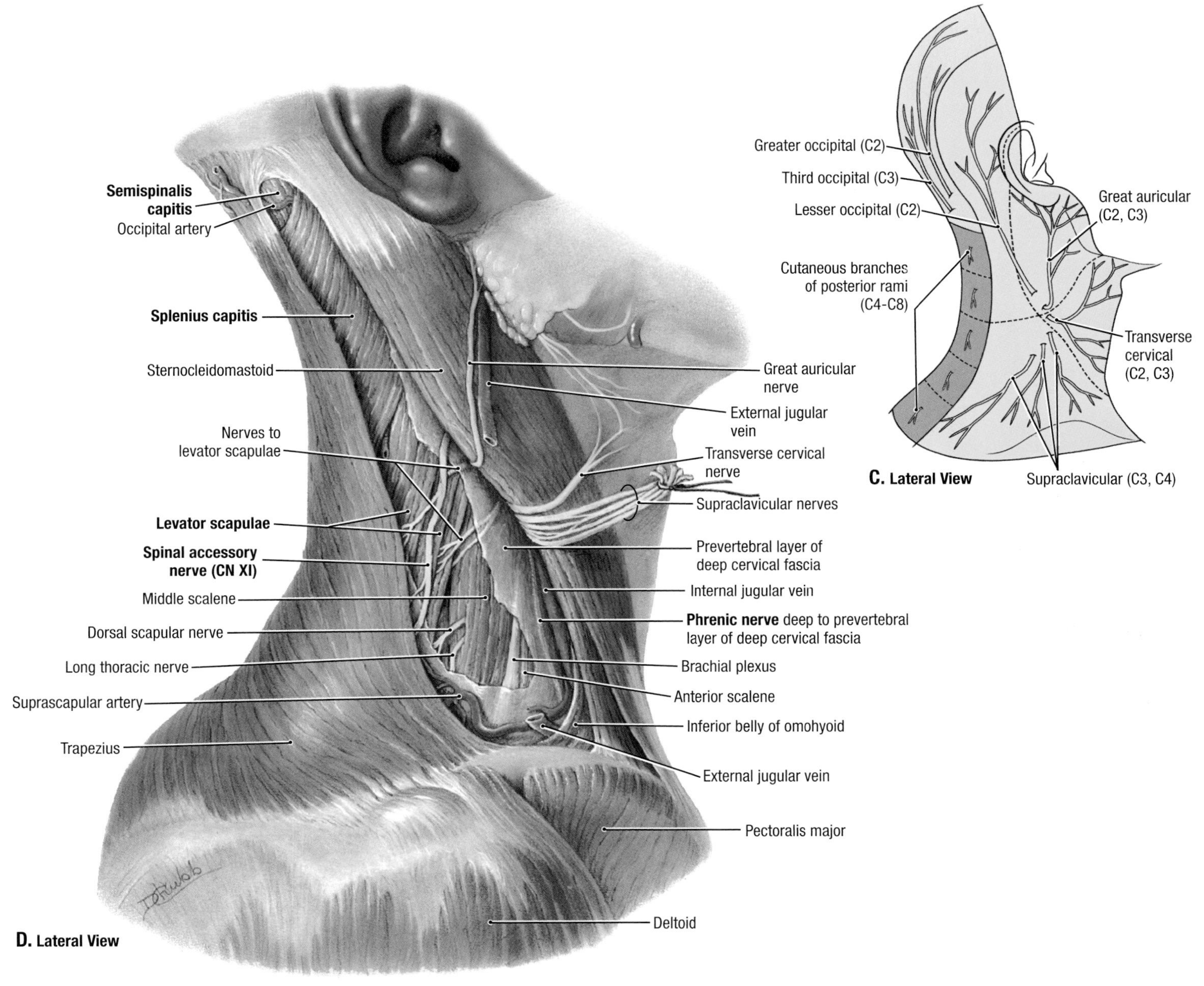
Semispinalis capitis
Occipital artery
Splenius capitis
Sternocleidomastoid
Nerves to levator scapulae
Levator scapulae
Spinal accessory nerve (CN XI)
Middle scalene
Dorsal scapular nerve
Long thoracic nerve
Suprascapular artery
Trapezius
Great auricular nerve
External jugular vein
Transverse cervical nerve
Supraclavicular nerves
Prevertebral layer of deep cervical fascia
Internal jugular vein
Phrenic nerve deep to prevertebral layer of deep cervical fascia
Brachial plexus
Anterior scalene
Inferior belly of omohyoid
External jugular vein
Pectoralis major
Deltoid
D. Lateral View
Greater occipital (C2)
Third occipital (C3)
Lesser occipital (C2)
Cutaneous branches of posterior rami (C4-C8)
Great auricular (C2, C3)
Transverse cervical (C2, C3)
Supraclavicular (C3, C4)
C. Lateral View

## 8.5 Serial dissection of lateral cervical region *(continued)*

**D.** Muscles forming the floor of the lateral cervical region. The prevertebral layer of deep cervical fascia has been partially removed, and the motor nerves and most of the floor of the region are exposed.

- The spinal accessory nerve (CN XI) supplies the SCM and trapezius muscles; between them, it courses along the levator scapulae muscle but is separated from it by the prevertebral layer of deep cervical fascia.
- The phrenic nerve (C3, C4, C5) supplies the diaphragm and is located deep to the prevertebral layer of deep cervical fascia on the anterior surface of the anterior scalene muscle.

Severance of a phrenic nerve results in an ipsilateral paralysis of the diaphragm. A phrenic nerve block produces a short period of paralysis of the diaphragm on one side (e.g., for a lung operation). The anesthetic agent is injected around the nerve where it lies on the anterior surface of the anterior scalene muscle.

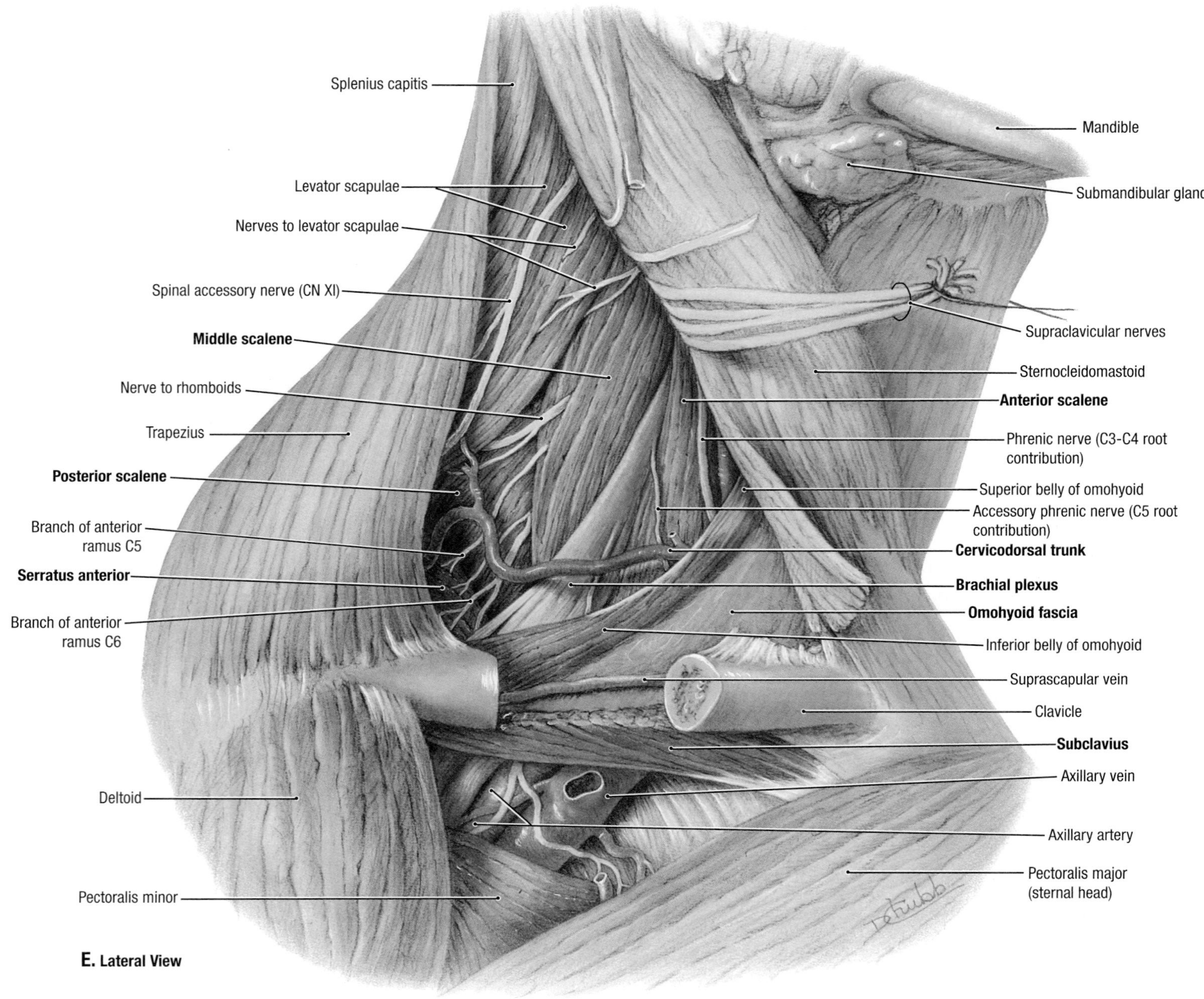
Splenius capitis
Mandible
Submandibular gland
Levator scapulae
Nerves to levator scapulae
Spinal accessory nerve (CN XI)
Supraclavicular nerves
Middle scalene
Sternocleidomastoid
Nerve to rhomboids
Anterior scalene
Trapezius
Phrenic nerve (C3-C4 root contribution)
Posterior scalene
Superior belly of omohyoid
Accessory phrenic nerve (C5 root contribution)
Branch of anterior ramus C5
Cervicodorsal trunk
Serratus anterior
Brachial plexus
Branch of anterior ramus C6
Omohyoid fascia
Inferior belly of omohyoid
Suprascapular vein
Clavicle
Subclavius
Axillary vein
Deltoid
Axillary artery
Pectoralis major (sternal head)
Pectoralis minor
E. Lateral View

## 8.5 Serial dissection of lateral cervical region *(continued)*

**E.** Vessels and motor nerves of the lateral cervical region. The clavicular head of the pectoralis major muscle and part of the clavicle have been removed.

The muscles that form the floor of the region are the semispinalis capitis, splenius capitis and levator scapulae superiorly and the anterior middle and posterior scalenes and serratus anterior inferiorly.

- The brachial plexus emerges between the anterior and middle scalene muscles.

A supraclavicular brachial plexus block may be utilized for anesthesia of the upper limb. The anesthetic agent is injected around the supraclavicular part of the brachial plexus. The main injection site is superior to the midpoint of the clavicle.

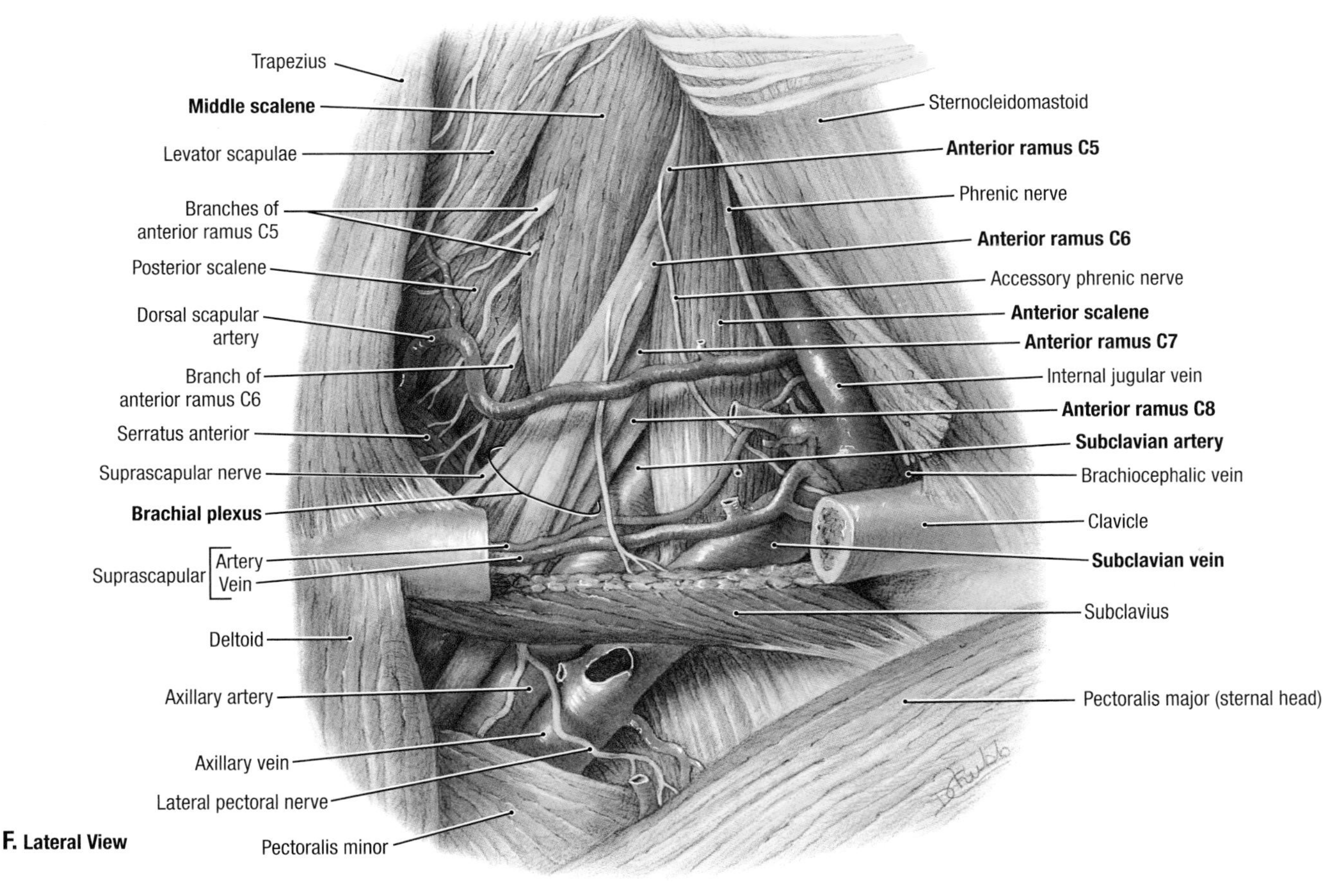
Trapezius
Middle scalene
Levator scapulae
Branches of anterior ramus C5
Posterior scalene
Dorsal scapular artery
Branch of anterior ramus C6
Serratus anterior
Suprascapular nerve
Brachial plexus
Suprascapular Artery
Vein
Deltoid
Axillary artery
Axillary vein
Lateral pectoral nerve
Pectoralis minor
Sternocleidomastoid
Anterior ramus C5
Phrenic nerve
Anterior ramus C6
Accessory phrenic nerve
Anterior scalene
Anterior ramus C7
Internal jugular vein
Anterior ramus C8
Subclavian artery
Brachiocephalic vein
Clavicle
Subclavian vein
Subclavius
Pectoralis major (sternal head)

**F. Lateral View**

## 8.5 Serial dissection of lateral cervical region *(continued)*

**F.** Structures of the omoclavicular (subclavian) triangle. The omohyoid muscle and fascia have been removed, exposing the brachial plexus and subclavian vessels.

- The anterior rami of C5–T1 form the brachial plexus (the anterior ramus of T1 lies posterior to the subclavian artery.
- The brachial plexus and subclavian artery emerge between the middle and anterior scalene muscles.
- The anterior scalene muscle lies between the subclavian artery and vein.

The right or left subclavian vein is often the site of placement for a central venous catheter, used to insert intravenous tubes ("central venous lines") for the administration of parenteral nutritional fluids or medications, for testing blood chemistry or central venous pressure, or inserting electrode wires for heart pacemaker devices. The relationships of the subclavian vein to the sternocleidomastoid muscle, clavicle, sternoclavicular joint and 1st rib are of clinical importance in line placement, and there is danger of puncture of the pleura or subclavian artery if the procedure is not performed correctly.

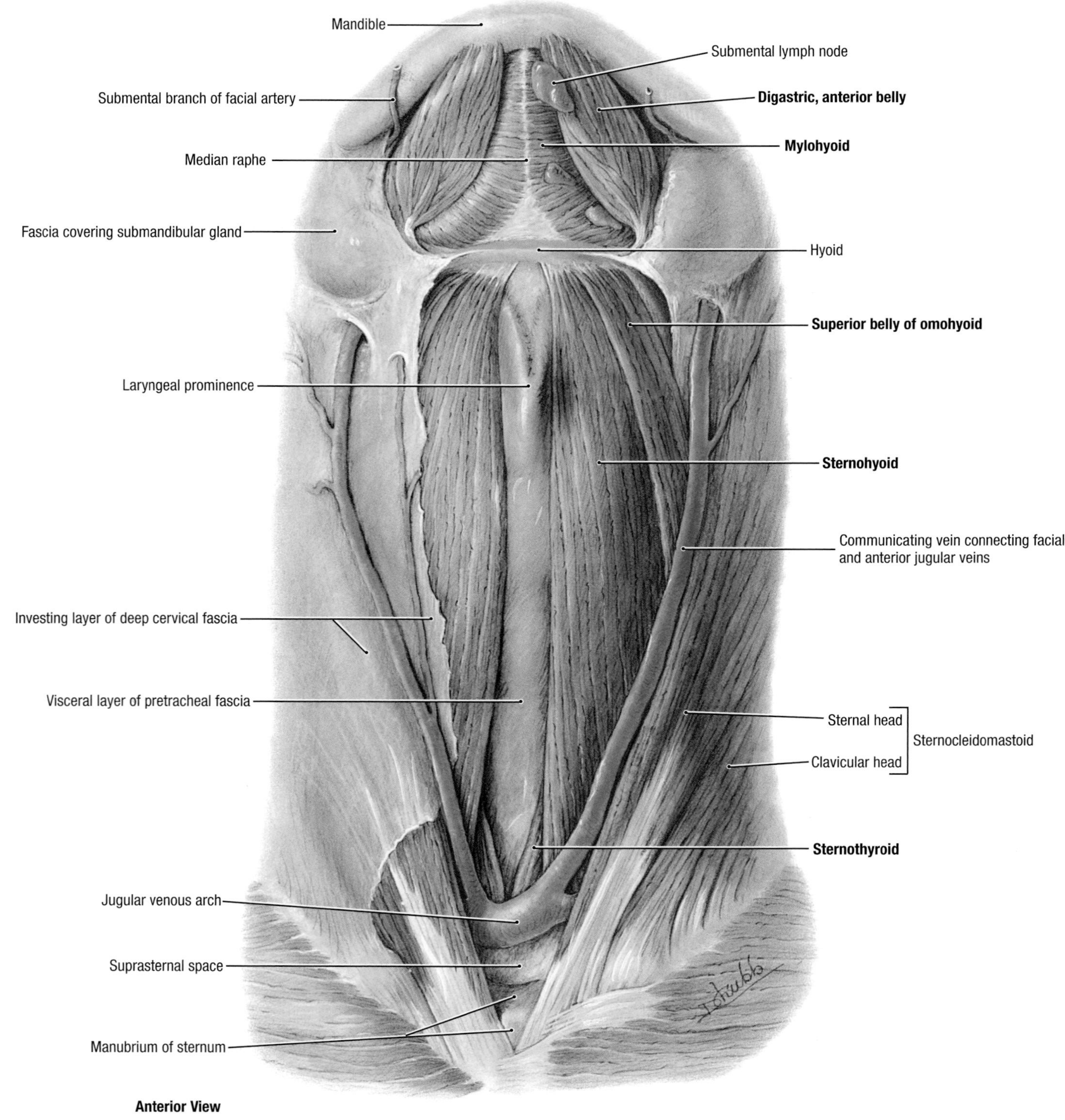

Mandible
Submental lymph node
Submental branch of facial artery
Digastric, anterior belly
Median raphe
Mylohyoid
Fascia covering submandibular gland
Hyoid
Superior belly of omohyoid
Laryngeal prominence
Sternohyoid
Communicating vein connecting facial and anterior jugular veins
Investing layer of deep cervical fascia
Visceral layer of pretracheal fascia
Sternal head
Sternocleidomastoid
Clavicular head
Sternothyroid
Jugular venous arch
Suprasternal space
Manubrium of sternum
Anterior View


## 8.6 Supra- and infrahyoid muscles

Much of the investing layer of deep cervical fascia has been removed.

- The anterior bellies of the digastric muscles form the sides of the suprahyoid part of the anterior cervical region, or submental triangle (floor of mouth). The hyoid bone forms the triangle's base, and the mylohyoid muscles are its floor.
- The infrahyoid part of the anterior cervical region is shaped like an elongated diamond bounded by the sternohyoid muscle superiorly and sternothyroid muscle inferiorly.

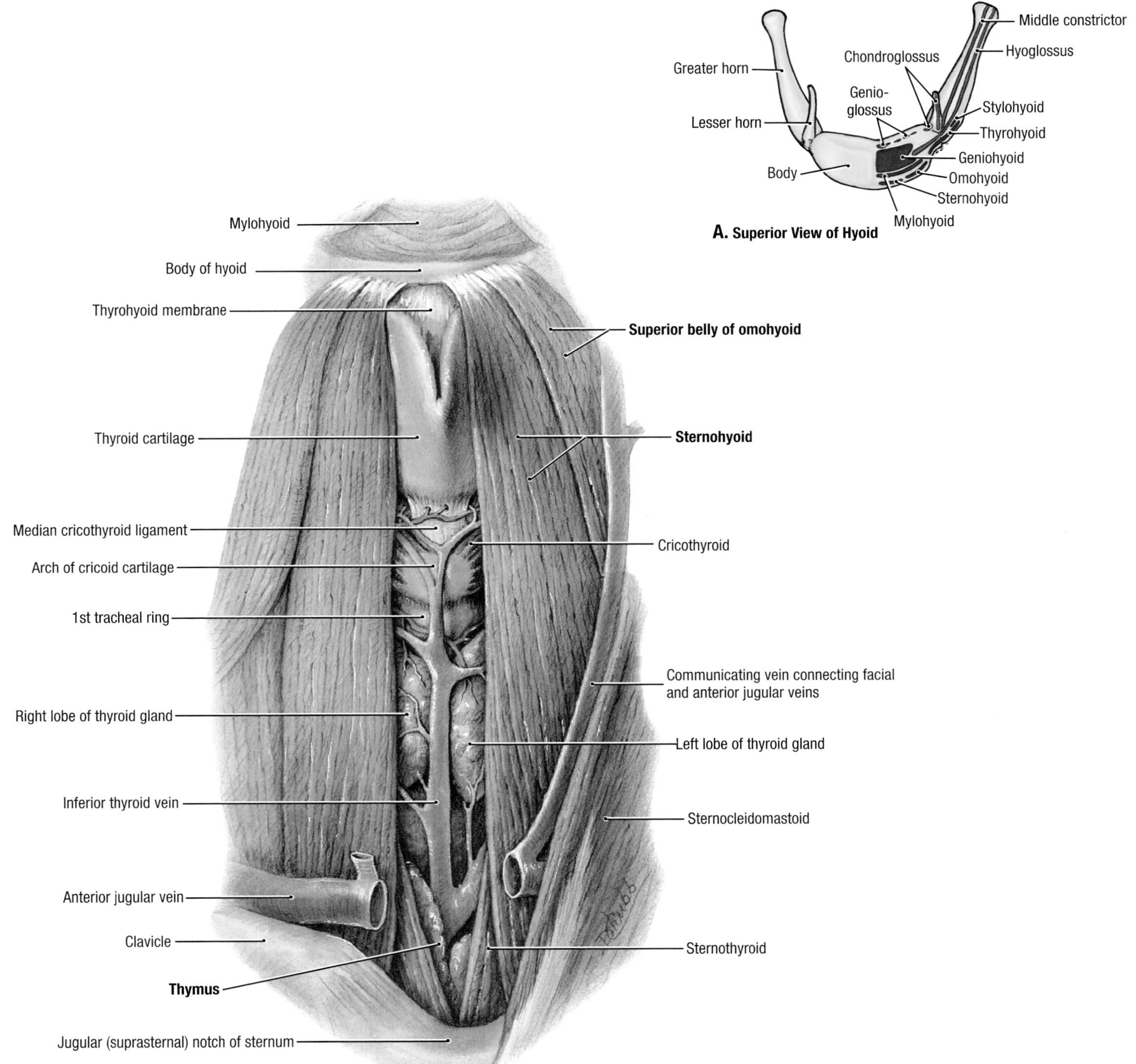
Middle constrictor
Hyoglossus
Chondroglossus
Greater horn
Genio-
glossus
Lesser horn
Stylohyoid
Thyrohyoid
Geniohyoid
Body
Omohyoid
Sternohyoid
Mylohyoid
A. Superior View of Hyoid
Mylohyoid
Body of hyoid
Thyrohyoid membrane
Superior belly of omohyoid
Thyroid cartilage
Sternohyoid
Median cricothyroid ligament
Cricothyroid
Arch of cricoid cartilage
1st tracheal ring
Communicating vein connecting facial
and anterior jugular veins
Right lobe of thyroid gland
Left lobe of thyroid gland
Inferior thyroid vein
Sternocleidomastoid
Anterior jugular vein
Clavicle
Sternothyroid
Thymus
Jugular (suprasternal) notch of sternum
B. Anterior View

## 8.7 Infrahyoid region, superficial muscular layer

**A.** Muscular attachments onto the hyoid bone.

**B.** The pretracheal fascia, right anterior jugular vein, and jugular venous arch have been removed.

- A persistent thymus projects superiorly from the thorax.
- The two superficial depressors of the larynx ("strap muscles") are the omohyoid (only the superior belly of which is seen here) and sternohyoid.

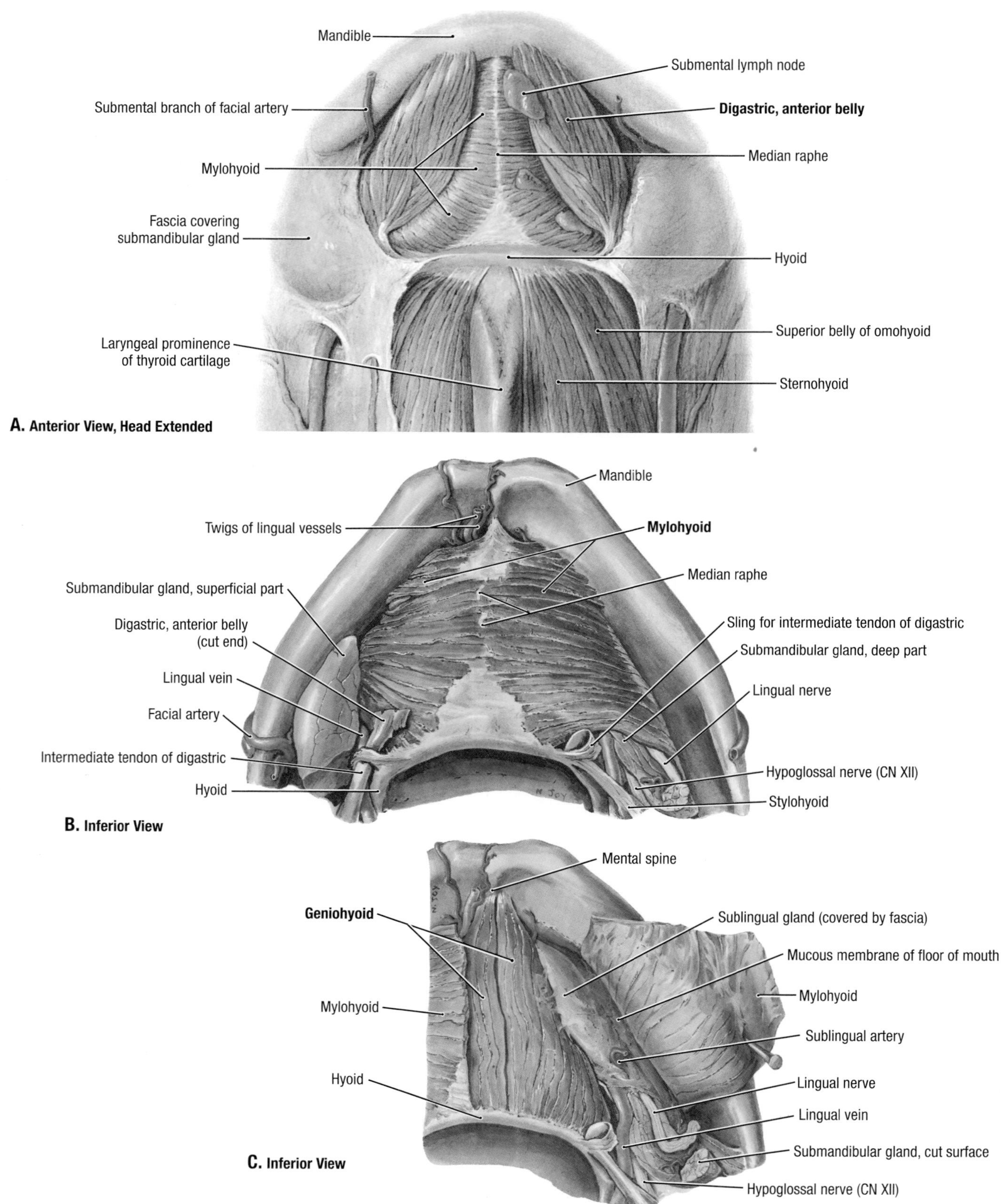
Mandible
Submental lymph node
Submental branch of facial artery
Digastric, anterior belly
Mylohyoid
Median raphe
Fascia covering submandibular gland
Hyoid
Superior belly of omohyoid
Laryngeal prominence of thyroid cartilage
Sternohyoid
A. Anterior View, Head Extended
Mandible
Twigs of lingual vessels
Mylohyoid
Median raphe
Submandibular gland, superficial part
Digastric, anterior belly (cut end)
Sling for intermediate tendon of digastric
Submandibular gland, deep part
Lingual vein
Lingual nerve
Facial artery
Intermediate tendon of digastric
Hypoglossal nerve (CN XII)
Hyoid
Stylohyoid
B. Inferior View
Mental spine
Geniohyoid
Sublingual gland (covered by fascia)
Mucous membrane of floor of mouth
Mylohyoid
Mylohyoid
Sublingual artery
Hyoid
Lingual nerve
Lingual vein
Submandibular gland, cut surface
Hypoglossal nerve (CN XII)
C. Inferior View

## 8.8 Suprahyoid region (submental triangle)

**A.** Superficial layer—anterior belly of digastric. **B.** Intermediate layer—mylohyoid muscles. **C.** Deep layer—geniohyoid muscles.

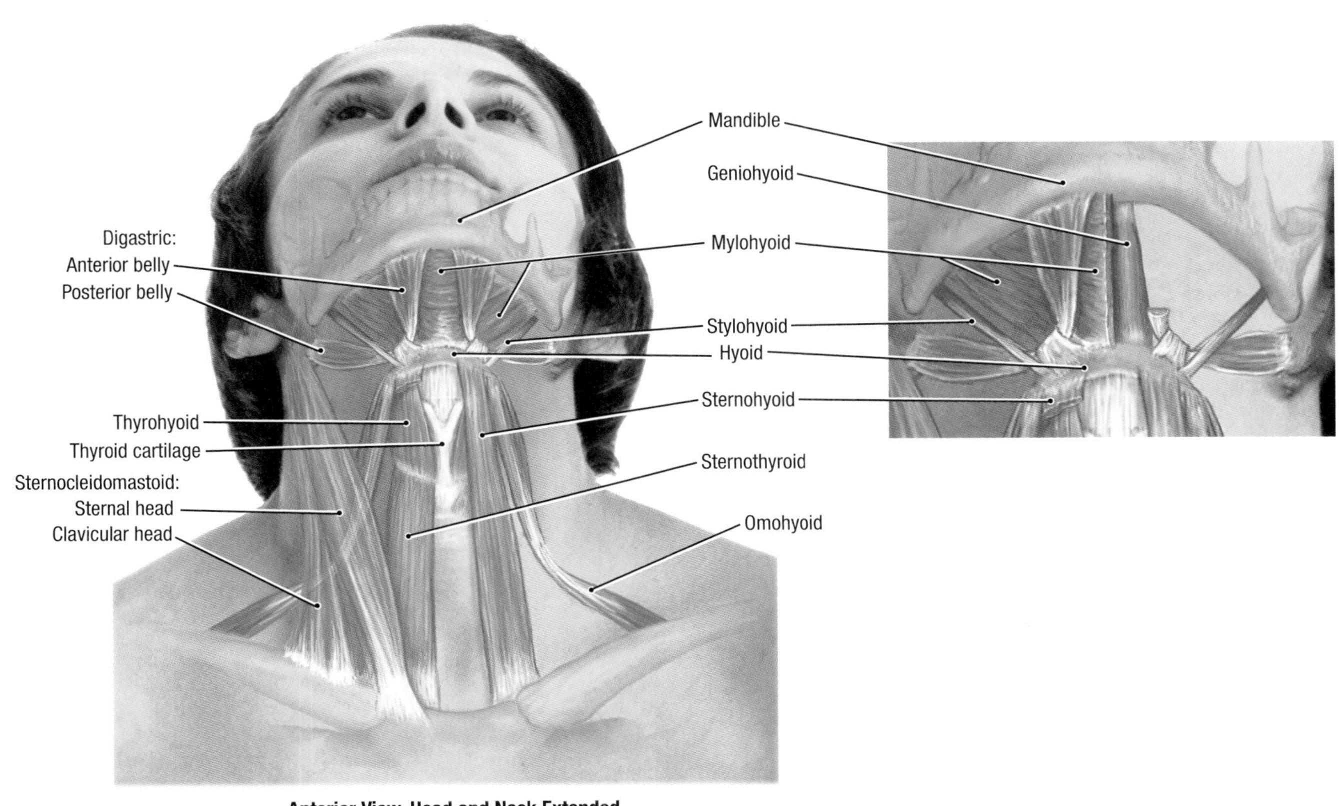
Digastric:
Anterior belly
Posterior belly
Thyrohyoid
Thyroid cartilage
Sternocleidomastoid:
Sternal head
Clavicular head
Mandible
Geniohyoid
Mylohyoid
Stylohyoid
Hyoid
Sternohyoid
Sternothyroid
Omohyoid

Anterior View, Head and Neck Extended

### TABLE 8.4 SUPRAHYOID AND INFRAHYOID MUSCLES

| Muscle | Origin | Insertion | Innervation | Main Action |
|---|---|---|---|---|
| **Suprahyoid muscles** | | | | |
| Mylohyoid | Mylohyoid line of mandible | Raphe and body of hyoid bone | Nerve to mylohyoid, a branch of inferior alveolar nerve (CN $V^3$) | Elevates hyoid bone, floor of mouth and tongue during swallowing and speaking |
| Digastric | *Anterior belly:* digastric fossa of mandible<br>*Posterior belly:* mastoid notch of temporal bone | Intermediate tendon to body and greater horn of hyoid bone | *Anterior belly:* nerve to mylohyoid, a branch of inferior alveolar nerve (CN $V^3$)<br>*Posterior belly:* facial nerve (CN VII) | Elevates hyoid bone and steadies it during swallowing and speaking; depresses mandible against resistance |
| Geniohyoid | Inferior mental spine of mandible | Body of hyoid bone | C1 via the hypoglossal nerve (CN XII) | Pulls hyoid bone anterosuperiorly, shortens floor of mouth, and widens pharynx |
| Stylohyoid | Styloid process of temporal bone | | Cervical branch of facial nerve (CN VII) | Elevates and retracts hyoid bone, thereby elongating floor of mouth |
| **Infrahyoid muscles** | | | | |
| Sternohyoid | Manubrium of sternum and medial end of clavicle | Body of hyoid bone | C1–C3 by a branch of ansa cervicalis | Depresses hyoid bone after it has been elevated during swallowing |
| Omohyoid | Superior border of scapula near suprascapular notch | Inferior border of hyoid bone | | Depresses, retracts, and steadies hyoid bone |
| Sternothyroid | Posterior surface of manubrium of sternum | Oblique line of thyroid cartilage | C2 and C3 by a branch of ansa cervicalis | Depresses hyoid bone and larynx |
| Thyrohyoid | Oblique line of thyroid cartilage | Inferior border of body and greater horn of hyoid bone | C1 via hypoglossal nerve (CN XII) | Depresses hyoid bone and elevates larynx |

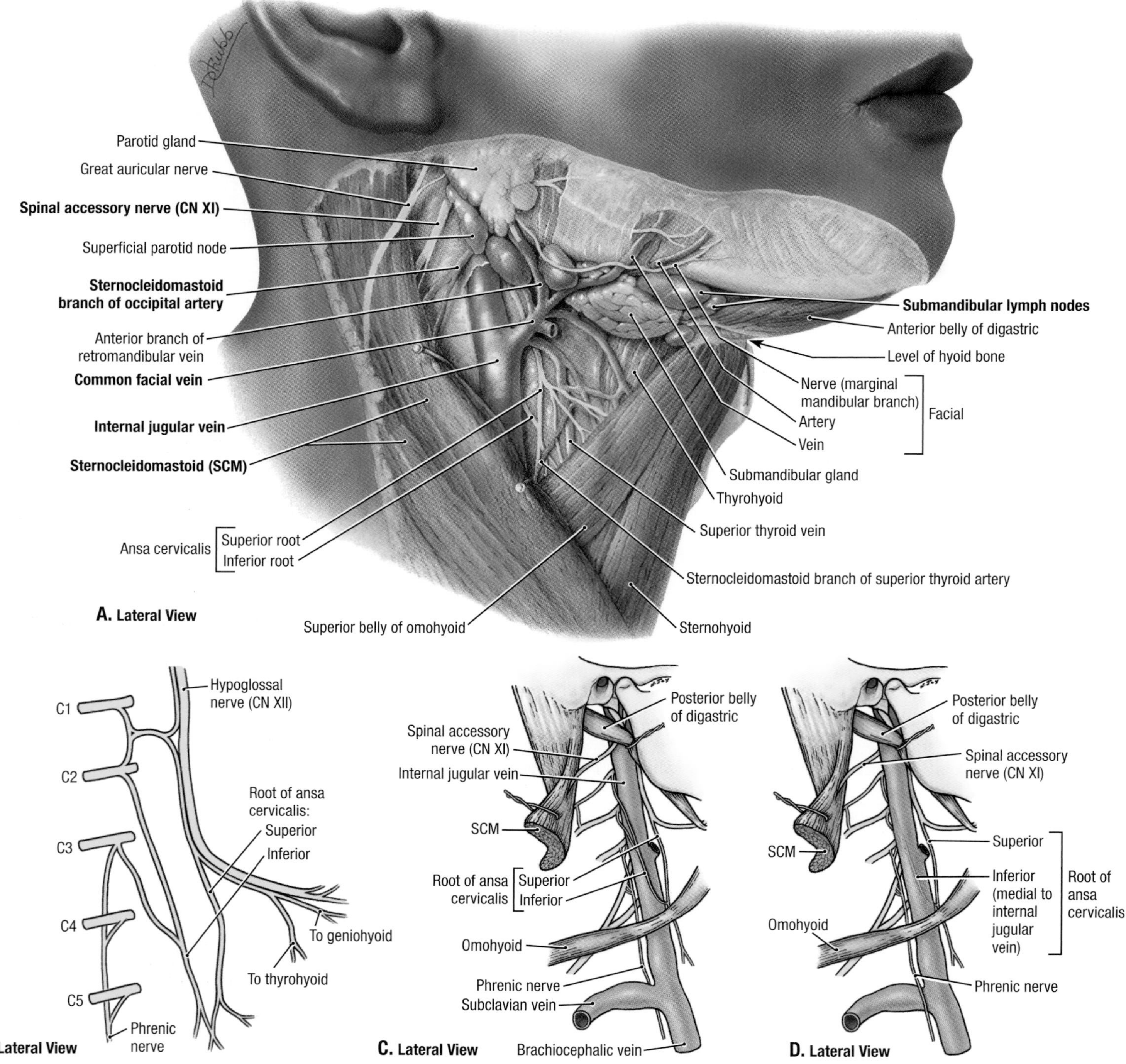
Parotid gland
Great auricular nerve
Spinal accessory nerve (CN XI)
Superficial parotid node
Sternocleidomastoid branch of occipital artery
Anterior branch of retromandibular vein
Common facial vein
Internal jugular vein
Sternocleidomastoid (SCM)
Ansa cervicalis
Superior root
Inferior root
A. Lateral View
Superior belly of omohyoid
Submandibular lymph nodes
Anterior belly of digastric
Level of hyoid bone
Nerve (marginal mandibular branch)
Artery
Vein
Facial
Submandibular gland
Thyrohyoid
Superior thyroid vein
Sternocleidomastoid branch of superior thyroid artery
Sternohyoid
C1
C2
C3
C4
C5
Hypoglossal nerve (CN XII)
Root of ansa cervicalis:
Superior
Inferior
To geniohyoid
To thyrohyoid
Phrenic nerve
B. Lateral View
Spinal accessory nerve (CN XI)
Internal jugular vein
Posterior belly of digastric
SCM
Root of ansa cervicalis
Superior
Inferior
Omohyoid
Phrenic nerve
Subclavian vein
Brachiocephalic vein
C. Lateral View
Posterior belly of digastric
Spinal accessory nerve (CN XI)
SCM
Superior
Inferior (medial to internal jugular vein)
Root of ansa cervicalis
Omohyoid
Phrenic nerve
D. Lateral View

## 8.9 Superficial dissection of carotid triangle

**A.** The skin, subcutaneous tissue (with platysma), and the investing layer of deep cervical fascia, including the sheaths of the parotid and submandibular glands, have been removed.

- The spinal accessory nerve (XI) enters the deep surface of the sternocleidomastoid muscle and is joined along its anterior border by the sternocleidomastoid branch of the occipital artery.
- The (common) facial vein joins the internal jugular vein near the level of the hyoid bone; here, the facial vein is joined by several other veins.
- The submandibular lymph nodes lie deep to the investing layer of deep cervical fascia in the submandibular triangle; some of the nodes lie deep in the submandibular gland.

**B.** Diagram of the motor branches of cervical plexus.

**C.** Typical relationships of ansa cervicalis, spinal accessory nerve (CN XI), and phrenic nerve to the internal jugular and subclavian veins.

**D.** Atypical relationships.

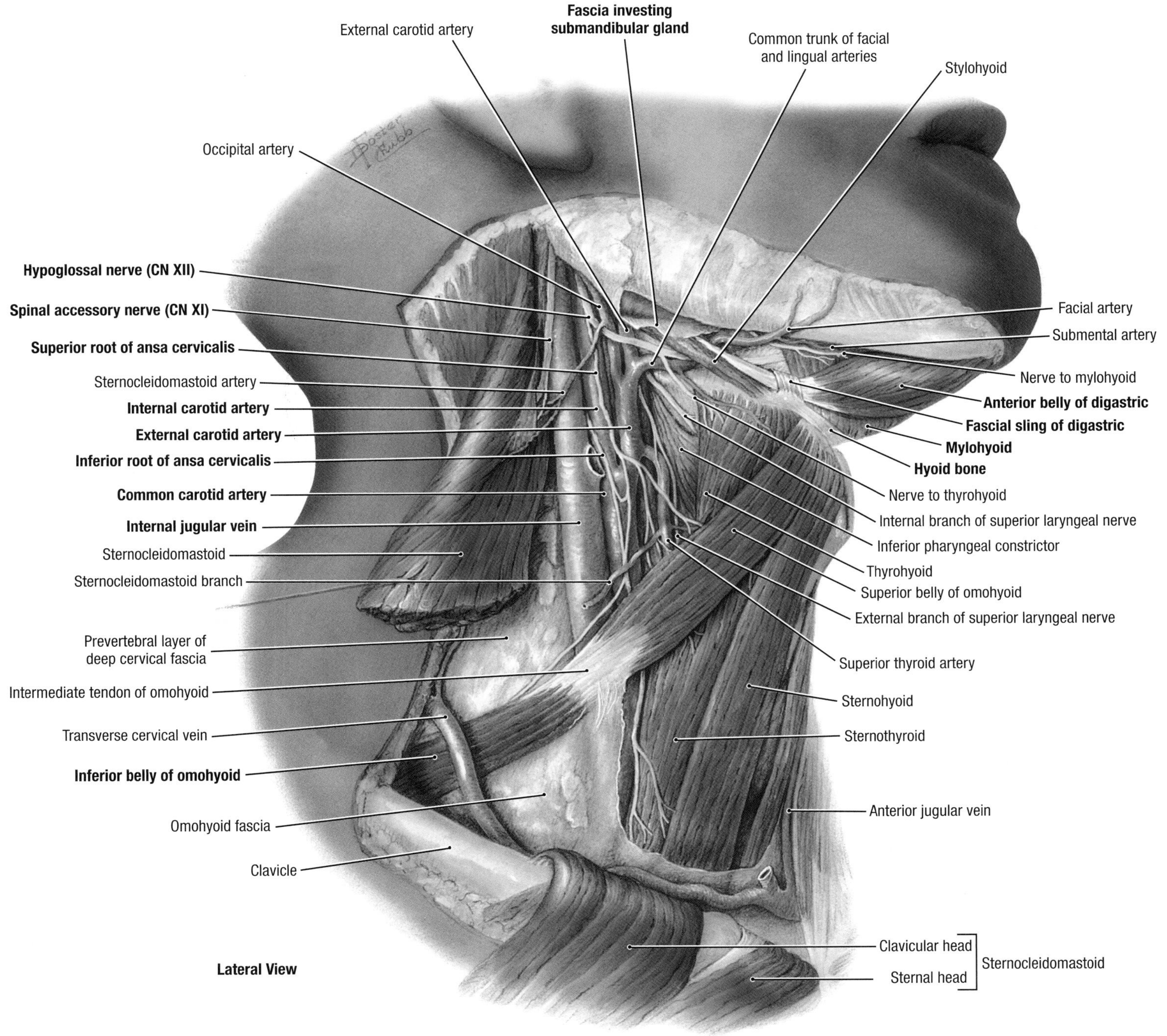
External carotid artery
Fascia investing submandibular gland
Common trunk of facial and lingual arteries
Stylohyoid
Occipital artery
Hypoglossal nerve (CN XII)
Spinal accessory nerve (CN XI)
Superior root of ansa cervicalis
Sternocleidomastoid artery
Internal carotid artery
External carotid artery
Inferior root of ansa cervicalis
Common carotid artery
Internal jugular vein
Sternocleidomastoid
Sternocleidomastoid branch
Prevertebral layer of deep cervical fascia
Intermediate tendon of omohyoid
Transverse cervical vein
Inferior belly of omohyoid
Omohyoid fascia
Clavicle
Lateral View
Facial artery
Submental artery
Nerve to mylohyoid
Anterior belly of digastric
Fascial sling of digastric
Mylohyoid
Hyoid bone
Nerve to thyrohyoid
Internal branch of superior laryngeal nerve
Inferior pharyngeal constrictor
Thyrohyoid
Superior belly of omohyoid
External branch of superior laryngeal nerve
Superior thyroid artery
Sternohyoid
Sternothyroid
Anterior jugular vein
Clavicular head
Sternal head
Sternocleidomastoid

## 8.10 Deep dissection of carotid triangle

The sternocleidomastoid muscle has been severed; the inferior portion reflected inferiorly and superior portion posteriorly.

- The tendon of the digastric muscle is connected to the hyoid bone by a fascial sling derived from the muscular part of the pretracheal layer of deep cervical fascia; the tendon of the omohyoid muscle is similarly tethered to the clavicle.
- In this specimen, the facial and lingual arteries arise from a common trunk and pass deep to the stylohyoid and digastric muscles.
- The hypoglossal nerve (CN XII) crosses the internal and external carotid arteries and gives off two branches, the superior root of the ansa cervicalis and the nerve to the thyrohyoid, before passing anteriorly deep to the mylohyoid muscle. In this specimen, the inferior root of the ansa cervicalis lies deep to the internal jugular vein and emerges at its medial aspect.

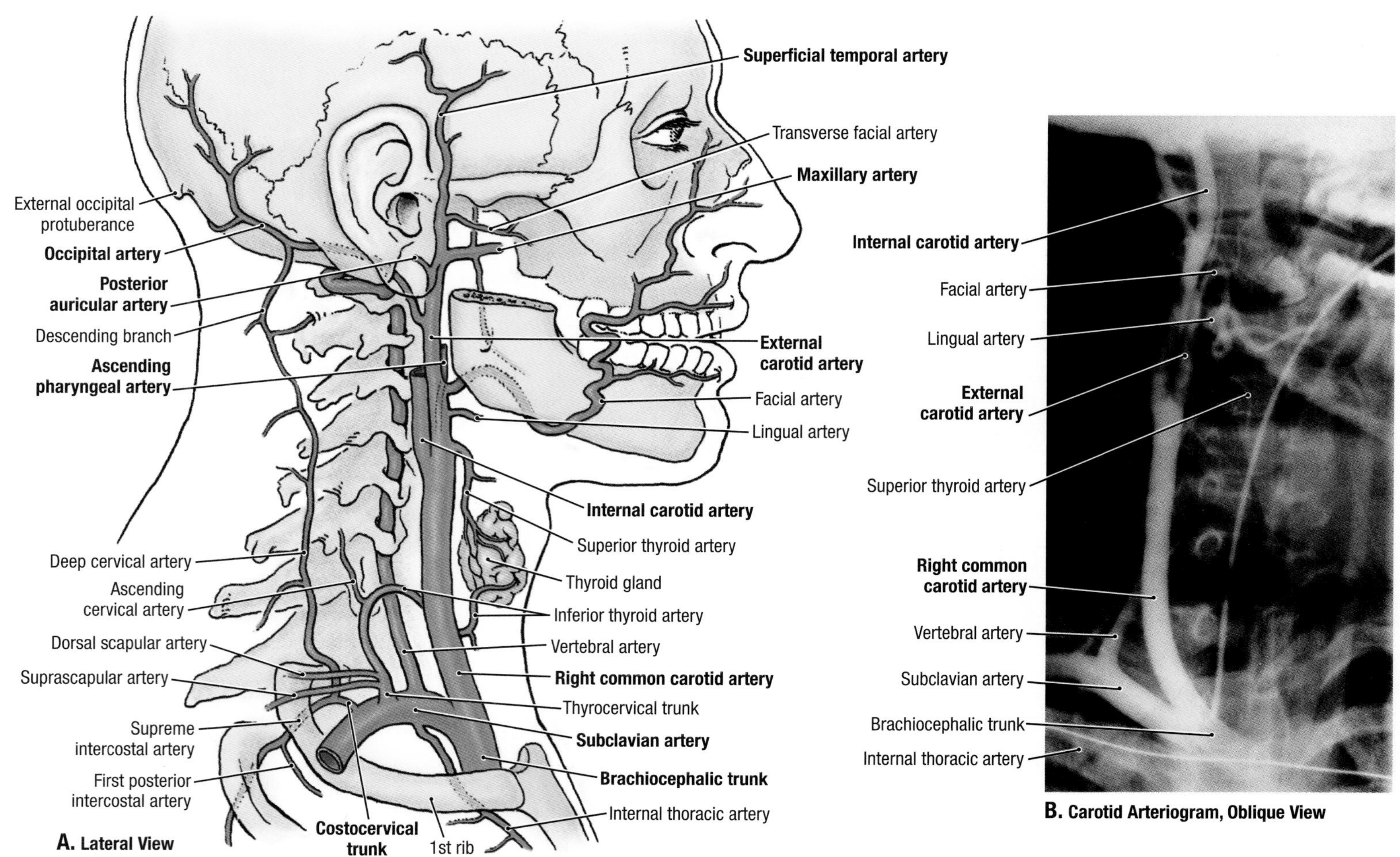
Superficial temporal artery
Transverse facial artery
Maxillary artery
External occipital protuberance
Occipital artery
Posterior auricular artery
Descending branch
Ascending pharyngeal artery
External carotid artery
Facial artery
Lingual artery
Internal carotid artery
Superior thyroid artery
Thyroid gland
Inferior thyroid artery
Vertebral artery
Right common carotid artery
Thyrocervical trunk
Subclavian artery
Brachiocephalic trunk
Internal thoracic artery
Deep cervical artery
Ascending cervical artery
Dorsal scapular artery
Suprascapular artery
Supreme intercostal artery
First posterior intercostal artery
Costocervical trunk
1st rib
Internal carotid artery
Facial artery
Lingual artery
External carotid artery
Superior thyroid artery
Right common carotid artery
Vertebral artery
Subclavian artery
Brachiocephalic trunk
Internal thoracic artery

**A.** Lateral View

**B.** Carotid Arteriogram, Oblique View

**TABLE 8.5 ARTERIES OF THE NECK**

| Artery | Origin | Course and Distribution |
|---|---|---|
| **Right common carotid** | Bifurcation of brachiocephalic trunk | Ascends in neck within carotid sheath with the internal jugular vein and vagus nerve (CN X). Terminates at superior border of thyroid cartilage (C4 vertebral level) by dividing into internal and external carotid arteries |
| **Left common carotid** | Arch of aorta | |
| **Right and left internal carotid** | Right and left common carotid | No branches in the neck. Enters cranium via carotid canal to supply brain and orbits. Proximal part location of carotid sinus, a baroreceptor that reacts to change in arterial blood pressure. The carotid body, a chemoreceptor that monitors oxygen level in blood, is located in bifurcation of common carotid |
| **Right and left external carotid** | | Supplies most structures external to cranium; the orbit, part of forehead, and scalp are major exceptions (supplied by ophthalmic artery from intracranial internal carotid artery) |
| **Ascending pharyngeal** | External carotid | Ascends on pharynx to supply pharynx, prevertebral muscles, middle ear, and cranial meninges |
| **Occipital** | | Passes posteriorly, medial and parallel to the posterior belly of digastric, ending in the posterior scalp |
| **Posterior auricular** | | Ascends posteriorly between external acoustic meatus and mastoid process to supply adjacent muscles, parotid gland, facial nerve, auricle, and scalp |

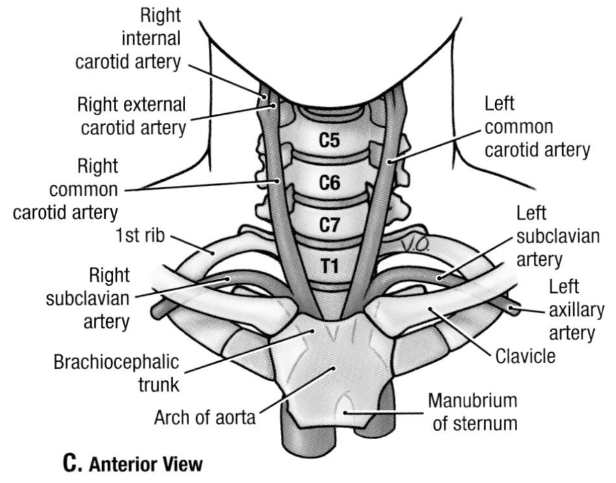
Right internal carotid artery
Right external carotid artery
Right common carotid artery
1st rib
Right subclavian artery
Brachiocephalic trunk
Arch of aorta
C5
C6
C7
T1
Left common carotid artery
Left subclavian artery
Left axillary artery
Clavicle
Manubrium of sternum

C. Anterior View

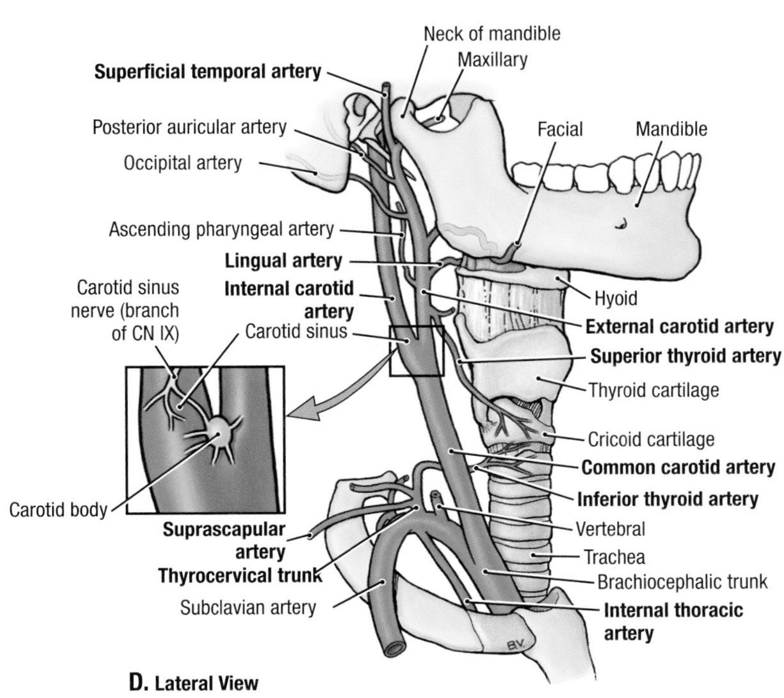
Neck of mandible
Maxillary
Superficial temporal artery
Posterior auricular artery
Occipital artery
Facial
Mandible
Ascending pharyngeal artery
Lingual artery
Carotid sinus nerve (branch of CN IX)
Internal carotid artery
Carotid sinus
Hyoid
External carotid artery
Superior thyroid artery
Thyroid cartilage
Cricoid cartilage
Common carotid artery
Inferior thyroid artery
Carotid body
Suprascapular artery
Thyrocervical trunk
Subclavian artery
Vertebral
Trachea
Brachiocephalic trunk
Internal thoracic artery

D. Lateral View

**TABLE 8.5 ARTERIES OF THE NECK *(continued)***

| Artery | Origin | Course and Distribution |
|---|---|---|
| **Superior thyroid** | External carotid | Runs anteroinferiorly deep to infrahyoid muscles to reach thyroid gland. Supplies thyroid gland, infrahyoid muscles, SCM, and larynx via *superior laryngeal artery* |
| **Lingual** | | Lies on middle constrictor muscle of pharynx; arches superoanteriorly and passes deep to CN XIII, stylohyoid muscle, and posterior belly of digastric then passes deep to hyoglossus, giving branches to the posterior tongue and bifurcating into *deep lingual* and *sublingual arteries* |
| **Facial** | | After giving rise to *ascending palatine artery* and a tonsillar branch, it passes superiorly under cover of the angle of the mandible. It then loops anteriorly to supply the submandibular gland and give rise to the *submental artery* to the floor of the mouth before entering the face |
| **Maxillary** | Terminal branches of external carotid | Passes posterior to neck of mandible, enters infratemporal fossa then pterygopalatine fossa to supply teeth, nose, ear, and face |
| **Superficial temporal** | | Ascends anterior to auricle to temporal region and ends in scalp |
| **Vertebral** | Subclavian | Passes through the transverse foramina of the transverse processes of vertebrae C1–C6, runs in a groove on the posterior arch of the atlas, and enters the cranial cavity through the foramen magnum |
| **Internal thoracic** | | No branches in neck; enters thorax |
| **Thyrocervical trunk** | | Has two branches: the *inferior thyroid artery*, the main visceral artery of the neck; the cervicodorsal trunk sending branches to the lateral cervical region, trapezius, and medial scapular arteries |
| **Costocervical trunk** | | Trunk passes posterosuperiorly and divides into *superior intercostal* and *deep cervical arteries* to supply the 1st and 2nd intercostal spaces and posterior deep cervical muscles, respectively |

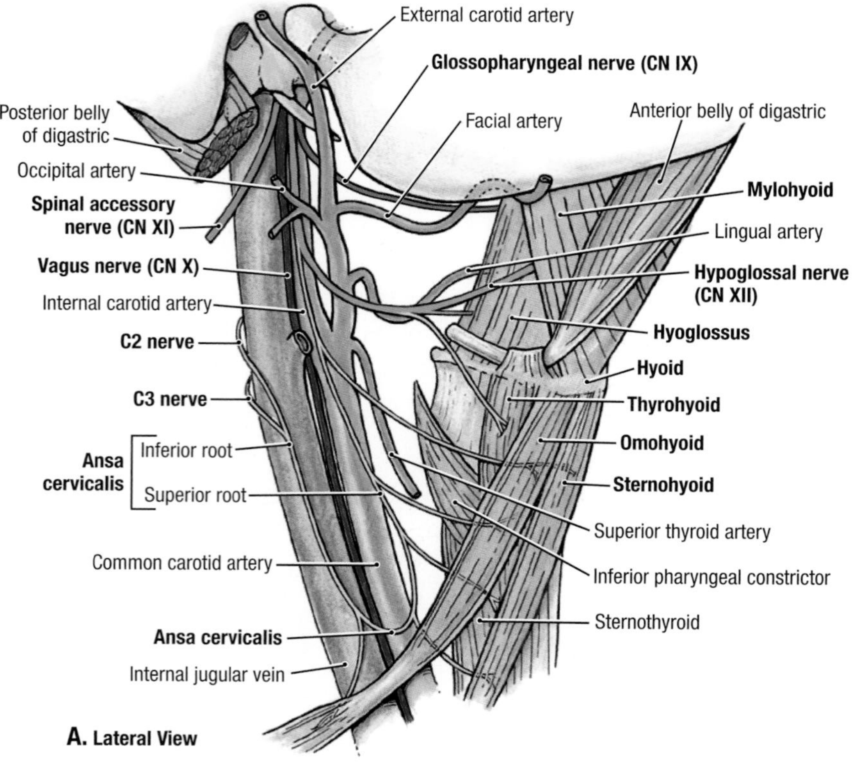
External carotid artery
Glossopharyngeal nerve (CN IX)
Facial artery
Anterior belly of digastric
Posterior belly of digastric
Occipital artery
Spinal accessory nerve (CN XI)
Vagus nerve (CN X)
Internal carotid artery
C2 nerve
C3 nerve
Ansa cervicalis
Inferior root
Superior root
Common carotid artery
Ansa cervicalis
Internal jugular vein
Mylohyoid
Lingual artery
Hypoglossal nerve (CN XII)
Hyoglossus
Hyoid
Thyrohyoid
Omohyoid
Sternohyoid
Superior thyroid artery
Inferior pharyngeal constrictor
Sternothyroid
A. Lateral View

| Glossopharyngeal—CN IX | Vagus—CN X |
|---|---|
| **Motor:** stylopharyngeus, parotid gland<br>**Sensory:** taste: posterior third of tongue; general sensation: pharynx, tonsillar sinus, pharyngotympanic tube, middle ear cavity | **Motor:** palate, pharynx, larynx, trachea, bronchial tree, heart, GI tract to left colic flexure<br>**Sensory:** pharynx, larynx; reflex sensory from tracheobronchial tree, lungs, heart, GI tract to left colic flexure |
| **Spinal accessory—CN XI** | **Hypoglossal—CN XII** |
| **Motor:** sternocleidomastoid and trapezius | **Motor:** all intrinsic and extrinsic muscles of tongue (excluding palatoglossus—a palatine muscle) |

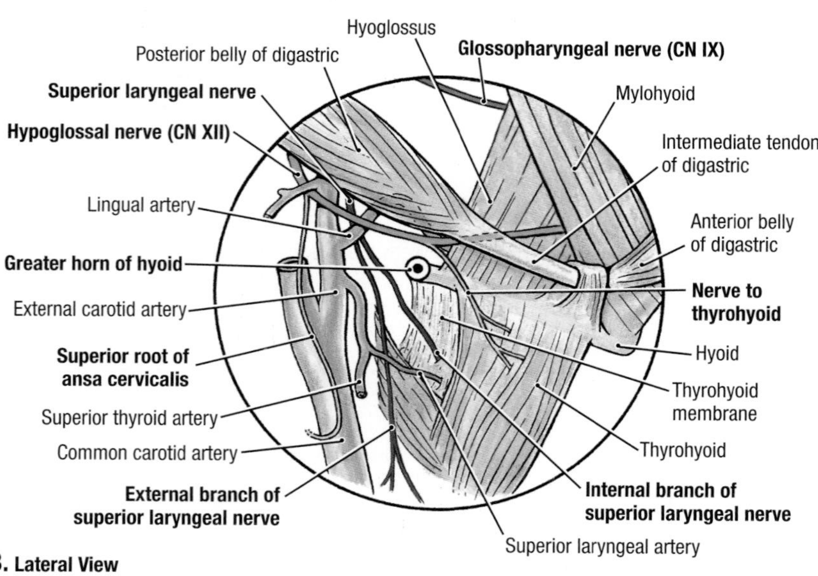
Hyoglossus
Posterior belly of digastric
Glossopharyngeal nerve (CN IX)
Superior laryngeal nerve
Mylohyoid
Hypoglossal nerve (CN XII)
Intermediate tendon of digastric
Lingual artery
Anterior belly of digastric
Greater horn of hyoid
Nerve to thyrohyoid
External carotid artery
Hyoid
Superior root of ansa cervicalis
Thyrohyoid membrane
Superior thyroid artery
Common carotid artery
Thyrohyoid
External branch of superior laryngeal nerve
Internal branch of superior laryngeal nerve
Superior laryngeal artery
B. Lateral View

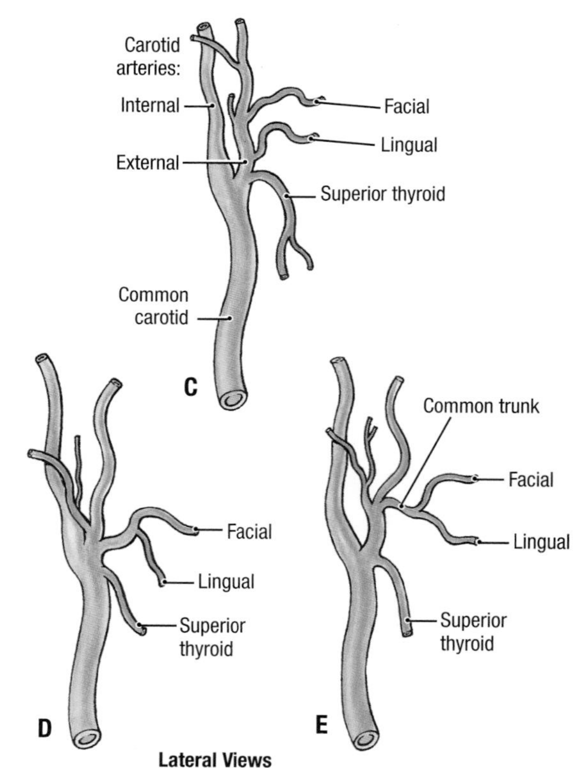
Carotid arteries:
Internal
External
Facial
Lingual
Superior thyroid
Common carotid
C
Facial
Lingual
Superior thyroid
D
Common trunk
Facial
Lingual
Superior thyroid
E
Lateral Views

## 8.11 Relationships of nerves and vessels in the carotid triangle of the neck

**A.** Ansa cervicalis and the strap muscles. **B.** Hypoglossal nerve (CN XII) and internal and external branches of superior laryngeal nerve (CN X). The tip of the greater hyoid bone, indicated with a *circle* is the reference point for many structures. **C–E.** Variation in the origin of the lingual artery as studied by Dr. Grant in 211 specimens. In 80%, the superior thyroid, lingual, and facial arteries arose separately **(C)**; in 20%, the lingual and facial arteries arose from a common stem inferiorly **(D)** or high on the external carotid artery **(E)**. In one specimen, the superior thyroid and lingual arteries arose from a common stem.

*Carotid occlusion,* causing stenosis (narrowing) can be relieved by opening the artery at its origin and stripping off the atherosclerotic plaque with the artery's lining (intima). This procedure is called carotid endarterectomy. Because of the relationships of the internal carotid artery, there is a risk of cranial nerve injury during the procedure involving one or more of the following nerves: CN IX, CN X (or its branch, the superior laryngeal nerve), CN XI, or CN XII.

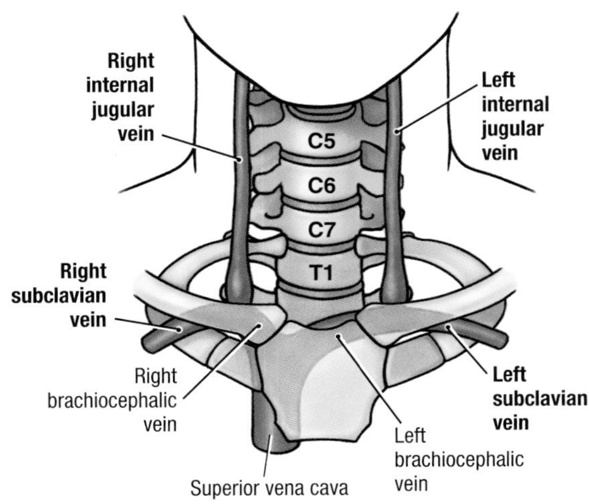
Right internal jugular vein
Left internal jugular vein
C5
C6
C7
T1
Right subclavian vein
Right brachiocephalic vein
Left subclavian vein
Left brachiocephalic vein
Superior vena cava
**A. Anterior View**

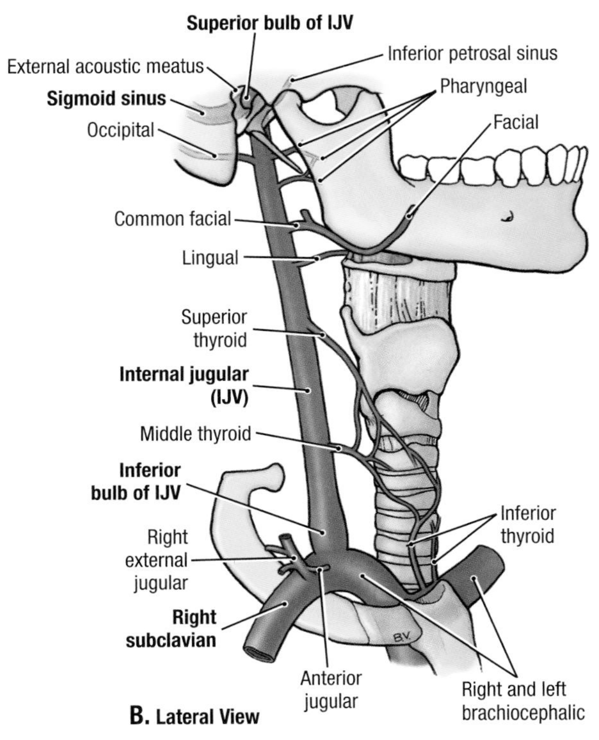
Superior bulb of IJV
External acoustic meatus
Inferior petrosal sinus
Sigmoid sinus
Pharyngeal
Occipital
Facial
Common facial
Lingual
Superior thyroid
Internal jugular (IJV)
Middle thyroid
Inferior bulb of IJV
Inferior thyroid
Right external jugular
Right subclavian
Anterior jugular
Right and left brachiocephalic
**B. Lateral View**

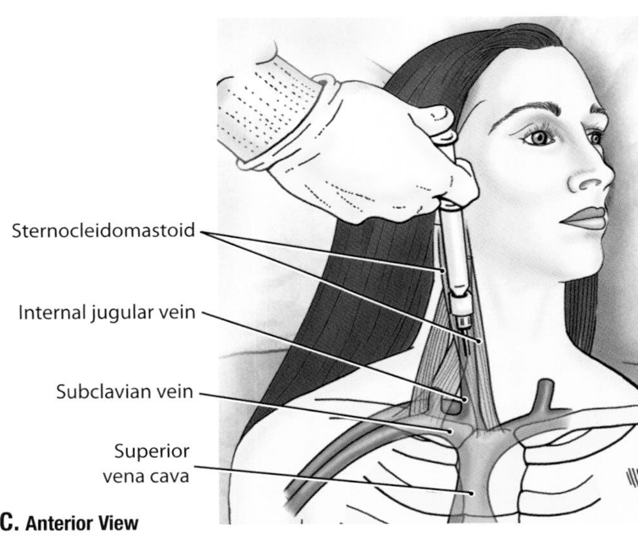
Sternocleidomastoid
Internal jugular vein
Subclavian vein
Superior vena cava
**C. Anterior View**

## 8.12 Deep veins of the neck

**A.** Internal jugular and subclavian veins. **B.** Tributaries of the internal jugular vein (IJV). The IJV begins at the jugular foramen as the continuation of the sigmoid sinus. From a dilated origin, the superior bulb of the IJV, the vein runs inferiorly through the neck in the carotid sheath. Posterior to the sternal end of the clavicle the vein merges perpendicularly with the subclavian vein, forming the "venous angle" that marks the origin of the brachiocephalic vein. The inferior end of the IJV dilates superior to its terminal valve, forming the inferior bulb of the IJV. The valve permits blood to flow toward the heart while preventing backflow into the IJV.

**C.** Internal jugular vein puncture. A needle and catheter may be inserted into the IJV for diagnostic or therapeutic purposes. The right internal jugular vein is preferable because it is usually larger and straighter. During this procedure, the clinician palpates the common carotid artery and inserts the needle into the IJV just lateral to it at a 30° angle, aiming at the apex of the triangle between the sternal and clavicular heads of the SCM. The needle is then directed inferolaterally toward the ipsilateral nipple.

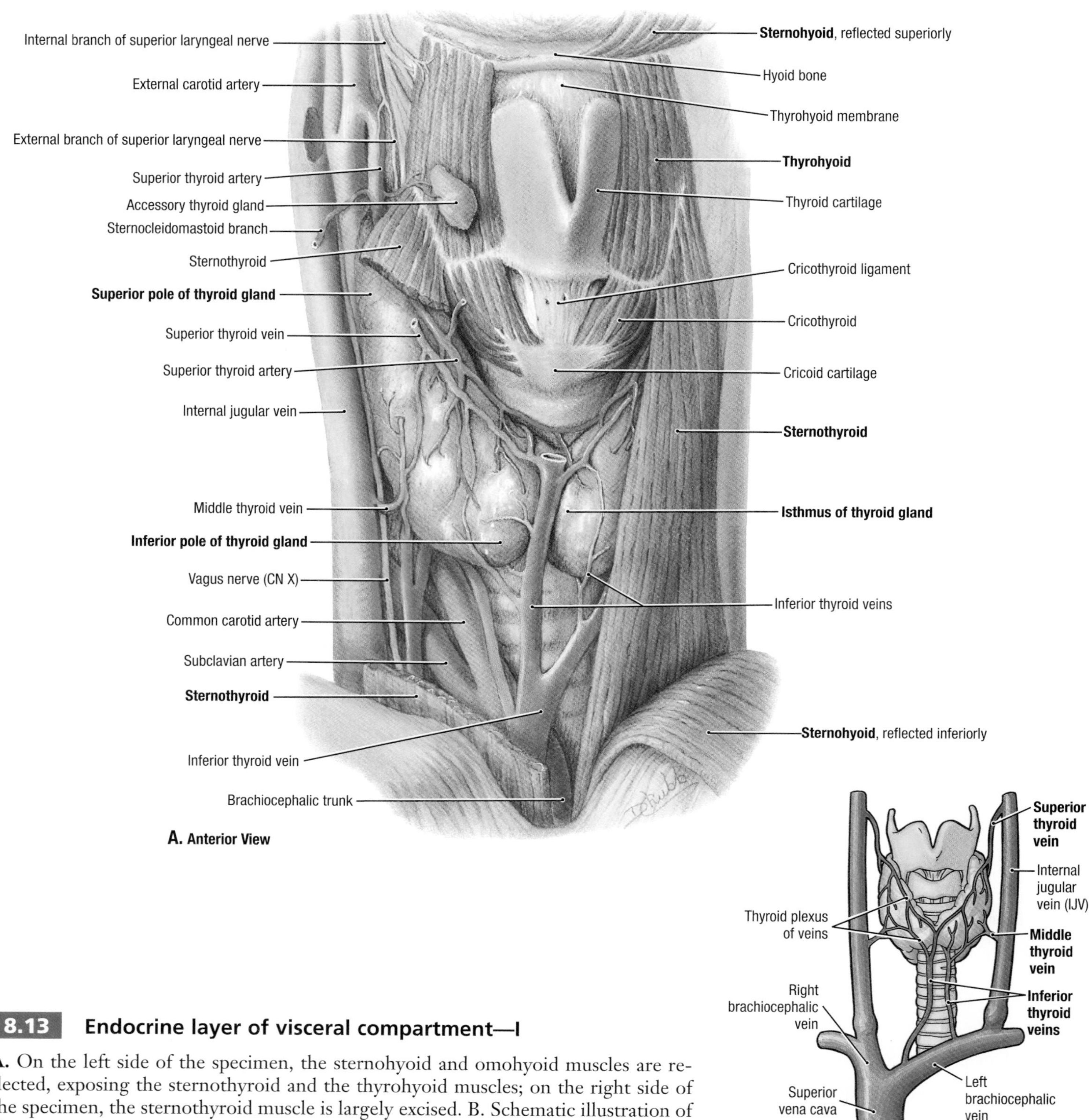
Internal branch of superior laryngeal nerve
External carotid artery
External branch of superior laryngeal nerve
Superior thyroid artery
Accessory thyroid gland
Sternocleidomastoid branch
Sternothyroid
Superior pole of thyroid gland
Superior thyroid vein
Superior thyroid artery
Internal jugular vein
Middle thyroid vein
Inferior pole of thyroid gland
Vagus nerve (CN X)
Common carotid artery
Subclavian artery
Sternothyroid
Inferior thyroid vein
Brachiocephalic trunk
Sternohyoid, reflected superiorly
Hyoid bone
Thyrohyoid membrane
Thyrohyoid
Thyroid cartilage
Cricothyroid ligament
Cricothyroid
Cricoid cartilage
Sternothyroid
Isthmus of thyroid gland
Inferior thyroid veins
Sternohyoid, reflected inferiorly
A. Anterior View
Superior thyroid vein
Internal jugular vein (IJV)
Thyroid plexus of veins
Middle thyroid vein
Right brachiocephalic vein
Inferior thyroid veins
Superior vena cava
Left brachiocephalic vein
B. Anterior View

## 8.13 Endocrine layer of visceral compartment—I

**A.** On the left side of the specimen, the sternohyoid and omohyoid muscles are reflected, exposing the sternothyroid and the thyrohyoid muscles; on the right side of the specimen, the sternothyroid muscle is largely excised. B. Schematic illustration of the venous drainage of the thyroid gland. Except for the superior thyroid veins, the thyroid veins are not paired with arteries of corresponding names.

The carotid pulse (neck pulse) is easily felt by palpating the common carotid artery in the side of the neck, where it lies in a groove between the trachea and the infrahyoid muscles. It is usually easily palpated just deep to the anterior border of the SCM at the level of the superior border of the thyroid cartilage. It is routinely checked during cardiopulmonary resuscitation (CPR). Absence of a carotid pulse indicates cardiac arrest.

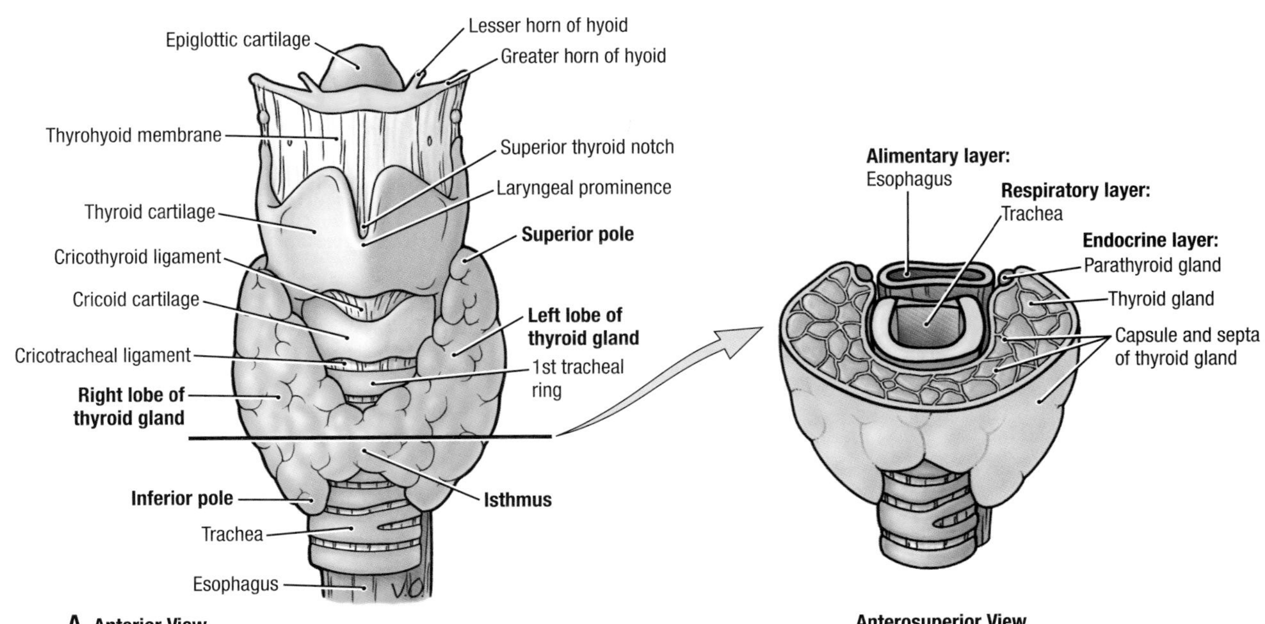

Epiglottic cartilage
Lesser horn of hyoid
Greater horn of hyoid
Thyrohyoid membrane
Superior thyroid notch
Laryngeal prominence
Thyroid cartilage
Superior pole
Cricothyroid ligament
Cricoid cartilage
Left lobe of thyroid gland
Cricotracheal ligament
1st tracheal ring
Right lobe of thyroid gland
Inferior pole
Isthmus
Trachea
Esophagus
A. Anterior View
Alimentary layer:
Esophagus
Respiratory layer:
Trachea
Endocrine layer:
Parathyroid gland
Thyroid gland
Capsule and septa of thyroid gland
Anterosuperior View


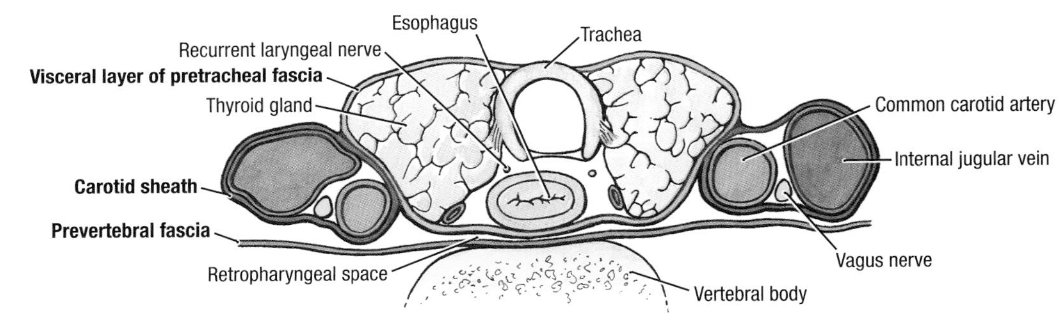

Esophagus
Trachea
Recurrent laryngeal nerve
Visceral layer of pretracheal fascia
Thyroid gland
Common carotid artery
Internal jugular vein
Carotid sheath
Prevertebral fascia
Vagus nerve
Retropharyngeal space
Vertebral body
B. Transverse Section, Inferior View


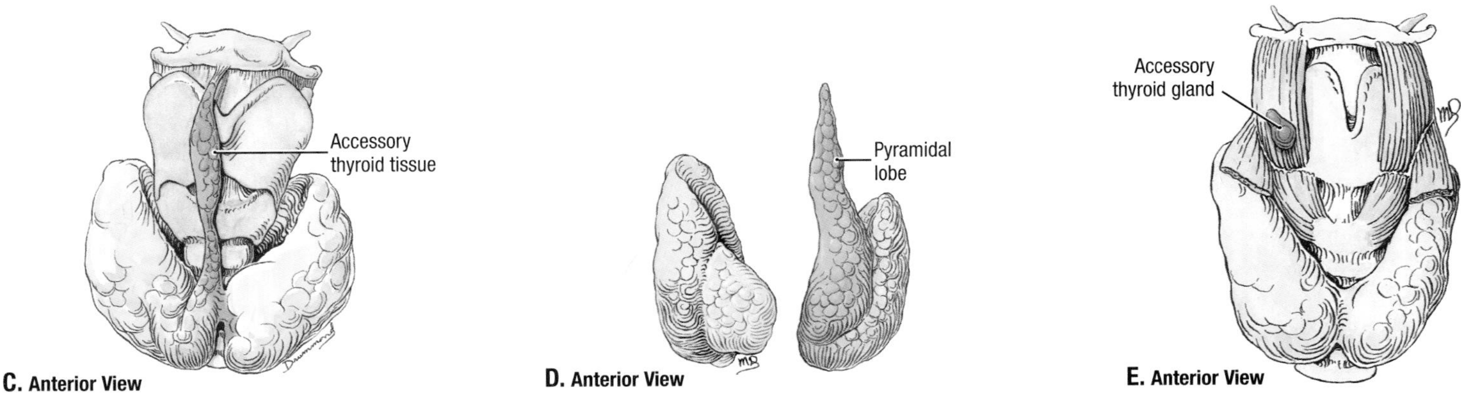

Accessory thyroid tissue
C. Anterior View
Pyramidal lobe
D. Anterior View
Accessory thyroid gland
E. Anterior View


## 8.14 Endocrine layer of visceral compartment—II

**A.** Relations of thyroid gland with transverse section showing alimentary, respiratory, and endocrine layers of visceral compartment. **B.** Fascia. **C.** Accessory thyroid tissue along the course of the thyroglossal duct. **D.** Approximately 50% of glands have a pyramidal lobe that extends from near the isthmus to or toward the hyoid bone; the isthmus is occasionally absent, in which case the gland is in two parts. **E.** An accessory thyroid gland can occur between the suprahyoid region and arch of the aorta (see Fig. 8.13A).

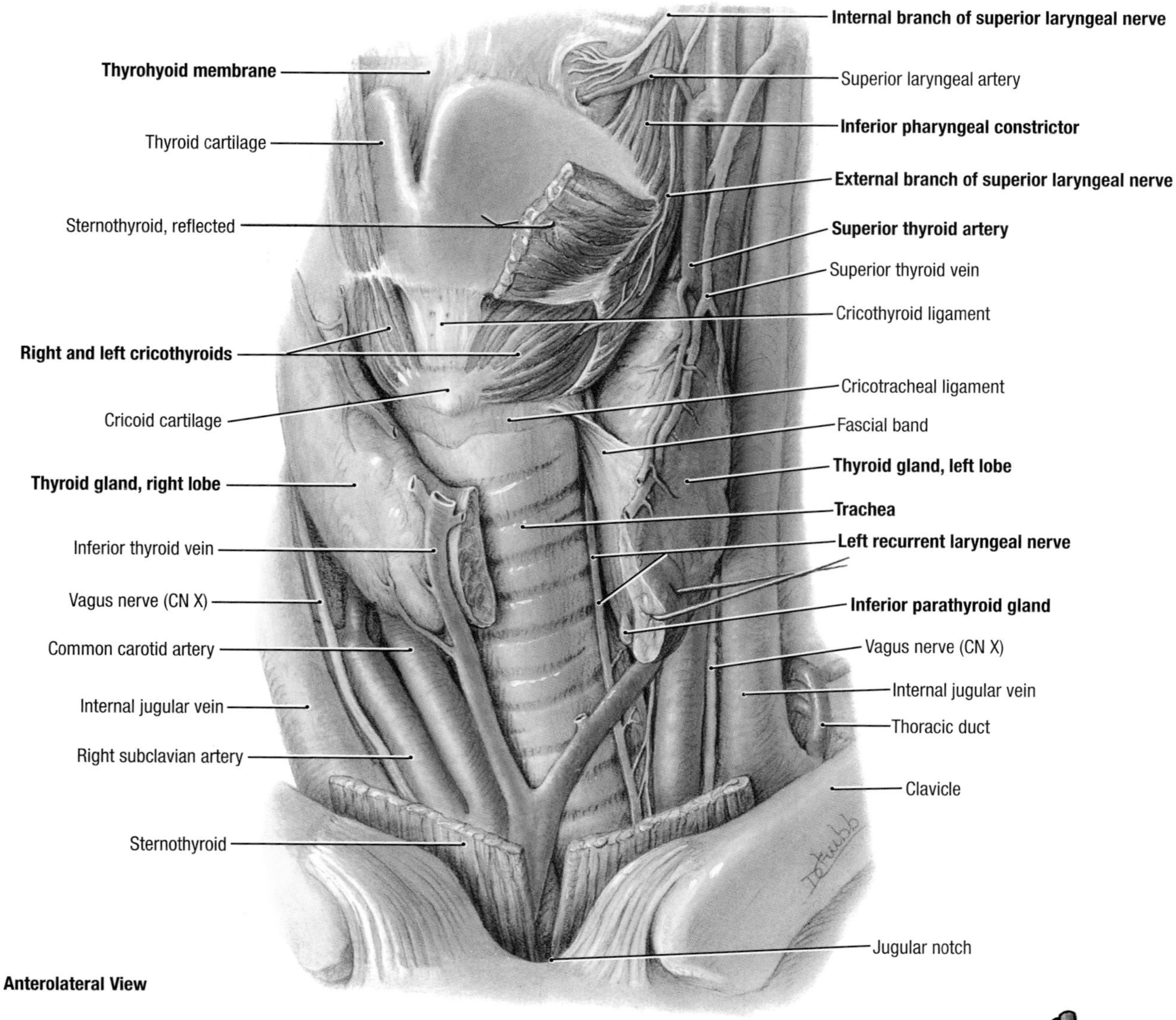

Internal branch of superior laryngeal nerve
Thyrohyoid membrane
Superior laryngeal artery
Thyroid cartilage
Inferior pharyngeal constrictor
External branch of superior laryngeal nerve
Sternothyroid, reflected
Superior thyroid artery
Superior thyroid vein
Cricothyroid ligament
Right and left cricothyroids
Cricotracheal ligament
Cricoid cartilage
Fascial band
Thyroid gland, right lobe
Thyroid gland, left lobe
Trachea
Inferior thyroid vein
Left recurrent laryngeal nerve
Vagus nerve (CN X)
Inferior parathyroid gland
Common carotid artery
Vagus nerve (CN X)
Internal jugular vein
Internal jugular vein
Thoracic duct
Right subclavian artery
Clavicle
Sternothyroid
Jugular notch

**A. Anterolateral View**

## 8.15 Respiratory layer of visceral compartment

**A.** The isthmus of the thyroid gland is divided, and the left lobe is retracted. The left recurrent laryngeal nerve ascends on the lateral aspect of the trachea between the trachea and esophagus. The internal branch of the superior laryngeal nerve runs along the superior border of the inferior pharyngeal constrictor muscle and pierces the thyrohyoid membrane. The external branch of the superior laryngeal nerve lies adjacent to the inferior pharyngeal constrictor muscle and supplies its lower portion; it continues to run along the anterior border of the superior thyroid artery, passing deep to the superior attachment of the sternothyroid muscle, and then supplies the cricothyroid muscle. **B.** Blood supply of the parathyroid glands and courses of the left and right recurrent laryngeal nerves.

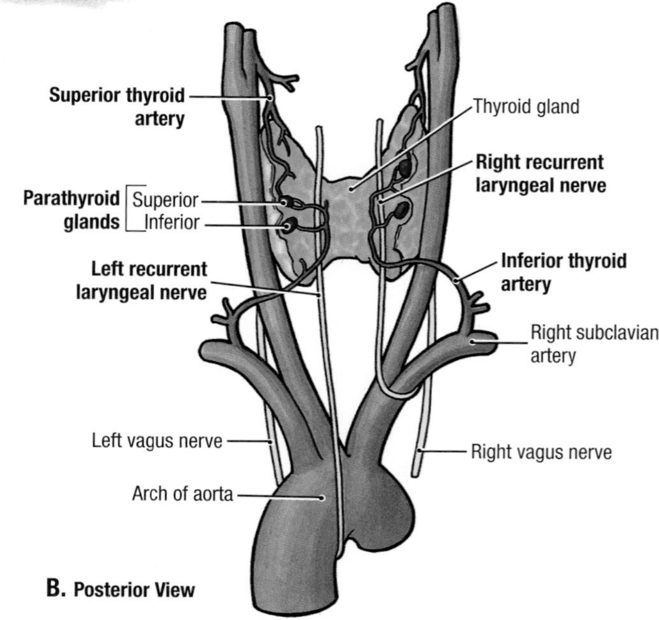
Superior thyroid artery
Thyroid gland
Right recurrent laryngeal nerve
Parathyroid glands
Superior
Inferior
Left recurrent laryngeal nerve
Inferior thyroid artery
Right subclavian artery
Left vagus nerve
Right vagus nerve
Arch of aorta

**B. Posterior View**

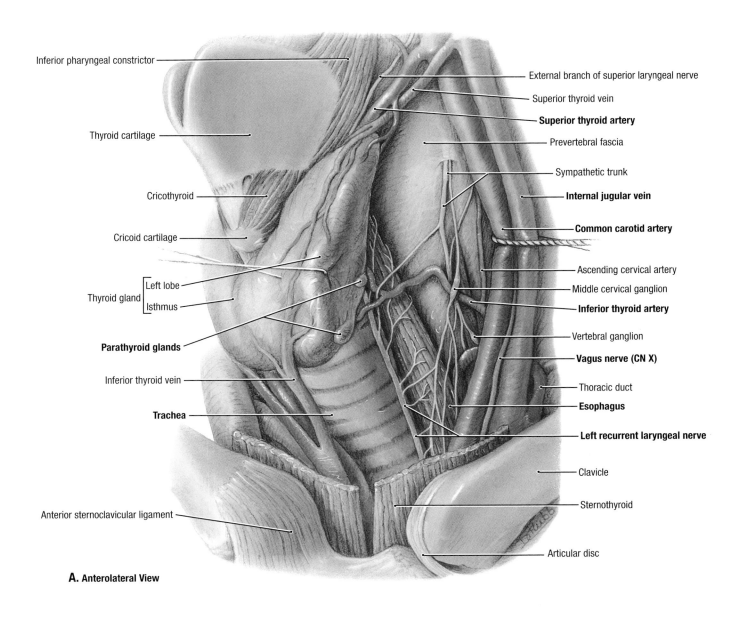

Inferior pharyngeal constrictor
Thyroid cartilage
Cricothyroid
Cricoid cartilage
Thyroid gland
Left lobe
Isthmus
Parathyroid glands
Inferior thyroid vein
Trachea
Anterior sternoclavicular ligament
External branch of superior laryngeal nerve
Superior thyroid vein
Superior thyroid artery
Prevertebral fascia
Sympathetic trunk
Internal jugular vein
Common carotid artery
Ascending cervical artery
Middle cervical ganglion
Inferior thyroid artery
Vertebral ganglion
Vagus nerve (CN X)
Thoracic duct
Esophagus
Left recurrent laryngeal nerve
Clavicle
Sternothyroid
Articular disc

**A. Anterolateral View**

## 8.16 Alimentary layer of visceral compartment

**A.** Dissection of the left side of the root of the neck. The three structures contained in the carotid sheath (internal jugular vein, common carotid artery, and vagus nerve) are retracted. The left recurrent laryngeal nerve ascends on the lateral aspect of the trachea, just anterior to the recess between the trachea and esophagus. **B.** Arterial supply of thyroid gland. The thyroid ima artery is infrequent (10%) and variable in its origin.

During a total thyroidectomy (e.g., excision of a malignant thyroid gland), the parathyroid glands are in danger of being inadvertently damaged or removed. These glands are safe during *subtotal thyroidectomy* because the most posterior part of the thyroid gland usually is preserved. Variability in the position of the parathyroid glands, especially the inferior ones, puts them in danger of being removed during surgery on the thyroid gland. If the parathyroid glands are inadvertently removed during surgery, the patient suffers from *tetany*, a severe convulsive disorder. The generalized convulsive muscle spasms result from a fall in blood calcium levels.

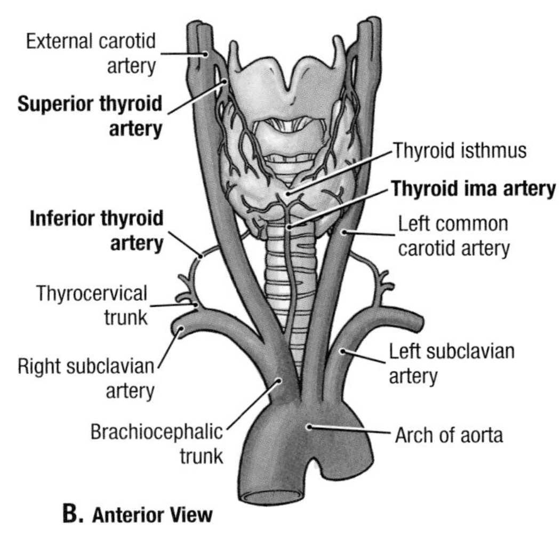
External carotid artery
Superior thyroid artery
Inferior thyroid artery
Thyrocervical trunk
Right subclavian artery
Brachiocephalic trunk
Thyroid isthmus
Thyroid ima artery
Left common carotid artery
Left subclavian artery
Arch of aorta

**B. Anterior View**

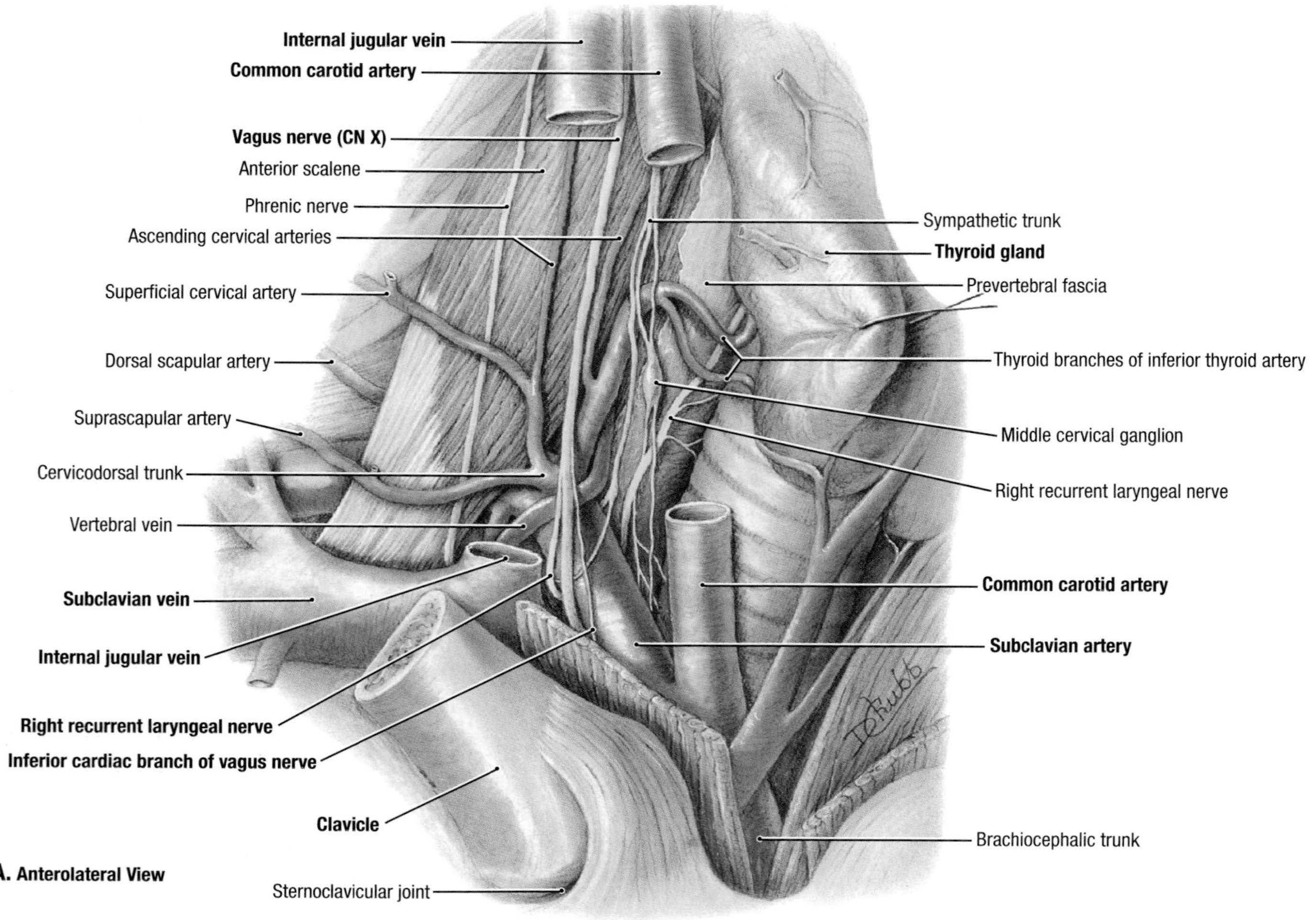
Internal jugular vein
Common carotid artery
Vagus nerve (CN X)
Anterior scalene
Phrenic nerve
Ascending cervical arteries
Superficial cervical artery
Dorsal scapular artery
Suprascapular artery
Cervicodorsal trunk
Vertebral vein
Subclavian vein
Internal jugular vein
Right recurrent laryngeal nerve
Inferior cardiac branch of vagus nerve
Clavicle
Sternoclavicular joint
Sympathetic trunk
Thyroid gland
Prevertebral fascia
Thyroid branches of inferior thyroid artery
Middle cervical ganglion
Right recurrent laryngeal nerve
Common carotid artery
Subclavian artery
Brachiocephalic trunk
A. Anterolateral View

## 8.17 Root of the neck

**A.** Dissection of the right side of the root of the neck. The clavicle is cut, sections of the common carotid artery and internal jugular vein are removed, and the right lobe of the thyroid gland is retracted. The right vagus nerve crosses the first part of the subclavian artery and gives off an inferior cardiac branch and the right recurrent laryngeal nerve. The right recurrent laryngeal nerve loops inferior to the subclavian artery and passes posterior to the common carotid artery on its way to the posterolateral aspect of the trachea.

- The recurrent laryngeal nerves are vulnerable to injury during thyroidectomy and other surgeries in the anterior cervical region of the neck. Because the terminal branch of this nerve, the inferior laryngeal nerve, innervates the muscles moving the vocal folds, injury to the nerve results in paralysis of the vocal folds.
- A non-neoplastic and noninflammatory enlargement of the thyroid gland, other than the variable enlargement that may occur during menstruation and pregnancy, is called a goiter. A *goiter* results from a lack of iodine. It is common in certain parts of the world where the soil and water are deficient in iodine and iodized salt is unavailable. The enlarged gland causes a swelling in the neck that may compress the trachea, esophagus, and recurrent laryngeal nerves. When the gland enlarges, it may do so anteriorly, posteriorly, inferiorly, or laterally. It cannot move superiorly because of the superior attachments of the sternothyroid and sternohyoid muscles. Substernal extension of a goiter is also common.

Esophagus
Sympathetic trunk
Ascending cervical artery
Carotid tubercle (C6 vertebra)
Anterior ramus C5
Vertebral artery
Anterior ramus C6
Inferior thyroid artery
Dorsal scapular artery
Anterior scalene
Anterior ramus C8
Phrenic nerve
Suprascapular artery
Right vagus nerve (CN X)
Right common carotid artery
1st rib
Cervical parietal pleura
Right brachiocephalic vein
Brachiocephalic trunk
Inferior thyroid vein
Thymic branch of inferior thyroid artery
Thyroid gland
Longus colli
Longus capitis
Phrenic nerve
Anterior vertebral vein
Middle scalene
Anterior scalene
Trachea
Dorsal scapular artery
Inferior thyroid artery
Thyrocervical trunk
Vertebral vein
Thoracic duct
Subclavian artery
Subclavian vein
Left subclavian artery
Left vagus nerve
Left common carotid artery
Internal jugular vein
Internal thoracic artery
Phrenic nerve
Internal thoracic vein
Left brachiocephalic vein

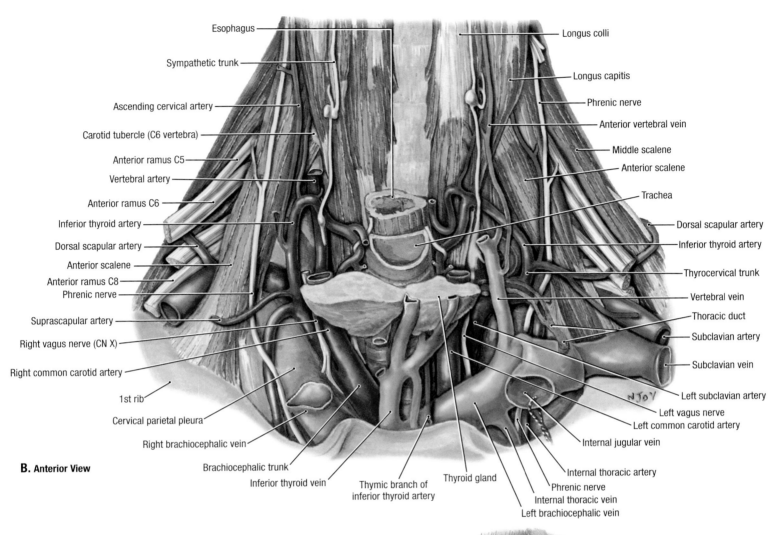

**B. Anterior View**

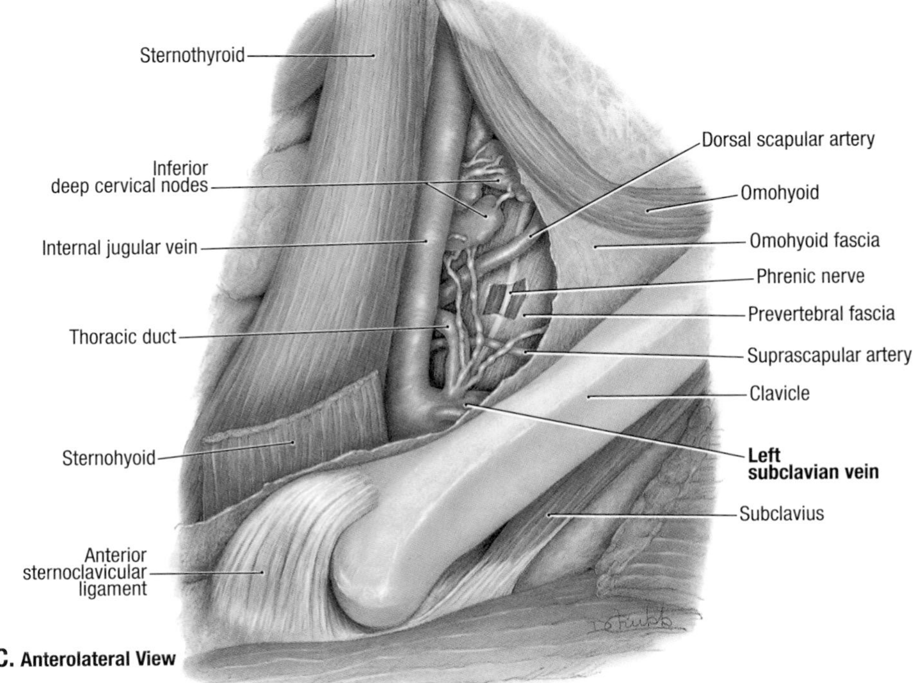
Sternothyroid
Inferior deep cervical nodes
Internal jugular vein
Thoracic duct
Sternohyoid
Anterior sternoclavicular ligament
Dorsal scapular artery
Omohyoid
Omohyoid fascia
Phrenic nerve
Prevertebral fascia
Suprascapular artery
Clavicle
Left subclavian vein
Subclavius

**C. Anterolateral View**

## 8.17 Root of the neck *(continued)*

**B.** Deep anterior dissection. **C.** Dissection of termination of the thoracic duct. The sternocleidomastoid muscle is removed, the sternohyoid muscle is resected, and the omohyoid portion of the pretracheal fascia is partially removed. The thoracic duct arches laterally in the neck, passing posterior to the carotid sheath and anterior to the vertebral artery, thyrocervical trunk, and subclavian arteries; it enters the angle formed by the junction of the left subclavian and internal jugular veins to form the left brachiocephalic vein (the left venous angle).

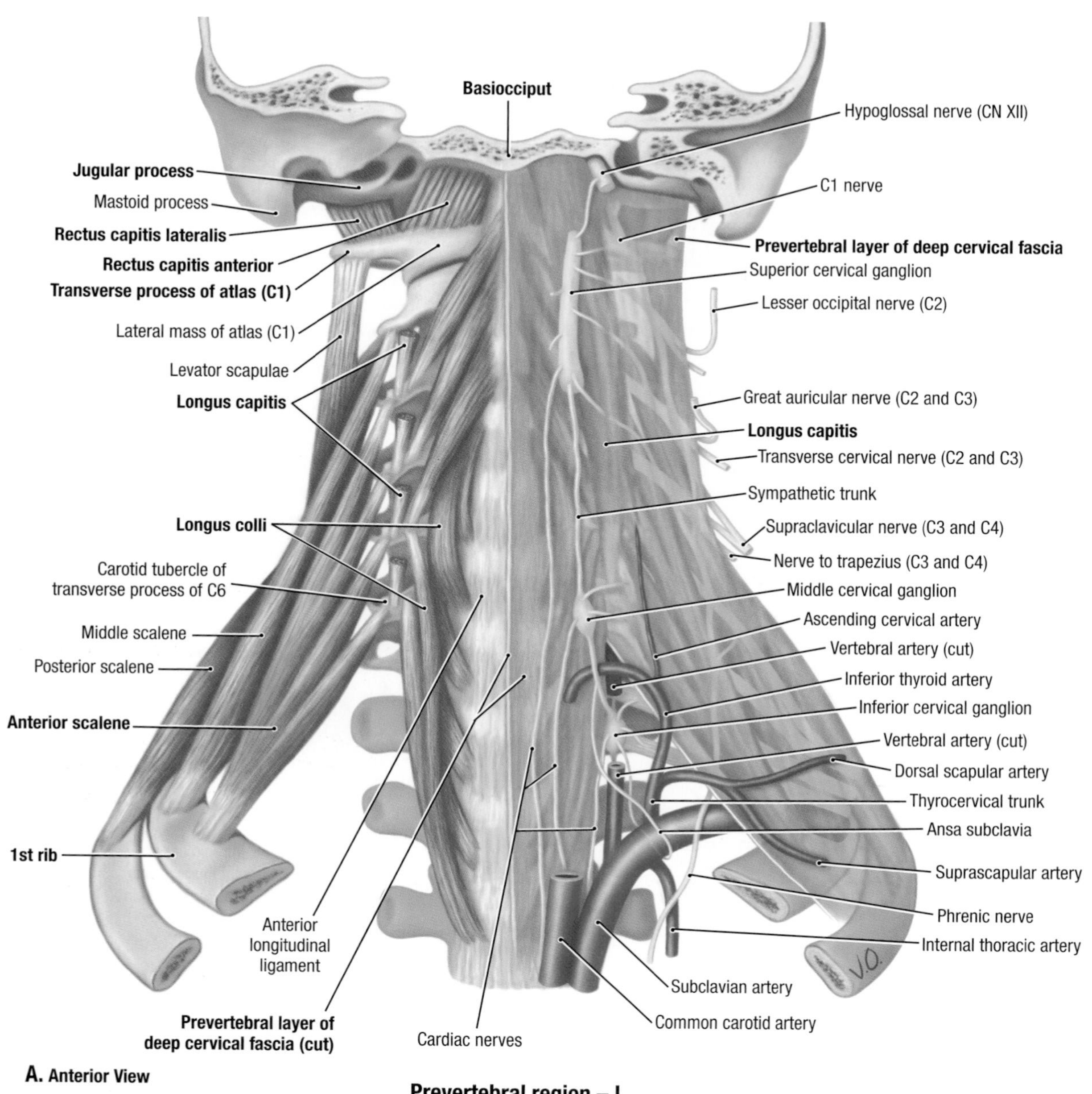
Basiocciput
Hypoglossal nerve (CN XII)
Jugular process
Mastoid process
C1 nerve
Rectus capitis lateralis
Prevertebral layer of deep cervical fascia
Rectus capitis anterior
Superior cervical ganglion
Transverse process of atlas (C1)
Lesser occipital nerve (C2)
Lateral mass of atlas (C1)
Levator scapulae
Longus capitis
Great auricular nerve (C2 and C3)
Longus capitis
Transverse cervical nerve (C2 and C3)
Sympathetic trunk
Longus colli
Supraclavicular nerve (C3 and C4)
Nerve to trapezius (C3 and C4)
Carotid tubercle of transverse process of C6
Middle cervical ganglion
Ascending cervical artery
Middle scalene
Vertebral artery (cut)
Posterior scalene
Inferior thyroid artery
Inferior cervical ganglion
Anterior scalene
Vertebral artery (cut)
Dorsal scapular artery
Thyrocervical trunk
Ansa subclavia
1st rib
Suprascapular artery
Phrenic nerve
Anterior longitudinal ligament
Internal thoracic artery
Subclavian artery
Common carotid artery
Prevertebral layer of deep cervical fascia (cut)
Cardiac nerves
A. Anterior View

**Prevertebral region – I**

**TABLE 8.6 ANTERIOR VERTEBRAL MUSCLES**

| Muscle | Superior Attachment | Inferior Attachment | Innervation | Main Action |
|---|---|---|---|---|
| **Longus colli** | Anterior tubercle of C1 vertebra (atlas); bodies of C1–C3 and transverse processes of C3–C6 vertebrae | Bodies of C5–T3 vertebrae, transverse processes of C3–C5 vertebrae | Anterior rami of C2–C6 spinal nerves | Flexes neck with rotation (torsion) to opposite side if acting unilaterally[a] |
| **Longus capitis** | Basilar part of occipital bone (basiocciput) | Anterior tubercles of C3–C6 transverse processes | Anterior rami of C1–C3 spinal nerves | Flexes head[b] |
| **Rectus capitis lateralis** | Jugular process of occipital bone | Transverse process of C1 vertebra (atlas) | From loop between C1 and C2 spinal nerves | Flexes head and helps to stabilize it[b] |

[a]Flexion of neck, anterior (or lateral) bending of cervical vertebrae C2–C7.
[b]Flexion of head, anterior (or lateral) bending of head relative to vertebral column at atlanto-occipital joints.

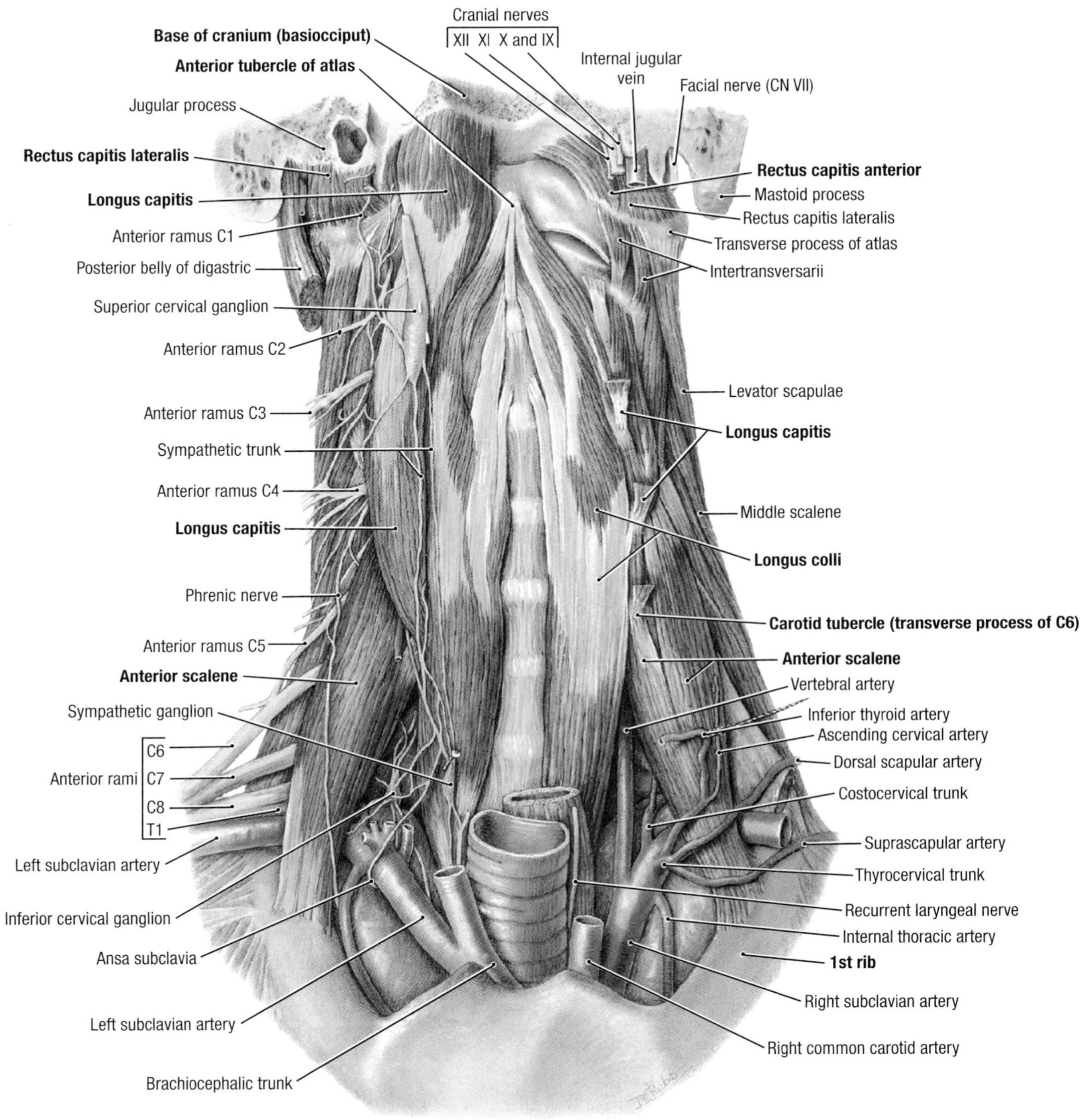
Cranial nerves
XII XI X and IX
Base of cranium (basiocciput)
Anterior tubercle of atlas
Internal jugular vein
Facial nerve (CN VII)
Jugular process
Rectus capitis lateralis
Longus capitis
Anterior ramus C1
Posterior belly of digastric
Superior cervical ganglion
Anterior ramus C2
Rectus capitis anterior
Mastoid process
Rectus capitis lateralis
Transverse process of atlas
Intertransversarii
Levator scapulae
Longus capitis
Anterior ramus C3
Sympathetic trunk
Anterior ramus C4
Longus capitis
Middle scalene
Longus colli
Phrenic nerve
Carotid tubercle (transverse process of C6)
Anterior ramus C5
Anterior scalene
Anterior scalene
Vertebral artery
Sympathetic ganglion
Inferior thyroid artery
Ascending cervical artery
Dorsal scapular artery
Anterior rami
C6
C7
C8
T1
Costocervical trunk
Left subclavian artery
Suprascapular artery
Thyrocervical trunk
Inferior cervical ganglion
Recurrent laryngeal nerve
Internal thoracic artery
Ansa subclavia
1st rib
Right subclavian artery
Left subclavian artery
Right common carotid artery
Brachiocephalic trunk

**B. Anterior View**

**Prevertebral region – II**

**TABLE 8.6 ANTERIOR VERTEBRAL MUSCLES (*continued*)**

| Muscle | Superior Attachment | Inferior Attachment | Innervation | Main Action |
|---|---|---|---|---|
| **Rectus capitis anterior** | Base of cranium, just anterior to occipital condyle | Anterior surface of lateral mass of atlas (C1 vertebra) | Branches from loop between C1 and C2 spinal nerves | Flexes head[b] |
| **Anterior scalene** | Anterior tubercles of transverse processes of C4–C6 vertebrae | 1st rib | Cervical spinal nerves C4–C6 | |

[a]Flexion of neck, anterior (or lateral) bending of cervical vertebrae C2–C7.
[b]Flexion of head, anterior (or lateral) bending of head relative to vertebral column at atlanto-occipital joints.

Sympathetic trunk
Vagus nerve (CN X)
Cervical cardiac branch
Middle scalene
Longus cervicis
Rami communicantes
Vertebral body C5
Vertebral artery
C5
Transverse process, C7
Cervicothoracic (stellate) ganglion:
1st rib
C6
Inferior cervical ganglion
1st thoracic ganglion
C7
Anterior rami
2nd rib
C8
Trunks of brachial plexus
T1
Trachea
Right common carotid artery
Dorsal scapular artery
Anterior scalene
Ansa subclavia
Pericardiacophrenic artery
Cervical parietal pleura
Subclavian artery
Right recurrent laryngeal nerve
NJoy

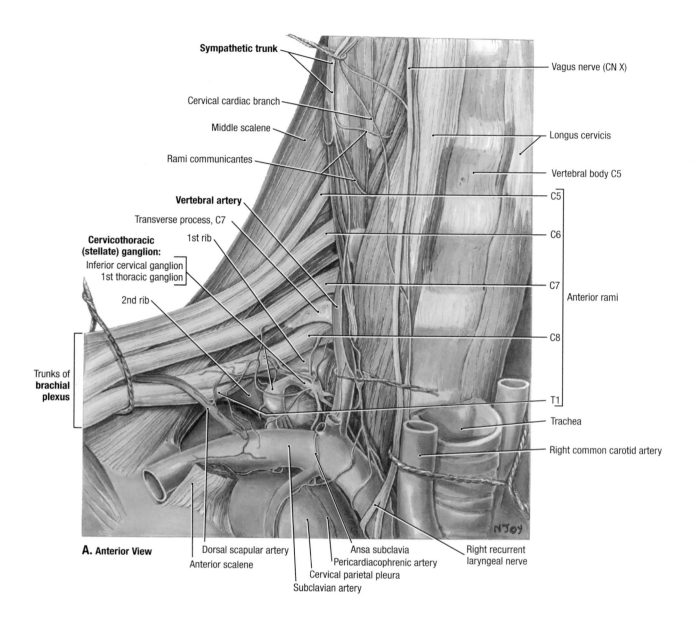

**A. Anterior View**

## 8.18 Brachial plexus and sympathetic trunk in the root of the neck

**A.** Dissection of right side of specimen. The pleura has been depressed, the vertebral artery retracted medially, and the brachial plexus retracted superiorly to reveal the cervicothoracic (stellate) ganglion (the combined inferior cervical and 1st thoracic ganglia). Anesthetic injected around the cervicothoracic (stellate) ganglion blocks transmission of stimuli through the cervical and superior thoracic ganglia. This ganglion block may relieve vascular spasms involving the brain and upper limb. It is also useful when deciding if surgical resection of the ganglion would be beneficial to a person with excess vasoconstriction of the ipsilateral limb. **B.** Relation of brachial plexus and subclavian artery to anterior and middle scalene muscles.

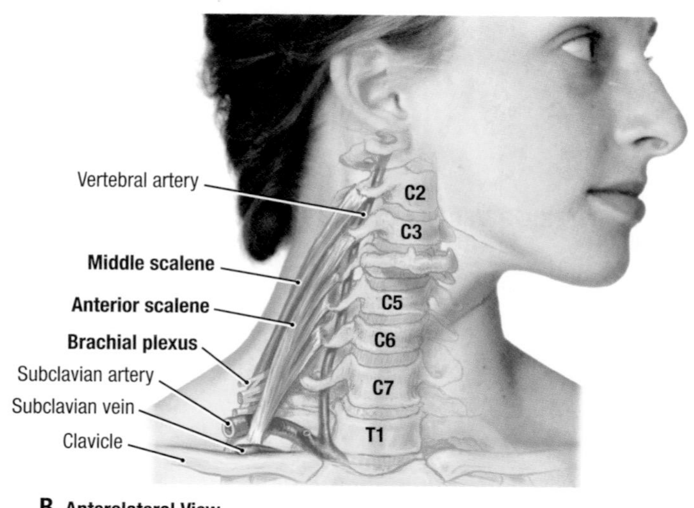
Vertebral artery
C2
C3
Middle scalene
Anterior scalene
C5
Brachial plexus
C6
Subclavian artery
C7
Subclavian vein
T1
Clavicle

**B. Anterolateral View**

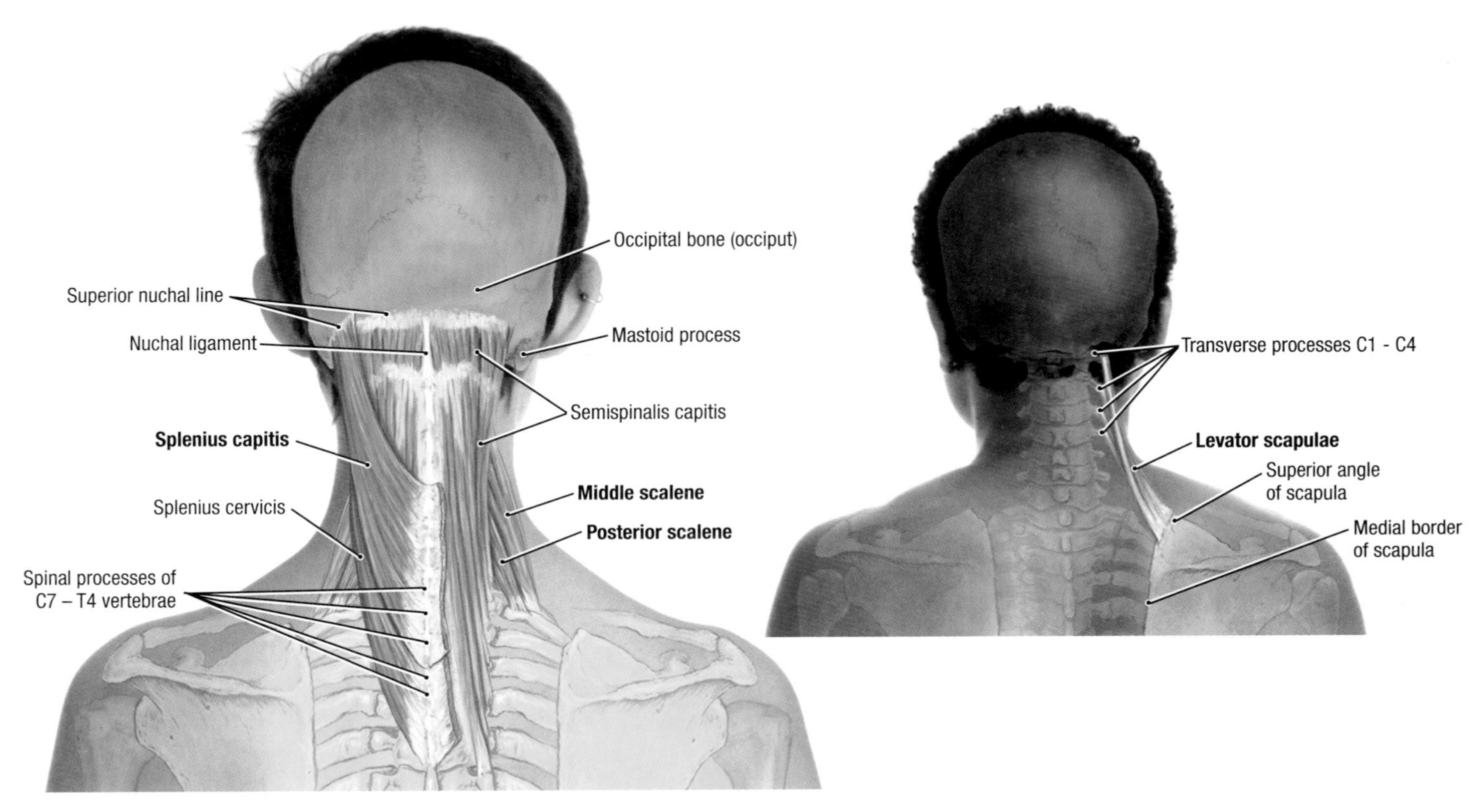
Occipital bone (occiput)
Superior nuchal line
Nuchal ligament
Mastoid process
Semispinalis capitis
Splenius capitis
Splenius cervicis
Middle scalene
Posterior scalene
Spinal processes of C7 – T4 vertebrae
Transverse processes C1 - C4
Levator scapulae
Superior angle of scapula
Medial border of scapula

## TABLE 8.7 LATERAL VERTEBRAL MUSCLES

| Muscle | Superior Attachment | Inferior Attachment | Innervation | Main Action |
|---|---|---|---|---|
| **Splenius capitis** | Inferior half of nuchal ligament and spinous processes of C7 and superior 3–4 thoracic vertebrae | Lateral aspect of mastoid process and lateral third of superior nuchal line | Posterior rami of middle cervical spinal nerves | Laterally flexes and rotates head and neck to same side; acting bilaterally, extend head and neck[a] |
| **Levator scapulae** | Posterior tubercles of transverse processes of C1–C4 vertebrae | Superior part of medial border of scapula | Dorsal scapular nerve (C5) and cervical spinal nerves C3 and C4 | Elevates scapula and tilts its glenoid cavity inferiorly by rotating scapula |
| **Middle scalene** | Posterior tubercles of transverse processes of C2–C7 vertebrae | Superior surface of 1st rib posterior to groove for subclavian artery | Anterior rami of cervical spinal nerves | Flexes neck laterally; elevates 1st rib during forced inspiration[b] |
| **Posterior scalene** | | External border of 2nd rib | Anterior rami of cervical spinal nerves C4 to C8 | Flexes neck laterally; elevates 2nd rib during forced inspiration[b] |

[a]Rotation of head occurs at atlantoaxial joints.
[b]Flexion of neck anterior (or lateral) bending of cervical vertebrae C2–C7.

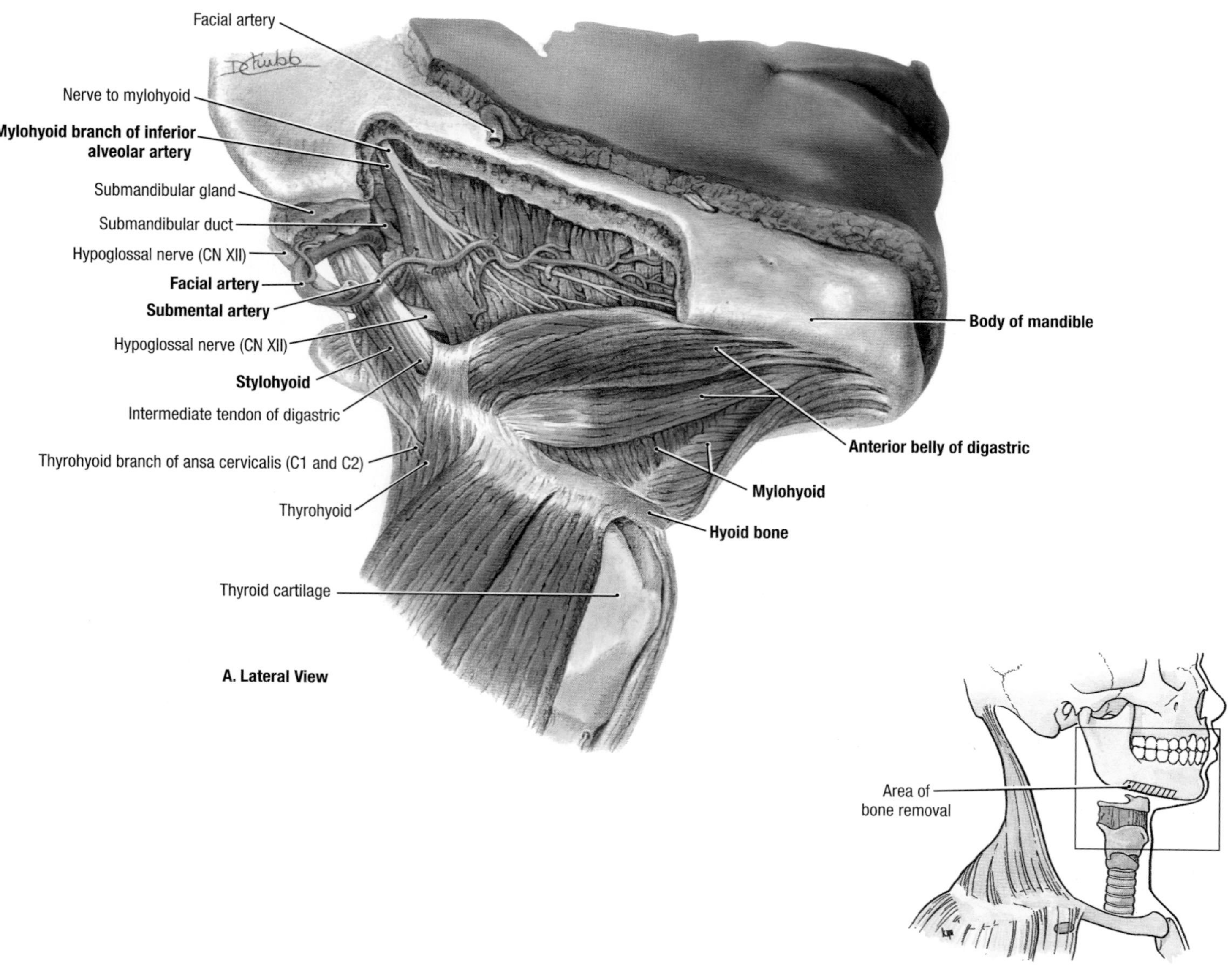
Facial artery
Nerve to mylohyoid
Mylohyoid branch of inferior alveolar artery
Submandibular gland
Submandibular duct
Hypoglossal nerve (CN XII)
Facial artery
Submental artery
Hypoglossal nerve (CN XII)
Stylohyoid
Intermediate tendon of digastric
Thyrohyoid branch of ansa cervicalis (C1 and C2)
Thyrohyoid
Thyroid cartilage
Body of mandible
Anterior belly of digastric
Mylohyoid
Hyoid bone
A. Lateral View
Area of bone removal

## 8.19 Serial dissection of submandibular region and floor of mouth—I

Mylohyoid and digastric muscles. **A.** Structures overlying the mandible and a portion of the body of the mandible have been removed.

- The stylohyoid and posterior belly and intermediate tendon of the digastric muscle form the posterior border of the submandibular triangle; the facial artery passes superficial to these muscles.
- The anterior belly of the digastric muscle forms the anterior border of the submandibular triangle. In this specimen, the anterior belly has an additional origin from the hyoid bone; the mylohyoid muscle forms the medial wall of the triangle and has a thick, free posterior border.
- The nerve to mylohyoid, which supplies the mylohyoid muscle and anterior belly of the digastric muscle, is accompanied by the mylohyoid branch of the inferior alveolar artery posteriorly and the submental artery from the facial artery anteriorly.

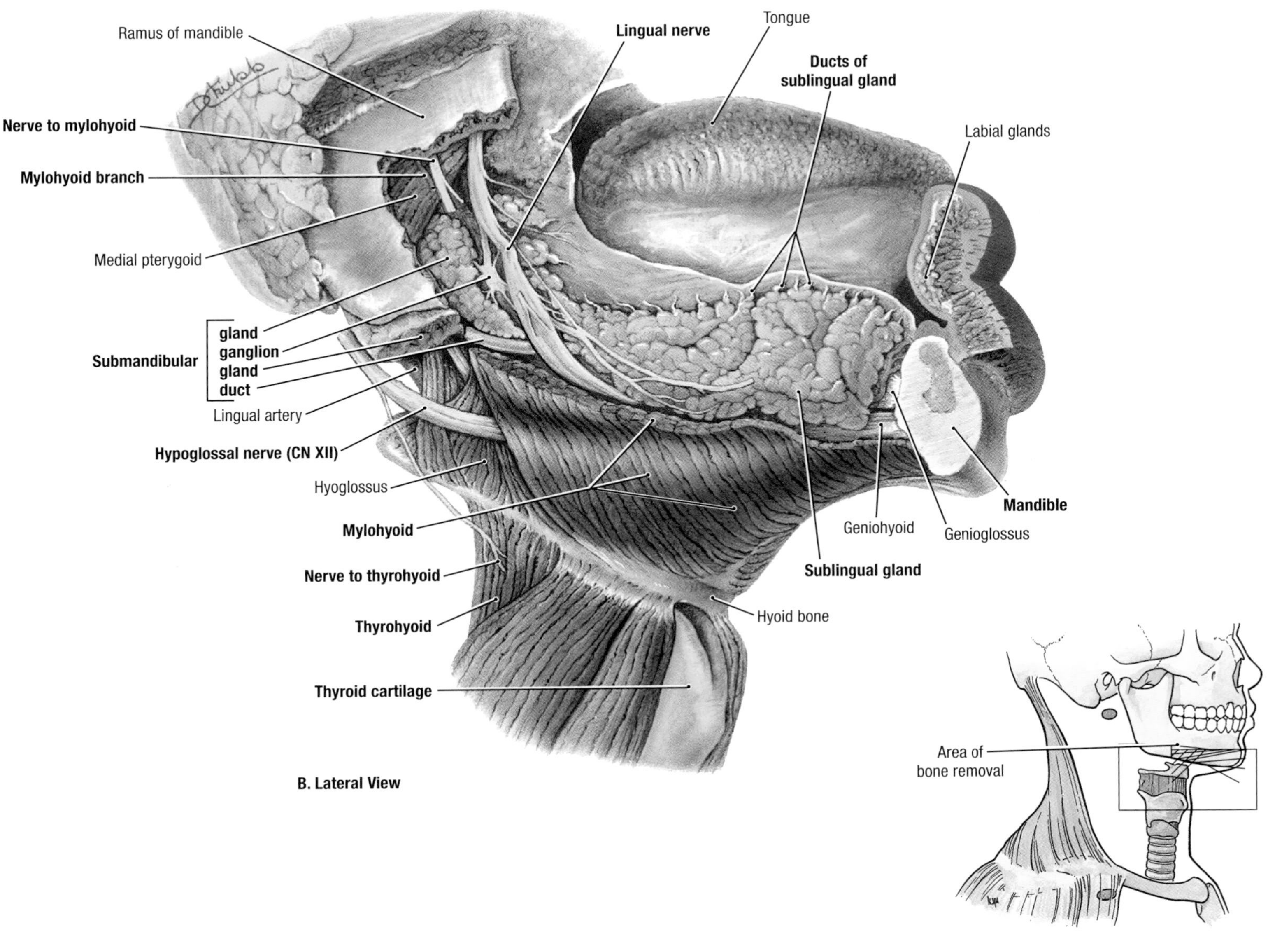
Ramus of mandible
Lingual nerve
Tongue
Ducts of sublingual gland
Labial glands
Nerve to mylohyoid
Mylohyoid branch
Medial pterygoid
Submandibular
gland
ganglion
gland
duct
Lingual artery
Hypoglossal nerve (CN XII)
Hyoglossus
Mylohyoid
Nerve to thyrohyoid
Thyrohyoid
Thyroid cartilage
Mandible
Geniohyoid
Genioglossus
Sublingual gland
Hyoid bone
Area of bone removal

B. Lateral View

## 8.19 Serial dissection of submandibular region and floor of mouth—II

**B.** Sublingual and submandibular glands. The body and adjacent portion of the ramus of the mandible have been removed.

- The sublingual salivary gland lies posterior to the mandible and is in contact with the deep part of the submandibular gland posteriorly.
- Numerous fine ducts pass from the superior border of the sublingual gland to open on the sublingual fold of the overlying mucosa.
- The lingual nerve lies between the sublingual gland and the deep part of the submandibular gland; the submandibular ganglion is suspended from this nerve.
- Spinal nerve C1 fibers, conveyed by the hypoglossal nerve (CN XII), pass to the thyrohyoid muscle before the hypoglossal nerve passes deep to the mylohyoid muscle.

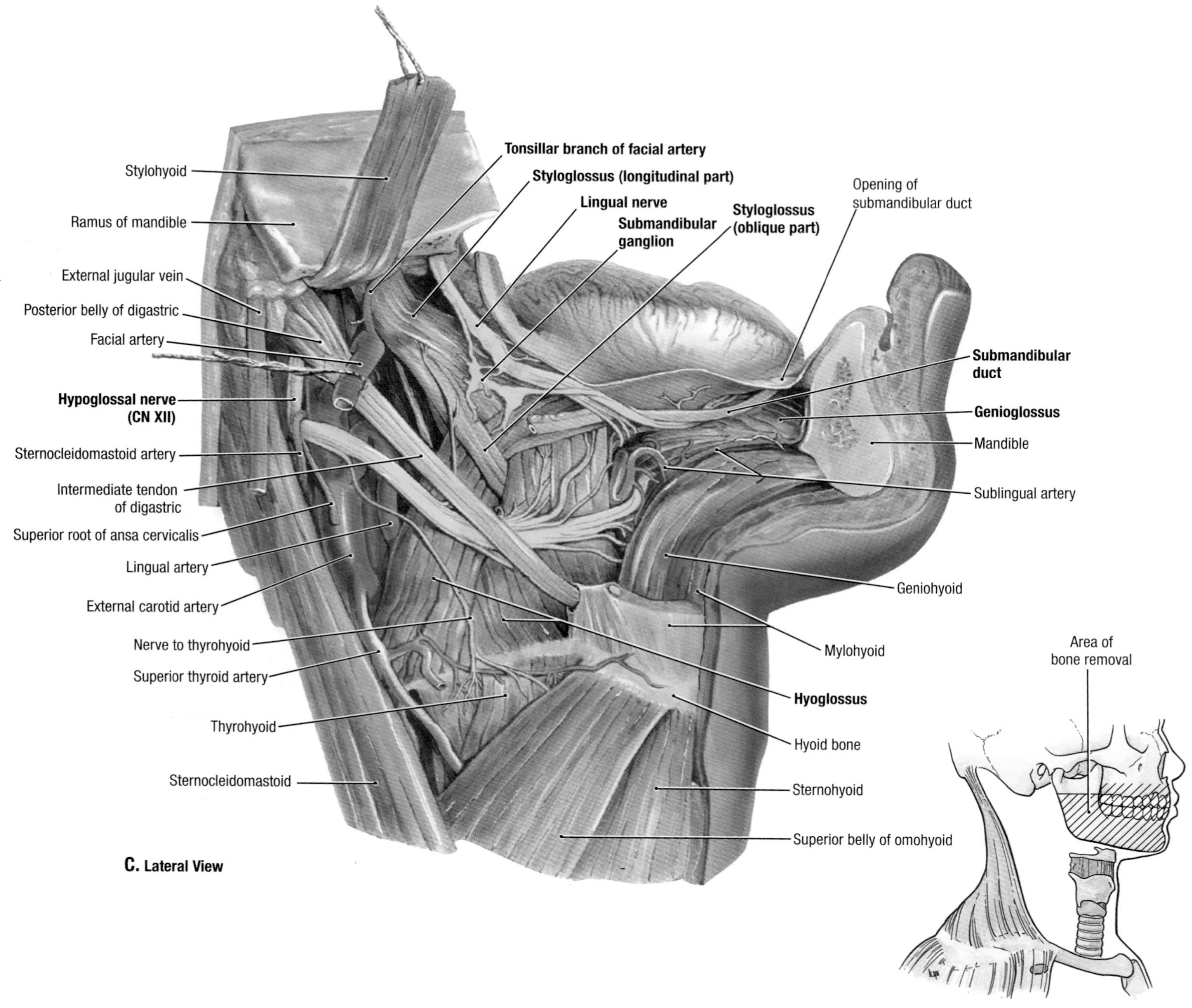

Stylohyoid
Ramus of mandible
External jugular vein
Posterior belly of digastric
Facial artery
Hypoglossal nerve (CN XII)
Sternocleidomastoid artery
Intermediate tendon of digastric
Superior root of ansa cervicalis
Lingual artery
External carotid artery
Nerve to thyrohyoid
Superior thyroid artery
Thyrohyoid
Sternocleidomastoid
Tonsillar branch of facial artery
Styloglossus (longitudinal part)
Lingual nerve
Submandibular ganglion
Styloglossus (oblique part)
Opening of submandibular duct
Submandibular duct
Genioglossus
Mandible
Sublingual artery
Geniohyoid
Mylohyoid
Hyoglossus
Hyoid bone
Sternohyoid
Superior belly of omohyoid
Area of bone removal

C. Lateral View

## 8.19 Serial dissection of submandibular region and floor of mouth—III

**C.** Hyoglossus muscle, lingual and hypoglossal nerves (CN XII). All of the right half of the mandible, except the superior part of the ramus, has been removed. The stylohyoid muscle is reflected superiorly, and the posterior belly of the digastric muscle is left in situ.

- The hyoglossus muscle ascends from the greater horn and body of the hyoid bone to the side of the tongue.
- The styloglossus muscle is crossed by the tonsillar branch of the facial artery posterosuperiorly, and its oblique part interdigitates with bundles of the hyoglossus muscle inferiorly.
- The hypoglossal nerve supplies all of the muscles of the tongue, both extrinsic and intrinsic, except the palatoglossus (a palatine muscle, innervated by CN X).
- The submandibular duct runs anteriorly in contact with the hyoglossus and genioglossus muscles to its opening on the side of the frenulum of the tongue.
- The lingual nerve is in contact with the mandible posteriorly, looping inferior to the submandibular duct and ending in the tongue. The submandibular ganglion is suspended from the lingual nerve; twigs leave the nerve to supply the mucous membrane.

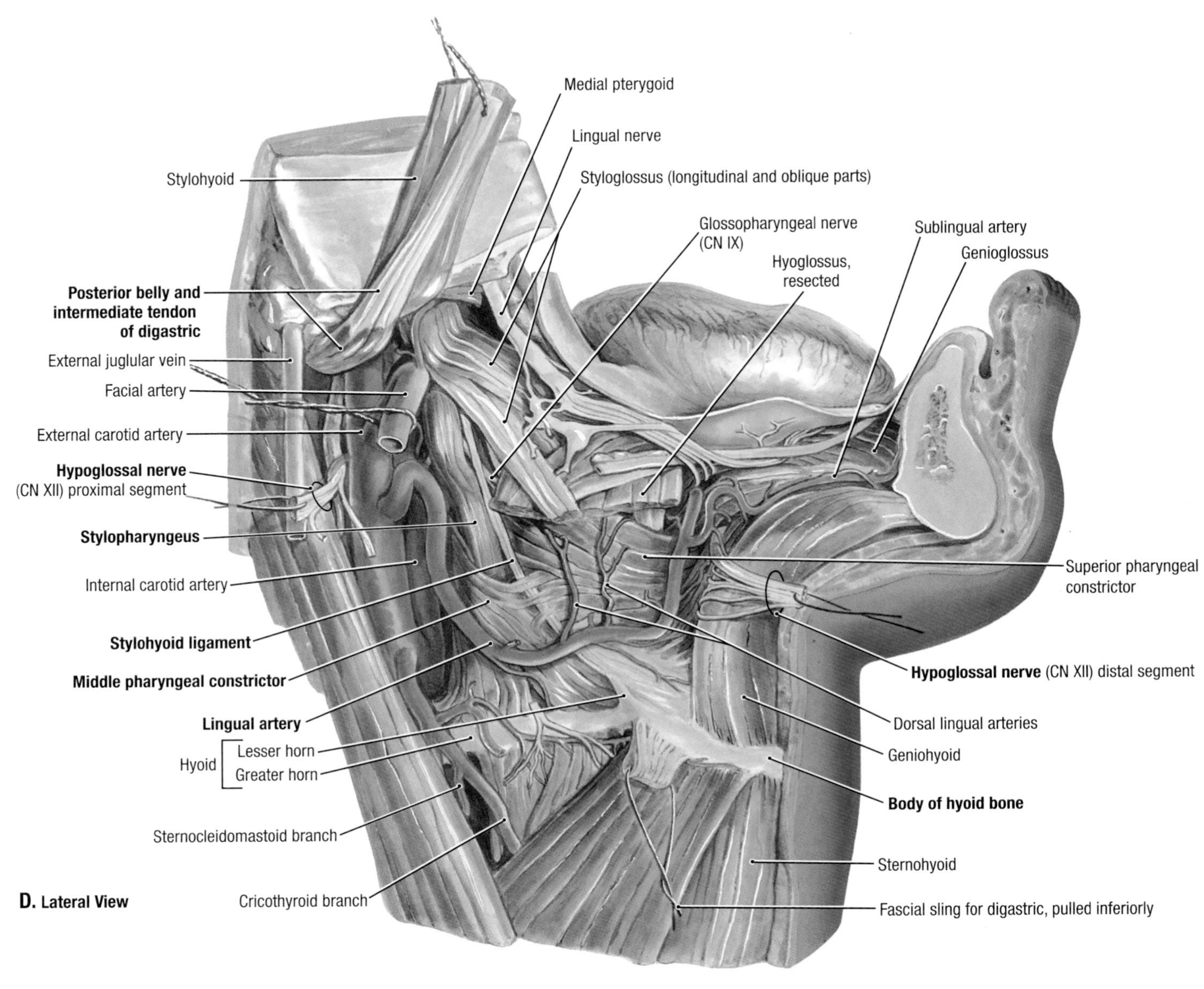
Medial pterygoid
Lingual nerve
Styloglossus (longitudinal and oblique parts)
Stylohyoid
Glossopharyngeal nerve (CN IX)
Sublingual artery
Genioglossus
Hyoglossus, resected
Posterior belly and intermediate tendon of digastric
External juglular vein
Facial artery
External carotid artery
Hypoglossal nerve (CN XII) proximal segment
Stylopharyngeus
Internal carotid artery
Superior pharyngeal constrictor
Stylohyoid ligament
Middle pharyngeal constrictor
Hypoglossal nerve (CN XII) distal segment
Lingual artery
Dorsal lingual arteries
Hyoid
Lesser horn
Greater horn
Geniohyoid
Body of hyoid bone
Sternocleidomastoid branch
Sternohyoid
D. Lateral View
Cricothyroid branch
Fascial sling for digastric, pulled inferiorly

## 8.19 Serial dissection of submandibular region and floor of mouth—IV

**D.** Genioglossus and geniohyoid muscles. The stylohyoid, posterior belly and intermediate tendon of the digastric muscle are reflected superiorly, the hypoglossal nerve is divided, and the hyoglossus muscle is mostly removed.

- The lingual artery passes deep to the hyoglossus muscle (resected here), close to the greater horn of the hyoid, and then passes lateral to the middle pharyngeal constrictor muscle, stylohyoid ligament, and genioglossus muscle and turns into the tongue as the deep lingual arteries.

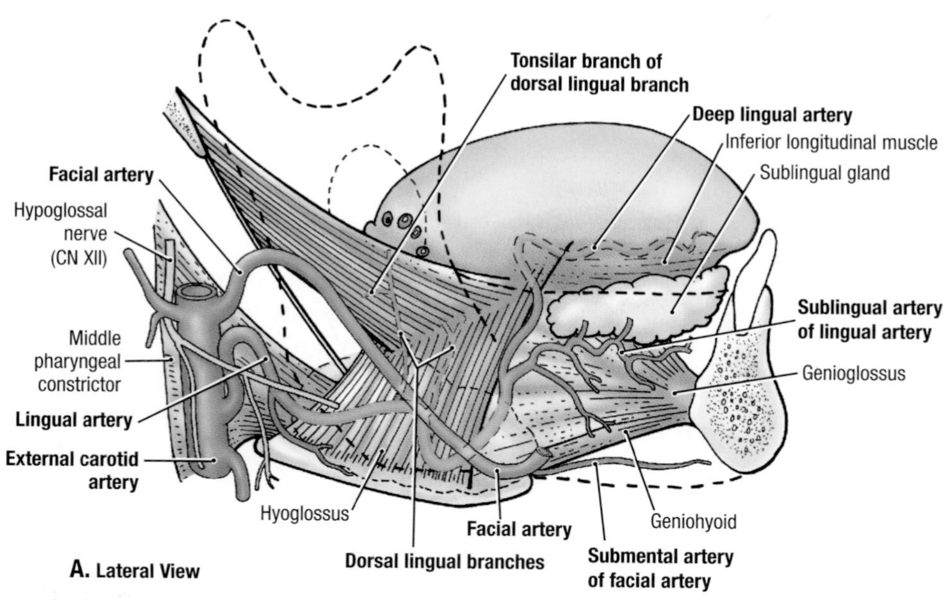
Tonsilar branch of dorsal lingual branch
Deep lingual artery
Inferior longitudinal muscle
Sublingual gland
Facial artery
Hypoglossal nerve (CN XII)
Sublingual artery of lingual artery
Middle pharyngeal constrictor
Genioglossus
Lingual artery
External carotid artery
Hyoglossus
Facial artery
Geniohyoid
Dorsal lingual branches
Submental artery of facial artery
A. Lateral View

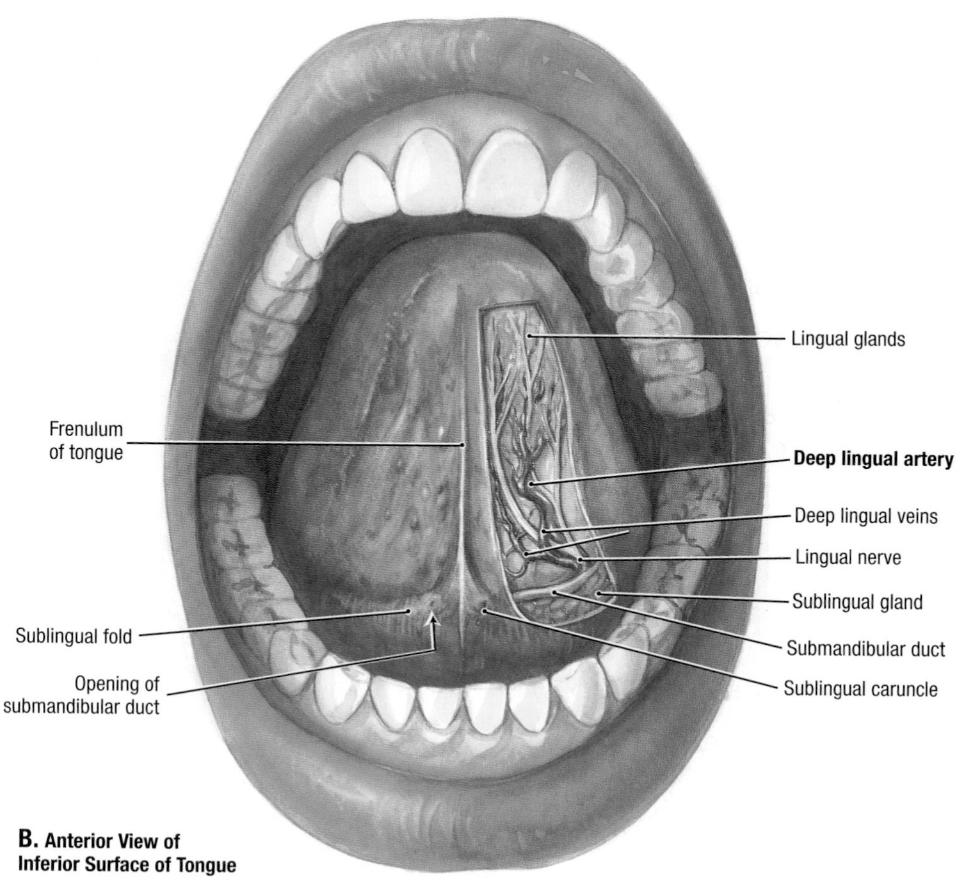
Lingual glands
Frenulum of tongue
Deep lingual artery
Deep lingual veins
Lingual nerve
Sublingual gland
Sublingual fold
Submandibular duct
Opening of submandibular duct
Sublingual caruncle
B. Anterior View of Inferior Surface of Tongue

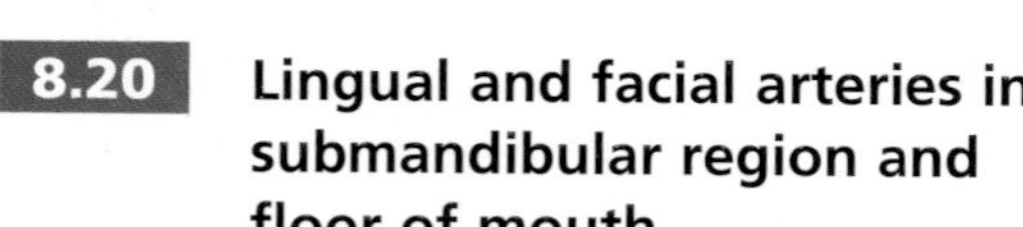

## 8.20 Lingual and facial arteries in submandibular region and floor of mouth

**A.** Course of the lingual artery. **B.** Inferior surface of the tongue and floor of the mouth.

In **A**:

- The dorsal lingual arteries supply the root of the tongue and palatine tonsil, the deep lingual artery supplies the body of the tongue, and the sublingual branch supplies the floor of the mouth.

In **B**:

- The inferior (sublingual) surface of the tongue is covered by a mucous membrane through which the underlying deep lingual veins can be seen.
- The sublingual caruncle, a papilla on each side of the frenulum, marks the location of the opening of the submandibular duct.

**Posterior Views**

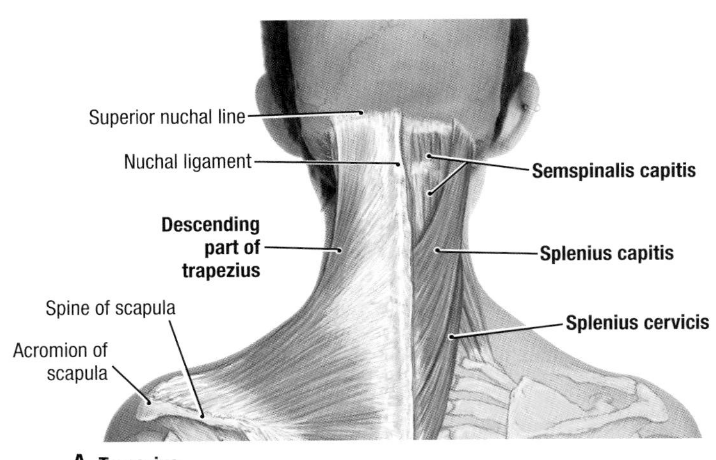

Superior nuchal line
Nuchal ligament
Descending part of trapezius
Spine of scapula
Acromion of scapula
Semspinalis capitis
Splenius capitis
Splenius cervicis


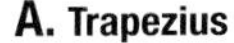

**A.** Trapezius

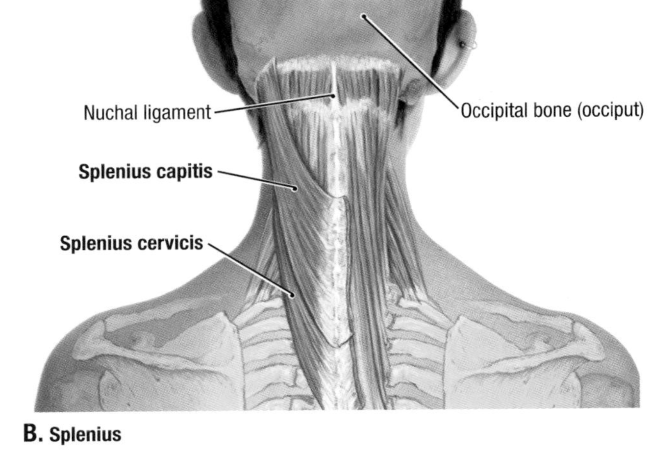

Nuchal ligament
Splenius capitis
Splenius cervicis
Occipital bone (occiput)


**B.** Splenius

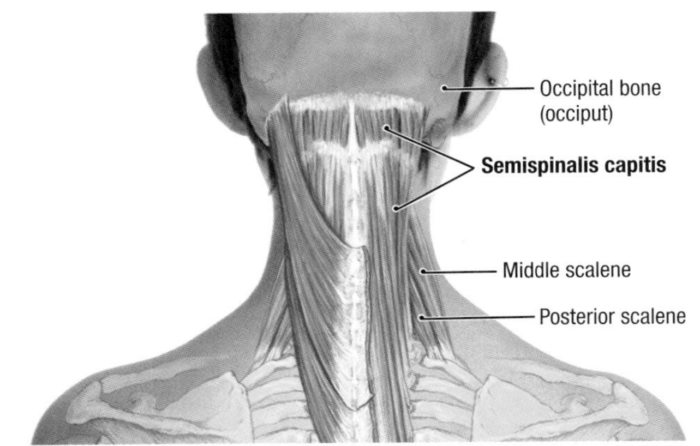

Occipital bone (occiput)
Semispinalis capitis
Middle scalene
Posterior scalene


**C.** Semispinalis

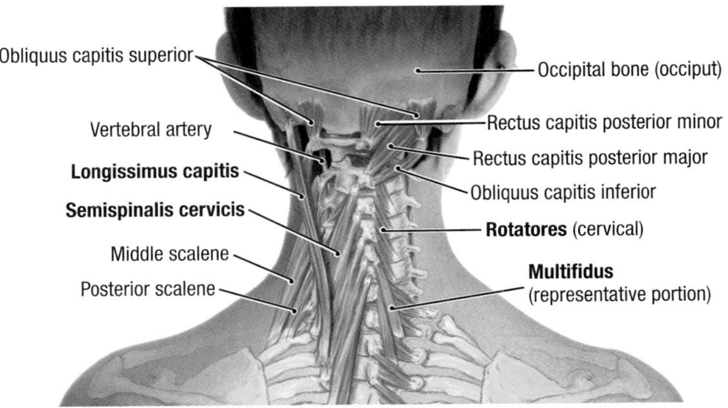

Obliquus capitis superior
Vertebral artery
Longissimus capitis
Semispinalis cervicis
Middle scalene
Posterior scalene
Occipital bone (occiput)
Rectus capitis posterior minor
Rectus capitis posterior major
Obliquus capitis inferior
Rotatores (cervical)
Multifidus (representative portion)


**D.** Deep posterior cervical muscles

## TABLE 8.8 MUSCLES OF POSTERIOR CERVICAL REGION

| Muscle | Superior Attachment | Inferior Attachment | Innervation | Main Action |
|---|---|---|---|---|
| **Extrinsic muscle of back (superior axioappendicular muscle)** | | | | |
| **Descending part of trapezius** | Medial third of superior nuchal line; external occipital protuberance; nuchal ligament | Lateral third of clavicle and lateral aspect of acromion of scapula | Spinal accessory nerve (CN XI) | Elevates scapulae and works with other parts of muscle to retract scapulae; with shoulder fixed, contributes to extension of head, side bending (lateral flexion) of neck |
| **Intrinsic muscles of back—superficial layer** | | | | |
| **Splenius** | Nuchal ligament and spinous processes of C7 toT3–T4 vertebrae | *Splenius capitis:* fibers run superolaterally to mastoid process of temporal bone and lateral third of superior nuchal line of occipital bone<br>*Splenius cervicis:* Tubercles of transverse processes of C1–C4 vertebrae | Posterior rami of spinal nerves | *Acting unilaterally:* laterally flex and rotate head to side of active muscle<br>*Acting bilaterally:* extend head and neck |
| **Intrinsic muscles of back—intermediate layer** | | | | |
| **Longissimus** | Transverse processes of T1–T5 vertebrae | *Longissimus capitis:* posterior mastoid process<br>*Longissimus cervicis:* transverse processes of C2–C6 | Posterior rami of spinal nerves | Extends vertebral column; longissimus capitis turns face ipsilaterally |
| **Intrinsic muscles of back—deep layer** | | | | |
| **Semispinalis** | Transverse processes of C4-T5 vertebrae | *Semispinalis capitis:* Superior nuchal line of occipital bone<br>*Semispinalis cervicis:* Spinous processes of cervical vertebrae | Posterior rami of spinal nerves | *Acting unilaterally:* contribute to contralateral rotation;<br>*Acting bilaterally:* extend head and neck |
| **Multifidus of cervical region** | Transverse processes of T1–T3<br>Articular processes of C4–C7 vertebrae | Spinous processes 2–4 segments inferior to attachment | | Stabilizes vertebrae during local movements of vertebral column |
| **Rotatores** | Transverse processes | Junction of lamina and transverse process, or spinous process of vertebra immediately (brevis) or two segments (longus) superior to origin | | Stabilize, assist with local extension and rotatory movements; may function as proprioceptive organs |

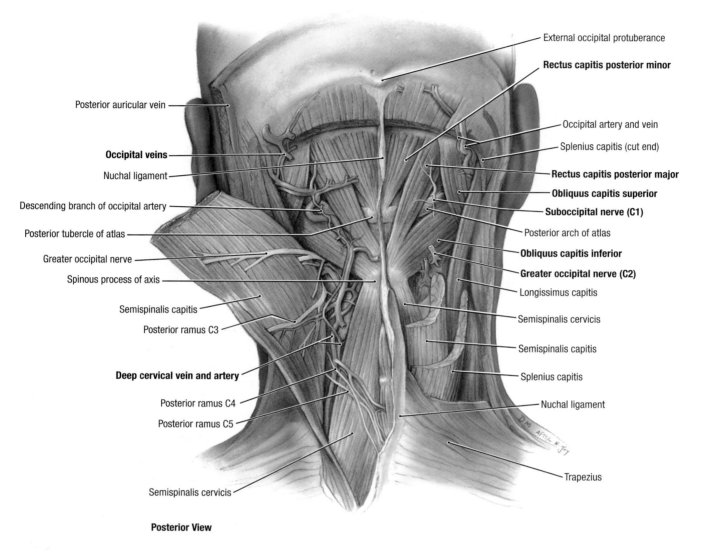

External occipital protuberance
**Rectus capitis posterior minor**
Posterior auricular vein
Occipital artery and vein
Splenius capitis (cut end)
**Occipital veins**
Nuchal ligament
**Rectus capitis posterior major**
**Obliquus capitis superior**
Descending branch of occipital artery
**Suboccipital nerve (C1)**
Posterior tubercle of atlas
Posterior arch of atlas
**Obliquus capitis inferior**
Greater occipital nerve
**Greater occipital nerve (C2)**
Spinous process of axis
Longissimus capitis
Semispinalis capitis
Semispinalis cervicis
Posterior ramus C3
Semispinalis capitis
**Deep cervical vein and artery**
Splenius capitis
Posterior ramus C4
Nuchal ligament
Posterior ramus C5
Trapezius
Semispinalis cervicis

**Posterior View**

## 8.21 Suboccipital region

**A.** Dissection. **B.** Schematic illustration.

- The suboccipital triangle is bounded by three muscles: obliquus capitis inferior and superior, and rectus capitis posterior major.
- The suboccipital nerve (posterior ramus of C1) emerges through the suboccipital triangle to innervate the muscles forming the triangle.

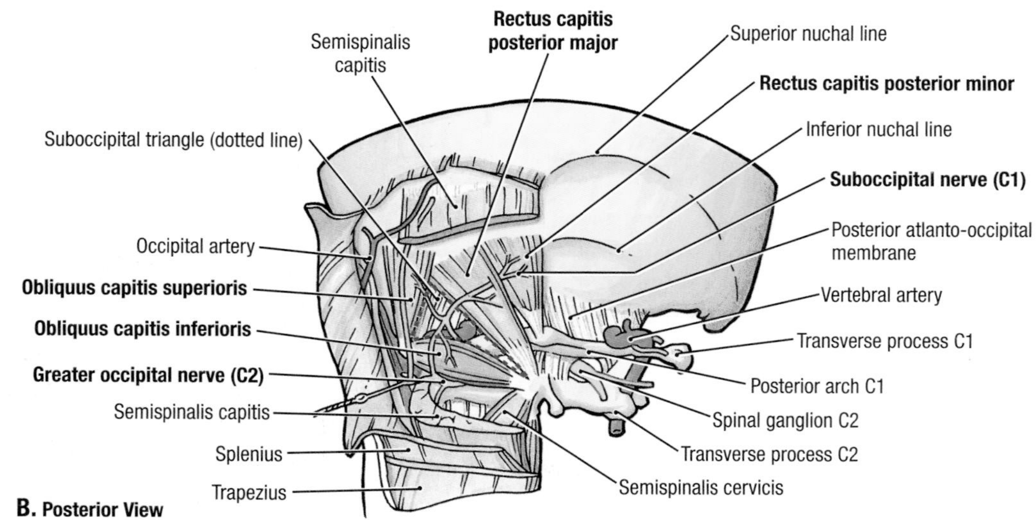
Semispinalis capitis
Rectus capitis posterior major
Superior nuchal line
Rectus capitis posterior minor
Inferior nuchal line
Suboccipital triangle (dotted line)
Suboccipital nerve (C1)
Occipital artery
Posterior atlanto-occipital membrane
Obliquus capitis superioris
Vertebral artery
Obliquus capitis inferioris
Transverse process C1
Greater occipital nerve (C2)
Posterior arch C1
Semispinalis capitis
Spinal ganglion C2
Splenius
Transverse process C2
Trapezius
Semispinalis cervicis

**B.** Posterior View

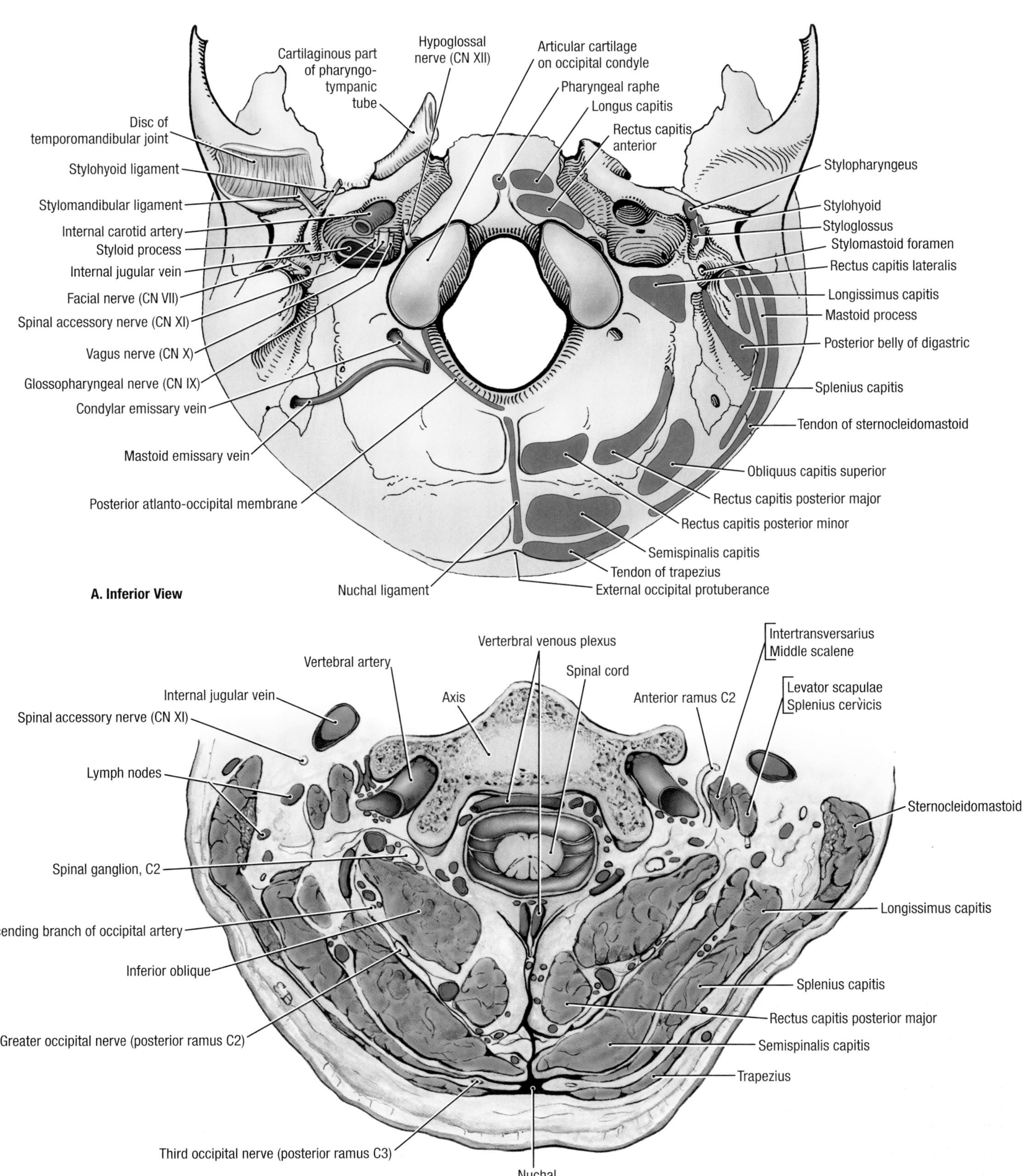
Cartilaginous part of pharyngo-tympanic tube
Hypoglossal nerve (CN XII)
Articular cartilage on occipital condyle
Pharyngeal raphe
Longus capitis
Rectus capitis anterior
Disc of temporomandibular joint
Stylohyoid ligament
Stylomandibular ligament
Internal carotid artery
Styloid process
Internal jugular vein
Facial nerve (CN VII)
Spinal accessory nerve (CN XI)
Vagus nerve (CN X)
Glossopharyngeal nerve (CN IX)
Condylar emissary vein
Mastoid emissary vein
Posterior atlanto-occipital membrane
Stylopharyngeus
Stylohyoid
Styloglossus
Stylomastoid foramen
Rectus capitis lateralis
Longissimus capitis
Mastoid process
Posterior belly of digastric
Splenius capitis
Tendon of sternocleidomastoid
Obliquus capitis superior
Rectus capitis posterior major
Rectus capitis posterior minor
Semispinalis capitis
Tendon of trapezius
External occipital protuberance
Nuchal ligament
A. Inferior View
Verterbral venous plexus
Vertebral artery
Spinal cord
Intertransversarius
Middle scalene
Levator scapulae
Splenius cervicis
Internal jugular vein
Spinal accessory nerve (CN XI)
Axis
Anterior ramus C2
Lymph nodes
Sternocleidomastoid
Spinal ganglion, C2
Longissimus capitis
Descending branch of occipital artery
Inferior oblique
Splenius capitis
Rectus capitis posterior major
Greater occipital nerve (posterior ramus C2)
Semispinalis capitis
Trapezius
Third occipital nerve (posterior ramus C3)
Nuchal ligament
B. Transverse Section

**8.22 Posterior cervical region—base of skull and transverse section**

**A.** Muscular attachments to and neurovascular relationships at the base of the skull. **B.** Transverse section through the axis (C2).

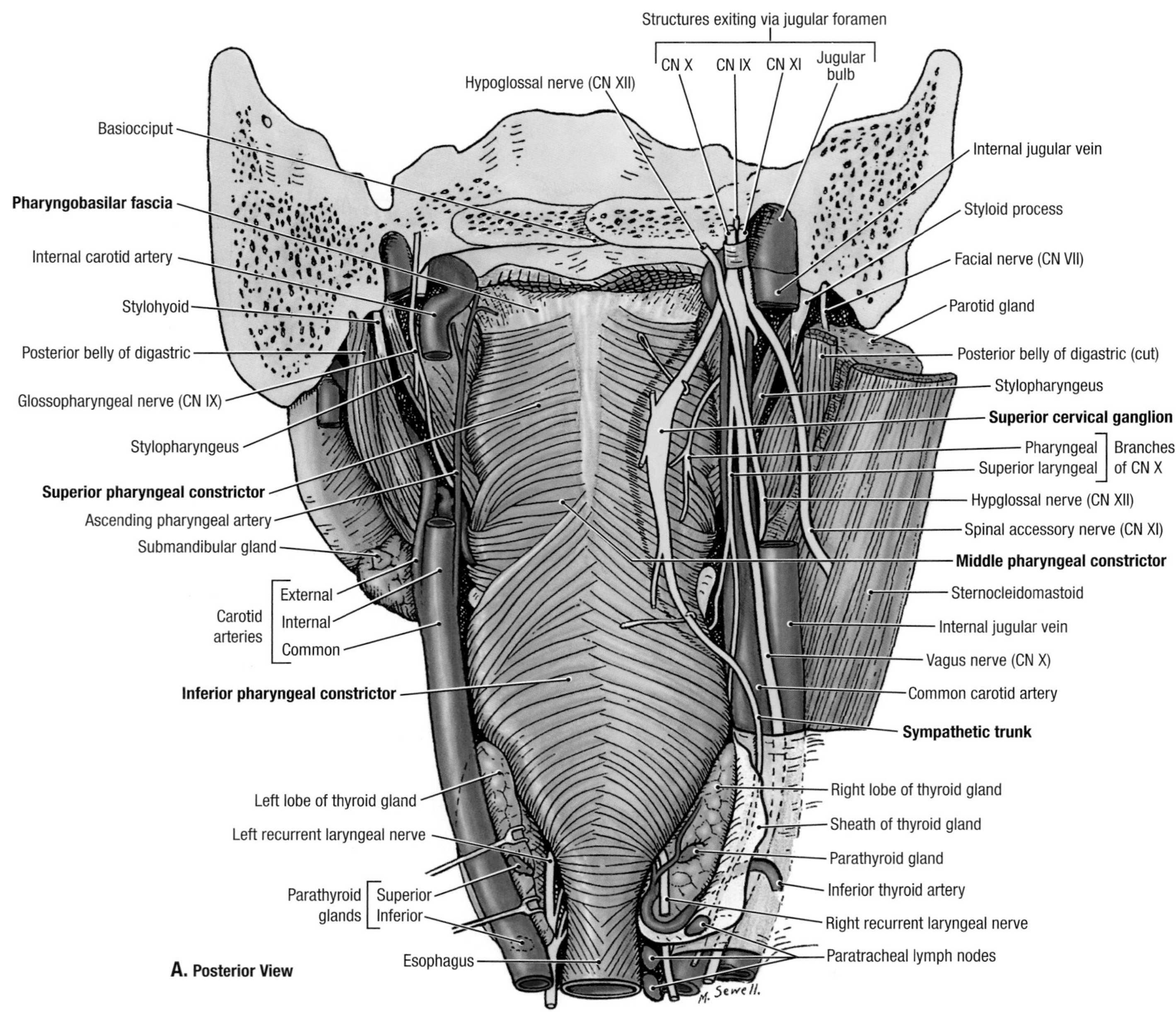
Structures exiting via jugular foramen
CN X
CN IX
CN XI
Jugular bulb
Hypoglossal nerve (CN XII)
Basiocciput
Pharyngobasilar fascia
Internal carotid artery
Stylohyoid
Posterior belly of digastric
Glossopharyngeal nerve (CN IX)
Stylopharyngeus
Superior pharyngeal constrictor
Ascending pharyngeal artery
Submandibular gland
Carotid arteries
External
Internal
Common
Inferior pharyngeal constrictor
Left lobe of thyroid gland
Left recurrent laryngeal nerve
Parathyroid glands
Superior
Inferior
Esophagus
A. Posterior View
Internal jugular vein
Styloid process
Facial nerve (CN VII)
Parotid gland
Posterior belly of digastric (cut)
Stylopharyngeus
Superior cervical ganglion
Pharyngeal
Superior laryngeal
Branches of CN X
Hypglossal nerve (CN XII)
Spinal accessory nerve (CN XI)
Middle pharyngeal constrictor
Sternocleidomastoid
Internal jugular vein
Vagus nerve (CN X)
Common carotid artery
Sympathetic trunk
Right lobe of thyroid gland
Sheath of thyroid gland
Parathyroid gland
Inferior thyroid artery
Right recurrent laryngeal nerve
Paratracheal lymph nodes
M. Sewell.

## 8.23 External pharynx—I

**A.** Illustration of a dissection similar to **B.** The sympathetic trunk (including the superior cervical ganglion), which normally lies posterior to the internal carotid artery, has been retracted medially.

- The pharyngobasilar fascia, between the superior pharyngeal constrictor muscle and the base of the skull, attaches the pharynx to the occipital bone and forms the wall of the noncollapsible pharyngeal recesses.
- As they exit the jugular foramen, CN IX lies anterior to CN X, and CN XI; CN XII, exiting the hypoglossal canal, lies medially.

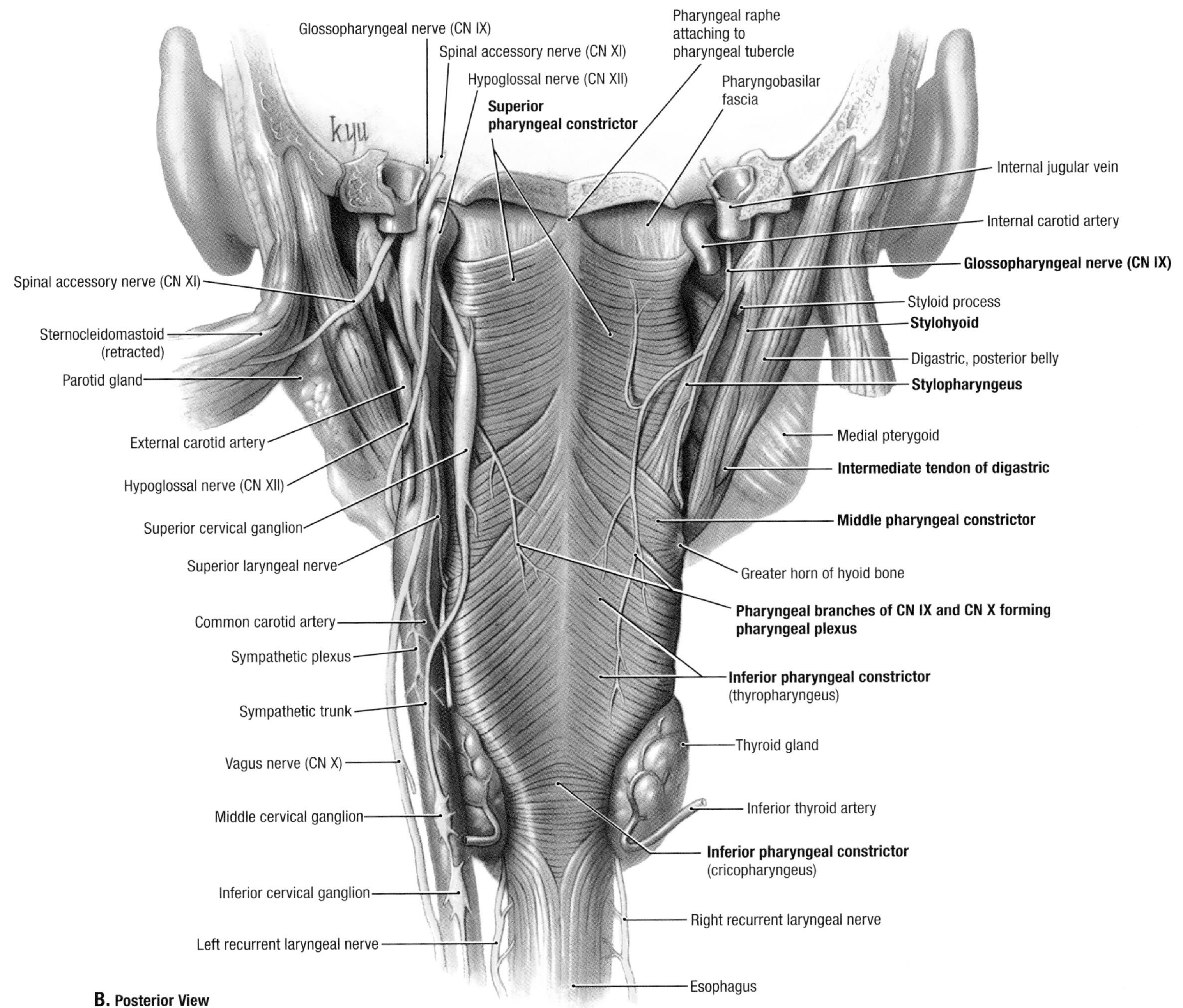
Glossopharyngeal nerve (CN IX)
Spinal accessory nerve (CN XI)
Hypoglossal nerve (CN XII)
Superior pharyngeal constrictor
Pharyngeal raphe attaching to pharyngeal tubercle
Pharyngobasilar fascia
kyu
Internal jugular vein
Internal carotid artery
Glossopharyngeal nerve (CN IX)
Spinal accessory nerve (CN XI)
Styloid process
Stylohyoid
Sternocleidomastoid (retracted)
Digastric, posterior belly
Parotid gland
Stylopharyngeus
Medial pterygoid
External carotid artery
Intermediate tendon of digastric
Hypoglossal nerve (CN XII)
Middle pharyngeal constrictor
Superior cervical ganglion
Greater horn of hyoid bone
Superior laryngeal nerve
Pharyngeal branches of CN IX and CN X forming pharyngeal plexus
Common carotid artery
Sympathetic plexus
Inferior pharyngeal constrictor (thyropharyngeus)
Sympathetic trunk
Thyroid gland
Vagus nerve (CN X)
Inferior thyroid artery
Middle cervical ganglion
Inferior pharyngeal constrictor (cricopharyngeus)
Inferior cervical ganglion
Right recurrent laryngeal nerve
Left recurrent laryngeal nerve
Esophagus

**B. Posterior View**

## 8.23 External pharynx—II

**B.** Dissection. A large wedge of occipital bone (including the foramen magnum) and the articulated cervical vertebrae have been separated from the remainder (anterior portion) of the head and cervical viscera at the retropharyngeal space and removed.

- The pharynx is a unique portion of the alimentary tract, having a circular layer of muscle externally and a longitudinal layer internally.
- The circular layer of the pharynx consists of the three pharyngeal constrictor muscles (superior, middle, and inferior), which overlap one another.
- On the right side of the specimen, the stylopharyngeus muscle and glossopharyngeal nerve (IX) pass from the medial side of the styloid process anteromedially through the interval between the superior and middle pharyngeal constrictor muscles to become part of the internal longitudinal layer. The stylohyoid muscle passes from the lateral side of the styloid process anterolaterally and splits on its way to the hyoid bone to accommodate passage of the intermediate tendon of the digastric.
- Pharyngeal branches of the glossopharyngeal nerve (CN IX) and the vagus nerve (CN X) form the pharyngeal plexus, which provides most of the pharyngeal innervation. The glossopharyngeal nerve supplies the sensory component, while the vagus supplies motor innervation.

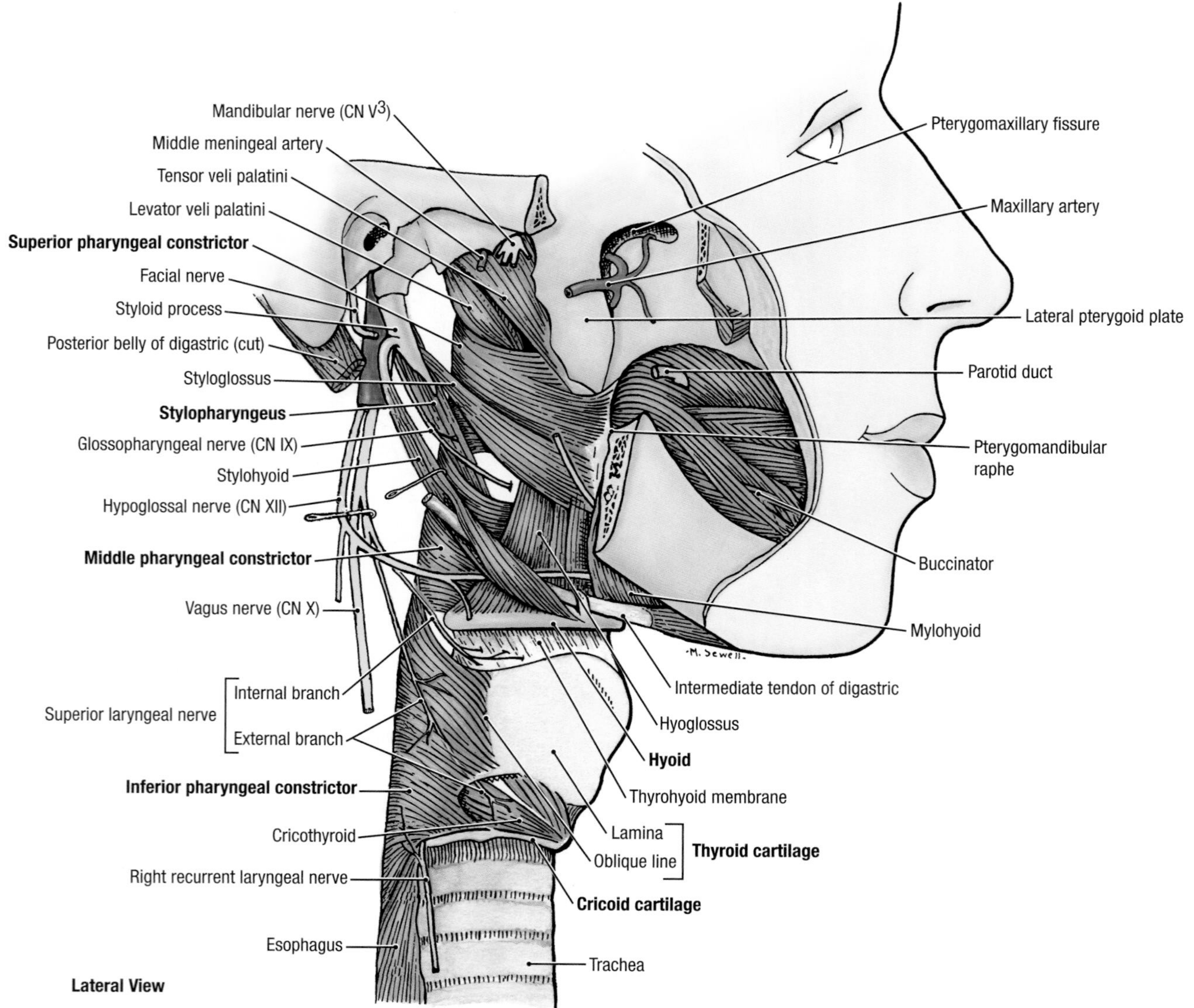

Mandibular nerve (CN V3)
Middle meningeal artery
Tensor veli palatini
Levator veli palatini
Superior pharyngeal constrictor
Facial nerve
Styloid process
Posterior belly of digastric (cut)
Styloglossus
Stylopharyngeus
Glossopharyngeal nerve (CN IX)
Stylohyoid
Hypoglossal nerve (CN XII)
Middle pharyngeal constrictor
Vagus nerve (CN X)
Superior laryngeal nerve
Internal branch
External branch
Inferior pharyngeal constrictor
Cricothyroid
Right recurrent laryngeal nerve
Esophagus
Lateral View
Pterygomaxillary fissure
Maxillary artery
Lateral pterygoid plate
Parotid duct
Pterygomandibular raphe
Buccinator
Mylohyoid
M. Sewell
Intermediate tendon of digastric
Hyoglossus
Hyoid
Thyrohyoid membrane
Lamina
Oblique line
Thyroid cartilage
Cricoid cartilage
Trachea


## TABLE 8.9 MUSCLES OF PHARYNX

<table>
<tr><th>Muscle</th><th>Origin</th><th>Insertion</th><th>Innervation</th><th>Main Action(s)</th></tr>
<tr><td>Superior pharyngeal constrictor</td><td>Pterygoid hamulus, pterygo-mandibular raphe, posterior end of mylohyoid line of mandible, and side of tongue</td><td rowspan="4">Pharyngeal raphe</td><td rowspan="4">Pharyngeal and superior laryngeal branches of vagus (CN X) through pharyngeal plexus</td><td rowspan="4">Constrict wall of pharynx during swallowing</td></tr>
<tr><td>Middle pharyngeal constrictor</td><td>Stylohyoid ligament and superior (greater) and inferior (lesser) horns of hyoid bone</td></tr>
<tr><td>Inferior pharyngeal constrictor</td><td></td></tr>
<tr><td>Thyropharyngeus</td><td>Oblique line of thyroid cartilage</td></tr>
<tr><td>Cricopharyngeus (see Fig. 8.20B)</td><td>Side of cricoid cartilage</td><td>Contralateral side of cricoid cartilage</td><td>Pharyngeal and superior laryngeal branches of vagus (CN X) through pharyngeal plexus + external laryngeal plexus</td><td>Serves as superior esophageal sphincter</td></tr>
<tr><td>Palatopharyngeus (see Fig. 8.21B)</td><td>Hard palate and palatine aponeurosis</td><td>Posterior border of lamina of thyroid cartilage and side of pharynx and esophagus</td><td rowspan="2">Pharyngeal and superior laryngeal branches of vagus (CN X) through pharyngeal plexus</td><td rowspan="3">Elevate pharynx and larynx during swallowing and speaking</td></tr>
<tr><td>Salpingopharyngeus (see Fig. 8.21B)</td><td>Cartilaginous part of pharyngotympanic tube</td><td>Blends with palatopharyngeus</td></tr>
<tr><td>Stylopharyngeus</td><td>Styloid process of temporal bone</td><td>Posterior and superior borders of thyroid cartilage with palato-pharyngeus</td><td>Glossopharyngeal nerve (CN IX)</td></tr>
</table>

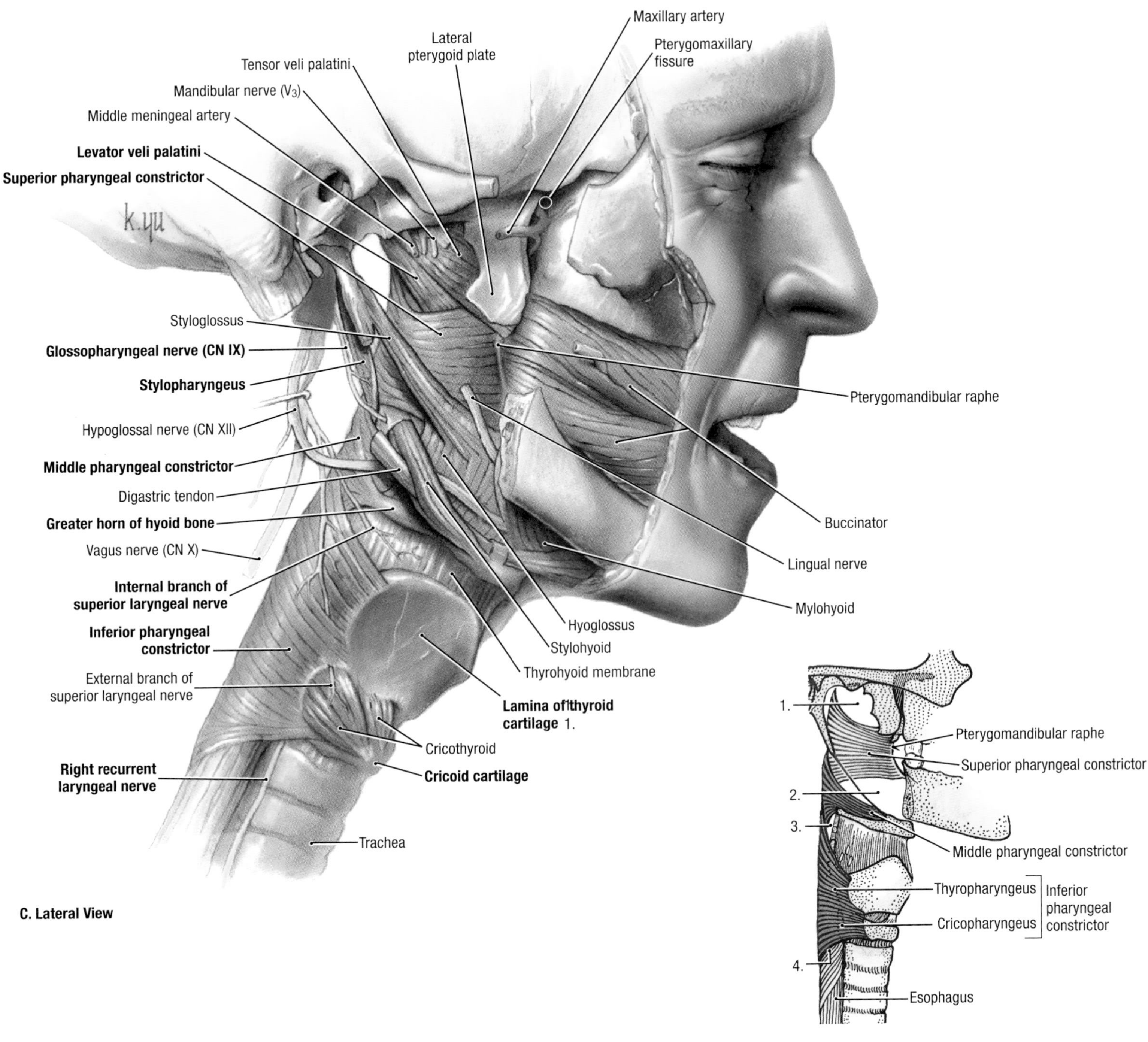
Maxillary artery
Lateral pterygoid plate
Pterygomaxillary fissure
Tensor veli palatini
Mandibular nerve (V3)
Middle meningeal artery
Levator veli palatini
Superior pharyngeal constrictor
Styloglossus
Glossopharyngeal nerve (CN IX)
Stylopharyngeus
Hypoglossal nerve (CN XII)
Middle pharyngeal constrictor
Digastric tendon
Greater horn of hyoid bone
Vagus nerve (CN X)
Internal branch of superior laryngeal nerve
Inferior pharyngeal constrictor
External branch of superior laryngeal nerve
Right recurrent laryngeal nerve
Trachea
Pterygomandibular raphe
Buccinator
Lingual nerve
Mylohyoid
Hyoglossus
Stylohyoid
Thyrohyoid membrane
Lamina of thyroid cartilage
Cricothyroid
Cricoid cartilage
C. Lateral View
1.
2.
3.
4.
Pterygomandibular raphe
Superior pharyngeal constrictor
Middle pharyngeal constrictor
Thyropharyngeus
Cricopharyngeus
Inferior pharyngeal constrictor
Esophagus
D. Lateral View

## 8.23 External pharynx—III

**C** and **D.** Observe that there are gaps in the pharyngeal musculature (1–4 in **D**) allowing the entry of structures:

1. Superior to the superior constrictor muscle: levator veli palatini muscle and pharyngotympanic (auditory) tube (see Fig. 8.24B)
2. Between the superior and middle constrictors: stylopharyngeus muscle, CN IX, and stylohyoid ligament
3. Between the middle and inferior constrictors: internal branch of superior laryngeal nerve and superior laryngeal artery and nerve (not shown)
4. Inferior to the inferior constrictor muscle: recurrent laryngeal nerve

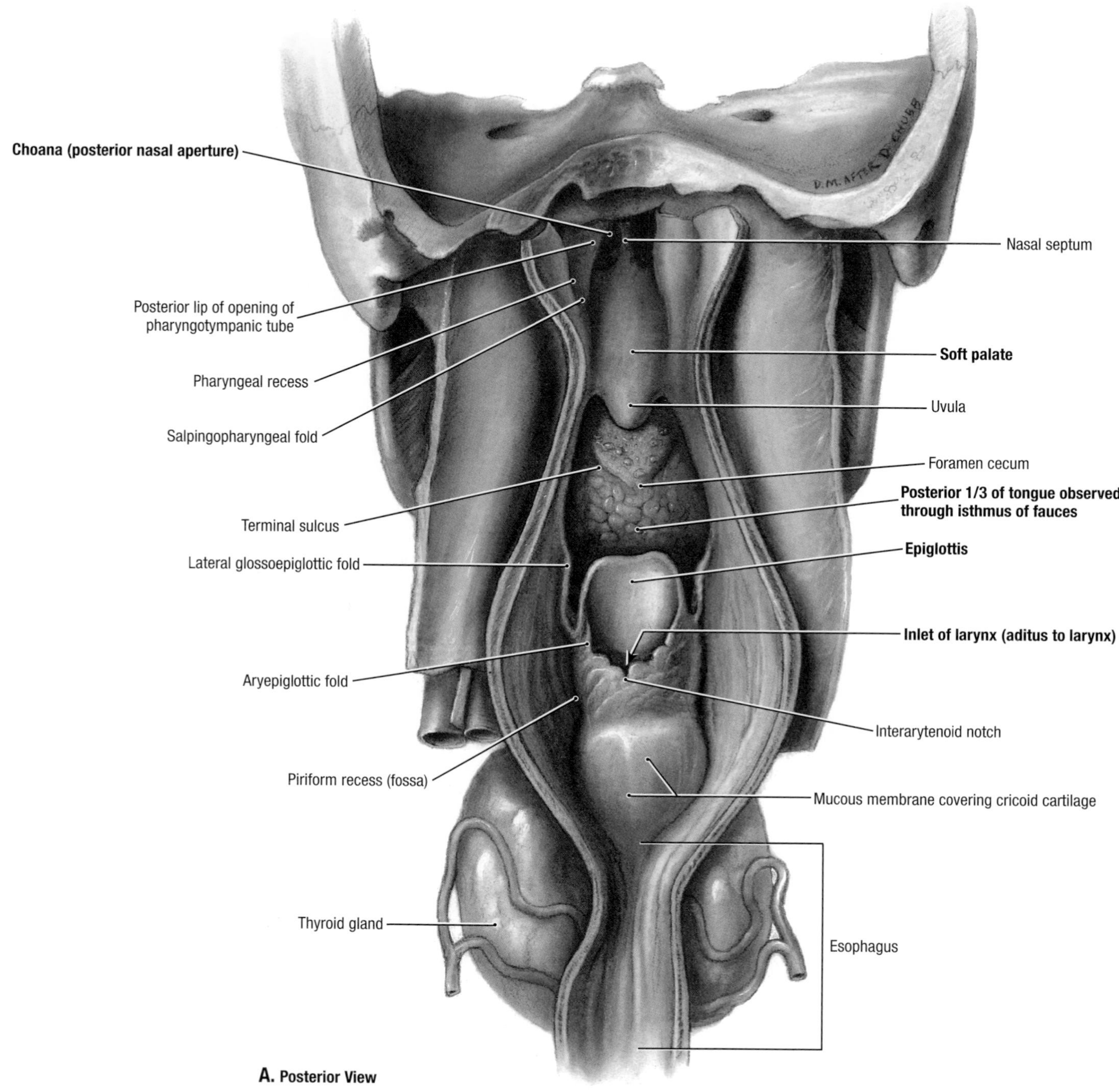
Choana (posterior nasal aperture)
Posterior lip of opening of pharyngotympanic tube
Pharyngeal recess
Salpingopharyngeal fold
Terminal sulcus
Lateral glossoepiglottic fold
Aryepiglottic fold
Piriform recess (fossa)
Thyroid gland
Nasal septum
Soft palate
Uvula
Foramen cecum
Posterior 1/3 of tongue observed through isthmus of fauces
Epiglottis
Inlet of larynx (aditus to larynx)
Interarytenoid notch
Mucous membrane covering cricoid cartilage
Esophagus
A. Posterior View

## 8.24 Internal pharynx—I

**A.** Dissection. The posterior wall of the pharynx has been split in the midline and the halves retracted laterally to reveal the internal aspect of the anterior wall of the pharynx, occupied by communications that define three parts of the pharynx: (1) the nasal part (nasopharynx), superior to the level of the soft palate, communicates anteriorly through the choanae with the nasal cavities; (2) the oral part (oropharynx), between the soft palate and the epiglottis, communicates anteriorly through the isthmus of the fauces with the oral cavity; and (3) the laryngeal part (laryngopharynx), posterior to the larynx, communicates with the vestibule of the larynx through the inlet of (aditus to) the larynx. The pharynx extends from the cranial base to the inferior border of the cricoid cartilage. Inferiorly, it is narrowed by the encircling cricopharyngeus.

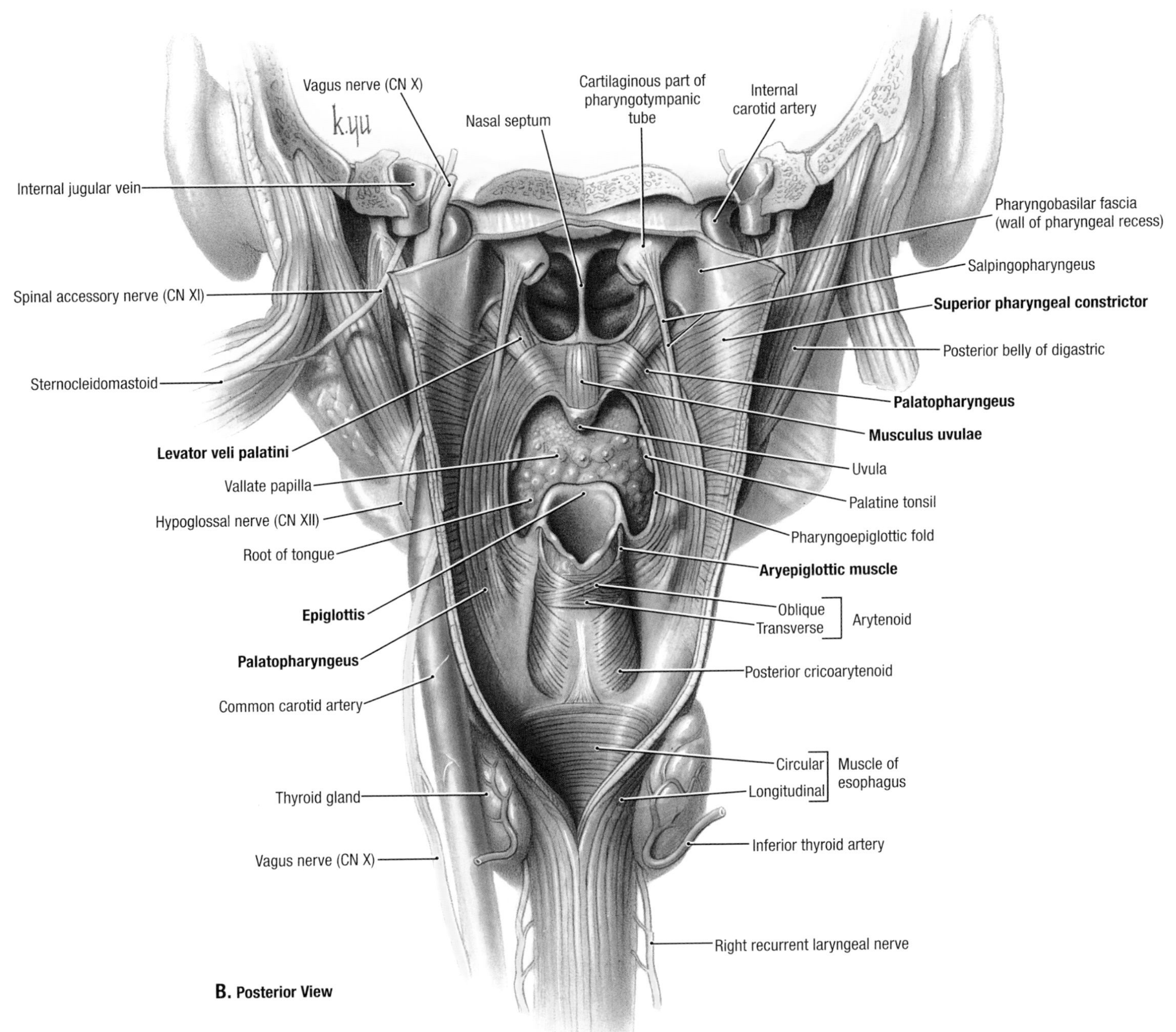
Vagus nerve (CN X)
Nasal septum
Cartilaginous part of pharyngotympanic tube
Internal carotid artery
Internal jugular vein
Pharyngobasilar fascia (wall of pharyngeal recess)
Salpingopharyngeus
Spinal accessory nerve (CN XI)
Superior pharyngeal constrictor
Posterior belly of digastric
Sternocleidomastoid
Palatopharyngeus
Musculus uvulae
Levator veli palatini
Uvula
Vallate papilla
Palatine tonsil
Hypoglossal nerve (CN XII)
Pharyngoepiglottic fold
Root of tongue
Aryepiglottic muscle
Oblique
Transverse
Arytenoid
Epiglottis
Palatopharyngeus
Posterior cricoarytenoid
Common carotid artery
Circular
Longitudinal
Muscle of esophagus
Thyroid gland
Inferior thyroid artery
Vagus nerve (CN X)
Right recurrent laryngeal nerve
B. Posterior View

## 8.24 Internal pharynx—II

**B.** Illustration. The posterior wall of the pharynx has been split in the midline and reflected laterally as in **A**; then, the mucous membrane was removed to expose the underlying musculature. The muscles of the soft palate, pharynx, and larynx work together during swallowing, elevating the soft palate, narrowing the pharyngeal isthmus (passageway between the nasal and oral parts of the pharynx) and laryngeal inlet, retracting the epiglottis, and closing the glottis, to keep food and drink out of the nasopharynx and larynx as they pass from oral cavity to esophagus. At other times, as when blowing one's nose, the palatopharyngeus muscles, partially encircling the opening to the oral cavity, constrict this opening and depress the soft palate, working with placement and expansion of the posterior tongue to direct expired air through the nasal cavity.

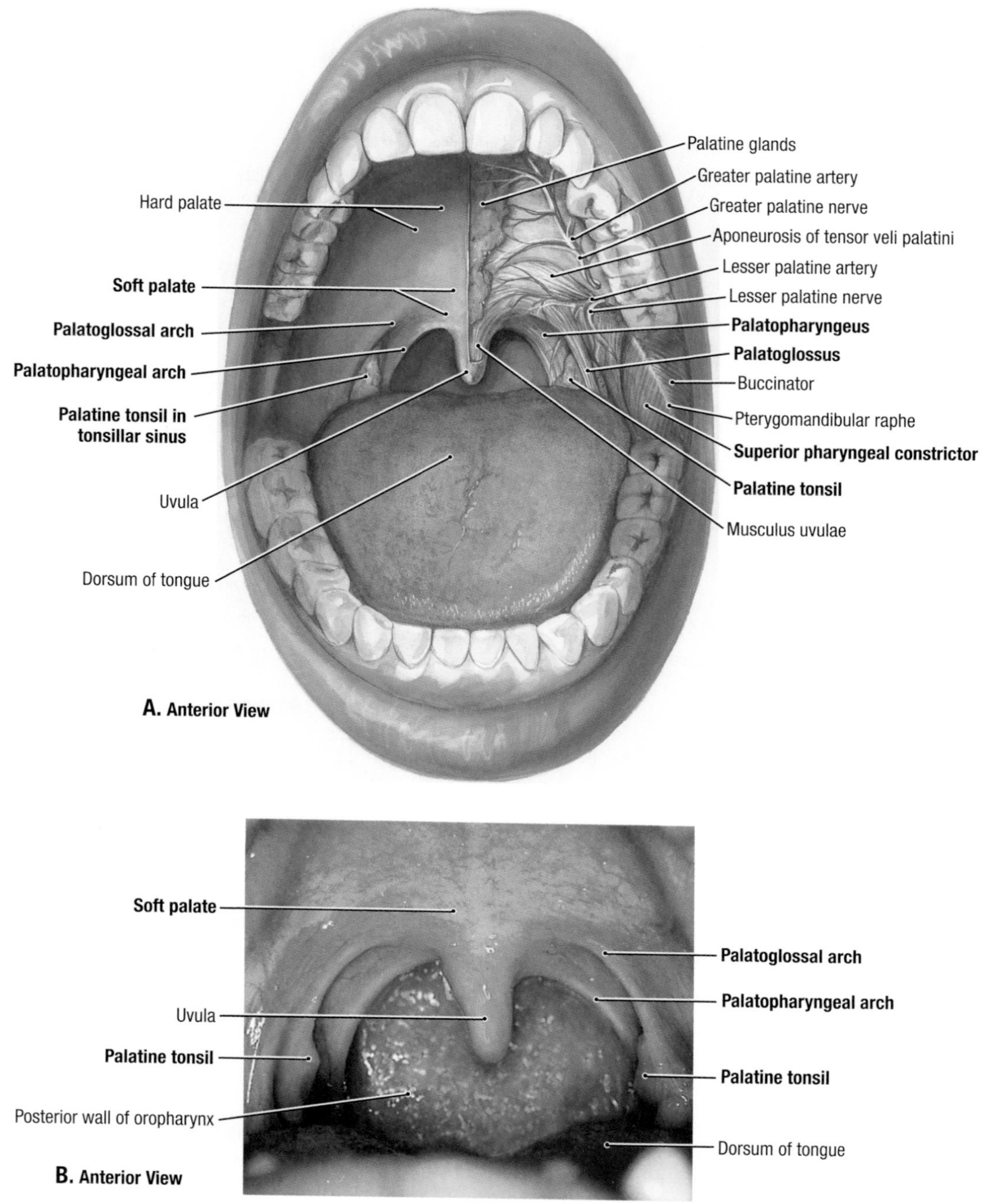
Hard palate
Soft palate
Palatoglossal arch
Palatopharyngeal arch
Palatine tonsil in tonsillar sinus
Uvula
Dorsum of tongue
Palatine glands
Greater palatine artery
Greater palatine nerve
Aponeurosis of tensor veli palatini
Lesser palatine artery
Lesser palatine nerve
Palatopharyngeus
Palatoglossus
Buccinator
Pterygomandibular raphe
Superior pharyngeal constrictor
Palatine tonsil
Musculus uvulae
A. Anterior View
Soft palate
Uvula
Palatine tonsil
Posterior wall of oropharynx
B. Anterior View
Palatoglossal arch
Palatopharyngeal arch
Palatine tonsil
Dorsum of tongue

## 8.25 Surface anatomy of isthmus of the fauces (oropharyngeal isthmus)

**A.** Oral cavity and isthmus demonstrating the sinus (bed) of the tonsils. **B.** Tonsillar sinuses with palatine tonsils in situ, and oropharynx.

- The fauces (throat), the passage from the mouth to the pharynx, is bounded superiorly by the soft palate, inferiorly by the root (base) of the tongue, and laterally by the palatoglossal and palatopharyngeal arches.
- The palatine tonsils are located between the palatoglossal and palatopharyngeal arches, formed by mucosa overlying the similarly named muscles; the arches form the boundaries, and the superior pharyngeal constrictor the floor, of the tonsillar sinuses.

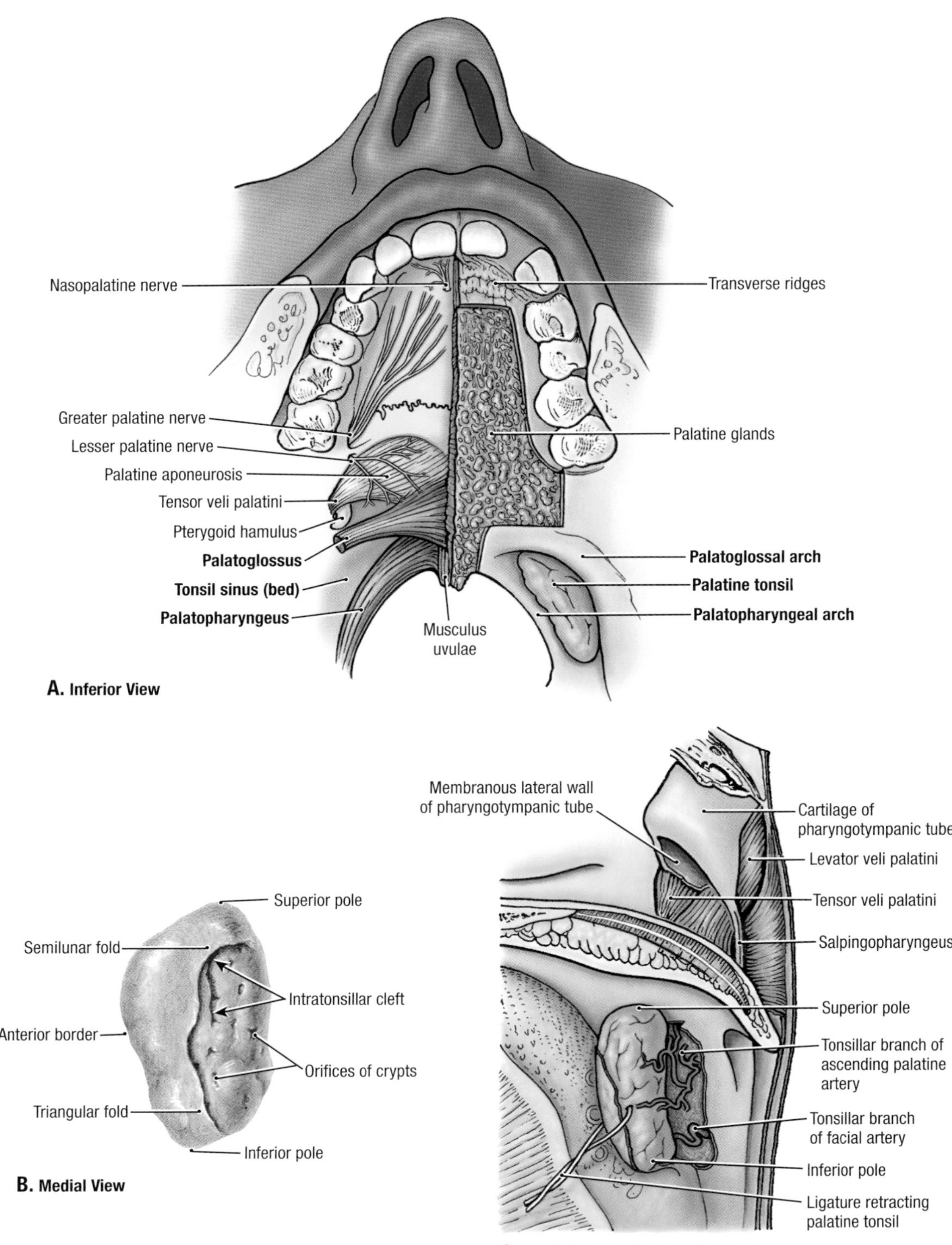
Nasopalatine nerve
Transverse ridges
Greater palatine nerve
Lesser palatine nerve
Palatine aponeurosis
Tensor veli palatini
Pterygoid hamulus
Palatoglossus
Tonsil sinus (bed)
Palatopharyngeus
Palatine glands
Palatoglossal arch
Palatine tonsil
Palatopharyngeal arch
Musculus uvulae
A. Inferior View
Membranous lateral wall of pharyngotympanic tube
Cartilage of pharyngotympanic tube
Levator veli palatini
Tensor veli palatini
Salpingopharyngeus
Superior pole
Tonsillar branch of ascending palatine artery
Tonsillar branch of facial artery
Inferior pole
Ligature retracting palatine tonsil
Superior pole
Semilunar fold
Intratonsillar cleft
Anterior border
Orifices of crypts
Triangular fold
Inferior pole
B. Medial View
C. Medial View of Right Half of Head

## 8.26 Palatine tonsil

**A.** Left side: Palatine tonsil in situ and glands of palatine mucosa. Right side: Palatine mucosa and tonsils removed demonstrating palatine nerves and muscles. **B.** Isolated palatine tonsil. **C.** Tonsillectomy. The procedure involves removal of the tonsil and the fascial sheet covering the tonsillar sinus. Because of the rich blood supply of the tonsil, bleeding commonly arises from the large external palatine vein or less commonly from the tonsillar artery or other arterial twigs. The glossopharyngeal nerve accompanies the tonsillar artery on the lateral wall of the pharynx and is vulnerable to injury because this wall is thin. The internal carotid artery is especially vulnerable when it is tortuous, as it lies directly lateral to the tonsil.

Middle nasal concha
Inferior nasal concha
Palatine bone
(bony palate)
Palatine glands
Palatoglossal
arch
Tonsillar fossa
Dorsum of tongue
Pharyngeal tonsil
Torus
Pharyngeal
opening
of pharyngotympanic tube
Ridge of levator veli palatini
Pharyngeal recess
Salpingopharyngeal fold
Soft palate
Uvula
Palatopharyngeal arch
Vallate papillae
Lingual follicles
Epiglottis

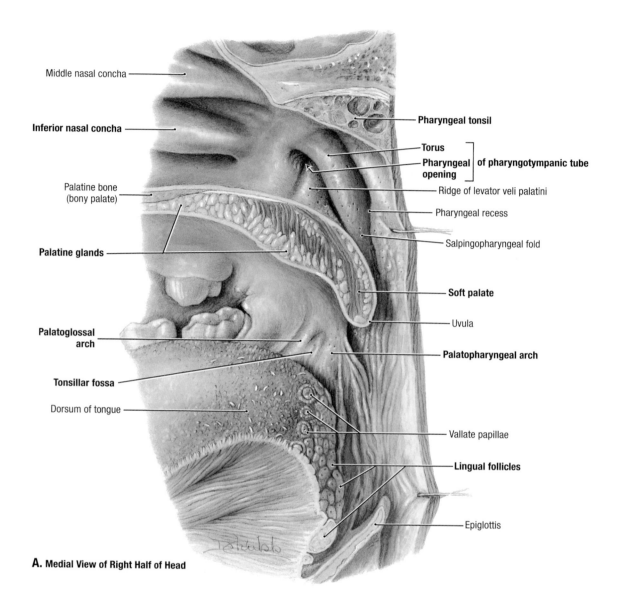

**A. Medial View of Right Half of Head**

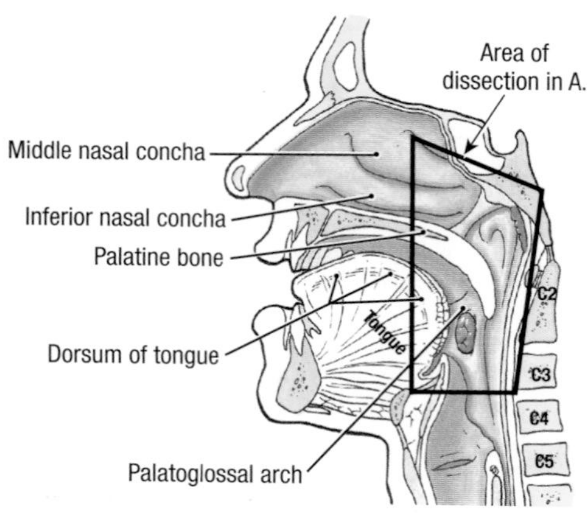
Area of
dissection in A.
Middle nasal concha
Inferior nasal concha
Palatine bone
Dorsum of tongue
Palatoglossal arch
Tongue
C2
C3
C4
C5

## 8.27 Serial dissection of isthmus of fauces and lateral wall of nasopharynx —I

- The pharyngeal opening of the pharyngotympanic tube is located approximately 1 cm posterior to the inferior concha.
- The numerous pinpoint orifices of the ducts of the mucous glands can be seen in the mucosa of the torus.
- The pharyngeal tonsil lies in the mucous membrane of the roof and posterior wall of the nasopharynx.
- The palatine glands lie in the soft palate.
- The palatine tonsil lies in the tonsillar sinus between the palatoglossal and palatopharyngeal arches.
- Each lingual follicle has the duct of a mucous gland opening onto its surface; collectively, the follicles are known as the lingual tonsil.

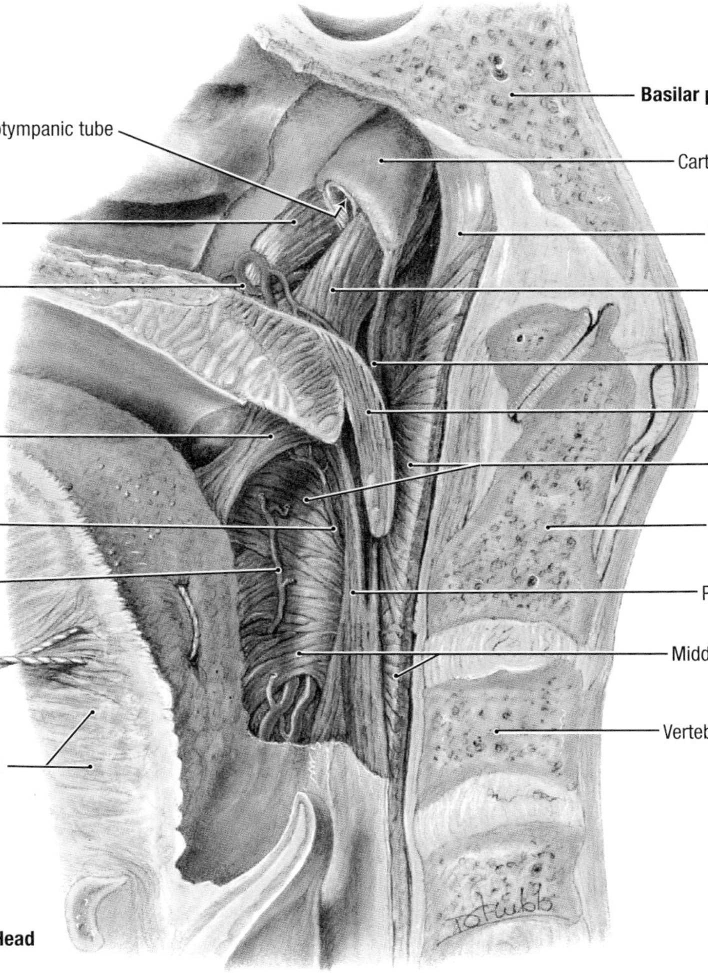

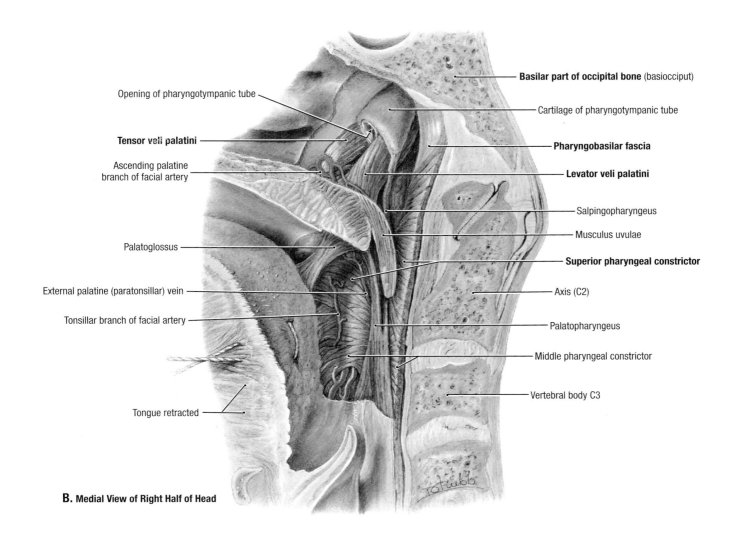

Opening of pharyngotympanic tube
Tensor veli palatini
Ascending palatine branch of facial artery
Palatoglossus
External palatine (paratonsillar) vein
Tonsillar branch of facial artery
Tongue retracted
Basilar part of occipital bone (basiocciput)
Cartilage of pharyngotympanic tube
Pharyngobasilar fascia
Levator veli palatini
Salpingopharyngeus
Musculus uvulae
Superior pharyngeal constrictor
Axis (C2)
Palatopharyngeus
Middle pharyngeal constrictor
Vertebral body C3

**B. Medial View of Right Half of Head**

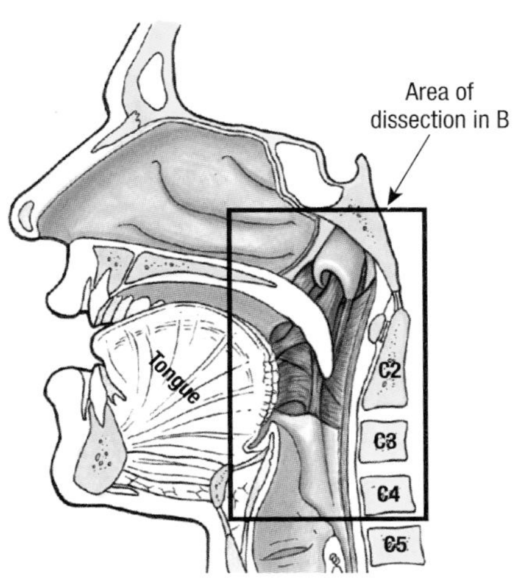
Area of dissection in B
Tongue
C2
C3
C4
C5

## 8.27 Serial dissection of isthmus of fauces and lateral wall of nasopharynx—II

Muscles underlying tonsillar sinus and wall of nasopharynx. The palatine and pharyngeal tonsils and mucous membrane have been removed. The pharyngobasilar fascia, which attaches the pharynx to the basilar part of the occipital bone was also removed, except at the superior, arched border of the superior pharyngeal constrictor.

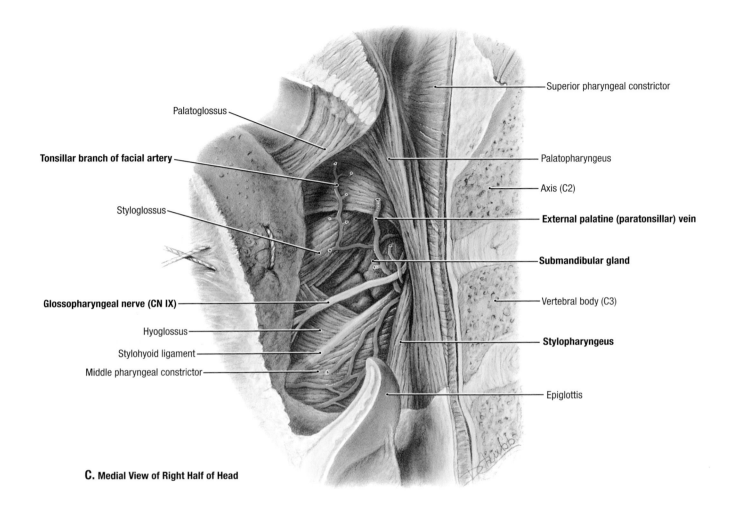

Superior pharyngeal constrictor
Palatoglossus
Tonsillar branch of facial artery
Palatopharyngeus
Axis (C2)
Styloglossus
External palatine (paratonsillar) vein
Submandibular gland
Glossopharyngeal nerve (CN IX)
Vertebral body (C3)
Hyoglossus
Stylopharyngeus
Stylohyoid ligament
Middle pharyngeal constrictor
Epiglottis

**C. Medial View of Right Half of Head**

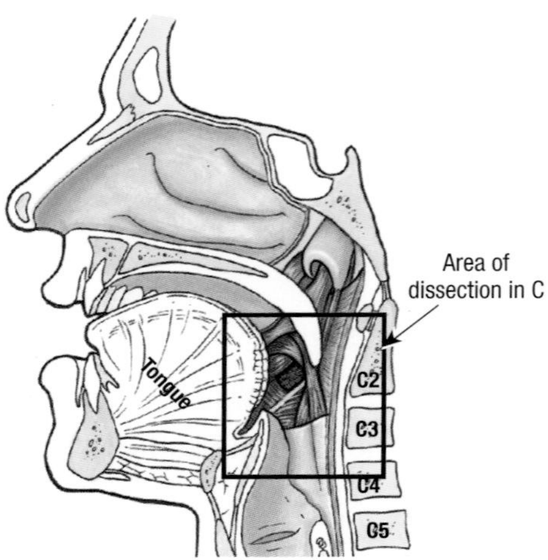
Area of dissection in C
Tongue
C2
C3
C4
C5

## 8.27 Serial dissection of isthmus of the fauces and lateral wall of nasopharynx—III

Neurovascular structures of tonsillar sinus and longitudinal muscles of the pharynx.

- In this deeper dissection, the tongue was pulled anteriorly, and the inferior part of the origin of the superior pharyngeal constrictor muscle was cut away.
- The glossopharyngeal nerve passes to the posterior one third of the tongue and lies anterior to the stylopharyngeus muscle.
- The tonsillar branch of the facial artery sends a branch (cut short here) to accompany the glossopharyngeal nerve to the tongue; the submandibular gland is seen lateral to the artery and external palatine (paratonsillar) vein.

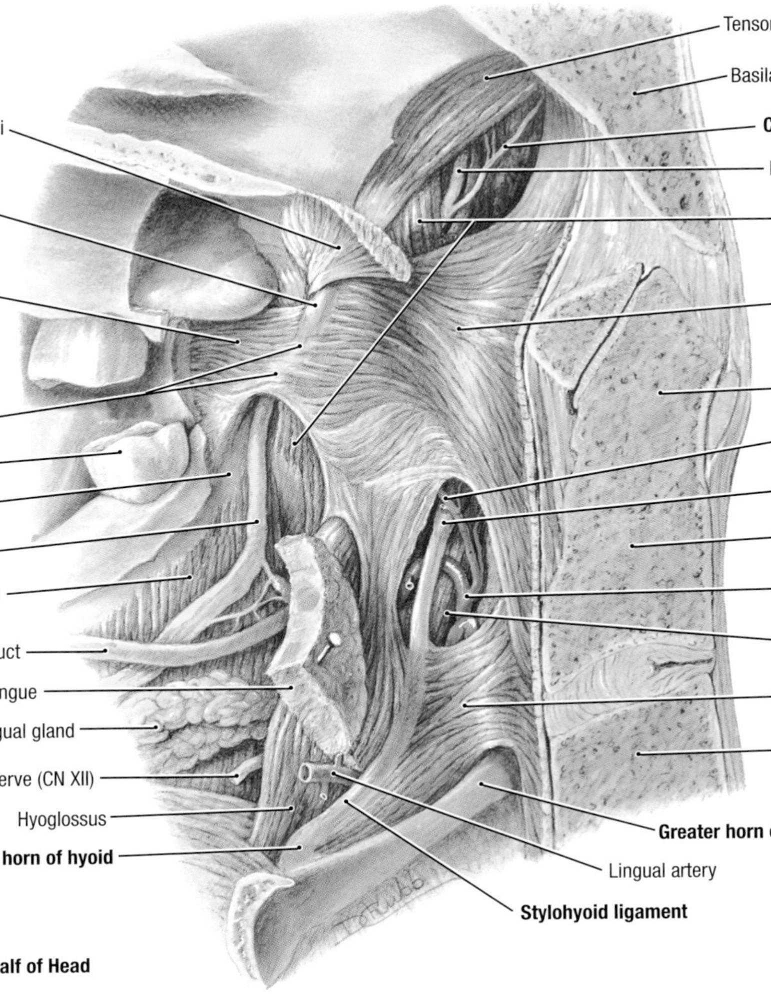

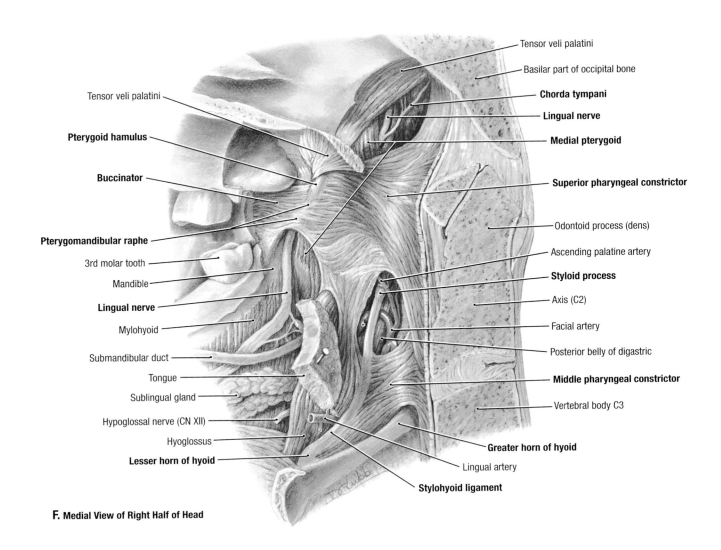

Tensor veli palatini
Pterygoid hamulus
Buccinator
Pterygomandibular raphe
3rd molar tooth
Mandible
Lingual nerve
Mylohyoid
Submandibular duct
Tongue
Sublingual gland
Hypoglossal nerve (CN XII)
Hyoglossus
Lesser horn of hyoid
Tensor veli palatini
Basilar part of occipital bone
Chorda tympani
Lingual nerve
Medial pterygoid
Superior pharyngeal constrictor
Odontoid process (dens)
Ascending palatine artery
Styloid process
Axis (C2)
Facial artery
Posterior belly of digastric
Middle pharyngeal constrictor
Vertebral body C3
Greater horn of hyoid
Lingual artery
Stylohyoid ligament

**F. Medial View of Right Half of Head**

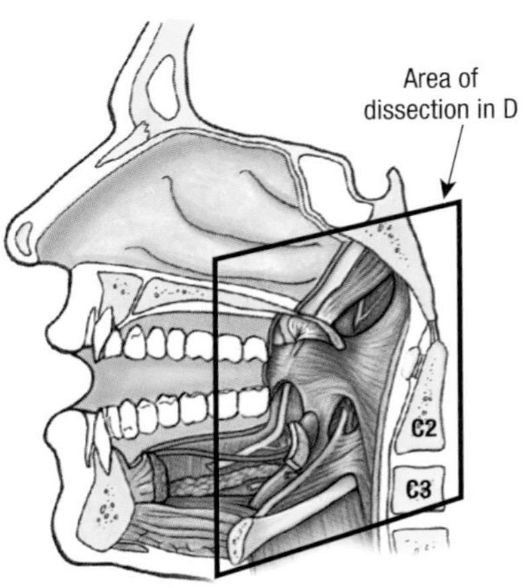
Area of dissection in D
C2
C3

## 8.27 Serial dissection of isthmus of the fauces lateral wall of nasopharynx—IV

- The superior pharyngeal constrictor muscle arises from (a) the pterygomandibular raphe, which unites it to the buccinator muscle; (b) the bones at each end of the raphe, the hamulus of the medial pterygoid plate superiorly and the mandible inferiorly; and (c) the root (posterior part) of the tongue.
- The middle pharyngeal constrictor muscle arises from the angle formed by the greater and lesser horns of the hyoid bone and from the stylohyoid ligament; in this specimen, the styloid process is long and, therefore, a lateral relation of the tonsil.
- The lingual nerve is joined by the chorda tympani, disappears at the posterior border of the medial pterygoid muscle, and reappears at the anterior border to follow the mandible.

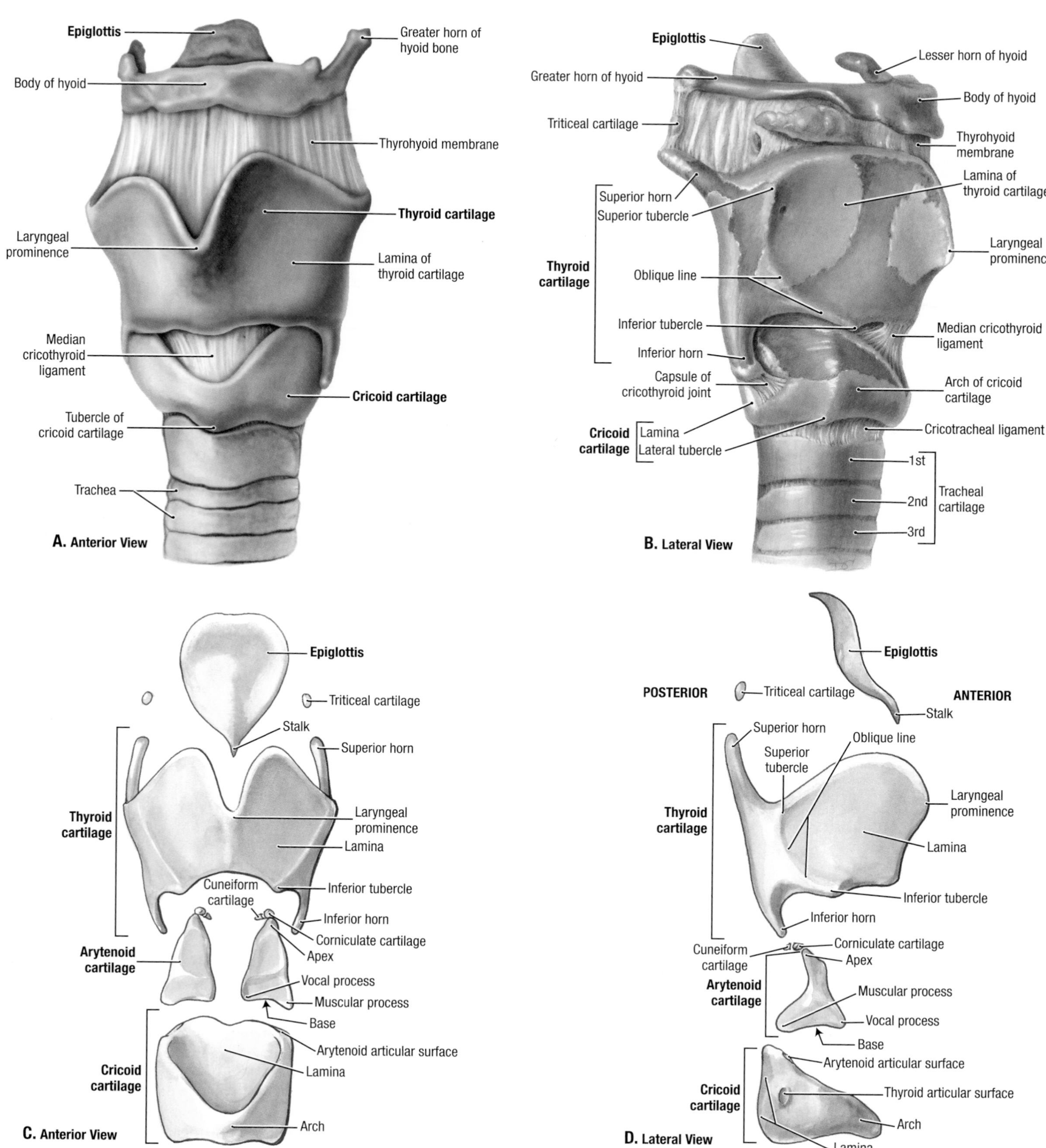
Epiglottis
Greater horn of hyoid bone
Body of hyoid
Thyrohyoid membrane
Thyroid cartilage
Laryngeal prominence
Lamina of thyroid cartilage
Median cricothyroid ligament
Cricoid cartilage
Tubercle of cricoid cartilage
Trachea
A. Anterior View
Epiglottis
Lesser horn of hyoid
Greater horn of hyoid
Body of hyoid
Triticeal cartilage
Thyrohyoid membrane
Lamina of thyroid cartilage
Superior horn
Superior tubercle
Thyroid cartilage
Laryngeal prominence
Oblique line
Inferior tubercle
Median cricothyroid ligament
Inferior horn
Capsule of cricothyroid joint
Arch of cricoid cartilage
Cricoid cartilage
Lamina
Lateral tubercle
Cricotracheal ligament
1st
2nd
3rd
Tracheal cartilage
B. Lateral View
Epiglottis
Triticeal cartilage
Stalk
Superior horn
Thyroid cartilage
Laryngeal prominence
Lamina
Cuneiform cartilage
Inferior tubercle
Inferior horn
Corniculate cartilage
Arytenoid cartilage
Apex
Vocal process
Muscular process
Base
Arytenoid articular surface
Cricoid cartilage
Lamina
Arch
C. Anterior View
Epiglottis
POSTERIOR
Triticeal cartilage
ANTERIOR
Stalk
Superior horn
Oblique line
Superior tubercle
Thyroid cartilage
Laryngeal prominence
Lamina
Inferior tubercle
Inferior horn
Cuneiform cartilage
Corniculate cartilage
Apex
Arytenoid cartilage
Muscular process
Vocal process
Base
Arytenoid articular surface
Cricoid cartilage
Thyroid articular surface
Arch
Lamina
D. Lateral View

**8.28 Cartilages of the laryngeal skeleton**

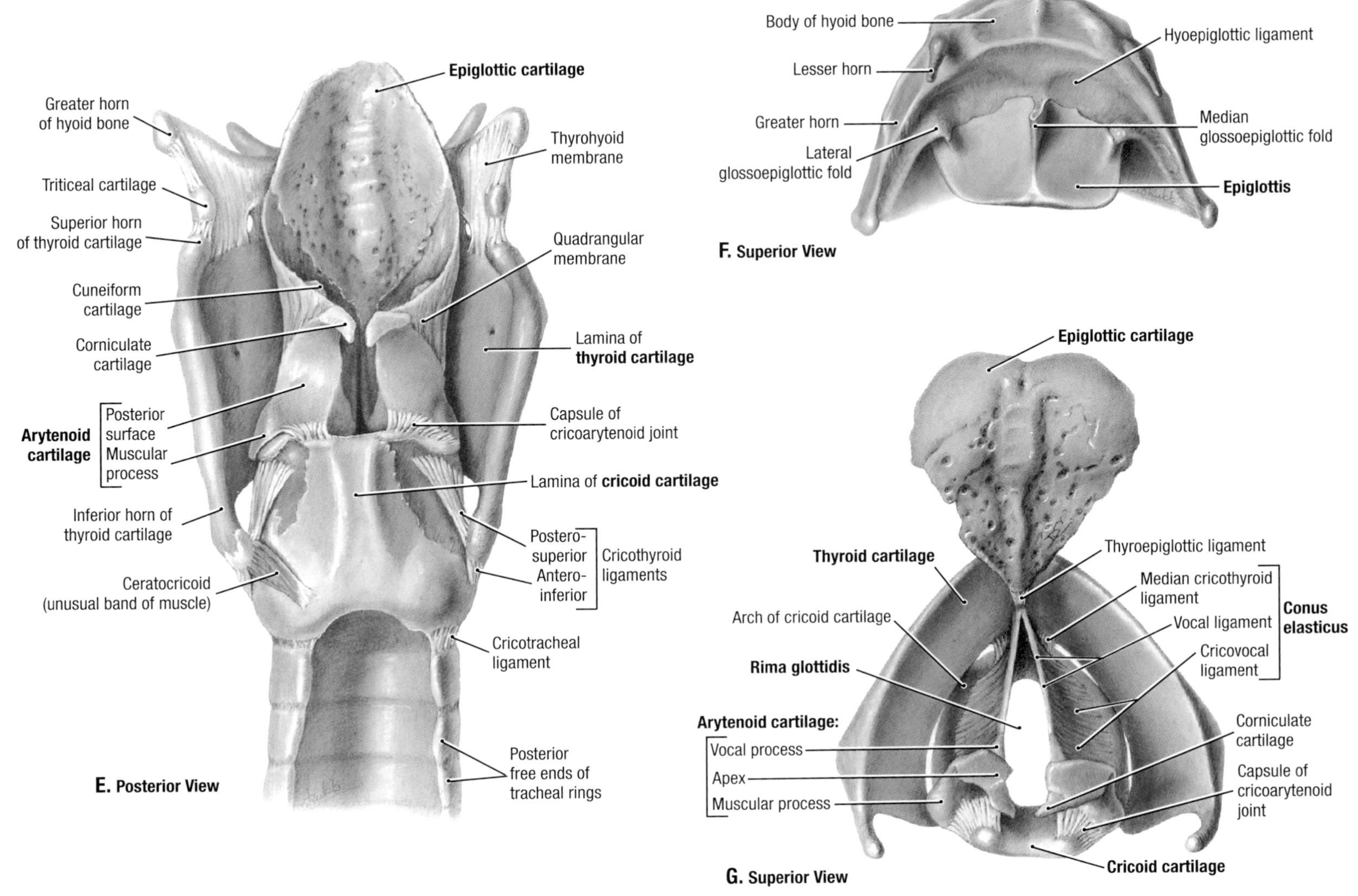
Epiglottic cartilage
Greater horn of hyoid bone
Thyrohyoid membrane
Triticeal cartilage
Superior horn of thyroid cartilage
Quadrangular membrane
Cuneiform cartilage
Corniculate cartilage
Lamina of thyroid cartilage
Arytenoid cartilage
Posterior surface
Muscular process
Capsule of cricoarytenoid joint
Lamina of cricoid cartilage
Inferior horn of thyroid cartilage
Postero-superior
Antero-inferior
Cricothyroid ligaments
Ceratocricoid (unusual band of muscle)
Cricotracheal ligament
Posterior free ends of tracheal rings
E. Posterior View
Body of hyoid bone
Lesser horn
Hyoepiglottic ligament
Greater horn
Median glossoepiglottic fold
Lateral glossoepiglottic fold
Epiglottis
F. Superior View
Epiglottic cartilage
Thyroid cartilage
Thyroepiglottic ligament
Median cricothyroid ligament
Vocal ligament
Cricovocal ligament
Conus elasticus
Arch of cricoid cartilage
Rima glottidis
Arytenoid cartilage:
Vocal process
Apex
Muscular process
Corniculate cartilage
Capsule of cricoarytenoid joint
Cricoid cartilage
G. Superior View

## 8.28 Cartilages of the laryngeal skeleton *(continued)*

**A, B,** and **E.** Articulated laryngeal skeleton. **C** and **D.** Cartilages disarticulated and separated. **F.** Epiglottis and hyoepiglottic ligament. **G.** Conus elasticus and rima glottidis.

- The larynx extends vertically from the tip of the epiglottis to the inferior border of the cricoid cartilage. The hyoid bone is generally not regarded as part of the larynx.
- The cricoid cartilage is the only cartilage that totally encircles the airway.
- The rima glottidis is the aperture between the vocal folds. During normal respiration, it is narrow and wedge shaped; during forced respiration, it is wide. Variations in the tension and length of the vocal folds, in the width of the rima glottidis, and in the intensity of the expiratory effort produce changes in the pitch of the voice.
- Laryngeal fractures may result from blows received in sports such as kickboxing and hockey or from compression by a shoulder strap during an automobile accident. Laryngeal fractures produce submucous hemorrhage and edema, respiratory obstruction, hoarseness, and sometimes a temporary inability to speak. The thyroid, cricoid, and most of the arytenoid cartilages often ossify as age advances, commencing at approximately 25 years of age in the thyroid cartilage.

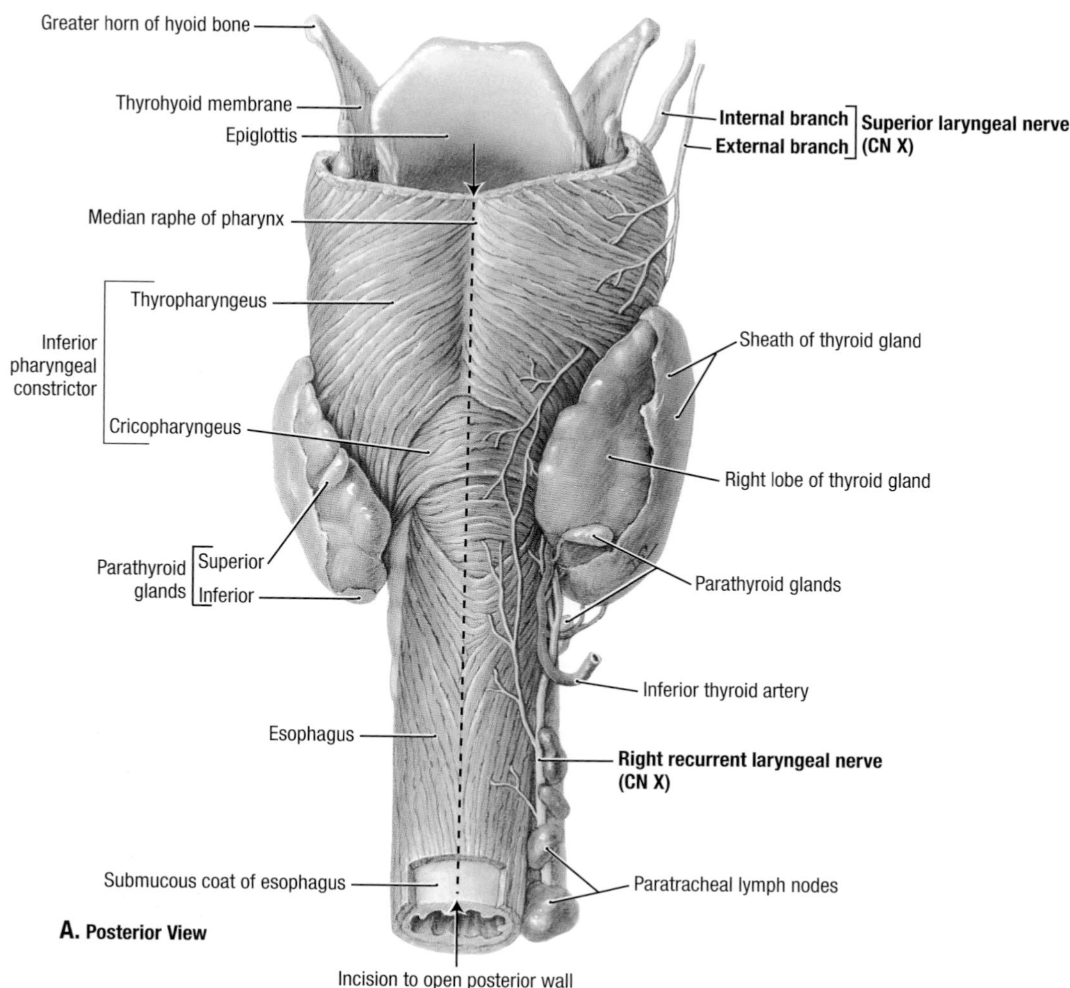
Greater horn of hyoid bone
Thyrohyoid membrane
Epiglottis
Internal branch
External branch
Superior laryngeal nerve (CN X)
Median raphe of pharynx
Thyropharyngeus
Inferior pharyngeal constrictor
Cricopharyngeus
Sheath of thyroid gland
Right lobe of thyroid gland
Parathyroid glands
Superior
Inferior
Parathyroid glands
Inferior thyroid artery
Esophagus
Right recurrent laryngeal nerve (CN X)
Submucous coat of esophagus
Paratracheal lymph nodes
Incision to open posterior wall of larynx and trachea (Fig. 8.30A)

**A. Posterior View**

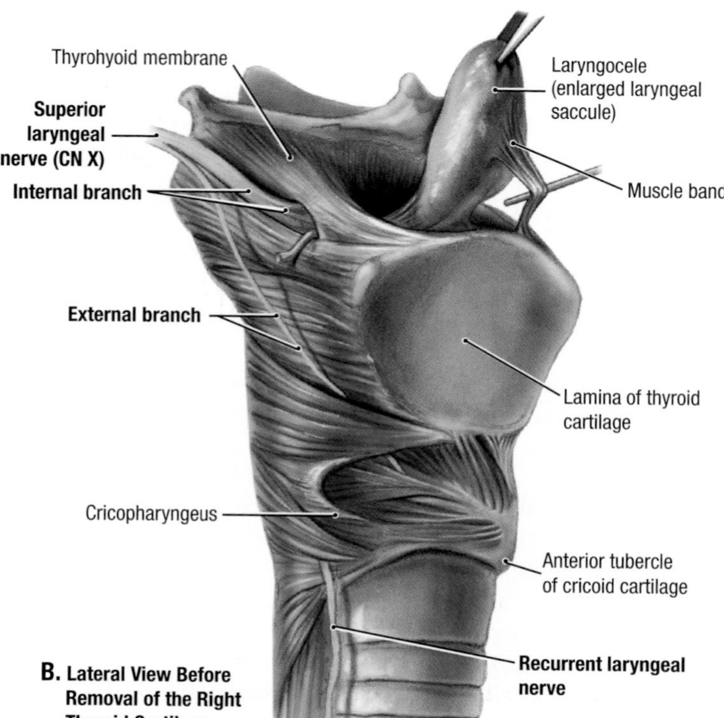
Thyrohyoid membrane
Superior laryngeal nerve (CN X)
Internal branch
External branch
Laryngocele (enlarged laryngeal saccule)
Muscle band
Lamina of thyroid cartilage
Cricopharyngeus
Anterior tubercle of cricoid cartilage
Recurrent laryngeal nerve

**B. Lateral View Before Removal of the Right Thyroid Cartilage**

## 8.29 External larynx and laryngeal nerves

**A.** Posterior aspect.

- The internal branch of the superior laryngeal nerve innervates the mucous membrane superior to the vocal folds, and the external laryngeal branch supplies the inferior pharyngeal constrictor and cricothyroid muscles.
- The recurrent laryngeal nerve supplies the esophagus, trachea, and inferior pharyngeal constrictor muscle. It supplies sensory innervation inferior to the vocal folds and motor innervation to the intrinsic muscles of the larynx, except the cricothyroid.

**B.** Laryngocele. A laryngocele (enlarged laryngeal saccule) projects through the thyrohyoid membrane and communicates with the larynx through the ventricle. This air sac can form a bulge in the neck, especially on coughing. The inferior laryngeal nerves are vulnerable to injury during operations in the anterior triangles of the neck. Injury of the nerve results in paralysis of the vocal fold. The voice is initially poor because the paralyzed fold cannot adduct to meet the normal vocal fold. In a bilateral paralysis, the voice is almost absent. Injury to the external branch of the superior laryngeal nerve results in a voice that is monotonous in character because the cricothyroid muscle is unable to vary the tension of the vocal fold. Hoarseness is the most common symptom of serious disorders of the larynx.

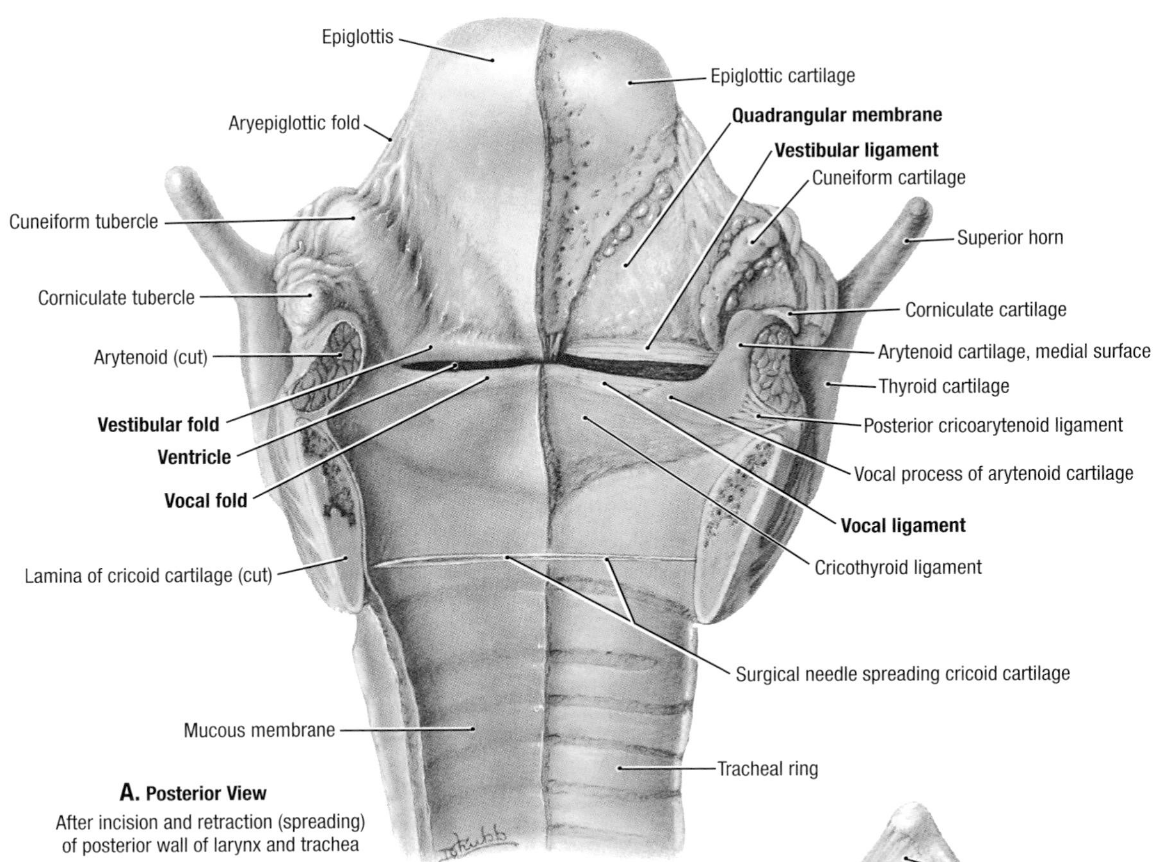
Epiglottis
Epiglottic cartilage
Aryepiglottic fold
Quadrangular membrane
Vestibular ligament
Cuneiform cartilage
Cuneiform tubercle
Superior horn
Corniculate tubercle
Corniculate cartilage
Arytenoid cartilage, medial surface
Arytenoid (cut)
Thyroid cartilage
Vestibular fold
Posterior cricoarytenoid ligament
Ventricle
Vocal process of arytenoid cartilage
Vocal fold
Vocal ligament
Cricothyroid ligament
Lamina of cricoid cartilage (cut)
Surgical needle spreading cricoid cartilage
Mucous membrane
Tracheal ring

**A.** **Posterior View**
After incision and retraction (spreading) of posterior wall of larynx and trachea

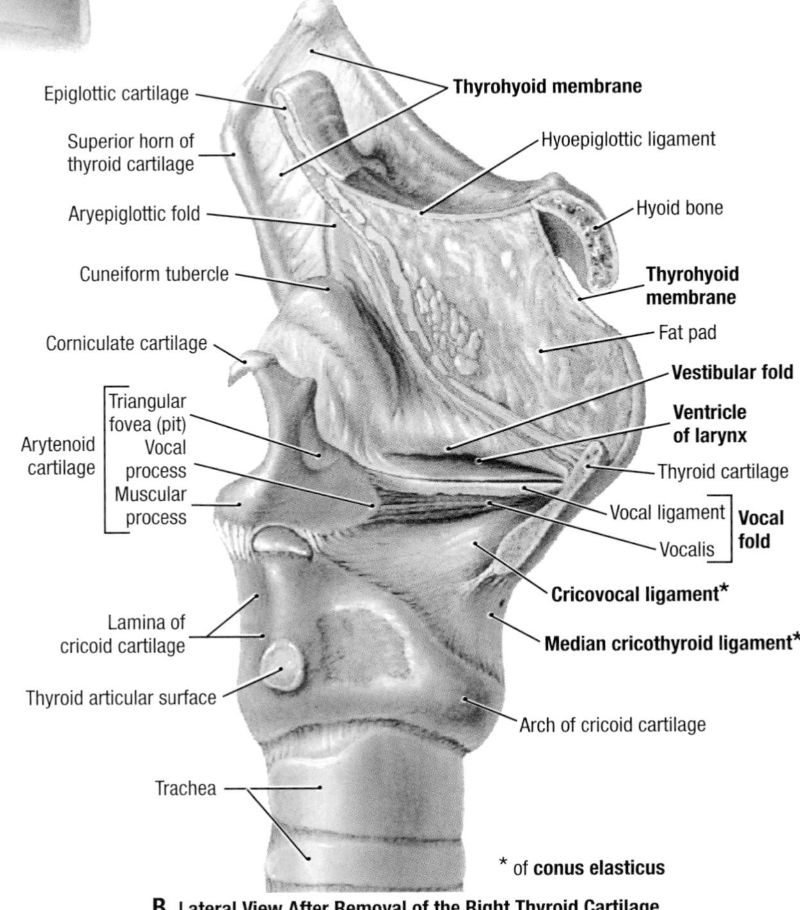
Thyrohyoid membrane
Epiglottic cartilage
Hyoepiglottic ligament
Superior horn of thyroid cartilage
Aryepiglottic fold
Hyoid bone
Cuneiform tubercle
Thyrohyoid membrane
Corniculate cartilage
Fat pad
Vestibular fold
Arytenoid cartilage
Triangular fovea (pit)
Vocal process
Muscular process
Ventricle of larynx
Thyroid cartilage
Vocal ligament
Vocalis
Vocal fold
Cricovocal ligament*
Lamina of cricoid cartilage
Median cricothyroid ligament*
Thyroid articular surface
Arch of cricoid cartilage
Trachea
* of conus elasticus

**B.** **Lateral View After Removal of the Right Thyroid Cartilage**

## 8.30 Internal larynx

**A.** The posterior wall of the larynx was split in the median plane (see Figure 8.29A), and the two sides held apart. On the left side of the specimen, the mucous membrane, which is the innermost coat of the larynx, is intact; on the right side of the specimen, the mucous and submucous coats were peeled off, and the next coat, consisting of cartilages, ligaments, and fibroelastic membrane, was uncovered. **B.** Interior of the larynx superior to the vocal folds. The larynx was sectioned near the median plane to reveal the interior of its left side. Inferior to this level, the right side of the intact larynx was dissected. The thyrohyoid membrane is intact; there is no laryngocele.

- The three compartments of the larynx are (a) the superior compartment of the vestibule, superior to the level of the vestibular folds (false cords); (b) the middle, between the levels of the vestibular and vocal folds; and (c) the inferior, or infraglottic, cavity, inferior to the level of the vocal folds.
- The quadrangular membrane underlies the aryepiglottic fold superiorly and is thickened inferiorly to form the vestibular ligament. The cricothyroid ligament (conus elasticus) begins inferiorly as the strong median cricothyroid ligament and is thickened superiorly as the vocal ligament. The lateral recess between the vocal and vestibular ligaments, lined with mucous membrane, is the ventricle.

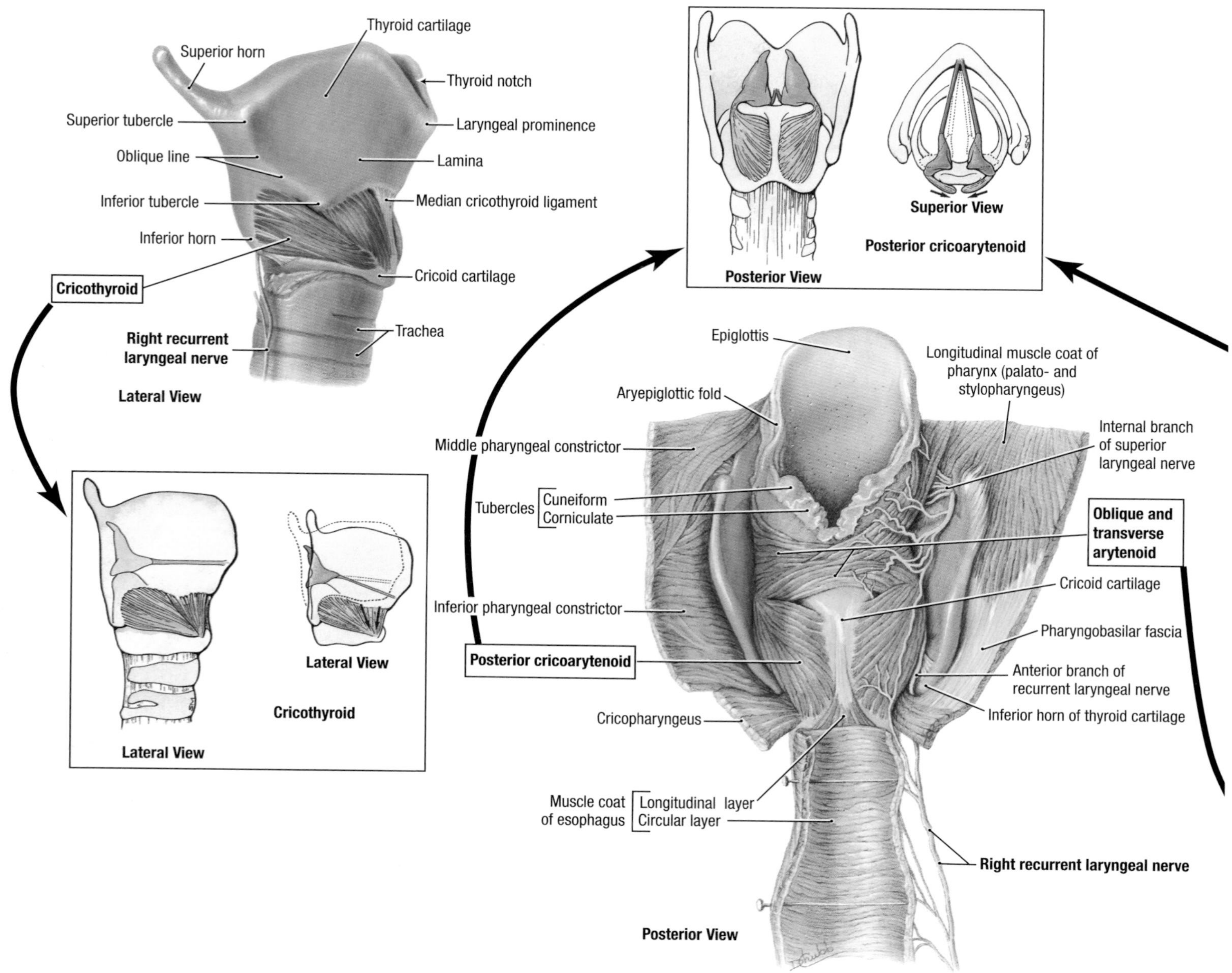
Thyroid cartilage
Superior horn
Thyroid notch
Superior tubercle
Laryngeal prominence
Oblique line
Lamina
Inferior tubercle
Median cricothyroid ligament
Inferior horn
Cricothyroid
Cricoid cartilage
Trachea
Right recurrent laryngeal nerve
Lateral View
Lateral View
Cricothyroid
Lateral View
Superior View
Posterior cricoarytenoid
Posterior View
Epiglottis
Longitudinal muscle coat of pharynx (palato- and stylopharyngeus)
Aryepiglottic fold
Internal branch of superior laryngeal nerve
Middle pharyngeal constrictor
Tubercles
Cuneiform
Corniculate
Oblique and transverse arytenoid
Cricoid cartilage
Inferior pharyngeal constrictor
Pharyngobasilar fascia
Posterior cricoarytenoid
Anterior branch of recurrent laryngeal nerve
Inferior horn of thyroid cartilage
Cricopharyngeus
Muscle coat of esophagus
Longitudinal layer
Circular layer
Right recurrent laryngeal nerve
Posterior View

## TABLE 8.10 MUSCLES OF LARYNX

| Muscle | Origin | Insertion | Innervation | Main Action(s) |
|---|---|---|---|---|
| **Cricothyroid** | Anterolateral part of cricoid cartilage | Inferior margin and inferior horn of thyroid cartilage | External branch of superior laryngeal nerve (CN X) | Tenses vocal fold |
| **Posterior cricoarytenoid** | Posterior surface of laminae of cricoid cartilage | Muscular process of arytenoid cartilage | Recurrent laryngeal nerve (CN X) | Abducts vocal fold |
| **Lateral cricoarytenoid** | Arch of cricoid cartilage | | | Adducts vocal fold |
| **Thyroarytenoid**[a] | Posterior surface of thyroid cartilage | | | Relaxes vocal fold |
| **Transverse and oblique arytenoids**[b] | One arytenoid cartilage | Opposite arytenoid cartilage | | Close inlet of larynx by approximating arytenoid cartilages |
| **Vocalis**[c] | Angle between laminae of thyroid cartilage | Vocal ligament, between origin and vocal process of arytenoid cartilage | | Alters vocal fold during phonation |

[a]Superior fibers of the thyroarytenoid muscle pass into the aryepiglottic fold, and some of them reach the epiglottic cartilage. These fibers constitute the thyroepiglottic muscle, which widens the inlet of the larynx.
[b]Some fibers of the oblique arytenoid muscle continue as the aryepiglottic muscle.
[c]This slender muscular slip is derived from inferior deeper fibers of the thyroarytenoid muscle.

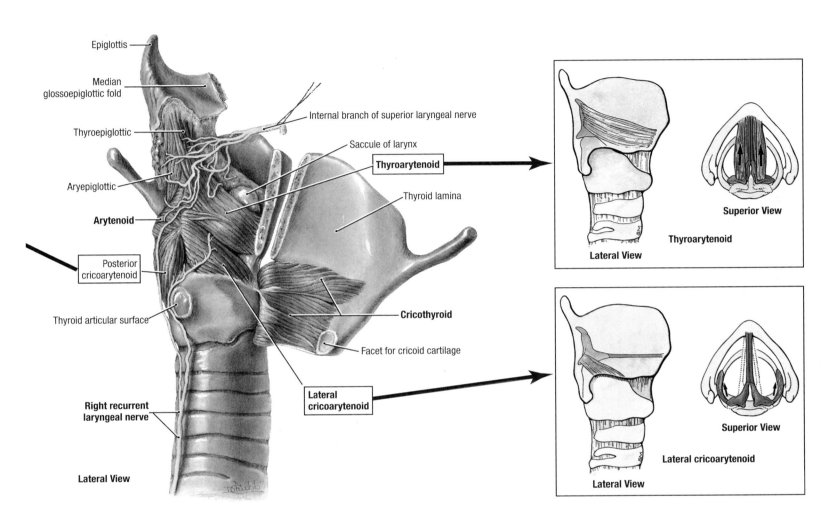

Epiglottis
Median glossoepiglottic fold
Internal branch of superior laryngeal nerve
Thyroepiglottic
Saccule of larynx
**Thyroarytenoid**
Aryepiglottic
Thyroid lamina
**Arytenoid**
Posterior cricoarytenoid
**Cricothyroid**
Thyroid articular surface
Facet for cricoid cartilage
**Lateral cricoarytenoid**
**Right recurrent laryngeal nerve**

**Lateral View**

**Superior View**
**Thyroarytenoid**
**Lateral View**

**Superior View**
**Lateral cricoarytenoid**
**Lateral View**

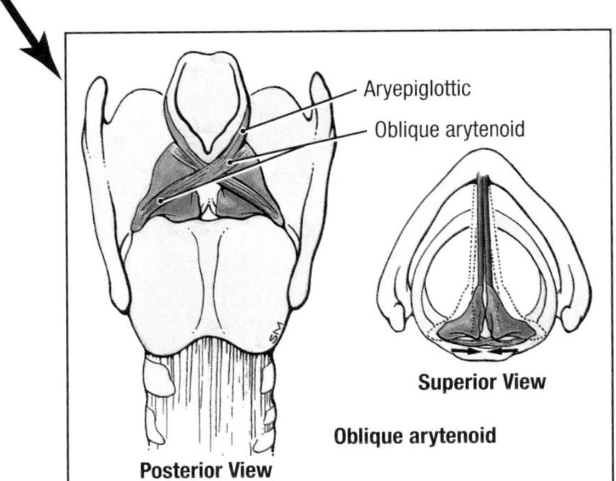
Aryepiglottic
Oblique arytenoid
Superior View
Oblique arytenoid
Posterior View

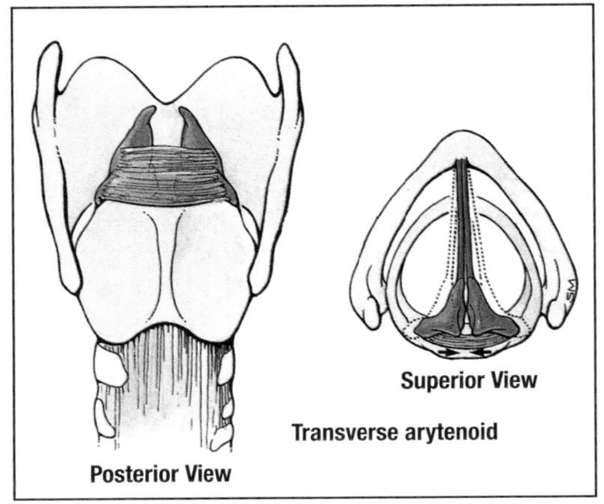
Superior View
Transverse arytenoid
Posterior View

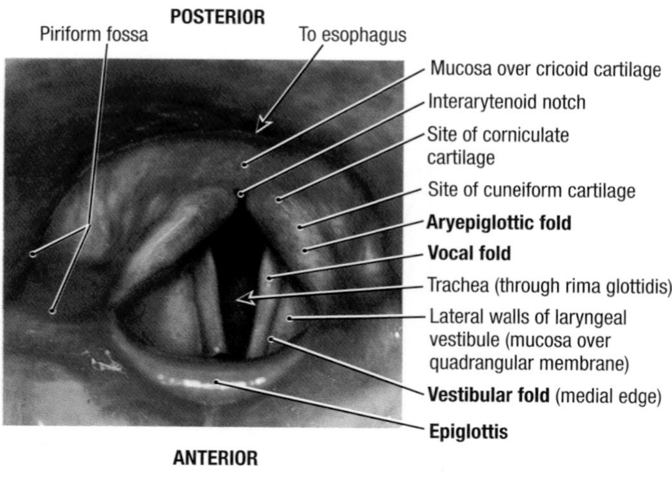
POSTERIOR
Piriform fossa
To esophagus
Mucosa over cricoid cartilage
Interarytenoid notch
Site of corniculate cartilage
Site of cuneiform cartilage
Aryepiglottic fold
Vocal fold
Trachea (through rima glottidis)
Lateral walls of laryngeal vestibule (mucosa over quadrangular membrane)
Vestibular fold (medial edge)
Epiglottis
ANTERIOR

**A.** Laryngoscopic Examination

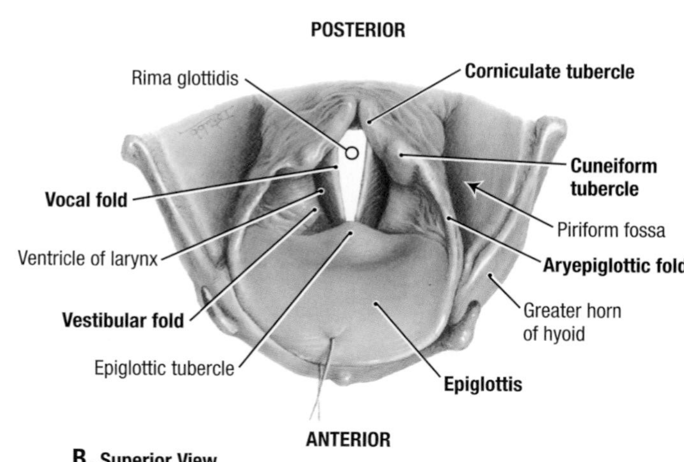
POSTERIOR
Rima glottidis
Corniculate tubercle
Cuneiform tubercle
Vocal fold
Piriform fossa
Ventricle of larynx
Aryepiglottic fold
Vestibular fold
Greater horn of hyoid
Epiglottic tubercle
Epiglottis
ANTERIOR

**B.** Superior View

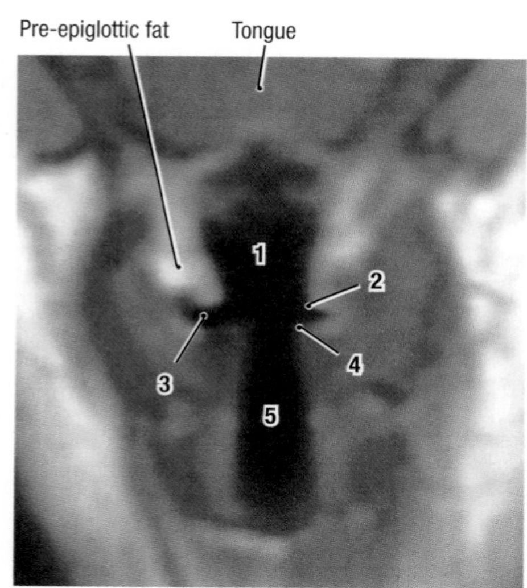
Pre-epiglottic fat
Tongue
1
2
3
4
5

**C.** Coronal MRI

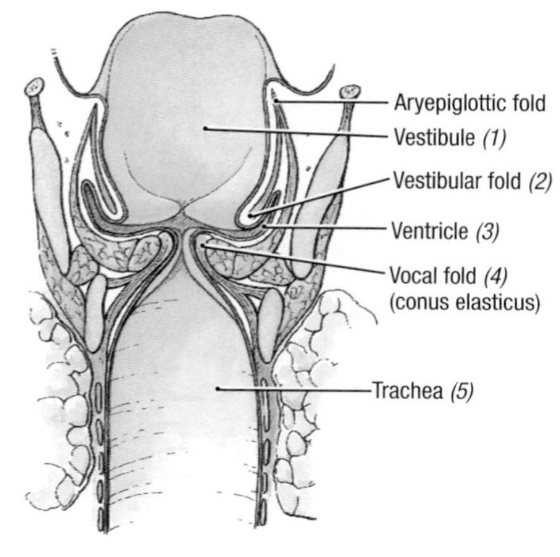
Aryepiglottic fold
Vestibule (1)
Vestibular fold (2)
Ventricle (3)
Vocal fold (4) (conus elasticus)
Trachea (5)

**D.** Posterior View

## 8.31 Laryngoscopic examination and MRI imaging of larynx

**A.** Laryngoscopic examination.
Laryngoscopy is the procedure used to examine the interior of the larynx. The larynx may be examined visually by indirect laryngoscopy using a laryngeal mirror or it may be viewed by direct laryngoscopy using a tubular and endoscopic instrument, a laryngoscope. The vestibular and vocal folds can be observed.

**B.** Vocal folds and rima glottidis.
The inlet, or aditus, to the larynx is bounded anteriorly by the epiglottis; posteriorly by the arytenoid cartilages, the corniculate cartilages that cap them, and the interarytenoid fold that unites them; and on each side by the aryepiglottic fold, which contains the superior end of the cuneiform cartilage.
**C.** Coronal MRI. **D.** Coronal section. Numbers in parentheses on diagram refer to numbered structures on MRI.

A foreign object, such as a piece of steak, may accidentally aspirate through the laryngeal inlet into the vestibule of the larynx, where it becomes trapped superior to the vestibular folds. When a foreign object enters the vestibule, the laryngeal muscles go into spasm, tensing the vocal folds. The rima glottidis closes and no air enters the trachea. Asphyxiation occurs, and the person will die in approximately 5 minutes from lack of oxygen if the obstruction is not removed. Emergency therapy must be given to open the airway. The procedure used depends on the condition of the patient, the facilities available, and the experience of the person giving first aid. Because the lungs still contain air, sudden compression of the abdomen (Heimlich maneuver) causes the diaphragm to elevate and compress the lungs, expelling air from the trachea into the larynx. This maneuver may dislodge the food or other material from the larynx.

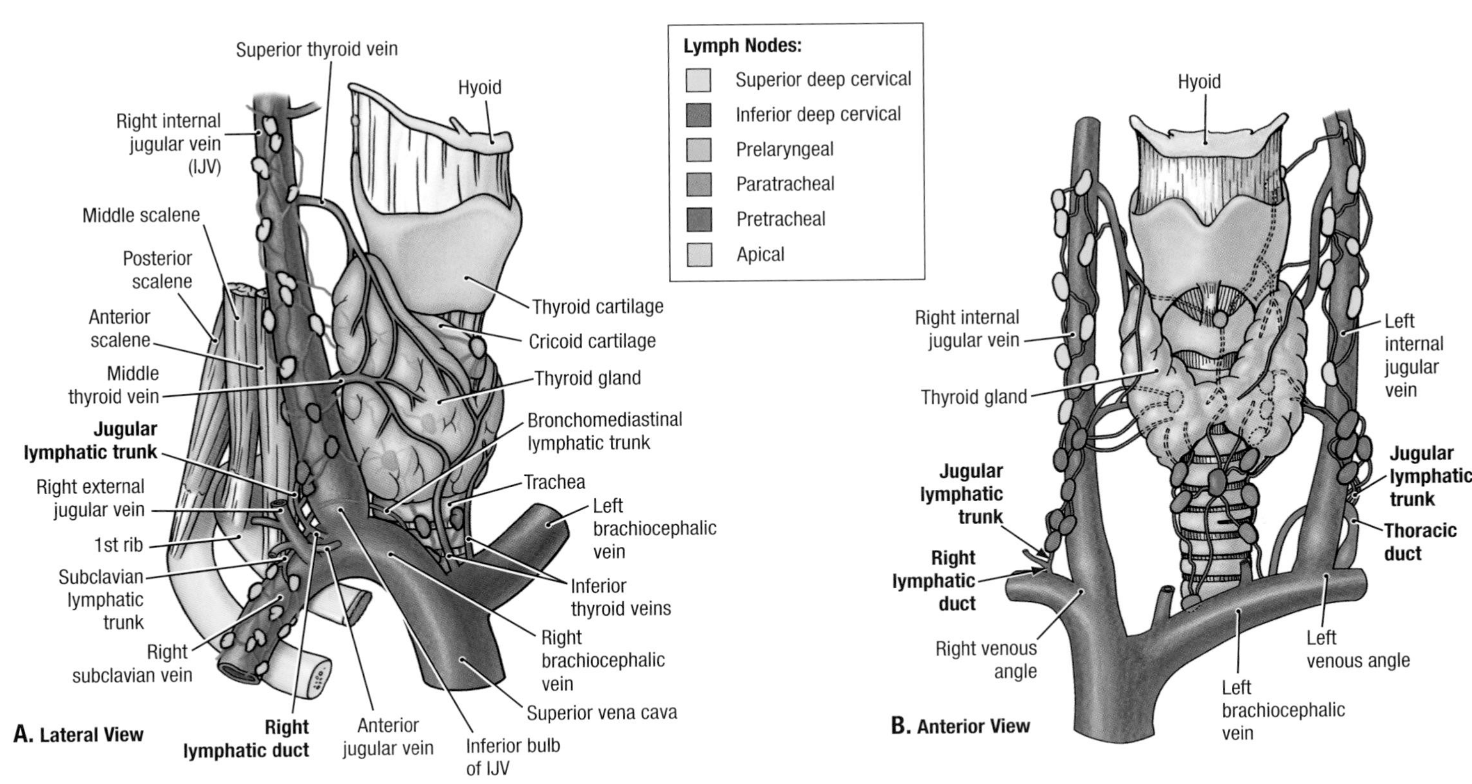
Lymph Nodes:
Superior deep cervical
Inferior deep cervical
Prelaryngeal
Paratracheal
Pretracheal
Apical
Superior thyroid vein
Hyoid
Right internal jugular vein (IJV)
Middle scalene
Posterior scalene
Anterior scalene
Middle thyroid vein
Jugular lymphatic trunk
Right external jugular vein
1st rib
Subclavian lymphatic trunk
Right subclavian vein
Thyroid cartilage
Cricoid cartilage
Thyroid gland
Bronchomediastinal lymphatic trunk
Trachea
Left brachiocephalic vein
Inferior thyroid veins
Right brachiocephalic vein
Superior vena cava
A. Lateral View
Right lymphatic duct
Anterior jugular vein
Inferior bulb of IJV
Hyoid
Right internal jugular vein
Thyroid gland
Jugular lymphatic trunk
Right lymphatic duct
Right venous angle
Left internal jugular vein
Jugular lymphatic trunk
Thoracic duct
Left venous angle
Left brachiocephalic vein
B. Anterior View

## 8.32 Lymphatic drainage of thyroid gland, larynx, and trachea

Radical neck dissections are performed when cancer invades the lymphatics. During the procedure, the deep cervical lymph nodes and the tissues around them are removed as completely as possible. Although major arteries, the brachial plexus, CN X, and the phrenic nerve are preserved, most cutaneous branches of the cervical plexus are removed. The aim of the dissection is to remove all tissue that contains lymph nodes in one piece.

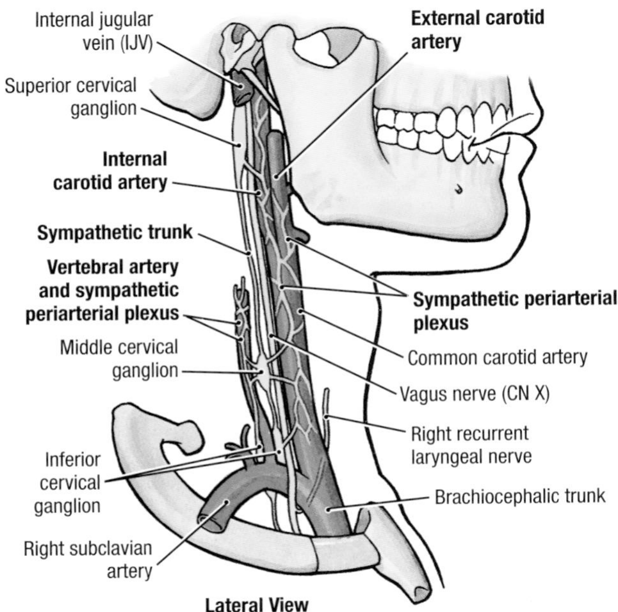
Internal jugular vein (IJV)
Superior cervical ganglion
Internal carotid artery
Sympathetic trunk
Vertebral artery and sympathetic periarterial plexus
Middle cervical ganglion
Inferior cervical ganglion
Right subclavian artery
External carotid artery
Sympathetic periarterial plexus
Common carotid artery
Vagus nerve (CN X)
Right recurrent laryngeal nerve
Brachiocephalic trunk
Lateral View

## 8.33 Sympathetic trunk and sympathetic periarterial plexus

A lesion of a sympathetic trunk in the neck results in a sympathetic disturbance called Horner syndrome, which is characterized by

- Pupillary constriction resulting from paralysis of the dilator pupillae muscle
- Ptosis (drooping of the superior eyelid), resulting from paralysis of the smooth (tarsal) muscle intermingled with striated muscle of the levator palpebrae superioris
- Sinking in of the eyeball (enophthalmos), possibly caused by paralysis of smooth (orbitalis) muscle in the floor of the orbit
- Vasodilation and absence of sweating on the face and neck (anhydrosis), caused by a lack of sympathetic (vasoconstrictive) nerve supply to the blood vessels and sweat glands

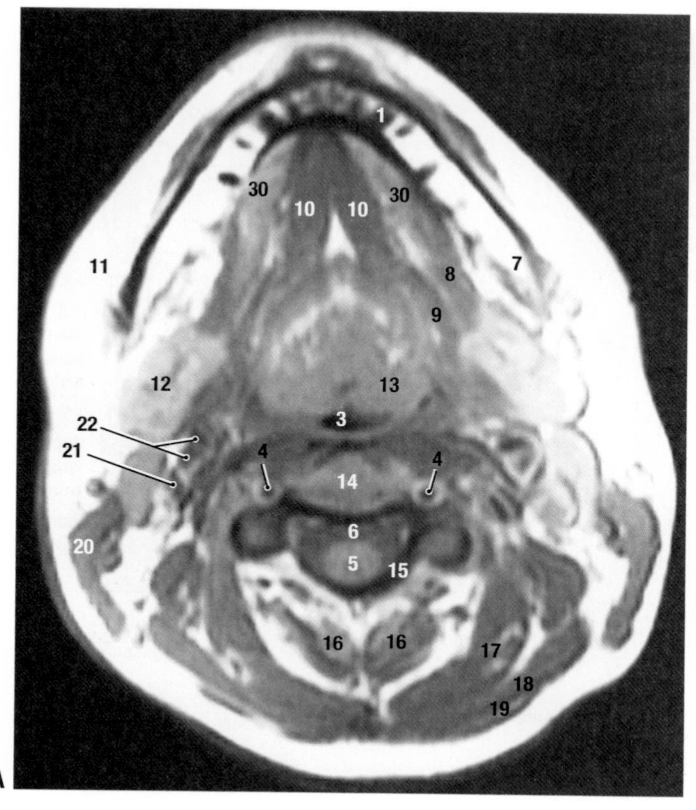
A

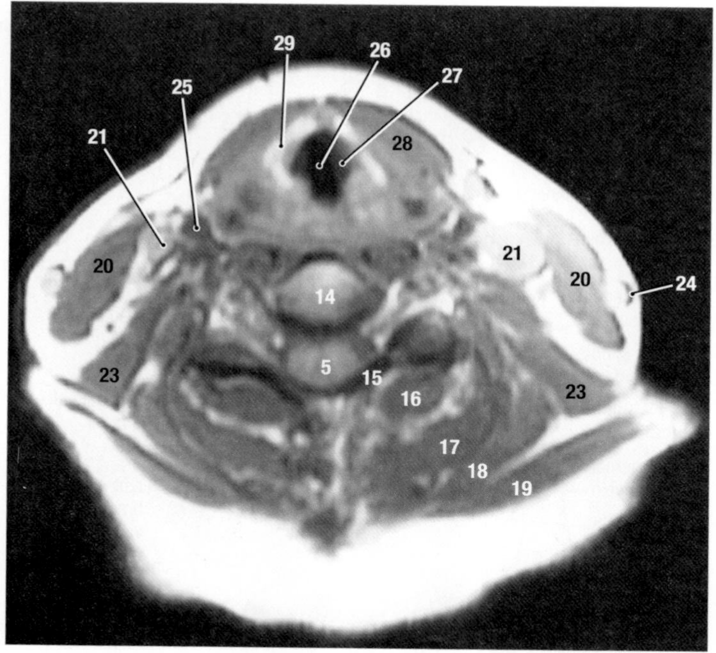
B

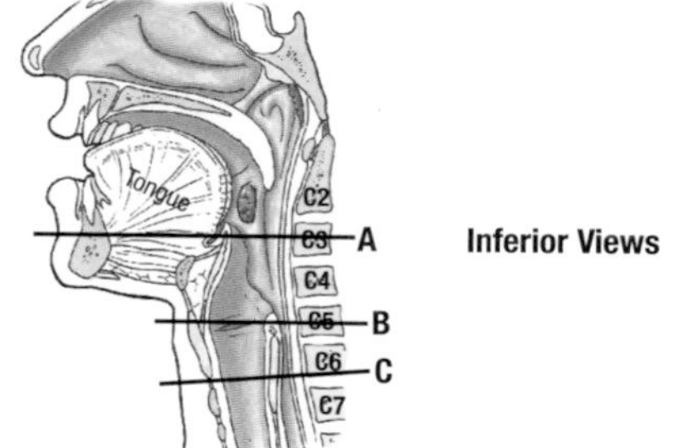
Tongue
C2
C3
C4
C5
C6
C7
A
B
C
Inferior Views

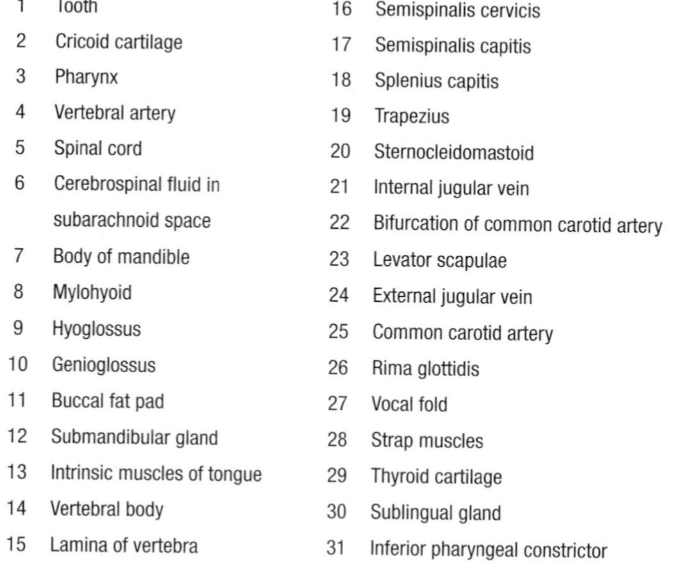

| | | | |
|---|---|---|---|
| 1 | Tooth | 16 | Semispinalis cervicis |
| 2 | Cricoid cartilage | 17 | Semispinalis capitis |
| 3 | Pharynx | 18 | Splenius capitis |
| 4 | Vertebral artery | 19 | Trapezius |
| 5 | Spinal cord | 20 | Sternocleidomastoid |
| 6 | Cerebrospinal fluid in subarachnoid space | 21 | Internal jugular vein |
| | | 22 | Bifurcation of common carotid artery |
| 7 | Body of mandible | 23 | Levator scapulae |
| 8 | Mylohyoid | 24 | External jugular vein |
| 9 | Hyoglossus | 25 | Common carotid artery |
| 10 | Genioglossus | 26 | Rima glottidis |
| 11 | Buccal fat pad | 27 | Vocal fold |
| 12 | Submandibular gland | 28 | Strap muscles |
| 13 | Intrinsic muscles of tongue | 29 | Thyroid cartilage |
| 14 | Vertebral body | 30 | Sublingual gland |
| 15 | Lamina of vertebra | 31 | Inferior pharyngeal constrictor |

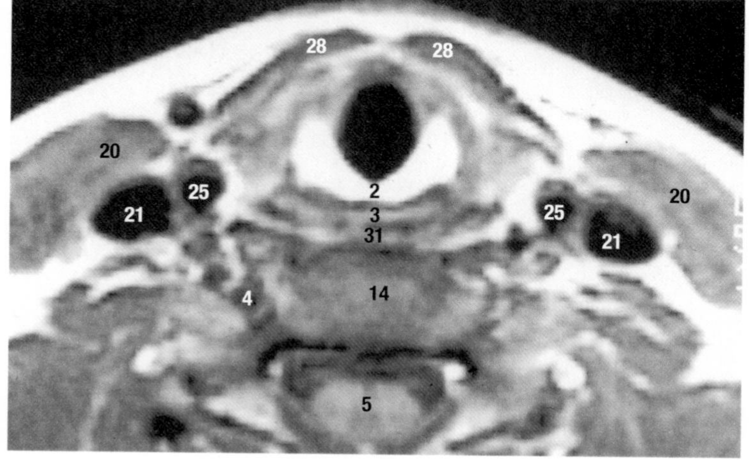
C

**8.34 Transverse MRIs of neck**

The orientation figure indicates the vertebral level of the MRI sections.

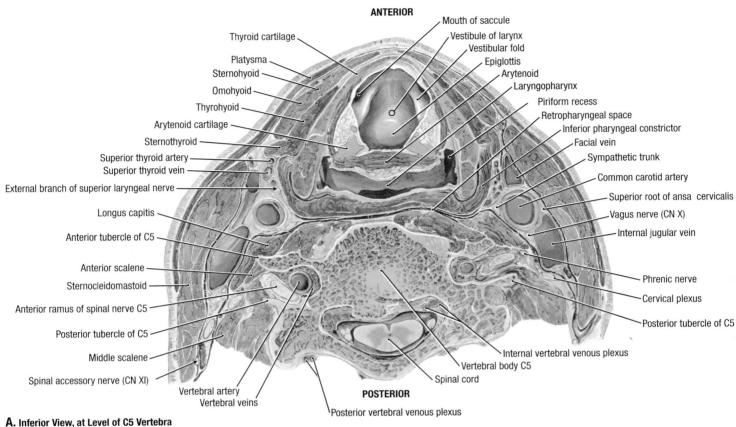
ANTERIOR
Mouth of saccule
Vestibule of larynx
Vestibular fold
Epiglottis
Arytenoid
Laryngopharynx
Piriform recess
Retropharyngeal space
Inferior pharyngeal constrictor
Facial vein
Sympathetic trunk
Common carotid artery
Superior root of ansa cervicalis
Vagus nerve (CN X)
Internal jugular vein
Phrenic nerve
Cervical plexus
Posterior tubercle of C5
Internal vertebral venous plexus
Vertebral body C5
Spinal cord
POSTERIOR
Posterior vertebral venous plexus
Thyroid cartilage
Platysma
Sternohyoid
Omohyoid
Thyrohyoid
Arytenoid cartilage
Sternothyroid
Superior thyroid artery
Superior thyroid vein
External branch of superior laryngeal nerve
Longus capitis
Anterior tubercle of C5
Anterior scalene
Sternocleidomastoid
Anterior ramus of spinal nerve C5
Posterior tubercle of C5
Middle scalene
Spinal accessory nerve (CN XI)
Vertebral artery
Vertebral veins

**A.** Inferior View, at Level of C5 Vertebra

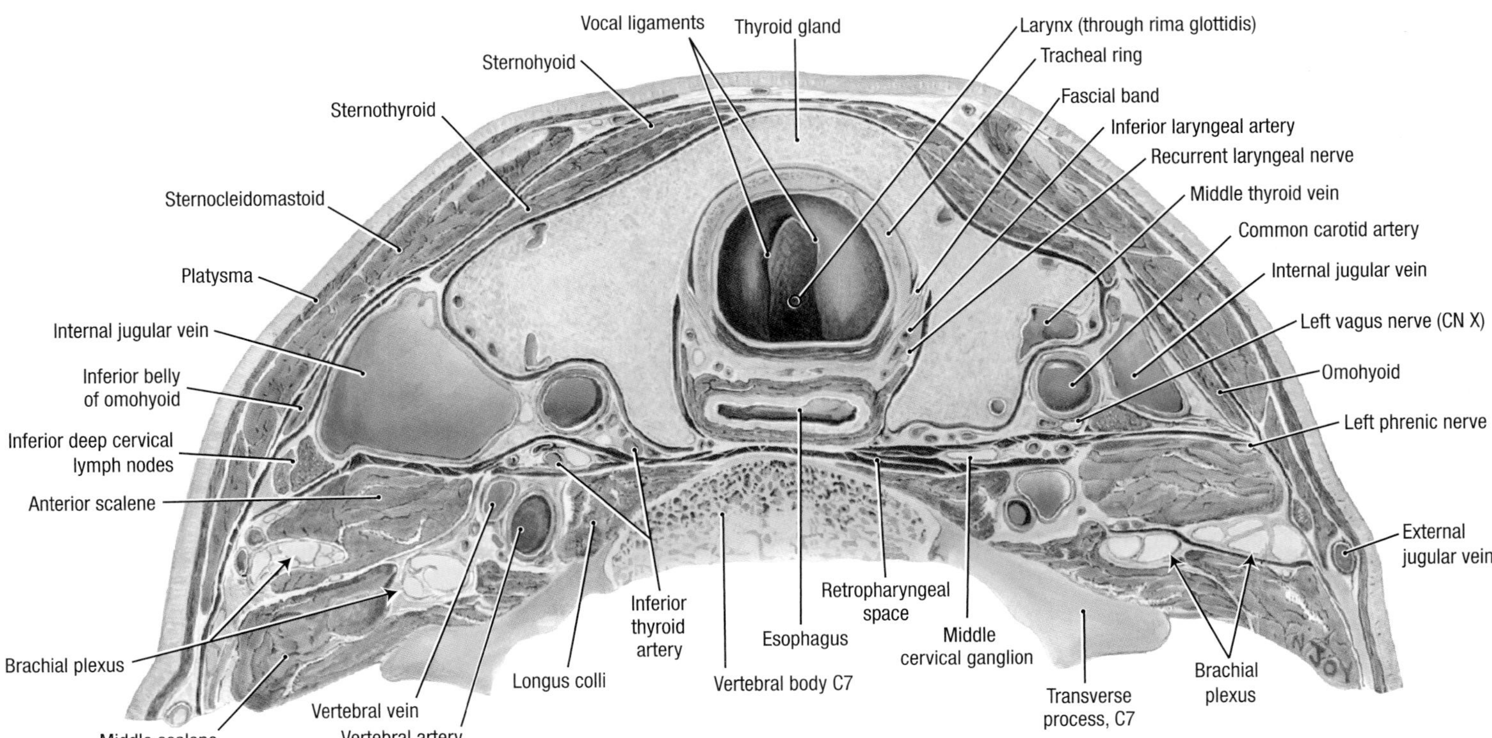
Vocal ligaments
Thyroid gland
Larynx (through rima glottidis)
Tracheal ring
Fascial band
Inferior laryngeal artery
Recurrent laryngeal nerve
Middle thyroid vein
Common carotid artery
Internal jugular vein
Left vagus nerve (CN X)
Omohyoid
Left phrenic nerve
External jugular vein
Brachial plexus
Transverse process, C7
Middle cervical ganglion
Retropharyngeal space
Esophagus
Vertebral body C7
Inferior thyroid artery
Longus colli
Vertebral artery
Vertebral vein
Middle scalene
Brachial plexus
Anterior scalene
Inferior deep cervical lymph nodes
Inferior belly of omohyoid
Internal jugular vein
Platysma
Sternocleidomastoid
Sternothyroid
Sternohyoid

**B.** Inferior View, at Level of C7 Vertebra

## 8.35 Transverse anatomical sections of neck

Level of C7 Vertebra

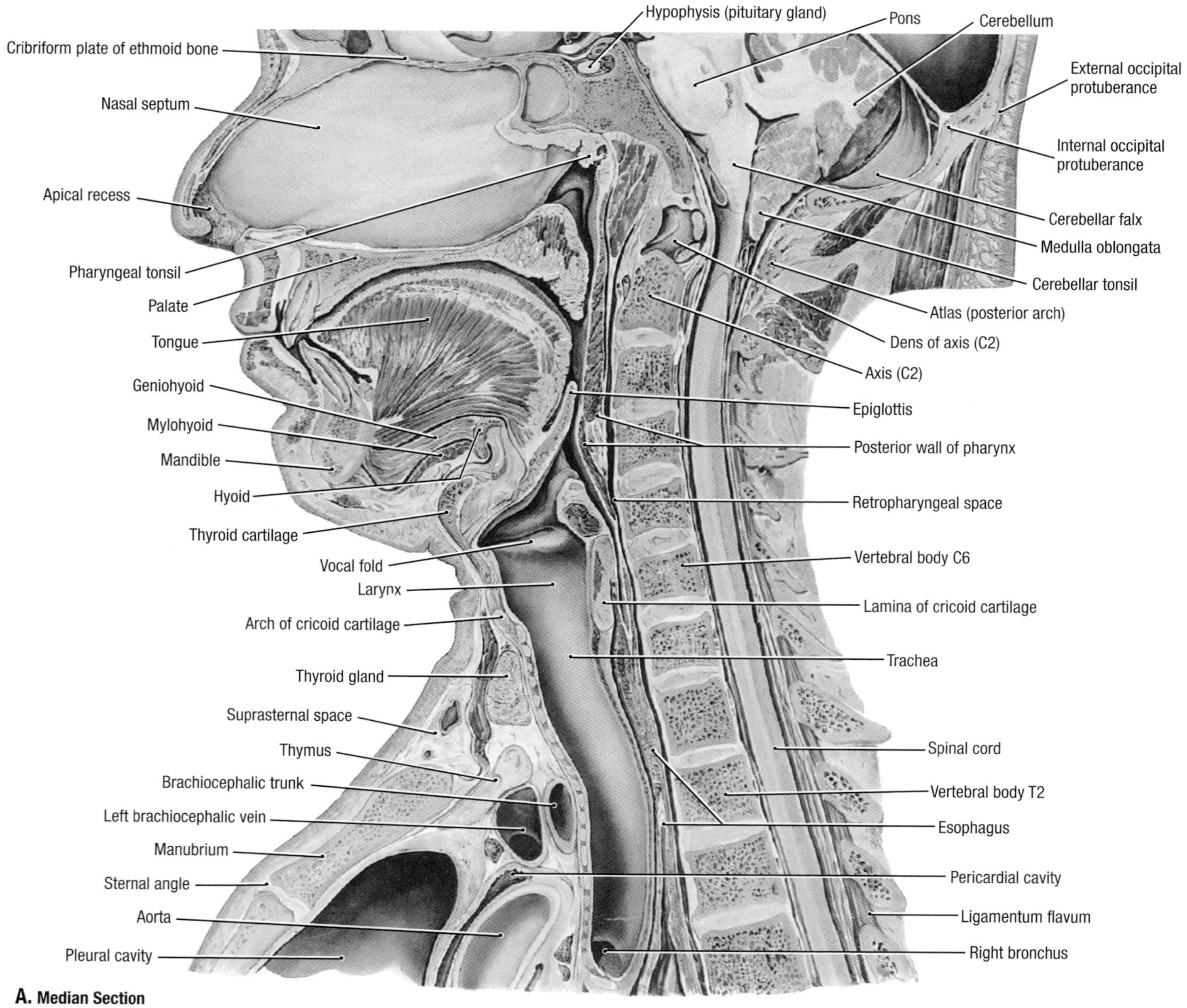

Hypophysis (pituitary gland)
Pons
Cerebellum
Cribriform plate of ethmoid bone
External occipital protuberance
Nasal septum
Internal occipital protuberance
Apical recess
Cerebellar falx
Medulla oblongata
Pharyngeal tonsil
Cerebellar tonsil
Palate
Atlas (posterior arch)
Tongue
Dens of axis (C2)
Axis (C2)
Geniohyoid
Epiglottis
Mylohyoid
Posterior wall of pharynx
Mandible
Hyoid
Retropharyngeal space
Thyroid cartilage
Vertebral body C6
Vocal fold
Larynx
Lamina of cricoid cartilage
Arch of cricoid cartilage
Trachea
Thyroid gland
Suprasternal space
Thymus
Spinal cord
Brachiocephalic trunk
Vertebral body T2
Left brachiocephalic vein
Esophagus
Manubrium
Sternal angle
Pericardial cavity
Aorta
Ligamentum flavum
Pleural cavity
Right bronchus

**A. Median Section**

## 8.36 Median section and MRI scan of head and neck

**A.** Median anatomical section.

**Swallowing.** (1) The bolus of food is squeezed to the back of the mouth by pushing the tongue against the palate. (2) The nasopharynx is sealed off, and the larynx is elevated, enlarging the pharynx to receive food. (3) The pharyngeal sphincters contract sequentially, squeezing food into the esophagus. The epiglottis deflects the bolus from but does not close the inlet to the larynx and trachea. (4) The bolus of food moves down the esophagus by peristaltic contractions.

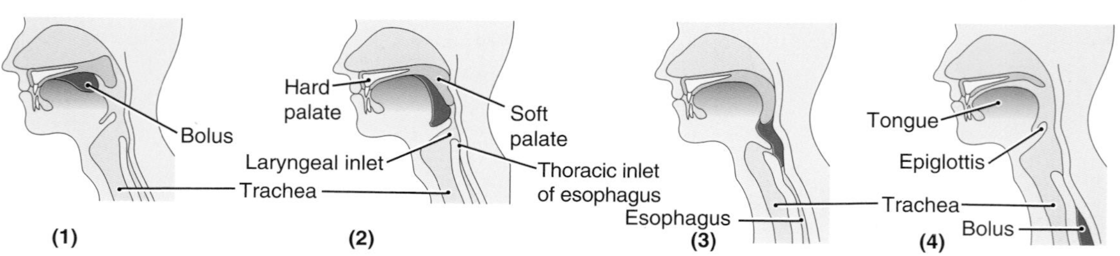
Bolus
(1)
Hard palate
Soft palate
Laryngeal inlet
Thoracic inlet of esophagus
Trachea
(2)
Esophagus
(3)
Tongue
Epiglottis
Trachea
Bolus
(4)

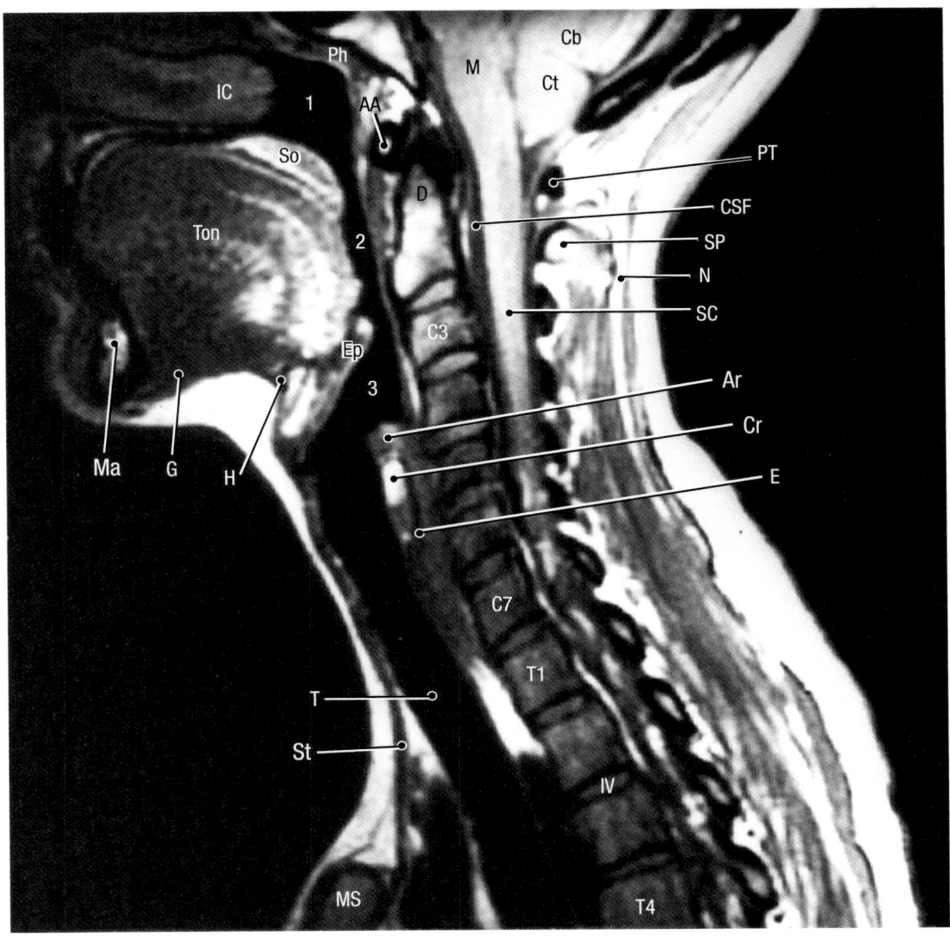
Ph
M
Cb
IC
1
AA
Ct
So
PT
CSF
Ton
2
D
SP
N
SC
C3
Ep
3
Ar
Cr
Ma
G
H
E
C7
T1
T
St
IV
MS
T4

**B. Median MRI Scan**

| | |
|---|---|
| 1 | Nasopharynx |
| 2 | Oropharynx |
| 3 | Laryngopharynx |
| AA | Anterior arch of C1 |
| Ar | Arytenoid cartilage |
| C3-T4 | Vertebral bodies |
| Cb | Cerebellum |
| Cr | Cricoid cartilage |
| CSF | Cerebrospinal fluid in subarachnoid space |
| Ct | Tonsil of cerebellum |
| D | Dens |
| E | Esophagus |
| Ep | Epiglottis |
| G | Genioglossus |
| H | Hyoid |
| IC | Inferior concha |
| IV | Intervertebral disc |
| M | Medulla oblongata |
| Ma | Mandible |
| MS | Manubrium of sternum |
| N | Nuchal ligament |
| Ph | Pharyngeal tonsil (adenoid) |
| PT | Posterior tubercle of C1 |
| SC | Spinal cord |
| So | Soft palate |
| SP | Spinous process |
| St | Strap muscles |
| T | Trachea |
| Ton | Tongue |

**8.36** Median section and MRI scan of head and neck *(continued)*

## 8.37 Doppler US color flow study of carotid artery

**Ultrasonography** is a useful diagnostic imaging technique for studying soft tissues of the neck. Ultrasound provides images of many abnormal conditions noninvasively, at relatively low cost, and with minimal discomfort. Ultrasound is useful for distinguishing solid from cystic masses, for example, which may be difficult to determine during physical examination. Vascular imaging of arteries and veins of the neck is possible using intravascular ultrasonography. The images are produced by placing the transducer over the blood vessel. Doppler ultrasound techniques help evaluate blood flow through a vessel (e.g., for detecting stenosis [narrowing] of a carotid artery).

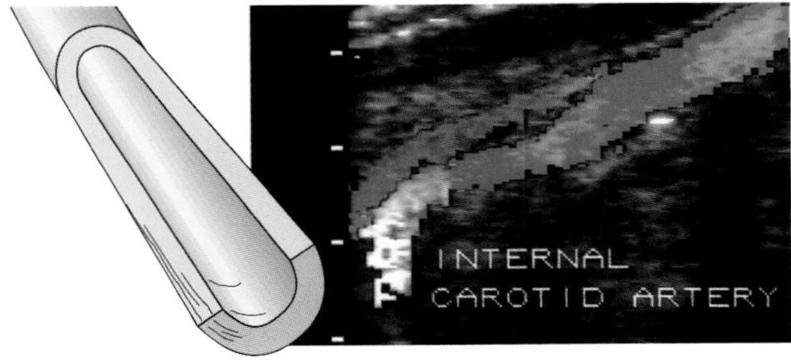
INTERNAL
CAROTID ARTERY

CHAPTER 9

# CRANIAL NERVES

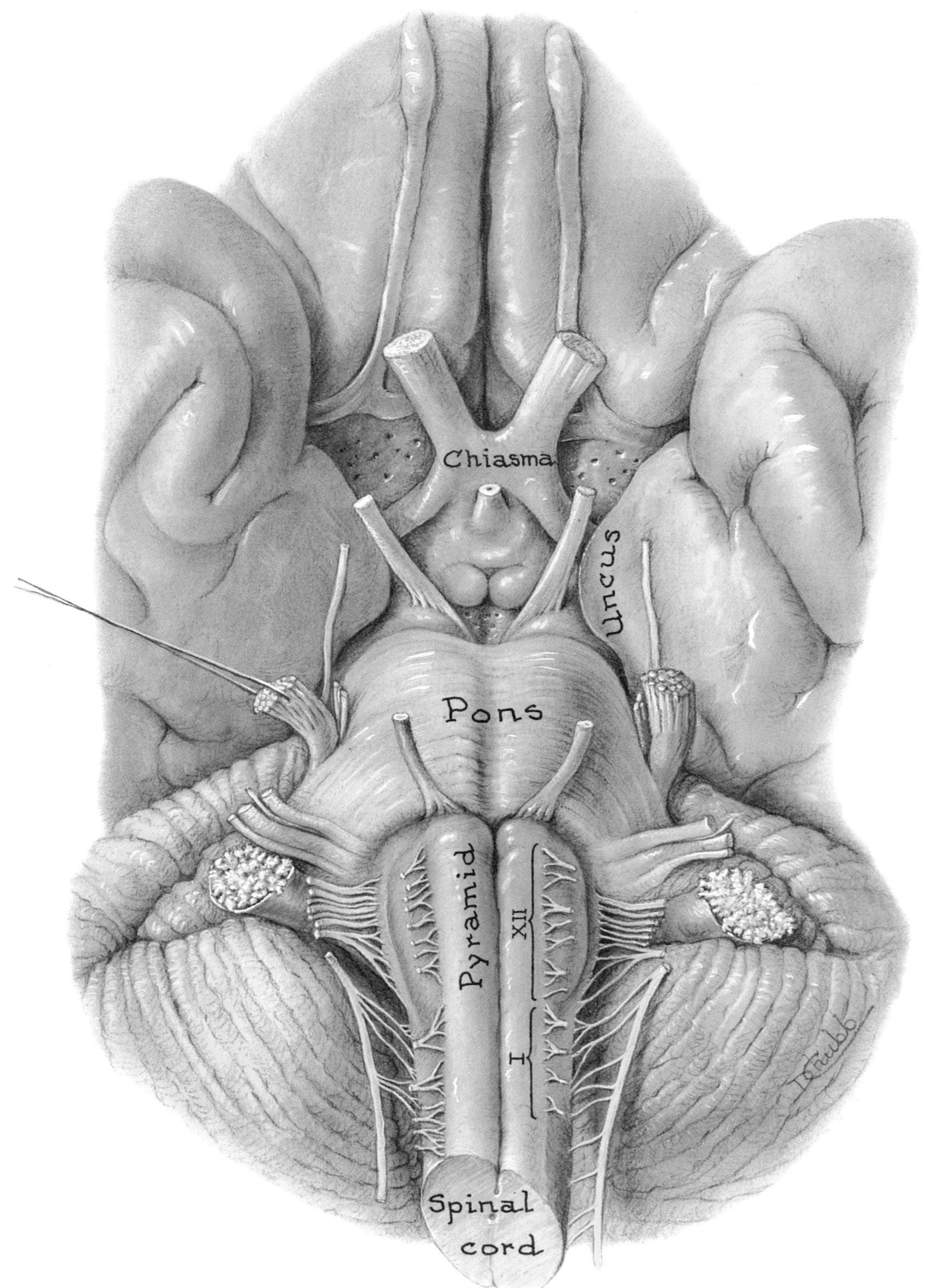
Chiasma
Uncus
Pons
Pyramid
XII
I
Spinal cord


- Overview of Cranial Nerves **812**
- Cranial Nerve Nuclei **816**
- Cranial Nerve I: Olfactory **818**
- Cranial Nerve II: Optic **819**
- Cranial Nerves III, IV, and VI: Oculomotor, Trochlear, and Abducent **821**
- Cranial Nerve V: Trigeminal **824**
- Cranial Nerve VII: Facial **830**
- Cranial Nerve VIII: Vestibulocochlear **832**
- Cranial Nerve IX: Glossopharyngeal **834**
- Cranial Nerve X: Vagus **836**
- Cranial Nerve XI: Spinal Accessory **838**
- Cranial Nerve XII: Hypoglossal **839**
- Summary of Autonomic Ganglia of Head **840**
- Summary of Cranial Nerve Lesions **841**
- Sectional Imaging of Cranial Nerves **842**

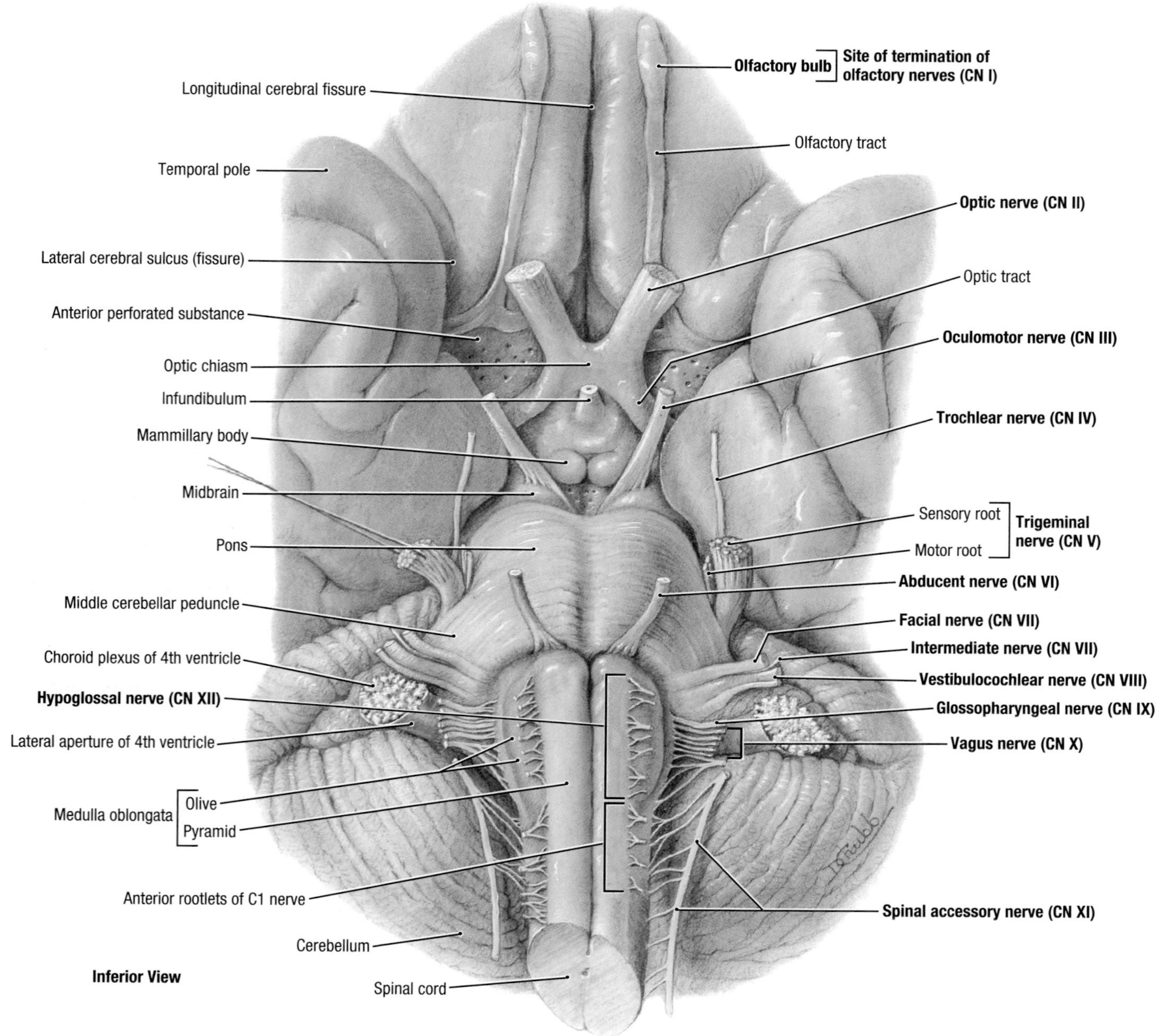
Olfactory bulb
Site of termination of olfactory nerves (CN I)
Longitudinal cerebral fissure
Olfactory tract
Temporal pole
Optic nerve (CN II)
Lateral cerebral sulcus (fissure)
Optic tract
Anterior perforated substance
Oculomotor nerve (CN III)
Optic chiasm
Infundibulum
Trochlear nerve (CN IV)
Mammillary body
Midbrain
Sensory root
Motor root
Trigeminal nerve (CN V)
Pons
Abducent nerve (CN VI)
Middle cerebellar peduncle
Facial nerve (CN VII)
Choroid plexus of 4th ventricle
Intermediate nerve (CN VII)
Vestibulocochlear nerve (CN VIII)
Hypoglossal nerve (CN XII)
Glossopharyngeal nerve (CN IX)
Lateral aperture of 4th ventricle
Vagus nerve (CN X)
Medulla oblongata
Olive
Pyramid
Anterior rootlets of C1 nerve
Spinal accessory nerve (CN XI)
Cerebellum
Inferior View
Spinal cord

## 9.1 Cranial nerves in relation to the base of the brain

Cranial nerves are nerves that exit from the cranial cavity through openings in the cranium. There are 12 pairs of cranial nerves that are named and numbered in rostrocaudal sequence of their superficial origins from the brain, brainstem, and superior spinal cord. The olfactory nerves (CN I, not shown) end in the olfactory bulb. The entire origin of the spinal accessory nerve (CN XI) from the spinal cord is not included here; it extends inferiorly as far as the C6 spinal cord segment.

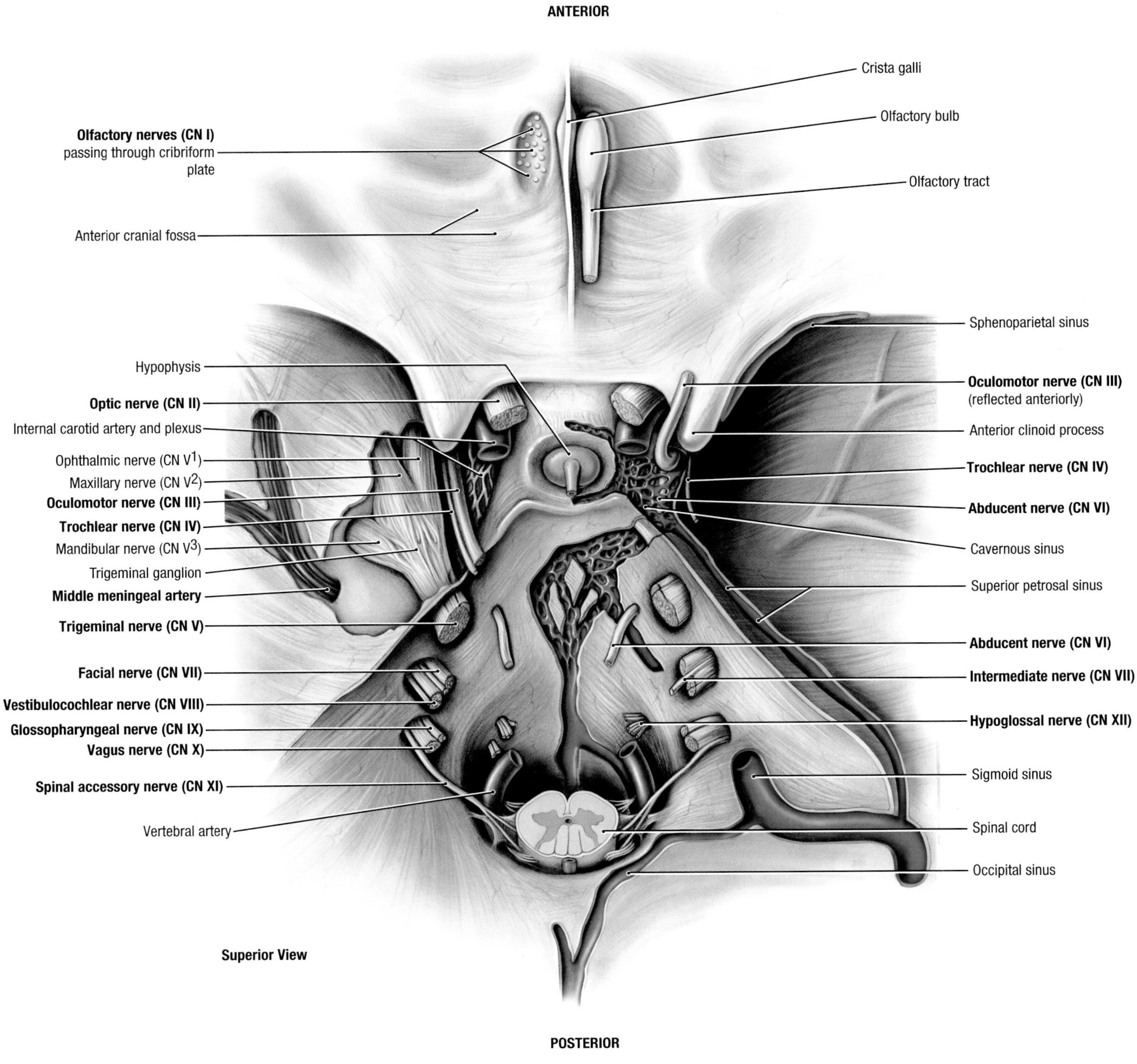

ANTERIOR
Crista galli
Olfactory bulb
Olfactory nerves (CN I) passing through cribriform plate
Olfactory tract
Anterior cranial fossa
Sphenoparietal sinus
Hypophysis
Oculomotor nerve (CN III) (reflected anteriorly)
Optic nerve (CN II)
Internal carotid artery and plexus
Anterior clinoid process
Ophthalmic nerve (CN V1)
Trochlear nerve (CN IV)
Maxillary nerve (CN V2)
Oculomotor nerve (CN III)
Abducent nerve (CN VI)
Trochlear nerve (CN IV)
Mandibular nerve (CN V3)
Cavernous sinus
Trigeminal ganglion
Middle meningeal artery
Superior petrosal sinus
Trigeminal nerve (CN V)
Abducent nerve (CN VI)
Facial nerve (CN VII)
Intermediate nerve (CN VII)
Vestibulocochlear nerve (CN VIII)
Glossopharyngeal nerve (CN IX)
Hypoglossal nerve (CN XII)
Vagus nerve (CN X)
Sigmoid sinus
Spinal accessory nerve (CN XI)
Vertebral artery
Spinal cord
Occipital sinus
Superior View
POSTERIOR

## 9.2 Cranial nerves in relation to the internal aspect of the cranial base

The venous sinuses have been opened on the right side. The ophthalmic division of the trigeminal nerve (CN $V^1$), and the trochlear (CN IV) and oculomotor (CN III) nerves have been dissected from the lateral wall of the cavernous sinus.

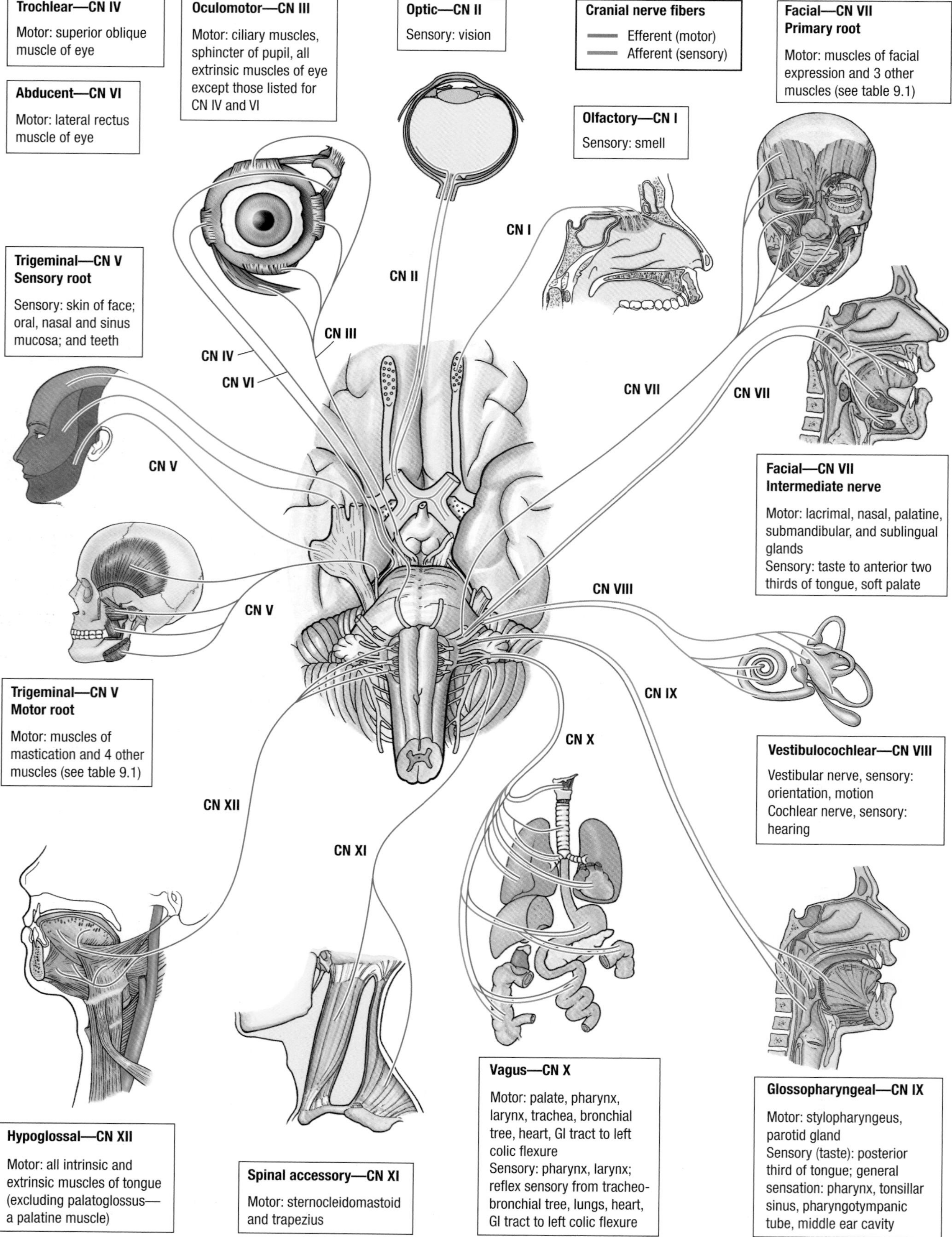
Trochlear—CN IV
Motor: superior oblique muscle of eye
Abducent—CN VI
Motor: lateral rectus muscle of eye
Oculomotor—CN III
Motor: ciliary muscles, sphincter of pupil, all extrinsic muscles of eye except those listed for CN IV and VI
Optic—CN II
Sensory: vision
Cranial nerve fibers
Efferent (motor)
Afferent (sensory)
Olfactory—CN I
Sensory: smell
Facial—CN VII
Primary root
Motor: muscles of facial expression and 3 other muscles (see table 9.1)
Trigeminal—CN V
Sensory root
Sensory: skin of face; oral, nasal and sinus mucosa; and teeth
CN I
CN II
CN III
CN IV
CN VI
CN VII
CN VII
CN V
Facial—CN VII
Intermediate nerve
Motor: lacrimal, nasal, palatine, submandibular, and sublingual glands
Sensory: taste to anterior two thirds of tongue, soft palate
CN VIII
CN V
CN IX
Trigeminal—CN V
Motor root
Motor: muscles of mastication and 4 other muscles (see table 9.1)
CN X
Vestibulocochlear—CN VIII
Vestibular nerve, sensory: orientation, motion
Cochlear nerve, sensory: hearing
CN XII
CN XI
Vagus—CN X
Motor: palate, pharynx, larynx, trachea, bronchial tree, heart, GI tract to left colic flexure
Sensory: pharynx, larynx; reflex sensory from tracheo-bronchial tree, lungs, heart, GI tract to left colic flexure
Glossopharyngeal—CN IX
Motor: stylopharyngeus, parotid gland
Sensory (taste): posterior third of tongue; general sensation: pharynx, tonsillar sinus, pharyngotympanic tube, middle ear cavity
Hypoglossal—CN XII
Motor: all intrinsic and extrinsic muscles of tongue (excluding palatoglossus—a palatine muscle)
Spinal accessory—CN XI
Motor: sternocleidomastoid and trapezius

**TABLE 9.1 SUMMARY OF CRANIAL NERVES**

| Nerve | Components | Location of Nerve Cell Bodies | Cranial Exit | Main Action |
|---|---|---|---|---|
| Olfactory (CN I) | Special sensory | Olfactory epithelium (olfactory cells) | Foramina in cribriform plate of ethmoid bone | Smell from nasal mucosa of roof of each nasal cavity, superior sides of nasal septum and superior concha |
| Optic (CN II) | Special sensory | Retina (ganglion cells) | Optic canal | Vision from retina |
| Oculomotor (CN III) | Somatic motor | Midbrain | Superior orbital fissure | Motor to superior, inferior, and medial rectus, inferior oblique, and levator palpebrae superioris muscle that raise upper eyelid and rotates eyeball superiorly, inferiorly, and medially |
| | Visceral motor (parasympathetic) | Presynaptic: midbrain; Postsynaptic: ciliary ganglion | | Secretomotor to sphincter pupillae and ciliary muscles that constrict pupil and accommodate lens of eye |
| Trochlear (CN IV) | Somatic motor | Midbrain | | Motor to superior oblique that assists in rotating eye inferolaterally |
| Trigeminal (CN V) Ophthalmic division (CN $V^1$) | General sensory | Trigeminal ganglion | | Sensation from cornea, skin of forehead, scalp, eyelids, nose, and mucosa of nasal cavity and paranasal sinuses |
| Maxillary division (CN $V^2$) | General sensory | Trigeminal ganglion | Foramen rotundum | Sensation from skin of face over maxilla including upper lip, maxillary teeth, mucosa of nose, maxillary sinuses, and palate |
| Mandibular division (CN $V^3$) | Branchial motor | Pons | Foramen ovale | Motor to muscles of mastication, mylohyoid, anterior belly of digastric, tensor veli palatini, and tensor tympani |
| | General sensory | Trigeminal ganglion | | Sensation from the skin over mandible, including lower lip and side of head, mandibular teeth, temporomandibular joint, and mucosa of mouth and anterior two thirds of the tongue |
| Abducent (CN VI) | Somatic motor | Pons | Superior orbital fissure | Motor to lateral rectus that rotates eye laterally |
| Facial (CN VII) | Branchial motor | Pons | Internal acoustic meatus, facial canal, and stylomastoid foramen | Motor to muscles of facial expression and scalp; also supplies stapedius of middle ear, stylohyoid, and posterior belly of digastric |
| | Special sensory | Geniculate ganglion | | Taste from anterior two thirds of tongue, floor of mouth, and palate |
| | General sensory | | | Sensation from skin of external acoustic meatus |
| | Visceral motor (parasympathetic) | Presynaptic: pons; Postsynaptic: pterygopalatine ganglion and submandibular ganglion | | Secretomotor to submandibular and sublingual salivary glands, lacrimal gland, and glands of nose and palate |
| Vestibulocochlear (CN VIII) Vestibular | Special sensory | Vestibular ganglion | Internal acoustic meatus | Vestibular sensation from semicircular ducts, utricle, and saccule related to position and movement of head |
| Cochlear | Special sensory | Spiral ganglion | | Hearing from spiral organ |
| Glossopharyngeal (CN IX) | Branchial motor | Medulla | Jugular foramen | Motor to stylopharyngeus that assists with swallowing |
| | Visceral motor (parasympathetic) | Presynaptic: medulla; Postsynaptic: otic ganglion | | Secretomotor to parotid gland |
| | Visceral sensory | Inferior ganglion | | Visceral sensation from parotid gland, carotid body and sinus, pharynx, and middle ear |
| | Special sensory | Superior ganglion | | Taste from posterior third of tongue |
| | General sensory | Inferior ganglion | | Cutaneous sensation from external ear |
| Vagus (CN X) | Branchial motor | Medulla | | Motor to constrictor muscles of pharynx, intrinsic muscles of larynx, muscles of palate (except tensor veli palatine), and striated muscle in superior two thirds of esophagus |
| | Visceral motor (parasympathetic) | Presynaptic: medulla; Postsynaptic: neurons in, on, or near viscera | | Motor to smooth muscle of trachea, bronchi, and digestive tract, moderates cardiac pacemaker and vasoconstrictor of coronary arteries |
| | Special sensory | Inferior ganglion | | Visceral sensation from base of tongue, pharynx, larynx, trachea, bronchi, heart, esophagus, stomach, and intestine |
| | General sensory | Superior ganglion | | Sensation from auricle, external acoustic meatus, and dura mater of posterior cranial fossa |
| | Somatic motor | Medulla | | Motor to striated muscles of soft palate, pharynx, and larynx |
| Spinal accessory nerve (CN XI) | Somatic motor | Cervical spinal cord | | Motor to sternocleidomastoid and trapezius |
| Hypoglossal (CN XII) | Somatic motor | Medulla | Hypoglossal canal | Motor to muscles of tongue (except palatoglossus) |

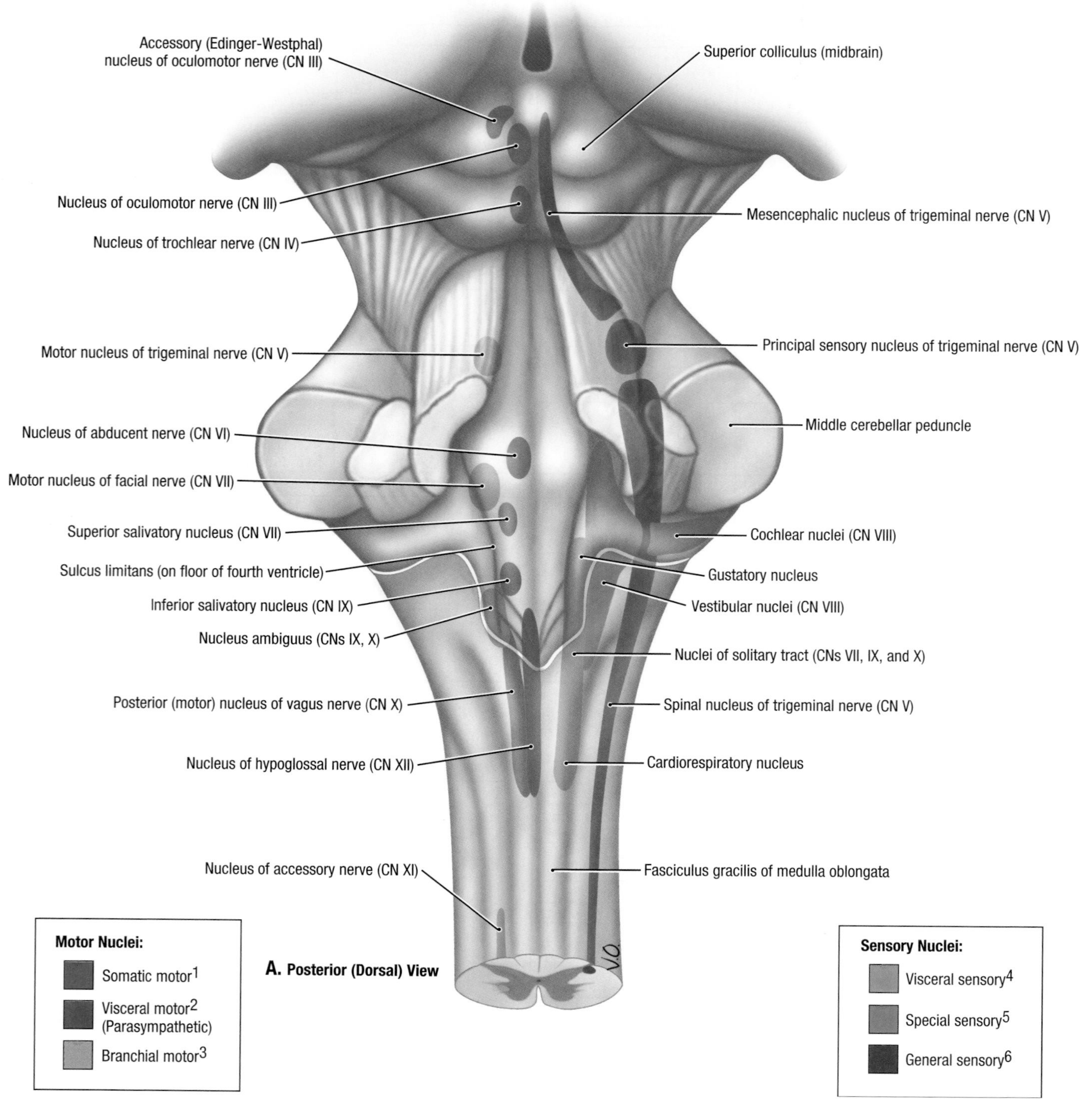
Accessory (Edinger-Westphal) nucleus of oculomotor nerve (CN III)
Superior colliculus (midbrain)
Nucleus of oculomotor nerve (CN III)
Mesencephalic nucleus of trigeminal nerve (CN V)
Nucleus of trochlear nerve (CN IV)
Principal sensory nucleus of trigeminal nerve (CN V)
Motor nucleus of trigeminal nerve (CN V)
Middle cerebellar peduncle
Nucleus of abducent nerve (CN VI)
Motor nucleus of facial nerve (CN VII)
Superior salivatory nucleus (CN VII)
Cochlear nuclei (CN VIII)
Sulcus limitans (on floor of fourth ventricle)
Gustatory nucleus
Inferior salivatory nucleus (CN IX)
Vestibular nuclei (CN VIII)
Nucleus ambiguus (CNs IX, X)
Nuclei of solitary tract (CNs VII, IX, and X)
Posterior (motor) nucleus of vagus nerve (CN X)
Spinal nucleus of trigeminal nerve (CN V)
Nucleus of hypoglossal nerve (CN XII)
Cardiorespiratory nucleus
Nucleus of accessory nerve (CN XI)
Fasciculus gracilis of medulla oblongata
Motor Nuclei:
Somatic motor1
Visceral motor2 (Parasympathetic)
Branchial motor3
Sensory Nuclei:
Visceral sensory4
Special sensory5
General sensory6
V.O.

**A. Posterior (Dorsal) View**

## 9.3 Cranial nerve nuclei

The fibers of the cranial nerves are connected to nuclei (groups of nerve cell bodies in the central nervous system), in which afferent (sensory) fibers terminate and from which efferent (motor) fibers originate. Nuclei of common functional types (motor, sensory, parasympathetic, and special sensory nuclei) have a generally columnar placement within the brainstem, with the sulcus limitans demarcating motor and sensory columns.

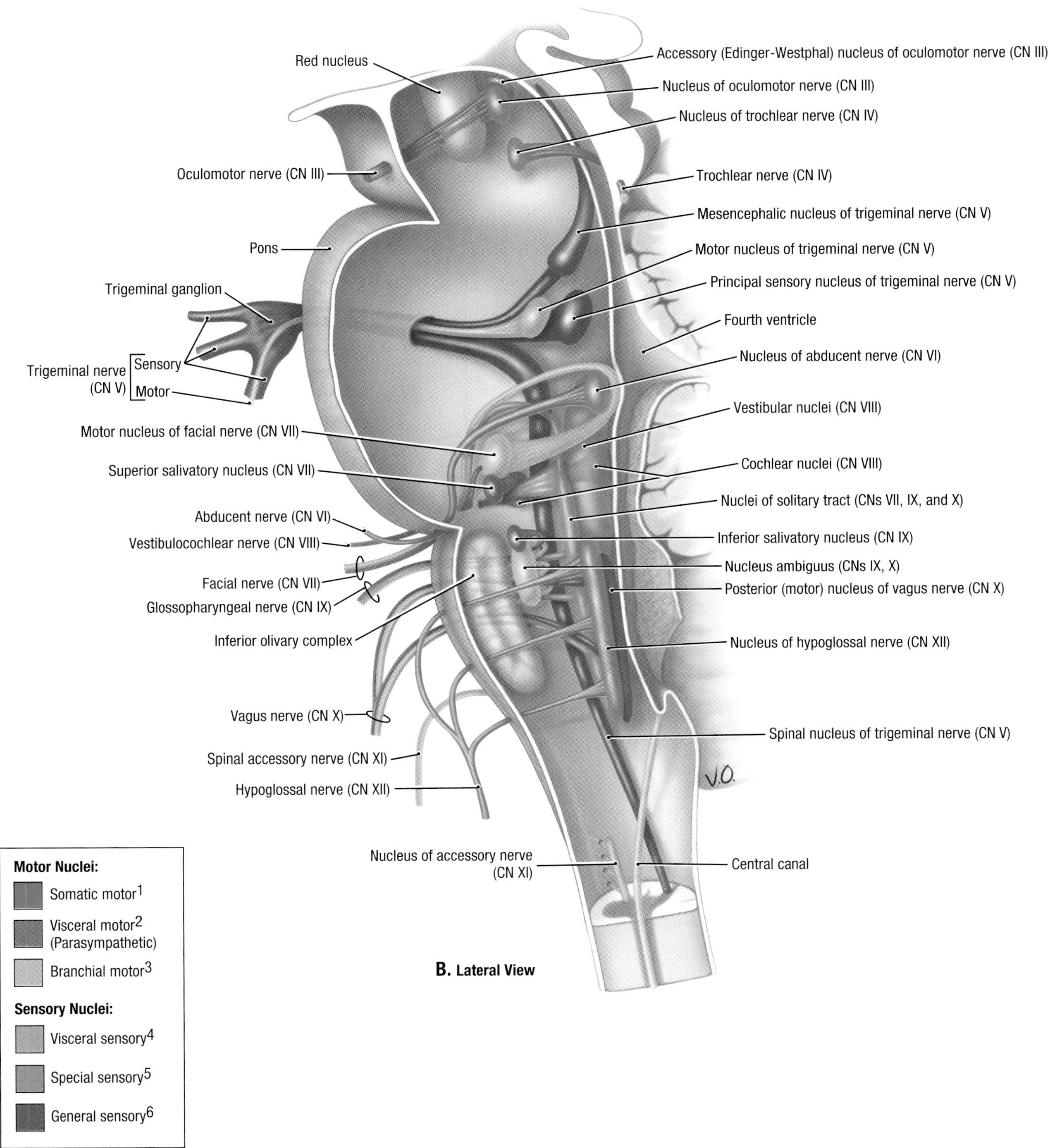
Red nucleus
Accessory (Edinger-Westphal) nucleus of oculomotor nerve (CN III)
Nucleus of oculomotor nerve (CN III)
Nucleus of trochlear nerve (CN IV)
Oculomotor nerve (CN III)
Trochlear nerve (CN IV)
Mesencephalic nucleus of trigeminal nerve (CN V)
Pons
Motor nucleus of trigeminal nerve (CN V)
Trigeminal ganglion
Principal sensory nucleus of trigeminal nerve (CN V)
Fourth ventricle
Trigeminal nerve (CN V)
Sensory
Motor
Nucleus of abducent nerve (CN VI)
Vestibular nuclei (CN VIII)
Motor nucleus of facial nerve (CN VII)
Cochlear nuclei (CN VIII)
Superior salivatory nucleus (CN VII)
Nuclei of solitary tract (CNs VII, IX, and X)
Abducent nerve (CN VI)
Inferior salivatory nucleus (CN IX)
Vestibulocochlear nerve (CN VIII)
Nucleus ambiguus (CNs IX, X)
Facial nerve (CN VII)
Posterior (motor) nucleus of vagus nerve (CN X)
Glossopharyngeal nerve (CN IX)
Inferior olivary complex
Nucleus of hypoglossal nerve (CN XII)
Vagus nerve (CN X)
Spinal nucleus of trigeminal nerve (CN V)
Spinal accessory nerve (CN XI)
Hypoglossal nerve (CN XII)
V.O.
Nucleus of accessory nerve (CN XI)
Central canal
Motor Nuclei:
Somatic motor1
Visceral motor2 (Parasympathetic)
Branchial motor3
Sensory Nuclei:
Visceral sensory4
Special sensory5
General sensory6

**B.** Lateral View

## 9.3 Cranial nerve nuclei *(continued)*

[1]General somatic efferent (GSE); [2]General visceral efferent (GVE); [3]Special visceral efferent (SVE); [4]Special/General visceral afferent (SVA/GVA); [5]Special somatic afferent; [6]General somatic afferent (GSA).

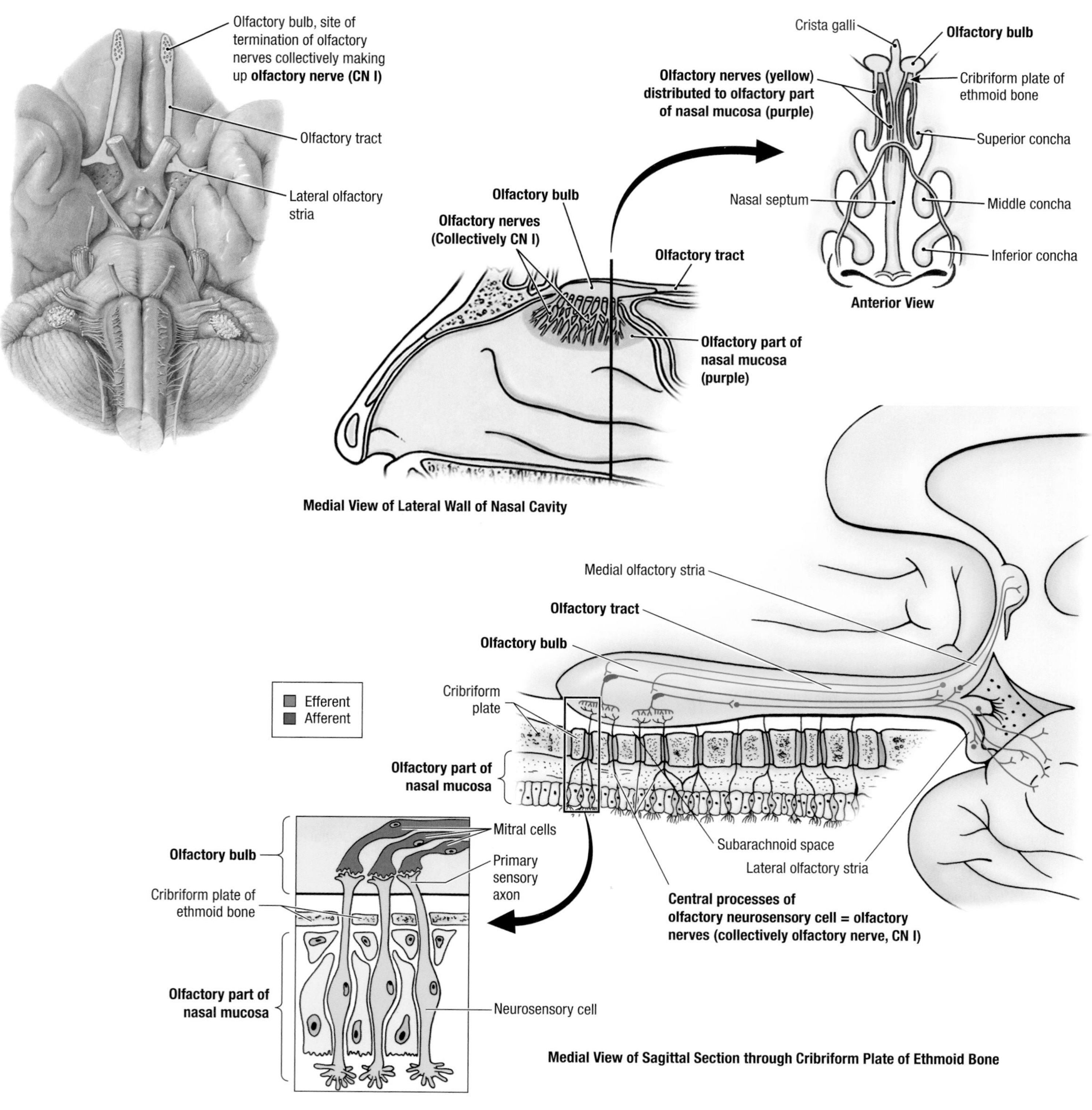
Olfactory bulb, site of termination of olfactory nerves collectively making up olfactory nerve (CN I)
Olfactory tract
Lateral olfactory stria
Crista galli
Olfactory bulb
Olfactory nerves (yellow) distributed to olfactory part of nasal mucosa (purple)
Cribriform plate of ethmoid bone
Superior concha
Nasal septum
Middle concha
Inferior concha
Anterior View
Olfactory bulb
Olfactory nerves (Collectively CN I)
Olfactory tract
Olfactory part of nasal mucosa (purple)
Medial View of Lateral Wall of Nasal Cavity
Medial olfactory stria
Olfactory tract
Olfactory bulb
Efferent
Afferent
Cribriform plate
Olfactory part of nasal mucosa
Subarachnoid space
Lateral olfactory stria
Central processes of olfactory neurosensory cell = olfactory nerves (collectively olfactory nerve, CN I)
Olfactory bulb
Mitral cells
Primary sensory axon
Cribriform plate of ethmoid bone
Olfactory part of nasal mucosa
Neurosensory cell
Medial View of Sagittal Section through Cribriform Plate of Ethmoid Bone

## TABLE 9.2 OLFACTORY NERVE (CN I)

| Nerve | Functional Components | Cells of Origin/ Termination | Cranial Exit | Distribution and Functions |
|---|---|---|---|---|
| **Olfactory** | Special sensory | Olfactory epithelium (olfactory cells/olfactory bulb) | Foramina in cribriform plate of ethmoid bone | Smell from nasal mucosa of roof and superior sides of nasal septum and superior concha of each nasal cavity |

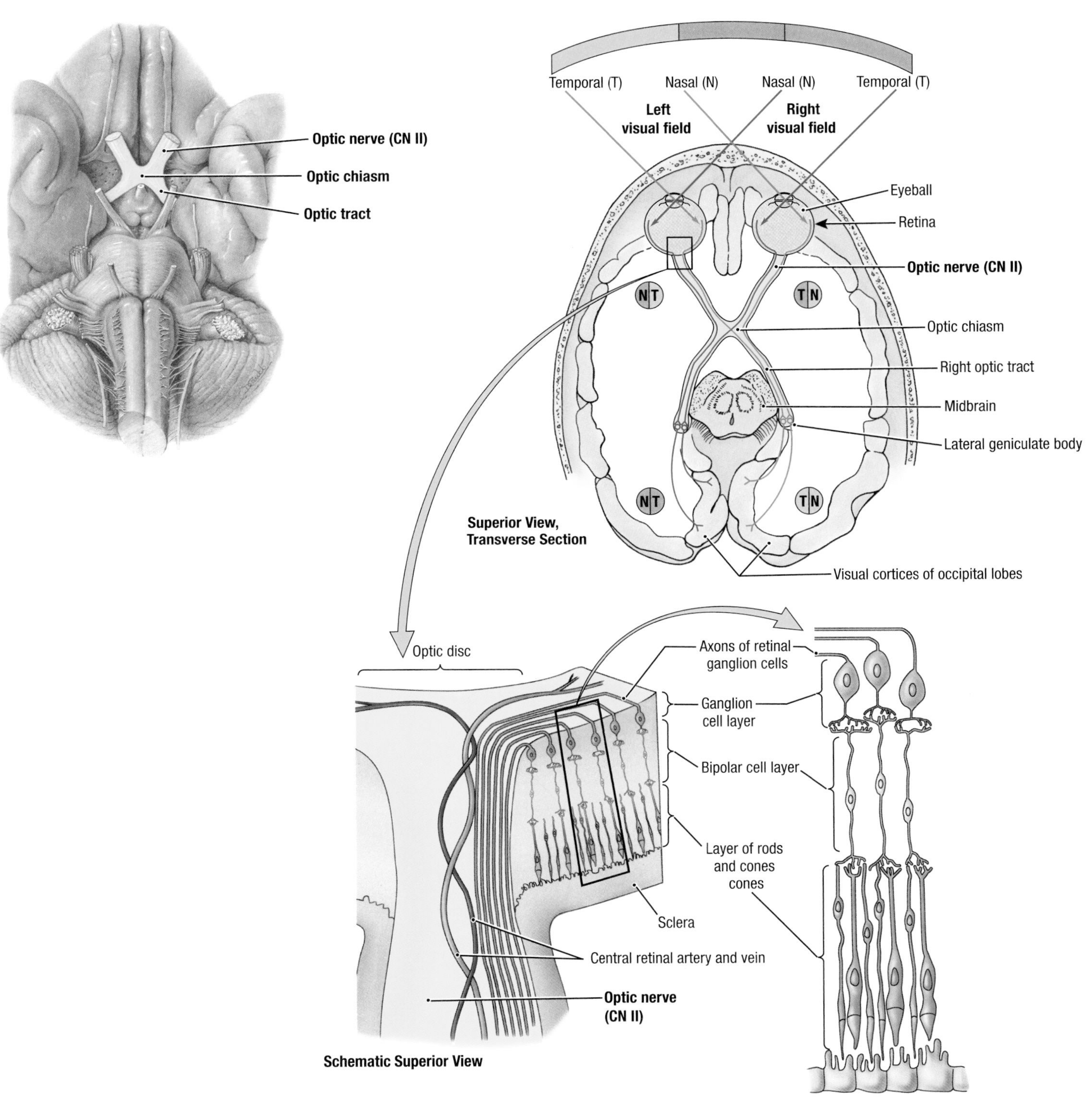
Optic nerve (CN II)
Optic chiasm
Optic tract
Temporal (T)
Nasal (N)
Nasal (N)
Temporal (T)
Left visual field
Right visual field
Eyeball
Retina
Optic nerve (CN II)
N T
T N
Optic chiasm
Right optic tract
Midbrain
Lateral geniculate body
N T
T N
Superior View, Transverse Section
Visual cortices of occipital lobes
Optic disc
Axons of retinal ganglion cells
Ganglion cell layer
Bipolar cell layer
Layer of rods and cones cones
Sclera
Central retinal artery and vein
Optic nerve (CN II)
Schematic Superior View

## TABLE 9.3 OPTIC NERVE (CN II)

| Nerve | Functional Components | Cells of Origin/ Termination | Cranial Exit | Distribution and Functions |
|---|---|---|---|---|
| **Optic** | Special sensory | Retina (ganglion cells)/ lateral geniculate body (nucleus) | Optic canal | Vision from retina |

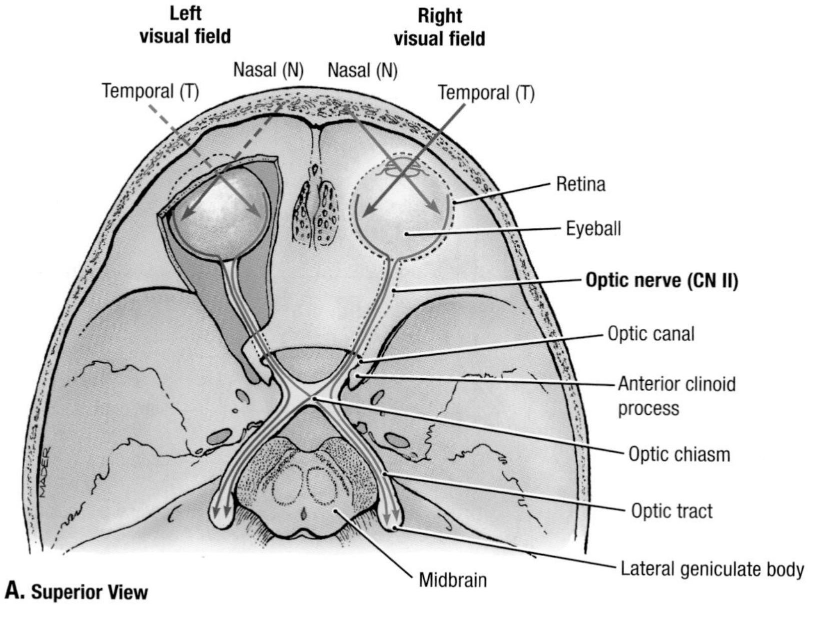
Left
visual field
Right
visual field
Nasal (N)
Nasal (N)
Temporal (T)
Temporal (T)
Retina
Eyeball
Optic nerve (CN II)
Optic canal
Anterior clinoid
process
Optic chiasm
Optic tract
Lateral geniculate body
Midbrain
A. Superior View

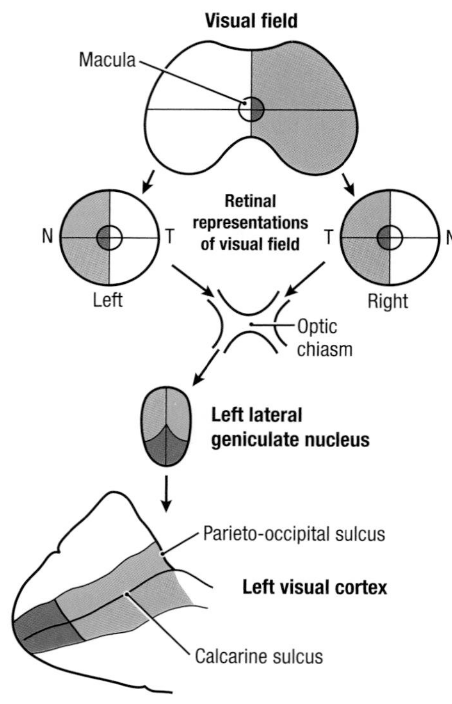
Visual field
Macula
Retinal
representations
of visual field
N
T
T
N
Left
Right
Optic
chiasm
Left lateral
geniculate nucleus
Parieto-occipital sulcus
Left visual cortex
Calcarine sulcus
B

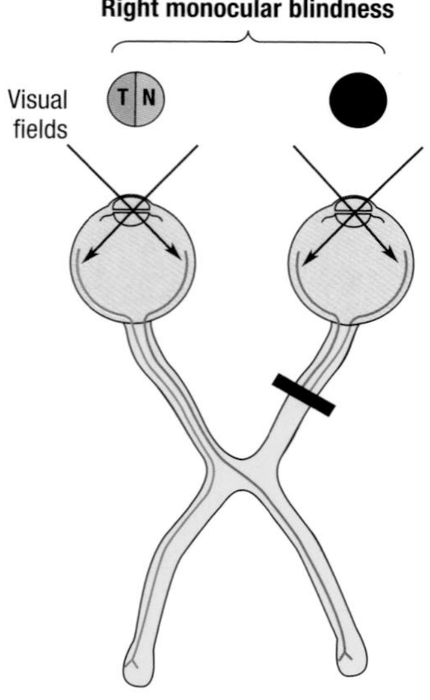
Right monocular blindness
Visual
fields
T
N
C. Section of Right Optic Nerve

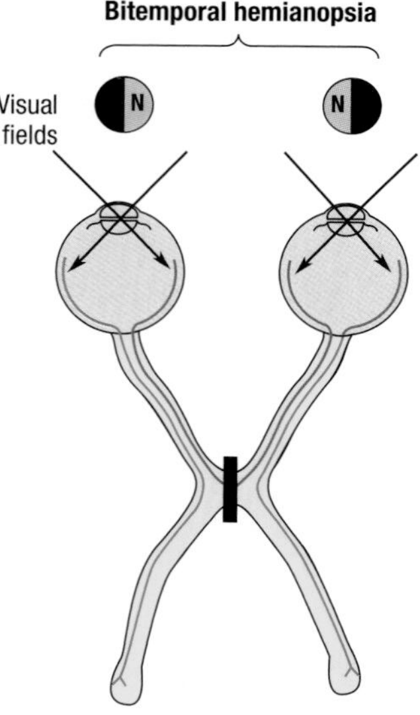
Bitemporal hemianopsia
Visual
fields
N
N
D. Section of Optic Chiasm

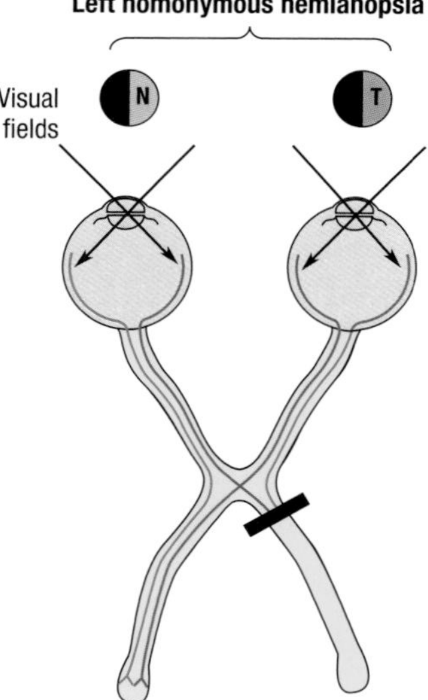
Left homonymous hemianopsia
Visual
fields
N
T
E. Section of Right Optic Tract

## 9.4 Visual pathway

A. The visual pathway in situ. B. Visual field representation on retinae, lateral geniculate nucleus, and visual cortex. C–E. Schematic illustrations of lesions of the visual pathway.

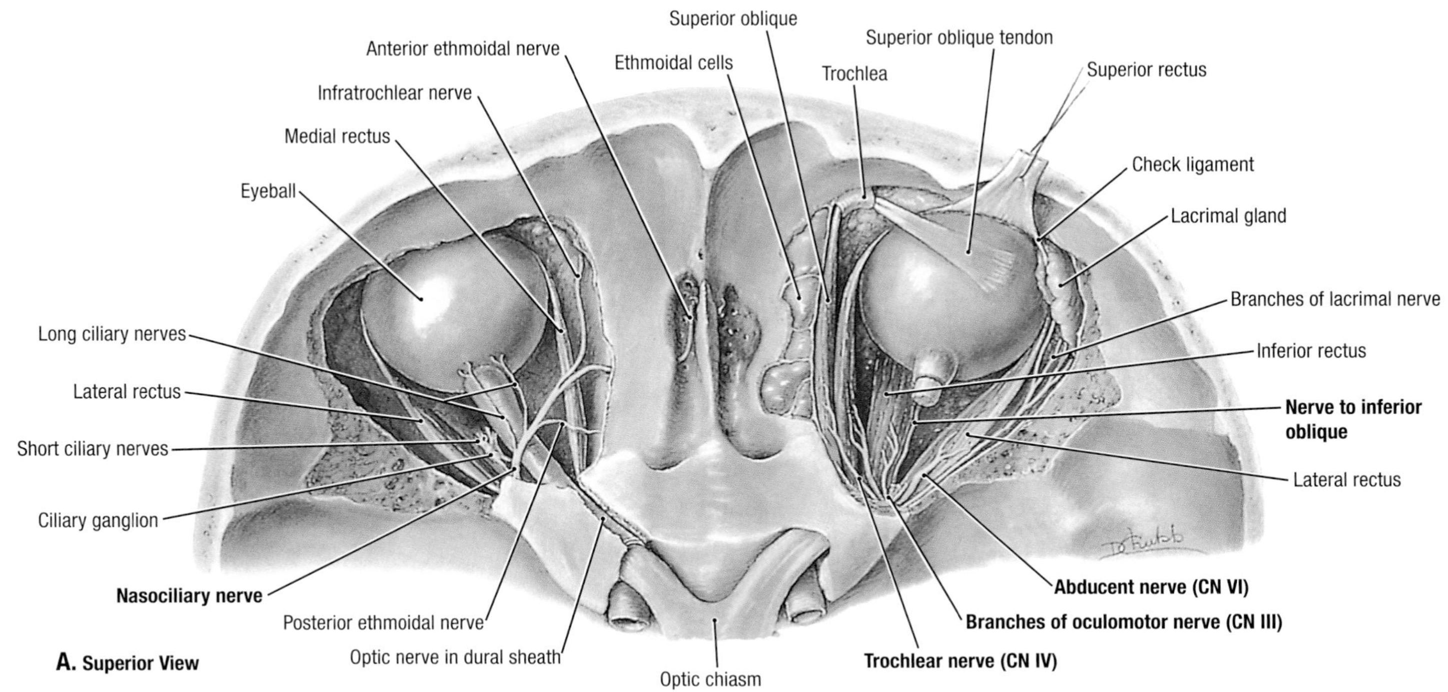

Superior oblique
Anterior ethmoidal nerve
Ethmoidal cells
Superior oblique tendon
Trochlea
Superior rectus
Infratrochlear nerve
Medial rectus
Check ligament
Eyeball
Lacrimal gland
Branches of lacrimal nerve
Long ciliary nerves
Inferior rectus
Lateral rectus
Nerve to inferior oblique
Short ciliary nerves
Lateral rectus
Ciliary ganglion
Abducent nerve (CN VI)
Nasociliary nerve
Posterior ethmoidal nerve
Branches of oculomotor nerve (CN III)
Optic nerve in dural sheath
Trochlear nerve (CN IV)
Optic chiasm
A. Superior View


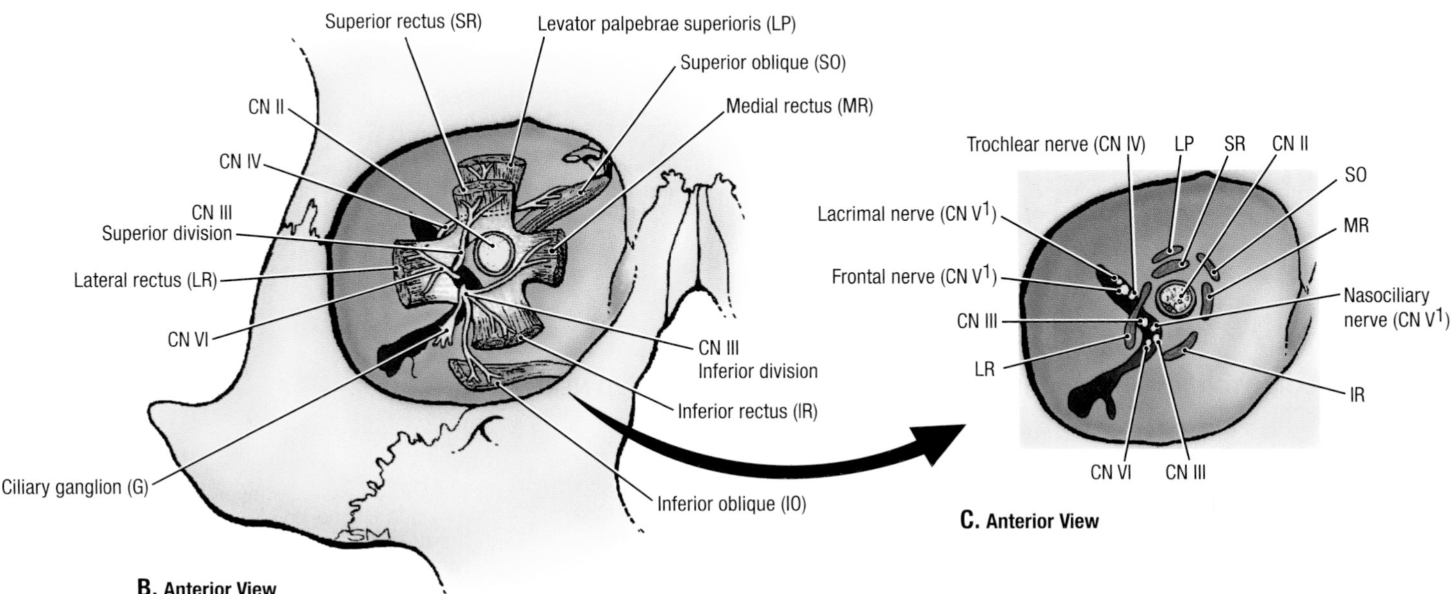

Superior rectus (SR)
Levator palpebrae superioris (LP)
Superior oblique (SO)
Medial rectus (MR)
CN II
CN IV
CN III
Superior division
Lateral rectus (LR)
CN VI
CN III
Inferior division
Inferior rectus (IR)
Ciliary ganglion (G)
Inferior oblique (IO)
B. Anterior View
Trochlear nerve (CN IV)
LP
SR
CN II
SO
Lacrimal nerve (CN V1)
MR
Frontal nerve (CN V1)
Nasociliary nerve (CN V1)
CN III
LR
IR
CN VI
CN III
C. Anterior View


## 9.5 Overview of muscles and nerves of orbit

**A.** Orbital cavities, dissected from a superior approach. **B.** Structures of apex of orbit. **C.** Relationship of muscle attachments and nerves at apex of orbit.

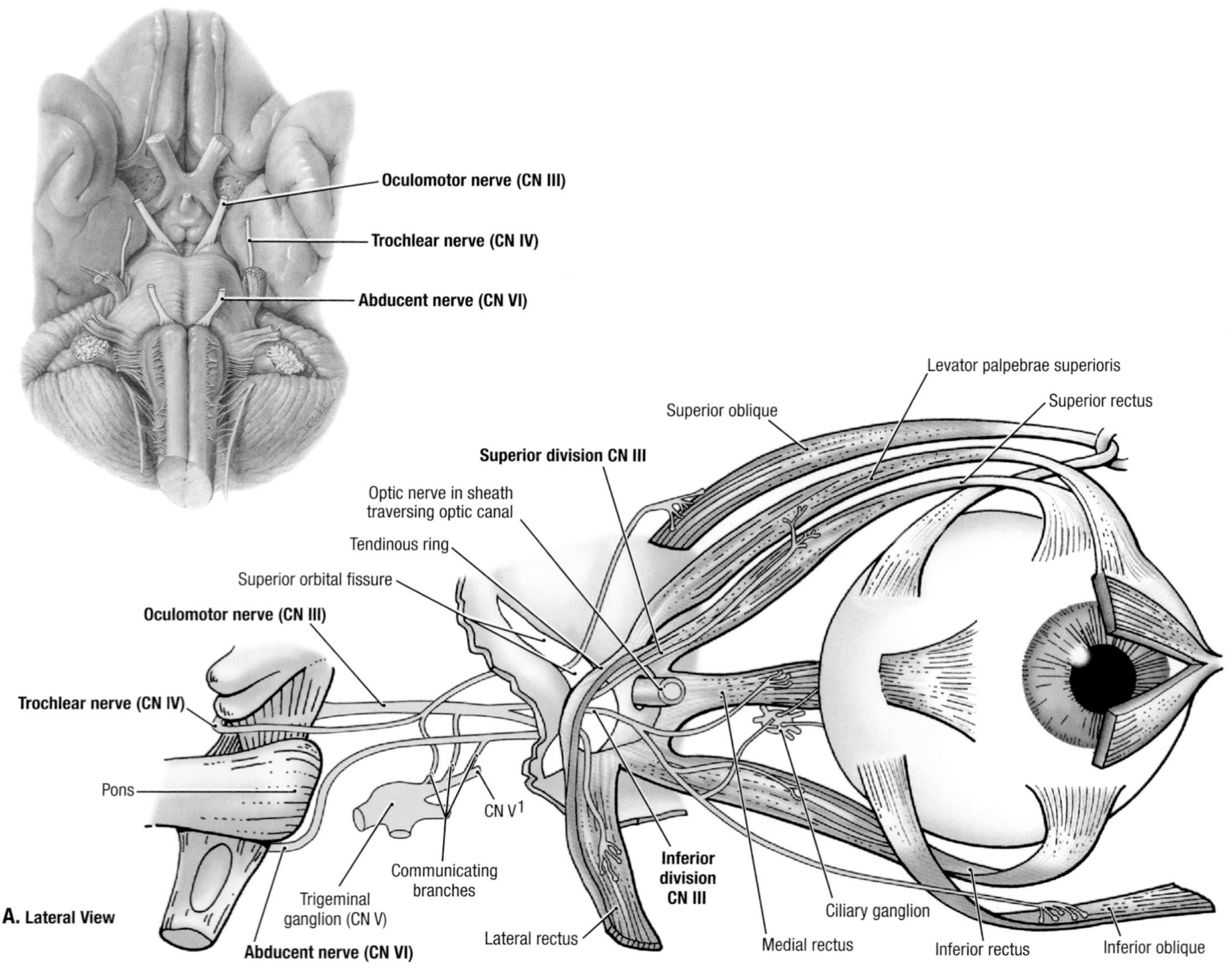
Oculomotor nerve (CN III)
Trochlear nerve (CN IV)
Abducent nerve (CN VI)
Levator palpebrae superioris
Superior rectus
Superior oblique
Superior division CN III
Optic nerve in sheath traversing optic canal
Tendinous ring
Superior orbital fissure
Oculomotor nerve (CN III)
Trochlear nerve (CN IV)
Pons
CN V1
Communicating branches
Trigeminal ganglion (CN V)
Abducent nerve (CN VI)
Lateral rectus
Inferior division CN III
Ciliary ganglion
Medial rectus
Inferior rectus
Inferior oblique

**A.** Lateral View

**TABLE 9.4 OCULOMOTOR (CN III), TROCHLEAR (CN IV), AND ABDUCENT (CN VI) NERVES[a]**

| Nerve | Functional Components | Cells of Origin/ Termination | Cranial Exit | Distribution and Functions |
|---|---|---|---|---|
| **Oculomotor** | Somatic motor | Oculomotor nucleus | Superior orbital fissure | Motor to superior, inferior, and medial recti, inferior oblique, and levator palpebrae superioris muscles; raises upper eyelid; rotates eyeball superiorly, inferiorly, and medially |
| | Visceral motor (parasympathetic) | Presynaptic: midbrain (Edinger-Westphal nucleus); Postsynaptic: ciliary ganglion | | Motor to sphincter pupillae and ciliary muscle that constrict pupil and accommodate lens of eyeball |
| **Trochlear** | Somatic motor | Trochlear nucleus | | Motor to superior oblique that assists in rotating eyeball inferolaterally |
| **Abducent** | Somatic motor | Abducent nucleus | | Motor to lateral rectus that rotates eyeball laterally |

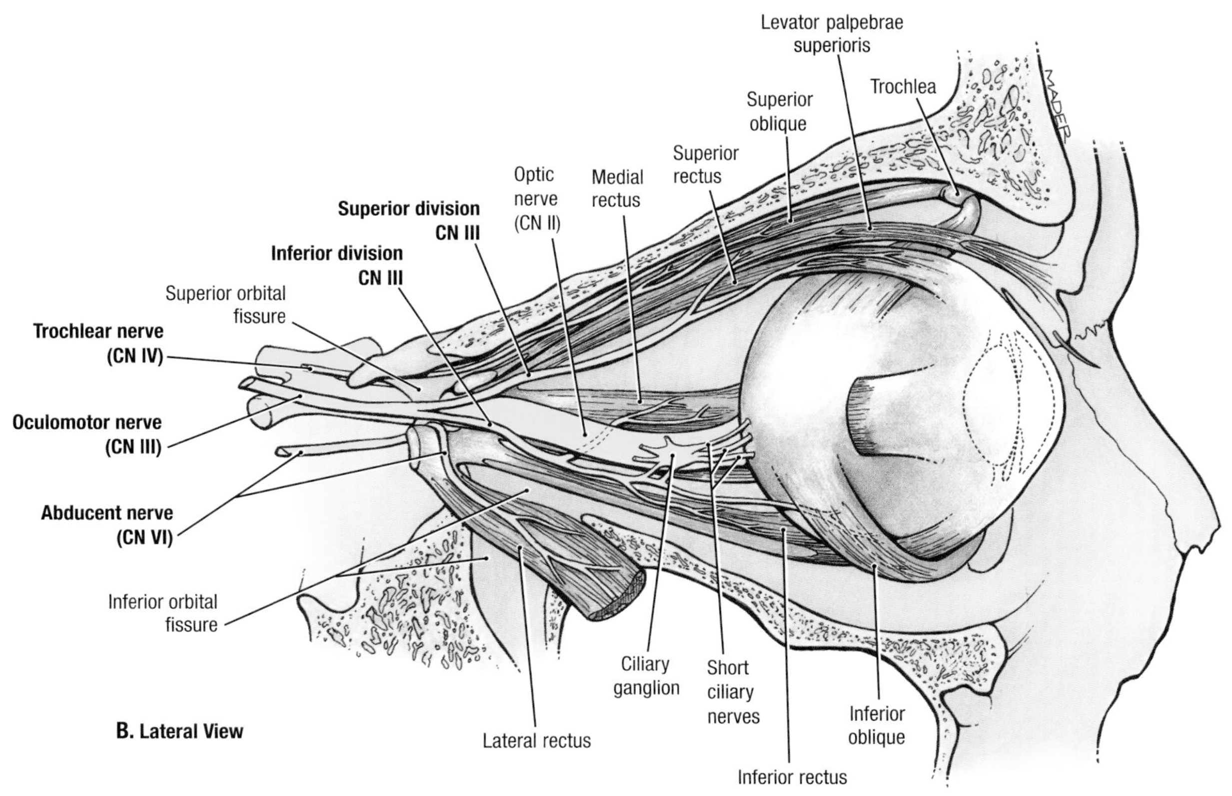
Levator palpebrae superioris
Trochlea
Superior oblique
Superior rectus
Medial rectus
Optic nerve (CN II)
Superior division CN III
Inferior division CN III
Superior orbital fissure
Trochlear nerve (CN IV)
Oculomotor nerve (CN III)
Abducent nerve (CN VI)
Inferior orbital fissure
Lateral rectus
Ciliary ganglion
Short ciliary nerves
Inferior rectus
Inferior oblique
MADER

**B. Lateral View**

CN II contains parasympathetic fibers originating from nerve cell bodies of the accessory (Edinger-Westphal) nucleus of the oculomotor nerve

Fibers synapse in the ciliary ganglion, consisting of post-synaptic parasympathetic nerve cell bodies associated with CN $V^1$

Short ciliary nerves (CN $V^1$) carry post-synaptic parasympathetic fibers to the ciliary and constrictor pupillae muscles.

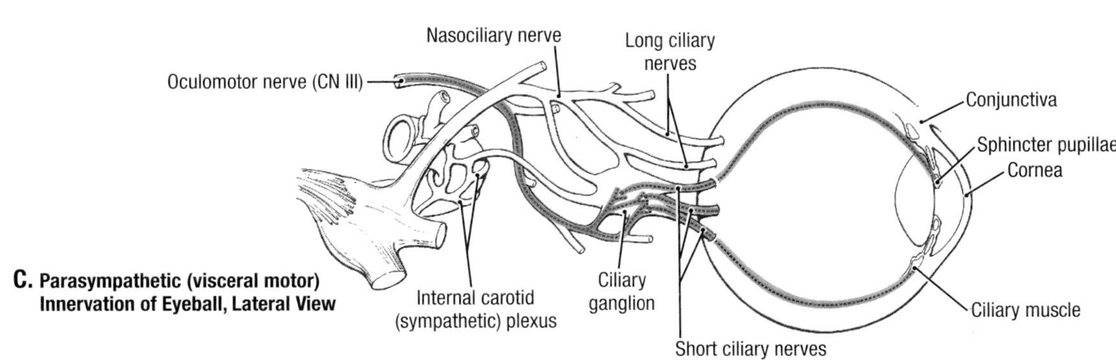
Oculomotor nerve (CN III)
Nasociliary nerve
Long ciliary nerves
Conjunctiva
Sphincter pupillae
Cornea
Internal carotid (sympathetic) plexus
Ciliary ganglion
Short ciliary nerves
Ciliary muscle

**C. Parasympathetic (visceral motor) Innervation of Eyeball, Lateral View**

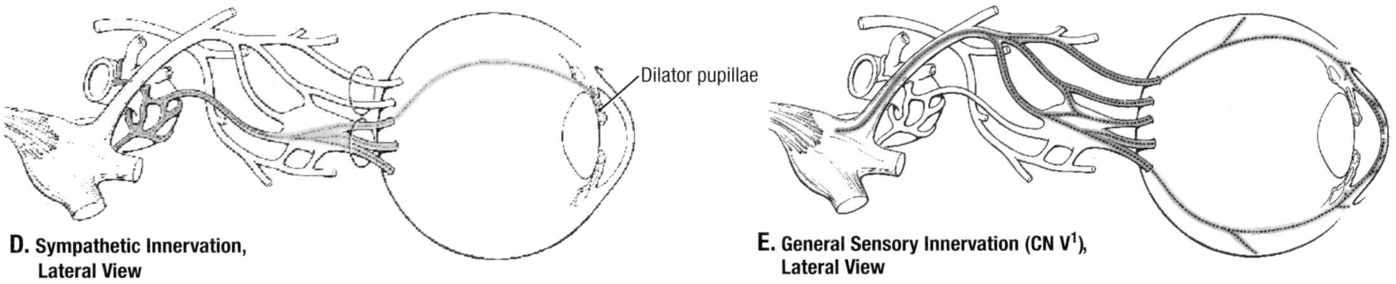
Dilator pupillae

**D. Sympathetic Innervation, Lateral View**

**E. General Sensory Innervation (CN $V^1$), Lateral View**

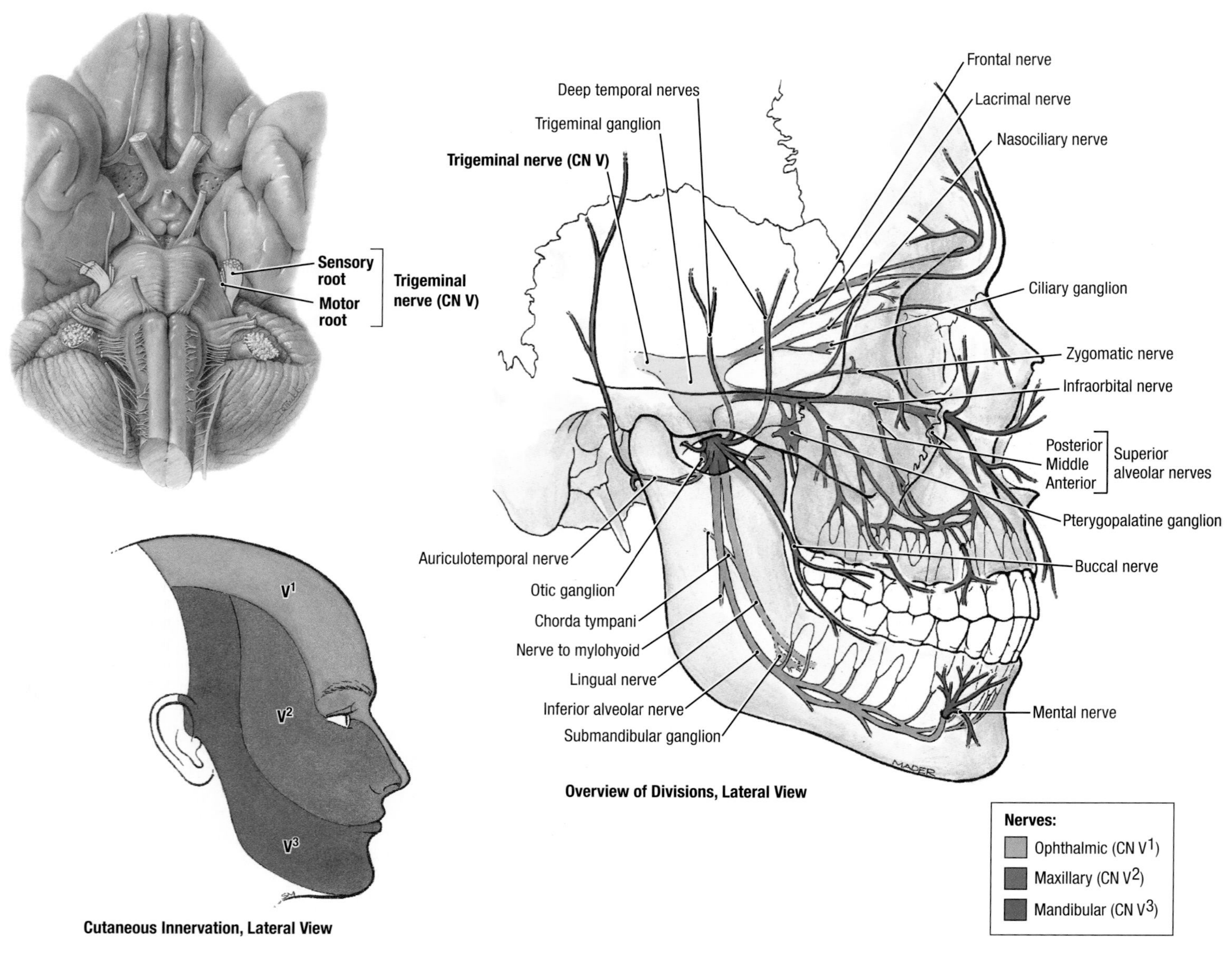
Sensory root
Motor root
Trigeminal nerve (CN V)
V1
V2
V3
Deep temporal nerves
Trigeminal ganglion
Trigeminal nerve (CN V)
Frontal nerve
Lacrimal nerve
Nasociliary nerve
Ciliary ganglion
Zygomatic nerve
Infraorbital nerve
Posterior
Middle
Anterior
Superior alveolar nerves
Pterygopalatine ganglion
Buccal nerve
Mental nerve
Auriculotemporal nerve
Otic ganglion
Chorda tympani
Nerve to mylohyoid
Lingual nerve
Inferior alveolar nerve
Submandibular ganglion
Nerves:
Ophthalmic (CN V1)
Maxillary (CN V2)
Mandibular (CN V3)

Cutaneous Innervation, Lateral View

Overview of Divisions, Lateral View

**TABLE 9.5 TRIGEMINAL NERVE (CN V)**

| Nerve | Functional Components | Cells of Origin/ Termination | Cranial Exit | Distribution and Functions |
|---|---|---|---|---|
| **Ophthalmic division (CN V¹)** | General sensory | Trigeminal ganglion/spinal, principal and mesencephalic nucleus of CN V | Superior orbital fissure | Sensation from cornea, skin of forehead, scalp, eyelids, nose, and mucosa of nasal cavity and paranasal sinuses |
| **Maxillary division (CN V²)** | | | Foramen rotundum | Sensation from skin of face over maxilla including upper lip, maxillary teeth, mucosa of nose, maxillary sinuses, and palate |
| **Mandibular division (CN V³)** | | | Foramen ovale | Sensation from the skin over mandible, including lower lip and side of head, mandibular teeth, temporomandibular joint, and mucosa of mouth and anterior two thirds of tongue |
| | Branchial motor | Trigeminal motor nucleus | | Motor to muscles of mastication, mylohyoid, anterior belly of digastric, tensor veli palatini, and tensor tympani |

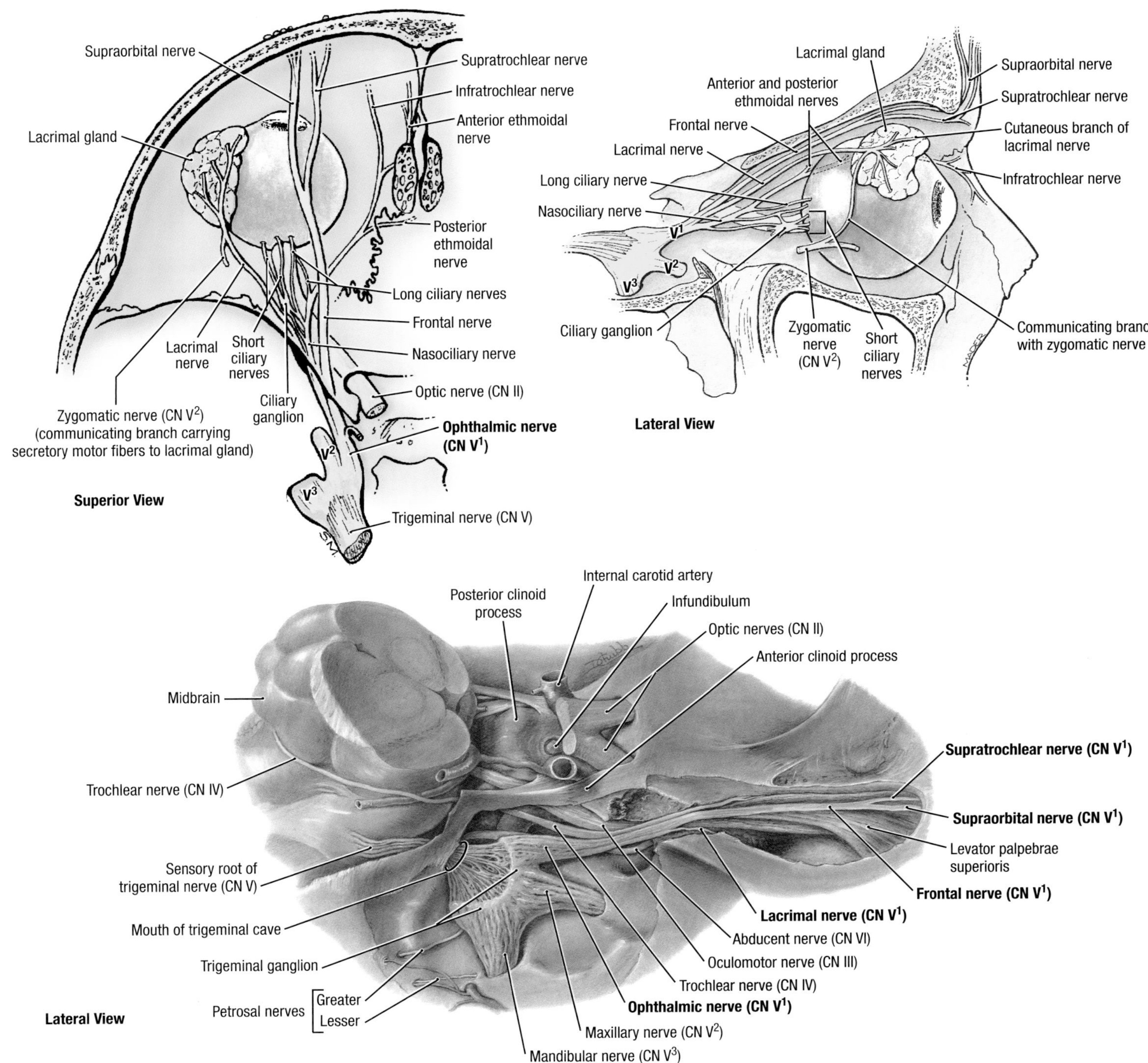
Supraorbital nerve
Supratrochlear nerve
Infratrochlear nerve
Anterior ethmoidal nerve
Lacrimal gland
Posterior ethmoidal nerve
Long ciliary nerves
Frontal nerve
Nasociliary nerve
Lacrimal nerve
Short ciliary nerves
Optic nerve (CN II)
Ciliary ganglion
Zygomatic nerve (CN V2) (communicating branch carrying secretory motor fibers to lacrimal gland)
Ophthalmic nerve (CN V1)
V2
V3
Superior View
Trigeminal nerve (CN V)
Lacrimal gland
Anterior and posterior ethmoidal nerves
Frontal nerve
Lacrimal nerve
Long ciliary nerve
Nasociliary nerve
V1
V2
V3
Supraorbital nerve
Supratrochlear nerve
Cutaneous branch of lacrimal nerve
Infratrochlear nerve
Ciliary ganglion
Zygomatic nerve (CN V2)
Short ciliary nerves
Communicating branch with zygomatic nerve
Lateral View
Internal carotid artery
Posterior clinoid process
Infundibulum
Optic nerves (CN II)
Anterior clinoid process
Midbrain
Supratrochlear nerve (CN V1)
Trochlear nerve (CN IV)
Supraorbital nerve (CN V1)
Levator palpebrae superioris
Sensory root of trigeminal nerve (CN V)
Frontal nerve (CN V1)
Lacrimal nerve (CN V1)
Mouth of trigeminal cave
Abducent nerve (CN VI)
Trigeminal ganglion
Oculomotor nerve (CN III)
Trochlear nerve (CN IV)
Greater
Petrosal nerves
Lesser
Ophthalmic nerve (CN V1)
Lateral View
Maxillary nerve (CN V2)
Mandibular nerve (CN V3)

## TABLE 9.6 BRANCHES OF OPHTHALMIC NERVE (CN $V^1$)

| Function | Branches |
|---|---|
| The ophthalmic nerve is a sensory nerve passing through the superior orbital fissure that supplies the eyeball and conjunctiva, lacrimal gland and sac, nasal mucosa, frontal sinus, external nose, upper eyelid, forehead, scalp, and central dura mater of anterior cranial fossa | Lacrimal nerve<br>Frontal nerve<br>  Supraorbital nerve<br>  Supratrochlear nerve<br>Nasociliary nerve<br>  Short ciliary nerves<br>  Long ciliary nerves<br>  Infratrochlear nerve<br>  Anterior and posterior ethmoidal nerves |

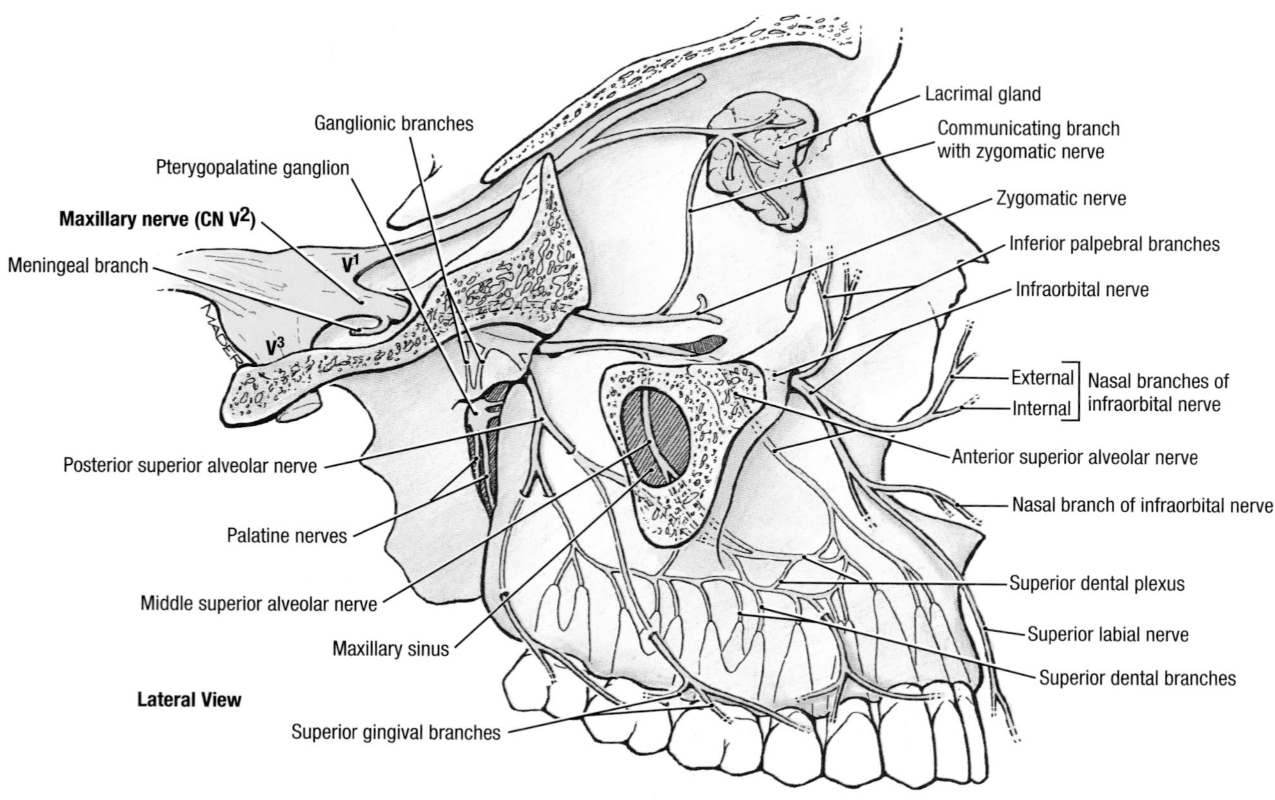
Ganglionic branches
Pterygopalatine ganglion
Maxillary nerve (CN V2)
Meningeal branch
V1
V3
Posterior superior alveolar nerve
Palatine nerves
Middle superior alveolar nerve
Maxillary sinus
Lateral View
Superior gingival branches
Lacrimal gland
Communicating branch with zygomatic nerve
Zygomatic nerve
Inferior palpebral branches
Infraorbital nerve
External
Internal
Nasal branches of infraorbital nerve
Anterior superior alveolar nerve
Nasal branch of infraorbital nerve
Superior dental plexus
Superior labial nerve
Superior dental branches

## TABLE 9.7 BRANCHES OF MAXILLARY NERVE (CN $V^2$)

| Function | Branches |
| --- | --- |
| The maxillary nerve is a sensory nerve passing through the foramen rotundum that supplies sensation to the face, upper teeth and gums, mucous membrane of the nasal cavity, palate and roof of the pharynx, maxillary, ethmoidal, and sphenoidal sinuses, and secretory fibers from the pterygopalatine ganglion, which pass with the zygomatic and lacrimal nerves to the lacrimal gland | Meningeal branch<br>Zygomatic nerve<br>  Zygomaticofacial nerve<br>  Zygomaticotemporal nerve<br>Posterior superior alveolar nerves<br>Infraorbital nerve<br>  Anterior and middle superior alveolar nerves<br>  Superior labial branches<br>  Inferior palpebral branches<br>  External and internal nasal branches<br>Greater palatine nerve<br>  Posterior inferior lateral nasal branches<br>Lesser palatine nerve<br>  Posterior superior lateral nasal branches<br>Nasopalatine nerve<br>Pharyngeal nerve |

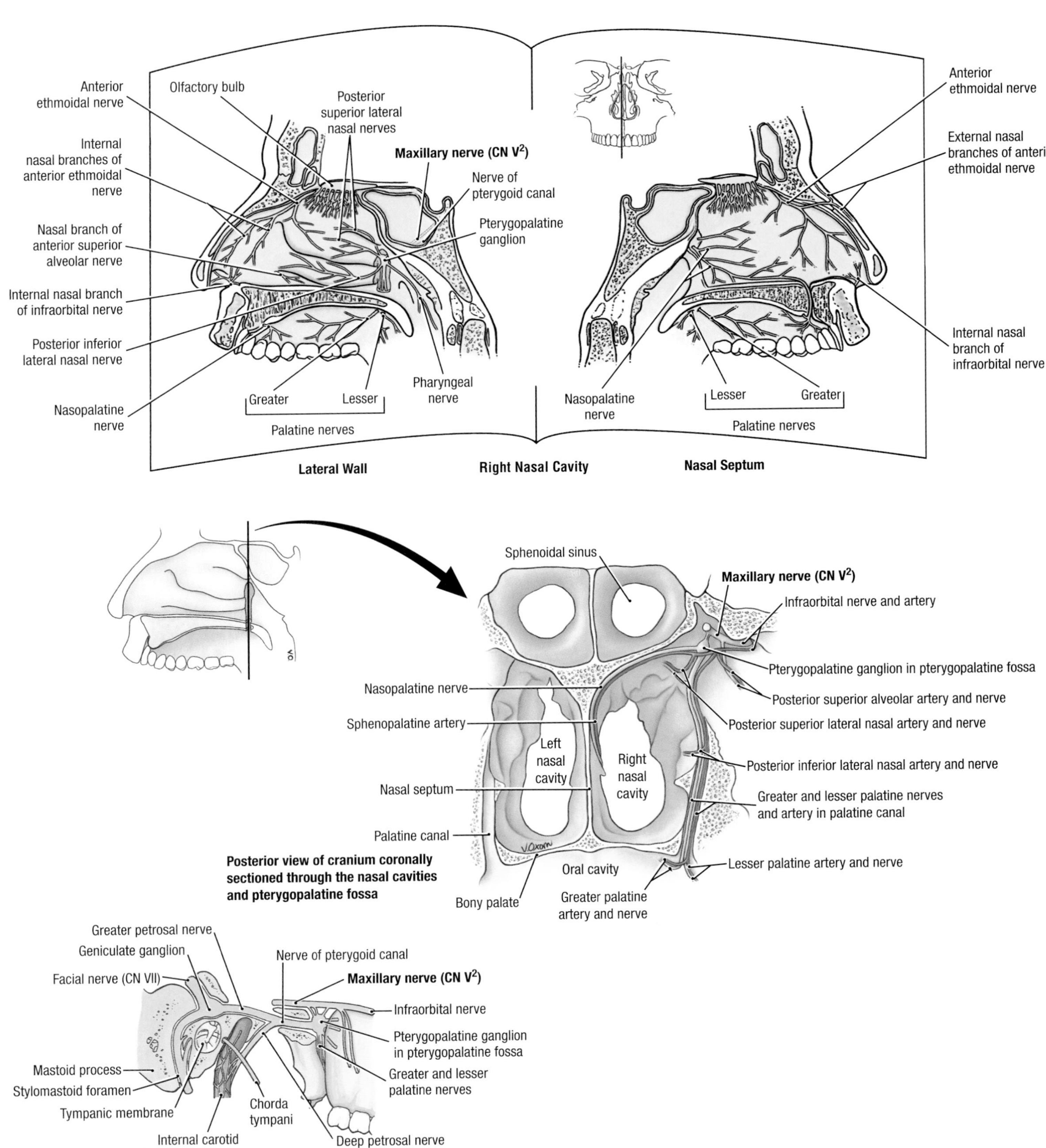
Anterior ethmoidal nerve
Olfactory bulb
Posterior superior lateral nasal nerves
Internal nasal branches of anterior ethmoidal nerve
Maxillary nerve (CN V²)
Nerve of pterygoid canal
Pterygopalatine ganglion
Nasal branch of anterior superior alveolar nerve
Internal nasal branch of infraorbital nerve
Posterior inferior lateral nasal nerve
Nasopalatine nerve
Greater
Lesser
Palatine nerves
Pharyngeal nerve
Lateral Wall
Right Nasal Cavity
Nasal Septum
Anterior ethmoidal nerve
External nasal branches of anterior ethmoidal nerve
Internal nasal branch of infraorbital nerve
Nasopalatine nerve
Lesser
Greater
Palatine nerves
Sphenoidal sinus
Maxillary nerve (CN V²)
Infraorbital nerve and artery
Pterygopalatine ganglion in pterygopalatine fossa
Nasopalatine nerve
Posterior superior alveolar artery and nerve
Sphenopalatine artery
Posterior superior lateral nasal artery and nerve
Left nasal cavity
Right nasal cavity
Posterior inferior lateral nasal artery and nerve
Nasal septum
Greater and lesser palatine nerves and artery in palatine canal
Palatine canal
Oral cavity
Lesser palatine artery and nerve
Bony palate
Greater palatine artery and nerve
Greater petrosal nerve
Geniculate ganglion
Nerve of pterygoid canal
Facial nerve (CN VII)
Maxillary nerve (CN V²)
Infraorbital nerve
Pterygopalatine ganglion in pterygopalatine fossa
Mastoid process
Greater and lesser palatine nerves
Stylomastoid foramen
Tympanic membrane
Chorda tympani
Internal carotid (sympathetic) plexus
Deep petrosal nerve
Lateral View

**Posterior view of cranium coronally sectioned through the nasal cavities and pterygopalatine fossa**

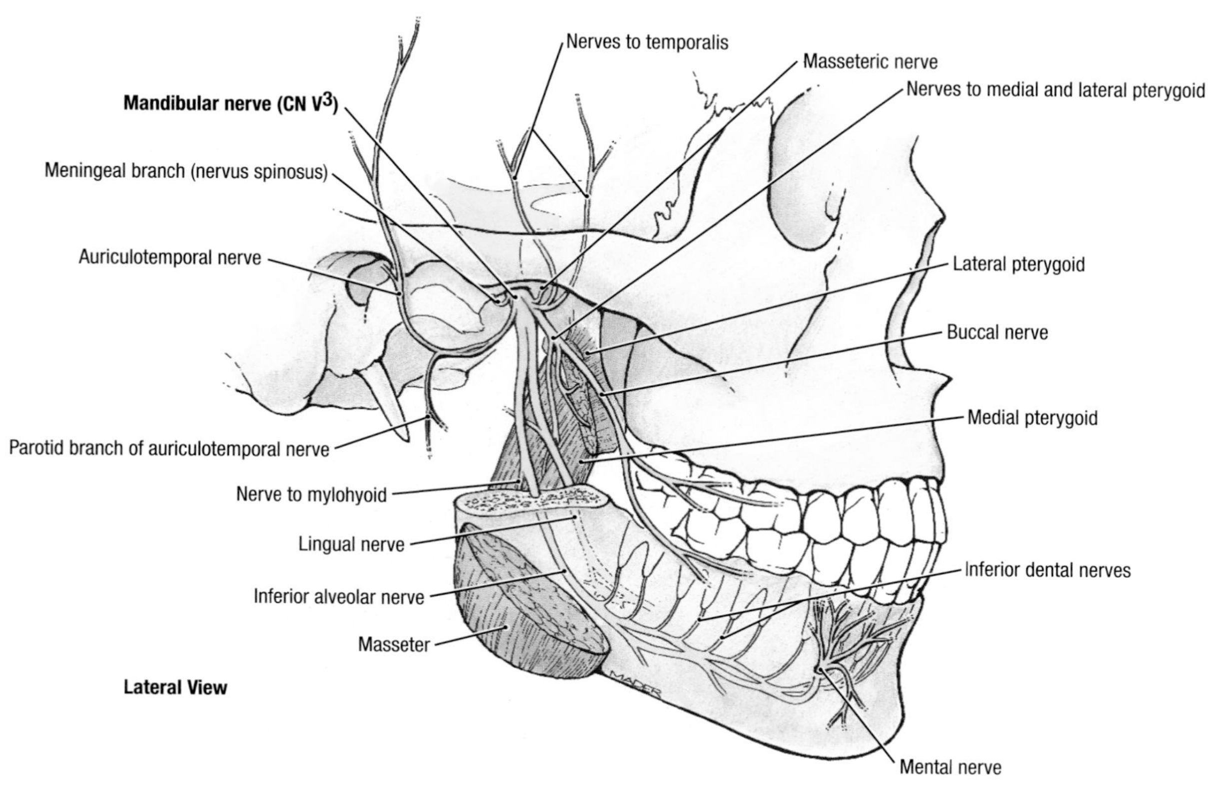
Nerves to temporalis
Masseteric nerve
Nerves to medial and lateral pterygoid
Mandibular nerve (CN V3)
Meningeal branch (nervus spinosus)
Auriculotemporal nerve
Lateral pterygoid
Buccal nerve
Medial pterygoid
Parotid branch of auriculotemporal nerve
Nerve to mylohyoid
Lingual nerve
Inferior alveolar nerve
Inferior dental nerves
Masseter
Lateral View
Mental nerve

## TABLE 9.8 BRANCHES OF MANDIBULAR NERVE (CN $V^3$)

| Function | Branches |
|---|---|
| The mandibular nerve is a sensory and motor nerve passing through the foramen ovale. General sensory branches supply the lower teeth, gums, lip, auricle, external acoustic meatus, outer surface of tympanic membrane, cheek, anterior two thirds of tongue, and floor of mouth. CN $V^3$ also conveys secretory fibers from the otic ganglion to the parotid gland. Taste from the anterior two thirds of the tongue and presynaptic secretomotor fibers to the submandibular ganglion are conveyed to the nerve by the chorda tympani. Postsynaptic fibers from the submandibular ganglion pass to the submandibular and sublingual glands | Meningeal branch<br>Buccal nerve<br>Auriculotemporal nerve<br>  Inferior alveolar nerve<br>  Inferior dental nerves<br>  Mental nerve<br>  Incisive nerve<br>Lingual nerve |
| Motor branches supply the muscles of mastication and other muscles derived from the first branchial arches | Masseter<br>Temporalis<br>Medial and lateral pterygoids<br>Tensor veli palatini<br>Mylohyoid<br>Anterior belly of digastric<br>Tensor tympani |

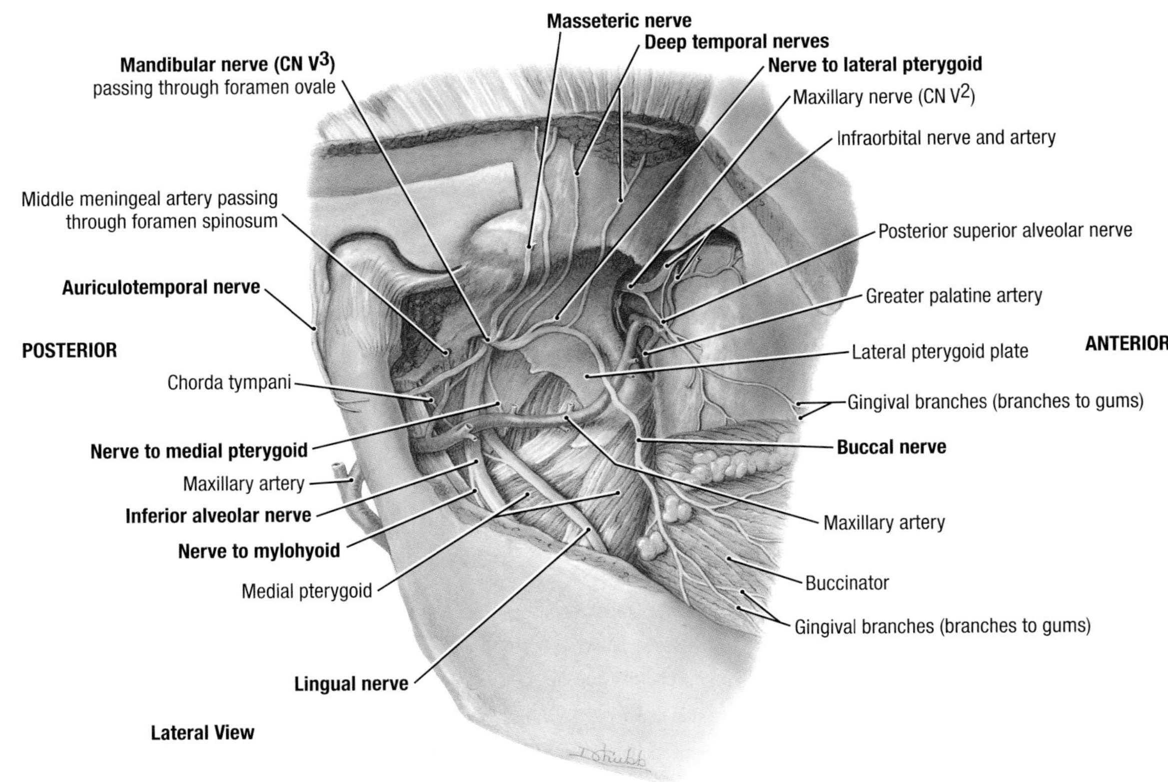
Masseteric nerve
Deep temporal nerves
Nerve to lateral pterygoid
Mandibular nerve (CN V3)
passing through foramen ovale
Maxillary nerve (CN V2)
Infraorbital nerve and artery
Middle meningeal artery passing
through foramen spinosum
Posterior superior alveolar nerve
Auriculotemporal nerve
Greater palatine artery
POSTERIOR
Lateral pterygoid plate
ANTERIOR
Chorda tympani
Gingival branches (branches to gums)
Nerve to medial pterygoid
Buccal nerve
Maxillary artery
Inferior alveolar nerve
Maxillary artery
Nerve to mylohyoid
Buccinator
Medial pterygoid
Gingival branches (branches to gums)
Lingual nerve
Lateral View

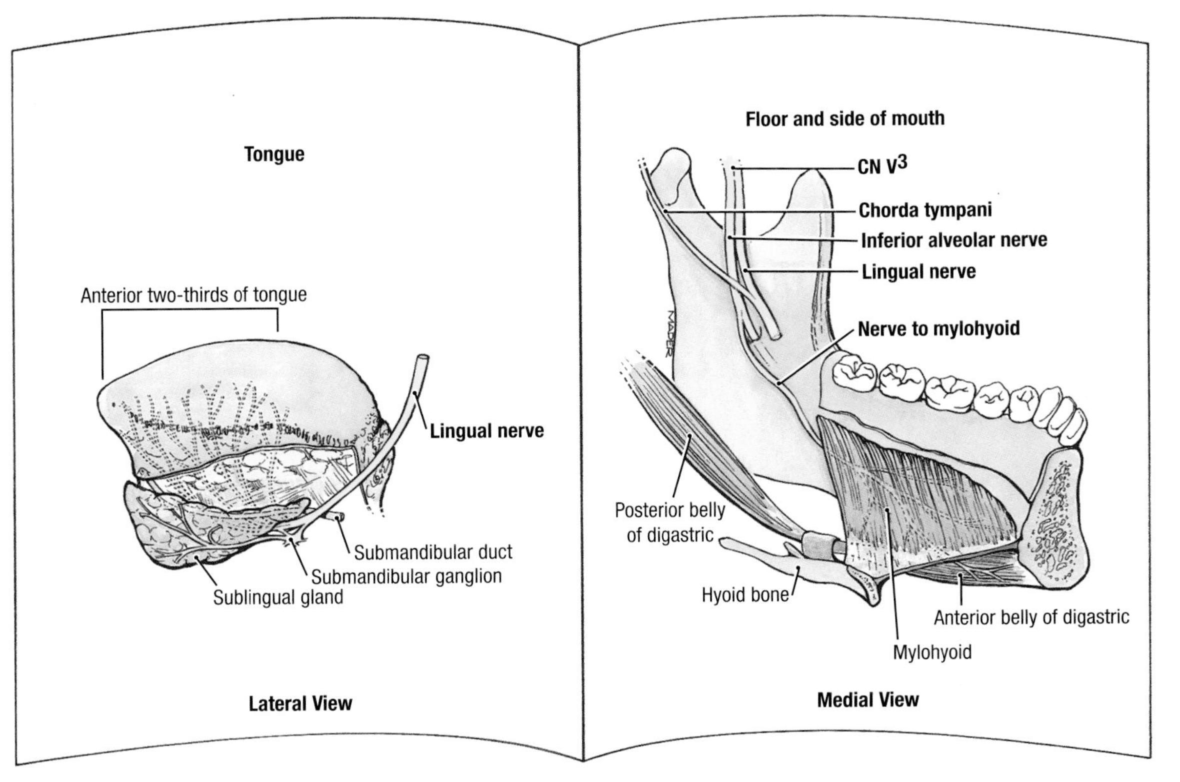
Tongue
Anterior two-thirds of tongue
Lingual nerve
Submandibular duct
Submandibular ganglion
Sublingual gland
Lateral View
Floor and side of mouth
CN V3
Chorda tympani
Inferior alveolar nerve
Lingual nerve
Nerve to mylohyoid
Posterior belly
of digastric
Hyoid bone
Anterior belly of digastric
Mylohyoid
Medial View

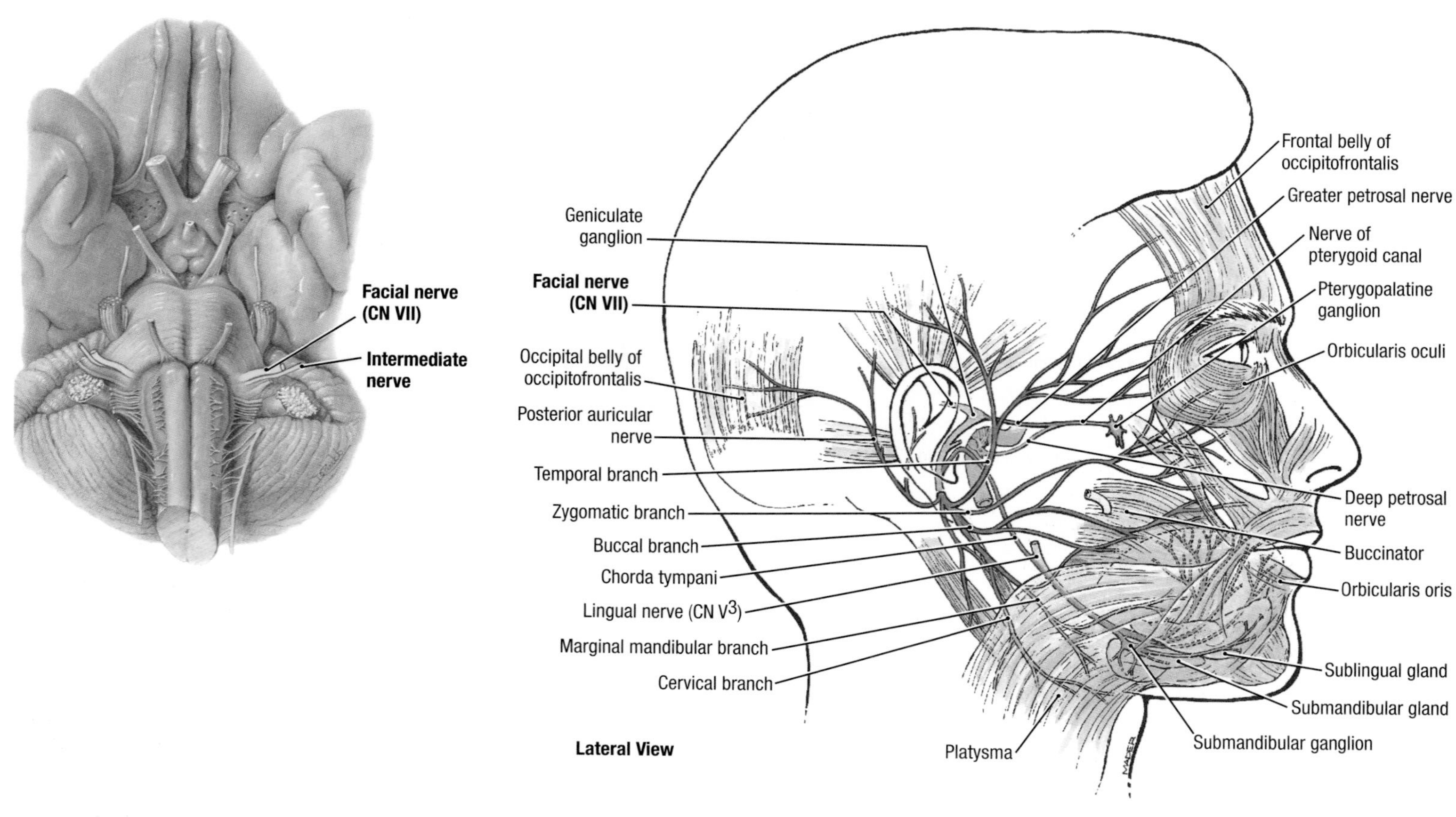
Facial nerve
(CN VII)
Intermediate
nerve
Geniculate
ganglion
Facial nerve
(CN VII)
Occipital belly of
occipitofrontalis
Posterior auricular
nerve
Temporal branch
Zygomatic branch
Buccal branch
Chorda tympani
Lingual nerve (CN V3)
Marginal mandibular branch
Cervical branch
Lateral View
Platysma
Frontal belly of
occipitofrontalis
Greater petrosal nerve
Nerve of
pterygoid canal
Pterygopalatine
ganglion
Orbicularis oculi
Deep petrosal
nerve
Buccinator
Orbicularis oris
Sublingual gland
Submandibular gland
Submandibular ganglion

### TABLE 9.9 FACIAL NERVE (CN VII), INCLUDING MOTOR ROOT AND INTERMEDIATE NERVE[a]

| Nerve | Functional Components | Cells of Origin/ Termination | Cranial Exit | Distribution and Functions |
|---|---|---|---|---|
| Temporal, zygomatic, buccal, mandibular, cervical, and posterior auricular nerves, nerve to posterior belly of digastric, nerve to stylohyoid, nerve to stapedius | Branchial motor | Facial motor nucleus | Stylomastoid foramen | Motor to muscles of facial expression and scalp; also supplies stapedius of middle ear, stylohyoid, and posterior belly of digastric |
| Intermediate nerve through chorda tympani | Special sensory | Geniculate ganglion/ solitary nucleus | Internal acoustic meatus/ facial canal/petro-tympanic fissure | Taste from anterior two thirds of tongue, floor of mouth, and palate |
| Intermediate nerve | General sensory | Geniculate ganglion/spinal trigeminal nucleus | Internal acoustic meatus | Sensation from skin of external acoustic meatus |
| Intermediate nerve through greater petrosal nerve | Visceral sensory | Solitary nucleus | Internal acoustic meatus/ facial canal/foramen for greater petrosal nerve | Visceral sensation from mucous membranes of nasopharynx and palate |
| Greater petrosal nerve Chorda tympani | Visceral motor (parasympathetic) | Presynaptic: superior salivatory nucleus; Postsynaptic: pterygopalatine ganglion (greater petrosal nerve) and submandibular ganglion (chorda tympani) | Internal acoustic meatus/ facial canal/foramen for greater petrosal nerve, (greater petrosal nerve) petrotympanic fissure (chorda tympani) | Secretomotor to lacrimal gland and glands of the nose and palate (greater petrosal nerve); sub-mandibular and sublingual salivary glands (chorda tympani) |

[a] See also Table 9.15.

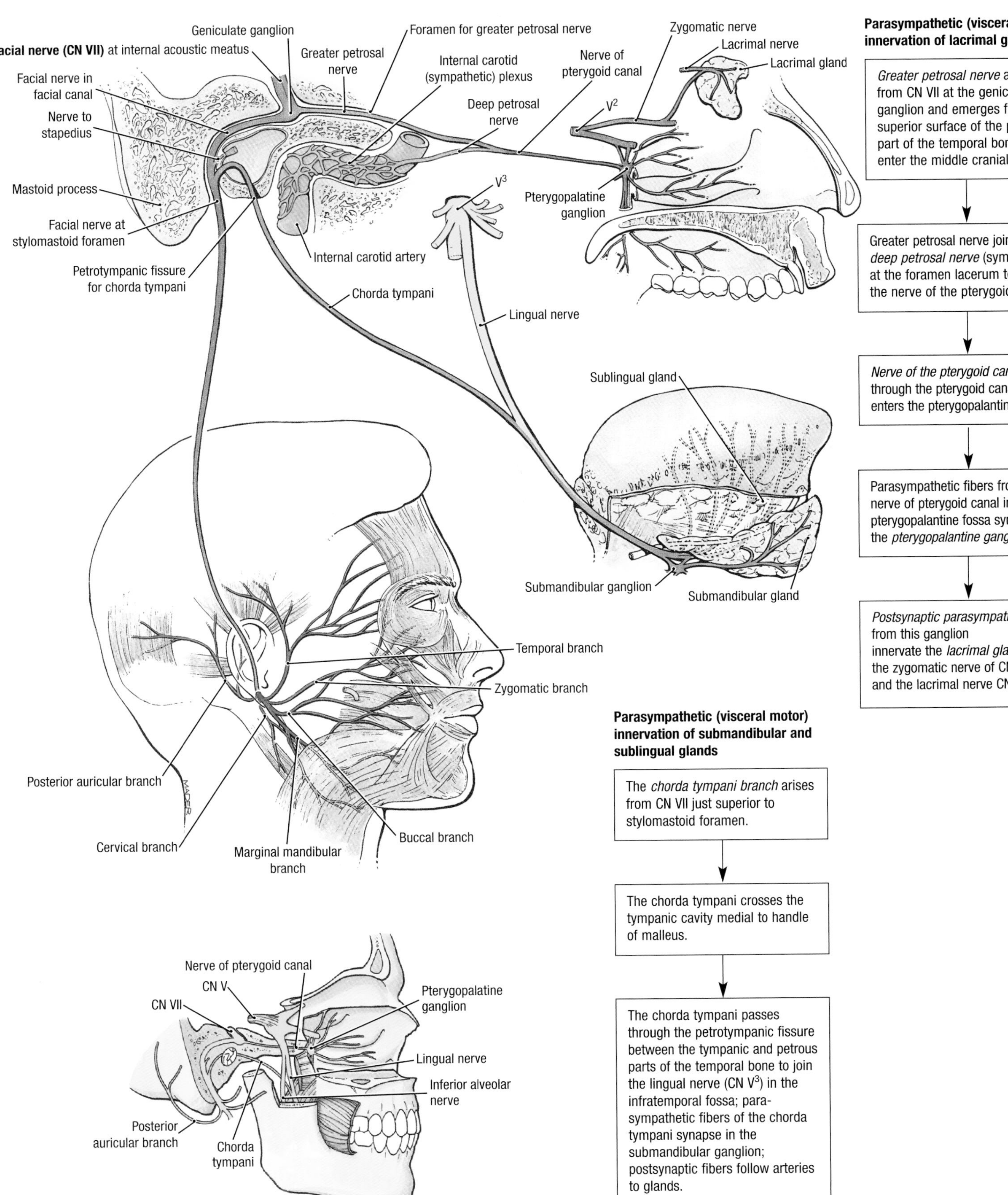
Geniculate ganglion
Foramen for greater petrosal nerve
Zygomatic nerve
Lacrimal nerve
Lacrimal gland
**Facial nerve (CN VII)** at internal acoustic meatus
Greater petrosal nerve
Internal carotid (sympathetic) plexus
Nerve of pterygoid canal
Facial nerve in facial canal
Deep petrosal nerve
V2
Nerve to stapedius
Mastoid process
V3
Pterygopalatine ganglion
Facial nerve at stylomastoid foramen
Internal carotid artery
Petrotympanic fissure for chorda tympani
Chorda tympani
Lingual nerve
Sublingual gland
Submandibular ganglion
Submandibular gland
Temporal branch
Zygomatic branch
Posterior auricular branch
Cervical branch
Marginal mandibular branch
Buccal branch
Nerve of pterygoid canal
CN V
CN VII
Pterygopalatine ganglion
Lingual nerve
Inferior alveolar nerve
Posterior auricular branch
Chorda tympani
**Parasympathetic (visceral motor) innervation of lacrimal gland**
*Greater petrosal nerve* arises from CN VII at the geniculate ganglion and emerges from the superior surface of the petrous part of the temporal bone to enter the middle cranial fossa.
Greater petrosal nerve joins the *deep petrosal nerve* (sympathetic) at the foramen lacerum to form the nerve of the pterygoid canal.
*Nerve of the pterygoid canal* travels through the pterygoid canal and enters the pterygopalantine fossa.
Parasympathetic fibers from the nerve of pterygoid canal in the pterygopalantine fossa synapse in the *pterygopalantine ganglion.*
*Postsynaptic parasympathetic* fibers from this ganglion innervate the *lacrimal gland* via the zygomatic nerve of CN V2 and the lacrimal nerve CN V1.
**Parasympathetic (visceral motor) innervation of submandibular and sublingual glands**
The *chorda tympani branch* arises from CN VII just superior to stylomastoid foramen.
The chorda tympani crosses the tympanic cavity medial to handle of malleus.
The chorda tympani passes through the petrotympanic fissure between the tympanic and petrous parts of the temporal bone to join the lingual nerve (CN V3) in the infratemporal fossa; parasympathetic fibers of the chorda tympani synapse in the submandibular ganglion; postsynaptic fibers follow arteries to glands.

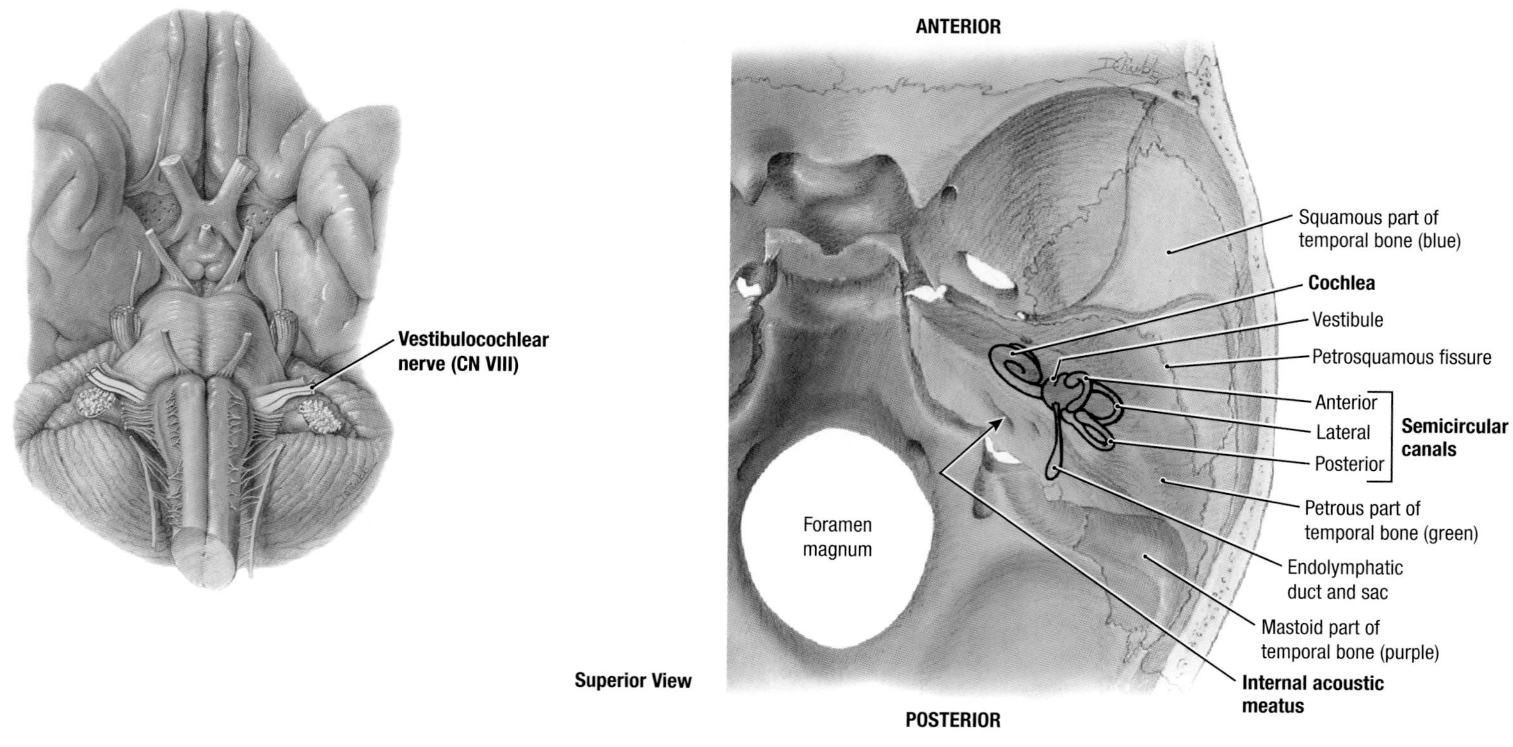
Vestibulocochlear nerve (CN VIII)
ANTERIOR
Squamous part of temporal bone (blue)
Cochlea
Vestibule
Petrosquamous fissure
Anterior
Lateral
Posterior
Semicircular canals
Petrous part of temporal bone (green)
Endolymphatic duct and sac
Mastoid part of temporal bone (purple)
Internal acoustic meatus
Foramen magnum
Superior View
POSTERIOR

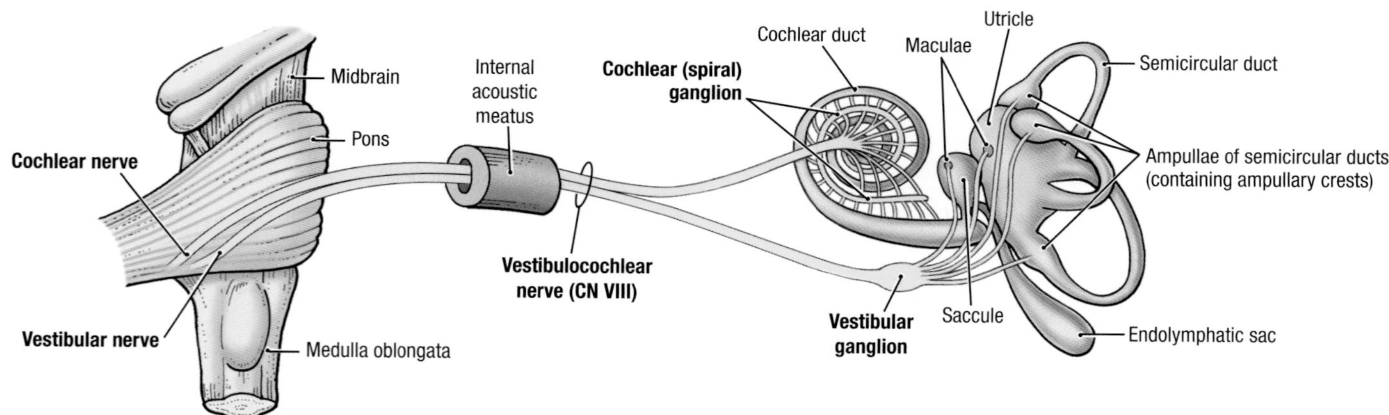
Midbrain
Pons
Cochlear nerve
Vestibular nerve
Medulla oblongata
Internal acoustic meatus
Cochlear (spiral) ganglion
Vestibulocochlear nerve (CN VIII)
Cochlear duct
Maculae
Utricle
Semicircular duct
Ampullae of semicircular ducts (containing ampullary crests)
Vestibular ganglion
Saccule
Endolymphatic sac

## TABLE 9.10 VESTIBULOCOCHLEAR NERVE (CN VIII)

| Part of Vestibuloccochlear Nerve | Functional Components | Cells of Origin/ Termination | Cranial Exit | Distribution and Functions |
|---|---|---|---|---|
| **Vestibular nerve** | Special sensory | Vestibular ganglion/ vestibular nuclei | Internal acoustic meatus | Vestibular sensation from semicircular ducts, utricle, and saccule related to position and movement of head |
| **Cochlear nerve** | Special sensory | Spiral ganglion/cochlear nuclei | Internal acoustic meatus | Hearing from spiral organ |

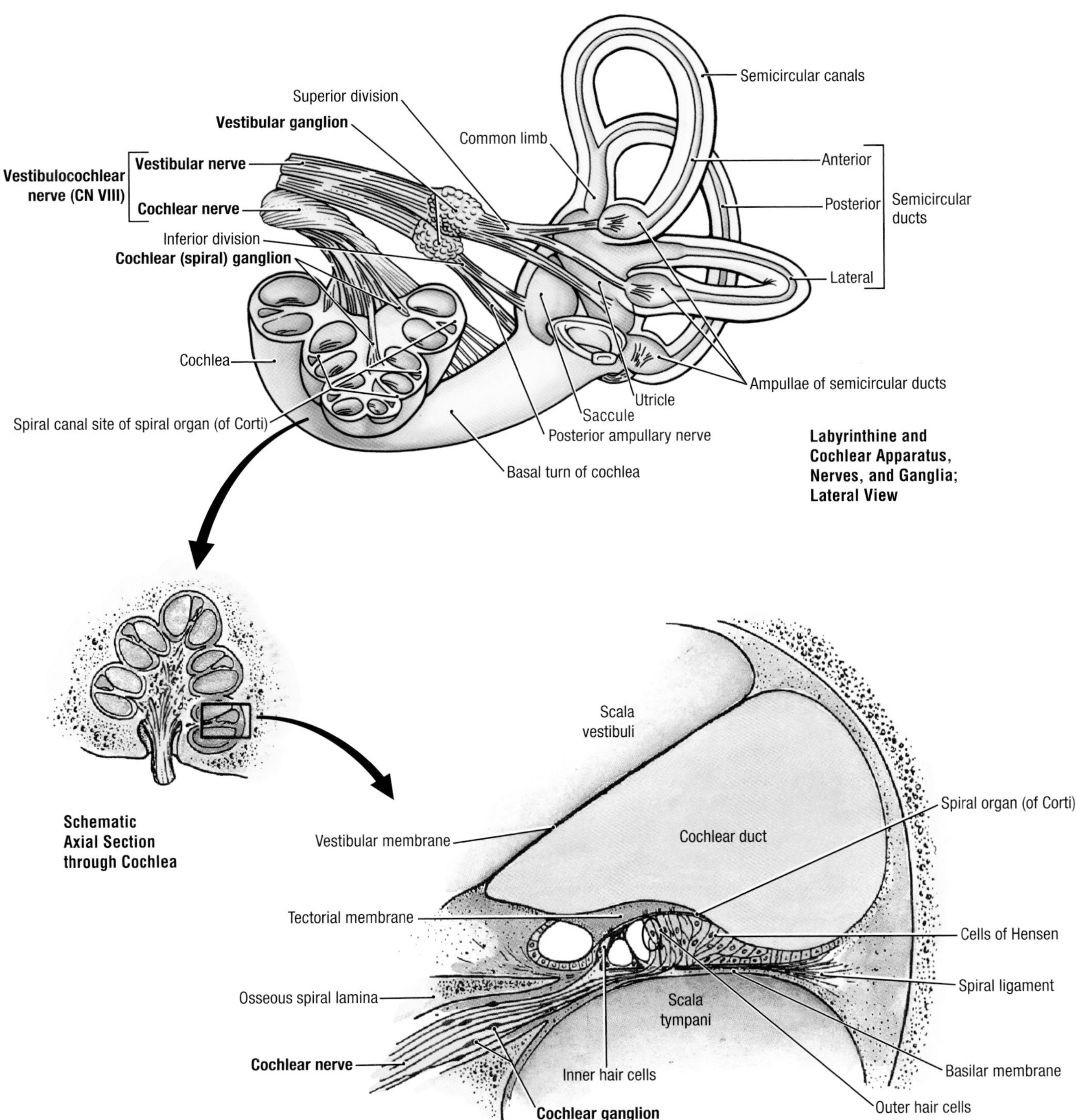
Semicircular canals
Superior division
Vestibular ganglion
Common limb
Vestibulocochlear nerve (CN VIII)
Vestibular nerve
Cochlear nerve
Anterior
Posterior
Lateral
Semicircular ducts
Inferior division
Cochlear (spiral) ganglion
Cochlea
Ampullae of semicircular ducts
Utricle
Saccule
Spiral canal site of spiral organ (of Corti)
Posterior ampullary nerve
Basal turn of cochlea
Labyrinthine and Cochlear Apparatus, Nerves, and Ganglia; Lateral View
Scala vestibuli
Spiral organ (of Corti)
Schematic Axial Section through Cochlea
Vestibular membrane
Cochlear duct
Tectorial membrane
Cells of Hensen
Spiral ligament
Osseous spiral lamina
Scala tympani
Cochlear nerve
Basilar membrane
Inner hair cells
Cochlear ganglion
Outer hair cells

Observe in the lower diagram:

- The cochlear duct is a spiral tube fixed to the internal and external walls of the cochlear canal by the spiral ligament.
- The triangular cochlear duct lies between the osseous spiral lamina and the external wall of the cochlear canal.
- The roof of the cochlear duct is formed by the vestibular membrane and the floor by the basilar membrane and osseous spiral lamina.
- The receptor of auditory stimuli is the spiral organ (of Corti), situated on the basilar membrane; it is overlaid by the gelatinous tectorial membrane.
- The spiral organ contains hair cells that respond to vibrations induced in the endolymph by sound waves.
- The fibers of the cochlear nerve are axons of neurons in the spiral ganglion; the peripheral processes enter the spiral organ (of Corti).

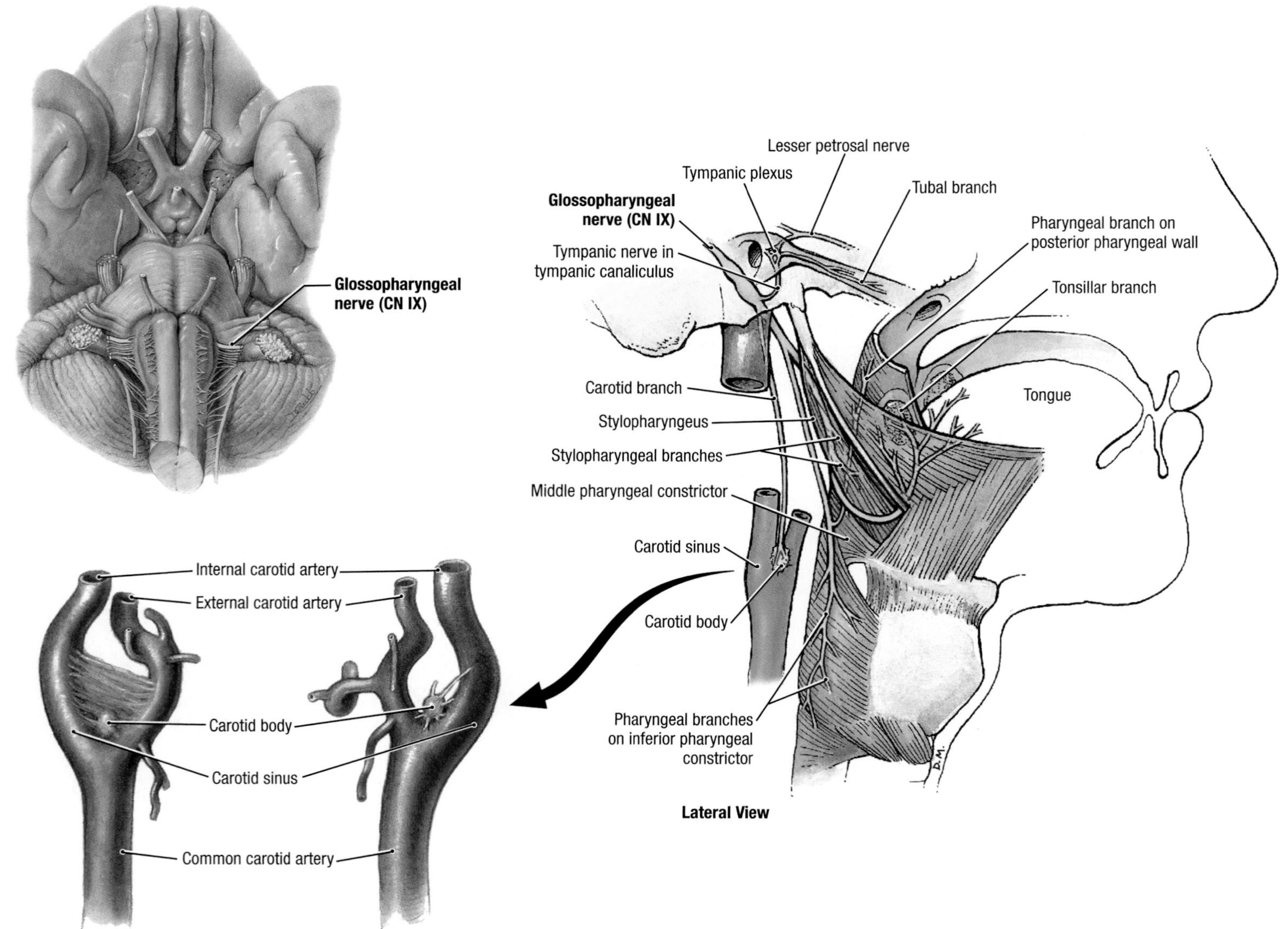
Glossopharyngeal nerve (CN IX)
Lesser petrosal nerve
Tympanic plexus
Tubal branch
Glossopharyngeal nerve (CN IX)
Pharyngeal branch on posterior pharyngeal wall
Tympanic nerve in tympanic canaliculus
Tonsillar branch
Tongue
Carotid branch
Stylopharyngeus
Stylopharyngeal branches
Middle pharyngeal constrictor
Carotid sinus
Carotid body
Pharyngeal branches on inferior pharyngeal constrictor
Lateral View
Internal carotid artery
External carotid artery
Carotid body
Carotid sinus
Common carotid artery
Posterior View

**TABLE 9.11 GLOSSOPHARYNGEAL NERVE (CN IX)[a]**

| Nerve Functions | Functional Components | Cells of Origin/ Termination | Cranial Exit | Distribution and Functions |
|---|---|---|---|---|
| **Glossopharyngeal** | Branchial motor | Nucleus ambiguus | Jugular foramen | Motor to stylopharyngeus that assists with swallowing |
| | Visceral motor (parasympathetic) | Presynaptic: inferior salivatory nucleus; postsynaptic: otic ganglion | | Secretomotor to parotid gland |
| | Visceral sensory | Solitary nucleus, spinal trigeminal nucleus/ inferior ganglion | | Visceral sensation from parotid gland, carotid body, carotid sinus, pharynx, and middle ear |
| | Special sensory | Solitary nucleus/inferior ganglion | | Taste from posterior third of tongue |
| | General sensory | Spinal trigeminal nucleus/ superior ganglion | | Cutaneous sensation from external ear |

[a] See also Table 9.15.

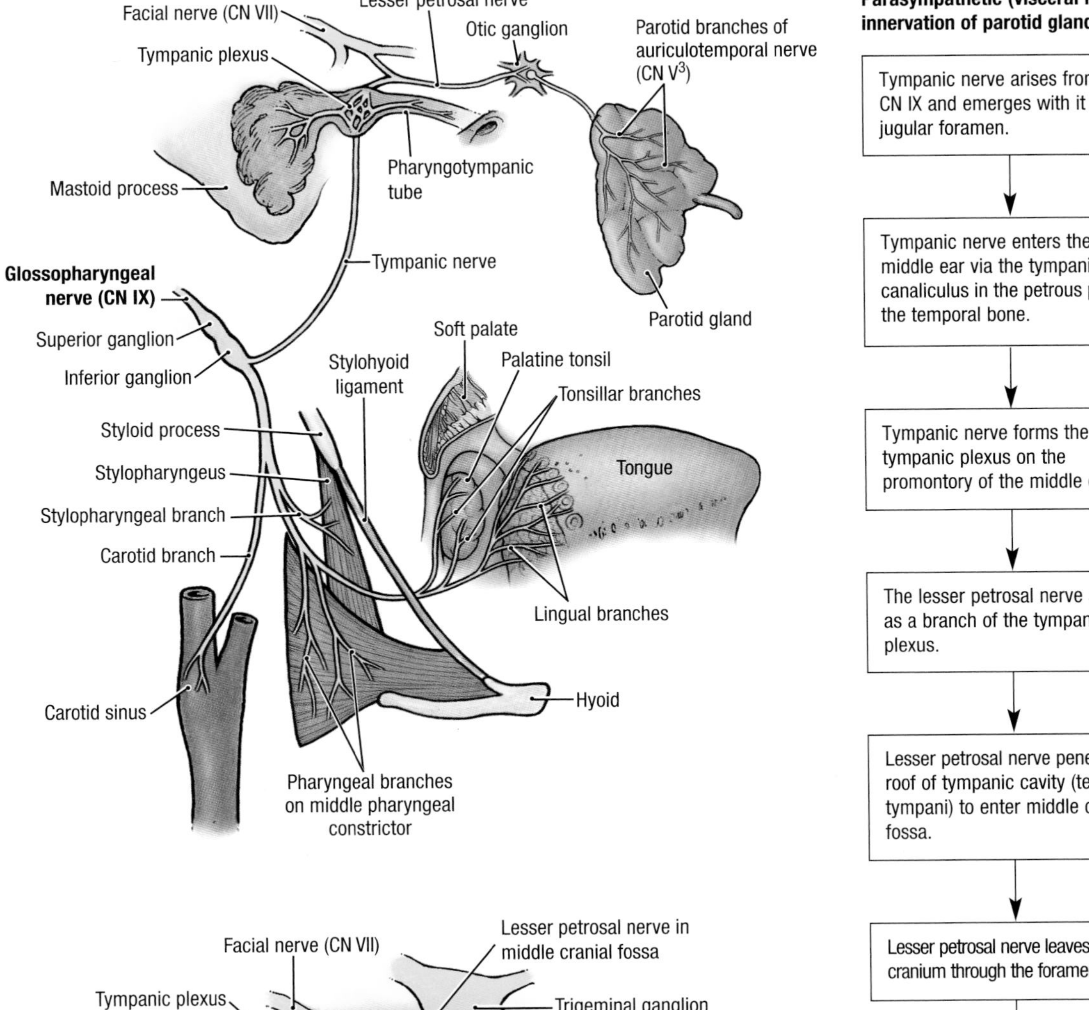
Facial nerve (CN VII)
Lesser petrosal nerve
Otic ganglion
Parotid branches of auriculotemporal nerve (CN V3)
Tympanic plexus
Mastoid process
Pharyngotympanic tube
Tympanic nerve
Glossopharyngeal nerve (CN IX)
Superior ganglion
Inferior ganglion
Parotid gland
Soft palate
Stylohyoid ligament
Palatine tonsil
Tonsillar branches
Styloid process
Tongue
Stylopharyngeus
Stylopharyngeal branch
Carotid branch
Lingual branches
Hyoid
Carotid sinus
Pharyngeal branches on middle pharyngeal constrictor

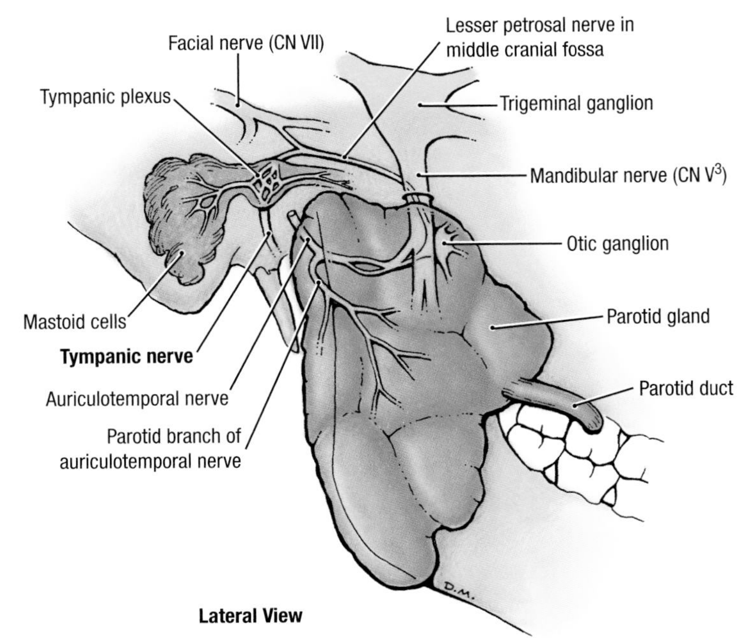
Facial nerve (CN VII)
Lesser petrosal nerve in middle cranial fossa
Tympanic plexus
Trigeminal ganglion
Mandibular nerve (CN V3)
Otic ganglion
Mastoid cells
Parotid gland
Tympanic nerve
Parotid duct
Auriculotemporal nerve
Parotid branch of auriculotemporal nerve
Lateral View

**Parasympathetic (visceral motor) innervation of parotid gland**

Tympanic nerve arises from CN IX and emerges with it from jugular foramen.

↓

Tympanic nerve enters the middle ear via the tympanic canaliculus in the petrous part of the temporal bone.

↓

Tympanic nerve forms the tympanic plexus on the promontory of the middle ear.

↓

The lesser petrosal nerve arises as a branch of the tympanic plexus.

↓

Lesser petrosal nerve penetrates roof of tympanic cavity (tegmen tympani) to enter middle cranial fossa.

↓

Lesser petrosal nerve leaves the cranium through the foramen ovale.

↓

Parasympathetic fibers synapse in the otic ganglion.

↓

Postsynaptic fibers pass to parotid gland via branches of auriculotemporal nerve (CN $V^3$).

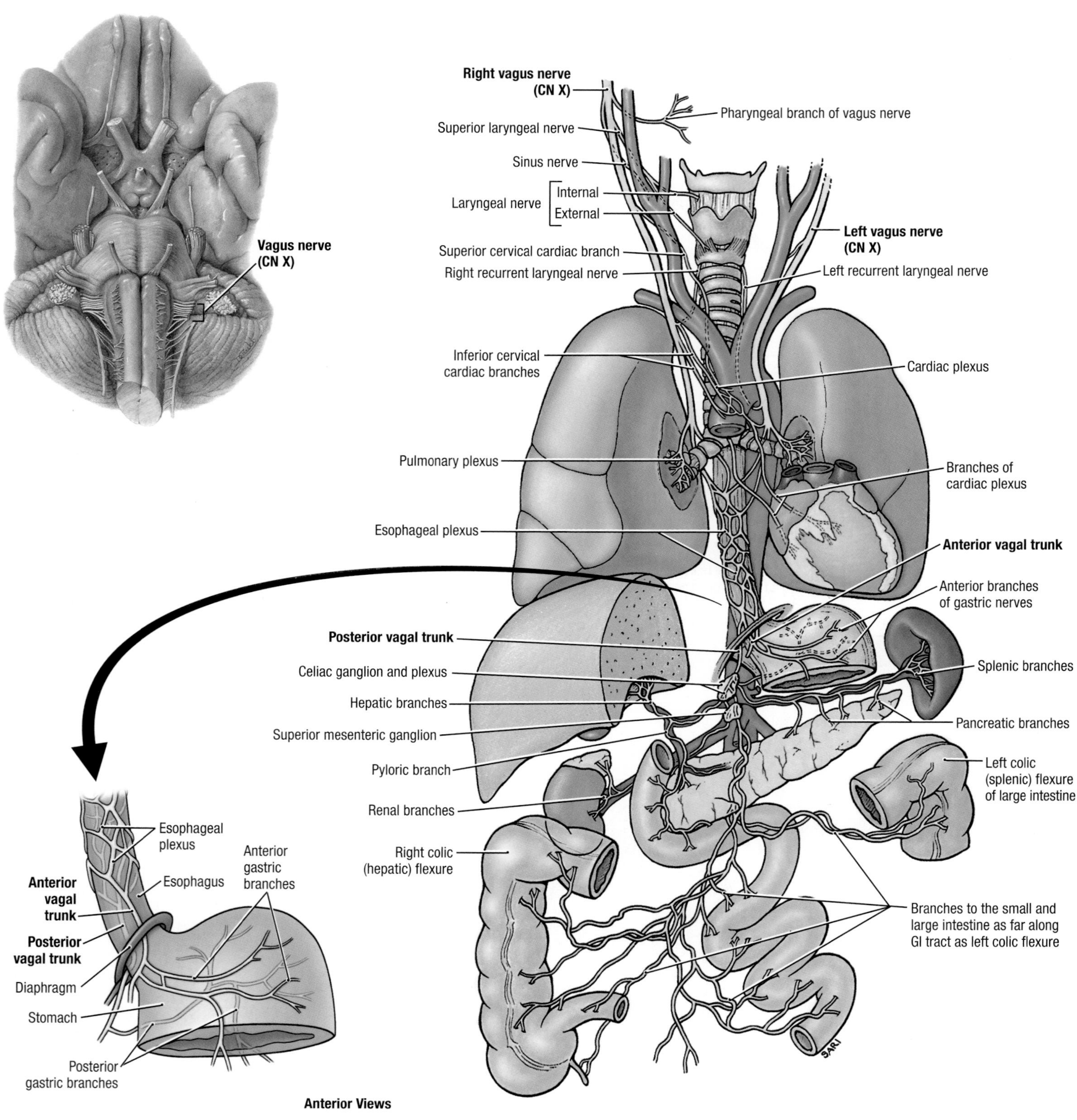
Vagus nerve
(CN X)
Right vagus nerve
(CN X)
Pharyngeal branch of vagus nerve
Superior laryngeal nerve
Sinus nerve
Laryngeal nerve
Internal
External
Left vagus nerve
(CN X)
Superior cervical cardiac branch
Right recurrent laryngeal nerve
Left recurrent laryngeal nerve
Inferior cervical
cardiac branches
Cardiac plexus
Pulmonary plexus
Branches of
cardiac plexus
Esophageal plexus
Anterior vagal trunk
Anterior branches
of gastric nerves
Posterior vagal trunk
Celiac ganglion and plexus
Splenic branches
Hepatic branches
Pancreatic branches
Superior mesenteric ganglion
Pyloric branch
Left colic
(splenic) flexure
of large intestine
Renal branches
Right colic
(hepatic) flexure
Branches to the small and
large intestine as far along
GI tract as left colic flexure
Esophageal
plexus
Anterior
gastric
branches
Esophagus
Anterior
vagal
trunk
Posterior
vagal trunk
Diaphragm
Stomach
Posterior
gastric branches
SARI

Anterior Views

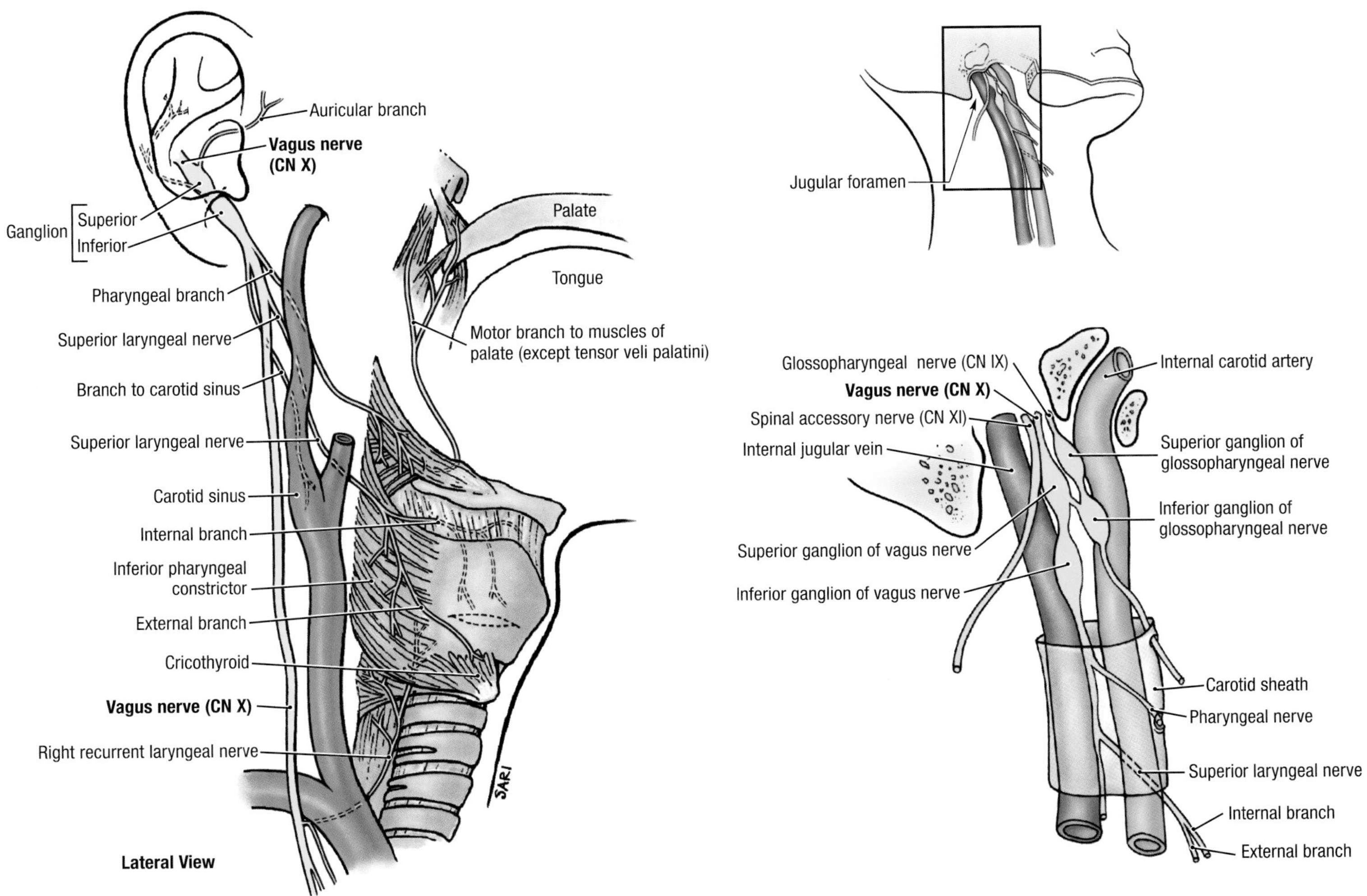
Auricular branch
Vagus nerve (CN X)
Ganglion
Superior
Inferior
Pharyngeal branch
Superior laryngeal nerve
Branch to carotid sinus
Superior laryngeal nerve
Carotid sinus
Internal branch
Inferior pharyngeal constrictor
External branch
Cricothyroid
Vagus nerve (CN X)
Right recurrent laryngeal nerve
Lateral View
Palate
Tongue
Motor branch to muscles of palate (except tensor veli palatini)
SARI
Jugular foramen
Glossopharyngeal nerve (CN IX)
Vagus nerve (CN X)
Spinal accessory nerve (CN XI)
Internal jugular vein
Superior ganglion of vagus nerve
Inferior ganglion of vagus nerve
Internal carotid artery
Superior ganglion of glossopharyngeal nerve
Inferior ganglion of glossopharyngeal nerve
Carotid sheath
Pharyngeal nerve
Superior laryngeal nerve
Internal branch
External branch

**TABLE 9.12 VAGUS NERVE (CN X)**

| Nerve Functions | Functional Components | Cells of Origin/ Termination | Cranial Exit | Distribution and Functions |
|---|---|---|---|---|
| **Vagus** | Branchial motor | Nucleus ambiguus | Jugular foramen | Motor to constrictor muscles of pharynx, intrinsic muscles of larynx, muscles of palate (except tensor veli palatini), and striated muscle in superior two thirds of esophagus |
| | Visceral motor (parasympathetic) | Presynaptic: dorsal vagal nucleus; Postsynaptic: neurons in, on, or near viscera | | Motor to smooth muscle of trachea, bronchi, and digestive tract; moderates cardiac pacemaker and vasoconstrictor of coronary arteries |
| | Visceral sensory | Solitary nucleus, spinal trigeminal nucleus/ inferior ganglion | | Visceral sensation from base of tongue, pharynx, larynx, trachea, bronchi, heart, esophagus, stomach, and intestine |
| | Special sensory | Solitary nucleus/inferior ganglion | | Taste from epiglottis and palate |
| | General sensory | Spinal trigeminal nucleus/ superior or inferior ganglion | | Sensation from auricle, external acoustic meatus, and dura mater of posterior cranial fossa |

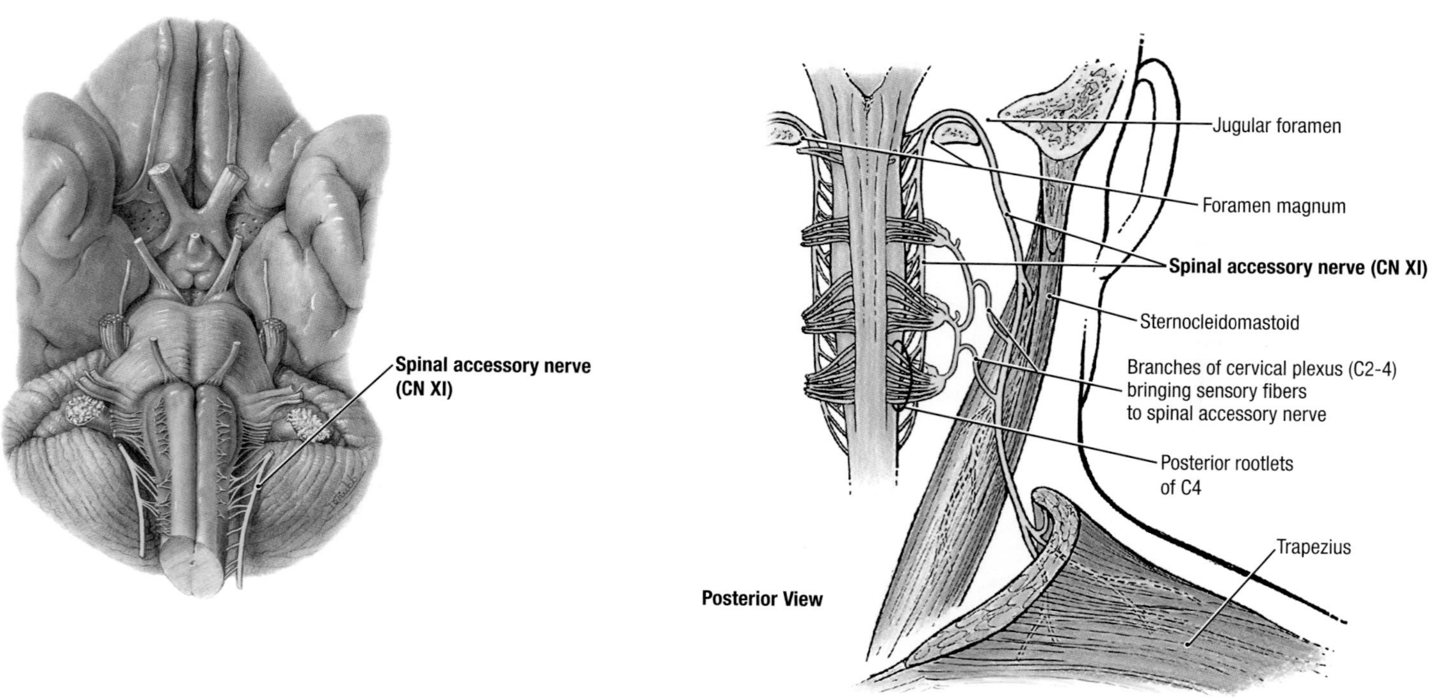
Spinal accessory nerve
(CN XI)
Jugular foramen
Foramen magnum
Spinal accessory nerve (CN XI)
Sternocleidomastoid
Branches of cervical plexus (C2-4)
bringing sensory fibers
to spinal accessory nerve
Posterior rootlets
of C4
Trapezius
Posterior View

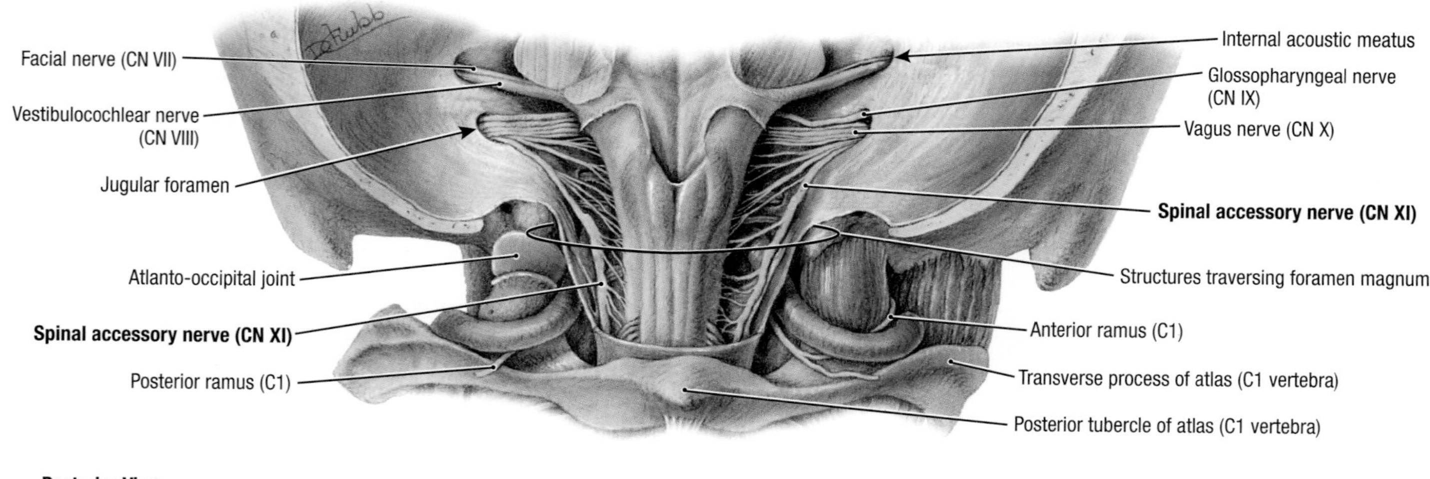
Facial nerve (CN VII)
Vestibulocochlear nerve
(CN VIII)
Jugular foramen
Atlanto-occipital joint
Spinal accessory nerve (CN XI)
Posterior ramus (C1)
Internal acoustic meatus
Glossopharyngeal nerve
(CN IX)
Vagus nerve (CN X)
Spinal accessory nerve (CN XI)
Structures traversing foramen magnum
Anterior ramus (C1)
Transverse process of atlas (C1 vertebra)
Posterior tubercle of atlas (C1 vertebra)

Posterior View

## TABLE 9.13 SPINAL ACCESSORY NERVE (CN XI)

| Nerve | Functional Components | Cells of Origin/ Termination | Cranial Exit | Distribution and Functions |
|---|---|---|---|---|
| **Spinal accessory** | Somatic motor | Accessory nucleus of spinal cord | Jugular foramen | Motor to sternocleidomastoid and trapezius |

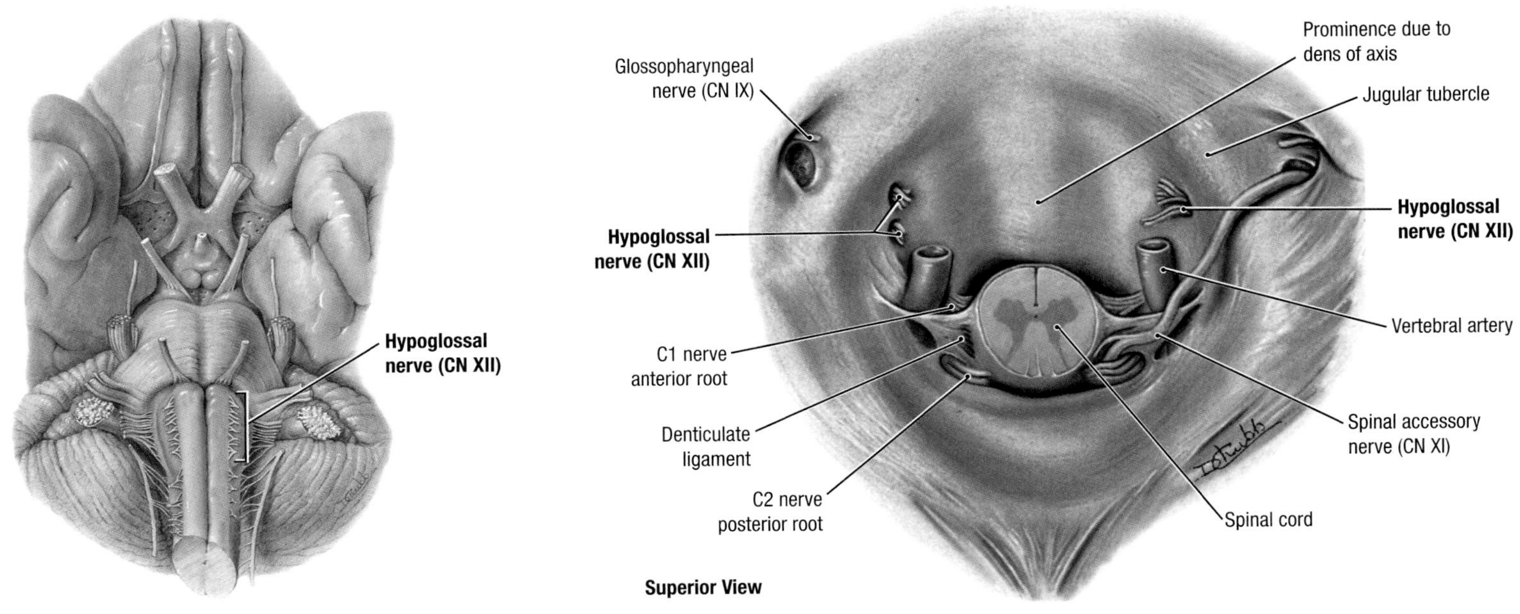
Hypoglossal nerve (CN XII)
Glossopharyngeal nerve (CN IX)
Hypoglossal nerve (CN XII)
C1 nerve anterior root
Denticulate ligament
C2 nerve posterior root
Superior View
Prominence due to dens of axis
Jugular tubercle
Hypoglossal nerve (CN XII)
Vertebral artery
Spinal accessory nerve (CN XI)
Spinal cord

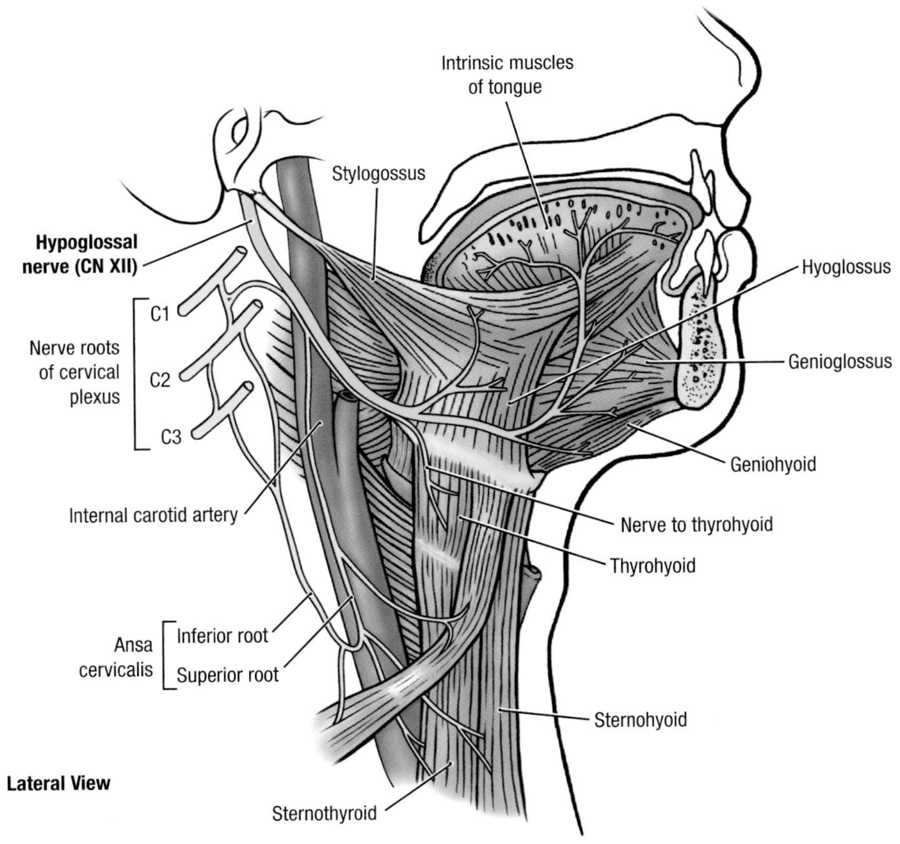
Intrinsic muscles of tongue
Stylogossus
Hypoglossal nerve (CN XII)
Nerve roots of cervical plexus
C1
C2
C3
Internal carotid artery
Ansa cervicalis
Inferior root
Superior root
Lateral View
Sternothyroid
Hyoglossus
Genioglossus
Geniohyoid
Nerve to thyrohyoid
Thyrohyoid
Sternohyoid

## TABLE 9.14 HYPOGLOSSAL NERVE (CN XII)

| Nerve | Functional Components | Cells of Origin/ Termination | Cranial Exit | Distribution and Functions |
|---|---|---|---|---|
| **Hypoglossal** | Somatic motor | Hypoglossal nucleus | Hypoglossal canal | Motor to muscles of tongue (except palatoglossus) |

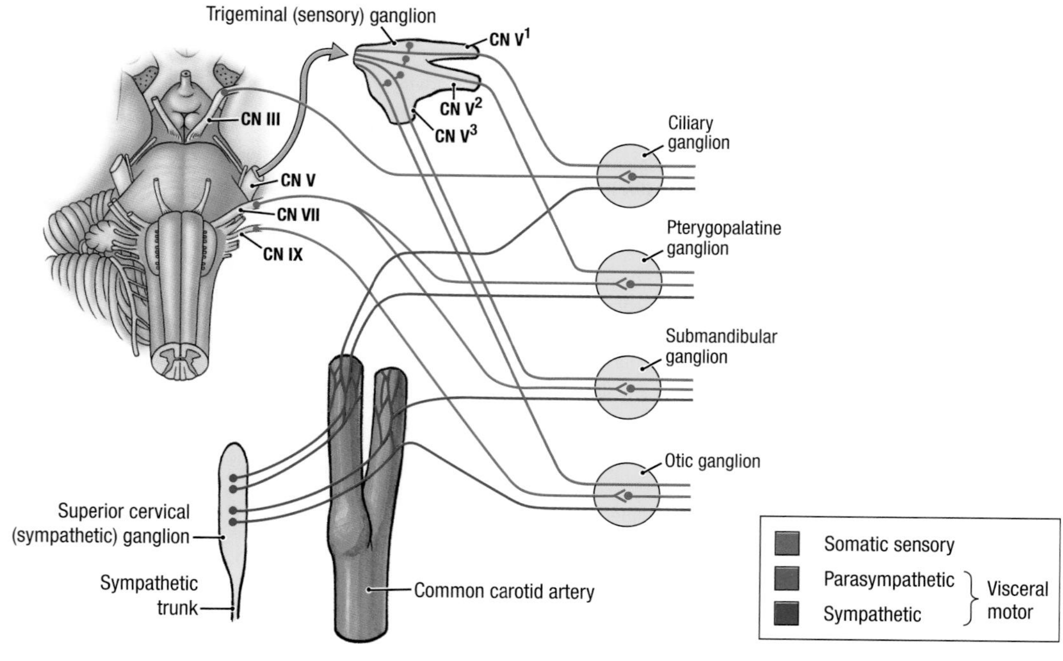
Trigeminal (sensory) ganglion
CN V1
CN V2
CN V3
CN III
CN V
CN VII
CN IX
Ciliary ganglion
Pterygopalatine ganglion
Submandibular ganglion
Otic ganglion
Superior cervical (sympathetic) ganglion
Sympathetic trunk
Common carotid artery
Somatic sensory
Parasympathetic
Sympathetic
Visceral motor

**TABLE 9.15 AUTONOMIC GANGLIA OF THE HEAD**

| Ganglion | Location | Parasympathetic Root (Nucleus of Origin) [a] | Sympathetic Root | Main Distribution |
|---|---|---|---|---|
| **Ciliary** | Between optic nerve and lateral rectus, close to apex of orbit | Inferior branch of oculomotor nerve (CN III) (Edinger-Westphal nucleus) | Branch from internal carotid plexus in cavernous sinus | Parasympathetic postsynaptic fibers from ciliary ganglion pass to ciliary muscle and sphincter pupillae of iris; sympathetic postsynaptic fibers from superior cervical ganglion pass to dilator pupillae and blood vessels of eye |
| **Pterygopalatine** | In pterygopalatine fossa, where it is attached by pterygopalatine branches of maxillary nerve; located just anterior to opening of pterygoid canal and inferior to CN V$^2$ | Greater petrosal nerve from facial nerve (CN VII) (superior salivatory nucleus) | Deep petrosal nerve, a branch of internal carotid plexus that is continuation of postsynaptic fibers of cervical sympathetic trunk; fibers from superior cervical ganglion pass through pterygopalatine ganglion and enter branches of CN V$^2$ | Parasympathetic postsynaptic fibers from pterygopalatine ganglion innervate lacrimal gland through zygomatic branch of CN V$^2$; sympathetic postsynaptic fibers from superior cervical ganglion accompany branches of pterygopalatine nerve that are distributed to the nasal cavity, palate, and superior parts of the pharynx |
| **Otic** | Between tensor veli palatini and mandibular nerve; lies inferior to foramen ovale | Tympanic nerve from glossopharyngeal nerve (CN IX); tympanic nerve continues from tympanic plexus as lesser petrosal nerve (inferior salivatory nucleus) | Fibers from superior cervical ganglion travel via plexus on middle meningeal artery | Parasympathetic postsynaptic fibers from otic ganglion are distributed to parotid gland through auriculotemporal nerve (branch of CN V$^3$); sympathetic postsynaptic fibers from superior cervical ganglion pass to parotid gland and supply its blood vessels |
| **Submandibular** | Suspended from lingual nerve by two short roots; lies on surface of hyoglossus muscle inferior to submandibular duct | Parasympathetic fibers join facial nerve (CN VII) and leave it in its chorda tympani branch, which unites with lingual nerve (superior salivatory nucleus) | Sympathetic fibers from superior cervical ganglion travel via the plexus on facial artery | Postsynaptic parasympathetic fibers from submandibular ganglion are distributed to the sublingual and submandibular glands; sympathetic fibers from superior cervical ganglion supply sublingual and submandibular glands |

[a] For location of nuclei, see Figure 9.3.

**TABLE 9.16 SUMMARY OF CRANIAL NERVE LESIONS**

| Nerve | Lesion Type and/or Site | Abnormal Findings |
|---|---|---|
| CN I | Fracture of cribriform plate | Anosmia (loss of smell); cerebrospinal fluid (CSF) rhinorrhea (leakage of CSF through nose) |
| CN II | Direct trauma to orbit or eyeball; fracture involving optic canal | Loss of pupillary constriction |
| | Pressure on optic pathway; laceration or intracerebral clot in temporal, parietal, or occipital lobes of brain | Visual field defects |
| | Increased CSF pressure | Swelling of optic disc (papilledema) |
| CN III | Pressure from herniating uncus on nerve; fracture involving cavernous sinus; aneurysms | Dilated pupil, ptosis, eye rotates inferiorly and laterally (down and out), pupillary reflex on the side of the lesion will be lost |
| CN IV | Stretching of nerve during its course around brainstem; fracture of orbit | Inability to rotate adducted eye inferiorly |
| CN V | Injury to terminal branches (particularly CN $V^2$) in roof of maxillary sinus; pathologic processes (tumors, aneurysms, infections) affecting trigeminal nerve | Loss of pain and touch sensations/paresthesia on face; loss of corneal reflex (blinking when cornea touched); paralysis of muscles of mastication; deviation of mandible to side of lesion when mouth is opened |
| CN VI | Base of brain or fracture involving cavernous sinus or orbit | Inability to rotate eye laterally; diplopia on lateral gaze |
| CN VII | Laceration or contusion in parotid region | Paralysis of facial muscles; eye remains open; angle of mouth droops; forehead does not wrinkle |
| | Fracture of temporal bone | As above, plus associated involvement of cochlear nerve and chorda tympani; dry cornea and loss of taste on anterior two thirds of tongue |
| | Intracranial hematoma ("stroke") | Weakness (paralysis) of lower facial muscles contralateral to the lesion, upper facial muscles are not affected because they are bilaterally innervated |
| CN VIII | Tumor of nerve | Progressive unilateral hearing loss; tinnitus (noises in ear); vertigo (loss of balance) |
| CN IX[a] | Brainstem lesion or deep laceration of neck | Loss of taste on posterior third of tongue; loss of sensation on affected side of soft palate; loss of gag reflex on affected side |
| CN X | Brainstem lesion or deep laceration of neck | Sagging of soft palate; deviation of uvula to unaffected side; hoarseness owing to paralysis of vocal fold; difficulty in swallowing and speaking |
| CN XI | Laceration of neck | Paralysis of sternocleidomastoid and superior fibers of trapezius; drooping of shoulder |
| CN XII | Neck laceration; basal skull fractures | Protruded tongue deviates toward affected side; moderate dysarthria (disturbance of articulation) |

[a] Isolated lesions of CN IX are uncommon; usually, CN IX, X, and XI are involved together as they pass through the jugular foramen.

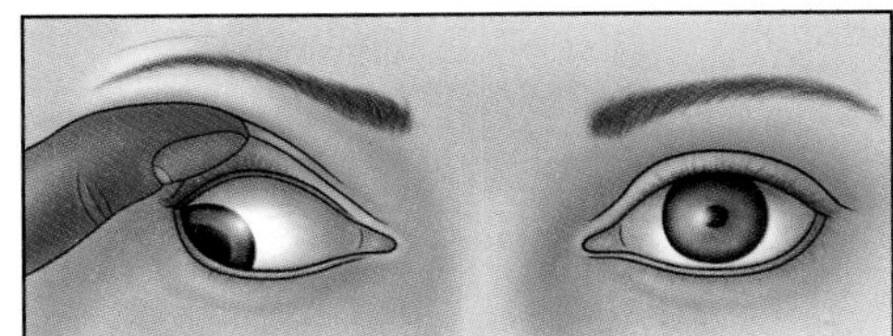
Right eye: Downward and outward gaze, dilated pupil, eyelid manually elevated due to ptosis
Left

**Right oculomotor (CN III) nerve palsy**

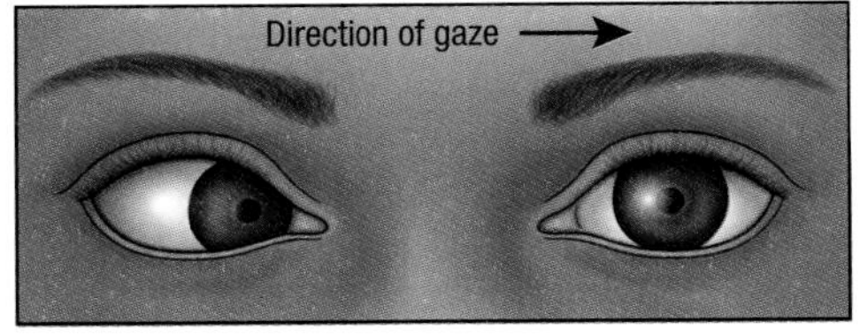
Direction of gaze
Right
Left eye: Does not abduct

**Left abducent (CN VI) nerve palsy**

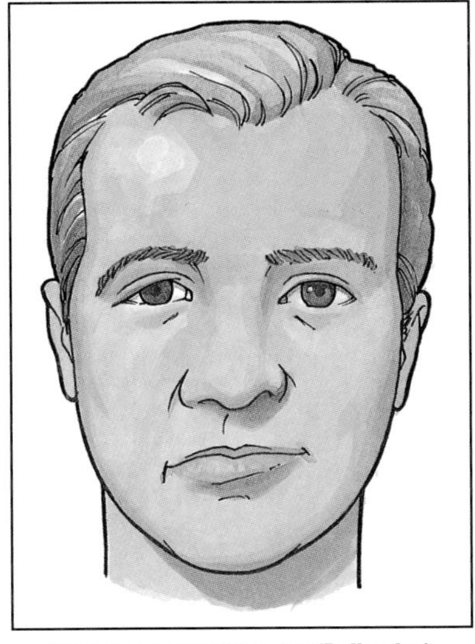

**Right facial (CN VII) palsy (Bell palsy)**

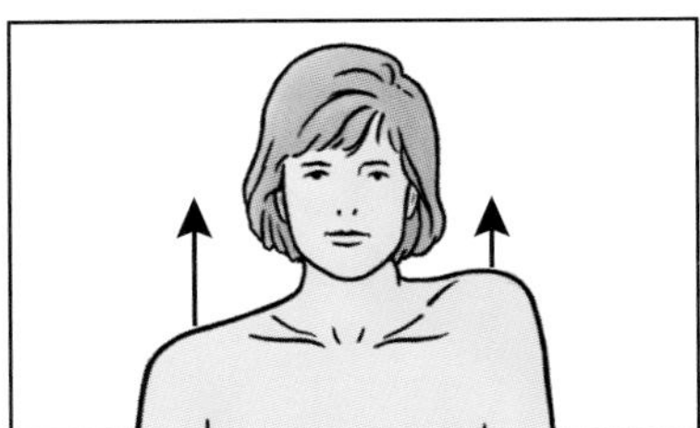

**Right CN XI lesion**

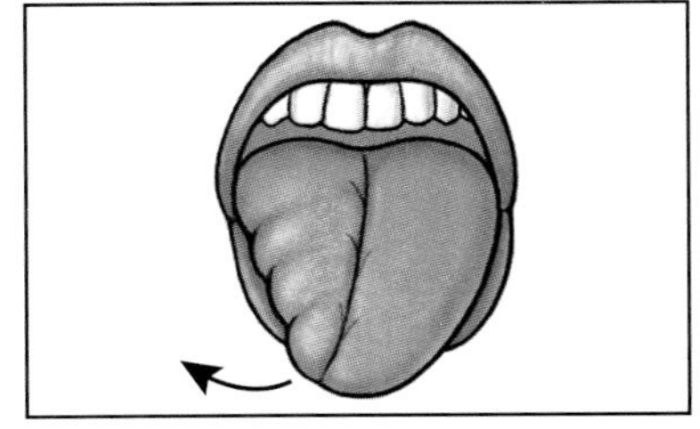

**Right CN XII lesion**

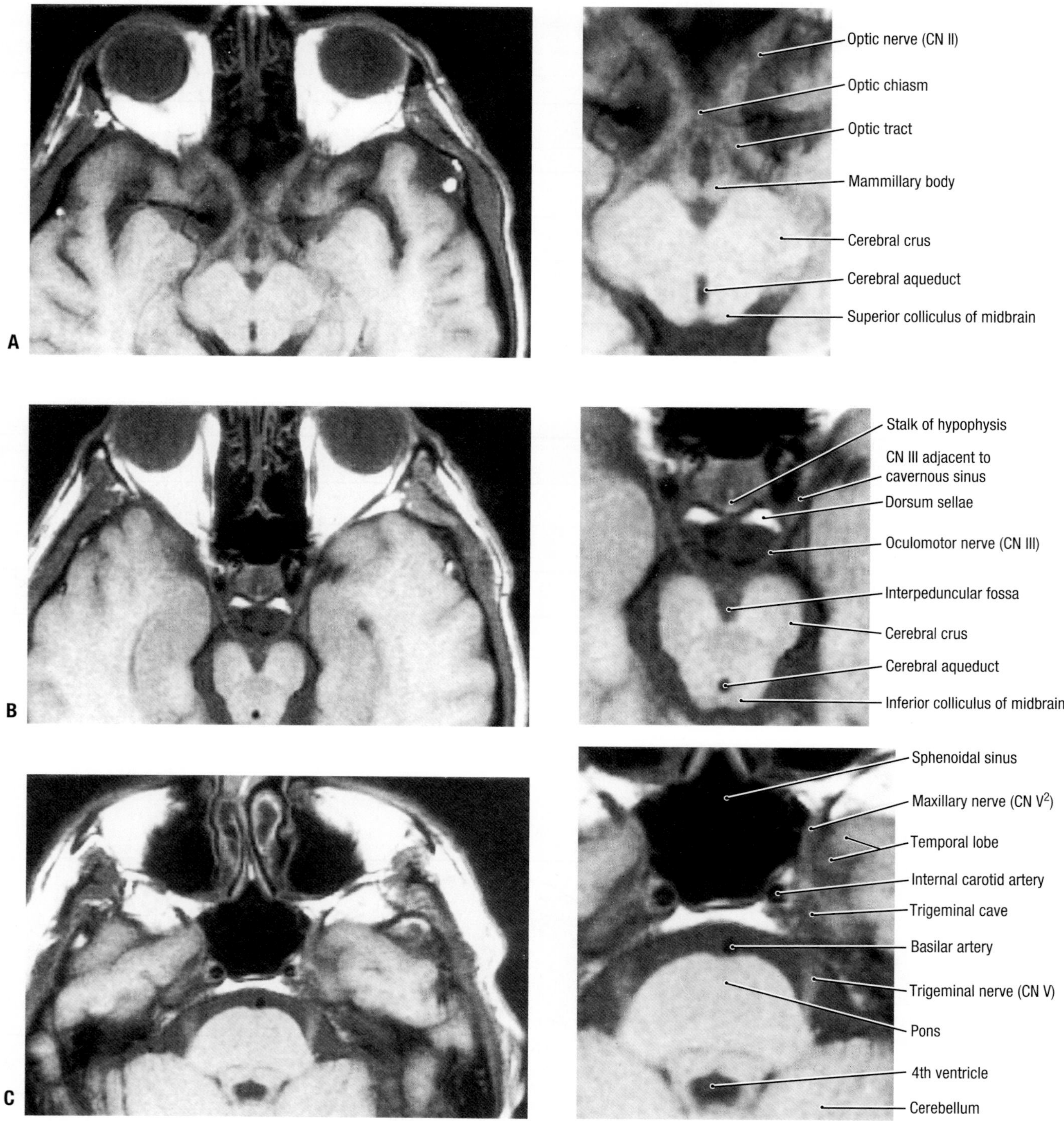
A
Optic nerve (CN II)
Optic chiasm
Optic tract
Mammillary body
Cerebral crus
Cerebral aqueduct
Superior colliculus of midbrain
B
Stalk of hypophysis
CN III adjacent to cavernous sinus
Dorsum sellae
Oculomotor nerve (CN III)
Interpeduncular fossa
Cerebral crus
Cerebral aqueduct
Inferior colliculus of midbrain
C
Sphenoidal sinus
Maxillary nerve (CN V2)
Temporal lobe
Internal carotid artery
Trigeminal cave
Basilar artery
Trigeminal nerve (CN V)
Pons
4th ventricle
Cerebellum

**9.6 Transverse MRIs through head, showing cranial nerves**

**A.** Optic nerve (CN II). **B.** Oculomotor nerve (CN III). **C.** Trigeminal nerve (CN V).

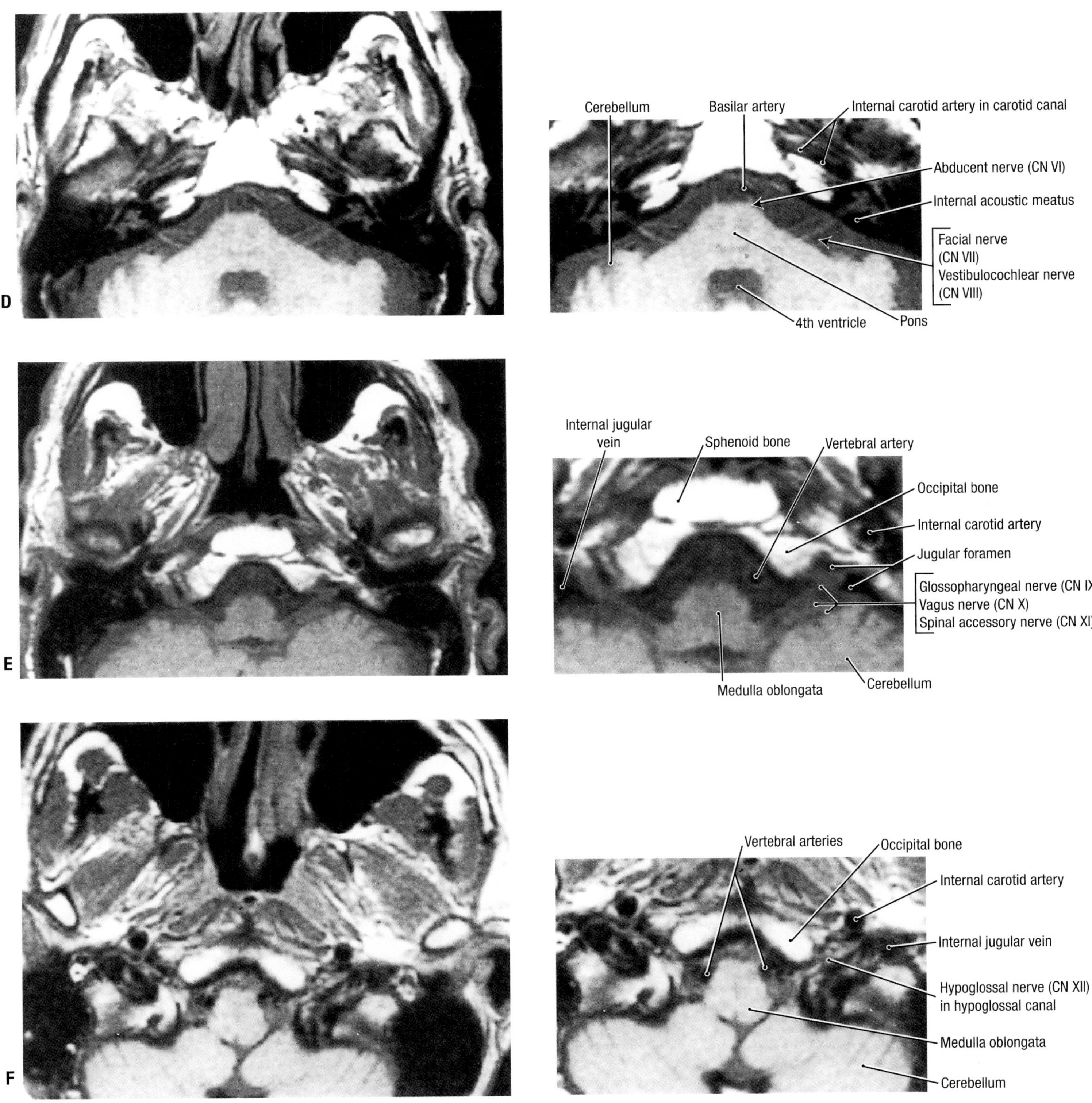
D
Cerebellum
Basilar artery
Internal carotid artery in carotid canal
Abducent nerve (CN VI)
Internal acoustic meatus
Facial nerve (CN VII)
Vestibulocochlear nerve (CN VIII)
4th ventricle
Pons
E
Internal jugular vein
Sphenoid bone
Vertebral artery
Occipital bone
Internal carotid artery
Jugular foramen
Glossopharyngeal nerve (CN IX)
Vagus nerve (CN X)
Spinal accessory nerve (CN XI)
Medulla oblongata
Cerebellum
F
Vertebral arteries
Occipital bone
Internal carotid artery
Internal jugular vein
Hypoglossal nerve (CN XII) in hypoglossal canal
Medulla oblongata
Cerebellum

**9.6 Transverse MRIs through head, showing cranial nerves *(continued)***

**D.** Abducent (CN VI), facial (CN VII), and vestibulocochlear (CN VIII) nerves. **E.** Glossopharyngeal (CN IX), vagus (CN X), and spinal accessory (CN XI) nerves. **F.** Hypoglossal nerve (CN XII).

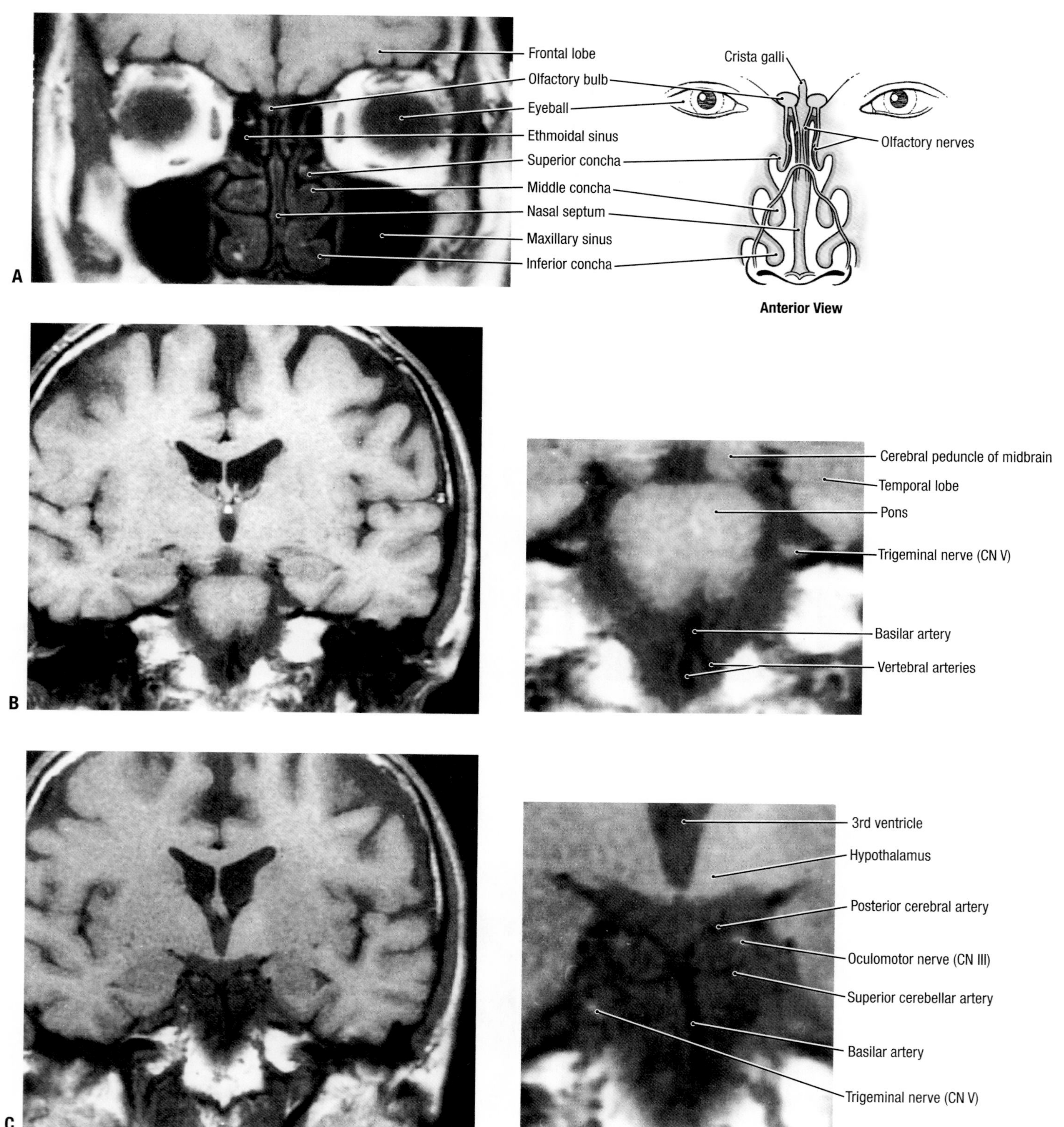
A
Frontal lobe
Olfactory bulb
Eyeball
Ethmoidal sinus
Superior concha
Middle concha
Nasal septum
Maxillary sinus
Inferior concha
Crista galli
Olfactory nerves
Anterior View
B
Cerebral peduncle of midbrain
Temporal lobe
Pons
Trigeminal nerve (CN V)
Basilar artery
Vertebral arteries
C
3rd ventricle
Hypothalamus
Posterior cerebral artery
Oculomotor nerve (CN III)
Superior cerebellar artery
Basilar artery
Trigeminal nerve (CN V)

**9.7 Coronal MRIs through head, showing cranial nerves**

**A.** Olfactory bulb. **B.** Trigeminal (CN V) nerve. **C.** Oculomotor (CN III) and trigeminal (CN V) nerves.

# INDEX

Note: Page numbers followed by t denote tables.


Abdomen
  autonomic innervation, 178, 179t
  contents, 119
  magnetic resonance imaging, 186–189, 191
  ultrasound, 190–191
  vagus nerves in, 181
  viscera, 96, 97, 162, 163
Abdominal wall
  anterior, 102–103, 152, 157
  anterolateral
    arteries, 101
    muscles, 104, 104t
    nerves, 101
    posterior aspect, 118
    structure, 105
    superficial dissection, 100
    surface anatomy, 98–99
  layers, 105
  posterior, 121, 162, 163, 172t
  subperitoneal fat, 164
Acetabular region, 396
Acetabulum, 196–199, 372, 380, 396–398
Acromion, 511, 518, 519, 527, 529, 533, 535–537, 598
Amnion, 239
Ampulla, 714
  ductus deferens, 216, 217, 220
  hepatopancreatic, 156
  phrenic, 132
  rectum, 208, 232
Anal column, 209, 211
Anastomosis
  genicular, 417
  knee, 416–417
  portal-systemic, 227
  transverse, 490
  upper limb, 486, 487
Anatomical snuff box, 580, 584, 585
Angiogram
  abdomen, 191
  aorta, 55, 70, 191
  head and neck, 649
  pelvis, 277
  thorax, 41, 92–93
Angle
  acromial, 519, 531
  of clitoris, 272
  costal, 13
  of eye, 650
  inferolateral, 313
  infrasternal, 10
  of mandible, 609, 610, 612, 664
  Q-, 407
  of scapula
    inferior, 11, 511, 518, 522, 523, 535
    superior, 511, 518, 523, 529, 536
  sternal, 12, 300, 499, 808
  subpubic, 196, 198, 199
  venous, 76, 716
Ankle, 354
  articular surfaces, 455
  coronal section, 456
  ligaments, 449, 452, 454
  magnetic resonance imaging, 456, 457
  medial aspect, 438, 439
  posterior aspect, 450
  posteromedial aspect, 451
  radiograph, 453, 454
  synovial sheaths and tendons, 430, 431
  transverse section, 457
Ankle region, 354
Ansa cervicalis, 762, 763, 766, 807
Antihelix, 703
Antrum
  mastoid, 713
  pyloric, 129, 132, 186, 189
Anulus fibrosus, 304–308
Anus, 161, 252, 271–274, 276–281
Aorta, 20, 29, 50, 57–59, 65, 73, 78, 83, 117, 120, 124, 130, 133, 137, 142, 144, 152–154, 157, 164, 165, 186, 188, 189, 215, 339, 808
  abdominal, 74, 85, 123, 163, 175, 191, 213
  ascending, 27, 41, 46, 49, 51, 59, 67, 70
    3-D volume reconstruction and CT angiogram, 92–93
    magnetic resonance imaging, 88–91
  bifurcation, 188
  branches, 174
  descending, 65, 67, 70, 71, 81, 351
    3-D volume reconstruction and CT angiogram, 92–93
    computed tomography, 6
    magnetic resonance imaging, 88–91
  dorsal, 67
  thoracic, 68, 69, 74–76, 82, 85
    descending, 119
  ultrasound, 190, 191
Aperture
  anterior nasal, 613
  lateral, 722, 724
  median, 723, 724
Aponeurosis
  bicipital, 522, 523, 525, 538, 539, 549
  epicranial, 330, 634, 743
  external oblique, 100, 102, 105–109, 111, 112, 372
  flexor carpi ulnaris with antebrachial fascia, 542
  gastrocnemius, 472
  internal oblique, 105, 107–109, 112
  levator palpebrae superior, 654
  palatine, 682, 684
  palmar, 554, 560–563, 566, 571, 606
  palmar carpal, 493
  plantar, 443–445, 456
  transversus abdominis, 109, 170, 322, 324
  triceps, 527
Appendices epiploicae, 144, 145
Appendix, 97, 128, 136, 139, 140, 160, 208, 232
  blood supply, 139
  of epididymis, 116
  omental, 136, 140
  of testis, 116
Aqueduct
  cerebral, 523, 723, 724, 729, 738, 739, 742
  vestibular, 714
Aqueous humor, 660, 661
Arachnoid granulations, 636–638, 724
Arachnoid mater, 334, 335, 338–340, 634, 636
Arch
  aortic, 25–27, 29, 39, 46, 47, 49, 52, 61, 68, 69, 72, 74, 75, 78, 81, 84, 85, 486
    branches, 70
    double, 71
    magnetic resonance imaging, 90, 91
    relationship to recurrent laryngeal nerve, 67
    variations, 70, 71
  carpal
    dorsal, 487, 573, 573t, 576
    palmar, 487, 570
  iliopectineal, 373
  longitudinal
    lateral, 466
    medial, 466
  neural, 290
  palatoglossal, 792–794
  palatopharyngeal, 792–794
  palmar
    deep, 486, 487, 550, 551, 570–573, 573t, 584
    superficial, 486, 487, 550, 551, 561, 566, 572, 573, 573t
  pancreaticoduodenal
    anterior, 135
    posterior, 135, 153
  plantar, 362, 440
    deep, 446
  pubic, 196, 198, 199
  superciliary, 611, 612
  transverse, 466
  venous
    deep palmar, 488
    dorsal, 363–365, 490
    dorsal digital, 490
    plantar, 363
    superficial palmar, 488
  vertebral, 16, 289
  zygomatic, 610, 612, 615, 666, 719
Areola, 4
Arm, 476, 477
  anterior aspect, 522, 523
  compartments, 521, 600
  lateral aspect, 524
  magnetic resonance imaging, 601
  medial aspect, 525
  muscles, 519
  posterior aspect, 526
Arteriogram
  axillary, 504
  brachial, 551
  carotid, 648
  celiac, 131
  coronary, 54
  hand, 572
  inferior mesenteric, 143
  popliteal, 440
  renal, 167
  superior mesenteric, 141
  vertebral, 648
Arteriole, inferior temporal retinal, 661
Artery
  acetabular, 401
  alveolar
    inferior, 670, 778
    posterior superior, 712
  anal, inferior, 261, 269
  angular, 632, 632t, 721
  appendicular, 139, 140
  arcuate, 362, 425, 427, 427t
  auricular
    deep, 670
    posterior, 632, 632t, 662, 764, 764t, 765
  axillary, 8, 22, 486, 487, 503, 508, 509
  basilar, 298, 341, 638, 640, 646, 647, 647t, 648, 649, 738, 739, 742
  brachial, 486, 487, 502, 539–541, 549–551
    deep, 504, 505t, 510, 521, 527, 600
  brachiocephalic, 66, 67
  bronchial, 35, 69, 75
  buccal, 668, 670
  calcaneal, medial, 457
  carotid
    common, 71, 738, 739, 763, 771, 772, 806, 807
      left, 46–49, 66, 67, 70, 71, 74, 81, 82, 88–91, 773
      right, 26, 48, 66, 67, 70, 71, 74, 88–90, 486, 764, 764t, 765, 773
    external, 662, 663, 667, 681, 713, 763, 764, 764t, 765
    internal, 350, 638, 640, 644–647, 647t, 648, 649, 662, 663, 667, 681, 710–713, 720, 721, 738–740, 763, 764, 764t, 765, 785, 809
  celiac, 78, 82, 130, 186, 188, 189
  central
    anteromedial, 731

Artery—*continued*
posterolateral, 731
posteromedial, 731
of retina, 657, 657t, 660, 661
cerebellar
anterior inferior, 647, 647t, 648
posterior, 648
posterior inferior, 647, 647t, 648, 740
superior, 341, 638, 647, 647t, 648, 740
cerebral
anterior, 638, 646, 647, 647t, 648, 649, 732, 733, 740, 742, 743
middle, 646, 647, 647t, 648, 649, 732, 733, 740, 742
posterior, 341, 638, 646, 647, 647t, 649, 738–740
cervical
ascending, 341, 772, 773
deep, 75, 331, 341, 784
superficial, 486, 772
ciliary
anterior, 657t, 661
long posterior, 657t, 661
short posterior, 657t, 661
circumflex femoral
lateral, 277, 362, 373, 382, 400, 401
medial, 277, 362, 373, 382, 400, 401
circumflex humeral
anterior, 486, 504, 505t, 509
posterior, 486, 504, 505t, 509, 510, 527, 528, 534, 536
circumflex iliac
deep, 101, 108, 109, 111, 112, 118, 224, 242, 362, 372
superficial, 101, 362, 370, 372
circumflex scapular, 487, 502, 504, 505t, 509, 510, 528
colic
left, 142, 143, 145
middle, 122, 126, 127, 134, 135, 140–142, 144, 145
accessory, 127
right, 127, 134, 140, 141, 145
collateral
medial, 486, 487
middle, 550
radial, 486, 487, 550
communicating
anterior, 646, 647, 647t, 649, 738–740
posterior, 638, 646, 647, 647t, 648, 649
coronary, 53, 59, 75
3-D volume reconstruction and CT angiogram, 92–93
anterior interventricular branch, 49
branches, 52
circumflex branch, 50
left, 46, 52, 54, 55, 63, 92–93
magnetic resonance imaging, 88–89
right, 46, 47, 49, 50, 52, 54, 55, 59, 63, 92–93
single, 55
cremasteric, 101, 108, 109, 112, 117
cystic, 130, 154, 155, 158
deep
of arm, 486, 487, 502, 509, 528, 550
of clitoris, 241
of thigh, 275, 362, 372, 373, 382, 400
digital
common palmar, 487, 561, 566, 569, 570, 572, 573t
dorsal, 362, 425, 487, 569, 573, 576
plantar, 362, 443, 446
proper palmar, 487, 561, 563, 569, 570, 572, 573t
dorsal
of clitoris, 241, 254, 272, 274
of foot, 362, 425–427, 427t, 431, 440, 441t
of penis, 116, 254, 264, 267
ductus deferens, 117, 216, 224, 225, 225t, 226
epigastric
inferior, 101, 103, 108, 109, 111, 112, 118, 136, 144, 208, 215, 218, 219, 224, 226, 232, 242, 362
superficial, 101, 102, 370
superior, 101, 103
esophageal, 65
ethmoidal
anterior, 657t, 693
posterior, 657t, 693
facial, 626, 627, 632, 632t, 662, 666, 667, 693, 721, 762–765, 765t, 766, 778, 780, 782, 796
groove, 664
transverse, 626, 627, 632, 632t, 662
femoral, 101, 109, 117, 118, 213, 222, 241, 250, 275, 277, 362, 370–373, 382, 399, 400, 440, 470
fibular, 362, 424, 427, 436, 437, 440, 441t
gastric
left, 75, 122, 126, 127, 129–131, 133–135, 154, 155, 162
posterior, 130, 135
right, 127, 129–131, 135, 154, 155
short, 129–131, 135
gastro-omental
left, 124–127, 129–131, 135
right, 124, 126, 127, 129–131, 134, 135
gastroduodenal, 130, 131, 133–135, 153–155, 174
genicular
descending, 362, 416
inferior lateral, 362, 404, 416, 417
inferior medial, 362, 404, 416, 417
lateral superior, 409
medial inferior, 408, 435, 440
medial superior, 408, 440
middle, 416
superior lateral, 362, 404, 416, 417
superior medial, 362, 404, 416, 417
gluteal
inferior, 212, 224, 225, 225t, 226, 242, 250, 277, 362, 393t
superior, 212, 224, 225, 225t, 226, 242, 277, 351, 362, 393t
gonadal, 165
hepatic, 124, 131, 147, 149–151, 154, 186
aberrant, 153, 155
accessory, 154
common, 123, 126, 127, 130, 131, 135, 153–155, 174, 186
proper, 122, 123, 130, 131, 133–135, 154, 155, 158, 174
variations, 158
ileal, 141, 145
ileocolic, 134, 139–141, 144, 145
iliac
common, 117, 142, 163, 165, 175, 188, 213, 215, 216, 224, 225, 225t, 226, 240–242, 277, 362
external, 101, 109, 111, 163, 175, 202, 212, 213, 215, 216, 218, 224, 225, 225t, 226, 240–242, 277, 362, 400
internal, 163, 165, 175, 202, 212, 213, 215, 216, 224, 225, 225t, 226, 240–242, 243t, 277, 351, 362
iliolumbar, 224, 225, 225t, 242, 243t
indicis
dorsalis, 576, 577, 584, 606
radialis, 561, 566, 570, 573, 573t, 577
infraorbital, 657t, 668, 670, 719, 720
intercostal, 341
anterior, 20, 22, 23
posterior, 17, 20, 75, 80–83, 101, 339, 341
supreme, 72, 75, 81
interosseous
anterior, 486, 487, 550, 550t, 551, 557, 573, 576, 602
common, 486, 487, 550, 550t, 551
posterior, 338–340, 487, 550, 550t, 551, 573, 577, 602, 634, 636
posterior recurrent, 577
recurrent, 487, 543, 550, 550t
interventricular, 66
anterior, 46, 47, 52
posterior, 47
jejunal, 135, 141, 145
labial
anterior, 241
inferior, 632, 632t
posterior, 241
superior, 632, 632t
lacrimal, 657t
laryngeal, inferior, 807
of ligament of head of femur, 401
lingual, 667, 680, 681, 763–765, 765t, 766, 781, 782
lumbar, 175, 341
malleolar
lateral, 362, 425, 427
medial, 362, 425, 427
marginal, 140–143
left, 46
right, 46, 55
maxillary, 384, 668–670, 681, 720, 764, 765, 765t
medullary
anterior segmental, 341
posterior segmental, 341, 342
meningeal, middle, 618, 635, 637, 640, 670, 712
mental, 632, 632t
mesenteric
inferior, 122, 133, 142–145, 163, 174, 175, 213, 215, 241
superior, 78, 82, 120, 122, 126, 127, 133–135, 140–142, 145, 153–156, 162, 163, 174, 175, 187–191
metacarpal
dorsal, 569, 573, 576
palmar, 487, 570, 572, 573
metatarsal, 427, 427t
dorsal, 362, 425
perforating branches, 425
plantar, 362, 444, 446
musculophrenic, 101
nasal
dorsal, 657t
lateral, 632, 632t
posterior lateral, 693
obturator, 118, 212, 224, 225, 225t, 242, 243t, 250, 277, 362, 396, 399, 401
anomalous, 226
occipital, 330, 331, 333, 632, 632t, 721, 762–764, 764t, 765, 785
ophthalmic, 648, 654, 657, 657t
ovarian, 233–235, 241, 243t
palatine
ascending, 693, 712
greater, 683, 693
lesser, 683
pancreatic
dorsal, 135
greater, 134, 135
inferior, 135
pancreaticoduodenal
anterior inferior, 134, 135
anterior superior, 134, 135, 145
posterior inferior, 134, 135, 153
posterior superior, 134, 135, 153
superior, 130
perforating, 362, 372, 393t, 427, 446, 576
pericardiacophrenic, 80
perineal, 202, 241
phrenic
inferior, 75, 163, 175
left inferior, 165
superior, 75
plantar
deep, 362, 427, 427t, 446
lateral, 362, 438, 440, 441t, 443, 446, 456
medial, 362, 438, 440, 441t, 443, 444, 446, 456
pollicis
dorsalis, 572, 573, 576, 577
princeps, 561, 572, 573, 573t, 606
pontine, 647, 647t
popliteal, 362, 402, 404, 416, 419, 420, 437, 440, 441t
pudendal
external, 102, 241, 269, 362, 370
internal, 212, 213, 218, 222, 224, 225, 225t, 226, 241, 242, 243t, 250, 274, 277, 393t

pulmonary, 27, 29, 34, 35, 68
3-D volume reconstruction and CT angiogram, 41, 92–93
left, 26, 27, 33, 41, 46, 47, 49, 52, 67, 68, 88–90
relationship to bronchi, 41
right, 33, 41, 46, 47, 68, 88–89, 91
radial, 486, 487, 540, 550, 550t, 551, 554, 558, 559, 561, 566, 570–573, 576, 577, 584, 585, 591, 602, 604, 605
dorsal branch, 582
dorsal carpal branch, 576
palmar branch, 572
palmar carpal branch, 570
recurrent, 486, 487, 540, 550, 550t, 551
superficial palmar branch, 566, 570
radicular
anterior, 341, 342
posterior, 341, 342
rectal
inferior, 202, 213, 241
middle, 212, 213, 224, 225, 225t, 226, 241, 242, 243t
superior, 142, 143, 213, 241
renal, 164, 166, 167
accessory, 164
left, 165, 174, 175, 188
right, 153, 174, 187–189
of round ligament, 110
sacral
lateral, 212, 224, 225, 225t, 241, 242, 243t, 277, 341
median, 175, 241
middle, 277
saphenous, 382
scapular, dorsal, 486, 487, 529, 772, 773
scrotal, posterior, 261
sigmoid, 142, 143, 145
sphenopalatine, 670, 693
spinal
anterior, 341, 342
posterior, 341, 342
splenic, 122, 123, 125–127, 130, 131, 133–135, 154, 155, 164, 174, 187–189
striate, anterolateral, 731
stylomastoid, 712
subclavian, 8, 23, 71, 72, 80, 511, 529, 757, 772, 773
left, 46, 47, 49, 66–68, 70, 71, 74, 81, 88–89, 91, 773
right, 25, 26, 66–68, 70, 71, 74, 84, 88–89, 486
subcostal, 75, 101, 163
submental, 763, 778
subscapular, 486, 487, 504, 505t, 509
sulcal, 342
supraduodenal, 130, 134
supraorbital, 632, 632t, 657t
suprarenal, 165, 167, 175
suprascapular, 486, 487, 504, 505t, 528, 529, 531, 537, 772, 773
supratrochlear, 632, 632t, 657t
tarsal
lateral, 362, 425, 427, 427t
medial, 362, 427
temporal
deep, 668, 670
superficial, 626, 627, 632, 632t, 662, 720, 721, 764, 765, 765t
testicular, 113, 116, 117, 145, 152, 153, 162, 163, 215, 216, 225t, 226, 264
thoracic, 175
internal, 8, 20, 22, 23, 48, 66, 67, 70, 72–74, 80, 81, 88–89, 486, 504, 505t, 529, 764, 765, 765t, 773
lateral, 8, 486, 502, 504, 505t, 509
superior, 509
supreme, 504, 505t
thoraco-acromial, 486, 500, 504, 505t, 508, 531
thoracodorsal, 487, 502, 504, 505t
thyroid
inferior, 75, 770–773, 807
superficial, 770, 771
superior, 762–765, 765t, 766, 807
thyroid ima, 749, 771
tibial
anterior, 362, 424, 425, 427, 437, 440, 441t, 457, 472
anterior recurrent, 362, 417, 425
posterior, 362, 436–438, 440, 441t, 443, 446, 451, 457, 458, 472
tympanic, anterior, 670
ulnar, 486, 487, 540, 550, 550t, 551, 555, 556, 558, 559, 566, 567, 570, 572, 573, 602, 604, 605
anterior recurrent, 550, 550t
deep branch, 567, 570, 572, 591
deep palmar branch, 572
dorsal carpal branch, 487, 566, 573, 576, 587
posterior recurrent, 542, 543, 550, 550t
superficial, 541
superior collateral, 486, 487, 504, 505t, 525, 539, 550
ulnar collateral, 521, 600
inferior, 486, 487, 504, 505t, 525, 539, 540, 550, 551
ulnar recurrent, 551
anterior, 486, 487
posterior, 486, 487
umbilical, 118, 144, 225, 225t, 241, 242, 243t
uterine, 212, 234, 235, 240–242, 243t
vaginal, 234, 235, 241, 242, 243t
vertebral, 74, 88–89, 297–299, 333, 335, 338, 341, 350, 352, 486, 529, 638, 640, 642, 646, 647, 647t, 648, 720, 721, 738–740, 764, 765, 765t, 773, 785, 806, 807
vesical, 277
inferior, 216, 226
superior, 224, 225, 225t, 226, 241, 242, 243t
of vestibule of vagina, 241
Asterion, 612
Atlas, 294–297, 350, 621, 720, 721, 743, 751, 808
anterior arch, 296, 297, 350, 750, 810
anterior tubercle, 742
posterior arch, 296, 297, 318, 331, 350, 750
Atrioventricular bundle, 55, 61, 64
Atrium, 694
left, 29, 47, 53, 58, 60, 64
3-D volume reconstruction and CT angiogram, 41, 92–93
interior, 57
magnetic resonance imaging, 88–91
radiograph, 27
right, 26, 27, 29, 46, 47, 49, 50, 53, 57, 60, 64, 84
3-D volume reconstruction and CT angiogram, 92–93
computed tomography, 6
interior, 56
magnetic resonance imaging, 88–91
Auricle, 721
of ear, 703, 704
left, 27, 46, 47, 49, 58, 60, 90
right, 46, 49, 60
Auscultation
of heart, 44
triangle of, 512, 514
Autonomic nervous system, 177, 346
Axilla, 497, 525
anterior wall, 500
contents, 502
medial wall, 509
posterior wall, 509, 510
structures, 508
veins, 501
walls, 502
Axis, 294–297, 333, 743, 751, 785, 808

Back
cutaneous nerves, 514
muscles, 321–329
cervical, 783, 783t
deep, 123, 171, 186, 189, 323, 325, 329t
intermediate, 322, 329t
magnetic resonance imaging, 88–89
superficial, 321, 329t, 513t
transverse section, 324
surface anatomy, 320, 512
Band
central, 569, 583
fascial, 807
lateral, 569, 583
spiral, 561
Bare area, 120, 122, 146, 147
Barium enema, 138
Barium swallow, 132
Basioccipital bone, 297
Bile duct, 122–124, 133, 134, 147, 149–159
Bladder, 96, 97, 118, 120–122, 128, 136, 165, 205, 208–210, 215, 276–283, 311, 470
female, 232, 233, 250
male, 216–222
trigone, 217, 221, 234
uvula, 221
Body
anococcygeal, 208, 232, 261, 262, 273, 275
ciliary, 661, 738, 739
erectile, 255, 266
geniculate
lateral, 734, 735
medial, 734, 735
mamillary, 639, 728, 729, 732–734, 742
perineal, 210, 253, 261–263, 273, 276, 277
pineal, 723, 742
restiform, 734
vertebral, 14–16, 72, 78, 88–90, 123, 288, 289, 301, 302, 310, 337, 743, 806–808, 810
vitreous, 660, 721, 738, 739
Brain
arterial supply, 647, 647t
coronal sections, 741
lobes, 722
frontal, 719, 722, 725, 726, 732, 733
occipital, 722, 725, 726, 728, 732, 733, 738, 739
parietal, 722, 725, 726
temporal, 722, 725, 726, 738–740
magnetic resonance imaging, 732–733, 738–740, 742
median section, 743
overview, 722–724
Brainstem, 722, 723, 734–735
Breast
anatomy, 4, 5
anterior view, 5
arterial supply, 8
axillary process (tail), 4
bed of, 7
imaging of, 6
lymphatic drainage, 9
sagittal view, 5
suspensory ligaments, 4–6
Bregma, 614
Bronchial tree, innervation, 84
Bronchogram, of tracheobronchial tree, 39–40
Bronchopulmonary segments, 36–37
Bronchus, 33, 71, 80, 81
anterior basal segmental, 40
anterior medial basal segmental, 40
anterior segmental, 40, 41
apical segmental, 39, 41
apicoposterior segmental, 39, 40
inferior lobar
left, 38, 39, 41, 74
right, 39, 41
intermediate, 38–40, 74
intrapulmonary, 69
left, 33, 36–38
lingular segmental
inferior, 41
superior, 41
lower lobar, right, 38
main
left, 28, 33, 35, 38, 41, 69, 74, 84
right, 28, 33, 34, 38, 69, 74, 84, 91
middle lobar, 41
left, 38
right, 39
relationship to pulmonary arteries, 41
right, 33, 36–38, 808
segmental, 36–38, 40, 41
superior lobar
left, 38, 39, 41, 74
right, 38, 39, 41, 74
superior segmental, 40

Bulb
of duodenum, 189
of internal jugular vein, 767
olfactory, 639, 719, 726, 818, 844
of penis, 209, 216, 217, 262, 266–268, 276, 277, 279
of vestibule, 272, 274
Bulla, ethmoidal, 695
Bundle, atrioventricular, 55, 61, 64
Bundle branch
left, 64
right, 64
Bursa
anserine, 415t
calcaneal, 438, 454, 457
gastrocnemius, medial semitendinous, 415, 415t
iliopectineal, 373
infrapatellar
deep, 415t, 421
subcutaneous, 415t, 421
obturator internus, 395, 399
olecranon, 544, 549
omental, 120, 121, 123–127, 162
popliteus, 415, 415t
prepatellar, subcutaneous, 410, 415t, 421
retromammary, 5
semimembranosus, 415, 415t
subacromial, 531, 534, 536, 537
subdeltoid, 503
subtendinous, 503, 532, 534, 537, 544, 574, 584
suprapatellar, 414, 415t, 420, 421

Calcaneus, 354, 430, 431, 437, 439, 442, 444, 448, 450, 452–454, 456, 458, 459, 461, 464–466
Calcarine spur, 727
Calices, renal, 165–167
Calvaria, 615, 636
Canal
adductor, 373
anal, 208, 210–212, 214, 232, 261, 268, 275
carotid, 616, 625, 645, 713
central, 723, 724
cervical, 238
condylar, 615
femoral, 371
gastric, 129
hypoglossal, 615, 619, 639
infraorbital, 650
inguinal, 103, 217
dissection, 112
structures forming, 108t
nasolacrimal, 695
obturator, 372
optic, 618, 619, 624, 639, 650
palatine, greater, 720
pterygoid, 617, 624, 702
nerve of, 701, 831
pudendal, 219, 261
pyloric, 124, 129
sacral, 197, 198, 202, 313, 316, 317
semicircular, 704, 709, 714, 738, 739, 832
vertebral, 296, 303
Canaliculus
bile, 151
cochlear, 625
lacrimal, 651
tympanic, 625
vestibular, 625
Canine teeth, 685, 688, 689t
Canthus, lateral, 651
Capillaries, lymphatic, 77
Capitate, 552, 574, 588, 589, 591, 593, 594, 599, 604, 605
Capitulum, 518, 544, 547, 549, 552, 598
Capsule
external, 726, 731–733, 741
extreme, 731–733, 741
internal, 727, 729–733, 740, 741
joint, 12
acromioclavicular, 535
glenohumeral (shoulder), 532, 533
hip, 390, 391, 398
knee, 410, 420, 421
temporomandibular, 674, 675
zygapophysial, 304, 305
renal, 171
synovial, 548
Caput medusae, 161
Cardiac cycle, 62
Carina, 38
Carpal bones, 476–479, 588, 589, 594, 599
Carpal tunnel, 493, 592, 593, 604, 605
Carpal tunnel syndrome, 567
Cartilage
articular, 410, 785
arytenoid, 798, 799, 807, 810
auricular, 703, 704
costal, 3, 10, 12, 22, 24, 48, 102, 103, 123, 124, 186, 499
cricoid, 749, 750, 788–790, 798, 799, 806, 808, 810
epiglottic, 799
nasal, 690
alar, 690, 691
septal, 690, 691
thyroid, 716, 743, 749, 750, 779, 788, 789, 798, 799, 806–808
triradiate, 397
vomeronasal, 691
Caruncle
hymenal, 253
lacrimal, 650, 651
sublingual, 782
Cauda equina, 334, 337, 351
Cave, trigeminal, 644
Cavity
abdominal, posterior, 144, 145
amniotic, 238
articular, 674, 675
glenoid, 533–535, 537
nasal, 28, 611, 691–693, 695–697
oral, 128, 697, 718–720, 792
orbital, 608, 611, 650–653
pericardial, 29, 53, 808
peritoneal, 121, 122
pleural, 28, 29, 72, 808
of temporomandibular joint, 674
tympanic, 705, 708, 710–713
Cecum, 96, 97, 122, 128, 136, 138–140, 144, 145, 160
Celiac arteriogram, 131
Cells
ethmoidal air, 621, 653, 695–698, 719, 721
hair, cochlear, 715
mastoid, 621, 711, 738, 739
Cerebellum, 639, 722, 723, 736–740, 742, 743, 808, 810
tonsil of, 736, 740, 808, 810
Cerebral hemispheres, 722, 723
Cerebrospinal fluid, 286, 352, 724, 738, 739, 806, 810
Cervical regions
anterior, 752, 752t, 753
lateral, 752, 752t, 753, 754–757
posterior, 783, 785
Cervix, 208, 232, 250
Chamber
anterior, 660, 721
posterior, 660
Chiasm, optic, 639, 721, 728, 734, 738, 739, 819, 820
Choana, 616, 790
Cholangiography, endoscopic retrograde, 156, 159
Chorda tympani, 681, 708, 711, 797, 831
Choroid, 660, 661
Cingulum, 728
Circle, cerebral arterial, 646, 649
Cistern
cerebral, 732, 733
chyle, 74, 76, 83, 117
collicular, 732, 733
interpeduncular, 738–740, 763
lumbar, 337
supracerebellar, 740
suprasellar, 738, 739
Claustrum, 726, 731–733, 741
Clavicle, 2–4, 8, 10–12, 24, 27, 39, 80, 96, 296, 476, 478, 479, 492, 494, 495, 498, 503, 511, 518, 519, 529–532, 535–537, 598, 763, 772
Cleft
gluteal, 261
intergluteal, 320
pudendal, 110
Clitoris, 273
angle of, 272
body, 255, 272
crus, 234, 272, 274, 275
deep artery, 241
dorsal artery, 241, 254, 272, 274
dorsal nerve, 254, 269, 270, 272, 274
frenulum, 271
glans, 253, 269, 271, 272
prepuce, 253, 269, 271, 274
suspensory ligament, 271
Clivus, 615, 619
Coccyx, 194–198, 202, 208–210, 216, 222, 232, 262, 273, 279, 312, 313
overview, 286, 288
tip, 263
Cochlea, 704, 714, 715, 832
Colliculus, 738, 739, 742
facial, 735, 738, 739
inferior, 734, 735
seminal, 221
superior, 730, 731, 734, 735, 816
Colon, 161
ascending, 96, 97, 119, 122, 128, 133, 136, 138, 140, 141, 143–145, 148, 160, 162, 186, 188
barium enema, 138
descending, 96, 97, 119, 122, 128, 133, 136–138, 142–145, 148, 160, 162, 163, 186, 188, 189
haustrum of, 139
sigmoid, 128, 137, 138, 142, 144, 145, 160, 163, 215, 233, 282
transverse, 96, 119, 121, 122, 124–126, 128, 136–138, 140–142, 145, 152, 187, 189
Commissure
anterior, 723, 727–729, 732–734, 740
habenular, 732, 733, 735
posterior, 728, 730, 741
Compartment(s)
adductor, 562
of arm, 521, 600
central, 562
infracolic, 122
of leg, 369
perineal, 254–255, 258, 259
supracolic, 122
thenar, 562
of thigh, 369
Compressor urethrae, 256t, 257, 260
Computed tomography
breast, 6
cervical vertebrae, 296, 350
cranium, 697
intervertebral disc, 305
lumbar vertebrae, 351
sacroiliac joint, 317, 351
Computed tomography angiogram
head and neck, 649
thorax, 41, 92–93
Concha, 705
inferior, 611, 690, 691, 694, 695, 700, 702, 719, 720, 738, 739, 810
inferior nasal, 794
middle, 690, 691, 694, 719, 720, 738, 739
superior, 691, 694, 719, 738, 739
Condyle
femoral, 419
lateral, 380, 381, 418
medial, 380, 381
lateral, 413
medial, 413
occipital, 614–617, 785
tibial
lateral, 380, 381, 418
medial, 380, 381, 418
Conjunctiva
bulbar, 650, 651
palpebral, 650
Conus arteriosus, 57
Conus elasticus, 799
Conus medullaris, 334, 337
Cornea, 660, 661, 721
Corona radiata, 725, 726
Coronary circulation, 55
Corpus callosum, 723, 728–730, 740–743
Cortex
cerebral, 634, 636
insular, 732, 733, 740, 742
renal, 166
visual, 820
Costovertebral articulations, 14
Cranial nerves
abducent (CN VI), 640, 644, 645, 652, 654, 656, 812–814, 815t, 821, 822, 822t, 823, 841, 841t, 843

facial (CN VII), 640–642, 663, 701, 708–713, 720, 734, 738, 739, 762, 812–814, 815t, 830, 831, 841, 841t, 843
branches, 627, 629, 634, 662
motor root, 830
glossopharyngeal (CN IX), 335, 640–642, 663, 680, 681, 720, 734, 766, 785–787, 789, 796, 812–814, 815t, 834–835, 841, 843
hypoglossal (CN XII), 335, 640, 641, 662, 663, 667, 680, 681, 720, 763, 766, 779, 780, 785, 786, 812–814, 815t, 839, 841, 841t, 843
lesions, 841, 841t
magnetic resonance imaging, 842–844
nuclei, 816–817
oculomotor (CN III), 640, 641, 643–645, 652, 654, 656, 734, 812–814, 815t, 821, 822, 822t, 823, 841, 841t, 842, 844
olfactory (CN I), 640, 692, 812–814, 815t, 818, 841
optic (CN II), 640, 641, 652, 653, 655–657, 660, 719, 727, 728, 732–734, 738, 739, 812–814, 815t, 819, 820, 841, 842
overview, 812–814
posterior exposures, 642
spinal accessory (CN XI), 333, 334, 511, 529, 642, 662, 663, 667, 720, 755, 762, 763, 766, 785, 807, 812–814, 815t, 838, 841, 841t, 843
summary, 815t
superficial origins, 641
trigeminal (CN V), 631, 631t, 640–643, 812–814, 815t, 824, 841, 842, 844
cutaneous branches, 630
groove for, 615
mandibular division, 824t, 828–829
maxillary division, 824t, 826–827
motor root, 645, 646, 734
ophthalmic division, 824t, 825
sensory root, 644–646, 734
spinal tract, 734
trochlear (CN IV), 640–645, 652, 656, 812–814, 815t, 821, 822, 822t, 823, 841
vagus (CN X), 181, 640–642, 662, 663, 667, 720, 766, 771, 772, 785, 807, 812–814, 815t, 836–837, 841, 843
in abdomen, 181
auricular branch, 703
inferior cardiac branch, 772
left, 25, 42, 48, 49, 65, 67–69, 81, 84, 85, 773, 836
right, 25, 42, 48, 67, 68, 72, 80, 84, 85, 773, 836
vestibulocochlear (CN VIII), 640–642, 709, 715, 734, 735, 738, 739, 812–814, 815t, 832–833, 841, 843
Cranium
base, interior, 618–619
of child, 608–609
computed tomography, 697
facial (frontal) aspect, 610–611
inferior aspect, 616–617
lateral aspect, 612–613
posterior view, 614–615
radiograph, 608, 609, 620–621, 697, 698
superior view, 614
Crest
frontal, 619
iliac, 104, 169, 194–198, 200, 311, 312, 354, 368, 380, 381, 390, 391, 397
infratemporal, 665
intertrochanteric, 381, 398
lacrimal, 613, 650
medial, 442
obturator, 396
occipital
external, 614, 615
internal, 619
pronator, 552
pubic, 106, 199, 380
sacral, 312, 313
median, 194, 195
supinator, 544
supramastoid, 613, 625
supraventricular, 57
urethral, 221
Crista galli, 618–620, 638, 697, 719
Crural region, 354
Crus
cerebral, 727, 729, 734, 735, 738, 739, 741
of clitoris, 234, 272, 274, 275
of diaphragm, 26, 74, 82, 85, 123, 172, 174, 186, 187, 352
lateral, 102, 106, 107, 110, 372
medial, 102, 106, 107, 110
of penis, 262, 266, 267, 276, 277
Cubital tunnel, 465, 542, 543
Cuboid, 427, 431, 444, 449, 453, 454, 458, 459, 461, 464, 466
Cuneiform, 453, 459, 462
first, 452, 465
lateral, 427, 431, 444, 449, 454, 458
medial, 427, 444, 449, 452, 458, 464
middle, 427, 431, 444, 452, 454
Cuneus, 728
Cusp
anterior, 63
commissural, 63
left, 60
posterior, 63
septal, 63

Decussation, ventral tegmental, 741
Dens, 296, 297, 299, 350, 352, 742, 810
of atlas, 750
of axis, 720, 721, 743, 808
Dermatomes, 348
of abdomen, 99
across bed of breast, 7
of lower limb, 360, 361
map, 348
of upper limb, 483
Diaphragm, 23–26, 28, 29, 40, 49, 73–76, 78, 80–83, 85, 118–124, 129, 132, 133, 147, 149, 163, 164, 172–174, 186, 189
central tendon, 24, 29, 73, 174
crura, 26, 74, 82, 85, 123, 172, 174, 186, 187, 352
left dome, 27, 48, 90, 125, 188
lymphatic drainage, 87
magnetic resonance imaging, 90
muscular part, 73
pelvic, 203, 254, 258, 259, 263
right dome, 27, 39, 48, 90, 96, 97, 125, 188
sellar, 643
surface markings, 45
vertebral attachment, 24, 172
Diaphragma sellae, 638, 740
Diastole, 62
Diencephalon, 723, 725–734
Digestive system, 128
Disc
articular, 12, 590, 591
radiocarpal joint, 592
sternoclavicular joint, 530
temporomandibular joint, 674, 675, 785
intervertebral, 286, 297, 300, 352, 810
computed tomography, 305
innervation, 304
ligaments, 306, 307
lumbar, 145, 324
movements, 307
optic, 660, 661
Diverticulum, ileal, 138, 139
Doppler ultrasound, internal carotid artery, 809
Dorsum sellae, 615, 618, 619, 624, 702, 738, 739
Duct
bile, 122–124, 133, 134, 147, 149–157, 159
cochlear, 714, 715, 833
collecting, 167
cystic, 123, 152–156, 159, 186
ejaculatory, 216, 217, 220
hepatic, 154, 155, 159
accessory, 159
common, 123, 152–154, 156, 158, 159, 186
radiograph, 158
variations, 159
lactiferous, 4–6
lymphatic
overview, 77
right, 9, 43, 76, 716, 805
nasolacrimal, 651, 695, 720
pancreatic
accessory, 133, 156, 157
development, 157
main, 133, 156, 157
papillary, 167
parotid, 627, 630, 662, 666, 668
semicircular, 714, 715
submandibular, 681, 779, 780
thoracic, 29, 69, 73–76, 79, 81–83, 117, 119, 123, 339, 716, 773, 805
vestibular, greater, 272, 274
Ductules
efferent, 217
prostatic, 220
Ductus deferens, 113, 116–118, 163, 210, 215–220, 222, 226, 264
ampulla, 216, 217, 220
Ductus reuniens, 714
Duodenal cap, 132
Duodenum, 96, 120–122, 126, 128, 129, 131, 135, 142, 144, 152–155, 158, 159, 162, 188, 189
ascending part, 133t, 156
blood supply, 135
bulb of, 189
descending part, 133t, 145, 156, 157, 186
inferior part, 133t, 145, 156, 186
parts, 133, 133t
radiograph, 132
relationships, 134
superior part, 133t, 156
Dura mater, 297, 335, 336, 338–340, 634, 636, 637–639

Ear
auricle of, 703, 704
external, 704, 705
inner, 704, 705, 709
middle, 704, 705, 709
ossicles, 704, 707
pharyngotympanic tube, 28, 615, 681, 695, 704, 705, 710–713, 720, 785, 790, 794
semicircular canals, 704, 709, 714, 738, 739, 832
tympanic cavity, 705, 708, 710–713
Ejaculatory duct, 216, 217, 220
Eminence
arcuate, 619, 625
frontal, 608, 609, 611, 613
iliopubic, 197, 198, 312, 372, 380
intercondylar, 418
parietal, 608, 609, 613, 614
thenar, 586
Endocardium, 53
Endometrium, 279, 282, 283
Endoscopic retrograde cholangiography and pancreatography, 156, 159
Epicardium, 53
Epicondyle
lateral, 380, 418, 518, 519, 523, 524, 542, 544, 547, 548, 552, 574
medial, 380, 491, 518, 519, 521, 523, 527, 538, 539, 542–544, 546, 548, 552, 574, 598, 600
Epididymis, 112, 113, 116, 117, 216, 217, 264
Epiglottis, 28, 743, 790, 791, 798, 799, 804, 807, 808, 810
Epiphyseal sites, upper limb, 598–599
Esophageal varices, 161
Esophagus, 29, 43, 65–67, 69, 71, 72, 74, 76, 80–82, 84, 85, 119, 122, 124, 127, 129, 161, 162, 174, 186, 188, 771, 773, 807, 808, 810
3-D volume reconstruction and CT angiogram, 92–93
abdominal, 128
arterial supply, 75
computed tomography, 6
lymphatic drainage, 87
magnetic resonance imaging, 88–89
radiograph, 132
thoracic, 128

Ethmoid bone, 610, 611, 613, 619, 623, 650, 690, 691, 695, 700
Expansion, extensor, 426, 427, 569, 574, 581–583, 585
Eye, surface anatomy, 650, 651
Eyeball, 653, 660, 661, 697, 719, 738, 739
Eyelid, 629, 650, 651, 654–655

Fabella, 420, 467
Facet
  articular, 442
    inferior, 300, 350
    superior, 14, 297, 300, 303, 338
  costal, 300
    superior, 14
    transverse, 14
  patellar, 411
  talar, 458
Falx cerebelli, 638, 639, 743, 808
Falx cerebri, 636, 638, 639, 732, 733, 743
Fascia
  abdominal, parietal, 219
  alar, 747
  antebrachial, 493, 542, 549, 602
  axillary, 492
  brachial, 492, 493, 539
  buccopharyngeal, 747
  cervical, 747
    deep, 492
    prevertebral layer, 763
  clavipectoral, 492, 500
  cribriform, 368
  crural, 368
  dartos, 113
  deep, 368, 369, 424, 436, 438
  deltoid, 493
  dorsal, 562
  endoabdominal, 219
  endopelvic, 248, 251, 279
  endothoracic, 72, 129
  extraperitoneal, 218
  gluteal, 383
  hypothenar, 560, 562, 563
  investing, 105, 171, 747
  lower limb, 368
  lumbar, 171
  obturator, 202–204, 212, 219, 258, 259, 262, 399
  omohyoid, 756, 763
  palmar, 560, 562
  pectineal, 373
  pectoral, 3, 4, 492–494
  pelvic
    diaphragmatic, 258, 259
    parietal, 219
    tendinous arch, 219
    visceral, 219, 220
  penile, 258, 265
  perineal, 258, 259
  pharyngobasilar, 786, 795
  plantar, 443
  popliteal, 405, 408, 409, 436
  pretracheal, 747, 769
  prevertebral, 678, 747, 769, 772, 774
  psoas, 163, 171, 202, 218, 310
  rectal, 259
  rectovesical, 209
  renal, 164, 171
  scrotal, 258
  spermatic, 108, 112, 113, 116, 264
  temporal, 634, 666
  thenar, 560, 562, 563
  thoracolumbar, 169, 171, 321, 324, 326, 512, 514
  umbilical, 251
  upper limb, 492, 493
  vesical, 251, 259
  visceral, 258
Fascia lata, 106, 112, 271, 274, 368, 470
  tensor, 250, 275, 368, 373, 375, 376, 377t, 381, 383, 385, 386t, 399, 470
Fascia transversalis, 101, 103, 105, 109, 111, 112, 118, 171
Fasciculus
  inferior fronto-occipital, 726
  lenticular, 741
  mammillothalamic, 729, 741
  superior longitudinal, 725
  uncinate, 726
Fasciculus cuneatus, 735
Fasciculus gracilis, 735, 816
Fat, 4, 453
  axillary, 536
  breast, 5
  encapsulated cushions, 456
  epidural, 286, 339
  extraperitoneal, 105, 109
  parapharyngeal, 738, 739
  perinephric, 171, 187
  perirenal, 152, 164, 171
  in popliteal fossa, 419–421
  prefemoral, 420
  renal, 123
  retrobulbar, 655, 721
  retroperitoneal, 187
  retropubic, 208, 232, 279
  subendocardial, 53
  subpericardial, 57
  subperitoneal, 164
  suprapatellar, 420
Fat body, ischioanal, 274
Fat pad, 73, 80, 81, 110, 111, 209, 443
  buccal, 630, 720, 806
  infrapatellar, 410, 420, 421
  synovial, 548
Fauces, isthmus of, 792–797
Femoral region, 354
Femur, 104, 200, 201, 275, 354, 355, 380, 381, 404, 418–420, 470, 471
  condyle, 419
    lateral, 380, 381, 418
    medial, 380, 381
  distal, 411
  head, 200, 222, 373, 380, 394, 399, 400, 470
    blood supply, 401
    ligament of, 222, 396, 399, 401
  neck, 250, 311, 381, 395, 400
  shaft, 400
Fetus, radiograph, 239
Fibers
  afferent, visceral, 246, 346
  efferent, visceral, 346
  intercrural, 102, 106, 110
  motor, somatic, 357
  parasympathetic, 230, 346, 717
  sympathetic, 230, 246, 346, 347, 717
Fibula, 354, 355, 380, 381, 420, 423, 429, 433, 436, 442, 448, 450, 453, 454, 472–473
  apex, 420
  head, 383, 406, 407, 419, 425, 433, 442, 472
  neck, 418, 425, 433
Filum terminale, 334, 336, 337
Finger pad, 588
Fissure
  calcarine, 731
  cerebral, 722
  horizontal, 25, 32, 34, 35
  lateral, 731–733, 740
  longitudinal, 740
  lung, 32, 96, 97
  oblique, 25, 32, 34, 35
  orbital
    inferior, 650
    superior, 615, 619, 624, 639, 650, 702
  parieto-occipital, 742
  petrotympanic, 625
Flexure
  left colic (splenic), 119, 122, 138, 187, 352
  right colic (hepatic), 119, 122, 126, 136, 138, 144
Flocculus, 736, 738, 739
Floor of mouth, 679, 681
Fold
  aryepiglottic, 790, 804
  axillary
    anterior, 2, 495, 497, 525
    posterior, 2, 495, 497, 512, 525
  conjunctival, semilunar, 650
  gastric, 132
  gastropancreatic, 126
  glossoepiglottic, lateral, 790
  gluteal, 195
  ileocecal, inferior, 139
  inguinal, 194, 195
  rectal, 213
    inferior transverse, 211
  rectouterine, 208, 232, 233, 280, 281
  sacrogenital, 215
  salpingopharyngeal, 790
  semilunar, 137
  sublingual, 681
  synovial, 454, 548, 549, 592, 593
    infrapatellar, 410
  umbilical
    lateral, 118, 219, 233
    medial, 218, 219, 226
    median, 118, 219
  vascular, of cecum, 139
  vesical, transverse, 233
  vestibular, 801, 804, 807
  vocal, 743, 801, 804, 806, 808
Follicle, 282, 283
  lingual, 794
Fontanelle
  anterior, 608, 609
  anterolateral, 608
  posterior, 609
  posterolateral, 608
Foot, 354
  arches, 466
  arteries, 441t
  dorsum, 426, 427, 427t, 449
  joints, 460t
  lateral aspect, 428, 429
  ligaments, 449, 464, 465
  medial, 439
  muscles, 428, 429, 444–447, 444t–447t
  postnatal development, 469
  radiograph, 453
  sole, 443–447, 464, 465
Foramen
  cribriform, 639
  ethmoidal
    anterior, 619, 650
    posterior, 619, 650
  incisive, 615
  infraorbital, 611, 612, 650
  interventricular, 724, 728–733
  intervertebral, 286, 302, 304, 339
  jugular, 615–617, 619, 639, 710
  lacrimal, 650
  mental, 611, 613, 664
  obturator, 196–199, 311, 312, 380
  omental, 120, 123, 124, 153, 162
  palatine, 682
    greater, 615
    lesser, 615
  parietal, 615
  sacral, 310, 313, 317, 334
    anterior, 200
    posterior, 201
  sciatic
    greater, 200–202, 390, 391
    lesser, 201, 202, 390
  sphenopalatine, 695, 699, 700
  sternal, 16
  stylomastoid, 616, 625, 785
  supraorbital, 611
  transverse, 16
  vertebral, 289, 297, 301
  zygomaticofacial, 611, 612, 650
Foramen cecum, 619, 676, 790
Foramen lacerum, 615, 619
Foramen magnum, 297, 334, 335, 350, 615, 617, 619, 639, 742, 743
Foramen ovale, 616, 619, 624, 639
Foramen rotundum, 619, 624, 639, 699, 702
Foramen spinosum, 616, 617, 619, 624
Foramen transversarium, 296, 297, 350
Forceps major, 729, 732, 733
Forceps minor, 729, 732, 733
Forearm, 476, 477
  arteries, 550, 550t, 551
  bones, 552, 574
  magnetic resonance imaging, 603
  muscles, 552, 553t, 554, 574, 575t, 576, 577
  radiograph, 545
  transverse section, 602
Foregut, 67
Fornix, 208, 232, 723, 727–735, 740–743
Fossa
  acetabular, 311, 398, 401
  axillary, 2
  canine, 611, 613
  cerebellar, 619
  coronoid, 518, 544
  cranial
    anterior, 641
    middle, 641, 644–645
    posterior, 641, 642
  cubital, 525, 538–540
  gallbladder, 154, 155
  glenoid, 503, 511, 536, 537
  hypophyseal, 619, 621, 624, 738, 739
  iliac, 196, 197, 200, 312, 373, 380
  incisive, 611, 682
  infraspinous, 519

infratemporal, 615, 622, 664, 665
inguinal
lateral, 219
medial, 118, 219
intercondylar, 381
interpeduncular, 738, 739
intrabulbar, 209
ischioanal, 118, 213, 218, 219, 222, 250, 258, 259, 261, 262, 268, 269, 271, 273–277, 280, 281
jugular, 625
malleolar, 455
mandibular, 615–617, 625, 674, 702
olecranon, 544
oval, 56, 58
pararectal, 215
paravesical, 215, 219, 233
perineal, parietal, 219
popliteal, 402–404, 416
fat in, 419–421
pterygoid, 615, 624, 702
pterygopalatine, 622, 699, 700–702
radial, 518, 544
scaphoid, 615, 624, 702
subarcuate, 625
subscapular, 518, 523
supinator, 544
supraclavicular, lesser, 752, 752t
supraspinous, 519
supravesical, 118, 208, 209, 219
temporal, 610, 612, 664, 665
tonsillar, 794
triangular, 703
Fossae ovalis, limbus, 56
Fovea, for ligament of head of femur, 311, 394, 398, 400
Frenulum
of clitoris, 271
labial, 253
of tongue, 782
Frontal bone, 608, 609, 611, 613, 614, 617–619, 622, 650, 651, 664, 691, 695, 699
Fundus
of gallbladder, 96, 119, 156, 159
ocular, 661
of stomach, 129, 132
of uterus, 234, 237, 279, 282
Furrow, posterior median, 320

Galactogram, 6
Gallbladder, 123, 124, 126–128, 132, 146–148, 150, 152, 153, 156, 157, 160, 186
body, 156, 159
endoscopic retrograde cholangiography, 159
folded, 159
fossa, 154, 155
fundus, 96, 119, 156, 159
lymphatic drainage, 185
mucous membrane, 156
neck, 156, 159
Ganglion
abdominopelvic, 176–178, 179t
aorticorenal, 177
celiac, 85, 163, 176, 177, 179, 181
cervical
middle, 68, 772, 807
superior, 786
cervicothoracic, 68, 72, 84, 85, 776
ciliary, 652, 653, 717, 840, 840t
cochlear, 715, 832
enteric, 214
geniculate, 709
mesenteric
inferior, 176, 177, 230
superior, 176, 177
otic, 681, 717, 840, 840t
parasympathetic, 230, 246
prevertebral, 214
pterygopalatine, 671, 699–701, 717, 831, 840, 840t
spinal, 17, 214, 246, 333, 334, 336, 642, 785
submandibular, 717, 779, 780, 840, 840t
sympathetic, 80–82, 173, 176, 177, 183, 230, 246, 717
thoracic, 68, 84, 85
trigeminal, 644, 717
vestibular, 832
Gas, in colon, 141, 143
Genital organs, female, 234
Genital system, autonomic stimulation effects, 230t
Genitalia, external
female, 253
male, 216
Genu, articularis, 380, 414
Gingiva
facial, 687
palatine, 687
Glabella, 610, 612
Gland
bulbourethral, 216–218, 254, 268
ciliary, 655
lacrimal, 630, 651–653, 701, 719, 831
mammary, 5
palatine, 682, 794
parathyroid, 770, 771
inferior, 770
parotid, 350, 627, 662, 663, 678, 716, 720, 721, 738, 739, 762
pineal, 728–731, 734, 735
prostate, 118, 209, 210, 216–220, 222, 223, 262, 263, 276–279
seminal, 118, 210, 216–220, 222, 276, 277, 279
sublingual, 681, 719, 779, 806, 831
submandibular, 666, 681, 762, 763, 779, 796, 806, 831
suprarenal, 183, 352
left, 97, 123, 125, 131, 133, 162, 163, 165, 181, 186
lymphatic drainage, 182
right, 97, 122, 123, 131, 133, 162–164, 181, 187
tarsal, 655
thyroid, 75, 716, 749, 759, 768–773, 790, 805, 807, 808
vestibular, greater, 272, 274
Glans penis, 116, 216, 217, 252, 264, 266–268
Globus pallidus, 732, 733, 740, 741
Gluteal region, 196
arteries, 393t
ligaments, 390, 391
muscles, 384, 385, 386t, 388, 389
nerves, 392t
Gonadal shield, 143
Gonads, descent, 114
Grasping movements, 596, 597
Gray matter, 732, 733, 738–740, 742
Great vessels, 46–47, 66
Groove
bicipital, 521, 525, 537, 600
carotid, 619, 702
costal, 13
deltopectoral, 525
facial artery, 664
fibularis brevis, 433, 450
fibularis longus, 427, 431, 433, 444, 447, 450
flexor digitorum longus, 433, 450
flexor hallucis longus, 433, 436, 444, 445, 450, 452, 455, 464
greater petrosal nerve, 619
infraorbital, 650
intertubercular, 503, 518
lacrimal, 650
meniscus
lateral, 411
medial, 411
middle meningeal, 621
middle meningeal artery, 625
middle temporal artery, 625
obturator, 197
occipital, 615
petrosal sinus, 618
prechiasmatic, 619
radial, 519
semimembranosus, 433
sigmoid sinus, 618, 625
superior petrosal sinus, 625
superior sagittal sinus, 618
tibialis posterior, 433, 450, 452
transverse sinus, 618, 619
trigeminal nerve, 615
ulnar nerve, 519
Gubernacular remnant, 116
Gutter, paracolic, 122
Gyrus
angular, 725
cingulate, 728
dentate, 729, 741
frontal
inferior, 725
middle, 725
superior, 725, 728
lingual, 728
occipitotemporal, 728
parahippocampal, 728, 729
postcentral, 722, 725
precentral, 722, 725
supramarginal, 725
temporal
inferior, 725
middle, 725
superior, 725
transverse, 725
Gyrus rectus, 732, 733

Hallux valgus, 463
Hamate, 552, 574, 587, 593, 594, 599, 604, 605
Hamulus, pterygoid, 615, 617, 624, 681, 702, 797
Hand, 476, 477
anastomoses, 487
arteries, 572–573, 573t, 576
bones, 552, 588, 589
cutaneous innervation, 578, 579
dorsal venous network, 491, 580
dorsum, 580–582
imaging of, 589
lateral aspect, 584–586
medial aspect, 587
muscles, 552
radiograph, 586, 589
surface anatomy, 560
Haustra, 136–140
Head
autonomic ganglia, 840, 840t
autonomic innervation, 717–718
blood supply, 649
lymphatic drainage, 716
magnetic resonance imaging, 718–721, 809
median anatomical section, 808
veins, 716
Heart, 40, 46–47
3-D volume reconstruction, 46, 47
apex, 26–28, 46, 58, 59, 96
auscultation, 44
circulation, 55
conduction system, 64, 129
coronal section, 28
crux, 52, 64
diaphragmatic surface, 55
excised, 60
fibrous skeleton, 61
innervation, 84
left, interior, 58, 59
lymphatic drainage, 86, 87
posterior relationships, 65
right, interior, 56, 57
sternocostal surface, 25, 49, 55
surface markings, 44, 45
Helix, 703
Hemivertebra, 318
Hepatocytes, 151
Hernia, inguinal, 115
Hiatus
aortic, 165, 174
esophageal, 74, 174
greater petrosal nerve, 625
sacral, 313
semilunar, 695, 696
urogenital, 254, 263
Hip bone, 194–196, 198, 286, 312, 316, 354, 355, 397
Hippocampus, 727, 729, 738–741
Hook of hamate, 571, 588, 589, 593, 594, 604, 605
Humerus, 476–479, 503, 518, 519, 521, 523, 534, 546–548, 600
anatomical neck, 533
capitulum, 523
distal, 598
head, 503, 534, 536, 537
lymph nodes, 9
proximal, 598
shaft, 598
supracondylar process, 541
surgical neck, 532, 533, 536
Hyoid bone, 681, 716, 743, 749–751, 759, 762, 763, 766, 778, 797, 808, 810
Hypophysis, 740, 742, 808
Hypothalamus, 723, 728, 742
Hysterosalpingogram, 284

Ileocecal region, 139
Ileum, 96, 121, 128, 136, 137, 139, 140, 144, 145
Ilium, 196, 311, 312, 316, 317, 373, 381, 390, 391, 397, 398
arcuate line, 199
articular surface, 312
body, 351
Incisor teeth, 685, 687, 688, 689t

Incisure, angular, 129, 132
Incus, 704, 706, 707, 709, 711
Infratemporal region, 668–669
Infundibulum, 639, 643, 729, 734, 738, 739, 742
  ethmoidal, 697
  pulmonary, 88–89
Inguinal region
  dissection, 112
  embryology, 114
  female, 110–112
  male, 106–109
Insula, 725, 731, 741
Intertendinous connection, 581, 582
Intestines, 136
Iris, 650, 651, 660, 661
Ischium, 196, 202, 222, 275, 312, 381, 391, 397
  body, 197, 312, 397
  ramus, 197, 199, 312, 397
Isthmus
  oropharyngeal, 792–797
  thyroid gland, 768

Jejunum, 96, 121, 128, 132, 134, 136, 137, 140, 144, 145, 162
Joint
  acromioclavicular, 519, 530, 531, 535, 536
  atlanto-occipital, 298, 299, 332t
  atlantoaxial, 297, 299, 332t
  calcaneocuboid, 430, 460t
  carpometacarpal, 571, 585, 590
  costochondral, 10
  costotransverse, 14, 15, 301
  craniovertebral, 298
  cubonavicular, 462
  cuneonavicular, 460t, 462
  elbow, 476, 477
    anastomoses, 487
    articular surfaces, 549
    bones, 544
    lateral aspect, 547
    magnetic resonance imaging, 546
    medial aspect, 546
    posterior aspect, 542, 543
    radiograph, 544, 547
    synovial capsule, 548
  glenohumeral (shoulder), 476, 477, 528, 530
    interior, 534, 535
    ligaments and articular capsule, 532, 533
    magnetic resonance imaging, 537
    radiograph, 536
    ultrasound, 537
  of head of rib, 14, 301
  hip, 250, 354, 390, 391, 394–395
    coronal section, 398
    magnetic resonance imaging, 399
    radiograph, 398
    transverse section, 399
  humeroulnar, 544
  intercarpal, 591
  interchondral, 12
  intermetatarsal, 460t
  interphalangeal, 460t, 552, 580
    distal, 552, 589, 595
    proximal, 552, 580, 589, 595
  manubriosternal, 10, 12, 48
  metacarpophalangeal, 552, 580, 589, 595
  metatarsophalangeal, 460t, 463
  midcarpal, 585, 593
  patellofemoral, 418
  radiocarpal, 590–592
  radioulnar
    distal, 545, 590, 591
    proximal, 544, 545
  sacrococcygeal, 196
  sacroiliac, 196–199, 310, 311
    articular surfaces, 316
    CT scan, 317, 351
    ligaments, 316
  sternoclavicular, 12, 88–89, 530, 772
  sternocostal, 12
  subtalar, 430, 458, 460t
  talocalcaneal, 459
  talocalcaneonavicular, 458, 460t
  tarsal, transverse, 458, 461
  tarsometatarsal, 460t, 462
  temporomandibular, 612, 663, 666
    movements, 673, 673t
    muscles acting on, 672, 672t
    sectional anatomy, 674–675
  tibiofibular
    proximal, 419
    superior, 442
  uncovertebral, 295, 296
  xiphisternal, 10, 12, 48
  zygapophysial, 296, 302, 304–306, 310
Junction
  anorectal, 211
  corneoscleral, 650
  costochondral, 26
  duodenojejunal, 122, 124, 135, 137, 144
  esophagogastric, 129
  gastroesophageal, 189
  ileocecal, 141
  neurocentral, 290
  xiphisternal, 499

Kidney, 145, 171
  anomalies, 168
  calices, 165–167
  cortex, 166
  ectopic pelvic, 168
  exposures, 169–171
  external features, 166
  hilum, 171
  horseshoe, 168
  left, 97, 122–125, 133, 162, 164, 165, 352
  magnetic resonance imaging, 187–189
  medulla, 166
  right, 97, 122–124, 126, 133, 152, 153, 162, 171, 352
  segments, 167
  structure, 166
  ultrasound, 191
Knee, 354
  anastomoses, 416–417
  anterior aspect, 406, 407
  articular surfaces, 411
  bursae, 415t
  cavity, 421
  coronal section, 419
  distended, 414, 415
  joint capsule, 410, 420, 421
  lateral aspect, 409
  ligaments, 411, 412
  magnetic resonance imaging, 419–421
  medial aspect, 408
  radiograph, 418, 420
  sagittal section, 420–421
Kyphosis
  sacral, 287
  thoracic, 287

Labium majus, 110, 208, 232, 253, 269, 280, 281
Labium minus, 208, 232, 253, 269, 273
Labrum
  acetabular, 394, 396, 398
  glenoid, 503, 533–535, 537
Labyrinth
  bony, 714
  membranous, 714
Lacrimal bone, 611–613, 650, 690, 691, 695, 700
Lambda, 612, 614
Lamina
  chorionic, 238
  of vertebra, 289, 296, 297, 301, 303, 310, 806
Large intestine, lymphatic drainage, 185
Laryngocele, 800
Laryngopharynx, 128, 790, 807, 810
Laryngoscopy, 804
Larynx, 28, 128, 807, 808
  external, 800
  inlet, 790, 804
  internal, 801
  lymphatic drainage, 805
  magnetic resonance imaging, 804
  muscles, 802, 802t
Leg, 354
  anterior aspect, 422–425
  arteries, 441t
  bones, 380, 381, 433
  deep vessels, 424, 425
  lateral aspect, 428, 429
  magnetic resonance imaging, 472–473
  muscles, 423t, 424, 428, 429
    deep, 425, 432t, 436, 437
    superficial, 422, 432t, 434, 435
  nerves, 424, 424t, 425
  posterior, 432–437
  proximal, 380, 381
  transverse sections, 472–473
Lemniscus
  lateral, 734, 735
  medial, 734, 735
Lens, 660, 721, 738, 739
Ligament
  acetabular, transverse, 396, 398
  acromioclavicular, 531
    superior, 530, 532
  alar, 299
  anococcygeal, 250
  anular, 543, 545–548, 551
  apical, 297
  arcuate
    lateral, 172, 174
    medial, 172, 174, 175
    median, 74
  bifurcate, 449, 454, 458
  broad, of uterus, 208, 233–237, 240, 282, 283
  calcaneocuboid
    dorsal, 454, 458
    medial, 454
    plantar, 464
  calcaneofibular, 430, 450, 451, 454, 458
  calcaneonavicular
    lateral, 454, 458
    plantar, 447, 452, 458, 464, 465
  calcaneotibial, 450
  carpal, palmar, 493
  collateral
    of digit, 571, 595
    fibular, 405, 409, 411, 412, 414, 419
    radial, 547, 548, 590
    tibial, 405, 408, 411, 412, 419
    ulnar, 546, 548, 549, 590
  commissural
    distal, 561
    proximal, 561
  conoid, 532
  coracoacromial, 523, 530–533, 535
  coracoclavicular, 529, 530, 532
  coracohumeral, 523, 535
  coronal, 408
  coronary, 120, 122, 146–148, 162, 411
  costoclavicular, 12, 530
  costotransverse, 15
    lateral, 15, 18, 327
    posterior, 327
    superior, 15, 17, 301, 327
  of costovertebral articulations, 15
  costoxiphoid, anterior, 12
  cricothyroid, median, 801
  cricovocal, 801
  cruciate
    anterior, 411–413, 419–421
    inferior longitudinal band, 297
    posterior, 411–413, 415, 419–421
    superior longitudinal band, 297
  cruciform, 299
  cuboideonavicular, dorsal, 458
  cubonavicular, plantar, 465
  cuneocuboid, plantar, 465
  cuneonavicular
    dorsal, 449
    plantar, 465
  deltoid, 438, 448–450, 452, 456
  denticulate, 334, 335
  falciform, 118, 119, 121–123, 126, 146–148, 152, 162, 186
  fundiform, of penis, 107
  gastrocolic, 119, 124–127, 129, 144
  gastrophrenic, 119
  gastrosplenic, 119, 123–125, 129, 131, 164
  glenohumeral
    inferior, 533, 534
    middle, 533, 534
    superior, 533, 534
  of head of femur, 222, 396, 399, 401
  of head of fibula, 442
  hepatoduodenal, 119, 126, 129, 154, 162
  hepatogastric, 119, 126, 129, 154
  humeral, transverse, 530, 532, 537
  hyoepiglottic, 799
  iliofemoral, 200, 201, 394–396, 399, 400
  iliolumbar, 200, 201, 314, 315
  of inferior vena cava, 146
  inguinal, 98, 101, 104, 106, 107, 109, 110, 200, 371–373, 400
  interchondral, 12
  interclavicular, 12, 530
  intermetatarsal

dorsal, 449
plantar, 464, 465
interspinous, 295, 297, 305, 308, 324
intra-articular, 12, 15, 301
ischiofemoral, 395
lacunar, 106, 202, 371–373, 399
lateral
of ankle, 451
of bladder, 220, 251
of temporomandibular joint, 674
longitudinal
anterior, 15, 17, 145, 200, 295, 297, 298, 301, 306, 308, 314, 339
posterior, 297, 306–308
medial, of ankle, 451, 452, 457, 458, 465
meniscofemoral, 419
posterior, 412
metacarpal
deep transverse, 571
interosseous, 590
superficial transverse, 561
metatarsal
deep transverse, 446
superficial transverse, 443
nuchal, 295, 328, 331, 333, 785, 810
of ovary, 233, 236, 237
palmar, 568, 571, 583, 591, 595
palpebral
lateral, 630
medial, 630
patellar, 374–376, 380, 383, 406, 408, 409, 411, 420–422, 424, 425
pectineal, 202, 371
perineal, transverse, 267
periodontal, 687
peritoneal, 120
phrenicocolic, 119, 122, 125
phrenicoesophageal, 129
pisohamate, 552, 570, 571, 587
pisometacarpal, 552, 571, 587
plantar, 446, 447
long, 447, 464
popliteal, oblique, 405
pubic, inferior, 202, 208, 232
pubofemoral, 200
puboprostatic, 209, 210, 263
pubovesical, 251
pulmonary, 34, 35
radiate, 15, 17, 301
sternocostal, anterior, 12
radiocarpal, palmar, 571
radioulnar, 551
retinacular, 583
round, 234
artery of, 110
of liver, 118, 119, 123, 146–148, 152, 154
of uterus, 110, 111, 122, 208, 232, 233, 248, 269, 271, 280, 281
sacrococcygeal
anterior, 200, 314
posterior, 201, 315
sacroiliac
anterior, 200, 314, 316
interosseous, 316, 317
posterior, 201, 315, 316, 390
sacrospinous, 200, 202, 222, 314–316, 390, 391
sacrotuberous, 200–202, 212, 262, 263, 273, 314–316, 390, 391
scapular, superior transverse, 517, 529
skin, 561, 567
sphenomandibular, 674, 681
splenorenal, 122–124, 127, 131, 162, 164
sternoclavicular, anterior, 12, 530
sternohyoid, 350
stylohyoid, 681, 721, 785, 797
stylomandibular, 674, 785
supraspinous, 201, 295, 300, 305, 308, 315
suspensory
of axilla, 492
of breast, 4–6
of clitoris, 271
of lens, 660
of ovary, 208, 232, 233, 236, 237, 248
of penis, 112, 116, 264
talocalcanean
interosseous, 448, 449, 454, 456, 458
lateral, 454
talofibular
anterior, 430, 448, 449, 454
posterior, 450, 451, 456, 457
posterior inferior, 450
talonavicular, dorsal, 449, 452, 454
tarsometatarsal
dorsal, 449
plantar, 464, 465
thyrohyoid, 801
tibiocalcanean, 450, 451
tibiofibular
anterior, 442
anterior inferior, 430, 448, 449, 454
interosseous, 456
posterior, 442, 450
posterior inferior, 450, 451
tibiotalar, posterior, 450–452
transverse, 297, 299, 350, 721
inferior, 442
trapezoid, 532
triangular, 122, 125–127, 146–148, 162
umbilical
medial, 208, 218, 219, 224, 225, 225t, 232, 233, 238, 242
median, 218, 219
uterosacral, 251
vestibular, 801
vocal, 807
Ligamentum arteriosum, 41, 46, 47, 49, 51, 67–69, 75, 81, 409
Ligamentum flavum, 297, 304–306, 308, 338, 808
Ligamentum venosum, 147, 154
Line
arcuate, 103, 118, 199, 219, 312
epiphyseal, 419
of Gennari, 731
gluteal
anterior, 381, 390, 397
inferior, 381, 390, 397
posterior, 381, 390, 397
intertrochanteric, 311, 380, 394
nuchal
inferior, 614, 615, 617
superior, 328, 330, 613–615
oblique, 611, 613
anterior, 544, 552
posterior, 544, 574
pain, pelvic, 230, 231
pectinate, 211
pectineal, 381
soleal, 381, 433
spiral, 381
supracondylar
lateral, 381
medial, 381
temporal, 610
inferior, 613, 614
superior, 613, 614
vertical, 433
Linea alba, 2, 98, 102, 103, 105–107, 351
Linea aspera, 381
Linea semilunaris, 98, 497
Lingula, 26, 35, 41
Lips, 128
Liver, 96, 97, 121, 124, 125, 127, 128, 152, 161, 352
anterior surface, 146
caudate lobe, 123, 125–127, 146–148, 150, 151, 151t, 152, 162, 186
computed tomography, 6
flow of blood and bile in, 151
lobes, 119, 123–126, 146–148, 150, 151, 151t, 160, 162
lobules, 151
lymphatic drainage, 185
magnetic resonance imaging, 187–189
posterior relations, 148
quadrate lobe, 126, 147, 154, 155
segments, 150, 151, 151t
superior surface, 146
visceral (posteroinferior) surface, 147
Lobes
of brain, 722
frontal, 719, 722, 725, 726, 732, 733
occipital, 722, 725, 726, 728, 732, 733, 738, 739
parietal, 722, 725, 726
temporal, 722, 725, 726, 738–740
of liver, 119, 123–126, 146–148, 150, 151, 151t, 160, 162
caudate, 123, 125–127, 146–148, 150, 151, 151t, 152, 162, 186
quadrate, 126, 147, 154, 155
of lung, 28, 32
left, 32, 33, 41
inferior, 25, 186, 188, 189
superior, 25
right, 32, 33, 41
inferior, 83, 187–189
middle, 25
superior, 83
Lobule
of auricle, 703
fat, 5
inferior parietal, 725
liver, 151
paracentral, 728
Lordosis
cervical, 287
lumbar, 287
Lower limb
arteries, 362
bones, 354, 355
bony anomalies, 467
cutaneous nerves, 359
dermatomes, 360, 361
fascia, 368
fascial compartments, 369
joints, 354
lymphatic drainage, 366
motor nerves, 356
myotatic (deep tendon) reflexes, 357
myotomes, 357
postnatal development, 468–469
regions, 354
veins
deep, 363
superficial, 364, 365
Lunate, 552, 574, 586–589, 591–594, 599
Lung, 147
apex, 32, 34, 35
cardiac notch, 26, 32, 96
coronal section, 28
costal surface, 25
extent of, 30–31
fissures, 32, 96, 97
innervation, 42
left, 28, 29, 48, 65, 68, 69, 96, 352
apex, 25, 26
bronchi, 33, 36–38
computed tomography, 6
inferior lobe, 25, 186, 188, 189
lobes, 32, 33, 41
magnetic resonance imaging, 88–91
mediastinal surface and hilum, 35
superior lobe, 25
lobes, 28, 32
lymphatic drainage, 43, 87
mediastinal surface, 25, 34–35
right, 28, 29, 65, 68, 69, 352
apex, 39, 96
bronchi, 33, 36–38
computed tomography, 6
inferior lobe, 83, 187–189
lobes, 32, 33, 41
magnetic resonance imaging, 88–91
mediastinal surface and hilum, 34
middle lobe, 25
superior lobe, 83
root, 25, 28, 48, 81
surface markings, 31t, 45
topography, 26
Lymph nodes, 68, 134, 275, 333
aortic arch, 43
apical, 9
appendicular, 185
auricular, posterior, 662
axillary, 9, 503
apical, 489
central, 489
humeral, 489
pectoral, 489
subscapular, 489
bronchopulmonary, 35, 43
celiac, 182, 184, 185
central, 9
cervical
deep, 676
inferior, 43, 716
superior, 716
superficial, 716
colic, 185

Lymph nodes—*continued*
cubital, 489, 538
cystic, 185
diaphragmatic
inferior, 185
superior, 86, 185
epicolic, 185
gastro-omental, 184
hepatic, 185
humeral, 9
ileocolic, 185
iliac
common, 182, 228, 229, 229t, 244, 245, 245t
external, 182, 228, 229, 229t, 244, 245, 245t
internal, 182, 228, 229, 244, 245
infraclavicular, 9, 489
infrahyoid, 676, 716
inguinal, 107, 117
deep, 109, 228, 229, 244, 245, 366
superficial, 228, 229, 229t, 244, 245, 245t, 366, 367, 370
interpectoral, 9
jugulo-omohyoid, 676, 716
jugulodigastric, 676, 716
lumbar, 117, 183, 185, 228, 229, 244, 245
mastoid, 716
mediastinal, posterior, 76
mesenteric
inferior, 182, 185, 228, 229, 244, 245
superior, 182, 184, 185
occipital, 716
overview, 77
pancreatic, 184
pancreaticoduodenal, 153, 184
paracolic, 145, 185
paraesophageal, 185
pararectal, 228, 229, 244, 245
parasternal, 9, 22, 86, 185
paratracheal, 716
parotid, 662, 716
pectoral, 9
popliteal, 366
preauricular, 662
prelaryngeal, 716
pretracheal, 716
pulmonary, 43
retroauricular, 716
retropharyngeal, 676, 716
sacral, 228, 229, 229t, 244, 245, 245t
splenic, 184
submandibular, 676, 716, 762
submental, 676, 716
subpyloric, 184
subscapular, 9
supraclavicular, 9
suprapyloric, 184
thoracic, 86, 87
tracheal, 43
tracheobronchial, 74
inferior, 43
superior, 43
Lymphatic drainage, 131
breast, 9
gallbladder, 185
head and neck, 716
large intestine, 185
larynx, 805
liver, 185
lower limb, 366
lung, 43, 87
overview, 77
pancreas, 184
pelvis and perineum
female, 244–245, 245t
male, 228–229, 229t
scrotum, 117
small intestine, 184
spleen, 184
stomach, 184
suprarenal gland, 182
testis, 117
thorax, 86–87
tongue, 676
trachea, 805
upper limb, 489

Macula, 661, 715
Macula lutea, 660
Magnetic resonance imaging
abdomen, 186–189, 191
ankle, 456, 457
arm, 601
brain, 732–733, 738–740, 742
cranial nerves, 842–844
elbow joint, 546
forearm, 603
glenohumeral (shoulder) joint, 537
head, 718–721, 809
hip joint, 399
knee, 419–421
larynx, 804
leg, 472–473
nasopharynx and oral cavity, 718–720
oropharynx, 721
patellofemoral joint, 418
pelvis and perineum, 276–282
teeth, 806
thigh, 470–471
thorax, 88–91
through carpal tunnel, 604, 605
through palm, 606
vertebrae
cervical, 352
lumbar, 343
thoracic, 300, 352
vertebral artery, 88–89
Malleolus
lateral, 354, 422, 426, 427, 429, 430, 433, 448–451, 453–457
medial, 354, 422, 426, 427, 433, 436, 438, 448–452, 454, 456, 457, 464, 472
Malleus, 704–709, 711
Mammogram, 6
Mandible, 608, 611, 613, 614, 620, 622, 664, 719, 738, 739, 743, 779, 808, 810
body, 609, 611, 612, 666, 778, 806
head, 664, 674
inferior border, 610, 612
internal surface, 665
medial aspect, 681
neck, 664, 720
ramus, 721
Mandibular teeth, 611
Manubrium, 10, 12, 21, 24, 29, 40, 48, 88–89, 499, 530, 808, 810
Margin
costal, 10, 24
infraorbital, 611
sphenoid, 625
supraorbital, 611
Mass
fatty, 350
lateral, 297, 350
Mater
arachnoid, 334, 335, 338–340, 634, 636
dura, 297, 335, 336, 338–340, 634, 636, 637–639
pia, 339, 573, 634, 636
Maxilla, 608, 609, 611, 613, 617, 622, 650, 664, 691, 695, 721, 738, 739
Maxillary teeth, 611
Meatus
acoustic
external, 612, 617, 625, 666, 703–706, 712
internal, 615, 619, 625, 639, 705, 712, 738, 739, 832
inferior, 694, 697, 720
middle, 694, 697
superior, 694
Mediastinum, 28
anterior, 29
inferior, 29
left side, 81
middle, 29
posterior, 29
innervation, 84
lymphatic drainage, 87
structures, 82–83
right side, 80
subdivisions, 29
superior, 29, 67–69, 72
innervation, 84
root of neck, 67
superficial dissection, 66
topography, 26
Medulla oblongata, 352, 722, 723, 734, 738, 739, 743, 808, 810
Membrane
areolar, 152, 153
atlanto-occipital
anterior, 297, 298
posterior, 295, 297, 298, 785
costocoracoid, 492
intercostal
external, 20–22
internal, 17, 18
interosseous, 369, 425, 442, 449, 472, 493, 546, 547, 551, 591, 602
obturator, 196, 202, 250, 372, 396
perineal, 202, 209, 210, 217, 218, 258, 259, 261, 262, 267, 268, 271, 272, 274, 280–282
quadrangular, 801
synovial, 12, 396, 398, 410, 421, 592
tectorial, 297–299
thyrohyoid, 770, 807
tympanic, 608, 703–706, 708, 711–713
Meninges, 335, 636
Meniscus
lateral, 409, 411–413, 419
medial, 408, 410–413, 419, 420
Mesentery, 120–122, 134, 137, 144, 148, 157, 162
Mesoappendix, 139
Mesocolon
sigmoid, 122, 137, 144, 145, 212, 215, 233
transverse, 120–122, 125, 126, 144, 145, 148, 162
Mesoesophagus, 73
Mesosalpinx, 236, 237
Mesotendon, 569
Mesovarium, 236
Metacarpals, 476–479, 552, 574, 582, 589, 590, 594, 595, 598, 599, 606
fifth, 587, 588, 594
first, 585, 586, 588, 594, 606
Metatarsals, 427, 431, 444, 453, 462, 464–466
fifth, 430, 431, 465
first, 439, 449, 452, 463, 465
heads, 443, 447
Meyer loop, 726
Midbrain, 639, 643, 723, 734, 738–740, 742, 743
Molar teeth, 685, 687, 688, 689t, 719
Mons pubis, 253, 269, 271
Mucosa, nasal, 818
Muscle
abdominal, posterior, 147
abductor brevis, 447
abductor digiti minimi, 430, 444, 444t, 445, 447, 456, 458, 552, 564, 565t, 566, 567, 570, 587, 606
abductor hallucis, 438, 444, 444t, 445, 447, 451, 452, 456
abductor pollicis
brevis, 552, 561, 564, 565t, 566, 567, 570, 606
longus, 481, 552, 566, 567, 571, 574, 575t, 576, 577, 581, 582, 584–586, 602, 604, 605
adductor brevis, 222, 375, 378t, 380–382, 396, 447, 447t, 470
adductor hallucis, 447
oblique head, 446, 446t
transverse head, 446, 446t
adductor longus, 222, 372–375, 378t, 379–382, 396, 470
adductor magnus, 375, 378t, 379–382, 384, 385, 388, 389, 396, 405, 408, 470
adductor pollicis, 480, 552, 564, 565t, 566, 567, 577, 584–586, 606
oblique head, 570
transverse head, 570
anconeus, 481, 519, 542, 543, 549, 574, 575t, 576, 577
ansa subclavia, 72
aryepiglottic, 791
arytenoid, 807
oblique, 802, 802t
transverse, 802, 802t
auricular, posterior, 662
axioappendicular, 499t
biceps brachii, 480, 491, 510, 521–525, 538–540, 552, 600
attrition of long head, 541
long head, 22, 502, 503, 508, 520, 520t, 521–523, 525, 530, 533, 537, 600
short head, 22, 499, 502, 503, 508, 518, 520, 520t, 521–523, 525, 530, 534, 600
third head, 541

biceps femoris, 380, 402, 403, 406, 407, 409, 419, 421, 434, 435, 437, 470
long head, 381, 383–385, 387t, 388, 389, 396, 470
short head, 381, 383–385, 387t, 388, 389, 470
brachialis, 480, 499, 502, 510, 518–520, 520t, 521–525, 527, 539, 540, 549, 552, 600
brachioradialis, 481, 518, 522, 524, 526, 527, 539, 540, 542, 546, 549, 552, 554, 556, 559, 571, 574, 575t, 576, 577, 581, 585, 602
buccinator, 626, 629t, 630, 662, 666, 668, 678, 712, 716, 721, 797
bulbospongiosus, 209, 210, 218, 255, 256t, 257, 260, 261, 271, 272
coccygeus, 203, 203t, 204, 210, 212, 254, 263, 273
nerve to, 206, 207, 207t
compressor urethrae, 254
coracobrachialis, 22, 480, 499, 502, 503, 508, 510, 518, 520, 520t, 521, 522, 525, 541, 600
corpus cavernosum, 216, 255, 261, 266–268, 276–279
corpus spongiosum, 216, 217, 255, 261, 266–268, 278, 279
corrugator supercilii, 626, 630
cremaster, 107, 108, 111–113, 116
cricoarytenoid
lateral, 802, 802t, 803
posterior, 802, 802t, 803
cricopharyngeus, 788, 788t
cricothyroid, 759, 770, 802, 802t, 803
dartos, 113
deltoid, 2, 4, 481, 490, 491, 495, 499–503, 508, 517–519, 522, 523, 525–529, 531, 534, 536, 537
acromial part, 513, 513t, 514, 524
clavicular part, 513, 513t, 521, 524, 600
spinal part, 320, 512, 513, 513t, 514, 521, 524, 600
depressor anguli oris, 626, 630, 662, 746
depressor labii inferioris, 626, 746
digastric, 330
anterior belly, 681, 758, 760, 761, 761t, 762, 763, 778
fascial sling, 763
posterior belly, 333, 350, 666, 667, 681, 721, 761, 761t, 785
nerve to, 662
erector spinae, 123, 171, 320, 323, 324, 328, 329t, 351
extensor carpi radialis
brevis, 481, 540, 574, 575t, 576, 577, 581, 582, 584, 585, 602, 604, 605
longus, 481, 518, 524, 527, 540, 542, 549, 552, 574, 575t, 576, 577, 581, 582, 584–586, 602, 604, 605
extensor carpi ulnaris, 481, 543, 552, 574, 575t, 576, 577, 581, 582, 587, 602, 604, 605
extensor digiti minimi, 481, 574, 575t, 576, 577, 581, 582, 602, 604, 605
extensor digitorum, 431, 481, 569, 574, 575t, 576, 577, 580–582, 585, 602, 604, 605
brevis, 422, 424–428, 430
longus, 422, 423, 423t, 424, 426, 428–431, 436, 457, 472
extensor hallucis
brevis, 422, 426–428, 431
longus, 422, 423, 423t, 424, 426–428, 431, 457, 472
extensor indicis, 481, 574, 575t, 576, 577, 581, 582, 602, 604, 605
extensor pollicis
brevis, 481, 574, 575t, 576, 577, 580–582, 584–586, 602, 604, 605
longus, 481, 574, 575t, 576, 577, 580–582, 584–586, 602, 604–606
extensor retinaculum, 368, 458, 576, 577, 581, 582, 587
facial expression, 626, 628–629, 629t, 634
fibularis brevis, 422–425, 427–429, 429t, 430, 431, 433–435, 439, 449, 454, 456, 457, 472
fibularis longus, 422–425, 428, 429, 429t, 430, 431, 434, 435, 439, 447, 454, 456–458, 472
fibularis tertius, 422, 423, 423t, 424, 426, 427, 429–431, 457
flexor carpi
radialis, 480, 540, 552, 553t, 554, 568, 570, 571, 585, 593, 602, 604, 605
ulnaris, 480, 543, 549, 552, 553t, 554–556, 559, 566, 570, 571, 574, 587, 593, 602
flexor digiti minimi, 446, 446t, 447
brevis, 552, 564, 565t, 567, 570
flexor digitorum
brevis, 438, 444, 444t, 445, 447, 456
longus, 432t, 433–439, 443, 445, 447, 448, 451, 456–458, 472
profundus, 480, 543, 552, 553t, 556, 557, 568, 570, 571, 574, 602, 604–606
superficialis, 480, 518, 543, 552, 553t, 555, 558, 566, 568, 570, 571, 602, 604–606
flexor hallucis
brevis, 439, 445, 446, 446t, 447, 452
longus, 432t, 433, 435–439, 443, 445, 447, 448, 456–458, 472
flexor pollicis
brevis, 552, 561, 564, 565t, 566, 567, 570, 606
longus, 480, 552, 553t, 555–557, 568, 602, 604–606
flexor retinaculum, 434, 436–438, 493, 554, 564, 567, 568, 570, 571, 591–593, 604, 605
frontalis, 634
gastrocnemius, 408, 409, 435
lateral head, 381, 383–385, 402, 403, 405, 409, 419, 421, 428, 432t, 433–435, 472
medial head, 381, 384, 385, 402, 403, 405, 419, 420, 422, 432t, 433–435, 472
gemellus, 381
inferior, 385, 386t, 388, 389, 391
nerve to, 206, 207, 207t
superior, 222, 385, 386t, 388, 389, 391, 399
genioglossus, 677, 677t, 678, 679, 681, 719, 780, 781, 806, 810
geniohyoid, 678, 679, 681, 743, 760, 761, 761t, 781, 808
gluteus maximus, 202, 222, 250, 261, 262, 268, 273, 275, 320, 351, 368, 381, 383, 385, 386t, 388, 389, 399, 470, 472, 514
gluteus medius, 202, 320, 351, 381, 384, 385, 386t, 388, 389, 399
gluteus minimus, 351, 380, 381, 386t, 389, 396
gracilis, 372, 373, 375, 378t, 379, 380, 382, 384, 389, 396, 408, 434, 437, 470, 472
hamstring, 384, 385, 387t, 388, 389
hyoglossus, 677, 677t, 681, 766, 780, 806
hypothenar, 480, 604, 605
iliacus, 118, 163, 172, 172t, 173, 212, 218, 250, 317, 373, 375, 376, 377t, 380, 382
iliococcygeus, 203, 203t, 204, 212, 254, 262, 263
iliocostalis, 18, 323, 324, 351
cervicis, 323
lumborum, 323, 328
thoracis, 323, 328
iliopsoas, 351, 372, 373, 375, 376, 377t, 380, 381, 399
infraspinatus, 481, 503, 512, 516, 517, 517t, 519, 526–528, 537
intercostal, 164
external, 17–21, 21t, 22, 24, 83, 327, 334
innermost, 17–21, 21t, 83, 334
internal, 18–21, 21t, 22–24, 72, 83
interosseous
dorsal, 447, 447t, 480, 564, 565, 565t, 566, 574, 576, 577, 580–582, 584–586, 606
palmar, 480, 564, 565, 565t, 606
plantar, 447, 447t
interspinales, 329t, 330
intertransversarius, 324, 326, 328, 329t, 333, 785
ischiocavernosus, 255, 256t, 257, 261, 271, 276, 277
laryngeal, 802, 802t
latissimus dorsi, 4, 7, 73, 100, 123, 169–171, 320, 321, 324, 351, 481, 496, 497, 499, 502, 509, 510, 512, 513, 513t, 514, 518, 521–523, 525, 526, 600
levator anguli oris, 626, 630, 721
levator ani, 118, 203, 203t, 204, 205, 208, 209, 211–213, 216, 218, 220, 232, 250, 261, 268, 272, 273, 276–278, 280, 281
nerve to, 206, 207, 207t, 210
tendinous arch, 218, 219
levator costarum, 327, 328, 329t
levator labii superioris, 626, 629t, 630
levator labii superioris alaeque nasi, 630
levator palpebrae superioris, 630, 652, 654, 658, 658t, 719
levator prostatae, 263
levator scapulae, 321, 322, 333, 481, 511, 513, 513t, 514, 518, 519, 529, 755, 777, 777t, 806
levator veli palatini, 684, 684t, 712, 713, 789, 791, 795
levatores costarum, 18, 21, 21t
longissimus, 18, 323, 324, 351, 783, 783t
capitis, 328, 330, 331, 333, 350, 785
cervicis, 328
thoracis, 323, 328
longitudinal
inferior, 677t
superior, 677, 677t, 679
longus capitis, 332, 333, 350, 721, 773, 774, 774t, 775, 785, 807
longus colli, 69, 80, 350, 721, 773, 774, 774t, 775, 807
lumbrical, 439, 445, 445t, 480, 556, 563–565, 565t, 566, 567, 571, 606
masseter, 630, 662, 666, 667, 672, 672t, 719–721, 738, 739
mastication, 672, 672t
mentalis, 626, 629t, 630, 746
multifidus, 324, 325, 328, 351, 783, 783t
mylohyoid, 678, 679, 681, 743, 758, 760, 761, 761t, 763, 766, 778, 779, 806, 808
nerve to, 681, 763, 778, 779, 828, 829
nasalis, 626, 629t
oblique
external, 2, 3, 7, 19, 22, 24, 73, 98, 100–104, 104t, 105–109, 111, 112, 118, 119, 123, 163, 169–171, 188, 320, 324, 351, 496, 497, 514
inferior, 651, 654, 658, 658t, 659, 659t, 719
nerve to, 651, 654, 821
internal, 19, 24, 101, 103, 104, 104t, 105, 107–109, 111, 112, 118, 119, 163, 169–171, 188, 324, 351, 382, 785
superior, 330, 651, 652, 658, 658t, 659, 659t, 719

Muscle—*continued*
obliquus capitis
inferior, 330–333, 350, 784
superior, 330–333, 350, 784, 785
obturator externus, 222, 250, 268, 273, 275, 378t, 380, 391, 394, 396, 470
obturator internus, 118, 202, 203, 203t, 204, 212, 213, 218, 219, 222, 250, 275, 278, 280–282, 385, 386t, 388, 391
nerve to, 206, 207, 207t, 392t
occipitalis, 330, 634
occipitofrontalis, 626, 629t, 630
omohyoid, 492, 518, 529, 758, 759, 761, 761t, 762, 766
opponens brevis, 614
opponens digiti minimi, 552, 565t, 567, 570, 587, 606
opponens pollicis, 552, 564, 565t, 567, 570, 585
orbicularis oculi, 626, 628, 629t, 655, 662, 666, 721
orbicularis oris, 626, 629t, 630, 721
palatoglossus, 677, 677t, 684, 684t, 721, 792, 793
palatopharyngeus, 684, 684t, 721, 788, 788t, 791–793
palmaris
brevis, 480, 561, 563, 566
longus, 480, 553t, 554, 559, 566, 570, 602, 604, 605
papillary, 58
anterior, 57, 59, 63, 64
magnetic resonance imaging, 88–89
posterior, 57, 59, 63
septal, 57, 63
pectinate, 56
pectineus, 222, 250, 275, 372, 373, 375, 378t, 380–382, 396, 399
pectoralis major, 4, 7, 22, 100, 103, 490, 492, 496, 499, 502, 503, 508–510, 518, 522, 523
abdominal part, 494–498, 499t
clavicular head, 2, 3, 494, 495, 497–499, 499t, 500
magnetic resonance imaging, 88–89
sternocostal head, 2, 3, 494, 495, 497–499, 499t, 500, 508
pectoralis minor, 492, 498, 499, 499t, 500–503, 508, 510, 518, 523, 530
perineal
deep transverse, 209, 216, 254, 256t, 257, 263
superficial, 268
superficial transverse, 255, 256t, 257, 261, 271
pes anserinus, 379, 408, 437
pharyngeal, 681, 788, 788t, 797
piriformis, 202, 203, 203t, 204, 212, 385, 386t, 388–391
nerve to, 206, 207, 207t
plantaris, 381, 385, 405, 432t, 433
platysma, 3, 494, 626, 629t, 630, 746, 746t, 807
popliteus, 381, 385, 404, 405, 414, 420, 421, 432t, 433, 435–437, 472
procerus, 626, 629, 630
pronator quadratus, 480, 552, 553t, 555–557, 571, 592
pronator teres, 480, 518, 522, 523, 539, 549, 552, 553t, 554, 555, 557, 574, 577, 602
deep head, 540
superficial head, 540
ulnar head, 518, 552
psoas, 133, 144, 145, 153, 163, 187, 188, 212, 215, 218, 317, 324, 352, 372, 373
psoas major, 171, 172, 172t, 173, 250, 334, 351, 375, 376, 377t
psoas minor, 172, 375
pterygoid
lateral, 668, 672, 672t, 720, 721, 738, 739
nerve to, 828, 829
medial, 672, 672t, 681, 720, 797
deep head, 668, 669
nerve to, 669, 828, 829
superficial head, 668, 669
pubococcygeus, 202, 203, 203t, 204, 210, 212, 254, 260, 262, 263
puboprostaticus, 203, 204, 260
puborectalis, 203, 203t, 204, 209–212, 222, 260, 263, 275–277
pubovaginalis, 203, 205, 260, 273
quadratus femoris, 375, 376, 377t, 381, 385, 386t, 390, 396
nerve to, 206, 207, 207t, 392t
quadratus lumborum, 153, 163, 171, 172, 172t, 173, 174, 187, 324, 326, 351
quadratus plantae, 438, 439, 445, 445t, 451, 452, 456
rectovesicalis, 260
rectus
inferior, 651, 653–655, 658, 658t, 659, 659t, 719
lateral, 652–654, 658, 658t, 659, 659t, 719, 721
medial, 651–653, 658, 658t, 659, 659t, 660, 697, 719, 721
superior, 651, 652, 654, 655, 658, 658t, 659, 659t, 660, 719
rectus abdominis, 2, 19, 22, 24, 98, 102–104, 104t, 118, 119, 123, 136, 187, 189, 209, 218, 219, 222, 279, 351
rectus capitis anterior, 332, 333, 774, 775, 775t, 785
rectus capitis lateralis, 333, 350, 681, 774, 774t, 775, 785
rectus capitis posterior
major, 330–333, 350, 784, 785
minor, 330–333, 350, 784, 785
rectus femoris, 250, 372–376, 377t, 380–383, 395, 396, 399, 406, 407, 470
rhomboid, 481, 512, 526
rhomboid major, 321, 322, 513, 513t, 514, 519, 527
rhomboid minor, 321, 322, 513, 513t, 514, 519, 529
rotator cuff, 516–517, 517f, 534, 535
rotatores, 328, 351, 783, 783t
brevis, 327
longus, 327
salpingopharyngeus, 788, 788t
sartorius, 250, 372–376, 377t, 379–382, 399, 406, 408, 434, 437, 470
scalene
anterior, 22–24, 72, 80, 82, 511, 756, 772–774, 774t, 775, 776, 807
middle, 22, 24, 72, 333, 511, 756, 776, 777, 777t, 785, 807
posterior, 22, 24, 756, 777, 777t
scalenus minimus, 72
semimembranosus, 379, 381, 384, 385, 387t, 388, 389, 396, 402, 403, 405, 408, 420, 421, 433–437, 470
semispinalis, 18, 325
capitis, 325, 328, 330–333, 350, 755, 783, 783t, 785, 806
cervicis, 328, 330, 331, 783, 783t, 806
semitendinosus, 379, 381, 384, 385, 387t, 388, 389, 396, 402, 403, 408, 419, 420, 434, 435, 437, 470
serratus anterior, 2–4, 7, 22, 98, 100, 102, 103, 494–499, 499t, 502, 503, 508–511, 518, 526, 527, 529, 756
nerve to, 510
serratus posterior
inferior, 21, 21t, 73, 169, 170, 322, 511
superior, 21, 21t, 24, 322
soleus, 381, 385, 402, 405, 422, 428, 432t, 433–437, 439, 472
spinalis, 323, 351
spinalis thoracis, 328
splenius, 329t
capitis, 323, 328, 331–333, 350, 755, 777, 777t, 783, 783t, 785, 806
cervicis, 323, 328, 333, 783, 783t, 785
sternocleidomastoid, 22, 332, 333, 350, 352, 499, 518, 662, 666, 716, 753, 753t, 759, 762, 763, 807
artery, 763, 785, 806
clavicular head, 24, 763
sternal head, 24, 763
sternohyoid, 22, 23, 350, 758, 759, 761, 761t, 762, 763, 766, 768, 785, 807
sternothyroid, 22, 23, 758, 759, 761, 761t, 763, 807
strap, 806, 810
styloglossus, 350, 677, 677t, 681, 780, 785
stylohyoid, 713, 721, 761, 761t, 763, 778, 787
stylopharyngeus, 350, 681, 713, 720, 785, 787, 788, 788t, 789, 796
subclavius, 22, 492, 498, 499t, 508–510, 756
subcostales, 17, 21, 21t
subscapularis, 481, 499, 502, 503, 508–511, 516, 517, 517t, 518, 522, 523, 525, 527, 530, 534, 537
nerve to, 502
supinator, 481, 540, 543, 552, 555, 557, 574, 575t, 577
supraspinatus, 481, 499, 516, 517, 517t, 518, 519, 522, 523, 528, 529, 531, 537
suspensory, 133
temporalis, 634, 666, 667, 672, 672t, 719–721, 738, 739
nerve to, 828, 829
tensor fascia lata, 250, 275, 368, 373, 375, 376, 377t, 381, 383, 385, 386t, 399, 470
tensor tympani, 711, 713
tensor veli palatini, 681, 684, 684t, 702, 720, 795
teres major, 320, 481, 499, 502, 509–512, 516, 517, 517t, 518, 521–523, 525–528, 534, 600
nerve to, 502
teres minor, 481, 503, 516, 517, 517t, 519, 527, 528, 537
thenar, 480, 604, 605
thyroarytenoid, 802, 802t, 803
thyrohyoid, 761, 761t, 762, 763, 766, 768, 779
nerve to, 763, 766, 779
thyropharyngeus, 788, 788t
tibialis anterior, 422, 423, 423t, 424, 426, 428, 431, 439, 447, 449, 452, 454, 457, 464, 472
tibialis posterior, 432t, 433–439, 447, 448, 451, 452, 456–458, 464, 472
of tongue, intrinsic, 806
transverse, 677t
transversospinalis, 329t
transversus abdominis, 19, 22–24, 101, 103, 104, 104t, 105, 108, 109, 111, 112, 118, 119, 163, 170–172, 188, 334, 351
transversus thoracis, 20, 21, 21t, 23, 73
trapezius, 321, 331–333, 350, 499, 513, 513t, 514, 518, 519, 537, 753, 753t, 785, 806
ascending part, 320, 321, 512, 514, 529
descending part, 320, 321, 512, 514, 526, 529, 783, 783t
transverse part, 320, 321, 512, 514, 529
triceps brachii, 502, 519, 527, 543, 546, 547, 574
lateral head, 481, 519, 520, 520t, 521, 523, 524, 526–528, 600
long head, 481, 509–511, 518–520, 520t, 521–528, 534, 535, 600
medial head, 481, 499, 510, 519, 520, 520t, 521–523, 525–527, 600
uvular, 260, 684, 684t, 791
vastus intermedius, 374–376, 377t, 380–382, 470
vastus lateralis, 250, 275, 373–376, 377t, 380–383, 406, 409, 470
vastus medialis, 375, 376, 377t, 380–382, 385, 406–408, 419–421, 434, 470
nerve to, 373, 382

vertical, 677t
zygomaticus major, 626, 662, 721
zygomaticus minor, 630
Myelogram, 337
Myocardium, 53, 58, 61
Myometrium, 279–283
Myotome, 348, 349

Nail bed, nerve to, 578
Nasal bone, 611–613, 622, 650, 690, 691, 695, 699, 721
Nasion, 610, 612
Nasopharynx, 128, 621, 718–720, 790, 794–797, 810
Navicular, 427, 431, 449, 454, 459, 461, 462, 464–466
fossa, 267, 444, 452, 453, 458
tuberosity, 439
Neck
arteries, 764, 764t–765t, 765
blood supply, 649
bones, 750, 751
cartilage, 749–751
Doppler ultrasound, 809
fascia, 747
lymphatic drainage, 716
magnetic resonance imaging, 806, 809
median anatomical section, 808
regions, 752, 752t
root of, 67, 772–773
transverse anatomical sections, 807
veins, 716
deep, 767
superficial, 748
Nephron, 167
Nerve
abducent, 640, 644, 645, 652, 654, 656, 812–814, 815t, 821, 822, 822t, 823, 841, 841t, 843
alveolar
anterior superior, 692, 826, 827
inferior, 669, 681, 687, 828, 829
middle superior, 826, 827
posterior superior, 671, 826, 827
superior, 687
anal, inferior, 214, 231, 261, 269, 270
anococcygeal, 206
auricular
great, 627, 662, 754, 762
posterior, 186, 189, 629, 662
auriculotemporal, 631t, 662, 663, 668, 828, 829
axillary, 345, 481, 506, 507t, 509, 510, 527, 528, 534, 536
buccal, 629, 630, 631t, 662, 668, 669, 828, 829
calcaneal, medial, 457
cardiac, 67
cervical, 68
inferior, 68, 84
middle, 68
cavernous, 231
cervical, 629, 639
transverse, 746, 754
ciliary
long, 652, 825
short, 652, 825
clunial
inferior, 270, 359, 392t
medial, 359, 392t
superior, 359, 392t
coccygeal, 206, 207, 207t
cochlear, 709, 715, 734, 735, 832–833
cranial. *See* Cranial nerves
cutaneous
of abdomen, lateral, 7
of arm
inferior lateral, 484, 485t, 527
medial, 484, 485t, 506, 507t
posterior, 484, 485t, 509, 510, 525
superior lateral, 484, 485t, 528
of forearm
lateral, 484, 485t, 521, 538, 539, 549, 579, 600
medial, 484, 485t, 506, 507t, 508, 521, 538, 600
posterior, 484, 485t, 521, 527, 578, 579, 600
lateral dorsal, 359
of lower limb, 359
pectoral
anterior, 3
lateral, 3, 7
perforating, 207, 207t
superficial back, 514
of thigh
anterior, 372
lateral, 163, 172, 173, 359, 372
posterior, 218, 250, 261, 269, 270, 359, 392t, 399
of upper limb, 484, 485t
dental, inferior, 828, 829
digital
common palmar, 566, 567, 569
common plantar, 444
plantar, 443
proper palmar, 561, 563, 566, 567, 569
proper plantar, 444
dorsal
of clitoris, 254, 269, 270, 272, 274
of penis, 116, 202, 231, 254, 264, 265, 267
ethmoidal
anterior, 638, 653, 692, 825
posterior, 638, 653, 825
facial, 640–642, 663, 701, 708–713, 720, 734, 738, 739, 762, 812–814, 815t, 830, 831, 841, 841t, 843
branches, 627, 629, 634, 662
motor root, 830
femoral, 118, 163, 172, 173, 212, 218, 222, 250, 275, 345, 356, 358t, 359, 372, 373, 382, 399
femoral cutaneous, posterior, 206, 207, 207t
fibular
common, 345, 356, 358t, 402, 403, 409, 424, 424t, 425, 428, 434–437
deep, 218, 270, 345, 356, 358t, 359, 424, 424t, 425, 426, 431, 457, 472
superficial, 270, 345, 356, 358t, 359, 424, 424t, 425, 428, 429
frontal, 631t, 656, 825
genitofemoral, 116, 163, 172, 173, 215
femoral branch, 109, 112, 359
genital branch, 110–112, 359
glossopharyngeal, 335, 640–642, 663, 680, 681, 720, 734, 766, 785–787, 789, 796, 812–814, 815t, 834–835, 841, 843
gluteal
inferior, 206, 207, 207t, 250, 392t
superior, 206, 207, 207t, 392t
hypogastric, 230, 231, 249
hypoglossal, 335, 640, 641, 662, 663, 667, 680, 681, 720, 763, 766, 779, 780, 785, 786, 812–814, 815t, 839, 841, 841t, 843
iliohypogastric, 100, 101, 103, 107, 108, 112, 163, 170–173, 359, 382, 496
ilioinguinal, 101–103, 107, 110–112, 116, 163, 172, 173, 264, 359, 382
incisive, 828, 829
infraorbital, 629, 630, 651, 671, 692, 700, 719, 720, 826, 827
infratrochlear, 629, 630, 631t, 653, 825
intercostal, 17, 19, 20, 22, 23, 72, 80–83, 85, 334, 339
collateral branches, 17, 18
lateral cutaneous branch, 19, 502, 511
lateral pectoral cutaneous branch, 494
posterior, 18
intercostobrachial, 3, 7, 100, 484, 485t, 494, 496, 502, 509, 511
intermediate, 709, 830
interosseous
anterior, 480, 557, 602
posterior, 345, 481, 543, 577, 602
labial
anterior, 270
posterior, 270
lacrimal, 629, 630, 631t, 652, 656, 701, 825
laryngeal
recurrent, 67, 807
left, 42, 49, 67–69, 81, 84, 85, 770, 771
relationship to aortic arches, 67
right, 42, 68, 72, 84, 85, 770, 772, 789, 800
superior, 763, 766, 770, 789, 800, 807
lingual, 669, 680, 681, 779, 780, 797, 828, 829
mandibular, 638, 640, 644, 645, 669, 671, 681, 687, 720, 824t, 828–829
marginal, 629
masseteric, 828, 829
maxillary, 638, 640, 644, 645, 671, 692, 699–701, 824t, 826–827
median, 345, 480, 484, 485t, 502, 508, 521, 525, 539–541, 549, 555, 556, 558, 559, 567, 570, 571, 579, 591, 593, 600, 602, 604, 605
lateral root, 508
medial root, 508
palmar branch, 579
palmar cutaneous branch, 559
palmar digital branches, 484, 578
recurrent branch, 559, 561, 563, 566, 567
meningeal, recurrent, 304
mental, 629, 631t, 828, 829
musculocutaneous, 345, 480, 502, 506, 507t, 508, 510, 521, 525, 540, 600
mylohyoid, 681, 763, 778, 779, 828, 829
nasal, external, 631t
nasociliary, 652–654, 656, 825
nasopalatine, 683, 692, 702, 826, 827
obturator, 118, 172, 173, 202, 205, 212, 250, 345, 356, 358t, 359, 372, 382, 394, 399
occipital, 333, 785
greater, 330, 331, 333, 784
lesser, 754
oculomotor, 640, 641, 643–645, 652, 654, 656, 734, 812–814, 815t, 821, 822, 822t, 823, 841, 841t, 842, 844
olfactory, 640, 692, 812–814, 815t, 818, 841
ophthalmic, 640, 644, 824t, 825
optic, 640, 641, 652, 653, 655–657, 660, 719, 721, 727, 728, 732–734, 738, 739, 812–814, 815t, 819, 820, 841, 842
palatine
greater, 671, 683, 692, 702, 826, 827
lesser, 671, 683, 692, 702, 826, 827
pectoral
lateral, 500, 503, 506, 507t, 508, 509
medial, 500, 503, 506, 507t, 508, 509
perineal, 202, 231, 265, 269
petrosal
deep, 701, 831
greater, 701, 831
lesser, 834, 835
pharyngeal, 692, 826, 827
phrenic, 67, 72, 80, 755, 762, 772, 773, 807
left, 25, 42, 48, 73, 81
right, 25, 42, 48, 73
plantar, 451
lateral, 345, 356, 359, 438, 443, 446, 456, 458
medial, 345, 356, 359, 438, 443, 446, 456, 458
pterygopalatine, 700–702
pudendal, 206, 207, 207t, 212, 214, 218, 222, 230, 231, 246, 250, 265, 269, 270, 274, 392t, 399
radial, 345, 481, 502, 506, 507t, 509, 510, 521, 527, 528, 540, 549, 579, 600
deep branch, 481, 540, 555–557, 577
dorsal digital branch, 569, 578
superficial branch, 481, 484, 485t, 540, 555–557, 559, 578, 582, 584, 602

Nerve—*continued*
rectal
inferior, 202, 278
superior, 214
saphenous, 345, 359, 373, 382, 438, 457
scapular, dorsal, 506, 507t, 529
sciatic, 172, 173, 206, 207, 207t, 212, 216, 218, 222, 230, 250, 268, 275, 345, 356, 358t, 390, 391, 392t, 399, 470
scrotal, posterior, 231, 261
spinal, 123, 169, 334, 336, 338–340, 343, 344, 352, 481
spinal accessory, 333, 334, 511, 529, 642, 662, 663, 667, 720, 755, 762, 763, 766, 785, 807, 812–814, 815t, 838, 841, 841t, 843
splanchnic, 17, 85, 123, 125
greater, 73, 80–83, 85, 176–178, 179t, 183
least, 176–178, 179t
lesser, 82, 176–178, 179t, 183
lumbar, 176–178, 179t, 214, 230, 231, 246
pelvic, 176–178, 179t, 206, 207, 207t, 210, 214, 230, 231, 246, 249
sacral, 176–178, 179t, 231
subclavian, 506, 507t
subcostal, 85, 100, 101, 163, 170–173, 359, 496
suboccipital, 330, 331, 784
subscapular
lower, 506, 507t, 508–511
upper, 503, 506, 507t, 509–511
supraclavicular, 3, 484, 485t, 494, 746, 754
supraorbital, 629, 630, 631t, 651, 825
suprascapular, 481, 509, 510, 528, 529, 537
supratrochlear, 629, 630, 631t, 651, 825
sural, 359, 403, 430, 457
sural cutaneous
lateral, 359
medial, 359, 434
temporal, 629
deep, 668
tentorial, 638
thoracic, 17, 112
lateral, 508
long, 7, 100, 496, 502, 503, 506, 507t, 508, 509, 511
posterior ramus, 18
thoracoabdominal, 100–102, 496
thoracodorsal, 502, 506, 507t, 508–510
tibial, 345, 356, 358t, 359, 402, 403, 434–438, 443, 451, 457, 472
anterior recurrent, 425
posterior, 269
trigeminal, 631, 631t, 640–643, 812–814, 815t, 824, 841, 842, 844
cutaneous branches, 630
groove for, 615
mandibular division, 824t, 828–829
maxillary division, 824t, 826–827
motor root, 645, 646, 734
ophthalmic division, 824t, 825
sensory root, 644–646, 734
spinal tract, 734
trochlear, 640–645, 652, 656, 812–814, 815t, 821, 822, 822t, 823, 841
tympanic, 710, 834–835
ulnar, 345, 476, 477, 480, 484, 485t, 502, 506, 507t, 508, 521, 525, 527, 540, 542, 543, 549, 555, 556, 558, 559, 566, 571, 579, 600, 602, 604, 605
communicating branch, 567
deep branch, 480, 567, 570, 571, 591
dorsal branch, 484, 559, 578, 582, 587
dorsal cutaneous branch, 566
dorsal digital branch, 578
palmar branch, 579
palmar digital branch, 578
superficial branch, 484, 567, 571
ulnar collateral, 525
vagus, 181, 640–642, 662, 663, 667, 720, 766, 771, 772, 785, 807, 812–814, 815t, 836–837, 841, 843
in abdomen, 181
auricular branch, 703
inferior cardiac branch, 772
left, 25, 42, 48, 49, 65, 67–69, 81, 84, 85, 773, 836
right, 25, 42, 48, 67, 68, 72, 80, 84, 85, 773, 836
vestibular, 709, 715, 734, 735, 832–833
vestibulocochlear, 640–642, 709, 715, 734, 735, 738, 739, 812–814, 815t, 832–833, 841, 843
zygomatic, 630, 631t, 700, 701, 826, 827
zygomaticofacial, 630
Nerve blocks, during pregnancy, 247
Nerve point of neck, 754
Nipple, 5–7, 100, 496, 497
Node
atrioventricular, 64
lymph. *See* Lymph nodes
sinoatrial, 64
superficial parotid, 762
Nose
bones, 690
cartilage, 690
lateral wall, 623
surface anatomy, 690
Nostril, 690
Notch
acetabular, 396
cardiac, 26, 32, 34, 35, 96
cardial, 129
clavicular, 12
costal, 12
fibular, 652
interarytenoid, 790
intertragic, 703
jugular, 10, 12, 499
mandibular, 612, 664
mastoid, 615, 625
notch, 625
pterygoid, 624
radial, 544, 548
sacrococcygeal, 313
sciatic
greater, 197, 312, 381, 397
lesser, 197, 202, 312, 381, 397
supraorbital, 650
suprascapular, 518, 532
suprasternal, 2, 495
tentorial, 643
trochlear, 544, 546, 547
ulnar, 589
vertebral, 289, 302
Nuchal region, 333
superior, 350
Nucleus
amygdaloid, 726, 727, 729, 741
caudate, 727, 729–734, 740–742
cingulate, 742
cochlear, 735
cranial nerve, 816–817
dentate, 740
geniculate
lateral, 741, 820
medial, 741
habenular, 731
lentiform, 726, 727, 730–734, 740, 741
red, 732, 733, 738, 739, 741
reticular, 741
thalamic
anterior, 741
lateral, 741
medial, 741
vestibular, 735
Nucleus pulposus, 306–308

Occipital bone, 350, 608, 609, 613, 617, 619, 664, 738, 739
basilar part, 617, 618, 795
lateral part, 618
squamous part, 614, 617, 618
Olecranon, 519, 521, 524, 526, 527, 542–544, 546–549, 574, 600
Olive, 639, 734
Omentum
greater, 119–121, 124, 136, 137
lesser, 119–121, 123–126, 147, 148
Opening
aortic, 172, 173
coronary sinus, 56, 64
esophageal, 125, 172
saphenous, 103, 107, 112, 368, 370, 371
Ora serrata, 660
Orbicular zone, 395
Orbit
arteries, 657, 657t
lateral aspect, 654–655
muscles, 658–659, 658t, 659t, 821
nerves, 656, 821
veins, 656
Orifice
of appendix, 139
atrioventricular
left, 58, 59
right, 56
cardial, 129
ileocecal, 139
maxillary, 695, 696
pyloric, 129
ureteric, 234
urethral, 271–273
external, 216, 253, 255
internal, 216
vaginal, 255, 271–273
Oropharynx, 128, 721, 790, 810
Os trigonum, 467
Ossicles, 704, 707
Otolith, 715
Ovary, 208, 232, 234, 240, 280–283
fetal, 114
left, 122

Pain, referred, 180
Palate, 28, 682–684, 808
hard, 623, 682, 684t, 697, 719, 721, 743
soft, 682, 684t, 713, 721, 743, 790, 792, 794, 810
Palatine bone, 617, 623, 664, 682, 691, 695, 700, 702
horizontal plate, 615, 682
orbital process, 650
pyramidal process, 682
Palm
compartments, 562
deep dissection, 570–571
fascia, 560, 562
muscular layers, 564
spaces, 562
superficial dissection, 566–567
synovial sheaths, 568
Pancreas, 96, 97, 120–122, 125–128, 131, 135, 145, 152, 154, 155, 160, 162, 188
blood supply, 135
body, 125, 133, 134, 156, 187
dorsal, 157
head, 127, 133, 134, 153, 156, 187, 189
lymphatic drainage, 184
neck, 127, 133, 156
relationships, 134
tail, 125, 133, 134, 156, 162, 164, 187, 189
artery to, 135
ultrasound, 190
uncinate process, 187, 189
ventral, 157
Papilla
inferior lacrimal, 651
lingual, 676
major duodenal, 133, 156
minor duodenal, 133, 156
renal, 166, 167
Paracolic gutter, 122
Parietal bone, 609, 611, 613, 614, 617, 619, 634, 636
Parotid bed, 666
Parotid region, 662–663
Pars tensa, 706
Patella, 354, 355, 374, 375, 380, 406, 407, 410, 411, 420–422
bipartite, 467
radiograph, 418
Pecten, anal, 211
Pectoral girdle, 530
Pectoral region
female, 4
male, 2–3, 494, 495
superficial dissection, 3, 4
surface anatomy, 2
Pedicle, 289, 296, 301–303, 310, 334, 337
Peduncle
cerebellar, 734, 735, 737–739, 816
cerebral, 732, 733, 742
Pelvic brim, 200
Pelvic girdle, 197
female, 195, 198t–199t
male, 194, 198t–199t

Pelvis
anatomical position, 197
angiography, 277
bifid, 168
bones, 196, 311
divisions, 196
female, 205, 208, 232–251
arteries, 241–243, 243t
autonomic nerves, 248–249
hysterosalpingogram, 284
innervation, 246–249
laparoscopic view, 233
lymphatic drainage, 244–245, 245t
magnetic resonance imaging, 279–282
organs, 232–239
subperitoneal region, 250–251
supporting and compressor/sphincteric muscles, 260
transverse section, 249
ultrasound, 282–283
veins, 242
vessels, 240–243
floor, 203–205, 203t
greater, 128
ligaments, 200, 201, 314, 315
male, 204, 209, 216–231
arteries, 224, 225, 225t, 226
innervation, 230–231
lymphatic drainage, 228–229, 229t
magnetic resonance imaging, 276–279
organs, 216–223
posterior view, 218–219
supporting and compressor/sphincteric muscles, 260
transrectal ultrasound, 223
transverse sections, 222
veins, 224, 227
vessels, 224–227
posterior, neurovascular structures, 212
radiograph, 311
renal, 143, 165, 166, 187
viscera, 246, 247, 251
walls, 203t, 204–205
Penis, 264
body, 252, 264, 266, 268
bulb of, 209, 216, 217, 262, 266–268, 276, 277, 279
corona, 252, 264
cross sections, 267
crura, 262, 266, 267, 276, 277
distal, urethral aspect, 268
dorsal artery, 116, 254, 264, 267
dorsal nerve, 116, 202, 231, 254, 264, 265, 267
dorsal vein, 116, 216, 224, 254, 264, 267, 268
fascia, 258, 265
fundiform ligament, 107
glans, 116, 216, 217, 252, 264, 266–268
layers, 265
nerves, 265
prepuce, 264, 265
root, 252, 264, 266, 268, 276, 277
septum, 267
subcutaneous tissue, 258
surface anatomy, 264
suspensory ligament, 112, 116, 264
Perforated area
anterior, 734
posterior, 734
Pericardium, 48–51, 53, 67
fibrous, 25, 29, 51, 65, 66
magnetic resonance imaging, 88–89, 91
posterior relationships, 65
relationship to sternum, 48
serous, 29, 50, 51
parietal layer, 25, 51, 65
visceral layer, 25, 50
subdivisions, 29
Pericranium, 634, 636, 743
Perilymph
cochlear, 738, 739
vestibular, 738, 739
Perineum, 196
compartments, 254–255, 258, 259
female, 269–275
compartments, 259
fascia, 259
innervation, 270
lymphatic drainage, 244–245, 245t
magnetic resonance imaging, 279–282
surface anatomy, 253
male
compartments, 258
dissection, 261–263
fascia, 258
innervation, 230–231
lymphatic drainage, 228–229, 229t
magnetic resonance imaging, 276–279
surface anatomy, 252
muscles, 256t–257t, 257
Peripheral nerves, 345
Peristaltic wave, 132
Peritoneum, 129, 152, 153, 157, 212, 218, 219
female pelvis, 208
male pelvis, 209
parietal, 105, 118, 120, 121, 124, 136, 164
of posterior abdominal cavity, 144
visceral, 120, 121, 124, 164
Perpendicular plate of ethmoid bone, 610, 690
Pes hippocampi, 741
Phalanx, 431, 476–479, 574, 598
distal, 427, 444, 466, 552, 574, 586, 588, 589, 595, 599
middle, 427, 444, 466, 552, 588, 589, 595, 599
proximal, 427, 444, 466, 552, 569, 574, 586, 588, 589, 595, 599
Pharyngeal constrictor
inferior, 770, 786–788, 788t, 789, 806, 807
middle, 786–788, 788t, 789
superior, 712, 713, 786–788, 788t, 789, 791, 792, 795, 797
Pharyngotympanic tube, 28, 615, 681, 695, 704, 705, 710–713, 720, 785, 790, 794
Pharynx, 28, 128, 738, 739, 742, 743, 790–791, 806, 808
cavity, 678
external, 786–787, 789
internal, 790–791
muscles, 681, 788, 788t, 797
Pinching movements, 596, 597
Pinna, 738, 739
Pisiform, 552, 558, 559, 566, 571, 587–589, 591–594, 599, 604
Placenta, 238, 239
Plane
interspinous, 128
orbitomeatal, 612, 613
transpyloric, 128
Plate
cribriform, 618, 619, 743, 808
horizontal, 615, 617, 682
perpendicular, of ethmoid bone, 610, 690
pterygoid
lateral, 617, 624, 702, 712, 720
medial, 617, 624, 702
tarsal
inferior, 629, 630
superior, 629, 630
tympanic, 615
Plateau, tibial, 411
Pleura, 129
cervical, 66–69
costal, 73
diaphragmatic, 73
mediastinal, 73
parietal, 20, 28, 72, 78, 83, 123, 334
cervical, 773
costal part, 80, 81
extent of, 30–31
mediastinal part, 25, 80, 81
sternal reflection, 72
surface markings, 31t, 45
visceral, 28, 31t
Plexus
abdominopelvic, 176–178, 179t
aortic, 84, 85, 230
arterial, pial, 342
brachial, 22, 82, 503, 756, 757, 776, 807
branches, 507t
illustration, 506
inferior trunk, 72
lateral cord, 508, 510
medial cord, 508, 510
posterior cord, 509, 510
cardiac, 68, 84
carotid
external, 717
internal, 701, 717
celiac, 176, 177, 181
cervical, 762, 807
choroid, 639, 727, 729, 731–733, 740
coccygeal, 206, 207, 207t
esophageal, 42, 65, 80, 85
hypogastric
inferior, 176, 177, 214, 230, 231, 246, 249
superior, 145, 214, 215, 230, 231, 246
intermesenteric, 176, 177
lumbar, 172
nerves, 173
lymphatic
deep, 43
of palm, 489
subareolar, 9
subpleural, 43
mesenteric
inferior, 176, 177
superior, 176, 177
ovarian, 246
para-aortic, 214, 246
pelvic, 214, 246
periarterial, sympathetic, 805
pharyngeal, 787
phrenic, inferior, 163
prostatic, 230, 231
pulmonary, 42, 67
anterior, 49, 68
left, 84
right, 84
renal, 176, 177
sacral, 205, 206, 207t, 214, 246
subtrapezial, 514
suprarenal, 176, 177
tympanic, 834–835
ureterovaginal, 249
uterine, 246
uterovaginal, 246
venous
basilar, 639
pampiniform, 113, 116, 216, 264
pial, 342
prostatic, 222, 224, 279
pterygoid, 639
rectal, 211, 224
uterine, 242
vaginal, 242
vertebral, 309, 333, 339, 342, 639, 785, 807
vesical, 224, 242
vesical, 230, 231
Plica semilunaris, 651
Pole
frontal, 728, 742
occipital, 728, 742
temporal, 639, 742
Pons, 639, 722, 723, 734, 738–740, 742, 743, 808
Popliteal region, 354, 405
Porta hepatis, 124, 147, 154, 155
Portacaval system, 161
Portal confluence, 187, 189
Portal triad, 123–125, 134, 147, 149–153, 162
Pouch
rectouterine, 120, 208, 232, 233, 238, 250
rectovesical, 121, 209, 215–217, 219, 279
superficial perineal, 258, 259
vesicouterine, 208, 232, 279
Precuneus, 728
Pregnancy, pelvic visceral innervation during, 247
Process
accessory, 300, 303
acromion, 532, 535
alveolar
of mandible, 611, 613, 664
of maxilla, 611, 613, 617, 721
articular, 289
inferior, 296, 297, 300, 302, 303, 310
superior, 15
axillary, of breast, 4
caudate, 147, 148
ciliary, 660
clinoid
anterior, 618, 619, 624, 702
posterior, 615, 618, 619, 624, 643, 702
condylar, of mandible, 612

Process—*continued*
coracoid, 27, 498, 508, 511, 518, 522, 523, 525, 530–532, 535, 536, 598
coronoid, 544, 546, 548, 549, 552, 613, 667, 720
digital, of fat, 269, 271, 274
frontal
of maxilla, 611, 613, 650, 690, 721
of zygomatic bone, 611, 613
jugular, 617
lateral, 433, 444, 450, 690
mamillary, 300, 303
mastoid, 350, 352, 609, 612, 614–617, 711–713, 720, 750, 785
medial, 433, 444, 450, 456
palatine, 615, 650, 682
pterygoid, 624, 699, 701
spinous, 11, 14, 88–89, 123, 187, 286, 288, 289, 295–297, 300–303, 310, 311, 330, 331, 350, 351, 750, 751, 810
styloid, 552, 574, 585, 587, 589–592, 612, 614–617, 625, 663, 681, 712, 713, 720, 785, 797
superior articular, 197, 296, 300, 302, 303, 310, 338
supracondylar, 541
transverse, 14–18, 187, 288–290, 295–297, 300–303, 310–313, 324, 339, 350, 351, 751, 807
atlas, 750
lumbar, 171, 200
vertebral, 132
uncal, 296
uncinate, 127, 133, 134, 187, 189, 295, 296
vaginal, 624
xiphoid, 2, 10, 12, 29, 48, 98, 128, 187, 300, 499
zygomatic, 611, 613, 617, 625, 664
Prominence, laryngeal, 749
Prominens, vertebral, 512
Promontory, 708, 710
sacral, 196, 197, 199, 313
Protrusion, synovial, 395
Protuberance
external occipital, 295, 328, 330, 331, 350, 613–615, 617, 743, 750, 785, 808
internal occipital, 618, 619, 621, 743, 808
mental, 610, 612, 664
Pterion, 612, 635
Pubic bone, 234, 280, 281
Pubis, 196, 197, 202, 222, 250, 312, 397
anterior aspect, 197
body, 197, 311, 312, 380
pecten, 197–199, 312, 380
ramus, 380
inferior, 197, 199, 397
superior, 106, 197, 198, 311, 312, 380, 396
Pulp, tooth, 687
Pulse, carotid, 768
Pulvinar, 730, 732, 733, 735
Punctum, inferior lacrimal, 651
Pupil, 650, 651, 660
Putamen, 732, 733, 740, 741
Pyelogram, 165
Pylorus, of stomach, 96, 125, 128, 129, 132, 134, 156, 189
Pyramid, 639, 708, 734, 738–740
renal, 166

Radiations, optic, 726, 728, 729, 732–734
Radiograph
ankle, 453, 454
biliary passages, 158
chest, 27
colon, 138
cranium, 608, 609, 620–621, 697, 698
duodenum, 132
elbow joint, 544, 547
esophagus, 132
foot, 453
forearm, 545
glenohumeral (shoulder) joint, 536
hand, 586, 589
hip joint, 398
hyoid bone, 750
knee, 418, 420
pelvis, 311
pregnant uterus, 239
stomach, 132
teeth, 685
uterus and uterine tube, 284
vertebrae
cervical, 292, 296, 297, 750
lumbar, 293, 302, 310
thoracic, 310
Radius, 476–479, 518, 519, 523, 545, 548, 552, 557, 574, 586, 590, 591, 593, 594, 598, 602
distal end, 592, 598
dorsal tubercle, 574, 581, 586
dysplasia, 131
head, 518, 519, 544, 546, 547, 549, 552, 574
neck, 544, 546, 547
proximal, 598
styloid process, 552, 574, 585, 589–592
ulnar notch, 589
Ramus
anterior, 17, 20, 333, 336, 338, 339, 345, 351, 352, 511, 642, 757, 773, 785
anterior abdominal branches, 103
sacral, 202, 205, 210, 212, 249
ischiopubic, 197–199, 263, 267, 273, 311, 312, 380
of ischium, 197, 199, 312, 397
of mandible, 350, 608, 610–613, 664
posterior, 17, 20, 83, 304, 327, 330, 331, 334, 336, 338, 339, 345, 352, 514, 642
pubic, 380
inferior, 197, 199, 397
superior, 106, 197, 198, 311, 312, 380, 396
Ramus communicans, 17, 20, 80, 81, 83, 334, 339
gray, 173, 230
white, 230
Raphe
perineal, 252
pharyngeal, 333, 785
pterygomandibular, 797
scrotal, 252
Recess
anterior, of ischioanal fossa, 118
apical, 808
articular, superior, 312, 313
costodiaphragmatic, 27, 28, 73, 78, 90, 118, 119, 123–125, 163, 164
costomediastinal, 29, 73
epitympanic, 708
hepatorenal, 123, 147, 152
ileocecal
inferior, 139
superior, 139
pharyngeal, 713, 720, 790
piriform, 790, 807
sacciform, 548, 591
spheno-ethmoidal, 694, 696
splenic, 164
subphrenic, 147
superior, 148
suprapineal, 741
Rectum, 97, 120–122, 128, 138, 160, 205, 209, 212, 216, 222, 233, 250, 254, 275–281
ampulla, 208, 232
autonomic stimulation effects, 230t
innervation, 214
in situ, 215
vasculature, 213
Referred pain, 180
Reflex
calcaneal (Achilles), 357
quadriceps, 357
Renal column, 166
Renal corpuscle, 167
Renal medulla, 166, 167
Respiration, muscles of, 24, 24t
Respiratory system, 28
Rete testis, 117
Retina, 660
Retinaculum, 398
extensor, 368, 458, 576, 577, 581, 582, 587
inferior, 422, 424, 426, 430, 431
superior, 422, 425
fibular
inferior, 425, 430
superior, 430, 434
flexor, 434, 436–438, 493, 554, 564, 567, 568, 570, 571, 591–593, 604, 605
patellar, 410
lateral, 375, 406
medial, 375, 406
Retroinguinal passage, 372, 373
Rib, 123, 290
anomalies, 16
atypical, 13
bicipital, 16
bifid, 16
cervical, 16
costovertebral articulations, 14
eighth, 10, 11, 13, 18, 26, 511
eleventh, 10, 11, 13, 164, 165
facets, 13, 14
fifth, 10, 11
first, 10, 11, 13, 23, 24, 26, 27, 39, 66–69, 75, 508, 530, 536, 773
floating, 11
fourth, 10, 11, 22, 26, 511
head, 13–15, 88–89
neck, 13
ninth, 10, 11, 19, 164
second, 10, 11, 13, 23, 24, 511
seventh, 10, 11, 14, 18, 124, 301
shaft, 13
sixth, 10, 11, 13, 14, 26
tenth, 10, 11, 26, 124, 163, 164
third, 10, 11
tubercle, 13, 14
twelfth, 10, 11, 13, 164, 165, 169–172, 174, 310
typical, 13
Ridge
supraepicondylar, 547
lateral, 519, 544, 552, 574
medial, 518, 544, 552
transverse, 12
Rima glottidis, 799, 804, 806
Ring
femoral, 371, 372
fibrous, 59
inguinal
deep, 108, 109, 111, 112, 118, 233
superficial, 102, 106, 107, 110, 116, 264, 372, 373
tendinous, common, 656
tracheal, 749, 807
umbilical, 105

Sac
dural, 83, 300, 334, 336–337
endolymphatic, 714
greater, 120, 122, 123
lacrimal, 651
pericardial, 51, 73, 80, 81, 119
Saccule, 714, 715, 807
Sacrum, 165, 194–198, 202, 208–210, 232, 278–282, 312, 313, 316
ala, 196–198, 310, 311, 313, 317
body, 197, 198
cornu, 194, 195
overview, 286, 288
promontory, 196, 197, 199
Scalp, 634, 636
Scaphoid, 552, 559, 574, 585, 586, 588, 589, 591–594, 599
Scapula, 10, 11, 97, 476–479, 503, 518, 519, 537, 598
anastomoses, 487
coracoid process, 498, 518
inferior angle, 11, 511, 518, 522, 523, 535
lateral border, 535, 536
medial border, 512, 522
movements, 515
spine, 11, 518, 519, 527, 529, 532, 536
superior angle, 511, 518, 523, 529, 536
superior border, 536
vertebral border, 536
Scapular region
dorsal, 528
surface anatomy, 526
Sclera, 661
Scrotum, 113, 117, 216, 252, 264
fascia, 258
lymphatic drainage, 117
Seminal vesicle, 118, 278
Seminiferous tubule, 117
Septum
interatrial, 58, 61
intermuscular
anterior, 369, 472
anteromedial, 470

fascial, 457
lateral, 409, 470, 493, 521, 543, 600
medial, 493, 521, 525, 540, 543, 600
posterior, 369, 437, 470, 472
posteromedial, 470
transverse, 369, 436–438
interventricular, 57, 58
inferior, 3-D volume reconstruction and CT angiogram, 92–93
magnetic resonance imaging, 88–89
membranous part, 59, 61
muscular part, 59, 64
membranous, 63
nasal, 690–693, 697, 719–721, 738, 739, 743, 790, 808
orbital, 630
inferior, 629, 630
superior, 629, 630
rectovesical, 216, 263
prostatic, 220
Septum pellucidum, 723, 727–733, 740, 743
Sesamoid, 443, 445, 447, 463, 589, 606
anomalous, 467
lateral, 439
medial, 439, 452
Sheath
arachnoid, 655
axillary, 502, 503
carotid, 678, 747, 769
digital, fibrous, 443, 446, 561, 566–569, 571
dural, 655
femoral, 112, 371, 373
hypogastric, 218, 251
pial, 655
rectus
anterior, 102–104, 107, 496, 497
layers, 105
posterior, 101, 103, 112, 118
synovial, 561, 568
tendon, intertubercular, 532
Shoulder region, 476, 477
Sialogram, 680
Sinus
aortic, 55, 59
cavernous, 639, 644, 740
confluence of, 724
coronal, 50
coronary, 47, 53
opening, 56, 64
valve of, 56
frontal, 620, 638, 695–698, 743
intercavernous, 639
lactiferous, 4, 5
maxillary, 620, 621, 691, 695–698, 700, 719, 720, 738, 739
occipital, 639
pericardial
oblique, 29, 60
anterior wall, 50
posterior wall, 51
transverse, 29, 49–51, 60
petrosal
groove, 618
inferior, 615, 639
superior, 615, 639
renal, 166, 171
sagittal
inferior, 636, 638, 639
superior, 618, 636–639, 724, 738–740, 743
sigmoid, 615, 619, 639, 713, 767
sphenoidal, 621, 624, 695–698, 702, 713, 721
sphenoparietal, 639
straight, 638, 639, 724, 732, 733, 738–740, 742
tonsil, 792, 793
transverse, 619, 639, 742
groove, 618, 619
right, 639
venous, scleral, 660
Sinus venarum, 56
Sinusoids, 151
Siphon, carotid, 740
Skin, 105, 743
Skull base, 350, 785
Small intestine, 96, 97, 128, 162, 187–189, 352
interior, 136
lymphatic drainage, 184
Smooth muscle, 256t, 257, 274
Somatic nervous system, 343
Space
infracolic, 122
intercostal
contents, 20
eighth, 10
inferior, 18, 19
ninth, 11
vertebral ends, 17, 18
intervertebral disc, 302
lateral pharyngeal, 713, 720
midpalmar, 562, 606
palmar, 606
perivertebral, 218
quadrangular, 510, 527, 528, 537
retromammary, 5
retropharyngeal, 350, 678, 807, 808
retropubic, 208, 209, 216, 218–220, 232
subaponeurotic areolar, 606
subarachnoid, 286, 337, 352, 655, 724, 738, 739, 806, 810
subhepatic, 121, 147
suprasternal, 808
thenar, 562
triangular, 528
Speech area, 722
Spermatic cord, 102, 106, 107, 109, 113, 216, 222, 268
coverings, 103, 112, 113
dissection, 116
internal spermatic fascia covering, 108
Sphenoid bone, 609, 611, 613, 614, 617, 619, 624, 650, 664, 691, 695, 701, 702, 721
body, 618, 701
greater wing, 613, 618, 624, 650, 701, 702, 721
lesser wing, 618, 620, 624, 650, 701, 702
spine, 615, 624
Sphincter
anal
external, 209–213, 216, 256t, 257, 261–263, 273
internal, 209–211, 216, 262, 263
pyloric, 129
urethral
external, 202, 209, 210, 216, 220, 254, 256t, 257, 260
internal, 209, 210, 216, 260, 282
urethrovaginal, 254, 256t, 257, 260, 273
Spinal cord, 83, 123, 187, 286, 300, 334–342, 350, 352, 639, 721, 742, 806–808, 810
blood supply, 341–342
cervical, 334, 338, 340
developmental changes, 344
lumbar, 334, 340
magnetic resonance imaging, 88–89
rootlets, 334, 335, 337, 339, 340
sacral, 340
termination, 337
thoracic, 340
Spine
ethmoidal, 619, 624
iliac
anterior inferior, 196–198, 200, 312, 380, 396, 397
anterior superior, 96, 98, 100–103, 106, 109, 110, 128, 194–198, 200, 311, 312, 354, 372, 373, 380, 382, 396, 397, 496, 497
posterior inferior, 197, 311, 312, 320, 381, 390, 391, 397
posterior superior, 194, 195, 197, 201, 312, 381, 390, 397, 512
ischial, 196, 197, 199, 202, 311, 312, 315, 381, 390, 397
nasal
anterior, 610, 612, 690
posterior, 615
scapular, 11, 518, 519, 527, 529, 532, 536
Spiral organ (of Corti), 715, 833
Spleen, 96, 97, 119, 124, 127, 128, 130, 133, 135, 160, 162–164, 187–189, 352
blood supply, 135
lymphatic drainage, 184
surface anatomy, 131
Spondylolisthesis, 319
Spondylolysis, 319
Spur, bony, 318
Stapes, 704, 706, 707, 710
Sternum, 12, 23, 29, 72, 174
3-D volume reconstruction and CT angiogram, 92–93
anatomy, 10
anomalies, 16
body, 10, 12, 21, 48, 300, 497–499
magnetic resonance imaging, 88–89
manubrium, 24, 498, 810
ossification, 16
Stomach, 82, 96, 119, 121, 123–128, 132, 135, 148, 154, 157, 160–162, 164, 187–189, 352
air-fluid level, 186
anterior view, 129–130
body, 129
greater curvature, 124, 125, 129, 132
lesser curvature, 124, 129
lymphatic drainage, 184
muscular layers, 129
pylorus of, 96, 125, 128, 129, 132, 134, 156, 189
radiograph, 132
Stria medullaris thalami, 728
Subcallosal region, 728, 729
Subcutaneous triangular area, 449
Subdeltoid region, 528
Suboccipital region, 330–333
Substantia nigra, 738–741
Sulcus
calcarine, 723, 728, 729, 742
callosal, 728
carotid, 624
central, 722, 725
cingulate, 728, 742
collateral, 728
coronary, 46
frontal, superior, 742
hippocampal, 728, 729
hypothalamic, 728
interatrial, 50
intraparietal, 725
lateral, 722, 725
marginal, 728
parieto-occipital, 723, 725, 728
postcentral, 725
precentral, 725
prechiasmatic, 624
temporal, superior, 742
terminal, 49, 676, 790
Sulcus limitans, 735
Suprascapular region, 529
Sustentaculum tali, 433, 438, 444, 445, 447, 448, 450, 452, 453, 456, 458, 464, 465
Sutural bone, 613, 614
Suture
coronal, 609, 613, 614
frontal, 608–610
frontonasal, 690
infraorbital, 650
intermaxillary, 608, 610
internasal, 608, 610
lambdoid, 609, 613, 614
median palatine, 682
occipitomastoid, 614
palatine, 617
parietomastoid, 614
sagittal, 609, 614, 615
Swallowing, 808
Symphysis
mandibular, 608–610
pubic, 98, 106, 120, 194, 196–200, 202, 208, 210, 217, 222, 232, 250, 263, 267, 272, 273, 275, 278, 279, 311, 354, 380
Synchondrosis, sternocostal, 10
Syndesmosis, tibiofibular, 442
Synostosis, 318
Systole, 62

T tube, 158
Taenia coli, 136, 137, 139, 140, 144
Talus, 427, 430, 431, 442, 450, 453–457, 459, 461, 466, 472
head, 444, 448, 452, 454, 455, 459
medial tubercle, 433, 438, 452
neck, 448, 452, 455, 459
Tapetum, 729
Tarsal bones, 459
Tarsal tunnel, 453
Teeth
canine, 685, 688, 689t
incisor, 685, 687, 688, 689t
innervation, 687
magnetic resonance imaging, 806
mandibular, 686, 688

Teeth—*continued*
maxillary, 686, 688
molar, 685, 687, 688, 689t, 719
permanent, 685–686
primary, 688, 689t
secondary, 689t
Tegmen tympani, 712, 713
Telencephalon, 722, 723, 725–733
Temporal bone, 133, 608, 609, 611, 613, 614, 617, 619, 625, 702
mastoid part, 613
petrous part, 618, 620, 621, 625, 714
squamous part, 613, 618, 625, 664, 721
tympanic part, 613, 625, 664
zygomatic process, 613, 664
Tendinous cords, 57–59, 63
Tendon
abductor pollicis longus, 558, 559, 591
Achilles, 453
biceps brachii, 522, 523, 539, 540, 546, 549, 557
biceps femoris, 409, 428
calcaneal, 428, 430, 433–439, 450–452, 454, 458, 472
central, 24, 29, 73, 174
common extensor, 518, 542, 549, 552, 574
common flexor, 518, 549, 552
conjoint, 103, 107–109, 111, 112
digastric, 787
extensor digitorum longus, 422
extensor hallucis longus, 422
fibularis brevis, 431
fibularis longus, 431
flexor carpi radialis, 558, 592
flexor carpi ulnaris, 558
flexor digitorum longus, 445
flexor digitorum profundus, 557, 569
flexor digitorum superficialis, 559, 569
flexor hallucis brevis, 447
flexor hallucis longus, 445, 446, 451
flexor pollicis longus, 559, 570
long head of biceps brachii, 531, 532, 534, 535, 537
obturator internus, 389, 395
palmaris longus, 558, 559, 561, 563, 566
pectoralis minor, 522
peroneus longus, 464
popliteus, 409
quadriceps, 376, 420, 421
rotator cuff, 534
sartorius, 406
subscapularis, 532–534
supraspinatus, 517, 531, 532, 534
synovial covering, 569
tensor tympani, 708
terminal, 583
tibialis anterior, 422, 424
tibialis posterior, 429
triceps, 524, 526–528, 542
Tenia coli, 122
Tentorium cerebelli, 638, 639, 740, 743
Terminale, filum, 334, 336, 337
Terminalis
crista, 56
lamina, 728
stria, 729, 731, 741
sulcus, 49, 676, 790
Testis, 116, 209, 210, 216, 217, 264
blood supply, 117
coverings, 112, 113
fetal, 114
lymphatic drainage, 117
rete, 117
Thalamus, 728, 730–733, 735, 740–742
Thigh, 354
anteromedial aspect, 382
arteries, 393t
bones, 380, 381
lateral aspect, 383
magnetic resonance imaging, 470–471
muscles
anterior, 375, 376, 377t
medial, 375, 376, 378t, 379
posterior, 384, 385, 387t, 388, 389
posterior aspect, 384, 385, 387t, 388, 389
surface anatomy, 374
transverse sections, 470–471
Thoracic cage, 128
Thoracic wall
anterior, internal aspect, 23
external aspect, 22
muscles, 21, 21t
Thorax
3-D volume reconstruction and CT angiogram, 92–93
autonomic innervation, 84–85
bony, 10–11
contents, 25
lymphatic drainage, 86–87
magnetic resonance imaging, 88–91
viscera, 96, 97
3-D volume reconstruction
heart, 46, 47
thorax, 41, 92–93
Thumb, movements, 596, 597
Thymus, 88–89, 749, 759, 808
Thyroid disease, 773
Tibia, 354, 355, 380, 381, 410, 419, 420, 422, 423, 425, 429, 433, 442, 448, 450, 453–455, 472–473
Tibiofibular syndesmosis, 442
Tissue
areolar, 108
loose, 634, 636
glandular, 5
subcutaneous, 3–5, 370, 494, 743
cervical, 747
fatty layer, 102, 105, 106, 110, 258, 259
membranous layer, 102, 105, 106, 110, 111, 258, 259, 261
Tongue, 28, 128, 676–677, 677t, 678–680, 719, 721, 738, 739, 743, 782, 790, 808, 810, 829
Tonsil
cerebellar, 736, 740, 808, 810
cerebral, 742
lingual, 676
palatine, 712, 716, 792, 793
pharyngeal, 716, 720, 743, 794, 808, 810
Trabecula, septomarginal, 57, 64
Trabeculae, 398
Trabeculae carneae, 57–59
Trachea, 25, 28, 29, 38–40, 43, 48, 66–69, 71, 72, 74, 75, 82, 84, 128, 300, 716, 750, 770, 773, 808, 810
arterial supply, 75
autonomic innervation, 84
bifurcation, 69
general anatomy, 39–40
lymphatic drainage, 805
magnetic resonance imaging, 88–90
relationship to great vessels, 66
Tracheobronchial tree, 39–40
Tracheostomy, 749
Tract
corticospinal, 740
iliotibial, 368, 369, 372, 373, 380, 383–385, 399, 406, 409, 419, 422, 425, 428, 470
olfactory, 639, 726, 728, 818
optic, 639, 721, 727, 732–734, 740, 741, 819, 820
upper respiratory, 694
urinary, autonomic stimulation effects, 230t
Tragus, 703
Trapezium, 552, 570, 571, 574, 586, 589, 591, 593, 594, 599, 604, 605
tubercle, 588, 591, 593
Trapezoid, 552, 574, 586, 588, 589, 593, 594, 599, 604, 605
Triangle
anal, 255, 273
of auscultation, 512, 514
carotid, 752, 752t, 762, 763, 766
clavipectoral, 3, 490, 491, 494, 495
cystohepatic, 154
femoral, 372, 373
lumbar, 514
muscular, 752, 752t
occipital, 752, 752t
omoclavicular, 752, 752t, 757
submandibular, 752, 752t
submental, 752, 752t, 760
suboccipital, 784
urogenital, 255, 273
vertebrocostal, 174
Triangular interval, 510, 528
Trigone
bladder, 217, 221, 234
collateral, 727
habenular, 730, 735
hypoglossal, 735
vagal, 735
Triquetrum, 552, 574, 587–589, 591–594, 599
Trochanter
greater, 311, 354, 380, 381, 390, 391, 394, 395, 398, 399
lesser, 311, 354, 380, 381, 390, 391, 394, 398
Trochlea, 41, 518, 544, 546, 549, 552, 598, 651
fibular, 431
Trunk
anterolateral aspect, 497
brachiocephalic, 29, 46–49, 68, 70, 74, 80, 82, 90, 486, 772, 773, 808
celiac, 75, 85, 120, 123, 127, 130, 131, 133–135, 154, 163, 174, 175, 184, 185, 190
cervicodorsal, 486, 529, 772
costocervical, 74, 75, 764, 765, 765t
lumbosacral, 172, 173, 202, 206, 207, 212, 230, 231
lymphatic
bronchomediastinal, 9, 43, 76, 716
intestinal, 182, 184
jugular, 9, 76, 716, 805
lumbar, 182, 184
subclavian, 9, 76, 716
pulmonary, 26, 41, 42, 46, 49–52, 57–59, 61, 65, 68, 84
3-D volume reconstruction and CT angiogram, 92–93
magnetic resonance imaging, 88–89
subclavian, 43
superficial dissection, 496
sympathetic, 17, 20, 72, 73, 80–85, 163, 172, 183, 212, 230, 231, 249, 334, 339, 720, 772, 773, 776, 786, 805, 807
left, 123
lumbar, 214, 246
thyrocervical, 70, 74, 486, 504, 505t, 529, 764, 765, 765t, 773
vagal, 181, 836
anterior, 85
posterior, 85, 163
Tube, left uterine, 122
Tubercle, 301
adductor, 373, 380, 381, 385, 433
anterior, 296, 297, 350, 444, 465, 730, 742, 807
articular, 617, 625, 675
of auricle, 703
carotid, 750, 773, 775
corniculate, 804
cuneate, 734, 735
cuneiform, 466, 804
dorsal, 574, 581, 586
gracile, 734, 735
greater, 503, 517–519, 522, 532, 536, 537
infraglenoid, 536
jugular, 335, 615, 619
lateral, 431, 455, 457
lesser, 518, 537
medial, 433, 438, 452, 455, 457
mental, 610, 613, 664
pharyngeal, 617, 721
posterior, 296, 297, 330, 331, 350, 807, 810
postglenoid, 675
pubic, 106, 108–111, 194–200, 311, 372, 373, 380, 397
of rib, 13, 14
of scaphoid, 559, 588, 591
of trapezium, 588, 593
Tuberculum cinereum, 732, 733
Tuberculum sellae, 619, 624
Tuberosity
biceps brachii, 544
calcaneal, 427, 443–445, 447, 457, 464
cuboid, 444
deltoid, 518, 519
gluteal, 381
iliac, 197, 312

Teeth—*continued*
maxillary, 686, 688
molar, 685, 687, 688, 689t, 719
permanent, 685–686
primary, 688, 689t
secondary, 689t
Tegmen tympani, 712, 713
Telencephalon, 722, 723, 725–733
Temporal bone, 133, 608, 609, 611, 613, 614, 617, 619, 625, 702
mastoid part, 613
petrous part, 618, 620, 621, 625, 714
squamous part, 613, 618, 625, 664, 721
tympanic part, 613, 625, 664
zygomatic process, 613, 664
Tendinous cords, 57–59, 63
Tendon
abductor pollicis longus, 558, 559, 591
Achilles, 453
biceps brachii, 522, 523, 539, 540, 546, 549, 557
biceps femoris, 409, 428
calcaneal, 428, 430, 433–439, 450–452, 454, 458, 472
central, 24, 29, 73, 174
common extensor, 518, 542, 549, 552, 574
common flexor, 518, 549, 552
conjoint, 103, 107–109, 111, 112
digastric, 787
extensor digitorum longus, 422
extensor hallucis longus, 422
fibularis brevis, 431
fibularis longus, 431
flexor carpi radialis, 558, 592
flexor carpi ulnaris, 558
flexor digitorum longus, 445
flexor digitorum profundus, 557, 569
flexor digitorum superficialis, 559, 569
flexor hallucis brevis, 447
flexor hallucis longus, 445, 446, 451
flexor pollicis longus, 559, 570
long head of biceps brachii, 531, 532, 534, 535, 537
obturator internus, 389, 395
palmaris longus, 558, 559, 561, 563, 566
pectoralis minor, 522
peroneus longus, 464
popliteus, 409
quadriceps, 376, 420, 421
rotator cuff, 534
sartorius, 406
subscapularis, 532–534
supraspinatus, 517, 531, 532, 534
synovial covering, 569
tensor tympani, 708
terminal, 583
tibialis anterior, 422, 424
tibialis posterior, 429
triceps, 524, 526–528, 542
Tenia coli, 122
Tentorium cerebelli, 638, 639, 740, 743
Terminale, filum, 334, 336, 337
Terminalis
crista, 56
lamina, 728
stria, 729, 731, 741
sulcus, 49, 676, 790
Testis, 116, 209, 210, 216, 217, 264
blood supply, 117
coverings, 112, 113
fetal, 114
lymphatic drainage, 117
rete, 117
Thalamus, 728, 730–733, 735, 740–742
Thigh, 354
anteromedial aspect, 382
arteries, 393t
bones, 380, 381
lateral aspect, 383
magnetic resonance imaging, 470–471
muscles
anterior, 375, 376, 377t
medial, 375, 376, 378t, 379
posterior, 384, 385, 387t, 388, 389
posterior aspect, 384, 385, 387t, 388, 389
surface anatomy, 374
transverse sections, 470–471
Thoracic cage, 128
Thoracic wall
anterior, internal aspect, 23
external aspect, 22
muscles, 21, 21t
Thorax
3-D volume reconstruction and CT angiogram, 92–93
autonomic innervation, 84–85
bony, 10–11
contents, 25
lymphatic drainage, 86–87
magnetic resonance imaging, 88–91
viscera, 96, 97
3-D volume reconstruction
heart, 46, 47
thorax, 41, 92–93
Thumb, movements, 596, 597
Thymus, 88–89, 749, 759, 808
Thyroid disease, 773
Tibia, 354, 355, 380, 381, 410, 419, 420, 422, 423, 425, 429, 433, 442, 448, 450, 453–455, 472–473
Tibiofibular syndesmosis, 442
Tissue
areolar, 108
loose, 634, 636
glandular, 5
subcutaneous, 3–5, 370, 494, 743
cervical, 747
fatty layer, 102, 105, 106, 110, 258, 259
membranous layer, 102, 105, 106, 110, 111, 258, 259, 261
Tongue, 28, 128, 676–677, 677t, 678–680, 719, 721, 738, 739, 743, 782, 790, 808, 810, 829
Tonsil
cerebellar, 736, 740, 808, 810
cerebral, 742
lingual, 676
palatine, 712, 716, 792, 793
pharyngeal, 716, 720, 743, 794, 808, 810
Trabecula, septomarginal, 57, 64
Trabeculae, 398
Trabeculae carneae, 57–59
Trachea, 25, 28, 29, 38–40, 43, 48, 66–69, 71, 72, 74, 75, 82, 84, 128, 300, 716, 750, 770, 773, 808, 810
arterial supply, 75
autonomic innervation, 84
bifurcation, 69
general anatomy, 39–40
lymphatic drainage, 805
magnetic resonance imaging, 88–90
relationship to great vessels, 66
Tracheobronchial tree, 39–40
Tracheostomy, 749
Tract
corticospinal, 740
iliotibial, 368, 369, 372, 373, 380, 383–385, 399, 406, 409, 419, 422, 425, 428, 470
olfactory, 639, 726, 728, 818
optic, 639, 721, 727, 732–734, 740, 741, 819, 820
upper respiratory, 694
urinary, autonomic stimulation effects, 230t
Tragus, 703
Trapezium, 552, 570, 571, 574, 586, 589, 591, 593, 594, 599, 604, 605
tubercle, 588, 591, 593
Trapezoid, 552, 574, 586, 588, 589, 593, 594, 599, 604, 605
Triangle
anal, 255, 273
of auscultation, 512, 514
carotid, 752, 752t, 762, 763, 766
clavipectoral, 3, 490, 491, 494, 495
cystohepatic, 154
femoral, 372, 373
lumbar, 514
muscular, 752, 752t
occipital, 752, 752t
omoclavicular, 752, 752t, 757
submandibular, 752, 752t
submental, 752, 752t, 760
suboccipital, 784
urogenital, 255, 273
vertebrocostal, 174
Triangular interval, 510, 528
Trigone
bladder, 217, 221, 234
collateral, 727
habenular, 730, 735
hypoglossal, 735
vagal, 735
Triquetrum, 552, 574, 587–589, 591–594, 599
Trochanter
greater, 311, 354, 380, 381, 390, 391, 394, 395, 398, 399
lesser, 311, 354, 380, 381, 390, 391, 394, 398
Trochlea, 41, 518, 544, 546, 549, 552, 598, 651
fibular, 431
Trunk
anterolateral aspect, 497
brachiocephalic, 29, 46–49, 68, 70, 74, 80, 82, 90, 486, 772, 773, 808
celiac, 75, 85, 120, 123, 127, 130, 131, 133–135, 154, 163, 174, 175, 184, 185, 190
cervicodorsal, 486, 529, 772
costocervical, 74, 75, 764, 765, 765t
lumbosacral, 172, 173, 202, 206, 207, 212, 230, 231
lymphatic
bronchomediastinal, 9, 43, 76, 716
intestinal, 182, 184
jugular, 9, 76, 716, 805
lumbar, 182, 184
subclavian, 9, 76, 716
pulmonary, 26, 41, 42, 46, 49–52, 57–59, 61, 65, 68, 84
3-D volume reconstruction and CT angiogram, 92–93
magnetic resonance imaging, 88–89
subclavian, 43
superficial dissection, 496
sympathetic, 17, 20, 72, 73, 80–85, 163, 172, 183, 212, 230, 231, 249, 334, 339, 720, 772, 773, 776, 786, 805, 807
left, 123
lumbar, 214, 246
thyrocervical, 70, 74, 486, 504, 505t, 529, 764, 765, 765t, 773
vagal, 181, 836
anterior, 85
posterior, 85, 163
Tube, left uterine, 122
Tubercle, 301
adductor, 373, 380, 381, 385, 433
anterior, 296, 297, 350, 444, 465, 730, 742, 807
articular, 617, 625, 675
of auricle, 703
carotid, 750, 773, 775
corniculate, 804
cuneate, 734, 735
cuneiform, 466, 804
dorsal, 574, 581, 586
gracile, 734, 735
greater, 503, 517–519, 522, 532, 536, 537
infraglenoid, 536
jugular, 335, 615, 619
lateral, 431, 455, 457
lesser, 518, 537
medial, 433, 438, 452, 455, 457
mental, 610, 613, 664
pharyngeal, 617, 721
posterior, 296, 297, 330, 331, 350, 807, 810
postglenoid, 675
pubic, 106, 108–111, 194–200, 311, 372, 373, 380, 397
of rib, 13, 14
of scaphoid, 559, 588, 591
of trapezium, 588, 593
Tuberculum cinereum, 732, 733
Tuberculum sellae, 619, 624
Tuberosity
biceps brachii, 544
calcaneal, 427, 443–445, 447, 457, 464
cuboid, 444
deltoid, 518, 519
gluteal, 381
iliac, 197, 312

fascial, 457
lateral, 409, 470, 493, 521, 543, 600
medial, 493, 521, 525, 540, 543, 600
posterior, 369, 437, 470, 472
posteromedial, 470
transverse, 369, 436–438
interventricular, 57, 58
inferior, 3-D volume reconstruction and CT angiogram, 92–93
magnetic resonance imaging, 88–89
membranous part, 59, 61
muscular part, 59, 64
membranous, 63
nasal, 690–693, 697, 719–721, 738, 739, 743, 790, 808
orbital, 630
inferior, 629, 630
superior, 629, 630
rectovesical, 216, 263
prostatic, 220
Septum pellucidum, 723, 727–733, 740, 743
Sesamoid, 443, 445, 447, 463, 589, 606
anomalous, 467
lateral, 439
medial, 439, 452
Sheath
arachnoid, 655
axillary, 502, 503
carotid, 678, 747, 769
digital, fibrous, 443, 446, 561, 566–569, 571
dural, 655
femoral, 112, 371, 373
hypogastric, 218, 251
pial, 655
rectus
anterior, 102–104, 107, 496, 497
layers, 105
posterior, 101, 103, 112, 118
synovial, 561, 568
tendon, intertubercular, 532
Shoulder region, 476, 477
Sialogram, 680
Sinus
aortic, 55, 59
cavernous, 639, 644, 740
confluence of, 724
coronal, 50
coronary, 47, 53
opening, 56, 64
valve of, 56
frontal, 620, 638, 695–698, 743
intercavernous, 639
lactiferous, 4, 5
maxillary, 620, 621, 691, 695–698, 700, 719, 720, 738, 739
occipital, 639
pericardial
oblique, 29, 60
anterior wall, 50
posterior wall, 51
transverse, 29, 49–51, 60
petrosal
groove, 618
inferior, 615, 639
superior, 615, 639
renal, 166, 171
sagittal
inferior, 636, 638, 639
superior, 618, 636–639, 724, 738–740, 743
sigmoid, 615, 619, 639, 713, 767
sphenoidal, 621, 624, 695–698, 702, 713, 721
sphenoparietal, 639
straight, 638, 639, 724, 732, 733, 738–740, 742
tonsil, 792, 793
transverse, 619, 639, 742
groove, 618, 619
right, 639
venous, scleral, 660
Sinus venarum, 56
Sinusoids, 151
Siphon, carotid, 740
Skin, 105, 743
Skull base, 350, 785
Small intestine, 96, 97, 128, 162, 187–189, 352
interior, 136
lymphatic drainage, 184
Smooth muscle, 256t, 257, 274
Somatic nervous system, 343
Space
infracolic, 122
intercostal
contents, 20
eighth, 10
inferior, 18, 19
ninth, 11
vertebral ends, 17, 18
intervertebral disc, 302
lateral pharyngeal, 713, 720
midpalmar, 562, 606
palmar, 606
perivertebral, 218
quadrangular, 510, 527, 528, 537
retromammary, 5
retropharyngeal, 350, 678, 807, 808
retropubic, 208, 209, 216, 218–220, 232
subaponeurotic areolar, 606
subarachnoid, 286, 337, 352, 655, 724, 738, 739, 806, 810
subhepatic, 121, 147
suprasternal, 808
thenar, 562
triangular, 528
Speech area, 722
Spermatic cord, 102, 106, 107, 109, 113, 216, 222, 268
coverings, 103, 112, 113
dissection, 116
internal spermatic fascia covering, 108
Sphenoid bone, 609, 611, 613, 614, 617, 619, 624, 650, 664, 691, 695, 701, 702, 721
body, 618, 701
greater wing, 613, 618, 624, 650, 701, 702, 721
lesser wing, 618, 620, 624, 650, 701, 702
spine, 615, 624
Sphincter
anal
external, 209–213, 216, 256t, 257, 261–263, 273
internal, 209–211, 216, 262, 263
pyloric, 129
urethral
external, 202, 209, 210, 216, 220, 254, 256t, 257, 260
internal, 209, 210, 216, 260, 282
urethrovaginal, 254, 256t, 257, 260, 273
Spinal cord, 83, 123, 187, 286, 300, 334–342, 350, 352, 639, 721, 742, 806–808, 810
blood supply, 341–342
cervical, 334, 338, 340
developmental changes, 344
lumbar, 334, 340
magnetic resonance imaging, 88–89
rootlets, 334, 335, 337, 339, 340
sacral, 340
termination, 337
thoracic, 340
Spine
ethmoidal, 619, 624
iliac
anterior inferior, 196–198, 200, 312, 380, 396, 397
anterior superior, 96, 98, 100–103, 106, 109, 110, 128, 194–198, 200, 311, 312, 354, 372, 373, 380, 382, 396, 397, 496, 497
posterior inferior, 197, 311, 312, 320, 381, 390, 391, 397
posterior superior, 194, 195, 197, 201, 312, 381, 390, 397, 512
ischial, 196, 197, 199, 202, 311, 312, 315, 381, 390, 397
nasal
anterior, 610, 612, 690
posterior, 615
scapular, 11, 518, 519, 527, 529, 532, 536
Spiral organ (of Corti), 715, 833
Spleen, 96, 97, 119, 124, 127, 128, 130, 133, 135, 160, 162–164, 187–189, 352
blood supply, 135
lymphatic drainage, 184
surface anatomy, 131
Spondylolisthesis, 319
Spondylolysis, 319
Spur, bony, 318
Stapes, 704, 706, 707, 710
Sternum, 12, 23, 29, 72, 174
3-D volume reconstruction and CT angiogram, 92–93
anatomy, 10
anomalies, 16
body, 10, 12, 21, 48, 300, 497–499
magnetic resonance imaging, 88–89
manubrium, 24, 498, 810
ossification, 16
Stomach, 82, 96, 119, 121, 123–128, 132, 135, 148, 154, 157, 160–162, 164, 187–189, 352
air-fluid level, 186
anterior view, 129–130
body, 129
greater curvature, 124, 125, 129, 132
lesser curvature, 124, 129
lymphatic drainage, 184
muscular layers, 129
pylorus of, 96, 125, 128, 129, 132, 134, 156, 189
radiograph, 132
Stria medullaris thalami, 728
Subcallosal region, 728, 729
Subcutaneous triangular area, 449
Subdeltoid region, 528
Suboccipital region, 330–333
Substantia nigra, 738–741
Sulcus
calcarine, 723, 728, 729, 742
callosal, 728
carotid, 624
central, 722, 725
cingulate, 728, 742
collateral, 728
coronary, 46
frontal, superior, 742
hippocampal, 728, 729
hypothalamic, 728
interatrial, 50
intraparietal, 725
lateral, 722, 725
marginal, 728
parieto-occipital, 723, 725, 728
postcentral, 725
precentral, 725
prechiasmatic, 624
temporal, superior, 742
terminal, 49, 676, 790
Sulcus limitans, 735
Suprascapular region, 529
Sustentaculum tali, 433, 438, 444, 445, 447, 448, 450, 452, 453, 456, 458, 464, 465
Sutural bone, 613, 614
Suture
coronal, 609, 613, 614
frontal, 608–610
frontonasal, 690
infraorbital, 650
intermaxillary, 608, 610
internasal, 608, 610
lambdoid, 609, 613, 614
median palatine, 682
occipitomastoid, 614
palatine, 617
parietomastoid, 614
sagittal, 609, 614, 615
Swallowing, 808
Symphysis
mandibular, 608–610
pubic, 98, 106, 120, 194, 196–200, 202, 208, 210, 217, 222, 232, 250, 263, 267, 272, 273, 275, 278, 279, 311, 354, 380
Synchondrosis, sternocostal, 10
Syndesmosis, tibiofibular, 442
Synostosis, 318
Systole, 62

T tube, 158
Taenia coli, 136, 137, 139, 140, 144
Talus, 427, 430, 431, 442, 450, 453–457, 459, 461, 466, 472
head, 444, 448, 452, 454, 455, 459
medial tubercle, 433, 438, 452
neck, 448, 452, 455, 459
Tapetum, 729
Tarsal bones, 459
Tarsal tunnel, 453
Teeth
canine, 685, 688, 689t
incisor, 685, 687, 688, 689t
innervation, 687
magnetic resonance imaging, 806
mandibular, 686, 688

ischial, 194, 195, 197, 201, 202, 250, 261–263, 268, 272, 273, 311, 312, 354, 368, 380, 381, 390, 391, 396, 397
maxillary, 702
navicular, 439, 452
pronator, 552, 574
radial, 544, 546, 547, 552
sacral, 312, 313, 316
subtendinous bursa, 544
tibial, 406, 420–422, 425
ulnar, 518, 544, 552
Tubule
convoluted
distal, 167
proximal, 167
seminiferous, 117
Tunica albuginea, 117
Tunica vaginalis, 112, 113, 116, 117

Ulna, 478, 479, 518, 519, 523, 544–548, 552, 557, 574, 590, 591, 593, 594, 598, 602
distal, 598
head, 552, 574, 580, 589, 590
proximal, 598
styloid process, 552, 574, 587, 589–592
subcutaneous part, 587
Ultrasound
abdomen, 190–191
glenohumeral (shoulder) joint, 537
hepatic veins, 149
internal carotid artery, 809
pelvis
female, 282–283
male, 223
Umbilical cord, 239
Umbilicus, 98, 100, 106, 118, 161, 219, 238, 496, 497
Uncus, 728, 729, 738, 739
Upper limb
arteries and arterial anastomoses, 486, 487
bones, 476–479, 598–599
cutaneous nerves, 484, 485t
deep fascia, 492, 493
dermatomes, 483
epiphyseal sites, 598–599
joints, 476, 477
lymphatic drainage, 489
motor innervation, 480, 481
myotatic (deep tendon) reflexes, 482
myotomes, 482
proximal
arteries, 504, 505t
bones, 518–519
regions, 476, 477
veins
deep, 488
superficial, 489–491
Ureter, 97, 118, 145, 152, 153, 162–166, 202, 212, 215–220, 226, 233, 240
anomalies, 168
bifid, 168
intramural part, 217
left, 133, 165
magnetic resonance imaging, 186–187
pelvic part, 217
relationship to uterine artery, 240
retrocaval, 168
right, 122, 133, 143
Urethra, 120, 165, 208, 217, 219, 222, 232, 250, 254, 255, 268, 275–278, 280–282
compressor, 202
intermediate, 209, 216, 217, 220, 268
intramural, 217
muscles compressing, 260
prostatic, 209, 216, 217, 221, 263, 268
spongy, 209, 216, 217, 267, 268
Urinary bladder, 96, 97, 118, 120–122, 128, 136, 165, 205, 208–210, 215, 276–283, 311, 470
female, 232, 233, 250
male, 216–222
trigone, 217, 221, 234
Urogenital system, male, 266
Uterine tube, 208, 232–234, 284
Uterus, 120, 122, 208, 232, 280–283
adnexa, 237
bicornate, 284
blood supply, 235
body, 279
cervix, 237, 279
fundus, 234, 237, 279, 282
pregnant, 238, 239
radiograph, 284
Utricle, 714, 715
prostatic, 220, 221
Uvula, 221, 790

Vagina, 120, 205, 208, 232, 250, 254, 275, 279–282
muscles compressing, 260
posterior fornix, 208, 232
vestibule, 269, 273, 280, 281
wall, 272, 273
Valve
aortic, 29, 55, 59, 60, 63, 88–89
atrioventricular, 63
during cardiac cycle, 62
coronary sinus, 56
heart
auscultation, 44
surface markings, 44
mitral, 58, 59, 61, 63
3-D volume reconstruction and CT angiogram, 92–93
pulmonary, 57, 60, 61
semilunar, 63
tricuspid, 57, 61, 63
Vasa recta, 140, 141
Vasa recta duodeni, 135
Vein
acetabular, 401
anal, inferior, 269
angular, 633, 633t, 656
appendicular, 160
auricular, posterior, 331, 662, 716, 748
axillary, 22, 488, 489, 501, 503, 508
azygos, 29, 73, 75, 76, 80, 82, 83, 119, 123, 161, 175, 186, 227, 339
3-D volume reconstruction and CT angiogram, 92–93
arch, 47, 49, 68, 69, 74, 80
magnetic resonance imaging, 88–90
overview, 78–79
basilic, 488–491, 501, 502, 509, 521, 525, 538, 539, 587, 600, 602
basivertebral, 309, 342
brachial, 488, 489, 501, 502, 539
deep, 488, 521, 600
brachiocephalic, 23, 748
left, 29, 46, 48, 66, 67, 76, 78, 80, 81, 91, 488, 716, 749, 773, 808
right, 46, 48, 49, 66, 67, 72, 76, 78, 80, 88–90, 488, 773
cardiac, 53
anterior, 46, 49, 53
great, 46, 47, 49, 50, 53, 58
middle, 47, 50, 53
small, 46, 47, 50, 53
smallest, 53
central, 151
cephalic, 3, 4, 488–491, 494, 500–502, 508, 521, 538, 584, 600, 602
cerebral
anterior, 649
deep middle, 649
great, 638, 639, 649, 724, 732, 733, 740, 743
internal, 727, 741
superior, 638, 743
cervical
deep, 330, 331, 784
transverse, 763
ciliary
anterior, 661
long posterior, 661
short posterior, 661
circumflex femoral
lateral, 363
medial, 363, 373
circumflex fibular, 363
circumflex humeral
anterior, 488
posterior, 488
circumflex iliac
deep, 108, 109, 111, 118, 224, 242, 363
superficial, 364, 370
circumflex scapular, 488
colic, 161
left, 160
middle, 122, 126, 127, 160
right, 127, 134, 160, 188
collateral, of elbow, 488
communicating
anterior, 649
posterior, 649
cremasteric, 108
cubital, median, 489–491, 538
cystic, 154, 160
anterior, 154
posterior, 154
digital
dorsal, 364, 490, 582
palmar, 488, 490
plantar, 363
diploic, 634
dorsal
of penis, 116, 216, 224, 254, 264, 267, 268
superficial, 272, 490, 491
emissary, 712
condylar, 785
mastoid, 785
epigastric, 161, 227
inferior, 108, 109, 111, 118, 218, 219, 224, 242, 363
superficial, 102, 364, 370
esophageal, 161, 227
facial, 627, 633, 633t, 639, 656, 662, 666, 716, 721, 748, 762, 807
common, 748, 762
deep, 633, 633t
femoral, 109, 118, 222, 250, 275, 363, 364, 370–373, 382, 399, 470
fibular, 363, 365
gastric
left, 126, 127, 129, 134, 154, 155, 160, 161, 227
right, 127, 129, 154, 155, 160
short, 129, 131, 160
gastro-omental
left, 126, 127, 129, 160
right, 126, 127, 129, 130, 160
genicular
descending, 363
lateral inferior, 363
lateral superior, 363
medial inferior, 363, 435
medial superior, 363
gluteal
inferior, 224, 242, 363
superior, 224, 242, 351, 363
gonadal, 175
hemiazygos, 78, 79, 81, 83, 175, 186, 339, 352
accessory, 78, 79, 81
magnetic resonance imaging, 88–89
hepatic, 146, 149, 150, 163, 175
intermediate, 186
left, 186
middle, 188, 189
right, 187
ileal, 160
ileocolic, 127, 134, 160
iliac
common, 79, 145, 163, 175, 216, 224, 242, 363
external, 109, 111, 163, 175, 202, 213, 215, 216, 218, 224, 225, 225t, 226, 242, 363
internal, 175, 216, 224, 226, 242, 351, 363
iliolumbar, 79
infraorbital, 656
intercostal
anterior, 22, 23
left superior, 67, 76, 78, 79, 81
posterior, 17, 79–83, 175, 339
right posterior, 78
superior, 72
internal, thoracic, 23
interosseous, anterior, 488
intervertebral, 342, 740
jejunal, 160
jugular, 713
anterior, 716, 748, 763
external, 488, 501, 662, 716, 748, 754, 806, 807
internal, 333, 350, 488, 501, 662, 663, 667, 681, 710–713, 716, 720, 721, 738, 739, 748, 762, 763, 767, 771–773, 785, 806, 807
confluence, 88–89

Vein—*continued*
inferior bulb, 767
left, 9, 43, 48, 76, 88–89, 716, 767
right, 26, 43, 48, 76
superior bulb, 767
lumbar, 79, 175
marginal, 53
maxillary, 639, 748
median, of forearm, 490, 491, 538
meningeal, middle, 637
mesenteric
inferior, 122, 127, 133, 134, 160, 161, 163, 174, 186, 215, 227
superior, 122, 126, 127, 133, 134, 145, 156, 160–162, 187–189, 227
oblique, 47, 50, 53, 79
obturator, 118, 224, 242, 250, 363, 399
occipital, 331, 784
ophthalmic
inferior, 639, 656
superior, 639, 656
ovarian, 233
palatine
ascending, 712
external, 796
pancreatic, 160
pancreaticoduodenal, 160
posterior superior, 154
paraumbilical, 118, 161, 227
perforating, 363, 365, 538, 539, 584
phrenic, inferior, 175
plantar, 365
popliteal, 363, 365, 402, 419, 420, 435, 437
portal, 160, 188, 189, 227
hepatic, 122–124, 126, 127, 133, 134, 147, 149–155, 160, 161, 187
pudendal
external, 269, 364, 370
inferior, 213
internal, 213, 222, 224, 242, 250, 274, 363
pulmonary, 34, 35, 81
imaging of, 41, 92–93
inferior, 80
left, 29, 33, 46, 47, 50, 51, 64, 65, 88–89
left inferior, 58, 68, 92–93
left superior, 41, 58, 60, 68, 92–93
right, 29, 33, 46, 47, 50–52, 58, 60, 65, 88–89
right inferior, 58, 68, 92–93
right superior, 41, 58, 68, 92–93
radial, 488
rectal
inferior, 161
middle, 213, 224, 242
portal and systemic, 227
superior, 160, 161, 213
recurrent
radial, 488
ulnar, 488
renal, 162, 164, 166
left, 78, 79, 127, 175, 186, 188, 189
right, 153, 175, 187
retinal, central, 660, 661
retromandibular, 350, 633, 633t, 662, 716, 720, 721, 748, 762
retroperitoneal, 161, 227
sacral
lateral, 224, 242
median, 175
saphenous, 382
great, 102, 103, 112, 275, 363–367, 370, 372, 382, 438, 457, 470, 472
small, 364, 430, 457, 472
scapular, dorsal, 488, 501
sigmoid, 160
spinal
anterior, 342
posterior, 342
splenic, 122, 125, 127, 134, 160, 161, 164, 187–189, 227
subclavian, 22, 80, 488, 501, 511, 748, 757, 762, 772, 773
left, 43, 48, 76, 81, 716, 767, 773
right, 26, 43, 48, 76, 716, 767
subcostal, 79
subscapular, 488
supraorbital, 633, 633t, 639, 656
suprarenal, 175
suprascapular, 488, 501, 748
supratrochlear, 633, 633t
temporal, superficial, 633, 633t, 662, 716, 721, 748
testicular, 113, 127, 145, 152, 153, 162, 163, 215, 226
thalamostriate, 730
of thigh
deep, 363, 373
lateral cutaneous, 364
medial cutaneous, 364
thoracic
internal, 22, 66, 72, 80, 81, 88–89, 773
lateral, 488
superior, 488
thoraco-acromial, 488, 500
thoracodorsal, 488
thymic, 66
thyroid
inferior, 66, 749, 768, 773
middle, 768, 807
superior, 762, 768, 807
tibial
anterior, 363, 437, 472
posterior, 363, 365, 451, 472
ulnar, 488
uterine, 242
varicose, 365
ventricular, left posterior, 47, 53
vertebral, 772, 773, 807
anterior, 773
vesical, 224, 242
inferior, 224
vorticose, 656, 660, 661
Velum, medullary
inferior, 735
superior, 742
Vena cava
inferior, 46, 47, 50, 51, 56, 58, 65, 73, 76, 78–80, 82, 119, 122–124, 133, 146–150, 152–154, 157, 160–163, 165, 174, 175, 186, 188, 189, 215, 227, 351, 363
computed tomography, 6
magnetic resonance imaging, 90, 91
radiograph, 27
tributaries, 175
valve of, 56
superior, 41, 46, 47, 49–52, 56–58, 60, 64, 65, 67, 72, 76, 78–80, 488, 716
3-D volume reconstruction and CT angiogram, 92–93
magnetic resonance imaging, 88–91
radiograph, 27
Venae cordis minimae, 53
Ventricle
of brain, 724
fourth, 723, 724, 738–740, 742, 743
of larynx, 801
lateral, 724, 727, 729–733, 738–742
left, 27, 29, 46, 47, 49, 50, 53, 58–60, 84
3-D volume reconstruction and CT angiogram, 92–93
computed tomography, 6
interior, 58, 59
magnetic resonance imaging, 90, 91
wall, 64
radiograph, 27
right, 29, 46, 47, 49, 50, 53, 59, 60, 84
3-D volume reconstruction and CT angiogram, 92–93
interior, 57
magnetic resonance imaging, 90, 91
wall, 64
third, 723, 724, 728, 730–733, 735, 740, 741
Venule, inferior temporal retinal, 661
Vermis
inferior, 738–740
superior, 736, 738–740
Vertebrae
3-D volume reconstruction and CT angiogram, 92–93
anomalies, 318
cervical, 16, 290, 291. *See also* Atlas; Axis
CT scan, 296, 350
features, 751
lower, 338
magnetic resonance imaging, 352
movements, 292
overview, 286, 288, 294, 294t
radiograph, 292, 296, 297, 750
typical, 294, 294t
homologous parts, 290
levels, 133
lumbar, 145, 171, 290, 291, 351
CT scan, 351
magnetic resonance imaging, 343
movements, 293
overview, 286, 288, 302–303, 302t
radiograph, 293, 302, 310
lumbosacral, transitional, 318
movements, 291
sacral, 290, 351
spondylolisthesis, 319
spondylolysis, 319
thoracic, 10, 11, 290, 291
magnetic resonance imaging, 300, 352
overview, 286, 288, 300–301, 300t
radiograph, 310
typical, 289
Vertebral column
curvatures, 287
imaging of, 350–352
lumbar region, 308, 337
overview, 286, 288
Vestibule, 234, 714
aortic, 59
bulb of, 272, 274
nasal, 694
vaginal, 269, 273, 280, 281
Viscera
abdominal, 96, 97, 162, 163
pelvic, 246, 247, 251
peritoneal, 120, 121, 124, 164
pleural, 28, 31t
thoracic, 96, 97
Visual pathway, 820
Vocalis, 802, 802t
Vomer, 610, 611, 613, 615, 617, 690, 691, 702, 720

White matter, 732, 733, 738–740, 742
Window
oval, 714
round, 710, 714
Wrist, 476, 477
anterior aspect, 558, 559
coronal section, 590
imaging of, 589
lateral aspect, 584–586
medial aspect, 587
surface anatomy, 560

Zygomatic bone, 608, 609, 611, 613, 617, 650, 651, 664, 699


CCS0409